modern NUTRITION in health and disease

EDITORS

MAURICE E. SHILS, M.D., Sc.D.

Adjunct Professor (Nutrition)
Department of Public Health Sciences
Bowman Gray School of Medicine
Wake Forest University
Winston-Salem, North Carolina
Professor Emeritus of Medicine
Cornell University Medical College
Formerly, Director of Clinical Nutrition
Memorial Sloan-Kettering Cancer Center
New York, New York

JAMES A. OLSON, Ph.D.

Distinguished Professor of Liberal Arts and Sciences
Department of Biochemistry and Biophysics
Iowa State University
Ames, Iowa

MOSHE SHIKE, M.D.

Director of Clinical Nutrition
Memorial Sloan-Kettering Cancer Center
Associate Professor of Clinical Medicine
Cornell University Medical College
New York, New York

modern NUTRITION in health and disease

EIGHTH EDITION

VOLUME 2

Lea & Febiger
PHILADELPHIA · BALTIMORE · HONG KONG
LONDON · MUNICH · SYDNEY · TOKYO
A WAVERLY COMPANY

Williams & Wilkins
Rose Tree Corporate Center, Building II
1400 North Providence Road, Suite 5025
Media, PA 19063-2043 USA

Executive Editor—R. Kenneth Bussy
Development Editor—Tanya Lazar
Project Editor—Dorothy DiRienzi
Production Manager—Samuel A. Rondinelli

First Edition, 1955
Second Edition, 1960 Reprinted August, 1961
Third Edition, 1964 Reprinted February, 1966
Four Edition, 1968 Reprinted March, 1970
Reprinted July, 1971
Fifth Edition, 1973 Reprinted September, 1974
Reprinted April, 1975
Reprinted June, 1976
Reprinted November, 1977
Sixth Edition, 1980 Reprinted July, 1980
Reprinted November, 1981
Reprinted August, 1984
Reprinted May, 1986
Seventh Edition, 1988
Eighth Edition, 1994

Library of Congress Cataloging-in-Publication Data

Modern nutrition in health and disease / edited by Maurice E. Shils,
James A. Olson, Moshe Shike.—8th ed.
p. cm.
Includes bibliographical references and index.
ISBN 0-8121-1485-X (set)
1. Nutrition. 2. Diet therapy. I. Shils, Maurice E. (Maurice Edward), 1914- . II. Olson, James A. III. Shike, Moshe.
[DNLM: 1. Diet Therapy. 2. Nutrition. WB 400 M689]
QP141.M64 1993
613.2—dc20
DNLM/DLC
for Librairy of Congress 92-49855
CIP

NOTE: Although the author(s) and the publisher have taken reasonable steps to ensure the accuracy of the drug information included in this text before publication, drug information may change without notice and readers are advised to consult the manufacturer's packaging inserts before prescribing medications.

PRINTED IN THE UNITED STATES OF AMERICA

Print No. 5 4 3

ISBN 0-8121-1752-2

IN MEMORIAM

Robert Stanley Goodhart, M.D.,D.M.S. (1909–1992)

Pioneer in clinical nutrition, ardent supporter of clinical nutrition research and education, founder with Matthew Wohl, M.D. of *Modern Nutrition in Health and Disease* and an editor of its first six editions. He established the standards we strive to emulate.

Maurice E. Shils
James Allen Olson
Moshe Shike

PREFACE

The eighth edition of *Modern Nutrition in Health and Disease* is published 38 years after its first edition appeared. Its new format of two volumes reflects the increasing information in all aspects of its field and the inclusion of many new topics, and will, we hope, permit easier use by the reader.

Its objective remains unchanged: to serve as a major authoritative textbook and reference source in basic and clinical nutrition for students and practitioners in the various aspects of biomedical research and education, medicine, dentistry, osteopathy, dietetics, nursing, pharmacy, and public health. This has been achieved by selecting authors who are authorities in their topic areas in large part as the result of their important personal contributions. These 133 authors of 98 chapters and subsections, representing 10 different countries and many scientific disciplines, are truly the source and strength of this publication.

Approximately one third of the chapters are devoted to energy and specific dietary components. The role of nutrition is then reviewed in relation to integrated biologic systems extending from the cell, to various organ systems, and to intact individuals in situations of physiologic and environmental stresses. Methods of nutritional assessment of the individual are followed by 25 chapters on dietary and nutritional interrelations with diseases, and then by chapters on nutrition support modalities and ethics and by a major section on diet and nutrition in the health of populations.

For the convenience of the reader this edition is in two volumes, each containing a full table of contents, index, and appendices.

When indicated, we have expressed quantitative data both in conventional units and in international system (SI) units. The widespread use of the SI units in major biomedical journals and publications in the United States and other countries makes this dual unitage useful to readers.

We are indebted to members of the Lea & Febiger staff who are identified on the copyright page. Our interactions have been mainly with R. Kenneth Bussy, Senior Executive Editor, and Samuel A. Rondinelli, Production Manager, and we greatly appreciate their cooperation and understanding. Thanks also to Mrs. Holly Lukens, project editor, and her copy editor colleagues for their meticulous work. Maggie Wheelock, Beverly A. Thomas, and Betty Bell Shils have enabled us to manage the enormous amount of communications, record-keeping, and paper work involving the editors, the many authors, the publisher's staff, and the copy editors. To our wives, Betty, Giovanna, and Sherry goes our appreciation for their understanding of the further demands on our time required in the preparation of this book. The senior editor expresses his appreciation to Curt Furberg, M.D., Ph.D. for his support.

Winston-Salem, North Carolina
Ames, Iowa
New York, New York

Maurice E. Shils
James Allen Olson
Moshe Shike

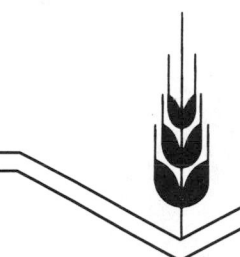

CONTRIBUTORS

PHYLLIS B. ACOSTA, Dr. P.H.
Director, Metabolic Diseases
Ross Laboratories
Columbus, Ohio

LINDSAY H. ALLEN, Ph.D., R.D.
Alumni Distinguished Professor of Nutritional Sciences
University of Connecticut
Storrs, Connecticut

G. HARVEY ANDERSON, Ph.D.
Acting Dean of Medicine
Professor of Nutritional Sciences, Medical Sciences, and Physiology
Faculty of Medicine
University of Toronto
Toronto, Canada

JAMES W. ANDERSON, M.D.
Professor of Medicine and Clinical Nutrition
College of Medicine
University of Kentucky
Chief of Endocrine-Metabolic Section
Veterans Affairs Medical Center
Lexington, Kentucky

HAROLD M. AUKEMA, Ph.D.
Research Associate
Department of Animal Science
Texas A&M University
College Station, Texas

LYNNE M. AUSMAN, D.Sc.
Scientist I
United States Department of Agriculture
Human Nutrition Research Center on Aging
Tufts University
Boston, Massachusetts

STEPHEN BARRETT, M.D.
Instructor of Health Education
Pennsylvania State University
State College, Pennsylvania

J. CHRISTOPHER BAUERNFEIND, Ph.D.
Formerly, Director of Agrochemistry and Nutrition and Research Coordinator
Hoffmann-LaRoche
Gainesville, Florida

GEORGE H. BEATON, Ph.D.
Professor of Nutritional Sciences
Faculty of Medicine
University of Toronto
Toronto, Canada

ABBY STOLPER BLOCH, M.S., R.D.
Coordinator of Clinical Nutrition Research
Memorial Sloan-Kettering Cancer Center
New York, New York

ALFRED JAY BOLLETT, M.D.
Clinical Professor of Medicine
School of Medicine
Yale University
New Haven, Connecticut
Vice President for Academic Affairs
Danbury Hospital
Danbury, Connecticut

IRWIN G. BRODSKY, M.D., M.P.H.
Research Assistant Professor
Clinical Associate Physician
College of Medicine
University of Vermont
Burlington, Vermont

HARRY P. BROQUIST, Ph.D.
Professor of Biochemistry Emeritus
Vanderbilt University
Nashville, Tennessee
Adjunct Professor
Utah State University
Logan, Utah

RAYMOND F. BURK, M.D.
Professor of Medicine
Chief of Gastroenterology
School of Medicine
Vanderbilt University
Nashville, Tennessee

FRANCISCO CHEW, M.D.
Medical Officer
Division of Nutrition and Health
Instituto de Nutrición de Centro América y Panamá (INCAP)
Gastroenterology Associate
Department of Pediatrics
Hospital Roosevelt
Guatemala City, Guatemala

ROBERT CHIN, JR., M.D.
Assistant Professor of Medicine
Section on Pulmonary and Critical Care Medicine
Bowman Gray School of Medicine
Wake Forest University
Winston-Salem, North Carolina

GRAEME A. CLUGSTON, M.B., D.C.H., PH.D.
Nutrition Section
World Health Organization
Geneva, Switzerland

J. JOSEPH CONNON, M.D.
Professor of Medicine
Faculty of Medicine
University of Toronto
Physician-in-chief
St. Michael's Hospital
Toronto, Canada

MARILYN C. CRIM, M.D., PH.D.
Assistant Professor
School of Nutrition
Assistant Professor
School of Medicine
Scientist II
United States Department of Agriculture
Human Nutrition Research Center on Aging
Tufts University
Boston, Massachusetts

KRISHNAMURTI DAKSHINAMURTI, PH.D.
Professor of Biochemistry and Molecular Biology
Faculty of Medicine
University of Manitoba
Winnipeg, Manitoba, Canada

KSHITISH C. DAS, M.D., PHD.
Professor and Head of Hematology
Faculty of Medicine
Kuwait University
Safat, Kuwait

EARL B. DAWSON, PHD.
Associate Professor of Obstetrics and Gynecology
University of Texas Medical Branch
Galveston, Texas

BESS DAWSON-HUGHES, M.D.
Chief of Calcium and Bone Metabolism Laboratory
United States Department of Agriculture
Human Nutrition Research Center on Aging
Tufts University
Boston, Massachusetts

DOMINICK P. DEPAOLA, D.D.S., PH.D.
President and Dean
Baylor College of Dentistry
Dallas, Texas

JOHN T. DEVLIN, M.D.
Associate Professor of Medicine
University of Vermont
Burlington, Vermont
Medical Director, Diabetes Center
Maine Medical Center
Portland, Maine

PIERRE M. DREYFUS, M.D.
Professor Emeritus of Neurology and Pediatrics
School of Medicine
University of California
Davis, California

JOHANNA T. DWYER, D.SC.
Professor of Medicine (Nutrition) and Community Health, School of Medicine
Tufts University
Director, Frances Stern Nutrition Center
New England Medical Center Hospitals
Boston, Massachusetts

LOUIS J. ELSAS, II, M.D.
Professor and Acting Chairman of Human Genetics
School of Medicine
Emory University
Atlanta, Georgia

JOHN W. ERDMAN, JR., PH.D.
Director of Nutritional Sciences
Professor of Food Science
University of Illinois
Urbana, Illinois

MARY P. FAINE, M.S., R.D.
Assistant Professor
Director of Nutrition Education
Department of Prosthodontics
School of Dentistry
University of Washington
Seattle, Washington

VIRGIL F. FAIRBANKS, M.D.
Consultant, Mayo Clinic
Professor of Medicine and Laboratory Medicine
Mayo Clinic and Mayo Foundation
Rochester, Minnesota

MICHAEL D. FALLON, M.D.†
Formerly, Associate Professor of Pathology
Jefferson Medical College
Thomas Jefferson University
Philadelphia, Pennsylvania

PHILIP M. FARRELL, M.D., PH.D.
Professor and Chairman of Pediatrics
Affiliate Faculty of Nutritional Sciences
University of Wisconsin
Madison, Wisconsin

†Deceased

LAWRENCE FEINMAN, M.D.
Chief of Gastroenterology
Veterans Affairs Medical Center
Bronx, New York
Associate Professor of Medicine
Mount Sinai School of Medicine
New York, New York

ELAINE B. FELDMAN, M.D.
Professor of Medicine, Physiology, and Endocrinology
Chief of Nutrition
Medical College of Georgia
Augusta, Georgia

ANN FOGELMAN, R.D., M.P.H.
Senior Research Associate
Department of Obstetrics and Gynecology
University of Texas Medical Branch
Galveston, Texas

ALLAN L. FORBES, M.D.
Medical Consultant (Foods and Nutrition)
Rockville, Maryland
Formerly, Director of Office of Nutrition and Food Sciences
Center for Food Safety and Applied Nutrition
Food and Drug Administration
Washington, D.C.

GILBERT B. FORBES, M.D.
Professor of Pediatrics and Biophysics
School of Medicine and Dentistry
University of Rochester
Rochester, New York

PATTI BAZEL GEIL, M.S., R.D.
Nutrition Coordinator
Metabolic Research Group
Adjunct Professor of Clinical Nutrition
University of Kentucky
Lexington, Kentucky

BARRY R. GOLDIN, Ph.D.
Associate Professor of Community Health
School of Medicine
Tufts University
Boston, Massachusetts

ELIZABETH J. GONG, M.P.H., M.S., R.D.
Nutrition Research Associate
Office of the President
University of California
Oakland, California

ALAN G. GOODRIDGE, Ph.D.
Professor and Head of Biochemistry
University of Iowa
Iowa City, Iowa

SHERWOOD L. GORBACH, M.D.
Professor of Community Health
School of Medicine
Tufts University
Boston, Massachusetts

HARRY L. GREENE, M.D.
Director of Nutritional Sciences
Mead Johnson Research Center
Evansville, Indiana

LOUIS E. GRIVETTI, Ph.D.
Professor of Geography and Nutrition
University of California
Davis, California

HERMAN GROSSMAN, M.D.
Professor of Radiology and Pediatrics
Duke University Medical Center
Durham, North Carolina

EDWARD H. HAPONIK, M.D.
Professor of Medicine
Section on Pulmonary and Critical Care Medicine
Bowman Gray School of Medicine
Wake Forest University
Winston-Salem, North Carolina

ALFRED E. HARPER, Ph.D.
E. V. McCollum Professor of Nutritional Sciences Emeritus
University of Wisconsin
Madison, Wisconsin

ROGER C. HARRIS, Ph.D.
Department of Comparative Physiology
Animal Health Trust
Newmarket, Suffolk, England

JOHN N. HATHCOCK, Ph.D.
Chief of Experimental Nutrition Branch
Division of Nutrition
Food and Drug Administration
Washington, D.C.

KENNETH C. HAYES, D.V.M., Ph.D
Professor of Biology (Nutrition)
Director of Foster Biomedical Research Laboratory
Brandeis University
Waltham, Massachusetts

FELIX P. HEALD, M.D.
Professor of Pediatrics
Director, Division of Adolescent Medicine
School of Medicine
University of Maryland
Baltimore, Maryland

WILLIAM C. HEIRD, M.D.
Professor of Pediatrics
Children's Nutrition Research Center
Baylor College of Medicine
Houston, Texas

VICTOR HERBERT, M.D., J.D.
Professor of Medicine
Mount Sinai School of Medicine
New York, New York
Chief of Hematology and Nutrition Laboratory
Veterans Affairs Medical Center
Bronx, New York

BASIL S. HETZEL, M.D.
Executive Director
International Council of Iodine Deficiency Disorders
Adelaide, Australia

STEVEN B. HEYMSFIELD, M.D.
Associate Professor of Medicine
College of Physicians and Surgeons
Columbia University
Director of Human Body Composition Laboratory
Director of Outpatient Obesity Research
Obesity Research Center
St. Luke's-Roosevelt Hospital
New York, New York

L. JOHN HOFFER, M.D., Ph.D.
Associate Professor of Medicine and Dietetics and Human Nutrition
Associate Director of McGill Nutrition and Food Science Centre
McGill University
Associate Physician
Royal Victoria Hospital
Montreal, Canada

MICHAEL F. HOLICK, Ph.D., M.D.
Professor of Medicine, Dermatology, and Physiology
School of Medicine
Boston University
Chief of Endocrine Section
Boston City Hospital
Boston, Massachusetts

BRUCE J. HOLUB, Ph.D.
Professor of Nutritional Sciences
University of Guelph
Guelph, Ontario, Canada

ERIC HULTMAN, M.D.
Professor of Clinical Chemistry
Karolinska Institutet
Huddinge, Sweden

DIANE M. HUSE, R.D., M.S.
Assistant Professor of Nutrition
Mayo Medical School
Dietician, Clinical Dietetics
Division of Endocrinology, Metabolism, and Internal Medicine
Mayo Clinic and Mayo Foundation
Rochester, Minnesota

ROBERT A. JACOB, Ph.D.
Research Chemist
United States Department of Agriculture
Western Human Nutrition Research Center
Presidio of San Francisco, California

KHURSHEED N. JEEJEEBHOY, M.B.B.S., Ph.D.
Professor of Medicine
Faculty of Medicine
Member, Institute of Medical Science
University of Toronto
Staff Gastroenterologist, St. Michael's Hospital
Toronto, Canada

ALEXANDRA L. JENKINS, R.D.
Research Associate
Department of Nutritional Sciences
University of Toronto
Senior Research Associate
Clinical Nutritional and Risk Factor Modification Centre
St. Michael's Hospital
Toronto, Canada

DAVID J.A. JENKINS, M.D., Ph.D.
Professor of Nutritional Sciences and Medicine
Faculty of Medicine
University of Toronto
Staff Physician
Division of Endocrinology and Metabolism
St. Michael's Hospital
Associate Physician
Division of Gastroenterology
Toronto General Hospital
Toronto, Canada

ERIC JÉQUIER, M.D.
Professor
Institut de Physiologie
Faculty of Medicine
University of Lausanne
Lausanne, Switzerland

MORLEY R. KARE, Ph.D.†
Formerly, Director
Monell Chemical Senses Center
Philadelphia, Pennsylvania

†Deceased

CARL L. KEEN, Ph.D.
Professor of Nutrition
University of California
Davis, California

GERALD T. KEUSCH, M.D.
Professor of Medicine
Division of Geographic Medicine and Infectious Diseases
New England Medical Center Hospitals
Boston, Massachusetts

JANET C. KING, Ph.D.
Professor of Nutritional Sciences
University of California
Berkeley, California

JOEL D. KOPPLE, M.D.
Professor of Medicine and Public Health
University of California
Los Angeles, California
Chief of Nephrology and Hypertension
Harbor-UCLA Medical Center
Torrance, California

MARK A. KORSTEN, M.D.
Associate Professor of Medicine
Mount Sinai School of Medicine
New York, New York
Assistant Chief of Medicine
Veterans Affairs Medical Center
Bronx, New York

JANE MORLEY KOTCHEN, M.D., M.P.H.
Professor of Medicine
School of Medicine
West Virginia University
Morgantown, West Virginia

THEODORE A. KOTCHEN, M.D.
E. B. Flink Professor and Chairman of Medicine
School of Medicine
West Virginia University
Morgantown, West Virginia

ELIZABETH A. KRALL, Ph.D.
Assistant Professor of Nutrition
School of Nutrition
Scientist II
United States Department of Agriculture
Human Nutrition Research Center on Aging
Tufts University
Boston, Massachusetts

MARIE FANELLI KUCZMARSKI, Ph.D., R.D.
Associate Professor of Nutrition and Dietetics
College of Human Resources
University of Delaware
Newark, Delaware

ROBERT J. KUCZMARSKI, Dr.P.H., R.D.
Nutritionist
United States Department of Health and Human Services
Centers for Disease Control
National Center for Health Statistics
Hyattsville, Maryland

PAUL A. LACHANCE, Ph.D.
Professor and Chairman of Food Science
Cook College
Rutgers University
New Brunswick, New Jersey

JAMES E. LEKLEM, Ph.D.
Professor of Nutrition and Food Management
Oregon State University
Corvallis, Oregon

ORVILLE A. LEVANDER, Ph.D.
Research Chemist
United States Department of Agriculture
Human Nutrition Research Center
Beltsville, Maryland

ALICE H. LICHTENSTEIN, D.Sc.
Assistant Professor
United States Department of Agriculture
Human Nutrition Research Center on Aging
Tufts University
Boston, Massachusetts

CHARLES S. LIEBER, M.D.
Professor of Medicine and Pathology
Mount Sinai School of Medicine
New York, New York
Director of Alcohol Research Center
Veterans Affairs Medical Center
Bronx, New York

WILLEM G. LINSCHEER, M.D., Ph.D.
Professor of Medicine
State University of New York
Chief of Gastroenterology
Veterans Affairs Medical Center
Syracuse, New York

ALEXANDER R. LUCAS, M.D.
Professor of Psychiatry
Mayo Medical School
Consultant, Section of Child and Adolescent Psychiatry
Mayo Clinic
Rochester, Minnesota

DONALD B. McCORMICK, Ph.D.
Fuller E. Callaway Professor and Chairman of Biochemistry
Emory University
Atlanta, Georgia

IAN MACDONALD, M.D., D.Sc.
Emeritus Professor of Applied Physiology
Guy's Hospital
University of London
London, England

WILLIAM J. McGANITY, M.D.
Ashbel Smith Professor of Obstetrics and Gynecology
University of Texas Medical Branch
Galveston, Texas

DONALD S. MCLAREN, M.D., Ph.D.
Honorary Head of Nutritional Blindness Prevention Programme
Institute of Ophthalmology
London, England

DONALD J. McNAMARA, Ph.D.
Professor of Nutrition and Food Science
University of Arizona
Tucson, Arizona

JOEL B. MASON, M.D.
Assistant Professor of Clinical Nutrition and Gastroenterology
School of Medicine
Scientist II
United States Department of Agriculture
Human Nutrition Research Center on Aging
Tufts University
Boston, Massachusetts

RICHARD D. MATTES, M.P.H., Ph.D., R.D.
Associate Member
Monell Chemical Senses Center
Adjunct Assistant Professor of Nutrition in Medicine
School of Medicine
University of Pennsylvania
Philadelphia, Pennsylvania

KATHLEEN SHIVE MATTHEWS, Ph.D.
Wiess Professor of Biochemistry and Cell Biology
Rice University
Houston, Texas

JAMES H. MEYER, M.D.
Chief of Gastroenterology
Sepulveda Veterans Affairs Medical Center
Sepulveda, California

MORTON A. MEYERS, M.D.
Professor of Radiology
State University of New York
Stony Brook, New York

J. ROBERTO MORAN, M.D.
Director of Pediatric Nutrition, Gastroenterology, and Allergy
Mead Johnson Research Center
Evansville, Indiana
Associate Clinical Professor
School of Medicine
Indiana University
Bloomington, Indiana

HAMISH N. MUNRO, M.D., D.Sc.
Professor, School of Nutrition
Professor, School of Medicine
Tufts University
Boston, Massachusetts

QUENTIN N. MYRVIK, Ph.D.
Vice President and Senior Scientist
Musculoskeletal Sciences Research Institute
Herndon, Virginia
Formerly, Professor of Microbiology and Immunology
Bowman Gray School of Medicine
Wake Forest University
Winston-Salem, North Carolina

FORREST H. NIELSEN, Ph.D.
Center Director and Research Nutritionist
United States Department of Agriculture
Grand Forks Human Nutrition Research Center
Grand Forks, North Dakota

MAN S. OH, M.D.
Professor of Medicine
Health Science Center at Brooklyn
State University of New York
Brooklyn, New York

JAMES A. OLSON, Ph.D.
Distinguished Professor of Liberal Arts and Sciences
Department of Biochemistry and Biophysics
Iowa State University
Ames, Iowa

ROBERT E. OLSON, M.D.
Professor of Medicine Emeritus
School of Medicine
Consulting Physician
University Hospital
State University of New York
Stony Brook, New York

MICHAEL W. PARIZA, Ph.D.
Director of Food Research Institute
Professor and Chairman of Food Microbiology and Toxicology
University of Wisconsin
Madison, Wisconsin

F. XAVIER PI-SUNYER, M.D.
Professor of Medicine
College of Physicians and Surgeons
Columbia University
Director, Division of Endocrinology, Diabetes, and Nutrition
Director of Obesity Research Center
St. Luke's-Roosevelt Hospital
New York, New York

NORA PLESOFSKY-VIG, Ph.D.
Research Associate
Departments of Genetics and Cell Biology and Plant Biology
University of Minnesota
St. Paul, Minnesota

ANGELA G. PONEROS-SCHNEIER, M.S.
Associate Program Coordinator in Food Science
University of Illinois
Urbana, Illinois

JEANNE I. RADER, Ph.D.
Chief of Nutrient Toxicity Section
Division of Nutrition
Food and Drug Administration
Washington, D.C.

ROBERT J. ROBERTS, M.D.
Chairman of Pediatrics
Children's Medical Center
University of Virginia
Charlottesville, Virginia

DAPHNE A. ROE, M.D.
Professor of Nutrition
Cornell University
Ithaca, New York

IRWIN H. ROSENBERG, M.D.
Professor of Medicine and Nutrition
School of Medicine
Director
United States Department of Agriculture
Human Nutrition Research Center on Aging
Tufts University
Boston, Massachusetts

ROBERT RUCKER, Ph.D.
Professor of Nutrition and Biological Chemistry
University of California
Davis, California

ROBERT M. RUSSELL, M.D.
Professor of Medicine and Nutrition
School of Medicine
Associate Director
United States Department of Agriculture
Human Nutrition Research Center on Aging
Tufts University
Boston, Massachusetts

HUGH A. SAMPSON, M.D.
Professor of Pediatrics
School of Medicine
Director of Pediatric Clinical Research Center
Johns Hopkins University
Baltimore, Maryland

BARBARA O. SCHNEEMAN, Ph.D.
Professor and Chair of Nutrition
University of California
Davis, California

YVES SCHUTZ, M.P.H., Ph.D.
Institut de Physiologie
Faculty of Medicine
University of Lausanne
Lausanne, Switzerland

MASUD SEYAL, M.D., Ph.D.
Associate Professor of Neurology
University of California
Davis, California

MOSHE SHIKE, M.D.
Director of Clinical Nutrition
Memorial Sloan-Kettering Cancer Center
New York, New York

MAURICE E. SHILS, M.D., Sc.D.
Adjunct Professor (Nutrition) of Public Health Sciences
Bowman Gray School of Medicine
Wake Forest University
Winston-Salem, North Carolina

WILEY W. SOUBA, JR., M.D., Sc.D.
Associate Professor of Surgery
Director of Surgical Metabolism
College of Medicine
University of Florida
Gainesville, Florida

LAWRENCE L. SPRIET, Ph.D.
Assistant Professor of Human Biology
University of Guelph
Guelph, Ontario, Canada

FRANCENE M. STEINBERG, R.D., Ph.D.
Research Fellow in Nutrition
University of California
Davis, California

MARIAN E. SWENSEID, Ph.D.
Professor Emerita of Community Health Sciences
School of Public Health
University of California
Los Angeles, California

VICHAI TANPHAICHITR, M.D., Ph.D.
Professor of Medicine
Director of Research Center
Faculty of Medicine
Ramathibodi Hospital
Bangkok, Thailand

JAMES A. THOMAS, Ph.D.
Professor of Biochemistry
Iowa State University
Ames, Iowa

JANET TIETYEN, M.S., R.D.
Graduate Research Assistant
Department of Grain Science and Industry
Kansas State University
Manhattan, Kansas

ANN TIGHE, M.S., R.D.
Research Dietitian
Obesity Research Center
St. Lukes-Roosevelt Hospital College of Physicians and Surgeons
Columbia University
New York, New York

BENJAMÍN TORÚN, M.D., Ph.D.
Senior Scientist and Head
Program of Clinical Nutrition and Metabolism
Instituto de Nutrición de Centro América y Panamá (INCAP)
Professor of Basic and Human Nutrition
University of San Carlos de Guatemala
Guatemala City, Guatemala

ELKE A. TRAUTWEIN, Ph.D.
Postdoctoral Fellow in Nutrition
Department of Biology
Foster Biomedical Research Laboratory
Brandeis University
Waltham, Massachusetts

A. STEWART TRUSWELL, M.D.
Boden Professor of Human Nutrition
University of Sydney
Sydney, Australia

JUDITH R. TURNLUND, Ph.D., R.D.
Research Nutrition Scientist
United States Department of Agriculture
Western Human Nutrition Research Center
Presidio of San Francisco, California

PENNY S. TURTEL, M.D.
Special Fellow
Memorial Sloan-Kettering Cancer Center
New York, New York
Clinical Professor
Robert Wood Johnson Medical School
University of Medicine and Dentistry of New Jersey
Piscataway, New Jersey

ANTOINE J. VERGROESEN, M.D., Ph.D.
Professor Emeritus of Nutrition
Erasmus University
Rotterdam, The Netherlands

RICHARD I. VOGEL, D.M.D.
Professor and Chairperson of Oral Pathology, Biology, and Diagnostic Sciences
New Jersey Dental School
University of Medicine and Dentistry of New Jersey
Newark, New Jersey

ZI-MIAN WANG, M.S.
Research Associate
Obesity Research Center
St. Lukes-Roosevelt Hospital
College of Physicians and Surgeons
Columbia University
New York, New York

ROBIN C. WATSON, M.D.†
Formerly, Professor of Radiology
Cornell University Medical College
Formerly, Chairman of Medical Imaging
Memorial Sloan-Kettering Cancer Center
New York, New York

ELSIE M. WIDDOWSON, D.Sc.
Department of Medicine
Addenbrookes Hospital and Medical Research Council
Cambridge, England

DOUGLAS W. WILMORE, M.D.
Frank Sawyer Professor of Surgery
Harvard Medical School
Boston, Massachusetts

THOMAS M.S. WOLEVER, M.D., Ph.D.
Associate Professor of Nutritional Sciences
University of Toronto
Toronto, Canada

RICHARD J. WOOD, Ph.D.
Scientist I
United States Department of Agriculture
Human Nutrition Research Center on Aging
Tufts University
Boston, Massachusetts

STEVEN H. ZEISEL, M.D., Ph.D.
Professor and Chairman of Nutrition
Professor of Pediatrics and Medicine
Schools of Public Health and Medicine
University of North Carolina
Chapel Hill, North Carolina

†Deceased

CONTENTS

Volume 1

part I • SPECIFIC DIETARY COMPONENTS

A. Major Dietary Constituents and Energy Needs

B. Minerals

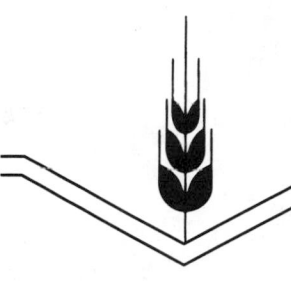

B. Physiologic and Metabolic Considerations

C. Nutrition in Growth and Aging

D. Other Diseases, Disorders and Conditions

E. Systems of Nutritional Support

D. Food Technology and Toxicology

E. Nutrition Policy

APPENDICES

INDEX

PART IV

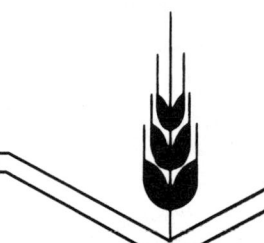

Diet and Nutrition in Disease

CHAPTER 56

Starvation

L. John Hoffer

Starvation refers to the physiologic state that results when food intake is chronically inadequate. The manifestations of fully developed starvation disease are those of energy and protein deficiency, hence the term "protein-energy malnutrition."[1] Because the emphasis of this chapter is on the physiologic and biochemical effects of food deprivation, the broader concept of starvation is retained in the discussion that follows. Also, it is important to bear in mind that starvation is almost always the result of a deprivation of all food, not just of protein and energy, so the clinical disease is frequently associated with deficiencies of micronutrients as well as the macronutrients.[2–4]

The physiology of starvation is central to human nutrition and relevant to many areas of metabolism and medicine. Chapter 57 deals with the clinical manifestations and treatment of protein-energy malnutrition. A major aim of this chapter, in addition to providing a general overview of starvation, is to establish links between aspects of basic nutritional biochemistry and areas of applied clinical nutrition that are covered in other chapters in this text, including, among others, body composition, protein and energy metabolism, physiologic stress, and obesity.

COMPOSITION OF WEIGHT LOSS DURING STARVATION

An energy-deficient diet is one that provides less usable food energy than the body expends. As a consequence, endogenous fuels must be oxidized to make up the energy deficit, and body substance is lost. However, the changes of body composition that occur in starvation are more complicated than this simple thermodynamic equation implies. In the late 1940s, Ancel Keys and his co-workers made detailed observations of human starvation in an experiment in which 32 young men volunteered to live on the campus of the University of Minnesota and consume a diet providing approximately 1600 kcal per day, about two thirds of their normal energy requirement.[5] Figure 56–1*B* illustrates the cardinal features of the protein-energy malnutrition that resulted.

The Minnesota volunteers lost an average of 23% of their initial body weight. Body composition measurements indicated that more than 70% of body fat was lost in the process. As evident from Figure 56–1, a large amount of muscle was lost as well: in all, they lost 24% of their "active tissues," the fat-free, metabolically active lean tissues of the body. The lean tissues comprise the skeletal muscles (the "peripheral" proteins, making up about 80% of the total) plus the defatted visceral organs, the cells of the blood and bone marrow, and the immune system ("central" proteins that make up the remaining 20%). "Body cell mass" is another term that refers, in a general sense, to the same tissues.[6,7] The total lean tissue content of the body is to be distinguished from its lean

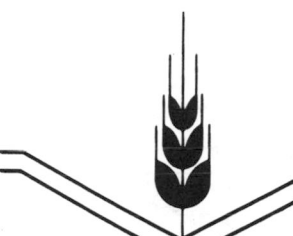

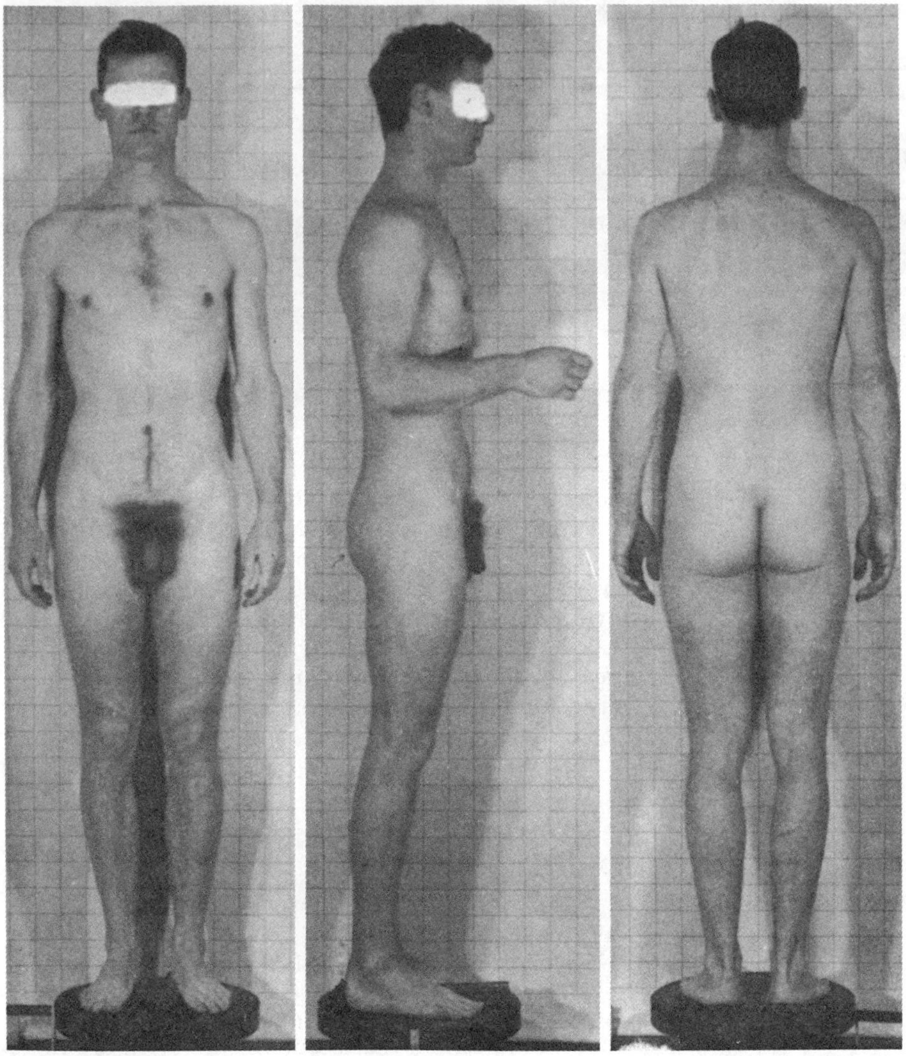

FIGURE 56–1. The Minnesota experiment. *A*, Three views of subject No. 20 before starvation.

body mass,[8] which is simply total body mass minus the contribution of pure fat (see Chap. 49).

Fat loss is detected easily because its percentage depletion is so great, but loss of the active, lean tissues is responsible for most of the weight loss of nonobese starving individuals. Table 56–1 provides details of the contributions of the different body compartments to the weight loss of the Minnesota volunteers. It illustrates that lean tissue loss (24% in this example) is directly proportional to weight loss (23%). Therefore, lean tissue depletion of nonobese starving adults can be estimated with reasonable accuracy by simply measuring weight loss. Table 56–1 also shows that measuring body weight alone underestimates the sum of fat and active tissue losses, because in starvation the extracellular fluid volume increases. In extreme cases (and especially in the presence of other diseases associated with water retention), this volume increase leads to obvious fluid swelling within the skin and subcutaneous tissues, called "hunger edema." The presence of edema makes an assessment of the severity of lean tissue depletion more difficult.[9]

The lean tissues are the site of about half the body's N; extracellular proteins, chiefly collagen, account for the other half. Little or no change occurs in extracellular N in adult starvation,[10] so despite important changes in the structure and biochemical composition of starving human muscle,[11] the rate of body N loss provides reasonably accurate information about the rate of depletion or regain of the lean tissues.[12]

ADAPTATION TO STARVATION: NUTRITIONAL FACTORS

Early in starvation weight loss is rapid, but it gradually slows even if no change occurs in the starvation diet. After 24 weeks of starvation, body weight of the Minnesota volunteers had reached a plateau. This life-saving

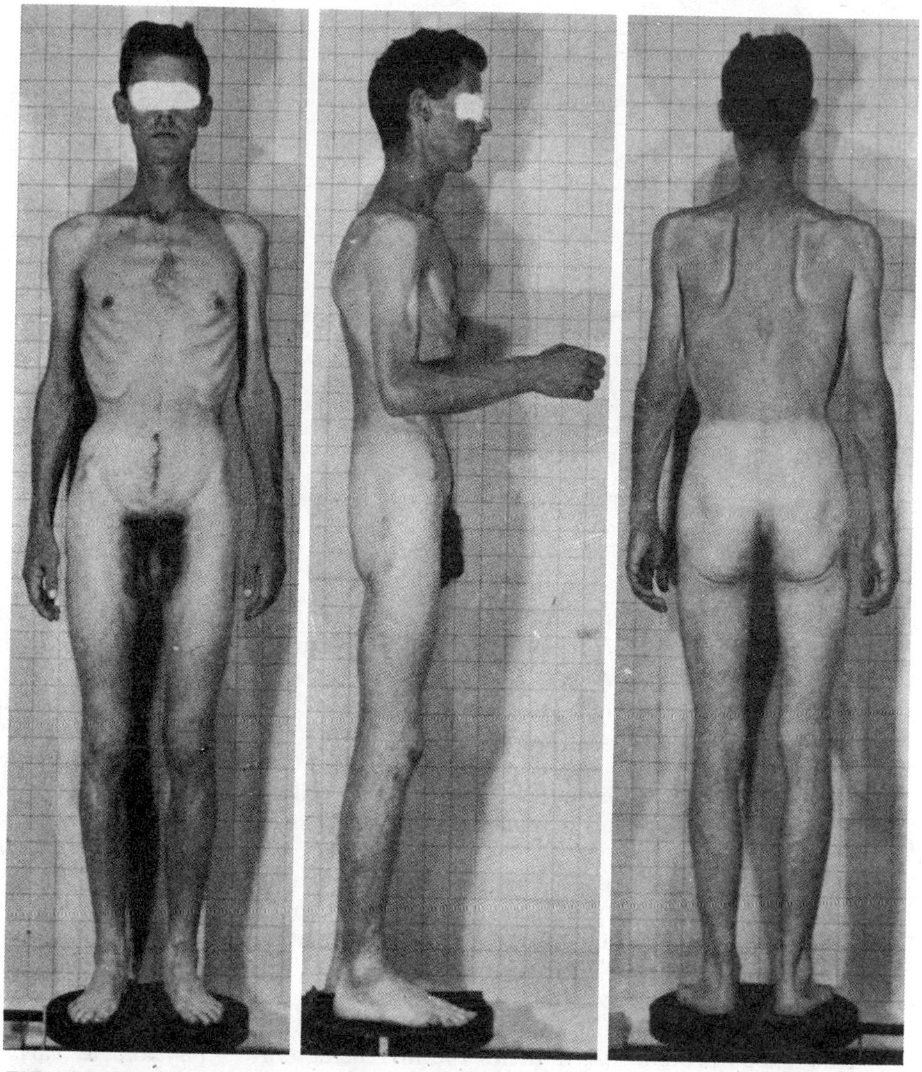

FIGURE 56–1. (Continued) *B*, The last of 24 weeks of starvation. Illustrated are the cardinal features of protein-energy malnutrition: depletion of subcutaneous fat stores and generalized muscle wasting. (From Keys, A., Brozek, J., Henschel, A., et al.: The Biology of Human Starvation. Minneapolis, University of Minnesota Press, 1950.)

adaptation involved the cessation of losses of both fat (energy) and lean tissue (protein).

DECREASED ENERGY EXPENDITURE

The basal metabolic rate is responsible for two thirds to three quarters of total energy expenditure. The basal metabolic rate of the Minnesota volunteers decreased by 40% after 24 weeks of starvation, thus coming approximately into line with their low energy intake. This decrease in resting energy expenditure was largely the result of a diminished lean tissue mass, which is responsible for most of the metabolic processes that determine energy expenditure.[13] The metabolic rate also decreased per unit of remaining lean tissue (Fig. 56–2). As well, energy expenditure over the day decreases in starvation, because smaller meals mean a smaller thermic effect of food, a lighter body weight requires less work of moving, and starving individuals voluntarily diminish their spontaneous movements.[5,14,15] These adjustments, when successful, bring starving individuals back into energy equilibrium.

OBLIGATORY PROTEIN LOSS

To reduce energy expenditure, the starving body must decrease its lean tissue mass. However, it cannot lose so much lean tissue that the adverse metabolic consequences of protein deficiency become intolerable. Successful adaptation is a process of controlled protein loss that is terminated when just enough has been jettisoned to re-establish zero energy balance. N equilibrium is

TABLE 56–1. BODY COMPOSITION CHANGES AFTER 24 WEEKS OF STARVATION

COMPONENT	CONTROL (%)	24 WEEKS (%)	CHANGE (%)
Total weight	100	100	−23
Fat	14	5	−71
Active tissue mass	57	56	−24
Extracellular fluid	24	34	+4

Body composition of normal men before and after 24 weeks of a diet providing approximately 50 g protein and 1600 kcal per day. Fat was determined by underwater weighing; extracellular fluid was measured as the thiocyanate space; and the active tissue mass was taken as the difference between body weight and the sum of fat, extracellular fluid, and bone mineral masses. Initial body weight was 69.5 kg. Total weight loss was 15.9 kg, fat loss was 6.9 kg, and "active tissue" loss, equivalent to lean tissue mass, was 9.7 kg. Note that fat and active tissue loss exceed the total weight loss. (Data from Keys, A., Brozek, J., Henschel, A., et al.: The Biology of Human Starvation. Minneapolis, University of Minnesota Press, 1950.)

re-established under these conditions by an adaptation that may be separated conceptually into two components: decreased endogenous N loss and increased efficiency of dietary protein retention (see Fig. 56–3). As starvation proceeds, the amount of lean tissue left to be lost is decreasing, which accounts for the observation that the change of lean tissue mass follows "first-order" kinetics and displays an exponential "decay" over time.[16] As well, changes that occur in cellular metabolism reduce the rate of endogenous amino acid oxidation.[17] Simultaneously, the efficiency of retention of exogenous (dietary) proteins increases. This phenomenon of increased "avidity" of starving tissues for dietary protein has long been recognized.[12,18] As shown in Figure 56–3, net body protein loss continues until the slowing of endogenous protein loss matches the increasing efficiency of dietary protein retention and a new state of protein equilibrium is established.

DETERMINANTS OF PROTEIN CONSERVATION

Because the starving individual is obliged to sacrifice a certain amount of protein to re-establish zero energy balance, protein loss must be regarded as beneficial during prolonged starvation because it allows the organism to survive.[19] However, energy intake is only one of several factors that affect the rate at which N is lost during starvation and the amount of lean tissue that must be sacrificed to re-establish N equilibrium. These factors include energy balance, protein intake, protein-nutritional state, biologic individuality, and possibly obesity.

Energy Balance. In the Minnesota study, the protein intake was close to the amount recommended as safe for normal adults (0.75 g/kg body weight), but extensive protein wasting still occurred. This effect may be understood teleologically as a lifesaving adaptation to reduce energy expenditure. However, the concept can also be expressed (and tested) quantitatively: energy deficiency impairs the efficiency with which the body retains its protein store. Results of many studies have shown that N balance at a constant protein intake is improved by an increase and worsened by a decrease in energy intake.[20,21] The energy effect is most potent in the modestly submaintenance range of both protein and energy intakes.[22] Under most circumstances, the source of the fuel (carbohydrate or fat) is immaterial.[23]

Kinney and Elwyn emphasized the importance of measuring the energy balance (the difference between exogenous energy ingested and energy expended), and not simply energy intake.[24,25] Because it is the amount of dietary energy in surplus or in deficit after accounting for expenditure, energy balance is probably the specific physiologic variable that when negative worsens N balance and when positive improves it. Direct measure-

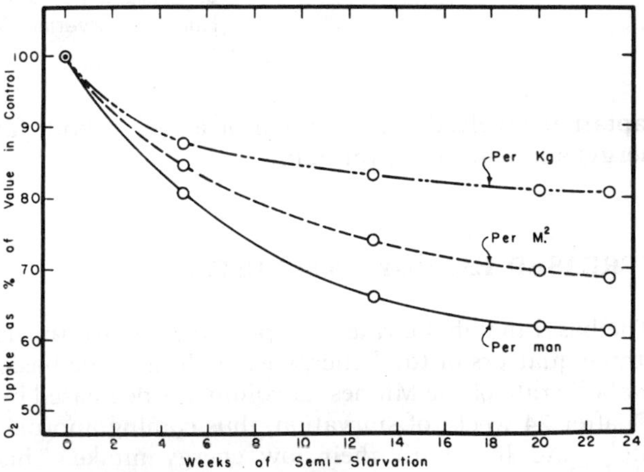

FIGURE 56–2. Mean basal metabolism for 32 men before and during 24 weeks of starvation. All values are expressed as percentage of the prestarvation values for the oxygen uptake per man, per square meter of body surface, and per kg of body weight. (From Keys, A., Brozek, J., Henschel, A., et al.: The Biology of Human Starvation. Minneapolis, University of Minnesota Press, 1950.)

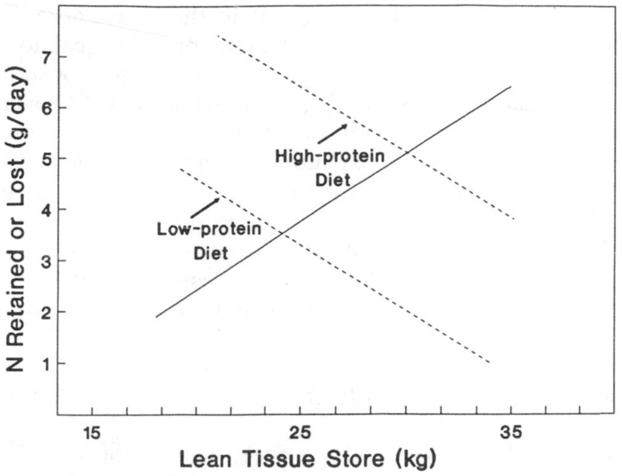

FIGURE 56–3. A hypothetic scheme to account for adaptation to starvation in the adult. A first-order (linear) relationship exists between the amount of lean tissue and the rate at which it is depleted. This is indicated by the solid line. An *inverse* relationship exists between the amount of lean tissue and the efficiency of retention of protein in the diet. This relationship is affected by the concentration of protein in the diet, resulting in a family of curves (dashed lines). As starvation progresses and the lean tissue store diminishes, the rate of protein depletion slows as the amount of protein retained from each meal increases. At the crossover point a new equilibrium is established and lean tissue loss ceases. The "price" paid to achieve this physiologic accommodation is a diminished lean tissue store. This scheme illustrates that a high-protein diet may permit protein equilibrium after only moderate lean tissue wasting; a low-protein diet may also be compatible with protein equilibrium, but the cost, in terms of protein wasting, will be greater.

ment of energy balance may be particularly important in hospitalized patients in whom energy expenditure rates vary considerably.[24]

Protein Intake. In clinical starvation, total food, not just energy, is eaten in inadequate amounts. The coexistence of energy and protein deficiency leads to a greater loss of body protein than necessary simply to reduce energy expenditure. Over a wide range of energy intakes, N balance is improved by increasing protein intake.[20] This effect is most significant for increases from low to moderate levels of protein intake. As protein intake increases into the maintenance range (and at maintenance energy), improvements in N balance continue but do not keep pace, indicating less efficient retention of dietary protein in the high range of protein intakes.[26,27] The effects of energy and protein intake on N balance are interactive. Thus, the effect of an increase in energy intake to improve N balance can be prevented by an inadequate protein intake. Conversely, an increase in protein intake may compensate for a negative energy balance.[20,28–30] This last interaction is illustrated in Figure 56–3. When the lean tissues are depleted, the fractional retention of the protein in a given meal becomes greater, so it is predictable that (over an appropriate range of protein intakes) a meal high in protein will be associated with a greater absolute r tion of protein than one low in protein. This explains a high-protein starvation diet is likely to result in pro equilibrium after only moderate lean tissue wastin low-protein starvation diet may be compatible w protein equilibrium, but the ultimate protein-wast will be greater. During refeeding after starvation, higher protein intake for any given level of ener promotes more rapid repletion of body protein.[29] How ever, in clinical practice, even a modest protein intak accomplishes nutritional rehabilitation as long as it i accompanied by adequate energy.[3]

Protein Nutritional Status. The efficiency of N retention at a given intake of protein and energy is increased by prior protein depletion,[31] in part because of the diminished mass of active body protein: the maintenance protein requirement of a slight individual is less than that of a large, muscular one. However, cellular adaptations also occur in the protein-deficient patient to improve the efficiency of amino acid use (see subsequent discussion). The influence of protein-nutritional status is implicit in the scheme shown in Figure 56–3, in which a given lean tissue mass (as indicated on the horizontal axis) has an important effect on both endogenous protein loss and dietary protein avidity.

Biologic Individuality. This is a convenient label for internal factors, presently unknown, that result in a large individual variation in the response to a given diet. When unexpected responses are observed, attention should always be directed to correctable factors such as malabsorption, the adequacy of micronutrient provision,[32] or the possible presence of physiologic stress (e.g., to cold, infection, or trauma). These influences are considered in detail in a subsequent section. However, even when all such factors are controlled, the variation in individual responses to starvation is wide.[33] This statement is consistent with the scope of biochemical individuality[34] and, specifically, with the wide variation in individual amino acid requirements of normal men.[35]

Obesity. The potential effect of increased adiposity to modify body protein losses during starvation is discussed elsewhere in this chapter.

BIOCHEMICAL ADAPTATION

The foregoing discussion highlighted nutritional factors that influence the physiologic adaptation to starvation. This section focuses on the hormonal and biochemical mechanisms that could mediate this adaptation.

ENERGY METABOLISM

The resting metabolic rate decreases within days of eating a starvation diet.[16,36,37] This early response occurs too soon to be caused by lean tissue loss alone, although lean tissue loss is plainly responsible for further decreases in the metabolic rate as starvation continues. The early, adaptive component of starving hypometabolism appears to be caused by alterations in catecholamine turnover and action, and in the peripheral metabolism of thyroxine (T_4), the hormone secreted by the thyroid gland. Serum levels of free T_4 and of thyrotropin (the pituitary hormone that regulates T_4 secretion) remain normal, but the peripheral conversion of T_4 to the active hormone triiodothyronine (T_3) decreases within a few days (or even hours) of initiating a starvation diet.[38] Both energy intake and, specifically, the amount of carbohydrate consumed affect this conversion process, apparently through their effect on insulin secretion.[30,38] Although an association between decreased circulating T_3 and lowered resting energy expenditure during starvation clearly exists, the precise nature of the relationship is not well understood,[36,38] nor is T_3 the only modulating factor. Thus, a carbohydrate-free diet that provides maintenance energy decreases T_3 levels, but the resting metabolic rate does not decrease.[39] Poorly controlled diabetes mellitus is associated with decreased serum T_3 levels, but the metabolic rate increases.[40]

In uncomplicated starvation, catecholamine secretion and turnover decrease, as measured in the blood and urine of humans and in the organs of laboratory animals.[14,19] The blood pressure, heart rate, and core temperature of starving patients are reduced as is their thermic response to cold or to a norepinephrine infusion. Pupil size, an indicator of basal sympathetic tone, is diminished.[5,14,41] As with T_4-to-T_3 conversion, both energy balance and carbohydrate intake, at least in part because of their effect on insulin release, appear to be important regulators of these effects. The thyroid and catecholamine effects are interconnected.[19] T_3 increases the number of tissue norepinephrine receptors, and in its absence, the number decreases.[42]

The energy cost of maintaining the normal transcellular gradient of sodium and potassium could make up a large component of total resting energy expenditure.[43] Because the activity of the sodium pump (Na,K-ATPase) is affected by levels of insulin, catecholamines, and T_3,[44] all of which change during starvation, slowing of the activity of the sodium pump could be an important means by which resting energy expenditure adaptively decreases, at least in severe starvation.[41] Considerable evidence exists[44–46] (although not all of it is consistent[47]) that pumping of sodium out of blood cells is decreased in advanced starvation, resulting in increased intracellular sodium and decreased intracellular potassium content, and a slower metabolic rate. Because the muscles, gut, and liver are responsible for most of the total resting energy expenditure, it would be important to show that Na,K-ATPase decreases in these tissues during starvation. Some evidence suggests that this is the case.[43]

Finally, body protein turnover decreases in starvation (described subsequently), and this change affects resting energy expenditure. The precise determinants of the energy cost of protein synthesis in the intact organism are not fully defined.[48] Furthermore, protein breakdown, although thermodynamically favored, also consumes energy because it is a highly regulated process.[49] Several authors have noted a relationship among N loss, protein turnover, and energy expenditure, and the energy cost of whole body protein turnover may play a role in that relationship.[25] Different commentators have speculated that protein turnover could be responsible for as little as 5% or as much as 30% of human resting energy expenditure.[50–54] The actual value is unknown.

PROTEIN METABOLISM

Liver and Muscle. In the rat, the feeding of a protein-deficient diet results in adaptive changes in the activities of amino acid-metabolizing enzymes in the liver and elsewhere,[55,56] altered protein turnover, and a decrease of liver weight and protein content.[57–60] The protein-deprived liver is also depleted of the tissue-protective free thiol, glutathione.[61] Protein deficiency decreases the synthesis of protein in the liver,[57,60,62] consistent with in vitro findings that protein synthesis increases and decreases in response to fluctuations in the amino acid supply comparable to those normally encountered during ingestion of protein meals.[63] Increased protein synthesis by delivery of amino acids can be evoked in the isolated perfused liver, showing that the hormonal responses evoked during meal absorption are not essential for liver protein synthesis.[63,64] Synthesis of albumin decreases promptly in protein deficiency.[57,58,65] Early in the feeding of a protein-deficient diet, liver protein breakdown rates are maintained or increase.[66–68] This finding, together with evidence for slowed protein synthesis,[60,62] accounts for the rapid loss of liver substance in early protein depletion. In contrast to liver, muscle protein mass is relatively well preserved in the earliest stages of protein deficiency. It is not yet clear whether muscle proteolysis remains constant or decreases at this stage.[69] However, protein synthesis decreases promptly[70] and in established starvation, both synthesis and proteolysis clearly are decreased.[50,62,71,72]

Whole-Body Studies. Dynamic studies of protein metabolism in the whole body of the intact animal or human provide important information about the regulation of protein metabolism. To carry out these studies, a tracer amino acid (usually an isotope of the essential amino acid leucine) is administered at a constant rate until its concentration in blood reaches a steady state. The extent of tracer "dilution" by influx into the blood of unlabeled leucine permits a calculation of the turnover, or "flux" of leucine into and through the bloodstream, which (when no leucine is being eaten) indicates the rate of whole-body protein breakdown. In steady state, the rate of appearance of leucine must equal its rate of removal from the circulation. Removed leucine is either taken up for new protein synthesis or oxidized. The rate of leucine oxidation can be inferred from the rate ofappearance, in expired air, of labeled carbon dioxide released upon oxidation of leucine labeled at the carboxyl carbon. (For the model to be valid, leucine oxidation must correspond to urea synthesis or N excretion over the same time period.) When the leucine oxidation value is then subtracted from the total flux, a measure of the rate of leucine uptake into newly synthesized protein is obtained.[73]

Another useful tracer method involves the use of ^{15}N-glycine to determine whole-body N turnover. The labeled N distributes widely among the free amino acids and ultimately equilibrates in the pools of urea and ammonia, the excretion end products of amino acid oxidation. By measuring ^{15}N enrichment in these pools, it is possible to calculate whole-body N flux, protein breakdown, and protein synthesis by using the same arguments as in the previous paragraph.[74] In this case, total amino acid oxidation is measured directly as urinary N excretion rather than inferred from appearance of tracer carbon in expired carbon dioxide.

This simplified protein-turnover model has important conceptual and practical limitations.[73,74] One limitation embedded in the concept of whole-body turnover is that it is an integrated value for all the proteins in all the tissues of the body. It cannot separate those that are turning over rapidly or slowly, nor will it be sensitive to situations in which turnover could be changing in opposite directions in different organs or tissues.[75] A second problem relates to the validity of the leucine turnover model when food is taken by mouth. The simplest and most widely used model assumes that food-derived amino acids are presented to the central sampling pool in the blood in a way that permits whole-body proteolysis to be calculated as the total flux through the circulation minus the rate of dietary amino acid intake. This calculation is not likely to be correct because it ignores "first-pass" events occurring in the splanchnic tissues which are critical in regulating amino acid retention or oxidation.[68,76] Even when amino acids are administered intravenously into the central pool, investigators have yet to show that whole-body leucine appearance from proteolysis necessarily equals the difference between the calculated total turnover and intake rates.[77,78] However, these limitations are more than compensated by the potential of the method to provide insight into dynamic aspects of protein and amino acid metabolism in the intact organism.

A useful feature of tracer-determined protein turnover, either in the whole organism or in individual tissue beds, is its ability to depict metabolic changes that are not apparent when studied by simple balance techniques. The rate of protein synthesis and protein breakdown (proteolysis) may be partly or wholly independent of the rate of amino acid uptake or release from the whole tissue. Thus, a tissue may be in negative amino acid balance with an unchanged or decreased rate of proteolysis if protein synthesis falls to a slower rate than breakdown. Indeed, this pattern is characteristic of chronic starvation. The distinction between "proteolysis" (which designates the absolute rate of protein breakdown) and "net proteolysis" (protein breakdown minus protein synthesis) must be considered.[71]

When assessed on a whole-body basis by means of tracer leucine infusions, protein synthesis, oxidation, and breakdown decrease during protein deficiency in rats[72] and in humans.[75,79] During the high-energy refeeding of previously starved patients, body protein turnover may increase to above-normal values at the same time that N balance becomes positive.[80] Hypocaloric protein refeeding is also associated with positive N balance, but protein turnover (both synthesis and breakdown) remains depressed.[31] Even late in refeeding and when the characteristically low serum levels of most essential amino acids are near normal, the postabsorptive release of many amino acids from peripheral tissues remains depressed,[12] indicating a continuing predominance of protein synthesis over breakdown.

Because protein synthesis is energetically expensive, an important question is whether the continuous recycling of body proteins in a seemingly "futile cycle" provides any biologic advantage. Newsholme has shown that substrate cycles at regulation points in metabolic pathways permit a finely tuned control of metabolite flow.[81] Does the recycling of entire proteins similarly allow a rapid remodeling of body protein distribution and function in times of need? If so, then slowed rates of protein turnover characteristic of adapted starvation could be bad for the organism.[59] Sukhatme and Margen carried out a detailed analysis of the patterns of N balance of normal men on maintenance diets with different protein contents.[82] Their observations indicated the presence of nonrandom cyclic fluctuations in N excretion with a periodicity of days, increasing in amplitude with increasing protein intake. Although not yet confirmed by other observers,[83] the concept emphasizes that the body's protein content is closely regulated, and the amplitude of fluctuations in N excretion could provide insight into the "feedback" characteristics of the process. It is apparent that the greater the protein intake, the coarser (and perhaps, therefore, less efficient) the regulation.[30,84] This phenomenon of a changing amplitude of N excretion with different protein intakes could relate to the interaction between energy and protein turnover in determining N balance during starvation. When the protein intake is high, protein turnover is maximal and dietary protein use as a consequence is inefficient. This state is associated with wide fluctuations in N excretion. When the protein intake is low, protein turnover rates are slowed to maximize amino acid reutilization, a state manifested by low fluctuations in N excretion.[84,85] Starvation is associated with a slower rate of body protein turnover, because (1) slower rates of turnover may be energy conserving, and (2) rapid flux through the free amino acid pools is incompatible with the finest regulation (and efficiency) of amino acid oxidation. The effect of exogenous energy provision might be to increase the efficiency of amino acid conservation at any rate of turnover.[86]

Hormonal Effects on Protein Turnover. Starvation is associated with many hormonal changes,[87,88] but little is known about the way they bring about adaptation. Considerable evidence exists that T_3 regulates muscle metabolism, but its precise effects in starvation are not yet well defined.[30,38] T_3 levels decrease early in starvation, and T_3 administration to fasting obese subjects increases their body N losses,[38] suggesting that the decreased T_3 is important (at least permissively) for successful adaptation. It has been noted, however, that the doses of T_3 administered in those studies were physiologically excessive.[36] Moreover, the relationship between T_3 and N balance apparent in total fasting studies is less clear when the study includes patients on hypocaloric diets.[36]

Circulating levels of growth hormone frequently are increased in starvation, but those of its target hormone, insulin-like growth factor-1 (IGF-1) are subnormal. IGF-1 release by the liver into the circulation is controlled by nutrition as well as by growth hormone.[89] In human studies, both protein and total energy intake affect IGF-1 levels. When dietary energy is severely restricted, the amount of carbohydrate eaten becomes a major determinant of the circulating IGF-1 response to growth hormone stimulation.[89,90] Structurally related to insulin, IGF-1 stimulates net protein synthesis in cultured cells and in isolated muscle in a manner similar to insulin.[49] Refeeding starving patients increases IGF-1 blood levels dramatically in association with improved N retention.[89,91] Because T_3 potentiates growth hormone-induced expression of mRNA for IGF-1[92] and stimulates IGF-1 release from the liver,[93] the refeeding effect could be mediated by insulin-stimulated rises in T_3.[30] Other data indicate that pharmacologic doses of growth hormone increase N retention in humans on hypocaloric[94] or hyponitrogenous diets.[95] One paradoxic effect of growth hormone in this setting is to prevent the expected decline in T_3 levels, perhaps by inducing insulin resistance causing a secondary rise in insulin secretion.[38,94]

Insulin stimulates protein synthesis and inhibits its breakdown in muscle and in liver.[49,68,96,97] Abnormalities of insulin release and its peripheral actions occur in protein-energy malnutrition.[87] Even in advanced protein-energy malnutrition, carbohydrate intake is sufficient to prevent the catabolic state characteristic of severe insulin deficiency,[12,98] but a starvation diet may stimulate an insulin response that, although adequate to prevent acute proteolysis, is still subnormal.[99] Such diminished insulin secretion could act together with decreased dietary amino acid delivery to curtail protein synthesis[60] and, secondarily, protein breakdown.[30] Such a combined insulin-amino-acid cellular action could be expressed both directly on the cells and indirectly, by diminishing the peripheral action of thyroid hormone.[30]

MUSCLE FUNCTION

In a variety of states of negative whole-body energy balance, abnormalities occur in the amount of tension developed by intact skeletal muscle in response to varying frequencies of electrical stimulation of its motor nerves (the force-frequency curve). Also, a pronounced slowing of the rate of muscular relaxation occurs after stimulation ceases. This general effect can be demonstrated early in starvation and even in well-nourished individuals on weight-reduction diets. It is promptly reversed by refeeding, before any increase in body protein content.[46,100] Biochemically, short-term or moderate starvation is associated with a decreased rate of glycolysis and a fall in muscle creatine phosphate content.[101] These changes may be the result of a limitation of the maximum rate of glucose oxidation owing to decreased activities of the glycolytic enzyme phosphofructokinase and of the Krebs cycle oxidative enzyme succinic dehydrogenase.[46,101] More severe abnormalities in muscle biochemistry occur in advanced protein-energy malnutrition.[11,102]

Metabolic changes induced in early starvation may especially affect the fast-twitch muscle fibers that are specialized for anaerobic glycolysis,[103] and, although muscle is globally lost in significant starvation, a selectively greater loss may be noted in the fast-twitch fibers.[104] It has also been suggested that the rate of heat production by resting muscle is decreased under these conditions, possibly because of decreased substrate cycling at the phosphofructokinase step.[105] Decreased T_3 presence or cellular action could account for the acute effect of energy deprivation on muscle function and contribute to the atrophy that occurs in prolonged starvation[30] by decreasing protein turnover directly[69,105] or indirectly by decreasing muscle tone through central nervous system effects.

The extent of muscle function derangement has been associated with both the severity of human protein-energy malnutrition and patient outcome after surgery.[106] Although these associations are presumably related to a combination of chronic starvation and current energy deficit, they are important because they suggest that muscle function testing could provide a valuable prognostic test. Moreover, the possibility emerges that brief nutritional "priming" of some starving patients, perhaps even those individuals not conventionally considered malnourished, could improve outcome during disease or postoperatively.

Even ample nutrition does not prevent atrophy if muscle is not exercised.[25,104] Muscle atrophy occurs after central or peripheral motor neuron destruction and even with extended bed rest or weightlessness in space.[104] Changes in protein turnover in muscle are evident within hours of immobilizing the limbs of animals,[104] although these effects have proven difficult to demonstrate in the whole bodies of normal men paid to stay in bed.[107] Unlike starvation, the atrophy of immobilization appears to affect the antigravity slow-twitch fibers more than the fast-twitch fibers, at least in animals.[104]

LABILE PROTEIN

In 1866, Carl Voit first demonstrated the existence of a small protein store the amount of which was determined by the protein content of the diet, and that was excreted during the first several days of fasting or on changing from a higher to a lower protein intake. This protein store is now known to be an example of a general phenomenon of rapid body protein gain or loss in response to variations in the protein intake level, energy level, or to a variety of hormonal and physiologic stimuli.[20] When a normal human is fed a low-protein or protein-free diet, urinary N excretion remains considerable for 3 to 5 days before it diminishes to a minimum steady-state value of approximately 2 or 3 g per day, the so-called "obligatory" or "endogenous" rate of urinary N loss.[20,108] When the former protein intake is resumed, N balance becomes positive until the previous losses are made up (Fig. 56–4). This protein readily gained or lost from the body has been termed "storage" or "labile" protein.[20,51,108] It is said to constitute about 3% of body protein in well-nourished rats or humans.[20] This figure is insignificant in terms of total body N economy, but important for understanding the adaptive response to starvation.

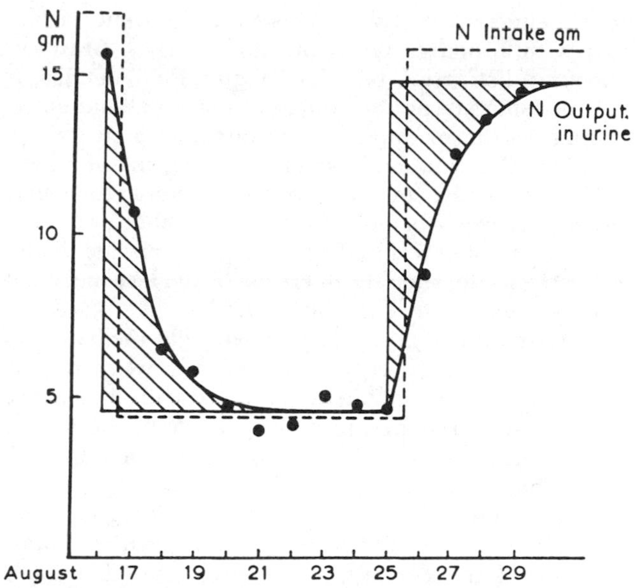

FIGURE 56–4. Labile protein. The solid line indicates the N excretion of a human subject abruptly changed to a low-protein diet. The dashed line indicates the level of N intake. Initially, N intake approximates its excretion and the subject is close to N equilibrium. On switching to the lower N intake, N loss exceeds intake for several days until equilibrium is reestablished. The N lost from the body during this period is shown in the first shaded area. On resuming former intake, the subject stores N, as shown by the second shaded area. The two shaded areas are approximately equal. (From Munro, H.N.: General aspects of the regulation of protein metabolism by diet and hormones. *In* Mammalian Protein Metabolism. Vol. 3. Edited by H.N. Munro and J.B. Allison. New York, Academic Press, 1964, pp. 381–481.)

METABOLIC SIGNIFICANCE

Although small, the amount of labile protein in the body is larger than the free amino acid pool, which makes up only about 0.5 to 1.0% of the body's amino acids and an even smaller percentage of the essential ones.[109,110] The free amino acid pool, because of its small size and rapid turnover, can be assumed to play an essential role in the regulation of tissue protein synthesis and breakdown.[110] Because labile protein undergoes the most rapid exchange with the free amino acid pool, it must be important in determining the extent of oxidation of amino acids, particularly those newly entering from the diet.[20]

After a loss of labile protein in response to dietary protein deprivation, body protein loss ceases if the new level of intake is compatible with homeostasis, or continues at a lower rate from less readily mobilized "endogenous" sources, leading to sustained lean tissue loss.[20] In the protein-deficient or fasted rat, the greatest acute loss of protein is from the liver, with the other visceral organs making up large contributions as well. This finding is in accord with the more rapid turnover rates of proteins in these organs.[62] With prolongation of the protein-deficient diet, subsequent losses occur as well from muscle, quantitatively the major nonstructural protein store.[20]

To distinguish the effects of acute changes in labile protein from the sustained, nutritionally significant effects of a dietary change, studies on the effects of starvation must allow a period of several days for the body to come into a new adapted state. During this time, the content of amino acid-transporting and metabolizing enzymes alters in the liver and other tissues to reestablish optimal metabolism of the amino acids and energy substrates in the new diet.[17,59] Allowance for adaptation to occur is important not only for N balance experiments, but also for studies that examine the effects of diet, hormones, or other treatments on body protein turnover. A changing mass of even a small pool of rapidly turning-over proteins could cause a significant change in total body protein turnover that has little to do with the sustained effect of the diet, drug, or hormone being tested.[75]

Although the biochemical adaptation to a new diet may require only a few days, even more rapid changes occur every day because food usually is consumed intermittently. When food is eaten, the free amino acid and protein content of the tissues undergo cyclic oscillations within hours. Waterlow and Garlick draw an important distinction between "regulation," defined as the usual short-term adjustments to internal and external changes (for example, to the intake of a customary meal), and "adaptation," which is the setting of a new, oscillating steady state (as in the response to a new dietary pattern). When observations are made at a given moment, the long-term effects of a diet must be distinguished from the short-term effects of the last meal and even the interval since the last meal.[111]

Moreover, although it is self-evident that the body can gain in protein (and energy) stores only when food is consumed, the fate of dietary amino acids—a choice between uptake into new protein synthesis or catabolism with elimination of the N as urea or ammonium—is decided not only during and shortly after their initial absorption into the body, but also throughout the interval between meals. Studies involving direct catheterization of the portal and hepatic veins of animals demonstrate a large postprandial increase in urea output in association with the hepatic uptake of amino acids derived from large protein meals,[112] and increases in plasma urea and urinary urea excretion immediately after protein consumption by humans.[113] However, urea synthesis in the postabsorptive state remains considerable, demonstrating a pattern that reflects both the protein and nonprotein content of the diet.[85,114] Thus, the acute urea response is smaller after carbohydrate-containing protein meals than those without it,[20,115,116] indicating (for an organism in N equilibrium) that carbohydrate delays amino acid oxidation, urea synthesis, or both.

Plasma concentrations of the essential amino acids are perturbed only modestly during protein meals despite the large influx of amino acids in relation to the size of the body's free amino acid pools.[97,117] This relative stability of the free amino acid pools could be achieved by an increase in protein synthesis (accelerating removal of amino acids from their free pools), by a decrease in endogenous protein breakdown (decreasing entry into the pools), or by an increase in amino acid oxidation. In this setting, oxidation may be considered an overflow device that eliminates surfeit essential amino acids from the body. Meal-related enhancement of protein synthesis and diminished protein breakdown, particularly in the splanchnic tissues,[97] would divert amino acids from oxidation by limiting the increase in the size of the free amino acid pools. The result is a transient increase in the body's protein content—labile protein. The amount of labile protein present at any moment is determined by the activity of the amino acid-metabolizing enzymes as programmed by the preceding habitual diet. In the interval between meals, a finer-tuned regulation occurs, as some of the amino acids in the labile proteins accumulated acutely during the dietary influx are released and redistributed for the synthesis of more slowly-turning over proteins.[20] Because amino acid oxidation remains considerable during this period, the body still has an opportunity to retain or discharge some body protein.

ADAPTATION AND ACCOMMODATION

Protein intake is below the minimum nutritional requirement when, on introduction in the diet, it results in a sustained negative N balance and body protein loss.[27] Eventually, a new steady state is established at which N equilibrium is restored but at the cost of surviving with a lower lean tissue store. Waterlow has drawn attention to the important difference, when assessing the nutritional value of diets, between "adaptation," which occurs within the acceptable range of protein intakes, and the protein-sacrificing response to an inadequate protein intake, which he has termed "accommodation."[58,59,83] This distinction is important because adaptation is understood to be an aspect of normal physiology that involves at most a nutritionally insignificant change in the labile protein mass. Accommodation implies a physiologic compromise with adverse health consequences.

Recognition of overt starvation in a clinic or ward patient residing in a wealthy society requires only physician or nutritionist awareness, because the diagnosis is readily made on the basis of a food-intake and body-weight history, physical examination, and a record of weight over time.[106] However, the definition of what constitutes the minimum acceptable food intake in societies in which food is scarce can be a difficult problem.[19,118,119] The existence of N equilibrium, although necessary, is insufficient proof that a diet is nutritionally adequate, because the successful attainment of zero N balance may have required accommodation, not merely adaptation.

The concept of a labile protein pool of varying size can be used to explain the changes in efficiency of body protein retention that normally occur when tissue protein needs change, as occurs during growth, muscular hypertrophy, and atrophy. Its depletion could also account for the increased efficiency of dietary protein retention that occurs in response to a decrease of dietary protein intake within the normal adaptive range. It is unclear to what extent a depletion of labile protein accounts for the increased retention of dietary protein that is part of the accommodation to starvation. It is also uncertain whether a decrease in whole-body protein turnover, comprised as it may be of a loss of labile protein mass and a true slowing of the turnover rate of other, long half-life proteins, is a sign of "normal" adaptation within an acceptable range of nutrient intake, or whether it indicates that accommodation was necessary, and therefore incriminates the diet under examination as inadequate.[59,84] It could even be argued that an optimum protein intake is one that maximizes the size of the labile protein pool (and hence maximizes the rate of whole body postabsorptive protein turnover), which allows for the most rapid transfer of amino acids among the tissues in response to changing metabolic needs.[83]

CLINICAL CHARACTERISTICS OF ACCOMMODATION

Accommodation has "succeeded" when energy equilibrium is re-established through a process of controlled lean tissue wasting that is arrested before the adverse consequences of protein deficiency become intolerable. The organism survives, but a metabolic and functional price must be paid.[58] The most apparent deficits are the loss of insulating fat and of muscle mass with its associated loss of physical power. A hypometabolic state of unwellness is induced reminiscent of (but not identical to) hypothyroidism.[38] Starving patients are hypothermic and do not mount an appropriate thermic response to environmental cold.[41] The loss of muscle mass diminishes the body's protein reserve and, together with slower protein turnover in the remaining muscle,[50] reduces the body's options for protein "remodeling" in response to changing metabolic needs. Thus, starving animals[120] and patients[121] mount a blunted rise of protein turnover and a smaller catabolic response during metabolic stress. The physical appearance of patients with protein-energy malnutrition is reminiscent of advanced aging, and indeed, some similarities of body composition exist (see Fig. 56–1).[122]

In addition to the loss of peripheral proteins, deficits in central protein occur as well. The anatomic and functional consequences of severe human starvation are covered in clinical depictions[5,123,124] and medical reviews.[3,125–128] These effects include anemia, altered heart muscle mass and function, decreased pulmonary mechanical function and a diminished response to stimuli to breathe, altered gut anatomy and mildly impaired absorptive function, impaired healing,[129] altered metabolism of many drugs,[61,130–132] and immunodeficiency.[8,133,134]

Immune competence is crucial for long-term survival, yet the precise nature of immune dysfunction in human starvation remains poorly understood. In both animals and humans, advanced protein-energy malnutrition results in a variety of immune deficits, especially of cell-mediated immunity (demonstrated clinically by anergy, the loss of delayed cutaneous hypersensitivity).[8,134] However, the clinical importance of immune deficiency in moderate starvation[135] and the possible additive effect of concurrent micronutrient deficiency at this stage are not well known.[3,41,136,137] A potential broad area of interaction is in cytokine production or release, which is independently impaired in protein-energy malnutrition and in numerous micronutrient deficiencies.[138,139] More information is needed to define the indications for initiating nutritional support, and the forms of support to give in moderate protein-energy malnutrition.

Successful accommodation to starvation requires relative preservation of the mass and function of the critical visceral or "central" proteins despite large fractional losses of "peripheral" skeletal muscle protein. Even though important deficits in organ function are apparent in patients who have successfully accommodated to starvation, weight loss is arrested and homeostasis is preserved; as long as nothing new supervenes (as will be described), they may remain in their fragile accommodated state indefinitely.[140] Weight-stable anorexia nervosa in an otherwise healthy young individual is in some ways a clinical paradigm for this condition.[135] More complex examples can be observed daily in any outpatient chronic disease clinic, and in broad segments of the population of many parts of the world. The key features of successful accommodation are a less-than-critical total lean tissue depletion and weight stability, the presence of a normal plasma albumin level, a normal peripheral blood total lymphocyte count, and intact delayed cutaneous hypersensitivity.[140,141]

As part of the accommodation to starvation, amino acids released during peripheral protein wasting are preferentially captured by the central lean tissues. However, when accommodation fails because of terminal depletion of the peripheral stores, metabolic stress, or for other reasons, proteins are lost from both the central and peripheral compartments (Fig. 56–5). Stress-induced central protein deficiency may occur because hyperglycemia induced by stress hormones stimulates insulin

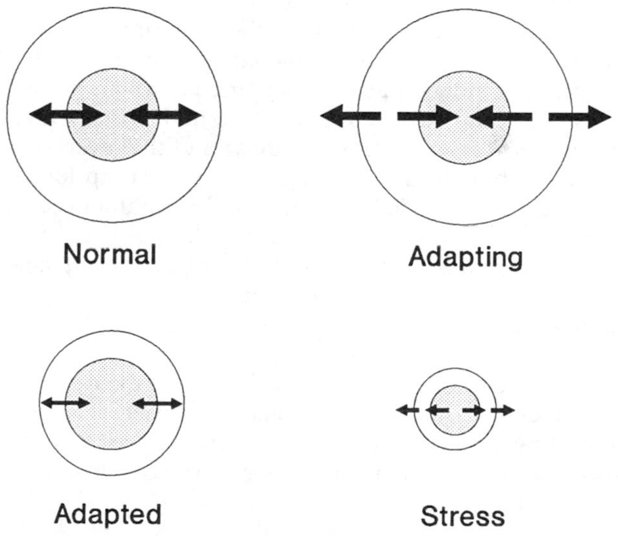

FIGURE 56–5. Adaptation to starvation. The outer circles represent the mass of peripheral, metabolically active proteins. The inner circles represent the central (visceral) proteins. The arrows represent N transfer. In normal life, protein equilibrium exists. During adaptation to starvation, N is lost from the body but there is a relative sparing of the central proteins. When accommodation is successful, equilibrium is reestablished at a major cost to peripheral proteins, but at a relatively minor cost to central proteins. Stress (or other reversal of accommodation) causes a loss of both central and peripheral N.

release, which drives scarce amino acids into the insulin-sensitive peripheral proteins at the expense of the insulin-insensitive central proteins.[20,140] A similar phenomenon occurs after prolonged administration of high-carbohydrate, amino acid-free intravenous infusions to unstressed patients. By contrast, the stress response in the well-nourished organism frequently is characterized by a mobilization of peripheral proteins to the center.[142]

The development of "central" protein deficiency, as manifested by anergy and hypoalbuminemia (with resultant edema) indicates a more advanced and dangerous condition.[140] Parallels have been drawn between simple, well-accommodated adult protein-energy malnutrition and childhood marasmus, and between central protein malnutrition in the adult and kwashiorkor, which may also be precipitated by stress or a high-energy, low-protein intake.[143] However, starvation in the chronically ill adult is only approximately similar to childhood marasmus or kwashiorkor,[41,144] and many observers disagree about the precise pathogenesis of kwashiorkor.[143] Most often, advanced protein-energy malnutrition in the adult has a mixture of "central" and "peripheral" features that tends toward one end of a spectrum or the other.

RECOGNITION OF FAILED ACCOMMODATION

Such failure should be suspected when a malnourished patient develops metabolic stress, as indicated by fever or a rapid heart rate. However, these responses to stress may be blunted in starving patients, and their absence does not rule out stress nor does it exclude factors other than stress that reverse accommodation. A more reliable sign of stress-induced protein wasting is an inappropriate rise in serum urea concentration and urinary urea excretion. By far, the simplest indicator of the reversal of accommodation from any cause is the resumption of weight loss in a previously weight-stable, malnourished patient, or the failure to gain weight despite the development of edema. Either situation indicates that new lean tissue loss is occurring. Factors that can impair accommodation and therefore should alert the clinician to its possible failure include further diminution of food intake, worsening of the primary disease or the development of one of its complications, the onset of a new disease that imposes a metabolic stress, or the administration of a treatment that alters protein or energy metabolism.

Metabolic Stress. The hypermetabolic, protein-catabolic response to severe infection, trauma, or major surgery reverses the accommodation to starvation.[140,145,146] Food intake previously compatible with homeostasis is now inadequate. Additionally, the starving patient tolerates stress poorly, moving rapidly into a state of central protein deficiency because peripheral and central protein reserves have previously been depleted.

Micronutrient Deficiency. Coexistent micronutrient deficiencies, particularly those of potassium,[32,147] phosphorus,[32] zinc,[148,149] and presumably magnesium, prevent maximal protein-sparing and an appropriate anabolic response to refeeding.

Metabolic Disease or the Administration of Hormones or Antimetabolites. Hyperthyroidism, pheochromocytoma, glucagonoma, poorly controlled diabetes mellitus, and states of glucocorticoid excess[150] are all associated with protein wasting. The existence of any of these diseases or its new development in starving patients calls for attention to the patient's nutritional status, because protein-energy malnutrition may develop rapidly, or the accommodation to pre-existing starvation may be reversed, progressing rapidly to an advanced stage. Some evidence reveals that the efficiency of protein metabolism remains abnormal even with appropriate insulin treatment of insulin-dependent diabetes.[151] Malnourished diabetic patients may therefore be at increased risk of severe protein depletion even when their blood glucose control is adequate.

Glucocorticoids or antimetabolites used to treat inflammatory conditions, or chemotherapeutic agents and extensive radiotherapy used in cancer therapy, may impair the accommodation to starvation. Anorexia is a systemic manifestation of certain malignancies, including those of the pancreas, stomach, and liver. Together with the anorexia induced by many chemotherapeutic agents,[152] abdominal radiation, and psychologic factors, food intake may be seriously impaired. This reduced intake adds to the metabolic effects of fever and infection, which are common in leukopenic and immunosuppressed individuals.

Food Restriction too Severe. The most common lethal maladaptation to starvation should not be described as maladaptation at all, but is merely the consequence of food restriction too severe for accommodation to succeed. The result is persistent weight loss until death occurs.

DEATH

Fat is the major storage fuel of animals, and in starvation, the size of the fat store determines the length of survival.[154] If energy expenditure is assumed to be 2000 kcal per day, the energy stored in the fat of a normal adult provides about 60 to 70 days of fuel. This amount coincides roughly with the length of survival of nonobese fasting individuals.[154] The expanded fat store of obese individuals permits longer survival. One grossly obese patient survived a fast of 310 days.[155] Unlike fat and carbohydrate, even a relatively moderate depletion of the lean tissue store has important adverse consequences. Because only moderately severe starvation largely depletes the fat store of nonobese individuals (see

Table 56–1), further weight loss by chronically starving patients even more so represents lean tissue wasting.

Adult body protein content is normally about 12 kg. About half of it is located in the active lean tissues. In total, this quantity of protein could theoretically supply only about 2 weeks of energy, but lean tissue loss in the range of 50% is incompatible with survival.[8,125,156,157] Because the previous normal weight of a patient is not always known, an even more precise predictor of the certainty of death from starvation may be the body mass index (body weight in kilograms divided by the square of height in meters). Data analyzed by Henry[158] indi-cate that death is certain when the body mass index falls to 13.

Terminal Causes of Death. In developed countries where severe starvation is almost always associated with a primary medical or surgical disease, the immediate causes of death are infectious pneumonia (related to decreased ventilatory mechanical function and drive, lung stasis, and ineffective cough); skin breakdown with local and systemic infection (related to inactivity, skin thinning, and edema); sepsis spreading from intravenous infusion catheters; diarrhea with dehydration; or synergistic worsening of the primary disease. Contributing to all these causes is starvation-induced immunodeficiency, itself the result of decreased mobilizable protein stores, hypothermia, anemia, and any of several possible micronutrient deficiencies.[2,137] In some patients, death is attributed to a cardiac arrhythmia.[5,159]

Although the nature of the primary disease influences the likelihood of death when starvation is only moderate, the dictum that death is increasingly certain when lean tissue depletion exceeds about 40% can be stated as a thermodynamic law, unaffected by the number of diagnostic procedures, operative interventions, or antibiotic combinations administered unless they are combined with nutritional therapy. It is possible occasionally to plot the weight loss velocity of patients maladapted to starvation and thereby to predict their date of death with an accuracy that is astonishing to physicians who failed to include the concept of maladapted starvation in their clinical evaluation.[160]

Descriptions of needless death from starvation evoke feelings of dismay in most commentators. Particularly moving are the writing of Fliederbaum, whose observations carried out in the Warsaw ghetto constitute probably the best clinical description of the effects of severe starvation ever published:[124]

". . . boys and girls from blooming like roses change into withered old people. One of the patients said, 'Our strength is vanishing like a melting wax candle.' Active, busy, energetic people are changed into apathetic, sleepy beings, always in bed, hardly able to get up to eat or to go to the toilet. Passage from life to death is slow and gradual, like death from physiological old age. There is nothing violent, no dyspnea, no pain, no obvious changes in breathing or circulation. Vital functions subside simultaneously. Pulse rate and respiratory rate get slower and it becomes more and more difficult to reach the patient's awareness, until life is gone. People fall asleep in bed or on the street and are dead in the morning. They die during physical effort, such as searching for food, and sometimes even with a piece of bread in their hands."

PROLONGED FASTING

It is important to know the precise meaning of the terms used by authors discussing metabolism in starvation or fasting. In this chapter, starvation refers to any prolonged submaintenance food intake, and fasting to the total denial of all food energy. A prolonged fast is one that extends for several days or longer. However, for many authors, starvation means total food energy deprivation (i.e., a fast). For other authors, fasting refers to the metabolic condition of any person after the overnight sleep (before "breakfast"), while others consider a fast to be any diet that is restricted to only a few nutrients, such as a "juice fast."

Metabolism during prolonged fasting is dominated by the low-insulin state that results when the body's limited carbohydrate store is exhausted (see Chapter 40). Fasting metabolism is characterized by a variety of features that result from insulin deficiency, including ketoacidosis. Because a carbohydrate intake of as little as 150 g per day elevates insulin levels enough to abolish ketosis,[98] only rarely are patients with even advanced protein-energy malnutrition in ketosis or do they manifest a hormonal and metabolic profile of prolonged fasting.[12] Insulin (and its lack) has enormous effects on all aspects of intermediary metabolism, so it is critical to know, when interpreting the results of biochemical studies of starvation, whether the nutritional manipulations involved severe insulin deficiency (as in fasting or diabetes), protein deficiency in the presence of adequate carbohydrate energy, or gradations between these extremes.

Despite its rarity as a clinical entity, and its inappropriateness in many respects as a clinical model of protein-energy malnutrition, the physiology of prolonged fasting has a long tradition in human nutrition research. Investigations of fasting metabolism have led to important insights into the hormonal regulation of fuel and protein metabolism, and a better understanding of diabetes mellitus. The major emphasis of this section is on body protein metabolism in prolonged fasting. For details of other fasting responses, the reader is referred to review articles on endocrinologic,[161] metabolic,[162] fuel-metabolic,[128,163] fluid and electrolyte,[164] and the clinical[165] aspects of prolonged fasting.

COMPARISON OF THE FED AND POSTABSORPTIVE STATES

A lucid description of fasting best proceeds from the last meal before the fast begins. Characteristic of the fed state are increased blood concentrations of glucose, fats (and their metabolic intermediates), and amino acids. Another characteristic is insulin secretion induced by the absorbed nutrients as well as by neural and gut hormone signals. Insulin regulates the disposition of the absorbed nutrients, by stimulating glucose incorporation into glycogen in the liver, glucose transport and glycogen synthesis in muscle, triglyceride synthesis, and amino acid transport and synthesis into proteins in the insulin-sensitive peripheral tissues (mainly muscle). Glucagon levels are unchanged or decreased during meals containing carbohydrate, but a protein meal low in carbohydrate stimulates glucagon secretion. This effect directs the liver to continue glycogen breakdown and glucose synthesis, thereby maintaining glucose levels in spite of the concurrent insulin stimulation driving glucose and amino acids into the peripheral tissues.

The fed state ends with disposal of the last absorbed nutrient and the transition to endogenous fuel consumption begins. The state, approximately 12 hours from the previous meal (corresponding to the condition following an overnight fast), has been found convenient for study and is termed the "postabsorptive state." It is characterized by the release, interorgan transfer, and oxidation of endogenous fatty acids, glucose from liver glycogen, and muscle amino acids, all a result of (or facilitated by) relatively low levels of circulating insulin. Even with high carbohydrate diets, the major postabsorptive fuel is fat, with two thirds of the resting energy expenditure provided by fat oxidation.[166]

KEY ROLE OF GLUCOSE

In normal postabsorptive man, the plasma glucose appearance rate is about 8 to 10 g per hour.[161] The free glucose pool of the body, about 16 g, is thus replaced every 2 hours. If the circulating glucose concentration falls rapidly below a critical value, altered mentation and coma result almost immediately, and prolonged hypoglycemia may destroy brain tissue. Given the fixed glucose requirement of the brain, no room for error is possible in the regulation of glucose delivery to the bloodstream by the liver. Indeed, in the healthy organism, blood glucose concentrations are tightly regulated within a narrow range by the action of at least three control systems. First, high insulin levels promote the uptake of glucose into muscle and fat and stimulate hepatic glycogen synthesis while inhibiting its breakdown, thereby decreasing the release of newly synthesized glucose molecules from the liver. All of these actions decrease circulating glucose levels. Low insulin levels allow blood glucose levels to rise by increasing net hepatic glycogen conversion to glucose while limiting glucose uptake into muscle and fat. Second, glucagon stimulates hepatic glycogen breakdown and gluconeogenesis, thereby increasing blood glucose concentrations. Third, an autonomic nervous and hormonal counter-regulatory system is activated in response to brain glucose deprivation, stimulating rapid glycogen breakdown and a rise in the blood glucose concentration.

In the postabsorptive state, liver glucose release equals its rate of use by the brain and other tissues, a total of about 200 to 250 g per day.[161] A large fraction of the glucose released by the postabsorptive liver is derived from glycogen, the remainder being formed from noncarbohydrate sources.[161] A major source of glucose precursors is the pool of three-carbon intermediates: glycerol derived from triglyceride hydrolysis, and lactate and pyruvate derived from the Embden-Meyerhof glycolytic pathway. Because this source of lactate and pyruvate is pre-existing glucose, their biotransformation into glucose molecules in the liver constitutes a substrate cycle (known as the Cori cycle in the case of lactate), the activity of which results in no net increase or decrease in the amount of glucose in the organism.

Action of the Cori cycle may account for about 40% of normal plasma glucose turnover.[167] The advantages of this cycle are as follows: (1) tissues that derive energy only by means of the anaerobic Embden-Meyerhof pathway (such as blood cells) may operate without causing a loss to the body of precious glucose molecules; the lactate and pyruvate molecules produced as end products of glycolysis are returned to the liver for resynthesis into new glucose molecules, the energy cost of this process being borne by fatty acid oxidation in the liver; and (2) muscle tissue cannot release stored glucose, because it lacks glucose-6-phosphatase; glucose-6-phosphate derived from muscle glycogen breakdown is metabolized to lactate and pyruvate, which may then leave that tissue to be used as a precursor for gluconeogenesis in the liver. The newly synthesized glucose is now available for use in the brain. Under usual dietary conditions, the brain oxidizes glucose completely to CO_2 and water and therefore irreversibly drains the body glucose pool. In the absence of dietary glucose or endogenous glycogen stores, the source of substrate to make up this requirement must come from elsewhere—from amino acids (except leucine, whose carbon atoms cannot be converted into glucose) and from glycerol derived from triglyceride hydrolysis. Although glycogen breakdown largely meets the needs of brain glucose oxidation postabsorptively, total body glycogen stores are inadequate to meet this requirement for more than 3 days. Brain glucose needs must therefore increasingly be met through amino acid conversion to glucose. A typical observation in early fasting is an abrupt and sustained loss of body N of about 12 g per day.[168]

Changes in insulin and glucagon orchestrate the process by which increasing amounts of muscle amino acids are made available for conversion to glucose in the liver. In the first days of a fast, the insulin level drops while that of glucagon remains constant or increases modestly and transiently. This combination primes enzymes in the liver to inhibit glycolysis and to convert gluconeogenic three-carbon intermediates into glucose, while blocking their oxidation through the Krebs cycle. The lowered insulin level allows for mobilization of free fatty acids from adipose tissue triglyceride and of free amino acids from muscle,[49] while the lowered insulin-glucagon ratio activates the liver for fatty acid oxidation. Once the liver is activated in this way, its rate of fatty acid oxidation is determined by the rate at which fatty acids are presented to it.[169] Thus, along with diminished conversion of glucose and glucose precursors to acetyl coenzyme A (the entry substrate for the Krebs cycle) there is an increase in acetyl coenzyme A production derived from fatty acid oxidation. Although some acetyl coenzyme A produced from fatty acid oxidation presumably is terminally oxidized through the intrahepatic Krebs cycle, most is converted to acetoacetate, which in turn gives rise reversibly to β-hydroxybutyrate and to a lesser extent (irreversibly) to acetone. The appearance in the circulation of these three substrates, collectively known as "ketone bodies," is the hallmark of a low insulin-to-glucagon ratio and rapid hepatic fatty acid oxidation.

Although small amounts of acetoacetate are produced and used in the liver even in the fed state,[170] circulating ketone body concentrations are almost unmeasurably low under these conditions (0.1 mM), and the export of ketone bodies from the liver is probably negligible. In the early days of fasting, the rate of acetoacetate synthesis increases greatly, and all, or almost all, synthesized acetoacetate and β-hydroxybutyrate leaves the liver to be used as a fuel substrate in the other tissues, including muscle and brain. As ketone body concentrations rise, they replace glucose as a brain fuel, and the rate of brain glucose oxidation decreases substantially.

In a study carried out in 5-week fasting humans, glucose uptake by the brain was equivalent to only 40 g per day, less than one half the normal rate. Moreover, only 60% of the glucose taken up by the brain was oxidized to CO_2 and water; the remainder was returned to the circulation as reusable lactate and pyruvate.[171] This adaptation permits a 75% reduction in the irreversible loss of glucose through brain oxidation with a concurrent decrease in the need for gluconeogenesis from amino acids and glycerol. More recently, positron-emission tomography studies in fully conscious humans have confirmed a dramatic decrease of glucose use in all brain regions after 3 weeks of fasting.[172]

Historically, the recognition that the glucose requirement of the brain can also be met by ketone bodies came by a different route. It was known that the early stages of fasting are accompanied by glycogen depletion, followed by a rise in body N loss, and carbohydrate provision early in the fast prevents these changes. In living animals, Lusk demonstrated the efficient conversion of protein to glucose. No similar conversion of fat to glucose occurred and, as predicted, if glucose was the energy source specifically required, equivalent amounts of fat had no protein-sparing effect.[166] Thus, it was apparent that glucose was required in early fasting, and in the absence of glycogen, the need was met by protein conversion to glucose. When the obligate glucose requirement of the brain was understood, the maximum possible rate of gluconeogenesis (as calculated from body N and glycerol loss) fell far short of the presumed brain metabolic needs during fasting.[168] Finally, the human study described by Owen and co-workers in 1967 demonstrated both ketone body use and decreased glucose oxidation in the prolonged fasting human brain.[171] Results of biochemical studies in the rat confirmed that brain tissues readily metabolize ketone bodies at a rate controlled by the prevailing ketone body concentration.[173]

PROTEIN METABOLISM

Several investigators have measured the response of whole-body protein turnover to prolonged fasting. Plasma branched-chain amino-acid concentrations increase greatly and leucine turnover increases modestly after 1 to 3 days of fasting (together with increased oxidation of the tracer). This response is prevented by the administration of carbohydrate,[174] and probably represents increased muscle proteolysis resulting from insulin deficiency.[49] The true increase of muscle proteolysis at this stage of fasting is probably underestimated by the whole-body leucine turnover measurement, which indicates the combined and opposite effects of increased muscle proteolysis and a diminished absolute breakdown rate of labile protein (related to a depletion of its total mass).[75] The urinary excretion of 3-methylhistidine, an indicator of myofibrillar protein breakdown, also appears to increase in the first few days of fasting.[75,175] By the end of the first week, these acute increases in protein turnover are followed by decreased leucine[75,174] or lysine[176] turnover with maintained oxidation[75] as body protein losses remain considerable. However, by 3 weeks, N excretion has clearly diminished, and protein turnover measured at this time has fallen even further than after 7 to 10 days of fasting,[31,177] along with decreased 3-methylhistidine excretion.[31] When small amounts of carbohydrate are provided at this time, leucine turnover decreases even further, in association with decreased leucine oxidation and diminished urinary N loss. By contrast, after 1 week of hypocaloric protein refeeding, N balance is positive despite the energy deficit, but leucine turnover remains as low as during the preceding total fast.[31]

MECHANISM FOR DIMINISHED PROTEIN LOSSES

The ability of the brain to use ketone bodies in place of glucose has been used to explain much of the adaptation to fasting. In a fast lasting more than 2 weeks, rates of urinary N loss diminish to 4 to 6 g per day, one half to one third those at the beginning. The adaptation is even more impressive, for about 50% of urinary N at this time is in ammonium excreted to buffer the protons generated by ketoacid production, and it can be eliminated by administering bicarbonate.[163,178,179] Some authors propose that this lifesaving slowing of body N loss occurs because ketone bodies increasingly displace glucose as brain fuel, thereby diminishing the need for gluconeogenesis from amino acids and sparing body protein.

Unexplained in this concept is the signal, after about 2 weeks of fasting, that "tells" the proteins catabolized as a result of insulin deficiency that they need no longer be broken down to provide carbons for gluconeogenesis. Much research has been conducted to address this question because of its relevance to clinical situations in which the sparing of body protein could be lifesaving.

In the postabsorptive state, muscle is in negative amino acid balance.[180] The release of alanine and glutamine far exceeds that of the other amino acids, and indeed, it can be estimated that only about one third of the alanine released from postabsorptive muscle is derived from the alanine of muscle protein itself.[181] The source of the alanine is pyruvate and N, but uncertainty exists both about the source of the pyruvate carbon skeleton and the amino group with which it condenses. According to one view, the pyruvate is derived almost entirely from glucose molecules. Alanine released by muscle, taken up by the liver, and converted into glucose would not then provide new glucose molecules to the body, but is recirculated in a cycle termed the "glucose-alanine cycle."[182,183] New glucose molecules would be synthesized when amino acid carbon skeletons are delivered intact to the liver, or after their conversion within the muscle to glutamine. Another view maintains that most amino acids are converted within muscle tissue into pyruvate, then aminated to alanine and released to the liver.[162,184] According to the latter view, alanine is largely an amino acid-derived gluconeogenic precursor and is not part of a substrate cycle. The N of alanine could be derived from the branched chain amino acids,[184] a view consistent with the glucose-alanine cycle or, alternatively, alanine could be a carrier to the liver of N removed from all amino acids catabolized to pyruvate within muscle.

In addition to alanine, postabsorptive muscle is in a negative balance of similar magnitude for glutamine.[97,185] Because each glutamine molecule contains two N atoms, glutamine is quantitatively a more important transporter of N from the muscle than alanine.[97,185] In the rat, a large proportion of muscle-exported glutamine is taken up by the intestinal tissues and oxidized as a fuel substrate.[186] Another important site of glutamine uptake is the kidney, where it is used as a substrate for renal ammonia production.[181] Interorgan glutamine traffic is altered dramatically during fasting, in part as a consequence of the metabolic acidosis that accompanies ketosis.[178]

The transiently increased muscle proteolysis and decrease in muscle protein synthesis that make free amino acids available for catabolism are probably the result of the combined effect of absent exogenous amino acids and insulin deficiency (and possibly a secondary decrease in IGF-1[49]). Both factors individually are known to inhibit muscle protein synthesis.[187] The liver during fasting is already primed for gluconeogenesis by the altered insulin-glucagon ratio. In early fasting, plasma alanine levels actually fall, despite their augmented muscle release. Findings of balance studies confirm that this decrease occurs because of exceptionally avid liver alanine uptake and conversion to glucose.[161] In prolonged fasting, the avidity of the liver for gluconeogenic precursors is unaltered. The protein-sparing mechanism of prolonged fasting appears therefore to reside in muscle, for as a fast is extended, muscle output of all the amino acids decreases (and especially of alanine and glutamine).[97,161] The question then becomes: What "tells" net muscle protein breakdown to diminish in prolonged fasting, thereby diminishing the rate of whole body protein loss?

After the brain has adapted to ketone body oxidation, it no longer uses as much glucose; the need for amino acid catabolism to provide gluconeogenic precursors therefore decreases. It might appear that the brain somehow "signals" muscle to decrease its rate of net proteolysis, but decreased brain glucose oxidation is not linked closely in time to the curtailment of N loss, which becomes evident only after about 2 weeks of fasting. Brain glucose oxidation probably declines as soon as a few days after fasting begins. The ketone-oxidizing enzymes in the brain are already active after an overnight fast,[161] and it is likely that blood ketone body levels of 2 mM (which may be achieved within 48 hours of fasting) permit efficient ketone body use.[188] Human studies with tracer glucose demonstrate a 40 to 50% decrease in plasma glucose turnover within a few days of fasting.[168,189] Under these conditions, glucose use is entirely attributable to oxidation and recycling; because the Cori cycle is quantitatively unchanged even in prolonged fasting,[190] the decrease in glucose turnover in early fasting is probably related to decreased oxidation. Indeed, even the large losses of body N of 12 g per day that may occur during the first week of fasting represent a loss to the body of only about 75 g of protein (lean tissue protein is 16% N by weight). This amount could generate a maximum of 45 g of new glucose per day,[191] which is inadequate to meet usual brain requirements once all glycogen is used. Therefore, brain fuel consumption has probably switched substantially to ketone oxidation by, at the latest, 1 week of fasting, at a time when body protein catabolism is still nearly maximal.

If a diminution of brain glucose oxidation does not signal the muscles to diminish amino acid oxidation, what may do so? During a fast, blood ketone body levels rise rapidly for about 7 to 10 days, followed by a more gradual rise to a plateau of 6 to 8 mM after 2 to 3 weeks. Liver ketone body production is already maximal by day 3 or 4, so the continuing rise in their blood levels must result from decreased use or excretion. In fact, both occur. In the first 3 to 10 days of fasting, the efficiency of renal conservation of ketone bodies increases, thus limiting their losses in the urine. In later fasting, muscle ketone body oxidation is largely replaced by fatty acid oxidation. In the face of continuing ketogenesis, this decrease in oxidation has the effect of raising the blood ketone body concentration.[161] One suggestion is that hyperketonemia itself may provide a protein-sparing signal to muscle.[192,193] Another possibility is that the process by which muscle metabolism switches from ketone body oxidation to fatty acid oxidation, as fasting progresses, is intimately involved in the decreased protein breakdown. Perhaps increased muscle fatty acid oxidation spares the branched chain amino acids (which have structural similarity to fatty acids) and these spared branched chain amino acids (or their metabolites) bring about diminished proteolysis.[163] This possibility is attractive because of evidence that these molecules, particularly leucine, have protein-sparing effects.[68,194] Finally, ketone bodies probably stimulate insulin secretion.[195] Even though circulating insulin levels remain low in prolonged fasting, hyperketonemia might stimulate a rise in insulin levels too slight to be measured consistently with methods now available.[129,169,195] A slight rise in insulin levels under these conditions could have an important effect in the body to spare proteins.

In summary, the major unanswered question in the physiology of human fasting is the identity of the hormone, fuel, or mechanism that arises to counteract the accelerated net muscle proteolysis induced by insulin deficiency. As already indicated, some of the N loss in late fasting is in ammonium needed to eliminate the protons generated by ketogenesis. Apart from these features, the adaptation to fasting (including an early loss of labile protein[75]) is probably the same as adaptation to starvation in general, depending on both intact hormonal signals and the sensitivity of the protein synthetic and degradative machinery of the individual tissues to amino acid delivery, as described previously.[30]

WEIGHT-REDUCTION DIETS AND STARVATION (SEE ALSO CHAP. 59)

Conventional weight-reduction diets used for the treatment of obesity are associated with an adaptation no different from the one that occurs in starving nonobese patients. Thus, weight-reducing obese patients may experience an adaptively lowered basal metabolic rate and lean tissue wasting, particularly when the energy deficiency imposed by the diet is severe[196] or if the protein intake is insufficient.[36] These adaptations are contrary to the goals of obesity therapy. The metabolic ideal during weight reduction is an acceptably rapid decrease of the fat store together with preservation of the lean tissue store to sustain fitness and the nutritional reserve, as well as to prevent a fall in the basal metabolic rate. To accomplish these goals, patients are counseled to be physically active. It is important also to bear in mind that protein use is impaired when the energy balance is negative, so to compensate for this fact, the protein intake should be higher than the normal recommendation.[197]

Differences in starvation-metabolism of obese and nonobese individuals have been described. For example, the energy intake of nonobese individuals can be reduced so greatly that no physiologic accommodation will lower energy expenditure enough to re-establish energy equilibrium. Under these circumstances, both fat and lean tissues continue to be lost (although at gradually decreasing rates) until death occurs, no matter how high the protein intake. Yet obese patients routinely achieve a state of continuing fat loss at the expense of only slight or acceptable lean tissue losses. In fact, the sparing of body proteins that occurs in obesity-starvation is the reason why energy expenditure remains high and the energy balance remains negative.

Such considerations, as well as comparisons of N excretion by lean and obese individuals involved in different starvation studies, have led to the conclusion that the excess fat store of weight-reducing obese individuals permits them to conserve their body protein more efficiently than starving nonobese individuals.[5,198,199] Indeed, in the rat, a short-term protein-sparing effect of obesity is suggested.[153] However, a problem arises with the human studies. Starving nonobese subjects observed in detail have invariably been men whose protein intake was relatively low, whereas obese subjects have predominantly been healthy women eating large amounts of protein. In those few human studies designed specifically to examine the effect of adiposity on protein loss in starvation, eliminating the effects of sex, diet composition, and prior protein depletion, no important differences in protein conservation have been observed.[200]

As described previously, the rate of weight loss and N loss during severe energy restriction is directly proportional to body weight and the lean tissue mass.[128,201,202] In agreement with this concept, N losses of starving obese individuals on diets of fixed protein intake vary directly with the urinary excretion of creatinine,[200,203,204] a measure of the lean tissue mass. To the extent that the lean tissue mass is increased in obese individuals, their absolute rate of N loss will actually be greater than that of leaner individuals.[165,204] Because somewhat similar rates of N loss occur in obese fasting individuals and in most normal-weight fasting individuals, both in early and adapted total fasting,[166,200] it is possible that relative to the total amount of lean tissue present, the fractional N loss could be somewhat slower in obesity.[199] However, clear-cut confirmation of this relationship is lacking.

Several factors could explain a protein-sparing effect of human obesity, if it exists. First, the maximum potential whole-body flux of free fatty acids released during lipolysis is greater in obesity because more triglyceride is available for lipolysis. Perhaps this higher flux (it must be higher in starving obesity because the metabolic rate is higher) in some manner more closely approximates the protein-sparing condition that exists when exogenous fuel is consumed. Second, obese individuals have a degree of peripheral insulin resistance, and therefore secrete more insulin than normal. Higher levels of circulating insulin could conceivably produce a more efficient recycling of body proteins. A problem with both these explanations is the lack of a dose-response relationship showing greater protein-sparing associated with increasing adiposity. Individuals with mild, and sometimes even trivial obesity are frequently in N equilibrium on high-protein weight-reduction diets.[200] Finally, the higher level of physical activity and greater amount of work performed by otherwise healthy, motivated, and cheerful obese patients could have a protein-sparing effect, when compared with physically inactive famine patients or the chronically ill. Clinical experience does show that therapeutic starvation as occurs in weight reduction is psychologically better tolerated by obese individuals than enforced starvation of lean individuals.[5]

USE OF VERY LOW-ENERGY DIETS FOR WEIGHT REDUCTION

Physician-supervised diets providing 600 kcal per day or less are in wide use because they are easy to follow and result in rapid short-term weight loss. Only brief observations of relevance to starvation metabolism in obesity are presented here, but excellent clinical and theoretic reviews are available.[36,205,206] First, zero N balance can be achieved within 2 or 3 weeks in some, but not all, obese patients. The initial pattern is an abrupt loss of body N, followed, over the ensuing 1 to 3 weeks, by improved N balance. However, individual variability is great, with some patients never attaining zero N balance over the period of observation. N losses continue more frequently in men than women, and in those with the greatest degree of overweight, presumably because of their greater initial lean tissue mass. Some body N losses are inevitable during weight reduction in extreme obesity, because loss of body fat decreases the need for extra muscles to move about and for extra supporting tissues to maintain the adipose tissue.[36,128] Because energy restriction is severe, it is even more important than with conventional dieting to provide a high intake of protein of high biologic value together with all the other nutrients required for lean tissue synthesis.[36]

Unlike prolonged fasting,[31,177] protein turnover is reasonably well maintained with very low-energy diets, provided enough protein is eaten.[177,197] At a low-protein intake or during the ingestion of a low-quality protein, protein turnover is dramatically reduced.[174,207] With intermediate protein intakes, evidence for a lowering of protein turnover is inconclusive.[197,207,208]

Because carbohydrate intake is limited, often to zero, all very low-energy diets are mildly to moderately ketogenic and are metabolically similar to a total fast, hence the term "protein-sparing modified fast" introduced by Bistrian and Blackburn in reference to the high-protein, carbohydrate-free diets they studied.[209] As implied by this name, the weight loss pattern differs from that in total fasting. The absolute rate of weight loss is slower, but the rate of fat loss is remarkably similar, because the decrease in metabolic rate characteristic of fasting is less intense when the lean tissues are spared. Thus, fasting, quite apart from its potential hazards, has the disadvantage that weight regain is obligatory during refeeding (to restore the depleted lean tissue store) and the greatly slowed metabolic rate promotes undesirable fat regain. The theoretic calculations in Table 56–2 demonstrate this phenomenon and provide a mathematic approach that can be used to monitor patients on very low-energy diets.[210–213] Sustained rates of weight loss faster than appropriate for the degree of negative energy balance are a danger sign, indicating maladaptation to the diet because of such factors as dietary noncompliance, micronutrient deficiency, or metabolic stress.

TABLE 56–2. WEIGHT LOSS BY AN OBESE PATIENT AFTER 3 WEEKS OF A TOTAL FAST OR A PROTEIN-SPARING MODIFIED FAST

	DIET	FAST
Energy expenditure		
R.M.R.	−10%	−25%
Activity factor	+50%	+25%
T.E.F. (kcal/day)	50	0
Ketonuria (kcal/day)	50	100
Total (kcal/day)	2260	1600
Energy intake (kcal/day)	500	100
Energy balance (kcal/day)	−1760	−1500
Weight loss (g/day)		
Adipose tissue	219	187
Lean tissue	0	125
Total	219	312

Calculated changes in body composition of a 35 year-old, 112-kg woman with a resting metabolic rate (R.M.R.) of 1600 kcal per day[210] after 3 weeks of a 420-g per day lean-meat diet (80 g protein and 20 g fat) or a total fast. By this time she is in zero N balance on the meat diet, but losing 4 g N per day after adaptation to the fast. To make these calculations, the thermic effect of the food (T.E.F.) is taken as 10% of its total energy; mixed body proteins are 16% N, and the lean tissues 20% protein by weight;[211] the energy stored in endogenous fat is 9.45 kcal/g; 85% of the weight lost when adipose tissue is dissipated is pure fat.[212,213] Note that loss of body protein provides the fasting patient with about 100 kcal per day usable energy. These predicted values for weight loss come close to those observed clinically.

METABOLIC SIGNIFICANCE OF KETOSIS

The mention of ketosis and ketoacidosis most often brings diabetes mellitus to mind. In the most severe form of diabetes, destruction or absence of the beta cells of the pancreas produces a state of severe insulin deficiency. The result is increased mobilization of fatty acids and a priming of the liver for ketone body production and gluconeogenesis.[214] Without insulin, little glucose is removed by muscle and adipose tissue, with the result that the blood glucose concentration rises to high levels. In the normal fasting individual, a sufficiently high circulating level of the ketone bodies probably stimulates insulin secretion.[195] The released insulin both inhibits ketogenesis and enhances peripheral ketone body use, with the result that ketone body levels do not rise above 6 to 8 mM. In severe diabetes, this feedback mechanism is unavailable and ketone body levels may rise to 12 to 14 mM, imposing an acid load too great for the buffering system to handle. A life-threatening fall in pH occurs if insulin therapy is unavailable.

Prolonged fasting is characterized not by a high, but by a low blood glucose concentration, because gluconeogenesis occurs slowly and peripheral glucose removal is unimpaired. The insulin level is low, not because of insulin deficiency as in diabetes, but because the low blood glucose concentration leaves insulin unstimulated; the feedback mechanisms that permit euglycemia and control of the ketone body level are intact. Ketosis in fasting is physiologic and is a manifestation of proper metabolic regulation; it does not lead to the severe condition typical of diabetic ketoacidosis.[161,169]

The ingestion of glucose stimulates insulin secretion and thereby prevents or abolishes ketosis; glucose therefore is said to be antiketogenic.[169] Dietary protein is also antiketogenic, although its effect in humans is less potent than that of glucose.[166] The blood ketone body concentration of an individual on a high-protein, carbohydrate-free diet is typically 2 to 3 mM, less than one half that found in association with prolonged fasting.[39,197,215] The switch from a carbohydrate-rich to a carbohydrate-free diet results in a transient loss of body protein and the development of sustained, mild ketosis.[39] After the period of adaptation, a carbohydrate-free diet, as long as it is adequate in protein and total energy, is compatible with normal protein economy.[23,39] On the other hand, a diet providing as little as 100 to 150 g of glucose per day is not typically ketogenic, yet it results in a sustained loss of body substance. It is apparent, then, that ketosis is not a sensitive or specific marker for starvation or a necessary condition for fat mobilization. It is best considered simply as the manifestation of the low-insulin state that occurs (in the absence of a pathologic insulin deficiency) when the diet is low in carbohydrate.

REFERENCES

1. Jelliffe, D.B.: J. Pediatr., *54:*227–256, 1959.
2. Golden, M.H.N., Jackson, A.A.: Chronic severe undernutrition. *In* Present Knowledge in Nutrition. 5th Ed. Edited by R.E. Olson, H.P. Brosquist, C.O. Chichester, et al. Washington, D.C., Nutrition Foundation, 1984, pp. 57–67.
3. Rivers, J.P.W.: The nutritional biology of famine. *In* Famine. Edited by G.A. Harrison. Oxford, Oxford University Press, 1988, pp. 57–106.
4. Bachrach, L.K., Katzman, D.K., Litt, I.F., et al.: J. Clin. Endocrinol. Metab., *72:*602–606, 1991.
5. Keys, A., Brozek, J., Henschel, A., et al.: The Biology of Human Starvation. Minneapolis, University of Minnesota Press, 1950.
6. Moore, F.D.: JPEN J. Parenter. Enteral Nutr., *4:*228–260, 1980.
7. Hill, G.L., Beddoe, A.H.: Dimensions of the human body and its compartments. *In* Nutrition and Metabolism in Patient Care. Edited by J.M. Kinney, K.N. Jeejeebhoy, G.L. Hill, et al. Philadelphia, W.B. Saunders, 1988, pp. 89–118.
8. Roubenoff, R., Kehayias, J.J.: Nutr. Rev., *49:*163–175, 1991.
9. Kotler, D.P., Wang, J., Pierson, R.N., Jr.: Am. J. Clin. Nutr., *42:*1255–1265, 1985.
10. James, H.M., Dabek, J.T., Chettle, D.R., et al.: Clin. Sci., *67:*73–82, 1984.
11. Heymsfield, S.B., Stevens, V., Noel, R., et al.: Am. J. Clin. Nutr., *36:*131–142, 1982.
12. Smith, S.R., Pozefsky, T., Chhetri, M.K.: Metabolism, *230:*603–618, 1974.
13. Ravussin, E., Lillioja, S., Anderson, T.E., et al.: J. Clin. Invest., *78:*1568–1578, 1986.
14. Shetty, P.S., Kurpad, A.V.: Eur. J. Clin. Nutr., *44 (Suppl. 1):*47–53, 1990.
15. Minghelli, G., Schutz, Y., Charbonnier, A., et al.: Am. J. Clin. Nutr., *51:*563–570, 1990.
16. Grande, F.: Man under caloric deficiency. *In* Handbook of Physiology. Section 4: Adaptation to the Environment. Edited by D.B. Dill. Washington, D.C., American Physiological Society, 1964, pp. 911–937.
17. Young, V.R., Moldawer, L.L., Hoerr, R., et al.: Mechanisms of adaptation to protein malnutrition. *In* Nutritional Adaptation in Man. Edited by K. Blaxter, J.C. Waterlow. London, John Libbey, 1985, pp. 189–217.
18. Lusk, G.: Physiol. Rev., *1:*523–552, 1921.
19. Shetty, P.S.: Nutr. Res. Rev., *3:*49–74, 1990.
20. Munro, H.N.: General aspects of the regulation of protein metabolism by diet and hormones. *In* Mammalian Protein Metabolism. Vol. 3. Edited by H.N. Munro, J.B. Allison. New York, Academic Press, 1964, pp. 381–481.
21. Elwyn, D.H., Gump, F.E., Munro, H.N., et al.: Am. J. Clin. Nutr., *32:*1597–1611, 1979.
22. Calloway, D.H.: Energy-protein relationships. *In* Protein Quality in Humans: Assessment and In Vitro Estimation. Edited by C.E. Bodwell, J.S. Adkins, D.T. Hopkins. Westport, CT, Avi Publishing Co., 1981, pp. 148–168.
23. Munro, H.N.: Physiol. Rev., *31:*449–488, 1951.
24. Elwyn, D.H.: Repletion of the malnourished patient. *In* Amino acids: Metabolism and Medical Applications. Edited by G.L. Blackburn, J. Grant, V.R. Young. Boston, John Wright PSG, Inc., 1983, pp. 359–375.
25. Kinney, J.M., Elwyn, D.H.: Annu. Rev. Nutr., *3:*433–466, 1983.
26. Joint Food and Agriculture Organization/World Health Organization Expert Committee: Energy and Protein Requirements. WHO Technical Report Series No. 522. Geneva, World Health Organization, 1973.

27. Food and Agriculture Organization/World Health Organization/United Nations University Expert Consultation: Energy and Protein Requirements. Technical Report Series No. 724. Geneva, World Health Organization, 1985.
28. Greenberg, G.R., Jeejeebhoy, K.N.: JPEN J. Parenter. Enteral Nutr., *3*:427–432, 1979.
29. Shaw, S.N., Elwyn, D.H., Askanazi, J., et al.: Am. J. Clin. Nutr., *37*:930–940, 1983.
30. Millward, D.J.: Clin. Nutr., *9*:115–126, 1990.
31. Hoffer, L.J., Forse, R.A.: Am. J. Physiol., *258*:E832–E840, 1990.
32. Rudman, D., Millikan, W.J., Richardson, T.J., et al.: J. Clin. Invest., *55*:94–104, 1975.
33. Passmore, R., Strong, J.A., Ritchie, F.J.: Br. J. Nutr., *12*:113–122, 1958.
34. Williams, R.J.: Biochemical Individuality. New York, John Wiley & Sons, 1956.
35. Hegsted, D.M.: Fed. Proc., *22*:1424–1430, 1963.
36. Gelfand, R.A., Hendler, R.: Diabetes Metab. Rev., *5*:17–30, 1989.
37. Fricker, J., Rozen, R., Melchior, J.-C., et al.: Am. J. Clin. Nutr., *53*:826–830, 1991.
38. Danforth, E., Jr., Burger, A.G.: Annu. Rev. Nutr., *9*:201–227, 1989.
39. Phinney, S.D., Bistrian, B.R., Wolfe, R.R., et al.: Metabolism, *32*:757–768, 1983.
40. Pittman, C.S., Suda, A.D., Chambers, J.B., Jr., et al.: Metabolism, *28*:333–338, 1979.
41. Golden, M.H.N.: Marasmus and kwashiorkor. *In* Nutrition and the Clinical Management of Disease. 2nd Ed. Edited by J.W.T. Dickerson, M.A. Lee. London, Edward Arnold, 1988, pp. 88–109.
42. Bilezikian, J.P., Loeb, J.N.: Endocr. Rev., *4*:378–388, 1983.
43. Milligan, L.P., McBride, B.W.: J. Nutr., *115*:1374–1382, 1985.
44. Clausen, T.: Physiol. Rev., *66*:542–580, 1986.
45. Willis, J.S., Golden, M.H.N.: Eur. J. Clin. Nutr., *42*:635–645, 1988.
46. Jeejeebhoy, K.N.: The functional basis of assessment. *In* Nutrition and Metabolism in Patient Care. Edited by J.M. Kinney, K.N. Jeejeebhoy, G.L. Hill, et al. Philadelphia, W.B. Saunders, 1988, pp. 739–751.
47. Harper, M.E., Patrick, J., Willis, J.S.: Eur. J. Clin. Nutr., *44*:549–558, 1990.
48. Flatt, J.P.: The biochemistry of energy expenditure. *In* Advances in Obesity Research. II. Edited by G. Bray. Westport, CT, Food and Nutrition Press, 1978, pp. 211–228.
49. Kettelhut, I.C., Wing, S.S., Goldberg, A.L.: Diabetes Metab. Rev., *4*:751–772, 1988.
50. Millward, D.J.: Proc. Nutr. Soc., *38*:77–88, 1979.
51. Jackson, A.A.: Nutritional adaptation in disease and recovery. *In* Nutritional Adaptation in Man. Edited by K. Blaxter and J.C. Waterlow. London, John Libbey, 1985, pp. 111–126.
52. Reeds, P.J., Wahle, K.W.J., Haggarty, P.: Proc. Nutr. Soc., *4*:155, 1982.
53. Reeds, P.J., Fuller, M.F., Nicholson, B.A.: Metabolic basis of energy expenditure with particular reference to protein. *In* Substrate and Energy Metabolism in Man. Edited by J.S. Garrow, D. Halliday. London, John Libbey, 1985, pp. 46–56.
54. Waterlow, J.C., Millward, D.J.: Energy cost of turnover of protein and other cellular constituents. *In* Energy Transformations in Cells and Organisms. Edited by W. Weisser, E. Graiger. Stuttgart, Thieme, 1989, pp. 277–282.
55. Schimke, R.T.: J. Biol. Chem., *237*:1921–1924, 1962.
56. Block, K.P., Aftring, R.P., Mehard, W.B., et al.: J. Clin. Invest., *79*:1349–1358, 1987.
57. Oratz, M., Rothschild, M.A.: The influence of alcohol and altered nutrition on albumin synthesis. *In* Alcohol and Abnormal Protein Synthesis. Edited by M.A. Rothschild, M. Oratz, S.S. Schreiber. New York, Pergamon Press, 1975, pp. 343–372.
58. Waterlow, J.C.: Annu. Rev. Nutr., *6*:495–526, 1986.
59. Young, V.R., Marchini, J.S.: Am. J. Clin. Nutr., *51*:270–289, 1990.
60. Eisenstein, R.S., Harper, A.E.: J. Nutr., *121*:1581–1590, 1991.
61. Albrecht, R., Pelissier, M.A., Miladi, N., et al.: Ann. Nutr. Metab., *30*:73–80, 1986.
62. McNurlan, M.A., Pain, V.M., Garlick, P.J.: Biochem. Soc. Trans., *8*:283–285, 1980.
63. Munro, H.N., Hubert, C., Baliga, B.S.: Regulation of protein synthesis in relation to amino acid supply—a review. *In* Alcohol and Abnormal Protein Biosynthesis. Edited by M.A. Rothschild, M. Oratz, S.S. Schreiber. New York, Pergamon Press, 1975, pp. 33–66.
64. Jefferson, L.S., Flaim, K.E.: Role of amino acid availability in the regulation of liver protein synthesis. *In* Amino Acids: Metabolism and Medical Applications. Edited by G.L. Blackburn, J.P. Grant, V.R. Young. Boston, John Wright PSG, 1983, pp. 167–182.
65. Strauss, D.S., Takemoto, C.D.: Endocrinology, *127*:1849–1860, 1990.
66. Conde, R.D., Scornik, O.A.: Biochem. J., *158*:385–390, 1976.
67. Mortimore, G.E., Khurana, K.K.: Int. J. Biochem., *22*:1075–1080, 1990.
68. McNurlan, M.A., Garlick, P.J.: Diabetes Metab. Rev., *5*:165–189, 1989.
69. Sugden, P.H., Fuller, S.J.: Biochem. J., *273*:21–37, 1991.
70. Garlick, P.J., Millward, D.J., James, W.P.T., et al.: Biochim. Biophys. Acta, *414*:71–84, 1975.
71. Rennie, M.J., Harrison, R.: Lancet, *1*:323–325, 1984.
72. Laurent, B.C., Moldawer, L.L., Young, V.R., et al.: Am. J. Physiol., *246*:E444–E451, 1984.
73. Bier, D.M.: Diabetes Metab. Rev., *5*:111–132, 1989.
74. Slevin, K., Jackson, A.A., Waterlow, J.C.: Proc. R. Soc. Lond. [Biol.], *243*:87–92, 1991.
75. Lariviere, F., Wagner, D.A., Kupranycz, D., et al.: Metabolism, *39*:1270–1277, 1990.
76. Hoerr, R.A., Matthews, D.E., Bier, D.M., et al.: Am. J. Physiol., *260*:E111–E117, 1991.
77. Anonymous: Nutr. Rev., *48*:380–382, 1990.
78. Louard, R.J., Gelfand, R.A.: Diabetes, *39 (Suppl. 1)*:27A, 1990.
79. Motil, K.J., Matthews, D.E., Bier, D.M., et al.: Am. J. Physiol., *240*:E712–E721, 1981.
80. Golden, M.H.N., Waterlow, J.C., Picou, D.: Clin. Sci., *53*:473–477, 1977.
81. Newsholme, E.A., Stanley, J.C.: Diabetes Metab. Rev., *3*:295–305, 1987.
82. Sukhatme, P.V., Margen, S.: Am. J. Clin. Nutr., *31*:1237–1256, 1978.
83. Young, V.R.: Am. J. Clin. Nutr., *46*:709–725, 1987.
84. Millward, D.J., Rivers, J.P.W.: Eur. J. Clin. Nutr., *42*:367–393, 1988.

85. Price, G., Millward, D.J.: Proc. Nutr. Soc., *49:*194A, 1990.
86. Hoffer, L.J., Bistrian, B.R., Phinney, S.D., et al.: Whole body protein turnover, studied with ^{15}N-glycine, during weight reduction by moderate energy restriction. *In* Amino Acids: Metabolism and Medical Applications. Edited by G.L. Blackburn, J. Grant, V.R. Young. Boston, John Wright, 1983, pp. 48–54.
87. Crim, M.C., Munro, H.N.: Protein-energy malnutrition and endocrine function. *In* Endocrinology. Edited by L.J. DeGroot, G.F. Cahill, Jr., W.D. Odell, et al. New York, Grune & Stratton, 1979, pp. 1987–2000.
88. Becker, D.J.: Annu. Rev. Nutr., *3:*187–212, 1983.
89. Clemmons, D.R., Underwood, L.E.: Annu. Rev. Nutr., *11:*393–412, 1991.
90. Snyder, D.K., Clemmons, D.R., Underwood, L.E.: J. Clin. Endocrinol. Metab., *69:*745–752, 1989.
91. Donahue, S.P., Phillips, L.S.: Am. J. Clin. Nutr., *50:*962–969, 1989.
92. Tollet, P., Enberg, B., Mode, A.: Mol. Endocrinol. *4:*1934–1942, 1990.
93. Ikeda, T., Fujiyama, K., Hoshino, T., et al.: Ann. Nutr. Metab., *34:*8–12, 1990.
94. Snyder, D.K., Clemmons, D.R., Underwood, L.E.: J. Clin. Endocrinol. Metab., *67:*54–61, 1988.
95. Lundeberg, S., Belfrage, M., Wernerman, J., et al.: Metabolism, *40:*315–322, 1991.
96. Jefferson, L.S., Flaim, K.E., Peavy, D.E.: Protein metabolism. *In* Diabetes Mellitus, Theory and Practice. 12th Ed. Edited by M. Ellenberg, H. Rifkin. New Hyde Park, Medical Examination Publishing Co., 1983, pp. 47–59.
97. Abumrad, N.N., Williams, P., Frexes-Steed, M., et al.: Diabetes Metab. Rev., *5:*213–226, 1989.
98. Aoki, T.T., Muller, W.A., Brennan, M.F., et al.: Am. J. Clin. Nutr., *28:*507–511, 1975.
99. Hoogwerf, B.J., Laine, D.C., Greene, E.: Am. J. Clin. Nutr., *43:*350–360, 1986.
100. Shizgal, H.M., Vasilevsky, C.A., Gardiner, P.F., et al.: Am. J. Clin. Nutr., *44:*761–771, 1986.
101. Pichard, C., Vaughan, C., Struk, R., et al.: J. Clin. Invest., *82:*895–901, 1988.
102. Kinney, J.M., Furst, P., Elwyn, D.H., et al.: The intensive care patient. *In* Nutrition and Metabolism in Patient Care. Edited by J.M. Kinney, K.N. Jeejeebhoy, G.L. Hill, et al. Philadelphia, W.B. Saunders, 1988, pp. 656–671.
103. Russell, D.McR., Walker, P.M., Leiter, L.A., et al.: Am. J. Clin. Nutr., *39:*503–513, 1984.
104. Musacchia, X.J., Steffen, J.M., Fell, R.D.: Exerc. Sport Sci. Rev., *16:*61–87, 1988.
105. Henriksson, J.: Eur. J. Clin. Nutr., *44 (Suppl. 1):*55–64, 1990.
106. Jeejeebhoy, K.N., Detsky, A.S., Baker, J.P.: JPEN J. Parenter. Enteral Nutr., *14:*193S–196S, 1990.
107. Stuart, C.A., Shangraw, R.E., Peters, E.J., et al.: Am. J. Clin. Nutr., *52:*509–514, 1990.
108. Peret, J., Jacquot, R.: Nitrogen excretion on complete fasting and on a nitrogen-free diet—endogenous protein. *In* Protein and Amino Acid Functions. Edited by E.J. Bigwood. Oxford, Pergamon Press, 1972, pp. 73–118.
109. Munro, H.N.: Free amino acid pools and their regulation. *In* Mammalian Protein Metabolism. Vol. 4. Edited by H.N. Munro. New York, Academic Press, 1970, pp. 299–386.
110. Waterlow, J.C.: Free amino acid pools and their regulation. *In* Nitrogen Metabolism in Man. Edited by J.C. Waterlow, J.M.L. Stephen. London, Applied Science Publishers, 1981, pp. 1–16.
111. Waterlow, J.C., Garlick, P.J.: Metabolic adaptions to protein deficiency. *In* Alcohol and Abnormal Protein Synthesis. Edited by M.A. Rothschild, M. Oratz, S.S. Schreiker. New York, Pergamon Press, 1975, pp. 67–94.
112. Elwyn, D.H.: The role of the liver in regulation of amino acid and protein metabolism. *In* Mammalian Protein Metabolism. Vol. 4. Edited by H.N. Munro. New York, Academic Press, 1970, pp. 523–558.
113. Raforth, R.J., Onstad, G.R.: J. Clin. Invest., *56:*1170–1174, 1975.
114. Wannemacher, R.W., Jr., Dinterman, R.E.: Biochem. J., *190:*663–671, 1980.
115. Larson, P.S., Chaikoff, I.L.: J. Nutr., *13:*287–304, 1937.
116. Owen, O.E., Mozzoli, M.A., Boden, G., et al.: Metabolism, *29:*511–523, 1980.
117. Wahren, J., Felig, P., Hagenfeldt, L.J.: J. Clin. Invest., *57:*987–999, 1976.
118. James, W.P.T., Ferro-Luzzi, A., Waterlow, J.C.: Eur. J. Clin. Nutr., *42:*969–981, 1988.
119. Garby, L.: World Rev. Nutr. Diet., *61:*173–208, 1990.
120. Munro, H.N., Chalmers, M.F.: J. Exp. Pathol., *26:*396–404, 1945.
121. Tomkins, A.M., Garlick, P.J., Schofield, W.N., et al.: Clin. Sci., *65:*313–324, 1983.
122. Lipschitz, D.A., Mitchell, C.O.: Nutritional assessment of the elderly—special considerations. *In* Nutritional Assessment. Edited by R.A. Wright, S. Heymsfield. Boston, Blackwell Scientific, 1984, pp. 131–139.
123. Helweg-Larsen, P., Hoffmeyer, H., Kieler, J., et al.: Acta Med. Scand. *144 (Suppl. 274):*1–460, 1952.
124. Fliederbaum, J.: Clinical aspects of hunger disease in adults. *In* Hunger Disease: Studies by the Jewish Physicians in the Warsaw Ghetto. Edited by M. Winick. New York, John Wiley & Sons, 1979, pp. 11–44.
125. Grant, J.P.: Clinical impact of protein malnutrition on organ mass and function. *In* Amino Acids: Metabolism and Medical Applications. Edited by G.L. Blackburn, J.P. Grant, V.R. Young. Boston, John Wright, 1983, pp. 347–358.
126. Heymsfield, S.B., Hoff, R.D., Gray, T.F., et al.: Heart Diseases. *In* Nutrition and Metabolism in Patient Care. Edited by J.M. Kinney, K.N. Jeejeebhoy, G.L. Hill, et al. Philadelphia, W.B. Saunders, 1988, pp. 477–509.
127. Silberman, H.: Parenteral and Enteral Nutrition. 2nd Ed. Norwalk, Appleton & Lange, 1989.
128. Owen, O.E.: Starvation. *In* Endocrinology. 2nd Ed. Edited by L.J. DeGroot, G.M. Besser, G.F. Cahill, Jr., et al. Philadelphia, W.B. Saunders, 1989, pp. 2282–2293.
129. Biden, T.J., Taylor, K.W.: Biochem. J., *212:*371–377, 1983.
130. Varma, D.R.: Drug. Dev. Res., *1:*183–198, 1981.
131. Anderson, K.E.: Clin. Pharmacokinet., *14:*325–346, 1988.
132. Krishnaswamy, K.: Clin. Pharmacokinet., *17 (Suppl. 1):*68–88, 1989.
133. Alexander, J.W.: Nutritional management of the infected patient. *In* Nutrition and Metabolism in Patient Care. Edited by J.M. Kinney, K.N. Jeejeebhoy, G.L. Hill, et al. Philadelphia, W.B. Saunders, 1988, pp. 625–634.
134. Fischer, J.E., Ghory, M.J.: Protein depletion and immunity in the hospitalized patient. *In* Nutritional Assessment. Edited by R.A. Wright, S. Heymsfield. Boston, Blackwell Scientific, 1984, pp. 111–129.

135. Wade, S., Bleiberg, F., Mosse, A., et al.: Am. J. Clin. Nutr., *42:*275–280, 1985.
136. Buzina, R., Bates, C.J., van der Beek, J., et al.: Am. J. Clin. Nutr., *50:*172–176, 1989.
137. Chandra, R.K.: Am. J. Clin. Nutr., *53:*1087–1101, 1991.
138. Meydani, S.N.: Nutr. Rev., *48:*361–369, 1990.
139. Grimble, R.F.: Nutr. Res. Rev., *3:*193–210, 1990.
140. Bistrian, B.R.: Nutritional assessment of the hospitalized patient: A practical approach. *In* Nutritional Assessment. Edited by R.A. Wright, S. Heymsfield. Boston, Blackwell Scientific, 1984, pp. 183–205.
141. Blackburn, G.L., Bistrian, B.R., Maini, B.S., et al.: JPEN J. Parenter. Enteral Nutr., *1:*11–22, 1977.
142. Moldawer, L.L., Lowry, S.F.: Annu. Rev. Nutr., *8:*585–609, 1988.
143. Latham, M.C.: Protein-energy malnutrition. *In* Present Knowledge in Nutrition. 6th Ed. Edited by M.L. Brown. Washington, International Life Sciences Institute-Nutrition Foundation, 1990, pp. 39–46.
144. Bistrian, B.R.: JPEN J. Parenter. Enteral Nutr., *14:*329–334, 1990.
145. Goldstein, S.A., Elwyn, D.H.: Annu. Rev. Nutr., *9:*445–473, 1989.
146. Long, C.L., Lowry, S.F.: JPEN J. Parenter. Enteral Nutr., *14:*555–562, 1990.
147. Knochel, J.P.: Adv. Intern. Med., *30:*317–335, 1984.
148. Wolman, S.L., Anderson, G.H., Marliss, E.B., et al.: Gastroenterology, *76:*458–467, 1979.
149. Khanum, S., Alam, A.N., Anwar, I., et al.: Eur. J. Clin. Nutr., *42:*709–714, 1988.
150. Garrel, D.R., Delmas, P.D., Welsh, C., et al.: Metabolism, *37:*257–262, 1988.
151. Lariviere, F., Chiasson, J.-L., Hoffer, L.J.: Clin. Res., *38:*294A, 1990.
152. Ollenschlaeger, G., Konkol, K., Wickramanayake, P.D., et al.: Am. J. Clin. Nutr., *50:*454–459, 1989.
153. Goodman, M.N., Lowell, B., Belur, E., et al.: Am. J. Physiol., *246:*E383–E390, 1984.
154. Leiter, L.A., Marliss, E.B.: JAMA, *248:*2306–2307, 1982.
155. Barnard, D.L., Ford, J., Garnett, E.S., et al.: Metabolism, *18:*564–569, 1969.
156. Garrow, J.S., Fletcher, K., Halliday, D.: J. Clin. Invest., *44:*417–425, 1965.
157. Heymsfield, S.B., McManus, C.B., III., Seitz, S.B., et al.: Anthropometric assessment of adult protein-energy malnutrition. *In* Nutritional Assessment. Edited by R.A. Wright, S. Heymsfield. Boston, Blackwell Scientific, 1984, pp. 27–82.
158. Henry, C.J.K.: Eur. J. Clin. Nutr., *44:*329–335, 1990.
159. Isner, J.M., Roberts, W.C., Heymsfield, S.B., et al.: Ann. Intern. Med., *102:*49–52, 1985.
160. Kotler, D.P., Tierney, A.R., Wang, J., et al.: Am. J. Clin. Nutr., *50:*444–447, 1989.
161. Felig, P.: Starvation. *In* Endocrinology. Edited by L.J. DeGroot, G.F. Cahill, Jr., W.D. Odell, et al. New York, Grune & Stratton, 1979, pp. 1927–1940.
162. Levenson, S.L., Seifter, E.: Starvation: Metabolic and physiologic responses. *In* Surgical Nutrition. Edited by J.E. Fischer. Boston, Little, Brown, 1983.
163. Cahill, G.F., Jr.: Clin. Endocrinol. Metab., *5:*397–415, 1976.
164. Drenick, E.J.: The effects of acute and prolonged fasting and refeeding on water, electrolyte, and acid-base metabolism. *In* Clinical Disorders of Fluid and Electrolyte Metabolism. Edited by M.H. Maxwell, C.R. Kleeman. New York, McGraw-Hill, 1980, pp. 1481–1501.
165. Drenick, E.J.: Weight reduction by prolonged fasting. *In* Obesity in Perspective: John E. Fogarty International Center for Advanced Study in the Health Sciences. D.H.E.W. Publication no. NIH 75-708. Edited by G.A. Bray. Bethesda, MD, National Institutes of Health, 1973, pp. 341–360.
166. Lusk, G.: The Science of Nutrition. 4th Ed. Philadelphia, W.B. Saunders, 1928.
167. Hoffer, L.J.: JPEN J. Parenter. Enteral Nutr., *14:*646–648, 1990.
168. Cahill, G.F., Jr., Herrera, M.G., Morgan, A.P., et al.: J. Clin. Invest., *45:*1751–1769, 1966.
169. Foster, D.W., McGarry, J.D.: N. Engl. J. Med., *309:*159–169, 1983.
170. Endemann, G., Goetz, P.G., Edmond, J., et al.: J. Biol. Chem., *257:*3434–3440, 1982.
171. Owen, O.E., Morgan, A.P., Kemp, H.G., et al.: J. Clin. Invest., *46:*1589–1595, 1967.
172. Redies, C., Hoffer, L.J., Beil, C., et al.: Am. J. Physiol., *256:*E805–E810, 1989.
173. Williamson, D.H., Bates, M.W., Page, M.A., et al.: Biochem. J., *121:*41–47, 1971.
174. Vasquez, J.A., Morse, E.L., Adibi, S.A.: J. Clin. Invest., *76:*737–743, 1985.
175. Giesecke, K., Magnusson, I., Ahlberg, M., et al.: Metabolism, *38:*1196–1200, 1989.
176. Henson, L.C., Heber, D.: J. Clin. Endocrinol. Metab., *57:*316–319, 1983.
177. Winterer, J., Bistrian, B.R., Bilmazes, C., et al.: Metabolism, *29:*575–581, 1980.
178. Abumrad, N.N., Yazigi, N., Cersosimo, E., et al.: JPEN J. Parenter. Enteral Nutr., *14:*71S–76S, 1990.
179. Sapir, D.G., Chambers, N.E., Ryan, J.W.: Metabolism, *25:*211–220, 1976.
180. Felig, P.: Annu. Rev. Biochem., *44:*933–955, 1975.
181. Felig, P.: Inter-organ amino acid exchange. *In* Nitrogen Metabolism in Man. Edited by J.C. Waterlow, J.M.L. Stephen. London, Applied Science Publishers, 1981, pp. 45–62.
182. Felig, P.: Metabolism, *22:*179–207, 1973.
183. Chang, T.W., Goldberg, A.L.: J. Biol. Chem., *253:*3677–3684, 1978.
184. Snell, K., Duff, D.A.: Branched chain amino acids and muscle alanine synthesis. *In* Metabolism and Clinical Implications of Branched Chain Amino and Ketoacids. Edited by M. Walser, J.R. Williamson. New York, Elsevier North Holland, 1981, pp. 251–256.
185. Marliss, E.B., Aoki, T.T., Pozefsky, T., et al.: J. Clin. Invest., *50:*814–817, 1971.
186. Windmueller, H.B., Spaeth, A.E.: J. Biol. Chem., *253:*69–76, 1978.
187. Jefferson, L.S.: Diabetes, *29:*487–496, 1980.
188. Flatt, J.P., Blackburn, G.L., Randers, G., et al.: Metabolism, *23:*151–158, 1974.
189. Nair, K.S., Woolf, P.D., Welle, S.L., et al.: Am. J. Clin. Nutr., *46:*557–562, 1987.
190. Streja, D.A., Steiner, G., Marliss, E.B., et al.: Metabolism, *26:*1089–1098, 1977.
191. Wolman, S.L., Fields, A.L.A., Cheema-Dhadli, S., et al.: JPEN J. Parenter. Enteral Nutr., *4:*487–489, 1980.
192. Palaiologos, G., Felig, P.: Biochem. J., *154:*709–716, 1976.

193. Nair, K.S., Welle, S.L., Halliday, D., et al.: J. Clin. Invest., *82:*198–205, 1988.
194. May, M.E., Buse, M.G.: Diabetes Metab. Rev., *5:*227–245, 1989.
195. Balasse, E.O., Fery, F.: Diabetes Metab. Rev., *5:*247–270, 1989.
196. Foster, G.D., Wadden, T.A., Feurer, I.D., et al.: Am. J. Clin. Nutr., *51:*167–172, 1990.
197. Hoffer, L.J., Bistrian, B.R., Young, V.R., et al.: J. Clin. Invest., *73:*750–758, 1984.
198. Van Itallie, T.B., Yang, M.U.: Nitrogen balance during weight reduction: Effect of body stores of protein and fat. *In* Recent Advances in Obesity Research: II. Edited by G.A. Bray. London, Newman Publishing, 1978, pp. 379–384.
199. Forbes, G.B.: Nutr. Rev., *45:*225–231, 1987.
200. Hoffer, L.J., Bistrian, B.R.: J. Obesity Weight Reduct., *3:*35–47, 1984.
201. Forbes, G.B.: Am. J. Clin. Nutr., *23:*1212–1219, 1970.
202. Forbes, G.B., Drenick, E.J.: Am. J. Clin. Nutr., *32:*1570–1574, 1979.
203. Forbes, G.B., Bruining, G.J.: Am. J. Clin. Nutr., *29:*1359–1366, 1976.
204. Henry, R.R., Wiest-Kent, T.A., Scheaffer, L., et al.: Diabetes, *35:*155–164, 1986.
205. Atkinson, R.L.: Med. Clin. North Am., *73:*203–215, 1989.
206. Fugate, L., Kaye, G., Perrin, D., et al.: Very Low Calorie Diets in the Management of Obesity. Columbus, Ohio, Ross Laboratories, 1990.
207. Garlick, P.J., Clugston, G.A., Waterlow, J.C.: Am. J. Physiol., *238:*E235–E244, 1980.
208. Bistrian, B.R., Sherman, M., Young, V.: J. Clin. Endocrinol. Metab., *53:*874–878, 1981.
209. Bistrian, B.R., Blackburn, G.L., Stanbury, J.B.: N. Engl. J. Med., *296:*774–779, 1977.
210. Owen, O.E., Kavle, E., Owen, R.S., et al.: Am. J. Clin. Nutr., *44:*1–19, 1986.
211. Reifenstein, E.C., Jr., Albright, F., Wells, S.L.: J. Clin. Endocrinol., *5:*367–395, 1947.
212. Grande, F., Keys, A.: Body weight, body composition and calorie status. *In* Modern Nutrition in Health and Disease. 6th Ed. Edited by R.S. Goodhart, M.E. Shils. Philadelphia, Lea & Febiger, 1980, pp. 3–34.
213. Garrow, J.S.: Am. J. Clin. Nutr., *35:*1152–1158, 1982.
214. McGarry, J.D., Woeltje, K.F., Kuwajmi, M., et al.: Diabetes Metab. Rev., *5:*271–284, 1989.
215. Marliss, E.B., Murray, F.T., Nakhooda, A.F.: J. Clin. Invest., *62:*468–479, 1978.

SELECTED READINGS

Felig, P.: Starvation. *In* Endocrinology. 1st Ed. Edited by L.J. DeGroot, G.F. Cahill, Jr., W.D. Odell, et al. New York, Grune & Stratton, 1979, pp. 1927–1940.

Helweg-Larson, P., Hoffmeyer, H., Kilder, J., et al.: Famine disease in German concentration camps: Complications and sequels. Acta Med. Scand., *144 (Suppl. 274):*1–460, 1952.

Hunger Disease: Studies by the Jewish Physicians in the Warsaw Ghetto. Edited by M. Winick. New York, John Wiley & Sons, 1979.

Nutritional Adaptation in Man. Edited by K. Blaxter, J.C. Waterlow. London, John Libbey, 1985.

Waterlow, J.C.: Metabolic adaptation to low intakes of energy and protein. Annu. Rev. Nutr., *6:*495–526, 1986.

CHAPTER 57

Protein-Energy Malnutrition

Benjamín Torún and Francisco Chew

Protein-energy malnutrition (PEM) results when the body's needs for protein, energy fuels, or both cannot be satisfied by the diet. It includes a wide spectrum of clinical manifestations conditioned by the relative intensity of protein or energy deficit, the severity and duration of the deficiencies, the age of the host, the cause of the deficiency, and the association with other nutritional or infectious diseases. Its severity ranges from weight loss or growth retardation to distinct clinical syndromes, frequently associated with deficiencies of minerals and vitamins.

Dietary energy and protein deficiencies usually occur together, but sometimes one predominates and, if severe enough, may lead to the clinical syndrome of *kwashiorkor* (predominant protein deficiency) or *marasmus* (mainly energy deficiency). *Marasmic kwashiorkor* is a combination of chronic energy deficiency and chronic or acute protein deficit. It is difficult to recognize which deficit predominates in milder forms of the disease.

The origin of PEM can be *primary,* when it is the result of inadequate food intake, or *secondary,* when it is the result of other diseases that lead to low food ingestion, inadequate nutrient absorption or utilization, increased nutritional requirements, and/or increased nutrient losses. Its onset can be relatively fast, as in starvation due to abrupt withholding of food, or gradual. This chapter discusses primary PEM of a relatively gradual onset, in which the metabolic alterations and clinical characteristics of protein and/or energy deficits predominate. PEM secondary to other diseases and the metabolic and clinical manifestations of starvation and of specific vitamin and mineral deficiencies are described in other chapters.

HISTORICAL BACKGROUND

It has long been recognized that inadequate food intake produces weight loss and growth retardation and, when severe and prolonged, leads to body wasting and emaciation. It took much longer to understand the nature of the edematous forms of PEM, probably because they could be found among children who were not starving and in families in good socioeconomic position. Descriptions of the disease in the early part of this century paid special attention to dermatologic signs and led to the belief that the disease was caused by tropical parasites or a vitamin deficiency.[1–7] This was questioned by various authors in the late 1920s and 1930s. The real nature of the disease was studied more carefully after Cicely Williams' descriptions in the mid-1930s of "kwashiorkor."[8,9] This term, used by the Ga tribe in the Gold Coast (now Ghana) for "the sickness the older child gets when the next baby is born," already suggested that the disease could be associated with an inadequate diet during the weaning period.

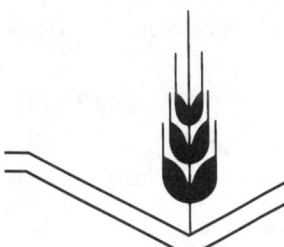

Other pediatricians who worked in tropical countries in the 1930s showed that the edematous disease could be cured by feeding milk or other high-protein foods.[10,11] In the 1940s, researchers showed that most patients had low concentrations of serum proteins and that this could also be related to the quality of dietary proteins.[12]

The nature and importance of this disease gained worldwide recognition in the 1950s, partly owing to publications such as those of Brock and Autret,[13] Autret and Behar,[10] and Trowell, Davies, and Dean.[11] By then, more than 40 names had been given to this clinical syndrome.[11] Some of them, such as "síndrome policarencial de la infancia" (infantile pluricarential syndrome), indicated that young children were mainly affected and that a deficit of various nutrients was involved. Others, such as "Mehlnahrschade" ("damage by cereal flours"), "starch edema," and "sugar babies" indicated that it was caused by the intake of foods with high carbohydrate and low protein contents. Today, the more comprehensive term of "protein-energy (or protein-calorie) malnutrition" is universally accepted,[14] and its severe forms are most often called "marasmus," "kwashiorkor," and "marasmic kwashiorkor." The term "malnutrition" is usually used in lay language for PEM.

Studies done in the last 25 years have shown that marasmus and kwashiorkor have distinct metabolic features, that some manifestations, such as anemia and reduced physical activity, are partly due to adaptive mechanisms, that the immune response of severely malnourished patients is impaired, and that physical and emotional stimulation are important elements in treating malnourished children. These findings are the basis of current therapeutic measures.

ETIOLOGY AND EPIDEMIOLOGY

Protein-energy malnutrition is the most important nutritional disease in developing countries because of its high prevalence and its relationship with child mortality rates, impaired physical growth, and inadequate social and economic development. Associated deleterious effects on mental growth and maturation have been demonstrated in experimental animals and they seem to occur in humans, but it has not been possible to disassociate completely the nutritional factors from other environmental conditions, or to ascertain the irreversibility of the nutritional mental damage. PEM occurs more frequently when infections impose additional demands, induce greater losses of nutrients, or produce metabolic alterations.

MAGNITUDE OF THE PROBLEM

Most malnourished persons live in developing countries, about 30% each in Africa and the Far East and 15% each in Latin America and the Near East. It was estimated that in 1990, one of every three children under the age of 5 in the developing world—or 177 million children— were or had been malnourished, based on a weight for age lower than two standard deviations below desirable values.[15] This prevalence ranged from 14% in the Americas to 47% in South Asia. Based on a country's dietary energy supplies and an energy intake of 1.4 times the basal metabolic rate as the minimum requirement for adults and adolescents, the United Nations's Food and Agriculture Organization estimated that in the mid-1980s more than 20% of the population of 98 developing countries was undernourished, and that 512 million persons, or 21% of the people in the developing world, were affected.[16] This proportion ranged from 11% in the Near East and 14% in Latin America, to 22% in the Far East and 32% in Africa.

A long-term analysis shows a trend for a decade-by-decade gradual improvement in the prevalence of child malnutrition, if countries are not disturbed by natural and man-made disasters such as droughts, desertification, wars, and economic crisis.[17] However, the total number of malnourished children has not decreased because of the rise in population in the countries where malnutrition is highly prevalent.

In industrialized countries, primary PEM is seen mainly among young children of the lower socioeconomic groups, the elderly who live alone, and adults addicted to alcohol and drugs.

CAUSES

Social, economic, biologic, and environmental factors may be underlying causes for the insufficient food intake or ingestion of foods with proteins of poor nutritional quality that lead to PEM.

Social and Economic Factors. *Poverty* that results in low food availability, overcrowded and unsanitary living conditions, and improper child care is a frequent cause of PEM.

Ignorance, by itself or associated with poverty, leads to poor infant- and child-rearing practices, misconceptions about the use of certain foods, inadequate feeding conducts during illnesses, and improper food distribution within the family members. A decline in the practice and duration of breast-feeding, combined with *inadequate weaning practices* when breast milk is withdrawn or when it can no longer provide sufficient dietary energy and protein to the infant, is associated with growing rates of infantile PEM.

Social problems such as child abuse, maternal deprivation, abandonment of the elderly, alcoholism, and drug addiction can result in PEM. *Cultural and social practices* that impose food taboos, some food and diet fads, particularly popular among adolescents and women, and the migration from traditional rural settings to urban slums can also contribute to, or precipitate, the appearance of PEM.

Biologic Factors. *Maternal malnutrition* prior to and/or during pregnancy is more likely to produce an underweight newborn baby.[18] This intrauterine malnutrition can be compounded after birth by insufficient food to satisfy the infant's needs for catch-up growth, resulting in PEM.

Infectious diseases are major contributing and precipitating factors in PEM. Diarrheal disease, measles, and respiratory and other infections frequently result in negative protein and energy balance due to anorexia (reduced food intake), vomiting, decreased absorption (increased nutrient losses), and catabolic processes (increased requirements and metabolic losses). Intestinal parasites have little or no effect unless the infection is extensive and causes anemia or diarrhea.[19]

Diets with low concentrations of proteins and energy, as occur with overdiluted milk formulas or bulky vegetable foods that have low nutrient densities, can lead to PEM in young children whose gastric capacity does not allow the ingestion of large amounts of food and in elderly persons with anorexia or difficulty in eating without assistance. Diets poor in protein and rich in carbohydrates are particularly likely to produce kwashiorkor.

Environmental Factors. *Overcrowded and/or unsanitary living conditions* lead to frequent infections. This is an important cause of PEM, especially among weanlings who develop severe or frequent episodes of diarrhea.

Agricultural patterns, droughts, floods, wars, and forced migrations lead to cyclic, sudden, or prolonged food scarcities and can cause PEM among whole populations. Post-harvest losses of food due to bad storage conditions and inadequate food distribution systems contribute to PEM, even after periods of agricultural plenty.

AGE OF THE HOST

PEM can affect all age groups but it is more frequent among infants and young children whose growth increases nutritional requirements, who cannot obtain food by their own means and who, when living under poor hygienic conditions, frequently become ill with diarrhea and other infections. Infants who are weaned prematurely from the breast or who are breast-fed for a prolonged time without adequate complementary feeding practices become malnourished for lack of adequate energy and protein intake.

The long-term intake of insufficient food can result in marasmus, which is the most common form of severe PEM before 1 year of age. Kwashiorkor, the edematous form of the disease, is more frequent after 18 months of age and typically occurs in children with diets consisting of starchy gruels, diluted cereal-based beverages, and vegetable foods rich in carbohydrates but almost devoid of proteins of good nutritional quality (i.e., lacking one or more essential amino acid). Most often, the severe protein deficit is associated with chronic dietary energy deficit and results in a combined form of marasmic kwashiorkor. The appearance of edema is frequently preceded or accompanied by acute diarrhea or other infectious disease.

Older children usually have milder forms of PEM because they can cope better with social and food availability constraints. Infections and other precipitating factors become less severe, and early survival may imply a natural selection of the more fit.

Pregnant and lactating women can also have PEM due to the increases in nutritional requirements. However, the consequences of the dietary deficiencies affect mainly the growth, nutritional status, and survival rates of their fetuses, newborn babies, and infants.

The elderly who are unable to care properly for themselves tend to suffer from PEM. Gastrointestinal alterations can be an important contributing factor.

Adolescents, adult men, and nonpregnant, nonlactating women usually have the lowest prevalence and the mildest forms of the disease because of greater opportunities to obtain food and cultural practices that protect the productive members of the family. Weight-reducing diets and food fads can predispose them to, or actually produce, some degree of PEM.

PATHOPHYSIOLOGY AND ADAPTIVE RESPONSES

PEM develops gradually in weeks or months. This allows a series of metabolic and behavioral adjustments that result in decreased nutrient demands and a nutritional equilibrium compatible with a lower level of cellular nutrient availability. If the supply of nutrients becomes persistently lower, the patient can no longer adapt and may even die. Metabolic disruptions can be due to severe nutrient deficit, complications (such as infections), or inadequate treatment (such as abrupt administration of large amounts of dietary energy or protein).

Patients whose PEM develops slowly—as is usually the case in marasmus—are better adapted to their current nutritional status and maintain a less fragile metabolic equilibrium than those with more acute PEM, as in kwashiorkor of rapid onset.

ENERGY MOBILIZATION AND EXPENDITURE

A decrease in energy intake is quickly followed by a decrease in energy expenditure, accounting for shorter periods of play and physical activity in children[20] and for longer rest periods and less physical work in adults.[21] When the decrease in energy expenditure cannot compensate for the insufficient intake, body fat is mobilized with a decrease in adiposity and weight loss.[22] Lean body mass diminishes at a slower rate, mainly as a consequence of muscle protein catabolism with increased efflux of amino acids, primarily alanine, that contribute to the energy sources. As the cumulative energy deficit becomes more severe, subcutaneous fat is markedly reduced, and protein catabolism leads to muscular wasting. Visceral protein is preserved longer, especially in the marasmic patients.

In marasmus, these alterations in body composition lead initially to increased basal oxygen consumption (i.e., basal metabolic rate) per unit of body weight, and it decreases in more severe stages.[23,24] In kwashiorkor, the severe dietary protein deficit leads to an earlier visceral depletion of amino acids that affects visceral cell function and reduces oxygen consumption; therefore, basal energy expenditure decreases per unit of lean or total body mass.

Blood glucose concentration remains normal, mainly at the expense of gluconeogenic amino acids and glycerol from fats, and it falls in severe PEM or when complicated by serious infections or fasting.

PROTEIN BREAKDOWN AND SYNTHESIS

The poor availability of dietary proteins reduces protein synthesis.[25] Adaptations lead to the sparing of body protein and the preservation of essential protein-dependent functions. The gradual and inevitable loss of body protein as a result of long-term dietary protein deficit is primarily from skeletal muscle. Table 57–1 illustrates some enzymatic changes that favor muscle protein breakdown and liver protein synthesis, as well as energy mobilization from fat depots. Some visceral protein is lost in the early development of PEM but then becomes stable until the nonessential tissue proteins are depleted; the loss of visceral protein then increases, and death may be imminent unless nutritional therapy is successfully instituted.

Under normal conditions about 75% of the free amino acids that enter the body pool from dietary and tissue proteins are recycled or reutilized for protein synthesis, and 25% are broken down for other metabolic purposes. When protein intake is reduced, there is not so much a decrease in total nitrogen or amino acid turnover, but an adaptive increase to 90 to 95% in the proportion that is recycled for synthesis and a proportional decrease in amino acid catabolism.[25,26] The latter markedly reduces urea synthesis and urinary nitrogen excretion.

The half-lives of several proteins increase. The rate of albumin synthesis decreases initially, but after a time lag of a few days the rate of breakdown also falls and its half-life increases. In addition to this, a shift of albumin from the extravascular to the intravascular pool assists in maintaining adequate levels of circulating albumin in the face of reduced synthesis. When protein depletion becomes too severe, the adaptive mechanisms fail and the concentration of serum proteins, and especially albumin, decreases. The ensuing reduction in intravascular oncotic pressure and outflow of water into the extravascular space contribute to the development of the edema of kwashiorkor.

TABLE 57–1. SELECTED ENZYME ACTIVITY CHANGES IN PROTEIN-ENERGY MALNUTRITION

CELLS	ENZYME ACTIVITY
Muscle and leukocytes	↓ Aldolase
	↓ Amino acid dehydrogenases
	↓ Pyruvic kinase
	↑ Aminotransferases
Liver	↓ Phenylalanine hydroxylase
	↓ Urea cycle enzymes
	↑ Amino acid activating enzymes

↓, ↑ = decrease or increase in activity.
(Adapted from Viteri, F.E.: Primary protein-energy malnutrition: clinical, biochemical, and metabolic changes. *In* Textbook of Pediatric Nutrition. Edited by R.M. Suskind. New York, Raven Press, 1981.)

ENDOCRINE CHANGES

Hormones are important in the adaptive metabolic processes. However, circulating levels of hormones do not always explain endocrine changes in PEM, because cellular responses to hormonal stimulation may also be altered. Table 57–2 summarizes the main changes in hormonal activity seen in patients with severe energy or protein deficiencies. They contribute to the maintenance of energy homeostasis through increased glycolysis and lipolysis; increased amino acid mobilization; preservation of visceral proteins through increased breakdown of muscle proteins; decreased storage of glycogen, fats, and proteins; and decreased energy metabolism. These effects can be summarized as follows (Fig. 57–1): (1) The decreased food intake tends to reduce plasma concentrations of glucose and free amino acids which, in turn, reduce insulin secretion and increase glucagon and epinephrine release; the latter further reduces insulin secretion; (2) the low plasma amino acid levels, seen mainly in kwashiorkor, also stimulate the secretion of human growth hormone and reduce somatomedin activity; this produces a further increase in growth hormone levels because of the absence of feedback inhibition; the increased levels of growth hormone and epinephrine influence the reduction of urea synthesis, thereby favoring amino acid recycling; (3) the stress induced by the low food intake and further amplified by fever, dehydration, and other manifestations of the infections that frequently accompany PEM also stimulates epinephrine release and corticosteroid secretion, more so in marasmus than in kwashiorkor, probably because of the greater severity in energy deficit that characterizes marasmus; resistance to the peripheral action of insulin increases, probably from the increase in plasma free fatty acid concentration resulting from the lipolytic activity of growth hormone, glucocorticoids, and epinephrine; (4) the low levels of circulating insulin and high levels of circulating cortisol may further reduce the

TABLE 57–2. SUMMARY OF SELECTED HORMONAL CHANGES USUALLY SEEN IN SEVERE PEM AND THEIR MAIN METABOLIC EFFECTS

HORMONE	INFLUENCED IN PEM BY	HORMONAL ACTIVITY IN: ENERGY DEFICIT	HORMONAL ACTIVITY IN: PROTEIN DEFICIT	EFFECTS OF ABNORMALITY IN PEM
Insulin	Low food intake (↓ glucose) (↓ amino acids)	Decreased	Decreased	↓ Muscle protein synthesis ↓ Lipogenesis ↓ Growth
Growth hormone (GH)	Low protein intake (↓ amino acids) Reduced somatomedin synthesis	Variable	Increased	↑ Visceral protein synthesis ↓ Urea synthesis ↑ Lipolysis ↓ Glucose uptake by tissues
Somatomedins (insulin-like growth factors)	Low protein intake Low circulating insulin High circulating cortisol	Variable	Decreased	↓ Muscle and cartilage protein synthesis ↓ Collagen synthesis ↓ Lipolysis ↓ Growth ↑ Production of growth hormone
Epinephrine	Stress of food deficiency, infections (↓ glucose)	Normal but can increase	Normal but can increase	↑ Lipolysis ↑ Glycogenolysis inhibits insulin secretion
Glucocorticoids	Stress of hunger Fever (↓ glucose)	Increased	Normal or increased	↑ Muscle protein catabolism ↑ Visceral protein turnover ↑ Lipolysis ↑ Gluconeogenesis ↓ Somatomedin-dependent actions of GH
Renin-aldosterone	↓ Blood volume ↑ Extracellular K? ↓ Serum Na?	Normal	Increased	↑ Sodium retention and ↑ Water retention contribute to appearance of edema
Thyroid hormones	↓ 5′-deiodinase (↑ reverse T_3) Defect in I uptake?	T_4 normal or decreased; T_3 decreased	T_4 usually decreased; T_3 decreased	↓ Glucose oxidation ↓ Basal energy expenditure ↑ Reverse T_3
Gonadotropins	Low protein intake? Low energy intake?	Decreased	Decreased	Delayed menarche

↓ = low or reduced ↑ = high or increased

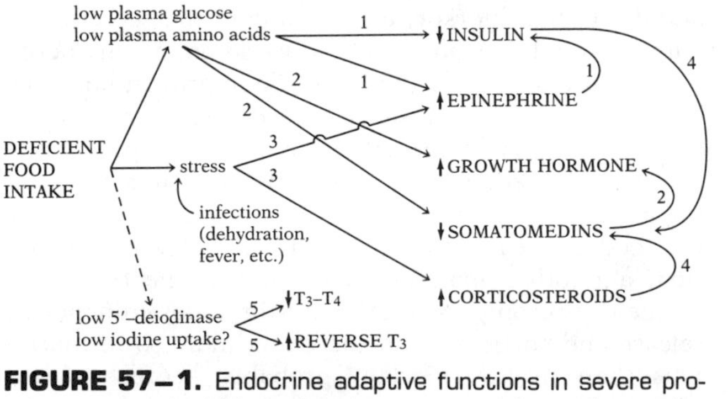

FIGURE 57–1. Endocrine adaptive functions in severe protein-energy malnutrition related to energy and protein metabolism. See the text for an explanation of the numbered events.

secretion of somatomedins; (5) a decrease in the activity of 5′-monodeiodinase reduces the production of triiodothyronine with a concomitant increase in the inactive reverse T_3; thyroxine levels are also reduced, possibly by a decrease in iodine uptake by the thyroid; the reduction in active thyroid hormone levels decreases thermogenesis and oxygen consumption, leading to energy conservation.

The secretion of hormones involved in nonvital growth-related functions, such as gonadotropins, decreases; the functional capacities of the hypothalamic-pituitary axis and adrenal medulla are preserved, thus allowing endocrine and metabolic responses to stress conditions. Some investigators have postulated that the evolution of PEM into either kwashiorkor or marasmus may be partly related to differences in adrenocortical response, whereby the better response will preserve visceral proteins more efficiently and lead to the better-adapted syndrome of marasmus.[28]

HEMATOLOGY AND OXYGEN TRANSPORT

The reduction in hemoglobin concentration and red cell mass that almost always accompanies severe PEM is, at least in part, an adaptive phenomenon related to tissue oxygen needs.[29] The reduction in lean body mass and the lower physical activity of malnourished patients lead to lower oxygen demands. The simultaneous decrease in dietary amino acids results in reduced hematopoietic activity, which spares amino acids for synthesis of other more necessary body proteins. As long as the tissues' needs for oxygen are satisfied by the existing capacity for oxygen transport, this should be considered an adaptive response and not a "functional" anemia (i.e., with tissue hypoxia). When tissue synthesis, lean body mass, and physical activity begin improving with dietary treatment, there is a rise in oxygen demands calling for accelerated hematopoiesis. If iron, folic acid, and vitamin B_{12} are not available in sufficient amounts, functional anemia with tissue hypoxia will develop.

Figure 57–2 shows that the administration of hematinics to a severely malnourished patient will not induce a hematopoietic response until dietary treatment produces an increase in lean body mass. Figure 57–3 shows that the reticulocyte response is related to the amount of protein intake when erythropoietic substances are not limiting.[27]

The severely malnourished patient may have relatively high body iron stores[30] and retains the ability to produce erythropoietin and reticulocytes in response to acute hypoxia.[31,32] Nevertheless, these patients are prone to develop functional, severe anemia if there is a superimposed dietary deficiency of iron or folic acid, or a chronic blood loss, as in hookworm infection.

OTHER PHYSIOLOGIC AND METABOLIC CHANGES

Not all pathophysiologic changes lead to advantageous adjustments. Certain functions are affected and some nutrient reserves decrease, making the malnourished individuals more susceptible to injuries that a well-nourished individual can withstand with little repercussion.

Cardiovascular and Renal Functions. Cardiac output, heart rate, and blood pressure decrease, and central circulation takes precedence over peripheral circulation.[33–35] Cardiovascular reflexes are altered, leading to postural hypotension and diminished venous return. In severe PEM, peripheral circulatory failure comparable to hypovolemic shock may occur. Hemodynamic compensation occurs primarily from tachycardia rather than

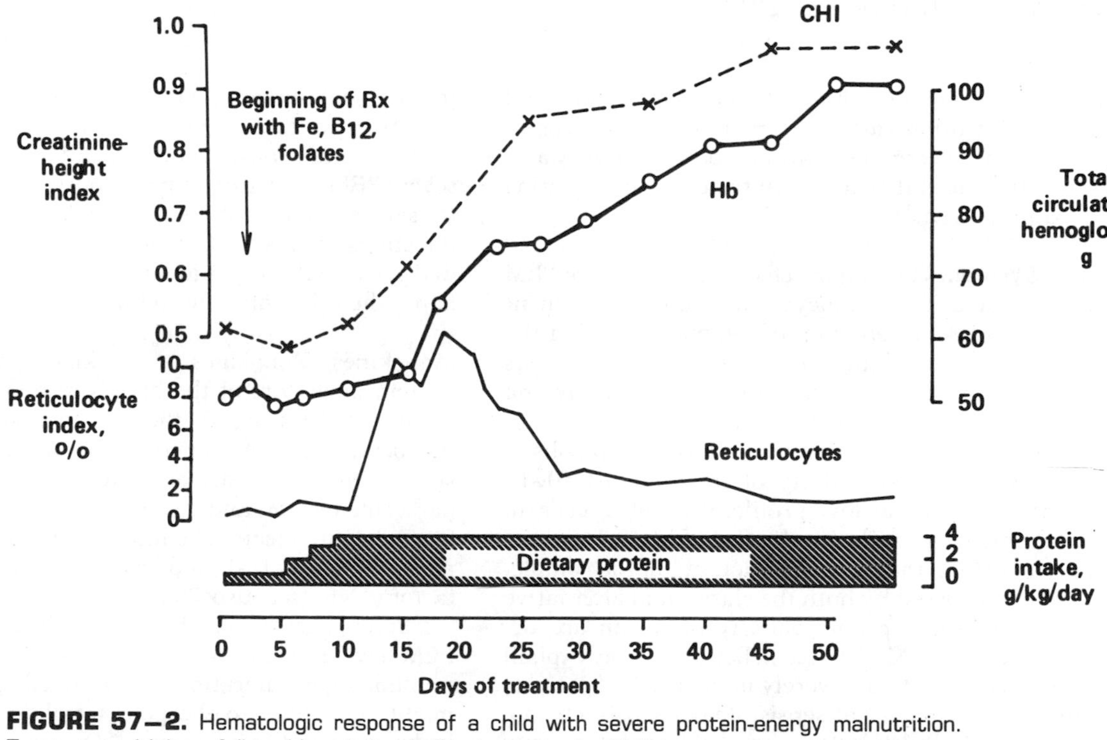

FIGURE 57–2. Hematologic response of a child with severe protein-energy malnutrition. Treatment with iron, folic acid, and vitamin B_{12} began on day 2; dietary energy and proteins were increased gradually to 150 kcal and 4 g protein/kg per day on day 9. No reticulocyte or hemoglobin response occurred until lean body mass, assessed by the creatinine-height index, began increasing.

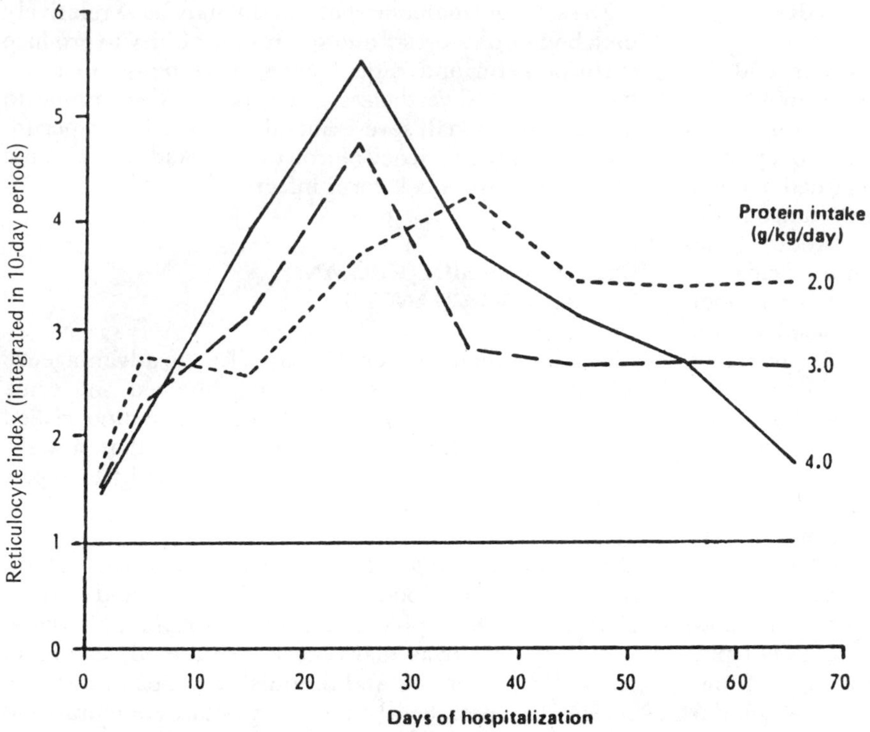

FIGURE 57–3. Reticulocyte response of children treated for severe protein-energy malnutrition with different amounts of dietary proteins and adequate amounts of dietary energy and hematinics. (From Viteri, F.E.: Primary protein-energy malnutrition: Clinical, biochemical, and metabolic changes. *In* Textbook of Pediatric Nutrition. Edited by R.M. Suskind. New York, Raven Press, 1981.)

from increased stroke volume. Renal plasma flow and glomerular filtration rates may be reduced as a consequence of the decreased cardiac output, but water clearance and the ability to concentrate and acidify urine appear unimpaired.[36–38]

Immune System. The major defects seen in severe PEM seem to involve T lymphocytes and the complement system.[39] A marked depletion of lymphocytes from the thymus and atrophy of the gland occur. In addition, cells from the T-lymphocyte regions of the spleen and lymph nodes are depleted, probably owing to decrease in thymic factors.[40,41] Alteration in monokine metabolism, particularly decreased activity of interleukin-1 (IL-1), may contribute to the low proliferation of T cells in severe malnutrition.[42] The production of several complement components, the functional activity of the complement system assessed by both the classic and alternative pathways, and the opsonic activity of serum are depressed in severe PEM.[43] These deficiencies may explain the high susceptibility of severely malnourished patients to gram-negative bacterial sepsis. Phagocytosis, chemotaxis, and intracellular killing are also impaired, partly because of the defects in opsonic and complement functional activities. The B-lymphocyte areas of spleen and lymph nodes and the circulating levels of B cells and immunoglobulin are relatively normal, but there may be defects in antibody production, such as secretory IgA.[39]

The overall consequences of all these alterations in severe PEM are a greater predisposition to infections and to severe complications of otherwise less important infectious diseases. The defects in immune functions disappear with nutritional rehabilitation, except perhaps when they are due to intrauterine malnutrition.[40]

Monokines. Monokines or cytokines are peptide/glycoprotein mediators of the body's response to injury (see Chap. 41). They are synthesized primarily by activated monocytic and phagocytic cells lining the liver and spleen. These peptides activate neighboring tissue in a paracrine fashion and also enter the circulation to exert more-distant effects. The most extensively characterized monokines are IL-1 and cachectin or tumor necrosis factor (TNF) (see also Chap. 69).

Macrophages from children with severe edematous PEM have decreased activity of IL-1.[42] In addition to the immunologic alterations mentioned previously, this might contribute to the poor febrile response and low leukocyte count in infections.[44] On the other hand, serum levels of TNF seem to be increased in severe malnutrition.[45] This could be associated with the anorexia and the muscle wasting and lipid abnormalities of PEM.

Electrolytes. Total body potassium decreases in PEM because of the reduction in muscle proteins and loss of intracellular potassium. The low insulin action and diminished intracellular energy substrates reduce the availability of adenosine triphosphate (ATP) and phosphocreatine. This process probably alters the cellular exchange of sodium and potassium, leading to potassium loss and increased intracellular sodium.[46] Water accompanies the sodium influx, and although total body intracellular water is decreased because of the loss in lean body mass, there may be intracellular overhydration. These alterations in cell electrolytes and energy sources may explain, at least in part, the increased fatigability and reduced strength of skeletal muscle.[47]

Gastrointestinal Functions. Impaired intestinal absorption of lipids and disaccharides and a decreased rate of glucose absorption occur in severe protein deficiency. The greater the protein deficit, the greater the functional impairment. A decrease in gastric, pancreatic, and bile production is also observed, with normal to low enzyme and conjugated bile acid concentrations.[48-50] These alterations further impair the absorptive functions. Nevertheless, the ingestion of nutrients in high therapeutic amounts usually allows for their uptake in sufficient quantity to permit nutritional recovery.[51] Malnourished persons, however, are prone to have diarrhea because of these alterations and possibly also because of irregular intestinal motility and gastrointestinal bacterial overgrowth. Diarrhea aggravates the malabsorption and can further impair nutritional status. Malabsorption disappears with nutritional recovery unless there is an underlying food or nutrient intolerance unrelated to primary PEM.

Central and Peripheral Nervous System. Individuals who suffer severe PEM at an early age may have decreased brain growth, nerve myelination, neurotransmitter production, and velocity of nervous conduction. The long-term functional implications of these alterations have not been clearly demonstrated, and they cannot be correlated with later behavior and the level of intelligence.[52] In the human, it is impossible to separate nutrition from other factors that can affect gross and fine motor skills, intelligence, and behavior. Factors that can lead either to a good or to a poor developmental outcome include the severity, timing, and duration of nutritional deprivation, the quality of nutritional rehabilitation and psychosocial support, the degree of family stimulation, and a host of positive and negative environmental factors.

FACTORS LEADING TO KWASHIORKOR

The concept that marasmus or kwashiorkor is the end result of either severe energy or protein deficiency is too simplistic. Nevertheless, the classic theory of a dietary cause of kwashiorkor and marasmus, which states that a diet deficient in protein and with a low protein-to-energy ratio is an important (perhaps even principal) factor in the production of kwashiorkor, still is valid. The deficiency of vitamins and minerals associated with food sources of protein, and the variability in nutrient requirements between children, may explain why some children develop the edematous and others the nonedematous form of the disease. It also explains, at least in part, some epidemiologic features of PEM, such as the predominance of marasmus in infants under 1 year of age and the predominance of either marasmus, kwashiorkor, or marasmic-kwashiorkor in different parts of the world and in urban or rural areas.

Other factors such as overloading a severely malnourished person with carbohydrates, or metabolic changes induced by infections, may cause or contribute to the appearance of kwashiorkor with its characteristic edema, hypoalbuminemia, and enlarged fatty liver. Some investigators have postulated that the evolution of PEM into either kwashiorkor or marasmus may be partly related to differences in adrenocortical response, whereby a greater response preserves visceral proteins more efficiently and leads to the better-adapted syndrome of marasmus.[28,53] Others have proposed that kwashiorkor results from aflatoxin poisoning,[54,55] but there is no clear difference in the amounts of aflatoxins or its metabolites in the diet, urine, or tissues of children with kwashiorkor and marasmus.

Golden and his colleagues have developed the theory that kwashiorkor results from an imbalance between the production of toxic free radicals and their safe disposal.[56-58] Among the factors that would increase free radicals are infections, toxins, sunlight, trauma, and catalysts such as iron. Formation of free radicals is decreased by the antioxidant function of vitamins A (or β-carotene), C, and E, by ceruloplasmin and transferrin that bind free iron and favor its oxidation, and by zinc-metallothionein, which acts as a free radical sink. Free radicals and the peroxides they generate are removed through reactions catalyzed by enzymes in which glutathione and trace minerals play an important role, such as Cu-Zn and Mn superoxide dismutase, and Se glutathione peroxidase. The toxic effects of free radicals would be responsible for cell damage leading to the alterations seen in kwashiorkor, such as edema, fatty liver, and skin lesions. This theory, however, has not been firmly established or subjected to the test of animal experiments. Nevertheless, it has drawn attention to factors and processes in the pathogenesis of severe PEM that have previously been neglected, and it may have important implications for treatment.[59]

When there is a severe lack of food, endocrine adjustments mobilize fatty acids from adipose tissue and amino acids from muscle tissue; plasma protein concentration remains normal, and hepatic gluconeogenesis is enhanced.[60] An increase in carbohydrate intake when protein intake is very low can produce a breakdown of those adjustments, as follows: (1) Carbohydrate intake induces insulin release and a reduction in the production of epinephrine and cortisol.[61,62] (2) Lipolysis decreases and the action of insulin is enhanced because of the suppression of the inhibitory effects of free fatty acids on the peripheral action of insulin.[63] (3) Muscle protein breakdown is reduced and the body pool of free amino acids decreases. The decreased supply of muscle amino acids to the other organs results in less visceral protein synthesis.[64–66] (4) The decreased synthesis of plasma proteins in the liver, particularly albumin, reduces intravascular oncotic pressure. Plasma water decreases and accumulates in extravascular tissues, tissue pressure rises, and cardiac output diminishes. This contributes to the appearance or increase of edema, as discussed later. (5) Increased hepatic fatty acid synthesis from the excess carbohydrate, impaired lipolysis, and reduced production of apo-β-lipoproteins for lipid transport lead to fatty infiltration of the liver and hepatomegaly.

Infections in undernourished children also can precipitate the onset of kwashiorkor. The process by which this occurs has not been satisfactorily explained, but the following mechanisms may be involved: (1) Infections might divert the meager amino acid pool to the production of globulins and acute phase reactant proteins (AP), instead of albumin and transport proteins. (2) The increase of AP that are proteinase inhibitors, such as α_1-antitrypsin and α_1-antichymotrypsin, may impair muscle protein breakdown.[67] (3) An impaired production and utilization of ketone bodies for energy during infections might lead to the use of more amino acids for gluconeogenesis.[68] (4) Protein catabolism and nitrogen losses are enhanced by many viral and febrile infections, probably through increased epinephrine and cortisol actions.[69,70] Regardless of the mechanisms involved, protein losses during severe infections can amount to as much as 2% of muscle protein per day.[71] (5) Leukocytes stimulated by infectious organisms produce large quantities of superoxide and hydrogen peroxide.[72] These are released into the surrounding medium and contribute to the production of kwashiorkor, according to the free-radical theory.[56,57]

The pathogenesis of edema in severe PEM has aroused much discussion. It is an important issue because of the key role of edema in the diagnosis of kwashiorkor and because it may give clues about the patient's dietary background and other precipitating factors of the disease. The edema of kwashiorkor has been classically linked to hypoalbuminemia through a reduction in colloid osmotic pressure of the plasma, which leads to outflow of fluid from the capillaries into the interstitial space. There is, however, an overlap in serum albumin levels between edematous and nonedematous PEM in children and adults; experimental studies on dogs fed a low-protein diet showed that many animals with plasma albumin below 20 g/L did not have edema, whereas almost all edematous dogs had albumin levels below that value.[73] Furthermore, the edema of kwashiorkor is reduced on treatment with protein-free or low-protein diets that contain potassium and other minerals, and moderate amounts of carbohydrates. All this suggests that hypoalbuminemia may be a necessary but not a sufficient cause for edema, and that some other factors may be needed, at least in some cases.[59] These factors include potassium deficiency, which promotes water and sodium retention,[74] excessive administration of water and sodium, and extravasation of fluid due to increased capillary permeability in infection.

A theory that became widely accepted for the production of edema in severe PEM involved a reduction in renal blood flow (RBF) and glomerular filtration rate (GFR) due to decreased plasma volume and decreased cardiac output as consequence of hypoalbuminemia; the decrease in RBF and GFR would result in sodium retention and production of renin and aldosterone which, in turn, would increase the tubular reabsorption of sodium and water, leading to edema.[75] However, there is conflicting evidence about the changes in plasma volume in kwashiorkor, and aldosterone activity may increase in children with marasmus as well as in children with edema.[76,77] Other theories include an increase in ferritin that stimulates production of antidiuretic hormone by the posterior pituitary,[78,79] energy deficiency that does not allow adequate function of the sodium pump and restoration of intracellular potassium,[80] and, more recently, leakiness of cell membranes caused by the damaging effects of free radicals.[56–58] None of these theories have been fully demonstrated, and some of them are supported by conflicting evidence. It is possible that the pathogenesis of edema in PEM is not a single entity and that it differs in accordance with the multiple nutritional deficiencies, the age of the patients, and other concomitant conditions. However, except for iatrogenic water overload, hypoproteinemia—especially hypoalbuminemia—is an essential component.

DISRUPTION OF ADAPTATION

When the supply for tissue and cell energy can no longer be maintained by patients with severe energy deficiency, a serious decompensation occurs causing hypoglycemia, hypothermia, impaired circulatory and renal functions, acidosis, coma, and death. These events can occur within a few hours. Metabolic decompensation due to severe protein deficiency, in addition to the changes discussed in the onset of kwashiorkor, may include hemorrhagic diathesis and jaundice due to failure by the liver to synthesize several clotting factors and transport proteins; various degrees of renal failure with acidosis and water and sodium retention; decreased cardiac work, pulmonary congestion, and increased susceptibility to pulmonary infections; coma; and death.

A high-carbohydrate, low-protein diet is not the only iatrogenic cause of serious metabolic disruption in patients who have or are prone to develop edematous PEM. The abrupt administration of too much protein to patients with edematous PEM can also have serious, life-threatening consequences. When such patients have been eating minute amounts of protein or none at all, and they are suddenly fed large amounts of proteins or given large transfusions of plasma or blood, they may experience a rapid increase in intravascular protein concentration and entry of extracellular fluid into the vascular compartment leading to cardiovascular insufficiency and pulmonary edema. In fact, premature introduction of a high-energy or high-protein diet may be fatal to a severely malnourished patient.[81,82]

DIAGNOSIS

The clinical, biochemical, and physiologic characteristics of PEM vary according to the severity of the disease, the patient's age, the presence of other nutritional deficits and infections, and the predominance of energy or protein deficiency.

CLASSIFICATION OF PEM

The classification scheme shown in Table 57–3 is useful for the diagnosis and treatment of PEM, and for the application and evaluation of public health measures. *Severity* is determined mainly by anthropometry, because other clinical findings and biochemical indexes usually do not show changes unless the disease is well advanced. More accurate measurements, such as assessment of body composition, are not practical or feasible in most of the settings in which primary PEM occurs, and they are usually used for research rather than for clinical purposes. The so-called functional indicators are not as yet well standardized, can be influenced by deficits of more than one single nutrient, or may be too complex to measure routinely.[83] Classification of the *course* or *duration* of the disease as acute, chronic, or acute with a chronic background is also done by anthropometry to assess current nutritional status and degree of growth retardation in children. Dietary history is useful, especially in adults, as are dietary surveys in population groups. The relative contributions of dietary *protein and energy deficits* in the mild and moderate forms of PEM are assessed mainly by the individual's dietary history or the population's dietary habits and food availability. Clinical characteristics and biochemical data confirm the diagnosis in severe PEM.

TABLE 57–3. CLASSIFICATION OF PEM ACCORDING TO SEVERITY OF DISEASE, ITS COURSE OR DURATION, AND PREDOMINANT NUTRIENT DEFICIENCY

SEVERITY	COURSE	MAIN DEFICIT
Mild	Acute	Energy
Moderate	Chronic	Protein
Severe	Both	Both

ANTHROPOMETRIC MEASUREMENTS

The choice of anthropometric measurements depends on their simplicity, accuracy, and sensitivity; on the availability of measuring instruments; and on the existence of reference standards for comparison.

To allow international comparisons, it is sensible to use the same standard of reference for various populations. International or universal standards based on reliable anthropometric data can be used because (1) most children have similar growth potentials, regardless of ethnic background,[84,85] (2) the relationship of various anthropometric measurements, especially weight and height, is relatively constant in normal, healthy individuals of all age groups, (3) the reference standards are merely for purposes of comparison and do not necessarily represent and ideal or a target, and (4) the interpretation of the comparison (i.e., the values that separate "normal" from "deficient" and further divide the latter into "mild," "moderate," and "severe" forms) is a matter of judgment that comes into play when deciding whether the expected normal value for a given population should be 100%, 90%, or another proportion of the standard. Setting different cut-off points relative to a single standard is more practical than constructing local standards that, in a country with heterogeneous population groups, may pose the same problem as a "foreign" commonly used reference. At present, the World Health Organization recommends the data from the United States National Center for Health Statistics (NCHS)[86] as reference for weight and height.[87]

The best anthropometric assessment of nutritional status and PEM is based on measurements of weight and height or length, and records of age, to calculate two indexes: *weight for height,* as an index of current nutritional status, and *height for age,* as an index of past nutritional history. Deficient height for age may represent a short period of growth failure at an early age or a longer period at a later age. Waterlow suggested the terms *wasting* for a deficit in weight for height and *stunting* for a deficit in height for age.[88] Patients may then fall into four categories: (1) normal, (2) wasted but not stunted (suffering from acute PEM), (3) wasted and stunted (suffering from acute and chronic PEM), and (4) stunted but not wasted (past PEM with present adequate nutrition, or "nutritional dwarfs"). The intensity of wasting and stunting can be graded by calculating weight as a percentage of the reference median weight for height, and height as a percentage of the reference median height for age, as follows:

$$\begin{matrix}\text{\% weight-for-height} \\ \text{(or height-for-age)}\end{matrix} = \frac{\text{observed weight (or height)}}{\begin{matrix}\text{reference weight for patient's ht} \\ \text{(or reference height for patient's age)}\end{matrix}} \times 100$$

The use of centiles or standard deviations from the mean, instead of percent deviations from the median, is statistically more adequate. However, percent deviations are easier to understand by the general public and to calculate by field workers. The grading shown in Table 57–4 is suggested for most countries, although some might find it convenient to use different cut-off points for specific groups. For example, the normal height for age in populations that are genetically short could be less than 95% of the reference. Color-coded charts and graphs have been devised to simplify the measurements and their interpretation.[89,90]

The *body mass index* (BMI, or Quetelet's index), weight/height^2, is recommended for adolescents and adults. Table 57–5 shows the criteria for classification of chronic energy deficiency in adults proposed by an international working party.[91] We suggest using the same BMI criteria to classify current PEM in adults. There will be a greater amount of body fat in women than in men at all three cut-off points, but the greater body fat found in women is an intrinsic biologic phenomenon. Therefore the same cut-off points can be used for both sexes.[91]

Based on data for whites and blacks in the United States,[92] we also suggest that the diagnosis of PEM in adolescents can be based on a BMI *below 15.0 at ages 11 to 13 years*, and *below 16.5 at ages 14 to 17 years*. As in adults, the same cut-off points can be used for boys and girls. Criteria have not been established to classify the severity of PEM in adolescents.

The use of deficit in weight for age does not differentiate between a truly underweight child (current PEM) and one who is short in stature but well proportioned in weight (past PEM); furthermore, the information about chronologic age is not always reliable. However, the classification of PEM as grades I (75 to 90% of reference weight for age), II (60 to 74%), and III (less than 60%), is useful in public health and epidemiologic studies, because it indicates the proportion of children in a population group who at some time in their lives have had malnutrition.[93]

Use of the upper arm circumference has been advocated under field conditions without access to a weighing scale. It is not a sensitive index, but it allows differentiating between a moderate-to-severe malnourished child and one with better nutritional condition.

TABLE 57–5. CLASSIFICATION OF INTENSITY OF PROTEIN-ENERGY MALNUTRITION IN ADULT MEN AND WOMEN

BODY MASS INDEX (BMI)	PEM
≥18.5	Normal
17.0–18.4	Mild
16.0–16.9	Moderate
<16.0	Severe

(Based on the classification proposed for chronic energy deficiency in James, W.P.T., Ferro-Luzzi, A., Waterlow, J.C.: Eur. J. Clin. Nutr., *42*:969–981, 1988.)

MILD AND MODERATE PEM

The main clinical feature of mild and moderate PEM is weight loss. A decrease in subcutaneous adipose tissue may become apparent. When PEM is chronic, children show growth retardation in terms of height (stunting). Groups of populations in whom PEM is highly prevalent or "endemic" show slow weight gains, as illustrated in Figure 57–4.

Physical activity and energy expenditure of children decrease.[20,94–96] Other functional indicators of immunocompetence, gastrointestinal functions, and behavior may be altered, but their assessment is not yet practical for diagnostic purpose.[24,27,40,97] Nonspecific manifestations include more-sedentary behavior, frequent episodes of diarrhea, and apathy, lack of liveliness, and short attention spans.

In adults, mild to moderate PEM results in leanness with reduction in subcutaneous tissue. The most common change in body composition is a reduction of adiposity below 12 and 20% in men and women, respectively. Capacity for prolonged physical work is reduced, but this change is usually apparent only in persons engaged in intense, energy-demanding occupations.[21,98] Malnourished women have a higher probability of giving birth to infants with low birth weights.[99] As in children, there may be other functional alterations not yet well characterized.

Biochemical information is not consistent in mild and moderate PEM. Laboratory data related to low protein intakes may include low urinary excretion of creatinine,

TABLE 57–4. CLASSIFICATION OF SEVERITY OF CURRENT ("WASTING") AND PAST OR CHRONIC ("STUNTING") PEM IN INFANTS AND CHILDREN, BASED ON WEIGHT-FOR-HEIGHT AND ON HEIGHT-FOR-AGE

	NORMAL	MILD	MODERATE	SEVERE
Weight for height (deficit = wasting)	90–110* (±1 Z)†	80–89 (−1.1 to −2 Z)	70–79 (−2.1 to −3 Z)	<70, or with edema (<−3 Z)
Height for age (deficit = stunting)	95–105 (±1 Z)	90–94 (−1.1 to −2 Z)	85–89 (−2.1 to −3 Z)	<85 (<−3 Z)

*Percentage relative to the median NCHS standards.[86,87]

†In parentheses: Standard deviations from the NCHS median, or "Z scores."[87]

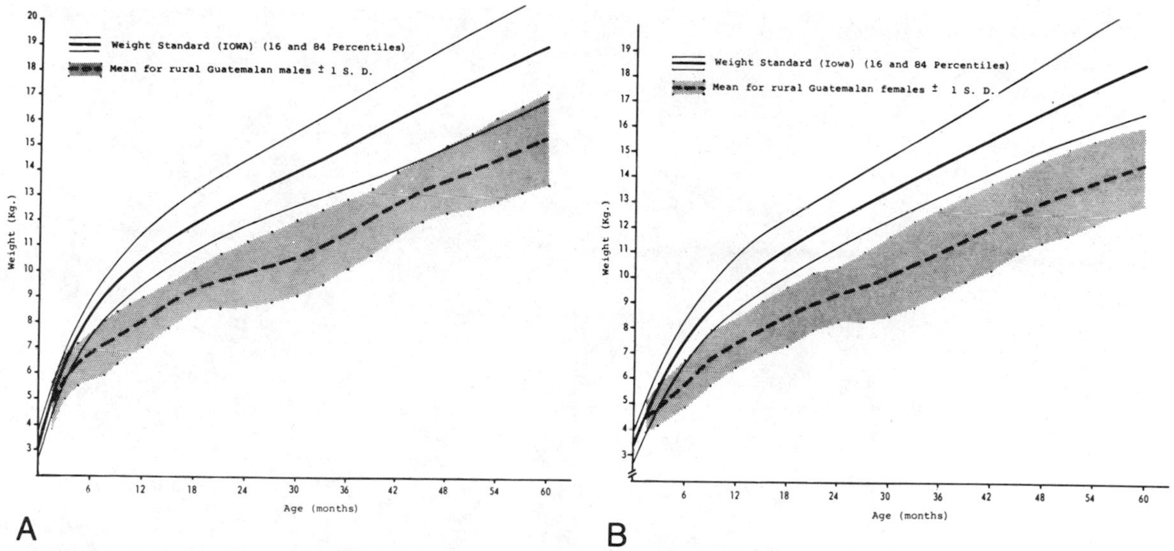

FIGURE 57–4. Pattern of weight gain, from birth to 5 years, in 431 boys *(A)* and 436 girls *(B)* from low-income families in rural Guatemala. (From INCAP: Evaluación Nutricional de la Población de Centro América y Panamá: Guatemala. Guatemala, Instituto de Nutrición de Centro América y Panamá, 1969.)

leading to a low creatinine-height index in children,[100] low urinary urea nitrogen and hydroxyproline excretions, altered plasma patterns of free amino acids with a decrease in branched-chain essential amino acids, slight decreases in serum transferrin and albumin, and a reduced number of circulating lymphocytes.

SEVERE PEM

The diagnosis is principally based on dietary history and clinical features. Marasmus is usually associated with severe food shortage, prolonged semistarvation, early weaning, or infrequent feeding of infants, and kwashiorkor with late weaning and poor protein intakes. Chronic or recurrent diarrhea and infections are common features.

MARASMUS

Generalized muscular wasting and absence of subcutaneous fat give the patient with severe, nonedematous PEM a "skin and bones" appearance (Figs. 57–5 and 57–6). Marasmic patients frequently have 60% or less of the weight expected for their height, and children have marked retardation in longitudinal growth. The hair is sparse, thin, and dry, without its normal sheen; it is easily pulled out without causing pain. The skin is dry, thin with little elasticity, and wrinkles easily. Patients are apathetic but usually aware and have a look of anxiety on their face. These features and the sunken cheeks caused by disappearance of the Bichat fat pads, which are among the last subcutaneous adipose depots to disappear, give the marasmic child's face the appearance of a monkey's or an old person's face.

Some patients are anorexic whereas others are ravenously hungry, but they seldom tolerate large amounts of food and they vomit easily. Diarrhea may be present. There is marked weakness and children frequently cannot stand without help. Heart rate, blood pressure, and body temperature may be low, but tachycardia may be present. Hypoglycemia can occur, especially after fasting for 6 or more hours, and is often accompanied by hypothermia of 35.5° C or less. The viscera are usually small. Abdominal distention may be present. The lymph nodes are easily palpable.

Differential diagnosis must be made from the secondary PEM of acquired immunodeficiency syndrome (AIDS) and other body-wasting diseases; dietary history plays an important role.

Common complicating features are acute gastroenteritis, dehydration, respiratory infections, and eye lesions due to hypovitaminosis A. Systemic infections lead to septic shock or intravascular clotting with high mortality rates.

KWASHIORKOR

The predominant feature is soft, pitting, painless edema, usually in the feet and legs, but extending to the perineum, upper extremities, and face in severe cases (Fig. 57–7). Most patients have skin lesions, often confused with pellagra, in the areas of edema, continuous pressure (e.g., at the buttocks and back), or frequent irritation (e.g., in the perineum and thighs). The skin may be erythematous, and it glistens in the edematous

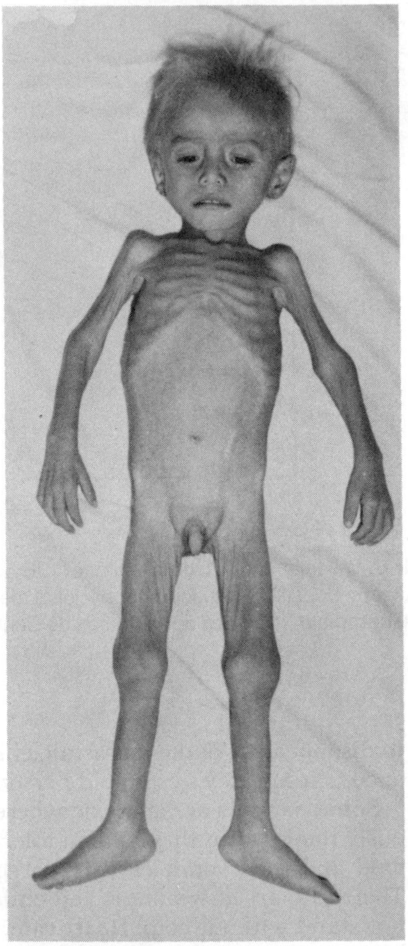

FIGURE 57–5. Marasmus in a 21-month-old child. (From Viteri, F.E.: Primary protein-energy malnutrition: clinical, biochemical, and metabolic changes. *In* Textbook of Pediatric Nutrition. Edited by R.M. Suskind. New York, Raven Press, 1981.)

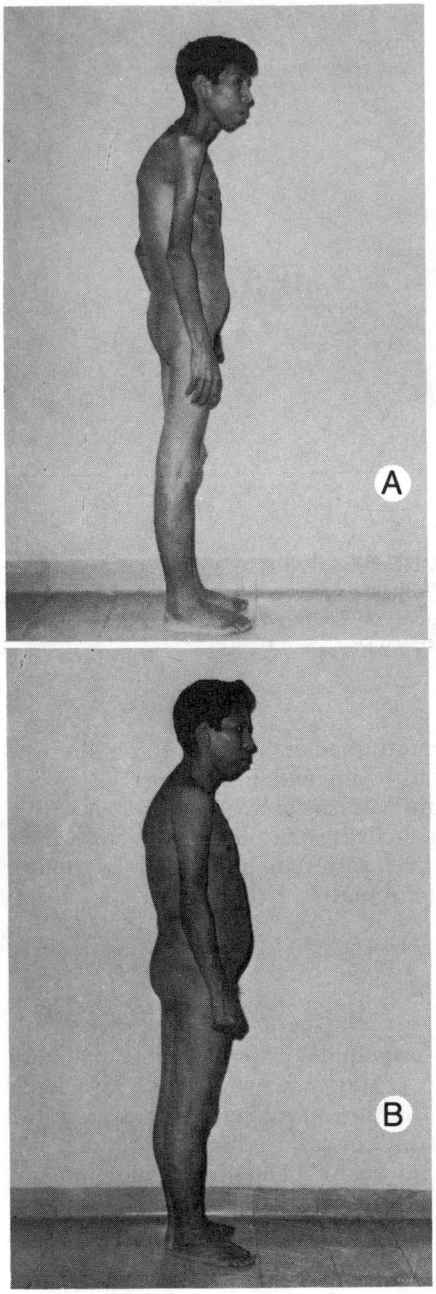

FIGURE 57–6. *A*, Marasmic protein-energy malnutrition in a 29-year-old man. *B*, The same patient after 3 months of treatment.

regions with zones of dryness, hyperkeratosis, and hyperpigmentation, which tend to become confluent. The epidermis peels off in large scales, exposing underlying tissues that are easily infected. Subcutaneous fat is preserved, and there may be some muscle wasting. Weight deficit, after accounting for the weight of edema, is usually not as severe as in marasmus. Height may be normal or retarded, depending on the chronicity of the current episode and on past nutritional history.

The hair is dry, brittle, and without its normal sheen, and can be pulled out easily without pain. Curly hair becomes straight, and the pigmentation usually changes to dull brown, red, or even yellowish white. Alternating periods of poor and relatively good protein intake can produce alternating bands of depigmented and normal hair, which have been termed the "flag sign" (Fig. 57–8).

The patients may be pale, with cold and cyanotic extremities. They are apathetic and irritable, cry easily, and have an expression of misery and sadness. Anorexia (sometimes necessitating nasogastric tube feeding), postprandial vomiting, and diarrhea are common. These conditions improve without specific gastrointestinal treatment as nutritional recovery progresses. Hepatomegaly with a soft, round edge caused by severe fatty infiltration is usually present. The abdomen is frequently protruding because of distended stomach and intestinal loops. Peristalsis is irregular and frequently slow. Muscle tone and strength are greatly reduced. Tachycardia is

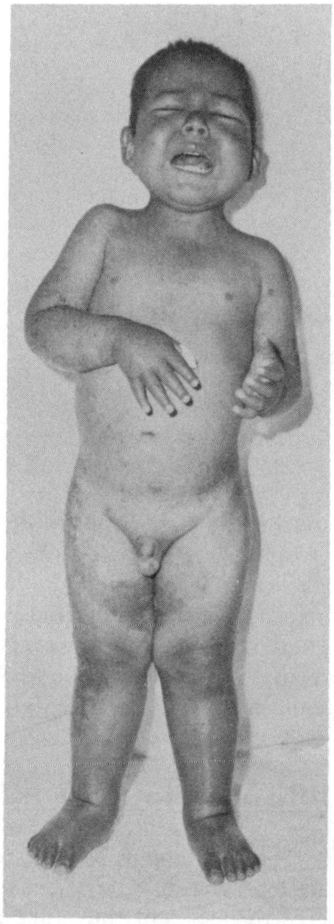

FIGURE 57–7. Kwashiorkor in a 36-month-old child. Note that subcutaneous tissues were preserved in the trunk and face.

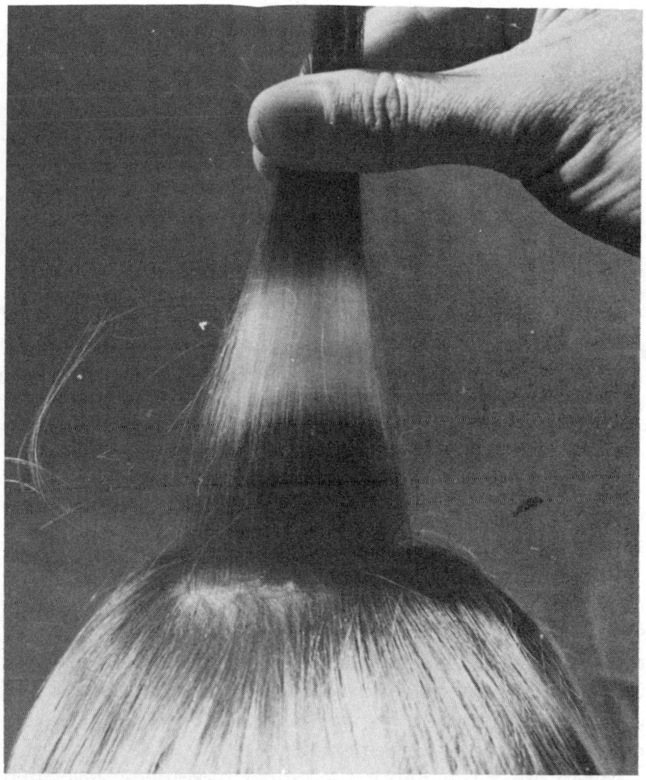

FIGURE 57–8. "Flag sign": bands of depigmented and normal hair caused by alternating periods of poor and relatively good protein intake. (From Torún, B., Viteri, F.E.: Protein-energy malnutrition. *In* Tropical and Geographical Medicine. 2nd Ed. Edited by K.S. Warren and A.A.F. Mahmoud. New York, McGraw-Hill, 1990.)

common. Both hypothermia and hypoglycemia can occur after short periods of fasting.

Differential diagnosis must be made from other causes of edema and hypoproteinemia, and from secondary PEM due to impairment in protein absorption or metabolism.

The same complications occur as in marasmus, but diarrhea and respiratory and skin infections are more frequent and severe. Serious, fatal infections may occur, frequently without fever, tachycardia, respiratory distress, or appropriate leukocytosis. The most common causes of death are pulmonary edema with bronchopneumonia, septicemia, gastroenteritis, and water and electrolyte imbalances.

MARASMIC KWASHIORKOR

This form of edematous PEM combines clinical characteristics of kwashiorkor and marasmus. The main features are the edema of kwashiorkor, with or without its skin lesions, and the muscle wasting and decreased subcutaneous fat of marasmus (Figs. 57–9 and 57–10). When edema disappears during early treatment, the patient's appearance resembles that of marasmus. Biochemical features of both marasmus and kwashiorkor are seen, but the alterations of severe protein deficiency usually predominate.

BIOCHEMICAL AND HISTOPATHOLOGIC FEATURES OF SEVERE PEM

The most common biochemical findings are the following: (1) serum concentrations of total proteins, and specially albumin, are markedly reduced in edematous PEM, and normal or moderately low in marasmus; (2) hemoglobin and hematocrit are usually low, more so in kwashiorkor than in marasmus; (3) the ratio of nonessential to essential amino acids in plasma is elevated in kwashiorkor and usually normal in marasmus; (4) serum levels of free fatty acids are elevated, particularly in kwashiorkor; (5) blood glucose level is normal, or low after fasting 6 or more hours; (6) urinary excretions of creatinine, hydroxyproline, 3-methylhistidine, and urea nitrogen are low. Edematous children have markedly reduced urinary creatinine excretions in relation to their height, leading to a low creatinine-height index,[100]

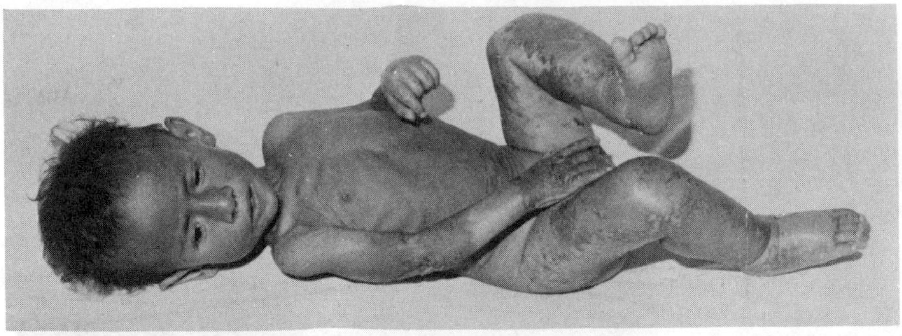

FIGURE 57–9. Marasmic kwashiorkor in a 22-month-old child. Note the edema in the lower part of the body, the emaciated upper part, and the skin lesions. (From Torún, B., Viteri, F.E.: Protein-energy malnutrition. *In* Tropical and Geographical Medicine. 2nd Ed. Edited by K.S. Warren and A.A.F. Mahmoud. New York, McGraw-Hill, 1990.)

whereas marasmic children may have a normal or somewhat low index.

Plasma levels of other nutrients vary and tend to be moderately low. They do not necessarily reflect the body stores. For example, serum iron and retinol may be normal with almost depleted body stores, or in kwashiorkor they may be relatively low with adequate stores because of alterations in the transport proteins, transferrin and retinol-binding protein.

Many other biochemical changes have been described in severe PEM; some of them were discussed in the section "Pathophysiology and Adaptive Responses." Others are listed in Table 57–6. Although they have little practical importance in diagnosing the disease, they allow better understanding of the pathophysiologic modifications.

Body protein decreases at a slow rate, most of it from muscle, and the greater loss of adipose tissue results in a relative increase of total body water (i.e., per unit of body mass), mainly as intracellular water. In severe protein deficiency (kwashiorkor) extracellular water also increases. The intracellular concentrations of potassium and magnesium decrease and that of sodium increases, although the serum concentrations of electrolytes do not necessarily reflect these alterations.[101]

Histopathologic studies show nonspecific atrophy, mainly in tissues with greater cell turnover rates, such as intestinal mucosa, red bone marrow, and testicular epithelium; intestinal villi are flattened and enterocytes lose their columnar appearance. In marasmus there is generalized atrophy of skeletal muscle. The skin changes consist of dermal atrophy, ecchymosis, ulcerations, and hyperkeratotic desquamation, seen primarily in areas subjected to irritation and not necessarily restricted to exposed areas, as in the case of pellagra. The liver in individuals with kwashiorkor is enlarged with fatty infiltration; periportal fat appears first and advances centripetally as severity increases. Other histologic analyses, special staining techniques, and electron microscopy reveal more alterations, not all of which result specifically from primary PEM. All do reflect generalized atrophy, however. Lesions due to superimposed infections and other nutrient deficiencies often are evident macroscopically and upon histopathologic examination. These changes usually revert to normal with nutritional recovery, although some residual lesions may persist for some time.

PROGNOSIS AND RISK OF MORTALITY

Treatment of mild and moderate PEM corrects the acute signs of the disease, but children's catch-up growth in height may take a long time or might never be achieved. These children have been deprived not only of food but also of opportunities for development, and they may have missed the critical periods for harmonic physical, mental, and social maturation. Weight for height can be restored easily, but the child may remain stunted and a small body size may influence his maximal working capacity as an adult. Many severely malnourished children appear to have residual behavioral and mental problems in terms of creativity and social interaction. However, the causal roles of malnutrition and a poor living environment are difficult to disassociate, and there is no irrefutable evidence that the damage cannot be corrected in a good, stimulating environment.

Anthropometric characteristics are associated with mortality rates, as in the classification of severe PEM into first, second, or third degrees, based on weight-for-age.[93] A higher mortality rate is associated with severe anthropometric deficits but not with mild or moderate deficiencies.[102] Mortality rate in severe PEM can be as high as 40% but adequate treatment can reduce it to less than 10%; the immediate causes of death are usually infections. Table 57–7 lists the characteristics that generally indicate a poor prognosis. Mortality rate can decrease to 10% or less with the prevention and adequate treatment of infections and other complications, together with adequate dietary therapy.

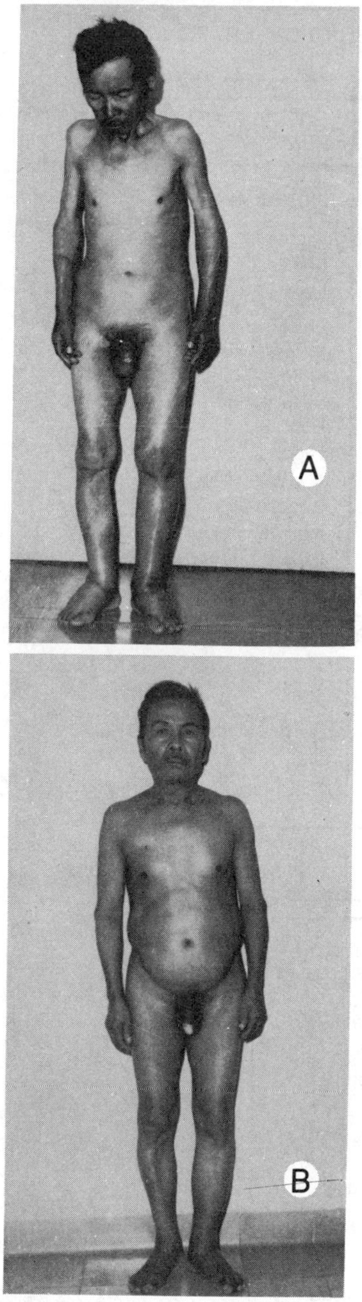

FIGURE 57–10. *A*, Edematous protein-energy malnutrition in a 46-year-old man. *B*, The same patient after 3 months of treatment.

TREATMENT

SEVERE PEM

Patients with uncomplicated PEM should be treated outside the hospital whenever possible. Hospitalization increases the risk of cross-infections, and the unfamiliar setting may increase apathy and anorexia in children, making feeding more difficult. Severely malnourished children with signs of a poor prognosis (Table 57–7) or other life-threatening complications, and those who live under deplorable social conditions that do not permit adequate medical and nutritional treatment as outpatients, must be hospitalized.

Treatment strategy can be divided into three stages: (1) resolving life-threatening conditions, (2) restoring nutritional status without disrupting homeostasis, and (3) ensuring nutritional rehabilitation.

RESOLVING LIFE-THREATENING CONDITIONS

Restoration of nutrition should start as soon as possible, but it can be delayed until life-threatening conditions are solved. The most frequent life-threatening conditions follow.

Fluid and electrolyte disturbances. The assessment of dehydration is not easy in severe PEM, because classic signs of dehydration, such as sunken eyeballs and decreased skin turgor, are frequently found in well-hydrated patients, whereas hypovolemia may coexist with subcutaneous edema, and irritability or apathy makes assessment of the mental state difficult. Useful signs are thirst, dry mouth and tongue, low urinary output, weak and rapid pulse, low blood pressure, cool and moist extremities, and a declining state of consciousness. The therapeutic approach differs from that in well-nourished patients because of water and electrolyte peculiarities of severe PEM, namely (1) hypo-osmolality with moderate hyponatremia, (2) mild-to-moderate metabolic acidosis, which decreases or disappears when the patient receives dietary or parenteral energy and when electrolyte balance is reestablished, (3) high tolerance to hypocalcemia, partly because the acidosis produces a relative increment in ionized calcium and partly because hypoproteinemia makes less protein available to bind calcium ions, (4) decreased body potassium without hypokalemia, and (5) decreased body magnesium, with or without hypomagnesemia.

Fluid repletion should allow a diuresis of at least 200 ml in 24 hours in children and 500 ml in adults, or a micturition every 2 to 3 hours. Whenever possible, oral or nasogastric rehydration should be used. The oral rehydration salt (ORS) solution currently recommended by the World Health Organization (WHO) can be used.[103] One liter of this solution contains 3.5 g NaCl, 2.9 g Na citrate (or 2.5 g Na bicarbonate), 1.5 g KCl, and 20 g glucose (or 40 g sucrose). It has an osmolality of 310 mOsm/L; it contains 90 mmol Na/L, 20 mmol K/L, and 111 mmol glucose/L. Some pediatricians believe that rehydration solutions for severely malnourished children should provide more potassium and, especially for edematous PEM, less sodium. However, there is clinical evidence that the use of the WHO solution is safe, and no controlled clinical trials show a clear advantage for the use of solutions with more K and less Na. Nevertheless, when dehydration is corrected, supplemental potassium

TABLE 57–6. ADDITIONAL SELECTED BIOCHEMICAL CHANGES OBSERVED IN SEVERE PEM

	MARASMUS	EDEMATOUS PEM
Body composition		
Total body water	High	High
Extracellular water	High	Higher
Total body potassium	Low	Lower
Total body protein	Low	Low
Serum or plasma		
Transport proteins*	Normal or low	Low
Branched-chain amino acids	Normal or low	Low
Tyrosine/phenylalanine ratio	Normal or low	Low
Enzymes (in general)†	Normal	Low
Transaminase	Normal or high	High
Liver		
Fatty infiltration	Absent	Severe
Glycogen	Normal or low	Normal or low
Urea cycle and other enzymes‡	Low	Lower
Amino acid synthesizing enzymes	High	Not as high

*For example, transferrin, ceruloplasmin, retinol-, cortisol-, and thyroxine-binding proteins, α- and β-lipoproteins,

†For example, amylase, pseudocholinesterase, alkaline phosphatase.

‡For example, xanthine oxidase, glycolic acid oxidase, cholinesterase.

(From Torún, B., Viteri, F.E.: Protein-energy malnutrition. *In* Tropical and Geographical medicine. 2nd Ed. Edited by K.S. Warren and A.A.F. Mahmoud. New York, McGraw-Hill, 1990.)

TABLE 57–7. CHARACTERISTICS THAT INDICATE POOR PROGNOSIS IN PATIENTS WITH PEM

Age less than 6 months
Deficit in weight-for-height greater than 30%, or in weight-for-age greater than 40%
Stupor, coma, or other alterations in mental status and consciousness
Infections, particularly bronchopneumonia or measles
Petechiae or hemorrhagic tendencies (purpura is usually associated with septicemia or a viral infection)
Dehydration and electrolyte disturbances, particularly hypokalemia, and severe acidosis
Persistent tachycardia, signs of heart failure, or respiratory difficulty
Total serum proteins below 30 g/l
Severe anemia with clinical signs of hypoxia
Clinical jaundice or elevated serum bilirubin
Extensive exudative or exfoliative cutaneous lesions, or deep decubitus ulcerations
Hypoglycemia or hypothermia

must be added to the diet to provide a total of about 6 to 10 mmol K per kg body weight per day, including the potassium in the diet.

The ORS solution should be given *orally* in small quantities (a teaspoonful or sips from a cup) every few minutes to provide between 70 and 100 ml per kg body weight over a period of 12 hours to children with mild-to-moderate dehydration. This is slower than customary for less undernourished, dehydrated children.[103] Breast-feeding should continue during the period of rehydration, approximately every half-hour. *Patients must be evaluated every hour.* Additional ORS solution should be given to compensate for the losses of diarrhea and vomiting. As soon as the patient improves, usually 4 to 6 hours after beginning rehydration, small amounts of liquid dietary formula with potassium, calcium, magnesium, and other electrolytes should be offered every 2 to 3 hours. If signs of dehydration are still present after 12 hours but the condition is improving, another 70 to 100 ml ORS/kg can be given over the next 12 hours. If the child's eyelids become puffy or edema increases, plain water or breast milk should be given instead of ORS.

Children who vomit constantly or cannot be fed orally should be rehydrated by *nasogastric tube*, giving 3 to 4 ml of ORS solution/kg slowly or drop by drop every half-hour. In addition to what was described for oral rehydration, the following actions must be taken based on frequent evaluations: if there is repeated vomiting or increasing abdominal distention, give the fluid more slowly and in smaller portions; if hydration is not improving after 4 hours, begin intravenous rehydration; when vomiting ceases and hydration improves, give ORS by mouth and, if the child tolerates oral solutions for the next 2 hours, remove the nasogastric tube.

Intravenous fluids must be used when there is repeated vomiting or persistent abdominal distention, and in severe dehydration with hypovolemia and impending shock. Hypo-osmolar solutions (200 to 280 mOsm/L) must be used. Potassium (when urinating) and sodium should not exceed 6 and 3 mmol/kg per day, respectively, and glucose must provide at least 63 to 126 kJ (15 to 30 kcal)/kg per day. Solutions that have been successfully used include a 1:1 mixture of 10% dextrose in water (D/W) either with isotonic saline (i.e., 5% glucose in 0.5 N saline) or with Darrow's solution; a 1:2:3 mixture of 0.17 sodium lactate:isotonic saline:10% D/W; or Hartmann's solution (Ringer's lactated solution). One of these should be infused *during the first hour* at a rate of 10 to 30 ml/kg, depending on the patient's condition. After that, 5% glucose in 0.2 N saline (800 ml of 5% D/W, 20 ml of 50% D/W, and 200 ml of isotonic saline), or a 1:2:6 mixture of lactate:isotonic saline:5% glucose with 50 ml of 50% D/W added to each 500 ml, should be infused at a rate of 5 to 10 ml/kg per hour, based on hourly evaluations of the patient, until oral therapy is initiated. When the patient is urinating, 2 g KCl (27 mmol K) is added to each liter of the infusion solution.

Increases in pulse and respiratory rate with weight gain after accounting for weight of excreta, pulmonary rales, and appearance or exacerbation of edema indicate overhydration. An increase in pulse and respiratory rate with weight loss, low urine output, and continuing losses from diarrhea and vomiting suggest insufficient fluid therapy.

Patients with severe hypoproteinemia (less than 30 g/L), anuria, and signs of hypovolemia or impending circulatory collapse should be given 10 ml plasma per kg in 1 to 2 hours, followed by 20 ml/kg per hour of a mixture of two parts of 5% dextrose and one part of isotonic saline for 1 or 2 hours. This will increase plasma protein concentration by about 5 to 10 g/L and help prevent the rapid exit of water from the intravascular compartment. If diuresis does not improve, the dose of plasma can be repeated 2 hours later. Further treatment is similar to that of well-nourished patients. Unless the patient is at risk of imminent death, only plasma tested to be human immunodeficiency virus (HIV)-negative should be used.

Hypocalcemia may occur secondary to magnesium deficiency. When the patient has symptoms of hypocalcemia and serum magnesium determinations are not available, it is essential not only to give calcium infusion but also to give magnesium intravenously or intramuscularly. When the serum concentration of calcium rises to normal level or, in the absence of laboratory data, when the symptoms of hypocalcemia disappear, calcium infusion may be discontinued. Intramuscular or oral magnesium supplementation should follow the initial parenteral magnesium until the patient is repleted with this ion as indicated by maintenance of serum and urine magnesium concentrations. When there are no laboratory facilities to monitor Mg concentrations, a general therapeutic guideline is to give magnesium intramuscularly as a 50% solution of magnesium sulfate in doses of 0.5, 1, and 1.5 ml for patients who weigh less than 7, between 7 and 10, and more than 10 kg, respectively. The dose can be repeated every 12 hours until there is no recurrence of the hypocalcemic symptoms and oral magnesium supplementation of 0.25 to 0.5 mmol mg (0.5 to 1 mEq) kg per day can be given, as described later. Certain antibiotics, such as amphotericin, can cause loss of magnesium and potassium into the urine, increasing the need for both ions.

Infections. Malnourished patients are particularly prone to infections, which are frequently the immediate cause of death in severe PEM (see also Chap. 69). Paradoxically, clinical manifestations may be mild, and the classic signs of fever, tachycardia, and leukocytosis may be absent. Antigen-antibody reactions are often impaired, and skin tests such as tuberculin, often give falsely negative results.

When an infection is suspected, appropriate antibiotic therapy must be started immediately, even before obtaining the results of microbiologic cultures. The choice of drug will vary with the suspected etiologic agent, the severity of the disease, and the pattern of drug resistance in that area. Although antibiotics should not be used prophylactically, when patients cannot be monitored closely by experienced personnel for signs of infection, as is often the case in rural hospitals of developing countries, it is safer to assume that all ill and severely malnourished patients have a bacterial infection, and to treat them with antibiotics to cover both gram-positive and gram-negative microorganisms; the latter are particularly common in PEM. When septicemia is suspected, a broad-spectrum antibiotic or a combination such as ampicillin and gentamicin (two inexpensive antibiotics generally available in developing countries) is usually given intravenously. Other supportive treatment may also be necessary, such as treatment for respiratory distress, hypothermia, and hypoglycemia.

However, clinicians should be aware that drug metabolism is likely to be altered and that detoxification mechanisms are likely to be compromised in severe PEM as a result of delayed absorption, abnormal intestinal permeability, reduced protein-binding, changes in the volume of distribution, decreased conjugation or oxidation in the liver, and decreased renal clearance.[104,105] For example, in malnourished children the half-lives of chloramphenicol,[106] sulfadiazine,[107] and gentamicin[104] are increased and their clearance is decreased. For this same reason, treatment for intestinal parasites, which is rarely urgent, should be deferred until nutritional rehabilitation is underway. This will decrease the risks of potential toxicity, including the possibility of absorbing drugs normally not absorbed by a healthy intestine.

Hemodynamic Alterations. Cardiac failure may develop when there is severe anemia, during or after administration of intravenous fluids, or shortly after the introduction of high-protein and high-energy feedings, leading to pulmonary edema and frequent secondary pulmonary infection. These alterations may be the result of impaired cardiac function, sudden expansion of the intravascular fluid volume, severe hypoxia, or impaired membrane function. Diuretics such as furosemide (10 mg intravenously or intramuscularly, repeated as necessary) should be given, and other supportive measures should be taken. Many clinicians advocate the use of digoxin (0.03 mg/kg intravenously, every 6 to 8 hours). *The use of diuretics merely to accelerate the disappearance of edema in kwashiorkor is contraindicated.*

Severe anemia. The routine use of blood transfusions endangers the patient; hemoglobin levels will improve with proper dietary treatment supplemented with hematinics. Therefore, blood transfusions should be given only in cases of severe anemia with less than 40 g hemoglobin/L, or with clinical signs of hypoxia or impending cardiac failure. In many developing countries with high prevalence of infection with HIV and few or no resources for screening the blood supply, the risk of transmission of HIV is significant; the use of transfusion should be restricted except in life-threatening situations. Whole blood (10 ml/kg) can be used in marasmic patients, but it is better to use packed red blood cells (6 ml/kg) in edematous PEM. The transfusion should be given slowly, over 2 to 3 hours and repeated if necessary after 12 to 24 hours.

Hypothermia and hypoglycemia. Body temperature below 35.5° C and plasma glucose concentration below 3.3 mmol/L (60 mg/dl) can be due to either impaired thermoregulatory mechanisms, reduced fuel substrate availability, or severe infection. Asymptomatic hypoglycemia can be treated (and prevented) by the frequent feeding of small volumes of glucose- or sucrose-containing diets and solutions. Severe symptomatic hypoglycemia must be treated intravenously with 10 to 20 ml of 50% glucose solution followed by oral administration of 25 to 50 ml of 5% glucose solution at 2-hour intervals for 24 to 48 hours.

Body temperature usually rises in the hypothermic patient with frequent feedings of glucose-containing diets or solutions. Patients must be closely monitored when external heat sources such as heavy clothing, heat lamps, and radiators are used to reduce the loss of body heat, because they may rapidly become hyperthermic. It is best to keep the seminude patients in an ambient temperature of 30 to 33° C.

Severe vitamin A deficiency. Severe PEM is often associated with vitamin A deficiency. A large dose of vitamin A should be given on admission, because ocular lesions can develop as a result of increased demands for retinol when adequate protein and energy feeding begins. Water-miscible vitamin A as retinol should be given orally or intramuscularly on the first day at a dose of 52 to 105 μmol (15,000 to 30,000 μg or 50,000 to 100,000 IU) for infants and preschool children, or 105 to 210 μmol (30,000 to 60,000 μg or 100,000 to 200,000 IU) for older children and adults, followed by 5.2 μmol (1500 μg or 5000 IU) orally each day for the duration of treatment. The initial dose should be repeated for 2 more days in symptomatic patients. Corneal ulcerations should be treated with ophthalmic drops of 1% atropine solution and antibiotic ointments or drops until the ulcerations heal.

HOMEOSTATIC RESTORATION OF NUTRITIONAL STATUS

The next objective of therapy is to replace nutrient tissue deficits as rapidly and safely as possible. This should start as soon as the measures to manage the life-threatening conditions have been established. Based on the premise that the patient is adapted to the malnourished state, nutritional treatment must begin slowly to avoid deleterious metabolic disruptions. Various regimens provide a diet that meets daily maintenance requirements for a few days, followed by a gradual increase in nutrient delivery. It is best to begin with a liquid formula fed orally or by nasogastric tube, divided equally into 6 to 12 feedings per day, depending on the patient's age and general condition. This frequent feeding of small volumes, which must be given around the clock to avoid fasting for more than 4 hours, prevents vomiting and the development of hypoglycemia and hypothermia. For older children and adults with good appetite, the liquid formula can be partly substituted with solid foods that have a high density of good-quality, easily digestible nutrients. The same diet can be used to treat marasmic and edematous patients. The only difference is that the marasmic patient may require larger amounts of dietary energy after 1 or 2 weeks of dietary treatment, which can be provided by adding vegetable oil to increase the diet's energy density. Diets that derive as much as 60 to 75% of their energy from fats are usually well tolerated; there may be some steatorrhea without profuse diarrhea, and 85 to 92% of the fat is absorbed.[51]

Intravenous alimentation is rarely justified in primary PEM and can increase mortality rates.[108]

The diet must be supplemented to provide 6 to 10 mmol (mEq) K, 3 to 5 mmol (mEq) Na, 4 mmol (8 mEq) Ca, and 0.5 to 1 mmol (1 to 2 mEq) Mg/kg of body weight per day. This can be accomplished by giving 3 mmol (mEq) of supplemental K/kg per day to children fed exclusively with milk formulas, or by adding appropriate amounts of the mineral mixture shown in Table 57–8 to most other diets. Additional supplements should include daily doses of 1 to 2.1 mmol (60 to 120 mg) elemental iron, 0.15 mmol (10 mg) elemental zinc, 1.2 mmol (0.3 mg) folic acid, 5.2 μmol (1500 μg or 5000 IU) vitamin A, and other vitamins and trace elements in the doses provided by most commercial preparations, which should be higher than the daily recommended allowances for well-nourished persons. It is best to withhold treatment with supplemental iron until 1 week after starting dietary therapy. Earlier administration of iron will not elicit a hematologic response (Fig. 57–2); it might facilitate bacterial growth in the organism and, if the free-radical theory is true, it might produce metabolic disturbances, especially in patients who have or may develop edematous PEM.

The protein source must be of high biologic value and easily digested. Cow's milk is frequently available, but some clinicians worry about the possibility of lactose malabsorption in severe PEM. However, cow's milk usually is well tolerated and assimilated by severely malnourished children and can be safely advocated.[109,110] Goat's, ewe's, buffalo's, and camel's milk can also be used. Human, mare's, and ass's milk, however, have very low protein concentrations. Cow's dried skimmed milk has very low energy density, which must be restored adding sugar and/or vegetable oil. Eggs, meat, fish, soy isolates, and some vegetable protein mixtures are also sources of good protein. Most vegetable mixtures have protein digestibilities that are 10 to 20% lower than those of animal proteins, making it necessary to feed larger amounts. Their bulk might pose a problem in feeding small children, but energy density can be increased by adding sugar and/or vegetable oil. The latter will also provide the essential fatty acids needed.

Some clinicians advocate feeding from the beginning of the dietary treatment ad libitum amounts of a liquid formula that provides about 30 g protein and 4200 kJ (1000 kcal)/L. It is expected that intake will be low at the beginning because of anorexia, and that it will gradually increase as appetite improves.

A more conservative strategy, which avoids the danger of initial excessive intakes by hungry patients and that can be applied to extremely anorexic patients who must be fed by nasogastric tube, is based on a more rigid dietary regimen that delivers small amounts of nutrients initially and increases them gradually every 2 to 3 days. A practical way to do this is based on the preparation of a *basic liquid food* with high protein concentration and high energy density; Table 57–9 gives several examples. Delivery of proteins and energy is gradually increased using different concentrations of the basic food, as shown in Table 57–10; the additional sugar compensates for the dilution of dietary energy. The liquid preparations must be fed at a dose of 100 ml/kg per day. *Additional water* must be given to provide at least 1 ml of total fluids per kilocalorie in the diet. After day 7, the patient can be allowed larger amounts of food (ad libitum). The intervals for the dietary increments in Table 57–10 can be lengthened to 3 to 5 days in severely malnourished children, especially those with plasma proteins less than 30g/L or with serious metabolic disturbances. The energy density of the diet of marasmic patients who are not gaining weight at an adequate rate by the second week (an average of at least 5 g/kg per day) should be increased at 5- to 7-day intervals by adding vegetable oil (Table 57–10).

Therapeutic diets for older children and adults must be adjusted to their age. Initial treatment should provide average energy and protein requirements, followed by a gradual increase to about 1.5 times the energy and 3 to 4 times the protein requirements by the seventh day. Dietary energy delivery to marasmic patients may have to be increased further.

The attitude of the person who feeds the patient and the appearance, color, and flavor of the foods are important to overcome the patient's lack of appetite.

The initial response to the diet is either no change in weight or a decrease caused by loss of edema, accompanied by large diuresis (Fig. 57–11). After 5 to 15 days, there is a period of rapid weight gain or "catch-up." The rate of catch-up usually is slower in marasmus than in kwashiorkor. In children, the rate of catch-up weight

TABLE 57–8. MINERAL MIXTURE TO COMPLEMENT LIQUID FORMULAS

SALT	AMOUNT (G)	1 G OF THE MIXTURE PROVIDES		
			MEQ	MMOL
KCl	26	K^+	5	5
NaCl	5	Na^+	2	2
Na_2HPO_4	4	Ca^{2+}	0.8	1.6
$CaCO_3$	3	Mg^{2+}	0.5	1
$MgSO_4$ $7H_2O$	4	HPO_4^{2-}	0.7	1.4

TABLE 57–9. FORMULATIONS FOR HIGH-PROTEIN, HIGH-ENERGY LIQUID FOODS (3–4 G PROTEIN AND 565 TO 605 KJ (135–145 KCAL) PER 100 ML

FOOD USED AS PROTEIN SOURCE	AMOUNT, G	SUCROSE, G	OIL,* G	WATER, ML
Cow's milk, full-cream powder	140	100	40	900
Cow's milk, skimmed powder	110	100	70	900
Cow's, goat's, or camel's milk, fresh	1000	100	40	—
Buffalo's or ewe's (sheep's) milk, fresh	850	100	15	150
Yogurt (cow's or goat's milk)	900	100	40	—
ICSM†	170	100	40	900
Incaparina‡	140	100	55	900

*Amount of vegetable oil can be substituted for up to one-half with isoenergetic amounts of sugar.

†Mixture of 63% cornmeal, 24% defatted soy flour, 5% skimmed milk powder, 5% soy oil, and 3% vitamin and mineral mix, distributed by U.S. AID and CARE.

‡Mixture of 58% lime-treated corn flour, 38% cottonseed flour, and 4% vitamin, mineral, and lysine mix, developed by INCAP.

(From Torún, B., Viteri, F.E.: Protein-energy malnutrition. *In* Tropical and Geographical medicine. 2nd Ed. Edited by K.S. Warren and A.A.F. Mahmoud. New York, McGraw-Hill, 1990.)

TABLE 57–10. EXAMPLE OF A DIETARY THERAPEUTIC REGIMEN FOR CHILDREN BASED ON DILUTIONS OF THE BASIC HIGH-ENERGY FOODS SHOWN IN TABLE 57–9*

DAYS FROM BEGINNING OF TREATMENT	PROPORTIONS OF BASIC FOOD + WATER	ADDITIONAL SUGAR, G/100 ML	ADDITIONAL OIL, ML/100 ML	100 ML WILL PROVIDE	
				PROTEIN, G	ENERGY, KCAL
1	1 + 2	10	—	1–1.3	85–90
3	1 + 1	10	—	1.5–2	110–115
5	3 + 1	5	—	2.3–3	120–130
7	Undiluted	—	—	3–4	135–145
Marasmus†					
12	Undiluted	—	3	3–4	160–170
17	Undiluted	—	6	3–4	185–195
22	Undiluted	—	9	3–4	210–220
etc.	Undiluted	—	†	3–4	†

*The formulas must be fed at 100 ml/kg per day. They must be supplemented with adequate amounts of vitamins, minerals, and electrolytes. Additional water must be given to provide at least 1 ml of total fluids per kcal in the diet.

†Marasmic patients may require more dietary energy; 2 to 3 ml (half a teaspoon) of vegetable oil per 100 ml of liquid diet should be added at 5-day intervals until the rate of weight gain becomes adequate.

(From Torún, B., Viteri, F.E.: Protein-energy malnutrition. *In* Tropical and Geographical Medicine. 2nd Ed. Edited by K.S. Warren and A.A. F. Mahmoud. New York, McGraw-Hill, 1990.)

gain generally is 10 to 15 times that of a normal child of the same age, and it can be as high as 20 to 25 times greater. Some patients only show a fourfold or fivefold increase in catch-up. Most often this is associated with insufficient energy intakes (e.g., because of inadequately prepared formula, insufficient amounts of formula given at each feeding, too few feedings per day, anorexia, or lack of patience of the person who feeds the child) or with overt or asymptomatic infections; urinary infections and tuberculosis are the most commonly seen asymptomatic diseases.

ENSURING NUTRITIONAL REHABILITATION

This last stage of treatment may begin in the hospital and continue on an outpatient basis, but the patient must continue to eat adequate amounts of protein, energy, and other nutrients, especially when traditional foods are introduced into the diet. Emotional and physical stimulation must be provided, and persistent diarrhea, intestinal parasites, and other minor complications must be treated. Children should be vaccinated during this period as well.

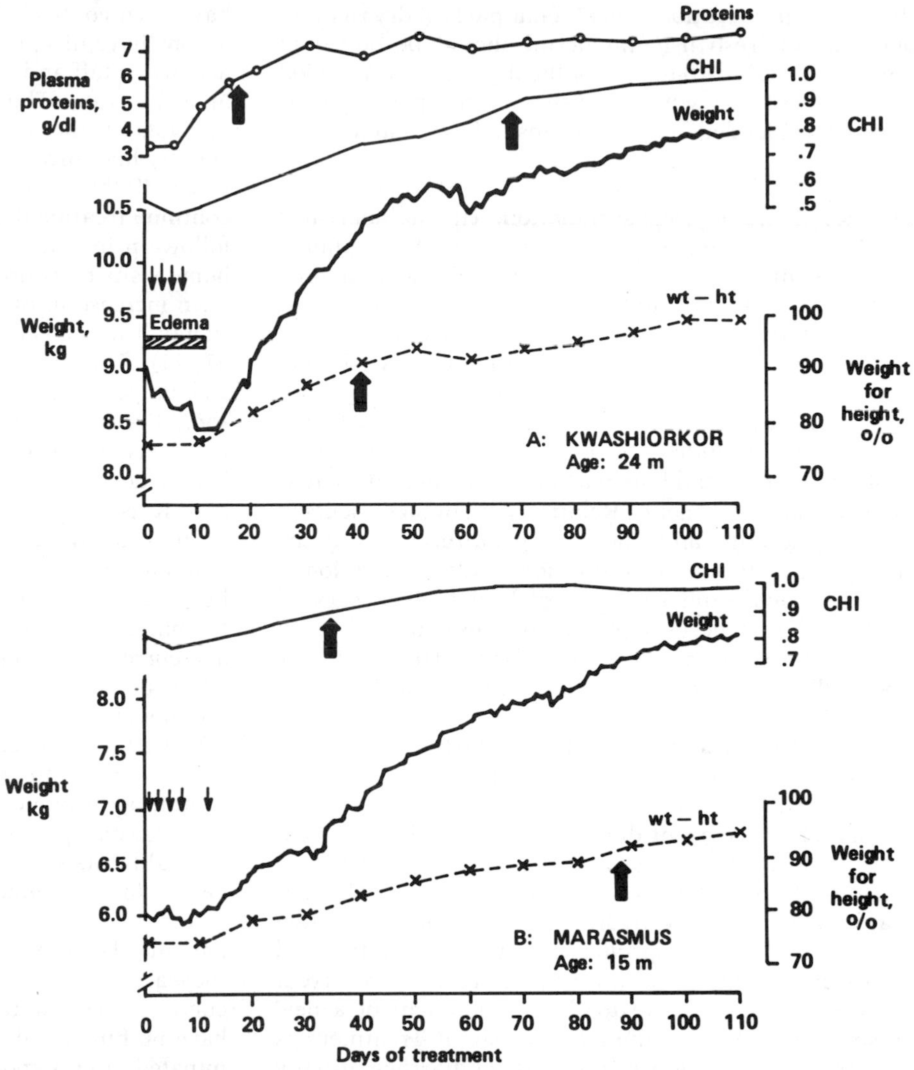

FIGURE 57–11. Weight gain and improvement in weight for height, creatinine-height index (CHI), and plasma protein concentration of two children treated at INCAP for kwashiorkor (child A) and marasmus (child B). The thin, downward arrows indicate gradual increments in dietary proteins and energy, as described in Table 57–10. The thick, upward arrows indicate the day when the lower limit of normal values was reached. The marasmic child had a normal plasma protein concentration on admission. Weight for height was calculated on child A on admission, after correcting for the weight of edema. Dietary energy was reduced on days 60 and 80 for child A and on day 100 for child B.

Introduction of traditional foods. Other foods, especially those available at home, are gradually introduced into the diet in a combination with the high-energy, high-protein formula. This step should be taken when edema has disappeared, the skin lesions are notably improved, the patient becomes active and interacts with the environment, the appetite is restored, and adequate rates of catch-up growth have been achieved. For children, a daily minimum intake of 3 to 4 g of protein and 500 to 625 kJ (120 to 150 kcal)/kg of body weight (or more in marasmus) must be ensured. To achieve this, the energy density of solid foods must be increased with oil, and protein density and quality must be high, using animal proteins, soybean protein preparations, and good vegetable protein mixtures. Local traditional foods can be used in appropriate combinations[111-113] *in addition to the liquid formula,* as in the following examples: (1) One part of a dry pulse or its flour (e.g., black beans, soybeans, kidney beans, cowpeas) and three parts of a dry cereal or flour (e.g., corn, rice, wheat); fat or oil should be added to the mashed or strained pulse during or after cooking in amounts equal to the weight of the dry pulse or flour, and to the cereal preparations in amounts of 10 to 30 ml oil/100 g dry cereal product, depending on the type of preparation; and (2) Four parts of dry rice and one part of fresh fish; fat or oil should be added in amounts equal to 20 to 40% of the dry weights. The food can be served as separate dishes or the parts can be mashed or blended and fed as paps to infants and young children.

Emotional and physical stimulation. The malnourished child needs affection and tender care from the beginning of treatment. This requires patience and understanding by the hospital staff and the relatives. Involvement of parents or relatives is usually helpful. Hospitals should be brightly colored and cheerful, with auditory stimulation such as music. As soon as the child can move without assistance and is willing to interact with the staff and other children, he or she must be encouraged to explore, to play, and to participate in activities that involve body movements. Relatively small increments in physical activity and energy expenditure during the course of nutritional rehabilitation result in faster longitudinal growth and accretion of lean body tissues.[114] Parents should be encouraged to stimulate and teach their children by playing and talking. Toys and play materials can often be made from discarded local articles.

Adult patients should exercise regularly with gradual increments in cardiorespiratory workload.

Persistent or recurrent diarrhea and other health problems. Mild diarrhea does not interfere with nutritional rehabilitation as long as fluid and electrolyte intakes maintain satisfactory hydration. This condition often disappears without specific treatment as nutritional status improves.[115] However, persistent or recurrent diarrhea can contribute to the development of a new episode of PEM and should be treated. Treatment is determined by the underlying cause of diarrhea, usually intestinal infections, excessive bacterial flora in the upper gut that ferment food substrates and deconjugate bile salts, intestinal parasites (particularly giardiasis, cryptosporidiosis, and trichiuriasis), and intolerance to food components.

As for food intolerances, lactose, milk protein, and gluten have commonly been held responsible. However, the apparent high prevalence of lactose malabsorption and intolerance in PEM is often founded on inadequate diagnostic procedures (e.g., intolerance to 2 g lactose/kg in aqueous solution, rather than to the 7 to 15 g lactose contained in a milk meal).[49] When food intolerance is suspected, the diet should be modified, taking care to preserve its nutritional quality and density. Before branding a patient intolerant to a given food, the food should be reintroduced into the diet to confirm the diagnosis, and adequate diagnostic tests should be done.

Criteria for recovery. Treatment until full recovery *should not* be in a hospital. Ideally, the patient should be referred to a nutrition clinic or rehabilitation center to continue treatment after all life-threatening conditions have been controlled, appetite is good, edema and skin lesions have disappeared, and the patient smiles, interacts with staff and other patients, and is gaining weight at a fast rate. The child's mother or caretaker must understand the importance of continuing the high-energy, high-protein diet until full recovery has taken place. If this can be done at home, the patient can continue treatment on an outpatient basis with regular follow-up in a nutrition clinic or its equivalent, or by home visits by trained personnel.

An increase in plasma protein or albumin concentration indicates a good response but not full recovery (Fig. 57–11). The most practical criterion for recovery is weight gain, and almost all fully recovered patients should reach the weight expected for their height (see later). As shown in Figure 57–11, however, weight for height does not necessarily indicate protein repletion, and it is best to use it in conjunction with body composition indices. If urine can be collected for 24 to 72 hours in children, the creatinine-height index (CHI) can be used as an indicator of body protein repletion. Premature termination of treatment increases the risk of a recurrence of malnutrition. As a general guideline, when body composition cannot be assessed, dietary therapy should continue for 1 month after the patient admitted with edematous PEM reaches an adequate weight for height without edema and his clinical and overall performances are adequate, or for 15 days after the marasmic patient reaches that weight. The minimum normal limits should be 92% of the weight expected for height (or 1 standard deviation below the reference median) and, especially in children, a CHI of 0.9. Some patients, however, do not reach those values because they are in the lower end of the normal distribution curve. If they continue growing at a normal rate and have no functional impairments, treatment can be terminated after 1 month of adequate dietary intake and weight for height and CHI stabilization. Specific treatment of other nutritional problems (e.g., iron deficiency) sometimes must be prolonged beyond discharge for PEM.

Before being discharged, patients or their parents must be taught about the causes of PEM, emphasizing rational and nutritious use of household foods, personal and environmental hygiene, appropriate immunizations, and early treatment—including dietary management—of diarrhea and other diseases.

MILD AND MODERATE PEM

The less severe forms of PEM should be treated in an ambulatory setting, supplementing the home diet with easily digested foods that contain proteins of high biologic value, a high energy density, and adequate amounts of micronutrients. In some instances, therapy can be achieved merely by instructing the adult patient about adequate eating habits and a better use of food resources, or by instructing mothers in improved child-feeding practices and in more nutritious culinary habits. It is almost always necessary, however, to provide both nutritious food supplements and instructions for their use.

The quantity of food supplements will vary depending on the degree of malnutrition and the relative deficit of proteins and energy. As a general guideline, the goal should be to provide a total intake, including the home diet, of *at least* twice the protein and 1.5 times the energy requirements. For preschool children, this would signify a daily intake of about 2 to 2.5 g of high-quality protein and 500 to 625 kJ (120 to 150 kcal)/kg of body weight, and for infants under 1 year, about 3.5 g protein and 625 kJ (150 kcal)/kg per day.

The ingestion of the food supplement by the malnourished person must be ensured. This is more likely to occur if it is appetizing to both the child and the mother, if it is ready-made or easy to prepare, if additional amounts are provided to feed other children living in the same household, and if it does not have an important commercial value outside the home that would make it easy and profitable for the family to sell the item for cash. A substitution effect on the home diet (i.e., a decrease in the usual food intake) is almost always unavoidable, but it can be reduced by using low-bulk supplements with high protein and energy concentrations. Special attention should be given to avoid a decrease in breast-feeding. The supplements for breast-fed infants should be paps or solid foods that will not quench the infant's thirst and thus not change the infant's demand or the mother's attitude toward lactation.

Adequate amounts of vitamins and minerals must be assured, although mild deficiencies can be overcome by the micronutrients in the food or by use of fortified vehicles such as iron-enriched bread or sugar fortified with retinol.

PREVENTION AND CONTROL OF PEM

Poverty, ignorance, frequent infections, cultural customs, cyclic climatic conditions, and natural and man-made disasters are among the main causes of PEM. Therefore, its control and prevention require multisectoral approaches that include food production and distribution, preventive medicine, education, social development, and economic improvement. At a national or regional level, control and prevention can only be achieved through short- and long-term political commitments and effective actions to enforce the measure to eradicate the underlying causes of malnutrition.

Nevertheless, the physician, nutritionist, public health worker, and educator *can and must* play an active role in the prevention of PEM, even though prevention is aimed at smaller population groups or individuals. If they have to attend only those at higher risk to develop PEM due to limited resources, a profile of risk factors is useful. The most likely victims are children under 2 years of age from low socioeconomic strata whose parents have misconceptions concerning the use of foods, who come from broken or unstable families, whose families have a high prevalence of alcoholism, who live under poor sanitary conditions, in urban slums, or in rural areas frequently subject to droughts or floods, and whose societal beliefs prohibit the use of many nutritious foods.

Special attention must be given to the availability and rational use of foods that optimize nutrient utilization, the control or reduction of infections, and health and nutrition education programs for the individual, the family, and the community.

FOOD AVAILABILITY

Animal foods are the best protein sources but they tend to be expensive, not always available, or prohibited by religious practices. Under such circumstances, the staple vegetable foods can be complemented with other vegetable foods combined in culturally acceptable ways to permit a good essential amino acid complementation and improve the biologic value of dietary protein. For example, corn and black bean combinations that provide proteins in a proportion of about 60:40, equivalent to about three parts of dry corn and one part of dry beans, have an excellent amino acid composition and permit adequate growth and function.[116] The same is true of a series of other combinations of grains and pulses.[111–113] The relatively low nitrogen digestibility of these vegetable sources must be considered in recommending the amounts to be eaten. Energy density can be increased by adding fats or carbohydrates.

It is often necessary to convince parents about the safety of using foods which, in some cultures, are fed only to adults and older children. This is especially true of foods used to complement mother's milk or to wean infants from the breast. Breast-fed infants from populations at risk of PEM should start receiving at 4 months of age commercial preparations of cooked rice, oat, or wheat, or home-made paps prepared by mashing boiled rice, bread soaked in about 50% water, or cooked corn products (e.g., tamale, tortilla). At 6 months of age, fish, egg, or minced meat, or one part of a cooked pulse (e.g., kidney beans, soybeans, chick peas) should be added for every three parts of rice, corn, or bread to provide a better protein mixture. If the child is underweight, 1 teaspoon of vegetable oil or 2 teaspoons of sugar can be added to every 2 to 3 ounces of pap. Trials at the Instituto de Nutrición de Centro América y Panamá (INCAP) have shown that it is feasible to feed paps based on black beans (Phaseolus vulgaris), a cereal, and vegetable oil to babies as young as 3 months of age without intestinal discomfort and without decreasing breast milk intakes. Examples of such paps are shown in Table 57–11.

Children who are fully weaned or only occasionally breast-fed must receive adequate amounts of energy- and protein-rich staples and, ideally, animal foods to satisfy their nutritional needs and allow adequate growth.

It is also important to convince parents that food

TABLE 57–11. PAPS TO COMPLEMENT BREAST MILK, USING COMMON FOODS AND BASED ON COMBINATIONS OF A LEGUME WITH A CEREAL OR POTATO, AND VEGETABLE OIL*

	A	B	C	D
Cooked beans (60% water)†	25 g	25 g	25 g	25 g
Corn dough (57% water)	75 g	—	—	—
White bread (50% water)	—	75 g	—	—
Boiled rice (55% water)	—	—	75 g	—
Boiled potatoes (33% water)	—	—	—	75 g
Water	25 ml	25 ml	25 ml	25 ml
Vegetable oil	10 ml	10 ml	10 ml	15 ml
Protein, g/100 g‡	3.6	4.8	3.4	2.2
Energy, kcal/100 g‡	176	176	183	147

*Modified from unpublished observations by F.E. Viteri, B. Garcia, and B. Torún. Black beans (Phaseolus vulgaris) cooked, mashed, and strained. Corn dough cooked with limestone, according to Guatemalan customs. White bread soaked in equal weight of water.

†In parentheses: proportion of water added to prepare 100 g.

‡Protein and energy content of 100 g of pap, ready to eat.

should not be withheld when a child has diarrhea, because in many developing countries children under 5 years of age have loose stools 15 to 20% of the time. It has been shown that many local foods of vegetable origin that are rich in fiber can be safely used and may even shorten the duration of diarrhea.[117]

REDUCING INFECTIONS

This is a logical consequence of the interactions of nutrition with infection. Because young children are at a greater risk of malnutrition, high priority must be given to immunizations, sanitary measures to reduce fecal contamination, and early oral rehydration and feeding of children with diarrhea.[117]

EDUCATION

The presence of a malnourished child in a family indicates that something is wrong in that family and suggests that other members of the household might also be at risk of malnutrition. Therefore, nutritional and health education must not be restricted to the rehabilitation of the index case, but should include the prevention of nutritional deterioration of other family members, especially siblings and pregnant and lactating women. Similarly, a high prevalence of children with malnutrition or growth retardation indicates that the entire community is at some risk of impaired nutrition. Consequently, education programs must be devised for community leaders, civic action groups, and the community as a whole. Such programs must emphasize promotion of breast-feeding, appropriate use of weaning foods, nutritional alternatives using traditional foods, personal and environmental hygiene, feeding practices during illness and convalescence, and early treatment of diarrhea and other diseases. Personal and communal involvement should be pursued through commitments to apply the recommendations. Toward this aim, it is important that all educational programs incorporate the community's own assessment of their nutritional problems and their feelings toward personal participation in solving these problems.

REFERENCES

1. Patron-Correa, J.P.: Rev. Med. Yucatán (Mexico), *3*:89–96, 1908.
2. Normet, L.: Bull. Soc. Pathol. Exot., *19*:207–213, 1926.
3. Kerandel, J.: Bull. Soc. Pathol. Exot., *19*:302–311, 1926.
4. McConnell, R.E.: Uganda Ann. Med. San. Report, Appendix 2. Entebbe, Government Printer, 1918.
5. Procter, R.A.W.: Kenya Med. J., *3*:264, 1927.
6. Mann, W.L., Helm, J.B., Brown, C.J.: JAMA, *75*:1416–1418, 1920.
7. Payne, G.C.: Payne, F.K.: Am. J. Hyg., *7*:73–83, 1927.
8. Williams, C.D.: Arch. Dis. Child., *8*:423–433, 1923.
9. Williams, C.D.: Lancet, *2*:1151–1152, 1935.
10. Autret, M., Behar, M.: Síndrome Policarencial Infantil (Kwashiorkor) and its Prevention in Central America. FAO Nutrition Studies No. 113. Rome, Food and Agriculture Organization, 1954.
11. Trowell, H.C., Davies, J.N.P., Dean, R.F.A.: Kwashiorkor. London, Edward Arnold, 1954.
12. Hegsted, D.M., Tsongas, A.G., Abbott, D.B., et al.: J. Lab. Clin. Med., *31*:261–284, 1946.

13. Brock, J.F., Autret, M.: Kwashiorkor in Africa. FAO Nutrition Studies No. 8. Rome, Food and Agriculture Organization, 1952.
14. Jelliffe, D.B.: J. Pediatr., *54*:227–256, 1959.
15. UNICEF: The State of the World's Children 1991. Oxford, Oxford University Press, 1991.
16. Food and Agriculture Organization: The State of Food and Agriculture 1990. FAO Agriculture Series No. 23. Rome, Food and Agriculture Organization, 1991.
17. United Nations ACC/SCN: Update in the Nutrition Situation. Recent Trends in Nutrition in 33 Countries. Geneva, World Health Organization, 1989.
18. Villar, J., Rivera, J.: Pediatrics, *81*:51–57, 1988.
19. Chagas, C., Keusch, G.T. (eds.): The Interaction of Parasitic Diseases and Nutrition. Pontificiae Academiae Scientiarum Scripta Varia No. 61. Vatican, Pontifical Academy of the Sciences, 1986.
20. Torún, B.: Short and long-term effects of low or restricted energy intakes on the activity of infants and children. *In* Activity, Energy Expenditure and Energy Requirements of Infants and Children. Edited by B. Schurch and N.S. Scrimshaw. Lausanne, International Dietary Energy Consulting Group, 1990, pp. 335–359.
21. Viteri, F.E., Torún, B.: Bol. Of. Sanit. Panam., *78*:58–74, 1975.
22. Torún, B., Viteri, F.E.: United Nations Univ. Food Nutr. Bull. Suppl., *5*:229–241, 1981.
23. Kerpel-Fronius, E., Vargas, F., Kun, K.: Ann. Pediatr. (Basel), *183*:1–28, 1954.
24. Viteri, F.E., Alvarado, J.: Rev. Col. Med. (Guatemala), *21*:175–230, 1970.
25. Waterlow, J.C., Garlick, P.J., Millward, J.D.: Protein Turnover in Mammalian Tissues and in the Whole Body. Oxford, North Holland, 1978.
26. Tomkins, A.M., Garlick, P.J., Schofield, W.N., Waterlow, J.C.: Clin. Sci., *65*:313–324, 1983.
27. Viteri, F.E.: Primary protein-energy malnutrition: clinical, biochemical, and metabolic changes. *In* Textbook of Pediatric Nutrition. Edited by R.M. Suskind. New York, Raven Press, 1981.
28. Reddy, V.: Protein-energy malnutrition; An overview. *In* Nutrition in Health and Disease and Industrial Development. Edited by A.E. Harper and G.K. Davis. New York, Alan R. Liss, 1981, pp. 227–235.
29. Viteri, F.E., Alvarado, J., Luthringer, D.G., et al.: Vitam. Horm., *26*:573–615, 1968.
30. Caballero, B., Solomons, N.W., Batres, R., et al.: J. Pediatr. Gastroenterol. Nutr., *4*:97–102, 1985.
31. MacDougall, L.G., Moodley, G., Eyberg, C., Quirk, M.: Am. J. Clin. Nutr., *35*:229–235, 1982.
32. Wickramasinghe, S.N., Mary-Cotes, P., Gill, D.S., et al.: Br. J. Haematol., *60*:515–524, 1985.
33. Viart, P.: Am. J. Clin. Nutr., *30*:334–348, 1977.
34. Viart, P.: Am. J. Clin. Nutr., *31*:911–926, 1978.
35. Heymsfield, S.B., Bethel, R.A., Ansley, J.D., et al.: Am. Heart J., *95*:584–594, 1978.
36. Alleyne, G.A.O.: Pediatrics, *39*:400–411, 1967.
37. Paniagua, R., Santos, D., Muñoz, R., et al.: Pediatr. Res., *14*:1260–1262, 1980.
38. Mahakur, A.C., Mishra, A.C., Panda, S.N., et al.: J. Assoc. Physicians India, *31*:79–81, 1983.
39. Keusch, G.T.: Malnutrition, infection and immune function. *In* The Malnourished Child. Edited by R.M. Suskind, and L. Lewinter-Suskind. Nestlé Nutrition Workshop Series, Vol. 19. New York, Raven Press, 1990, pp. 37–59.
40. Chandra, R.K.: Am. J. Clin. Nutr., *53*:1087–1101, 1991.
41. Olusi, S.O., Thurman, G.B., Goldstein, A.L.: Clin. Immunol. Immunopathol., *15*:687–691, 1980.
42. Bhaskaram, R., Siwakumar, B.: Arch. Dis. Child, *61*:182–185, 1986.
43. Keusch, G.T., Torún, B., Johnson, R.B., et al.: J. Pediatr., *105*:434–436, 1984.
44. Kauffman, C.A., Jones, R.G., Kluger, M.J.: Am. J. Clin. Nutr., *44*: 449–452, 1986.
45. Cerami, A., Ikeda, Y., LeTrang, N., et al.: Immunol. Lett., *11*:173–175, 1985.
46. Nichols, B.L., Alvarado, J., Hazlewood, C.F., et al.: J. Pediatr., *80*:319–330, 1972.
47. Lopes, J., Russell, D.M., Whitwell, J., et al.: Am. J. Clin. Nutr., *36*: 602–610, 1982.
48. Viteri, F.E., Schneider, R.: Med. Clin. North Am., *58*:1487–1505, 1974.
49. Torún, B., Solomons, N.W., Viteri, F.E.: Arch. Latinoam. Nutr., *29*:445–494, 1979.
50. Lifshitz, F., Teichber, S., Wapnir, R.A.: Malnutrition and the intestine. *In* Nutrition and Child Health: A Perspective for the 1980's. Edited by R.C. Tsang and B.L. Nichols. New York, Alan R. Liss, 1981.
51. Torún, B.: Nutrient absorption in malnutrition. *In* The Interactions of Parasitic Diseases and Nutrition. Edited by C. Chagas and G.T. Keusch. Scripta Varia No. 61. Vatican, Pontifical Academy of the Sciences, 1986.
52. Winick, M.: J. Pediatr. Gastroenterol. Nutr., *6*:833–835, 1987.
53. Jaya-Rao, K.S.: Lancet, *1*:709–711, 1974.
54. Hendrickse, R.G.: Trans. R. Soc. Trop. Med. Hyg., *78*:427–435, 1984.
55. Coulter, J.B.S., Suliman, G.I.: Eur. J. Clin. Nutr., *42*:787–796, 1988.
56. Golden, M.H.N.: The consequences of protein deficiency in man and its relationship to the features of kwashiorkor. *In* Nutritional Adaptation in Man. Edited by K.L. Blaxter and J.C. Waterlow. London, John Libby, 1985, pp. 169–188.
57. Golden, M.H.N., Ramdath, D.: Proc. Nutr. Soc., *46*:53–68, 1987.
58. Golden, M.H.N., Ramdath, D., Golden, B.E.: Free radicals and malnutrition. *In* Trace Elements, Micronutrients and Free Radicals. Edited by I.E. Dreosti. Clifton, NJ, Humana Press, 1990.
59. Waterlow, J.C.: Causes of oedema and its relation to kwashiorkor. Submitted for publication.
60. Olson, R.E.: Am. J. Clin. Nutr., *28*:626–637, 1975.
61. Alleyne, G.A.O., Trust, P.M., Flores, H., et al.: Br. J. Nutr., *27*:585–592, 1972.
62. Munro, H.N.: General aspects of the regulation of protein metabolism by diet and by hormones. *In* Mammalian Protein Metabolism, Vol 1. Edited by H.N. Munro and J.B. Allison. New York, Academic Press, 1964.
63. Felig, P.: N. Engl. J. Med., *283*:149–159, 1970.
64. Arroyave, G., Wilson, D., Funes, C., et al.: Am. J. Clin. Nutr., *11*: 517–524, 1962.
65. Holt, L.E., Snyderman, S.E., Norton, P.M., et al.: Lancet, *2*:1343–1348, 1963.
66. Vis, H.L.: Aspects de mecanismes des hyperaminoaciduries de l'enfance. Paris, Editions Arsica, 1963.
67. Schelp, F.P., Migasena, P., Pongpaew, P., et al.: Am. J. Clin. Nutr., *31*:451–456, 1978.
68. Neufeld, H.A., Pace, J.A., White, F.E.: Metabolism, *25*:877–884, 1976.

69. Beisel, W.R., Sawyer, W.D., Ryll, E.D., et al.: Ann. Intern. Med., *67:*744–779, 1967.
70. Beisel, W.R., Am. J. Clin. Nutr., *30:*1236–1247, 1977.
71. Powanda, M.C.: Am. J. Clin. Nutr., *30:*1254–1268, 1977.
72. Gabig, T.G., Babior, B.M.: Oxygen-dependent microbial killing by neutrophils. *In* Superoxide Dismutase, Vol. 2. Edited by L.W. Oberly. Boca Raton, FL, CRC Press, 1982, pp. 1–15.
73. Weech, A.A.: Bull. N.Y. Acad. Med., *15:*63–91, 1939.
74. Walter, S.J., Shore, A.C.: Clin. Sci., *75:*621–628, 1988.
75. Klahr, S., Alleyne, G.A.O.: Kidney Int., *3:*129–141, 1973.
76. Migeon, C.J., Beitins, I.Z., Kowarski, A., Graham, G.G.: Plasma aldosterone concentration and aldosterone secretion rate in Peruvian infants with marasmus and kwashiorkor. *In* Endocrine Aspects of Malnutrition. Edited by L.I. Gardner and P. Amacher. Santa Ynez, CA, Kroc Foundation, 1973, pp. 399–424.
77. Beitins, I.Z., Graham, G.G., Kowarski, A., et al.: J. Pediatr., *84:*444–451, 1974.
78. Srikantia, S.G., Gopalan, C.: Am. J. Appl. Physiol., *14:*829–833, 1959.
79. Srikantia, S.G., Mohanham, S.: J. Clin. Endocrinol., *31:*312–314, 1970.
80. Golden, M.H.N.: Lancet, *1:*1261–1265, 1982.
81. Torún, B., Viteri, F.E.: Rev. Col. Med. (Guatemala), *27:*43–62, 1976.
82. Patrick, J.: Br. Med. J., *1:*1051–1054, 1977.
83. Benjamin, D.R.: Ped. Clin. North Am., *36:*139–161, 1989.
84. Habicht, J.P., Martorell, R., Yarborough, C., et al.: Lancet, *1:*611–615, 1974.
85. Graitcer, P.L., Gentry, E.M.: Lancet, *2:*297–299, 1981.
86. United States Dept. of Health, Education and Welfare (DHEW): NCHS Growth Curves for Children from Birth to 18 Years. Publication PHS 78–1650. Hyattsville, MD, DHEW, 1970.
87. WHO: Measuring Change in Nutritional Status. Geneva, World Health Organization, 1983.
88. Waterlow, J.C.: Classification and definition of protein-energy malnutrition. *In* Nutrition in Preventive Medicine. Edited by G.H. Beaton and J.M. Bengoa. Geneva, World Health Organization, 1976.
89. Nabarro, D., McNab, S.: J. Trop. Med. Hyg., *83:*21–33, 1980.
90. Torún, B., Samayoa, C.: Un sistema sencillo para evaluar el estado nutricional de niños, con participación comunitaria. *In* Proceedings 9th Latin American Congress of Nutrition, San Juan, PR, 1991, p. 159.
91. James, W.P.T., Ferro-Luzzi, A., Waterlow, J.C.: Eur. J. Clin. Nutr., *42:*969–981, 1988.
92. Cronck, C.E., Roche, A.F.: Am. J. Clin. Nutr., *35:* 347–354, 1982.
93. Gomez, F., Ramos-Galvan, R., Frenk, S.: Adv. Pediatr., *7:*131–169, 1955.
94. Rutishauser, I.H.E., Whitehead, R.G.: Br. J. Nutr., *28:*145–152, 1972.
95. Viteri, F.E., Torún, B.: Nutrition, physical activity and growth. *In* The Biology of Normal Human Growth. Edited by M. Rizen, A. Aperia, K. Hall, et al. New York, Raven Press, 1981.
96. Spurr, G.B., Reina, J.C.: Eur. J. Clin. Nutr., *42:*819–834, 1988.
97. Allen, L.H.: Clin. Nutr., *3:*169–175, 1984.
98. Viteri, F.E., Torún, B., Immink, M.D.C., et al.: Marginal malnutrition and working capacity. *In* Nutrition in Health and Disease and International Development. Edited by A.E. Harper and G.K. Davis. New York, Alan R. Liss, 1981.
99. Habicht, J.P., Lechtig, A., Yarborough, C., et al.: Maternal nutrition, birth weight and infant mortality. *In* Size at Birth. Edited by J. Elliott and J. Knight. Ciba Foundation Symposium 27. Amsterdam, Associated Scientific Publishers, 1974.
100. Viteri, F.E., Alvarado, J.: Pediatrics, *46:*696–706, 1970.
101. Parra, A., Garza, C., Garza, Y., et al.: J. Pediatr., *82:*133–142, 1973.
102. Chen, L.C., Chowdry, A.K.M.A., Hoffman, S.L.: Am. J. Clin. Nutr., *33:* 1838–1845, 1980.
103. WHO: A Manual for the Treatment of Diarrhea. Programme for the control of Diarrhea Disease, WHO/CDD/SER/80.1 Rev. 1 1990. Geneva, World Health Organization, 1990.
104. Krishnaswamy, K.: Clin. Pharmacokinet., *17 (Suppl. 1):*68–88, 1989.
105. Mehta, S.: Drug metabolism in the malnourished child. *In* The Malnourished Child. Edited by R.M. Suskind and L. Lewinter-Suskind. Nestlé Nutrition Workshop Series, Vol. 19. New York, Raven Press, 1990, pp. 329–338.
106. Mehta, S., Nain, C.K., Kalso, H.K., Mathur, V.S.: Indian J. Med. Res., *74:*244–250, 1981.
107. Mehta, S., Naim, C.K., Sharma, B., Mathur, V.S.: Pharmacology, *21:*369–374, 1980.
108. Janssen, F., Bouton, J.M., Vuye, A., et al.: J. Parenter. Enteral Nutr., *7:*26–36, 1983.
109. Solomons, N.W., Torún, B., Caballero, B., et al.: Am. J. Clin. Nutr., *40:*591–600, 1984.
110. Torún, B., Solomons, N.W., Caballero, B., et al.: Am. J. Clin. Nutr., *40:*601–610, 1984.
111. Cameron, C., Hofvander, Y.: Manual on Feeding Infants and Young Children. 2nd Ed. New York, United Nations Protein-Calorie Advisory Group, 1976.
112. Torún, B., Young, V.R., Rand, W.M. (eds.).: Protein-Energy Requirements of Developing Countries: Evaluation of New Data. Tokyo, United Nations Univ. Food Nutr. Bull. *(Suppl. 5)* 1981.
113. Rand, W.M., Uauy, R., Scrimshaw, N.S. (eds.): Protein-Energy Requirement Studies in Developing Countries: Results of International Research. Tokyo, United Nations Univ. Food Nutr. Bull. *(Suppl. 10)* 1984.
114. Torún, B., Schutz, Y., Bradfield, R.B., et al.: Effect of physical activity upon growth of children recovering from protein-calorie malnutrition (PCM). *In* Proceedings 10th International Congress Nutrition, Kyoto, Victory-sha Press, 1976.
115. Torún, B.: Alimentación de niños con desnutrición proteínico-energética y diarrea, con énfasis en las experiencias del INCAP. *In* Pan Am Health Organization Meeting on Feeding of Children Ill with Diarrhea. Washington, D.C., Pan American Health Organization, 1983.
116. Viteri, F.E., Torún, B., Arroyave, G., et al.: Food Nutr. Bull., *(Suppl. 5)* 202–209, 1981.
117. Torún, B., Chew, F.: Trans. R. Soc. Trop. Med. Hyg., *85:*12–17, 1991.
118. INCAP: Evaluación nutricional de la población de Centro América y Panamá: Guatemala. Guatemala, Instituto de Nutrición de Centro América y Panamá, 1969.
119. Torún, B., Viteri, F.E.: Protein-energy malnutrition. *In* Tropical and Geographical Medicine. 2nd Ed. Edited by K.S. Warren and A.A.F. Mahmoud. New York, McGraw-Hill, 1990.

CHAPTER **58**

Behavioral Disorders Affecting Food Intake: Anorexia Nervosa and Bulimia Nervosa

Alexander R. Lucas and Diane M. Huse

Eating disorders are deviations in eating behavior that lead to disease or disability. Mild deviations are extremely common and occur with great variation at any age. They may be classified on the basis of their visible end result, i.e., extreme thinness or fatness, or on the basis of variations in eating patterns (fasting, food restriction, binge eating). The most common eating disorder, obesity, is discussed elsewhere (see Chap. 59). This chapter deals with those disorders in which eating behavior is grossly disturbed: anorexia nervosa and bulimia nervosa.

Anorexia nervosa is characterized by self-imposed weight loss, endocrine dysfunction, and a distorted psychopathologic attitude toward eating and weight. The illness typically occurs in girls shortly after puberty or later in adolescence, but onset can be premenarchal or later in life. Rarely, the illness occurs in males.

Bulimia nervosa is a severe disorder characterized by frequent binge eating and purging associated with loss of control over eating and a persistent overconcern about body shape and weight. The disorder occurs predominantly in young adult women. Milder forms of binge eating and purging are common in normal-weight women.

HISTORICAL NOTE

Medical descriptions of anorexia nervosa exist from many centuries ago. The disease was formally identified simultaneously by Sir William Gull in England and by Charles Lasègue in France. These authors recognized a psychologic cause, but for many years, no effective treatments existed. Bruch, in the 1960s, elucidated psychologic manifestations of the disorder and developed effective psychotherapeutic techniques. Recent research has focused on physiologic concomitants of the disorder and on the development of multifaceted treatment approaches.[1]

The historical meaning of bulimia is ravenous appetite manifested by voracious eating. It was described in conditions of hypothalamic dyscontrol. In 1979, Russell described bulimia nervosa as a distinct syndrome and serious variant of anorexia nervosa.[2] Subsequently, much attention has been given to the many variants of eating disorders manifested by binge eating, self-induced vomiting, and other forms of purging.

PATHOPHYSIOLOGY

The pathophysiologic changes seen in anorexia nervosa are similar to those observed in other states of semistarvation. For the most part, they are adaptive responses that allow the individual to survive a decreased dietary intake of sources of energy. Such adaptations, however, are not without their "cost": functional impairment in other systems that limit the capacity of an individual to perform normal physical and mental activities. Many of the symptoms and signs of anorexia nervosa can be understood within the context of "normal" adaptations to semistarvation.[3]

Starvation is associated with energy conservation, adaptations that spare glucose and protein while favoring use of fat, often dramatic shifts in fluid and electrolyte balances, and alterations in hypothalamic-pituitary function that result especially in amenorrhea and infertility. These adaptive changes may not account for all of the decrease in energy use. Diminished protein synthesis and turnover probably also contribute substantially. However, the known alterations in insulin, thyroid, and catecholamine metabolism provide a framework for understanding some of the signs and symptoms experienced by semistarved patients, including the reductions in pulse rate, respiratory rate, blood pressure, oxygen consumption, carbon dioxide production, cardiac output, gut motility, and other autonomic nervous system responses.

The alterations in thyroid hormone and catecholamine metabolism may also contribute to cold intolerance, dry skin, dry hair, hypercarotenemia, hypercholesterolemia, prolongation of ankle reflexes, constipation, and other symptoms of semistarvation. A more detailed discussion of fasting diuresis and refeeding edema, energy conservation, and endocrine adaptations in fasting and semistarvation, delineated in the classic studies by Benedict and Keys et al., is published elsewhere.[3]

The hypothalamic responses to energy deprivation are also adaptive, allowing the organism to survive better than would be the case if such adaptations failed to occur. The most obvious example is the alteration in control of secretion of pituitary gonadotropins, resulting in disruption of normal cyclic patterns and producing anovulation, amenorrhea, infertility, and reduced libido. Such adaptations decrease the likelihood of becoming pregnant and also preserve the iron and protein stores that normally would be lost during menstrual flow.

To the extent that semistarvation is a feature in bulimic syndromes, changes similar to those seen in anorexia nervosa occur. The diversity of eating patterns that is seen among patients with bulimic syndromes, however, makes it impossible to generalize regarding their physiologic changes. Like anorexia nervosa, the bulimic syndromes have multiple determinants. A depressive diathesis has been suggested because of favorable response to antidepressant medication in some patients. One study showed an impairment in cholecystokinin metabolism and reduced postprandial satiety.[4] Studies of normal-weight bulimic women indicate that they are in a state of semistarvation because they had once maintained a higher weight, and being in the statistically "normal" weight range was suboptimal for them. They tended to have had greater maximum weights than control subjects, and to have had weight fluctuations with periods of low weight. Resting metabolic rate was lower in this group of women than in controls, but much individual variation was noted.[5]

ETIOLOGY AND PATHOGENESIS

The prevailing view is that eating disorders have multiple interacting causes. The biopsychosocial conceptualization identifies roots in three spheres—biologic, psychologic, and social. This model suggests a unique interaction of variables for each individual. An as yet unexplained physiologic predisposition with possible genetic determinants leads to a variable degree of biologic vulnerability in persons at risk to develop eating disorders. Specific early experiences and family influences may create intrapsychic conflicts that determine the psychologic predisposition.[1] Despite the studies by Minuchin et al. delineating certain "psychosomatic" family patterns,[6] evidence has accumulated that a considerable variety of psychodynamic patterns exists in the families of patients with anorexia nervosa.[7,8]

Social influences and expectations that exert special pressures on modern women play an important role in the development of eating disorders.[9] The biologic factors that initiate anorexia nervosa may be mediated by pubertal endocrine changes. Psychologic conflicts lead to personality and behavioral changes that promote and support dieting. The social climate, such as the cultural obsession with thinness, tends to reinforce the psychologic motivation. Each of the three factors has greater or lesser importance for particular individuals who develop the disease. Thus, some appear to have a strong innate tendency to develop the disorder, despite a supportive family environment; others are reacting particularly to conflicted family experiences; and still others are reacting primarily to the pressures of society.[1]

Most commonly, the process of dieting begins at puberty, shortly after menarche. Sensitive about her developing figure and rapid weight gain associated with puberty, a girl who develops anorexia nervosa typically restricts her food intake by eliminating sweets, snacks, and high-calorie foods. This effort may at first seem like the innocent dieting so common among her peers. However, her efforts persist and become increasingly intense. Weight loss prompts further efforts at food restriction and the setting of lower and lower weight goals. Excessive exercise becomes ritualized. She becomes more and more compulsive, secretive, and idiosyncratic about her diet habits. Physical and mental signs of starvation begin to develop. The latter are often ignored or actively denied. She withdraws increasingly from social interaction, becomes quiet and seclusive, immerses herself in achievement-oriented activities, persists in dieting, and becomes increasingly active. Eventually, she becomes irritable and hostile toward her family. School performance may decline, despite excessive hours of studying, as she becomes distractible and preoccupied and, ultimately, depressed and apathetic.

Unsuppressible hunger may supervene as a reaction to chronic semistarvation. This urge may be suppressed for months or even years, or it may lead to rapid weight gain and obesity. Often, it results in bulimic behavior with episodes of binge eating. If the bulimic individual clings tenaciously to her pursuit of thinness, she will resort to vomiting or purging through laxative and diuretic abuse to maintain low body weight. This practice leads to chronic anorexia nervosa and bulimia nervosa.

Binge eating and purging also occur in normal-weight individuals who have never had anorexia nervosa. Some may be overweight or may desire a much slimmer figure. A pattern characterized by meal skipping often starts the process.

EPIDEMIOLOGY

Anorexia nervosa most commonly begins in the second decade of life. Fewer than 10% of patients have premenarchal onset. Among females, more than one half the cases begin before age 20 years and about three quarters before age 25 years (Fig. 58–1). The disorder occurs 8 to 12 times more frequently in females than in males. The prevalence in Rochester, Minnesota was 0.3% for females and 0.02% for males in 1985.[10] Among 15- to 19-year-old girls, the prevalence was 0.5%. Among the 15-year-old girls in Göteborg, Sweden, the prevalence was 0.84%.[11]

Estimates of the annual incidence in Western countries based on hospitalized patients and psychiatric case registers have shown an apparent increase from 0.5 per 100,000 population in 1950 to 5.0 per 100,000 in the 1980s.[12] In a population-based study from 1935 to 1984, a higher average incidence rate of 8.2 per 100,000 (14.6 for females and 1.8 for males) was found. No change occurred over time in the rates for females age 20 years and over, or for males. For females 15 through 24 years old, the most suspectible group, a linear increase was noted, with rates rising from 13.4 per 100,000 during 1935 to 1939 to 76.1 per 100,000 during 1980 to 1984.[10]

The severe form of the disorder is still relatively rare. Suggestions have arisen from results of the population-based study that the occurrence of this form of the disorder has not varied over time. Anorexia nervosa is thought to be more frequent in higher socioeconomic classes, but it is doubtful that data from population-based studies will bear this out. Confirmed cases are not reported from underdeveloped nations, but they would be difficult to identify among other forms of malnutrition. The disorder is rare in black individuals, perhaps related to biologic factors affecting vulnerability.

Studies of the epidemiology of bulimic syndromes have focused on the prevalence of the disorders. The reliability and validity of many of the studies is questionable because of great variation in the diagnostic criteria used and because many of the studies are based on questionnaires and self-reports. Nonetheless, evidence is accumulating that when strict criteria for bulimia nervosa are used, with interviews, the prevalence rate among adolescent and young adult women is 1 to 2%. It is virtually nonexistent among males. When broader criteria for bulimia are used and data are based on self-reports, the prevalence rates are higher, from 3 to 9%. With broader criteria for binge eating, more males are included.[13] Because bulimic syndromes were widely recognized only recently, incidence studies do not yet exist.

CLINICAL ASPECTS AND COMPLICATIONS

The signs and symptoms, as well as laboratory findings, in anorexia nervosa and in bulimic syndromes are understood most easily in the context of the stage of the illness and the diet pattern that has been followed. At the

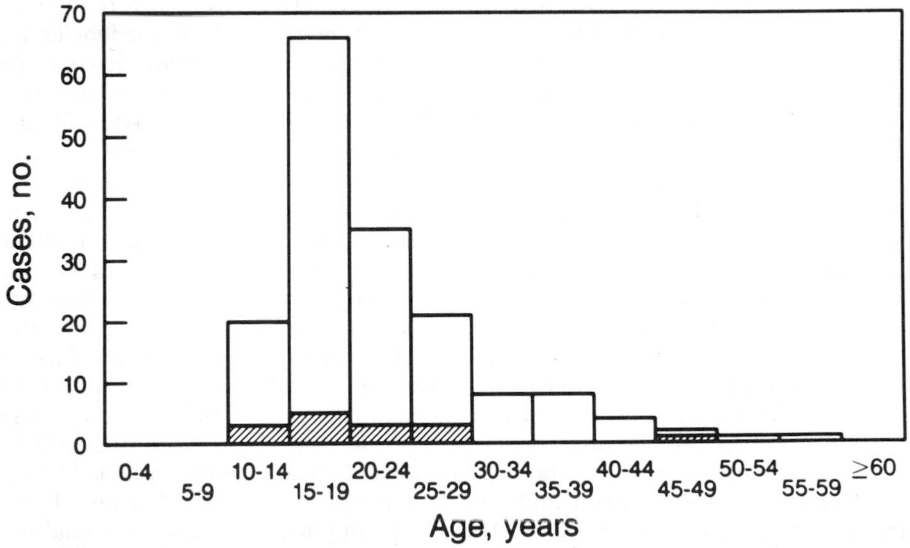

FIGURE 58–1. Distribution of age at diagnosis of anorexia nervosa in Rochester, Minnesota, from 1935 to 1984. Open bars, females (n = 166); hatched bars, males (n = 15). (Adapted from Lucas, A.R., Beard, C.M., O'Fallon, W.M., et al.: Am. J. Psychiatry, *148*:917–922, 1992.)

onset of the illness, and for a considerable time thereafter, the patient may have no observable signs other than depletion of adipose tissue, and no abnormalities on laboratory tests. The negative findings are simply confirmation that in a previously healthy individual, even starvation is compensated for by the homeostatic mechanisms of the body. The absence of abnormal findings tends to reinforce the patient's conviction that nothing is wrong. Bulimia (ravenous appetite) may lead to obesity. Occasional binge eating may be seen in normal-weight individuals without complications. Bulimia alternating with prolonged fasting, vomiting, or purging leads to serious complications. Bulimia also occurs in certain forms of morbid obesity, notably Prader-Willi syndrome.[14]

Many clinicians thought that patients with anorexia nervosa have similar diet patterns characterized by specific carbohydrate avoidance. A study of the diet patterns in 96 patients indicated much diversity.[15] All restricted their calorie intake, but 38% maintained satisfactory quality in the selection of their diets. Of the 62% whose diets were unsatisfactory in quality, most had irregular meal patterns, and many in this group indulged in binge eating, vomiting, or fasting. Recognition of the great variability in diet preferences among anorexic patients has implications for planning individualized treatment.

Physical signs in anorexia nervosa include dry, thin skin, a sallow complexion, and loss of body fat. Bradycardia, hypotension, hypothermia, and cold intolerance occur. Often, patients experience abdominal pain and a sensation of fullness. Constipation is common. Amenorrhea is a constant feature in females; males experience an analogous loss of sexual interest. Excessive loss of scalp hair may occur and eventually fine downy hair (lanugo) may appear on the body and face.

Personality features include model behavior, compliance, perfectionism, and high academic achievement. The patient usually presents a rigid, unspontaneous demeanor and is unusually serious and polite but inhibited and brief in responses. Excessive activity occurs but may be concealed. Sleep disturbance is common. Eventually, manifestations of depression appear.

Among normal-weight individuals with bulimia, binge eating generally occurs frequently, at least several times a week. Usually, the episodes tend to last less than 2 hours, although they may last for many hours at a time. High-calorie, easily ingested foods such as ice cream, bread products, and candy tend to be eaten during binges. Vomiting is often a part of the syndrome, and patients with the disorder may also abuse laxatives and diuretics. Personality features differ from those in patients with anorexia nervosa who restrict intake. Depressive symptoms are common and suicide attempts are frequent among bulimic patients. Many have impulse-control problems in other areas of their lives. Shoplifting (frequently of food) is reported, as well as other forms of stealing. The positive association among substance abuse, alcoholism, and bulimia is being recognized more frequently.

A person with bulimia may demonstrate no physical signs until damaging eating and vomiting behaviors have appeared. Nonpainful swelling of salivary glands is suggestive of extreme variability in quantity of food intake. Erosion of dental enamel occurs with frequent vomiting, and calluses of the knuckles proclaim self-induced vomiting.

Laboratory studies are of greatest help in documenting the degree of physiologic adaptation to undernourishment, documenting complications of anorexia nervosa and bulimia, and identifying other illnesses resembling eating disorders. No laboratory profile is diagnostic. When a patient has physical signs and laboratory findings not usually associated with anorexia nervosa, such as increased heart rate, erythrocyte sedimentation rate, or leukocyte count, the physician should be alert to a possible medical complication or the presence of another disorder.[16]

The laboratory profile varies considerably from normal to severely deranged and gives only a picture of these variables at the time of the test. In an illness that may last for many years, its stage is an important consideration in evaluating the laboratory findings. Abnormalities may not be observed until the illness is in an advanced stage. Serum electrolyte values usually are in the normal range, except in cases in which vomiting or laxative or diuretic abuse is a feature. The reported values may be high because of dehydration. The hematologic picture is variable because of changes in hydration. Anemia is a frequent finding in moderately severe cases, but it may be masked by hemoconcentration.

Dietary deficiencies lead to nutritional anemia in some patients. A peculiar morphologic change of erythrocytes resembling acanthocytosis is frequently present. The erythrocyte sedimentation rate usually is low. Leukopenia with relative lymphocytosis is common. Overt vitamin deficiencies are rare.[17] Serum protein values tend to remain normal until the patient achieves advanced stages of starvation. The serum cholesterol level is increased in about one third of patients, and the serum carotene value may be high.

Little documentation of the long-term complications exists in the literature, although various cardiovascular and renal complications can ensue. Demineralization of bone (osteoporosis) can be a long-range consequence.[18] Kidney stones can occur. During the acute or subacute phases, gastrointestinal complications, including decreased motility and atonic gut resembling paralytic ileus, may occur. Pancreatitis has been reported but, like sialadenosis, its mechanism is not known.[19,20]

Vomiting and laxative and diuretic abuse may be accompanied by serious electrolyte imbalances, notably hypokalemia, leading to cardiac arrhythmias, muscular weakness, renal impairment, and even death.

Although mortality rates of up to 21.5% have been reported, rates were less than 5% in over one half of outcome studies.[21] Death from inanition is rare. It most often occurs from electrolyte disturbance or by suicide in individuals with longstanding bulimia nervosa, but it also has been attributed to overwhelming infection and to cardiopulmonary complications. Death has also been attributed to overzealous refeeding, specifically, aspiration during tube feeding, and fluid and electrolyte imbalance during intravenous therapy.[22]

DIAGNOSIS AND DIFFERENTIAL DIAGNOSIS

ANOREXIA NERVOSA

The diagnosis of this condition is not difficult. It should be suspected when significant weight loss cannot be explained by physical illness. The physician then should inquire about whether weight loss was intentional. Psychologic characteristics, including the fear of becoming fat and misperception of body image, often are features of the illness. Three major features are required to make the diagnosis: (1) self-inflicted severe loss of weight by avoiding foods considered to be fattening, by self-induced vomiting or abuse of purgatives, or by excessive exercise; (2) a secondary endocrine disorder of the hypothalamus-anterior pituitary-gonad axis manifested in the female by amenorrhea and in the male by a dimunition of sexual interest and activity; and (3) a psychologic disorder that has as its central theme a morbid fear of being unable to control eating and becoming too fat, either specified or implied by the eating behavior. Loss of appetite is not a usual feature of anorexia nervosa; rather, it involves an aversion to eating and to gaining weight.

Other disorders associated with weight loss must be differentiated from anorexia nervosa. The chief physical diseases to be differentiated are gastrointestinal diseases involving malabsorption. Among psychiatric disorders, depression often manifests with true loss of appetite and weight loss. In schizophrenia, bizarre eating habits and delusions about food can lead to a clinical picture resembling anorexia nervosa.

BULIMIA NERVOSA

Diagnostic criteria for bulimia nervosa include the essential features of episodic binge eating, fear of not being able to stop eating voluntarily, self-induced vomiting, use of laxatives or diuretics, fasting, or vigorous exercise to prevent weight gain, and persistent overconcern with body shape and weight. Bulimia nervosa is a frequent sequel to anorexia nervosa. It also occurs in individuals who have always been normal in weight and occasionally in overweight individuals. It is associated with frequent weight fluctuations. Conditions to be differentiated include rumination syndrome in adolescence and involuntary vomiting.

TREATMENT

Although many cases of anorexia nervosa and bulimic syndromes can be managed by the family physician, internist, or pediatrician, they do take time and sincere interest on the part of the physician. Patients mildly affected often respond to concerned counseling about adolescent growth, normal nutrition, and the consequences of starvation, binging, and purging. It has become customary to refer most patients to psychiatrists familiar with the treatment of eating disorders. Severe disorders are best managed by someone particularly experienced in treating the disorder. These patients need to be followed for a long time with various combinations of support, psychologic counseling, and diet counseling. When these syndromes are so severe that precipitous weight loss, binging, or purging continue despite outpatient treatment efforts, intensive hospital treatment is required.

Regardless of whether the patient remains at home or is hospitalized, the general principles of treatment involve education about the physiologic and psychologic consequences of starvation, encouragement to begin eating a healthy diet and controlling fasting, binging, and purging behavior, and emotional support for the patient and the family.

DIETARY TREATMENT

Treatment of anorexia nervosa and bulimic syndromes involves the joint efforts of a physician and a dietitian; they meet separately with the patient periodically, usually once a week, after the comprehensive evaluation. With anorexia nervosa patients, the dietitian deals with the effects of starvation, energy, and nutrient needs (including growth needs), and the specifics of diet modification to encourage the resumption of normal eating patterns and the restoration of normal weight, both of which are central to recovery. Starvation, nutrient needs, and specifics of diet modification are addressed by the dietitian with bulimic syndrome patients also. These patients must also understand that their initial goal is weight stabilization until eating behaviors are well regulated with additional emphasis on control of binging and purging.

ANOREXIA NERVOSA

As in restoration of weight in other conditions involving starvation, a valid physiologic approach to treatment in anorexia nervosa is to encourage the cessation of weight loss initially, to improve the nutritional state while low weight is maintained for a time, and then to encourage the gradual increase of weight through normal self-feeding. The use of supplemental food products or parenteral feeding are not necessary. Contrary to the ideas espoused by some authors, clinicians do not need to encourage anorexic patients to consume above-average quantities of food. On the contrary, because of the low body weight and hypometabolic state, unusually small quantities are necessary at first (see Appendix Table A–8f). Estimated basal calorie requirements should be adjusted on the basis of the measured basal metabolic rate. The initial use of small quantities meets the psychologic needs of the patient, who is fearful of gaining weight rapidly and of becoming fat. Because some of the anorexic patients are realistically guarding against over-eating, encouraging them to eat large quantities and high-calorie snacks is countertherapeutic. As the patient becomes less fearful of weight gain, physiologically acceptable weight goals can be set based on the patient's height, body build, and weight history.

Treatment involves several phases: obtaining a detailed diet history, determining the calorie content of the initial diet, designing an appropriate diet plan, planning gradual progression in the diet, considering weight gain expectations, and, finally, designing a diet plan for weight maintenance. Specifics of this approach have been described in more detail elsewhere.[23]

BULIMIA NERVOSA

The initial goal of the dietary guidelines in bulimic syndromes is for the patient to gain control of eating binges by encouraging regularity in eating habits, to minimize the likelihood of the eating binges, and to avoid periods of fasting that may contribute to the binging, purging, and fasting cycle. Emphasis during the initial stages usually is on stabilizing weight while more acceptable eating patterns are being established.

For weight stabilization, the kilocalorie level of the initial diet can be identified by determining the patient's basal calorie needs for (see Appendix Table A–8f) present weight. A diet planned at this calorie level usually results in weight stabilization. If the patient is active, a kilocalorie allowance for activity should be added.

During the last phases of treatment, when the patient has regulated the dietary intake and is feeling more confident with the ability to control eating behaviors while keeping weight relatively stable, the need for a gradual weight loss program can be reassessed.

Treatment phases used in anorexia nervosa can be adapted for use in bulimia nervosa. Treatment should begin with a frank educational discussion about nutritional and health consequences of bulimic behaviors.

Additional information needed when using anorexia nervosa treatment phases for bulimia nervosa is the identification of factors that trigger binges for patients as well as how frequently binging and vomiting occur. What types of foods are eaten during a binge and what the patient identifies as a binge is useful information for treatment. The frequency and duration of fasting should also be determined.

Follow-up support and nutrition counseling needs to continue even after weight has been stabilized and eating behaviors are regulated.

OUTPATIENT TREATMENT

In addition to the dietary aspects of treatment aimed at normalizing eating patterns and weight, outpatient treatment deals with all aspects of the patient's functioning. Fears and misconceptions surrounding eating are addressed. Psychotherapy focuses on personal, family, and social conflicts that exist. With younger patients who are still living in their parental home, parents must be involved in the treatment either with supportive counseling or in family therapy. A variety of individual and family treatment techniques have been developed, but the superiority of any one technique has not been established. These techniques have been described in detail.[24,25] Qualities in the therapist as well as characteristics of the illness and the patient are important in determining response to treatment. The individual needs of the patient are the most important considerations in planning a treatment program.

HOSPITAL TREATMENT

The decision regarding hospitalization is based on the severity and rapidity of weight loss; the degree of malnutrition; the inability to control vomiting, laxative abuse, and other self-destructive behaviors; the presence of electrolyte disturbance or other hazardous complications; serious depression; suicidality; destructive family conflicts unresponsive to outpatient treatment; and the patient's lack of motivation for change. Hospital treatment requires a well-coordinated effort by the physician and hospital personnel on a unit that is geared to meeting the special needs of patients with eating disorders, not necessarily an "eating disorders unit." This may be a pediatric ward, an adolescent unit, a general medical ward, or a psychiatric unit for adolescents or adults. Essential considerations are that the staff should have experience in treating patients with eating disorders and that patients be grouped by age. School-age children and adolescents need the opportunity to continue their education in the hospital.[26]

MEDICATION

No evidence exists that neuroleptic or antidepressant medications either shorten the course of anorexia nervosa or improve the chance of recovery. Trials of medication have focused on their effect on short-term weight gain, but rapid weight gain bears no relationship to long-term outcome. On the other hand, antidepressant medications can reduce the frequency of binging and purging in bulimia nervosa over the short term, apparently independent of an antidepressant effect.[25]

OUTCOME

The course and outcome of anorexia nervosa are extremely variable. Meaningful conclusions as to outcome require follow-up of at least 4 years. In reviewing such studies, Hsu found that between 50 and 60% of patients were at normal weight and about one half were having normal menses. Between 11 and 20% of the patients were still underweight. Mortality rate was 0 to 5%.[25] Findings from the longest-term studies in which investigators have observed patients for several decades underscore the fact that even after 6 years, some patients recover and others have recurrences. After 6 years of illness, about 50% of the patients had recovered. As the observation time extended, more patients recovered, but also more died. Twelve years after the onset of the illness, 75% had recovered. The remainder developed chronic illness, some with bulimic forms. Death from complications of starvation or from suicide continued to occur. Recovery after more than 12 years of illness was uncommon. After 33 years, 6% had poor outcome and 18% had died.[27]

Outcome studies of bulimia nervosa are still rare and in few has follow-up been more than 1 year. Hsu was encouraged about the short-term outcome in these studies. Two thirds of patients no longer had symptoms of the disorder. Cautious optimism is justified until longer follow-up becomes available. Outcome will likely vary greatly, with many patients recovering fully and others developing severe chronicity and complications.[25]

REFERENCES

1. Lucas, A.R.: Mayo Clinic Proc., *56:*254–264, 1981.
2. Russell, G.: Psychol. Med., *9:*429–448, 1979.
3. Lucas, A.R., Callaway, C.W.: Anorexia nervosa and bulimia. *In* Bockus Gastroenterology. 4th Ed. Edited by J.E. Beck. Philadelphia, W.B. Saunders, 1984.
4. Geracioti, T.D., Liddle, R.A.: N. Engl. J. Med., *319:*683–688, 1988.
5. Devlin, M.J., Walsh, T., Kral, J.G., et al.: Arch. Gen. Psychiatry, *47:*144–148, 1990.
6. Minuchin, S., Rosman, B.L., Baker, L.: Psychosomatic Families: Anorexia Nervosa in Context. Cambridge, MA, Harvard University Press, 1978.
7. Garfinkel, P.E., Garner, D.M.: Anorexia Nervosa: A Multidimensional Perspective. New York, Brunner/Mazel, 1982.
8. Strober, M.: An empirically derived typology of anorexia nervosa. *In* Anorexia Nervosa: Recent Developments in Research. Edited by P. Darby, D.M. Garner, P.F. Garfinkel. New York, Alan R. Liss, 1983.
9. Bruch, H.: Eating Disorders: Obesity and Anorexia Nervosa. New York, Basic Books, 1973.
10. Lucas, A.R., Beard, C.M., O'Fallon, W.M., et al.: Am. J. Psychiatry, *148;*917–922, 1992.
11. Råstam, M., Gillberg, C., Garton, M.: Br. J. Psychiatry, *155:*642–646, 1989.
12. Lucas, A.R., Beard, C.M., O'Fallon, W.M., et al.: Mayo Clin. Proc., *63:*433–442, 1988.
13. Fairburn, C.G., Beglin, S.J.: Am. J. Psychiatry, *147:*401–408, 1990.
14. Holm, V.A., Sulzbacher, S., Pipes, P.L.: Prader-Willi Syndrome. Baltimore, University Park Press, 1981.
15. Huse, D.M., Lucas, A.R.: Am. J. Clin. Nutr., *40:*251–254, 1984.
16. Lucas, A.R.: Mayo Clinic Proc., *52:*748–750, 1977.
17. Casper, R.C., Kirschner, B., Sandstead, H.H., et al.: Am. J. Clin. Nutr., *33:*1801–1808, 1980.
18. Rigotti, N.A., Nussbaum, S.R., Herzog, D.B., et al.: N. Engl. J. Med., *311:*1601–1606, 1984.
19. Nordgren, L., von Schéele, C.: Biol. Psychiatry, *12:*681–686, 1977.
20. Schoettle, U.C.: J. Am. Acad. Child Adolesc. Psychiatry, *18:*384–390, 1979.
21. Hsu, L.K.: Arch. Gen. Psychiatry, *37:*1041–1046, 1980.
22. Drossman, D.A., Ontjes, D.A., Heizer, W.D.: Gastroenterology, *77:*1115–1131, 1979.
23. Huse, D.M., Lucas, A.R.: J. Am. Diet. Assoc., *83:*687–690, 1983.
24. Bruch, H.: The Golden Cage. Cambridge, MA, Harvard University Press, 1978.
25. Hsu, L.K.G.: Eating Disorders. New York, Guilford Press, 1990.
26. Lucas, A.R., Duncan, J.W., Piens, V.: Am. J. Psychiatry, *133:*1034–1038, 1976.
27. Theander, S.: J. Psychiatr. Res., *19:*493–508, 1985.

SELECTED READINGS

Bruch, H: Eating Disorders: Obesity and Anorexia Nervosa. New York, Basic Books, 1973.

Cahill, G.F., Jr., Aoki, T.T., Rossini, A.: Metabolism in obesity and anorexia nervosa. *In* Disorders of Eating and Nutrients in Treatment of Brain Diseases. Vol. 3. Edited by R.J. Wurtman, J.J. Wurtman. New York, Raven Press, 1979.

Garfinkel, P.E., Garner, D.M.: Anorexia Nervosa. New York, Brunner/Mazel, 1982.

Hsu, L.K.G.: Eating Disorders. New York, Guilford Press, 1990.

Keys, A., Brožek, J., Henschel, A., et al.: The Biology of Human Starvation. Vols. 1 and 2. Minneapolis, University of Minnesota Press, 1950.

Stunkard, A.J., Stellar, E.: Eating and Its Disorders. (Association for Research in Nervous and Mental Disease.) Vol. 62. New York, Raven Press, 1984.

CHAPTER 59

Obesity

F. Xavier Pi-Sunyer

DEFINITION AND CLASSIFICATION

Obesity, characterized by an excess accumulation of fat, is a detriment to good health and well-being. It is easy for individuals to take on excess fat as soon as enough food and leisure are available in a society, causing an imbalance between energy intake and energy expenditure. Although there continues to be disagreement as to which side of this energy equation is more important in the epidemic of obesity, both sides certainly play a role.

CRITERIA FOR WEIGHT NORMALITY

A population cannot be precisely divided into normal and obese, because with a gradually increasing fat accumulation, there is not a biphasic distribution with a "normal" and an "abnormal" group, nor is there a normal bell-shape curve of weights in Western industrialized societies. Rather, the curve is skewed to the right, with a trailing out of excess weights.

Even in a genetically homogenous population, weight is variable. In the modern world, with the great intermixing of ethnic and racial groups, wide genetic heterogeneity exists. The heterogeneity is manifested by differing heights, body circumferences (chest, waist, hips), and heaviness of frame. It is undesirable to focus on a single number of kilograms for height in centimeters as the "normal" weight. This is particularly evident because it is not clear what the criterion for "normal" weight should be. Should it be low mortality, low morbidity, a combination of the two, or should it be the longest extended "optimal health" or "well-being" of the individual?

For lack of a better data base, life insurance industry statistics have been used widely to develop tables of normality. These tables give weight ranges for height and frame size and are associated with the greatest longevity in individuals who were healthy at the time of initial examination when their height and weight were measured (see Appendix Table A–11 for further discussion).

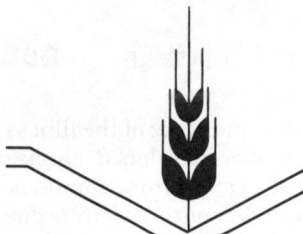

Although these are the best data available, they are inadequate in several ways. They predominantly reflect data from upper middle class white groups. They are sex- and height-specific but not age-specific. As such, they provide data on the basis of the predictive longevity of young persons weighed in their early twenties and followed to their death. The tables have been used on the assumption that whatever weight is desirable at age 21 years is also desirable at age 45 or 65. Yet, in Western society, weight changes with age in a normal population, with a gradual increase in women from 20 to 60 and a more gradual increase for men from 20 to 50, with a fall after that.[1] In addition, body composition changes with age, with the gradual accretion of fat and loss of lean body mass. Therefore, it is unclear whether the "normal" weight should be the same as age advances or whether it should rise as the percentage of body adipose tissue increases.

In an effort to clarify the confusion about how to classify overweight, Garrow proposed a classification that is useful clinically.[2] It is based on two simple measurements: height without shoes and weight with minimal clothing. The weight/height^2 (W/H^2), called the body mass index (BMI), is then calculated, with weight expressed in kilograms and height in meters. The population, whether male or female, can be divided for degree of obesity as follows:

Grade III: W/H^2 >40
II: W/H^2 30 to 40
I: W/H^2 25 to 29.9
O: W/H^2 20 to 24.9

The major weakness of the use of W/H^2 (originally proposed by Quetelet in 1871) is that some muscular individuals may be classified as obese when they are not.[3] These numbers will be small, however. BMI is the relative weight index that shows the highest correlation with independent measures of body fat.[4] The BMI range of 20 to 24.9, classified as normal, coincides well with the normal mortality ratio derived from life insurance tables. The mortality ratio begins to increase at BMI levels above 25, and it is here that health professionals should be concerned.

Although the increase in mortality in grade I obesity (W/H^2 = 25 to 29.9) is not great, it is of importance because it is transitional to grades II and III, which truly create health risks for the individual.

Figure 59–1 presents a diagram of this classification by height and weight.[2] A nomograph for estimating BMI is given in Appendix Table A–11i.

OTHER RELATIVE WEIGHT MEASURES

Another relative weight index, W/H, has been suggested, but it correlates less well with body fat.[4,5] In addition, neither the ponderal index, the cube root of the weight divided by height ($W^{0.33}/H$), nor the Rohrer index (W/H^3) has been helpful because neither is independent enough of height to accurately reflect overweight.

SKINFOLDS

Over half the fat in the body is deposited under the skin, and the percentage increases with increasing weight. The thickness of this subcutaneous fat can be measured at various sites with the use of standardized skin calipers. The distribution and amount of subcutaneous fat change with age and are also quite different by sex. One difficulty with skinfold measurement is that there is no agreement on the number and sites that best reflect actual body fat content. Another is that it is easy to make large errors if the observer is inexperienced or careless.

Data on skinfolds for children are less reliable than for adults. They have been obtained on cross-sectional population studies. Arbitrary definitions of obesity (such as 85th percentile and above of weight) have been set. Sex differences in percentage total body fat occur early in life, so that by 5 years of age different standards are necessary for males and females. In adults, sex differences are marked. Subcutaneous fat is about 11% of body weight in men and 18% in women.[6] Tables are available for triceps and subscapular percentile distributions for boys and girls (see Appendix Table A–14a) and for adult men and women (see Appendix Table A–14b)[7] with provisional data for the elderly (see Appendix Table A–14d).

Because the amount of fat distributed from place to place in the body varies, some investigators have suggested that using the sum of skinfolds from different areas will better reflect total body fat. Durnin and Womersley derived tables, for instance, using the sum of four skinfolds (biceps, triceps, subscapular, and suprailiac) and related them to the fat content of the body[8] (see Appendix Table A–15 and Chap. 49).

OTHER BODY FAT MEASUREMENTS

Other measurements that can be used for measuring body fat and other body compartments are more difficult, expensive, and time-consuming and have generally been used for research purposes. These include indirect measurements of body fat done by measuring the fat-free compartment and subtracting this amount from total body weight to derive the weight of fat.

For instance, total body water can be measured by dilution of tritiated (^3H_2O) or deuterated (D_2O) water. Both deuterium and tritium oxides rapidly equilibrate in body water, so the test can be done in 2 to 3 hours. Deuterium is nonradioactive and therefore is preferentially used in children and women of childbearing age. Water is then assumed to be a fixed proportion of fat-free mass (FFM), that is, FFM = water mass/0.73. The calculated FFM is subtracted from total body weight to obtain total body fat.[9] Alternatively, the naturally occurring ^{40}K in the body can be counted in a whole body counter. Total body ^{40}K can be measured as an index of lean body mass because potassium is present only in the fat-free compartments of the body. ^{40}K makes up 0.012% of the total potassium and since it is radioactive it can be detected by a sensitive counter. Using an estimated value

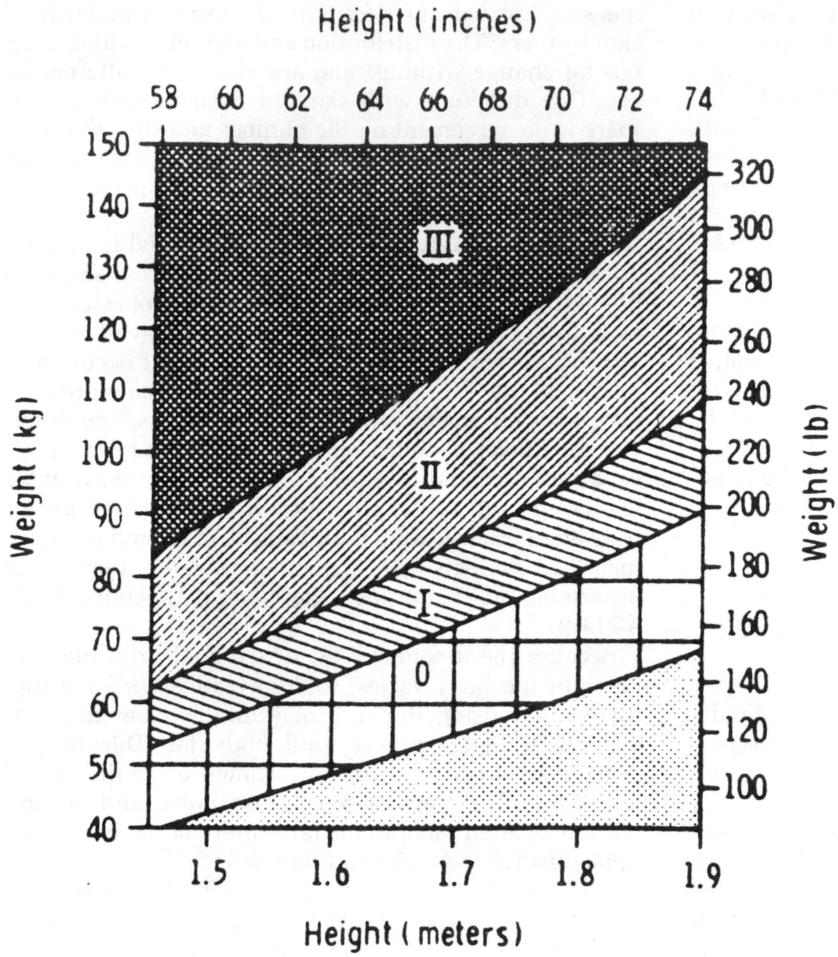

FIGURE 59—1. Relation of weight to height defining the desirable range (O), and grades I, II, and III obesity, marked by the boundaries W/H^2 = 25 to 29.9, 30 to 40, and over 40 respectively. (From Garrow, J.S., Treat Obesity Seriously. Edinburgh, Churchill Livingstone, 1981, p. 3, with permission of Churchill Livingstone.)

for the meq of K in lean body, one can calculate the lean body mass and once again derive total body fat [10] (see also Chap. 49).

BODY DENSITY

The density of the whole body is derived from the density of the various body components (bone, water, fat, protein), which are all slightly different. It is easier to think of the body as divided into a fat and a fat-free mass, with fat having a density of 0.900 g/ml and the fat-free mass a density of 1.100 g/ml. Therefore, as the proportion of fat in the body increases, the density will decrease. The amount of fat in the body can be determined by measuring the density of the entire body. This requires total submersion of an individual and accurate correction for lung and abdominal air.[11]

FAT-SOLUBLE GASES

The most tedious method for estimating fat is to use an inert gas, such as krypton or xenon, which is soluble in fat but poorly soluble in water. The gas must be breathed for several hours so equilibration with tissues can occur. The proportion of gas retained reflects the amount of fat in the body.[12]

PREVALENCE

STANDARDS OF NORMALITY

Efforts to produce standards of obesity for the population against which individuals can be compared have generally concentrated on weight and have taken two forms. The first is the use of "desirable" weight, which is weight (stratified for sex and height and frame size) that is correlated to the greatest longevity. These weights come from life insurance data. The 1983 Tables of the Metropolitan Life Insurance Company[13] are presented in Appendix Table A–11c. The second is the use of average weights of subsamples of a general population stratified by sex, age, and height. The data for these populations are often given in percentiles. Examples are the Health and Nutrition Examination Survey (HANES) tables produced by the National Center for Health Statistics in 1960 to 1962,[1] 1971 to 1974, and 1976 to 1980.[14] The data are presented in Table A–13a to d, in six age groupings from 18 to 74 years and by sex for the years 1976 to 1980.[15] In these tables, it becomes necessary to define at what percentile level values will be considered abnormal. The National Center for Health Statistics defines overweight as a BMI greater than or equal to the 85th percentile and severe overweight as greater than or equal to the 95th percentile.[16] Age-adjusted percentages of overweight persons by ethnicity and sex in the United States are shown in Table 59–1.

Two points are evident from the Metropolitan Life tables and the HANES tables. The first is that, as a rule, the desirable weights of the insurance tables are lower than the average weights descriptive of the United States population, although this is less true using the 1983 Metropolitan Life Tables, which were set considerably higher than the 1959 tables. The second is that the HANES data show an increase of weight by age from 18 years to 54 years, with a plateau and then a fall after that. This shows that, in the United States population, weight is not static with age once maturity is reached, but is actually a function of age.

The insurance companies used the terms "ideal weight" or "desirable weight" to describe weights that actuarially were associated with the least mortality. In subsequent usage of these tables, the definition of overweight has been accepted as 10% above an ideal or desirable weight and of obesity as 20% or more above this point. Using such criteria, researchers found a high incidence of overweight in the HANES Survey of 1960 to 1962.[1] Data of the HANES Survey of 1971 to 1974 show that United States adults measured at that time were comparably obese.[14] The latest survey available (1976 to 1980) determined a continuing obesity trend.[15] These latest data are shown in Table 59–2.

The tables make clear that an alarming percentage of Americans are overweight. This percentage increases with age, particularly among women. What constitutes "healthy weight" at various ages is controversial. It has been suggested that, as a person ages, some increase in weight is acceptable and not harmful.[17] The NIH geriatrics tables allow for such an increase,[18] and they are printed in Appendix A–11h. The 1989 weight guidelines of the National Academy of Sciences,[19] which reflect this point of view, are also shown in Appendix A–11j, expressed as BMI units. Such more liberal tables have been vigorously attacked, however.[20]

OBESITY IN CHILDREN

The prevalence of obesity in the Western world begins with infancy. Studies available, though imperfect, suggest that one third or more of infants in the Western industrialized world are too heavy.[21–23] Data for schoolchildren are less available and estimates have varied between 6 and 15%.[21,24,25] Adolescent obesity rates have been calculated at the 20 to 30% rate.[23,25–27] The studies suggest that young women are more likely to be obese than are young men. The prevalence of obesity seems to be relatively constant throughout childhood.

Whether obesity in childhood leads to obesity in the adult has been widely debated. Some retrospective studies have suggested that there is a direct progression from a fat child to a fat adult.[28] Rimm and Rimm report that 50% of adult women in every age group with

TABLE 59–1. AGE-ADJUSTED PERCENTAGES OF OVERWEIGHT AND SEVERELY OVERWEIGHT PERSONS AGED 20 TO 74 YEARS FROM THE NATIONAL HEALTH AND NUTRITION EXAMINATION SURVEY (NHANES) II AND THE NHANES BY ETHNICITY AND SEX

	MALE		FEMALE	
	Overweight (%)	Severe overweight (%)	Overweight (%)	Severe overweight (%)
White	24.4	7.8	24.6	9.6
Black	26.3	10.4	45.1	19.7
Mexican	31.2	10.8	41.5	16.7
Cuban	28.5	10.3	31.9	6.9
Puerto Rican	25.7	7.9	39.8	15.2

(From Kuczmarski, R.J.: Am. J. Clin. Nutr., *55*:495S–502S, 1992, with permission of the American Society for Clinical Nutrition.)

TABLE 59–2. AGE-ADJUSTED PERCENTAGES OF OVERWEIGHT PERSONS AGED 20 TO 74 YEARS BY RACE AND SEX IN THE UNITED STATES

	WHITE			BLACK		
	1960–1962	1971–1974	1976–1980	1960–1962	1971–1974	1976–1980
Both sexes	24.1	24.8	25.1	32.6	35.7	37.7
Male	23.5	24.3	24.9	21.7	25.0	27.7
Female	24.4	25.0	25.2	42.9	44.5	46.1

(From Kuczmarski, R.J.: Am. J. Clin. Nutr., *55*:495S–502S, 1992, with permission of the American Society for Clinical Nutrition.)

weights greater than 18% of ideal body weight had been obese adolescents.[29] In addition, it has been stated that 30% of adults who are obese become obese during childhood. About 80% of obese adolescents become obese adults,[30] and they have been reported to be fatter than those who become obese as adults.[29] Of obese infants and children, 26.5% were still obese two decades later, compared with the 15% expected by chance.[31] The more severe the disease in childhood, the greater the likelihood of persistence to adulthood.[32]

SOCIOECONOMIC INFLUENCE

Epidemiologic studies have shown a strong association between socioeconomic status and the prevalence of obesity. This relationship is much stronger in women.

The effect of social environment on obesity was investigated in the "Midtown Manhattan Study," which studied a population with both high- and low-income groups. Socioeconomic status and the prevalence of obesity were found to be inversely related.[33] As many as 30% of women of lower socioeconomic class were obese, 16% of middle-status women, and 5% of upper status. Men showed similar but less exaggerated trends. Similar socioeconomic trends have been found in other countries.[34,35] Obesity was also related in the Manhattan study to ethnicity[36] with Eastern Europeans being particularly heavy. Others have also found ethnicity to be an important variable.[37] In addition, religious affiliation was important, with the prevalence being higher among Jews, followed by Catholics, and lowest among Protestants.[38]

Although a relationship exists in the United States between increasing prevalence of obesity and socioeconomic status, it is not all clear-cut. For example, an English study showed that the prevalence of overweight was low in males of lower socioeconomic status engaged in heavy manual labor.[39]

Race also affects obesity. In the United States, for instance, black women have a higher prevalence of obesity than white women and black men have a higher prevalence than white men.[40] The reasons for this finding are not at present evident.

MORTALITY AND MORBIDITY

Overweight has been associated with excess mortality in many studies.[41–44] Table 59–3 summarizes mortality data for three such studies, the Build and Blood Pressure Study of 1959,[43] the American Cancer Society Study,[45] and the Build and the Blood Pressure Study of 1979.[44] All three studies show increasing mortality with increasing overweight, with higher mortality risks in men than in women.

The American Cancer Society Study, which was not an insurance study, counteracts the objections that insured lives are not typical of the general population because insured individuals tend to be richer and predominantly white, and that it is not valid to use weight at insurance to relate to death some 35 years afterward. Because the results of the American Cancer Society data are similar to the insured data, they validate the use of the actuarial data of insured lives.

Because insurance companies relate only to healthy persons, their data generally exclude ill people. The American Cancer Society study in all likelihood overstated the mortality of underweight persons because it only lasted 12 years, and the general population it studied no doubt included some persons with illnesses and weight loss that could have caused early death.

The mortality rate increase is not linear with increasing weight. An accelerated mortality occurs as people get heavier, particularly for males.[46] In addition, in the insurance data, the relative mortality is higher in males who are overweight than in females, whereas this is not so in the general population, as reflected by the American Cancer Society Study. Many studies do not show increased risk of mortality at relative weights up to 20% above desirable level.[46–50] In the extensive Norwegian study, where weights and heights were taken in a large proportion of the population between 1963 and 1975, relative mortality showed an increase as the BMI increased above 27.[51]

Evidence now exists that the relationship between weight and mortality is different at different times of life. The Whitehall study of 18,000 English civil servants showed that the relationship between weight quintile and mortality changes with age, so for the youngest men, coronary heart disease mortality shows a linear increase

TABLE 59–3. MORTALITY RATIOS ACCORDING TO VARIATIONS IN WEIGHT*

	BUILD AND BLOOD PRESSURE STUDY 1959		AMERICAN CANCER SOCIETY STUDY		BUILD AND BLOOD PRESSURE 1979	
Weight Group	Male	Female	Male	Female	Male	Female
20% Underweight	95	87	110	110	105	110
10% Underweight	90	89	100	95	94	97
10% Overweight	113	109	107	108	111	107
20% Overweight	125	121	121	123	120	110
30% Overweight	142	130	137	138	135	125
40% Overweight	167		162	163	153	136
50% Overweight	200		210		177	149
60% Overweight	250				210	167

*Each study measured departures from its own set of average weights, where mortality would be 100.
(From Van Itallie. T.B.: Am. J. Clin. Nutr., *32*:2723–2733, 1979, with permission of the American Society for Clinical Nutrition.)

TABLE 59–4. MORTALITY RATIOS (FACTOR OF INCREASED RISK)*

	MEN 20% ABOVE AVERAGE WEIGHT		MEN 40% ABOVE AVERAGE WEIGHT	
Cause of Death	Build Study 1979	American Cancer Society	Build Study 1979	American Cancer Society
Coronary heart disease	118	128	169	175
Cerebral "hemorrhage" (stroke)	110	116	164	191
Cancer	100	105	105	124
Diabetes	250	210	500	300
Digestive diseases	125	168	220	340
All causes	120	121	150	162

*Each study measured departures from its own set of average weights, where mortality would be 100.
(From Van Itallie, T.B.: Am. J. Clin. Nutr., *32*:2723–2733, 1979, with permission of the American Society for Clinical Nutrition.)

from lowest weight quintile to highcst, whereas for the oldest men, no relationship is evident.[52]

Three other studies have investigated this relation of weight to mortality in the elderly. All seem to agree on a protective effect of increased weight in old age.[53–55]

The finding of a relationship between obesity and increased mortality at a young age and no such relationship at an older age implies that it is continuous obesity over many years that affects health and can lead to death. Moreover, as people grow older, other risk factors for death take on increased importance.

The data on the relationship of obesity and mortality may be obscured by the fact that fatness may relate to the type of death as well as to overall mortality. That is, with increasing obesity, individuals are at a greater risk of death from cardiovascular disease and diabetes, but not from cancer.[56] Thus, it may not be possible to assign a single optimum weight or an optimum level of fatness. There may be "different optima for different causes of death at different time periods and . . . no single value of weight or fatness is optimal for all."[57]a

CAUSES OF DEATH AND MORBIDITY

The causes of death in men 20 and 40% above average weight as derived from the data of the American Cancer Society Study[58] and the Build Study of 1979[59] are shown in Table 59–4.

Cardiovascular Disease. Prospective studies of cardiovascular morbidity and mortality have shown an association with obesity. In studies where smoking has been controlled for, lowest mortality is in the leanest weight category.[60,61] The effect of obesity on cardiovascular disease has not always been independent, but has generally been through exacerbation of other risk factors such as hypertension, diabetes, and hyperlipidemia.[62] This finding is not surprising, because blood pressure, blood lipids, and glucose values increase when individuals gain substantial weight.[63] This predictable increase in cardiovascular risk factors by increasing weight has been well quantified in the Framingham study. For every 10% rise in relative weight, systolic blood pressure rises

6.5 mm, plasma cholesterol 12 mg/dl, and fasting blood glucose 2 mg/dl.[64] Although the association of these cardiovascular risk factors is not as strong in women as in men, the association of obesity to cardiovascular disease is as strong in women as in men.[65]

Evidence indicates that obesity, when it occurs at an earlier age (20 to 40 years), has a greater influence on cardiovascular disease than later-onset obesity.[66] The Manitoba Study, which compared the 26-year incidence of coronary heart disease (CHD) and had a young average entry age of 30.8 years, found that body mass index was significantly related to CHD.[67] Myocardial infarction, sudden death, and coronary insufficiency were all associated with a high BMI. This association was not evident until the tenth year of follow-up. This was also true of the Framingham study, where the effect of risk of obesity on cardiovascular mortality increased with time of follow-up.[68] Thus, short-term studies, or studies concentrating on older individuals, may not show an independent effect of obesity because they are too short or have not focused on the correct age group.

Similarly, studies by Chapman et al. using ponderal index as a measure of obesity found a higher rate of myocardial infarction in men under age 40 and not in those older.[69] In the Whitehall study, the 10-year coronary heart disease mortality showed an increase from the lowest- to the highest-weight quintiles for the younger men, but no effect of weight in the older men.[52] In addition, the effect of weight is small when blood pressure, cholesterol, and smoking are accounted for. For the older men, the highest mortality is in the lowest-weight quintile.

Numerous studies now show that the pattern of fat distribution affects morbidity and mortality from cardiovascular disease.[70] In fact, this risk factor is an important as smoking, hypertension, and hypercholesterolemia.[71] The effect is more important at younger ages and tends to lose importance after the seventh decade.[71]

Blood Lipids. Although hypertriglyceridemia has been associated with obesity,[72] the association is not strong. Triglycerides are transported predominantly as very low density lipoproteins (VLDL).[73] Hypertriglyceridemia may be related to the insulin resistance and consequent hyperinsulinemia of obesity,[74] which increases plasma triglyceride secretion.[73,75] In addition, because FFA levels are raised in obesity, the increased hepatic uptake of FFA may increase the secretory rate of triglyceride.[76] Enhanced triglyceride production may also come from more glucose precursors extracted by the liver.[76] Despite this increased triglyceride production, the level of triglycerides in obese persons is often normal or only slightly elevated. Because lipoprotein lipase activity is elevated in obesity,[77] and rises higher after weight loss,[78,79] it is possible that this activity enhances VLDL clearance at the periphery. After weight reduction, plasma triglycerides that were high tend to fall.[73] This change is associated with a decreased VLDL-triglyceride production and a decreased insulinemia.[73] In families carrying the combined hyperlipidemia trait, obese relatives tend to manifest high levels of VLDL, whereas the nonobese individuals show elevated low density lipoproteins (LDL).[80]

Much less evidence exists of cholesterol elevation in obesity. Only marginally significant correlations have been shown.[81,82] High-density lipoprotein (HDL) cholesterol is usually low in obesity, and because of this, the ratio of LDL to HDL is elevated. The elevation of this ratio enhances the risk of CHD. Low HDL cholesterol concentrations are a risk factor for CHD, independent of the concentration of LDL cholesterol.[83,84]

Diabetes Mellitus. A strong association exists between obesity and diabetes mellitus. In fact, obesity can be considered the most important "environmental" determinant in the manifestation of diabetes. In epidemiologic studies including many geographic areas, races, and cultures, West et al. noted a marked correlation between prevalence of diabetes and overweight.[85] This also has been shown in other, more recent studies.[86] Even moderate obesity can raise the risk of diabetes tenfold.[86] In the Framingham study, women in the upper quintile of weight were four times as likely to develop glucose intolerance as women in the lower quintile.[87]

Body fat distribution has been implicated as a predictor of glucose intolerance and hyperinsulinemia.[88–91] It is also a predictor of frank diabetes.[92,93] The size of fat cells in the abdominal area is related to metabolic disturbance; this is not so in the thigh area.[90,91] This increased risk with abdominal fat suggests that a "male" pattern of fat distribution poses a greater risk for diabetes than a "female" pattern. The important factor is intra-abdominal or visceral obesity.[70]

Obesity is associated with hyperinsulinemia,[94] and, in general, the fatter an individual, the higher will be the basal or fasting insulin.[74] In addition, in nondiabetics, the height of the insulin response to glucose or other stimuli is related to basal insulin and therefore is closely correlated with the degree of obesity.[74] In obese subjects with an abnormal glucose tolerance, however, the percentage increase of insulin over basal values is actually decreased in comparison to lean subjects. Thus, the impairment of glucose disposal can often be explained by an accompanying impairment of insulin secretion. This impairment is first observed in the early phase of insulin response, but as carbohydrate tolerance deteriorates, the entire time course of the insulin response is affected.

Insulin Resistance. The phenomenon of excessive blood insulin levels in obesity, both basal and after stimuli, demonstrates that an insulin resistance or insensitivity is present. This is manifested by a tissue resistance at the muscle and liver level, decreasing glucose uptake at the periphery and increasing hepatic glucose output.[95,96] Adipose tissue sensitivity remains high, and it is possible that nutrients are therefore shunted to this tissue for storage.[96]

Insulin Receptor and Postreceptor Defects. The first step in the action of insulin on the cell is the binding of the hormone to a specific receptor on the outer plasma membrane. This process then initiates a series of "postreceptor" biochemical events, such as glucose and amino acid transport, stimulation of protein synthesis, activation of certain enzymes, inhibition of others, stimulation of certain gene transcription, and inhibition of others.[97] Generally, where high levels of insulin prevail in the blood, low levels of insulin receptors are present. This self-regulation of the membrane insulin receptor, so high insulin levels cause a lowering of insulin receptor number, is called down-regulation.[98] It now seems clear that cells from obese humans have a decreased number of insulin receptors.[99,100]

Although part of the insulin resistance in obesity can be attributed to changes in insulin receptor number and/or receptor affinity for insulin, the tissues of obese animal models show intracellular postreceptor defects in glucose metabolism that account for the major part of insulin resistance.

In obese humans, the degree of insulin resistance is much greater than can be predicted from the magnitude of the decrease of insulin receptors. Using the euglycemic glucose clamp technique, researchers can study in vivo insulin dose-response curves. The least hyperinsulinemic, least insulin-resistant patients show only a receptor defect, whereas the most hyperinsulinemic show the largest postreceptor defect.[101] The nature of the postreceptor defect is being actively investigated. The β subunit of the receptor, which faces inward, when stimulated by insulin, expresses kinase activity towards its tyrosine residues.[102,103] This tyrosine phosphorylation may be faulty, causing defective signaling within the cell. The postreceptor defect could also be due to an abnormality in the glucose transporter system within the affected cells. Because levels of glucose transporter protein and mRNA are normal in skeletal muscle cells of insulin resistant persons, the defect may rest in the functional activity or insulin-mediated translocation of the transporters.[104]

Significance of Hyperinsulinemia. The production of excessive quantities of insulin for a prolonged period may lead to pancreatic exhaustion in those who are genetically predisposed.[105] Eventually, insulin response can decrease, resulting in metabolic decompensation.[106] Support for this position comes from data suggesting that the duration of obesity rather than the degree can be best correlated with carbohydrate intolerance in obese adults.

Hypertension. Blood pressure elevation is a common concomitant of obesity.[107–109] The causes of the association of obesity and hypertension are not clear. A relationship between weight gain and increase in blood pressure is well documented.[110–111] In hypertensive patients, weight reduction reduces blood pressure,[112–114] and weight regain raises pressure. The fall in blood pressure with weight reduction is associated with a decrease in blood volume, cardiac output, and sympathetic activity.[115]

The cardiac output and the peripheral vascular resistance are the most important determinants of the blood pressure. These, in turn, are affected by the total body sodium content and by neurohumoral factors. Data by Dahl et al. incriminated sodium loss rather than weight loss as the cause of the lowered blood pressure with caloric restriction.[116] Others, however, have reported that it is weight reduction that is important.

Insulin may play a role in the hypertension of obesity,[117] because changes in the plasma insulin concentration can affect sodium transport in the human kidney.[118] Insulin reduces sodium excretion independent of changes in plasma glucose. This effect can be noted without concurrent changes in filtered load of glucose, glomerular filtration rate, renal blood flow, and plasma aldosterone levels.[119] Natriuresis occurs during fasting or hypocaloric diets, when insulin levels fall, and antinatriuresis occurs with refeeding, when insulin rises again.[120] The hyperinsulinemia of obesity may raise the blood pressure by increasing renal sodium absorption, which in turn expands the extracellular fluid volume, raising cardiac output, peripheral resistance, and blood pressure.[117]

Whether catecholamines play a role in the hypertension of obesity is unclear, although Landsberg and Young reported a decreased sympathetic nervous system activity during weight loss diets and an increase during refeeding.[121]

The distribution of fat in the body may have an important effect on blood pressure risk, as it does in diabetes, with central fat or upper body fat being more likely to raise blood pressure than the lower body fat of the gluteal and thigh region.[122,123] The reasons for this tendency are not clear.

Respiratory Problems. As an individual becomes more obese, the muscular work required for ventilation increases. If the limitation of movement of the chest wall is great enough, CO_2 retention occurs. This condition can lead to lethargy and somnolence. The CO_2 narcosis can also lead to periods of apnea that usually occur during sleep and exacerbate the problem of CO_2 retention. In addition, polycythemia may occur, which can enhance thrombosis. In severe cases of respiratory disease, pulmonary hypertension, cardiac enlargement, and congestive heart failure may develop.

Gallbladder Disease. The risk for gallbladder disease is higher as obesity increases and is greater for women than for men.[124–127] An increased body fat reservoir is associated with certain conditions that predispose individuals to gallstone formation. There is a supersaturation of the cholesterol in bile[128,129] and increased cholesterol excretion.[130] Hypomotility of the gallbladder also occurs, allowing for pooling and nucleation of stones.[131] As a result, cholesterol stone formation is enhanced.[132]

Arthritis. The clinical impression is that the incidence of osteoarthritis of the weight-bearing joints is higher in obese than in lean persons and that this condition tends to become worse with higher weight.[133] No good prevalence studies are available, however.

Gout. The cause for the rise in uric acid levels with increasing weight is unclear. Usually, this uric acid elevation is asymptomatic, but the occurrence of gouty attacks is higher in obese than in lean individuals, particularly when overweight reaches 30% above ideal.

Cancer of the Breast and Endometrium. Obesity has been implicated as a risk factor in the development of certain cancers. In a large prospective study, the mortality ratio for cancer in persons who were more than 40% overweight was 1.33 for men and for women 1.55.[134] In men, the higher mortality was for colorectal and prostate cancer, and in women, for endometrial, gallbladder, cervical, ovarian, and breast cancers.[134] Cancer of the endometrium has been particularly implicated.[135–137] It is possible that this association is related to endocrine abnormalities, and an increased conversion of estrone to androstenedione in adipose tissue has been implicated. In addition, obesity is correlated with increasing estrogenicity of cervical smears.[138] Although such increased estrogen activity could cause the increased risk of breast cancer reported in postmenopausal women,[139–141] no proof of this effect is available.

GENETICS AND ENVIRONMENT

Twin studies have been pursued to try to determine the relative importance of genetic inheritance versus environmental influences in obesity. The weights of identical twins raised in separate homes have been reported to be similar,[142] thereby suggesting that heredity contributes significantly to weight. Although Newman et al. showed a greater difference in twins raised apart than in twins raised together, thereby implicating environment, they also found that fraternal twins raised apart showed a greater weight difference than did identical twins, suggesting a strong genetic component.[143] The role of inherited factors in the origin of obesity is not well defined. Whereas clear genetic effects exist, these are modified by environmental and behavioral factors. To add to the complexity, there is not one obesity syndrome but several. Thus, geneticists are not dealing with a single disorder, but with a series of disorders. Studies of twins by Stunkard et al. reinforce the importance of heredity.[144,145] Using a model of path analysis, Bouchard studied BMI and reported a total transmissible variance across generations of about 35%, but a genetic effect of only 5%.[146] The heritability of body fat distribution, and particularly of the central or visceral fat, has also been studied.[147] Some reports have stated that the abdominal depot is determined partly by genotype. The response to overfeeding in a group of pairs of identical twins has been studied. The intrapair resemblance was high, and the resemblance between pairs varied much more.[148] Thus, the genotype seems important with regard to weight gain during overfeeding.

The Ten-State Nutrition Study suggests that environmental factors may be most important in the obesity found in families. Skinfold thicknesses were compared in 429 adoptive parent-child pairs and in 198 genetically unrelated siblings. In addition, 6372 pairs of biologic parent-child pairs and 3713 biologic pairs of siblings were measured. No difference was found between the correlations for biologic sibling pairs as compared to genetically unrelated siblings.[149] In addition, the correlations in skinfolds between parents and children were high.[150] If parents were divided into lean, medium, or obese and placed in appropriate mother-father combinations (lean-lean, lean-obese, obese-lean, obese-obese), the children were fatter as the parents increased in fatness. This latter finding, however, does not prove a genetic risk; in households with fatter parents, food may be more plentiful and may lead to fatness in the children.

Studying adoptive parent-child pairs, Withers could find no evidence that the correlation of fatness between a parent and an adopted child was different from that between a parent and a biologic child.[151] However, Biron et al. studied 374 families with one or more adopted children.[152] No correlation was found in weight between adopted children and their adoptive parents and siblings.

Common environment seems to have less influence as children grow older. Rao et al., studying 1068 families in Brazil, found that the influence of shared family environment on weight could account for only 18% of the variance.[153]

Thus, the relative importance of genetics and environment on weight is still unclear. To date, no specific genetic marker of obesity has been found.

PATHOGENESIS

ENDOCRINOPATHY IN OBESITY

Although popular thought ascribes obesity to glandular troubles, in actuality endocrinopathy is a rare cause of obesity. Overactivity of the adrenal gland, leading to Cushing's syndrome, causes central obesity. Why in this condition adipocytes located at the center of the body are stimulated to multiply and fill, whereas those at the extremities are not, is unclear. The central obesity is associated with hypertension and diabetes.

In severe hypothyroidism, some increased adipose mass may occur, but most of the increased weight is water. Few obese patients suffer from hypothyroidism.

Hypogonadism is sometimes associated with mild obesity, although the reason is not clear. Women with polycystic ovarian syndrome are generally overweight. Although the origin of this syndrome is unclear, investigators have documented that the ovaries are the major source of androgens in PCOS.[154] Not only are excess androgens produced, but in obesity, sex-hormone binding globulin is decreased,[155] so less of the androgens are bound. These women have significant insulin resistance.[154] The relationship between the increased androgens and the insulin resistance is not clear.

A hypothalamic lesion caused by tumor, infection, or, rarely, trauma may lead to obesity. This is secondary to damage of nerve fibers coursing through the ventromedial area, which are important in food intake regulation.

In children, obesity may be seen with certain congenital syndromes. The cause of these obesities is unknown. They include Prader-Willi syndrome, Laurence-Moon-Biedl syndrome, adiposogenital dystrophy (Fröhlich's syndrome), Bongiovanni-Eisenmenger syndrome, and pseudohypoparathyroidism.

Whereas the cause of obesity is seldom a hormonal abnormality, obesity may lead to abnormalities of hormone levels.[156] Owing to the development of insulin resistance, insulin levels in the blood rise, as has already been discussed. Triiodothyronine (T_3) rises in conditions of high caloric intake with adequate carbohydrate (though not to abnormal levels). Thyroxine levels are normal. The urinary excretion of free cortisol and of hydroxycorticoids, sometimes elevated in obesity, is probably related to an increase in cortisol turnover. These changes are related to the higher lean body mass in the obese. Blood cortisol levels are usually in the normal range in obesity, and diurnal patterns are generally normal. Growth hormone levels are in the low-normal range. Stimulatory tests with arginine, insulin hypoglycemia, or L-dopa demonstrate a poor growth hormone response. This growth hormone response reverts toward normal with weight loss.

THERMOGENESIS

Obese individuals have been described as utilizing energy calories more "efficiently" than lean subjects. They have been characterized as requiring fewer calories per unit of lean body mass. If they eat a number of calories equal to those eaten by a lean subject, more of the calories will be available as extra energy to be deposited as fat. This subject, however, is extremely controversial.

The expenditure of energy takes three forms: basal metabolic rate (BMR), activity, and the thermic effect of food.

Basal Metabolic Rate. The BMR is that energy required for the basic maintenance of the cells of the body and body temperature. In most sedentary adults, the BMR makes up about 60 to 70% of total energy expenditure.[157] Fat-free mass, fat mass, sex, and age explain about 80% of the variance in BMR.[158] Because the metabolic rate is defined primarily by the cell mass of the body, it is reasonable to express it in terms of the lean body mass (LBM). The contribution of the LBM to the BMR is much greater per kilogram than that of body fat.[159,160] The correlation of BMR with LBM explains why men have higher metabolic rates than women and why metabolic rates decrease with age. The high metabolic rate of children can be ascribed to the energy cost of growth.[161,162]

There is, however, a difference in metabolic rate in individuals matched for age, sex, and LBM.[163] These differences can be as high as 30%. As a result, at a given fixed intake per kg LBM, one individual may gain weight while the other does not. Thus, different people will maintain weight on different caloric intakes.

The BMR of obese persons is higher than that of lean individuals.[164,165] Because obese people have a higher LBM than lean people, this finding is not surprising. The obese often have a BMR lower than that of lean individuals if it is expressed per kilogram of body weight. This phenomenon is reasonable because per unit of weight they have a relatively lower amount of metabolizing cell mass. If one expresses BMR as total energy expended per unit time, the obese expend more calories than lean people. Recent studies have reported that individuals with a low relative metabolic rate will be at risk for gaining weight and becoming obese.[166–168] Further studies are necessary to confirm this interesting phenomenon, which proposes one mechanism by which individuals may be gaining weight. Moreover, a high 24-hour respiratory quotient, which is an index of carbohydrate/fat oxidation, has been shown to predict weight gain,[169] and insulin resistance has predicted a low rate of weight gain.[170]

Thermic Effect of Foods. The rise of metabolic rate above basal after eating has been called the thermic effect of food (TEF). About 10% of the ingested diet that can be metabolized is lost as heat, which is used up in the intermediary metabolism of substrates, in the utilization of ATP, and in the formation of ATP from reduced coenzymes by oxidative phosphorylation.

Although some studies have suggested that obese people have a lower TEF than lean people,[171–173] others have reported no difference.[174–176]

Insulin may be required for a full diet-induced thermogenic effect.[177] Insulin deficiency and/or resistance leads to defective glucose oxidation and impaired thermogenesis.[178] Thus, whether obese individuals show an impaired or delayed TEF depends on their insulin sensitivity or insulin response.[179] The TEF seems to be diminished in the obese as a function of insulin resistance,[178,179] although an independent effect of obesity has also been described.[180] The decreased TEF in obese subjects, however, seems to be secondary to obesity rather than primary.[181] Thus, an impaired TEF is unlikely to play a role in the development of obesity. In addition, even in those studies showing a decreased TEF, if it is added to the elevated BMR all obese persons manifest, the total energy expenditure (BMR and TEF) is elevated over that of lean persons.

Thermogenesis and Overfeeding. Neumann suggested 90 years ago that if a lean individual overate, the excess calories eaten were dissipated as heat (luxus consumption) and normal weight was maintained.[182] Garrow summarized the results of 15 studies in which lean and obese subjects were overfed.[183] Most show fairly conclusive evidence that significant overfeeding (2000 + extra calories per day) for at least 10 days leads to some energy wastage. In the 4 studies in which obese subjects were evaluated, however, no evidence of luxus consumption was found. Thus, it is possible that the lean people are more adept at burning off excess ingested energy than are the obese. Even in lean people, however, instances of caloric wastage have only been documented with very large caloric overeating, much higher than is usual.

The case for deficient ability to increase thermogenesis with overingestion in obese humans has been attractive because it has been documented in genetically obese rodents.[184] This finding has been ascribed to brown fat activity, but there is doubt whether enough brown fat is available in adult man to produce such excess heat. The extrapolation of small animal data to man is not valid at this time.

Exercise. Does exercise potentiate TEF? Again, the data are contradictory. Some studies support this theory,[185,186] others do not.[187–189] Overfeeding did not potentiate the effect of exercise in two studies,[190,191] and even in studies suggesting a potentiating effect of exercise on food, the effect is small.[192] If a difference is present between lean and obese individuals, it is smaller still.

In summary, the experimental evidence suggests a difference in lean and obese individuals in wasteful energy production to any stimulant. There are two exceptions. First, it is probable that with great overfeeding (2000 kcal or more above the usual intake) for a long period of time (10 days or more) some wasteful energy production will occur and that this may be greater in the lean than the obese person. Second, it is possible that obese patients with insulin resistance or insulin deficiency, having a defective glucose disposal system, have a depressed TEF.

FAT CELLS

Fat cells or adipocytes are distributed throughout the body. They form a reservoir depot of energy that is elastic, being able to expand and contract to accommodate the energy balance of the organism. The depot can expand in two ways: by increasing the size of the fat cells or by increasing their number. Although the size of the fat cell is generally between 0.3 and 0.9μg, the number is more expandable, averaging from as low as 2×10^{10} to as high as 16×10^{10}.[193] Thus, enormous flexibility exists for expansion of the adipose reservoir.

Fat cells develop from fat cell precursors called preadipocytes. It is unclear what stimulus activates the preadipocyte to differentiate into an adipocyte and begin to accumulate lipid. The size of adipocytes gradually increases if energy balance continues to be positive until a cell size of about 1.0 μg is reached. At this point, it does not seem possible for the adipocyte to enlarge further.

If positive energy balance then persists, a trigger for adipocyte proliferation occurs, and cell number begins to rise. Because the expansivity of numbers is virtually unlimited, the adipose reservoir can reach huge dimensions if caloric intake remains high.

Key time periods of adipose cell proliferation have been a controversial subject. It was initially reported that an increase in rat fat cell number occurred in the preweaning phase,[194] and not in the postweaning phase.[195] However, others have since shown that rat fat cells can proliferate in the postweaning period.[196–198] Although the data in humans are more sparse, evidence indicates an increase in fat cell size in the initial year of life with a rise in fat cell number subsequently,[199] so fat cell number increases fivefold between 1 and 22 years of age.

Fat cell number may continue to increase as long as nutritional excess occurs. Thus, excess storage energy is accommodated by enhancing fat cell number. Once fat cells are formed, however, it seems to be difficult to dedifferentiate them. The number seems to remain fixed even if weight is lost,[200] although some contraction of number with weight loss has been reported. The net effect of weight loss is then to bring fat cell size down toward normal and eventually, if enough weight is lost, to below normal.

If maximum fat cell size is attained by infants at 1 year of age and then additional fat reserves are created by increasing fat cell number, the child overfed on a long-term basis will develop an excess number of fat cells (hyperplasia). This condition has been well documented. This hyperplastic child is not, however, destined inevitably to become a hyperplastic adult. Obesity at age 2 or 3 is not necessarily predictive of obesity at age 21. Even though a child who is hyperplastic has a greater number of fat cells than his lean contemporary, he has a lower total number than a lean adult. Thus, he may "grow out" of his obesity by retaining his greater number of fat cells, which, if not increasing as he grows older, may gradually approach normality.

In summary, obesity can be classified as hypertrophic or as both hypertrophic and hyperplastic. Obese patients are not hyperplastic without being hypertrophic unless they have lost weight by dieting or illness. This classification may be important prognostically in treatment. Hypertrophic obese patients have been reported to maintain weight loss better than hyperplastic ones.[201] This possibility requires further investigation.

LIPOPROTEIN LIPASE

Adipose tissue lipoprotein lipase (LPL) is an enzyme that determines the rate of uptake by fat cells of circulating plasma triglyceride. It originates in adipocytes and muscle cells and then is secreted to the capillary endothelium where it acts on circulating VLDL triglyceride. Activated LPL enhances the breakdown of triglycerides to glycerol phosphate and free fatty acids, which smaller molecular weight substances can enter adipose cells, be re-esterified, and be stored as triglyceride.

Adipose tissue LPL activity is elevated in human obesity.[77,202] When adipose LPL is expressed per cell, it correlates significantly with fat cell size and with percent desirable weight.[77,202,203] This correlation is not true of postheparin LPL, muscle LPL, or hepatic lipase.[202] Racial differences also seem to exist in LPL. For instance, Pima Indians, a group renowned for their high prevalence of obesity, have lower levels than obese Caucasians.[203]

Obese individuals could have elevated LPL as a primary defect that enhances their ability to "pull" triglyceride into cells, or obesity could develop from some other cause and the enhanced LPL activity could be secondary to the enlarged fat cells. Schwartz and Brunzell have suggested that the first hypothesis is correct, and that the LPL activity rises further with weight loss and returns to lower (though elevated) values with weight regain.[204,205] The further elevation of LPL with any weight drop tends to enhance lipid clearance, to raise stored triglyceride levels, and to restore the obese state.[78,79]

Although this hypothesis is attractive, recent data do not confirm it. Two studies have shown that after stabilized significant weight reduction, the elevated adipose tissue LPL activity drops,[202,206] whereas other tissues lipases are not affected.[202] In addition, with refeeding, the LPL activity rises rapidly to above previous baseline levels.[206] Thus, this change may enhance the capacity of storing triglycerides that are circulating owing to the enhanced food intake. It may therefore contribute to the efficient regain of weight in a refeeding obese patient who was previously on a hypocaloric regimen.

WEIGHT REGAIN

Of patients who lose significant amounts of weight, 80 to 90% regain it. The explanation for this dismal record is not readily evident, but a few hypotheses bear mentioning.

The first is that a reducing obese patient has decreased energy requirements. Patients while on a reducing diet experience a significant drop of 15 to 30% in their metabolic rate.[207,208] As a result, it is more difficult for them to lose weight on the same hypocaloric diet in the second month than in the first, and in the third than the second.[207] This reduced metabolic rate also may make it easier to regain weight on returning to a more normal diet. After a fast or a hypocaloric diet, refeeding is associated with a supranormal tissue response to nutrients. This response is characterized by a "repletion reaction" that includes a generalized increased substrate utilization with an adaptive hyperlipogenesis in adipose tissue and liver. In adipose tissue, this hyperlipogenesis is characterized by a marked production of triglyceride and CO_2 from glucose.[209,210] The rapid transfer of glucose into the tissues, enhanced by increased insulin levels plus greater tissue insulin sensitivity, may cause enhanced lipogenesis and may also lead to lower blood glucose levels that may enhance hunger and stimulate greater food intake.[210]

The increased efficiency of rats after fasting has been documented. Animals fasted for 4 days and then refed could maintain their new lower weight (90% of baseline) if fed only 60% of the original daily calories.[211] In addition, fasted rats refed their original daily caloric intake could regain their lost weight without overeating. These reports suggest that during the refeeding period, animals are more efficient at utilizing the same number of calories.[212]

Suggestive evidence of a similar phenomenon is beginning to emerge from human studies. In morbidly obese patients whose weight was significantly reduced (from an average 152 to 100 kg), 7-day energy intake requirements to maintain weight dropped from 1432 to 1021 kcal/m^2/day.[213] The figure of 1021 kcal/m^2/day was significantly lower than the value of 1341 kcal/m^2/day found in normal lean individuals weighing a mean of 63 kg. Because this weight loss was recent, a second metabolic study was executed with reduced obese patients who had maintained their weight loss for 4 to 6 years. These 4 women also showed kilocalorie requirements averaging 1031/m^2/day to maintain their weight.

This finding suggests that at least some reduced obese individuals have lowered caloric requirements that may persist for years and that if caloric intake is increased above the 1000 kcal/m^2/day range, weight regain will occur. This theory may help to explain the poor record in maintaining weight loss after dieting.

The regulation of adipose tissue mass may occur by an ability of the organism to sense the filling of adipose cells with triglyceride. That is, weight regain in a refeeding animal seems to continue until fat cells have once again returned to their original size. Some investigators have suggested that in this way adipose tissue exerts a regulatory function on energy intake and energy balance.[214] This process could explain why reduced obese patients have such difficulty staying on hypocaloric diets after they have dropped to a certain weight. At that point, their fat cells are at lower limits of normal size. To drop weight further, these cells would need to reduce to an abnormally low size. If hyperplastic obese persons do succeed in lowering their weight to an extent where fat cell size is below normal, they will be unable to remain at that weight, regain will occur, and fat cells will be filled to at least a "normal" size.[215]

The role of the fat cell in energy regulation is intriguing, and more investigative studies in this area are necessary.

THERAPY FOR OBESITY

DIETARY MANAGEMENT

Many strategies for losing weight have been tried over the years because, as a rule, losing weight and keeping the weight off are extremely difficult. This is particularly true for those individuals who are 25% or more overweight.

Impaired Absorption. Impairment of intestinal absorption of ingested calories has been a suggested strategy. Fiber has been particularly touted in this regard. There is, however, little evidence that fiber significantly affects total intestinal absorption.[216]

Nondigestible fat substitutes have been developed. An example is sucrose polyester, which can be used in the diet as a replacement for fat. Perfluoroactyl bromide, an inert synthetic product, can coat the gastrointestinal tract and prevent some caloric absorption. Also being developed are agents that slow the natural breakdown of macromolecular nutrients into the smaller absorbable molecules. An example is the glucosidase inhibitor acarbose, which inhibits hydrolysis of carbohydrate.[217] These "starch-blockers," however, have only been shown to delay absorption, not to inhibit it. As a result, no weight loss has been documented.

Because of the noxious side effects of fat and carbohydrate malabsorption, the acceptability and marketability of malabsorptive products have been low.

Unbalanced Low-Calorie Diets. These diets all have a marked imbalance of macronutrients that can also cause an imbalance of micronutrients. They emphasize particular food groups (carbohydrate, protein, or fat) and prohibit or deemphasize others. Because of their focused nature, they are easier for individuals to follow and this makes them popular.

They can be divided into different types. The ketogenic diets are high-protein, high-fat, low-carbohydrate diets. The carbohydrate generally makes up less than 20% of the calories. Proponents suggest that the ketosis causes appetite suppression. The effectiveness of ketones in inhibiting food intake has not been effectively demonstrated, however.

Such diets tend to be low in vitamin C. Enhanced calcium loss can occur. The high uric acid produced may be dangerous for those predisposed to gout. These diets have a high cholesterol content, dangerous for people with hypercholesterolemia.[218] They often cause nausea, hypotension, and fatigue.[218]

The aforementioned diets have been modified to be high-protein (40 to 45%), low-fat (30 to 35%), and low-carbohydrate (20 to 25%). These diets tend to be lower in calories by the limiting of fat, a high-calorie item. They are still ketogenic, with the same side effects of nausea, hypotension, and fatigue. They tend to be high in saturated fats and cholesterol and low in vitamin A, C, thiamin, and iron. The amount of cholesterol may be triple that in a regular diet.[219]

A radically different type of diet is one that is high in carbohydrate, low in protein (35 g/day), and low in fat (as low as 10%).[220] The emphasis is on fruits, vegetables, breads, and cereals. No table fats, oil, or dairy products except skim milk are allowed. Often these diets prohibit sugar. If taken faithfully, such diets may be low in salt, iron, essential fatty acids, and fat-soluble vitamins. Most commonly used today are diets relatively low in fat (20 to 30% of calories) that are also hypocaloric and have adequate protein. Such diets have been shown to be successful in inducing weight loss.[221–223]

Total and Modified Fasts. Some physicians have proposed total fasting as a way of losing weight.[224,225] Advocates have used it intermittently in treating obese type 2 diabetics. The problem with a total fast is that not only fat, but also much lean body mass, is lost.[226] Particularly in older individuals, lean body mass is difficult to regain. In addition, because of the diuresis induced, significant mineral losses occur.

Because of the deficiencies of total fasting, regimens called protein-supplemented modified fasts (PSMF) have become popular.[227] These severely limited diets of 400 to 700 calories generate a rapid weight loss. The protein is given in the form of either formula or natural foods such as lean meat, fowl, or fish. These diets have been given for extensive periods of time, although the consensus is that it is dangerous to allow them for longer than 16 weeks.[228]

Patients lose 1.5 to 2.3 kg a week on these diets. The protein that the patients take needs to be of high biologic quality to help prevent the loss of body protein that occurs during a standard fast.[227]

In a fasting subject, the nitrogen excretion is initially high (11 to 23 g/per day).[229] Nitrogen loss decreases steeply in the first few days to a nadir of obligate nitrogen excretion.[230] With total fasting, a cumulative nitrogen loss of 154 g of nitrogen or 963 g of protein occurs after 15 days.[231] Simply adding 100 g of carbohydrate per day decreases nitrogen loss by 40%.[232] Administering 55 g of high-quality protein per day causes negative nitrogen balance to occur initially for the first 10 days, but many patients achieve balance at about 20 days.[233] These low-calorie diets were given large-scale trials by 3 groups.[234–236] All required vitamin and mineral supplements daily as well as essential fatty acids.[235] They reported little morbidity. Vertes et al., with 1200 outpatient years of experience, had 4 deaths, which they describe as less than expected for the population treated.[237]

It has been hypothesized that these diets spare protein by decreasing insulin level and enhancing ketonemia.[238] The ketonemia will, in turn, inhibit release of amino acids from muscle.[239] Little experimental evidence indicates that this hypothesis is correct, because insulin levels are not absolute determinants of protein sparing.[240,241]

With the popularization of these PSMF diets, numerous commercial preparations of liquid protein have become available for over-the-counter purchase. Fifty-eight deaths were associated with the use of these formulas in the 1970s.[242] Although the reason for these deaths is unclear, 17 of them have been investigated.[243,244] Patients seem to develop refractory ventricular arrhythmias. Whether this condition is secondary to myocardial protein atrophy, myocarditis, potassium deficiency, or other mineral losses is unclear.[243,245,246]

These deaths have been attributed to poor-quality protein in the commercial-formula diets. The proteins eaten in a regular diet, such as dairy products, meat, fish, and poultry, and grain and cereal products, provide about 87% of the calcium, 80% of the phosphorus, 60% of the magnesium, 74% of the iron, 80% of the zinc, 57% of the copper, 80% of the manganese, and 100% of the selenium in a usual diet. Many of the poor-quality hydrolyzed protein diets did not adequately replace these minerals and others. The more recent formula preparations have used high-quality protein (casein or soy protein), have replaced micronutrients adequately, and have not led to untoward events.[247]

Besides mortality, morbidity also occurs with these diets. Orthostatic hypotension may be a problem with the sodium diuresis and volume depletion that occur.[248] This condition is probably secondary to the natriuretic effect of hyperketonemia[249] and the impaired norepinephrine secretion associated with it.[248] Other symptoms and signs include dehydration, cold intolerance, fatigue, dry skin, hair loss, and menstrual irregularities. Cholecystitis, pancreatitis, and peroneal nerve palsy occasionally have been reported.

Although it is true that nitrogen balance is better with PSMF than with starvation, there is little evidence that PSMF is better than a mixed diet. Comparisons of an 800-kcal mixed diet and an 800-kcal all-protein ketogenic diet and starvation in obese subjects have shown that, whereas starvation gives the most negative nitrogen balance, nitrogen loss is less and not much different between the mixed and the all-protein diet.[250] Over a 10-day period, 2.8 kg of weight are lost with a mixed diet and 4.7 kg with the ketogenic diet, but all the extra weight lost with the ketogenic diet is water.[250] Longer 60-day studies show no difference in nitrogen balance between a mixed diet and a ketogenic diet.[251]

Balanced Hypocaloric Diets. In view of the aforementioned risks and problems of unbalanced diets, and the prolonged periods of time that restricted diets must be followed, a well-balanced mixed diet seems a sensible approach. Diets in the 1100- to 1200-kcal range can include appropriate macro- and microelements, vitamins, and protein.[252] They can be followed for months without specific supplements. The nutrients most likely to be deficient are iron, folacin, vitamin B_6, and zinc.[252] In such a diet, the percentage of protein is raised, so at least 240 calories or about 60 g per day are as protein. The protein should be of high quality and should make up about 25% of calories. At least 20% of the rest of the diet should be carbohydrate and at least 20% fat. In this way, fat-soluble vitamins and essential fatty acids will be available from fat and fiber and antiketogenic effect from carbohydrate. If diets of 800 to 1100 kcal are used, they must be supplemented with vitamins and minerals. In general, the caloric deficit should not exceed 500 to 1000 kcal per day and should not be below a total of 800 kcal unless the individual is under tight medical surveillance.

In formulating a balanced diet for micronutrients and vitamins, one should use food items from the four food groups: (1) meat, fish, poultry, and meat substitutes; (2) milk and milk products; (3) cereals and cereal products; and (4) vegetables and fruits. The nutrients obtained are: (1) protein, fat, niacin, iron, and thiamin; (2) vitamins A and D, calcium, magnesium, and zinc; (3) carbohydrates, fat, phosphorus, magnesium, zinc, and copper; and (4) carbohydrate, vitamins A and C, iron, and magnesium.[252]

Because obese individuals need to be on a diet for a long time, it is crucial that the diet be acceptable. The diet must therefore fit the tastes and habits of the individual and be flexible enough to allow eating outside the home as well as in.

EXERCISE

The therapeutic use of exercise to reverse obesity has been widely hailed. As has been previously mentioned, body weight is determined by a balance between energy intake and energy expenditure. If the energy expenditure can be increased by incremental physical activity and if energy intake is kept constant, weight will drop. A number of points must be emphasized. The first is that it requires a significant amount of physical effort to expend a significant number of calories. Calorie charts for expenditure are usually listed as the total caloric expenditure for a given period of time. It is clear, however, that an individual not doing the activity would not revert to an expenditure of zero calories but would expend at somewhat above basal levels (sitting, standing, or walking). For example, an obese woman exercising on a treadmill at 4 MPH would expend about 7.0 kcal per minute or 210 calories if she were to continue this exercise for 30 minutes. Sitting in a chair, such a woman would expend about 1.3 kcal per minute, or 39 kcal over 30 minutes. Thus, her exercise-induced expenditure would not be 210 kcal but 210 minus 39 or 171 kcal. Therefore, in looking at expenditure tables, one must always subtract between 1 and 1.5 kcal per minute for the resting or sitting metabolic expenditure that would occur anyway.

The second point that must be clarified is the purported prolonged elevation of oxygen consumption for long periods after exercise. Such a sustained effect of exercise lasting for 7 to 48 hours has been described, but two reviews of the literature have concluded that no sustained increase could be demonstrated after exercise.[253,254] Studies have supported a lack of a sustained effect, using exercise levels that would be realistic for individuals on weight-control programs.[255–258] Because little appreciable caloric loss occurs beyond that generated by the exercise period itself, claims for sustained effects of exercise on resting metabolic rate in weight-control programs are unwarranted.

The third point relates to the effect of exercise on food intake. Although it has been generally suggested that exercise inhibits food intake, this phenomenon has not been documented. In lean individuals, exercise generally leads to an increased energy intake and a maintenance of body weight.[259] This tendency is true with both mild (about 400 kcal/day) or moderate (about 775 kcal/day) exercise.[260] In obese individuals, it may be that in response to exercise, weight is defended to the same degree as in lean persons.

Most of the studies of the effect of exercise on obese subjects have only measured weight or body fat; they have not measured food intake. As mentioned previously, if expenditure is increased and food intake remains stable, weight loss will be commensurate with the increased expenditure. Such a result has been described.[261] Other studies, however, have documented amounts of weight loss that suggest that food intake was curtailed.[262,263] Some studies show no effect of exercise on weight at all.[264] Two metabolic ward studies over long periods of time, 19-day intervals[255] or 57-day intervals,[256] suggest that obese women tend to fix on an intake and remain at that intake even if the amount of activity is changed. The changes in intake seemed to relate more to the gustatory characteristics of the diet provided than to whether exercise was high or low.[264] Prospective epidemiologic studies have shown a lower risk for overweight in the more physically active persons.[265] With regard to weight loss, one review describes a modestly greater effect of diet and exercise over diet alone,[266] but the effect is not great. A beneficial effect of exercise can best be documented in the weight maintenance phase, predicting greater success.[267]

Although exercise is not invested with magical powers in sustaining an enhanced metabolic rate or in inhibiting food intake, every calorie expended can help in the net battle to utilize significantly more calories than are ingested. Moreover, exercise will help maintain weight loss while allowing less stringent diets—a more acceptable regimen to many patients.

PHARMACOLOGIC TREATMENT

Although the most widely used drugs for weight control are appetite suppressants, others have been tried that attack the food intake and metabolizing pathway at other sites, such as at digestion, absorption, lipid synthesis, or thermogenesis. The anorectic agents, which suppress appetite, will be discussed first.

The first, and a successfully marketed drug for many years, was amphetamine. Amphetamine is a β-phenethylamine and seems to induce anorexia via brain catecholamines, specifically norepinephrine and dopamine, although the relative importance of each in man is not yet clear. It causes not only anorexia, but also many other effects, among which are central stimulation, mood enhancement, cardiovascular excitation, and a selective effect on certain normal transmitter agents, especially catecholamines. Some of these effects can lead susceptible individuals to abuse.[268] In addition, in a few patients, discontinuing the drug seems to be associated with onset of depression.

Five anorexic drugs that seem to have fewer side effects and induce less dependence than amphetamine are most commonly used: diethylpropion, mazindol, fenfluramine, phentermine, and phenylpropanolamine.

Diethylpropion seems to have little effect on sleep and infrequent addiction has been reported. It is closest in structure to amphetamine, being modified by addition of a keto group on the β carbon and of ethyl groups on the N terminal. Mazindol is thought to act by prolonging the action of norepinephrine. It also causes central nervous system stimulation.[269] It is a tricyclic compound with a long plasma half-life (33 to 55 hours). Fenfluramine has an ethyl group on the N terminal and a CF_3 on the phenyl ring. Its action is thought to be mediated by a central serotonergic system. It has no central stimulant effect.[270] Phentermine resin has had methyl groups substituted on the α carbon. The stimulant properties of this drug are less than those of amphetamine and yet it seems to be as effective; however, dry mouth, tachycardia, and increased blood pressure often occur. Phenylpropanolamine is a derivative of amphetamine, having an extra hydroxyl group. It is available over the counter and as a result is widely used, but its effect is generally modest.[271,272]

Although we do not know enough yet to classify obesity in terms of etiology, it probably has differing causes. The drugs available are also different. It is not surprising, therefore, that the response is different from person to person.

These drugs may be a useful adjunct for treatment of obesity in some patients. The widespread belief in some medical circles that all appetite-suppressant drugs are useless and that tolerance quickly develops are not necessarily true. In addition, although side effects are common if excess dosage is taken, they do not necessarily occur at recommended dosage. An anorectic agent can be helpful in some people. One must remember, however, that the drug will be ineffective unless appropriate dosage is given and blood levels are adequate. It is also wise to individualize use to a patient's dietary habits. One would not administer a relatively short-acting drug in the morning if a patient eats no breakfast and is an evening and night eater. Recently, the suggestion has been put forward that long-term drug therapy for obesity should be considered.[273] Certain experimental studies have reported moderate success with long-term therapy.[274] Further studies seem warranted.

Anorectic drugs will not work alone. Other therapy, such as diet and exercise, must also be stressed. Drugs may be helpful not only during weight loss but also in the difficult period of weight maintenance when many obese patients have their hardest time.

Although other pharmacologic agents have been tried, none has been shown to be successful enough to be marketed. These include inhibitors of dietary lipid absorption and inhibitors of lipid synthesis. An effort to develop thermogenic agents is underway, but no satisfactory drug is available to date.

Thyroid preparations, digitalis, or human chorionic gonadotrophin have no place in the treatment of obesity. Diuretics are rarely necessary, and certainly should never be used in combination with low-calorie diets.

Bulking agents, such as methylcellulose and other fibers, have been touted as aids in weight loss, but no evidence of this is available. They do not cause malabsorption and have not been shown to decrease food intake.[275]

In summary, though drugs may be helpful in some individuals at some periods in the weight loss and the weight maintenance periods, they do not hold first rank in any therapeutic program.

PSYCHOTHERAPY

The psychologic treatment of obesity has not enjoyed much success. Although a few optimistic reports have stated the effect of psychoanalysis in producing weight loss,[276,277] particularly in adolescents,[276] therapeutic failure is the common result. Many obese patients may have emotional problems, but these vary. Some have anxiety, some are depressed, but some have no evident psychiatric problems at all, except for overeating and/or underactivity.[278] There is no particular personality type who is obese.

Although some investigators have suggested that obesity may be protective for underlying neurotic behavior, this possibility has not been confirmed by patients undergoing surgical treatment of obesity. Some psychiatrists predicted that morbidly obese individuals would develop other addictive tendencies or overt neurotic or psychotic traits as weight loss occurred. This has not happened. Patients either have had no psychiatric change or have improved, but few have deteriorated.[279]

A distortion of body image does seem to exist in a minority of obese patients with an overestimation of body size.[278] In a study of morbidly obese subjects whose weight was reduced enough to have significant changes in body size, the distortion of body image was persistent, particularly in those obese from childhood.[280]

Some psychiatrists have even reported evidence of low anxiety and depression in obese individuals,[281] and epidemiologic evidence suggests that they have a lower incidence of suicide than the general population.

Because no evidence indicates that all or even most obese subjects are neurotic, it is incumbent on health professionals to individually evaluate each patient.

Some persons who wish to lose weight are binge eaters. If they have true bulimia nervosa, with vomiting, laxative use, and electrolyte changes, this condition should be addressed by a psychiatrically trained professional. If an obese person engages in binge eating without purging, it seems wise to direct therapy to the binge eating first, before attempting weight loss.[282]

BEHAVIOR MODIFICATION

Because of the poor record in the treatment of obesity by classic psychoanalysis and psychotherapy, behavior modification has grown in favor. Behavior modification programs grew out of the hypothesis that the obese overeat because they are stimulus-bound, and that environmental food-relevant cues controlled eating rather than any psychogenic neurotic states.[283] This "externality theory" suggested that external environmental stimuli overrode whatever internal hunger or satiety cues generally caused lean individuals to initiate or stop eating.[284] This theory differentiating obese from lean is now questioned because others have not been able to duplicate these differences in the two groups.[285]

Nevertheless, the theory won wide recognition and stimulated interest in behavior modification programs to control food intake. Programs evolved whose intention was to greatly diminish the number of external cues that led to overeating.[286]

As a first step in a behavior modification program, the eating and activity patterns of an individual must be identified. As a result, careful diaries are kept. Patients record not only when and what was eaten, but where, with whom, how (sitting, standing, walking), their feelings, and hunger. In addition to the diary of food-related behavior, a diary of all activity-related behavior is kept, including when, with whom, where, and feelings at the time. Food management behavior must also be itemized, including buying, storing, preparing, serving, and cleaning up food. These diaries are analyzed to identify possible clues, whether environmental (such as television) or emotional (such as depression), that lead to overeating, so that these may be recognized and controlled. Once these cues have been identified, then techniques are invoked to try to control or evade them. Environmental stimuli to eating are controlled. Food shopping habits, visual cues, food preparation habits, and food storage habits are changed.

In addition, techniques to control the act of eating are also controlled. These include always eating in the dining room, sitting, concentrating on eating (no reading or watching television), eating more slowly, taking more and smaller bites, putting utensils down between bites, not skipping meals, not taking snacks, changing high-calorie foods for low-calorie ones, and eating at prescribed times only.

Besides these efforts to diminish environmental cues, new discriminative stimuli are introduced to develop new eating patterns. These include distinctive sites for eating, new and smaller plates, and eating with others as often as possible.

Finally, behavior modification programs try to change the consequences of eating. A reward system is introduced for changing behavior. The rewards are generally immediate and may be monetary or social feedback. Family, friends, group members, and group leaders can all contribute.

Mahoney outlined the assumptions under which the behavior modification movement operates. They are

(1) Obesity is a learning disorder, created by and amenable to principles of conditioning; (2) obesity is a simple disorder resulting from excess calorie intake; (3) the obese individual is an overeater; (4) obese persons are more sensitive to food stimuli than are nonobese individuals; (5) there are important differences in the "eating style" of obese and nonobese persons; (6) training an obese person to behave like a nonobese one will result in weight loss.[287]

Many, if not all, of these assumptions are now considered to be untrue, so many of the strategies for weight loss in behavioral modification programs are founded on false assumptions. It can be argued, however, that though the theoretic background may be incorrect, the strategy developed is nevertheless effective. This argument is probably true. Stunkard reviewed 30 controlled trials and found that behavioral treatment was more successful in producing weight loss than a variety of other treatments.[288] Compared to group psychotherapy, nutrition education, and relaxation training, the behavior modification programs seemed to be more successful. That success is not universal, however, and some patients do well and others poorly. To date, it has not been possible to identify the characteristics that determine success.

Although some weight has been lost, it has not been impressive. Jeffrey et al. reviewed 21 studies and found a mean weight loss of 11.5 lb.[289] This amount, although a loss, is not enough to be clinically of much importance. In addition, the success in maintaining weight loss in the long term has been minimal. Not many persons have lost weight after termination of the program,[290] and maintenance of weight loss in the longterm has been poor.[291]

In summary, it is difficult to be certain at this point whether behavioral treatment is better, and if so, how much better, than other forms of treatment. Well-controlled follow-up studies suggest that the same problem in recidivism that is true of other weight-control programs may be true of behavior modification programs.

SURGICAL TREATMENT

The refractoriness of many patients with morbid obesity to diet, psychotherapy, behavior modification, drugs, and exercise programs has led to a pessimistic outlook on the part of physicians concerning the likelihood of long-term therapeutic success. As a result, surgical treatment has been attempted. The surgical treatment is based on one of two principles: (1) a short bowel is created to produce malabsorption of ingested calories and (2) a small stomach is created so the reduced reservoir for food will prevent much caloric intake at any one time.

Short Bowel Procedure. There were many variations of the jejunoileal bypass procedure.[292] These depended on how much jejunum and how much ileum was bypassed. The earliest procedure connected 12 to 15 in. of jejunum to 4 to 8 in. of ileum. Connections were end to end or end to side. The bypass loop was either left to drain where it was (end to side) or was reconnected to drain somewhere in the ascending or transverse colon (end to end). Various-sized segments were left in continuity (14 to 4 in., 10 to 10 in., 14 to 8 in.). Weight loss did generally occur, although it was variable, and few patients lost only a small amount of weight. The bypass procedure created malabsorption of both exogenous nutrients and endogenous gastrointestinal secretions. Complications made this procedure unacceptable.[292] These included hypokalemia, hypocalcemia, vitamin B_{12} deficiency, hepatic toxicity, renal calculi, and polyarthritis. In addition were operative risks, including pulmonary embolus, pneumonia, wound infections, wound dehiscence, and phlebitis. Because of all these problems, this procedure was discontinued.

Gastric Surgery. The gastric bypass operation was first described by Mason and Ito in 1967.[293] In this operation, the stomach was transected (or stapled), so a small upper pouch (30 to 50 ml) was created. This pouch was anastomosed to a loop of jejunum. The opening between pouch and jejunum was 9 to 11 mm in diameter. This operation made a blind loop of much of the stomach, the duodenum, and the proximal jejunum.

More commonly now, a modification of this operation, the gastroplasty, is done. The stomach is stapled across, creating a small 50- to 60-ml reservoir on top and a small 1-cm outlet to the rest of the stomach on the lesser, middle, or greater curvatures.

Another recent procedure is the vertical banded gastroplasty.[294] In this procedure, a 20- to 30-ml stomach pouch is made by two longitudinal staple lines. In addition, wrapping of the pouch with Teflon mesh can be undertaken to prevent pouch distention and stoma widening.

These operations have been associated with considerably less morbidity than the intestinal operations.[295] The problems are generally postoperative and include anastomotic leaks, transient gastrojejunostomy obstruction, and intra-abdominal abscess. Wound infection, dehiscence, pulmonary embolism, and atelectasis can also occur.

Subsequent to these early problems, late morbidity is greatly dependent on how much education the patient is given and how compliant he or she is. Vomiting is frequent if the speed or amount of eating is too great. Late complications consist primarily of revisions caused by suture-line disruption or channel size problems. If chronic vomiting persists, esophagitis, hypokalemia, and malnutrition with dehydration can occur.

The success rate with gastroplasty has been variable, depending greatly on the surgeon. It is difficult to construct a stoma small enough to inhibit too rapid a transit from the small reservoir to the large, yet not so small that it will cause obstructive symptoms. Whereas Mason and Ito reported a 36-kg average weight loss in 3 years, others have not done as well.[293]

In addition, patients can ensure failure by consuming high-caloric-density liquid or semisolid food that can easily pass through the small stoma.

Lipectomy. This treatment is not for obesity. It is surgical removal of adipose tissue for cosmetic purposes. Not enough fat can be removed to make a real impact on obesity, and it should not be performed for this reason. Lipectomy may be used to treat localized unsightly adiposity. A recent modification of this procedure is suction lipectomy. Long-term results of this procedure are unavailable.

WEIGHT CYCLING

In recent years, data have suggested that weight cycling, that is, gaining and losing weight several times, may be detrimental. Although some studies have suggested increased morbidity and mortality,[296,297] others have not.[298,299] Further studies will be necessary before this issue is resolved.

REFERENCES

1. National Center for Health Statistics, Roberts, J.: Weight by Height and Age of Adults. United States, 1960–62. Vital and Health Statistics. Series 11, No. 14. PHS Pub. No. 1000. Public Health Service, Washington, D.C., U.S. Government Printing Office, 1966.
2. Garrow, J.S.: Treat Obesity Seriously. Edinburgh, Churchill Livingstone, 1981, p. 3.
3. Simopolous, A.P., VanItallie, T.B. Ann. Intern. Med., *100:*285–295, 1984.
4. Womersley, J., Durnin, J.V.G.A.: Br. J. Nutr., *38:*271–284, 1977.
5. Keys, A., Fidanza, F., Karvonen, M.J., et al.: J. Chronic Dis., *25:*329–343, 1972.
6. Wilmer, H.A.: Proc. Soc. Exp. Biol. Med., *43:*386–388, 1940.
7. National Center for Health Statistics: Basic Data on Anthropometric Measurements and Angular Measurements of the Hip and Knee Joints for Selected Age Groups 1–74 years of Age, U.S. 1971–1975. Vital and Health Statistics. DHHS Publication No. (PH) 81–1669, Series 11, No. 219. Hyattsville, MD, 1981. See also, Bishop, E.W., Bowen, P.E., Ritchey, S.J.: Am. J. Clin. Nutr. *34:*2530–2539, 1981.
8. Durnin, J.V.G.A., Womersley, J.: Br. J. Nutr., *32:*77–97, 1974.
9. Pace, N., Rathbun, E.: J. Biol. Chem., *158:*685–691, 1945.
10. Smith, T., Hesp, R., Mackenzie, J.: Phys. Med. Biol., *24:*171–175, 1979.
11. Behnke, A.R., Wilmore, J.H.: Evaluation of Body Build and Composition. Englewood Cliffs, NJ, Prentice Hall, 1974.
12. Lesser, G.T., Deutsch, S., Markofsy, J.: Metabolism, *20:*792–804, 1971.
13. 1983 Metropolitan Height and Weight Tables: Stat. Bull Metropolitan Life Insurance Co., *64:*2–9, 1984.
14. National Center for Health Statistics, Abraham, S., Johnson, C.L. and Najjar, M.F.: Weight by Height and Age for Adults 18–74 years, United States, 1971–74. Vital and Health Statistics. Series 11, No. 208. DHEW Pub. No. (PHS) 79–1656. Public Health Service, Washington, D.C. U.S. Government Printing Office, 1979.
15. Najjar, M.F., Rowland, M.: Anthropometric Data and Prevalence of Overweight, United States: 1976–1980. Vital and Health Statistics, Series 11, No. 238. Washington, D.C., U.S. Government Printing Office, 1987.
16. Kuczmarski, R.J.: Am. J. Clin. Nutr., *55:*495S–502S, 1992.
17. Andres, R., Elahi, D., Tobin, J.D., et al.: Ann. Intern. Med. *103:*1030–1033, 1985.
18. Andres, R.: Mortality and obesity: the rationale for age-specific height-weight tables. *In* Principles of Geriatric Medicine. Edited by E.L. Bierman and W.R. Hazzard. New York, McGraw-Hill, 1985, pp. 311–318.

19. National Research Council Committee on Diet and Health: Diet and Health: Implications for Reducing Chronic Disease Risk. Washington, D.C., National Academy Press, 1989, pp. 563–592.
20. Willett, W.C., Stampfer, M., Manson, J., et al.: Am. J. Clin. Nutr., *53:*1102–1103, 1991.
21. Taitz, L.S.: Br. Med. J., *1:*315–316, 1971.
22. Shukla, A., Forsyth, H.A., Anderson, C.M., et al.: Br. Med. J., *4:*507–515, 1972.
23. Jelliffe, D.B., Jelliffe, E.F.: Environ. Child Health Monogr., *41:*124–159, 1975.
24. Johnson, M.L., Burke, B.S., Mayer, J.: Am. J. Clin. Nutr., *4:*231–238, 1956.
25. Hathaway, M.L., Sargent, D.W.: J. Am. Diet. Assoc., *40:*511–515, 1962.
26. Garn, S.M., Clark, D.C.: Pediatrics, *57:*443–456, 1976.
27. Colley, J.R.T.: Br. J. Prev. Soc. Med., *28:*221–225, 1974.
28. Mossberg, H.: Acta Paediatr. Scand., *35 (Suppl. II):*1–122, 1948.
29. Rimm, I.J., Rimm, A.A.: Am. J. Public Health, *66:*479–481, 1976.
30. Abraham, S., Nordsieck, M.: Public Health Rep., *75:*263–273, 1960.
31. Garn, S.M., LaVelle, M.: Am. J. Dis. Child., *139:*181–185, 1985.
32. Borjeson, M.: Acta Paediatr, *51(Suppl. 132):*1–76, 1962.
33. Goldblatt, P.B., Moore, M.E., Stunkard, A.J.: Social factors in obesity. JAMA, *192:*1039–1044, 1965.
34. Baird, I.M., Silverstone, J.T., Grimshaw, J.J., et al.: Practitioner, *212:*706–714, 1974.
35. Noppa, H., Bengston, C.: J. Epidemiol. Community Health, *34:*134–142, 1978.
36. Stunkard, A.J.: Fed. Proc., *27:*1367–1373, 1968.
37. Ross, C.E., Mirowsky, J.: J. Health Soc. Behav., *24:*288–296, 1983.
38. Moore, M.E., Stunkard, A.J., Srole, L.: JAMA, *181:*962–966, 1962.
39. Silverstone, J.T., Gordon, R.P., Stunkard, A.J.: Practitioner, *202:*682–688, 1969.
40. Height and Weight of Adults Ages 18–74 Years by Socioeconomic Status and Geographic Variables, United States. DHHS Publication No (PHS) 81–1674, National Center for Health Statistics, Hyattsville, MD, 1981.
41. Armstrong, D.B., Dublin, L.I., Wheatley, G.M., et al.: JAMA, *147:*1007–1014, 1951.
42. Lew, E.A.: J. Am. Diet. Assoc., *38:*323–327, 1961.
43. Build and Blood Pressure Study, 1959, Vol 1. Chicago, Society of Actuaries, 1960.
44. Build Study 1979. Chicago, Society of Actuaries and Association of Life Insurance Medical Directors, 1980.
45. Lew, E.A., Garfinkel, L.: J. Chronic Dis., *32:*563–576, 1979.
46. Belloc, N.B.: Prev. Med., *2:*67–81, 1973.
47. Andres, R., Elahi, D., Tobin, J.D., et al.: Int. J. Obes., *4:*381–386, 1980.
48. Dyer, A.R., Stamler, J., Berkson, D.M., et al.: J. Chronic Dis., *28:*109–123, 1975.
49. Keys, A., Aravanis, C., Blackburn, G., et al.: Ann. Intern. Med., *77:*15–27, 1972.
50. Keys, A.: Nutr. Rev., *38:*297–307, 1980.
51. Waaler, H.T.: Acta Med. Scand., *(Suppl.) 679:*1–56, 1984.
52. Jarrett, R.J., Shipley, M.J., Rose, G.: Br. Med. J., *285:*535–537, 1982.
53. Libow, L.S.: Geriatrics, *29:*75–88, 1974.
54. Milne, J.S., Lauder, I.J.: Age Ageing, *7:*129–137, 1978.
55. Burr, M.I., Lennings, C.I., Milbank, J.E.: Age Ageing, *11:*249–255, 1982.
56. Rissanen, A., Heliovaara, M., Knekt, P., et al.: J. Clin. Epidemiol., *42:*781–789, 1988.
57. Garn, S.M., Hawthorne, V.M., Pilkington, J.J., et al.: Am. J. Clin. Nutr., *38:*313–319, 1983.
58. Build Study 1979. Chicago, Society of Actuaries and Association of Life Insurance Medical Directors, 1980.
59. Lew, E.A., Garfinkel, L.: J. Chronic Dis., *32:*563–576, 1979.
60. Lindsted, K., Tonstad, S., Kuzma, J.W.: Int. J. Obes., *15:*397–406, 1990.
61. Sidney, S., Friedman, G.D., Siegelaub, A.B.: Am. J. Public Health, *77:*317–322, 1987.
62. Keys, A.: Overweight and the Risk of Heart Attack and Sudden Death. Vol. 2. *In* Obesity in Perspective. Edited by G.A. Bray. Washington, D.C., Dept. of Health, Education and Welfare. NIH Publication No. 75–708, 1976, pp. 215–223.
63. Kannel, W.B., LeBauer, E.J., Dawber, T.R., et al.: Circulation, *35:*734–744, 1967.
64. Kannel, W.B., Gordon, T.: Physiological and medical concomitants of obesity: the Framingham study. *In* Obesity in America. Edited by G.A. Bray. Washington, D.C., Dept. of Health, Education and Welfare. NIH Publication No 79–359, 1979, pp. 125–163.
65. Manson, J.E., Colditz, G.A., Stampfer, M.J., et al.: N. Engl. J. Med., *372:*882–889, 1990.
66. Ostfeld, A.M., Gibson, D.C.: Epidemiology of Aging. Washington, D.C., Dept. of Health, Education and Welfare. NIH Publication No. 75–711, 1975, pp. 217–219.
67. Rabkin, S.W., Mathewson, F.A.L., Hsu, P.H.: Am. J. Cardiol., *39:*452–458, 1977.
68. Feinlieb, M.: Ann. Intern. Med., *103:*1019–1024, 1985.
69. Chapman, J.M., Coulson, A.H., Clark, V.A., et al.: J. Chronic Dis., *23:*631–645, 1971.
70. Bouchard, C., Bray, G., Hubbard, V.S.: Am. J. Clin. Nutr., *52:*946–950, 1990.
71. Larsson, B., Svardsudd, K., Welin, L., et al.: Br. Med. J., *289:*1257–1261, 1984.
72. Albrink, M.H., Meigs, J.W.: Am. J. Clin. Nutr., *15:*255–261, 1964.
73. Olefsky, J., Reaven, G.M., Farquhar, J.W.: J. Clin. Invest., *53:*64–76, 1974.
74. Bagdade, J.D., Bierman, E.L., Porte, D., Jr.: J. Clin. Invest., *46:*1549–1557, 1967.
75. Olefsky, J.M., Farquhar, J.W., Reaven, G.M.: Am. J. Med., *57:*551–560, 1974.
76. Havel, R.J., Kane, J.P., Balasse, E.O., et al.: J. Clin. Invest., *49:*2017–2035, 1970.
77. Pykalisto, O.J., Smith, P.H., Brunzell, J.D.: J. Clin. Invest., *56:*1108–1117, 1975.
78. Eckel, R.H., Yost, T.J.: J. Clin. Invest., *80:*992–997, 1987.
79. Kern, P.A., Ong, J.M., Saffari, B., et al.: N. Engl. J. Med., *322:*1053–1059, 1990.
80. Brunzell, J.D., Hazzard, W.R., Motulsky, A.G., et al.: Clin. Res., *22:*462a, 1974.
81. Rifkind, B.M., Begg, T.: Br. Med. J., *2:*208–210, 1966.
82. Montoye, H.J., Epstein, F.H., Kjelsberg, M.O.: Am. J. Clin. Nutr., *18:*397–406, 1966.
83. Kannel, W.B., Castelli, W.P., Gordon, T.: Ann. Intern. Med., *90:*85–91, 1979.
84. Yaari, S., Doldbourt, U., Even-Zohar, S., et al.: Lancet, *1:*1011–1015, 1981.

85. West, K.M., Kalbfkeisch, J.M.: Diabetes, *20:*99–108, 1971.
86. Hartz, A.J., Rupley, D.C., Kalkhoff, R.D., et al.: Prev. Med., *12:*351–357, 1983.
87. Kannel, W.B.: Health and obesity: An overview. *In* Health and Obesity. Edited by H.L. Conn, Jr., E.A. DeFelice and P. Kuo. New York, Raven Press, 1983.
88. Feldman, R., Sender, A.J., Siegelaub, A.B.: Diabetes, *18:*478–486, 1969.
89. Hartz, A.J., Rupley, D.C., Kalkhoff, R.D., et al.: Prev. Med., *2:*351–357, 1983.
90. Kissebah, A.H., Vydelingum, N., Murray, R.: J. Clin. Endocrinol. Metab., *54:*254–260, 1982.
91. Krotkiewski, M., Bjorntorp, P., Sjostrom, L., et al.: J. Clin. Invest., *72:*1150–1162, 1983.
92. Ohlson, L.O., Larsson, B., Svardsudd, K., et al.: Diabetes, *34:*1055–1058, 1985.
93. Haffner, S.M., Stern, M.P., Hazuda, H.P., et al.: JAMA, *263:*2893–2898, 1990.
94. Karam, J.H., Grodsky, G.M., Forsham, P.H.: Diabetes, *12:*197–204, 1963.
95. DeFronzo, R.A.: Diabetes, *37:*667–687, 1988.
96. Caro, J.F., Dohm, L.G., Pories, W.J., et al.: Diabetes Metab. Rev., *5:*665–689, 1989.
97. Granner, D.K., O'Brien, R.M.: Diabetes Care, *15:*369–395, 1992.
98. Kahn, C.R., Neville, D.M., Jr., Roth, J.: J. Biol. Chem., *248:*244–250, 1973.
99. Archer, J.A., Gorden, P., Roth, J.: J. Clin. Invest., *55:*166–174, 1975.
100. Olefsky, J.M.: J. Clin. Invest., *57:*1165–1172, 1976.
101. Roth, J., Kahn, C.R., Lesniak, M.A., et al.: Recent Prog. Horm. Res., *31:*95–126, 1976.
102. Kahn, C.R., White, M.F.: J. Clin. Invest., *82:*1151–1154, 1988.
103. Rosen, O.M.: Diabetes, *38:*1508–1514, 1989.
104. Garvey, W.T.: Diabetes Care, *15:*396–417, 1992.
105. Pfeifer, M.A., Halter, J.B., Porte, D., Jr.: Am. J. Med., *70:*579–588, 1981.
106. DeFronzo, R.A., Bonadonna, R.C., Ferrannini, E.: Diabetes Care, *15:*318–368, 1992.
107. Berchtold, P., Sims, E.A., Horton, E.S., et al.: Biomed. Pharmacother., *37:*251–258, 1983.
108. Stamler, J., Stamler, R., Romberg, A., et al.: J. Chronic Dis., *28:*499–525, 1975.
109. Tobian, L.: N. Engl. J. Med., *298:*46–48, 1978.
110. Johnson, B.C., Karunas, T.M., Epstein, F.H.: Clin. Sci. Mol. Med., *45(Suppl. 1):*355–455, 1973.
111. Kannel, W.B., Brand, N., Skinner, J.J.: Ann. Intern. Med., *67:*48–59, 1967.
112. Oberman, A., Lane, N.E., Harlan, W.R., et al.: Circulation, *36:*812–822, 1967.
113. Tyroler, H.A., Heyden, S., Harnes, C.G.: Weight and hypertension: Evans County studies of blacks and whites. *In* Epidemiology and Control of Hypertension. Edited by O. Paul. New York, Stratton Intercontinental Medical Book, 1975, pp. 177–201.
114. Reisin, E., Abel, R., Modan, et al.: N. Engl. J. Med., *298:*1–6, 1978.
115. Reisen, E., Frolich, E.D., Messerli, F.H., et al.: Ann. Intern. Med., *98:*315–319, 1983.
116. Dahl, L.K., Silver, L., Christie, R.W.: N. Engl. J. Med., *258:*1186–1192, 1958.
117. DeFronzo, R.A.: Insulin and renal sodium handling: clinical implications. *In* Recent Advances in Obesity Research. III. Edited by P. Bjorntorp, M. Cairella, and A.N. Howard. London, John Libbey, 1980, pp. 32–41.
118. DeFronzo, R.A., Goldberg, M., Agus, Z.: J. Clin. Invest., *58:*83–89, 1976.
119. DeFronzo, R.A., Cooke, C.R., Andres, R., et al.: J. Clin. Invest., *55:*845–855, 1975.
120. Kolanowski, J., Bodson, A., Desmecht, P., et al.: Eur. J. Clin. Invest., *8:*277–282, 1978.
121. Landsberg, L., Young, J.B.: N. Engl. J. Med., *298:*1295–1301, 1978.
122. Weinsier, R.L., Norris, D.J., Birch, R., et al.: Hypertension, *7:*578–585, 1985.
123. Bjorntorp, P.: Ann. Intern. Med., *103:*994–995, 1985.
124. Rimm, A.A., White, P.L.: Obesity: Its risks and hazards. *In* Obesity in America. Edited by G.A. Bray. Washington, D.C., NIH Publication No. 79–359, 1979, pp. 103–124.
125. GREPCO: The Rome Group for Epidemiology and Prevention of Cholelithiasis: Hepatology, *129:*587–595, 1988.
126. Jorgensen, T.: Gut, *30:*528–534, 1989.
127. Maclure, K.M., Hayes, K.C., Colditz, G.A., et al.: N. Engl. J. Med., *321:*563–569, 1989.
128. Bennion, L.J., Grundy, S.M.: J. Clin. Invest., *56:*996–1011, 1975.
129. Reuben, A., Qureshi, Y., Murphy, G.M., et al.: Eur. J. Clin. Invest., *16:*133–142, 1985.
130. Miettinen, T.A.: Horm. Metab. Res., *14:*37–44, 1974.
131. Marzio, L., Capone, F., Neri, M., et al.: Dig. Dis. Sci., *33:*4–9, 1988.
132. Grundy, S.M., Metzger, A.L., Adler, R.D.: J. Clin. Invest., *51:*3026–3043, 1972.
133. Leach, R.E., Baumgard, S., Broom, J.: Clin. Orthop., *93:*271–273, 1973.
134. Garfinkel, L.: Overweight and cancer. Ann. Intern. Med., *103:*1034–1036, 1985.
135. Blitzer, P.H., Blitzer, E.C., Rimm, A.A.: Prev. Med., *5:*20–31, 1976.
136. McMahon, B.: Gynecol. Oncol., *2:*122–129, 1974.
137. Dunn, L.J., Bradbury, J.T.: Am. J. Obstet. Gynecol., *97:*465–471, 1967.
138. DeWaard, F., Baanders-Van Halewijn, E.A.: Acta Cytol., *13:*675–678, 1969.
139. DeWaard, F.: Cancer Res., *35:*3351–3356, 1975.
140. Wynder, E.L., Bross, I.J., Hirayama, T.: Cancer, *13:*559–601, 1960.
141. Beer, A.E., Billingham, R.E.: Lancet, *1:*296, 1978.
142. Shields, J.: Monozygotic Twins Brought Up Apart and Brought Up Together. London, Oxford University Press, 1962.
143. Newman, H.H., Freeman, F.N., Holzinger, K.J.: Twins: A Study of Heredity and Environment. Chicago, University of Chicago Press, 1937.
144. Stunkard, A.J., Foch, T.T., Hrubec, Z.: JAMA, *256:*51–54, 1986.
145. Stunkard, A.J., Harris, J.R., Pedersen, N.L., et al.: N. Engl. J. Med., *322:*1438–1487, 1990.
146. Bouchard, C.: Inheritance of human fat distribution. *In* Fat Distribution During Growth and Later Health Outcomes. Edited by C. Bouchard and F.E. Johnston. New York, Alan Liss, 1988.
147. Bouchard, C.: Acta Med. Scand., *(Suppl.)723:*135–141, 1988.
148. Bouchard, C., Tremblay, A., Despres, J.P., et al.: N. Engl. J. Med., *322:*1477–1482, 1990.

149. Garn, S.M., Bailey, S.M.: Am. J. Clin. Nutr., *29:*1067–1068, 1976.
150. Garn, S.M., Clark, D.C.: Pediatrics, *57:*443–455, 1976.
151. Withers, R.F.J.: Eugenic Rev., *56:*81–90, 1964.
152. Biron, P., Mongeau, J.G., Bertrand, D.: J. Pediatr., *91:*555–558, 1977.
153. Rao, D.C., MacLean, C.J., Morton, N.E., et al.: Am. J. Hum. Genet., *27:*509–520, 1975.
154. Dunaif, A., Givens, J.R., Haseltine, F., et al.: The Polycystic Ovary Syndrome. Cambridge, MA, Blackwell Scientific, 1991.
155. Plymate, S.R., Fariss, B.L., Bassett, M.L., et al.: J. Clin. Endocrinol. Metab., *52:*1246–1248, 1981.
156. Sims, E.A.H., Danforth, E., Jr., Horton, E.J., et al.: Recent Prog. Horm. Res., *29:*457–476, 1973.
157. Ravussin, E., Lillioja, S., Anderson, T.E., et al.: J. Clin. Invest., *78:*1568–1578, 1986.
158. Bogardus, C., Lillioja, S., Ravussin, E., et al.: N. Engl. J. Med., *315:*96–100, 1986.
159. Bernstein, R.S., Thornton, J.C., Yang, M.U., et al.: Am. J. Clin. Nutr., *37:*595–602, 1983.
160. Zurlo, F., Larson, K., Bogardus, C., et al.: J. Clin. Invest., *86:*1423–1427, 1990.
161. Millward, D.J., Garlick, P.J.: Proc. Nutr. Soc., *35:*339–349, 1976.
162. Spady, B.W., Payne, P.R., Picou D., et al.: Am. J. Clin. Nutr., *29:*1073–1088, 1976.
163. Boothby, W.M., Berkson, J., Dunn, H.L., et al.: Am. J. Physiol., *116:*468–484, 1936.
164. James, W.P.T., Trayhurn, P.: Br. Med. Bull., *37:*43–48, 1981.
165. Ravussin, E., Burnand, B., Schutz, Y., et al.: Am. J. Clin. Nutr., *35:*566–573, 1982.
166. Roberts, S.B., Savage, J., Coward, W.A., et al.: N. Engl. J. Med., *318:*461–466, 1988.
167. Griffiths, M., Payne, P.R., Stunkard, A.J., et al.: Lancet, *336:*76–77, 1990.
168. Ravussin, E., Lillioja, S., Knowler, W.C., et al.: N. Engl. J. Med., *318:*467–472, 1988.
169. Zurlo, F., Lillioja, S., Esposito-Del Puente, A., et al.: Am. J. Physiol., *259:*E650–E657, 1990.
170. Swinburn, B.A., Nyomba, B.L., Saad, M.F.: J. Clin. Invest., *88:*168–173, 1991.
171. Shetty, P.S., Jung, R.T., James, W.P.T., et al.: Clin. Sci., *60:*519–525, 1981.
172. Pittet, P., Chappuis, P., Acheson, K., et al.: Br. J. Nutr., *35:*281–288, 1976.
173. Ravussin, E., Bogardus, C., Schwartz, R.S., et al.: J. Clin. Invest., *72:*893–902, 1983.
174. Strang, J.M., McClugage, H.B.: Am. J. Med. Sci., *182:*79–81, 1931.
175. Clough, D.P., Durnin, J.V.G.A.: J. Physiol., *207:*89P, 1970.
176. Felig, P., Cunningham, J., Levitt, M., et al.: Am. J. Physiol., *244:*E45–51, 1983.
177. Rothwell, N.J., Stock, M.J.: Metabolism, *30:*673, 678, 1981.
178. Golay, A., Schutz, Y., Meyer, H.U., et al.: Diabetes, *31:*1023–1028, 1982.
179. Segal, K.R., Lacayanga, I., Dunaif, A., et al.: Am. J. Physiol., *256:*E573–579, 1988.
180. Segal, K.R., Albu, J., Chun, A., et al.: J. Appl. Physiol., *71:*2402–2411, 1991.
181. Thorne, A.: Acta Chir. Scand., *(Suppl.) 558:*6–59, 1990.
182. Neumann, R.O.: Arch. Hyg., *45:*1–87, 1902.
183. Garrow, J.S.: The regulation of energy expenditure in men. *In* Recent Advances in Obesity Research. Vol 2. Edited by G.A. Bray. London, Newman, 1978, pp. 200–210.
184. James, W.P.T., Trayhurn, P.: Obesity in mice and men. *In* Nutritional Factors: Modulating Effects on Metabolic Processes. Edited by R.F. Beers and E.G. Barrett. New York, Raven Press, 1981, pp. 123–138.
185. Bradfield, R.B., Curtis, D.E., Margen, S.: Am. J. Clin. Nutr., *21:*1208–1210, 1968.
186. Segal, K.R., Gutin, B.: Metabolism, *32:*581–589, 1983.
187. Swindells, Y.E.: Br. J. Nutr., *27:*65–73, 1972.
188. Hansen, J.J.: J. Appl. Physiol., *35:*587–591, 1973.
189. Warnold, I., Lenner, R.A.: Am. J. Clin. Nutr., *30:*304–315, 1977.
190. Strong, J.A., Shirling, D., Passmore, R.: Br. J. Nutr., *21:*909–919, 1967.
191. Sims, E.A.H., Goldman, R.F., Gluck, C.M., et al.: Trans. Assoc. Am. Physicians, *81:*153–170, 1968.
192. Segal, K.R., Pi-Sunyer, F.X.: Med. Clin. North Am., *73:*217–236, 1989.
193. Sjostrom, L.: Fat cells and body weight. *In* Obesity. Edited by A.J. Stunkard. Philadelphia, W.B. Saunders, 1980.
194. Knittle, J.L., Hirsch, J.: J. Clin. Invest., *47:*2091–2098, 1968.
195. Hirsch, J., Han, P.W.: J. Lipid Res., *10:*77–82, 1969.
196. Braun, T., Kazdova, L., Fabry, P., et al.: Metab. Clin. Exp., *17:*825–832, 1968.
197. DiGirolamo, M., Mendlinger, S.: Am. J. Physiol., *221:*859–864, 1971.
198. Lemmonier, D.: J. Clin. Invest., *51:*2907–2915, 1972.
199. Hager, A., Sjostrom, L., Arvidsson, B., et al.: Metabolism, *26:*607–614, 1977.
200. Hager, A., Sjostrom, L., Arvidsson, B., et al.: Am. J. Clin. Nutr., *31:*68–75, 1978.
201. Krotkiewski, M., Sjostrom, L., Bjorntorp, P., et al.: Int. J. Obes., *1:*395–416, 1977.
202. Lithell, H., Boberg, J. Hellsing, K., et al.: Ups. J. Med. Sci., *83:*45–52, 1978.
203. Reitman, J.S., Kosmakos, F.C., Howard, B.V., et al.: J. Clin. Invest., *70:*791–797, 1982.
204. Schwartz, R., Brunzell, J.: Lancet, *1:*1230–1231, 1978.
205. Schwartz, R., Brunzell, J.: J. Clin. Invest., *67:*1425–1430, 1981.
206. Rebuffe-Scrive, M., Basdevant, A., Guy-Grand, B.: Am. J. Clin. Nutr., *37:*974–980, 1983.
207. Apfelbaum, M., Bostsarron, J., Lacatis, D.: Am. J. Clin. Nutr., *24:*1405–1409, 1971.
208. Grande, F., Anderson, J.T., Keys, A.: J. Appl. Physiol., *12:*230–238, 1958.
209. Owens, J.L., Thompson, D., Shah, N.: J. Nutr., *109:*1584–1591, 1979.
210. Bjorntrop, P., Enzi, G., Karlsson, M., et al.: Int. J. Obes., *4:*11–19, 1980.
211. DiGirolamo, M., Smith, U., Bjorntorp, P.: Refeeding effects on adipocyte metabolism. *In* Recent Advances in Obesity Research. Edited by P. Bjorntorp, M. Cairella, and A.N. Howard. London, John Libbey, 1980, pp. 99–105.
212. Bjorntorp, P., Yang, M.U.: Am. J. Clin. Nutr., *36:*444–449, 1982.
213. Leibel, R.L., Hirsch, J.: Metabolism, *33:*164–170, 1984.
214. Faust, J.M., Johnson, P.R., Hirsch, J.: Science, *197:*393–396, 1977.
215. Krotkiewski, M., Sjostrom, L., Bjorntorp, P.: Int. J. Obes., *1:*395–416, 1977.

216. Van Itallie, T.B.: Am. J. Clin. Nutr., *31:*543–552, 1978.
217. Caspary, W.F.: Lancet, *1:*1231–1233, 1977.
218. Council on Foods and Nutrition: JAMA, *224:*1415–1419, 1973.
219. Rickman, F., Mitchell, N., Dingman, J., et al.: JAMA, *228:*54–58, 1974.
220. Pritikin, N.: Live Longer Now: The First One Hundred Years of Your Life. New York, Grosset and Dunlap, 1974.
221. Lissner, L., Levitsky, D.A., Strupp, B.J., et al.: Am. J. Clin. Nutr., *46:*886–892, 1987.
222. Kendall, A., Levitsky, D.A., Strupp, B.J., et al.: Am. J. Clin. Nutr., *53:*1124–1129, 1991.
223. Weinsier, R.L., Johnston, M.H., Doleys, D.M., et al.: Br. J. Nutr., *47:*367–379, 1982.
224. Thompson, T.J., Runcie, J., Miller, V.: Lancet, *2:*992–996, 1966.
225. Drenick, E.J., Swendseid, M.E., Blahd, W.H., et al.: JAMA, *187:*100–105, 1964.
226. Felig, P., Owen, O.E., Wahren, J., et al.: J. Clin. Invest., *48:*584–594, 1969.
227. Lindner, P.G., Blackburn, G.L.: Obes. Bariatric Med., *5:*198–216, 1976.
228. Wadden, T.A., Stunkard, A.J., Brownell, K.D.: Ann. Intern. Med., *99:*675–684, 1983.
229. Owen, O.E., Felig, P., Morgan, A.P., et al.: J. Clin. Invest., *48:*574–583, 1969.
230. Calloway, D.H., Odell, A.C.F., Margen, S.: J. Nutr., *101:*775–786, 1971.
231. Felig, P., Owen, O.E., Wahren, J., et al.: J. Clin. Invest., *48:*584–594, 1969.
232. Consolazio, C.F., Matoush, L.O., Johnson, H.L., et al.: Am. J. Clin. Nutr., *21:*803–812, 1968.
233. Apfelbaum, M., Bostsarron, J., Brigant, L., et al.: Gastroenterologia, *108:*121–134, 1967.
234. Bistrian, B.R., Winterer, J., Blackburn, G., et al.: J. Lab. Clin. Med., *89:*1030–1035, 1977.
235. Baird, I.M., Parsons, R.L., Howard, A.N.: Metabolism, *23:*645–657, 1974.
236. Genuth, S.M., Castro, J.H., Vertes, V.: JAMA, *230:*987–991, 1974.
237. Vertes, V., Genuth, S.M., Hazelton, I.M.: JAMA, *238:*2151–2153, 1977.
238. Flatt, J.P., Blackburn, G.L.: Am. J. Clin. Nutr., *27:*175–187, 1974.
239. Sherwin, R.S., Hendler, R.G., Felig, P.: J. Clin. Invest., *55:*1382–1390, 1975.
240. Marliss, E.B., Murray, F.T., Nakhooda, A.F.: J. Clin. Invest., *62:*468–479, 1978.
241. Landau, R.L., Rochman, H., Blix-Gruber, P., et al.: Am. J. Clin. Nutr., *34:*1300–1304, 1981.
242. Frattali, V.P.: FDA By-Lines *9:*179, 1979.
243. Sours, H.E., Frattali, V.P., Brand, C.D., et al.: Am. J. Clin. Nutr., *34:*453–461, 1981.
244. Singh, B.N., Gaarder, T.D., Kanegae, T., et al.: JAMA, *240:*115–119, 1978.
245. Van Itallie, T.B.: JAMA, *240:*144–145, 1978.
246. Jones, A.O.L., Jacobs, R.M., Fry, B.E., et al.: Am. J. Clin. Nutr., *33:*2545–2550, 1980.
247. Pi-Sunyer, F.X.: Am. J. Clin. Nutr., *56:*240s–243s, 1992.
248. DeHaven, J., Sherwin, R., Hendler, R., et al.: N. Engl. J. Med., *302:*477–482, 1980.
249. Sigler, M.H.: J. Clin. Invest., *55:*377–387, 1975.
250. Yang, M.U., Van Itallie, T.B.: J. Clin. Invest., *58:*722–730, 1976.
251. Yang, M., Barbosa-S, J.L., Pi-Sunyer, F.X., et al.: Int. J. Obes., *5:*231–236, 1981.
252. Pi-Sunyer, F.X.: Obesity. *In* Conn's Current Therapy. Edited by R.E. Rackel. Philadelphia, W.B. Saunders, 1985.
253. Steinhaus, A.H.: Physiol. Rev., *13:*103–147, 1983.
254. Karpovitch, P.V.: Res. Q., *12:*423–431, 1941.
255. Woo, R., Garrow, J.S., Pi-Sunyer, F.X.: Am. J. Clin. Nutr., *36:*470–477, 1982.
256. Woo, R., Garrow, J.S., Pi-Sunyer, F.X.: Am. J. Clin. Nutr., *36:*478–484, 1982.
257. Freedman-Akabas, S., Colt, E., Kissileff, H.R., et al.: Am. J. Clin. Nutr., *4:*545–549, 1985.
258. Adams, R.P., Welch, H.G.: J. Appl. Physiol., *49:*863–868, 1980.
259. Passmore, R., Thomson, J.G., Warnock, G.M.: Br. J. Nutr., *6:*253–264, 1952.
260. Woo, R., Pi-Sunyer, F.X.: Metabolism, *34:*836–841, 1985.
261. Dempsey, J.A.: Res. Q., *35:*275–287, 1964.
262. Williams, B.T.: J. Am. Geriatr. Soc., *16:*794–797, 1968.
263. Boileau, R.A., Buskirk, E.R., Horstman, D.H., et al.: Med. Sci. Sports, *3:*183–189, 1971.
264. Pi-Sunyer, F.X., Woo, R.: Am. J. Clin. Nutr., *42:*983–990, 1985.
265. Rissanen, A., Heliovara, M., Knekt, P., et al.: Eur. J. Clin. Invest., *45:*419–430, 1991.
266. King, A.C., Tribble, D.L.: Sports Med., *11:*331–349, 1991.
267. Pavlou, K.N., Krey, S., Steffee, W.P.: Am. J. Clin. Nutr., *49:*1115–1123, 1989.
268. Craddock, D.: Obesity and Its Management. 3rd Ed. Edinburgh, Churchill Livingstone, 1978, pp. 92–109.
269. Evans, E.R., Wallace, M.G.: Curr. Med. Res. Opin., *4:*132–137, 1975.
270. Sullivan, A.C., Cheng, L.: Appetite regulation and its modulation by drugs. *In* Nutrition and Drug Interrelations. Edited by J.N. Hathcock and J. Coon. New York, Academic Press, 1978.
271. Griboff, S.L., Berman, R., Silverman, H.I.: Curr. Ther. Res. Clin. Exp., *17:*535–543, 1975.
272. Hoebel, B.G., Krauss, I., Cooper, J., et al.: Obes. Bariatric Med., *4:*200–206, 1975.
273. Bray, G.A.: Ann. Intern. Med., *115:*152–153, 1991.
274. Weintraub, M., Sundaresan, P.R., Madan, M., et al.: Clin. Pharmacol. Ther., *51:*581–642, 1992.
275. Van Itallie, T.B.: Am. J. Clin. Nutr., *32:*2723–2733, 1979.
276. Bruch, H.: Eating Disorders: Obesity, Anorexia Nervosa and the Person Within. New York, Basic Books, 1973.
277. Rand, C.S., Stunkard, A.J.: J. Am. Acad. Psychoanal., *5:*459–497, 1977.
278. Powers, P.S.: Obesity, the Regulation of Body Weight. Baltimore, Williams & Wilkins, 1980.
279. Halmi, K.A., Stunkard, J.A., Mason, E.E.: Am. J. Nutr., *33:*446–451, 1980.
280. Glucksman, M.L., Hirsch, J.: Psychosom. Med., *31:*1–7, 1969.
281. Crisp, A.H., McGuiness, B.: Br. Med. J., *1:*7–9, 1975.
282. Telch, C.F., Agras, W.S., Rossiter, E., et al.: J. Consult. Clin. Psychol., *58:*629–635, 1990.
283. Schachter, S.: Am. Psychol., *26:*129–144, 1971.
284. Schachter, S.: Emotion, Obesity and Crime. New York, Academic Press, 1971.
285. Rodin, J.: The externality theory today. *In* Obesity. Edited by A.J. Stunkard. Philadelphia, W.B. Saunders, 1980.
286. Stuart, R.B.: Behav. Res. Ther., *5:*357–365, 1967.

287. Mahoney, M.J.: Psychiatr. Clin. North Am., *1*:651–660, 1978.
288. Stunkard, A.J.: Int. J. Obes., *2*:237–249, 1978.
289. Jeffrey, R.W., Thompson, P.D., Wing, R.R.: Behav. Res. Ther., *16*:363–370, 1978.
290. Stalonas, P.M., Johnson, W.G., Christ, M.: J. Consult. Clin. Psychol., *46*:463–469, 1978.
291. Wadden, T.A., Sternberg, J.A., Letizia, K.A., et al.: Int. J. Obes., *13*:39–46, 1989.
292. Pi-Sunyer, F.X.: Am. J. Clin. Nutr., *29*:409–416, 1976.
293. Mason, E.E., Ito, C.: Surg. Clin. North Am., *47*:1345–1351, 1967.
294. Tretbar, L.L., Sifers, E.C.: Int. J. Obes., *5*:538, 1981.
295. Kral, J.: Surgical treatment of obesity. *In* Obesity. Edited by P. Bjorntorp and B.M. Brodoff. Philadelphia, J.B. Lippincott, 1992.
296. Lissner L., Odell, P.M., D'Agostino, R.B.: N. Engl. J. Med., *324*:1839–1844, 1991.
297. Hamm, P., Shekele, R.B., Stamler, J.: Am. J. Epidemiol., *129*:312–318, 1989.
298. Wing, R.R.: Ann. Behav. Med., *14*:113–119, 1992.
299. Jebb, S.A., Goldberg, G.R., Coward, W.A., et al.: Int. J. Obes., *15*:367–374, 1991.

CHAPTER 60

Nutrition In Relation To Dental Medicine

Dominick P. DePaola, Mary P. Faine, Richard I. Vogel

CELLULAR AND STRUCTURAL CHARACTERISTICS OF THE ORAL TISSUES

Distinctive characteristics of oral tissues may render them particularly sensitive to nutritional extremes. For example, the inability of enamel to remodel, coupled with the high turnover rate of oral mucosa, makes oral tissues a unique indicator of physiologic perturbations.

In the same vein, nutrition and oral health and disease transcend the relationship between fermentable carbohydrates and dental caries. The oral cavity is the site of chronic disease (e.g., caries, periodontal disease(s), AIDS, herpes, salivary gland disorders, cancer), and congenital anomalies (such as cleft lip and palate), which could relate to nutritional status. Nutrients interact with physiologic systems in the oral cavity, such as cell replication, cell repair, and immune response mechanisms, in such a manner as to increase or decrease the risk of disease. Thus, the oral tissues constitute a major site of interactions between nutritional factors and the physiologic systems, a relationship that makes oral health no less vulnerable to the effect of nutrition than general health. It is imperative, therefore, to consider the unique cellular and structural characteristics of the oral tissues to understand the oral diseases related to nutritional abnormalities.

Teeth are specialized structures vital for the initial processing of food composed of three mineralized tissues, enamel, dentin, and cementum, which encase the highly vascular dental pulp or "nerve." These relationships can be seen in the schematic cross section of a tooth in Figure 60–1. The teeth are retained in their bony sockets by means of a fibrous structure termed the periodontal membrane or ligament. Influences that affect the integrity of this structure and bone surrounding the socket result in periodontal disease that may progress sufficiently to cause loosening and loss of the teeth.[1]

Each tooth develops from a tooth bud or germ located in the jaws. The bud consists of an epithelial component that arises as an invagination from the surface and produces enamel. The mesenchymal component consists of the dental papilla, which produces the tooth pulp and dentin, and the dental follicle, which produces the cementum and periodontal ligament once the tooth has formed. Table 60–1 details the chronology of the human dentition. The primary teeth begin forming about 6 weeks in utero when cells in the primitive oral cavity differentiate to form the dental lamina, which is the site of tooth bud development. The formation of the crown of the tooth begins with the secretion of a dentin matrix containing collagen fibrils. Mineral ions then enter the

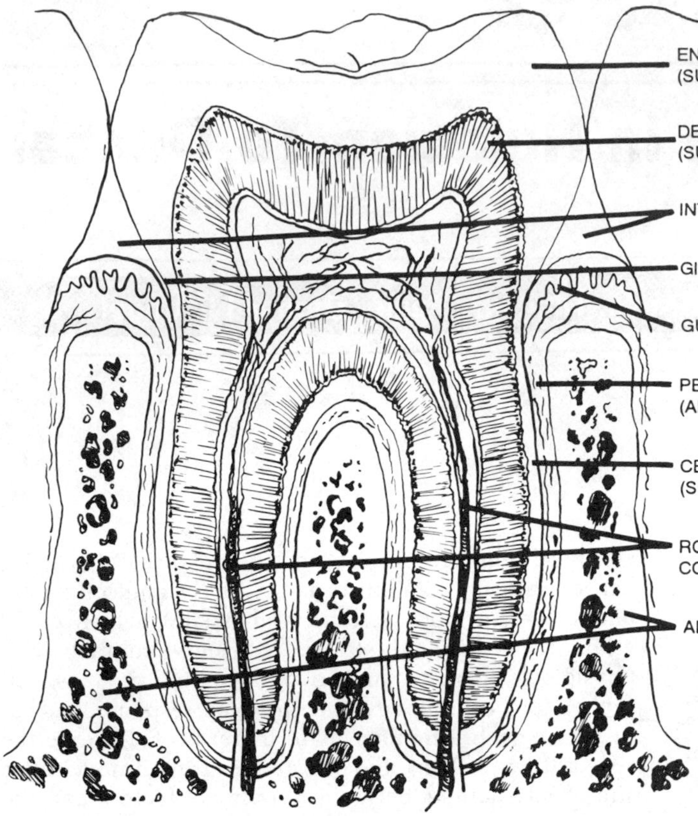

FIGURE 60–1. Schematic illustration of teeth in contact with the alveolar bone.

matrix to form small crystals on or between the collagen fibrils. Enamel formation begins as soon as the first dentin layer has been laid down. This mineralization process constitutes the maturation of enamel and continues after all the matrix is formed. As can be seen in Table 60–1, the mineralization process begins as early as 4 months in utero and continues into late adolescence. After the tooth erupts into the oral cavity, it continues to incorporate minerals (including fluoride) into its structure from saliva, food, and drinking fluids.[2]

The life history of a tooth may be divided into three main eras: (1) the period during which its crown is forming and mineralizing in the jaw; (2) the period of maturation when the tooth is erupting into the oral cavity and its root or roots are forming; and (3) the maintenance period while it is functioning in the oral cavity.[1]

During the pre-eruptive period, the developing enamel and dentin are subject to nutritional deficiencies or imbalances in the same manner as any other developing tissues. Indeed, nutrient deficiencies can affect either the secretory or the maturation stage of enamel formation. For example, hypoplastic lesions in the enamel reflect disturbances affecting the secretory process, whereas hypomineralized defects reflect interference with the maturation process. These are systemic effects of nutrient imbalances. Of course, both hypoplasia and hypocalcification can be induced by other environmental stresses, such as febrile episodes, genetic defects, and chemical toxicants. Following eruption into the oral cavity, the enamel is bathed in saliva and is exposed to oral micro-organisms and their by-products as well as food, so nutritional deficiencies or excesses and dietary habits may affect teeth in a totally different or more local manner.[2]

At least three striking differences exist between the mineralized tissues of the teeth and the other tissues of the body. First, enamel contains no capillary or lymphatic vessels to act as transport systems; however, the intimate relationships between the organic and the inorganic components of enamel suggest that pathways in the enamel exist for diffusion of ions and small molecules from saliva, and possibly from blood. Although the dentin likewise contains no formed vascular elements, it is more readily permeable to the passage of extracellular fluids from the blood, by reason of the dentinal tubules that traverse the dentin. The interchange between elements in the enamel takes place through the bathing of its external surface with saliva. In contrast, the interchange in the dentin occurs by reason of the ions present in the blood supply to the pulp or periodontal membrane.[1]

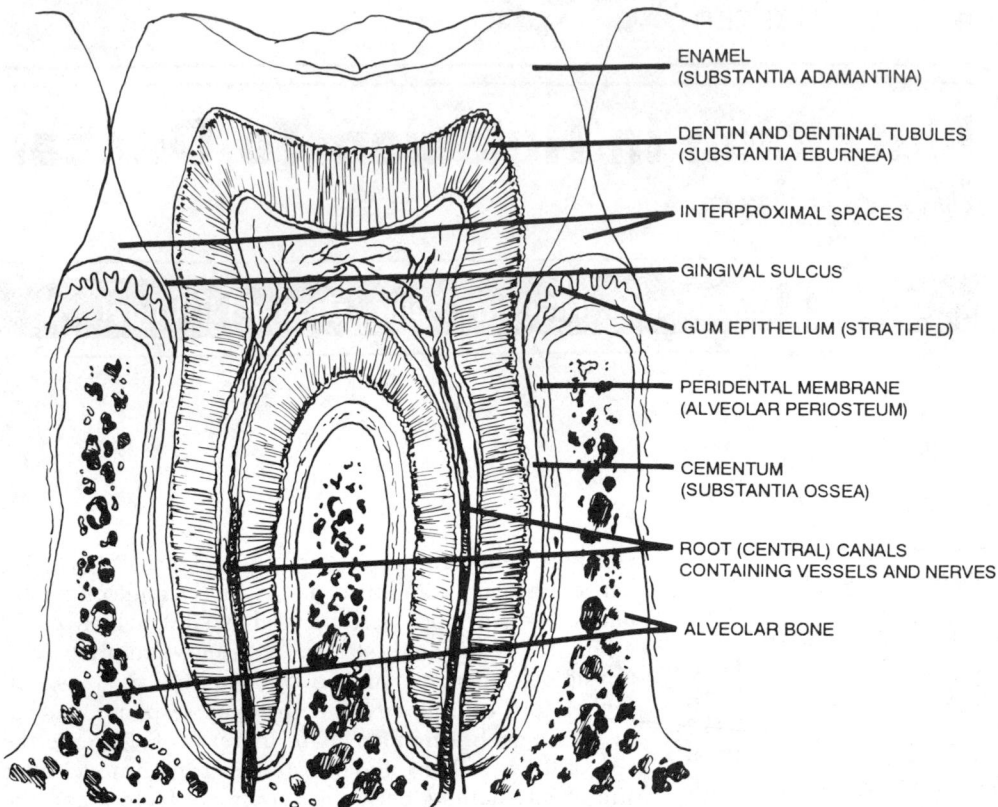

Second, owing to the absence of cells, mineralized dental tissues do not have a microscopically or chemically detectable ability to repair improperly formed or mineralized areas, and the tooth does not have the ability to repair itself after a portion has been destroyed

TABLE 60–1. CHRONOLOGY OF DEVELOPMENT OF THE HUMAN DENTITION

TOOTH	HARD TISSUE FORMATION BEGINS	AMOUNT OF ENAMEL FORMED AT BIRTH	ENAMEL COMPLETED	ERUPTION	ROOT COMPLETED
Primary Dention					
Maxillary					
Central incisor	4 mo in utero	Five sixths	1½ mo	7½ mo	1½ yr
Lateral incisor	4½ mo in utero	Two thirds	2½ mo	9 mo	2 yr
Cuspid	5 mo in utero	One third	9 mo	18 mo	3¼ yr
First molar	5 mo in utero	Cusps united	6 mo	14 mo	2½ yr
Second molar	6 mo in utero	Cusp tips still isolated	11 mo	24 mo	3 yr
Mandibular					
Central incisor	4½ mo in utero	Three fifths	2½ mo	6 mo	1½ yr
Lateral incisor	4½ mo in utero	Three fifths	3 mo	7 mo	1½ yr
Cuspid	5 mo in utero	One third	9 mo	16 mo	3¼ yr
First molar	5 mo in utero	Cusps united	5½ mo	12 mo	2¼ yr
Second molar	6 mo in utero	Cusp tips still isolated	10 mo	20 mo	3 yr
Permanent Dentition					
Maxillary					
Central incisor	3–4 mo	—	4–5 yr	7–8 yr	10 yr
Lateral incisor	10–12 mo	—	4–5 yr	8–9 yr	11 yr
Cuspid	4–5 mo	—	6–7 yr	11–12 yr	13–15 yr
First bicuspid	1½–1¾ yr	—	5–6 yr	10–11 yr	12–13 yr
Second bicuspid	2–2¼ yr	—	6–7 yr	10–12 yr	12–14 yr
First molar	at birth	Sometimes a trace	2½–3 yr	6–7 yr	9–10 yr
Second molar	2½–3 yr	—	7–8 yr	12–13 yr	14–16 yr
Mandibular					
Central incisor	3–4 mo	—	4–5 yr	6–7 yr	9 yr
Lateral incisor	3–4 mo	—	4–5 yr	7–8 yr	10 yr
Cuspid	4–5 mo	—	6–7 yr	9–10 yr	12–14 yr
First bicuspid	1¾–2 yr	—	5–6 yr	10–12 yr	12–13 yr
Second bicuspid	2¼–2½ yr	—	6–7 yr	11–12 yr	13–14 yr
First molar	at birth	Sometimes a trace	2½–3 yr	6–7 yr	9–10 yr
Second molar	2½–3 yr	—	7–8 yr	11–13 yr	14–15 yr

(Adapted and slightly modified by Massler and Shour) from Logan, W.A.G., Kronfeld, R.: J. Am. Dent. Assoc., *20*:420, 1933.

by tooth decay or mechanical injury. An exception is the remineralization of slightly demineralized, superficial areas of the enamel where the organic matrix and surface integrity are still intact, commonly referred to as "white spots." In addition, secondary dentin is formed by the odontoblasts, which persist throughout life on the pulpal surface of the dentin, in response to chemical stimuli from an advancing carious lesion in an effort to wall off the noxious influence. Lack of ability to repair dental tissues is in direct contrast to bone, with its continual turnover and ability to remodel.[1]

Third, unlike other tissues, the mineralized tissues of teeth have a partial change of environment midway in their life. When the tooth begins to emerge into the oral cavity, the vascular supply to the enamel organ is severed, and the enamel surface comes in contact with a complex mixture of saliva, micro-organisms, food debris, and epithelial remnants. Thus, instead of a pure systemic environment, the erupted tooth has, in addition, an oral or external environment. As a consequence, the enamel and cementum surfaces on which carious lesions are initiated by microbial action are largely outside the influences of humoral immune systems, so immune relationships with the caries process are primarily limited to those in saliva.[1]

The development and maintenance of the soft tissues and bone that support the teeth are also subject to nutrient defects. The periodontium, as seen in Figure 60–1, comprises the gingiva, the periodontal ligament (peridental membrane), which joins the root cementum to the alveolar bone, the root cementum, which is a specialized, mineralized tissue similar to bone that covers the root of the tooth, and the alveolar bone, which forms and supports the sockets of the teeth. The alveolar bone grows in response to dental eruption, is modified by dental changes, and resorbs when teeth are lost. The finite space between the tooth and the gingiva, known as the gingival sulcus, is lined by a nonkeratinized epithelium. In addition, dental plaque, one of the primary agents responsible for the initiation of both dental caries and gingivitis, contains a high concentration of bacteria, which, in the gingival sulcus, is juxtaposed with a "naked" epithelium. Thus, bacteria and their by-products or antigens can permeate the gingival epithelium and precipitate a classic inflammatory response that denotes periodontal disease(s). In fact, an intact immune system, which is highly dependent on nutrient status, is vital to maintain periodontal health. In this same vein, another unique characteristic of the oral soft tissues is that they undergo rapid turnover rates; thus, continued optimum levels of nutrients are necessary to promote oral health and to prevent disease. Indeed, the diversity of hard and soft tissues that comprise the oral structures and the distinctive nutritional needs of each contribute to the uniqueness of the mouth as an external reflection of past and present nutritional problems.[3]

ROLE OF NUTRITION IN CRANIOFACIAL AND ORAL TISSUE DEVELOPMENT

Many severe and even moderate nutrient deficits can result in defects in tooth development. The most commonly studied nutrients and conditions that have affected tooth integrity, enamel solubility, and salivary flow and composition in animal models include protein/calorie malnutrition, ascorbic acid, vitamin A, vitamin D, calcium/phosphorus, iron, zinc, and fluoride. Only protein/calorie malnutrition, deficiencies of vitamin A, ascorbic acid, vitamin D, and iodine, and fluoride excess have been demonstrated to affect the human dentition. See Table 60–2.

Characteristically, enamel hypoplastic defects and hypomineralization have been the hallmarks of under- or overnutrition during tooth development. For example, Sweeney et al. noted that 73% of Guatemalan children with third-degree malnutrition and 43% of children with second-degree malnutrition had hypoplasia of enamel formed prior to the diagnosis of malnutrition.[4] Data on 45 malnourished children in a marginal population supported the findings of Sweeney.[5]

Vitamin A deficiency has been implicated as a critical factor because it frequently accompanies protein/calorie malnutrition and is known to affect epithelial tissue development, tooth morphogenesis, and odontoblast differentiation.[6] Protracted vitamin A deficiency during tooth development results in atrophy of the enamel organ, metaplasia of the ameloblasts, and defective apposition and calcification of dentin.[3] The interference with calcification is expressed clinically by enamel hypoplasia.[7]

Vitamin D, calcium, and phosphorus deficiencies all result in significant effects on tooth development and resistance to the caries challenge. Vitamin D deficiency appears to exert its metabolic effect through lowering plasma calcium levels; it has been difficult to localize vitamin D metabolites in target tooth and bone cells.[8] Leaver has demonstrated that extreme calcium and phosphorus deficiencies may result in hypomineralization of developing teeth.[9] The deficit must be severe enough to reduce plasma levels of calcium and phosphorus. This finding suggests that the occurrence of this

TABLE 60–2. EFFECTS OF NUTRIENT DEFICIENCIES ON TOOTH DEVELOPMENT

NUTRIENT	EFFECT ON TISSUE	EFFECT ON CARIES	HUMAN DATA
Protein/calorie malnutrition	Tooth eruption delayed Tooth size decreased Enamel solubility decreased Salivary gland dysfunction	Yes	Yes
Vitamin A	↓ Epithelial tissue development Tooth morphogenesis dysfunction ↓ Odontoblast differentiation ↑ Enamel hypoplasia	Yes	Yes
Vitamin D/calcium/ phosphorus	Lowered plasma calcium Hypomineralization (hypoplastic defects) Tooth integrity compromised (decreased mineral concentration) Delayed eruption patterns	Yes	Yes
Acorbic acid	Dental pulpal alterations Odontoblastic degeneration Aberrant dentin	No	No
Fluoride	Increase in stability of enamel crystal (enamel formation) Inhibition of demineralization Stimulation of remineralization Mottled enamel (excess) Inhibition of bacterial growth	Yes	Yes
Iodine	Delayed tooth eruption Altered growth patterns Malocclusion?	No	Yes
Iron	Slow growth Salivary gland dysfunction	Yes	No

mechanism in the human population is unlikely, because of the highly effective homeostatic mechanisms that mobilize calcium from the skeleton to maintain normal plasma calcium levels. Bawden postulates that vitamin D hypovitaminosis may be more important in considering hypomineralization due to inadequate calcium transport into developing dental tissues.[10] Vitamin D deficiency has also been shown to affect tooth structure and to delay eruption patterns of teeth.[11]

In childhood vitamin D deficiency, the teeth are characterized microscopically by a widened layer of predentin, by the presence of interglobular dentin, and by interference with enamel formation (hypoplastic defects).[12] Young children with rickets have delayed eruption of the deciduous teeth, and the sequence of eruption is altered.[3] The permanent incisors, cuspids, and first molars are usually affected because their development coincides with the age at which rickets is most common.[3] Vitamin D-resistant rickets result in more frequent and severe tooth defects relative to primary rickets, including large pulps with developmental "exposures" of the pulp.

Vitamin C deficiency has also been demonstrated to affect tooth development and eruption. Deciduous and permanent teeth of scorbutic infants contain minute pulpal hemorrhages attributable to vitamin C deficiency. In older vitamin C-deficient children, the dental pulp undergoes hyperemia, edema, necrosis, and aberrant calcification, whereas the dentin shows odontoblastic degeneration and irregular formation.[13] The relation of vitamin C deficiency to dental caries is poorly defined, however. Indeed, although it is likely that the primary mechanism of vitamin C deficiency-induced tooth, gingival, and bone disease is mediated through the disruption of collagen biosyntheses, no study has clearly demonstrated the relationship between scurvy and dental caries.[14]

In areas where goiter is endemic, children born to mothers with severe iodine deficiency are characterized by marked mental and physical growth retardation. Eruption of the primary and secondary teeth is often greatly delayed and precluded. Malocclusion is relatively common because of the altered patterns of craniofacial growth and development.[3]

Perhaps the most intriguing and important data on nutritional status during development and oral disease come from observations on malnutrition and dental caries. Several studies have demonstrated that tooth eruption is delayed, tooth integrity is compromised (especially enamel surface solubility), and dental caries is increased in animals and in chronically malnourished children.[15,16] A study in Lima, Peru demonstrated significant delays in tooth eruption and exfoliation in three groups of malnourished children; such delays were associated with and appeared to be the direct cause of a significant temporal delay in caries development in the primary teeth.[106] These data support previous studies on malnourished children in India and Guatemala.[17,18]

Clearly, the development of teeth and salivary glands is intimately associated with the nutrient supply. Teeth subjected to nutritional insult during critical stages of development show a diminished ability to withstand caries and thus are at a higher risk. In many studies, impaired salivary function has accompanied the morphologic changes in teeth, which may be a primary factor in the subsequent increase in caries susceptibility.[19] These data also explain the positive association between socioeconomic status and the prevalence of dental caries in deciduous but not permanent teeth.[16] Nutritional injuries early in life may affect tooth formation and may result in increased caries susceptibility, whereas chronic malnutrition is associated with delayed tooth emergence and a shift of the curve for caries prevalence versus age.[16] Thus, in understanding any cross-sectional survey on caries prevalence, the nutritional history must be taken into account.

On a broader scale, 7% of babies born in the United States each year have some mental or physical defect evident at birth or later.[20] Prominent among these defects are structural, functional, or biochemical abnormalities involving the craniofacial complex. The most common of these malformations are cleft lip and cleft palate, affecting 1 out of 600 white infants, with the incidence higher among Asians, Native Americans, and Eskimos and lower among blacks.[20] One out of 1600 babies born alive suffers from craniofacial anomalies other than cleft lip or palate, including jaw deformities, defects in ossification, malformed or missing teeth, facial asymmetries, and defects that are a component of other syndromes, such as fetal alcohol syndrome.[20] Fetal alcohol syndrome consists primarily of small size for gestational age, dysmorphism (especially of the face and eyes, heart, joints, and internal genitalia), and mental deficiency. Of particular interest are the facial aberrant growth patterns, which include a low nasal bridge, short palpebral fissures, indistinct philtrum of the lip, thin upper lip, short nose, small midface, epicanthic folds, and small head circumference.[21]

In addition, certain other craniofacial oral-dental disorders such as craniosynostosis, hemifacial microsomia, anodontia, amelogenesis imperfecta, dentinogenesis imperfecta, osteogenesis imperfecta, chondrodystrophies, and juvenile periodontitis represent major challenges to human oral health.[22] Many of these malformations and disorders have a genetic basis or an environmental cause. Certain nutrients given in excess, especially early in pregnancy (e.g., retinoic acid, and other lipophilic molecules such as vitamins K and E) are known to induce craniofacial oral-dental malformations. Therapeutic doses of 13-cis retinoic acid administered to treat cystic acne have resulted in significant craniofacial oral-dental malformations when the agent is taken during the first trimester of pregnancy. The molecular mechanisms during these genetic-environmental interactions are not known.[22]

A small proportion of craniofacial malformities can be traced to specific genetic or chromosomal disorders, whereas another group can result from environmental factors, such as malnutrition, maternal disease, exposure to drugs, and obstetric problems. Most investigators believe, however, that craniofacial malformations have a multifactorial basis, in which particular genes alter the ability of the developing fetus to adapt to environmental factors.[20] Indeed, evidence from studies of identical twins clearly establishes the role of environmental and genetic factors in cases of isolated cleft lip or cleft palate.[20]

The regulatory genes and gene products functioning as transcriptional factors for the branchial arches that give rise to the midface and lower face are being discovered, and their interactions with nutrients (e.g., retinoic acid via its specific receptors) has been found to be critical to craniofacial oral-dental morphogenesis.[23] A superfamily of genes is now considered to interact with nutrients during instructive stages of craniofacial development in the mammalian embryo (i.e., at about 19 to 26 days of gestation in the human embryo). Endogenous retinoic acid appears to function as a developmental organizer during limb development and limb regeneration. Excess exogenous retinoic acid produces significant craniofacial malformations associated with clefting, dental development, hemifacial microsomia, spina bifida, eye defects, and limb morphogenesis.[24] What the function is of endogenous retinoic acid in craniofacial development and how excess levels of retinoic acid might produce congenital malformations are two central questions in this area[25] (see also Chap. 16 on differentiation and morphogenesis). A striking illustration of the need to understand the effects of nutrition on birth defects is the recent datum that demonstrated that folate supplements provided around the time of conception significantly reduced the recurrence of neural tube defects among high-risk individuals in the United Kingdom.[26]

Dietary advice following thorough diagnostic endeavors can materially benefit the expectant mother, lactating woman, or infant. The dependence of proper oral tissue development on adequate nutrient supply is clear. When dietary advice is provided during such critical development times, it is appropriate to consult with other professionals, including physicians, dietitians, and nutritionists, to ensure reasonable and substantive therapy. Most important, appropriate dietary counseling, particularly with reference to critical developmental times, and intake of essential nutrients, can ensure optimal oral health. Clearly, this knowledge base has profound implications for the continuing advancement of nutrition in the education of the dental health-care professional and in integrating dentistry more closely with medicine and the health-care delivery system.

NUTRITION AND DENTAL CARIES

Dental caries is a preventable infectious disease of the oral cavity and is a major cause of tooth loss in children and adults in the United States. Caries has declined among children (Fig. 60–2), however. A measure of the level of dental caries in a population is the decayed-missing-filled-surface (DMFS) rate. This represents the

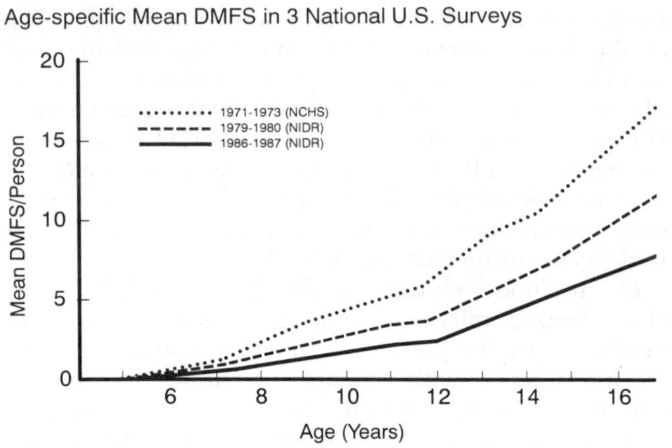

FIGURE 60–2. Age-specific mean decayed, missing, and filled surfaces (DMFS) index in three national United States surveys. (From National Institute of Dental Research: The National Survey of U.S. School Children: 1986–1987. NIH Publication No. 89-2247. Washington D.C., United States Government Printing Office, 1989.)

sum of the number of permanent tooth surfaces (out of a possible 128 surfaces on 32 teeth) that are decayed, missing, or filled. A national survey conducted in 1986 and 1987 of United States children aged 5 to 17 showed that approximately half of all subjects examined had a caries-free dentition; however, the mean DMFS rate was 3.07 per child.[27] In comparison, in 1979 and 1980, 37% of school children examined had no caries in their permanent teeth, and the mean DMFS rate was 4.77.[28] This marked decline in caries is primarily attributed to the widespread use of fluorides. However, dental decay increases with age, so by 17 years of age, only 15.6% of United States teens studied in the latest survey were caries free (Fig. 60–3). Cavitation occurs most frequently (58%) on the occlusal or chewing surface of the tooth. Importantly, decay on the smooth surfaces of teeth has declined 34% since 1980, whereas interproximal caries has nearly been eradicated in the younger age groups.[27]

Based on data collected in the National Institute of Dental Research (NIDR) Oral Health Survey of Adults and Seniors in 1985 to 1986, the incidence of dental caries in adults in the United States appears to be rising.[29] The oldest employed adults surveyed had a mean of 29 decayed and filled tooth surfaces. In adults 60 years of age or older who were examined, 2 to 3% were caries free and 41% were edentulous.[29] In a longitudinal study of older adults, examiners found a mean annual rate of 1.36 new decayed and filled surfaces per 100 surfaces at risk.[30] If the caries rate is based on the number of teeth at risk, caries incidence was as high in adults as in 7- to 12-year-old children. Many adults have had fluoride exposure for part of their lives; as a result, teeth are retained longer. Root carious lesions in the area below the crown of the tooth are primarily a disease of the older population. In the NIDR survey, root surface lesions were found in 67% of men and in 61% of women

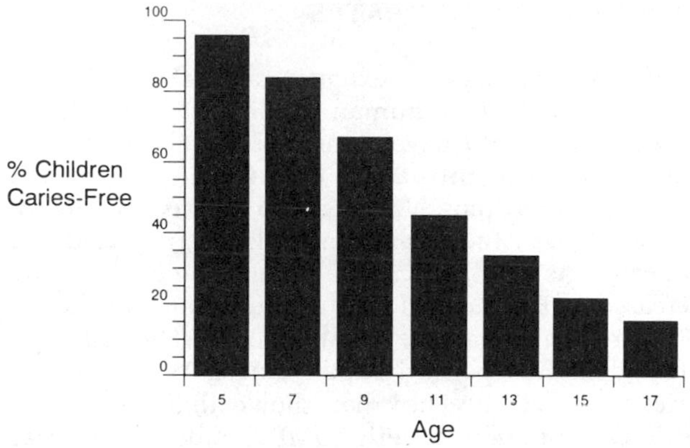

FIGURE 60–3. Percentage of United States children who were caries-free in their permanent dentition by age. (From National Institute of Dental Research: The National Survey of U.S. School Children: 1986–1987. NIH Publication No. 89-2247. Washington D.C., United States Government Printing Office, 1989.)

65 years of age or older. The mean number of decayed-filled root surfaces in the 1985 to 1986 retired group was 3.2; only about half of the lesions had been filled.[29] Older adults at greatest risk of developing root caries include persons with coronal caries, gingival recession, low saliva flow, low fluoride exposure, and frequent intake of fermentable carbohydrates.

The decline in caries prevalence does not imply that caries is no longer a public health problem. Eighty percent of the dental caries is seen in 20% of the children. Even the most optimistic data indicate that 50% of children still have the disease. The target group for intervention, including dietary intervention, has shifted, however, to individuals at high risk, such as persons of lower socioeconomic status, immigrants to the United States from developing countries, developmentally disabled individuals, persons undergoing head and neck radiation, and individuals in the latter cases with compromised host defenses because of complicating medical or pharmacy regimens that affect the oral tissues.

For many years, dental caries was thought to be irreversible. Recently, it was determined that caries is a dynamic process that has three phases: (1) demineralization; (2) equilibrium; and (3) remineralization of tooth enamel. With frequent fermentable carbohydrate exposure and poor oral hygiene, incipient lesions may develop rapidly. In this early stage of tooth decay, the process can be reversed. During periods when no bacterial fermentation is occurring, calcium, phosphorus, and fluoride that have been released from the tooth enamel can be redeposited in the enamel to remineralize the tooth. A clinical cavity (caries) is the final stage in the disease process. The average time for progression of incipient caries to a carious lesion in children is about 18 ± 6 months.

ETIOLOGY OF DENTAL CARIES

The direct relationship between diet and dental caries is clearly established. Dental caries results from the interaction of four factors in the genetically susceptible host mouth: (1) cariogenic plaque bacteria; (2) fermentable substrate; (3) fluoride and other minerals; and (4) saliva (Fig. 60–4). These factors must be present simultaneously in the oral cavity for a sufficient length of time to interact.

Dental plaque is a sticky, gelatinous mass composed of gram-positive bacteria, extracellular polysaccharides, proteins of salivary and dietary origins, and lipids. Without effective oral hygiene, plaque may cover all surfaces of the teeth. When foods are ingested, plaque bacteria metabolize the carbohydrate component to form organic acids—lactic, butyric, acetic, formic, and proprionic—on the surfaces of the teeth. This fermentation begins immediately and may continue for hours. These acids cause the plaque pH to fall and can dissolve tooth structure. The pH at which demineralization of enamel is thought to occur is between 5.3 and 5.7. Stephan proposed that a pH of 5.5 be used as the "critical pH" when measuring the cariogenicity of a food. Frequent intake of foods that depress the plaque pH below 5.5 can cause repeated "acid attacks."[31] When substrate is exhausted, acid production stops and the plaque pH

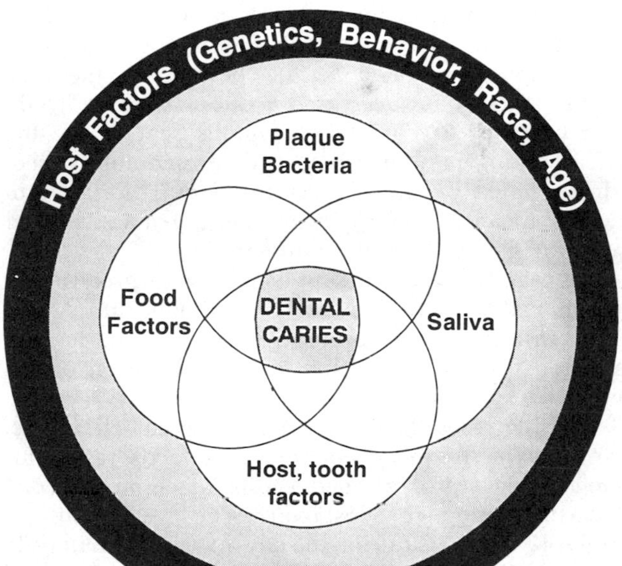

FIGURE 60–4. Major factors that interact in the dental caries process. (Adapted From United States Department of Health and Human Services, Public Health Service, National Institute of Dental Research: Broadening the Scope. Long Range Research Plan for the 1990's. NIH Publication No. 90-1188. Washington D.C., United States Government Printing Office, 1990.)

returns to a resting state. Measuring changes in human plaque pH in situ has been used to estimate the cariogenic potential of foods and snacks.

Dental caries is the most common chronic infectious disease in humans. In 1960, Fitzgerald and Keyes demonstrated that, when germ-free animals were fed a high-sucrose diet, no caries developed.[32] When sucrose-fed animals were inoculated with mutans streptococci or exposed to infected animals, however, they developed smooth-surface and fissure caries. Elevated numbers of mutans streptococci are found in children, teens, and adults with high rates of dental caries. Six genetically distinct species of mutans streptococci are now recognized.[33] Streptococcus mutans (serotype C) has been identified as the principal organism responsible for the initial destruction of enamel and the underlying dentin in North American populations. The ability to survive and metabolize carbohydrate in the low-oxygen, acidic environment of dental plaque is a unique property of S. mutans. In addition to streptococci, species of actinomyces and lactobacilli are linked to dental caries.

Human clinical trials to measure the effect of dietary habits on the development of caries or to confirm the findings of epidemiologic studies are considered unethical and are prohibited today. Thus, rats, hamsters, and monkeys have been widely used in caries research and for testing foods for cariogenicity. Rats have been used most extensively because the etiologic agents are essentially the same as in man.[34] Caries can be produced within a few weeks in rats, whereas it takes 6 to 18 months for caries to develop in monkeys or in humans. Although tooth morphology and salivary composition differ, lesions develop in the pits, fissures, smooth surfaces, and roots of rodents' teeth. As in humans, Streptococcus mutans species are the critical cariogenic microbes, and fermentable carbohydrates must be present. Essential nutrition is provided by means of gastric intubation to bypass the oral cavity, or by orally giving animal chow, or by orally feeding a gelled nutrient supplement. Poor growth and high mortality have occurred in animals undergoing gastric intubation, however, so this technique is used less often than the provision of an oral noncariogenic diet.

To enable researchers to monitor the caloric intake, quantity, and frequency of intake of foods tested for cariogenicity, a programmed feeding machine is used.[35] A measured amount of a test food can be given to animals at up to 17 intervals during the day. At approximately 35 days, the animals are sacrificed, and the teeth are scored for carious lesions. By using the feeding machine, researchers have shown that caries activity is linked to the quantity and frequency of fermentable carbohydrate intake.[34] The results of animal trials cannot be extrapolated directly to humans, but they provide supportive evidence of the probable role of carbohydrates in the human mouth.

ROLE OF CARBOHYDRATES

Epidemiologic surveys, extensive animal experiments, and early controlled human studies have all linked carbohydrates to the development of dental caries. When refined sugar was introduced into the diets of populations such as Eskimos, New Zealand Maoris, and Australian aborigines, their caries prevalence increased dramatically. As the per capita consumption of sucrose increased in England and the United States in the last 100 years, the prevalence of caries rose. When sugar was rationed in Europe and Japan during World War II, caries rates fell. Sreenby has shown that the average decayed-missing-filled-teeth (DMFT) index in 12-year-old children in 47 countries was highly correlated with the grams of sugar available per capita on a daily basis.[36] In the United States today, added sugars constitute 13 to 14% of children's total calorie intake. Most dietary sugars are added to manufactured foods rather than added to foods by the consumer at home.

In rodents, monkeys, and humans, the presence of sucrose in the mouth increases the volume and rate of plaque formation. Sucrose has a unique role in permitting bacteria to colonize on the teeth. When high concentrations of sucrose are present, Streptococcus mutans is able to produce extracellular polysaccharides, glucans, which form an organic matrix on the tooth's surface. These insoluble, sticky polymers permit bacterial colonies to adhere to the tooth. In addition to glucans, S. mutans produces intracellular polysaccharides, primarily fructans, from sucrose that are stored and used in glycolysis when dietary carbohydrates are unavailable. Figure 60–5 is a schematic illustration of the relationship between nutritive and nonnutritive sweeteners with plaque micro-organisms.

The critical concentration of carbohydrate in a food that will cause caries in man is unknown; however, foods with 15% sugars by weight are considered high-sugar foods. In animals, caries scores increase as the sugar content increases.[37] The Hopewood House Study showed that children eating diets containing complex carbohydrates but few refined sugars had low caries increments.[38] In a longitudinal study of school children in England where the fluoride level in the drinking water was low, the relation of sugar intake to caries increment was examined; the greatest correlation was between grams of sugar eaten daily and caries experience.[39] The weak correlations found between food habits and caries increment can be attributed to several factors: a low level of caries in all the children, a high intake of sugary foods by all children, and the widespread use of topical fluorides.

The other mono- and disaccharides—glucose, fructose, maltose, and lactose—found in fruits, dairy products, and processed foods are also readily used by oral micro-organisms. These sugars diffuse rapidly through dental plaque to become available for bacterial fermentation. Within a few minutes of ingestion, fructose and

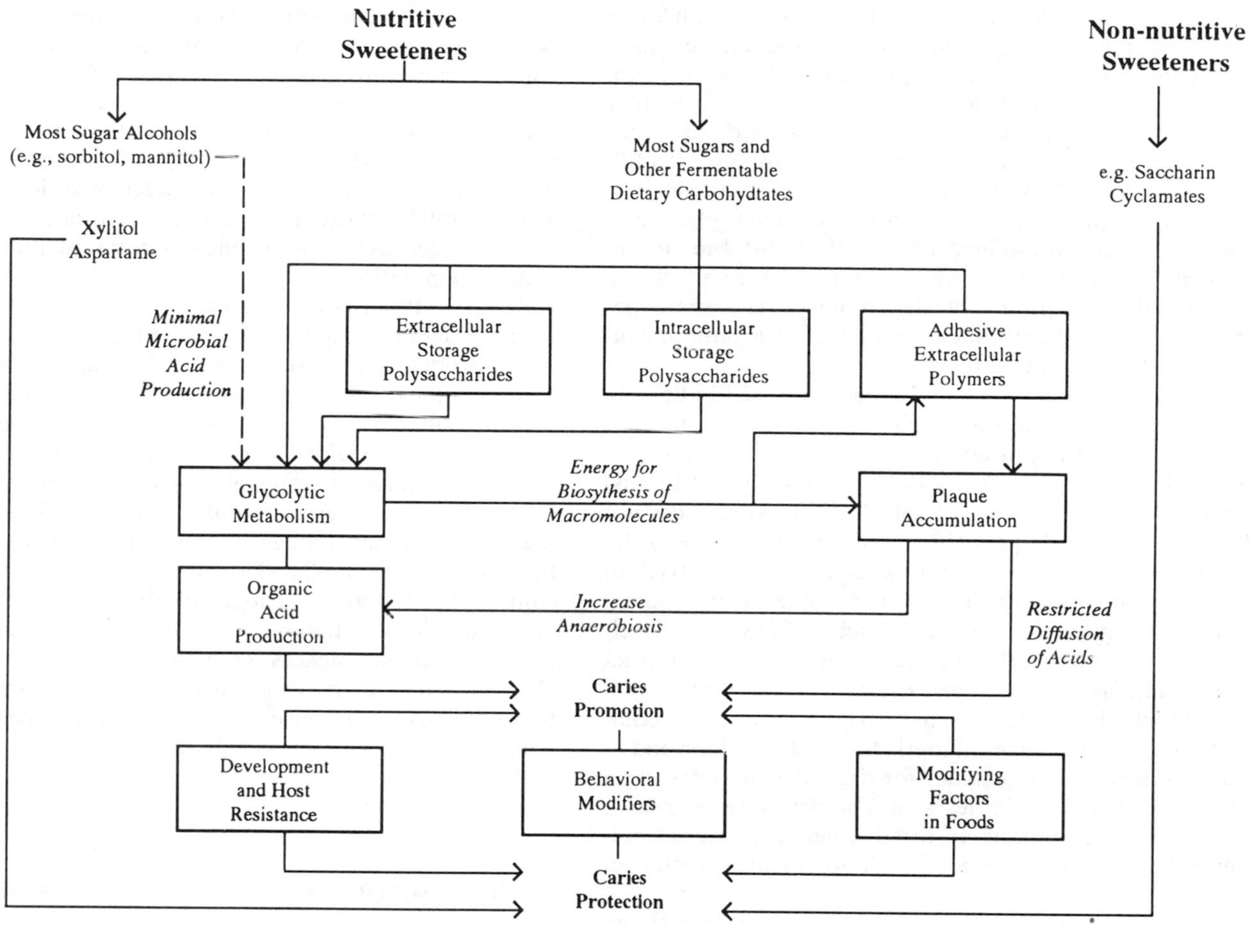

FIGURE 60–5. The relationship of nutritive and nonnutritive sweeteners to oral microbial metabolism and dental caries. (Adapted from Alfano, M.C.: Food Technol., *34*:70–74, 1980.)

glucose cause falls in plaque pH similar to sucrose; thus, they are considered as cariogenic as sucrose.

When eaten with meals, fresh fruits are of low cariogenic potential. This is attributed to the high water content and the presence of citric acid, which stimulates saliva secretion. Fresh fruits vary in sucrose content from 10 to 15% by weight in apples, bananas, and some grapes, 7 to 8% in citrus fruits, to 2% in berries, cherries, and pears. However, daily intake of large quantities of apples and grapes by orchard workers resulted in a high caries rate.[40] Foods of high acid content, such as lemons and oranges, may prevent bacterial fermentation, but they cause enamel erosion.

Sugars in solution have been considered less harmful to teeth than solid sweets because beverages clear the mouth quickly. In the 1940s, however, Stephan showed that a 10% glucose rinse lowered the plaque pH below 5.5.[31] The total amount of sugars in carbonated beverages, fruit drinks, and fruit juices is about 10%, and sport drinks contain about 4.4% total sugars. Based on sugar content, acidity, and changes in plaque pH after rinsing with these beverages, all of them appear to have similar cariogenic potential.[41] Analysis of dental data from the 1971 to 1974 National Health and Nutrition Examination Survey (NHANES II) showed that frequent between-meal intake of sweetened beverages was associated with increased caries.[42] Teenagers and young adults who used sugar-sweetened soft drinks three or more times between meals on a daily basis increased their odds of having a high DMFT score by 179%. Since that time, food manufacturers have replaced some of the sucrose in beverages with high-fructose corn syrup, saccharin, or aspartame. Whether these new beverage formulations are less cariogenic is unknown. Substitution of sport drinks or ion drinks for carbonated beverages or fruit drinks was associated with decalcification of Japanese children's teeth.[43] Most of these drinks have a pH below 4. Slowly drinking sugar-sweetened tea or coffee may also lead to enamel dissolution.

Extensive studies of sugar alcohols show that they result in limited acid production by plaque bacteria. Plaque bacteria are able to ferment sorbitol and mannitol, but at too slow a rate to induce dental caries in most people. If sorbitol-sweetened products are used frequently, some evidence suggests that bacterial adaptation may occur.[44] After several weeks of regular sorbitol mouth rinses, increased acid production has been measured in adults when they are given additional sorbitol. However, acid production may be clinically significant only in xerostomic patients who are at high risk of developing caries. If sorbitol-mannitol-sweetened gums and candies are used regularly to relieve the symptoms of dry mouth, xerostomic patients should be cautioned about the cariogenic potential of these products.[45]

Xylitol, a five-carbon sugar alcohol, is used in Canada and Europe to replace sucrose in candies, gum, and medicines. In the United States, it is approved for use in special dietary products by the Food and Drug Administration (FDA). Ingestion of solutions of xylitol does not cause a drop in plaque pH because oral bacteria lack the enzymes to ferment xylitol. A 2-year clinical trial in Finland, known as the Turku study, showed that young adults using foods sweetened solely with xylitol developed no new caries,[46] whereas groups assigned to fructose and sucrose developed caries. Xylitol, however, is not widely used because it is costly to produce. Saccharin, found in beverages, dietetic foods, dentifrices, and in tablets as a table sweetener for diabetics, inhibits tooth decay in rats. Low caries scores and low recoveries of Streptococcus mutans resulted when rats were challenged with a cariogenic diet supplemented with saccharin.[47]

Aspartame does not support the growth of Streptococcus mutans, acid production in the mouth, or plaque formation. Frequent rinsing with aspartame was no more cariogenic in rats than distilled water.[48] Because soft drinks are a popular cariogenic snack, the use of aspartame in these beverages is safer for teeth.

Frequent use of chewing gum sweetened with xylitol or xylitol-sorbitol mixtures causes significant reductions in dental plaque, as well as plaque and saliva levels of Streptococcus mutans.[49] The Turku chewing gum study showed that chewing four sticks of xylitol gum daily reduced dental decay by 80% when compared to subjects chewing sucrose-sweetened gum.[50] Gum chewing stimulates salivary flow and pushes saliva into the interproximal area where salivary buffers can neutralize bacterial acids. Chewing also removes food particles from plaque and the soft tissues. The net result is that the stimulation of salivary flow caused by the physical act of chewing, coupled with the helpful effects of a noncalorie sweetener, can be beneficial to dental health by "neutralizing" the plaque bacteria's acid response to fermentable carbohydrate-containing foods.

The effect of starch-containing foods on teeth is dependent on the form, on whether the starch is raw or cooked, and on whether sucrose is present. Vegetables lacking sugars do not cause intraoral acid production or demineralization of enamel in man. Adults with hereditary fructose intolerance are a unique study group who consistently avoid fruits, table sugar, and refined starches containing sucrose because they cause nausea, but these persons often eat wheat, rice, potatoes, and root vegetables. An examination of the caries status of these young adults showed that 15 of 27 adults examined were caries free and the remainder had low DMFT scores. Siblings without the inborn error of metabolism had a higher caries prevalence, similar to that of the general population.[51]

Because starch is a large molecule, it cannot diffuse through dental plaque. When cereal grains are refined in the production of breads or crackers and are cooked, however, they are more easily hydrolyzed by salivary and plaque amylases. Fermentation of the resulting sugar, maltose, yields acids that demineralize enamel rapidly. Mixtures of starches and sugars in ready-to-eat breakfast cereals, pastries, and many convenience foods are often retained longer in the interproximal plaque than high-sugar foods. This may make sugar-starch combinations more cariogenic than sugar alone.[52] Foods previously thought to be of low cariogenicity—breads, muffins, crackers, chips—are no longer considered safe for teeth, especially when they are eaten between meals, because of their retentive properties and their ability to act as substrates for plaque microbial fermentation.

OTHER FACTORS AFFECTING CARIOGENICITY

Sugars and starch are not the only factors that determine the cariogenic potential of a food. Frequency of intake, physical consistency, and position of a food in the meal are also important. In rats, the intervals between eating snacks or meals has a profound effect on the number of Streptococcus mutans in plaque and the number of cavities formed. Little caries develops in rats fed a cariogenic diet two or three times a day. As the frequency of sugar exposures increases, however, the number of carious lesions increases. In the 1950s, the classic human intervention trial, the Vipeholm study, was conducted in Sweden.[53] Institutionalized adults were fed an adequate diet and were either supplemented with retentive, sweet foods (chocolate, toffees, and caramels) between meals or nonsticky, sweet foods at meal time. When the subjects were provided up to ten times the sucrose at meals, they did not experience a significant increase in caries relative to the control subjects. However, the group receiving between-meal retentive sweets developed more caries than subjects receiving sugar at mealtimes. In the same way, an analysis of the NHANES I data, obtained in a cross-sectional survey, revealed that individuals with high DMFT scores were more frequent consumers of table sugars, syrups, sugary desserts, and snacks than persons with low DMFT scores.[54] In a 3-year longitudinal study of Michigan children, those subjects who developed the most caries tended to derive more calories from snack carbohydrates and sugars than children with low caries increments.[55] In rat experiments, granola cereal, French fries, bananas, cupcakes, and raisins had a cariogenic potential equal to or greater than sucrose.[52]

The sequence of eating foods in a meal affects the magnitude of a drop in plaque pH. If a piece of aged cheese is eaten following an acidogenic food such as canned pears in syrup, the plaque pH will rise above the danger zone immediately.[56] The pH drop in response to sugared coffee will be rapid but will rise if followed by an unsweetened food. If sugared coffee is drunk at the end of a meal, however, a prolonged drop in plaque pH will occur. By placing acidogenic items between other foods, the risk of demineralization is lessened.

Saliva and protective components in foods modify the effect of fermentable carbohydrates on the teeth.[57] The importance of saliva in caries prevention is perhaps best demonstrated by the rampant caries that develop in xerostomic patients. Saliva flow is stimulated by mastication of foods, by citric acid in fruits, and by sugars. The composition of saliva is also influenced by dietary components.

Four protective mechanisms of saliva are important in preventing caries. First, saliva prevents the aggregation of bacteria on the tooth's surface and speeds the clearance of food particles and sugars from the mouth. A second mechanism is the buffering action of proteins, bicarbonates, and phosphates in saliva that dilute and neutralize plaque acids. Third, immunoglobulins present in saliva protect the teeth by depressing bacterial activity. Finally, the presence of calcium, phosphate, and fluoride ions in saliva promotes the remineralization of tooth enamel.

Food components can have protective effects on tooth enamel. Some foods decrease the solubility of enamel (demineralization), and other foods stimulate salivary secretion or remineralization. Substances that make the enamel less soluble include fluoride in tea, an unidentified factor in cocoa, phytate, oxalate, and proteins in milk. Citric acid found in citrus fruits stimulates saliva production and thereby increases the amount of bicarbonate and phosphate buffers in the mouth.

Much research has been done on the effects of cheese on plaque pH. Over 21 aged cheeses have been identified that do not cause the pH in plaque to fall.[58] These cheeses have hypoacidogenic and anticariogenic activity because fermentable carbohydrate-laden foods when ingested after cheese do not result in a plaque pH drop. The protective properties of these cheeses are attributed to their texture, which stimulates salivary flow, and their protein, calcium, and phosphorus content which neutralize plaque acids. The cheese seems to prevent demineralization and to increase remineralization.[59] Some speculation also exists that a "protective pH rise factor" is present, but it has yet to be isolated.

MEASURING THE CARIOGENIC POTENTIAL OF HUMAN FOOD

The results of three indirect types of tests[60] when taken together on a variety of commonly consumed foods reveal that the foods with high cariogenic potential are those high in fermentable carbohydrate content, eaten frequently, and adherent to the teeth. These tests also demonstrated that the following foods cause the pH at interproximal sites to fall below pH 5.5, implying that, if they are ingested frequently, the risk of caries will substantially increase: dried fruits, breads, cereals, cookies, snack crackers, and potato chips.[61] Foods that are noncariogenic (do not drop the plaque pH below 5.5) include some vegetables, meats, fish, aged cheeses, and nuts. These tests are useful predictors of cariogenicity, but additional factors will determine whether caries actually develop. They include the following: host susceptibility, genetic predisposition, virulence of the oral bacteria, how frequently a food is eaten, the sequence in which foods are eaten in a meal, and the interactions among foods eaten concurrently.

In addition to the continuing concern regarding food cariogenicity and caries prevalence and experience in the so-called normal population, two other specific groups have been targeted as high-risk groups, primarily because of eating and social behavioral patterns. These two groups include the infant/toddler, at risk of "baby bottle" caries, and the elderly, at risk of developing root surface caries.

BABY BOTTLE CARIES

Inappropriate feeding practices can result in rampant caries in infants and toddlers. Baby bottle tooth decay (BBTD) usually occurs between 1 and 2 years of age, develops rapidly, involves many teeth, and can cause severe pain. Early decay of the primary dentition is attributed to exposing the teeth to sugary liquids for long periods of time. When a child falls asleep with a bottle, sweetened liquids pool around the teeth, leading to demineralization of the enamel. The same disease condition may result from prolonged breast-feeding. Breast-fed infants with rampant decay have reportedly been allowed to sleep with the mother and nurse at will during the night. During sleep, the protective action of saliva is greatly reduced by diminished flow rates. Severity of the disease is linked to the number of feedings per day and to the duration of bottle or breast-feeding.

Surveys show that 50% of Native American 1 to 3 year olds have severe dental caries. Fifteen percent of Head Start children in cities with fluoridated water and 20% of children in cities with nonfluoridated water had BBTD.[62] Initially, the facial surfaces of the four maxillary incisor teeth are involved, and later, decalcification of the maxillary and mandibular molars and canines occurs. The tongue protects the lower anterior four incisors. Early white-spot lesions on the teeth go undetected by parents. That stage is followed by a dull white band of demineralization that develops rapidly along the gum line of the upper incisors. If the disease progresses further, a brown or black collar encircles the necks of the teeth. The four maxillary incisors may be completely destroyed, so only brownish root stumps remain.

Streptococcus mutans is not part of the indigenous flora of the oral cavity at birth. When the deciduous teeth erupt, at about 6 months of age, bacterial colonies begin to form in the mouth. S. mutans is believed to be transmitted to infants by caregivers. If mothers have high levels of S. mutans, their infants will be at greater risk of implanting elevated levels of these cariogenic organisms in their plaque. To prevent BBTD, all caregivers—parents, grandparents, and daycare workers—must be counseled about the proper use of the nursing bottle. Nap or nighttime bottle feeding should be discouraged. If a bedtime bottle is offered, the only safe liquid is water.

ROOT CARIES

Dietary factors are also important in the initiation and progression of root caries. When gingival tissues recede, the root surfaces of teeth are exposed to the oral environment. Because roots lack the protective enamel layer, they are highly susceptible to dental caries. High levels of Streptococcus mutans are found in adults with root caries.[63] Examination of ancient skulls and dentition of members of primitive societies revealed that root caries was more common than coronal caries. Because these groups consumed starches but not refined sugars, complex carbohydrates are implicated in the development of root caries. Adults who have periodontitis or have had periodontal surgery resulting in exposed root surfaces frequently develop root caries if their intake of fermentable carbohydrates is high.[64] A high daily intake of liquid-solid and slow-dissolving fermentable foods such as ice cream, gelatin, hard candies, and antacids was positively correlated with root caries in a cross-sectional study of healthy, free-living elderly persons.[65]

In a 2-year, longitudinal study of elderly Bostonians, subjects in the highest quintile for root caries had significantly higher intakes of sweetened liquids, solid fermentable carbohydrates, and starches than adults who were free of root caries.[66] Adults who were caries free ate 50% more cheese and 25% more milk than persons with caries. Because root caries develop more rapidly than coronal caries, preventive measures are critical. Nutrition counseling, home oral care, and fluoride therapy should be provided to older adults with gingival recession.

FLUORIDE

The decline in coronal caries in industrialized countries during the past 40 years is primarily attributed to the widespread use of fluorides. Currently, the primary sources of fluorides for humans are community water supplies, foods, beverages, dentifrices and other dental products. The ionic fluoride ingested in water has a systemic effect prior to tooth eruption and a topical effect after eruption. Dietary fluoride supplements are prescribed for children when fluoride is lacking in the water supply. Professionally applied topical applications of fluoride in higher concentrations are used to protect erupted teeth and are not swallowed. The preventive benefits of fluoride depend upon the concentration of fluoride used, whether it is given systemically or topically, and the type of agent used, whether in water, tablet, drops, a rinse, or a gel. The caries-preventive properties of systemic and topical fluoride are additive. Fluoride is more effective in the prevention of smooth-surface than occlusal caries.

MECHANISMS OF ACTION

Although the cariostatic properties of fluoride are widely recognized, the protective role of fluoride in the oral environment is not fully understood. At least three mechanisms of action are recognized.[67] First, fluoride ions replace some of the hydroxyl groups of the hydroxyapatite in developing teeth to form fluoridated hydroxyapatite. This increases the stability of the enamel crystals because fluoridated hydroxyapatite is less soluble to organic acids than hydroxyapatite. Fluoride uptake by calcified tissues is high in infancy but decreases with age. Second, low concentrations of fluoride in the saliva and plaque fluids can inhibit demineralization and enhance remineralization of early lesions. Third, fluoride has direct effects on the acidogenic plaque bacteria. In higher concentrations, fluoride inhibits growth of Streptococcus mutans found in dental plaque and in low concentrations inhibits bacterial enzymes, reducing acid production from catabolism of fermentable carbohydrates.

WATER FLUORIDATION

Fluoridation of community water supplies is the most effective method of providing fluoride to large populations. Through extensive epidemiologic studies of communities with naturally fluoridated water in the United States in the 1930s, the protective properties of fluoride in the prevention of dental caries were fully recognized.[68] In 21 United States cities, an inverse relationship was shown between caries prevalence in children and the fluoride content of the drinking water at an optimal range (Fig. 60–6).

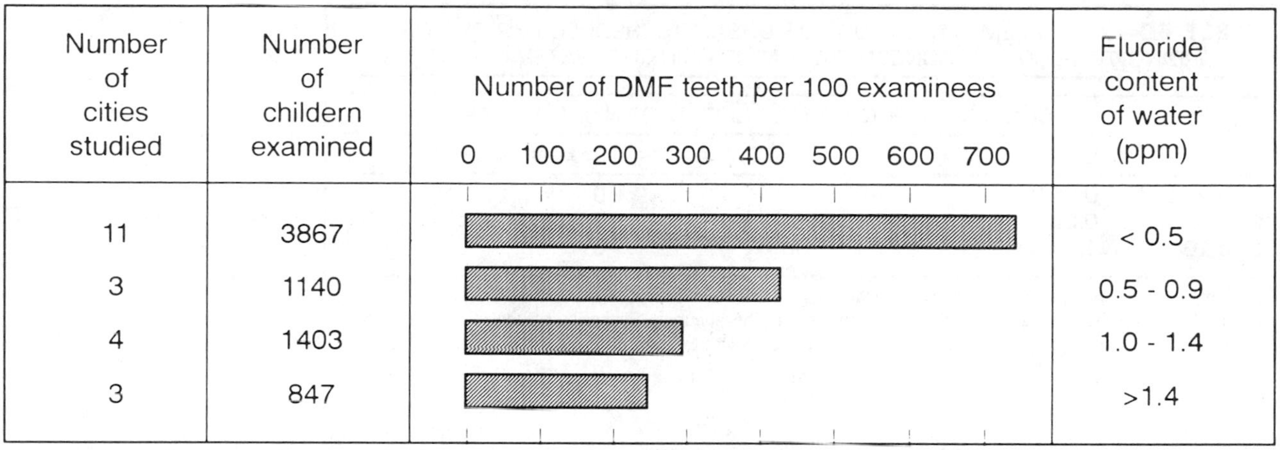

Number of cities studied
Number of childern examined
Number of DMF teeth per 100 examinees
0 100 200 300 400 500 600 700
Fluoride content of water (ppm)
11
3867
< 0.5
3
1140
0.5 - 0.9
4
1403
1.0 - 1.4
3
847
>1.4

FIGURE 60–6. The relationship between caries prevalence and fluoride content of drinking water in 21 cities. (From Newbrun, E.: Fluorides and Dental Caries. 3rd Ed. Springfield, IL, Charles C Thomas, 1986.)

In 1945, Grand Rapids, Michigan, became the first city in the world to fluoridate the drinking water. Between 1950 and 1980, clinical studies conducted in 20 countries showed that adding fluoride to community water supplies resulted in a 40 to 50% caries reduction in primary teeth and a 50 to 60% reduction in dental caries in permanent teeth.[69] Recent comparisons of caries in United States children who had always lived in communities with optimally fluoridated water with children never exposed to fluoridated drinking water revealed 25% lower DMFS scores in the fluoridated group.[70] The decline in caries prevalence among children living in communities with nonfluoridated water is attributed to intake of foods processed in fluoridated water, the use of fluoride-containing dentifrices, and the use of topical fluorides in the dental office and at home. Adults also experience benefits from the consumption of fluoridated water. The prevalence of coronal and root caries seems to be 20 to 30% lower in adults living in communities with optimally fluoridated water than in adults residing in cities with lower levels of fluoride in the water supply.[71]

According to the United States Public Health Service, the desirable fluoride concentration for dental caries prevention is about 1 part per million (0.7 to 1.2 ppm, based on climactic temperature). By 1990, 42 of the 50 largest cities in the United States had fluoridated their water supplies. Currently in the United States, approximately 130.5 million people, or 53% of the population, drink water with 0.7 ppm or higher levels of fluoride.[74] This includes 9 million people who drink water with natural fluoride at optimal levels. Continuous exposure to fluoride is desirable. In communities where water fluoridation has been interrupted or eliminated, a significant increase in dental caries has been observed.[71]

Water fluoridation is the most cost-effective method of preventing tooth decay in the United States. The current average cost for delivering fluoride in the drinking water is less than a dollar per person per year. Even though scientists, health professionals, and the courts generally agree that community water fluoridation is safe, effective, economical, and legally valid, some members of the mass media and public remain confused about fluoride's safety. Opponents to fluoridation have attempted to link it to AIDS, Alzheimer's disease, and cancer, but they have provided no scientific evidence to support their claims. Over 50 epidemiologic studies have demonstrated no association between water fluoridation and the risk of cancer.[67] In addition, animal studies have failed to establish a relationship between fluoride and cancer. Water fluoridation cannot be taken for granted. Health professionals—nutritionists, physicians, dentists, pharmacists, nurses, and public health specialists—have a responsibility to educate patients and the public about the health and economic benefits of fluoridation.

DIETARY SUPPLEMENTATION

Children living in cities and rural areas with suboptimal water fluoridation can receive the caries-preventive benefits of fluoride by taking a prescribed fluoride supplement. When children are given fluoride drops or tablets daily from birth through the early teenage years, a low prevalence of caries is found. The level of dietary supplementation is determined by the age of the child and the concentration of fluoride in the water supply. Well water should be tested for fluoride concentration by a local water district or the county or state health department. Table 60–3 presents the recommended levels of daily fluoride supplementation as approved by the American Dental Association (ADA) Council on Dental Therapeutics and the American Academy of Pediatrics. The optimal fluoride intake for children appears to

TABLE 60–3 SUPPLEMENTAL FLUORIDE DOSAGE SCHEDULE (MG PER DAY*) ACCORDING TO FLUORIDE CONCENTRATION OF DRINKING WATER

	CONCENTRATION OF FLUORIDE IN DRINKING WATER (PPM)		
Age (yr)	Less than 0.3	0.3 to 0.7	Greater than 0.7
Birth to 2	0.25	0	0
2 to 3	0.50	0.25	0
3 to 16	1.00	0.50	0

*2.2 mg sodium fluoride contains 1 mg fluoride.
(From American Dental Association Council on Dental Therapeutics: Prescribed fluoride supplements. *In* American Dental Association Accepted Dental Theraputics. 40th Ed. Chicago, American Dental Association, 1984.)

be 0.05 mg/kg body weight. Future dosage schedules may be based on body weight rather than age.

Liquid fluoride supplements (drops) are recommended for infants and young children. Fluoride drops or tablets alone are as effective as fluoride-vitamin supplements. A list of accepted fluoride supplements is published regularly by the ADA Council on Dental Therapeutics.[72] Fluoride-vitamin supplements are not recommended by the ADA because, when vitamins are discontinued, the use of fluorides may also cease. Few healthy, full-term, formula-fed infants require a vitamin-mineral supplement. The fluoride present when commercial formula is diluted with fluoridated water is 95 to 100% available. If infant formula is prepared with nonfluoridated water, however, fluoride drops should be prescribed. The fluoride concentration of breast milk is low (0.1 ppm). Full-term infants, if exclusively breast-fed, should receive fluoride drops at 6 months of age, even though they live in a community with fluoridated water.

For older children, fluoride tablets are available in the following doses: 0.25, 0.5, or 1 mg F. Tablets are formulated with neutral sodium fluoride or acidulated phosphate fluoride (APF). The caries-preventive effects of neutral fluoride tablets is similar to that of APF tablets. Chewable fluoride tablets seem to have topical as well as systemic benefits. Patients should be instructed to allow the tablet to dissolve by chewing before swallowing. A child may ingest fluoride from multiple sources; therefore, dentists and physicians should consider this possibility when prescribing fluoride supplements. Administering the appropriate dosage of fluoride preparations should be carefully explained to parents because excess fluoride intake may lead to dental fluorosis.

Other countries have incorporated fluoride into the food supply by fluoridating salt, milk, flour, or sugar. If community water fluoridation is impractical, these foods appear to be possible vehicles for fluoride. Unfortunately, individual intake of these foods varies widely, so formulating a dosage regimen is difficult.

Primary tooth development begins before birth; therefore, the efficacy of prenatal fluoride supplementation is of interest.[73] During pregnancy, fluoride diffuses across the placental barrier and is incorporated into fetal bones and teeth. The concentration of fluoride in fetal blood appears to be about 25% of fluoride concentration of maternal blood. Although prenatal supplements are considered safe for the mother and fetus, the benefits of supplementation in reducing caries are inconclusive.

DENTAL FLUOROSIS

Fluorosis is characterized by white opaque flecks, white or brown staining, or in severe cases, pitting of the tooth enamel. This condition develops only during the period of enamel formation when the daily fluoride ingestion is greater than 2 ppm. Because the crowns of all permanent teeth are forming between birth and 14 years of age, the effects of excess systemic fluoride are limited to this age group. Fewer than 2% of school children in the 1986 to 1987 NIDR survey had moderate to severe fluorosis.[74] An increase in the prevalence of mild dental fluorosis has been observed in communities with both fluoridated and nonfluoridated water in recent years, however (Fig. 60–7). This problem is primarily cosmetic and does not increase the teeth's susceptibility to caries.

Exposure to multiple sources of fluoride increases a child's risk of developing fluorosis.[75,76] The relative importance of fluoride supplements and fluoride dentifrices in the development of fluorosis is unclear. If a child is receiving optimal amounts of fluoride from dietary sources of fluoridated water and swallows large amounts of dentifrice, fluorosis can occur. Ninety percent of all toothpastes in the United States contain fluoride, which is readily absorbed when ingested. Approximately 25% of the fluoride in toothpastes is swallowed by children prior to 6 years of age. Therefore, parents should dispense a small amount of toothpaste for young children to prevent excess intake of fluoride.

Substantial amounts of fluoride can be introduced into the infant's diet through food processing. In the 1970s, it was discovered that infant formulas contained variable and often high levels of fluoride. To reduce the risk of infants' receiving too much fluoride, beginning in 1979, infant formula manufacturers greatly reduced the amount of fluoride in formulas. Soy-based formulas appear to have higher fluoride levels than milk-based

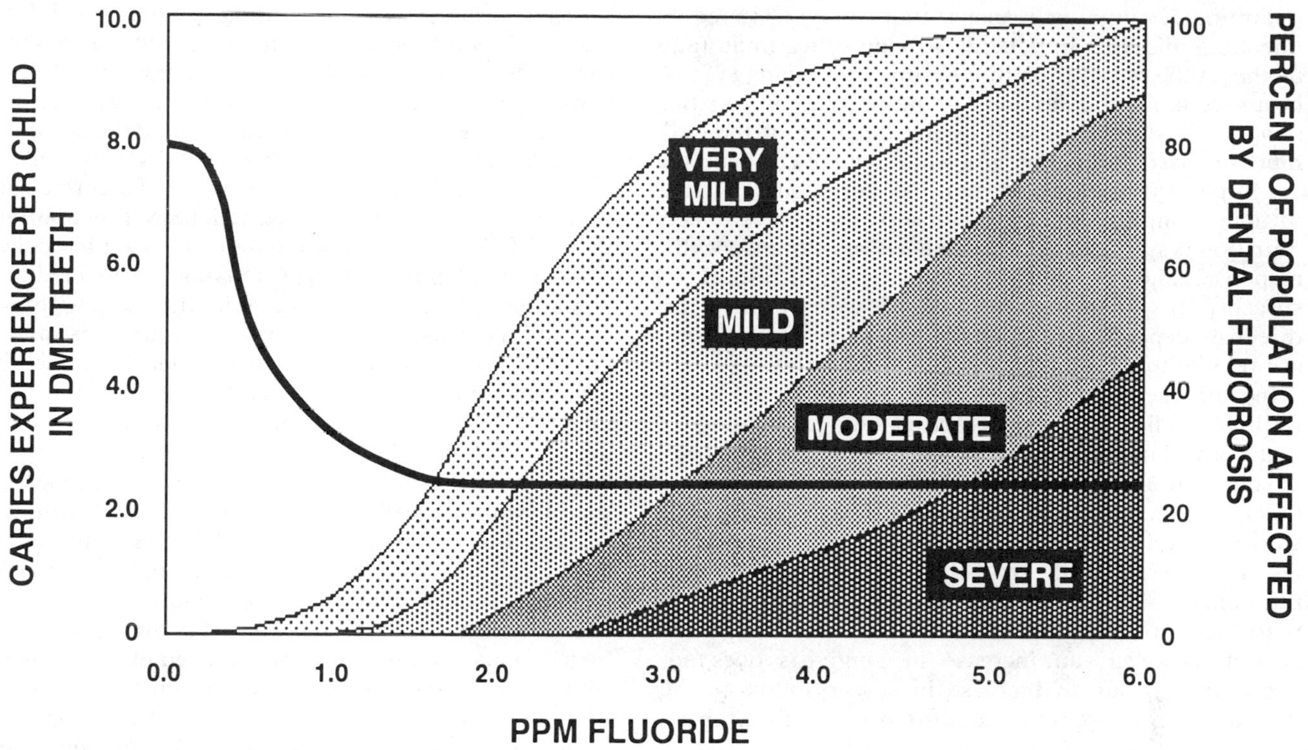

FIGURE 60–7. Prevalence of dental caries and dental fluorosis in relation to fluoride in drinking water. (From United States Department of Health and Human Services, Public Health Service: Review of Fluoride Benefits and Risks. Report of the Ad Hoc Subcommittee on Fluoride of the Committee to Coordinate Environmental Health and Related Programs. Washington D.C., United States Government Printing Office, 1991.)

formulas because the soy products contain components that bind fluoride. Continued monitoring of the fluoride content of a "market basket" of infant and toddler foods in the United States is needed to ensure that fluoride intake remains within safe limits. When the pathogenesis of enamel fluorosis is better understood, the appropriateness of the current fluoride supplementation schedule can be determined.

NUTRITION AND PERIODONTAL DISEASE

The periodontium comprises those soft and hard tissues surrounding the individual teeth. The gingival unit consists of that part of the oral mucosa that covers the root and the apical portion of the crown, whereas the attachment apparatus comprises the ligamentous attachment of the tooth to the surrounding alveolar bone.

Periodontal disease, a general term, describes a bacterial infection of either the gingival unit or both the gingival unit and the attachment apparatus. If the infection is confined to the gingival unit, the resulting disease is called gingivitis. If the infection involves the destruction of the attachment apparatus, the disease is termed periodontitis. Current evidence indicates that the two diseases are not a continuum of the same process, but are in fact two separate diseases, each associated with a different plaque flora. Most forms of periodontitis result in a slow loss of attachment of the tooth to the surrounding alveolar bone. This loss of attachment is not a continuous process but is characterized by periods of destructive activity followed by periods of remission. When tissue destruction will occur cannot be predicted at present. Though most individuals have some degree of periodontal disease, severe periodontal destruction is confined to approximately 24% of the adult population.[29]

The etiology of gingivitis is relatively simple, i.e., a pathologic bacterial flora; however, the etiology of periodontitis is extremely complex. Though bacterial plaque is the major etiologic agent, other local and systemic factors, many unidentified, play a large role as well. For example, several sites within the same patient often harbor similar pathologic flora and similar patterns of other identified local co-etiologic factors, and yet the degree or even the presence of periodontitis differs.

During the past decade, the oral microbes primarily responsible for the initiation and progression of periodontal diseases have been characterized. In addition, reaction of the periodontal tissues to microbial antigens and by-products has been found to be a classic chronic inflammatory-immune response that can be observed in infectious diseases in general. Among other important factors is the recognition that optimal functioning of the host's cellular and humoral immune system and the phagocytic system, as well as the integrity of the oral mucosa (particularly the gingival sulcular epithelium), are important to the maintenance of periodontal health. Although important scientific observations have linked nutritional status to the immune system, to phagocytic response, and to mucosal integrity with respect to susceptibility to many infectious disease states, little direct evidence indicates that these same mechanisms are related to the human periodontal diseases.

In both the animal model and man, numerous longitudinal studies have been carried out, attempting to make associations between either nutritional deficiency or nutrient supplementation and gingivitis. Unfortunately, the majority of these studies were poorly controlled. The few animal and human longitudinal studies that were well controlled have demonstrated relationships of deficiencies of ascorbate and folate with severity of gingivitis.[77–79] As previously discussed, however, an increase in gingivitis does not necessarily mean an increase in susceptibility to the destructive disease that compromises tooth support, namely, periodontitis.

In 1976, Alfano concluded that evidence linking diet and nutritional factors to periodontitis is meager and frequently controversial.[80] Considering the inability to determine whether or not a period of active destruction of the attachment apparatus is occurring until after the fact, and considering the complex nature of the disease with yet unknown local and systemic contributing etiologic factors, it is not surprising that this data base has not dramatically increased in the ensuing years.

Epidemiologic studies have attempted to link periodontitis to nutrition by looking at the degree of periodontal destruction in societies where malnutrition is pervasive or by attempting to evaluate intake of specific nutrients as assessed at one time to the degree of periodontal destruction in well-nurtured societies.[81,82] The former studies generally demonstrate a greater degree of periodontal destruction in malnourished populations as compared to well-nourished societies. The role of nutrition as a contributing factor is unclear, however, because these populations consistently demonstrate poor oral hygiene resulting in massive pathogenic plaque accumulation, which would lead to greater loss of attachment with or without the possible effects of malnutrition. In the latter studies, the periodontal destruction measured is the result of previous disease, and an attempt to correlate this with present nutritional intake is obviously problematic.

Nutrition does play a role in the pathogenesis of destructive periodontal disease. By extrapolating known data about the importance of various aspects of the host's defense mechanism to the pathogenesis of the disease and by further extrapolating known relationships between nutrition and these defense mechanisms, rational assumptions for testing can be made. For example, it has been well documented that patients with deficiencies of polymorphonuclear neutrophil leukocytes (PMN) have increased susceptibility to destructive periodontal disease.[83] Although little direct evidence of the interrelationships of nutrition and PMN function and periodontitis exists, chronic deficiencies of ascorbate and iron are associated with impaired PMN function, and these deficiencies could contribute to an altered host response to plaque pathogens, making the affected individual more susceptible to periodontitis. Likewise, several animal and human studies have demonstrated a positive correlation between nutrient deficits of ascorbic acid, iron, folate, and zinc and the permeability or integrity of the gingival sulcular epithelium compromising an additional host defense mechanism. More globally, because periodontitis is an infection and because the literature is replete with references indicating that malnutrition has almost always a synergistic interaction with infection, one could hypothesize that malnutrition would in general render the host more susceptible to destructive periodontal disease. This susceptibility to infection may be even more pronounced in the periodontium because these tissues are constantly exposed to toxic and antigenic challenges from the omnipresent bacterial plaque and thus are in a state of continuous repair.

In fact, some evidence indicates that these tissues may be susceptible to end-organ deficiencies.[84] Such a deficiency connotates that though systemic levels of a specific nutrient as measured biochemically in serum may be within normal limits, increased challenges at a local site may be such that levels normally considered adequate may be inadequate for the maintenance of optimal health at the local site. Such end-organ deficiencies have been reported in other organ systems.[85]

One of the more dramatic clinical signs of destructive periodontal disease is resorption of alveolar bone. The literature contains much speculation that calcium deficiency is a major etiologic factor in periodontitis, and periodontal disease may be a harbinger of systemic metabolic bone disorders. No evidence indicates that individuals with destructive periodontal disease have any greater disposition to metabolic bone disorders. Similarly, the literature does not support the premise that calcium deficiency predisposes the periodontium to destructive disease.

EFFECTS OF ORAL HEALTH AND DISEASE ON SYSTEMIC NUTRITION

Oral lesions may adversely affect systemic nutrition. This relationship, though obvious, is often ignored by members of both the medical and the dental professions, and very little in the literature explores this relationship. Either thermal or mechanical stimuli may cause tooth pain and may thus alter an individual's selection of food. Gingival recession is a common clinical finding in middle-aged and older adults, with thermal sensitivity (more to cold than to heat) a common sequela. Other causes of thermal and mechanical sensitivity include cervical abrasion and erosion of teeth, caries, and sequelae of certain components of periodontal therapy, such as root planing and surgery. Tooth sensitivity can be corrected by the use of over-the-counter dentifrices containing either strontium chloride or potassium nitrate, professional application of fluoride, tooth sealants, and resin dental restorations.

Although an intact dentition is not necessarily required to maintain nutritional health, loss of teeth or of the supporting periodontium can affect food selection. Though the majority of people in the Western World receive routine dental therapy, a large percentage of individuals in the lower socioeconomic strata do not. Large carious lesions and considerable loss of periodontal attachment resulting in mobile teeth leads to a preference for soft foods of lower nutrient density and an avoidance of hard or fibrous foods that require chewing. The number of missing teeth also affects masticatory efficiency and selection of food.[86] The biting force and the ability to chew a food to a particle size that can be swallowed is reduced in partially (fewer than 10 to 13 teeth per side of mouth) or fully edentulous individuals.[87] In fact, the average denture wearer's masticatory efficiency is thought to be about 20% of the dentate adults.[88] Thus, it is not surprising that adults with compromised dentitions are overrepresented in groups with poor-quality diets.

The consumption of essential nutrients by individuals with one or two complete (upper and lower) dentures is reduced approximately 20%, as compared to individuals with partial dentures or individuals with an intact dentition.[89] Considering that approximately 40% of the population of the United States 65 years of age or older is edentulous, this problem is relatively common. If the dentally impaired are counseled to eat more slowly and to chew longer, they can enjoy a wide variety of foods with texture. Alternately, they should be encouraged to consume cooked fruits and vegetables or bite-sized raw fruits and vegetables. Longer cooking will tenderize fibrous meats to facilitate chewing and provide protein. Totally edentulous individuals seem to increase calorie intake after dentures are inserted and patients adjust to the new prosthesis.

Saliva is a primary factor in both the function and maintenance of the oral cavity. In addition to being important in speech and deglutition, certain antimicrobial and nonantimicrobial systems in saliva protect both the hard and soft tissues of the mouth. Cessation or severe decrease of salivary flow from such causes as surgical removal of salivary glands, radiation therapy, and Sjögren's syndrome can lead to microbial infection of the oral cavity, rampant caries, and loss of taste acuity, as well as inability to lubricate, masticate, and swallow food. All these conditions have a profound effect on selection and ingestion of foods and thus on systemic nutrition. In fact, significant deficiencies of fiber, vitamin B_6, iron, calcium, and zinc were found in xerostomic older adults.[90] The use of artificial saliva, though not a panacea, may be beneficial to some of these patients. To prevent rampant caries in such individuals, aggressive home care emphasizing effective oral hygiene and daily fluoride application is usually recommended. Comfort in wearing dentures depends on lubrication of the soft tissues by saliva. Patients with oral dryness have poor retention of their dentures and may develop ulcerations at denture borders, making mastication difficult and painful.

It was once believed that the aging process brought with it a "natural" reduction of salivary flow, but, in fact, salivary flow in healthy individuals does not decrease with age.[91] Nearly 50% of elderly subjects are taking medications that diminish salivary flow, however[92] (Table 60–4). Though salivary flow is decreased in these individuals, it generally still does not interfere with either deglutition or the maintenance of hard and soft tissues. Nonetheless, these patients often feel as if their mouths are dry and frequently use hard candies or gum to stimulate salivary flow throughout the day. Because most of the candies and gum used contain fermentable carbohydrates, the constant exposure may result in rampant caries and altered food intake because of discomfort or loss of integrity of the dentition. Patients taking xerostomia-producing drugs should be counseled about side effects and should be advised to use candies and gums containing relatively nonfermentable sugar alcohols such as sorbitol, mannitol, or xylitol.

It was also believed, on the basis of threshold studies, that advancing age produced taste loss as well, which could also contribute to decreased nutrient intake. However, these elevations in threshold are relatively small and have few clinical effects. The hypogeusia observed in some elderly individuals is possibly associated with specific disorders leading to taste loss, rather than a normal component of the aging process.[93]

The oral cavity is a principal site of lesions associated with human immunodeficiency virus (HIV) infection, which are often painful and drastically limit the intake of nutrients at a time when nutrition is extremely important. These lesions include HIV-associated gingivitis and periodontitis, oral candidiasis, recurrent herpes simplex infection, xerostomia, and Kaposi's sarcoma. Curative or

TABLE 60—4. XEROSTOMIA-INDUCING DRUGS BY CLASS

Analgesics	Anti-inflammatory agents
Anticholinergics	Antiparkinson agents
Antidepressants	Antipsychotic agents
Antihypertensives	Decongestants
Systemic antihistamines/ decongestants	Diuretics
Systemic bronchodilators	Gastrointestinal agents

(Adapted from Levy, S.M., Baker, K.A., Semla, T.P., et al.: Gerodontics, *4*:121, 1988.)

palliative therapy for these lesions is relatively successful in allowing the normal ingestion of nutrients. Excellent reviews on the management of these lesions are available.[94,95] The occurrence of many of these lesions can be drastically curtailed or their severity reduced by the use of prophylactic regimens. Unfortunately, oral manifestations of HIV are often ignored until they reach crisis proportion and thus contribute to the "wasting" of the patient.

Some of the same oral lesions associated with HIV infections are also seen in cancer patients undergoing chemotherapy (see Chap. 73). The antimetabolic activity of these drugs often induces a mucositis, rendering the tissues more susceptible to physical trauma from sharp tooth edges and hard bits of food. Ulceration, secondary infection, and painful stomatitis may result. Generally, the more intense the cytotoxic therapy, the more common the oral complications. Through the use of proper prophylactic therapy prior to chemotherapy, many lesions can be prevented or minimized, with the result of fewer problems in ingesting needed nutrients.[96]

In 1987, 9742 Americans died of oral cancers. The 5-year relative survival rate for persons with oral cancers is 52%, among the lowest survival rates of the major cancers. The majority of these malignant neoplasms are squamous cell carcinomas. Tobacco use and heavy alcohol consumption are the primary causative agents of oral cancers. Surveys show that about 60% of head and neck cancer patients are nutritionally compromised at the time of initial diagnosis. The amount of weight loss that occurs prior to surgery is a good predictor of the risk of developing postoperative complications. Postsurgically, depending on the nature of the surgical procedure, food intake may be severely compromised and should be closely monitored throughout treatment. The least invasive method of providing essential nutrients to maintain weight should be used. Blended foods given by mouth are tolerated by some patients. If adequate calories cannot be obtained orally, tube or parenteral feeding must be provided; however, oral feedings should resume as soon as possible in oral cancer patients.

Radiation therapy for head and neck cancers causes several conditions that can adversely affect systemic nutrition[97] (see Chap. 62C). If not treated prior to irradiation, chronic pulpal and periodontal infections can become acute because of radiation-associated changes and can lead to osteoradionecrosis. These lesions are extremely painful and difficult to treat and can impair systemic nutrition for months. Radiation therapy can also lead to oral mucositis with complications similar to those previously described for the chemotherapeutic patient. In addition, if the radiation beam passes through the major salivary glands, fibrosis of the gland occurs, with all the resultant problems associated with xerostomia. If the salivary glands are not the primary foci of irradiation, lead shields can be individually fabricated for the patient, to protect the glands from unnecessary irradiation. If the radiation beam is aimed through the muscles of mastication, fibrosis of the musculature may occur. This fibrosis results in limitation of mandibular movement called trismus, which usually becomes evident 3 to 6 months after irradiation. This trismus makes it difficult for patients to consume a normal diet. Though it will not stop the fibrosis of the musculature, physiotherapy, such as range-of-motion and isometric exercises starting prior to the onset of the fibrosis, can decrease the extent of mandibular immobility.[98]

EFFECT OF NUTRIENT DEFICIENCIES ON ORAL TISSUES

The oral cavity is one of the first regions of the body to exhibit clinical signs of malnutrition. Virtually every classic nutrition deficiency disease, including scurvy, beriberi, and pellagra, has signs and symptoms in the oral cavity and surrounding structures. The lips, tongue, oral mucosa, and gingiva may all reflect nutritional deficiencies. The oral mucosa is susceptible to physiologic or anatomic changes resulting from nutritional deficit for two major reasons. First, the turnover rate of oral mucosal cells is relatively rapid. For example, gingival sulcular epithelial cells have a turnover rate of 3 to 7 days. The clear implication is that sufficient nutrients must be available at the appropriate times and in the correct concentration so DNA replication, protein synthesis, and cell/tissue maturation can occur, consistent with the tissues' physiologic needs. Second, as stated earlier, the oral epithelium acts as an effective barrier against the invasion of toxic substances, particularly antigens derived from oral microbes, into the underlying collagenous connective tissue. Inadequate nutrition can cause the oral epithelia to either break down or to be compromised, to increase the tissue's susceptibility to infectious disease.

The manifestation of systemically induced oral changes include anatomic lesions, color changes, functional changes (e.g., burning mouth and tongue), textural changes, and inflammation of the lips, oral mucosa, corners of the mouth, tongue, and gingiva[3] (see Chap. 55). The rule of thumb is that no simple clinical sign is of any real significance by itself; usually, several etiologic factors are suspected in ascertaining a differential diagnosis. Painful oral lesions resulting from nutrient deficiency can alter a patient's food selection and oral hygiene behavior, thus increasing the risk of oral disease and other systemic diseases. Cheilosis, inflammation of the lips, or angular stomatitis, inflammation of the corners of the mouth, vertical fissuring of the lips, cracks at the corners of the mouth, dryness and peeling of the lips, or bleeding when the lips are irritated are changes associated with riboflavin, iron, or protein deficiency. However, inflammation or cracking of the lips may also be due to non-nutritional factors, such as allergies, licking of the lips, or drooling. Loss of vertical dimension occurs in long-time denture wearers, resulting in overclosure of the jaw. Skin folds develop at the corners of the mouth, providing a moist area where bacterial or fungal infections may develop.

The dorsum of the tongue may undergo changes in size or color; taste changes may result from atrophy or hypertrophy of the tongue papillae. Inflammation, a burning sensation, and tenderness of the tongue or palate may be caused by a deficiency of vitamin B complex, protein, or iron. In one study, clinical symptoms of burning mouth syndrome were diagnosed to be associated with vitamin B-complex deficiencies based on biochemical tests.[99] When a vitamin B-complex supplement was given, clinical symptoms were resolved in 24 of 28 subjects. Long-standing nutrient deficiencies may lead to atrophy of the papillae and denudation of the dorsum. For example, a bright red, painful tongue and swelling of the oral mucosa may be early symptoms of pernicious anemia resulting from a lack of Vitamin B_{12}.

Changes in the oral mucosa may also be due to diabetes, food allergies, aphthous ulcers, or nutritional deficiencies. For example, one variety of gingivitis is the oral manifestation of ascorbic acid deficiency; initially, the interdental papillae are red, and the marginal and attached gingiva become inflamed and swollen. Ultimately, the gingiva becomes boggy and bleeds easily. A bright red, inflamed mucosa, from a vitamin B-complex deficiency, may be seen in long-term alcoholics. The mucosa may become pale because of iron-, folic acid-, or vitamin B_{12}-induced anemia.

ALVEOLAR OSTEOPOROSIS

The alveolar process on the crest of the maxilla and mandible is composed primarily of trabecular bone. Histologically, it is the same type of bone found in the distal radius, neck of the femur, and vertebrae. When negative calcium balance occurs in the body, calcium is more easily mobilized from skeletal sites consisting of trabecular than cortical bone. Thus, the alveolar bone provides a potential labile source of calcium available to meet other tissue needs. In fact, the alveolar process is thought to undergo resorption prior to other bones; therefore, changes detected in the alveolar process may be used for early diagnosis of osteoporosis. Edentulous subjects with severe alveolar resorption were found to have low bone density of the radius,[100] and mandibular bone mass correlated with total body calcium and bone mass of the radius and vertebrae in dentate and edentulous postmenopausal women with osteoporosis.[101] The highest correlation was between total body calcium and mandibular bone mass. Thus, the mandible seems to reflect the mineral status of the entire skeleton. Calcium intake in postmenopausal osteoporotic women was correlated with mandibular density; thus, low calcium intake may reduce bone density.

Resorption of the alveolar process is a widespread problem among patients with dentures. Remodeling of the alveolar bone occurs in response to occlusal forces associated with chewing. With the loss of teeth, the alveolar bone is no longer required for tooth support; as a consequence, bone resorption is accelerated and bone height is diminished. Bone loss is greatest during the first 6 months following tooth extractions. The reduction in residual ridge height is more pronounced in women than in men; and resorption is greater in the mandible than in the maxilla. Severe mandibular resorption makes it difficult to construct a mandibular denture with good stability and retention. A low calcium intake may compound bone loss in denture wearers.[102] In a small group of edentulous adults, those with the greatest loss of vertical height had lower calcium intakes. Calcium supplementation for new denture wearers may help maintain calcium balance and may slow the rate of alveolar resorption. Positive calcium balance may be especially important to help preserve the integrity of the residual ridges of edentulous postmenopausal women.

DENTAL MANAGEMENT OF EATING DISORDERS

Long-term, self-induced vomiting may result in permanent damage to the teeth of patients with eating disorders. The extent of oral tissue damage depends on the frequency of the purging and the cariogenicity of the diet. Because they are often the first health-care providers to see these patients, dentists may make an early diagnosis of an eating disorder. Some symptoms that may cause these patients to seek dental treatment are sensitivity to hot and cold temperatures or to air or dental pain, as well as concern about the appearance of their teeth.

The most obvious clinical symptom of bulimia nervosa is loss of tooth enamel (perimylosis) and dentin on the lingual and incisal surfaces of anterior teeth and occlusal surfaces of posterior teeth. Enamel erosion is primarily caused by chronic regurgitation of the acidic contents of the stomach. Erosion may also result from frequent intake of fruit juices high in citric acid, sucking on chewable vitamin C tablets, disulfiram (Antabuse) therapy for alcoholism, or exposure to industrial acids. Contact and thermal hypersensitivity occurs when the dentin is exposed. The acidic oral environment causes irritation of the oral mucosa including the gingiva, palate, and pharynx. With repeated vomiting, esophageal tears may develop. The lips may become cracked, and fissures may develop at the corners of the mouth. Enlargement of the parotid glands, which are painful to palpation, may occur 2 to 6 days after vomiting. When compared to normal adults, low resting salivary flow rates have been found in patients with eating disorders. This may result in xerostomia.[103] The dental caries profile and periodontal status of bulimia nervosa patients is similar to those of healthy young adults without eating disorders.[104] Low levels of dental caries, dental plaque, and gingival recession have been reported; however, high intakes of fermentable carbohydrates during binges may cause caries.

Dental treatment must be coordinated with the primary health-care provider. Definitive restorative treatment cannot occur until the vomiting behavior is under control. Temporary restorations are placed on eroded tooth surfaces to prevent further loss of enamel and to prevent hypersensitivity. The patient is encouraged to practice meticulous oral hygiene. Patients are cautioned against brushing immediately after vomiting, to prevent further erosion of dental enamel. Instead, a sodium bicarbonate or magnesium hydroxide rinse is recommended to neutralize acid in the mouth. Neutral pH sodium fluoride rinses (0.5%) or the home application of stannous fluoride gels (0.4%) in custom trays will prevent dental erosion and will enhance remineralization of teeth.[105] Patients should be counseled to limit fruit juices with high citric acid content and to avoid sticky, sweet foods between meals. Foods of low cariogenicity—nuts, seeds, cheese, and vegetables—are desirable snacks. If dry mouth is a problem, chewing paraffin wax, sugarless chewing gum, or sugar-free lemon drops may be used to stimulate saliva flow.

CONCLUSION

In conclusion, earlier epidemiologic studies could not identify clear relationships between dietary intake patterns and the prevalence of oral disease. Careful review of the literature reveals that, among other things, the measures of dietary intake and nutritional status used in those studies lacked adequate sensitivity. Therefore, a great need exists to update these epidemiologic data to identify profiles of food intake and the risk of disease using more accurate, contemporary indices of dietary intake and nutritional status.

Nevertheless, the observations made in the past decade suggest that diet and nutrition are intimately linked to general and oral tissue health promotion and disease prevention. The discovery that people can change their eating behavior as a consequence of aggressive health promotion and disease prevention programs, and that better, more sensitive measures of nutritional status exist, will have a major impact on our understanding of nutrient-oral tissue relationships and subsequent dietary intervention programs. In this regard, the Surgeon General's recent report on nutrition and health places nutrition and oral health in the appropriate context, articulating that life style is associated with oral health. The impact of nutrition on dental education and clinical practice will be profound, provided appropriate academic programs are implemented to train investigators and clinicians in nutrition and oral health science. The consequences will be nothing short of integrating dentistry more closely into the health-care delivery system and of improving public health and welfare.

REFERENCES

1. Shaw, J.H., Sweeney, E.A. Nutrition in relation to dental medicine. In Modern Nutrition in Health and Disease. 7th Ed. Edited by M.E. Shils and V.R. Young. Philadelphia, Lea & Febiger, 1988, pp. 1070–1071.
2. Surgeon General's Report on Nutrition and Health: Dental Diseases. U.S. Department of Health & Human Services, Publ. No. 88-50210. Washington, D.C., United States Government Printing Office, 1988, pp. 345–380.
3. Dreizen, S.: Pediatrician, *16:*139–146, 1989.
4. Sweeney, E.A., Saffir, A.J., deLeon, R.: Am. J. Clin. Nutr., *4:*29–31, 1971.
5. Sawyer, D.R., Kwoku A.L.: J. Dent. Child., *54:*141–145, 1985.
6. Punysingh, J.T., Hoffman, S., Harris, S.S., et al.: J. Oral Pathol., *13:*40–57, 1984.
7. Boyle, P.E.: J. Dent. Res., *13:*139–150, 1933.
8. Kim, Y.S., Stumpf, W.A., Clark, S.A., et al.: J. Dent. Res., *62:*58–59, 1983.
9. Leaver, A.G.: Clin. Orthop., *78:*90–107, 1971.
10. Bawden, J.W.: Anat. Rec., *224:*226–233, 1989.
11. Mellanby, M.: Br. Dent. J., *44:*1031–1041, 1923.
12. Wolf, J.J.: Am. J. Dis. Child., *49:*905–911, 1935.
13. Boyle, P.E.: J. Dent. Res., *14:*172, 1934.
14. Schiltz, J.R., Rosenbloom, J., Levinson, G.E.: J. Embryol. Exp. Morphol., *37:*49–57, 1977.
15. Alvarez, J.O., Eguren, J.C., Caleda, J., et al.: J. Dent. Res., *69:*1564–1566, 1990.
16. Alvarez, J.O., Navia, J.M.: Am. J. Clin. Nutr., *49:*417–426, 1989.
17. Rami-Reddy, V., Vijayalakshmi, P.B., Chandrasekhar-Reddy, B.K.: Odont. Pediatr., *7:*1–5, 1986.
18. Delgado, H., Habicht, J.P., Yarbrough, C., et al.: Am. J. Clin. Nutr., *38:*216–224, 1975.
19. Menaker, L., Navia, J.M.: J. Dent. Res., *52:*688–691, 1973.
20. National Institute of Dental Research: Mineralized tissues, craniofacial development, dentofacial malrelations and trauma. *In* Broadening the Scope: Long-Range Research Plan for the Nineties. NIH Publ. No. 90–1188. Washington, D.C., United States Government Printing Office, 1990.
21. Iber, F.L.: Nutr. Today, *15:*5, 1980.
22. Slavkin, H.C.: Cleft Palate J., *27:*101–109, 1990.
23. Akam, M.: Cell, *57:*347–349, 1989.
24. Lammer, E.J., Chen, D.T., Hoar, R.M., et al.: N. Engl. J. Med., *313:*837–841, 1985.
25. Slavkin, H.C.: Personal communication, 1992.
26. MRC Vitamin Study Research Group: Lancet, *338:*131–137, 1991.
27. National Institute of Dental Research: Oral Health of United States Children: The National Survey of Dental Caries in U.S. School Children: 1986–1987. NIH Publ. No.

89–2247. Washington D.C., United States Government Printing Office, 1989.
28. National Institute of Dental Research: The Prevalence of Dental Caries in United States Children, 1979–1980. NIH Publ. No. 82–2245. Bethesda, MD, United States Government Printing Office, 1981.
29. National Institute of Dental Research: Oral Health of U.S. Adults: The National Survey of Oral Health in United States Employed Adults and Seniors: 1985–1986. NIH Publication No. 87–2868. Washington D.C., United States Government Printing Office, 1987.
30. Glass, R.L., Alman, J.E., Chauncey, H.H.: Caries Res., *21:*360–367, 1987.
31. Stephan, R.M.: J. Am. Dent. Assoc., *23:*257–266, 1944.
32. Fitzgerald, R.J., Keyes, P.H.: J. Am. Dent. Assoc., *61:*9–19, 1960.
33. Loesche, W.: Microbiol. Rev., *50:*353–380, 1986.
34. Tanzer, J.M.: J. Dent. Res., *65(Spec. Iss.):*1491–1497, 1986.
35. Konig, K.G., Schmid, P., Schmid, R.: Arch. Oral Biol., *13:*13–26, 1968.
36. Sreenby, L.M.: Commun. Dent. Oral Epidemiol., *10:*1–7, 1982.
37. Ishii, T., König, K.G., Mühlemann, H.R.: Helv. Odontol. Acta, *12:*41–47, 1968.
38. Harris, R.: J. Dent. Res., *42:*1387–1399, 1963.
39. Rugg-Gunn, A.J., Hackett, A.F., Appleton, D.R.: Caries Res., *21:*464–478, 1987.
40. Grobler, S.R., Blignaut, J.B.: Clin. Prevent. Dent., *11:*8–12, 1989.
41. Birkhed, D.: Caries Res., *18:*120–127, 1984.
42. Ismail, A.I., Burt, B.A., Eklund, S.A.: J. Am. Dent. Assoc., *109:*241–245, 1984.
43. Motokawa, W., Mraham, R., Ishii, K., et al.: Quintessence Int., *21:*983–987, 1990.
44. Mäkinen, K.K., Isokogas, P.: Prog. Food Nutr. Sci., *12:*73–109, 1988.
45. Kalfas, S., Svanäter, D., Birkhed, D., et al.: J. Dent. Res., *69:*442–446, 1990.
46. Scheinen, A., Mäkinen, K.K.: Acta Odontol. Scand., *34:*179–216, 1975.
47. Tanzer, J.M., Slee, A.M.: J. Am. Dent. Assoc., *106:*331–333, 1983.
48. Lout, R.K., Messer, L.B., Soberay, A., et al.: Caries Res., *22:*237–241, 1988.
49. Söderling, E., Mäkinen, K.K., Chen, C.Y.: Caries Res., *23:*378–384, 1989.
50. Scheinen, A., Mäkinen, K.K., Larmas, M.: Acta Odontol. Scand., *39:*269–278, 1975.
51. Newbrun, E., Hoover, C., Mettrauz, G., et al.: J. Am. Dent. Assoc., *101:*619–626, 1980.
52. Mundorff, S.A., Featherstone, J.D.B., Bibby, B.G., et al.: Caries Res., *24:*344–355, 1990.
53. Gustaffsson, B., Quensel, S.E., Svenander-Lanke, L., et al.: Acta Odontol. Scand., *11:*232–264, 1954.
54. Ismail, A.I.: J. Dent. Res., *65:*1435–1440, 1986.
55. Burt, B.A., Eklund, S.A., Morgan, K.J., et al.: J. Dent. Res., *67:*1422–1429, 1988.
56. Rugg-Gunn, A.J., Edgar, W.M., Jenkins, G.N.: J. Dent. Res., *60:*867–872, 1981.
57. Tabak, L.A., Bowen, W.H.: J. Dent. Res., *68:*1560–1566, 1989.
58. Jensen, M.E., Harlander, S.K., Schachtell, C.F., et al.: Evaluation of the acidogenic and antacid properties of cheeses by telemetric recording of dental plaque. *In* Food, Nutrition and Dental Health. Vol. V. Edited by J.J. Hefferen, H.M. Koehler, and J.C. Osborn. Park Forest South, IL, Pthotox, 1984.
59. Silva, M.F., Jenkins, G.N., Burgess, R.C., et al.: Caries Res., *20:*263–269, 1986.
60. DePaola, D.P.: J. Dent. Res., *65(Spec. Iss.):*1540–1543, 1986.
61. Schachtele, C.F., Harlander, S.K.: J. Can. Dent. Assoc., *50:*213–219, 1984.
62. Ripa, L.W.: Baby Bottle Tooth Decay: A Comprehensive Review. Atlanta, Centers for Disease Control: Dental Disease Prevention Activity, DDPA, 1988.
63. Van Houte, J., Jordan, R., Laraway, R., et al.: J. Dent. Res., *69:*1463–1468, 1990.
64. Havald, N., Hamp, S.E., Birkhed, D.: J. Clin. Periodont., *13:*758–767, 1986.
65. Papas, A.S., Palmer, C.A., McGandy, R., et al.: Gerodontics, *3:*30–37, 1987.
66. Papas, A.S., Palmer, C.A., Rounds, M.C., et al.: Ann. N.Y. Acad. Sci., *561:*124–142, 1989.
67. Department of Health & Human Services, Public Health Service: Review of Fluoride Benefits and Risks. Report of the Ad Hoc Subcommittee on Fluoride of the Committee to Coordinate Environmental Health & Related Programs. Washington, D.C., United States Government Printing Office, 1991.
68. Dean, H.T.: Epidemiological Studies in the United States. *In* Dental Caries and Fluoride. Edited by F.R. Moulton. Washington, D.C., American Association of Advancement of Science, 1946.
69. Murray, J.J., Rugg-Gunn, A.J.: Fluorides and Dental Caries. 2nd Ed. Bristol, England, John Wright & Sons, 1982.
70. Brunelle, J.A., Carlos, J.P.: J. Dent. Res., *69(Spec. Iss):* 723–727, 1990.
71. Newbrun, E.: J. Public Health Dent., *49:*279–289, 1989.
72. American Dental Association: Prescribed fluoride supplements. *In* American Dental Association Accepted Dental Therapeutics. 40th Ed. Chicago, American Dental Association, 1984.
73. Kula, K., Wei, S.H.Y.: Fluoride supplements and dietary sources of fluoride. *In* Clinical Uses of Fluoride. Edited by S.H.Y. Wei. Philadelphia, Lea & Febiger, 1985.
74. Brunelle, J.A.: J. Dent. Res., *68:*995, 1989.
75. Levy, S.M., Zavash, Zarei-M.: J. Dent. Child., *58:*467–473, 1991.
76. Pendrys, D.G., Stamm, J.W.: J. Dent. Res., *69(Spec. Iss.):*529–538, 1990.
77. Alvares, O., Siegel, I.: J. Oral Pathol., *10:*40–48, 1981.
78. Alvares, O., Altman, L.C., Springmeyer, S., et al.: J. Periodont. Res., *16:*628–636, 1981.
79. Leggott, P.J., Robertson, P.B., Rothman, D.C., et al.: J. Periodontol., *57:*480–485, 1986.
80. Alfano, M.C.: Dent. Clin. North Am., *20:*519–548, 1976.
81. Russell, A.L.: J. Dent. Res., *42:*233–247, 1963.
82. Burt, B.A., Eklund, S.A., Landis, J.R., et al.: A Study of Dietary Intake Food Patterns and Dental Health. Analysis of Data from the HANES I Survey. Ann Arbor, MI, University of Michigan, 1980.
83. Genco, R.J., Wilson, M.E., DeNardin, E.: Peridontal complications and neutrophil abnormalities. *In* Contemporary Periodontitis. Edited by R. Genco, H. Goldman, and D.W. Cohen. St. Louis, C.V. Mosby, 1990.

84. Malleck, H.M.: An Investigation of the Role of Ascorbic Acid and Iron in the Etiology of Gingivitis in Humans. Doctoral Thesis. Cambridge, MA, Institute Archives, Massachusetts Institute of Technology, 1978.
85. Whitehead, N., Ryner, F., Lindenbaum, J.: JAMA, *226:*1421–1424, 1973.
86. Chauncy, H.H., Muench, M.E., Kapur, K.K., et al.: Int. Dent. J., *34:*98–104, 1984.
87. Wayler, A.H., Muen, C.H., Kapur, K.K., et al.: J. Gerontol., *39:*284–289, 1984.
88. Kapur, K.K., Soman, K.K.: J. Prosthet. Dent., *14:*1054–1064, 1964.
89. McGrandy, R.B., Russell, R.M., Hartz, S.C.: Nutr. Res., *6:*785–798, 1986.
90. Rhodus, N.L., Brown, J.: J. Am. Diet. Assoc., *90:*1688–1692, 1990.
91. Heft, M.W., Baum, B.J.: J. Dent. Res., *63:*1182–1185, 1984.
92. Beck, J.D., Hunt, R.J.: J. Dent. Educ., *49:*407–425, 1985.
93. Bartoshuk, L.M.: Chemical sensation: taste. *In* Nutrition in Oral Health and Disease. Edited by R. Pollack and R. Kravitz. Philadelphia, Lea & Febiger, 1985.
94. Robertson, P.B., Greenspan, J.S.: Oral Manifestations of Aids: Diagnosis and Management of HIV-Associated Infections. Littleton, MA, PSG Publishing, 1988.
95. Winkler, J.R., Murray, P.A., Grassi, M., et al.: J. Am. Dent. Assoc., *119*(Suppl.):25–40, 1989.
96. Toth, B.B., Martin, J.W., Flemming, R.J.: Clin. Periodont., *17:*508–515, 1990.
97. Nikoskelainen, J.: J. Clin. Periodont., *17:*504–507, 1990.
98. Montgomery, M.T.: Irradiation. *In* Internal Medicine for Dentistry. Edited by L. Rose and D. Kaye. St. Louis, C.V. Mosby, 1990.
99. Lamey, P.J., Allam, B.F.: Br. Dent. J., *160:*81–83, 1986.
100. Bays, R.A., Weinstein, R.S.: J. Oral Maxillofac. Surg., *40:*270–272, 1982.
101. Kribbs, P.J., Chestnut, C.H., Ott, S., et al.: J. Prosthet. Dent., *62:*703–707, 1989.
102. Wical, K.E., Swoope, C.C.: J. Prosthet. Dent., *32:*13–22, 1974.
103. Tylenda, C.A., Robert, M.W., Elin, R.J.: J. Am. Dent. Assoc., *122:*37–41, 1991.
104. Roberts, M.W., Li, S.H.: J. Am. Dent. Assoc., *115:*407–410, 1987.
105. Gross, K.B.W., Brough, K.M., Randolph, P.M.: J. Dent. Child. *53:*378–381, 1986.
106. Alvarez, J.O., Lewis, C.A., Saman, C., et al.: Am. J. Clin. Nutr., *48:*368–372, 1988.

SELECTED READINGS

Curzon M.E.J., tenCate J.M. (eds.): Diet, nutrition and dental caries: Proceedings of the Second European Congress on Diet, Nutrition and Dental Caries. Caries Res., *24(Suppl. 1):*1–79, 1990.
National Research Council: Diet and Health: Implications for Reducing Chronic Disease Risk. Washington D.C., National Academy Press, 1989.
Newbrun, E.: Cariology. 3rd Ed. Chicago, Quintessence, 1989.
Nizel A.E., Papas A.S.: Nutrition in Clinical Dentistry. 3rd Ed. Philadelphia, W.B. Saunders, 1989.
Pollack, R.L., Kravitz E.: Nutrition in Oral Health & Disease. Philadelphia, Lea & Febiger, 1985.

CHAPTER 61

The Stomach and Nutrition

James H. Meyer

THE STOMACH AS A DIGESTIVE ORGAN

Clinical observations indicate that the stomach plays several roles in normal alimentation. All patients who have had a surgical removal of the whole stomach or the distal stomach (removal of the antrum at subtotal gastrectomy) malabsorb food to some degree. Whenever they eat, some patients with total or subtotal gastrectomy experience a variety of gastrointestinal symptoms that prevent them from eating enough. As a result of both malabsorption and early satiety, many patients are undernourished after these operations. Some are malnourished, exhibiting iron deficiency, and/or loss of bone mass.[1] After total gastrectomy, B_{12} deficiency ensues in 3 to 5 years unless the vitamin is given parenterally. These observations indicate that the stomach is an organ that is not necessary for long survival but one that greatly facilitates the efficient digestion and absorption of nutrients.

The stomach secretes intrinsic factor, acid, and enzymes important to normal digestion and absorption. It grinds coarse pieces of solid food into fine, easily digestible particles before passing them on into the small intestine. The stomach stores food, not only prolonging the time for intragastric digestion, but also limiting the rates at which nutrients enter the duodenum to those optimal for enzymatic degradation, solubilization, and intestinal absorption.

GASTRIC SECRETION AND INTRAGASTRIC DIGESTION

The acid-secreting or oxyntic mucosa lies mostly in the fundus or proximal stomach, extending from the level of the gastroesophageal junction to the antrum. The sight or smell of food and distention of the stomach trigger nervous reflexes that stimulate acid secretion from the parietal cells. Caffeine and other alkaloids in coffee, ethanol, calcium ions, high intragastric pH, and proteins that have been digested partially by pepsin release the hormone, gastrin, when they contact the antral mucosa. Gastrin stimulates acid secretion. On reaching the small intestine, dietary proteins also stimulate gastric secretion, while fats in the small intestine inhibit this action.[2] As a result of these stimuli, acid secretion rapidly rises to a peak at about 90 minutes after ingestion of the meal and is sustained for 3 to 4 hours above basal rates of output. Intragastric pH has a variable time course: if the meal contained much dissolved protein (as in a milkshake), much of the initially secreted acid is buffered so the pH falls more slowly than after a meal of solid, undissolved protein.[3]

Hydrochloric acid is a major component of normal gastric secretion. Under fasting conditions, high gastric acidity kills bacteria and parasites, greatly increasing the size of an inoculum needed to infect the individual. After meals, gastric acid also plays important roles in digestion. Gastric acid solubilizes inorganic iron (iron salts). For example, patients who have had subtotal gastric resections secrete acid at rates less than 20% of normal. Iron salts added to food are poorly absorbed by these individuals, and likewise, iron salts are poorly absorbed from meals after normal subjects have had their acid secretion suppressed by the H_2 secretory antagonist, cimetidine.[1] Ferric salts are insoluble at pH 4 to 6, but ferrous salts are about 100 times more soluble in this pH range.[4] Dissolution of ferric salts at low pH in the stomach allows their reduction to ferrous salts before they enter the duodenum where ferrous salts are sufficiently soluble for intestinal absorption. Acidity also dissociates vitamin B_{12} from proteinaceous foods and promotes its complex formation with intrinsic factor.[1]

Intrinsic factor is similarly secreted from fundic parietal cells in response to gastrin and neural stimuli, but over a shorter time course.[3] The major proteases secreted by the stomach are pepsinogens I and II. Both are secreted from the chief and mucous neck cells in the oxyntic mucosa in response to gastrin and neural stimuli. The less prominent pepsinogen II is also secreted by pyloric gland cells in the antrum. Gastric lipase is secreted in response to gastrin by the chief cells in the fundic mucosa in which pepsin and lipase are located together.[5] In addition, both salivary amylase and traces of a pharyngeal lipase are swallowed and remain active to some degree in the stomach.

Intrinsic factor has a high affinity and a high specificity for cyanocobalamin.[6] It normally is secreted in great excess from the oxyntic mucosa—estimated at 100 times what is needed to facilitate adequate absorption of dietary B_{12}.[7] Thus, B_{12} deficiency is uncommon after subtotal gastrectomy, an operation during which the antrum is removed but 10 to 20% of the oxyntic mucosa is left in the fundus; but, B_{12} deficiency develops in 3 to 5 years after total gastrectomy (an operation during which all source of intrinsic factor is removed), unless the vitamin is given parenterally. Patients who have intact stomachs but spontaneously develop pernicious anemia usually have atrophic gastritis, a common condition in older individuals. The fundic mucosa becomes inflamed and atrophies. Even so, some nests of parietal cells remain, so that most older individuals with atrophic gastritis still have enough intrinsic factor to absorb vitamin B_{12} normally. Those few who acquire pernicious anemia have an inherited, autoimmune disease in which antibodies are formed to intrinsic factor, to parietal cells, and frequently to other tissues, such as thyroid. The antibodies block the ability of remaining intrinsic factor to bind B_{12} or to attach to the ileal transporter of B_{12}.[8]

Pepsinogens are converted to active pepsins after a small peptide spontaneously separates from the main molecule in the presence of acid. Pepsins have proteolytic activity below pH 4.5. They are endopeptidases with broad, but highest activities against bonds adjacent to aromatic amino acids, cleaving proteins into polypeptides (almost no free amino acids are found in gastric contents after a protein meal). Only about 10 to 15% of peptide bonds are broken by peptic digestion of protein in the stomach.[9,10] Nevertheless, this small amount of peptic hydrolysis renders proteins more rapidly digestible by pancreatic endo- and exopeptidases in the duodenum,[10] because even this small amount of hydrolysis denatures or uncoils protein to make it more accessible to attack by endopeptidases and because peptic hydrolysis increases the number of C-terminal amino acids susceptible to attack by pancreatic carboxypeptidases. Also, the peptic formation of polypeptides converts native proteins to stimuli of acid and pancreatic secretion.[2,10]

Both gastric and pharyngeal (salivary) lipases differ from pancreatic lipase, having lower molecular weights, a lower pH optimum (4 to 6 vs 6 to 8), and greater stability at pH 3. In humans, most acidic lipase in the stomach is secreted from the fundus,[5] but in rodents, most comes from salivary glands. These lipases are important in the hydrolysis of triglycerides in milk during early infancy, when the secretion of pancreatic lipase is not fully developed; but scientists estimate that even in the adult, as much as 10 to 15% of ingested fat may be partially hydrolyzed in the stomach.[11,12] Liberation of small amounts of free fatty acids in the stomach accelerates subsequent lipolysis by pancreatic lipase in the small intestine,[12] because the lipolytic products formed promote the emulsification of the remaining triglyceride and the binding of colipase to the surfaces of the oil droplets formed.

Swallowed salivary amylase is destroyed at gastric pH of less than 3. Nevertheless, gastric pH is above 3 for a substantial period after the meal, during which time salivary amylase remains active.[13] Moreover, the pH in the stomach is not uniform, remaining much closer to 7 in saliva floating in the fundus, while falling below 3 in the antrum. Also, salivary amylase may remain inside balls of chewed and swallowed bread at more neutral pH, while the pH of aqueous contents of the stomach around the bread is lower. As a consequence of these sequestrations, as much as 60% of swallowed bread or rice (simple starches) may be digested by salivary amylase during residence in the stomach.[9]

GASTRIC GRINDING AND SIEVING OF SOLID FOOD

Chewed, solid food often is swallowed as pieces considerably larger than 1 cm; but more than 95% of particles of meat or bread emptying from the stomach are smaller than 1 mm.[14] One half are smaller than 0.06 mm. The stomach grinds or triturates the larger chunks of food into the tiny particles and also selectively retains or sieves out the larger ones, so that only the smallest particles pass into the duodenum. Grinding, sieving, and propulsion from the stomach appear to be separate processes, because they can be dissociated from one another to some degree. For example, when 0.25-mm particles of liver radiolabeled with one nuclide were ingested simultaneously with 10-mm particles of liver labeled with another nuclide, the 0.25-mm particles passed promptly from the stomach, whereas the 10-mm pieces did not begin to empty for 30 minutes or so, while they were being ground to a smaller size.

Some of the grinding and/or sieving of particles of solid food reside in the most distal stomach, as the size of particles that pass from the stomach is sharply increased if the pylorus and more than 4 cm of terminal antrum are surgically removed. Thus, 30% of ingested radiolabeled meat emptied as particles larger than 1 mm in animals or human patients who had undergone distal gastric resection, a common operation for peptic ulcer.

The distal two thirds of the stomach (antrum and distal body) undergoes vigorous peristalsis; that is, up to three times a minute, powerful rings of contractions sweep aborally over the distal stomach to the pylorus. These peristaltic contractions push fluid and suspended food toward the duodenum. Early in each cycle, some of the gastric contents are forced through the open pylorus; but the pylorus closes sometime before the advancing contraction wave reaches the end of the antrum. Thus, in the terminal phase of the contraction cycle, the antrum continues to narrow its lumen while the closed pyloric valve prevents gastric contents from escaping into the duodenum. As the antral lumen is obliterated by a terminal antral contraction, gastric contents, no longer able to exit, are suddenly retropelled into the more proximal stomach. This sequential to-and-fro movement of gastric contents has been visualized with cineradiographic or real-time ultrasonographic studies. It is believed that the sudden to-and-fro motions of gastric contents tumble and eventually sheer large pieces of food into small particles.[14] Peptic digestion facilitates the grinding process, but normally most of the fracturing of meat into small particles appears to be achieved mechanically through gastric motor activity.

Most particles of food emptying from the stomach are considerably smaller than 1 mm and thus are smaller than minimum pyloric diameter of about 2.5 mm. Therefore, the selective emptying of tiny particles by the stomach does not likely depend only on pyloric size. The current idea is that sieving is accomplished by hydrodynamic forces. According to one hypothesis, the smallest particles with the least inertia are accelerated much ahead of the larger particles, as a contraction wave advances over the antrum toward the pylorus; and with each cycle, only the smallest particles travel across the pylorus into the duodenum before reversal of flow. Two observations strongly support the idea of hydrodynamic selection. First, small plastic spheres more dense than water empty more slowly than other spheres of the same size but with a density equal to that of water. The denser spheres have greater inertia. Second, increasing the viscosity of gastric contents shifts the distribution of emptied particles to larger sizes. For example, adding the viscous, gel-forming, polysaccharide guar to a meal resulted in the gastric emptying of large pieces of meat from the normal canine stomach. By increasing the fluid drag on food particles, especially on those of larger diameter or cross-sectional area, increasing viscosity would reduce the sensitivity of the selection of particles by inertial properties. Both observations are thus consistent with the idea that a hydrodynamic process selects the smallest food particles for expulsion.

The normal ability of the stomach to grind and empty only the small particles greatly enhances digestion in the small intestine, because the smaller particles of food have a large ratio of surface to mass. Pancreatic enzymes in the aqueous contents of the small intestine can attack solid nutrients only at the particle surfaces. This idea is supported by results of an experiment in which dogs with intact stomachs and dogs with distal gastric resections were fed meals that contained ^{14}C-triolein, either as a liquid fat in margarine or as a part of solid food after its incorporation into the cells of chicken liver.[15] The investigators measured the amount of radiotriolein that was digested and absorbed by midintestine. The dogs with intact stomachs digested and absorbed the triolein about as well from the liquid oil as from the solid liver (Fig. 61–1). The dogs that had undergone distal gastric resection absorbed the liquid triolein normally but malabsorbed much of the radiotriolein from the solid liver. Almost all the unabsorbed triolein in these dogs resided in abnormally large particles of liver, which emptied from the resected stomachs and remained still undigested by the time they reached the mid-small intestine.

After subtotal gastric resection for ulcer disease or cancer, ordinary meals of solid food are emptied at rates that range from about one fourth to about twice as fast as normal. Although rapid gastric emptying of food may account for maldigestion and malabsorption of nutrients in some of these patients (discussed further subsequently), even those patients who empty their stomachs slowly malabsorb fat. The inability to digest abnormally large pieces of food that empty from the resected stomach likely accounts for much of the malabsorption among those with slow gastric emptying.

DYNAMICS OF FOOD STORAGE IN THE STOMACH

In contrast to the antrum, the proximal third of the stomach does not undergo peristalsis. This part of the stomach relaxes its muscular tone to accommodate incoming meal volume, and thus serves as a reservoir for both solid and liquid food.[14] Relaxation is mediated in part by vagal reflexes, which initially are triggered as food is swallowed and distends the throat and esophagus. The proximal stomach slowly presses liquid or solid foods into the distal stomach, where vigorous peristalsis grinds the solid food and propels both liquids and solid particles into the duodenum. Of course, the liquid components of the meal flow with gravity. Furthermore, high tonic pressures caused by distention of the proximal stomach with meals of large volume generate substantial fluid pressure gradients between stomach and duodenum. Sometimes, gravitational and/or tonic pressure gradients may suffice to propel fluids across the antrum into the duodenum without much antral peristalsis. At other times, for example, when intragastric volume is low, tonic or gravitational pressures are so low that fluids must be pumped from the stomach by antral peristalsis.

The speed of emptying of stored food is tightly regulated so that the rate of duodenal entry of nutrients is held constant despite a wide range of intake.[16,17] Chem-

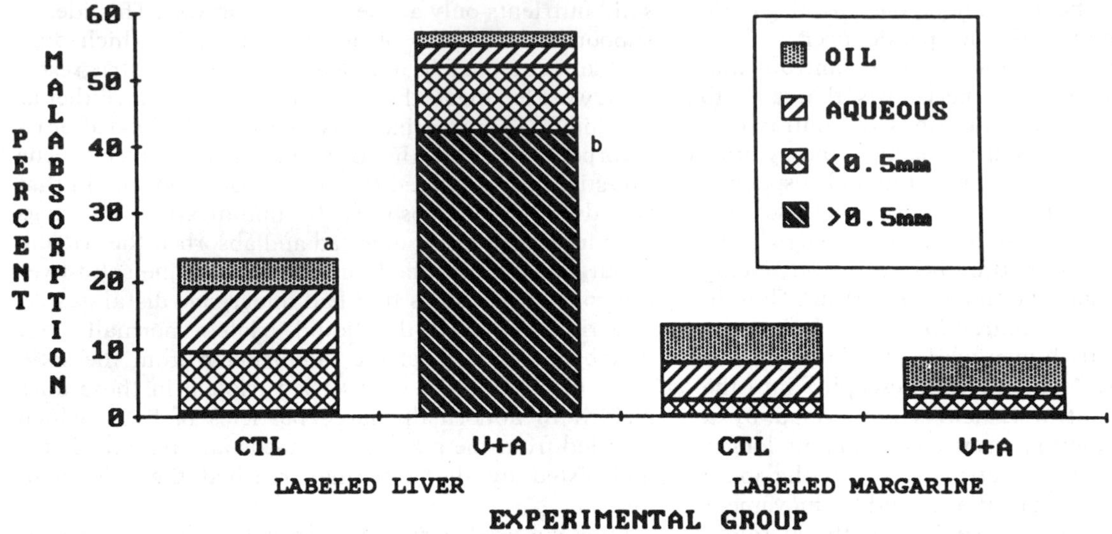

FIGURE 61–1. Percentage of ^{14}C-triolein still unabsorbed (i.e., "malabsorbed") by midgut in normal dogs (CTL) and in dogs with vagotomy + antrectomy (V+A), that is, with removal of the distal 40% of the stomach. The ^{14}C-triolein was incorporated into margarine or was inserted intracellularly into live chicken livers that were later removed, cooked, and fed to the dogs. In the control animals, as well as in the dogs with distal gastric resection, only 10 to 15% of the triolein in the margarine remained unabsorbed by the time the chyme reached midintestine. In the normal dogs, about 80% of the triolein in the solid chicken liver was absorbed by midintestine, so digestion and absorption were nearly as efficient when the triolein was consumed as a liquid fat as when it was consumed within pieces of solid food. In the normal dogs, almost all the remaining solid food reached the midintestine as particles<0.5 mm in diameter. By contrast, the dogs with antrectomy absorbed only 40% of the radiotriolein that had been ingested in the chicken liver. Almost all this unabsorbed triolein resided in particles of food (liver) that were abnormally large, that is, >0.5 mm. (From Doty, J.E., Meyer, J.H.: Gastroenterology, *94*:50–56, 1988.)

ical sensors in the intestine detect the presence of digestive products and inhibit gastric emptying. Many sugars (including glucose, sucrose, lactose, maltose, and maltotriose), fatty acids, monoglycerides, a few amino acids, and titratable acidity trigger feedback inhibition from the small intestine. With all of these substances, the degree of inhibition is directly proportional to the speed at which the digestive product arrives in the small bowel. This precise regulation is achieved through the summation of sensory input along a length of intestine. The length of intestine contacted by a nutrient and the concentration profile of the nutrient along that length are determined by a balance between the speed of inflow and the rate of absorption.

For example, glucose meals begin to inhibit gastric emptying at concentrations exceeding 200 mmol/L and maximally inhibit emptying at 1000 mmol/L concentrations well above the maximum for the glucose transporter in the intestine. Therefore, at concentrations above 200 mmol/L, the amount of glucose absorbed per centimeter is constant, and the faster glucose enters the duodenum, the longer the length of bowel required for absorption. At these high luminal concentrations, the strength of the feedback signal from a short length of bowel is independent of concentration; but the longer the length of intestinal mucosa contacted, the greater the total inhibiting signal. Maximum inhibition requires about 50% of small bowel length.

As a result of this metering system, the rate of glucose entry is held to about 0.2 mmol per minute when glucose drinks range from 200 to 1000 mmol/L. Because intestinal absorptive capacity, not the hydrolytic capacity of pancreatic or mucosal enzymes, is rate limiting for absorption of most polymeric nutrients, the length of intestine contacted by maltose and maltotriose (ultimately glucose after hydrolysis at the brush border) will be about the same after starch drinks as with drinks that contain amounts of starch isocaloric with glucose. Thus, isocaloric meals of starch or glucose empty from the stomach at about the same speed.

In contrast to glucose, which is actively transported, fatty acids are absorbed from the intestine by passive diffusion. The rate of absorption is therefore not constant, but it is proportional to luminal concentrations (normally 5 to 25 mmol/L after a meal), and the rates of absorption of fatty acid are slower than that of glucose. As a result, more than one half of the small intestine (that is, the length capable of signaling maximal inhibition) is contacted by fatty acid whether the concentration is 3 or 27 mmol/L. However, within this range of concentrations, the intensity of feedback inhibition depends greatly on concentrations of fatty acid. Thus, metering is achieved through the sensing of varying concentrations along the length of bowel that has maximal inhibiting capacity.[33]

Inhibiting signals from the small intestine can act at a variety of sites to slow gastric emptying. Thus, they can relax the proximal stomach, thereby reducing the rate at which food is pressed into the antrum. They can completely inhibit antral peristalsis, eliminating propulsive activity and/or the trituration of solid food. They can stimulate the pylorus to contract, increasing the resistance to gastric outflow of liquids. They can narrow duodenal caliber and increase nonpropulsive duodenal contractility, thereby reducing duodenal receptive capacity and increasing duodenal resistance to gastric outflow. Nutrients in the small intestine trigger combinations of these actions. The responses are mediated by both nervous signals and release of hormones from the small intestine.

Precise control of gastric emptying by nutrients in the small intestine ensures their efficient digestion, absorption, and metabolism. Thus, nutrients normally enter the duodenum at rates below total intestinal absorptive capacity. Additionally, a controlled rate of duodenal entry assures that polymeric nutrients enter the duodenum slowly enough to be completely hydrolysed by pancreatic and mucosal enzymes before reaching distal intestine. Normally, the rate of entry of nutrients is slow enough to ensure that about 85% of food is digested and absorbed by mid-small intestine.[11]

Digestive derangements after subtotal gastrectomy illustrate the importance of normal regulation of gastric emptying. The partially resected stomach is less capable of controlling the rate of emptying, so that nutrient-containing liquid meals empty rapidly. When gastrectomy patients consumed a liquid meal that contained glucose, fat, and protein, a large percentage of the protein and fat was still unabsorbed by the time it reached the terminal ileum, but the glucose was still mostly absorbed by mid-intestine. Secretion of pancreatic enzymes in such patients is normal, but enzyme concentration is low because of dilution by rapidly emptying meal volume. The poor digestion and absorption of the protein and fat was most likely the outcome of an imbalance between substrate and enzyme concentrations and the rapid intestinal transit that diminished time for hydrolysis within the small intestine. That glucose was absorbed efficiently despite its rapid rate of entry into the duodenum testifies to the large capacity of the small intestine for active absorption. On the other hand, the rapid emptying and subsequently rapid absorption of the glucose in such patients frequently leads to transitory hyperglycemia and glucosuria, and sometimes to subsequent rebound hypoglycemia.[1] Obviously, the glucosuria and perhaps the subsequent glycogenolysis needed to defend against rebound hypoglycemia are examples of poor nutrient use as a direct outcome of uncontrolled gastric emptying. Finally, the abnormally rapid entry of nutrients and/or the abnormal spread of unabsorbed nutrients along nutrient-sensing, small intestine triggers a variety of symptoms (known collectively as the "dumping syndrome") which include early satiety, or even nausea, that may prevent the individual from eating enough.[1]

DIET IN GASTROESOPHAGEAL DISEASES

DIET IN GASTROESOPHAGEAL REFLUX DISEASE

Excessive reflux of gastric contents into the esophagus leads to peptic esophagitis and heartburn or, in severe cases, to the complications of esophageal ulcers or esophageal strictures. The pathogenesis of these disorders is a weak or ineffective lower esophageal sphincter (LES), which permits acidic and peptic gastric contents to bathe and erode the lower esophageal mucosa. Also contributing is a delay in the esophageal propulsion of refluxed gastric contents back into the stomach, a situation that is common at night while the recumbent patient sleeps. With such a delay in clearance, the prolonged contact of gastric juices promotes digestion and erosion of the esophageal mucosa.[18]

Patients who frequently experience heartburn claim that peppers, spicy foods, fatty foods, citrus fruits or juices, alcoholic beverages, and coffee characteristically provoke this condition, although the list of offending foods may be long.[19] Little scientific evidence supports these claims.

Specific foods may exacerbate heartburn in patients with reflux esophagitis in three ways. First, because of its high tonicity, astringency, or acidity,[20] the food may stimulate irritable sensory nerves in an inflamed mucosa, producing the pain of heartburn, much in the same way that dilute hydrochloric acid reproduces heartburn when it is dripped onto the inflamed mucosa in patients who have esophagitis (Bernstein test). This mechanism of direct chemical irritation probably accounts for common complaints about spicy or citrus foods. Second, the offending food is a powerful stimulus of gastric secretion, so that it promotes the esophageal reflux of especially acidic and peptic juices in patients who have an ineffective LES. This mechanism has been established for coffee. In normal individuals, coffee increases the contraction of the LES in a dose-related manner,[21] but it has no such effect in patients who have heartburn associated with an impaired LES because the weak LES cannot respond to the coffee. However, it is a powerful stimulus of gastric secretion. The heartburn that coffee evoked in patients with an impaired LES was abolished by predosing the patients with cimetidine, an antisecretory drug.[22] Third, through the release of gastrointestinal hormones or the triggering of neural reflexes, foods may relax the

LES and thus the barrier to gastroesophageal reflux. Fat,[23,24] chocolate syrup, and high doses (180 to 300 ml of whiskey) of alcohol[25,26] appear to have these properties. Additionally, alcohol is a powerful stimulus of gastric secretion, so that the increase in episodes of low esophageal pH it induced in normal volunteers could have resulted from both its effect on the LES and its stimulation of acid secretion in the stomach.

Because of these observations, dietary advice given to patients suffering from frequent heartburn is to avoid large meals (especially before retiring for the night) and to refrain from ingesting alcohol, chocolate, coffee, or excessively fatty foods.[18] Large meals taken shortly before lying down for the night may promote reflux of retained food and acidic gastric contents. Nevertheless, the scientific certainty is not high. Only a few studies document the effects of foods on LES function. Most of these studies were performed in the early 1970s, before technical difficulties of measuring pressures in the eccentric and narrow LES were recognized. The technical difficulties, the lack of dose-response data in some reports, and the absence of a number of confirmatory studies make this body of information scientifically weak.

DIET IN PEPTIC ULCER DISEASES

Throughout most of this century, physicians have prescribed diets to treat peptic ulcers. Undoubtedly, the practice arose from frequent clinical observations that feeding often ameliorates ulcer pain and from laboratory analyses showing that food, especially protein, buffers acid. Dietary therapy for acute exacerbations of ulcer disease was rationalized[27] to small, frequent feedings—frequent, to provide more or less constant buffering, and small, to limit the amount of gastric distention and thus stimulation of acid secretion. Feedings often consisted of milk or eggs (for buffering capacity) with or without cream (for inhibition of acid secretion and of gastric emptying) or of pureed foods. Both milk and pureed foods were thought to be mechanically soft and not physically irritating to the raw ulcer surface. On recovery, other mechanically soft, proteinaceous foods (chicken, fish) were administered as a "bland diet." Patients frequently were advised to abstain from coffee and alcohol (gastric secretagogues), as well as peppers and spicy foods (chemical irritants of a raw ulcer).

Such dietary treatment was discredited by a few randomized, controlled trials in the 1950s, the results of which showed no differences between regular (i.e., unrestricted) and therapeutic diets with regard to time to healing of the ulcer (by radiographic criteria) or to remission of symptoms.[26–30] Furthermore, proteinaceous foods, especially milk,[30] which possessed the most buffering capacity, were also found to be the most powerful stimuli of acid secretion,[31] so their frequent feeding may actually result in an increase in the amount of acid flowing over the ulcer in a 24-hour period. Buffering by food elevates intragastric pH but does not neutralize acid, like antacids do. Although it is unknown whether acid at low pH is more injurious than titratable acidity at higher pH, the negative clinical trials of diet on ulcer healing suggest that the underlying premises are wrong about the utility of buffering gastric acid with foods. The need for dietary buffering of acid has virtually disappeared with the discovery of powerful antisecretory drugs. Finally, a somewhat increased prevalence of atherosclerosis in ulcer patients who took frequent feedings with milk, eggs, or meats[27] casts further doubt on the desirability of this approach.

Still, the idea lingers that foods somehow may affect the course of peptic ulcer disease. In rats, fiber (i.e., cellulose or sawdust) or coarse foods were observed to influence the distribution of ulcerations induced by indomethacin. In humans, a controlled trial of a high-fiber versus a low-fiber diet did not support the idea that dietary fiber affects the healing of gastric ulcers. Capsaicin, the biologically active ingredient in chile peppers, has been shown to have important effects on mucosal nerves, including those that regulate mucosal blood flow. A number of investigations in rats suggest that capsaicin affects susceptibility to experimentally induced ulcers, but this area of investigation is just emerging.

STARVATION FROM ANOREXIA NERVOSA AND GASTRIC FUNCTION

During starvation, the loss of visceral protein from gastric muscle parallels similar losses from cardiac and skeletal muscles. Just as cardiac output drops in parallel to loss of cardiac muscle, gastric emptying (of aqueous suspensions of barium sulfate) slowed in semistarved volunteers, suggesting diminished work by wasted gastric muscle.[32]

In anorexia nervosa with profound weight loss, gastric emptying of solid foods usually is abnormally slow;[33] this abnormality correlates with diminished contractility of the antrum. Some of these patients exhibit abnormal electrical activity from antral muscle. The disturbances in gastric motor function improve or may even disappear entirely when patients with anorexia nervosa recover and regain weight. However, gastric emptying is normal in patients with other gastrointestinal diseases with comparable amounts of weight loss.

These observations in anorexia nervosa can be interpreted in two ways. One is that the disturbed gastric motor function is the outcome of wasting of gastric muscle. The other is that signals from the brain in this psychosis alter gastric function. At this time, little evidence exists to support one interpretation over the other.

REFERENCES

1. Meyer, J.H.: Chronic morbidity after ulcer surgery. *In* Gastrointestinal Disease: Pathophysiology-Diagnosis-Management. Edited by M.H. Sleisenger and J.S. Fordtran. Philadelphia, W.B. Saunders, 1989, pp. 962–987.
2. Grossman, M.I.: Regulation of gastric acid secretion. *In* The Physiology of the Digestive Tract. Edited by L.R. Johnson, J. Christensen, and M.I. Grossman, et al. New York, Raven Press, 1981, pp. 659–671.
3. Malagelada, J.R., Go, V.L.W., Summerskill, W.H.J.: Dig. Dis. Sci., *24:*101–110, 1979.
4. Conrad, M.E.: Factors affecting iron absorption. *In* Iron Deficiency. Pathogenesis. Clinical Aspects. Therapy. Edited by L. Halberg, H.G. Harworth and A. Vannotti. New York, Academic Press, 1970, pp. 87–115.
5. Moreau, H., Bernadac, A., Gargouri, Y. et al.: Histochemistry, *91:*419–423, 1989.
6. Donaldson, R.M.: Intrinsic factor and transport of Cobalamin. *In* The Physiology of the Digestive Tract. Edited by L.R. Johnson, J. Christensen, M.I., et al.: New York, Raven Press, 1981, pp. 641–658.
7. Ardeman, S., Chaarin, I., Doyle, J.C.: Studies on secretion of gastric intrinsic factor. Br. Med. J., *2:*600. 1964.
8. Weinstein, W.M.: Gastritis. *In* Gastrointestinal Disease: Pathophysiology, Diagnosis, Management. 4th Ed. Edited by M.H. Sleisenger and J.S. Fordtran. Philadelphia, W.B. Saunders, 1989, pp. 792–813.
9. James, A.H.: The nature of the gastric contents in man. *In* The Physiology of Gastric Digestion. London, Edward Arnold, 1957, pp. 1–24.
10. Meyer, J.H., Kelly, K.A.: Am. J. Physiol., *231:*682–691, 1976.
11. Borgstrom, B., Dahlquist, Lundh, G., et al.: J. Clin. Invest., *36:*1521–1536, 1957.
12. Carey, M.C., Small, D.M., Bliss, C.M.: Lipid digestion and absorption. Annu. Rev. Physiol., *45:*651–77, 1983.
13. Fried, M., Abramson, S., Meyer, J.H.: Passage of salivary amylase through the stomach in humans. Dig. Dis. Sci., *32:*1097–1103, 1987.
14. Meyer, J.H.: Gastric motility and gastric emptying. *In* Textbook of Gastroenterology. Edited by T. Yamada, D.H. Alpers, C. Owyang, et al.: Philadelphia, J.B. Lippincott, pp. 137–157.
15. Doty, J.E., Meyer, J.H.: Gastroenterology, *94:*50–56, 1988.
16. Hunt, J.N., Stubbs, D.F.: J. Physiol. (Lond.), *215:*209–225, 1975.
17. McHugh, P.R., Moran, T.H.: Am. J. Physiol., *236:*R254–R260, 1979.
18. Hogan, W.J., Dodds, W.J.: Gastroesophageal reflux disease (reflux esophagitis). *In* Gastrointestinal Disease: Pathophysiology, Diagnosis, Management. 4th Ed. Edited by M.H. Sleisenger and J.S. Fordtran. Philadelphia, W.B. Saunders, 1989, pp. 594–619.
19. Lloyd, D.A., Borda, I.T.: Gastroenterology, *80:*740–1, 1981.
20. Price, S.F., Smithson, K.W., Castell, D.O.: Gastroenterology, *75:*240–243, 1978.
21. Cohen, S., Booth, G.H.: N. Engl. J. Med., *293:*897–899, 1975.
22. Cohen, S.: N. Engl. J. Med., *303:*122–5, 1980.
23. Nebel, O.T., Castell, D.O.: J. Appl. Physiol., *35:*6–8, 1973.
24. Babka, J.C., Castell, D.O.: Dig. Dis. Sci., *18:*391–397, 1973.
25. Hogan, W.J., Viegas de Andrade, S.R., Winship, D.H.: J. Appl. Physiol., *32:*755–760, 1972.
26. Kaufman, S.E., Kaye, M.D.: Gut, *19:*336–338, 1978.
27. Bockus, H.L.: Management of uncomplicated peptic ulcer. *In* Gastroenterology. 2nd Ed. Edited by H.L. Bockus. Philadelphia, W.B. Saunders, 1964, pp. 527–564.
28. Lawrewnce, J.S.: Lancet, *1:*482–485, 1952.
29. Doll, R.: Lancet, *1:*5–9, 1956.
30. McArthur, K., Hogan, D., Isenberg, J.I.: Gastroenterology, *83:*199–203, 1982.
31. Saint-Hilaire, S., Lavers, M.K., Kennedy, J., et al.: Gastric acid secretory value of different foods. Gastroenterology, *39:*1–16, 1960.
32. Keys, A., Brozek, J., Henschel, A., et al.: The Biology of Human Starvation. Minneapolis, University of Minnesota Press, 1950, pp. 587–600.
33. Lin, H.C., Meyer, J.H.: Disordered gastric emptying or motility. *In* Textbook of Gastroenterology. Edited by T. Yamada, D.H. Alpers, C. Owyang, et al. Philadelphia, J.B. Lippincott, pp. 1213–1240.

This work was supported by research funds from the United States Veterans Administration.

CHAPTER 62

Intestinal Disorders

A. SHORT BOWEL SYNDROME

Khursheed N. Jeejeebhoy

The short bowel syndrome refers to the clinical effects of extensive small bowel resection. It includes diarrhea, fluid and electrolyte disturbances, and malabsorption associated with malnutrition. To understand the effects of the short bowel syndrome, it is important to review some essential aspects of gastrointestinal physiology.

PHYSIOLOGIC CONSIDERATIONS

GASTRIC EMPTYING

The rate at which a meal enters the intestine is regulated by the rate of gastric emptying. Gastric emptying of liquids depends on their osmolarity. For digestible solids, the emptying is regulated by the particle size. However, of greater importance in relation to the short bowel syndrome is that chyme entering the distal intestine inhibits gastric emptying.[1]

SMALL BOWEL

Small bowel motility is three times slower in the ileum than in the jejunum.[2] In addition, the ileocecal valve may slow transit, especially when the ileum has been resected.[3]

The small bowel receives about 5 to 6 L of endogenous secretions and 2 to 3 L of exogenous fluids per day. It reabsorbs most of this volume in the small bowel. The amount reabsorbed in the small intestine depends on the nature of the meal.[4] With a meat and salad meal, most of the fluid was absorbed in the jejunum, whereas with a milk and doughnut meal, less was absorbed proximally and more distally. In addition, the absorptive processes are different in the jejunum as compared with the ileum. These differences depend in part on the nature of the electrolyte transport processes and in part on the permeability of the intercellular junctions. In general, water absorption is a passive process resulting from the active transport of nutrients and electrolytes. The transport of sodium creates an electrochemical gradient and also drives the uptake of sugars and amino acids across the intestinal mucosa. In addition, neutral sodium chloride absorption occurs in the ileum. However, the net absorption depends not only on these processes but also on the extent of back diffusion of the transported material into the intestinal lumen through "leaky" intercellular junctions. In the jejunum, these junctions are very leaky and thus, jejunal contents are always isotonic. Fluid absorption in this region of the bowel is inefficient when compared with that in the ileum. It has been estimated that the efficiency of water absorption is 44 and 70% of the ingested load in the jejunum and ileum, respectively. For sodium, the corresponding estimates are 13 and 72%.[5] Hence, the ileum is important in the conservation of fluid and electrolytes.

COLON

The colon has the slowest transit, varying between 24 and 150 hours. The intercellular junctions are the tightest in this part of the bowel and the efficiency of water and salt absorption in the colon exceeds 90%.[5] In addition, carbohydrate is fermented in the colon to short-chain fatty acids (SCFA) that have two important actions. First, SCFA enhance salt and water absorption.[6] Second, the energy content of malabsorbed carbohydrates is salvaged by being absorbed as SCFA. Our recent data suggest that this salvage in short bowel patients may be greater than that in normal subjects.[7] Thus, the colon becomes an important organ for fluid and electrolyte conservation and for the salvage of malabsorbed energy substrates in patients with a short bowel.

ILEUM

The ileum uniquely absorbs vitamin B_{12} and bile salts. Bile salts are essential for the efficient absorption of fats and fat-soluble vitamins. Normally, the demand for bile salts imposed by fat absorption cannot be met by synthesis alone. This full need is only met by ileal resorption of bile salts, which are then recycled into the intestine. With ileal resection, the loss of bile salts increases and is not met by an increase in synthesis. The bile salt pool is depleted and fat absorption is reduced. In addition, loss of bile salts into the colon reduces the ability of the colon to reabsorb salt and water, resulting in increased diarrhea. In the colon, bile salts are also dehydroxylated to deoxy bile salts, which induce colonic water secretion.

EFFECTS OF INTESTINAL RESECTION

MOTILITY

Gastric motility is enhanced by small bowel resection.[8] Whereas proximal resection does not increase the rate of intestinal transit, ileal resection prompts significant acceleration.[8,9] In this situation, the colon aids in slowing intestinal transit, so that in patients with a short bowel without a colon, a marker fed by mouth was excreted completely in a few hours.[10]

ABSORPTION OF FLUID AND ELECTROLYTES

The effect of intestinal resection depends on the extent and site of resection. Proximal resection results in no bowel disturbance because the ileum and colon absorb the increased fluid and electrolyte load efficiently. The remaining ileum continues to absorb bile salts and thus scant amounts reach the colon to impede salt and water resorption. In contrast, when the ileum is resected, the colon receives a larger load of fluid and electrolytes and also receives bile salts that reduce its ability to absorb salt and water, resulting in diarrhea. In addition, if the colon is resected, the ability to maintain fluid and electrolyte homeostasis is severely impaired.[11]

ABSORPTION OF NUTRIENTS

Nutrient absorption occurs throughout the small bowel and the removal of the jejunum alone results in the ileum taking over most of the lost function. In this situation, there is no malabsorption.[12] In contrast, even a loss of 100 cm of ileum causes steatorrhea.[13] The degree of malabsorption increases with the length of resection, and the variety of nutrients malabsorbed increases.[14,15] Balance studies of energy absorption showed that the absorption of fat and carbohydrate were reduced equally to between 50 and 75% of intake.[16] However, nitrogen absorption was reduced to a lesser extent, to 81% of intake. In the study of Ladefoged et al.,[15] the degree of calcium, magnesium, zinc, and phosphorus absorption were reduced but did not correlate with the remaining length of bowel. The authors recommended that parenteral nutrition be mandatory in these patients. Our studies showed similar reduction in absorption, but only one half of our patients required parenteral replacement. The data taken as a whole suggest it is easier to meet needs for energy and nitrogen by increasing oral intake than the needs for electrolytes and divalent ions. A review of the literature before the availability of parenteral nutrition shows that resections of as much as 33% result in no malnutrition, those up to 50% could be tolerated without special aids, but those in excess of 75% require nutritional support to avoid severe malnutrition.[17–27]

ADAPTATION OF THE INTESTINE

After resection, the remaining small bowel hypertrophies and increases absorptive function.[28–31] This process enhances the ability of the remaining bowel to recover the lost function and is thus an important compensatory process. The factors that influence this adaptation are complex and are discussed subsequently, as are the effects of total parenteral nutrition (TPN).

Eating exposes the gastrointestinal tract to a unique set of stimuli that does not occur when it is kept constantly empty; this process is bowel rest. The advent of TPN resulted in the ability to rest the bowel for short or long periods of time without causing malnutrition, a situation that had not been possible previously. This process nourished the body but excluded the gut from nutrient and hormonal stimuli that occur during the ingestion of an oral diet. The advent of defined formula diets (DFD) without residue and diets composed of monomers such as glucose instead of polymeric starch modified the stimuli received by the gut when exposed to a normal diet. It should also be recognized that because nutrients are absorbed progressively along the length of the bowel, the jejunum is exposed to a higher concentration of nutrients than the ileum. Resection of the proximal bowel results in the ileum receiving more nutrients. Resection of the ileum, on the other hand, does not alter the jejunal nutrient load, but it may reduce stimuli from hormones released by the ileum.

Effect of Excluding Food from the Bowel Lumen. The most obvious change that occurs, in laboratory animals, is hypoplasia of the mucosa. At the same time, body composition can be maintained simultaneously by the use of TPN. These facts have been documented extensively and the interested reader is referred to a recent review by Lo and Walker.[32]

In growing or neonatal animals, TPN and bowel rest maintain normal body growth but result in reduced bowel length and gastric and pancreatic hypoplasia.[33–36] Despite the occurrence of mucosal hypoplasia, the development of disaccharidase enzymes and glucose transport is accelerated, and mucosal levels of these enzymes increase in neonatal animals receiving TPN.[34,36] Hypoplasia occurs mainly in the proximal small bowel and is less evident distally.[35] In adult animals, the effect of TPN and bowel rest diminishes mucosal mass but stimulates glucose absorption per milligram of mucosal protein.[37] In addition, TPN and bowel rest increase intestinal permeability[38] and alter the response to endotoxin.[39]

Does Enteral Nutrition Cause Hypoplasia? It is not simply the lack of food but also the nature of the diet that influences mucosal bulk. In neonatal studies, mother's milk is no better than formula.[35] However, refined intragastric liquid feeds cause relative hypoplasia as compared with a solid diet.[33,40]

Factors Influencing Bowel Atrophy. The decreased digestive and absorptive activities of the mucosa during bowel rest appear to be the major reasons for hypoplasia. This concept is supported by the fact that simply increasing the tonicity of the bowel contents results in an increase of the mucosal mass.[41] Absorption of amino acids results in a nonspecific increase of mucosal function and mass.[42] Finally, disaccharide hydrolysis followed by absorption stimulates mucosal growth to a greater extent than equivalent monosaccharide absorption.[43]

Another factor appears to be biliary-pancreatic secretion. Transplantation of the ampulla causes mucosal hypoplasia, whereas infusion of cholecystokinin and secretin stimulate mucosal growth.[44,45] Recently, SCFA were shown to prevent or reduce mucosal atrophy in animals receiving TPN and bowel rest, even when given parenterally.[46–48] Dietary fiber is the main source of colonic fermentable substrate for SCFA production. Therefore, fiber in the diet aids the maintenance of mucosal mass and DFD are not quite as good as a solid diet in this regard. Glutamine is a nutrient for the bowel mucosa, and the supplementation of TPN with glutamine preserves gastric and colonic mass in TPN-fed animals but does not preserve small bowel mucosal height.[49]

Does Bowel Rest Induce Gut Atrophy in Man? In the rat, bowel rest with TPN causes atrophy in days,[50] but in man, even after 21 days of bowel rest with TPN, no change was noted in gut hormone production after a meal[51] and no histologic atrophy was identified.[52] However, investigators did note a reduction in the size of the microvilli and a fall in brush border enzyme activity.[52]

In summary, animal data suggest that when the bowel is not used, it atrophies. Mucosal atrophy results from a combination of the lack of functional stimulation and the absence of biliary and pancreatic secretion. The only convincing trophic factors are SCFA and perhaps glutamine. Finally, the dramatic mucosal atrophy seen in animals on bowel rest while receiving TPN does not occur in humans even after a few weeks of bowel rest. Thus, few data are available to suggest that patients on TPN for short periods need to be fed progressively to avoid malabsorption.

COMPLICATIONS

GASTRIC HYPERSECRETION AND PEPTIC ULCERATION

Gastric hypersecretion occurs immediately after intestinal resection and tends to be transient. In some patients, however, peptic ulceration may occur. Treatment with H_2 blockers has been successful.[53,54]

CHOLELITHIASIS

After ileal resection, the enterohepatic cycle of bile salts is interrupted. In consequence, bile salt loss occurs in excess of the ability of the liver to increase synthesis and the bile salt concentration in bile falls. The reduction of the concentration of chenodeoxycholate in the bile increases cholesterol secretion.[55] This combination makes the bile lithogenic. In this situation an increased incidence of gallstones has been observed clinically.[56] A study in laboratory animals has shown an increased incidence of pigment stones.[57]

RENAL STONES

Hyperoxaluria occurs in short bowel patients because of increased absorption of oxalate by the colon.[58] Bile salts in the colon increase oxalate absorption.[59] Hyperoxaluria is associated with renal stone formation and the propensity to form stones is decreased by reduced citrate.[60] Treatment involves following a low-oxalate diet, taking cholestyramine to bind bile salts, and using citrate to prevent stone formation.

D-LACTIC ACIDOSIS

In some patients with a short bowel, a syndrome of slurred speech, ataxia, and altered affect occur in episodes.[61] Superficially, the patient appears "drunk." The cause of this syndrome is fermentation of malabsorbed carbohydrate in the colon to D-lactate and absorption of this metabolite.[62] The treatment of this condition involves the use of a low-carbohydrate diet.[63]

NUTRITIONAL TREATMENT

On the basis of considerations already discussed, the approach to a patient with intestinal resection depends on the extent of the resection, the presence of continuing intestinal disease that reduces the functional length of the intestine, the site of resected bowel, and time for adaptation. The progress of the patient with time will lead to modifications of therapy. However, several therapeutic avenues are applicable to all patients. These general approaches are considered and then the specific applications are discussed.

GENERAL THERAPEUTIC APPROACHES

Initially, an assessment is made to determine whether the patient has had a resection that is unlikely to cause serious malabsorption, a jejunal resection leaving an intact ileum and colon. Such patients need observation and are likely to recover full bowel function without the need for nutritional or other therapeutic support. Others who have had a resection of less than 100 cm of terminal ileum require only the use of a bile salt binder, cholestyramine (4 to 12 g per day) to control bile salt-induced diarrhea. In addition, they require periodic parenteral vitamin B_{12} therapy. The remaining patients with a greater length of resection should be treated as follows.

CONTROL OF DIARRHEA

Diarrhea results from a combination of increased secretions, increased motility, and osmotic stimulation of water secretion because of malabsorption of luminal contents. Initially, diarrhea is controlled by keeping the patient from taking anything orally to reduce any osmotic component. Gastric hypersecretion can be controlled by the continuous infusion of 1200 mg of cimetidine per day. In addition, loperamide can be used to slow gastric and intestinal transit. If loperamide does not work, codeine or phenoxylate are logical choices.

INTRAVENOUS FLUIDS

In the immediate postoperative period, all patients require intravenous fluids and electrolytes to replace losses. Sodium and potassium chloride as well as magnesium are the most important ions to be replaced and plasma levels of the ions should be monitored frequently. Fluid is infused according to measured losses and to maintain a urine output of about 2 L per day. The infusion is tapered as oral intake is increased.

ORAL FEEDING

The next consideration is to determine the nature of oral feeds. In patients who have more than 60 to 80 cm of bowel left, refeeding should be progressive, with a view ultimately to feeding a normal oral diet. By contrast, in patients who have little small bowel left, the initial target should be small volume isotonic feeds containing a glucose-electrolyte content similar to the oral rehydration solutions (see Chap. 37). The composition of this solution should be glucose 3.4% with sodium (85 to 90 mmol/L), potassium (12 mmol/L), bicarbonate (9 mmol/L), and chloride (80 to 90 mmol/L). Such a solution avoids osmotic stimulation of secretion and yet stimulates the bowel to absorb, thus promoting adaptation. For patients with intermediate lengths of bowel, progressive feeding should be attempted with the following plan. The same carbohydrate-electrolyte feeds as just described should be started. A mixture of a similar composition has been shown to be well absorbed by patients with massive resection who have previously been dependent on intravenous fluids.[64] The diet should be lactose-free, because lactase levels in such patients are reduced.[65] Vitamin B_{12} absorption should be measured. If subnormal, injections of 200 micrograms per month are instituted.

Although it is popular to try DFD in these patients, studies by McIntyre have shown that they are not absorbed better than a solid diet.[66]

Early observations had suggested that a lowfat diet with medium-chain triglyceride (MCT) and containing a high-carbohydrate content was better for patients with a short bowel.[67–69] The theory behind these suggestions was the finding that malabsorbed long-chain fatty acids (LCT) can cause colonic water secretion resulting in higher fecal output with steatorrhea and consequently greater loss of divalent ions. However, such studies were not controlled and MCT can also cause osmotic diarrhea. Using a controlled crossover design in two studies,[10,16] we showed that a high-fat diet was comparable to a high-carbohydrate diet in regard to total fluid, energy, nitrogen, sodium, potassium, and divalent ion absorption. Therefore, we recommend a low-lactose diet containing high calories from both fat and carbohydrate and a high-nitrogen intake. We aim to increase intake gradually to about 252 kJ/kg (60 kcal/kg) body weight to provide sufficient calories despite malabsorption. The rationale for this approach is discussed by Woolf et al.[16] Supplements of potassium, magnesium, and zinc are given while monitoring serum levels.

PARENTERAL NUTRITION

In patients with less than 60 cm of remaining small bowel and in those with a combined small bowel and colon resection, parenteral nutrition is lifesaving. It is started in such patients within a few days of the resection, and initially 32 kcal/kg of a mixed energy substrate and 1 g/kg amino acids is infused with sodium (150 to 200 mmol), potassium (60 to 100 mmol), calcium (9 to 11 mmol), magnesium (7 to 15 mmol), and zinc (70 to 100 μmol) per day. Among trace elements, zinc is the most important, as we found large losses in patients with a high endogenous output of intestinal fluids. Oral feeds are started simultaneously and attempts are made to reduce parenteral feeding as oral feeds are increased. It becomes apparent whether the patient needs parenteral feeding on a long-term basis. If so, the patient begins a program of home parenteral nutrition. We have found that as the bowel adapts over months and even years, the patient requires less parenteral feeding and, ultimately, in about 30% of our patients, home parenteral nutrition can be replaced by 2 L of oral rehydration solution, a high-calorie diet, and supplements of potassium, magnesium, calcium, fat-soluble vitamins, and zinc. They are monitored regularly until the weight is stable and they are in electrolytes balance. Hypomagnesemia is particularly a serious problem in these patients. Ingestion of magnesium salts orally enhances diarrhea and therefore magnesium supplements often become difficult to use. The author has had success in using magnesium glucoheptonate (Magnesium Rougier) for this purpose. This preparation is available as a palatable liquid that is added to the gastrolyte supplement in quantities of 30 mmol per day. If this approach is not successful, magnesium sulfate is injected intramuscularly in doses of 12 mmol one to three times per week to supplement the oral intake.

Vitamin supplementation needs comment. These patients can absorb water-soluble vitamins but have difficulty absorbing fat-soluble vitamins. They require large doses of vitamin A, D, and E to maintain normal levels. Also, pills often pass out whole in these patients, necessitating the use of liquid preparations. The author recommends the measurement of these vitamin levels and supplementation with aqueous preparations of vitamin A and E (Aquasol A and E) and 1,25 dihydroxyvitamin D in doses that normalize the plasma levels. Normalization may not be possible with oral vitamins in some individuals, especially vitamin E levels.

In other individuals, an oral diet with intravenous fluid and electrolytes becomes necessary, and in the remainder, full parenteral nutrition is given.

SPECIAL CONSIDERATIONS

Somatostatin Analogue. Long-acting somatostatin analogue has become available and can be administered subcutaneously. Results of all studies have shown a reduction in the volume of output and an increase in sodium or chloride absorption.[70–72] However, the reduction did not seem to be sufficient to avoid using parenteral nutrition in patients who required it.[71]

Jejunal Resection With Intact Ileum and Colon. Patients in this category can be fed orally immediately and rarely have any problems.

Ileal Resection of Less than 100 cm With Colon Largely Intact. Patients in this category have so-called choleraic diarrhea, and are best helped by the administration of 4 g of cholestyramine three times per day to bind bile salts left unabsorbed by the resected ileum. Vitamin B_{12} absorption should be measured; if levels are low, patients should receive intramuscular injection in doses of 100 to 200 μg per month.

Ileal Resection of More Than 100 to 200 cm With Colon Largely Intact. These patients have little difficulty in maintaining nutrition with an oral diet, but they do have fatty acid diarrhea. For such patients, fat restriction is mandatory. With the larger resection, the bile salt pool is depleted and cholestyramine is no longer beneficial. Parenteral vitamin B_{12} replacement is required.

Resection in Excess of 200 cm of Small Bowel and Lesser Resection With Associated Colectomy. Patients of this class require the graduated adaptation program indicated previously under general considerations.

Resection Leaving Less Than 60 cm Small Bowel or Only Duodenum: Massive Bowel Resection. These patients need home parenteral nutrition indefinitely. Many patients, however, even in this category, may show a surprising degree of adaptation and require less parenteral nutrition and benefit from orally absorbed nutrients. The indication to reduce parenteral nutrition is weight gain beyond the desired limit and the fact that reduced infusion does not cause electrolyte imbalance and dehydration.

REFERENCES

1. Malagelada, J.-R.: Gastric, pancreatic and biliary response to a meal. *In* Physiology of the Gastrointestinal Tract. Edited by L.R. Johnson. New York, Raven Press, 1981.
2. Summers, R.W., Kent, T.H., Osborne, J.W.: Gastroenterology, *59:*731–739, 1970.
3. Ricotta, J., Zuidema, G.D., Gadacz, T.R., et al: Surg. Gynecol. Obstet., *152:*310–314, 1981.
4. Fordtran, J.S., Locklear, T.W.: Dig. Dis. Sci., *11:*503–521, 1966.
5. Powell, D.W.: Intestinal water and electrolyte transport. *In* Physiology of the Gastrointestinal Tract. 2nd Ed. Edited by L.R. Johnson. New York, Raven Press, 1987.
6. Binder, H.J., Mehta, P.: Gastroenterology, *96:*989–996, 1989.
7. Royall, D., Wolever, T.M., Jeejeebhoy, K.N.: Am. J. Gastroenterol., *85:*1307–1312, 1990.
8. Nylander, G.: Acta Chir. Scand., *133:*131–138, 1967.
9. Reynell, P.C., Spray G.H.: Gastroenterology, *31:*361–368, 1956.
10. Woolf, G.M., Jeejeebhoy, K.N.: Gastroenterology, *84:*823–828, 1983.
11. Cummings, J.H., James, W.P.T., Wiggins, H.S.: Lancet, *1:*344–347, 1973.
12. Booth, C.C., Aldis, D., Read, A.E.: *Gut, 2:*168–174, 1961.
13. Hoffman, A.F., Poley, J.R.: Gastroenterology, *62:*918–934, 1972.
14. Hylander, E., Ladefoged, K., Jarnum, S.: Scand. J. Gastroenterol., *15:*853–858, 1980.
15. Ladefoged, K., Nicolaidou, P., Jarnum, S.: Am. J. Clin. Nutr., *33:*2137–2144, 1980.
16. Woolf, G., Miller, C., Kurian, R., et al.: Dig. Dis. Sci., *32:*8–15, 1987.
17. Haymond, H.E.: Surg. Gynecol. Obstet., *61:*693–705, 1953.
18. McClenahan, J.E., Fisher, B.: Am. J. Surg., *79:*684–688, 1950.
19. Trafford, H.S.: Br. J. Surg., *44:*10–13, 1956.
20. West, E.S., Montague, J.R., Judy, F.R.: Dig. Dis. Sci., *5:*690–692, 1938.
21. Pilling, G.P., Cresson, S.L.: Pediatrics, *19:*940–948, 1957.
22. Martin, J.R., Patee, C.J., Gardner, C., et al.: Can. Med. Assoc. J., *69:*429–433, 1953.
23. Kinney, J.M., Goldwyn, R.M., Barr, J.S., et al.: JAMA, *179:*529–532, 1962.
24. Walker-Smith, J.: Med. J. Aust., *1:*857–860, 1967.
25. Clayton, B.E., Cotton, D.A.: Gut, *2:*18–22, 1961.
26. Anderson, C.M.: Br. Med. J., *5432:*419–422, 1965.
27. Meyer, H.W.: Surgery, *51:*755–759, 1962.
28. Flint, J.M.: Johns Hopkins Med. J., *23:*127–144, 1912.
29. Porus, R.L.: Gastroenterology, *48:*753–757, 1965.
30. Booth, C.C., Evans, K.T., Menzies, T., et al.: Br. J. Surg., *46:*403–410, 1959.
31. Althausen, T.L., Doig, R.K., Uyeyama, K., et al.: Gastroenterology, *16:*126–139, 1950.
32. Lo, C.W., Walker, W.A.: Nutr. Rev., *47:*193–198, 1989.
33. Goldstein, R.M., Hebiguchi, T., Luk, G., et al.: J. Pediatr. Surg., *20:*785–791, 1985.
34. Shulman, R.J.: Gastroenterology, *95:*85–92, 1988.
35. Morgan, W., Yardley, J., Luk, G., et al.: J. Pediatr. Surg., *22:*541–545, 1987.
36. Gall, D.G., Chung, M., O'Laughlin, E.V., et al.: Biol. Neonate, *51:*286–296, 1987.
37. Kolter, D.P., Levine, G.M., Shiau, Y.F.: Am. J. Physiol., *240:*432–436, 1981.
38. Purandare, S., Offenbartl, K., Westrom, B., et al.: Scand. J. Gastroenterol., *24:*678–682, 1989.
39. Fong, Y.M., Marano, M.A., Barber, A., et al.: Ann. Surg., *210:*449–456, 1989.
40. Hosoda, N., Nishi, M., Nakagawa, M., et al.: J. Surg. Res., *47:*129–133, 1989.
41. Weser, E., Babbitt, J., Vandeventer, A.: Dig. Dis. Sci., *30:*675–681, 1985.
42. Levine, G.M.: Gastroenterology, *91:*49–55, 1986.
43. Weser, E., Babbit, J., Vandeventer, A.: Gastroenterology, *91:*521–527, 1986.
44. Hughes, C.A., Bates, T., Dowling, R.H.: Gastroenterology, *75:*34–41, 1978.
45. Weser, E., Bell, D., Tawil, T.: Dig. Dis. Sci., *26:*409–416, 1981.
46. Koruda, M.J., Rolandelli, R.H., Bliss, D.Z., et al.: Am. J. Clin. Nutr., *51:*685–689, 1990.
47. Koruda, M.J., Rolandelli, R.H., Settle, R.G., et al.: Gastroenterology, *95:*715–720, 1988.
48. Kripke, S.A., Fox, A.D., Berman, J.M., et al.: J. Surg. Res., *44:*436–444, 1988.
49. Grant, J.P., Snyder, P.J.: J. Surg. Res., *44:*506–513, 1988.
50. Hughes, C.A., Prince, A., Dowling, R.H.: Clin. Sci., *59:*329–336, 1980.
51. Greenberg, G.R., Wolman, S.L., Cristofides, N.D., et al.: Gastroenterology, *80:*988–993, 1981.
52. Guedon, C., Schmitz, J., Lerebours, E., et al.: Gastroenterology, *90:*373–378, 1986.
53. Murphy, J.P. Jr., King, D.R., Dubois, A.: N. Engl. J. Med., *300:*80–81, 1979.
54. Cortot, A., Fleming, C.R., Malagelada, J.R.: N. Engl. J. Med., *300:*79–80, 1979.
55. Farkkila, M.A.: Surgery, *104:*18–25, 1988.
56. Roslyn, J.J., Pitt, H.A., Mann, L.L., et al.: Gastroenterology, *84:*148–154, 1983.
57. Pitt, H.A., Lewinski, M.A., Muller, E.L., et al.: Surgery, *96:*154–162, 1984.
58. Dobbins, J.W., Binder, H.J.: N. Engl. J. Med., *296:*298–301, 1977.
59. Chadwick, V.S., Gaginella, T.S., Carlson, G.L., et al.: J. Lab. Clin. Med., *94:*661–674, 1979.
60. Pak, C.Y.C., Peterson, R., Sakhaee, K., et al.: Am. J. Med., *79:*284–288, 1985.
61. Traube, M., Bock, J.L., Boyer, J.L.: Ann. Intern. Med., *98:*171–173, 1983.
62. Satoh, T., Narisawa, K., Konno, T., et al.: Eur. J. Pediatr., *138:*324–326, 1982.
63. Ramakrishnan, T., Stokes, P.: JPEN J. Parenter. Enteral Nutr., *9:*361–363, 1985.
64. Griffin, G.E., Fagan, E.F., Hodgson, A.J., et al.: Dig. Dis. Sci., *27:*902–908, 1982.
65. Richards, A.J., Condon, J.R., Mallinson, C.N.: Br. J. Surg., *58:*493–494, 1971.

66. McIntyre, P.B.: Br. J. Surg., *72:*S92–S93, 1985.
67. Andersson, H., Isaksson, B., Sjogren, B.: Gut, *15:*351–359, 1974.
68. Weser, E.: Gastroenterology, *71:*146–150, 1976.
69. Zurier, R.B., Campbell, R.G., Hashim, S.A.: N. Engl. J. Med., *274:*490–493, 1966.
70. Rodrigues, C.A., Lennard-Jones, J.E., Thompson, D.G., et al.: Aliment. Pharmacol. Ther., *3:*159–169, 1989.
71. Ladefoged, K., Christensen, K.C., Hegnhoj, J., et al.: Gut, *30:*943–949, 1989.
72. Dharmsathaphorn, K., Gorelick, F.S., Sherwin, R.S., et al.: J. Clin. Gastroenterol., *4:*521–524, 1982.

B. INFLAMMATORY BOWEL DISEASE

Irwin H. Rosenberg and Joel B. Mason

Inflammatory bowel disease (IBD) refers to idiopathic chronic inflammatory conditions of the intestine, principally ulcerative colitis and Crohn's disease. Ulcerative colitis is an inflammatory ulcerating process of the colon. Crohn's disease is a transmural granulomatous enteritis that may involve any part of the gastrointestinal tract, but primarily involves the distal small intestine and the colon.

Chronic IBD, ulcerative colitis and Crohn's disease, by their direct involvement of the gastrointestinal tract and their effects on food intake, are commonly associated with nutritional depletion. Proper management of these diseases requires persistent attention to nutritional maintenance and/or repletion, often concurrent with dietary restrictions designed to facilitate healing of the inflamed bowel.

NUTRITIONAL DEFICIENCIES

From Table 62B–1, the reader can appreciate the challenge to patients with IBD in maintaining an adequate nutritional state. Spontaneous oral intake is reduced in the presence of postprandial exacerbation of symptoms. Crohn's disease, by affecting the small bowel, may lead to malabsorption. Both Crohn's disease and ulcerative colitis may cause increased nutrient use in the face of heightened cell turnover and excessive enteric losses of protein, iron (bleeding), and zinc (diarrhea). Drugs may interfere with nutrient absorption or use.

A wide range of nutritional problems may develop in patients with IBD (Table 62B–2).[1] Most patients, especially those with Crohn's disease, suffer from some degree of calorie/protein depletion. Weight loss is reported in most individuals with Crohn's disease and in many with ulcerative colitis. Micronutrient depletion is less prevalent, but as diagnostic techniques improve, the risk of deficiency of fat-soluble vitamins and folate and of minerals and trace minerals, iron and zinc in particular, becomes apparent. The importance of maintaining adequate nutritional status in these diseases is emphasized by findings in those studies demonstrating such defects as impaired wound healing,[2] enhanced susceptibility to infection,[3] and defects in gastrointestinal function[4] related to protein-calorie malnutrition.

PRINCIPLES OF NUTRITION MANAGEMENT

The principle is to set dietary goals that are adequate for the nutritional needs of the patient and, at the same time, to minimize stress on the inflamed and often narrowed segments of bowel. Evidence of lactose intolerance should be documented when possible and dietary restriction should be imposed as needed. In many patients with intestinal cramping and diarrhea, decreasing the intake of dietary fiber or residue is beneficial. In those with steatorrhea, decreased fat intake may substantially improve diarrhea. Once these restrictions are imposed, it is important to replenish the diet with other foods that will provide sufficient calories, protein, vitamins, and minerals to restore and maintain desirable body weight and nutritional status. In some patients, this goal can be attained only by the use of vitamin, mineral, and caloric supplements.

In general, the diet should be liberal in protein with calories sufficient to maintain or restore weight, or to support growth in children and adolescents. The diet should be supplemented by a multivitamin preparation containing one to five times the normal recommended dietary allowances.[5] The higher (therapeutic) dose is indicated if clinical or laboratory evidence reveals deficiency of any of the several nutrients that may be poorly absorbed or whose requirements may be increased.

The techniques for identification of nutritional deficiencies and for monitoring efficacy of therapy are not unique to patients with IBD. Appropriate nutritional assessment and monitoring techniques are discussed elsewhere in this book.

RATIONALE FOR MODIFYING FOOD INTAKE

Nutritional maintenance by diet may be difficult at times of symptomatic activity of IBD. Most patients report postprandial worsening of symptoms. Diarrhea, which may lead to depletion of electrolytes and other micronutrients, is worsened by eating. Eating increases the likelihood of certain complications of IBD. The impaction of bulky food in a narrowed or inflamed loop of bowel in Crohn's disease may precipitate obstruction. Likewise, fistulas will not heal in the presence of active flow of bowel contents.

TABLE 62B–1. CAUSES OF MALNUTRITION IN INFLAMMATORY BOWEL DISEASE

ETIOLOGY	EXAMPLES
Decreased oral intake	Disease-induced (abdominal pain, diarrhea, nausea, anorexia)
	Iatrogenic (restrictive diets without supplementation)
Malabsorption	Decreased absorptive surface due to disease or resection
	Bile salt deficiency after ileal resection
	Bacterial overgrowth
	Drugs (see below)
Increased secretion and nutrient loss	Protein-losing enteropathy
	Electrolyte, mineral, and trace metal loss in diarrhea
	GI blood loss
Increased utilization and increased requirements	Inflammation, fever, infection
	Increased intestinal cell turnover
	Hemolysis (see sulfasalazine)
Drug interference	Corticosteroids and calcium absorption/protein metabolism
	Sulfasalazine and folate absorption/hemolysis
	Cholestyramine and fat-soluble vitamin absorption

TABLE 62B–2. REPORTED NUTRITIONAL DEFICIENCIES IN HOSPITALIZED PATIENTS WITH INFLAMMATORY BOWEL DISEASE

Calorie-protein deficiency
Iron deficiency anemia
Low serum vitamin B_{12}
Low serum folate
Low serum magnesium
Low serum potassium
Low serum vitamin A
Low serum vitamin C
Low serum 25-OH-vitamin D
Low serum zinc
Low serum copper
Metabolic bone disease
Pellagra
Hypoprothrombinemia (vitamin K deficiency)

(Modified from Driscoll, R.H., Rosenberg, I.H.: Med. Clin. North Am., *62*:185–201, 1978.)

To decrease these eating-associated symptoms and decrease bowel activity during healing, patients hospitalized for IBD are sometimes placed on a "bowel rest" program, with the reasoning that an elimination or reduction in oral intake, or a switch to a liquid formula diet containing no residue, can decrease the absorptive work of the bowel, minimize the mechanical trauma caused by food passage, and decrease diet-associated secretions and the inflammation that can be attributed in part to growth of bacterial organisms. In addition, because the pathogenesis of ongoing inflammation may involve continued antigenic stimulation in the gut, cessation or reduction in oral intake may be effective not only by decreasing luminal flora, but also by avoiding exposure to antigenically complex foodstuffs. Nevertheless, total cessation of enterally administered nutrients has not provided a therapeutic advantage over ongoing enteral intake when this issue has been examined in a prospective, controlled fashion.[6] Furthermore, results of both animal and human studies suggest that enteral, compared to parenteral, feeding reduces susceptibility to infection apparently by minimizing atrophy of the gastrointestinal epithelium, thereby reducing bacterial translocation across the gut wall.[7] Strong consideration of enteral feeding is therefore prudent unless the available evidence suggests that parenteral nutrition is necessary.

A diet that is highly restrictive in dietary residue owing to withdrawal of fruits, vegetables, and milk products is often inadequate in some B vitamins, folate, vitamin C, and calcium, unless these are provided specifically. Proper management of Crohn's disease or ulcerative colitis must accomplish both goals of lessening symptoms and maintaining nutritional adequacy.

SPECIAL DIETARY THERAPIES

Lactose Restriction. A substantial proportion of patients with IBD malabsorb lactose, and most such individuals develop symptoms of bloating, cramps, and diarrhea as a result. In a group of children and adolescents with

Crohn's disease, Kirschner et al. found that 34% failed to absorb physiologic doses (32 or 25 g) of lactose.[8] Nearly one half of black and Jewish children had positive tests. Not surprisingly, individuals with diffuse involvement of the small intestine had a particularly high prevalence of lactose malabsorption. In most such patients, elimination of dietary lactose decreases abdominal cramps and diarrhea.

It is prudent to document the presence of lactose intolerance before eliminating or reducing it in the diet, because the major dietary source of lactose (milk and milk products) is also the major source of calcium, and prolonged adherence to a milk-free diet may contribute to negative calcium balance.[9] Most patients with lactose malabsorption require only diminution of milk or ice cream to 1 cup per day. For the especially fastidious patient, guidelines for greater restriction of lactose are available elsewhere in this text (see Appendix Table A–35). In some, especially in growing children or adolescents, use of bacterial lactase (LactAid) to hydrolyze the lactose in milk may be indicated. LactAid-treated milk is now available in many food stores. Exogenous sources of lactase need not be incubated with milk overnight: lactase added at the time of the meal substantially reduces symptoms and lactose malabsorption in most lactase-deficient subjects.[10]

Low-Residue (Fiber) Diets. In patients with inflammatory narrowing of the lumen or chronic stenosis, the rationale for restricting dietary fiber is apparent: by avoiding substances that are not digested in the gastrointestinal tract, the probability of worsening symptoms of intestinal obstruction is reduced. In addition, physical irritation of the inflamed bowel should be lessened. The other physiologic effects of a low-residue diet include reduced stool weight and frequency and slower rate of intestinal transit.

Because available data on fiber content of food are incomplete, this diet usually is described in qualitative terms (see Chap. 4). Fiber intake can be reduced by avoiding coarse whole-grain breads and cereals, nuts, and most fruits and vegetables. As a result, this diet may be marginal in folic acid, ascorbic acid, other vitamins, and some minerals.

The benefits of a fiber-restricted diet are controversial. A retrospective study of 32 patients with Crohn's disease treated with an unrefined carbohydrate, fiber-rich diet failed to support the impression that dietary fiber worsens symptoms. Hospital admissions were significantly fewer and shorter in patients consuming fiber-enriched diets, and only one subject (versus five controls) required surgery during the study period.[11] No patient on the high-fiber diet developed obstruction. If a change in dietary fiber intake is recommended to patients, the change should be made carefully and gradually, and the response of the individual patient must guide continuing use of this aspect of diet management. Increased fiber intake usually is not appropriate for patients with evidence of intestinal narrowing.

Fat Restriction. Patients with Crohn's disease involving the small bowel, particularly with resections, have fat malabsorption of varying severity. Steatorrhea is a major factor in the diarrhea of these patients, with fatty acids and their hydroxylated derivatives exerting a cathartic effect on the colonic mucosa.[12] In addition, a direct correlation exists between loss of fat in stools and the loss of calcium, magnesium, and possibly zinc. Also related to the formation of fatty acid-calcium complexes in the stool is the excessive absorption of uncomplexed oxalate as well as the hyperoxaluria and increased risk of calcium oxalate stone formation in the urinary tract. Diarrhea with persistent serious fluid loss, if not adequately replaced, may lead to acidic concentrated urine and to systemic acidosis that predisposes also to urate stone formation.

Patients with steatorrhea experience symptomatic benefit from decreasing intake of dietary fat. Often, modifications of intake from the usual 100 to 120 g or more of fat in the Western diet to 70 to 80 g suffices to lessen diarrhea and improve calcium and magnesium balances without serious impairment of palatability. In patients with more severe malabsorption, especially those with short bowel syndrome, further reduction may be needed with consequent depressed palatability and total calorie intake. The calories lost by removal of calorie-dense fat from the diet must be replaced by more easily absorbed calorie sources if the diet is to remain adequate in energy. The most ready sources of calories for substitution are the carbohydrates-sugars and starches. Some patients benefit also from the use of medium-chain triglycerides (MCT) in substitution for some fat in the diet (salad dressing, some baked and cooked foods), because MCT are absorbed more efficiently. Similarly, calorie intake can be increased with commercially available carbohydrates derived from corn solids by partial hydrolysis (e.g., Polycose). The broader use of formula supplements to augment dietary intake or to provide a complete source of enteral nutrition in selected patients is discussed later.

Enteric Hyperoxaluria. Calcium oxalate kidney stones are a common complication in patients with Crohn's disease after ileal resection.[13] Such patients have increased urinary oxalate concentrations resulting from increased absorption of dietary oxalate.[14] Results of studies in both animals and man emphasize that the colon is the major site for oxalate absorption and that most oxalate is absorbed by passive diffusion. Steatorrhea increases enteric absorption of oxalate by two mechanisms: (1) the unabsorbed fatty acids bind calcium, and therefore more oxalate is free in solution and available for colonic absorption; and (2) studies in rats show that the fatty acids increase the colonic permeability to oxalate. Dietary fat restriction lessens steatorrhea and reduces absorption and urinary supersaturation with oxalate.[15] Alternative or adjunctive forms of therapy include the use of supplemental calcium taken along with meals, which appears to decrease the amount of free oxalate available for intestinal absorption, and increasing the urine volume by increasing the oral intake of fluids. Reducing the dietary sources of oxalate frequently imposes unreasonable limitations on the patient.

Drug-Nutrient Interactions. Special attention must be paid to patients who are taking drugs that interfere with the absorption or metabolism of certain nutrients. For example, sulfasalazine is a competitive inhibitor of intestinal folate absorption, and diminished folate status is common in patients taking this medication even while eating an unrestricted diet adequate in folate.[16] Folate deficiency in such a patient can be reversed or prevented by providing 1 mg of folic acid per day as a separate supplement or as part of a multivitamin. In patients with ulcerative colitis, folate supplementation may be associated with a decreased incidence of colonic dysplasia.[17]

The bile salt-binding resin cholestyramine, used in patients with ileal disease or resection with bile salt malabsorption and watery diarrhea, binds several nutrients such as folic acid and vitamin D,[18,19] and may increase steatorrhea. Osteomalacia has been described in patients with Crohn's disease and intestinal resections taking cholestyramine; it can be reversed by vitamin D treatment.[20] Similar effects on other fat-soluble vitamins may occur, but they have not been documented clearly. Patients taking large doses of cholestyramine must be monitored for the development of fat-soluble vitamin or folate deficiency, allowing supplementation as needed.

Corticosteroid therapy can lead to significant metabolic bone disease by interfering with many aspects of calcium and bone metabolism. Exogenous corticosteroids inhibit bone formation and vitamin D-mediated calcium absorption in the intestine, and increase urinary excretion of calcium.[21–23] Patients receiving long-term corticosteroid therapy should receive calcium supplements after ensuring that they are not hypercalciuric.

TREATMENT OF SPECIFIC DEFICIENCIES

In some patients, specific nutritional supplementation is necessary in addition to dietary change and multivitamins. Sometimes, this supplementation requires special enteral or intravenous formulas, which are discussed later, particularly when special problems arise in meeting calorie and protein requirements. When deficiencies in micronutrients are the concern, targeted regimens of supplementation may be indicated. For example, patients with extensive disease and/or resection of terminal ileum for Crohn's disease usually have a defect in vitamin B_{12} absorption. Such patients require supplementation with intramuscular vitamin B_{12} at a dose of 500 to 1000 μg at least every 3 months and, in some, every month. Patients with persistent watery diarrhea may have difficulty maintaining adequate zinc status by dietary means.[24] In such patients, supplementation with zinc at a usual dose of 60 mg per day of zinc as sulfate may be indicated.

Iron deficiency is a challenge in the presence of intermittent or chronic blood loss and altered absorption. Iron supplements in full therapeutic doses may exacerbate symptoms. Slower supplementation using ferrous salts containing 30 to 60 mg of elemental iron daily may be a useful strategy. A substantial increase in inorganic iron absorption can be effected by administering 500 mg of ascorbic acid along with the iron.

The causes of metabolic bone disease in patients with Crohn's disease, in particular, are multiple. Chronic corticosteroid therapy results in chronic negative calcium balance; malabsorption of vitamin D and calcium may result from small bowel disease. In such patients, measuring blood levels of 25-hydroxyvitamin D may be the best way to screen for deficiency. In most patients with low values, doses of oral vitamin D between 2000 and 10,000 IU daily will restore normal 25-hydroxyvitamin D levels and correct osteomalacia, as documented by bone biopsy.[25]

In some patients, protein deficits, which reflect enteric protein loss as much as dietary deficiency or malabsorption, can be reversed by selective increase in sources of high-quality protein (protein supplements).

INTENSIVE NUTRITIONAL SUPPORT

Thus far, this discussion has focused primarily on ambulatory patients who represent the majority of individuals with moderate to mild symptoms. For patients with more severe symptoms unresponsive to medical therapy, the challenge of medical management and consideration of surgery both increase. In that setting, more intensive nutritional support may be mandatory.

Liquid Formulas. Liquid formulas have been reported to be effective for some patients with ulcerative colitis or Crohn's disease, even with fistulas, growth retardation, or short bowel. Some enthusiastic proponents believe that the "partial bowel rest" provided by these nutritionally complete, minimal-residue, liquid diets, which involve considerably fewer risks and less expense than parenteral nutrition, may be the preferred form of management.[11] Using intensive enteral nutrition as a primary mode of therapy for active Crohn's disease instead of corticosteroids or other drugs is considerably more controversial: it has been shown to be effective in some settings[26] but not in others.[27] The use of defined liquid formulas is clearly an important adjunct in the treatment of inflammatory bowel disease; whether it can substitute for corticosteroids or other drugs continues to be a research question.

Either parenteral nutrition or liquid formula diets can be used to restore nutritional status and achieve weight gain, and each has particular advantages. Experience with such diets and total parenteral nutrition (TPN) is reviewed in the sections that follow.

Lactose-free, fiber-free nutritional liquid formulas can be administered by mouth as a complete diet or as a dietary supplement, or such formulas can be administered by feeding tube to meet calorie and nutritional goals. Administration of a total liquid formula diet by tube is well tolerated and can be performed at home for extended periods. Nutritional deficits can be reversed by such a regimen while symptoms are ordinarily kept in control with the additional use of drug therapy. A controlled trial of the use of liquid formula supplements in patients with Crohn's disease demonstrated a clear benefit over unsupplemented control subjects in measures of nutritional status including weight, arm circumferences, and albumin level.[28] However, the symptomatic response was similar in both supplemented and control groups.

Enteral formulas have been used successfully in the management of patients with fistulas in Crohn's disease with a clear decrease in fistula drainage and healing in some individuals. Enteral formula supplements have been used effectively to meet calorie requirements and to restore growth in children with growth retardation complicating Crohn's disease.[29]

Parenteral Nutrition. In the management of many hospitalized patients with severely active ulcerative colitis or Crohn's disease, physicians tend to place the patient on a nothing-by-mouth regimen, together with medications including corticosteroids, in an effort to control symptoms of diarrhea, abdominal pain, and sometimes fever. In such patients, TPN may be used for nutritional repletion and maintenance. In ulcerative colitis, the combined reported experience in uncontrolled studies demonstrates clinical remission in approximately one third of severely symptomatic patients who receive TPN, whereas the remainder usually require surgery eventually.[30] In one controlled study of patients with colitis comparing TPN with hospitalization and drug therapy alone, no greater incidence of remission was observed in those receiving parenteral nutrition.[31]

In Crohn's disease, the experience with the use of TPN is more extensive and more positive. About 70% of patients in reported series will undergo clinical remission while in the hospital, and reversal of nutritional deficits occurs regularly.[30] However, the duration of symptomatic remission is highly variable. More controlled studies comparing TPN to enteral nutrition and to other forms of hospital management are required. To date, such studies do not reveal an advantage to using TPN in this group as a whole,[6] although it does seem to confer advantages over an enteral route in carefully selected instances.

Often, TPN is used in patients with enterocutaneous fistulas from Crohn's disease. In the reported series of hospital patients, approximately one third of fistulas healed with the patient on such a regimen.[30]

The reinstitution of enteral feeding in a patient who has been on a prolonged course of TPN and bowel rest should be done gradually in deference to the structural and functional atrophy that the small intestinal mucosa undergoes during complete bowel rest.[31] Most brush border enzyme activities recover within 10 days after resumption of enteral feeding.

Glutamine is an important substrate for energy and protein metabolism in the gastrointestinal mucosa. Furthermore, increasing evidence indicates that, under conditions of systemic inflammation, glutamine becomes an essential amino acid.[32] Studies suggest that the integrity of the gastrointestinal mucosa is more effectively maintained, and better restored after injury, when glutamine is included in either enteral or parenteral feeding solutions.[33,34] Clinical studies are still lacking, but it seems likely that defined liquid formulas and TPN that contains glutamine will promote healing of the injured gut mucosa in patients with exacerbations of inflammatory bowel disease.

NUTRITIONAL MANAGEMENT OF GROWTH RETARDATION

When inflammatory bowel disease begins in childhood, persistently active disease may affect growth and sexual maturation in as many as one third of such children. Although retarded growth may reflect the chronic use of high daily doses of corticosteroids in some patients, the major cause of growth retardation is the calorie deficit, particularly in view of the increased caloric requirement for growth in children who modify their eating patterns to lessen postprandial symptoms. Consistently, growth-retarded children ingest less than two thirds of the projected requirements in calories.[29] Increased demand for protein because of high losses into the inflamed intestine must also be met. Vitamin deficiencies are not common in this population, and iron and zinc deficiencies are no more prevalent than in patients with normal growth.

Re-establishing growth and sexual maturation in the growth-retarded adolescent necessitates meeting nutritional needs, particularly those for adequate calories. In many patients, these goals can be met by aggressive attention to dietary caloric intake once symptoms are controlled by medication to the extent possible.[29] In some individuals, liquid dietary supplements are required in addition to foods. A small percentage of patients requires intensive nutritional support by nasoenteral tube feeding of defined formula diets or TPN. Dramatic improvements in growth retardation have been observed with nocturnal tube feedings:[35] for motivated patients, this supplementation can be an effective way of addressing this problem. When surgery is indicated, particularly for severe narrowing or obstruction in Crohn's disease, symptomatic improvement is associated with an improved dietary intake to meet the needs for growth. The principle is that growth retardation or arrest can be reversed if nutritional requirements are met. Sometimes, because of the delay in bone age that accompanies growth retardation, the adolescent growth spurt is delayed by as much as 2 or 3 years, and growth may continue well beyond the usual adolescent span.

HOME PARENTERAL NUTRITION

Experience is growing with the use of home TPN in the management of severe and intractable Crohn's disease. Home TPN was used first in such patients who had had recurrent and extensive small bowel resections and could not meet their nutritional requirements by diet alone.[36] As the technique of home TPN has become more available, this approach is sometimes used as a substitution for a bowel rest and an in-hospital TPN regimen for patients with uncontrolled disease or unhealing fistulas or for those requiring extensive nutritional repletion in preparation for surgery. Other patients who require this regimen are those with short bowel syndrome who cannot maintain a normal nutritional state by enteral means. A few series involving the use of such an approach have been published. Fleming et al. reported the largest experience: 123 patients with severe Crohn's disease receiving home TPN for an average of 58 months.[37] Significant improvements in nutritional status, frequency of hospital re-admissions, and physical rehabilitation were observed, as was significant reversal of growth retardation among adolescent patients. Kushner et al. reported a similarly salutory experience with 10 home TPN patients with severe Crohn's disease.[38] They also observed a significant decrease in corticosteroid requirements in these patients.

Complications of home TPN occur, although how the frequency of complications compares to that among in-patients is unclear. Findings of large series indicate that 0.25 to 0.63 admissions per patient per year are to be expected for TPN-related complications, principally catheter infections.[37,39] Experience with children with Crohn's disease in Los Angeles, CA demonstrated that home parenteral nutrition was capable of producing symptomatic remissions in most patients, but symptomatic recurrences required reinstitution of home therapy in many of these patients within 1 year.[40] After 10 years of experience,[41] these investigators observed that 13% of their 102 home-TPN pediatric patients died of TPN-related complications; 70% of these deaths were attributable to catheter infection. Home TPN, therefore, offers several advantages to carefully selected patients as an alternative to repeated hospitalizations, but it is not without its own problems.

REFERENCES

1. Driscoll, R.H., Rosenberg, I.H.: Med. Clin. North Am., *62:*185–201, 1978.
2. Haydock, D.A., Hill, G.L.: JPEN J. Parenter. Enteral Nutr., *10:*550–554, 1986.
3. Bistrian, B.R., Blackburn, G.L., Scrimshaw, N.S., et al.: Am. J. Clin. Nutr., *28:*1148–1155, 1975.
4. Viteri, F.E., Schneider, R.E.: Med. Clin. North Am., *58:*1487–1505, 1974.
5. Food and Nutrition Board, National Research Council: Recommended Dietary Allowances. 10th Ed. Washington, D.C., National Academy Press, 1989.
6. Greenberg, G.R., Fleming, C.R., Jeejeebhoy, K.N., et al.: Gut, *29:*1309–1315, 1988.
7. Moore, F.A., Moore, E.E., Jones, T.H. et al.: J. Trauma, *29:*916–923, 1989.
8. Kirschner, B.S., de Favara, M.V., Jensen, W.: Gastroenterology, *81:*829–832, 1981.
9. Meredith, S.C., Rosenberg, I.H.: Clin. Endocrinol. Metab., *9:*131–150, 1980.
10. Rosado, J.L., Solomons, N.W., Lisker, R., et al.: Gastroenterology, *87:*1072–1082, 1984.
11. Heaton, K.W., Thornton, J.R., Emett, P.M.: Br. Med. J., *2:*764–766, 1979.
12. Ammon, H., Phillips, S.F.: Gastroenterology, *65:*744–749, 1973.
13. Smith, L.H., Fromm, H., Hofmann, A.F.: N. Engl. J. Med., *286:*1371–1375, 1972.
14. Chadwick, V.S., Madha, K., Dowling, R.H.: N. Engl. J. Med., *289:*172–176, 1973.
15. Earnest, D.L., Johnson, G., Williams, H.E., et al.: Gastroenterology, *66:*1114–1122, 1974.
16. Franklin, J.L., Rosenberg, I.H.: Gastroenterology, *59:*567–574, 1973.
17. Lashner, B.A., Heidenreich, P.A., Su, G.L., et al.: Gastroenterology, *97:*255–259, 1989.
18. Roe, D.A.: Nutr. Rev., *42:*141–154, 1984.
19. Thompson, W.G., Thompson, G.R.: Gut, *10:*717–722, 1969.
20. Compston, J.E., Creamer, B.: Gut, *18:*171–175, 1977.
21. Baylink, D.J.: N. Engl. J. Med., *309:*306–308, 1983.
22. Hahn, T.J., Halsted, L.R., Baran, D.T.: J. Clin. Endocrinol. Metab., *52:*111–115, 1981.
23. McCann, V.J., Fulton, T.T.: J. Clin. Endocrinol. Metab., *40:*1038–104, 1975.
24. Wolman, S.L., Anderson, G.H., Marliss, E.B., et al.: Gastroenterology, *76:*458–468, 1979.
25. Driscoll, R.H., Jr., Meredith, S.C., Sitrin, M., et al.: Gastroenterology, *83:*1252–1258, 1982.
26. O'Morain, C., Segal, A.W., Levin, A.J.: Br. Med. J., *288:*1859–1862, 1984.
27. Lochs, H., Steinhardt, H.J., Klaus-Wentz, B., et al.: Gastroenterology, *101:*881–888, 1991.
28. Harries, A.D., Danis, V., Heatley, R.V., et al.: Lancet, *1:*887–890, 1983.

29. Kirschner, B.S., Klich, J.R., Kalman, S.S., et al.: Gastroenterology, *80:*10–15, 1981.
30. Bengoa, J.M., Rosenberg, I.H.: Year Book of Medicine. Chicago, Year Book, 1983, pp. 363–385.
31. Dickinson, R.J., Ashton, M.G., Axon, A.T.R., et al.: Gastroenterology, *79:*1199–1204, 1980.
32. Lacey, J.M., Wilmore, D.W.: Nutr. Rev., *48:*297–309, 1990.
33. O'Dwyer, S.T., Smith, R.J., Hwang, T.L., et al.: J. Parenter. Enteral Nutr., *13:*579–585, 1989.
34. Fox, A.D., Kripke, S.A., DePaula, J., et al.: J. Parenter. Enteral Nutr., *12:*325–331, 1988.
35. Aiges, H., Markowitz, J., Rosa, J., et al.: Gastroenterology, *97:*905–910, 1989.
36. Jeejeebhoy, K.N., Langer, B., Tsallas, G., et al.: Gastroenterology, *71:*943, 1976.
37. Fleming, C.R., Burnes, J.: Gastroenterology, *98:*A412, 1990.
38. Kushner, R.F., Shapir, J., Sitrin, M.D.: JPEN J. Parenter. Enteral Nutr., *10:*568–573, 1986.
39. Howard, L., Claunch, C., Fleming, R., et al.: Gastroenterology, *96:*A219, 1989.
40. Strobel, C.T., Byrne, W.J., Ament, M.E.: Gastroenterology, *77:*272, 1979.
41. Vargas, J.H., Ament, M.E., Berquist, W.E.: JPEN J. Parenter. Enteral Nutr., *6:*24–32, 1987.

C. DISEASES OF THE SMALL BOWEL

Penny S. Turtel and Moshe Shike

Crohn's disease (see Chap. 62B), the short bowel syndrome (see Chap. 62A), celiac disease (see Chap. 62D), and various intestinal parasite infections are the most common diseases of the small bowel that result in malabsorption and nutritional problems. This chapter addresses other, less common diseases that may also cause severe intestinal dysfunction, malabsorption, and malnutrition.

RADIATION ENTERITIS

Abdominal and pelvic radiation, commonly used in the treatment and palliation of various tumors, can cause major gastrointestinal morbidity. With the development of supervoltage techniques, high doses can be administered to the tumor without skin toxicity, making gastrointestinal tolerance the main dose-limiting factor. During the time of radiation, most patients experience acute radiation toxicity, manifested as nausea, vomiting, and diarrhea. This form of toxicity is self-limiting and usually subsides within weeks of ending the radiation therapy (RT). Chronic, late gastrointestinal complications occur less frequently and can cause major morbidity and mortality.

Risk factors predisposing to radiation injury of the small and large intestine include: previous abdominal surgery, thin physique, hypertension, diabetes mellitus, and pelvic inflammatory disease.[1] Concomitant chemotherapy, especially with actinomycin D, seems to compound the damage.[2] Total dose administered and volume of bowel irradiated are major determinants of late radiation damage. Significant injury generally occurs when more than 5000 rads are administered.[3] Appropriate fractionation of the total dose of radiotherapy helps to protect against injury.

PATHOLOGY

Acute Phase. Acute radiation changes are manifested primarily in the mucosal layer. Mitotic activity in the segment of irradiated intestinal epithelium decreases within 12 hours of the first treatment, continues to drop during the first week, and persists at low levels throughout treatment.[4] Mucosal injury occurs with shortening of villi, decrease in mucosal thickness, edema, erosions, inflammation, and ulcerations. Within 2 weeks after completion of therapy, the histologic picture returns to normal in most patients.[4]

Subacute Phase. Vascular and connective tissue damage become evident in the subacute period, from 2 to 12 months after radiation treatment. Large "foam cells" beneath the intima, abnormal fibroblasts, and submucosal fibrosis are characteristic. As a result, there is obliteration of venules and arterioles and progressive ischemia, which can then insidiously lead to clinically apparent chronic radiation enteritis (RE).

Chronic Phase. All layers of the gut wall and mesentery are involved in chronic radiation injury. Submucosal fibrosis, edema, lymphatic ectasia, and obliterative endarteritis are characteristic (Fig. 62C–1). These pathologic changes can result in ulcerations, perforations, strictures, and fistulas.

CLINICAL MANIFESTATIONS

Acute Phase. Acute gastroenterologic symptoms from abdominal RT are common. Most patients experience anorexia, nausea, and vomiting early in treatment, which seem to be mediated through the central nervous system. After 2 to 3 weeks of RT, abdominal cramping and watery diarrhea may occur. Weight loss is common. It occurs more frequently with abdominal than with pelvic RT,[5] and is attributed mainly to decreased food intake.

Malabsorption of water, fats, bile salts, carbohydrates, calcium, magnesium, iron, and vitamin B_{12} occurs commonly during RT.[6] It is generally most pronounced at midtreatment, and persists to the end of treatment.[6]

Malabsorbed bile salts and carbohydrates play a major role in acute radiation-induced diarrhea. Bile salts that normally are absorbed in the terminal ileum, reach the colon where they induce secretion of fluids and minerals, inhibit absorption, and stimulate peristalsis ("cholerrheic diarrhea"). Malabsorbed carbohydrates, presumably resulting from secondary brush border enzyme deficiencies, exert strong osmotic effects in the intestinal lumen, compounding the fluid losses.

In most patients, acute radiation symptoms resolve within several weeks after cessation of therapy.[7] In a small percentage, symptoms persist, and merge with those of chronic RE.

Chronic Phase. The relationship between acute and chronic RE is unclear. Absence of early symptoms does not guarantee protection from delayed morbidity. An estimated 5 to 15% of patients suffer late sequelae of radiation, with latency periods ranging from 1 year to over 20 years, commencing in most studies at 1 to 2 years.[8–10] These percentages represent reported series of patients with severe disease, and probably underestimate the incidence of chronic overall morbidity.[11] In one study of 17 woman with previous pelvic radiation, none of whom sought attention for gastroenterologic complaints, 12 reported a permanent change in bowel habits, 16 had abnormal cholylglycine breath tests, and 8 had abnormal small bowel radiologic studies.[12]

Colicky abdominal pain, diarrhea, steatorrhea, and weight loss are the most common clinical manifestations. Small bowel obstruction, fistulization, abscess formation, bleeding, and perforation are less frequent, but graver complications, often requiring operation, with its attendant high postoperative morbidity and mortality.[8,13] Gallstones and hyperoxaluria may develop as a consequence of ileal dysfunction.

Several factors contribute to the malabsorption that occurs in late radiation damage. These include: (1) bacterial overgrowth, secondary to strictures, fistulas, and stasis; (2) decreased available absorptive surface area because of radiation damage and resection; (3) chronic lymphatic obstruction causing steatorrhea and protein loss; (4) secondary disaccharidase deficiency and subsequent osmotic catharsis; (5) bile salt malabsorption leading to cholerrheic diarrhea; and (6) rapid intestinal transit.

MANAGEMENT

In general, nutrition is optimized by determining the elements contributing to malabsorption and correcting treatable factors. These measures include: broad-spectrum antibiotics for bacterial overgrowth; diet (lowfat, lactose free); cholestyramine for bile acid malabsorption; antidiarrhea medications for rapid transit; anticholinergic and antispasmodic preparations for pain and cramps. Dietary therapy can play a major role in both controlling symptoms and assuring adequate nutrition.

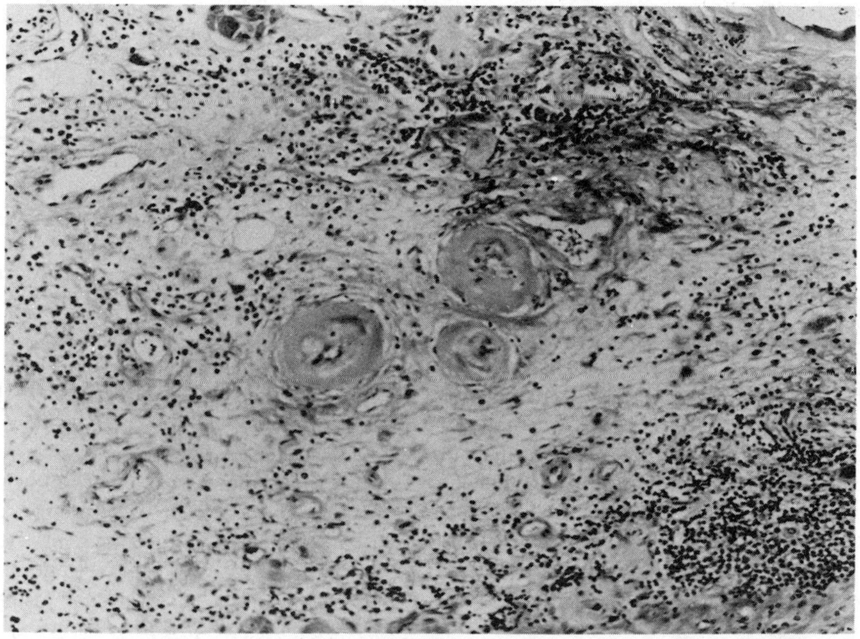

FIGURE 62C–1. Chronic radiation enteritis. Small bowel biopsy demonstrating (in the center) three blood vessels partially occluded by fibrosis and inflammation in the walls.

In addition, enteral and parenteral nutrition can be used in severe cases.

Acute Radiation Enteritis. During RT, control of diarrhea and prevention of weight loss constitute important goals. A diet low in lactose and fat is recommended, as transient ileal dysfunction and brush border enzyme deficiencies are highly prevalent, causing diarrhea and malabsorption.

Experimental evidence suggests that intraluminal contents, especially pancreatic secretions and bile acids, potentiate acute small intestinal radiation damage.[14] This finding has led to trials of enteral feeding with solutions containing amino acids or partially digested protein and very low fat content. These solutions are absorbed proximally in the small intestine, and are thought to stimulate less pancreatic, biliary, and salivary secretions compared to normal diets. Studies in which patients received only such enteral feeding during RT indeed demonstrate less diarrhea and weight loss, and less frequent interruption of the radiation schedule because of toxicity.[15,16] When used as dietary supplements, enteral nutrition solutions provide no clinical benefit.[17]

Despite data supporting the use of enteral feeding with partially or fully digested protein during RT, the transient nature of the acute injury, the inconvenience of limiting intake to these formulas, and their unpalatability requiring their administration through a tube make them impractical for general use. Such enteral feedings should be used in only those patients who develop severe acute toxicity, or who have pre-existing malnutrition.

Several studies have evaluated the role of total parenteral nutrition (TPN) during pelvic and abdominal RT. TPN clearly prevents weight loss, and in some causes, lessens gastrointestinal toxicity while enhancing the ability of the patient to tolerate RT on schedule.[18,19] Survival is not affected. Two randomized prospective trials concluded that TPN should be reserved only for those patients malnourished before starting a course of curative RT.[18,20] This conclusion is reasonable considering the complexity of TPN and the fact that acute RE is a transient disorder.

Chronic Radiation Enteritis. Assessment of the functional outcome of chronic RE should be the first step in management of this disorder. The nutritional status of the patient should be evaluated and a complete investigation for malabsorption and specific nutrient deficiencies should be performed. The investigation may include radiographic studies of the intestinal tract, absorption studies (D-xylose tolerance test, stool fat, and Schilling test) and assessment of blood levels of selected nutrients.

Dietary management is an effective way of dealing with both the diarrhea of chronic RE and nutritional deficiencies. Sequential restrictions of fat, fiber, lactose, and gluten may establish an optimal diet that provides symptomatic relief and improved nutrition. In addition, such an approach may clarify those pathophysiologic mechanisms that are salient in an individual patient. The histologic similarity between RE and other malabsorptive diseases, such as sprue, has led to trials using specific dietary therapy as the major form of treatment for RE. A diet free of gluten, cow's milk protein, and lactose, with low fat and fiber content was given to five children with severe, delayed injury manifested by small bowel obstruction after whole abdominal irradiation.[2] In all patients, clinical symptoms improved, and radiographic studies and histologic pictures normalized. After 1 to 2 years, the gradual addition of fiber, gluten, milk, and fat was well-tolerated by all. In another trial, dietary fat was restricted to 40 g per day in nine women with diarrhea after pelvic irradiation.[21] Three to 6 months later, fecal excretion of bile salts decreased, and diarrhea abated in eight of nine patients.

A trial of a lowfat, partially digested protein liquid formula given through a tube is the next step in patients who fail to improve with oral dietary therapy. Although several reports document significant reductions in fecal fluid, fat, and nitrogen with the use of enteral feedings,[22,23] other authors report no benefit.[10] Patients with limited absorptive capacity can benefit from enteral feedings given in a pump-controlled, slow infusion through a gastrostomy tube. This technique avoids the overwhelming of the limited absorptive capacity, which can occur in bolus feeding or oral feeding. Using this mode of nutrition, patients can be maintained in good nutritional state, avoiding the use of TPN.

In patients with severe RE who are unable to maintain their weight with oral or enteral diets, TPN is lifesaving. It achieves weight gain, improves overall nutrition, and may help in decreasing fistula drainage.[24,25] Some evidence also suggests a direct therapeutic role for TPN. In one trial, absorption tests (Schilling, D-xylose, and fecal fat) and radiographic studies normalized or improved after an 8-week course of TPN with nothing by mouth.[10] Several of these patients achieved prolonged remissions without further need for TPN.

Although these results are encouraging, most data indicate that the role of TPN is supportive, not therapeutic,[25] and that TPN should be reserved for those patients with nutritional failure refractory to dietary therapy and enteral feeding.

EOSINOPHILIC GASTROENTERITIS

Eosinophilic gastroenteritis (EGE) is a spectrum of disorders characterized by food-related gastrointestinal symptoms, peripheral eosinophilia, and eosinophilic infiltration of the gastrointestinal tract[26] (see also Chap. 77). Peak age of onset is in the third decade and children constitute approximately 20% of reported cases.[27] The disease shows a slight male predominance.[28,29]

The cause of EGE remains unknown. An allergic basis is believed most likely, supported by a frequent association with atopic disorders, such as asthma, dermatitis, eczema, allergic rhinitis, and bronchitis. The role of tissue eosinophilia remains unclear. Whether the eosinophils are mediating the injury or are responding to and modulating the inflammation is not known.

PATHOLOGY AND CLINICAL MANIFESTATIONS

Three clinicopathologic patterns of EGE have been described.[30]

Mucosal Layer-Predominant. This pattern is the most common, generally involving the stomach alone, or both the stomach and small intestine; rarely, the small intestine is involved alone. Presenting complaints include eating-related nausea, vomiting, and abdominal pain, occasionally with diarrhea.

Approximately 50% of patients have a history of allergic disorders. Edema, pallor, occult fecal blood, and, frequently, signs of allergic disease are present on physical examination. In children, growth retardation is prominent. Further evaluation typically reveals iron-deficiency anemia, peripheral eosinophilia (up to 55%), hypoproteinemia, and evidence of malabsorption. Protein-losing enteropathy is present, confirmed by chromium-labeled albumin studies. D-Xylose test typically is abnormal, reflecting small intestinal mucosal dysfunction, whereas the Schilling test for vitamin B_{12} absorption and the fecal fat test are variably abnormal. Radiographic and endoscopic studies reveal edematous, distorted, and sometimes nodular folds, irritability, and increased secretions.[31] Occasionally, ulcers are present, involving primarily the gastric antrum and proximal small intestine. The pathologic hallmark of the disease is eosinophilic infiltration and tissue edema without vasculitis.[30] Villous architecture varies from normal to complete flattening as seen in sprue. Involvement is patchy, and several biopsies may be required to confirm the diagnosis.[26]

Muscle-Layer-Predominant. Obstructive symptoms are more prominent. Radiographic studies reveal thickening and rigidity of the gut. Full-thickness biopsy often is needed to demonstrate eosinophilic infiltration through the muscularis propria.

Subserosa-Predominant. This pattern is the least common. Patients typically present with ascites, which contains high numbers of eosinophils. The subserosa is thickened and infiltrated with eosinophils. Mucosal and muscle layers are variably involved.

Exacerbations and remissions characterize the long-term course of most patients, often with no relationship to therapeutic interventions. Symptoms tend to recur in repetitive patterns in a particular individual.[30]

RELATIONSHIP TO FOOD ALLERGY

EGE is distinguished from "food allergy" by the inability in EGE to identify a specific offending dietary agent the withdrawal of which is associated with amelioration of symptoms and the reintroduction is associated with symptom recurrence. Many patients with EGE report intolerance to specific foods, most commonly beef, eggs, milk, and pork.[30] Blind food challenges, using nasogastric tube delivery, demonstrate precipitation of symptoms and an increase in white blood cells, IgE, and peripheral and tissue eosinophils in response to specific foods.[30,32–34] Yet, dietary manipulation is generally ineffective,[26] and patients with EGE are thus distinguished by their requirement for steroids to induce remission and by their chronicity.[28] Tube feeding with specific formulas devoid of the allergen as well as TPN can be used to treat patients who do not respond to dietary manipulation.

MANAGEMENT

Given the high prevalence of food intolerance in EGE, the first step in treatment should be a trial of eliminating the suspected offending agent. In the absence of a suspect agent, sequential elimination of milk, eggs, pork, beef, and gluten has been recommended.[35] Whereas some patients transiently respond to such measures, sustained response is rare.[26,28]

Corticosteroids are the mainstay of therapy. Although efficacy has not been documented in controlled clinical trials, anecdotally, they are highly effective, produce quick resolution of symptoms, and allow weight gain in most patients.[26,28,30] Many patients require small maintenance doses; others need dietary restriction and short courses of steroids for exacerbations only.

In severe cases in which patients fail to improve while receiving steroids and have exacerbation of symptoms with any oral intake (a rare occurrence), TPN and bowel rest may be necessary to provide nutrition and induce remission. In one such case, TPN and intravenous administration of steroids led to a decrease in eosinophilia and in symptoms. When oral feeding was resumed, the disease worsened, and the patient ultimately died.[36]

AMYLOIDOSIS

Amyloidosis is a multisystem pathologic complex characterized by extracellular deposition of amyloid. Amyloid consists of aggregated, linear glycoprotein fibrils arranged in a beta pleated sheet. Clinical classification is into two major groups. Primary amyloidosis, is associated with no preceding or coexisting disease, except in cases of multiple myeloma. Secondary amyloidosis is associated with underlying conditions, mainly chronic infections (osteomyelitis, tuberculosis) and chronic inflammatory disorders (rheumatoid arthritis, inflammatory bowel disease). Other forms include localized, heredofamilial, and senile amyloidosis.

The biochemical classification is based on the structure of the fibrils: immunoglobulin light chains in primary and in multiple myeloma-related amyloidosis (AL amyloid); protein A in secondary forms and in familial Mediterranean fever (AA amyloid); prealbumin in other familial forms (AF amyloid).[37] Typically, AL affects the gastrointestinal tract, nerves, skin, heart, and tongue, whereas AA more heavily involves liver, spleen, and kidneys.[37] Actually, overlap exists, and the gastrointestinal tract frequently is involved in both primary and secondary forms.[38]

PATHOLOGY

In the gastrointestinal tract, blood vessels are the earliest and most common site involved by amyloid deposition, usually at the submucosal level. Progression of vessel wall thickening and luminal narrowing may cause bowel ischemia and infarction.[38] Gastrointestinal smooth muscle is heavily infiltrated, leading to pressure atrophy and impaired motility. Only with massive deposition is mucosa invaded. Villous architecture in the small intestine most often is normal.[39,40] Mucosal atrophy and ulceration may result from vascular insufficiency. Neurons in the myenteric plexus and visceral nerve trunks may be damaged by direct pressure from deposition.[38]

On routine hematoxylin and eosin staining, amyloid appears pink and amorphous. Congo red staining viewed under polarized light reveals its unique apple-green birefringence. Electron microscopy demonstrates its fibrillar structure.

CLINICAL MANIFESTATIONS

Gastrointestinal symptoms may predominate in all forms of systemic amyloidosis, and are particularly prominent in the familial forms.[39-41] Constipation or diarrhea typically occur early in the course. Progression to severe, disabling diarrhea, often with incontinence, may occur subsequently.[40,41] Autonomic neuropathy of the gut nerves and direct muscle layer infiltration underlie these abnormalities, causing dysmotility, stasis, and, often, bacterial overgrowth.

Abdominal pain, infarction, perforation, and bleeding are less common manifestations, and reflect vascular insufficiency or direct invasion.[37,38] Mechanical obstructions may occur, usually from massive localized amyloid deposition or from ischemia-induced strictures, and must be differentiated from pseudoobstructions, which result from severe motility abnormalities, stasis, and dilatation.

Malabsorption may occur in all forms of amyloidosis, but it is particularly prominent in the familial forms, in which it is an important cause of cachexia and death.[39,40] Multiple factors are involved, including: bacterial overgrowth, direct mucosal and submucosal destruction, vascular insufficiency, and pancreatic insufficiency (from amyloid destruction of acini). In familial amyloidosis with polyneuropathy, the degree of steatorrhea and evolution of gastrointestinal symptoms has been correlated with severity of electromyographic changes in peripheral nerves,[41] implicating the neuropathy as a major factor in producing these symptoms.

Fecal weight and fat content are elevated in most patients with significant gastrointestinal involvement,[38-40] whereas D-Xylose absorption and results of Schilling and bile acid breath tests are variably abnormal. Prothrombin time may be elevated, and carotene levels often are depressed.[38] Hypocalcemia and hypokalemia occasionally occur. Anemia, when present, may reflect iron or B_{12} deficiency or the underlying chronic disease. Hypoalbuminemia and edema are common,[38] usually reflecting nephrotic syndrome (secondary to amyloid in the kidneys), hepatic dysfunction, malabsorption, and rarely, protein-losing enteropathy.[42]

The most common radiographic appearance is that of diffuse thickening of the small bowel valvulae conniventes without significant luminal fluid.[43] Other radiographic features include pseudonodularity, atypical large nodules, pseudo-obstruction, ischemic manifestations, dilation without thickening, and blunting of plical folds.[44,45]

The definitive diagnosis of amyloidosis is made by demonstrating amyloid on Congo red staining of a biopsy specimen. High-yield sites for biopsy include rectum, small bowel, and abdominal fat pad. Several biopsies should be performed, because amyloid deposition may be patchy.

MANAGEMENT

The use of broad-spectrum antibiotics for enteric bacterial overgrowth often alleviates diarrhea, steatorrhea, and bile acid deconjugation;[39] however, the effect is temporary, and repeated courses may be needed. In one patient with diarrhea refractory to all standard agents and to combination chemotherapy, the long-acting somatostatin analogue SMS 201-995 produced dramatic resolution of diarrhea.[46] Enterostomy may be beneficial in cases of intractable diarrhea with incontinence. Pancreatic enzymes are useful when massive acinar destruction contributes to the maldigestion. Sodium restriction is helpful in patients with edema, and dietary fat restriction is advisable for patients with significant steatorrhea. In managing the nutritional state, special attention should be paid to supplement fat-soluble vitamins, which can be severely malabsorbed in the presence of steatorrhea.

Both TPN and enteral feedings are useful in the nutritional support of the cachectic patient with severe wasting and malabsorption related to gastrointestinal amyloidosis.

Combination chemotherapy, with prednisone, melphalan, and colchicine, may halt progression of nephropathy in some patients with AL amyloid.[37,47] Treatment of the underlying inflammatory condition and adjunctive use of colchicine has been advocated in secondary amyloidosis.[37,48–50]

INTESTINAL LYMPHANGIECTASIA

Intestinal lymphangiectasia (IL) is a protein-losing enteropathy characterized by dilated small bowel lymphatic channels (Fig. 62C–2), obstruction to lymph flow, and leakage of protein and lymphocyte-rich chyle into the intestinal lumen. The primary form probably represents a congenital malformation of lymphatics, and generally presents in early childhood. Family history often is positive in these cases, and lymphatic abnormalities outside the gastrointestinal tract are common. Lymphatic blockage may occur in several locations—lamina propria, submucosa, serosa, and mesentery.[51] A transient, acquired type of primary IL has also been described. Secondary IL develops in a variety of disease states in which lymph flow is obstructed. These diseases include constrictive pericarditis, chronic congestive heart failure, left subclavian venous obstruction, retroperitoneal fibrosis or neoplasms, Crohn's disease, mesenteric diseases, tuberculosis, sarcoid, mesenteric panniculitis, RE, chronic pancreatitis, and after abdominal surgical procedures.

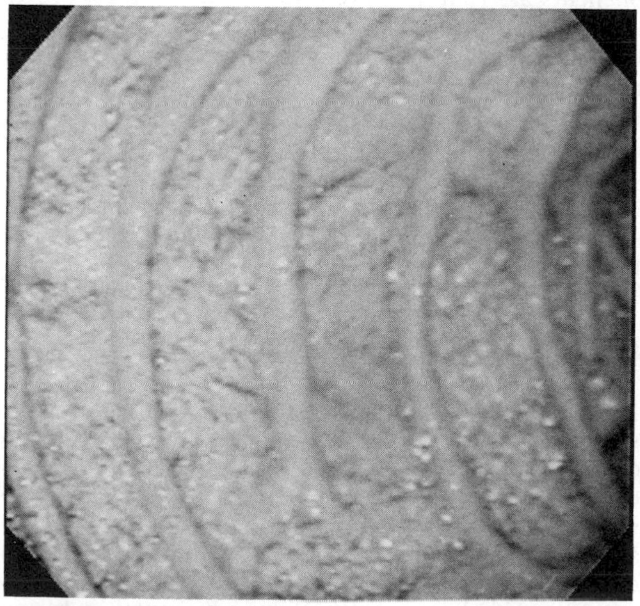

FIGURE 62C–2. Endoscopic picture of the small bowel mucosa of a patient with lymphangiectasia. Dilated lymphatic channels can be seen in the form of many nodules carpeting the mucosal surface.

PATHOLOGY

The histologic hallmark is dilatation of mucosal and submucosal lymph vessels (Fig. 62C–3). Foamy macrophages containing neutral lipids are found in the lymphatic channels, nodules, and lymph nodes. Mesenteric lymphatics are thickened by medial muscular hypertrophy, fibrosis, and elastosis.[52]

Grossly affected small bowel is edematous and slightly dilated with thickened folds. The serosal surface appears congested. Serosal lymphatics are dilated and may contain yellow nodules. Mesenteric lymph nodes are variably enlarged and yellow. "Enlarged, bleb-like tips" give the villous surface a pebbly, papillary appearance.[52]

CLINICAL MANIFESTATIONS

Edema is the typical presenting feature, and may be generalized or localized.[52,53] Diarrhea with variable steatorrhea, nausea, and vomiting occur at some time in most patients.[51] Chylous effusions and abdominal distention with ascites are common, but significant abdominal pain is unusual. Growth retardation may be prominent in children. Bacterial infections, related to lymphopenia and hypogammaglobulinemia, and hypocalcemic tetany owing to vitamin D malabsorption, may occur in severely affected patients.

Hypoproteinemia and lymphopenia are the salient laboratory features. Reduction in the serum albumin and globulin levels is pronounced, whereas those of other proteins are moderately reduced.[51] Coagulation formations usually are normal, as is the hemoglobin concentration, although iron deficiency may occur. The cholesterol level is low to normal; deficiencies of fat-soluble vitamins occur to a variable extent. Hypocalcemia, hypomagnesemia, and alkalosis may develop. Results of fecal fat studies range from upper normal to significant steatorrhea. D-Xylose absorption typically is normal.[52]

The typical radiographic feature is diffuse, symmetric thickening of folds with increased secretions. Less common findings include dilatation, spiculation, disorganization, punctate lucencies, and jejunization of ileum.[51] Lymphangiography, generally not needed for diagnosis, may be helpful in identifying discrete abnormalities amenable to surgical therapy.

Definitive diagnosis requires small bowel biopsy. The abnormally dilated submucosal lymphatics may be patchy; therefore, several biopsy samples should be obtained.[51]

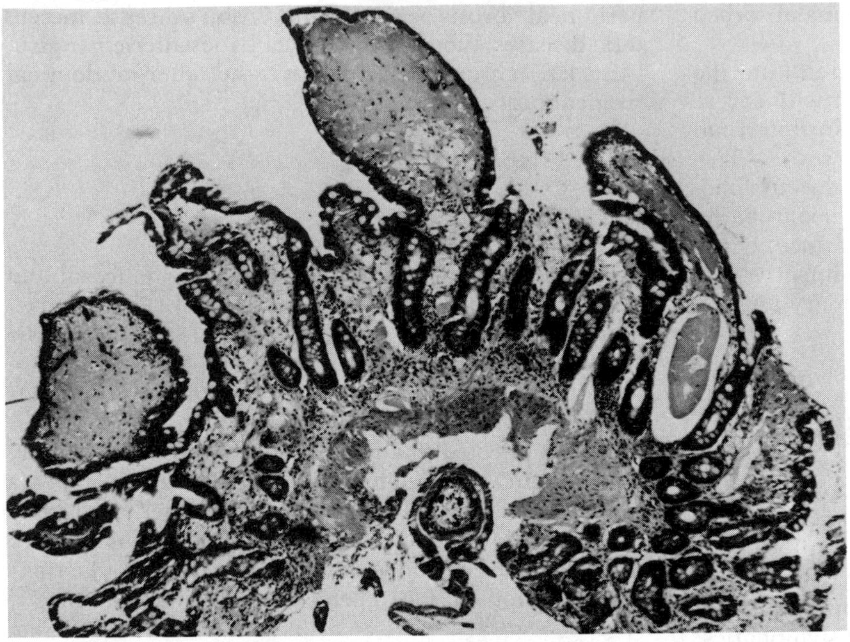

FIGURE 62C–3. Intestinal lymphangiectasia. Small bowel biopsy demonstrating dilated lymphatic channels with widened distorted villi.

MANAGEMENT

Diet clearly plays a crucial role in the management of IL. Intestinal lymph production is stimulated by long-chain fatty acids in the intestinal lumen. Decreased production may diminish local lymphatic pressure, resulting in less enteral chyle leakage. Indeed, restriction of fat to less than 5 g per day has been shown to increase serum albumin and albumin half-life, and to decrease diarrhea and steatorrhea.[54] A high-protein, fat-free diet with medium-chain triglyceride (MCT) supplements produced partial to complete remission in the majority of 15 patients.[51]

The MCT, containing C8-C10 fatty acids, are absorbed directly into the portal system and do not significantly increase lymph flow. When added to the fat-free diet of patients with IL, they enhance its palatability, while providing a good source of calories. In one report, all six children placed on a fat-free, MCT diet showed rapid and sustained long-term clinical improvement.[53] Relapse occurred with introduction of long-chain triglycerides, and responded to resumption of the previous diet. Despite clinical improvement, persistence of the underlying chyle leak was suggested by refractory lymphopenia and hypoglobulinemia. In several other reports, however, lymphocyte and globulin levels tended to parallel the disease course.[51,55]

Short periods of fasting and TPN have been advocated to allow distended lymphatics to collapse and edema to resolve, maximizing conditions for treatment with a fat-free, MCT diet.[56] This plan may be particularly useful for patients with severe diarrhea. In one patient treated in this way, abdominal pain, edema, and diarrhea subsided within 8 days, albumin levels rose, and radiography revealed mucosal edema was improved.[56] Provision of adequate amounts of the essential fatty acids must be assured.

Low-sodium diets, diuretics, and intravenous albumin infusions provide symptomatic relief. Oral vitamin supplements are routinely prescribed. For the rare, highly localized lesion, segmental intestinal resection may be beneficial. Corticosteroids, gluten-free diets, and gammaglobulin injections have repeatedly been ineffective.[52,53]

In most patients, the disease is permanent, and its course is marked by spontaneously fluctuating symptoms. Dietary management is successful, for the most part, in maintaining remission. Occasionally, the defect is transient and is completely reversible.[51,53,55]

ABETALIPOPROTEINEMIA

Abetalipoproteinemia (ABL) is a rare, autosomal recessive disorder characterized by: (1) abnormal lipid metabolism, (2) acanthocytosis (spiny or thorny red blood cells), (3) retinitis pigmentosa, and (4) progressive neurologic dysfunction. Failure of the intestinal mucosa to synthesize apoprotein B (apoB) is the basic defect. This apoprotein is essential for synthesis and structural integrity of chylomicrons (CM) and very low-density and low-density lipoproteins (VLDL, LDL). All of these lipoproteins are therefore absent in ABL. Defective CM formation leads to impaired transportation of fat out of enterocytes, and leads to malabsorption of fat-soluble vitamins. Acanthocytosis and lipid abnormalities are present from birth; neurologic and retinal findings generally develop in the second decade, perhaps reflecting deficiency states (vitamins E and A) rather than the underlying disease.

PATHOLOGY

Grossly, the mucosa has a diffuse yellow hue.[57] Histologic appearance is unique. Enterocytes appear distended and vacuolated because of engorgement with lipid droplets, even in the fasting state. Nuclei are pressed to the base of cells.[58] Villous structure is normal. In contrast to the enterocytes, the lacteals, submucosa, lamina propria, and lymphatics contain no fat. Immunofluorescence studies reveal absence of apoB in jejunal mucosa in the fasting state, and lack of apoB synthesis after fat feeding.[59]

CLINICAL MANIFESTATIONS

Gastrointestinal symptoms of diarrhea, steatorrhea, anorexia, vomiting, and growth retardation manifest in the first year of life. In many cases, the diagnosis is celiac sprue, and a gluten-free diet is administered, without relief. When the appropriate diagnosis is made and a lowfat diet is prescribed, clinical improvement ensues. Symptoms of fat intolerance tend to diminish with age,[58,60] perhaps as a result of increased use of the portal route of fat absorption.

Neurologic problems begin toward the end of the first decade, years after the onset of gastrointestinal symptoms. These include ataxia, intention tremors, clumsiness, and muscle weakness. Examination reveals abnormalities of the posterior columns, peripheral nerves, cerebellum, and muscles, similar to those in Friedrich's ataxia, which often is erroneously diagnosed. Visual complaints, scotomata and decreased acuity, are the last to develop. Ophthalmoscopic examination demonstrates fine mottling of the retina, consistent with atypical retinitis pigmentosa. Decreased photoreceptor response in both light and dark conditions may be demonstrated on physiologic testing (electroretinography). Untreated, the neurologic and retinal features progress relentlessly, and cause severe impairment.[61,62]

The biochemical hallmark of ABL is complete absence of apoB and undetectable or small amounts of β-lipoproteins—LDL, VLDL, and CM—on plasma lipid electrophoresis.[61,63] Serum cholesterol and triglyceride levels are low (0.78 to 2.07 mmol/L (30 to 80 mg/dl) and less than 0.11 mmol/L (10 mg/dl), respectively), and the triglyceride level fails to rise after fat ingestion.[63] Although linoleic acid levels are reduced in blood and in tissue, essential fatty acid (EFA) deficiency does not contribute significantly to the clinical picture.[63,64]

Fecal fat content is mildly to moderately increased. D-Xylose and Schilling absorption tests typically are normal, as are measurements of serum electrolytes and complete blood count. Examination of the blood smear preparations reveals spiny or thorn erythrocytes—acanthocytes. The lipid composition of the membranes of these red blood cells is abnormal, with a unique phospholipid distribution: decreased lecithin and increased sphingomyelin.[58] These changes may contribute to the abnormal configuration. Although acanthocytes function normally, increased autohemolysis and increased sensitivity to peroxide hemolysis, the latter of which is correctable with dietary vitamin E supplementation, are demonstrable.[58]

A combination of impaired vitamin E absorption and defective transport (because of the absence of apoB, its normal carrier) results in severe vitamin E deficiency.[61] Serum levels are undetectable; tissue levels are low.[65] Vitamin E deficiency likely contributes significantly, if not entirely, to the neurologic, and perhaps retinal, manifestations of ABL[60–62] (see Chap. 18).

Vitamin A is moderately to severely malabsorbed, and night blindness may compound the visual symptoms. Carotene levels are low.[63] Coagulopathy from vitamin K deficiency is mild or nonexistent,[58] whereas vitamin D deficiency has not been a clinical problem.

Thickened folds in the duodenum and jejunum, slight dilatation, and mild hypersecretion are seen radiographically.[66]

The clinical features of fat malabsorption, growth retardation, and neurologic and visual abnormalities, with acanthocytes on the blood smear and the absence of apoB strongly suggest the diagnosis. The histologic abnormality is diffuse, and small bowel biopsy is diagnostic. A normal biopsy result rules out ABL.[67]

TREATMENT

Oral supplementation with fat-soluble vitamins is the cornerstone of treatment. With high-dose oral supplementation (2.40 to 4.80 μmol of retinol [= 2286 to 4572 IU]/kg daily), normal vitamin A levels can be attained.[61,62] Abnormalities in dark adaptation response and in electroretinography generally improve with supplementation, although retinal degeneration is not prevented.[62] Massive oral doses of vitamin E (200 to 300 mg/kg daily) can produce detectable serum levels and correct in vitro red blood cell hemolysis.[61,65] Normal serum levels are rarely, if ever, attained.[58,61] The administration of vitamin E in the first few years of life may prevent retinopathy.[62] Given later in the course of the disease, vitamin E may halt or retard neurologic and retinal deterioration and may even lead to improvement in some patients.[61,62] Oral vitamin K, 5 mg twice a month, has been adequate in correcting the coagulopathy that seldom occurs.[57]

Moderate fat restriction, initially to approximately 10% of ingested calories ameliorates the gastrointestinal symptoms of diarrhea and steatorrhea and allows resumption of normal growth, and even "catch-up" growth.[61,62] With age, the capacity to absorb fat increases and patients should be encouraged to increase fat intake as tolerated.[58,64] Additional polyunsaturated fat as corn oil is sometimes recommended to correct the associated biochemical EFA deficiency.[64] The MCT are useful as a source of extra calories and clearly aid in weight gain; however, their potential to worsen long-chain fat malabsorption and to cause hepatic steatosis makes their use controversial.[61]

Gluten-free diets, steroids, and β-lipoprotein-rich plasma infusions have been administered without benefit.[58,63]

REFERENCES

1. Potish, R.A.: Am. J. Clin. Oncol., *5:*189–194, 1982.
2. Donaldson, S.S., Jundt, S., Ricour, JC., et al.: Cancer, *35:*1167–1178, 1975.
3. Earnest, D.L., Trier, J.S.: Radiation enteritis and colitis. *In* Gastrointestinal Disease. 4th Ed. Edited by M.H. Sleisinger, J.S. Fortran. Philadelphia, W.B. Saunders, 1989.
4. Trier, J.S., Browning, T.H.: J. Clin. Invest., *45:*194–204, 1966.
5. Pezner, R., Archambeau, J.O.: Cancer, *55:*263–267, 1985.
6. Dalla Palma, L.: Intestinal malabsorption in patients undergoing abdominal radiation therapy. *In* Gastrointestinal Radiation Injury. Report of a Symposium, Richland, Washington, Sept. 25–28, 1966. Edited by M.E. Sullivan. Amsterdam, Exerpta Medica Foundation, 1968, pp. 261–275.
7. Yeoh, E.K., Horowitz, M.: Surg. Gynecol. Obstet., *165:*373–379, 1987.
8. DeCosse, J.J., Rhodes, R.S., Wentz, W.B., et al.: Ann Surg., *170:*369–384, 1969.
9. Kinsella, T.J., Bloomer, W.D.: Surg. Gynecol. Obstet., *151:*273–284, 1980.
10. Loiudice, T.A., Lang, J.A.: Am. J. Gastroenterol., *78:*481–487, 1983.
11. Yeoh, E., Horowitz, M.: Br. J. Hosp. Med., *39:*498–504, 1988.
12. Newman, A., Katsaris, J., Blendis, L.M., et al.: Lancet, *2:*1471–1473, 1973.
13. Galland, R.B., Spencer, J.: Lancet, *1:*1257–1258, 1985.
14. Mulholland, M.W., Levitt, S.H., Song, C.W., et al.: Cancer, *54:*2396–2402, 1984.
15. Bounous, G., Lebel, E., Shuster, J.: Strahlenther. Onkol., *149:*476–483, 1975.
16. McArdle, A.H., Reid, E.C., Laplante, M.P., et al.: Arch. Surg., *121:*879–885, 1986.
17. Brown, M.S., Buchanan, R.B., Karran, S.J.: Clin. Radiol., *31:*19–20, 1980.
18. Kinsella, T.J., Malcolm, A.W., Bothe Jr., A., et al.: Int. J. Radiat. Oncol. Biol. Phys., *7:*543–548, 1981.
19. Valerio, D., Overett, L., Malcolm, A., et al.: Surg. Forum, *29:*145–148, 1978.
20. Donaldson, S.S., Welsey, M.N., Ghavimi, F., et al.: Med. Pediatr. Oncol., *10:*129–139, 1982.
21. Bosaeus, I., Andersson, H., Nystrom, C.: Acta Radiol. Oncol., *18:*460–464, 1979.
22. Beer, W.H., Fan, A., Halsted, C.H.: Am. J. Clin. Nutr., *41:*85–91, 1985.
23. Haddad, H., Bounous, G., Tahan, W.T., et al.: Dis. Colon Rectum, *17:*373–376, 1974.
24. Lavery, I.C., Steiger, E., Fazio, V.W.: Dis. Colon Rectum, *23:*91–93, 1980.
25. Miller, D.G., Ivey, M., Young, J.: Ann. Intern. Med., *91:*858–860, 1979.
26. Leinbach, G.E., Rubin, C.E.: Gastroenterology, *59:*874–889, 1970.
27. Heyman, M.B.: Food sensitivity and eosinophilic gastroenteropathies. *In* Gastrointestinal Disease. 4th Ed. Edited by M.H. Sleisinger, J.S. Fortran. Philadelphia, W.B. Saunders, 1989.
28. Katz, A.J., Twarog, F.J., Zeiger, R.S., et al.: J Allergy Clin. Immunol., *74:*72–78, 1984.
29. Talley, N.J., Shorter, R.G., Phillips, S.F., et al.: Gut, *31:*54–58, 1990.
30. Klein, N.C., Hargrove, L., Sleisinger, M.H., et al.: Medicine, *49:*299–319, 1970.
31. Marshak, R.H., Lindner, A., Maklansky, D., et al.: JAMA, *245:*1677–1680, 1981.
32. Caldwell, J.H., Tennenbaum, J.I., Bronstein, H.A.: N. Engl. J. Med., *292:*1388–1390, 1975.
33. Scudamore, H.H., Phillip, S.F., Swedlund, H.A., et al.: J. Allergy Clin. Immunol., *70:*129–138, 1982.
34. Greenberger, N.J. Tannenbaum, J.I., Ruppert, R.D.: Am. J. Med., *43:*777–784, 1967.
35. Cello, J.P.: Am. J. Med., *67:*1097–1104, 1979.
36. Tytgat, G.N., Grimj, R., Dekker, W., et al.: Gastroenterology, *71:*479–483, 1976.
37. Kyle, R.A., Greipp, P.R.: Mayo Clin. Proc., *58:*665–683, 1983.
38. Gilat, T., Spiro, H.M.: Dig. Dis. Sci., *13:*619–633, 1968.
39. Feurle, G.E.: Digestion, *36:*13–17, 1987.
40. Steen, L., Ek, B.: Acta Med. Scand., *214:*387–397, 1983.
41. Steen, L.E., Ek, B.O.: Scand. J. Gastroenterol., *19:*480–486, 1984.
42. Hunter, A.M., Borsey, D.Q., Campbell, I.W., et al.: Postgrad. Med. J., *55:*822–823, 1979.
43. Marshak, R.H., Lindner, A.E.: Amyloidosis. *In* Radiology of the Small Intestine. 2nd Ed. Philadelphia, W.B. Saunders, 1976.
44. Case Records of the MGH. Case 43-1985: N. Engl. J. Med., *313:*1070–1079, 1985.
45. Smith, T.R., Cho, K.C.: Am. J. Gastroenterol., *81:*477–479, 1986.
46. O'Connor, C.R., O'Dorisio, T.M.: Ann. Intern. Med., *110:*665–666, 1989.
47. Benson, M.D.: Arthritis Rheum., *29:*683–687, 1986.
48. Becker, S.A., Bass, D., Nissim, F.: J. Clin. Gastroenterol., *7:*296–300, 1985.
49. Meyers, S., Janowitz, H.D., Gumaste, V.K., et al.: Gastroenterology, *94:*1503–1507, 1988.

50. Edwards, P., Cooper, D.A., Turner, J., et al.: Gastroenterology, *95:*810–815, 1988.
51. Vardy, P.A., Lebenthal, E., Shwachman, H.: Pediatrics, *55:*842–851, 1975.
52. Waldmann, T.A., Steinfeld, J.L., Dutcher, T.F. et al.: Gastroenterology, *41:*197–207, 1961.
53. Tift, W.L., Lloyd, J.K.: Arch. Dis. Child., *50:*269–276, 1975.
54. Jeffries, G.H., Chapman, A., Sleisinger, M.H.: N. Engl. J. Med., *270:*761–767, 1964.
55. Orbeck, H., Larsen, T.E., Hovig, T.: Acta Paediatr. Scand., *67:*677–682, 1978.
56. Wagner, A.: Digestion, *2:*167–171, 1969.
57. Delpre, G., Kadish, U., Glantz, I., et al.: Endoscopy, *10:*59–62, 1978.
58. Kayden, H.J.: Annu. Rev. Med., *23:*285–296, 1972.
59. Glickman, R.M., Green, P.H., Lees, JR.S., et al.: Gastroenterology, *76:*288–292, 1979.
60. Muller, JD.P.R.: Clin. Gastroenterol., *11:*119–140, 1982.
61. Illingworth, D.R., Connor, W.E., Miller, R.G.: Arch. Neurol., *37:*659–662, 1980.
62. Muller, D.P.R., Lloyd, J.K., Bird, A.C.: Arch. Dis. Child., *52:*209–214, 1977.
63. Isselbacher, K.J., Scheig, R., Plotkin, G.R., et al.: Medicine, *43:*347–361, 1964.
64. Kayden, H.J.: Nutr. Rev., *38:*244–246, 1980.
65. Muller, D.P.R., Harries, J.T., Lloyd, J.K.: Gut, *15:*966–971, 1974.
66. Laufer, I., Herlinger, H.: Radiologic Features of Malabsorption Syndromes. *In* Bocchus Gastroenterology. 4th Ed. Edited by J.E. Berk. Philadelphia, W.B. Saunders, 1985.
67. Trier, J.S.: Hosp. Pract., *23:*195–211, 1988.

D. CELIAC DISEASE

J. Joseph Connon

HISTORICAL BACKGROUND

An illness resembling celiac disease was described as early as the first century A.D. by Aretaeus of Cappadocia.[1] In the nineteenth century, Dr. Samuel Gee provided an excellent clinical description and recommended dietary treatment of a diarrheal illness that he termed "the celiac affection."[2] Determination of the cause and dietary therapy of celiac disease, however, awaited the observations of W.R. Dicke, a Dutch pediatrician, who noted improvement followed by deterioration of his celiac patients as bread was first withdrawn and then reintroduced into their diets during and after the Second World War.[3] Further progress in understanding the disease was facilitated by the development of peroral intestinal biopsy devices by Shiner,[4] and by Crosby and Kugler,[5] which confirmed Paulley's observation ofintestinal mucosal flattening in surgically obtained specimens.[6]

PATHOLOGY

The normal small bowel mucosa is thrown up in a series of concertina-like folds called the valvulae conniventes. At a microscopic level, the absorptive surface of the mucosa is configured as millions of villi covered by columnar epithelial cells, whereas the secretory mucosa primarily consists of the crypts of Lieberkühn. In advanced celiac disease, the valvulae are thinner and more widely spaced than normal, and scalloping of their free margins has been described at endoscopy.[7,8] The microscopic changes are usually diffuse rather than focal and diminish in severity distally. Changes range in severity from intraepithelial lymphocytic infiltration to complete loss of villi, crypt hyperplasia, and infiltration of the lamina propria by plasma cells, lymphocytes, neutrophils, eosinophils, and mast cells.[9] The remaining absorptive cells are cuboidal and vacuolated. Occasionally, changes are patchy.[10]

Changes similar to those of celiac disease have been described in other local and systemic disorders that affect the intestinal mucosa. These include lymphoma, giardiasis, tropical sprue, bacterial overgrowth, viral gastroenteritis, cow's milk protein intolerance, and graft-versus-host disease.[11]

Dietary exclusion of gluten usually results in restoration of a more normal mucosal appearance within 2 to 3 months. In children, complete recovery may occur, but some residual villous blunting and lymphocytic infiltration are the rule.[12] If rechallenge with gluten is believed necessary to confirm the diagnosis, 10 g gluten per day should be added to the diet for up to 2 months, followed by another biopsy. Some patients will be unable to tolerate gluten for more than a few days because of nausea, bloating, and diarrhea. Occasionally, gluten challenge fails to cause typical histologic changes in patients who have a relapse years later.[13] The presence of a normal mucosa, even on a normal diet, does not exclude the eventual development of celiac disease.

PREVALENCE

Celiac disease has a worldwide distribution, but significant variations in prevalence exist, ranging from 1 in 300 in Ireland[14] to 1 in 3500 in Finland.[15] It is extremely rare in blacks, Chinese, and Japanese populations, but has been described in India.[16] Celiac disease is more common in women, especially during the reproductive years, but this may be an artifact related to increased case finding. The prevalence of celiac disease is higher in adults than in children, and the majority of such adults have no history of childhood symptoms. The peak prevalence in women occurs between 35 and 44 years of age.[17] In Scotland, the incidence of childhood celiac disease appears to have fallen since 1976, perhaps as a result of changes in weaning practice with the later introduction of cereal products to the infant diet. The incidence of celiac disease has not declined in Sweden, however, despite similar infant feeding practices.[18]

GENETICS

Strong evidence suggests an inherited predisposition to celiac disease.[19] It occurs up to 100 times more frequently in first-degree relatives of patients with the disease than in the general population. Studies of identical twins have shown a disease concordance of 70%.[20] This inherited susceptibility is closely associated with HLA-B8, HLA-DR3, and HLA-DQ alleles. The alleles encoding DQW2 are in linkage disequilibrium with B8 and DR3. More than 90% of celiac patients possess the HLA-DQW2 allele,[21] but the nature of the pathogenetic connections between the HLA type and gluten sensitivity remains unclear. Seventy percent of unaffected siblings have the same HLA-DR phenotypes as their affected sibling,[22] so some additional genetic or environmental factors appear necessary for gluten sensitivity to be manifest.

PATHOGENESIS

GLUTEN

Gluten is a component of wheats, oats, barley, and rye, all of which belong to the species Triticum aestivale. Gliadin, the toxic agent in gluten, is rich in proline and glutamine, hence the term prolamins for alcoholic extracts of gluten. Several subfractions of gliadin are known, the best studied being, α, β, γ, and ω. These have in turn been subfractionated, and all the gliadin moieties appear harmful to the intestinal mucosa.[23]

The causal relationship between dietary gluten and mucosal changes in susceptible patients is unquestioned; however, many questions remain regarding the mechanism whereby gluten exerts its harmful effects. Initially, it was suggested that incomplete brush border hydrolysis of gluten as a consequence of enzyme deficiency led to the formation of toxic products,[24] but inability to demonstrate abnormally low mucosal peptidase or carbohydrase activity following treatment with a gluten-free diet rendered this hypothesis untenable.[25]

ADENOVIRUS INFECTION

Kagnoff et al. have noted significant structural amino acid homology between a gliadin fragment and a nonstructural component, E1B of type 12 adenovirus. These investigators suggested that adenovirus infection of susceptible subjects brings about gluten sensitization through the process of molecular mimicry.[26,27] Although this group found a significant increase in the prevalence of antiadenovirus 12 antibodies in patients with untreated celiac disease, other workers have failed to confirm this finding.[28] The polymerase chain reaction technique, using primers specific for the EB1 gene, showed no evidence for persistent adenovirus infection in celiac disease.[29]

ANTIBODIES

A variety of antibodies directed against both dietary and self antigens have been found in serum and intestinal secretions of celiac patients.[30,31] Antigliadin IgA antibodies are found in up to 90% of untreated celiac patients, and their titer gradually diminishes on gluten withdrawal.[32] Other food-related antibodies such as antiovalbumin and anticasein have been described. It appears likely that antibody production is related to the increased paracellular intestinal permeability found in celiac disease. Although pathogenic mechanisms involving disordered immunity have been proposed, such as antibody-dependent cell-mediated cytotoxic effects and immune complex formation, the role of antibodies in causing villous damage remains conjectural.

IgA antibodies directed against specific tissue components have also been identified. These include antireticulin,[33] antijejunal,[34] and antiendomysial antibodies,[35] which can be detected by immunofluorescence techniques in both human and animal tissues. Antijejunal and antiendomysial antibodies likely recognize a common antigen.[36] The endomysium is a delicate connective tissue layer surrounding intestinal smooth muscle, and antiendomysial antibodies have been found in more than 95% of patients with celiac disease.[37] The antibody specificity of both antiendomysial and antigliadin antibodies is 90%. Antiendomysial antibody titers decrease after institution of a gluten-free diet. Measurement of antibody titers has been suggested as a screening test for celiac disease and as a means of evaluating dietary compliance in unresponsive patients.[13,38]

CLINICAL MANIFESTATIONS

The presentation of celiac disease is variable, ranging from mild, nonspecific features through monodeficiency states to a full-blown classic panmalabsorption syndrome.[39] The classic form of the disease is now the least common presentation, and several authors have emphasized the need to consider celiac disease in patients with irritable bowel-like features occurring in association with another trigger finding such as anemia, weight loss, or a monodeficiency state.[40,41]

DIARRHEA

Diarrhea is found in 70% of patients.[42] It is usually intermittent, occurs three to four times daily, and is of mushy consistency. Celiac patients often have crampy abdominal pain that, in association with diarrhea and bloating secondary to fermentation of lactose and other maldigested compounds, may simulate the irritable bowel syndrome. In a few patients, the diarrhea is more severe, and stools have the classic malabsorptive features of large volume, frothiness, offensive odor, greasy appearance, and a tendency to float. This last quality is the result of increased gaseous content, rather than fat concentration.

WEIGHT LOSS

Some weight loss is usual, but the amount is variable. Its degree is as much dependent on associated anorexia as on malabsorption. Patients with villous atrophy confined to the proximal small intestine may have no loss of weight.

MALAISE

A loss of general well-being is found in 80% of patients, but it is often so insidious in onset that its presence is only recognized retrospectively after the institution of a gluten-free diet.

MONODEFICIENCY SYNDROMES

Isolated, monomalabsorption of substances absorbed from the duodenum and proximal and midjejunum is well recognized.[43] This includes malabsorption of iron, vitamin D, vitamin K, calcium, magnesium, albumin, and folic acid.[11,44] A combination of iron and folate deficiency is not unusual. The increased metabolic demands of pregnancy may unmask marginal absorption, especially of iron and folate.

ASSOCIATED DISEASES

The clinical features of celiac disease may sometimes be overshadowed by the more dramatic manifestations of associated diseases, thus leading to a delay in diagnosis. Many of these diseases have an autoimmune basis. They include dermatitis herpetiformis,[45] intestinal lymphoma,[46] diabetes,[47] thyroid disease,[48] IgA deficiency,[49] cerebellar atrophy,[50] inflammatory bowel disease,[51] and sclerosing cholangitis.[52]

DERMATITIS HERPETIFORMIS

This disease causes pruritic, vesicular, and papular lesions with an erythematous background, primarily on the extensor surfaces of the limbs. The lesions demonstrate granular or linear deposition of IgA at the junction of dermis and epidermis.[53] Although intestinal symptoms are uncommon, virtually all patients with the granular pattern of IgA deposition show patchy mucosal changes identical to those of celiac disease. Linear deposition of IgA is not associated with celiac disease. Both the cutaneous and mucosal abnormalities respond to a gluten-free diet, and in some patients, dapsone therapy can be withdrawn.[54,55]

MALIGNANT DISEASES

Certain malignant disorders have been associated with celiac disease, notably small intestinal lymphoma. Celiac-associated lymphoma is generally accepted to be of T-cell origin, though it has been variously described as a B-cell tumor and as a malignant histiocytosis.[56] Although some investigators have suggested that the mucosal atrophy associated with this lymphoma is secondary to the lymphoma rather than vice versa,[57] many are reluctant to accept that the malignant features of lymphoma may be delayed for many years and that gluten exclusion would restore a normal mucosal appearance in intestinal lymphoma. Moreover, antigliadin antibodies have been noted in patients who develop lymphoma in the course of celiac disease, whereas these antibodies are absent in patients who are first seen with a lymphoma without a prior history of celiac disease.[58]

A variety of presentations have been noted, including diarrhea, intestinal obstruction, intestinal perforation, weight loss, abdominal pain, intestinal bleeding, fever, and finger clubbing. IgA levels may increase. Enteropathy-associated T-cell lymphoma (EATL) may be difficult to diagnose.[59] If routine investigations, including small bowel enema and abdominal computed tomography (CT) scan, are negative and the clinical picture is suspicious, a laparotomy with full-thickness biopsies should be done. Local resection is rarely possible, and response to systemic chemotherapy is poor.

Other cancers also occur with increased frequency in celiac disease, including esophageal and pharyngeal cancer, as well as small intestinal adenocarcinoma.[60] A reduced incidence of small bowel lymphoma has been reported in patients who adhere to a gluten-free diet.[61]

Several other diseases have also been linked with celiac disease. These include psychiatric disorders, farmer's lung, autoimmune thrombocytopenia, anemia, and Berger's disease, but the evidence is not conclusive.[62]

INVESTIGATIONS

HEMATOLOGY

Anemia is present in 40 to 80% of patients.[63] Unexplained iron or folate deficiency anemia rather than florid malabsorption raises the suspicion of celiac disease.[64] The simultaneous deficiency of both iron and folate produces a dimorphic blood picture, giving rise to an increased red cell distribution width (RDW). Hyposplenism is common in celiac disease and produces Howell-Jolly bodies.[65] Folate deficiency may cause a slightly low serum B_{12}, which responds to folate replacement. Rarely, mucosal atrophy extending to the terminal ileum or bacterial overgrowth secondary to celiac-associated intestinal stasis may produce B_{12} deficiency.

BIOCHEMISTRY

Biochemical abnormalities in celiac disease essentially reflect both the extent and duration of malabsorption and range from none to multiple changes involving fluids, minerals, proteins, fat, and gut hormones. The stool fat content is usually increased in celiac patients with diarrhea, but it may be normal in monosymptomatic patients whose presenting feature is iron, folate, or vitamin D deficiency.[66] Steatorrhea tends to be less marked in celiac disease than in chronic pancreatitis, and stool fat concentration is also relatively lower because of greater fluid losses in the celiac stool.[67] The importance of stool fat measurement has diminished in parallel with the increasing use of endoscopic small bowel biopsy.

D-Xylose is an inert sugar absorbed in the upper small intestine. Serum or urinary levels following oral administration provide a measure of jejunal absorptive capacity, but test reliability is influenced by variations in gastric emptying, age, and renal function.[68] Tests of selective mucosal absorption using probes of different molecular size have been used both in the diagnosis and the follow-up of celiac disease. These molecules include mannitol, lactulose, and lactobiose. In celiac patients, larger molecules are selectively absorbed probably by paracellular routes, and transcellular absorption of smaller molecules is diminished as a result of villous atrophy.[69] Although a high sensitivity and negative predictive value have been claimed for tests of differential urinary excretion, they have not yet gained wide acceptance.

RADIOLOGY

The primary role of radiology of the small bowel is exclusion of other diseases such as Crohn's disease, jejunal diverticulosis, strictures, or lymphoma, and barium studies are not routinely required. In celiac disease, the radiologic appearance is often normal, but it may show dilatation of the lumen and thickening of mucosal folds.

ANTIGLIADIN AND ANTIENDOMYSIAL ANTIBODIES

Increasing recognition of the subtle and atypical modes of presentation of celiac disease has underlined the importance of noninvasive screening tests. The finding of increased antigliadin and antiendomysial antibody titers has been described in up to 95% of celiac patients. Population studies have also demonstrated test specificity exceeding 95%. The greatest sensitivity and specificity are associated with IgA antiendomysial antibodies. Because biopsy of the intestine of all subjects, especially children, with chronic diarrhea is impractical, a good case can be made for screening for IgA antiendomysial antibodies in this group.

An enzyme-linked immunosorbent assay (ELISA) kit for home testing for the presence of gluten in food has been developed,[70] but further evaluation is necessary.

The use of serologic screening has identified asymptomatic subjects with typical mucosal changes of celiac disease. Whether a gluten-free diet is appropriate in this group is unclear.

INTESTINAL BIOPSY

Endoscopic biopsy of the second or third portions of the duodenum has largely replaced use of the Crosby or Watson capsule. Although these latter devices provide larger biopsy specimens, frustration with the technical difficulties associated with them compared with the ease of obtaining multiple, albeit smaller, endoscopic samples has led to a marked decline in their use. An immediate diagnosis of villous atrophy can be made by dissecting microscopic examination of the biopsy material. Recently, gastric antral histologic changes have been reported in celiac patients.[71]

Endoscopy may reveal macroscopic changes in some patients. These include thinning, wider separation, and scalloping of the margins of the valvulae conniventes.[7,8] En face, the mucosa may show a mosaic appearance enhanced when the mucosa is partially covered with blood following biopsy.

The biopsy appearance of celiac disease is nonspecific, and definitive diagnosis requires repeat biopsy to demonstrate histologic improvement on a gluten-free diet and reversion to abnormality after gluten challenge. In adults, the last step is frequently omitted.

TREATMENT

Dietary avoidance of gluten is central to the management of celiac disease. The majority of patients notice a significant symptomatic improvement within days. Changes in mucosal histology take longer. A reduction in intraepithelial lymphocyte infiltration occurs within a few weeks,[72] but recovery of the normal villous appearance usually takes 2 to 3 months. In some patients, full recovery never occurs even though they feel well.

The diet should be supplemented, initially, with appropriate vitamins and minerals in those patients with demonstrated deficiencies, but long-term supplementation is unnecessary.

Wheat, barley, rye, oats, and triticale are the main sources of gluten, and foodstuffs derived from these products must be excluded. Adherence to a strict gluten-free diet may be rendered difficult because of the presence of cereal products in a variety of prepared foods, but deliberate noncompliance is a much larger problem. Dietary surveys have shown that 30% of patients admit to taking gluten and remain asymptomatic.[73] In some patients, however, ingestion of even small amounts of gluten results in bloating and diarrhea. Attainment of expected adult stature may be compromised by gluten intake during childhood and adolescence.[74] The desirability of adhering to a gluten-free diet is heightened by a study demonstrating a reduction in the rates of intestinal lymphoma in compliant patients.[61]

Significant differences exist internationally in the constituents of a gluten-free diet. In Canada, the diet must not contain any wheat, barley, rye, oats, or triticale, whereas in many European countries, levels ranging from 5 to 50 μg gliadin per day are acceptable. The Celiac Sprue Association U.S.A., in addition to recommending complete exclusion of gluten-containing cereals, also advises avoidance of buckwheat and any foods using cereal mash in their manufacture. These include distilled alcoholic beverages and white vinegar, which contain no detectable gliadins. Beer contains 3 μg/L prolamin and probably should be avoided. For detailed information on gluten-free diet, see Appendix Table A–34.

TREATMENT FAILURE

In the event of failure to respond to treatment, it is important to consider deliberate or inadvertent intake of gluten as well as diagnostic error. If one is in any doubt about the adequacy of the original intestinal biopsies, further tissue should be obtained. Consideration must be given to other disorders associated with mucosal flattening, especially ulcerative jejunoileitis and lymphoma.

True failure to respond to dietary treatment is rare, and its pathogenesis is uncertain. Some patients respond successfully to corticosteroid treatment.[75] Rapidly metabolized "first-pass" steroids have been used to treat celiac disease instead of dietary therapy,[76] and such compounds may become the drugs of choice in unresponsive patients.

REFERENCES

1. Hude, C.: Aretaeus: Corpus Medicorum Graecorum II. 2nd Ed. Berlin, Academy of Sciences, 1958.
2. Gee, S.J.: St. Bartholomew's Hosp. Rep., *24:*17–20, 1888.
3. Dicke, W.K.: Coeliakie. Ph.D. thesis, University of Utrecht. Utrecht, 1950.
4. Shiner, M.: Lancet, 1:85, 1956.
5. Crosby, W.H., Kugler, H.W.: Am. J. Dig. Dis., *2:*236–241, 1957.
6. Paulley, J.W.: Proc. R. Soc. Med., *42:*241, 1949.
7. Jabbari, M., Wild, G., Goresky, C.A., et al.: Gastroenterology, *95:*1518–1522, 1988.
8. Brocchi, E., Corazza, G., Treggiari, E.A., et al.: N. Engl. J. Med., *319:*741–744, 1988.
9. Rubin, C.E., Brandborg, L.L., Phelps, P.C., et al.: Gastroenterology, *38:*28–49, 1960.
10. Scott, B.B., Losowsky, M.S.: Gut, *17:*984–992, 1976.
11. Cooke, W.T., Holmes, G.K.T.: Coeliac Disease. New York, Churchill Livingstone, 1984.
12. Rubin, C.E., Eidelman, S., Weinstein, W.M.: Gastroenterology, *58:*409–413, 1970.
13. Kuitunen, P., Savilahti, E., Verkasalo, M.: Acta Paediatr. Scand., *75:*340–342, 1986.
14. Mylotte, M., Egan-Mitchell, B., McCarthy, C.F., et al.: Br. Med. J., *1:*703–705, 1973.
15. Simila, S., Kokkonen, J., Voulukka, P., et al.: Lancet, *1:*494–495, 1981.
16. Misra, R.C., Kasthuri, D., Chuttani, H.K.: Br. Med. J., *2:*1230–1232, 1966.
17. Logan, R.A.F., Rifkind, E.A., Busuttil, A., et al.: Gastroenterology, *90:*334–342, 1986.
18. Ascher, H., Krantz, I., Kristiansson, B.: Arch. Dis. Child., *66:*608–611, 1991.
19. Mylotte, M., Egan-Mitchell, B., Fottrell, P.F., et al.: Q. J. Med., *43:*359–369, 1974.
20. Polanco, I., Biemond, I., van Leeuwen, A., et al.: *In* Genetics of Coeliac Disease: Proceedings of an International Symposium. Edited by R.D. McConnell. Lancaster, England, MTP Press, 1981.
21. Tosi, R., Vismara, D., Tanigaki, N., et al.: Clin. Immunol. Immunopathol., *28:*395–404, 1983.
22. Kagnoff, M.F., Harwood, J.I., Bugawan, T.L., et al.: Proc. Natl. Acad. Sci. U.S.A., *86:*6274–6278, 1989.
23. Ciclitira, P.J., Evans, D.J., Fagg, N.L.K., et al.: Clin. Sci., *66:*357–364, 1984.
24. Frazer, A.C., Fletcher, R.F., Ross, C.A.: Lancet, *2:*252–255, 1959.
25. Davidson, A.G.F., Bridges, M.A.: Clin. Chim. Acta, *163:*1–40, 1987.
26. Kagnoff, M.F., Austin, R.K., Hubert, J.J., et al.: J. Exp. Med., *160:*1544–1557, 1984.
27. Kagnoff, M.F., Paterson, Y.J., Kumar, P.J., et al.: Gut, *28:*995–1001, 1987.
28. Howdle, P.D., Blair Zajdel, M.E., Smart, C.J., et al.: Scand. J. Gastroenterol., *24:*282–286, 1989.
29. Mahon, J., Blair, G.E., Wood, G.M.: Gut, *32:*1114–1116, 1991.
30. Kenrick, K.G., Walker-Smith, J.A.: Gut, *11:*635–640, 1970.
31. Ferguson, A., Carswell, F.: Br. Med. J. (Clin. Res.), *1:*75–77, 1972.
32. Kelly, C.P., Feighery, C.F., Weir, D.G.: Gastroenterology, *94:*A221, 1988.
33. Mäki, M., Hällström, O., Vesikari, T., et al.: J. Pediatr., *105:*901–905, 1984.
34. Kárpáti, S., Török, E., Kosnaii, J.: Invest. Dermatol., *87:*703–706, 1986.

35. Volta, U., Molinaro, N., Fusconi, M., et al.: Dig. Dis. Sci., *36:*752–756, 1991.
36. Kárpáti, S., Meurer, M., Burgin-Wolff, A., et al.: Gut, *33:*191–193, 1992.
37. Kumar, V., Lerner, A., Valeski, J.E., et al.: Immunol. Invest., *18:*533–544, 1989.
38. Cacciari, E., Volta, U., Lazzari, R., et al.: Lancet, *1:*1469–1471, 1985.
39. Mann, J.G., Brown, W.R., Kern, F.: Am. J. Med., *48:*375–366, 1970.
40. Rifkind, E.A., Busuttil, A., Ferguson, A.: Br. Med. J., *281:*1637, 1980.
41. Swinson, C.M., Levi, A.J.: Br. Med. J., *281:*1258–1260, 1980.
42. Dawson, A.M.: Neth. J. Med., *31:*256–262, 1997.
43. Rossi, E.: Eur. J. Pediatr., *138:*4–5, 1982.
44. Weir, D.G., Hourihane, D.O'B.: Gut, *15:*450–457, 1974.
45. Marks, J., Shuster, S., Watson, A.J.: Lancet, *2:*1280–1282, 1966.
46. Holmes, G.K.T., Stokes, P.L., Sorahan, T.M., et al.: Gut, *17:*612–619, 1976.
47. Walker-Smith, J.A.: Arch. Dis. Child., *50:*668, 1975.
48. Midhagen, G., Järnerot, G., Kraaz, W.: Scand. J. Gastroenterol., *23:*1000–1004, 1988.
49. Mawhinney, H., Tomkin, G.H.: Lancet, *2:*121–124, 1971.
50. Finelli, P.F., McEntee, W.J., Ambler, M., et al.: Neurology, *30:*245–249, 1980.
51. Shah, A., Mayberry, J.F., Williams, G., et al.: Q. J. Med., *74:*283–288, 1990.
52. Hay, J.E., Wiesner, R.H., Shorter, R.G., et al.: Ann. Intern. Med., *109:*713–717, 1988.
53. Lawley, T.J., Strober, W., Yaoita, H., et al.: J. Invest. Dermatol., *74:*9, 1980.
54. Weinstein, W.M., Brow, J.R., Parker, F., et al.: *60:*362–369, 1971.
55. Fry, L., Seah, P.P., Riches, D.J., et al.: Lancet, *1:*288–291, 1973.
56. Isaacson, P.G., O'Connor, N.T., Spencer, J., et al: Lancet, *2:*688–691, 1985.
57. Wright, D.H., Jones, D.B., Clark, H., et al.: Lancet, *337:*1373–1374, 1991.
58. O'Farrelly, C., Feighery, C., O'Briain, D.S., et al.: Br. Med. J. (Clin. Res.), *293:*908–910, 1986.
59. Isaacson, P.G.: Coeliac disease: malignant lymphoma. *In* Topics in Gastroenterology. Vol. 14. Edited by D.P. Jewell and A. Ireland. Boston, Blackwell Scientific Publications, 1986.
60. Swinson, C.M., Slavin, G., Coles, E.C., et al.: Lancet, *1:*111–115, 1983.
61. Holmes, G.K.T., Prior, P., Lane, M.R., et al.: Gut, *30:*333–338, 1989.
62. Mulder, C.J., Tytgat, G.N.: Neth. J. Med., *31:*286–289, 1987.
63. Hoffbrand, A.V.: Clin. Gastroenterol., *3:*71–89, 1974.
64. Logan, R.A.F., Tucker, G., Rifkind, E.A.: Br. Med. J., *286:*95–97, 1983.
65. Ferguson, A., Hutton, M.M., Maxwell, J.D., et al.: Lancet, *1:*163–164, 1970.
66. McGuigan, J.E., Volwiler, W.: Gastroenterology, *47:*636–641, 1964.
67. Bow-Linn, G.W., Fordtran, J.S.: Gastroenterology, *87:*319–322, 1984.
68. Craig, R.M., Atkinson, A.J., Jr.: Gastroenterology, *95:*223–231, 1988.
69. Juby, L.D., Rothwell, J., Axon, A.T.: Gastroenterology, *96:*79–85, 1989.
70. Skerritt, J.H., Hill, A.S.: Lancet, *337:*379–382, 1991.
71. Wolber, R., Owen, D., Delbuono, L.: Gastroenterology, *93:*310, 1990.
72. Yardley, J.H., Bayless, T.M., Norton, J.H., et al.: N. Engl. J. Med., *267:*1173–1179, 1962.
73. Kumar, P.J., Clark, M.L., Dawson, A.M.: Q. J. Med., *57:*803, 1985.
74. Colaco, J., Egan-Mitchell, B., Stevens, F.M., et al.: Arch. Dis. Child., *62:*706–708, 1987.
75. Taylor, A.B., Wollaeger, E.E., Comfort, M.W.: Gastroenterology, *20:*203–228, 1952.
76. Mitchison, H.C., al Mardini, H., Gillespie, S., et al.: Gut, *32:*260–265, 1991.

CHAPTER **63**

Nutrition in Pancreatic and Liver Disorders

Mark A. Korsten and Charles S. Lieber

The functional integrity of the liver and pancreas is essential for optimal digestion and effective utilization of nutrients. Thus, disorders of these organs will have far-reaching effects on nutritional status. We will first delineate the role of these organs in normal digestive processes. Next, the nutritional complications of liver and pancreatic dysfunction and approaches for correcting nutritional deficiencies in these disorders will be assessed. Finally, nutritional factors that may themselves result in pancreatic or liver injury will be discussed.

LIVER AND PANCREAS IN NORMAL DIGESTION

LIVER

The liver influences nutritional status through its elaboration of bile salts and its role in intermediary metabolism of protein (amino acids), carbohydrate, fat, and vitamins.

BILE SALTS

Bile salts are synthesized in the liver from cholesterol, secreted in bile, and mixed with the intestinal contents in response to a meal. In the intestine, bile salts are active in the intraluminal phase of fat assimilation, its principal action being that of a detergent. Triglycerides enter the duodenum in the form of an emulsion. The surface of this emulsion is covered by a relatively polar layer of phospholipids and proteins that must be removed by bile salts before lipolysis via pancreatic lipase can proceed. However, clearance of these polar substances from the emulsion also separates glyceride in the emulsion from lipase in the water phase; lipolysis, as a result, becomes dependent on the presence of another enzyme, colipase, which is secreted with lipase in the pancreatic juice. By binding to lipase and altering its molecular conformation, colipase overcomes the inhibitory actions of bile salts on lipolysis.[1,2]

The products of lipolysis, such as fatty acids, monoglycerides, and small amounts of lysophospholipids form mixed micelles with bile salts. The intestinal uptake of long chain fatty acids depends on these mixed micelles. In contrast, the absorption of short and medium chain fatty acids proceeds in the absence of bile.[3] Following uptake of fatty acids, bile salts are conserved by being recycled through an enterohepatic circulation. Bile salts, especially conjugates of the trihydroxy bile acid, cholic acid, are reabsorbed from the distal small bowel by an active, sodium-dependent process. Dihydroxy bile salts are absorbed by passive diffusion from the proximal small bowel.[4] The liver extracts these reabsorbed bile salts from the portal vein blood and returns them to the biliary tree. Hepatic synthesis of bile salts replenishes the fraction of the bile salt pool that escapes reabsorption and is excreted in the feces.[5]

INTERMEDIARY METABOLISM

The liver plays a fundamental role in intermediary metabolism. This is a highly complex topic and is not covered here in an exhaustive manner. Instead, we review the highlights of this subject with the goal of providing an overall view for understanding the nutritional complications of liver injury.

Carbohydrates. The liver regulates carbohydrate metabolism by the synthesis, storage, and breakdown of glycogen. A polymeric form of glucose, large amounts of glycogen can be stored within the hepatocyte without major effects on the intracellular osmotic pressure. Glycogen is formed when the intake of glucose (or other gluconeogenic fuels) exceeds energy requirements; glycogen is broken down when intake lags behind energy needs. The principal enzymes controlling glycogenesis and glycogenolysis are glycogen synthase and phosphorylase, respectively. There is a reciprocal relationship between these two enzymes. Stimulation of glycogen synthase is usually accompanied by inhibition of phosphorylase; conversely, agents that stimulate phosphorylase inhibit glycogen synthase. Factors that control these enzymes include intracellular levels of glucose-6-phosphate and hormones such as epinephrine, glucagon, and insulin. Epinephrine and glucagon raise blood glucose levels by activating phosphorylase whereas insulin lowers blood glucose, in part, by stimulating glycogen synthase.

Hepatocytes also possess enzymes that enable them to synthesize glucose from various precursors such as amino acids, pyruvate, and lactate (gluconeogenesis). It is well established that hypoglycemia promotes this process. The link between hypoglycemia and gluconeogenesis is probably mediated by the secretion of cortisol from the adrenal medulla. Cortisol secretion is under pituitary control (adrenocorticotropic hormone, or ACTH) and is known to mobilize glycogenic amino acids from various tissues.

Fat. The liver is a major site of fatty acid breakdown and triglyceride synthesis. The breakdown of fatty acids provides an alternative source of energy when glucose is unavailable as during fasting or starvation. Triglyceride in adipose tissue is hydrolyzed to release fatty acids. Bound to albumin in the blood, the released fatty acids are rapidly removed by the hepatocyte and transported into the mitochondria by a carnitine-mediated process. Within the mitochondria, a number of enzymes degrade the fatty acid molecule to acetyl CoA fragments, a sequence known as β oxidation. In turn, acetyl CoA can enter the citric acid cycle and generate adenosine triphosphate (ATP) by oxidative phosphorylation. Triglyceride synthesis occurs when carbohydrate intake exceeds energy requirements; under such conditions, glucose may overwhelm the glycogen reservoir, and the acetyl CoA generated by glycolysis is not needed for oxidative phosphorylation. During such times of nutrient abundance, the energy charge inherent in acetyl CoA is conserved by its conversion to fatty acids and, ultimately, triglycerides. Synthesis of fatty acids involves repetitive additions of two carbon fragments (derived from acetyl CoA) to malonyl CoA. After reaction with α-glycerophosphate, the resulting triglycerides are transported to the adipose tissues as part of lipoproteins, specifically, the very low-density lipoproteins (VLDL).

Proteins. The liver plays a central role in the synthesis and degradation of protein. As such, it contains the enzymes necessary for the transamination and oxidative deamination of amino acids as well as the enzymes required for urea synthesis. As noted previously, amino acids can also participate in gluconeogenesis. Gluconeogenesis proceeds after conversion of deaminated amino acids to pyruvate or intermediates of the citric acid cycle. Plasma proteins including albumin, coagulation factors, transferrin, and ceruloplasmin constitute about one-half of the protein synthesized in the liver. Like pancreatic proteins (see later), these export proteins are synthesized on the rough endoplasmic reticulum and pass through intracellular pathways. Protein synthesis by the liver is influenced by the nutritional state as well as by hormones. Insulin, glucagon, and glucocorticoids are particularly relevant in this respect. Insulin and steroids stimulate the synthesis of hepatic proteins, whereas glucagon inhibits synthesis and promotes their degradation.

PANCREAS

COMPONENTS OF PANCREATIC JUICE

Three types of cells (centroacinar, ductular, and acinar) within the pancreas elaborate a juice rich in bicarbonate and enzyme proteins. Within centroacinar cells and ductular cells, carbonic anhydrase mediates production of bicarbonate. Bicarbonate in the pancreatic juice serves two functions: it neutralizes gastric acid delivered to the duodenum and, by maintaining the duodenal pH in the neutral to slightly basic range, permits optimal activity of digestive enzymes. Acinar cells secrete the latter in both active forms (e.g., lipase and amylase) and inactive forms (e.g., trypsinogen and chymotrypsinogen). These enzymes are synthesized on the ribosomes of the rough endoplasmic reticulum, penetrate into the cisternal space, and appear to remain largely segregated until stimulation results in their discharge from the cell (exocytosis). The latter process involves fusion of zymogen granules with the cell membrane. However, insofar as some degree of enzyme secretion persists even in the absence of zymogen granules, it has been suggested that enzymes may also traverse the cytosol without being membrane-bound.[6]

The quantitative significance of this transcytosolic pathway remains uncertain.

PANCREATIC SECRETAGOGUES

A number of hormones are known to modulate pancreatic secretion. Of these, secretin, vasoactive intestinal polypeptide (VIP), cholecystokinin (CCK), and gastrin are excitatory, whereas pancreatic polypeptide is inhibitory. Other hormones including peptide YY, somatostatin, and glucagon are suspected of having inhibitory effects but their physiologic relevance has been questioned. Secretin (and its structural analogue, VIP) stimulate water and bicarbonate secretion whereas cholecystokinin (and its structural analogue gastrin) increases the protein content of the juice. As mentioned above, pancreatic polypeptide has inhibitory effects on pancreatic secretion. The release of this as well as other inhibitory hormones may signal the pancreas to cease secretion after digestion is complete.[7,8]

PANCREATIC STIMULUS-SECRETION COUPLING

Two classes of hormone receptors have been found on acinar cells. These receptors are believed to link hormones to the intracellular events resulting in secretion (stimulus-secretion coupling). Separate classes of receptors have been identified for secretin (and its analogues) and for CCK (acetylcholine and bombesin also share this receptor class).[9] Receptors for CCK are further differentiated by their affinity (high versus low) for the hormone, the high affinity receptors most likely mediating the secretory response.[10] Regardless of the receptor involved, hormonal effects are mediated by the activation of protein kinases and the subsequent phosphorylation of regulatory proteins. However, the intermediary steps are different for the two classes of hormone receptors. Hormones that interact with secretin receptors result in the activation of intracellular adenylcyclase. The second messenger for these receptors is, therefore, cyclic adenosine monophosphate (cAMP). A different series of reactions takes place when CCK receptors are occupied. These receptors activate membrane-bound phospholipase C. The breakdown of phosphatidyl-inositol generates inositol triphosphate (IP_3), increased levels of which trigger the release of calcium from intracellular stores. Calmodulin, in turn, mediates the effects of intracellular calcium on protein kinases. Thus, activation of protein kinases is the final common pathway of both classes of receptors. This may explain why one stimulatory hormone can augment the actions of other hormonal stimuli.[11] For example, when secretin and CCK are administered together, the pancreatic response to the combination is greater than the sum of the individual responses.

Pancreatic secretion is also altered by neural mechanisms. It has been known for many years that vagal stimulation or administration of cholinergic agents increase the protein content of pancreatic juice. More recently, increased bicarbonate secretion after vagal stimulation has been ascribed to the release of VIP from intrapancreatic nerves.[12] Although it has long been established that cholinergic pathways play a role in the cephalic phase of pancreatic stimulation, recent work indicates that these pathways also mediate the intestinal phase of pancreatic stimulation (see later in the chapter).

CONTROL OF PANCREATIC SECRETION

Pancreatic stimulation has been divided into four components: basal, cephalic, gastric, and intestinal.[13] *Basal secretion* of the pancreas has been shown to be synchronized to the migrating myoelectric complex (MMC), and is maximal during phase III.[14] The coordination of the MMC and pancreatic secretion can be disrupted by atropine. The *cephalic phase* is initiated with the sight or smell of food. Like basal secretion, the pancreatic response to cephalic stimuli can be blocked by anticholinergic agents. The stomach (*gastric phase*) influences pancreatic secretion by a number of routes. Food in the gastric antrum induces pancreatic secretion by distension and gastrin release. Distension of the antrum is the afferent limb of a reflex that increases pancreatic secretion, while gastrin is a weak CCK-like secretagogue. Indirectly, the stomach may also alter pancreatic secretion by its production of acid and its partial breakdown of dietary protein and lipid. The *intestinal phase* of pancreatic stimulation results from the exposure of the proximal small bowel to hydrogen ions, fatty acids, and amino acids. In this scheme, hydrogen releases secretin from the gastrointestinal mucosa, while fatty acids and amino acids trigger release of CCK. Numerous in vivo perfusion experiments support this concept. However, studies on the effect of feeding per se on secretagogue levels have been less convincing in this respect. This is especially true for serum levels of secretin after a meal where, in contrast to acid perfusion experiments, increases are barely demonstrable and are transient.[15,16] The difference in secretin response to duodenal acid perfusion and feeding may involve the intensity and duration of acid exposure. Unlike direct instillation of acid, the postcibal decline in duodenal pH is minimal after a test meal. It has not yet been firmly established that small, short-lived spikes in secretin levels are physiologically relevant. However, it remains possible that small increases in secretin release may be significant, especially inasmuch as augmentation by other hormonal stimuli has been shown to occur (see earlier in the chapter). Pancreatic secretion per se, in part, may also modulate the release of secretagogues from the proximal small bowel. Data derived from a number of species indicates that trypsin inhibits release of CCK from the gut and that CCK release can be augmented by diversion or inhibition of trypsin.[17,18] In humans, the role of pancreatic trypsin in the control of CCK release has been questioned. Despite low levels of trypsin output, plasma levels of CCK are not consistently increased in patients with chronic pancreatic insufficiency,[19–21] nor are they decreased when the duodenum of normal volunteers is perfused with pure trypsin or pancreatic extract.[22]

PANCREAS IN NORMAL DIGESTION

Pancreatic enzymes are essential for the optimal digestion of dietary carbohydrate, lipid, and protein. The enzymes involved in breakdown of these nutrients include amylase, lipase, and trypsin, respectively. *Amylase* cleaves 1,4 linkages within straight chain polysaccharides to yield maltose and maltotetrose. Because 1,6 linkages are immune to amylolytic breakdown, branched-chain polysaccharides give rise to dextrins as well as maltose and maltotetrose. *Lipase* hydrolyzes triglycerides to fatty acids and monoglycerides at water-oil interfaces. By increasing the total surface area of this interface, bile salts improve the efficiency of this process. However, as previously pointed out, bile salts also inhibit lipase activity. This inhibition is reversed by colipase, another constituent of pancreatic juice. Phospholipases are also present in pancreatic secretion. In particular, phospholipase A_2 promotes the breakdown of phospholipids. *Trypsin* and a variety of other enzymes (chymotrypsin, elastase) reduce proteins into smaller oligopeptides and amino acids by cleaving bonds in the midportion of the peptide chain. Trypsin hydrolyzes peptide bonds in the vicinity of lysine or arginine, whereas chymotrypsin has specificity for bonds in the vicinity of aromatic residues (e.g., phenylalanine, tyrosine, and tryptophan). Another group of enzymes, the carboxypeptidases, breaks the first or last bond in the peptide chain. All these enzymes are secreted in large excess; therefore, pancreatic damage must be extensive before maldigestion becomes clinically apparent. However, when these nutritional complications do arise, their timely recognition can lead to effective therapeutic interventions.

NUTRITIONAL CONSEQUENCES OF LIVER AND PANCREATIC INJURY

LIVER

ACUTE LIVER INJURY

Regardless of cause, acute liver injury is often associated with anorexia, nausea, and vomiting. When the liver injury is due to alcohol, these symptoms may be exacerbated by concomitant alcoholic gastritis. Thus, acute liver injury is likely to decrease the oral intake of food but, if the illness is short-lived and self-limited, nutritional consequences are minimal. Both alcoholic and nonalcoholic acute liver injury may cause fasting hypoglycemia. This has been attributed to depleted liver glycogen reserves and a block in gluconeogenesis from amino acids.

CHRONIC LIVER INJURY

Nutritional complications are frequent when liver function becomes impaired in chronic liver injury, particularly cirrhosis. Regardless of cause, cirrhosis is likely to cause patients to have abnormal anthropometric measurements (i.e., muscle wasting) and to be anergic to common antigens on skin testing.[23] Circulating levels of both fat- and water-soluble vitamins are low in a high percentage of patients with alcoholic cirrhosis. Low serum levels of fat-soluble vitamins (rather than the water-soluble variety) are more characteristic of nonalcoholic cirrhosis.[24] These nutritional deficiencies arise as a result of one or more of the following factors: inadequate dietary intake, maldigestion, malabsorption, and defective metabolism. All these factors may converge, as exemplified by the decrease in hepatic total phospholipids and phosphatidylcholine after chronic alcohol consumption.[25] This may result not only from reduced dietary intake but also from maldigestion, malabsorption as well as some specific enzyme deficiencies; i.e., decreased activity of phosphatidylethanolamine methyltransferase.[26] Phospholipids play a key role, especially as the backbone of membranes, which are strikingly altered after chronic alcohol consumption.[27] Functional abnormalities include decreased cytochrome oxidase activity in hepatic mitochondria and their correction by phospholipids in vitro.[28] Supplementation with polyenylphospholipids in vivo results in striking protection against alcohol-induced fibrosis and cirrhosis in the baboon (Fig. 63–1),[25] possibly because of the correction of the abovementioned abnormalities and/or promotion of collagen breakdown by stimulation of collagenase activity.[25]

Dietary Intake. Inadequate intake of protein is common, especially among alcoholics with cirrhosis. Indeed, if the alcoholic patient continues to drink despite cirrhosis, protein intake may be low. Changes in mental status that result from hepatic encephalopathy may also contribute to the poor intake of patients with advanced liver disease. Hepatic coma, in turn, is likely to result in hospitalization, which may itself exacerbate nutritional deficiencies in these patients. Malnutrition in hospitalized patients arises as a result of both diagnostic (radiologic or endoscopic procedures) and therapeutic (e.g., variceal sclerotherapy) interventions.

Maldigestion and Malabsorption. Decreases in bile salt secretion and pool size have been demonstrated in patients with cirrhosis.[29] In light of the role of bile salts in fat digestion (see "Bile Salts" earlier) a contraction of the bile salt pool would be expected to impair micelle formation and lead to abnormalities of fat assimilation, especially in patients with underlying pancreatic insufficiency. Steatorrhea, in turn, causes deficiencies in fat-soluble vitamins with clinical manifestations such as night blindness, osteoporosis, and easy bruisability or hemorrhage.

Metabolic Changes. A number of defects in protein metabolism have been noted in patients with chronic liver failure. These include decreased hepatic synthesis of export proteins (albumin, coagulation factors), decreased urea synthesis,[30] and decreased metabolism of aromatic amino acids. The effect of advanced liver disease on protein catabolism is controversial. Using

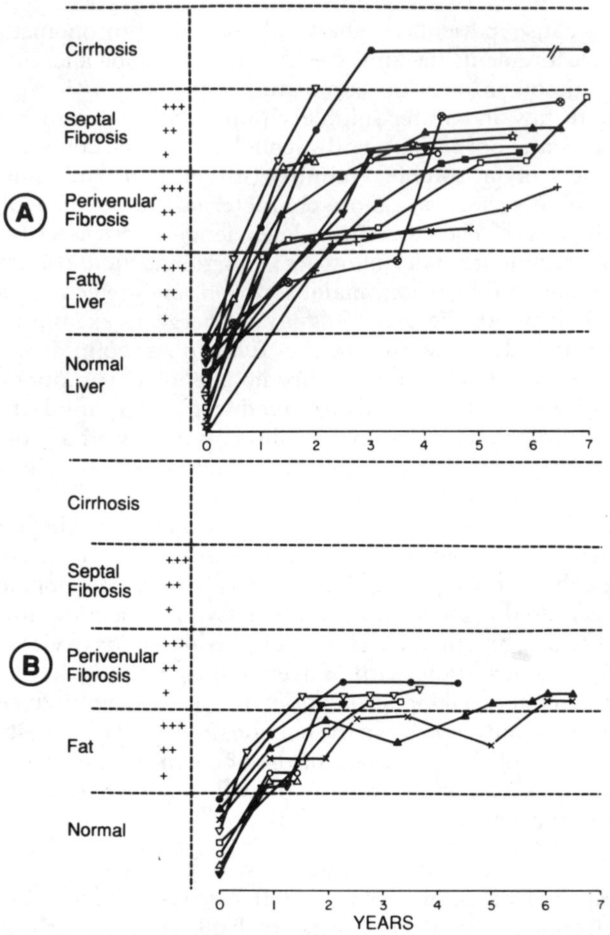

FIGURE 63–1. Sequential development of alcoholic liver injury in baboons fed ethanol with a normal diet (A) or the same diet supplemented with polyenylphosphatidylcholine (B), resulting in striking prevention of septal fibrosis and cirrhosis. (Modified from Lieber, C.S., et al., Gastroenterology *106:* 152–159, 1994.)

stable isotopes such as ^{13}C leucine, turnover studies indicate that protein degradation is normal in fasted cirrhotics.[31] However, after feeding, protein flux appears to be increased.[32] These alterations have important clinical consequences. Decreased synthesis of plasma proteins may lead to hypoalbuminemia and exacerbate the formation of ascites in patients with portal hypertension. Depressed levels of coagulation factors may predispose these patients to the risk of gastrointestinal (GI) hemorrhage. The failure to detoxify ammonia and the abnormal amino acid profile of patients with cirrhosis may, in part, increase the likelihood of hepatic encephalopathy. Despite these abnormalities in intermediary metabolism, overall nitrogen balance can be maintained at positive levels by amounts of dietary protein similar to the amount in the noncirrhotic individual (35 to 50 g per day).[33]

Glucose tolerance is frequently abnormal in the cirrhotic patient and has been linked to insulin resistance. The high fasting and postprandial insulin levels in these patients may relate to factors such as portosystemic shunting, increased levels of growth hormone, and depleted body stores of potassium.[34,35] Also, because glycogen stores are often depleted in the cirrhotic liver, fatty acid oxidation appears to supplant glucose as a source of fuel during fasting.[31,35–38] This is apparent when indirect calorimetry is performed, because stable cirrhotics have a respiratory quotient (RQ) significantly less than that of normal controls. Energy expenditure in chronic liver injury is comparable to that in controls,[36,37,39] making hypermetabolism per se an unlikely explanation for weight loss in these patients. A number of investigators have reported higher- than-predicted energy production rates in cirrhotic patients but have found this only when energy expenditure was related to urinary creatinine excretion.[38,40] However, as pointed out by Merli et al.[37] and Heymsfield et al.,[41] the use of urinary creatinine excretion as a measure of active cell mass is invalid in patients with cirrhosis because the hepatic production of creatine is depressed. Isotopic methods involving labeled water and potassium have been recommended for estimating the metabolically active body cell mass in patients with decompensated cirrhosis.[41]

Abnormalities of water- and fat-soluble vitamins are common in patients with cirrhosis. In the nonalcoholic with cirrhosis, deficiencies of fat-soluble vitamins are likely to arise from malabsorption. In part, abnormal bile salt metabolism and defective micelle formation limit the uptake of such vitamins in these patients. In the alcoholic, inadequate intake of vitamins, especially those that are water-soluble (thiamin and folic acid), is an important factor.

In addition to inadequate intake and decreased uptake, vitamin metabolism per se may be deranged in chronic liver injury. Defects have been described in the phosphorylation of thiamine by alcoholic cirrhotics,[42] in the synthesis of retinol-binding protein,[43] in the degradation of pyridoxal-5′-phosphate,[44] and in the conversion of vitamin D to its active form.[45] Hepatic vitamin A levels are depressed by both heavy alcohol consumption and drug use.[46,47] It is conceivable that part of the hepatic depletion may be due to mobilization inasmuch as hepatic lipoprotein secretion is increased by chronic alcohol consumption.[48] It is also possible that "induced" hepatic microsomes may enhance the degradation of both retinol and retinoic acid.[49–51] As a result of these derangements, vitamin repletion strategies require modification in patients with liver failure, as discussed later in this chapter.

PANCREAS

ACUTE INJURY

Acute pancreatitis is characterized by severe epigastric pain that radiates to the back. This is often accompanied by nausea and vomiting. A history of biliary tract disease can be elicited in many patients; other predisposing factors include medications (furosemide, 6-mercaptopurine, AZT), hyperlipidemia, hypercalcemia, abdominal operations, and certain viral infections (mumps, coxsackie, HIV). Fever, rebound tenderness, abdominal guarding, and decreased bowel sounds are typical features on physical examination. Severe cases are complicated by hypotension, oliguria, and dyspnea. Laboratory evaluation will usually reveal elevations of the serum amylase or lipase level. Additional findings may include leukocytosis, hyperglycemia, azotemia, and hypocalcemia. Additional assessment should include a flat plate of the abdomen and ultrasonic examination of the liver and pancreas. The initial approach to these patients should include vigorous fluid resuscitation, elimination of oral feeding, and analgesia. The majority of patients will recover quickly and uneventfully with this approach.

When pseudocysts, abscesses, or fistulas develop, a protracted course should be anticipated; it is in this setting that nutritional complications are most likely to arise. Patients with severe acute pancreatitis demonstrate increased rates of protein catabolism and negative nitrogen balances. The released amino acids are utilized for gluconeogenesis. However, unlike the situation in normal individuals, gluconeogenesis in the setting of pancreatitis is not completely suppressed by an intravenous infusion of glucose.[52]

Hypermetabolism is a consistent finding in patients with acute pancreatitis,[53,54] with measured energy expenditure ranging up to 14% above that predicted. In very ill patients, this phenomenon may be even more pronounced. Energy expenditure and other metabolic parameters were assessed by indirect calorimetry in mechanically ventilated patients with acute pancreatitis in one study.[55] Energy expenditure was 49% greater than predicted, much of the energy being derived from gluconeogenesis. These patients experienced negative nitrogen balance and exhibited a disparity between the amount of glucose administered and the glucose oxidation rate. This nutritional pattern is not specific for acute pancreatitis. Similar metabolic changes have been observed in septic patients and those with extensive burns.[56]

CHRONIC INJURY

In contrast to acute pancreatitis, chronic pancreatitis usually evolves insidiously over many years, and its likelihood of occurrence is strongly correlated with alcohol consumption. The disorder is characterized by recurrent attacks of abdominal pain and the development of pancreatic calcification and insufficiency (Fig. 63–2). Thus, the nutritional status of the patient with chronic pancreatitis is in jeopardy from two standpoints. During painful exacerbations, oral intake is limited either spontaneously by the patient or as part of a therapeutic regimen. Between flareups, absorption of foodstuffs may be marginal to the extent that synthesis and delivery of digestive enzymes is inadequate. Malabsorption of fat (steatorrhea) is clinically apparent because it produces diarrhea and causes the stool to become greasy and foul smelling. In contrast, poor absorption of protein (azotorrhea) and of carbohydrate are less obvious and less likely. There are several reasons for this difference: (1) The output of proteolytic enzymes persists longer than that of the lipolytic enzymes,[57] and (2) carbohydrate breakdown may proceed under the influence of extrapancreatic amylases (derived from the salivary glands, stomach, and duodenum).[58]

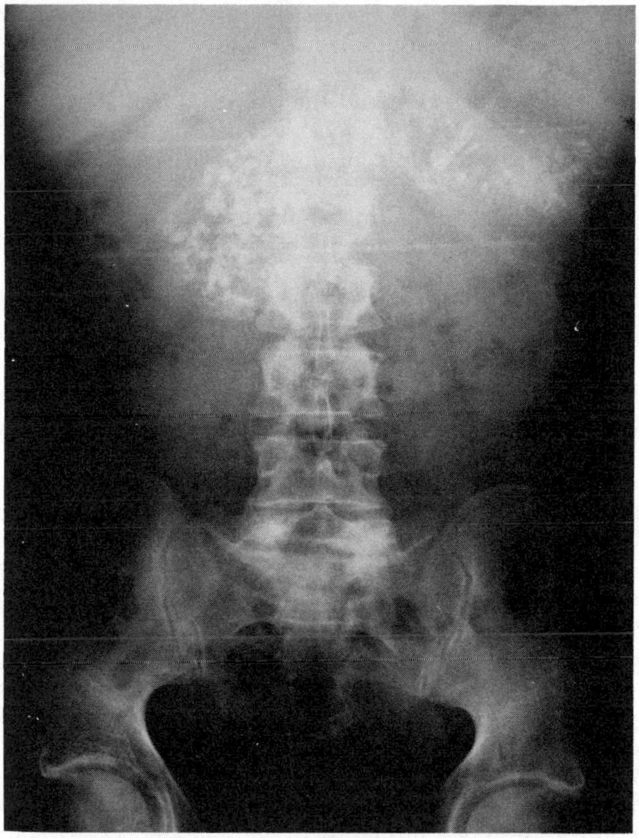

FIGURE 63–2. Plain radiograph of the abdomen in a patient with diabetes mellitus secondary to chronic pancreatitis. As a result of parenchymal calcification, the shape of the pancreas can be completely visualized. It extends from right of the midline (the head) to the left upper quadrant (body and tail).

The most apparent effect of pancreatic insufficiency is weight loss. This is a reflection of depleted fat stores and, later, muscle mass as well. Deficiencies of fat-soluble vitamins (A, D, and K) and minerals have also been identified in these patients. However, although deficiencies of fat-soluble vitamins are common in the course of pancreatic insufficiency, their occurrence may be clinically inapparent except under close scrutiny.

NUTRITIONAL THERAPY IN LIVER AND PANCREATIC DISORDERS

LIVER

PROTEIN AND AMINO ACIDS

To the extent that patients with liver injury, either acute or chronic, are in negative nitrogen balance, it has been assumed that liver regeneration will be delayed and that muscle wasting will be accelerated. However, when feeding protein or administering amino acids, one must be aware of the precarious balance between the need to restore protein intake and the potential risk of precipitating hepatic encephalopathy. There is often only a small margin of safety in this respect. The amount of dietary protein that can be tolerated will vary considerably. At times, only minimal amounts of protein can be ingested without altering the mental state. Under such circumstances, the breakdown of remaining protein stores can be minimized by the provision of calories in the form of fats and carbohydrates.

In acute liver injury, much work has focused on the role of protein or amino acid supplementation on the outcome of alcoholic hepatitis. Both enteral and parenteral routes have been employed in these investigations. In general, studies in patients with acute hepatitis have demonstrated that hepatic encephalopathy can usually be avoided by judicious titration of dietary protein, that relatively little dietary protein can be associated with positive nitrogen balance, and that symptomatic as well as biochemical improvement (if not prognosis) can be expected.[59–65]

Positive nitrogen balance can be attained in patients with chronic liver injury (cirrhosis) with daily amounts of dietary protein (0.74 g/kg) similar to that required by normal individuals.[33] Conflicting results have been obtained regarding the extent to which the source of the dietary protein (animal or vegetable) effects overall nitrogen balance.[66,67]

Attempts have been made to normalize the plasma amino acid pattern found in patients with cirrhosis. The ratio of branched-chain amino acids, or BCAA (isoleucine, leucine, valine, and lysine), to aromatic amino acids (phenylalanine, tryptophan, and tyrosine) is abnormally low in these patients, especially those who are malnourished. However, compared to standard mixtures of amino acids, administration of branched-chain-enriched amino acids has shown no significant advantage in terms of nitrogen balance.[68–71]

There was hope that correction of the abnormal amino acid profile in patients with cirrhosis would be beneficial in the treatment of hepatic encephalopathy. To this end, mixtures with high ratios of branched-chain amino acids (BCAA) to aromatic amino acids have been administered, and the source of protein (vegetable-derived protein is relatively lacking in aromatic amino acids) has been varied. A potential benefit seemed plausible in light of the false neurotransmitter hypothesis of Fischer and colleagues.[72] In this scheme, the entry of aromatic amino acids into the brain is favored by low plasma levels of BCAA. In the brain, sympathomimetic amines are generated from these aromatic amino acids, especially phenylalanine, the presence of which hinders neuronal transmission by competitive interactions with bona fide neurotransmitters at the receptor level. Initial studies in humans involving infusion of BCAA-enriched mixtures were encouraging, but these early clinical trials were not fully controlled or randomized.[73] Using tighter designs, a majority of subsequent studies have failed to confirm the efficacy of intravenous or orally administered branched-chain-enriched mixtures in treating acute hepatic encephalopathy.[23] Despite a recent meta-analysis that detected a trend favoring this therapy,[74] the evidence does not support the routine clinical use of these amino acid mixtures in acute encephalopathy.[75] However, it remains possible that a subset of protein-intolerant patients with chronic encephalopathy (and better liver function) might benefit from BCAA.[76]

Some success has been achieved in treating hepatic encephalopathy using protein derived from vegetable sources.[66,77] However, improvement in encephalopathy does not correlate with changes in the plasma amino acid profile. As a result, it has been suggested that the beneficial effects of vegetable protein are mediated by its fiber content rather than by its amino acid composition per se.[78] Fiber may increase the elimination of nitrogenous waste, but the high fiber content of these diets is poorly tolerated.

Dietary restrictions of amino acids or protein are important in a number of inherited liver abnormalities, including disorders of the urea cycle and hypertyrosinemia (see Chap. 67). Specifically, reduction in nitrogen intake is the cornerstone of therapy in hyperammonemia syndromes. In these disorders, the activity of urea cycle enzymes is diminished, ammonia accumulates in the blood, and central nervous system toxicity (lethargy, coma) develops. Depending on the specific location of the defect in the cycle, certain amino acids must also be supplemented. For example, in citrullinemia there is diminished conversion of citrulline to arginine as a result of a deficiency of argininosuccinic acid synthetase. Supplemental arginine bypasses this block and permits the urea cycle to proceed.[79] In hypertyrosinemia, there is a defect in the final step in the breakdown of tyrosine and phenylalanine.[80] This leads to high levels of tyrosine in the blood and urine, renal tubular dysfunction and, eventually, death from liver failure. Dietary restriction of tyrosine and phenylalanine may be helpful.[81]

CARBOHYDRATES

Cirrhotic patients are prone to develop diabetes. As already noted, insulin resistance appears to the account for this abnormality of glucose homeostasis. In patients with portal hypertension complicated by portosystemic shunting, an alteration in the metabolism of insulin may contribute to this resistance. Depleted body stores of potassium and elevated levels of growth hormone are probably additional significant factors. As in other patients with diabetes, nutritional management plays an important role in therapy. Specifically, provision of calories in the form of complex carbohydrates is effective in reducing insulin requirements. Increasing the intake of complex carbohydrate may also be advantageous in terms of hepatic encephalopathy because the nonabsorbable fiber found in such foods decreases colonic transit time and lowers colonic pH. Indeed, the efficacy of lactulose, one of the mainstays in the treatment of hepatic encephalopathy, has been related to these same effects.

Inherited disorders of hepatic carbohydrate metabolism may also benefit from dietary manipulation. This heterogeneous group of disorders, which includes galactosemia (see Chap. 67), glycogen storage disease, and fructose intolerance, can be traced to specific enzymatic deficiencies. These defects impair the orderly flow of substrates along pathways involved in anaerobic glycolysis. The accumulation of these substrates in various organs, especially the liver and muscle, results in organ injury and, frequently, hypoglycemia. Galactosemia can be successfully controlled by strict dietary exclusion of milk products containing galactose. Likewise, fruit, vegetables, and sucrose must be eliminated from the diet of children who are fructose-intolerant. At least in type I glycogen storage disease (von Gierke's disease), biochemical improvement can be expected when hypoglycemia is prevented with frequent feedings of glucose-rich formulas.[82]

FAT (FAT-SOLUBLE VITAMINS)

Poor dietary intake together with changes in bile salt metabolism and pancreatic function increase the likelihood of fat-soluble vitamin deficiency in patients with both alcoholic and nonalcoholic cirrhosis.

Vitamin A. It is recommended that the diet of the nonalcoholic with cirrhosis be supplemented with 5000 to 15,000 IU vitamin A. In patients with alcoholic cirrhosis, caution must be exercised in this respect because microsomal induction may increase the toxicity of this vitamin (Fig. 63–3).[83,84]

Vitamin D. Supplementation of the diet with this vitamin may fail to halt the progression of osteoporosis and osteopenia. However, there appears to be no hazard in recommending ingestion of additional 25-OH D_3 (100 to 300 nmol (40 to 120 μg per day)) when patients complain of bone pain or demonstrate pathologic fractures.[85]

Vitamin E. In children with biliary atresia and cholestasis, vitamin E deficiency may be associated with a number of neurologic alterations. Although such infants and children may benefit from supplementation, repletion of vitamin E stores in adults with liver injury is of no proven clinical efficacy.

Vitamin K. Deficiency of this vitamin leads to easy bruisability and, at times, to overt bleeding from esophageal varices or hemorrhoids. When the prothrombin time is lengthened, parenteral supplementation of vitamin K (10 mg per day for 3 days) will serve to discriminate between vitamin K deficiency and failure of the liver to synthesize normal coagulation factors. After vitamin K, an abnormal prothrombin time will be corrected in the former setting but not in the latter.

WATER-SOLUBLE VITAMINS AND TRACE MINERALS

Deficiencies of water-soluble vitamins (folic acid, thiamine, and pyridoxine) are most likely to occur in the malnourished alcoholic with advanced liver injury. In patients with Wilson's disease or those with chronic cholestasis (e.g., primary biliary cirrhosis), there is excessive copper accumulation in the liver.[86,87] Although chelation of copper by penicillamine is highly effective, it is also advantageous to reduce the intake of foods rich in this mineral. Foods rich in copper include chocolate, shellfish, and liver. Zinc deficiency occurs in alcoholics with liver injury and is discussed in Chapter 10.

PANCREAS

ACUTE PANCREATITIS

As noted previously (see "Acute Injury" under "Pancreas"), patients with acute pancreatitis are in a hypermetabolic, hypercatabolic state. In this setting, defective glucose oxidation can be demonstrated as can compensatory increases in gluconeogenesis and oxidation of BCAA by muscles. Malnutrition is common in patients with a protracted clinical course. In one study, 80% of patients with acute pancreatitis had decreased levels of albumin and transferrin and decreased numbers of lymphocytes.[88] Nutritional goals in this illness are the maintenance of a positive nitrogen balance, a reduction in the degree of pancreatic stimulation and, ultimately, an improvement in the prognosis. Enteral and parenteral infusates have been formulated to meet these goals. Regardless of the route, basal energy requirements must be met and the proportion of amino acids, carbohydrate, and fat must be adjusted for the severity of the illness. Energy requirements can be calculated in relationship to the weight, height, and age of the patient using the Harris-Benedict equation.[89] In life-threatening cases of acute pancreatitis, fats and amino acids are increased (at the expense of carbohydrates). This adjustment serves a number of purposes. Severely ill patients may lose, at times, more than 1071 mmol (15 g) per day) of nitrogen in the urine. By increasing the overall percentage of amino acids (as well as the relative amounts of BCAA) in the enteral and parenteral formulas, visceral protein breakdown may be prevented and the lean body mass repleted. Finally, a reduction of carbohydrate calories has been useful in patients with respiratory distress. The oxidation of carbohydrates generally proceeds with a higher RQ (ratio of CO_2 produced to O_2 consumed) than that of lipids. Therefore, by replacing carbohydrates with fat in the administered formulas, one strives to reduce the amount of CO_2 produced by oxidative pathways and to lessen the likelihood of CO_2 retention.

Enteral Feeding in Acute Pancreatitis. As already reviewed under "Control of Pancreatic Secretion," certain pancreatic secretagogues are released from the gas-

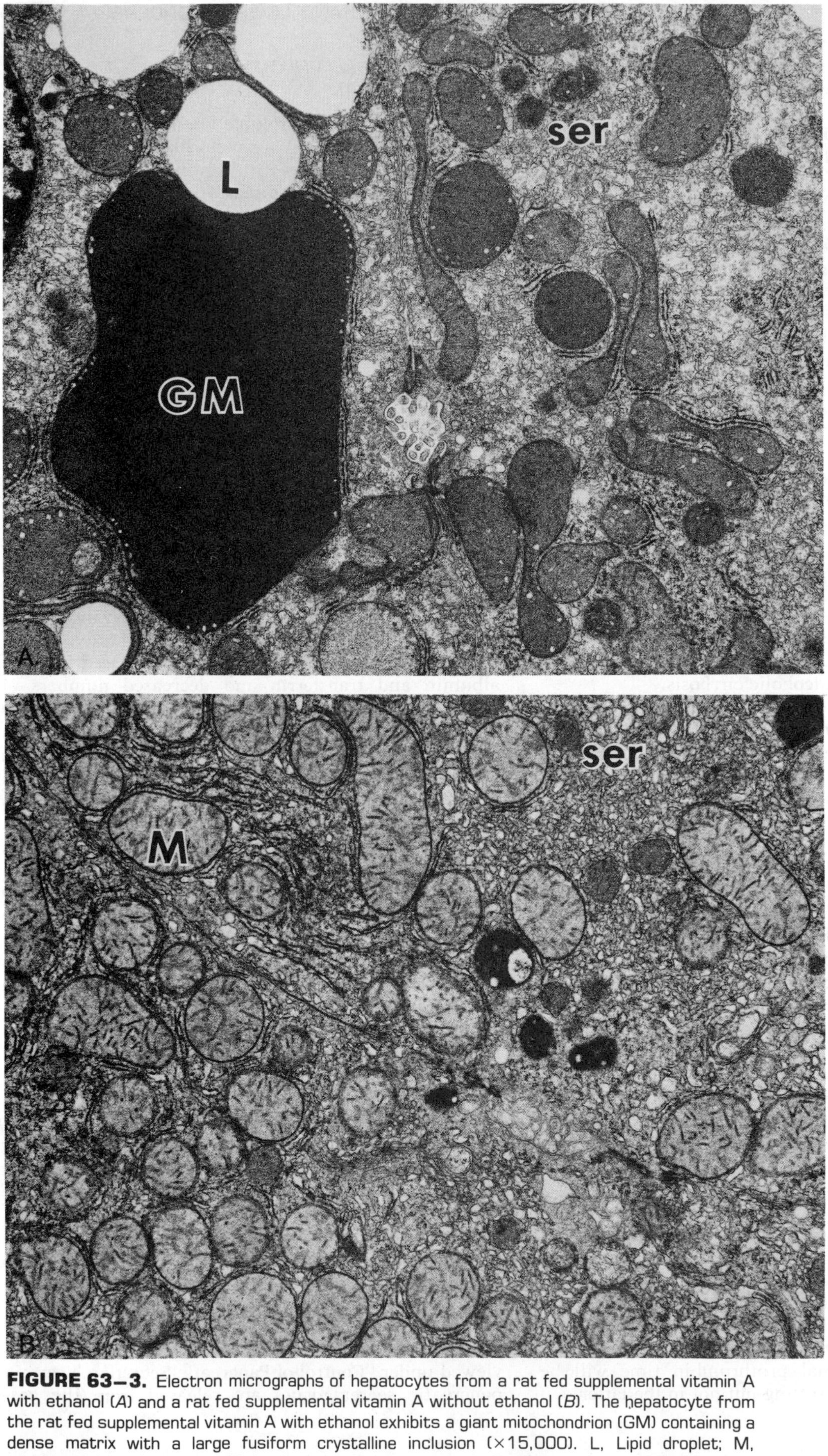

FIGURE 63–3. Electron micrographs of hepatocytes from a rat fed supplemental vitamin A with ethanol (*A*) and a rat fed supplemental vitamin A without ethanol (*B*). The hepatocyte from the rat fed supplemental vitamin A with ethanol exhibits a giant mitochondrion (GM) containing a dense matrix with a large fusiform crystalline inclusion (×15,000). L, Lipid droplet; M, mitochondrion. (From Leo, M.A., Arai, M., Sato, M. et al.: Gastroenterology, *82:*194–205, 1982.)

trointestinal mucosa upon exposure to nutrients (fatty acids and amino acids) and hydrogen chloride. A gradient exists within the small bowel in terms of the content and release of these hormones. Because secretagogue content is greater in the proximal small bowel (duodenum) than in the distal portions (jejunum and ileum), it is not surprising that the pancreatic response to enteral feeding will depend on the mode of its administration. At least in dogs, the greatest response was observed after oral feeding; an *equivalent* nutrient load infused into the jejunum produced the least exocrine output.[90,91] In humans, jejunal feeding of elemental diets offers an effective alternative to parenteral alimentation because there is minimal pancreatic stimulation when using low-fat formulations. However, this approach is only feasible when intestinal motility and absorptive surfaces remain intact. Unfortunately, this is not always the case in acute pancreatitis. Small bowel motility may be impaired in patients with acute pancreatitis for various reasons. The classic finding of a "sentinel loop" on plain films of the abdomen in close proximity to the pancreas indicates a nonmechanical obstruction of a portion of small bowel. More generalized distension of small bowel loops with multiple air-fluid levels may imply metabolic derangements such as hypokalemia. Differential air-fluid levels may suggest a mechanical obstruction as by an abscess or enlarging pseudocyst. In the presence of any of these complications, jejunal feeding is contraindicated because of the increased likelihood of aspiration.

Enteral feeding of elemental diets can achieve positive nitrogen balance in patients with acute pancreatitis.[92] However, it has yet to be demonstrated that enteral feeding has a favorable influence on prognosis. Patients who are well enough to tolerate enteral feeding are already likely to make a full recovery. Therefore, additional improvement in outcome as a result of nutritional support may be difficult to detect.

Parenteral Feeding in Acute Pancreatitis. Parenteral nutrition has been variously reported to increase,[93] decrease,[94] or have no effects[95–97] on pancreatic secretion in normal humans and laboratory animals. Despite these variable results, nutritional support (either lipid- or glucose-based) of patients with acute pancreatitis has generally been found to be safe and capable of sustaining positive nitrogen balance.

Certain issues arise regarding the caloric substrate in these patients. A significant percentage of patients with severe pancreatitis (27%) will not tolerate a glucose-based parenteral formula despite coverage with large amounts of insulin.[88] It has been recommended that individuals requiring more than 80 units per day of insulin receive lipid-based nutritional support. However, caution should be exercised when administering intravenous lipid to patients in whom acute pancreatitis is associated with hyperlipidemia. When hyperlipidemia is thought to be the cause of the pancreatitis, intravenous lipid should be used sparingly. Glucose, instead, should provide the bulk of calories in this setting. When there is uncertainty about the cause and effect relationship between pancreatitis and hyperlipidemia, a test dose of lipid in conjunction with frequent monitoring of the serum triglyceride level has been advocated.[98]

Although parenteral nutrition has positive effects on nitrogen balance, controlled studies in patients with acute pancreatitis receiving this form of support have not documented improved survival.[99] Others have argued that total parenteral nutrition (TPN) is useful in more severe forms of pancreatitis (Ranson scores greater than 2): in one such group of seriously ill patients, mortality was highest (21%) when nitrogen balance remained negative despite parenteral nutrition.[88] An alternative interpretation of this data is that nitrogen balance becomes worse as the severity of the underlying pancreatitis increases. These patients would also be expected to have the poorest prognosis with or without TPN. In any case, catheter-related sepsis is a hazard of parenteral alimentation. This potential complication must be balanced against the theoretical benefits of TPN on nutritional status.

CHRONIC PANCREATITIS

Abdominal pain, malabsorption, and diabetes mellitus are complications of chronic pancreatitis that affect nutritional status. In turn, the management of these complications often rests on nutritional manipulations.

Pain Relief. Abdominal pain in chronic pancreatitis is often intractable and debilitating. The cause of this pain remains unclear but has been related to increased intraductal and tissue pressure, parapancreatic neural irritation, and, most recently, pancreatic ischemia.[100] Food may be avoided to the extent that pain is precipitated by eating. This will lead to nutritional deficits even in the absence of malabsorption. Whenever possible, it is preferable to use non-narcotic analgesic medications (aspirin, acetaminophen, or nonsteroidal anti-inflammatory agents) for pain relief to minimize the likelihood of narcotic dependency. If such simple measures are ineffective, a therapeutic trial of pancreatic enzymes has been advocated. The use of pancreatic extracts is based on the assumption that proteolytic enzymes inhibit pancreatic secretion by negative feedback control of CCK release from the duodenum (see "Control of Pancreatic Secretion"). Although controlled studies related to the efficacy of enzyme preparations for treatment of abdominal pain have yielded mixed results,[101–103] subsets of patients more likely to respond have been identified. These include the alcoholic with mild pancreatic insufficiency and the female with idiopathic (nonalcoholic) chronic pancreatitis. Dietary reduction of fat may be beneficial in some patients, perhaps in part by decreasing CCK release from the duodenum. Apart from minimizing pancreatic stimulation, a low-fat diet may also reduce the degree of steatorrhea in maldigesting patients. However, unless nonfat calories are proportionally increased, restricting fat intake may exacerbate caloric deficits and, possibly, weight loss.

Percutaneous block of the celiac axis provides transient relief (usually less than 6 months) of abdominal pain with low morbidity. In patients who are not surgical candidates or who refuse surgical options, long-term control of abdominal pain can be achieved by this approach. In the alcoholic patient who remains abstinent, repetitive celiac block can forestall and, in some instances, preclude the need for surgery.[104,105] Surgery has traditionally been directed toward the decompression of the pancreatic duct with the rationale that increased pressure within the duct gives rise to abdominal pain. The duct is decompressed by anastomosing it to the jejunum in a variety of configurations. These operations effectively relieve pain in the majority (80%) of patients. However, this does not prove the validity of the underlying assumption that pain arises from ductal hypertension. When critically assessed, it has become apparent that pain relief after surgery does not correlate with patency of the decompressive anastomosis. In some cases, pain was absent despite endoscopic evidence of anastomotic closure; in other instances, pain persisted despite evidence that the anastomosis was open.[106] Endoscopic management of pancreatic pain is being assessed. Sporadic reports of endoscopic occlusion of the pancreatic duct,[107] endoscopic lithotomy,[108,109] and stent placement[110] are encouraging. However, these procedures have generally been applied to a limited number of patients in uncontrolled and nonrandomized studies.

In unusually severe cases, abdominal pain, anorexia, and weight loss may be severe enough to require administration of elemental diets by enteral or parenteral routes. In practice, however, this approach is only feasible over a short period. This approach might be applicable when preparing a severely malnourished patient for surgery.

Malabsorption. Pancreatic enzyme preparations will usually improve (but not completely correct) the steatorrhea of pancreatic insufficiency. In contrast, steatorrhea due to mucosal abnormalities (tropical sprue, gluten intolerance) will fail to respond to these extracts.

The therapeutic efficacy of pancreatic enzyme preparations depends on the efficiency with which an adequate amount of active enzyme (30,000 units in the case of lipase) can be delivered to the duodenum during the postprandial digestive period.[105] Delivery has been enhanced by measures that protect acid sensitive enzymes such as lipase from denaturation in the stomach (enteric coating, H_2 receptor antagonists), systems that allow rapid emptying of enzymes from the stomach (incorporation of enzymes into microspheres) and strategies that improve patient compliance with dosing regimens (higher potency preparations requiring fewer capsules per meal).

Steatorrhea can also be managed by modifying the fat content of the diet to include a higher percentage of medium-chain triglycerides (MCT). The latter can be absorbed directly into the portal system without lipolysis, but the hyperosmolarity of these preparations can result in cramps and diarrhea.[112]

Protein (azotorrhea) and carbohydrate malabsorption can usually be demonstrated in patients with steatorrhea but are less clinically overt. Nevertheless, azotorrhea can result in hypoalbuminemia, and carbohydrate malabsorption increases overall energy wastage. As fecal losses of protein and carbohydrate do not have the negative symptomatic consequences of excess stool fat, increasing the intake of dietary protein and carbohydrate is useful in terms of increasing absorption and is well tolerated. Given these considerations, a diet high in protein (2 g/kg per day) and carbohydrate (6 g/kg per day) but low in fat (limited to 20 to 25% of calories or titrated relative to symptoms) is generally recommended in patients with pancreatic insufficiency and steatorrhea. Fat-soluble vitamins and minerals are not routinely supplemented unless overt manifestations of deficiency are present or stool fat exceeds 20 g per day.[113]

Diabetes Mellitus. Management of diabetes in patients with pancreatic insufficiency presents unique challenges given their concurrent difficulties in carbohydrate digestion. Unpredictable insulin requirements further complicate the situation. At times, even small doses of insulin may predispose patients to hypoglycemia, a phenomenon attributed to coexisting glucagon deficiency. Ideally, carbohydrate intake should be limited in these patients; if possible, oral hypoglycemics should be employed rather than insulin to minimize the risks of hypoglycemia.

EFFECTS OF NUTRITION ON THE LIVER AND PANCREAS

LIVER

At least in children, protein deficiency (kwashiorkor) is associated with the development of fatty liver.[114,115] Studies performed during and after World War II also indicated that severe malnutrition could also lead to liver injury in adults.[116] These studies did not convincingly prove that malnutrition per se caused liver injury. Indeed, a number of other factors, including hepatotoxins (e.g., aflatoxin) and parasites (schistosomiasis) prevalent in war-ravaged or underdeveloped countries may have mediated the relationship between liver injury and poor nutrition.[117]

However, because malnutrition is also common in alcoholics, these early findings were used to bolster the argument that malnutrition, rather than alcohol per se, could explain the pathogenesis of alcohol-induced liver injury. Over the past three decades, a more balanced view has evolved. Based on studies in humans, subhuman primates, and rodents, it is now established that alcohol can cause liver damage in the absence of dietary deficits. Epidemiologic data also support this revised concept. In both France and Germany, a close correlation exists between per capita alcohol consumption and the likelihood of cirrhosis.[118,119] Furthermore, although the incidence of malnutrition among alcoholics has been decreasing, the number of deaths attributable to alcoholic liver injury has been rising.[120] Lastly, no relationship has been documented between nutritional status and the severity of alcohol-induced liver injury as defined histologically.[121] The above notwithstanding, it is now becoming clear that nutrition and the toxic effects of alcohol are often intertwined at the biochemical level. For example, by inducing microsomal cytochromes, chronic ethanol consumption is known to result in energy wastage, and to promote the breakdown of nutrients including retinol.[49–51]

PANCREAS

Perhaps more than any other organ, the pancreas responds to nutritional variation by changes in its functional capacity. Animal models have shown that the level of enzymes within the pancreas varies with dietary composition.[122,123] Similar results have been reported in human infants.[124] Under more extreme conditions, as in kwashiorkor or marasmus, morphologic changes are detected in the pancreas. The pancreas shrinks and its cells atrophy, becoming fat-filled and disorganized.[125,126] Functionally, pancreatic enzyme secretion ceases and fails to respond to secretagogue stimulation.[127,128] Tropical pancreatitis has also been linked to dietary deficiencies. This disorder occurs in area of India and Africa where protein-calorie deficiency is endemic. However, the illness can arise in the absence of kwashiorkor, and is rare in some areas despite widespread protein calorie malnutrition. Furthermore, certain histologic aspects of tropical pancreatitis such as pancreatic calculi are not seen in kwashiorkor. Therefore, other factors have been implicated in the cause of tropical pancreatitis. These include a high intake of cassava (which contains cyanogenic glycosides) and zinc and selenium deficiency.[129] It is also possible that nutrition may alter the pancreatic response to a broad range of insults. Indeed, animal data support such a concept. Diets that are abundant in fats were found to increase the severity of experimental pancreatitis in dogs.[130] Additionally, rats with experimentally induced pancreatitis exhibit an increased mortality rate when fed diets enriched in both fat and protein.[131,132]

Alcoholics with pancreatitis have been studied extensively in terms of their premorbid nutritional habits. In the United States, malnourished alcoholics appear to have an increased risk of chronic pancreatitis.[133] In contrast, in France,[134,135] West Germany,[136] Italy,[137] and Mexico,[138] alcoholic pancreatitis is more closely linked to nutritional excess than to deficits. It is not clear why enriched diets should increase the risk of chronic pancreatitis. However, to the extent that such diets enhance the enzyme content of the pancreas, the potential for deleterious episodes of autodigestion may also be favored. Recent studies in the rat support the concept that the effects of ethanol on the pancreas, at least in part, are mediated by the protein content of the diet. In rats receiving standard amounts of dietary protein, long-term administration of ethanol resulted in an increased pancreatic content and release of lipase. The stimulatory effect of ethanol on these parameters was abolished when ethanol was administered in animals receiving diets deficient in protein (Fig. 63–4).[139]

In summary, the liver, the pancreas, and nutrition interact at many levels. At the most basic level, the liver and pancreas are essential for efficient digestion of ingested foodstuffs. As a result, failure of the liver or pancreas inevitably leads to defects in the uptake and assimilation of nutrients. Because dysfunction of the liver and pancreas also alters the intermediary metabolism of protein, carbohydrate, and fat, efforts directed at nutritional repletion are often stymied. Finally, to the extent that malnutrition per se alters the structural integrity of the liver and pancreas, a vicious cycle may be perpetuated wherein organ failure leads to nutritional defects and these, in turn, engender further impairment in organ function.

In conclusion, the continuing challenge in patients with disorders of the liver or pancreas is to provide nutritional support that avoids complications and improves prognosis. This chapter has summarized some of the progress made toward these twin goals.

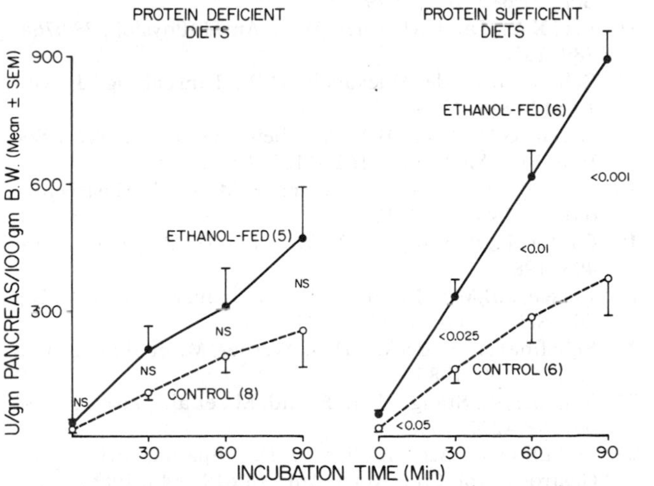

FIGURE 63–4. Combined effects of dietary protein and ethanol on cholecystoleinin (CCK)-induced lipase secretion of isolated rat pancreatic acini. Lipase units are expressed as μmol H^+ per minute. (From Korsten, M.A., Wilson, J.S., Lieber, C.S.: Gastroenterology, *99*:229–236, 1990.)

REFERENCES

1. Borgström, B., Erlanson, C.: Gastroenterology, *75:*382–386, 1978.
2. Borgström, B., Erlanson-Albertsson, C., Wielock, F.: J. Lipid Res., *20:*805–816, 1979.
3. Westergaard, H., Dietschy, J.M.: J. Clin. Invest., *58:*97–108, 1976.
4. Lock, L., Weiner, I.M.: Fed. Proc., *22:*1334–1338, 1963.
5. Carey, M.C.: The enterohepatic circulation. *In* The Liver: Biology and Pathobiology. Edited by I.M. Arias, H. Popper, D. Schacter, and D.A. Shafritz. New York, Raven Press, 1982, pp. 429–465.
6. Rothman, S.S.: Science, *190:*747–753, 1975.
7. Adrian, T.E., Besterman, H.S., Mallinson, C.N., et al.: Gut, *20:*37–40, 1979.
8. Taylor, I.L., Solomon, T.E., Walsh, J.H., et al.: Gastroenterology, *76:*524–528, 1979.
9. Gardner, J.D., Jensen, R.T.: *In* Physiology of the Gastrointestinal Tract. 2nd Ed. Vol. 2. Edited by J.R. Johnson, J. Christensen, M.J. Jackson, et al. New York, Raven Press, 1987, pp. 1109–1127.
10. Sankaran, H., Goldfine, I.D., Deveney, C.W., et al.: J. Biol. Chem., *255:*1849–1853, 1980.
11. Hootman, S.R., Williams, J.A.: Stimulus-secretion coupling in the pancreatic acinus. *In* Physiology of the Gastrointestinal Tract. 2nd Ed. Vol. 2. Edited by J.R. Johnson, J. Christensen, M.J. Jackson, et al. New York, Raven Press, 1987, pp. 1129–1146.
12. Fahrenkrug, J., Schaffalitzky de Muckadell, O.B., Holst, J., et al.: Am. J. Physiol., *237:*E535–E540, 1979.
13. Meyer, J.H.: Pancreatic physiology. *In* Gastrointestinal Disease—Pathophysiology, Diagnosis, Management. 4th Ed. Vol. 2. Edited by M.H. Sletsenger and J.S. Fordtran. Philadelphia, W.B. Saunders, 1989, pp. 1777–1788.
14. DiMagno, E.P., Hendricks, J.C., Go, V.L.W., et al.: Dig. Dis. Sci., *24:*689–693, 1979.
15. Lee, K.Y., Tai, H.H., Chey, W.Y.: Am. J. Physiol., *230:*784–789, 1976.
16. Schaffalitzky de Muckadell, O.B., Fahrenkrug, J.: Gut, *19:*812–818, 1978.
17. Green, G.H., Olds, B.A., Matthews, G., et al.: Proc. Soc. Exp. Biol. Med., *142:*1162–1167, 1973.
18. Folsch, U.R., Cantor, P., Wilms, H.M., et al.: Gastroenterology, *92:*449–458, 1987.
19. Cantor, P., Petronijevic, L., Worning, H.: Pancreas, *1:*488–493, 1986.
20. Jansen, J.B.M.J., Hopman, W.P.M., Lamers, C.B.H.W.: Dig. Dis. Sci., *24:*1109–1117, 1984.
21. Schafmayer, A., Becker, H.D., Werner, M., et al.: Digestion, *32:*136–139, 1985.
22. Mossner, J., Stange, J.H., Ewald, M., et al.: Gastroenterology, *98:*A227, 1990.
23. McCullough, A.J., Mullen, K.D., Smanik, E.J., et al.: Gastroenterol. Clin. North Am., *18:*619–643, 1989.
24. Mezey, E.: Liver and biliary system. *In* Clinical Nutrition. 2nd Ed. Edited by D.M. Paige. C.V. Mosby, St. Louis, 1988, pp. 186–197.
25. Lieber, C.S., Robins, S.J., Li, J.-J., et al.: Gastroenterology *106:*152–159, 1994.
26. Lieber, C.S., Robins, S.J., Leo, M.A.: Alcoholism: Clin Exp Res (*in press*).
27. Yamada, S., Mak, K.M., Lieber, C.S.: Gastroenterology, *88:*1799–1806, 1985.
28. Arai, M., Gordon, E.R., Lieber, C.S.: Biochim Biophys Acta, *797:*320–327, 1984.
29. Vhlachevic, Z.R., Buhac, I., Farrar, J.J., et al.: Gastroenterology, *60:*491–498, 1971.
30. Rudman, D., Di Fulco, T.J., Galambos, J.T., et al.: J. Clin. Invest., *52:*2242–2249, 1973.
31. Mullen, K.D., Denne, S.C., MuCullough, A.J., et al.: Hepatology, *6:*622–630, 1986.
32. Swart, G.R., Van DenBerg, J.W.O., Wahimena, J.L.D., et al.: Clin. Sci., *75:*101–107, 1988.
33. Gabuzda, G.J., Shear, L.: Am. J. Clin. Nutr., *23:*479–484, 1970.
34. Collins, J.R., et al.: Arch. Intern. Med., *126:*608–614, 1970.
35. Conn, H.O.: Am. J. Med., *259:*394–404, 1970.
36. Owen, O.E., Trapp, V.E., Reichard, G.A.: J. Clin. Invest., *72:*1821–1832, 1983.
37. Merli, M., Riggio, O., Romiti, A., et al.: Hepatology, *12:*106–112, 1990.
38. Schneeweiss, B., Graninger, W., Ferenci, P., et al.: Hepatology, *11:*387–393, 1990.
39. Jhongiani, S.S., Nanakram, A., Holmes, R., et al.: Am. J. Clin. Nutr., *44:*323–329, 1986.
40. Shanbhogue, R.L.K., Bistrian, B.R., Jenkins, R.L., et al.: JPEN J. Parentero. Enterol. Nutr., *11:*305–308, 1987.
41. Heymsfield, S.B., Waki, M., Reinus, J.: Hepatology, *11:*502–504, 1990.
42. Fennelly, J., Frank, O., Baker, H., et al.: Am. J. Clin. Nutr., *20:*946–949, 1967.
43. Russell, R.M., Morrison, S.A., Smith, F.R., et al.: Ann. Intern. Med., *88:*622–626, 1978.
44. Mitchell, D., Wagner, C., Stone, W.J., et al.: Gastroenterology, *71:*1043–1049, 1976.
45. Skinner, R.K., Sherlock, S., Long, R.G., et al.: Lancet, *1:*720–721, 1977.
46. Leo, M.A., Lieber, C.S.: N. Engl. J. Med., *307:*597–601, 1982.
47. Leo, M.A., Lowe, N., Lieber, C.S.: Am. J. Clin. Nutr., *40:*1131–1136, 1984.
48. Borowsky, S.A., Perlow, W., Baraona, E., et al.: Dig. Dis. Sci., *25:*22–27, 1980.
49. Sato, M., Lieber, C.S.: Arch. Biochem. Biophys., *213:*557–564, 1982.
50. Leo, M.A., Lieber, C.S.: J. Biol. Chem., *260:*5228–5231, 1985.
51. Leo, M.A., Lieber, C.S.: J. Nutr., *117:*70–76, 1987.
52. Shaw, J.H.F., Wolfe, R.R.: Ann. Surg., *204:*666–672, 1986.
53. Askanazi, J., Nordenstrom, J., Rosenbaum, S.H., et al.: Anesthesiology, *54:*373–377, 1981.
54. Mann, S., Westenskow, D.R., Houtchens, B.A.: Crit. Can. Med., *13:*173–177, 1985.
55. Bouffard, Y.H., Delafosse, B.X., Annat, G.J., et al.: JPEN J. Parenter. Enteral. Nutr., *13:*26–29, 1989.
56. Saffle, J.R., Medina, E., Raymond, J., et al.: J. Trauma, *25:*32–39, 1986.
57. DiMagno, E.P., Malagelada, J.R., Go, V.L.W.: Ann. N.Y. Acad. Sci., *252:*200–207, 1975.

58. Taubin, H.L., Spiro, H.M.: Am. J. Clin. Nutr., *26:*367–373, 1973.
59. Nasrallah, S.M., Galambos, J.T.: Lancet, *2:*1276–1277, 1980.
60. Smith, J., Horowitz, J., Henderson, J.M., et al.: Am. J. Clin. Nutr., *35:*56–72, 1982.
61. Calvey, H., Davis, M., Williams, R.J.: Hepatology, *1:*141–151, 1985.
62. Diehl, A.M., Boitnott, J.K., Herlong, H.F., et al.: Hepatology, *5:*57–63, 1985.
63. Naveau, S., Pelletier, G., Poynard, T., et al.: Hepatology, *6:*270–274, 1986.
64. Achord, J.L.: Am. J. Gastroenterol., *82:*871–875, 1987.
65. Simon, D., Galambos, J.T.: J. Hepatol., *7:*200–207, 1988.
66. Greenberger, N.J., Carley, J., Schenker, S., et al.: Dig. Dis. Sci., *22:*845–855, 1977.
67. Shaw, S., Worner, T.M., Lieber, C.S.: Am. J. Clin. Nutr., *38:*59–63, 1983.
68. Rocchi, E., Casaanelli, M., Gilbertini, P., et al.: JPEN J. Parenter. Enteral. Nutr., *9:*447–451, 1981.
69. Okuno, M., Nagayama, M., Takai, T.: J. Surg. Res., *39:*93–102, 1985.
70. Mendenhall, C., Bongiovanni, G., Goldberg, S., et al.: JPEN J. Parenter. Enteral. Nutr., *9:*590–596, 1985.
71. Kaneinatsu, T., Koyanagi, N., Matsumata, T., et al.: Surgery, *104:*482–488, 1988.
72. Fischer, J.E., Baldersarini, R.J.: Lancet, *2:*75–80, 1971.
73. Fischer, J.E., Yoshimura, N., Aguirri, A., et al.: Am. J. Surg., *127:*40–47, 1974.
74. Naylor, C.D., O'Rourke, K., Detsky, A.S., et al.: Gastroenterology, *97:*1033–1042, 1989.
75. Vilstrup, H., Gluud, C., Hardt, F., et al.: J. Hepatol., *10:*291–296, 1990.
76. Horst, D., Grace, N.D., Conn, H.O., et al.: Hepatology, *4:*279–287, 1984.
77. Uribe, M., Marquez, M.A., Ramos, G.G., et al.: Dig. Dis. Sci., *27:*1109–1116, 1982.
78. Weber, F.L., Minco, D., Fresard, K.M., et al.: Gastroenterology, *89:*538–544, 1985.
79. Brusilow, S.W.: J. Clin. Invest., *74:*2144–2148, 1984.
80. Lindblad, B.: Proc. Natl. Acad. Sci. U.S.A., *74:*4641–4645, 1977.
81. Scriver, C.R., Larochelle, J., Silverberg, M.: Am. J. Dis. Child, *113:*41–46, 1967.
82. Greene, H.L., Slonim, A.F., O'Neill, J.A., et al.: N. Engl. J. Med., *294:*423–425, 1976.
83. Leo, M.A., Sato, M., Lieber, C.S.: Gastroenterology, *84:*562–572, 1983.
84. Leo, M.A., Arai, M., Sato, M., et al.: Gastroenterology, *82:*194–205, 1982.
85. Long, R.G., Meinhard, E., Skinner, R.K., et al.: Gut, *19:*85–90, 1978.
86. Gibbs, K., Walshe, J.M.: Clin. Sci., *41:*189–202, 1971.
87. Walshe, J.M.: Semin. Liver Dis., *4:*252–263, 1984.
88. Sitzmann, J.V., Steinborn, P.A., Zinner, M.J., et al.: Surg. Gynecol. Obstet., *168:*311–317, 1989.
89. Roza, A.M., Shizgal, H.M.: Am. J. Clin. Nutr., *40:*168–182, 1984.
90. Ragins, H., Levenson, S.M., Signer, R., et al.: Am. J. Surg., *126:*606–614, 1973.
91. Cassim, M.M., Allardyce, D.B.: Ann. Surg., *180:*228–231, 1974.
92. Blackburn, G.L., Williams, L.F., Bistrian, B.R., et al.: Am. J. Surg., *131:*114–124, 1976.
93. Konturek, S.J., Tasler, J., Cieszkowski, M., et al.: Gastroenterology, *75:*817–824, 1978.
94. Klein, E., Shnebaum, S., Ben-Ari, G., et al.: Am. J. Gastroenterol., *78:*31–33, 1983.
95. Lawson, L.J.: Br. J. Surg., *52:*795–800, 1965.
96. Den Besten, L., Reyna, R., Connor, W., et al.: J. Clin. Invest., *75:*1384–1393, 1973.
97. Hughes, C.A., Prince, A., Dowling, R.H.: Clin. Sci., *59:*329–336, 1980.
98. Havala, T., Shrouts, E., Cerra, F.: Gastroenterol. Clin. North Am., *18:*525–542, 1989.
99. Sax, H.C., Werner, B.W., Talamini, M.A., et al.: Am. J. Surg., *153:*117–124, 1987.
100. Karanjia, N.D., Widdison, A.L., Leung, F.W., et al.: Gastroenterology, *98:*A221, 1990.
101. Isaksson, G., Ihse, I.: Dig. Dis. Sci., *28:*97–1002, 1983.
102. Slaff, J., Jacobson, D., Tillman, C.R., et al.: Gastroenterology, *87:*44–52, 1984.
103. Halgreen, H.: Scand. J. Gastroenterol., *21:*104–108, 1986.
104. Leung, J.W.C., Bowen-Wright, M., Aveling, W., et al.: Br. J. Surg., *70:*730–732, 1983.
105. DiMagno, E.P., Clain, J.E.: Chronic Pancreatitis. *In* The Exocrine Pancreas. Edited by V.L.W. Go, F.P. Brooks, E.P. DiMagno, et al. New York, Raven Press, 1986, pp. 541–575.
106. Kugelberg, C.H., Wehlin, L., Arnesjö, B., et al.: Gut, *17:*267–272, 1976.
107. Roesch, W., Demling, L.: Surg. Clin. North Am., *62:*845–852, 1982.
108. Tsurumi, T., Fujii, Y., Takeda, M., et al.: Acta Med. Okayama, *38:*169–174, 1984.
109. Cremer, M., Vandermeerin, A., Delhaye, M.: Gastroenterology, *94:*A80, 1988.
110. Kozarck, R.A., Patterson, D.J., Ball, T.J., et al.: Ann. Surg., *209:*261–266, 1989.
111. Regan, P.T., Malagelada, J.R., DiMagno, E.P., et al.: Gastroenterology, *77:*285–289, 1979.
112. Twersky, Y., Bank, S.: Gastroenterol. Clin. North Am., *18:*543–565, 1989.
113. Dutta, S.K., Bustin, M.P., Russell, R.M., et al.: Ann. Intern. Med., *97:*549–552, 1982.
114. Cook, G.C., Hutt, M.S.: Br. Med. J., *3:*454–457, 1967.
115. Ramalingaswami, V.: Nature, *201:*546–551, 1964.
116. Snapper, I.: Chinese Lessons to Western Medicine. 2nd Ed. New York, Grune & Stratton, 1965.
117. Conn, H.O., Atterbury, C.E.: Cirrhosis. *In* Diseases of the Liver. Edited by L. Schiff and E.R. Schiff. Philadelphia, J.B. Lippincott, 1987, pp. 725–864.
118. Pequinot, G., Chabert, C., Eydowx, et al.: Rev. Alcohol., *20:*191–202, 1974.
119. Lelbach, W.K.: Ann. N.Y. Acad. Sci., *252:*85–105, 1975.
120. Lieber, C.S.: Alc. Health Res. World, *13:*197–205, 1989.
121. Mills, P.R., Shankin, A., Anthony, R.S., et al.: Am. J. Clin. Nutr., *38:*849–859, 1983.
122. Grossman, M.I., Greengard, H., Ivy, A.C.: Am. J. Physiol., *138:*676–682, 1943.
123. Ben Aldeljlel, A., Visani, A.M., Desnuelle, P.: Biochem. Biophys. Res. Commun., *10:*112–116, 1963.
124. Zoppi, G., Andreotti, G., Pajno-Ferrara, F., et al.: Pediatr. Res., *6:*880–886, 1972.
125. Veghelyi, P.V., Kemeny, T.T., Pozsonyi, J., et al.: Am. J. Dis. Child., *79:*658–665, 1950.
126. Shaper, A.G.: Lancet, 1223–1224, 1960.
127. Thompson, M.D., Trowell, H.C.: Lancet, *1:*1032–1053, 1952.

128. Tandon, B.N., George, P.E., Sama, S.K., et al.: Am. J. Clin. Nutr., *22:*1476–1482, 1969.
129. McMillan, D.E., Guvarghese, P.J.: Diabetes Care, *2:*202–208, 1979.
130. Haig, T.H.B.: Surg. Obstet. Gynecol., *131:*914–918, 1970.
131. Ramo, O.J.: Gut, *28:*64–69, 1982.
132. Ramo, O.J., Apaja-Sarkkinen, M., Jalovaara, P.: Res. Exp. Med., *187:*33–41, 1987.
133. Mezey, E., Kolman, C.J., Diehl, A.M., et al.: Am. J. Clin. Nutr., *48:*148–151, 1988.
134. Sarles, H., Sarles, J.-C., Camatti, R., et al.: Gut, *6:*545–559, 1965.
135. Durbec, J.P., Sarles, H.: Digestion, *18:*337–350, 1978.
136. Goebell, H., Hotz, J.: Biol. Gastroenterol., *8:*365, 1975.
137. Vantini, I., Carrallini, G., Angelini, G., et al.: Rendic Gastroenterol., *9:*13–17, 1977.
138. Uscanga, L., Robles-Diaz, G., Sarles, H.: Dig. Dis. Sci., *30:*110–113, 1985.
139. Korsten, M.A., Wilson, J.S., Lieber, C.S.: Gastroenterology, *99:*229–236, 1990.

CHAPTER 64

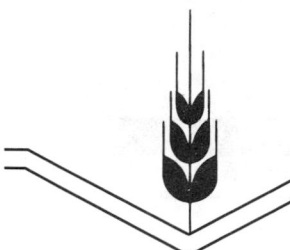

Nutrition And Diet In Alcoholism

Lawrence Feinman and Charles S. Lieber

The interactions between nutrition and alcoholism occur at many levels and are complex. Alcoholic beverages contain calories but almost no other useful constituents.[1] Ethanol-containing beverages alter appetite and affect the level of food intake and utilization. They displace required nutrients from the diet. Ethanol and nutrients have multiple interactions at almost every level of the gastrointestinal tract. Ethanol alters the storage, mobilization, activation, and metabolism of nutrients.

Ethanol is directly toxic to many body tissues. Ethanol's interplay with malnutrition in causing damage, particularly with respect to the liver, the predominant site of its metabolism, still needs clarification. Alcoholism remains one of the major causes of nutritional deficiency in the United States; alcohol-related illness poses an enormous medical burden and often entails complex nutritional therapy. Nutritional therapy is frequently a balance between maximizing recovery while avoiding iatrogenic complications. Encephalopathy, for example, may develop in patients with alcoholic liver disease despite dietary protein below the daily requirement; tolerance in a given patient may change rapidly, requiring daily evaluation.

NUTRITIONAL VALUE OF ALCOHOLIC BEVERAGES

Alcoholic beverages contain water, ethanol, variable amounts of carbohydrate, and little else of nutritive value. The carbohydrate content varies greatly: whiskey, cognac, and vodka have none, red and dry white wines have 2 to 10 g/L, beer and dry sherry have 30 g/L, and sweetened white and port wines have as much as 120 g/L.[2] Protein and vitamin content of these beverages is extremely low except for beer. Even if one used beer as a nutrient source, a liter would be necessary daily for nicotinic acid requirement, 15 to 20 L for protein, and 25 L for thiamin. Iron content may be appreciable, especially in wine.[2] The amounts of iron, lead, or cobalt may reach harmful levels. The significance of congener content is yet obscure.[1]

Americans probably consume 4.5% of total calories as ethanol,[3] and adult drinkers over 10%. Heavy drinkers may derive more than half their daily calories from ethanol. Combustion of ethanol in a bomb calorimeter yields 7.1 kcal/g; however, we know that its biologic value is probably less, compared to carbohydrates on a calorie basis. Lowered body weight in alcohol drinkers compared to nondrinkers is especially clear in women.[4] When subjects were given additional calories as alcohol under metabolic ward conditions they did not gain weight (Fig. 64–1).[5,6]

Hospitalized alcoholics on an open ward also gained no additional weight when 1800 calories from ethanol were added beyond their 2600-calorie diet.[7] Isocaloric substitution of ethanol for carbohydrate, as 50% of total calories in a balanced diet, conducted under metabolic ward conditions, resulted in a decline in body weight[8], when given as additional calories ethanol achieved less gain in weight than equivalent carbohydrate or fat (Figs. 64–2 and 64–3).[1,6] Others have found variable responses in weight to additional calories as ethanol.[9] Body composition measurements were not reported. The ability of ethanol to support body weight may vary according to the quality of carbohydrate fed with it.[10]

There is a good deal of evidence that ethanol increases metabolic rate, which would at least partly explain its reduced biologic energy value. Ethanol increases oxygen consumption in normal subjects, and does so to a greater degree in alcoholics.[11] Substitution of ethanol for carbohydrates increases metabolic rate in humans and rodents.[12,13] Thermogenesis increased by 15% in rats fed ethanol for only 10 days in one study.[12] Diet-induced thermogenesis (DIT) also increased in humans.[12] Only a small portion of the energy waste in rats could be attributed to brown fat thermogenesis.[14] It is theorized that energy waste during ethanol consumption may occur via oxidation without phosphorylation by the microsomal ethanol oxidizing system (MEOS).[6] The MEOS is inducible by chronic ethanol consumption, which aggravates energy waste.[15,16] Some[17] have implicated uncoupling of mitochondrial NADH (the reduced form of nicotinamide adenine dinucleotide) reoxidation, perhaps abetted by a hyperthyroid state or catecholamine release, to explain energy waste.[17] The hyperthyroid state has been questioned.[18]

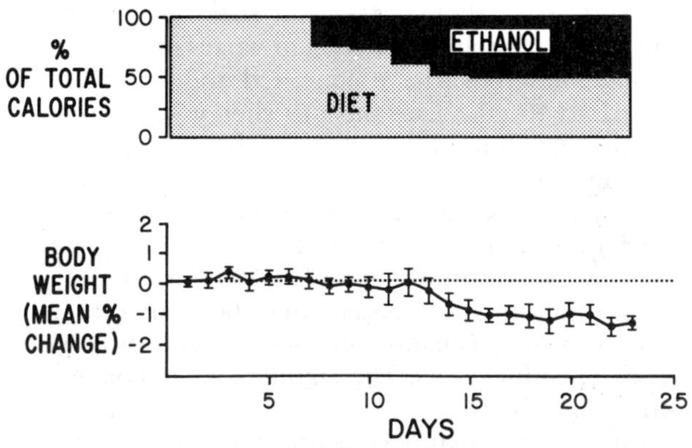

FIGURE 64–1. Effect of the isocaloric substitution of ethanol for carbohydrate calories on body weight. Substitution of ethanol as 50% of total calories results in body weight loss. (From Pirola, R.C., Lieber, C.S.: Pharmacology, 7:185, 1972.)

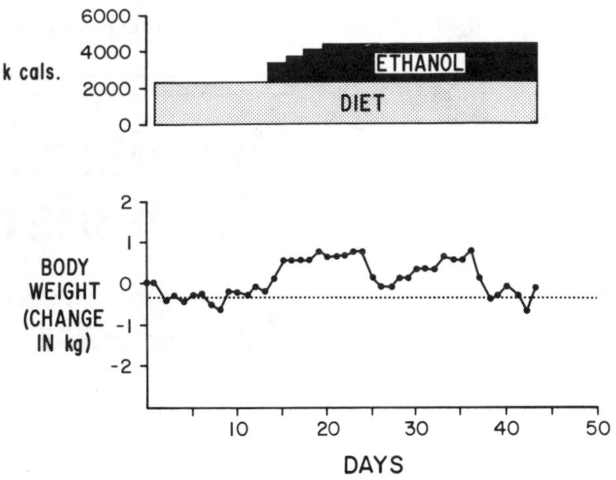

FIGURE 64–2. Effect on body weight of the addition of alcohol-derived calories to the diet. (From Pirola, R.C., Lieber, C.S.: Pharmacology, 7:185, 1972.)

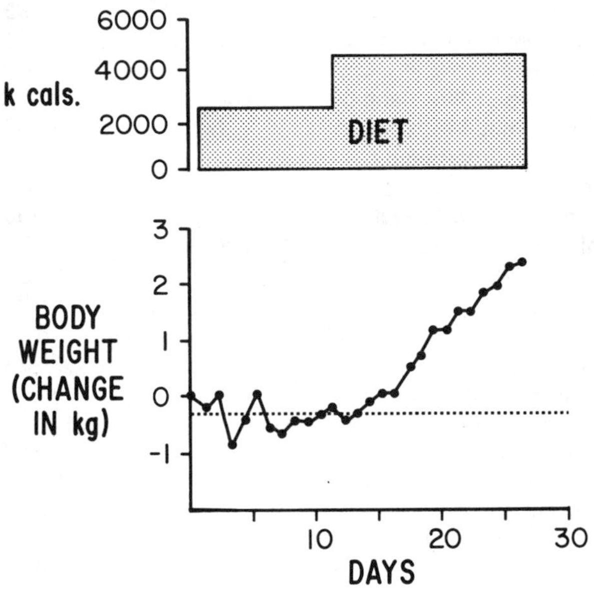

FIGURE 64–3. Effect of nonalcohol-derived calories. Supplementary calories from ethanol produced less weight gain than calorically equivalent carbohydrate. (From Pirola, R.C., Lieber, C.S.: Pharmacology, 7:185, 1972.)

NUTRITIONAL STATUS OF ALCOHOLICS

Alcoholism can undermine nutritional status. Not too long ago it was estimated that 20,000 alcoholics were suffering major illnesses due to malnutrition in the United States each year, accounting for 7½ million days of hospitalization.[19] The subgroup of alcoholics hospitalized for medical complications of alcoholism has the most severe malnutrition. These alcoholics have inadequate dietary protein,[20] signs of protein malnutrition,[19,21] and anthropomorphic measurements indicative of impaired nutrition: the height-to-weight ratio is lower,[22] muscle mass estimated by the creatinine-height index is reduced,[21,22] and triceps skin folds are thinner.[21-23] Continued drinking results in weight loss, whereas abstinence results in weight gain,[24,25] in patients with and without liver disease.[23]

Many patients who drink to excess are either not malnourished or are less malnourished than the group hospitalized for medical problems. Those with moderate alcohol intake,[26] even those admitted to hospital for alcohol rehabilitation rather than for medical problems,[27] hardly differ nutritionally from controls (matched for socioeconomic status and health history), except that the females have a lower level of thiamin saturation.[27]

The wide range in nutritional status of our alcoholic population surely reflects differences in what they eat. Moderate alcohol intake, alcohol accounting for 16% of total calories (alcohol included), is associated with slightly increased total energy intake.[28] Perhaps because of the energy considerations already discussed, this group with higher total caloric intake has no weight gain despite physical activity levels comparable to those of the non–alcohol consuming population. This level of alcohol intake, and even slightly higher levels (23%),[29] is associated with a substitution of alcohol for carbohydrate in the diet. In those individuals consuming more than 30% of total calories as alcohol, significant decreases in protein and fat intake occur too, and their intake of vitamins A, C, and thiamin may descend below the recommended daily allowances.[28] Calcium, iron, and fiber intake are also lowered.[29]

The mechanisms underlying the altered pattern of food intake are not exactly known. Suppression of appetite has been postulated[30] but has not been studied much. Depressed consciousness during inebriation, hangover, and gastroduodenitis due to ethanol partly explain the decreased food intake.

In summary, alcohol intake is associated with a wide spectrum of nutritional states; most of the alcohol-consuming public has slight if any detectable impairment, whereas those hospitalized for medical complications are likely to be severely malnourished. The contribution of subtle nutritional alterations produced by ethanol to the pathogenesis of ethanol-induced or other disease states is largely undetermined. Nutritional therapy per se for alcoholism has not been successful.[31]

EFFECTS OF ETHANOL ON DIGESTION AND ABSORPTION

Alcohol consumption is associated with motility changes in the gastrointestinal tract and affects the digestion and absorption of nutrients. Diarrhea and weight loss frequently occur in alcoholics. Ethanol effects may be direct or indirect, acute or chronic. One of the most intense changes, intestinal malabsorption secondary to folic acid deficiency, is not a direct effect of ethanol, but rather comes from diminished folic acid intake accompanying alcoholism.

GASTROINTESTINAL TRACT

Patients with cirrhosis of the liver due to alcohol have edema, interstromal fat infiltration and fibrosis of the parotid glands, decreased basal and citric acid stimulated salivary flows, and lower salivary concentrations of sodium, bicarbonate, and proteins.[32] Changes in esophageal peristalsis and lower esophageal sphincter pressure follow no consistent patterns[33-35] and usually do not lead to clinically significant dysphagia. However, the changes in saliva and esophageal motility and the direct effect of ethanol may be important in causing esophagitis and stricture, which are common in alcoholics and interfere dramatically with food intake.

Alcohol ingestion is a cause of acute gastritis and duodenitis.[36] These areas of the gut are exposed to the highest concentrations of ethanol for the longest times. Damage to the gastric mucosal "barrier" is important in making the mucosa more susceptible to acid and hyperosmolarity. Damage is probably due to a combination of diminished gastric mucus production, altered mucosal blood flow, inhibition of active transport, increased permeability due to mast cell release of histamine and leukotriene C_4, cell membrane disruption, hyperosmolarity, changes in prostaglandin and cyclic adenosine monophosphate (cAMP) content of mucosa, and lipoperoxidative mechanisms. Erosive gastritis occurs, as does nonerosive hemorrhagic gastritis consisting of subepithelial hemorrhage of the foveolar region with surrounding edema.[37] The effects of ethanol on gastric emptying of meals are concentration-dependent, higher concentrations causing more consistent delays of passage of solid contents[38] while even enhancing movement of liquid contents.[39]

Alcoholics frequently suffer from diarrhea[40] and malabsorption. Acute effects of ethanol on motility and acute and chronic effects on the mucosa are responsible. Concomitant nutrient deficiencies can contribute significantly to mucosal changes, particularly folate deficiency. In the jejunum ethanol decreases type I (impeding) waves, while in the ileum it increases type III (propulsive) waves. Decreases in villus height[41] and disaccharide activity[42,43] of mucosal biopsy specimens have been found in alcoholics with associated lactose intolerance, especially in black cirrhotics[43] (Figs. 64–4 to 64–6). The possibility of lactase deficiency must be considered in dietary treatment. Monosaccharide absorption is variably affected by ethanol; glucose is absorbed less well in rabbits after acute ethanol exposure,[44] but chronic ethanol exposure enhances galactose absorption in rats[45] and glucose absorption in humans.[46]

Acute depression of amino acid absorption can readily be demonstrated using high concentrations of ethanol

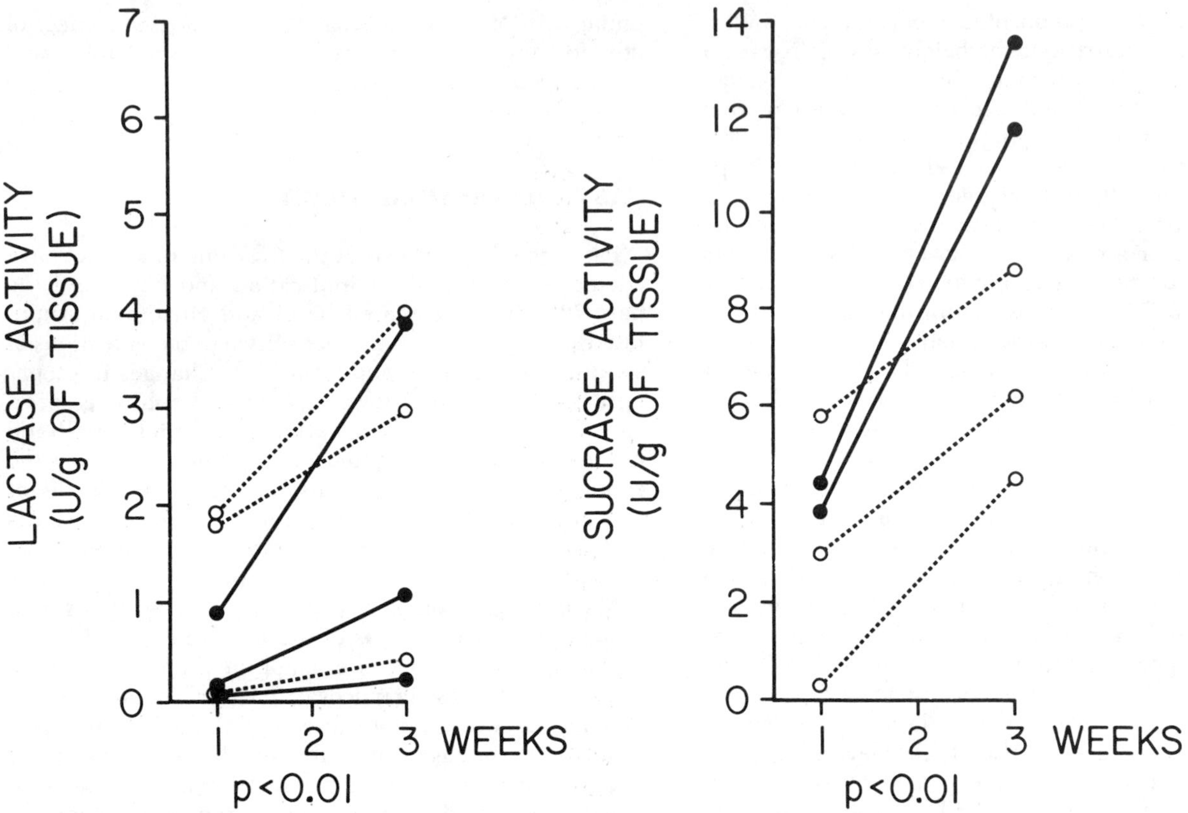

FIGURE 64–4. Effect of withdrawal from alcohol upon intestinal lactase. A significant increase in intestinal lactase was observed following 1 to 3 weeks of withdrawal from alcohol. A similar effect was noted for intestinal sucrase activity. (From Perlow, W., Baraona, E., Lieber, C.S.: Gastroenterology, *72*:680–684, 1977.)

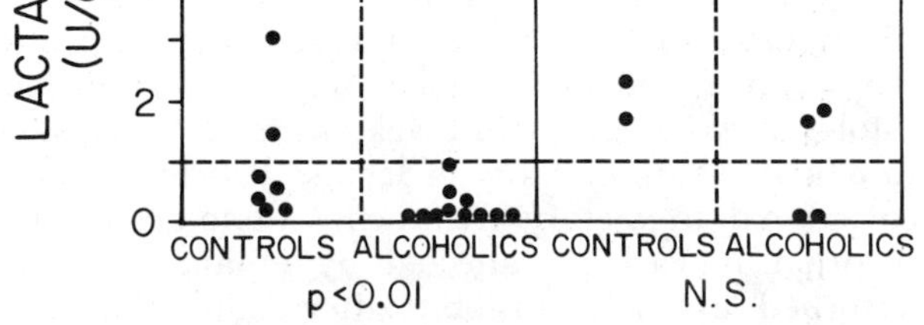

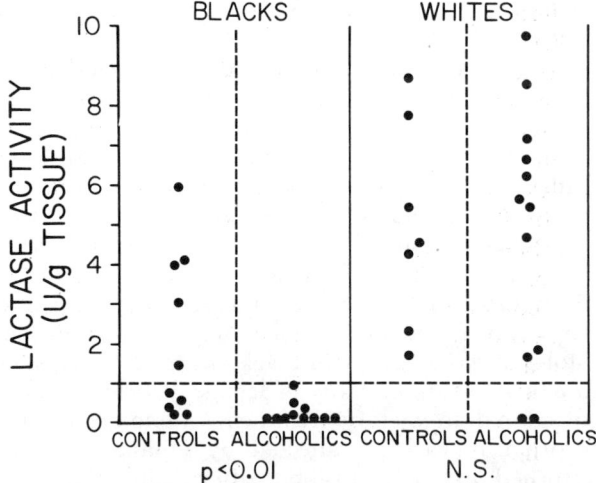

FIGURE 64–5. The effects of chronic alcohol consumption on lowering intestinal lactase activity. Black alcoholics were found to be especially sensitive. (From Perlow, W., Baraona, E., Lieber, C.S.: Gastroenterology, *72*:680–684, 1977.)

(0.5 to 3.0%) in experimental models of ethanol exposure, using short segments of gut perfused in vivo or gut sacs bathed in vitro. It has not been easy to demonstrate depressed absorption acutely using smaller concentrations of ethanol in whole intestines of living animals or in models fed ethanol chronically. A couple of relevant topics are virtually unstudied: the effect of ethanol on amino acid absorption from complex mixtures (including peptides), and the possible effect of local changes in amino acid absorption on body nitrogen utilization.

BILE SALTS

Steatorrhea, when it occurs in alcoholics, is mostly due to folic acid deficiency (see later) but may be contributed to by luminal bile salt deficiency. Intraluminal bile salts are decreased by acute ethanol administration.[47] In rodents, long-term ethanol administration delays the half-time excretion of cholic and chenodeoxycholic acids by decreasing the daily excretion and expanding the pool size slightly.[48] Alcoholic cirrhotic patients may have bile low in deoxycholic acid, possibly due to impaired conversion of cholate to deoxycholate by bacteria.[49]

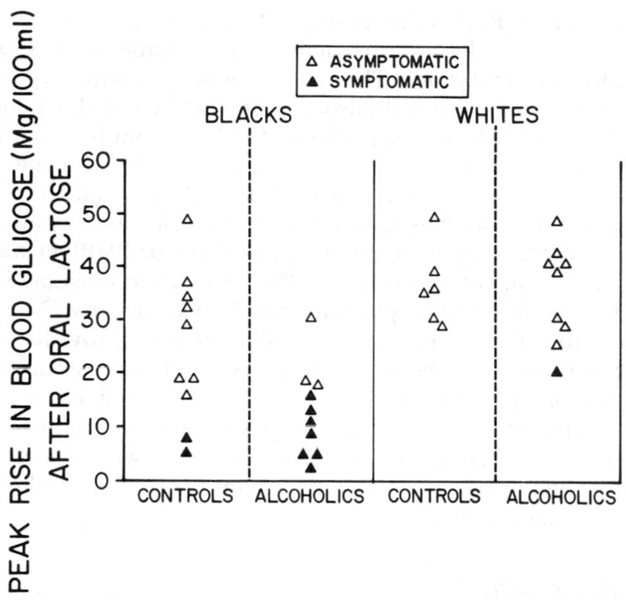

FIGURE 64–6. Effect of lactase deficiency on rise in serum glucose after oral lactase administration. Blood glucose rose the least in subjects with the most severe lactase deficiency. There was a good correlation between symptoms and the lack of rise in glucose. (From Perlow, W., Baraona, E., Lieber, C.S.: Gastroenterology, *72*:680–684, 1977.)

Thus, decreased cholic acid synthesis, decreased bile acid pool size,[50] low concentrations of bile salts in intestinal juice, and bacterial deconjugation of bile salts by altered intestinal flora all promote steatorrhea in cirrhotics. Pigmented gallstones are more frequent in cirrhotics.[51]

ALTERATIONS OF NUTRIENT METABOLISM

WATER-SOLUBLE VITAMINS

OVERALL CHANGES

Alcoholics tend to have clinical or laboratory signs of soluble vitamin insufficiency correlated with the increasing amount of alcohol they drink and a corresponding decrease in vitamin intake. This is true for thiamin, riboflavin, pyridoxine, folic acid, and ascorbic acid, but has not been demonstrated for vitamin B_{12}. Alcohol effects on absorption, activation, and storage must also be considered. Alcohol is clearly able to impair thiamin absorption in rodents; human thiamin absorption may not be susceptible to alcohol. Alcohol interferes with riboflavin absorption in rodents, but is not studied in humans. Alcohol impairs folic acid absorption in malnourished humans; the mechanism by which this happens is unclear. Some experimental animals, even with malnutrition, have impaired folic acid absorption by alcohol; others do not. The hepatic retention of folic acid is inhibited by alcohol, which also interferes with the hematologic utilization of folic acid and promotes urinary and fecal losses of folic acid. A role for alcohol interfering with the activation and storage of thiamin is controversial. Riboflavin and pyridoxine storage in the liver is adversely affected by alcohol, at least in experimental animals.

THIAMIN

Thiamin deficiency is most often present in alcoholics in our society and causes Wernicke-Korsakoff syndrome and beriberi heart disease, and probably contributes to polyneuropathy. Neuroanatomic lesions comparable to the human syndrome can be produced in rhesus monkeys upon prolonged thiamin deficiency without the need for alcohol intake.[51,52] There has been no confirmation of an inborn error of transketolase affinity for coenzyme in Wernicke-Korsakoff syndrome as was once claimed.[53] Thiamin intake will be insufficient for those relying on alcoholic beverages for their energy needs. When obvious deficiency is not present, decreases of blood transketolase activity with increases on in vitro addition of cofactor thiamin pyrophosphate (TPP) has been thought useful for diagnosis by some[54] but not by others.[55] It is postulated that profound thiamin deficiency, alcohol intake[56] or liver disease[57] may affect levels of apoenzyme transketolase or its binding to cofactor and thus prevent the TPP effect. Others have found that decreased erythrocyte transketolase activity alone correlates best with thiamin deficiency in patients with Wernicke's encephalopathy.[58] In any case, in experimental animals[59] and in well-nourished alcoholics who take in normal or greater amounts of thiamin, thiamin levels in the organs are maintained[60] and there is no abnormality in the relative amounts of phosphorylated species of thiamin.[61]

Hospitalized alcoholics were reported to have impaired thiamin absorption compared to control patients when tested by radioactive thiamin excretion,[62] a test also affected by steps not related to absorption. Also, folic acid deficiency was not adequately excluded as a cause of thiamin malabsorption in these studies. When refined testing is used, reduced thiamin absorption due to alcohol is seen in a minority of subjects.[63] Jejunal perfusion studies could not show an effect of 5% alcohol on thiamin absorption in man.[64] Interestingly, thiamin absorption is lower in middle-aged subjects (alcoholics and controls) than in younger individuals. Studies in rats have progressed further but they may not be relevant to human disease (discussed previously). In rodents, thiamin absorption is accomplished by an active system with a low K_m and a passive system with a higher K_m.[60] Alcohol interferes with thiamin absorption via the low concentration active pathway, and presumably (if humans are similarly constituted) is an important factor for alcoholics with marginal or low thiamin intake. The effects of alcohol on thiamin activation and storage in the liver are controversial.[60]

Thiamin is well absorbed from sorghum beer despite its 3% alcohol and liver yeast content.[64] Therefore, it is feasible to add thiamin to alcoholic beverages. Thiamin should be provided to all alcoholics because there is an appreciable incidence of thiamin deficiency in alcoholics, it is difficult to assess any but the most glaring thiamin deficiency syndromes, it is important to reverse early neurologic disease, and thiamin replacement is easy and safe. Thiamin should be given parenterally, 50 mg per day, until oral intake can be established, followed by 50 mg per day orally for weeks or longer if neurologic problems persist.

RIBOFLAVIN

When there is a general lack of B vitamin intake, riboflavin deficiency may be encountered. In one study deficiency was found in 50% of a small group of patients with medical complications severe enough to warrant hospital admission.[65] Although none of the patients exhibited classic signs of riboflavin deficiency, they had an abnormal activity coefficient (AC) that returned to normal 2 to 7 days after intramuscular replacement with 5 mg riboflavin daily. Activity coefficient is measured as the ratio of erythrocyte glutathione reductase activity upon addition of flavin adenine dinucleotide (FAD) to the activity with no additions. A study showed that riboflavin deficiency could be induced readily by alcohol feeding to the Syrian hamster; the most severe deficiency was seen in animals also restricted in riboflavin intake.[66] Ethanol also impaired hepatic accumulation of riboflavin in rats given vitamins and alcohol by acute gavage, with evidence that ethanol markedly inhibited the intestinal enzymes that hydrolyze the vitamin forms—flavin mononucleotide (FMN), phosphatase, FAD, pyrophosphatase—and may decrease vitamin absorption.

Riboflavin replacement is easy because absorption occurs readily, excess is excreted in the urine, and there is no known toxicity. It usually given to alcoholic patients as part of a multivitamin preparation.

PYRIDOXINE

Neurologic, hematologic, and dermatologic disorders can be caused in part by pyridoxine deficiency. Pyridoxine deficiency, as measured by low plasma pyridoxal-5'-phosphate (PLP), was reported in over 50% of alcoholics without hematologic findings or abnormal liver function tests.[67,68] Inadequate intake may partly explain low PLP, but increased destruction and reduced formation may also be important. PLP is more rapidly destroyed in erythrocytes in the presence of acetaldehyde, the first product of ethanol oxidation, perhaps by displacement of PLP from protein and consequent exposure to phosphatase.[67,69] Fairly high levels of acetaldehyde were used in the studies referred to, so the significance of the proposed mechanism is uncertain. Previous studies showed that chronic ethanol feeding lowered hepatic content of PLP by decreasing net synthesis from pyridoxine,[70–72] and that this depended in some studies on alcohol oxidation. The acetaldehyde produced was thought to enhance hydrolysis of PLP by cellular phosphatases.[67] Actual displacement of PLP from its binding protein by acetaldehyde has been shown in rat hepatocytes.[73] More recently in studies of mice[73] and rats[74] ethanol actually increased total hepatic levels of vitamin B_6 (PLP and pyridoxamine-5-phosphate, or PMP), primarily because of an increase in PMP. However, plasma PLP may be lowered by plasma phosphatase activity.[68]

Clinical management generally involves provision of pyridoxine in the usual multivitamin dosage unless neuropathy or pyridoxine-responsive anemia has been diagnosed. Because ataxia due to sensory neuropathy has been ascribed to toxicity from as little as 200 mg of pyridoxine per day, the indiscriminate use of large doses must be avoided.[75,76]

FOLIC ACID

Alcoholics tend to have low folic acid status when they are drinking heavily and their folic acid intake is reduced. A group of unselected alcoholics showed a 37.5% incidence of low serum folate levels and a 17.6% incidence of low red blood cell folate levels.[77] In monkeys folate deficiency can be created by ethanol feeding (50% of total calories) for over 2 years despite provision of an otherwise adequate diet: hepatic folate is low and there is evidence for decreased folate absorption.[78] In pigs fed ethanol for 11 months folic acid absorption is normal but jejunal folate hydrolase, an early enzyme of polyglutamate breakdown, is decreased.[79,80] In vitro preparations of rat intestine absorb folate less well when exposed to a variety of alcohols.[81] Malnourished alcoholics without liver disease also absorb folic acid less well compared to their better-nourished counterparts.[82] Folic acid absorption, usually increased by partial starvation, is less increased in rats when alcohol is ingested.[83] It has not been clearly shown, however, that either protein deficiency or alcohol[82,84] decreases folate absorption in vivo. Thus, it is still unclear what aspects of malnutrition adversely affect folate absorption and under what clinical circumstances alcohol may interfere with folate absorption.

Alcohol accelerates the production of megaloblastic anemia in patients with depleted folate stores[85] and suppresses the hematologic response to folic acid in folic acid–depleted patients.[86] Alcohol also has other effects on folate metabolism but their significance is not clear: alcohol given acutely causes a decrease in serum folate, which is partly explained by increased urinary excretion;[87] alcohol given chronically to monkeys decreases hepatic folate levels, partly because of the inability of the liver to retain folate,[88] and perhaps partly because of increased urinary and fecal losses.[89]

The clinical approach to folate deficiency without anemia is straightforward. A diet providing adequate folate, perhaps with additional folate, will replete stores in a matter of weeks. If malabsorption persists after this period, evaluation for causes other than folate deficiency should be instituted. When the patient is anemic the diagnostic evaluation is more complex.[85] In addition to folate deficiency, the direct effect of alcohol on the bone marrow, liver disease, hypersplenism, bleeding, iron deficiency, infection, and the use of anticonvulsants are all commonly encountered, and will exert separate and combined influences on the hematologic picture. It should be kept in mind, first, that in well-nourished alcoholics folic acid deficiency is a rare cause of anemia,[90] and second, that a search for folic acid deficiency (serum or red cell folate levels) as an explanation for anemia is unwarranted unless some or all of the morphologic features of the vitamin deficiency are present (macro-ovalocytes, hypersegmentation of polymorphonuclear leukocytes, megaloblastosis of the bone marrow). The following sequence has been proposed for the development of folic acid deficiency: negative folate balance (serum folate less than 3 ng/ml); folate depletion (red blood cell folate less than 160 ng/ml), serum folate less than 120 ng/ml, neutrophil lobe average greater than 3.5, liver folate less than 1.2 μg/g); folate deficient anemia (low hemoglobin, elevated mean corpuscular volume, macro-ovalocytosis).[91] When there is combined iron and folate deficiency the expression of macrocytosis will be modified or a dimorphic red blood cell population may occur. Hypersegmentation of leukocyte nuclei and macro-ovalocytosis may persist for several weeks after folate replacement has started.[85]

Some have proposed adding folate to alcoholic beverages because the taste of the beverage is not altered and vitamin absorption is adequate.[92]

VITAMIN B_{12}

Alcoholics do not commonly get vitamin B_{12} deficiency. Their serum levels are usually normal even when they are deficient in folate, whether they have cirrhosis[93,94] or not.[82,83] This is due to large body stores of vitamin B_{12} and reserve capacity for absorption, because there are several factors in the context of alcoholism that would promote vitamin depletion. Pancreatic insufficiency, for example, results in decreased vitamin B_{12} absorption as measured by the Schilling test. In this circumstance there is insufficient lumenal protease activity and alkalinity, which normally serve to release vitamin B_{12} from the "r" protein, which is secreted by salivary glands, intestines, and possibly the stomach.[95] Alcohol ingestion has also been shown to decrease vitamin B_{12} absorption in volunteers after several weeks of intake.[96] The alcohol effect may be in the ileum because co-administration of intrinsic factor or pancreatin does not correct the Schilling test results. It is controversial whether the binding of intrinsic factor-vitamin B_{12} complex to ileal sites is abnormal.[97,98]

VITAMIN C

The vitamin C status of alcoholic patients admitted to a hospital is lower than that of nonalcoholics as measured by serum ascorbic acid, peripheral leukocyte ascorbic acid, or urinary ascorbic acid after an oral challenge.[99] In addition to a lower mean ascorbic acid level, some 25% of patients with Laennec's cirrhosis in one study had serum ascorbic acid levels below the range of healthy controls.[99] Ascorbic acid status is low in alcoholic patients with and without liver disease. When alcohol intake exceeds 30% of total calories vitamin C generally falls below recommended dietary allowances.[100] Inadequate vitamin C intake provides only a partial explanation for low ascorbic acid status. It is unknown what the clinical significance might be for patients who have low ascorbic acid levels but who are not clearly scorbutic. Daily supplementation with 175 to 500 mg of ascorbic acid may be necessary for weeks or months to restore plasma and urinary ascorbate to normal.[99]

FAT-SOLUBLE VITAMINS

GENERAL CHANGES

Clinical or laboratory evidence of fat-soluble vitamin deficiency with increased alcohol intake and poor diet does not occur as readily as it does for water-soluble vitamins. Vitamins A and D are most likely to be insufficient, with diminished intake an important factor. Poor absorption may also contribute when steatorrhea is significant because of pancreatic insufficiency or advanced cholestasis and bile salt deficiency. Under such conditions vitamin K malabsorption may also occur. Vitamin A depletion from the liver is pronounced both in alcoholics with advancing liver disease and in experimental animals fed alcohol. Important mechanisms are increased vitamin A degradation and increased mobilization from the liver. In the case of vitamin D, hepatic storage is also interfered with in alcoholism, but depletion may depend on factors other than the direct influence of alcohol, such as calcium and phosphorus intake and absorption, and parathormone levels. Bone abnormalities, also profound in alcoholism, may not be due primarily to alcohol's interaction with vitamin D metabolism. Alcohol feeding increases the conversion of α-tocopherol to the quinone in the endoplasmic reticulum of the liver in experimental animals (see later in the chapter). The significance of this observation for possible impairment of vitamin E protection against oxidative liver injury is under study.

VITAMIN A

The interaction of alcoholism and vitamin A involves the intake, possibly the absorption of the vitamin, and its metabolism; there is evidence that alcohol may modulate the role of vitamin A in hepatotoxicity and carcinogenesis.

Vitamin A ingestion is not significantly below normal for Americans taking up to 400 kcal per day as alcohol (or less than 20% of total calories),[100] probably because the vitamin A density of the nonalcoholic portions of the diet is similar to that ingested by nonalcoholic populations. Americans taking 24% of total calories as alcohol ingest only 75% of the recommended dietary allowance (RDA) for vitamin A.[101] Probably those with intense alcoholism—that is, who ingest 50% or more of daily calories as alcohol—eat even less vitamin A. Chilean wine drinkers, for example, eat only 25% of the RDA for vitamin A when they take 150 g (1050 kcal) of alcohol per day.[102] Elderly American men who consume alcohol regularly have a lower vitamin A intake.[103] In a single study vitamin A absorption was diminished 17% by 120 ml of wine.[104] Chronic alcoholic pancreatic insufficiency may substantially reduce vitamin A absorption. Low blood β-carotene levels were found in 98% of chronic alcoholics (150g alcohol per day for 5 to 25 years) admitted to a hospital despite the lack of clinical signs of vitamin A deficiency.[104]

The effect of short-term ingestion of alcohol on vitamin A blood levels has been variously reported as unchanged in man,[105] increased in dogs,[106] or increased as retinol-bound lipoproteins in rats.[107] The effect of long-term alcohol consumption on hepatic vitamin A has been consistent and profound: hepatic vitamin A stores are diminished whether dietary vitamin A is low, normal, or high. Rodents fed alcohol repeatedly in one study had lower hepatic vitamin A;[108] 5/kg per day yielded a 20% decrease in the liver in another study.[109] Higher intakes of alcohol—36% of calories or about 14 g/kg per day—decreased hepatic vitamin A by 60% in 4 to 6 weeks and by 72% in 7 to 9 weeks, without changes in serum vitamin A or retinol binding protein (RBP) in a study.[107] Five times the usual amount of vitamin A was given, which still did not prevent hepatic depletion by alcohol. When baboons were fed 50% of calories as alcohol, a 60% decrease in hepatic vitamin A occurred after 4 months and a 95% decrease after 24 to 84 months.[107] Hepatic vitamin A levels show progressive decrease with increasing severity of lesions to include cirrhosis in humans (Fig. 64–7).[110] Enhancement of hepatic vitamin A degradation due to alcohol consumption is one likely explanation for the drop in vitamin content. Vitamin A degradation by metabolism of retinoic acid to 4-hydroxy and 4-oxoretinoic acid and other polar metabolites is catalyzed by microsomal enzymes inducible by ethanol consumption,[110] but these enzymes are not active enough to deplete vitamin A stores. A more likely candidate for depleting hepatic vitamin A is a newly discovered microsomal pathway for oxidation of retinol to polar metabolites,[111] it is also inducible by alcohol consumption.[112] In addition, alcohol promotes vitamin A mobilization from the liver.[112]

An important clinical consequence of low tissue vitamin A status is night blindness. A study showed that abnormal dark adaption occurred in 15% of alcoholics without cirrhosis and in 50% with cirrhosis.[113] One can exclude retinal dysfunction with 95% confidence when the serum vitamin A level is 1.4 μmol/L (42.9 IU) or higher.[114] The correlation of serum vitamin A with tissue stores is complicated by liver disease and protein deficiency.

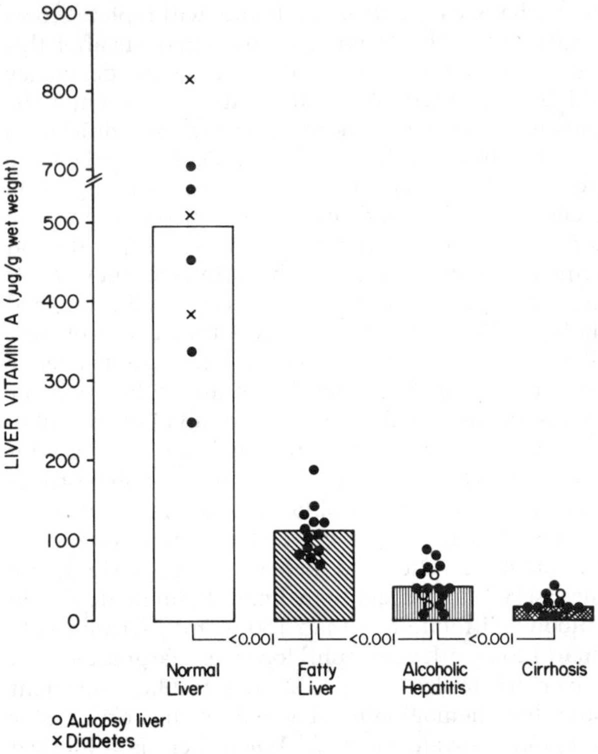

FIGURE 64–7. Hepatic vitamin A levels in subjects with normal livers, chronic persistent hepatitis, and various stages of alcoholic injury. (From Leo, M.A., Lieber, C.S.: N. Engl. J. Med., *37*:597–601, 1982, by permission of the New England Journal of Medicine.)

The effects of vitamin A status and its related disease are widespread throughout the body and are in turn affected by ethanol consumption. Hepatotoxicity from diminished vitamin A includes the presence of multivesicular lysosomes and is potentiated by concomitant alcohol intake.[115] Hepatotoxicity from increased vitamin A also includes fibrosis,[116,117] which also is potentiated by concomitant alcohol.[118] The squamous metaplasia of rodent trachea due to vitamin A depletion is also enhanced by ethanol.[119] Ethanol increases vitamin A in lung and esophagus.[120] The role of alcohol in increasing vitamin A content of some tissues while having the opposite effect in others, speeding or altering the conversion of vitamin A to metabolites, probably has important consequences for the hepatotoxicity, fibrosis, and squamous metaplasia described above. Alcohol-mediated alterations of vitamin A status could be relevant to the association of low vitamin A or carotene levels with malignant diseases.[120,121]

Several factors make vitamin A therapy a complicated affair in the setting of alcoholism: assessment of tissue stores of vitamin A is difficult, vitamin A in high doses is toxic, even usual doses of vitamin A are potentially toxic with continued intake of alcohol (or other microsome-inducing drugs), and monitoring vitamin A hepatotoxicity is difficult in the presence of continued alcohol intake. Vitamin A replacement must therefore be modest for patients who cannot be assured an alcohol- and drug-free environment. Replacement of vitamin A should be considered for patients who are confirmed as deficient and who can be assured abstinence from alcohol. Night blindness (or abnormal dark adaptation) with low serum vitamin A (<30 μg/dl, or 1.4 μM/L) may be considered evidence of deficiency. Vitamin A given at 2000 μg per day for several weeks should provide an adequate trial. A low serum zinc (>80 μg/dl) can be treated with doses of 600 μg $ZnSO_4$ per day, considering the interrelationship of vitamin A and zinc metabolism. Zinc therapy, therefore, might also be tried when vitamin A therapy fails. Documented fat malabsorption should prompt parenteral replacement of vitamin A. These recommendations appear reasonable, but are not based on extensive clinical trials.

VITAMIN D

Alcoholics have illness related to abnormalities of calcium, phosphorus, and vitamin D homeostasis. They have decreases in bone density[122] and bone mass,[123] increased susceptibility to fractures,[124] and increased osteonecrosis.[125] Low blood calcium, phosphorus, magnesium, and low, normal, or high vitamin D_3 levels have been reported, indicating disturbed calcium metabolism.[123]

In patients with alcoholic liver disease, vitamin D deficiency probably derives from too little vitamin D substrate, which results from poor dietary intake, malabsorption due to cholestasis or pancreatic insufficiency, and insufficient sunlight. The physiologic sequence is conversion of 7-dehydrocholesterol of animal origin to cholecalciferol (vitamin D_3) by photolysis, followed by hydroxylation to 25-hydroxycholecalciferol (25-OH vitamin D_3) by the liver, and finally hydroxylation to the most active compound, 1,25-dihydroxycholecalciferol (1,25-OH vitamin D_3) by kidney, bone, and placenta. Cholecalciferol absorption depends on intact absorption of fat. The status of 25 hydroxylation appears adequate even in advanced liver disease,[123,126,127] although some disagree.[128] There is a lower concentration of vitamin D binding globulin, a protein synthesized in the liver, in alcoholic liver disease,[126] but because of its excess of binding sites its decrease is an unlikely cause of 25-OH vitamin D_3 deficiency. Gascon-Barré says that although blood levels of 25-OH vitamin D_3 and 1,25-OH vitamin D_3 may be normal or even elevated in alcoholics, their stores of vitamin D_3 are often depleted, severely so in nutritionally depleted alcoholics.[123] Insufficient intake of calcium and phosphorus or decreased calcium absorption in the presence of normal or increased 1,25-OH vitamin D_3 (and parathormone) might accelerate bone loss in alcoholics.

The diagnosis of osteopenia in liver disease may require bone densitometry because other clinical parameters of liver disease correlate poorly with osteopenia.[129] Moreover, levels of free 25-OH vitamin D_3 may be normal in liver disease when total levels are low.[130] Bone disease in patients with liver disease should be treated by increasing intake of vitamin D_3, ultraviolet light therapy, and correction of fat malabsorption to keep plasma calcium and phosphorus normal. Of course, abstinence from alcohol is very important.

VITAMIN K

Vitamin K deficiency in alcoholism may arise when there is an interruption of fat absorption due to pancreatic insufficiency, biliary obstruction, or intestinal mucosal abnormality secondary to folic acid deficiency. Dietary vitamin K inadequacy is not a likely cause of clinical deficiency unless there is concomitant sterilization of the large gut, a reliable source of the vitamin. Alcohol-induced hepatocyte injury interferes with utilization of available vitamin K with a consequent drop in blood levels of clotting factors II, VII, IX, and X, whose syntheses depend on this vitamin. Vitamin K serves as a cofactor for the microsomal carboxylase that affects post-translational modification of these proteins, the conversion of glutamic acid (Glu) residues to γ-carboxyglutamic acid (Gla) residues, which is necessary for function. Abnormally high levels of inactive factor II (prothrombin) are found in the plasma in the presence of cirrhosis or vitamin K deficiency.[131] Vitamin K may be given intramuscularly to clinically test whether hepatocellular dysfunction or lack of availability of vitamin K to the liver is responsible for low levels of vitamin K–dependent clotting factors in the blood.[132]

VITAMIN E AND SELENIUM

Vitamin E and selenium serve protective roles as antioxidants and interact physiologically.[133–136] Vitamin E is a powerful antioxidant that prevents peroxidation of cellular and subcellular membrane phospholipids. Selenium is also involved in antioxidant functions and is a component of red blood cell glutathione peroxidase. Vitamin E and selenium function synergistically: vitamin E reduces selenium requirement, prevents its loss from the body, and maintains it in an active form; selenium spares vitamin E and reduces the requirement for the vitamin.[135]

Vitamin E deficiency is not a recognized complication of alcoholism, but has occurred in adults with diverse causes of fat malabsorption[133] and primary biliary cirrhosis.[137] Clinical manifestations include decreased erythrocyte survival and neurologic disturbances (areflexia, gait disturbance, decreased proprioception and vibratory sensation, ophthalmoplegia).

When rodents were fed ethanol repeatedly in one study their hepatic vitamin E levels, measured as α-tocopherol, were low[138]; this was accompanied by increased hepatic lipid peroxidation when alcohol was combined with a low–vitamin E diet.[139] The mechanism of hepatic vitamin E depletion by ethanol is probably enhanced oxidation of α-tocopherol (α-Toc) to α-tocopherol quinone (αTQ) in liver microsomes.[139] Alcohol-induced liver injury may be mediated, in part, by stress on cellular antioxidant mechanisms interrelated with vitamin E and selenium. Considering the findings in humans with fat malabsorption or severe cholestasis, and the evidence of vitamin E depletion by chronic alcohol feeding of experimental animals, it would seem that there is great potential for vitamin E deficiency in chronic alcoholics who may combine low vitamin E intake with steatorrhea from chronic pancreatitis or prolonged cholestasis. Indeed, in alcoholic patients with pancreatic insufficiency and fat malabsorption, low serum vitamin E levels were recently reported.[140]

Selenium metabolism is of great theoretic interest to hepatologists in view of the proposed lipoperoxidative mechanism of drug- and alcohol-induced liver injury.[141] Interestingly, serum selenium levels have been recorded as low in the alcoholic, especially in the presence of liver disease, but this may be a consequence of liver injury,[141] because other nonalcoholic patients with liver disease also have low levels. No recommendation for dietary modifications of vitamin E or selenium intake in alcoholism can yet be made.

WATER, MINERALS, ELECTROLYTES

SALT AND WATER RETENTION OF CIRRHOSIS

Alcoholics with chronic liver disease often have disorders of water and electrolyte balance. Sodium and water retention are clinically apparent as weight gain, peripheral edema, ascites, and pleural effusions. Patients may have respiratory difficulties or umbilical herniation as further complications. Not only is sodium retained avidly, but a water load cannot be excreted normally.[142] Low body potassium may result from vomiting, diarrhea, hyperaldosteronism, muscle wasting, renal tubular acidosis, or diuretic therapy. Potassium depletion may contribute to the appearance of renal vein ammonia and may worsen hepatic encephalopathy.[143]

The pathogenesis of fluid retention and ascites is complex. At the hepatic level, portal hypertension, hypoalbuminemia, and alteration of lymph flow are important factors for ascites formation.[144] Endocrine accompaniments and other phenomena suggest that the body is reacting to a diminished "effective circulating volume" (total blood volume is normal or elevated, but a disproportionately large fraction is sequestered in the splanchnic region)[145]: hyperreninemia, hyperaldosteronemia, increased blood norepinephrine, and reversal of salt and water retention by restoration of nonsplanchnic volume via head-out body immersion in water or via peritoneal venous (LeVeen) shunting of ascites. Additionally there may be a relative insufficiency of factors (or insensitivity to such factors) that promote salt loss by the kidneys, such as atrial natriuretic factor (ANF),[146] because ANF levels are raised[147,148] and there is an abnormality of renal hemodynamics based, in part, on alterations in renal prostaglandins.[146]

Patients with cirrhosis and fluid overload may require urgent relief, as when ascites and pleural effusion are causing respiratory difficulties or when imminent rupture of an umbilical hernia may result in lethal peritonitis. Thoracentesis, paracentesis, or both should be performed promptly. Usually, diuresis may be unhurried once a diagnostic tap has shown the fluid to be noninfected transudate. Treatment is aimed at preventing recurrence of fluid retention. Dietary management combines sodium and water restriction. It is difficult to provide a palatable diet on a long-term basis with less then 0.5 to 1 g of sodium and 1500 to 2000 ml of total fluid daily. These amounts are recommended with addition of spironolactone, followed, if necessary, by small doses of diuretics (hydrochlorothiazide or furosemide), to achieve an initial daily weight loss of no more than 0.5 kg.[149] More-rapid weight loss is probably safe when the patient has mobilizable peripheral edema, and when the patient can be observed carefully.[149] Accelerated diuresis risks renal failure. Use of prostaglandin inhibitors such as nonsteroidal anti-inflammatory drugs (NSAID) carries the potential risk of altering renal hemodynamics and precipitating renal failure. Careful monitoring for the development of hypokalemia (or hyperkalemia), hyponatremia, and renal failure must be undertaken. Recently, periodic large volume paracenteses have again been resorted to, with intravenous fluid and albumin, and seem to be as safe as diuretics.[150] For patients in whom a reasonable program of salt and water restriction and diuretic therapy is not successful, or for whom periodic paracentesis is cumbersome, a peritoneal-venous (LaVeen) shunt may be useful.[151–153] Best results have been obtained for patients without encephalopathy, coagulopathy, or severe jaundice.

MAGNESIUM

Neuromuscular excitability in acute alcohol withdrawal resembles that seen in magnesium deficiency. Therefore the status of magnesium in alcoholism has been investigated for some time. It was found that acute doses of ethanol caused magnesium loss in the urine,[154] although chronic ethanol feeding resulted in no change in urinary magnesium.[155] Flink has summarized much work in the field to show that alcoholism is associated with magnesium deficiency[156]: alcoholics have low blood magnesium and low body-exchangeable magnesium; symptoms in alcoholics resemble those in patients with magnesium deficiency of other causes; alcohol ingestion causes magnesium excretion; upon withdrawal from alcohol magnesium balance is positive; and hypocalcemia in alcoholics may only be responsive to magnesium repletion. The correlation of magnesium content of blood with that of other tissues and with the severity of clinical symptoms in individual cases is imperfect, although it is statistically obvious among groups. Magnesium replacement should be seriously considered for symptomatic patients with measurably low serum magnesium, for anorectic patients with low serum magnesium, and for hypocalcemic alcoholics who do not respond to calcium replacement. The majority of alcoholics will replete body stores of magnesium readily from normal dietary sources.

IRON

Iron metabolism is important in alcoholism in that there may be deficiency or there may be excess of iron in the body. The status of transferrin may provide a marker for chronic alcohol consumption.

Alcoholics may be iron-deficient as a result of the several gastrointestinal lesions to which they are prone and that may bleed (esophagitis, esophageal varices, gastritis, duodenitis). The usual laboratory indicators, red blood cell morphology (with alertness to altered morphology in the presence of folate deficiency), serum iron, and serum iron-binding capacity, are helpful. Iron therapy should be restricted to clearly diagnosed cases of deficiency.

There is an increased hepatic iron content in autopsy studies of most patients with early alcoholic cirrhosis.[157] Iron overload of the liver was described in Bantus who consumed alcoholic beverages prepared in iron containers that thereby contributed a large amount of elemental iron to their diet. In most alcoholics, the iron content of the liver is normal or only modestly elevated, although there may be stainable iron in reticuloendothelial cells, possibly due to hepatic necrosis or bouts of hemolysis. It is unclear whether increased intestinal absorption of iron due to alcohol[158] or hepatic uptake of iron from serum in established alcoholic liver disease[159] contributes significantly to an increase in hepatic iron. There should be little difficulty in distinguishing the hepatic iron increases of alcoholic liver disease from the much higher amounts characteristic of genetic hemochromatosis, using a measure of absolute iron content per gram of liver with upward adjustments for age.[160,161] Of great potential significance is the contribution hepatic iron may make to liver damage via its role in lipid peroxidation[162] (perhaps in conjunction with the effects of alcohol) and its possible role in promoting fibrogenesis.[163]

Alcoholism has been reported to result in qualitative changes in transferrin, the serum transport protein for iron: a higher fraction of molecules bear a reduced sialic acid content.[164,165] This provides a useful test for chronic alcohol consumption.[166,167] The synthesis of transferrin is decreased at the stage of alcoholic cirrhosis, as is serum transferrin concentration.[168] At the stage of alcoholic fatty liver the serum transferrin concentration is normal, although catabolic rate and presumably synthesis are both increased.[168] The significance of these changes in transferrin is not yet apparent.

ZINC

Zinc is an essential element for man; deficiency results in growth retardation, male hypogonadism, rough dry skin, disordered taste, poor appetite, and mental lethargy. It is absorbed from the small bowel. In the rat, the ileum has the greatest capacity for absorption[169] and appears to increase absorption when zinc deficiency is produced experimentally.[170] Among the enzymes that contain zinc are hepatic alcohol dehydrogenase (which converts ethanol to acetaldehyde), ocular retinol dehydrogenase (which converts retinol to retinal), and hepatic and erythrocyte superoxide dismutases (which serve to protect against oxidative damage). Zinc deficiency induced in rats results in poor growth and lowered hepatic alcohol dehydrogenase, with diminished rate of elimination of a test dose of ethanol.[171,172] Diminished capacity for conversion of retinol to retinal was found in the retinas of zinc-deficient rats in one study.[172] Hypogonadism in zinc-deficient rats is attributed to Leydig cell failure rather than to pituitary changes.[173]

Alcoholic cirrhosis is associated with abnormalities of zinc homeostasis, although the clinical implications are uncertain. Patients have low plasma zinc,[174] low liver zinc,[175] and an increase in urinary zinc.[175,176] Acute ethanol ingestion, however, does not cause zincuria.[177] The low zinc content of chronic alcoholics with cirrhosis is thought to be due to decreased intake and decreased absorption as well as increased urinary excretion. Many Americans have a diet that is marginal in zinc.[178] Alcoholics fall into several of those groups with marginal intake. It is interesting that zinc absorption has been shown to be low in alcoholic cirrhotics but not in patients with cirrhosis of other causes.[179] Some instances of night blindness not fully responsive to vitamin A replacement (see vitamin A discussion) have responded to zinc replacement. It is possible that human hypogonadism of alcoholism may involve pertubations of vitamin A and zinc interactions, but this is largely unstudied.

Currently the therapeutic use of zinc in alcoholism is restricted to the treatment of night blindness not responsive to vitamin A. Sullivan and his colleagues could not raise serum zinc in patients with alcoholic cirrhosis: zinc was increased in the urine.[180,181]

COPPER

Hepatic copper content is increased in advanced alcoholic cirrhosis.[157] Serum copper content has been reported to be elevated in alcoholics independent of the stage of liver disease,[182] but others have reported normal levels.[181] These findings have no known clinical significance.

TRACE METALS

Nickel is consistently increased in alcoholic liver disease; manganese and chromium are unchanged.[157] Intracellular shifts in trace metals have been described upon acute administration of alcohol.[183] These shifts, with possible effects on organelle function, may be important but are not revealed in measurement of whole organ content. Versiek reported increased serum molybdenum in patients with acute liver disease;[184] increased levels were not seen in those patients with cirrhosis. The clinical significance of trace metal changes is yet obscure, except for the cardiotoxicity ascribed long ago to alcoholic beverages with high cobalt content.

EFFECT OF ETHANOL ON METABOLISM OF CARBOHYDRATES, URIC ACID, LIPIDS, AND PROTEINS

CARBOHYDRATES

The clinical problems of carbohydrate metabolism include hyperglycemia (frequent, but rarely severe or life-threatening), hypoglycemia (infrequent, mostly occurring in conjunction with fasting or prolonged poor food intake, except in children, but which can be lethal), and disaccharide (mostly lactose) malabsorption.

In large population studies, alcohol intake correlates with hyperglycemia.[184] Except in patients with chronic pancreatitis and endocrine (insulin) insufficiency there had been no ready explanation for this until recently. The suspicion was that ethanol per se impaired glucose tolerance,[185,186] but this was difficult to prove because the elevated insulin levels that accompanied alcohol intake could have been a reflection of insulin resistance due to alcohol or to the augmentation of insulin release that alcohol itself causes.[187–189] Insulin resistance caused by alcohol has now been demonstrated in healthy subjects using the insulin clamp technique whereby glucose utilization is measured during glucose infusions at steady blood glucose and insulin levels.[190]

In the fed state, when liver glycogen is abundant, glycogenolysis supports blood glucose levels. In the fasting state, the following pathways that can support blood glucose are interfered with by concomitant metabolism of alcohol: glycogenesis from amino acids, formation of glucose from glycerol, lactate, and galactose.[191,192] Increase in the NADH/NAD ratio from hepatic metabolism of alcohol is partly responsible for these metabolic changes. Changes in enzyme activities relevant to various metabolic steps of gluconeogenesis[193,194] and lipogenesis[10] have also been described. Clinically, hypoglycemia must be suspected when an alcohol imbiber exhibits altered mental status (even in the fed state, especially in children). Provision of glucose, usually intravenously, is simple and effective.

Monosaccharide malabsorption due to alcohol can be demonstrated experimentally, but as a clinical problem in alcoholics it is probably restricted to those with folic acid deficiency. Malabsorption in alcoholics with folic acid deficiency can be documented by the xylose tolerance test.[195,196] Long-term ethanol ingestion depresses intestinal disaccharidase activities (sucrase, maltase, and lactase)[197] and is associated with lactose intolerance (see Figs. 64–4 to 64–6).[110,198]

URIC ACID

It is an old observation that drinking alcoholic beverages is associated with precipitation of acute gouty attacks. Hyperuricemia accompanying bouts of intense alcohol intake has been shown to occur in patients without known disorders of uric acid metabolism or renal function.[197] An important mechanism of alcoholic hyperuricemia is decreased urinary excretion of uric acid secondary to elevated serum lactate. This is illustrated in data from one patient in Figure 64–8.[197] Lactate is produced in the liver from pyruvate by the action of NADH generated in the metabolism of ethanol by alcohol dehydrogenase. Depending on the metabolic state of the liver, NADH generation either enhances hepatic lactate production or prevents the liver from completing the

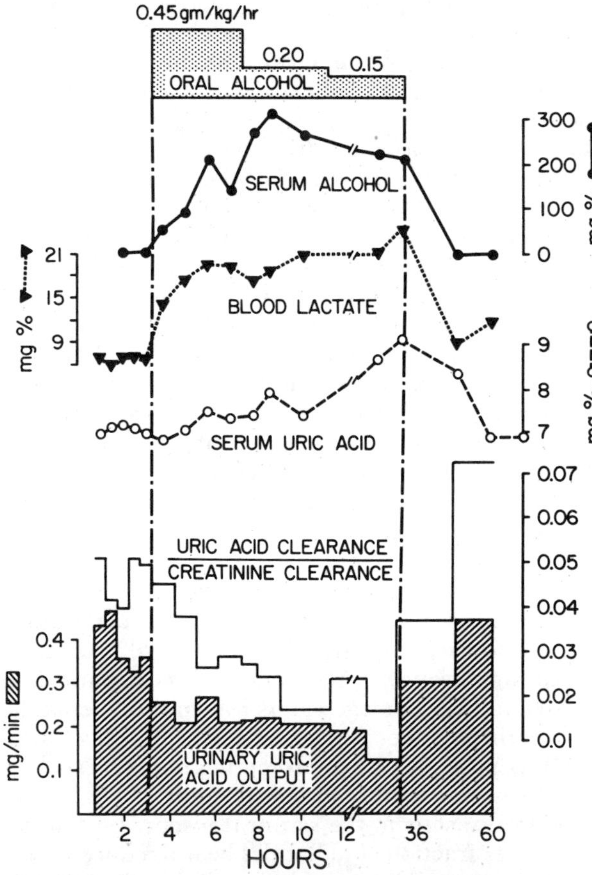

FIGURE 64–8. Effect of oral ethanol on blood and urine uric acid and lactate. (From Lieber, C.S., Jones, D.P., Losowsky, M.S., et al.: J. Clin. Invest., *41*:1863, 1962, by copyright permission of the American Society of Clinical Investigation.)

Cori cycle and utilizing lactate originating in peripheral tissues, especially lactate produced from muscle activity during alcohol withdrawal.[199] Alcohol-associated ketosis or starvation may also provoke hyperuricemia. The renal mechanism neither depends on pH of the urine[197] nor is abolished by probenecid[200]: it remains unexplained.

Increase in urate production partly due to increase in adenosine nucleotide turnover has caused hyperuricemia in gouty volunteers.[88] Urinary urate clearance was increased and urinary urate and oxypurines were higher in the study. This mechanism was demonstrated at lower blood alcohol levels than were achieved by those investigating the lactate-related renal mechanism, and the blood alcohol levels were also lower than those usually seen in patients with alcoholic hyperuricemia. The purine content (guanosine) of some beers may also be a contributing factor for hyperuricemia and gout in alcoholic subjects.[201]

Gouty patients should refrain from significant alcohol intake, especially of purine-containing beers. The hyperuricemia encountered in the recent drinker should be observed during several days to a week of abstinence, which will allow alcoholic hyperuricemia to recede; thus a costly work-up for other causes of hyperuricemia may be avoided.

LIPIDS, FATTY LIVER, HYPERLIPIDEMIA, KETOACIDOSIS

Alcohol ingestion is associated with fatty infiltration of the liver, hyperlipidemia, and ketosis, each of which is largely explained by the effects that alcohol has on the metabolism of lipids.[202]

Fatty liver is composed of triglycerides having fatty acids derived from dietary sources, when available, but of endogenously synthesized ones when dietary fatty acids are not available. High-fat diets increase the amount of fat that accumulates. Low-fat diets, high-protein diets, and even hypocaloric diets will lessen the amount of fat that accumulates because of alcohol, but will not completely prevent fatty liver. Dietary fat composed of triglycerides of medium chain length causes less hepatic fat accumulation than fat containing triglycerides of long-chain fatty acids. The increase in NADH/NAD ratio consequent to the oxidation of alcohol to acetaldehyde, by alcohol dehydrogenase (ADH), reduces NAD availability for fatty acid oxidation by the citric acid cycle and thereby depresses fatty acid oxidation. Because of structural damage to mitochondria, oxidation of 2 carbon fragments from all sources is inhibited. The major pathway of fatty acid synthesis, in the cytosol, is not increased. Fatty acid elongation by mitochondria is stimulated, probably by the increased NADH/NAD ratio. Glycerolipid synthesis is increased as a result of the greater availability of fatty acids (as described above), the conversion of dihydroxy acetone phosphate to glycerol-3-phosphate favored by the increased NADH/NAD ratio, and possibly the increased capacity of lipid-synthesizing mechanisms. There is increased activity both of the rate-limiting enzyme, phosphatidate phosphohydrolase, which removes phosphorus from phospatidic acid to form diacylglycerol, and of diacylglycerol acyl transferase, which catalyzes the formation of triglycerides. These enzymes are present in both endoplasmic reticulum and cytosol.

The administration of ethanol to man consistently results in hyperlipidemia; the extent is modified by associated dietary and pathologic conditions. The major elevation occurs in serum triglycerides with some cholesterol elevation; the involved lipoproteins are very low-density lipoproteins (VLDL) and chylomicrons, dietary particles formed by the intestines (Fig. 64–9). High-density lipoproteins (HDL) are also increased by ethanol. Alcoholic hyperlipemia is usually classified as type IV according to the International Classification of Hyperlipidemias and Hyperlipoproteinemias because it is composed mostly of VLDL, but may be classified as type V when chylomicrons are also present. About 6% of alcoholics have type II hyperlipidemia, hypercholesterolemia due to increased low-density lipoproteins (LDL). Alcohol-induced hyperlipemia may change rapidly in

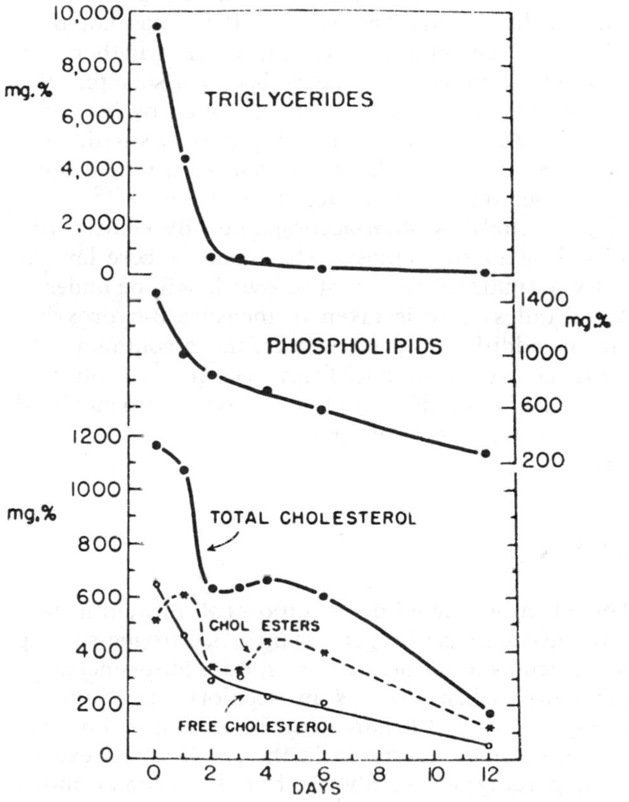

FIGURE 64–9. Serum lipids in the alcoholic and the effect of withdrawal from ethanol. Lipid fractions decrease at varying rates. (From Losowsky, M.S., Jones, D.P., Davidson, C.S., et al.: Am. J. Med., *35*:794, 1963.)

composition when clearing because of more-rapid clearing of triglycerides than of cholesterol and phospholipids. The postprandial hyperlipidemia is greatly exaggerated by fat-containing meals.[203] When alcohol is administered for several weeks at a dosage of 300 g per day the initial several-fold increase in triglycerides gradually returns to normal.[204] This may be due to liver damage or increased lipoprotein lipase activity. Hyperlipemia is usually absent with severe liver injury (e.g., cirrhosis), and hypolipemia may be present.[205–207]

Some patients may have marked hyperlipemia during alcohol ingestion. This most likely represents an underlying genetic defect in lipid metabolism in addition to the effects of alcohol, such as hyperchylomicronemia (type I) due to decreased postheparin lipoprotein lipase activity,[198] carbohydrate sensitive hyperlipidemia,[208] diabetes, obesity, pancreatitis, or other diseases.

The treatment of alcohol-induced hyperlipidemia consists of abstinence from alcohol and provision of a normal diet. A low-fat diet is unpalatable, may lead to inadequate energy intake,[209] and is not usually necessary. The lipemia should rapidly disappear. Associated factors such as obesity and diabetes should be appropriately treated. Persistent hyperlipemia requires investigation for genetic or other causes not related to alcohol.

Moderate alcohol intake is associated with an increase in the fasting levels of a species of high-density lipoprotein cholesterol (HDL_3) whose significance regarding risk for heart disease, unlike that for HDL_2, has not been established. Therefore, it is not clear whether any decreased risk for coronary heart disease associated with moderate alcohol intake can be explained by increased levels of HDL due to alcohol. HDL_2 increases with more substantial alcohol intake, but this level of intake is not cardioprotective and may even be deleterious.[210]

Alcohol intake is often accompanied by ketosis with minimal or absent acidosis. The blood glucose level is usually normal.[211] The extent of ketosis will be underestimated unless care is taken to measure β-hydroxybutyrate in addition to acetoacetate, more common with diabetic ketosis. Abstinence from alcohol and a return to normal diet is usually the only required treatment. Fluid and electrolytes may be given. Insulin is usually not required.

PROTEIN

The effect of ethanol per se on overall protein metabolism, measured as nitrogen balance, is nitrogen-sparing when given as additional calories, but causes increased urinary urea when given as an isocaloric substitute for carbohydrate.[212,213] Ethanol can be shown to interfere with amino acid absorption in the gut in many experimental paradigms (see above), but the ultimate nutritional consequences are unknown because gross malabsorption of protein has not been demonstrated. An increase in urea nitrogen could represent protein that has escaped small bowel absorption, has been converted to ammonia in the colon, and subsequently has been converted to urea by the liver.[213] As reviewed elsewhere,[214] ethanol given in single doses causes impaired hepatic amino acids uptake, decreased gluconeogenesis, increased serum branched chain amino acids, and impaired synthesis of lipoproteins[215] and albumin.[216,217] Given over time ethanol causes impaired protein secretion from the liver probably related to alterations in microtubles and retention of proteins in enlarged hepatocytes.[218] The importance of these effects on the hepatotoxicity of ethanol is being studied. Manipulation of dietary protein is not suggested during active alcoholism. The alterations in intermediary metabolism, including amino acids and nitrogen, in established cirrhosis and the implications for diet therapy will be dealt with in Chapter 63.

EFFECTS OF DIETARY FACTORS ON ETHANOL METABOLISM

Alcohol is metabolized to acetaldehyde predominantly by alcohol dehydrogenase (ADH), a cytosolic enzyme, and also by the microsomal ethanol oxiding system (MEOS) found in the endoplasmic reticulum. ADH is considered by some to be rate-limiting for the oxidation of ethanol.[219] Low-protein diets reduce hepatic ADH in rats[220] and lower ethanol oxidation rates in rats[220] and in man.[221] Prolonged fasting also decreases ethanol oxidation rates as shown in isolated rat liver cells. A mechanism for lowered metabolism of ethanol during fasting is the lack of available metabolites to shuttle reducing equivalents from ethanol oxidation into mitochondria.[222] For a given alcohol intake, malnourished alcoholics may develop higher blood alcohol levels and sustain them longer than normally nourished individuals,[223] with possible deleterous consequences. Other forms of ADH have recently been discovered in the stomach and are responsible for metabolism of ethanol before it reaches the portal circulation and the liver.[224,225] Gastric ADH is lower in women,[226] allowing for higher blood alcohol levels, for similar alcohol ingestion, than occurs in men. Gastric ADH is also inhibited by the histamine H_2-receptor antagonist cimetitidine taken orally.

A study showed that MEOS activity in the liver showed greater induction when given with a normal rather than a low-fat diet in rats, although induction of the P450IIE1 specific for ethanol metabolism was the same.[227]

ALCOHOL, NUTRITION, AND ORGAN DAMAGE IN THE ALCOHOLIC

LIVER

The role of nutrition in the pathogenesis of alcoholic liver injury (fatty liver, hepatitis, and cirrhosis) has been investigated from the perspectives of epidemiology, clinical therapeutic trials, and animal experimentation:

the direct toxic effect of ethanol in each case was considered.

Malnutrition was previously thought to be important for the development of alcoholic fatty liver: it is present in kwashiorkor (particularly in children); a highly visible subset of alcoholics with fatty liver is malnourished (the "skid row" denizens); and rodents could readily be given fatty livers when subjected to diets deficient in lipotropes (see below). Our current understanding is that alcohol per se, given in sufficient quantities, can cause fatty liver in man (and lower animals) despite the presence of an otherwise adequate diet.[228–232] The lipid and protein composition of the diet have modulating effects on the amount and types of fat that accumulate in the liver. Reduction of dietary fat to 10% of total calories (but not lower) greatly lessens, but does not completely eliminate, hepatic fat accumulation. Fatty acids of chain length found in the diet accumulate in the liver when available from the diet; otherwise endogenously synthesized fatty acids deposit. Long-chain fatty acids in the diet have a greater tendency than medium-chain fatty acids to promote fatty liver in the presence of ethanol. However, provision of higher than usually recommended dietary protein (25% of total calories) will not eliminate hepatic fat accumulation. The amount of fat accumulating in the ethanol-induced fatty liver is but one parameter of damage, and must be considered along with organelle dysfunction and metabolic imbalances.

Lipotrope deficiency (choline and methionine) can cause fatty liver in rats,[233] and so attention was first directed towards the possible relevance of such deficiency for human alcoholic liver disease. However, there is no evidence that dietary choline deficiency causes human liver disease or is a part of ethanol-induced liver disease. Additionally, choline therapy is not effective when alcohol intake is continued.[234–238] The difference in susceptibility to choline deficiency between rats and man is not surprising in view of the low choline oxidase activity in human liver.

The inappropriateness of the extrapolation of choline deficiency data in experimental animals to human alcoholic liver disease is also manifested by the differences between choline deficiency and ethanol-induced liver injury. The lesions differ ultrastructurally,[239] in the levels of hepatic carnitine with which they are associated (increased with ethanol[240] and decreased with choline deficiency[241]), in their response to orotic acid supplementation[242] and in the decrease in lipoprotein production and serum lipoproteins in choline deficiency[243,244] and the opposite changes due to alcohol.[245] Even in rats choline supplementation has failed to fully prevent ethanol-induced lesions.[226,247] Dietary supplementation with choline, at times to extraordinary levels, did not prevent ethanol-induced fatty liver, fibrosis, and ultrastructural lesions[248] and was associated with hepatotoxicity of its own at high levels. Side effects such as nausea, vomiting, salivation, sweating, and anorexia have been noted with choline supplementation.[249]

In summary, current evidence shows no relevance of choline deficiency hepatotoxicity to that induced by ethanol in humans or in experimental animals. Should a subtle interaction be proved in the future, it is unlikely that choline supplementation could be provided safely as treatment.

The role of nutrition in the pathogenesis of alcoholic hepatitis has been studied in much less detail. It is a lesion considered too severe to be induced in volunteers.

Alcoholic cirrhosis has been directly linked to the intensity of ethanol consumption by its drop in the United States during the prohibition era and during World War II when alcoholic beverages were rationed.[250,251] The studies of Lelbach also show the direct influence of intensity of alcohol consumption (g/kg per day × years) on the incidence of chronic liver disease in patients admitted to alcohol rehabilitation spas in Europe.[252] Neither the beverage source of ethanol nor concomitant malnutrition was noted to be an influence. These findings have been confirmed.[253] The implied direct effect of ethanol in causing hepatic fibrosis and cirrhosis has been confirmed in the baboon model of hepatic injury.[254–256]

The direct hepatotoxic effect of ethanol has been shown histologically (by light and electron microscopy) and biochemically in both alcoholics and nonalcoholics regardless of dietary variation in fat, protein, vitamins, and lipotropes.[237,257–260] The intimate mechanism of ethanol-related cell injury is under active investigation and includes consideration of alteration of the NADH/NAD ratio (a consequence of ethanol oxidation), alterations of calcium flux, and lipid peroxidation. Ethanol intake may influence lipid peroxidation via its induction of the endoplasmic reticulum, which contains relevant enzyme activities. Interactions of ethanol with selenium, iron, copper, and zinc, each of which is related to cellular control of peroxidation, are under study and have been reviewed.[141] Dietary imbalances are not inferred and dietary manipulations are not warranted from these very preliminary studies.

The role of nutrition in the recovery from alcoholic liver injury was studied by clinicians before the pathogenesis of the injury was understood. Patek et al.[261,262] and Morrison[263] demonstrated the efficacy of a normal-protein, normal-fat, vitamin-enriched diet in the treatment of cirrhosis as measured by clinical response and longevity. Erenoglu et al., extending previous work, treated cirrhotic patients with 198 ml of ethanol daily and an adequate diet; they found no adverse effects and a possible benefit from higher dietary protein.[264] This level of alcohol intake was much lower than that which many alcoholics ingest spontaneously. In view of the current appreciation of the direct toxicity of ethanol, and the lack of control that most alcoholics have in limiting their alcohol intake, strict abstinence from alcohol is recommended.

The significance of congeners,[265] moderate dosages of alcohol, genetic factors, and marginal nutritional deficiencies in alcohol-related tissue injury and in the recovery phase is under study.

There is no established prophylatic regimen except abstinence. As discussed previously, our best evidence indicates that acute liver damage consistently occurs if sufficient alcohol is ingested, and is not preventable by provision of a nutritious diet. There probably are safe levels of intake, although they have not been carefully established clinically. In any case, alcoholics are not usually able to control their drinking at lower levels. Chronic liver injury from alcohol also appears to be dose- and time-related with no indication that dietary manipulation will act as a preventative. Patients with precursor lesions, such as perivenular fibrosis,[141] require special attention, but the treatment approach is still abstinence. Efforts to define populations with varying degrees of susceptibility to ethanol-induced liver disease on the basis of genetics or viral exposure have not yet been convincing; however, females are more susceptible than males.[266,267] We cannot advise a different approach for any group. Nutritional treatment of cirrhosis and its complications is described in Chapter 63.

STROKE

The incidence of stroke is strongly associated with advancing age, black race, obesity, and hypertension. Moderate to heavy alcohol consumption, over 45 g per day, has been identified as an independent predictor of stroke after the increased risk due to hypertension and cigarette smoking were accounted for.[268] A reviewer of most of the English language literature concludes that moderate alcohol intake, less than 60 g per day, has a complex association with ischemic stroke in white populations (very low levels are possibly protective and higher levels are definitely deleterious), but little, if any, association in Japanese populations; by contrast, moderate drinking increases hemorrhagic stroke (intracerebral and subarachoid hemorrhage) in diverse populations.[269] Alcohol consumption may contribute to stroke by raising blood pressure to hypertensive levels as shown by most,[28,270–272] but not all,[273] studies. Sodium intake and phosphorus intake were also positively identified as nutrient predictors of hypertension.[28] Some authors have detected an immediacy of alcohol intake just prior to stroke[274] (although others have not[269]), which points to acute alcohol-induced changes that might precipitate stroke.[275] If true, this finding is encouraging in that abstinence might yield early benefits.

HEART

Acute and chronic alcohol consumption affects the heart in some ways that are understood and in others that are obscure. The acute effects of even small amounts of hard liquor (several ounces) include measureable myocardial depression,[276] effects such as a dose-dependent impairment of left ventricular emptying at rest,[277] and electrophysiologic effects such as slight delay in atrial conduction and shortening of both the atrioventricular conduction time and the effective ventricular myocardial refractory period.[278] These usually are not clinically apparent in people with normal hearts, especially because the impaired left ventricular emptying disappears with exercise.[277] Patients with angina pectoris, even with congestive failure, have responses in left ventricular performance similar to those seen in controls at blood alcohol levels of 100 mg/dl.[277] In patients with myocardial ischemia an unfavorable distribution of coronary blood flow away from ischemic areas may occur.[279] The result of alcohol intake is thus not always predictable because it depends on the relative influence of alcohol on peripheral vasodilatation, coronary blood flow, direct myocardial depression, electrophysiologic changes, and the extent of underlying cardiac reserve.[280] Patients with chronic alcoholism or heart disease[280] and even normal nonalcoholic patients may develop atrial arrhythmias after substantial acute alcohol ingestion.[281,282]

Chronic alcohol consumption may result in heart disease by its association with hypertension, as already discussed in relation to stroke, or by its association with severe thiamin deficiency in the beriberi heart syndrome. The relevance of alcohol-induced changes in serum HDL cholesterol to the appearance of heart disease is not established (see earlier discussion of lipemia). Most of the epidemiologic studies of alcohol intake and either coronary artery disease or, more usually, total cardiac death rate show a U-shaped relationship with an increase in disease in abstainers or near abstainers, the lowest incidence of disease in moderate drinkers (1 to 2 ounces of hard liquor or the equivalent per day), and the greatest incidence of disease in those who consume larger amounts of alcohol. These results may be found in the Hawaiian study,[283] the Milwaukee study,[284] and a study of the elderly in Massachusetts,[285] but not clearly in the Albany experience.[286]

A fairly characteristic syndrome known as alcoholic cardiomyopathy has been described in a subset of these individuals with alcoholism and heart disease. It is a congestive cardiomyopathy seen typically in men aged 30 to 55 years who have been drinking 30 to 50% of calories as alcohol for 10 to 15 years.[280] Arrhythmias are frequent. Coronary artery disease, hypertension, valvular abnormalities, and congenital heart disease must be excluded before the diagnosis of this disorder is made. Treatment with rest, diuretics, and abstention from alcohol may yield dramatic improvement,[287,288] but many times does not.

BLOOD AND BONE MARROW

In addition to the anemias due to blood loss and folic acid deficiency already discussed, alcohol has direct or at least unexplained effects on the blood elements. Alcohol ingestion is associated with vacuolization of erythroid precursors, which is not prevented by adequate diet and pharmacologic doses of folic acid.[289] Alcohol ingestion also causes granulocytopenia, probably mediated by nutritional inadequacy,[289] thrombocytopenia, and impairment of platelet function,[290,291] which are partly attributed to direct effects because they are not mediated by folic acid or other identifiable nutritional deficiencies.

NUTRITIONAL THERAPY IN ALCOHOLISM

Nutritional therapy in alcoholism is directed at the prevention of illness due to alcoholism, the treatment of documented or presumed deficiencies, and the management of complications of alcoholism. As discussed previously, individuals consuming over 30% of total calories as alcohol have a high probability of ingesting less than the recommended daily amounts of carbohydrate, protein, fat, vitamins A, C, and B (especially thiamin), and minerals such as calcium and iron. It is sensible to recommend a complete diet comparable to that of nonalcoholics to forestall deficiency syndromes, although some organ damage due to direct toxicity of alcohol (e.g., alcoholic liver disease) cannot thereby be fully prevented. The feasibility and desirability of adding thiamin and perhaps folic acid to alcoholic beverages has been discussed previously but has not yet been done.

The management of observed deficiencies of protein and calories is straightforward in the absence of organ damage. The treatment of gross malnutrition of proteins and calories in the context of severe acute and chronic liver disease is discussed in Chapter 63. Nervous system damage due to thiamin lack is serious and treatable with a great margin of safety; therefore thiamin deficiency should be presumed if not definitely disproved. Parenteral therapy with 50 mg of thiamin per day should be given until similar doses can be taken by mouth. Riboflavin and pyridoxine should be routinely given at the dosages usually contained in standard multivitamin preparations. Adequate folic acid replacement can be accomplished with the usual hospital diet. Additional replacement is optional unless deficiency is severe. Vitamin A replacement should only be given for well-documented deficiency, and to patients whose abstinence from alcohol is assured (see the earlier discussion on hepatotoxicity of hypervitaminosis A with alcohol). Vitamin A at doses of 2000 to 3000 μg per day may then be given. Zinc replacement should be given for night blindness unresponsive to vitamin A replacement. Magnesium replacement is recommended for symptomatic patients with low serum magnesium. Iron deficiency that has been clearly diagnosed may be replaced in the usual manner orally. Wernicke-Korsakoff syndrome requires at least 50 mg of thiamin daily (parenterally if necessary) for prolonged periods. Beriberi heart failure responds quickly to thiamin. Peripheral nerve damage will necessitate months or years of vitamin B therapy. Acute pancreatitis may require withholding oral feeding for prolonged periods, during which time central venous alimentation must be given (see Chap. 63). Chronic pancreatic exocrine insufficiency is treated by dietary manipulation (often decreases in fat) with oral pancreatic enzymes at mealtime (see Chap. 63). The nutritional management of acute and chronic liver disease due to alcoholism has the aim of defining feeding programs to reverse malnutrition, ameliorate liver disease, and decrease mortality, without promoting hepatic encephalopathy (see Chap. 63).

REFERENCES

1. Feinman, L., Lieber, C.S.: Alcoholism: Clin. Exp. Res., *12*:2–6, 1988.
2. Pekkanen, L., Forsander, O.: Nutr. Bull., *4*:91, 1977.
3. Scheig, R.: Am. J. Clin. Nutr., *23*:467, 1970.
4. Williamson, D.F, Forman, M.R., Binkin, N.J., et al.: Am. J. Public Health, *77*:1324–1330, 1987.
5. Lieber, C.S., Jones, D.P., DeCarli, L.M.: J. Clin. Invest., *44*:1009, 1965.
6. Pirola, R.C., Lieber, C.S.: Pharmacology, *7*:185, 1972.
7. Mezey, E., Faillace, L.A.: J. Nerv. Ment. Dis., *153*:445, 1971.
8. Pirola, R.C., Lieber, C.S.: Pharmacology, *7*:185, 1972.
9. Crouse, J.R., Grundy, S.M.: J. Lipid Res., *25*:486, 1984.
10. Guthrie, G.D., Myers, K.J., Gesser, E.J., et al.: Clin. Exp. Res., *14*:17–22, 1990.
11. Tremolieres, J., Carre, L.: Rev. Alcoolisme, *7*:202, 1961.
12. Stock, M.J., Stuart, J.A.: Nutr. Metabol., *17*:297, 1974.
13. Stock, A.L., Stock, M.J., Stuart, J.A.: Proc. Nutr. Soc., *32*:40A, 1973.
14. Rothwell, N.J., Stock, M.J.: Metabolism, *33*:768, 1984.
15. Pirola, R.C., Lieber, C.S.: J. Nutr., *105*:1544, 1975.
16. Pirola, R.C., Lieber, C.S.: Am. J. Clin. Nutr., *29*:90, 1976.
17. Israel, Y., Videla, L., Bernstein, L.: Fed. Proc., *34*:2052, 1975.
18. Teschke, R., Moreno, F., Heinen, E., et al.: Alcohol Alcohol., *18*:151, 1983.
19. Iber, F.L.: Nutr. Today, *6*:2–9, 1971.
20. Patek, A.J., Toth, E.G., Saunder, M.E., et al.: Arch. Intern. Med., *135*:1053–1057, 1975.
21. Mendenhall, C., Bongiovanni, G., Goldberg, S., et al.: J. Parenter. Enteral. Nutr., *9*:590–596, 1985.
22. Morgan, M.Y.: Acta Chir. Scand., *507 (Suppl.)*81–90, 1981.
23. Simko, V., Connell, A.M., Banks, B.: Am. J. Clin. Nutr., *35*:197–203, 1982.
24. World, M.J., Ryle, P.R., Jones, D., et al.: Alcohol Alcohol., *19*:281–290, 1984.
25. World, M.J., Ryle, P.R., Pratt, O.E., Thompson, A.D.: Alcohol Alcohol., *19*:1–6, 1984.
26. Bebb, H.T., Houser, H.B., Witschi, J.C., et al.: Am. J. Clin. Nutr., *24*:1042–1052, 1971.
27. Neville, J.N., Eagles, J.A., Samson, G., et al.: Am. J. Clin. Nutr., *21*:1329–1340, 1968.
28. Gruchow, H.W., Sobociaski, K.A., Barboriak, J.J.: JAMA, *253*:1567, 1985.
29. Hillers, V.N., Massey, L.K.: Am. J. Clin. Nutr., *41*:356–362, 1985.
30. Westerfeld, W.W., Schulman, M.P.: JAMA, *170*:197–203, 1959.

31. Hillman, R.W.: Alcoholism and Malnutrition. *In* Biology of Alcoholism. Vol. III. Edited by B. Kissin and H. Begleiter. New York, Plenum Press, 1974, pp. 513–560.
32. Datta, S.K., Dukehart, M., Narang, A., et al.: Gastroenterology, *96:*510–518, 1989.
33. Winship, D.H., Carlton, R.C., Zaboralskie, et al.: Gastroenterology, *55:*173–178, 1968.
34. Silver, L.S., Worner, T.M., Korsten, M.A.: Am. J. Gastroenterol., *81:*423–427, 1986.
35. Keshavarzian, A., Iber, F., Ferguson, Y.: Gastroenterology, *92:*621–657, 1987.
36. Gottfried, E.B., Korsten, M.A., Lieber, C.S.: Am. J. Gastroenterol., *70:*587–592, 1978.
37. Laine, L., Weinstein, W.M.: Gastroenterology, *94:*1254–1262, 1988.
38. Barboriak, J.J., Meade, R.C.: Am. J. Clin. Nutr., *23:*1151–1153, 1970.
39. Jian, R., Cortot, A., Ducrot, F., et al.: Dig. Dis. Sci., *31:*604–614, 1986.
40. Keshavarzian, A., Dangleis, M., Wobbleton, J., et al.: Gastroenterology, *88:*1444, 1985.
41. Hermos, J.A., Adams, W.H., Liu, Y.K., et al.: Ann. Intern. Med., *76:*957–965, 1972.
42. Madzarovova-Nonejlova: J. Biol. Gastroenterol., *4:*325, 1971.
43. Perlow, W., Baraona, E., Lieber, C.S.: Gastroenterology, *72:*680–684, 1977.
44. Thomson, A.B.R.: Dig. Dis. Sci., *29:*267–274, 1984.
45. Mazzanti, R., Debhaw, E.S., Jenkins, W.J.: Gut, *28:*56–60, 1987.
46. Green, P.H.R.: Am. J. Med., *67:*1066–1076, 1979.
47. Marin, G.A., Ward, N.L., Fischer, R.: Dig. Dis., *18:*825–833, 1973.
48. Lefevre, A., DeCarli, L.M., Lieber, C.S.: J. Lipid Res., *13:*48–55, 1972.
49. Knodell, R.G., Kinsey, D., Boedeker, E.C., et al.: Gastroenterology, *71:*196–201, 1976.
50. Vlahcevic, S.R., Juttijudata, P., Bell, C.C., et al.: Gastroenterology, *62:*1174–1183, 1972.
51. Nicholas, P., Rinaudo, P.A., Conn, H.D.: Gastroenterology, *63:*112–118, 1972.
52. Witt, E.D., Goldman-Rakic, P.S.: Ann. Neurol., *13:*396–401, 1983.
53. Blass, J.P., Gibson, G.E.: N. Engl. J. Med., *297:*1367–1370, 1977.
54. Somogyi, J.C.: Biblthca. Nutr. Diets, *23:*78–85, 1976.
55. Camilo, M.E., Morgan, M.Y., Sherlock, S.: Scand. J. Gastroenterol., *16:*273–279, 1981.
56. Bitsch, R., Hansen, J., Hotzel, D.: Int. J. Vitamin Nutr. Res., *52:*126–133, 1982.
57. Fennelly, J., Frank, O., Baker, H., et al.: Am. J. Clin. Nutr., *20:*946–949, 1967.
58. Wood, B., Breen, K.J., Penington, D.G.: Aust. N.Z. J. Med.: *7:*475–484, 1977.
59. Shaw, S., Gorkin, J., Lieber, C.S.: Am. J. Clin. Nutr., *34:*856–860, 1981.
60. Hoyumpa, A.M.: Alcoholism: Clin. Exp. Res., *7:*11–14, 1983.
61. Dancy, M., Evans, G., Gaitonde, M.K., et al.: Br. Med. J., *289:*79–82, 1984.
62. Thompson, A.D., Majumdar, S.K.: Clin. Gastroenterol., *10:*263–293, 1981.
63. Breen, L.J., Buttigieg, R., Iossifidis, S., et al.: Am. J. Clin. Nutr., *42:*121–126, 1985.
64. Katz, D., Metz, J., van der Westhuyzen, J.: Am. J. Clin. Nutr., *42:*666–670, 1985.
65. Rosenthal, W.S., Adam, M.F., Lopez, R., et al.: Am. J. Clin. Nutr., *26:*858–860, 1973.
66. Kim, C.-I., Roe, D.A.: Drug-Nutr. Interact., *3:*99–107, 1985.
67. Lumeng, L., Li, T.-K.: J. Clin. Invest., *53:*693–704, 1974.
68. Fonda, M.L., Brown, S.G., Pendleton, M.W.: Alcoholism: Clin. Exp. Res., *3:*804–809, 1989.
69. Lumeng, L.J. Clin. Invest., *62:*286–293, 1978.
70. Veitch, R.L., Lumeng, L., Li, T.K.: J. Clin. Invest., *55:*1056–1032, 1975.
71. Parker, T.H., Marshall, J.P., Roberts, R.K., et al.: Am. J. Clin. Nutr., *32* :1246 –1252, 1979.
72. Lumeng L., Schenker, S., Li, T.-K., et al.: J. Lab. Clin. Med., *103:*59–64, 1984.
73. Shane, B.: J. Nutr., *112:*610–618, 1982.
74. Liebman, D., Furth-Walker, D., Smolen, T.N., et al.: Alcohol, *7:*61–68, 1989.
75. Schaumberg, H., Kaplan, L., Windebank, A., et al.: N. Engl. J. Med., *309:*445–448, 1983.
76. Perry, G., Bredesen, D.E.: Neurology, *35:*1466–1468, 1985.
77. World, M.J., Ryle, P.R., Jones, D., et al.: Alcohol Alcohol., *19:*281–290, 1984.
78. Romero, J.J., Tamura, T., Halsted, C.H.: Gastroenterology, *80:*99–102, 1981.
79. Reisenauer, A.M., Buffington, C.A.T., Villanueva, J.A., et al.: Am. J. Clin. Nutr., *50:*1429 –1435, 1989.
80. Naughton, C.A., Chandler, C.J., Duplantier, R.B., et al.: Am. J. Clin. Nutr., *50:*1436–1441, 1989.
81. Said, H.M., Strum, W.B.: Digestion, *35:*129–135, 1986.
82. Halsted, C.H., Robles, E.Z., Mezey, E.: N. Engl. J. Med., *285:*701–706, 1971.
83. Racusen, L.C., Krawitt, E.L.: Am. J. Dig. Dis., *22:*915–920, 1977.
84. Lindenbaum, J., Lieber, C.S.: Effects of ethanol on the blood, bone marrow and small intestine of man. *In* Biological Aspects of Alcohol. Vol. III. Edited by M.K. Roach, W.M. McIsaac, and P.J. Cleaven. Austin, University of Texas Press, 1971, pp. 27–45.
85. Lindenbaum, J., Lieber, C.S.: Alcohol and the hematologic system. *In* Medical Disorders of Alcoholism. Pathogenesis and Treatment. Vol. 22. Edited by C.S. Lieber. Philadelphia, W.B. Saunders, 1982, pp. 313–362.
86. Sullivan, L.W., Herbert, V.: J. Clin. Invest., *43:*2048–2062, 1964.
87. Russell, R.M., Rosenberg, I.H., Wilson, P.D., et al.: Am. J. Clin. Nutr., *38:*64–70, 1983.
88. Tamura, T., Romero, J.J., Watson, J.E., et al.: J. Lab. Clin. Med., *97:*654–661, 1981.
89. Tamura, T., Halsted, C.H.: J. Lab. Clin. Med., *101:*623–628, 1983.
90. Eichner, E.R., Buchanan, B., Smith, J.W., et al.: Am. J. Med. Sci., *273:*35–42, 1972.
91. Herbert; V.: Book of Abstracts—XXI Congress, International Society of Haematology, Sydney, Australia, 1986, *11–12:*216.
92. Kaunitz, J.D., Lindenbaum, J.: Ann. Intern. Med., *87:*542–545, 1977.
93. Herbert, V., Zalusky, R., Davidson, C.S.: Ann. Intern. Med., *58:*977–988, 1963.
94. Klipstein, F.A., Lindenbaum, J.: Blood, *25:*443–456, 1965.
95. Herzlich, B., Herbert, V.: Am. J. Gastroenterol., *81:*678–680, 1986.
96. Lindenbaum, J., Lieber, C.S.: Ann. N.Y. Acad. Sci., *252:*228–234, 1975.

97. Findlay, J., Sellers, E., Forstner, G.: Can. J. Physiol. Pharmacol., *54:*469–476, 1976.
98. Lindenbaum, J., Saha, J.R., Shea, N., Lieber, C.S.: Gastroenterology, *64:*762, 1973.
99. Bonjour, J.P.: Int. J. Vitamin Nutr., *49:*434–441, 1979.
100. Gruchow. H.W., Sobovinski, K.A., Barboriak, J.J., et al.: Am. J. Clin. Nutr., *42:*289–295, 1985.
101. Hillers, V.N., Massey, L.K.: Am. J. Clin. Nutr., *41:*356–362, 1985.
102. Bunout, D., Gattas, V., Iturriaga, H., et al.: Am. J. Clin. Nutr., *38:*469–473, 1983.
103. Barboriak, J.J., Rooney, C.B., Leitschuh, T.H., et al.: J. Am. Diet. Assoc., *72:*493–495, 1978.
104. Althausen, T.L., Uyeyama, K., Loran, K.: Gastroenterology, *38:*942–945, 1960.
105. Russell, R.M., Giovetti, A., Garrett, M., et al.: Gastroenterology, *77:*A36, 1979.
106. Lee, M., Lucia, S.P.: J. Stud. Alcohol, *26:*1–8, 1965.
107. Sato, M., Lieber, C.S.: Gastroenterology, *79:*1123, 1980.
108. Blomstrand, R., Lof, A., Osterling, H.: Nutr. Metab., *21(Suppl. 1):*148 –151, 1977.
109. Nadkarni, G.D., Deshpande, U.R., Pahuja, D.N.: Experientia, *35:*1059–1060, 1979.
110. Leo, M.A., Lieber, C.S.: N. Engl. J. Med., *37:*597–601, 1982.
111. Leo, M.A., Lieber, C.S.: J. Biol. Chem., *260:*5228–5231, 1985.
112. Leo, M.A., Kim, C., Lieber, C.S.: Alcoholism: Clin. Exp. Res., *10:*487–492, 1986.
113. Bonjour, J.P.: Int. J. Vitamin. Nutr. Res., *51:*166–177, 1981.
114. Carney, E.A., Russel, R.M.: J. Nutr., *110:*552–557, 1980.
115. Leo, M.A., Sato, M., Lieber, C.S.: Gastroenterology, *84:*562–572, 1983.
116. Leo, M.A., Lieber, C.S.: Alcoholism: Clin. Exp. Res., *7:*15–21, 1983.
117. Leo, M.A., Lieber, C.S.: Hepatology, *3:*1–11, 1983.
118. Leo, M.A., Arai, M., Sato, M., et al.: Gastroenterology, *82:*194–205, 1982.
119. Mak, K.M., Leo, M.A., Lieber, C.S.: Trans. Assoc. Am. Phys., *98:*210–221, 1984.
120. Lieber, C.S.: Alcohol and the liver. *In* Liver Annual—VI. Edited by I.M. Arias, M.S. Frenkel, and J.H.P. Wilson. Amsterdam, Excerpta Media, 1987, pp. 163–240.
121. Anonymous: Lancet, *2:*325–326, 1985.
122. Saville, P.D.: J. Bone Joint Surg. [Am.], *47:*492–499, 1965.
123. Gascon-Barré, M.: J. Am. Coll. Nutr., *4:*565–574, 1985.
124. Nilsson, B.E.: Acta Chir. Scand., *136:*383–384, 1970.
125. Solomon, L.: J. Bone Joint Surg. [Br.], *55:*246–261, 1973.
126. Long, R.G.: Vitamin D in chronic liver disease. *In* Liver in Metabolic Diseases. Edited by L. Bianchi, W. Gerok, L. Landmann, et al. Boston, MTP Press, 1983, pp. 421–427.
127. Posner, D.B., Russell, R.M., Absood, S., Gastroenterology, *74:*866–870, 1978.
128. Jung, R.T., Davie, M., Hunter, J.O., et al.: Gut, *19:*290–293, 1978.
129. Bonkovsky, H.L., Hawkins, M., Steinberg, K., et al.: Hepatology, *12:*273–280, 1990.
130. Bikle, D.D., Halloran, B.P., Gee, E., et al.: J. Clin. Invest., *78:*748–752, 1986.
131. Blanchard, R., Furie, B.C., Jorgensen, M., et al.: N. Engl. J. Med., *305:*242–248, 1981.
132. Roberts, H.R., Cederbaum, A.I.: Gastroenterology, *63:*297–320, 1972.
133. Bieri, J.G., Corash, L., Hubbard, V.S.: N. Engl. J. Med., *308:*1063–1071, 1983.
134. Scott, M.L.: Fed. Proc., *39:*2736–2739, 1980.
135. Martin, D.W., Jr.: Fat-soluble vitamins. *In* Harper's Review of Biochemistry. 20th Ed. Edited by D.W. Martin Jr., P.A. Mayes, V.W. Rodwll, and D.K. Granner. Los Altos, CA, Lange Medical Publications, 1985, pp. 118–127.
136. Levander, O.A., Burk, R.F.: JPEN, *10:*545–549, 1986.
137. Knight, R.E., Bourne, A.J., Newton, M., et al.: Gastroenterology, *91:*209–211, 1986.
138. Bjorneboe, G.-E., Bjorneboe, A., Hagen, B.F., et al.: Biochim. Biophys. Acta, *918:*236–241, 1987.
139. Kawase, T., Kato, S., Lieber, C.S.: Hepatology, *10:*815–821, 1989.
140. Kalvaria, I., Labadarios, D., Shephard, G.S., et al.: Int. J. Pancreatol., *1:*119–128, 1986.
141. Lieber, C.S.: Alcohol and the liver. *In* Liver Annual VI. Edited by I.M. Arias, M.S. Frenkel, and J.H.P. Wilson. Amsterdam, Excerpta Medica, 1987, pp. 163–240.
142. Gabuzda, G.J.: Med. Clin. North Am., *54:*1455–1472, 1970.
143. Shear, L., Gabuzda, G.J., Shear, L., et al.: Am. J. Clin. Nutr., *23:*614–618, 1970.
144. Summerskill, W.H.J., Barnardo, D.E., Baldus, W.P.: Am. J. Clin. Nutr., *23:*499–507, 1990.
145. Epstein, F.H.: N. Engl. J. Med., *307:*1577–1578, 1982.
146. Epstein, F.H.: Hepatology, *6:*312–315, 1986.
147. Warner, L.C., Campbell, P.J., Morali, G.A., et al.: Hepatology, *12:*460–466, 1990.
148. Rector, W.G. Jr, Adair, O., Hossack, K.F., et al.: Gastroenterology, *99:*766–770, 1990.
149. Boyer, T.D.: Gastroenterology, *90:*2022–2023, 1986.
150. Kellerman, P.S.: Ann. Intern. Med., *112:*889–891, 1990.
151. LeVeen, H.H.: Annual review of medicine. *In* Selected Topics in Clinical Sciences. Vol. 36. Edited by W.P. Creger, C.H. Coggins, and E.W. Hancock. Palo Alto, CA, Annual Reviews Inc., 1985, pp. 453–469.
152. Smajda, C., Franco, D.: Ann. Surg., *201:*488–493, 1985.
153. Wapnic, S., Grossberg, S.J., Evans, M.I.: Br. J. Surg., *66:*667–670, 1979.
154. McColister, R., Prasad, A.S., Doe, R.P., et al.: J. Lab. Clin. Med., *52:*928–932, 1958.
155. McDonald, J.T., Morgen, S.: Am. J. Clin. Nutr., *32:*823–833, 1979.
156. Flink, E.B.: Alcoholism: Clin. Exp. Res., *10:*590–594, 1986.
157. Volini, F., de la Huerga, J., Kent, G., et al.: Trace metal studies in liver disease using atomic absorption spectroscopy. *In* Laboratory Diagnosis of Liver Disease. Edited by F.W. Sunderman and F.W. Sunderman, Jr. St. Louis, W.H. Green, 1968, pp. 199–206.
158. Chapman, R.W., Morgan, M.Y., Bell, R., et al.: Gastroenterology, *84:*143–147, 1983.
159. Chapman, R.W., Morgan, M.Y., Boss, A.M., et al.: Dig. Dis. Sci., *28:*321–327, 1983.
160. Bassett, M.L., Halliday, J.W., Powell, L.W.: Hepatology, *6:*24–29, 1986.
161. Olynk, J., Hall, P., Sallie, R., et al.: Hepatology, *12:*26–30, 1990.
162. Bacon, B.R., Britton, S.: Hepatology, *11:*127–137, 1990.
163. Chojkier, M., Houglum, K., Solis-Herruzo, J., et al.: J. Biol. Chem., *264:*16957–16962, 1989.
164. Stibler, H., Allgulander, C., Borg, S., et al.: Acta Med. Scand., *204:*49–56, 1978.
165. Stibler, H., Sydow, O., Borg, S.: Pharmacol. Biochem. Behav., *13(Suppl.):*47–51, 1990.
166. Behrens, U.J., Worner, T.M., Braly, L.F., et al.: Clin. Exp. Res., *12:*427–437, 1988.

167. Behrens, U.J., Worner, T.M., Lieber, C.S.: Alcoholism: Clin. Exp. Res., *12:*539–544, 1988.
168. Potter, G.J., Chapman, R.W.G., Nunes, R.M., et al.: Hepatology, *5:*714–721, 1985.
169. Antonson, D.L., Barak, A.J., Vanderhoff, J.A.: J. Nutr., *109:*142–147, 1979.
170. Smith, K.T., Cousins, R.J., Silbon, B.L., et al.: J. Nutr., *108:*1849–1857, 1978.
171. Anonymous: Nutr. Rev., *43:*158–159, 1985.
172. Huber, A.M., Gershoff, S.N.: J. Nutr., *105:*1486–1490, 1975.
173. McClain, C.J., Gavaler, J.S., Thiel Van, D.H.: J. Lab. Clin. Med., *104:*1007–1015, 1984.
174. Vallee, B.L., Wacker, W.E.C., Bartholomay, A.F., et al.: N. Engl. J. Med., *225:*403–408, 1956.
175. Vallee, B.L., Wacker, E.C., Bartholomay, A.F., et al.: N. Engl. J. Med., *257:*1055–1065, 1957.
176. Sullivan, J.F.: Gastroenterology, *42:*439–442, 1962.
177. Sullivan, J.F.: Q.J. Stud. Alcohol, *23:*216–220, 1962.
178. Sandstead, H.H.: Am. J. Clin. Nutr., *26:*1251–1260, 1973.
179. Valberg, L.S., Flanagan, P.R., Ghent, C.N., et al.: Dig. Dis. Sci., *30:*329–339, 1985.
180. Sullivan, J.E., Lankford, H.G.: Am. J. Clin. Nutr., *10:*153–157, 1962.
181. Sullivan, J.F., Williams, R.V., Burch, R.E.: Alcoholism: Clin. Exp. Res., *3:*235–239, 1979.
182. Hartoma, T.R., Sontaniemi, R.A., Pelkonen, O., et al.: Eur. J. Clin. Pharmacol., *12:*147–151, 1977.
183. Szutowski, M.M., Lipsaka, M., Bandolet, J.P.: Polish J. Pharmacol. Pharm., *28:*397–401, 1974.
184. Versieck, J., Hoste, J., Vanballenberghe, L., et al.: J. Lab. Clin. Med., *97:*535–544, 1981.
185. Phillips, G.B., Safrit, H.F.: JAMA, *217:*1513, 1971.
186. Rehfeld, J.F., Juhl, E., Hilden, M.: Gastroenterology, *64:*445–451, 1973.
187. Dornhorst, A., Ouyang, A.: Lancet, *2:*957, 1971.
188. Metz, R., Berger, S., Mako, M.: Diabetes, *18:*517, 1969.
189. Nikkilä, E.A., Taskin, M.R.: Diabetes, *24:*933, 1975.
190. Yki-Järvinen, H., Nikkilä, E.A.: Metabolism, *61:*941, 1985.
191. Krebs, H.A., Freedland, R.A., Hems, R., et al.: Biochem. J., *112:*117, 1969.
192. Madison, L.L., Lochner, A., Wulff, J.: Diabetes, *16:*252, 1967.
193. Duruibe, V., Tejwani, G.A.: Mol. Pharmacol., *20:*621, 1981.
194. Stiffel, F.B., Green, H.L., Lufkin, E.G., et al.: Biochim. Biophys. Acta, *428:*633, 1976.
195. Dinda, P.K., Beck, I.T.: Dig. Dis. Sci., *29:*46, 1984.
196. Halsted, C.H., Robles, E.A., Mezey, E.: Gastroenterology, *64:*526–532, 1973.
197. Lieber, C.S., Jones, D.P., Losowsky, M.S., et al.: J. Clin. Invest., *41:*1863, 1962.
198. Losowsky, M.S., Jones, D.P., Davidson, C.S., et al.: Am. J. Med., *35:*794, 1963.
199. Newcomb, D.S.: Metabolism, *21:*1193, 1972.
200. MacLachlan, M.J., Rodman, G.P.: Am. J. Med., *42:*38, 1967.
201. Gibson, T., Rodgers, A.V., Simmonds, H.A., et al.: Br. J. Rheumatol., *23:*203, 1984.
202. Maddrey, W.C., Weber, F.L., Coutler, A.W., et al.: Gastroenterology, *71:*190–195, 1976.
203. Wilson, D.A., Schreibman, P.H., Brewster, A.C., et al.: J. Lab. Clin. Med., *75:*264, 1970.
204. Lieber, C.S., Jones, D.P., Mendelson, J., et al.: Trans. Assoc. Am. Physicians, *76:*289, 1963.
205. Borowsky, S.A., Perlow, W., Baraona, E., et al.: Dig. Dis. Sci., *25:*22, 1980.
206. Guisard, D., Gonard, J.P., Laurent, J., et al.: Nutr. Metab., *13:*222–229, 1971.
207. Marzo, A., Ghiradi, P., Sardini, P., et al.: Klin. Wochenschr., *48:*949–950, 1970.
208. Ginsberg, H., Olefsky, J., Farquhar, J.W., et al.: Ann. Intern. Med., *80:*143–149, 1974.
209. Crews, R.H., Faloon, W.W.: JAMA, *181:*754, 1982.
210. Lieber, C.S.: N. Engl. J. Med., *311:*846–848, 1984.
211. McGhee, A., Henderson, M., Milikan, W.J., et al.: Ann. Surg., *197:*288, 1983.
212. Klatskin, G.: Yale J. Biol. Med., *34:*124, 1961.
213. Rodrigo, C., Antezana, C., Baraona, E.: J. Nutr., *101:*1307–1310, 1971.
214. Lieber, C.S.: Alcohol and the liver. *In* Liver Annual—VI. Edited by I.U. Arias, M.S. Frenkel, and J.H.P. Wilson. Amsterdam, Excerpta Medica, 1987, pp. 163–240.
215. Schapiro, R.H., Drummer, G.D., Shimuzu, Y., et al.: J. Clin. Invest., *43:*1338–1347, 1964.
216. Rothschild, M.A., Oratz, M., Mongelli, J., et al.: J. Clin. Invest., *50:*1812–1818, 1971.
217. Jeejeebhog, K.N., Phillips, M.J., Bruce-Robertson, A., et al.: Biochem. J., *126:*1111–1126, 1972.
218. Baraona, E., Leo, M.A., Borowsky, S.A., et al.: Science, *190:*794–795, 1975.
219. Crow, K.E., Cornell, N.W., Veech, R.L.: Clin. Exp. Res., *1:*143–47, 1977.
220. Bode, J.L., Goebell, H., Stahler, M.: Gesampte Exp. Med., *152:*111–124, 1970.
221. Bode, J.L., Buchwald, B., Goebell, H.: German Med. Mon., *1:*149–151, 1971.
222. Meijer, A.J., Van Woebkon, G.M., Williamson, J.R., et al.: Biochem. J., *150:*205–209, 1975.
223. Korten, M.A., Matsuzaki, S., Feinman, L., et al.: N. Engl. J. Med., *292:*386–389, 1975.
224. Caballeria, J., Baraona, E., Rodamilans, M., et al.: Gastroenterology, *96:*388–392, 1989.
225. Hernandez-Munoz, R., Caballeria, J., Baraona, E., et al.: Alcoholism: Clin. Exp. Res., *14:*946–950, 1990.
226. Frezza, M., Di Padova, C., Pozzato, G., et al.: N. Engl. J. Med., *322:*95–99, 1990.
227. Lieber, C.S., Lasker, J.M., DeCarli, L.M., et al.: Pharmacol. Exp. Ther., *247:*791–795, 1988.
228. Lieber, C.S.: Alcohol, protein nutrition and liver injury. *In* Nutrition and Drugs. Edited by M. Winick. New York, Wiley and Sons, 1983.
229. Klatskin, G., Krehl, W.A., Conn, H.O.: J. Exp. Med., *100:*605, 1954.
230. Lieber, C.S., DeCarli, L.M.: Am. J. Clin. Nutr., *23:*474, 1970.
231. Lieber, C.S., Spritz, N.: J. Clin. Invest., *45:*1400, 1966.
232. Lieber, C.S., Spritz, N., DeCarli, L.M.: J. Lipid Res., *10:*283, 1969.
233. Best, C.H., Hartroft, W.S., Lucas, C.C., et al.: Br. J. Med., *11:*10001, 1949.
234. Olsen, R.E.: Nutrition and alcoholism. *In* Modern Nutrition Health and Disease. Edited by M.G. Wohl and R.S. Goodhart. Philadelphia, Lea & Febiger, 1964.
235. Phillips, G.B., Davidson, C.S.: Ann. N.Y. Acad. Sci., *57:*812, 1954.
236. Post, J., Benton, J.G., Breakstone, R., et al.: Gastroenterology, *20:*403, 1952.
237. Rubin, E., Lieber, C.S.: N. Engl. J. Med., *278:*869, 1968.
238. Volwiler, W., Jones, C.M., Mallory, T.B.: Gastroenterology, *11:*164, 1948.
239. Iseri, O.A., Lieber, C.S., Gottlieb, L.S.: Am. J. Pathol., *48:*535, 1966.

240. Konrup, J., Grunnet, N.: Biochem. J., *132:*373, 1973.
241. Corredor, C., Mansbach, C., Bressler, R.: Fed. Proc., *26:*278, 1967.
242. Edreirta, J.G., Hirsch, R.L., Kennedy, J.A.: Q.J. Stud. Alc., *35:*20, 1974.
243. Chalvardian, A.: Can. Biochem. J., *48:*1234, 1970.
244. Haines, D.S.M.: Can. J. Biochem., *44:*45, 1966.
245. Baraona, E., Lieber, C.S.: J. Clin. Invest., *49:*769–778, 1970.
246. DiLuzio, N.R.: Am. J. Physiol., *194:*453, 1958.
247. Lieber, C.S., DeCarli, L.M.: Gastroenterology, *50:*316, 1966.
248. Lieber, C.S., Leo, M.A., Mak, K.M., et al.: Hepatology, *5:*561, 1985.
249. Wood, J.L., Allison, R.G.: Fed. Proc., *41:*3015, 1982.
250. Lederman, S.: Alcohol, alcoholisme, alcoholisation. Paris, Institut national d'études demographiques, travaux, et documents. Cahier No. 41, Presses Universitaires de France, 1964.
251. United States Bureau of the Census: Vital Statistics Rates in the United States, 1900–1940. Washington, D.C., Government Printing Office, 1943.
252. Lelbach, W.K.: Acta Hepatosphlenol. (Stutg.), *14:*9, 1967.
253. Tuyns, A.J., Esteban, J., Pequinot, G.: Br. J. Addict., *79:*389, 1984.
254. Lieber, C.S., DeCarli, L.M.: J. Med. Primatol., *3:*153–163, 1974.
255. Lieber, C.S., DeCarli, L.M., Rubin, E.: Proc. Natl. Acad. Sci. U.S.A., *72:*437–441, 1925.
256. Rubin, E., Lieber, C.S.: N. Engl. J. Med., *290:*128–135, 1974.
257. Lieber, C.S., Jones, D.P., DeCarli, L.M.: J. Clin. Invest., *44:*1009–1021, 1965.
258. Lane, B.P., Lieber, C.S.: Am. J. Pathol., *49:*593–603, 1966.
259. Lieber, C.S., Rubin, E.: Am. J. Med., *44:*200–206, 1968.
260. Rubin, E., Lieber, C.S.: Fed. Proc., *26:*1458, 1967.
261. Patek, J.A., Post, J.: J. Clin. Invest., *20:*481, 1941.
262. Patek, A.J., Post, J., Ratnoff, O.B., et al.: JAMA, *138:*543, 1948.
263. Morrison, L.M.: Ann. Intern. Med., *24:*465, 1946.
264. Erenoglu, E., Dereira, J.G., Patek, A.J. Jr.: Ann. Intern. Med., *60:*814, 1964.
265. Feinman, L., Lieber, C.S.: Alcoholism: Clin. Exp. Res., *12:*2–6, 1988.
266. Wilkinson, P., Santamaria, J.N., Rankin, J.G.: Aust. Ann. Med., *18:*222, 1969.
267. Morgan, M.Y., Sherlock, S.: Br. Med. J., *2:*939, 1972.
268. Gill, J.S., Sezulka, V., Shipley, M.J., et al.: N. Engl. J. Med., *315:*1041, 1986.
269. Camargo, C.A. Jr.: Stroke, *20:*1611–1626, 1989.
270. Blackwelder, W.C., Yano, K., Rhoads, G., et al.: Am. J. Med., *68:*164, 1980.
271. Klatsky, A.L., Friedman, G.D., Siegelaub, A., et al.: N. Engl. J. Med., *296:*1194, 1977.
272. Witteman, J.C.M., Willet, W.C., Stampfer, M.J., et al.: Am. J. Cardiol., *65:*633–637, 1990.
273. Coates, R.A., Corey, P.N., Ashley, M.J., et al.: Prev. Med., *14:*1, 1985.
274. Taylor, J.R., Combs-Orune, T., Anderson, E., et al.: Clin. Exp. Res., *8:*283–285, 1984.
275. Wolf, P.A.: N. Engl. J. Med., *315:*1085, 1986.
276. Lang, R.M., Borrow, K.M., Neumann, A., et al.: Ann. Intern. Med., *102:*742–747, 1985.
277. Kelbaek, H.: Prog. Cardiovasc. Dis., *32:*347–364, 1990.
278. Gould, L., Reddy, C.V.R., Becker, W., et al.: Electrocardiography, *11:*219–226, 1978.
279. Friedman, H.S., Neal, C., Dowd, A., et al.: Am. J. Cardiol., *47:*61, 1981.
280. Segel, L.D., Klausner, S.C., Gnadt, J.T.H., et al.: Med. Clin. North Am., *68:*147–161, 1984.
281. Anonymous: Lancet, *11:*1374, 1985.
282. Thornton, J.R.: Lancet, *2:*1013, 1984.
283. Kagan, A., Yano, K., Rhoad, G.G., et al.: Gut, *19:*290, 1978.
284. Barboriak, J.J., Anderson, A.J., Rimm, A.A., Tristani, F.E.: Alcoholism: Clin. Exp. Res., *3:*29, 1979.
285. Colditz, G.A., Branch, L.G., Lipnic, R.J., et al.: Prog. Cardiol., *109:*886–889, 1985.
286. Gordon, T., Doyle, J.T.: Am. Heart J., *110:*331–334, 1985.
287. Agatson, A.S., Snow, M.E., Samet, P.: Alcoholism: Clin. Exp. Res., *10:*386–387, 1986.
288. Kupari, M.: Postgrad. Med. J., *60:*151–154, 1984.
289. Lindenbaum, J., Lieber, C.S.: N. Engl. J. Med., *281:*333–338, 1969.
290. Haut, M.J., Cowan, D.H.: Am. J. Med., *56:*22–32, 1974.
291. Lindenbaum, J., Hargrove, R.L.: Ann. Intern. Med., *68:*526–532, 1968.

CHAPTER **65**

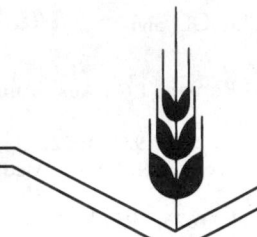

Nutrition, Diet, and the Kidney

Joel D. Kopple

KIDNEY FUNCTION

The kidney has three primary functions: excretory, endocrine, and metabolic. All three functions may be impaired in renal disease and may have an impact on the patient's nutritional status and management. When injury and necrosis of the renal parenchyma cause a loss of renal function, the quantity of the substances that are filtered by the kidney falls. However, many aspects of renal function undergo changes that preserve homeostasis and minimize the derangements in plasma and tissue concentrations of substances that normally are excreted by the kidney.

Many organic compounds accumulate in renal failure.[1] Most of these compounds are products of amino acid and protein metabolism. Quantitatively, the most prominent are urea, creatinine, other guanidine compounds and uric acid (Fig. 65–1). It is generally believed that some of these compounds are toxic in high concentrations. Low protein intakes reduce accumulation of many of these substances. Eventually, renal failure may become so severe that the aforementioned adaptive mechanisms are no longer adequate to maintain homeostasis, even with special dietary therapy that restricts the intake of fluid, electrolytes, and protein. The accumulation of these compounds, the endocrine and metabolic disturbances, and the clinical signs and symptoms that result from renal failure are referred to as uremia. If this condition is not treated by hemodialysis, peritoneal dialysis, or renal transplantation, death will eventually supervene.

Excretion and regulation of body water, minerals, and organic compounds are clearly the most important functions of the kidney. Without renal excretory function, patients rarely live longer than 4 to 5 weeks and often less than 10 days, particularly if they are hypercatabolic. In contrast, anephric patients can be kept alive for years with intermittent hemodialysis or peritoneal dialysis, even though endocrine and metabolic functions of the kidney are not replaced.

The kidney elaborates certain hormones that have diverse metabolic effects including 1,25-dihydroxycholecalciferol, erythropoietin, and kallikreins. These effects have been the subject of many excellent and comprehensive reviews.[2–5] The kidney plays an essential role in vitamin D metabolism.[4] Vitamin D_3 (cholecalciferol) is hydroxylated in the liver to form 25-hydroxycholecalciferol. This compound is then converted in the kidney to 1,25-dihydroxycholecalciferol (1,25-dihydroxyvitamin D). The actions of 1,25-dihydroxyvitamin D are discussed in Chapter 17. In renal failure, the impaired synthesis of 1,25-dihydroxyvitamin D contributes to a vitamin D-deficient state associated with impaired intestinal calcium absorption, hyperparathyroidism, and the development of renal osteodystrophy.

Erythropoietin is a glycoprotein with a molecular weight of 39 kd that stimulates erythropoiesis in bone marrow.[5,6] The anemia of chronic renal failure is primarily caused by impaired erythropoiesis. Decreased red cell formation is mainly due to reduced erythropoietin production in the diseased kidneys, although other compounds that accumulate in renal failure also may suppress erythropoiesis. A mild hemolysis often contributes to the anemia. Certain kidney diseases, such as kidney cysts or tumors, are occasionally associated with increased hemoglobin and hematocrit caused by increased synthesis of erythropoietin. Recombinant DNA-synthesized human erythropoietin is commonly used to increase the blood hemoglobin levels of patients who receive maintenance dialysis.[7]

INTERRELATIONSHIPS BETWEEN NUTRIENTS AND KIDNEY FUNCTION

Kidney function both regulates and is influenced by the body's pools and concentrations of water, minerals, and many other nutrients and their metabolites. The reader is referred elsewhere in the text for a discussion of the physiology of water, sodium, potassium, acids and bases (Chap. 6), calcium and phosphorus (Chap. 7), magnesium (Chap. 8), and trace elements (Chap. 15).

EFFECTS OF MALNUTRITION ON THE KIDNEY

Malnutrition can have important but usually reversible effects on renal function. In humans, malnutrition decreases the glomerular filtration rate (GFR),[8,9] as well as the capacity to concentrate and to acidify urine.[9–11] If nutritional intake improves, these functions may normalize. GFR falls reversibly in obese subjects placed on weight-reduction diets containing no protein or calories but providing water, vitamins, and small quantities of minerals. This phenomenon is at least partly due to a reduction in extracellular body water, circulating blood volume, and renal blood flow. Increased salt and water intake rapidly reverses this condition. The low or absent protein intake may possibly contribute to the lower renal blood flow and GFR.[8,9]

Ichikawa and co-workers investigated the mechanisms responsible for reduction in GFR with protein malnutrition.[12] These investigators found that in rats pair-fed a low-protein (6%) diet, as compared to an isocaloric high-protein (40%) diet, there was almost a 35% reduction in GFR. Increased resistance was evident in the arterioles leading into (afferent) and out of (efferent) the glomerulus. There was also about a 25% reduction in the glomerular capillary plasma flow rate and almost a 50% decrease in the glomerular capillary ultrafiltration coefficient. Glomerular transcapillary hydraulic pressure differences were similar in the two groups. A reduction in the intrarenal synthesis of insulin-like growth factor-I (IGF-I) may contribute to these changes.[13,14]

Malnourished individuals often have lower specific gravity in random urine specimens and increased daily urine volumes. Impaired concentrating ability probably contributes to the nocturia that occurs in malnutrition. The inability of the malnourished patient to concentrate urine normally appears to be due to their low protein intake and consequent low rate of urea synthesis.[10] Urea is critical for normal urinary concentration. Some urea filtered by the glomerulus is reabsorbed in the renal tubule and accumulates in the interstitium of the renal medulla. The loss of water from the collecting duct lumen increases the concentration of urine. When protein intake is low, urea synthesis falls and serum urea nitrogen (SUN) decreases; less urea is filtered by the glomerulus and reabsorbed into the renal medulla. Thus, medullary hypertonicity falls, and there is less tendency for water to move from the distal tubule and collecting duct to the medulla; hence maximum renal concentrating ability is reduced. Ingestion of urea or protein by subjects who are malnourished or who have low-protein diets improves renal concentrating ability.[10] The capacity to dilute urine is normal in malnutrition.

Malnourished subjects are more likely to develop acidosis after an acid load.[11] Urinary phosphate and ammonia are primary carriers of acid in the urine. Hydrogen ion secretion into the lumen of the distal nephron lowers the pH of tubular fluid and converts HPO_4^- to $H_2PO_4^-$ and ammonia to NH_4^+. In individuals who have a low phosphorus intake, the phosphate filtered in the kidney is largely reabsorbed to conserve body phosphate pools, and less is excreted in the urine. Thus, the capacity to excrete acid is reduced. Infusion of phosphate improves urinary excretion of titratable acid in malnourished patients.[11] In malnutrition, renal production and excretion of ammonia are also reduced, both under basal conditions and after an acid load.[11] Why this capacity of the kidney to synthesize and excrete ammonia is reduced is not clear.

During prolonged starvation, the kidney may account for up to 45% of endogenous glucose production, although part of the rise in the renal contribution to glucose synthesis is due to a fall in total body glucose production.[15] In extended starvation, net renal extraction of lactate, pyruvate, amino acids, and glycerol also occurs.[15] The carbon skeleton in these compounds is virtually completely converted into glucose. During prolonged starvation, free fatty acids and β-hydroxybutyrate are also extracted by the kidney, and acetoacetate is released.[15]

Acute starvation and other conditions associated with increased catabolism of nucleic acids, purines, and amino acids, such as chemotherapy of leukemias and certain other tumors, can cause a marked increase in uric acid production. Hyperuricemia with deposition of uric acid sludge in the kidney and lower urinary tract may occur and may cause acute renal failure. Treatment consists of allopurinol, which inhibits the synthesis of uric acid, maintenance of good hydration and a large urine flow, and alkalinization of the urine because urate is far more soluble in alkaline solutions.[16]

EFFECTS OF PROTEIN AND AMINO ACID INTAKE ON RENAL FUNCTION

Protein intake appears to engender both an immediate and a more long-term increase in renal blood flow and GFR in humans. A transient increase in renal blood flow and GFR of about 20 to 28% occurs following a protein meal.[17,18] The rise occurs about 2 hours after the meal and generally lasts about 1 hour. Renal blood flow and GFR also increase transiently following an intravenous infusion of a mixture of essential and nonessential amino acids,[19] or a 30-minute infusion of arginine hydrochloride.[20] Infusion of somatostatin blocks the rise induced by an amino acid infusion, indicating that peptide hormones may mediate the amino acid and protein enhancement of renal blood flow and GFR.[19] A glucagon infusion that raises blood glucagon levels similar to those observed after an amino acid load increases renal blood flow and GFR.[21] Hence glucagon may play a role in the amino acid or protein-induced increase in renal blood flow and GFR. Acromegalic patients have an abnormally high GFR,[22] and an injection of growth hormone into normal humans increases renal blood flow and GFR after several hours.[23] IGF-I appears to mediate the growth hormone-induced rise in renal hemodynamics.[13,24]

Most patients with renal insufficiency also demonstrate a protein or amino acid induced rise in renal blood flow and GFR.[17,18] This increase has been called the "renal functional reserve." Some investigators have suggested that the maximum renal blood flow and GFR after a protein or amino acid load in patients with renal disease, as compared to normal subjects, gives a better estimate of the magnitude of renal damage and scarring. This has not been confirmed because the maximum renal blood flow and GFR following a protein load appear to vary according to the individual's previous daily protein intake.

EFFECT OF NUTRITIONAL INTAKE ON THE RATE OF PROGRESSION OF RENAL FAILURE

EARLY EXPERIENCE

Physicians have known for many decades that patients with chronic renal disease who have sustained a substantial loss of GFR often continue to lose renal function inexorably until they develop terminal renal failure.[25–27] Although the rate of progression of renal failure varies among patients, in many individuals the decline in kidney function is linear.[25–27] The percentage of patients with renal insufficiency who will progress to renal failure is not known, but the suspicion is that most patients who sustain a loss of 50% in GFR will show continued progression of renal failure. Renal failure may progress because of continued activity of the underlying renal disease or because of superimposed disorders such as hypertension, kidney infection, obstruction, adverse effects of nephrotoxic medicines such as antibiotics or radiocontrast material, hypercalcemia, or hyperuricemia. However, in innumerable instances the progression continues even after the initial cause of the renal disease seems to have disappeared.[28–31] For example, this phenomenon may occur in patients who have relief of urinary tract obstruction, control of hypertension, discontinuance of nephrotoxic medications, or partial recovery from acute renal failure. Moreover, the continued progression of renal failure may occur when no associated causes of impaired renal function are identified. Several theories have been advanced to explain this phenomenon. These include the hypothesis that scarring and fibrosis of the diseased kidney cause obstruction of the renal tubules or small vessels, which in turn leads to intrarenal obstruction of tubular fluid and blood flow. Another suggestion is that the injured renal tissue elicits a secondary autoimmune response that causes further renal injury.[32] None of these theories have been confirmed.

Traditionally, dietary protein restriction has been used to minimize uremic toxicity.[33] In the first half of the twentieth century, research studies in rats indicated that protein restriction could retard progression of renal failure.[34–36] The experimental design of these studies was often faulty, and the data were not considered applicable to humans. Moreover, observations in humans with renal disease were not well controlled, and the results were inconsistent.

RECENT EXPERIMENTAL EVIDENCE

In the 1970s and 1980s, studies in both humans and rats indicated that dietary control can retard the state of progression of renal failure in a variety of renal diseases. In rats, several models of renal insufficiency were studied. These included surgical removal of the upper and lower poles of one kidney or ligation of about two thirds to three quarters of the arteries to one kidney; in both models, contralateral nephrectomy was performed. In some cases, experimental glomerulonephritis was created.[37–41] In these animal models, diets low in protein and/or phosphorus retard or prevent progression of renal failure.[37–41] In addition, a diet low or high in certain fats may retard progressive renal damage.[42–45] Moreover, administration of prostaglandins may affect the progression of chronic renal disease in animals.[46–48]

There is a rather common response to chronic loss of renal function that is, to a large degree, independent of the underlying type of kidney disease. When the loss of functioning nephrons becomes sufficient to cause renal insufficiency, the remaining individual functioning nephrons undergo an increase in the glomerular plasma flow and GFR and an enlargement in size of both the glomeruli and the tubules (i.e., nephron hypertrophy).[49,50] The capillary blood flow of the remaining glomeruli increases, as does the blood pressure gradient across the capillary wall.[50,51] In addition, the chemical and electrical as well as pore size barriers to the movement of plasma proteins across the glomerulus into the renal tubule are impaired.[52,53] Migration of leukocytes and monocytes, platelet aggregation, collagen deposition, cellular proliferation, and other inflammatory and scarifying changes may occur to a greater or lesser degree and may cause progressive renal damage.

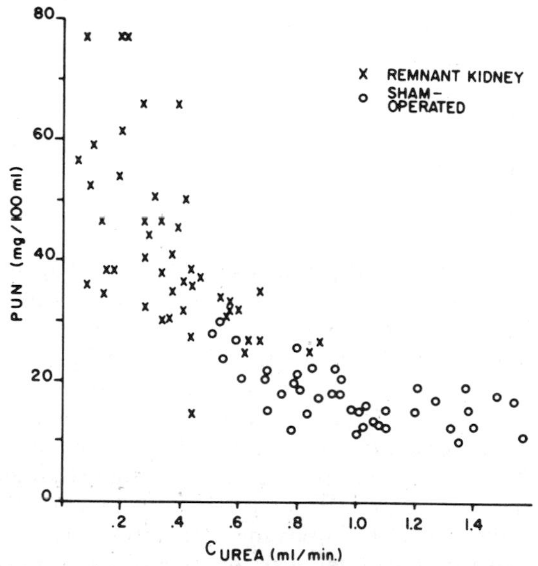

FIGURE 65–1. Relationship between the plasma urea nitrogen (PUN) and glomerular filtration rate, as indicated by the urea clearance, in Sprague-Dawley rats with chronic renal insufficiency and sham-operated controls. Chronic renal failure was produced by ligation of two thirds to three fourths of the arterial supply to the left kidney and contralateral nephrectomy. (From Kopple, J.D.: Nutrition and the kidney. *In* Human Nutrition: A Comprehensive Treatise. Vol. 4. Edited by R.B. Alfin-Slater and D. Kritchevsky. New York, Plenum Publishing, 1979, pp. 409–457, by permission of Plenum Publishing.)

Many of these changes, some of which could be considered adaptive, are believed to promote further renal injury and lead to progressive renal failure. It is possible that dietary therapy may reduce the rate of progression of renal failure by altering these processes. Current thinking regarding potential causes of progressive renal failure is summarized in Table 65–1.

Proteins. A high-protein diet stimulates the increase in glomerular filtration rate, glomerular capillary blood flow, blood pressure gradients across the glomerular capillary wall, and enlargement of individual nephrons, whereas a low-protein diet blunts or prevents this response.[50] Moreover, rats with renal injury who are fed a high-protein diet develop renal failure, and when such animals are fed a low-protein diet, the progression of renal failure is retarded or arrested.[35,36,40] A current theory postulates that a high protein intake, by increasing both glomerular capillary blood flow and transcapillary glomerular hydraulic pressure, causes progressive renal injury to the basement membrane (filtering wall) of the glomerulus. These alterations, in turn, increase capillary permeability, enhance movement of large molecules across the glomerular basement membrane, and cause deposition of these compounds in the mesangium, mesangial expansion, an inflammatory response in the glomerulus, scarring, and glomerulosclerosis.[50,54,55] A low-protein diet retards or stops progressive renal damage by preventing or reducing these high flow rates and pressures. Diets providing soya protein, a vegetable protein, as compared to casein, an animal protein, may be more effective in retarding the progression of kidney failure in rats with remnant kidneys.[56]

Diabetic rats with moderate hyperglycemia develop similar changes,[57] and similar abnormalities appear to occur in the intact kidney of humans with diabetes mellitus. Early during the course of diabetes mellitus, patients develop increased renal blood flow, increased GFR, and large kidneys.[58] Ultimately, in a large proportion of these individuals, glomerulosclerosis occurs and renal failure supervenes.[59,60]

Phosphorus and Calcium. As previously indicated, a low phosphorus intake independent of protein intake seems to retard progression of renal failure.[37] The mechanism of action of the low phosphorus intake is unclear. One theory is that a low phosphorus intake decreases the deposition of calcium phosphate in kidney tissue, which may cause further renal damage.[61,62] Indeed, in renal tissue obtained by biopsy or autopsy, a direct correlation exists between the calcium content and the serum creatinine concentration.[63] Moreover, in rats with chronic renal insufficiency, administration of the calcium-channel blocker verapamil retards the rate of progression of renal failure, as compared with treatment with an antihypertensive agent that does not impede the intracellular movement of calcium.[64] In general, the calcium concentration of renal tissue is increased in kidneys with severe renal histopathologic features.

TABLE 65–1. POTENTIAL CAUSES AND MECHANISMS OF PROGRESSIVE RENAL FAILURE*

CAUSES†
Continued activity of the underlying renal disease
Systemic hypertension
High-protein diet
High-phosphorus diet
High-total-fat or -cholesterol diet
High calcium-phosphorus product in sera
Vitamin D overdose (causing hypercalcemia)
High serum oxalate levels (can be enhanced by high ascorbic acid intake)
Hyperuricemia
Acidemia
Iron and or high (i.e., normal) hematocrit
Nephrotoxic medicines (e.g., radiocontrast material, aminoglycoside antibiotics)
MECHANISMS
Intraglomerular capillary pressure and capillary blood flow
Intraglomerular transcapillary hydraulic pressure
Glomerular hypertrophy
Lipoprotein and lipid deposition in glomerulus
Deposition of other proteins in glomerulus
Inflammatory response in kidney with release of cytokines and monokines
Platelet aggregation in kidney
Calcium phosphate or calcium oxalate deposition in the kidney
Release of growth factors in kidney
Increased mesangial matrix production
Enhanced renal tubular generation of ammonia leading to complement activation
Increased generation of oxidants and oxygen radicals in remaining functional nephrons
Urate deposition in the kidney
Lead, cadmium toxicity

*For many of these factors, evidence that they may cause progressive renal failure is derived from animal models or in vitro systems.

†Except for the first item, these causes of progressive renal failure may act through one or more of the mechanisms listed in the lower half of this table.

Lipids and Lipoproteins. Many animal studies suggest a pathogenetic role of dietary fat intake and hyperlipoproteinemia. Rats, rabbits, and guinea pigs fed a high-cholesterol diet developed hypercholesterolemia and progressive glomerulosclerosis and renal failure.[42,65,66] The lipid composition of renal cortical tissue is altered, and there is an increase in mesangial cellularity, as well as matrix formation.[65] Glomerular capillary pressure increases, even though systemic blood pressure is not extremely elevated. This finding suggests that glomerular hypertension may play a role in the loss of renal function in the dietary cholesterol or hypercholesterolemia model of renal insufficiency. The cholesterol-induced renal injury is much greater when cholesterol-supplemented rats have other underlying renal disease. Drugs that lower serum lipoprotein levels may also ameliorate glomerular injury in rats.[67]

Mesangial cells and monocytes have receptors for certain lipoproteins.[68] Monocytes may ingest low-density lipoprotein (LDL) cholesterol and other lipoproteins. These compounds, once ingested, may initiate a series of biochemical and physiologic processes that may induce injury. For example, monocytes from hypercholesterolemic animals have increased adherence of endothelial cells and migrate to the subendothelial spaces more effectively, as compared with normal monocytes.[69] Activated macrophages produce more toxic oxygen radicals. Moreover, rats made hypercholesterolemic by high-cholesterol diets show evidence of increased glomerular arteriole contractility, probably by oxidized lipoprotein activation of thromboxane.[70] Hypercholesterolemia may also alter the metabolism of certain fatty acids including arachidonic and linoleic acid.

The essential fatty acid linoleic acid can be metabolized in the kidney to several families of eicosanoids including prostaglandins. Prostaglandins have far-reaching effects on the blood flow and blood pressure inside the glomerulus, the propensity for platelets to clot in the glomerulus, and the inflammatory process. Certain eicosanoids have antagonistic effects; some increase glomerular blood flow and pressure and may impair platelet clotting, whereas others do the opposite. In renal insufficiency, elaboration of certain eicosanoids is increased in the kidney,[45,71] and they appear to play an important role in the complex adaptive processes undergone by the nephron as kidney function deteriorates.[2,72]

Experiments in which rats and mice with impaired renal function or renal disease were given supplemental dietary linoleic acid,[45] injections of prostaglandin E_1 or E_2 (PGE_1 or PGE_2), [46,47] drugs that inhibit synthesis of thromboxane, a prostaglandin that causes intrarenal vasoconstriction and platelet aggregation,[72] or anticoagulants that inhibit platelet clotting have reduced progressive renal injury and maintain a more normal GFR. These experimental studies suggest that eicosanoids may play an important role in the progression of renal failure.

Experimental studies in NZB/NZW mice also suggest that dietary manipulation may ameliorate a renal disease resembling lupus erythematosus that occurs in these animals. A diet fed to these mice that is restricted in essential fatty acids decreases the severity of glomerulonephritis, lowers serum antinuclear antibody and anti-DNA antibody levels, and prolongs life.[43,44,73] Diets deficient in essential fatty acids reduce synthesis of eicosanoid compounds, including PGE.[43] Subcutaneous injections of PGE_1 or PGE_2 in NZB/NZW mice also reduce the severity of renal disease, decrease the incidence of proteinuria, and prolong survival even though they do not alter serum immunoglobulin levels or antinuclear or anti-DNA antibodies.[46,47] Moreover, supplementing the diet with eicosapentaenoic acid reduces proteinuria and prolongs survival in these NZB/NZW F_1 mice.[74] The mechanism of action of eicosapentaenoic acid may be related to its propensity to impair platelet aggregation, which may, in turn, be due to the ability of this lipid to inhibit the synthesis of prostaglandins and thromboxanes from arachidonic acid.

McLeish and co-workers reported that injection of PGE_1 ameliorated the inflammatory and cellular response to immune-complex glomerulonephritis and may reduce deposition in the glomerulus of IgG and C_3, but not IgM.[48] The glomerular synthesis of leukotriene B_4, a lipoxygenase product of arachidonic acid released during inflammation, is increased in rats with immune-complex-mediated glomerulonephritis.[75] Preliminary evidence suggests that this compound may cause glomerular constriction and may participate in the reduced glomerular function that accompanies glomerular inflammatory injury.[76] In rats with Heymann nephritis, dietary protein restriction itself reduces eicosanoid synthesis.[77] Hence the beneficial effects of dietary protein restriction may possibly be partly related to its effects on eicosanoid production. Glomerular perfusion and pressure, platelet aggregation, and the inflammatory response each may be mediated by eicosanoid compounds. Hence the administration of diets or drugs that alter synthesis of various eicosanoids and anticoagulants may retard progressive renal disease.

Medicines. Although results of the foregoing studies in animals indicate an important role for dietary restriction of protein and phosphorus, and reduction or increase of certain fats to control progressive renal failure, there is evidence that certain medicines may be capable of substituting for the restriction of nutrients. Enalapril, a drug that decreases blood pressure by inhibiting the conversion of angiotensin I to angiotensin II, also lowers glomerular capillary blood flow and blood pressure gradients across the glomerular capillary wall in rats with renal insufficiency.[78] This agent also appears to retard progressive renal failure in these animals.[78,79] Several angiotensin-converting enzyme inhibitors reduce urinary protein excretion in patients with kidney disease.[80,81] The class of antihypertensive medicines that are calcium-channel blockers may also have a specific effect in inhibiting progressive renal failure.[82,83] Evidence also strongly suggests that blood pressure control, by itself, may retard progressive renal failure.[82–84]

As described earlier, certain prostaglandins, as well as drugs that prevent blood clotting or inhibit the synthesis of other eicosanoids, also seem to reduce scarring and loss of renal function in rats.[72,85] Moreover, medicines that bind phosphorus in the intestinal tract can enhance the effectiveness of dietary phosphorus restriction.[37,86] These last drugs are of particular value as a supplement to dietary phosphorus restriction because it is difficult to lower dietary phosphorus intake to necessary levels without making diets highly restrictive, unpalatable, and unconducive to adherence.

Human Studies. To what extent are animal data applicable to patients? From the mid-1970s to the present, virtually all dietary studies in humans with renal insufficiency have indicated that a low intake of dietary protein and phosphorus is effective in retarding the progression of renal failure.[87–96] Some evidence indicates that a low protein and phosphorus intake may each act separately to slow progressive renal failure.[97]

The earlier studies of this question in humans generally suffered from one or more major defects in experimental design, including small sample size, inadequate or absent control groups, poor documentation of patients' actual intake, and imprecise methods of measuring renal function. Some more recent clinical trials have used more effective research protocols. These later studies have generally compared a low-protein, low-phosphorus diet providing about 0.40 to 0.60 g protein/kg body weight per day or about 0.28 g protein/kg per day supplemented with essential amino acids or keto acids to a more liberal diet containing approximately 1.0 g protein/kg per day and more phosphorus or an ad libitum diet. Both nondiabetic patients and patients with insulin-dependent diabetes mellitus have been evaluated in different studies. These more recent studies also indicate that the low-protein, low-phosphorus diets do retard progression of renal failure in comparison with higher protein and phosphorus intakes.[95,96]

The very low-protein diet providing about 0.28 g/kg per day (e.g., about 16 to 25 g protein per day) is supplemented with 10 to 20 g per day of the nine essential amino acids or of mixtures of several essential amino acids, in some preparations several nonessential amino acids, and keto acid or hydroxyacid analogues of other essential amino acids.[87,89–92,94] The keto acid or hydroxyacid analogue is structurally identical to its corresponding essential amino acid, except the amino (NH_2) group attached to the second (α) carbon of the amino acid is replaced with a keto group or hydroxy group, respectively (Fig. 65–2).

The keto acid and hydroxyacid analogues can be transaminated in the body to the respective amino acids, although a proportion of the analogues are degraded rather than transaminated. Because the keto acids and hydroxyacids lack the nitrogen-containing amino group on the α carbon, these compounds provide the patient with a lesser nitrogen load. As they are degraded in the body, they should engender fewer waste products that will accumulate in renal failure. Keto acid analogues of the branched-chain amino acids, especially of leucine, may be particularly likely to promote protein anabolism, possibly by decreasing protein degradation.[98,99] Hence it is possible but not yet demonstrated that these keto acids may play a beneficial role in maintaining protein mass in patients with renal failure.

Walser et al. developed a mixture of keto acids, hydroxyacids, and amino acids that was fed to patients with chronic renal failure in association with a diet that provided about 0.28 g protein/kg per day.[92,94] This combined low-protein, keto acid, and amino acid diet appears to have a marked effect in retarding or stopping progression of renal failure for up to 3 years. Progression of renal failure was examined before and after starting these diets, and no concurrent control diet was evaluated in these studies. However, the results were dramatic enough to suggest that this diet may be more effective at arresting progressive renal failure than any other diet that has been evaluated. The nitrogen content of this keto acid-supplemented diet is not substantially lower than that of a 40-g protein diet. This finding suggests, but does not prove, that the keto acid diet may exert a specific protective effect on progression of renal failure that may be independent of its nitrogen content. The keto acid formulation used in these studies contains no phenylalanine and little or no tryptophan, which are both essential amino acids, although a substantial amount of tyrosine will replace most of the need for phenylalanine. Further investigation is necessary to determine the risks of malnutrition with these low-protein diets and how to minimize such risks.

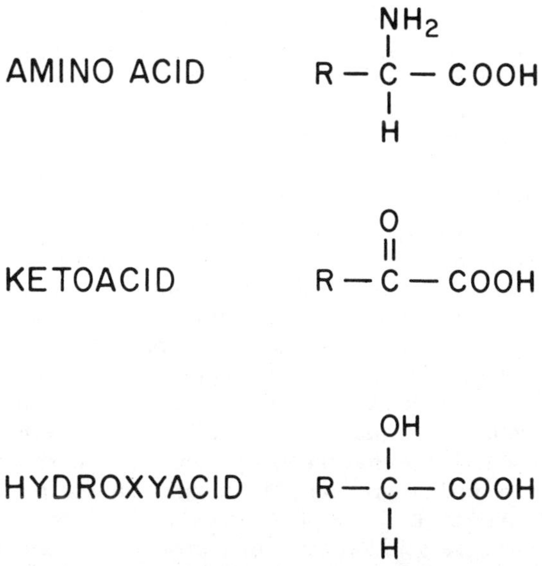

FIGURE 65–2. The prototype structure of an amino acid and of a keto acid and hydroxyacid analogue of the amino acid. R refers to the side chain, which is different for each individual compound.

An interesting sidelight to these studies of the effects of diet on progression of renal failure is the question whether diet may promote or retard the development of renal failure in individuals with no underlying renal disease. As indicated previously, very high-cholesterol diets may cause renal failure in animals. Rats without renal disease or with only one kidney that are allowed to eat ad libitum or are fed high-protein diets throughout life have a higher incidence of renal disease in old age.[100–103] In normal humans, after about the fourth decade of life, renal function falls progressively with age;[104] it is possible that high-protein diets may play a role in this phenomenon. In healthy young men and women, a high-protein intake increases renal blood flow and GFR.[8] Moreover, similarities exist between the type of scarring that occurs in normal aging human kidneys and the kidneys of rats fed high-protein diets. Adults who have had a congenital absence, failure of development, or surgical removal of one kidney during childhood have a small increase in the incidence of spontaneous glomerular scarring in the remaining kidney.[105] The cause of this phenomenon is not known. However, it is possible that the typical protein intake of Americans, which is considerably higher than the recommended dietary allowances for protein,[106] may increase glomerular capillary blood flow and pressure and may cause progressive renal injury.

NEPHROTIC SYNDROME

The nephrotic syndrome is a kidney disorder characterized by losses of large quantities of protein in the urine (at least 3.0 g per day), low serum albumin concentrations, high blood levels of certain fats, and accumulation of body water to form frank edema.[107] This condition is caused by diseases that affect the glomerulus and increase glomerular permeability to protein. Patients with the nephrotic syndrome are often wasted and debilitated. Because of their large protein losses and their frequently poor appetite, such patients often develop protein malnutrition. Because certain vitamins and most trace elements are protein bound in plasma, these individuals are also at risk for developing deficiencies of these nutrients. Vitamin D deficiency has been reported in patients with the nephrotic syndrome.[107,108] Wasting and malnutrition may occur in nephrotic patients even when they do not have advanced kidney failure.

Studies suggest that both protein-restricted diets and angiotensin-converting-enzyme inhibitors reduce proteinuria in nephrotic patients without causing a reduction in serum albumin levels or albumin pools.[80,109–111] Treating nephrotic syndrome patients with both an angiotensin-converting-enzyme inhibitor, which may decrease proteinuria, and a higher-protein diet, to increase protein synthesis, has been suggested as the most effective way to maintain a more normal albumin mass in these individuals.[80,111] This hypothesis has been demonstrated in one study in nephrotic rats but has not yet been tested in nephrotic patients.[111]

NUTRITIONAL AND METABOLIC CONSEQUENCES OF CHRONIC RENAL FAILURE

Chronic renal failure causes pervasive nutritional and metabolic disorders that may affect virtually every organ system. These abnormalities are reviewed briefly.

CLINICAL, NUTRITIONAL, AND METABOLIC DISORDERS

Patients with chronic renal failure develop azotemia and uremia. Azotemia refers to the accumulation of nitrogenous metabolites in the blood. Uremia is the combination of azotemia with the clinical signs and symptoms of advanced renal failure. Chronic advanced renal failure is a complex disorder caused by a marked reduction in the excretory, endocrine, and metabolic functions of the kidney.

The many symptoms of uremia include weakness, a feeling of ill health, insomnia, fatigue, loss of appetite, nausea, vomiting, diarrhea, itching, muscle cramps, hiccups, twitching or jerking of the extremities, fasciculations, tremors, emotional irritability, and decreased mental concentration and comprehension. A characteristic fetid breath is often present. The fluid and electrolyte disturbances associated with renal failure can lead to congestive heart failure and hypertension or, if excessive sodium depletion occurs, reduction in extracellular fluid volume and a fall in blood pressure.

Altered serum electrolyte concentrations and acidosis can also occur, and these complications can have profound and life-threatening effects on the physiologic processes and metabolism of the body. Abnormalities in water and electrolyte balance and acidosis are caused by impaired ability of the failing kidney to regulate the content of water, salts, and acids in the body. Most of these clinical and metabolic disorders can be controlled or prevented with dietary therapy or dialysis. When untreated, uremia can lead to lethargy, loss of consciousness, coma, convulsions, and death.

Chronic advanced renal failure causes pervasive alterations in the absorption, excretion, or metabolism of many nutrients. These disorders include the accumulation of chemical products of protein metabolism;[1,112] a decreased ability of the kidney either to excrete a large salt load or to conserve salt rigorously when dietary sodium is restricted;[113] impaired renal ability to excrete water, potassium, calcium, magnesium, phosphorus, trace elements, acids, and other compounds;[114] a tendency to retain phosphorus;[115] decreased intestinal absorption of calcium,[115,116] and possibly iron;[117] and a high risk for developing certain vitamin deficiencies, particularly vitamin B_6, vitamin C, folic acid, and the most potent known form of vitamin D, 1,25-dihydroxycholecalciferol.[115,118] The patient with chronic renal failure is also likely to accumulate certain potentially toxic chemicals, such as aluminum, that normally are ingested in small amounts and excreted in the urine.[119]

Uremia is also a polyendocrinopathy, and many of the metabolic and clinical manifestations of uremia are caused by the endocrine disorders. Many hormone concentrations are elevated in renal failure, particularly those of the peptide hormones, because of the impaired ability of the kidney to degrade peptides. These substances include parathyroid hormone, glucagon, insulin, growth hormone, prolactin, luteinizing hormone, often follicle-stimulating hormone (FSH), and gastrin.[115,120–128] Increased secretion of some hormones, such as insulin, may contribute to elevated plasma levels. Chronically uremic patients have altered thyroid hormone levels that are similar to the euthyroid sick syndrome, but hypothyroidism is not common.[129] Of the hormones elaborated by the kidney, plasma erythropoietin and 1,25-dihydroxycholecalciferol are reduced,[4–6,115] and plasma renin activity may be increased, normal, or decreased. Serum IGF-1 (somatomedin C) levels, measured by radioreceptor assay or radioimmunoassay, are usually reported to be normal in renal failure, but the biologic activity of IGF-1 may be inhibited by uremic sera.[130,131] There is increased sensitivity to the actions of glucagon, which is reversed by hemodialysis, although hyperglucagonemia persists.[121] Resistance to the peripheral action of insulin occurs.[132] These effects on insulin and glucagon contribute to the mild glucose intolerance usually present in chronic renal failure.[132]

The ability of the failing kidney to synthesize or to metabolize many compounds, including amino acids, is impaired. Thus, the failing kidney demonstrates reduced catabolism of glutamine, impaired synthesis of alanine, and decreased conversion of glycine to serine.[112,133,134]

Many products of metabolism accumulate in renal failure; the majority of these are derived from amino acids and proteins.[135] Most of these compounds accumulate as the result of decreased excretion, although in some instances enhanced synthesis or impaired degradation by the diseased kidney or other organs plays a role.[112] Abnormal metabolism in the gastrointestinal tract and probably the liver also contributes to increased levels of certain metabolites in renal failure.[112,136]

Quantitatively, the most important end product of nitrogen metabolism is urea.[135] In a clinically stable patient with chronic renal failure who eats at least 40 g of protein per day, the net quantity of urea produced each day contains an amount of nitrogen equal to about 80 to 90% of the daily nitrogen intake. Guanidines are the next most abundant end product of nitrogen metabolism. These compounds include creatinine, creatine, and guanidinosuccinic acid. The "middle molecules" are a class of compounds that are midway in size between the small, readily dialyzable substances that accumulate in renal failure and small proteins. Most middle molecules are considered to have molecular weights of approximately 300 to 2500 and contain amino acids. Some middle molecule compounds are increased in uremic sera.[135] Despite decades of study, the compounds that cause uremic toxicity are not well defined. Probably, many compounds contribute to uremic toxicity. Prime suspects for uremic toxins include urea, guanidine compounds, phenolic acids, middle molecules, and some of the hormones elevated in uremic plasma, especially parathyroid hormone and glucagon.[135]

Altered gastrointestinal function may affect nitrogen metabolism in uremic patients. The gastrointestinal tract metabolizes urea, uric acid, creatinine, and choline and synthesizes or releases from larger molecules dimethylamine, trimethylamine, ammonia, sarcosine, methylamine, and methylguanidine.[112] The gut metabolism or synthesis of many of these compounds is increased in renal failure, possibly because of the rise in the quantity of intestinal bacterial flora.[136]

Some of the metabolic alterations in uremia are adaptive homeostatic responses that offer both benefits and disadvantages to the patient. Hyperparathyroidism is an example. As the kidneys fail, impaired excretion of phosphorus leads to phosphorus retention. Concomitantly, the diseased and scarred renal parenchyma is less able to convert 25-hydroxycholecalciferol to the most potent metabolite of vitamin D, 1,25-dihydroxycholecalciferol.[115,116] Low plasma concentrations of 1,25-dihydroxycholecalciferol lead to an increase in parathyroid hormone secretion. In addition, deficiency of 1,25-dihydroxycholecalciferol both impairs intestinal calcium absorption and causes resistance to the actions of parathyroid hormone in bone. These alterations also promote hypocalcemia and lead to the development of hyperparathyroidism. The elevated serum parathyroid hormone reduces renal tubular reabsorption of phosphorus (enhancing urine phosphorus excretion), lowers serum phosphorus, promotes renal synthesis of 1,25-dihydroxycholecalciferol, mobilizes calcium from bone, and increases intestinal calcium absorption, although intestinal calcium absorption usually remains low or, in mild renal insufficiency, normal. The benefits derived from these homeostatic actions are that more normal concentrations of plasma phosphorus and calcium are maintained. The "trade-off" is the development of hyperparathyroidism.[137] Parathyroid hormone has been implicated as a pervasive uremic toxin that affects many organs and tissues and contributes to the uremic syndrome.[138]

With the institution of appropriate dietary therapy or treatment with hemodialysis or peritoneal dialysis, blood levels of many metabolic products that accumulate in uremic plasma decrease, and the patient may experience clinical improvement. Maintenance hemodialysis or peritoneal dialysis enables patients to live for many years with essentially no renal function. Despite such improvement, however, many clinical and metabolic disorders may persist or even progress. These include: (1) a type IV hyperlipidemia;[139] (2) a high incidence of cardiovascular disease;[140] (3) osteodystrophy with disordered bone architecture, osteoporosis, or osteomalacia (aluminum toxicity often contributes to the osteomalacia);[115,116,119] (4) anemia;[5,6,117] (5) mildly impaired peripheral and central nervous system function; (6) muscle weakness and atrophy; (7) frequent occurrence of viral hepatitis;[141] (8) sexual impotency and infertility; (9) generalized wasting and malnutrition;[112,142–154] (10) a general feeling of ill health or depression; and (11) poor rehabilitation.[155] Most of these complications can be aggravated by poor nutritional intake or improved with good nutrition. Anemia, which usually is primarily due to impaired erythropoiesis caused by deficiency of erythropoietin, can be treated effectively with this hormone. To reduce the risk of therapy, usually sufficient erythropoietin is given to raise the hematocrit only to about 33%. When kidney failure is a complication of an underlying systemic disease, such as diabetes mellitus, hypertension, or lupus erythematosus, other manifestations of these underlying diseases may also adversely affect the patient and may be progressive. All the foregoing problems do not seriously affect every patient, and many patients with chronic uremia and who undergo dialysis patients lead full and productive lives.

The foregoing considerations indicate that the intestinal absorption, excretion, and/or metabolism of virtually every nutrient may be altered in renal failure. In addition, the decreased intake of food and excessive intake of certain minerals, such as aluminum from the ingestion of aluminum phosphate binders, may alter nutritional status. Moreover, medicinal therapy may adversely affect nutrient metabolism in renal failure. For example, anticonvulsant medicines may cause deficiencies of vitamin D and folic acid; hydralazine, isoniazid, and other medicines may cause vitamin B_6 deficiency.[118] Part of the challenge of dietary therapy for patients with renal failure is to provide for the altered requirements of many nutrients that occur in this condition.

WASTING SYNDROME

The patient with chronic renal failure frequently shows evidence of wasting or protein-calorie malnutrition (Table 65–2).[112,142–154,156] Evidence includes decreased relative body weight (i.e., the patient's body weight divided by the weight of normal people of the same age range, height, sex, and skeletal frame size),

TABLE 65–2. EVIDENCE OF WASTING OR PROTEIN-CALORIE MALNUTRITION IN PATIENTS WITH ADVANCED CHRONIC RENAL FAILURE

ANTHROPOMETRY, BODY COMPOSITION, AND ISOTOPE DILUTION STUDIES*	BIOCHEMISTRY*
Decreased	Decreased
Body weight	Serum
Height (children)	Total protein
Growth (children)	Albumin
Body fat (skinfold thickness)	Transferrin
Fat-free solids	Prealbumin
Intracellular water	C3
Muscle mass (midarm muscle circumference)	C3 Activator
Total body potassium (nondialyzed patients)	Cholinesterase
Total body nitrogen (CAPD patients)	Pseudocholinesterase
Total albumin mass, synthesis, and catabolism	Plasma
Valine pools (nondialyzed patients)	Leucine
	Isoleucine
	Total tryptophan
	Valine
	Tyrosine
	Valine/glycine ratio
	Essential/nonessential ratio
	Muscle
	Alkali-soluble protein
	RNA:DNA ratio
	Valine
	Tyrosine
	Increased
	Plasma
	Glycine

*Patients with chronic renal failure may have normal values for these parameters, but statistical comparisons indicate that the levels are often abnormal in these individuals.

skinfold thickness (an estimate of total body fat), arm muscle mass, total body nitrogen, low growth rates in children, decreased serum concentrations of many proteins including albumin, transferrin, and certain complement proteins, and low muscle alkali-soluble protein. The plasma amino acid pattern, which is pathognomonic of renal failure, also has similarities to that found in malnutrition. Total body potassium is reported to be low in patients with chronic renal failure and normal in those undergoing long-term maintenance hemodialysis. The findings of wasting are sometimes observed in nondialyzed patients with chronic renal failure, but are more prevalent in patients undergoing maintenance hemodialysis or chronic peritoneal dialysis. Not every dialysis patient has evidence of these disorders; however, virtually every survey of maintenance dialysis patients indicates that, as a group, these patients show evidence of malnutrition. Wasting and malnutrition are only mild to moderate in most of these patients. About 8% of dialysis patients have evidence of severe wasting.

The causes of wasting in chronic renal failure are many.[112,154] First, dietary intake is often inadequate, particularly for energy requirements.[112,143,152,153] The low dietary intake is caused by anorexia because of uremic toxicity, the debilitating effects of chronic illnesses, depression, and the effects of acute superimposed illnesses on the patient's ability to eat or to accept tube feeding. In addition, the dietary prescription in renal failure, which is low in protein and other nutrients and which may be difficult to prepare or unpalatable, can lead to low nutrient intakes. Second, patients with renal failure have a high incidence of superimposed catabolic illnesses.[155–158] Third, the dialysis procedure itself may induce wasting. During hemodialysis and peritoneal dialysis, free amino acids, peptides or bound amino acids,[159–161] water-solute vitamins,[118] proteins (with peritoneal dialysis),[162] glucose (during hemodialysis with glucose-free dialysate),[160] and probably other bioactive compounds are lost. Hemodialysis also seems to increase net protein breakdown.[163] Fourth, patients with renal failure sustain blood losses. Because blood is a rich source of protein, these losses might contribute to protein depletion. The blood losses occur from frequent blood drawing for laboratory testing, occult gastrointestinal bleeding, which is common in renal failure, and sequestration of blood in the hemodialyzer and blood tubing.[164]

Other possible but unestablished causes of wasting include: (1) altered endocrine activity, particularly insulin resistance; hyperglucagonemia,[121] inhibition of IGF-1 activity;[131] hyperparathyroidism, and deficiency of 1,25-dihydroxycholecalciferol;[115] (2) endogenous uremic toxins; (3) exogenous uremic toxins, such as aluminum; and (4) loss of metabolic functions of the kidney. Because the kidney is a metabolic organ that synthesizes or degrades many biologically valuable compounds, including amino acids,[112] the loss of these activities in kidney failure could possibly disrupt the body's metabolism and promote wasting.

Several investigators have shown an inverse relationship between dietary protein consumption, as determined by the patient's urea nitrogen appearance or average blood urea nitrogen (BUN) level, and morbidity and mortality.[165,166] Moreover, a striking inverse relationship in these patients exists between their serum albumin level and their mortality rate.[167] These studies were not prospective with randomized assignment to different nutritional intakes, and it is likely that the patients' underlying illnesses contributed to both their high mortality and the low protein intake or serum albumin. Nonetheless, the data are consistent with the thesis that poor nutrient intake and malnutrition adversely affect prognosis in patients receiving long-term hemodialysis.

DIETARY MANAGEMENT OF CHRONIC RENAL DISEASE AND FAILURE

Recommended nutrient intake is given in Table 65–3 for patients with chronic renal failure who are not undergoing dialysis therapy as well as for patients undergoing maintenance hemodialysis or continuous ambulatory peritoneal dialysis. The following text explains my approach to the dietary management of these patients.

GENERAL PRINCIPLES OF DIETARY THERAPY

The widespread metabolic and nutritional disorders, frequent occurrence of protein-calorie malnutrition, and evidence that diet may retard the progression of renal failure indicate that nutritional management is a critical aspect of the treatment of chronic renal failure. The three goals of dietary therapy are: (1) to retard or to stop the rate of progression of renal failure; (2) to maintain good nutritional status; and (3) to prevent or to minimize uremic toxicity and the metabolic derangements of renal failure.

Adherence to specialized diets is difficult and stressful for most patients and their families. Generally, it requires patients to undergo a major change in their behavior patterns and to forsake many of their traditional sources of daily pleasure. The patient must procure special foods, prepare special recipes, usually forego or severely limit intake of many favorite foods, and often eat foods that are not desirable. Demands are made on the time, effort, and emotional support system of the family or close associates. Therefore, it is incumbent on the physician not to prescribe radical changes in dietary intake without a clear indication that such changes may be beneficial to the patient. To ensure successful dietary therapy, patients with renal failure must undergo extensive training in the principles of nutritional therapy and the design and preparation of diets, and they need continuous encouragement regarding dietary adherence. These patients must receive repeated retraining with regard to their nutritional therapy. When nutritional intake is not carefully monitored, patients tend to adhere poorly to dietary prescriptions. They may eat too little of certain nutrients rather than too much.

A team approach to dietary management may improve adherence to the special diet. The team should include the physician, dietitian, close family members, nursing staff, and, where available, psychiatrists or social workers. Diet plans should be designed specifically for the individual tastes of the patient. At each visit, the physician should monitor dietary intake and should discuss the results with the patient.

The physician must strongly support the dietitian's efforts to train and counsel the patient and to obtain dietary compliance. Generally, the patient's spouse or other close relatives or friends should work closely with the patient to provide moral support and to assist with acquisition and preparation of foods. To promote adherence to the diet, the entire medical team should assume an energetic, positive, and sympathetic approach.

Because the prescribed diets are often marginally low in some nutrients, such as protein, and high in others, such as calcium, and malnutrition is not infrequent, it is important periodically to evaluate the adequacy of the diet and the patient's nutritional status. Nutritional evaluation should include assessment of dietary intake by interviews, dietary diaries, and measurement of urea nitrogen appearances (UNA) and evaluation of nutritional status by anthropometry, biochemical measurements, bone radiography, and other parameters[146] (see Table 65–2). The dietitian is often best qualified to perform nutritional evaluation. In general, to maintain good dietary compliance and to monitor fluid and electrolyte disorders and clinical and nutritional status, patients with advanced renal failure should be seen monthly by the physician and the dietitian. Patients with slowly progressive mild or moderate renal insufficiency, under some circumstances, may see the physician less frequently, but should still see the dietitian approximately monthly to promote adherence to the diet.

Evidence suggests that chronically uremic patients are at greatest risk for wasting and malnutrition during the period when the GFR falls below 5 ml per minute and when the patient is commencing maintenance dialysis therapy.[154] Moreover, the nutritional status of patients at the onset of chronic dialysis treatment appears to be a good predictor of nutritional status 2 to 3 years later.[154,168] Hence particular effort should be made to preventing malnutrition as the patient approaches the time when dialysis should be instituted and during the first few weeks of chronic dialysis therapy. Such effort should be directed toward maintaining good nutritional

TABLE 65–3. RECOMMENDED NUTRIENT INTAKE FOR NONDIALYZED PATIENTS WITH CHRONIC RENAL FAILURE AND FOR PATIENTS UNDERGOING MAINTENANCE HEMODIALYSIS OR CHRONIC PERITONEAL DIALYSIS

	CHRONIC RENAL FAILURE[a,b]	HEMODIALYSIS (HD) OR CHRONIC PERITONEAL DIALYSIS (PD)
Protein source	Low-protein diet: 0.55–0.60 g/kg/day ≥0.35 g/kg/day of high-biologic-value protein Very low-protein diet: About 0.28 g/kg/day of protein of any protein of any biologic value supplemented with a ketoacid and amino acid mixture[d]	Hemodialysis[c] 1.0–1.2 g/kg/day ≥50% high-biologic-value protein PD 1.2–1.5 g/kg/day ≥50% high-biologic-value protein
Energy[e]	≥35 kcal/kg/day unless the patient's relative body weight is greater than 120% or the patient gains unwanted weight	
Fat (% of total energy intake)[fg]	30–40	30–40
Polyunsaturated: saturated fatty acid ratio[g]	1.0:1.0	1.0:1.0
Carbohydrate[h]	Rest of nonprotein calories	
Total fiber intake[g]	20–25 g	20–25 g
	Range of Intake	
Minerals		
sodium	1,000 to 3,000 mg/day[i]	750 to 1,000 mg/day[i]
potassium	40 to 70 mEq day	40 to 70 mEq/day
phosphorus	4 to 10 mg/kg/day[j,k]	8 to 17 mg/kg/day[k]
calcium	1,400 to 1,600 mg/day[l]	1,400 to 1,600 mg/day[l]
magnesium	200 to 300 mg/day	200 to 300 mg/day
iron	≥10 to 18 mg/day[m]	≥10 to 18 mg/day[m]
zinc	15 mg/day	15 mg/day
Water	up to 3,000 ml/day as tolerated[i]	usually 750 to 1,500 ml/day[i]
	Diets to be Supplemented with These Quantities	
Vitamins		
thiamin	1.5 mg/day	1.5 mg/day
riboflavin	1.8 mg/day	1.8 mg/day
pantothenic acid	5 mg/day	5 mg/day
niacin	20 mg/day	20 mg/day
pyridoxine HCl	5 mg/day	10 mg/day
vitamin B_{12}	3 μg/day	3 μg/day
vitamin C	60 mg/day	60 mg/day
folic acid	1 mg/day	1 mg/day
vitamin A	no addition	no addition
vitamin D	see text	see text
vitamin E	15 IU/day	15 IU/day
vitamin K	None[n]	None[n]

[a]GFR above 4–5 ml/min/1.73 m^2 and less than 15–25 ml/min/1.73 m^2.

[b]See text for discussion of dietary intake for patients with less severe renal insufficiency.

[c]Protein intake for hemodialysis patients generally should be closer to 1.2 g/kg/day; for PD patients who are not malnourished, it should be about 1.2–1.3 g/kg/day.

[d]There is no unanimity concerning the optimal quantity and formulation of the keto acid and amino acid supplements. The values listed here are representative of the amounts used by nephrologists working in this field.

[e]This includes energy intake from dialysate in the PD patients.

[f]Refers to percentage of total energy intake (diet plus dialysate); if triglyceride levels are elevated, the percentage of fat in the diet may be increased to about 40% of total calories; otherwise, 30% of total calories is preferable.

[g]These dietary recommendations are considered less crucial than the others, unless hyperlipemia is present (see text).

[h]Should be primarily complex carbohydrates, if tolerated by the patient.

[i]Can be higher in PD patients or in those nondialyzed patients with chronic renal failure and hemodialysis patients who have greater urinary losses.

[j]Phosphorus intake should be 4–9 mg/day for patients ingesting a very low-protein diet supplemented with keto acids and amino acids; with the 0.55 to 0.60-g protein/kg/day diet, a phosphorus intake of 5–10 mg/kg/day is more tolerable.

[k]Phosphate binders (aluminum carbonate or hydroxide, calcium carbonate, acetate, or citrate) are often needed as well.

[l]Dietary intake usually must be supplemented to provide these levels.

[m]≥10 mg/day for males and nonmenstruating females; ≥18 mg/day for menstruating females.

[n]Vitamin K supplements may be needed for patients who are not eating and who are receiving antibiotics.

intake during this period, rapidly instituting therapy for supervening illnesses, and maintaining good nutritional intake during such illnesses.

UREA NITROGEN APPEARANCE AND SERUM UREA NITROGEN: SERUM CREATININE RATIO

The control of protein intake is pivotal to the nutritional management of patients with acute or chronic renal failure. Hence one must accurately monitor nitrogen intake. Fortunately, this is possible for most patients. Those who are in nitrogen balance should have a total nitrogen output equal to nitrogen intake minus about 0.5 g nitrogen per day for unmeasured losses from growth of skin, hair, and nails and from sweat, respiration, flatus, and blood drawing.[169] For clinical purposes, a slightly positive or negative balance does not substantially alter the use of the nitrogen output to estimate intake. If patients are in very positive or negative balance, such as from pregnancy or severe infection, nitrogen output may not reflect intake. However, it is usually readily apparent to the clinician whether the patient is in very positive or negative balance and whether the nitrogen output will reflect intake.

The measurement of total nitrogen output is too laborious and expensive to be widely applied for clinical uses. However, because urea is the major nitrogenous product of protein and amino acid degradation, the UNA can be used to estimate total nitrogen output and hence nitrogen intake.[158,170,171] UNA refers to the amount of urea that appears or accumulates in body fluids and all outputs, such as urine, dialysate, and fistula drainage. The term UNA is used rather than urea production or generation because some urea is degraded in the gastrointestinal tract; the ammonia released from urea is largely transported to the liver and converted back to urea.[172,173] Thus, the enterohepatic urea cycle has little effect on urea or total nitrogen economy, and this cycle can be ignored without compromising the ability of the UNA to estimate total nitrogen output or intake accurately. Moreover, the recycling of urea cannot be measured without costly and time-consuming isotope studies.

UNA is calculated as follows:

Equation 1:

$$\text{UNA (g/day)} = \text{urinary urea nitrogen (g/day)} + \text{dialysate urea nitrogen (g/day)} + \text{change in body urea nitrogen (g/day)}$$

Equation 2:

$$\text{Change in body urea nitrogen (g/day)} = (\text{SUN}_f - \text{SUN}_i\text{, g/L/day}) \times \text{BW}_i\text{ (kg)} \times (0.60\text{ L/kg}) + (\text{BW}_f - \text{BW}_i\text{, kg/day}) \times \text{SUN}_f\text{ (g/L)} \times (1.0\text{ L/kg})$$

where i and f are the initial and final values for the period of measurement, SUN is serum urea nitrogen (grams per liter), BW is body weight (kilograms), 0.60 is an estimate of the fraction of body weight that is water, and 1.0 is the fractional distribution of urea in the weight that is gained or lost (i.e., 100%).

The estimated proportion of body weight that is water may be increased in patients who are edematous or lean and decreased in individuals who are obese or very young. Changes in body weight during the 1- to 3-day period of measurement of UNA are assumed to be due entirely to changes in body water. In patients undergoing hemodialysis or intermittent peritoneal dialysis, the urea concentration in dialysate is low and difficult to measure accurately, and UNA is usually calculated during the interdialytic interval and then normalized to 24 hours. Because many patients undergoing dialysis have little or no urinary excretion, the equation for calculating their UNA during the interdialytic interval often can be simplified to Equation 2.

In our metabolic studies, the relationship between UNA and total nitrogen output in chronically uremic patients not undergoing dialysis is as follows:

Equation 3:

$$\text{Total nitrogen output (g/day)} = 0.97\text{ UNA (g/day)} + 1.93$$

If the individual is more or less in neutral nitrogen balance, the UNA also will correlate closely with nitrogen intake. Equation 4 describes our observed relationships between UNA and dietary nitrogen intake in clinically stable nondialyzed chronically uremic patients.

Equation 4:

$$\text{Dietary nitrogen intake (g/day)} = 0.69\text{ UNA (g/day)} + 3.3$$

When both nitrogen intake and UNA are known, nitrogen balance can be estimated from the difference between nitrogen intake and nitrogen output estimated from the UNA. If the patient is pregnant, particularly in the later stages, Equation 4 will underestimate nitrogen intake. For patients who have large protein losses, such as from nephrotic syndrome or peritoneal dialysis, or who are acidemic and have sufficient kidney function to excrete large quantities of ammonia, Equations 3 and 4 will underestimate both nitrogen output and nitrogen intake. In most circumstances, however, these conditions are not present, and the UNA provides a powerful tool for monitoring nitrogen output and intake or estimating balance. Maroni et al. and Sargent and Gotch have described similar techniques for monitoring these parameters.[171,174]

The ratio of SUN to serum creatinine also correlates closely with dietary protein or amino acid intake in chronically uremic patients who are not undergoing dialysis treatment.[175] This relationship can be used to estimate the recent daily intake of such patients. Although this ratio is not as precise as the UNA and is influenced by certain clinical factors, it is easy and inexpensive to measure.

PROTEIN, AMINO ACID, AND KETO ACID INTAKE

GFR Higher than 70 ml/1.73 m² per minute. Virtually no data exist concerning the optimal dietary protein and phosphorus intakes for patients with chronic renal disease and mild impairment in renal function. As information becomes available, dietary guidelines doubtless will change. At present, my colleagues and I do not routinely restrict protein for patients with a GFR higher than 70 ml/1.73 m² per minute unless renal function is continuing to decline. In the latter case, the patient is treated as indicated in the next paragraph. (Note: When the recommended nutrient intake is given in terms of body weight, that body weight measurement refers to desirable body weight as determined from the 1983 Metropolitan Life Insurance Tables.[176])

GFR 25 to 70 ml/1.73 m² per minute. The studies indicating that low-protein, low-phosphorus diets may retard the rate of progression of renal failure are sufficiently convincing to warrant offering patients dietary therapy. Currently, my policy is to discuss with the patient the evidence that such diets retard progression and to indicate that the data justify undergoing dietary protein restriction. If the patient agrees to dietary therapy, a diet is offered providing 0.55 to 0.60 g protein/kg per day, of which at least 35 g/kg per day is high-biologic-value protein to ensure a sufficient intake of the essential amino acids. This quantity of protein should maintain neutral or positive nitrogen balance, and for many patients, it should not be excessively burdensome.

Chronic Renal Failure (GFR lower than 25 ml/1.73 m² per minute) without Dialysis: Role of Low-Protein Diets Supplemented with Amino Acids and Keto Acids. The amino acid- and keto acid-supplemented diets, as currently used, generally provide about 16 to 20 g protein per day (about 0.28 g protein/kg per day) supplemented with essential amino acids or mixtures of amino acids, keto acids, and sometimes hydroxyacids.[87,89–92,177–180] The quantity of essential amino acids or their keto acid or hydroxyacid analogues in the supplements is sufficiently great that it is not necessary to ingest food proteins of high biologic value. This allows patients greater freedom of food selection. The essential amino acid supplements are usually composed of the nine essential L-amino acids, including histidine, and usually are given in daily doses of 14 to 21 g.[89,177–180] Traditionally, the essential amino acids have been proportioned according to the Rose daily amino acid requirements for healthy young adults.[177,178,180] Amino acid formulations have been modified to normalize the concentrations of several plasma and muscle intracellular amino acids in patients with chronic renal failure.[179]

Furst reported, on the basis of ^{15}N studies, that patients with chronic renal failure may not be able to synthesize histidine, whereas normal adults can.[181] However, we have demonstrated that neither normal nor chronically uremic adults are able to synthesize sufficient histidine for their needs.[182] Moreover, we have not observed any difference in the metabolism of histidine in chronically uremic patients, as compared to normal individuals, although the renal histidine clearance is less in the uremic patients.[182–184]

The keto acid formulations have generally included mixtures of four essential L-amino acids (histidine, lysine, threonine, and tryptophan) and α-keto acid or α-hydroxyacid analogues of the five other essential amino acids.[87,89–92] The keto acids and hydroxyacids have the same structure as the respective essential amino acids, except the α-amino nitrogen is removed and a keto or a hydroxy group is substituted (see Fig. 65–2). The keto acids and hydroxyacids generally are formulated as calcium salts or are bound to certain nonessential amino acids, especially ornithine.[87,90–92]

The use of amino acid or keto acid formulations in patients with renal insufficiency has several potential advantages.[185] The relative quantities of these compounds can be modified to normalize both plasma or tissue amino acid concentrations[179] or to increase the content of one or more essential amino acids or amino acid precursors that may improve nitrogen balance.[98,186–188] Several studies have indicated that an increased daily intake of leucine or all three branched-chain amino acids or keto acid analogues may promote protein anabolism.[98,186,188–190] Because the keto acids and hydroxyacids lack the α-amino group, for the same intake of amino acid equivalents less nitrogen is provided and there is less generation of potentially toxic nitrogenous compounds. Another advantage of the amino acid and keto acid diets is that reducing the quantity of protein in the diet lowers the phosphorus intake.

No definitive evidence indicates whether one type of low-nitrogen intake is more likely to retard the progression of renal failure. Clinical trials indicate that the worsening of kidney failure can be slowed in patients prescribed diets providing about 0.40 to 0.60 g protein/kg per day,[88,93,95,96] about 16 to 20 g protein per day (0.28 g protein/kg per day) supplemented with essential amino acids,[89] or 16 to 20 g protein per day supplemented with keto acids.[90–92,94] There are few controlled comparisons among low-nitrogen diets. Jungers and colleagues found in a small number of patients that a keto acid-supplemented diet may retard progression more effectively than a dietary prescription of about 0.60 g protein/kg per day.[191] In addition, the studies of Mitch and co-workers using a low-protein diet and the keto acid-amino acid formulation referred to as EE showed a dramatic slowing of progression of renal failure.[92] Although the authors did not have a concurrent control group, their results with this keto acid-amino acid formulation were more striking than the published reports with other types of low-nitrogen diets. Moreover, in one study, several patients who showed progression of chronic renal failure while ingesting a diet supplemented with essential amino acids and very low in protein displayed substantial slowing of the disease's progression when they were changed to the keto acid-amino acid formulation EE.[94] Thus, it is likely, but not proved, that diets providing about 0.28 g protein/kg per day supplemented with certain keto acid mixtures may be more effective in lowering the rate of progression of renal failure. Prospective clinical trials are currently underway to test this hypothesis.

Based on the foregoing considerations, it seems reasonable that when the GFR decreases to about 25 ml/1.73 m^2 per minute, patients should be prescribed a diet providing 0.28 g protein/kg per day supplemented with a mixture of about 10 to 20 g of keto acids and amino acids (i.e., about 0.28 g/kg body weight per day) (Table 65–3). Because the foregoing evidence suggests that essential amino acid-supplemented very low-protein diets may not be as effective as the keto acid-supplemented diets in preventing progression of renal failure, the former supplements generally are not recommended. In the United States, keto acid supplements have not yet been approved for clinical use. Where keto acids are not available, patients may be prescribed 0.55 to 0.60 g protein/kg daily with at least 0.35 g/kg per day of high-biologic-value protein (Table 65–3). Both these diets generally maintain neutral or positive nitrogen balance and generate a low UNA.[87,177,180,186,192] The diet prescribed to patients with mild-to-severe renal failure should be increased by 1.0 g per day of high-biologic-value protein for each gram of protein excreted in the urine each day.

When the GFR falls below 5 ml/1.73 m^2 per minute, there is not conclusive evidence that patients fare as well with low-nitrogen diets as with regular dialysis and higher protein intakes. Because these patients may be at high risk for wasting or malnutrition,[112] it is recommended that maintenance dialysis treatment or renal transplantation be inaugurated at this time.

NEPHROTIC SYNDROME

Formerly, it was recommended that patients with the nephrotic syndrome be prescribed high-protein diets to prevent protein malnutrition.[193] The current evidence that a high protein intake may accelerate the progression of renal failure has caused a rethinking of the dietary protein prescription for nephrotic patients. Moreover, evidence now indicates that low-protein diets (e.g., 0.80 g protein/kg per day) may decrease urine protein excretion and may maintain or actually increase slightly the serum albumin levels.[109,110] Until more information is available, it is recommended that patients with the nephrotic syndrome be prescribed a diet containing about 0.70 g protein/kg per day and 1.0 g per day of high-biologic-value protein for each gram of urinary protein lost each day. The angiotensin-converting-enzyme inhibitors may reduce proteinuria[80] and therefore should be given preference in the treatment of hypertension in these patients. Patients with the nephrotic syndrome must be monitored closely for depletion of protein, vitamin D analogues, and trace elements.

MAINTENANCE DIALYSIS THERAPY

Although few studies of dietary protein requirements have been conducted in patients undergoing maintenance hemodialysis,[163,194] it seems clear that these patients have greater protein needs because of the removal of amino acids and peptides by dialysis procedures[159,160] and possibly because of other metabolic disorders that occur with end-stage renal disease, such as the catabolic stimulus of hemodialysis.[163] Based upon available evidence from nitrogen balance studies and clinical monitoring of outpatients, patients undergoing maintenance hemodialysis should receive 1.0 to 1.2 g protein/kg per day (Table 65–3). Because many patients receiving maintenance dialysis have evidence of protein wasting, a protein intake of 1.2 g/kg per day is preferable for most individuals.

Patients undergoing continuous ambulatory peritoneal dialysis (CAPD) lose about 9 g protein per day into dialysate as well as a small amount of peptides and about 2.5 to 4.0 g per day of amino acids.[161,162] Nitrogen balance studies suggest that patients undergoing CAPD should, in general, be prescribed 1.2 to 1.3 g protein/kg per day.[195] Patients undergoing CAPD who are protein depleted may be prescribed up to 1.5 g protein/kg per day. At least 50% of the daily protein intake of all patients undergoing maintenance dialysis should be of high biologic value. Several reports indicate that patients undergoing CAPD may maintain their body protein mass with lower dietary protein intakes (e.g., about 0.9 g protein/kg per day). The high incidence of protein malnutrition in these patients would suggest,[156] however, that until more well-controlled evidence is available, the higher protein intakes recommended in this chapter should be prescribed.

ENERGY

Studies in nondialyzed chronically uremic patients and in those undergoing maintenance hemodialysis indicate that energy expenditure is normal when patients are lying in bed and sitting, following ingestion of a standard meal, and during defined exercise.[196,197] Nitrogen balance studies in nondialyzed chronically uremic patients ingesting 0.55 to 0.60 g protein/kg per day indicate that the amount of energy intake necessary to ensure neutral or positive nitrogen balance is approximately 35 kcal/kg per day.[196] However, virtually every survey of energy intake in nondialyzed chronically uremic patients and in patients undergoing maintenance hemodialysis or CAPD indicates that, on average, the dietary intake is lower than this level and usually 30 kcal/kg daily or less.[112,143,146,153] In nondialyzed patients with advanced renal failure and in patients undergoing hemodialysis, the finding that decreased body fat is one of the more prominent alterations in nutritional status supports the contention that these patients require more energy than they usually ingest.[146,149,153] In contrast, patients undergoing CAPD not uncommonly gain fat, probably because of the additional energy intake from glucose absorbed through the peritoneum from dialysate.

Current recommendations are that nondialyzed chronically uremic patients and patients undergoing maintenance hemodialysis or CAPD should ingest at least 35 kcal/kg per day. Patients who are obese with an edema-free body weight greater than 120% of desirable body weight may be treated with lower calorie intakes. Some patients, particularly those with mild renal insufficiency and young or middle-aged women, may become obese on this energy intake or may refuse to ingest the recommended calories out of fear of obesity. These individuals may require a lower energy prescription to avoid alienation from the staff.

Many commercially available high-calorie foodstuffs are low in protein, phosphorus, sodium, and potassium. A nephrology dietitian can recommend these foodstuffs as well as other low-protein, high-calorie foods that can be prepared easily at home.

LIPIDS AND OBESITY

Nondialyzed chronically uremic patients and patients undergoing maintenance hemodialysis and CAPD have a high incidence of type IV hyperlipoproteinemia with increased serum triglyceride levels, elevated serum LDL and very LDL (VLDL), and a low serum high-density lipoprotein (HDL) cholesterol.[139,198] Serum VLDL cholesterol and total cholesterol may also be elevated in patients undergoing CAPD. One cause of these disorders is impaired clearance from blood of triglyceride-rich LDL and VLDL. In addition, because diets in patients with renal failure are usually restricted in protein, sodium, potassium, and water, it is often difficult to provide sufficient energy without resorting to a large intake of purified sugars that may increase triglyceride production. Activities of plasma and hepatic lipoprotein lipase and lecithin cholesterol acyltransferase (LCAT) are decreased.[199] Moreover, carnitine deficiency may sometimes be present.[200,201] Patients with the nephrotic syndrome have hypercholesterolemia, which is caused by increased hepatic apoprotein B and cholesterol synthesis and suppression of LDL-receptor synthesis. These changes are stimulated by hypoalbuminemia. Renal transplant recipients may have type IIb hyperlipidemia with high serum total cholesterol. Type IV hyperlipidemia also is often present after kidney transplantation, particularly if renal failure persists. Medicinal therapy (glucocorticoids, cyclosporine A, diuretics, antihypertensives), renal failure, fasting hyperinsulinemia, and obesity, which occurs frequently after renal transplantation, all may add to the high incidence of serum lipid disorders in renal transplant patients.

Because these abnormalities may contribute to the high incidence of atherosclerosis and cardiovascular disease in patients with chronic renal failure, those undergoing maintenance dialysis, and those receiving renal transplants, attention has been directed toward reducing serum cholesterol and triglycerides and increasing HDL cholesterol.

Serum triglycerides may be lowered by a diet in which the carbohydrate content is reduced to about 35% of total calories, the fat content is increased to about 55% of total calories, and the polyunsaturated:saturated fatty acid ratio is raised to about 1.5:1.0 (Table 65–3).[202,203] However, evidence suggesting that high cholesterol and fat intakes increase the risk of atherosclerotic vascular disease argues against using such diets, particularly because hypertriglyceridemia is not a strong risk factor for atherosclerotic vascular disease. Several investigators have reported that serum triglycerides may be decreased if dialysis patients take L-carnitine, a compound that is often low in their plasma and possibly muscle.[200,201] However, other investigators have not confirmed this effect.[199] Ingestion of activated charcoal may lower serum cholesterol and triglyceride levels in chronically uremic rats.[204] Clofibrate also lowers serum triglyceride levels in uremic patients, but owing to the altered pharmacokinetics of this drug in renal failure, the risk of developing myopathy or other toxicities is high.[205] Omega-3 fatty acids, such as eicosapentaenoic acid and docosahexaenoic acid which are found in fish oil, lower serum triglyceride and total cholesterol levels as well as phospholipids and may be tried.[206] Fish oil also decreases platelet aggregation and exerts anti-inflammatory effects.[207] Some evidence suggests that omega-3 fatty acids or fish oil may retard the progression of chronic renal failure.[208]

At present, I recommend an American Heart Association step I diet for patients with chronic renal failure, nephrosis, or renal transplants. This diet contains no more than 30% of total calories from fat, with saturated fat containing less than 10% of total calories and a cholesterol content of 300 mg per day or lower. My current policy is to treat hypertriglyceridemia by dietary modification when serum triglyceride levels are more than slightly elevated (for example, at least 50 mg/dl above the upper given limit of normal). In these cases, we recommend more energetically that dietary fat intake is not increased above 40% and preferably not above 30% of total calories, and as much as possible of the carbohydrate should be given as complex carbohydrates. Saturated fat should be less than 10% of total calories, polyunsaturated fat 10% or less of total calories, and monounsaturated fat 10 to 15% of calories. The patient's energy intake should be monitored with this diet to ensure that it does not fall. If serum triglyceride levels remain elevated, serum carnitine should be measured. If serum carnitine is low, 0.5 to 1.0 g per day orally may be given to nondialyzed patients with chronic renal failure and patients undergoing maintenance dialysis. Alternatively, patients undergoing hemodialysis may be given L-carnitine, 1.5 g orally or intravenously, at the end of each dialysis. Fish oil supplements may be tried for severe hypertriglyceridemia.[206] Fish oil also is reported to lower serum total cholesterol levels and diastolic blood pressure in hyperlipemic patients undergoing maintenance hemodialysis.[206] Hypercholesterolemia may be treated by giving more of the fatty acids as omega-6 (linoleic)[209] or using hydroxymethylglutaryl coenzyme A (HMGCoA) reductase inhibitors.

Renal transplant patients should be offered a dietary total fat, cholesterol, and saturated fatty acid intake as described previously. The stable renal transplant patient also can undergo a reduction in hyperlipidemia with such diets.[210,211] Pagenkemper et al. reported that a dose of fish oil providing 3 g per day of omega-3 fatty acids for 3 months is also reported to decrease serum triglyceride and VLDL cholesterol levels in hyperlipemic renal transplant recipients; there was no change in their serum total cholesterol or LDL cholesterol levels.[212] No established treatment exists for the low serum concentrations of HDL in uremic patients, although a small amount of alcohol (one glass of wine per day) and exercise may increase levels.[213]

It is uncommon for hemodialysis patients to gain substantial amounts of body fat. On the other hand, patients undergoing CAPD not uncommonly gain excessive body fat because of the additional 400 to 700 kcal they receive from the glucose absorbed from dialysate. Patients are particularly likely to become obese after a successful renal transplant, possibly because of the appetite-stimulating effects of prednisone as well as the rapid correction of uremia, which engenders anorexia. Obesity, defined as a body mass index greater than 30, is reported to increase morbidity and mortality in renal transplant patients.[214] Hence special efforts should be made to prevent or correct obesity in these patients by reducing dietary energy intake.

Few long-term data are available on the effects of dietary fat and carbohydrate intake, obesity, or changing serum lipid levels on the clinical course of patients with specific renal diseases, the nephrotic syndrome, renal failure, or renal transplantation. The recommendations given here are largely derived from data obtained from populations without renal disease, from the recognition that patients with renal disease or renal failure have a high incidence of abnormal serum lipid and lipoprotein levels and atherosclerotic vascular disease, and from studies in animals with renal disease that now indicate that high lipid intakes or elevated lipoprotein levels may accelerate the rate of progression of renal failure, as previously discussed.

CARBOHYDRATES

The patient should be encouraged to eat complex rather than purified carbohydrates to reduce triglyceride synthesis and, where pertinent, to improve glucose tolerance.

FIBER

Studies in the normal population suggest that high dietary fiber intake may reduce the incidence of constipation, irritable bowel syndrome, diverticulitis, and neoplasia of the colon.[215] Fiber may improve glucose tolerance in diabetic patients including those with chronic renal failure.[216] Soluble fiber, which is soluble in the intestinal lumen but is not absorbed, includes pectins, certain gums, and psyllium. Supplemental soluble dietary fiber may also reduce plasma total cholesterol and LDL cholesterol levels in hypercholesterolemic men[217] and may decrease serum fasting triglycerides in hypertriglyceridemic patients with diabetes mellitus.[218] A high dietary fiber intake also may reduce the SUN by decreasing colonic bacterial ammonia generation and enhancing fecal nitrogen excretion.[219] High fiber intakes may promote fecal losses of trace elements. Foods high in fiber are often high in potassium, phosphorus, and low-quality protein. Thus, caution must be exercised when prescribing high-fiber diets to patients with renal failure. Because patients with renal failure may benefit from fiber intake, we currently encourage them to eat 20 to 25 g of total fiber daily.

PHOSPHORUS

In patients with chronic renal failure, a high dietary phosphorus intake can lead to a high plasma phosphorus and calcium-phosphorus product with increased risk of calcium phosphate deposition in soft tissues.[220] As previously discussed, both animal and human studies indicate that a low phosphorus intake may reduce the progression of chronic renal failure.[61,62,97,221]

The optimal dietary phosphorus intake for patients with renal insufficiency has not been established. For the nondialyzed patient, one approach is to attempt to maintain normal renal tubular reabsorption of phosphorus to prevent elevated serum parathyroid hormone levels. This approach would require an extremely low phosphorus intake, lower than can usually be obtained with the combination of a low-phosphorus diet and phosphate binders, unless keto acid- or essential amino acid-supplemented very low-protein diets are used and the GFR is above 15 ml per minute (Table 65–3). At least, in both nondialyzed and dialyzed patients, the morning fasting serum phosphorus concentrations should always be maintained within the normal range. Because a rough correlation exists between the protein and the phosphorus content of the diet, it is easier to restrict phosphorus if protein intake is reduced.

For nondialyzed patients with a GFR below 25 ml/1.73 m^2 per minute who are prescribed a 0.55- to 0.60-g/kg per day protein diet, phosphorus intake generally can be decreased to 5 to 10 mg/kg per day. This may increase the burdensomeness of the diet, particularly at the lower phosphorus intakes. This level of dietary phosphorus restriction usually does not maintain serum phosphorus levels within normal limits in patients with a GFR under about 15 ml per minute, even with a reduction in the renal tubular reabsorption of phosphorus. Hence phosphate binders are also used. Traditionally, the two most commonly used phosphate binders have been aluminum carbonate and aluminum hydroxide. Usually, two to four 500-mg capsules taken three to four times per day are needed. Greater doses may be used if necessary. Evidence that aluminum-induced osteomalacia, anemia, and possibly dementia could be causally related to the intake of aluminum phosphate binders has made many nephrologists reluctant to use such binders.[222,223]

Several alkaline calcium salts are often used to bind phosphate. These include calcium carbonate, calcium acetate, and calcium citrate. Calcium acetate appears to be more potent than calcium carbonate at binding phosphate in the intestinal tract, whereas calcium citrate appears to be the least effective binder. Patients should not ingest calcium citrate if they are taking aluminum as well because the citrate anion may complex with aluminum and enhance its intestinal absorption. The calcium salts are taken in divided doses with meals and should not be given unless the serum phosphorus level is normal, to avoid precipitation of calcium phosphate in soft tissues. Thus, hyperphosphatemic patients may be treated with an aluminum binder of phosphate until serum phosphorus falls to within normal limits, and at that time, they may be changed to calcium carbonate or calcium acetate. Concern exists that calcium binder doses providing more than about 2.0 g calcium per day may cause excessive accumulation of calcium in soft tissues.

As previously indicated, one advantage of the diets providing amino acids or keto acids with about 0.28 g protein/kg per day is the greater ease with which the phosphorus intake can be lowered, often to as low as 4 to 6 mg/kg per day. If future studies confirm that these lower phosphorus intakes are both safe and beneficial for patients with mild or moderate renal insufficiency, this would provide additional justification for the use of these semisynthetic diets at earlier stages of renal failure.

For patients with a GFR between 25 and 70 ml/1.73 m^2 per minute or with a higher GFR and progressive loss of renal function, 7 to 12 mg phosphorus/kg per day may be prescribed with the 0.55- to 0.60-g protein/kg per day diet. Even this level of reduction in phosphorus intake is difficult for many patients to accept, and lower phosphorus intakes make the diet too restrictive for virtually all patients. These individuals generally are not given phosphate binders unless serum phosphorus levels rise above normal. The recommended phosphorus intake for the patient undergoing maintenance hemodialysis or CAPD is about 17 mg/kg per day or less. This higher upper limit was chosen because dialysis patients, with their greater protein intakes, cannot readily ingest less phosphorus without making the diet too restrictive. Patients undergoing maintenance dialysis usually require phosphate binders to prevent hyperphosphatemia.

At present, no lower safe limit for the serum phosphorus level in renal failure has been defined. Experience suggests that if the fasting serum phosphorus is maintained above the lower limit of normal, patients will not develop manifestations of phosphate depletion. More work is necessary to examine whether this perception is valid.

CALCIUM

Patients with chronic renal failure, including those undergoing maintenance dialysis therapy, usually have an increased dietary calcium requirement because they have both vitamin D deficiency and resistance to the actions of vitamin D. These disorders, which lead to impaired intestinal calcium absorption, are compounded by the low calcium content of diets for uremic patients. A 40-g protein, low-phosphorus diet, for example, generally provides only about 300 to 400 mg of calcium daily. Dietary calcium intake is low because many foods that are high in calcium are high in phosphorus, such as dairy products, and are therefore restricted for uremic patients.

Nondialyzed chronically uremic patients usually require 1200 to 1600 mg per day of calcium for neutral or positive calcium balance.[224] The current recommendation is to provide a total daily calcium intake (diet plus supplement) of 1400 to 1600 mg per day. Thus, low-protein diets need to be supplemented with 1000 to 1400 mg of elemental calcium daily. Supplemental calcium should not be initiated unless the serum phosphorus concentration is normal (2.5 to 4.5 mg/dl), to prevent calcium phosphate deposition in soft tissues. In addition, frequent monitoring of serum calcium is important because hypercalcemia may develop, particularly if serum phosphorus should fall to low-normal or low levels. Patients undergoing maintenance hemodialysis or peritoneal dialysis may require 1.0 g per day of supplemental calcium even with the net calcium uptake from dialysate. The supplemental calcium should be taken in two or three divided doses each day.

As indicated previously, the use of calcium binders of phosphate often results in a daily calcium intake that exceeds these levels. Whether these large intakes of calcium will cause hazardous calcium deposits in skeletal or soft tissues is not known. A syndrome called aplastic bone disease has been described predominantly in patients undergoing CAPD.[225] It is characterized by relatively low serum parathyroid hormone concentrations, decreased bone osteoblasts, and marked reduction in bone turnover. The syndrome appears to be new. Treatment with large doses of calcium binders of phosphate has been implicated as a cause of this disorder. Calcium comprises 40% of calcium carbonate, 25% of calcium acetate, and 21% of calcium citrate. Treatment with vitamin D analogues may decrease the daily calcium requirement by enhancing intestinal calcium absorption.

MAGNESIUM

In chronic renal failure, net absorption of approximately 50% of ingested magnesium from the intestinal tract occurs (net absorption is the difference between dietary intake and fecal excretion).[224] The absorbed magnesium is excreted primarily by the kidney. Hence, in renal failure, hypermagnesemia may occur.[226] Because the restricted diets of uremic patients are low in magnesium (usually about 100 to 300 mg per day for a 40-g protein diet), serum magnesium levels are usually normal or only slightly elevated unless the patient takes substances that are high in magnesium content, such as magnesium-containing antacids and laxatives.[224,226] Nondialyzed chronically uremic patients require about 200 mg per day of magnesium to maintain neutral balance.[224] The optimal dietary magnesium allowance for the patient undergoing dialysis has not been well defined.

SODIUM AND WATER

Sodium is freely filterable by the glomerulus. In the normal kidney, the renal tubules reabsorb well over 99% of the filtered sodium. As renal insufficiency progresses, both the glomerular filtration and fractional reabsorption of sodium fall progressively. Thus, many patients with renal failure are able to maintain sodium balance with a normal salt intake. Normally, only about 1 to 3 mEq per day of sodium are excreted in the feces, and in the nonsweating individual, only a few milliequivalents of sodium are lost through the skin each day. Despite an adaptive reduction in the renal tubular reabsorption of sodium when end-stage renal disease supervenes, patients may be unable to excrete the quantity of sodium ingested, and they may develop edema, hypertension, or congestive heart failure. This syndrome is particularly likely to occur when the GFR is below 4 to 10 ml per minute. When renal insufficiency is complicated by congestive heart failure, the nephrotic syndrome, or advanced liver disease, the propensity for sodium retention is increased. With decreased ability to excrete sodium, restriction of sodium and water intake and the use of diuretic medications may be necessary. In renal failure, hypertension often is more easily controlled with sodium restriction and may be accentuated with increased sodium intake, possibly because of expansion of the extracellular fluid volume.[227]

In addition, nondialyzed patients with chronic renal failure often have an inability to conserve sodium normally.[113] A low sodium intake may not be sufficient to replace urinary and extrarenal sodium losses, and the patient may develop sodium depletion, decreases in extracellular fluid volume, blood volume, and renal blood flow, and a further reduction in GFR. Volume depletion may be difficult to recognize. An unexplained weight loss or decrease in blood pressure may be signs of this condition. Nondialyzed patients with chronic renal failure who do not have evidence of fluid overload, hypertension, or heart failure may be cautiously given a greater sodium intake to determine whether their GFR can be improved slightly by extracellular volume expansion.

In general, when sodium balance is well controlled, thirst regulates water balance adequately. When the GFR falls below 2 to 5 ml per minute, however, there is a particular risk of overhydration. In diabetics, hyperglycemia may also increase thirst and enhance positive water balance. For patients with far-advanced renal failure whose total body water is at the desired level (as indicated by normal or near-normal blood pressure, absence of edema, and normal serum sodium), urine volume may be a good guide to water intake. The daily water intake should equal the urine output plus approximately 500 ml to replace insensible losses.

In most nondialyzed patients with advanced renal failure, a daily intake of 1000 to 3000 mg (40 to 130 mEq) of sodium and 1500 to 3000 ml of fluid will maintain sodium and water balance. The requirement for sodium and water varies, and each patient must be managed individually. Patients undergoing maintenance hemodialysis or peritoneal dialysis usually are oliguric or anuric. For hemodialysis patients, daily sodium and total fluid intake generally should be restricted to 1000 to 1500 mg and 700 to 1500 ml, respectively. Patients undergoing CAPD usually tolerate a greater sodium and water intake because salt and water can be easily removed by using hypertonic dialysate, which increases the flow of water from the body into the peritoneal cavity, where it can be drained. Maintaining a large dietary sodium and water intake allows the quantity of fluid removed from the CAPD patient, and hence the daily dialysate volume, to be increased. This increase may be advantageous because the daily clearance of small molecules with CAPD is directly related to the volume of dialysate outflow. In nondialyzed chronically uremic patients or in those undergoing maintenance dialysis who are not anuric and who gain excessive sodium or water despite attempts at dietary restriction, a potent diuretic, such as furosemide, may be tried to increase urinary sodium and water excretion.

POTASSIUM

Normally, the kidney provides the major route for potassium excretion. In renal failure, potassium retention may occur and may lead quickly to fatal hyperkalemia. Two factors may prevent this occurrence in renal failure. First, as long as daily urine output remains at approximately 1000 ml or more, tubular secretion of potassium in the remaining functioning nephrons will tend to be increased, and therefore the renal potassium clearance will not fall as markedly as the GFR. Second, fecal excretion of potassium is increased owing to enhanced intestinal secretion.[192] Thus, patients with chronic renal failure usually do not become hyperkalemic unless they have: (1) excessive intake of potassium; (2) acidosis, oliguria, or hypoaldosteronism (e.g., secondary to decreased renin secretion by the diseased kidney or renal tubular resistance to the actions of aldosterone); or (3) catabolic stress. Patients with chronic renal failure and those undergoing maintenance hemodialysis, in general, should receive no more than 70 mEq of potassium per day.

TRACE ELEMENTS

Dietary requirements for trace elements have not been well defined in uremic patients. It is likely that excesses and deficiencies of certain trace elements are prevalent in renal failure. The problem is compounded because, for many trace elements, it is difficult to ascertain in renal insufficiency whether body pools are adequate. Iron deficiency is common because intestinal iron absorption is sometimes impaired, substantial blood losses often occur, and iron may bind to the dialyzer membrane.[164,228] Both chronically uremic patients and those undergoing dialysis may be given oral iron supplements. Ferrous sulfate, 300 mg three times a day, half an hour after meals, may be used. In some patients, other oral iron salts are better tolerated. Patients who are intolerant to oral iron supplements or who have iron deficiency may be treated with intramuscular or intravenous iron.

Although the zinc content of most tissues is normal in renal failure,[229] serum and hair zinc levels may be low and red cell zinc is increased. Some reports indicate that dysgeusia, poor food intake, and impaired sexual function, which are common problems of uremic patients, may be improved by giving them zinc supplements.[230,231] Impaired intestinal absorption of zinc has been described in patients undergoing maintenance hemodialysis.[232] This finding suggests that the dietary requirement for zinc may be increased in patients with renal failure.[232,233]

As previously indicated, in nondialyzed chronically uremic patients and in those receiving maintenance dialysis, increased body burden of aluminum has been implicated as a cause of a progressive dementia syndrome (particularly in hemodialysis patients), osteomalacia, weakness of the muscles of the proximal limbs, and anemia.[119,234,235] Although contamination of dialysate with aluminum previously was the major source of aluminum toxicity in many dialysis centers, current methods of water treatment have removed virtually all aluminum from dialysate. At present, ingestion of aluminum binders of phosphate is probably the major cause of the excess body burden of aluminum. Consequently, many nephrologists now use aluminum binders more sparingly and rely more on low-phosphorus diets and nonaluminum phosphate binders, particularly calcium salts, to control serum phosphorus levels.[236] Aluminum toxicity may be treated by reduction of aluminum intake and by intravenous infusions of desferrioxamine, a chelator of aluminum.[119] This chelator can be removed from the body by hemodialysis or peritoneal dialysis. Because desferrioxamine may predispose patients to serious infections, nephrologists use this medicine infrequently.

Many trace elements are bound avidly to serum proteins, and when present even in small quantities in dialysate, they may be taken up into blood and cause toxicity. Therefore, as a routine practice, dialysate should be purified of trace elements prior to use. In certain circumstances, therapeutic doses of trace elements can be administered through dialysis, as has been done for zinc.[231]

VITAMINS

Chronically uremic patients are prone to develop deficiencies of water-soluble vitamins unless supplements are given. There are specific reasons for this tendency. First, vitamin intake is often low because of anorexia and poor food intake and also because many foods that are high in water-soluble vitamins are often restricted owing to the elevated potassium content. The typical diet for patients with nondialyzed chronic renal failure and those undergoing maintenance dialysis is frequently below the recommended dietary allowances for certain water-soluble vitamins.[118] Second, the metabolism of certain water-soluble vitamins tends to be altered in chronic renal failure.[237,238] Third, many medicines interfere with the intestinal absorption, metabolism, or actions of vitamins.[118] Vitamin B_6, vitamin C, and folic acid are the water-soluble vitamins most likely to be deficient in nondialyzed patients with chronic renal failure and in patients receiving maintenance dialysis. Vitamin B_{12} deficiency is uncommon in uremia because the daily requirement is small (2 μg/day for nonpregnant, nonlactating adults),[106] the body can store relatively large quantities of this vitamin, and vitamin B_{12} is protein bound in plasma and hence is poorly dialyzed.

Many of the studies that indicated a need for routine vitamin supplementation in patients with nondialyzed chronic renal failure or those undergoing maintenance dialysis were carried out in the 1960s and early 1970s, when the incidence of poor nutritional intake in these patients may have been greater than today.[118] Indeed, more recent studies have suggested that many patients receiving maintenance hemodialysis may subsist for months with no vitamin supplementation and without developing deficiencies of water-soluble vitamins.[239] However, these more recent studies have not demonstrated that a small but substantial proportion of patients will not develop water-soluble vitamin deficiencies, particularly after 1 or more years of dialysis treatment. Because water-soluble vitamin deficiencies have several different causes in these patients and because the water-soluble vitamin supplements are safe, it would seem prudent to continue to use them routinely until these issues are more completely resolved.

Daily supplements for most vitamins are not well defined in renal failure. Evidence indicates that, in addition to vitamin intake from foods, the following daily supplements of vitamins will prevent or correct vitamin deficiency (Table 65–3): pyridoxine hydrochloride, 5 mg in nondialyzed patients and 10 mg in maintenance hemodialysis or peritoneal dialysis patients; folic acid, 1 mg; and the recommended dietary allowance for normal individuals for the other water-soluble vitamins.[106] Patients with renal failure probably need less than 1.0 mg per day of folic acid; however, because this vitamin is safe and some evidence suggests that there may be competitive interference with its actions,[118,237] it may be advisable to prescribe this dose of folic acid until more definitive studies of the requirements are conducted. A supplement of only 60 mg per day of vitamin C (the recommended dietary allowance[106]) is advised because ascorbic acid can be metabolized to oxalate. Large doses of ascorbic acid have been associated with increased plasma oxalate levels in patients with renal failure.[240,241] Oxalate is highly insoluble, and concern exists that high plasma oxalate concentrations can lead to precipitation in soft tissues. Moreover, in the nondialyzed patient with chronic renal insufficiency, there is concern that oxalate deposition in the kidney might cause further impairment of renal function.

Because serum retinol-binding protein and vitamin A are elevated in uremia,[242] the routine use of supplemental vitamin A is not recommended, particularly because even relatively small doses of vitamin A (i.e., 7500 to 15000 IU per day) may cause bone toxicity.[243] Additional vitamin E and K are probably not necessary. However, patients who receive antibiotics for extended periods and who do not ingest foods containing vitamin K may need vitamin K supplements.[244]

Although, in renal failure, many of the beneficial effects of 1,25-dihydroxycholecalciferol can be reproduced by administration of other vitamin D analogues, such as dihydrotachysterol, cholecalciferol, or 25-hydroxycholecalciferol, 1,25-dihydroxycholecalciferol has the advantage that it is the most potent agent. Because it is given in smaller doses and has a shorter half-life, there is little storage of this compound. Hence it may be a safer agent to use. The high potency of 1,25-dihydroxycholecalciferol, however, increases the risk of hypercalcemia and hyperphosphatemia.[115,116]

Treatment with oral 1,25-dihydroxycholecalciferol increases intestinal calcium and phosphorus absorption, raises serum calcium, lowers serum parathyroid hormone, decreases serum alkaline phosphatase activity, reduces bone resorption, decreases endosteal fibrosis, and often improves osteomalacia.[115,116] Therapy with this substance is indicated for hyperparathyroidism, osteitis fibrosa, mixed osteomalacia, osteitis fibrosa, and severe hypocalcemia.[115] Some chronically uremic patients with vitamin D deficiency develop a myopathy, primarily of the proximal limb muscles, and may have presenting symptoms of severe weakness. Strength may improve with vitamin D therapy. 1,25-dihydroxycholecalciferol has many immunologic effects in vitro;[245] whether the treatment of patients with renal failure with this substance improves their immune function is not known.

Treatment with 1,25-dihydroxycholecalciferol usually is started at 0.25 to 0.50 μg per day. The serum calcium level must be monitored carefully, and if it is low and does not rise by at least 0.5 mg/dl with any particular dosage, the dose may be increased by 0.25 to 0.50 μg per day every 4 to 6 weeks. Hypercalcemia is treated by temporary withdrawal of the agent. Ultimately, the best criteria for effective treatment with this substance is improvement in bone anatomy as determined by bone histologic examination, radiographs, and densitometry. Improvement in muscle function or abolition of severe hypocalcemia also may indicate appropriate dosage. In time, the requirements and tolerance for this vitamin may decrease, and the maintenance dosage may have to be reduced. This change may occur after there has been sufficient bone healing, so the skeleton no longer serves as a sink for calcium and phosphorus. It is important that 1,25-dihydroxycholecalciferol not be started unless serum calcium and phosphorus are not elevated and the calcium-phosphorus product preferably is below 45. Serum calcium and phosphorus should be monitored during therapy to ensure that concentrations are normal.

Slatopolsky and Andress and their co-workers have reported that, in patients receiving maintenance hemodialysis, intravenous 1,25-dihydroxycholecalciferol suppresses the secretion and serum levels of parathyroid hormone and ameliorates osteitis fibrosa more effectively than the oral preparation.[246,247] The greater effect of the intravenous agent may occur because a lower fraction of the dose may be taken up by the small intestine, where it promotes calcium absorption and hypercalcemia. Because a lower fraction of infused 1,25-dihydroxycholecalciferol is bound by and acts upon the intestine, greater amounts can be administered safely. Hence, with intravenous treatment, higher blood concentrations of the vitamin can be obtained, and the parathyroid glands may be suppressed more readily. Experiments are currently in process concerning the effectiveness and safety of vitamin D-like compounds that suppress parathyroid hormone secretion but have little or no hypercalcemic effect.

Vitamin D analogues currently are administered routinely only to patients with chronic renal failure who have clinical signs or symptoms of vitamin D deficiency and to uremic children to promote growth. Eventually, all patients with renal insufficiency who have low vitamin D levels or hyperparathyroidism will probably be given these agents.

ACIDOSIS

Metabolic acidosis occurs frequently in nondialyzed patients with chronic renal failure because the ability of the kidney to excrete acidic metabolites is impaired. In the earlier stages of chronic renal failure, metabolic acidosis can also be caused by excessive renal losses of bicarbonate. The rate of acid production is probably normal or below normal in stable, chronically uremic patients. Acidosis is reported to cause bone reabsorption, net protein degradation,[248] and symptoms of lethargy and weakness. Ingestion of low-nitrogen diets may prevent or reduce the severity of the acidosis by decreasing the endogenous generation of acidic products of protein metabolism. Alkali supplements are usually effective for preventing or treating the acidosis of chronic renal failure. Calcium carbonate, 5 g per day, may correct mild acidosis, provide needed calcium, and reduce intestinal phosphate absorption. For more severe acidosis, sodium bicarbonate or citrate may be administered orally or intravenously. If the nondialyzed chronically uremic patient is not oliguric and is not likely to develop edema, sodium is usually readily excreted when administered as sodium bicarbonate or citrate. Alkali therapy should probably be initiated if the arterial pH is below 7.35 or the serum bicarbonate is less than 20 mEq/L. Before alkali therapy is implemented, one must ascertain that the low serum bicarbonate is not a compensatory response to chronic respiratory alkalosis. If acidosis is severe and not controlled by the foregoing measures, hemodialysis or peritoneal dialysis may be used.

PRIORITIZING DIETARY GOALS

The number and magnitude of dietary modifications for chronic uremia are so great that if they are all presented to the patient at one time, the patient is likely to become demoralized and noncompliant. Hence I often list goals for dietary treatment according to priority. Control of protein, phosphorus, sodium, energy, potassium, calcium, and magnesium intake generally is emphasized. On the other hand, unless the patient has a lipid disorder that carries a high risk of atherosclerotic disease, recommendations concerning the types and amounts of carbohydrates and fats ingested are usually given lower priorities. Moreover, a high dietary fiber intake is given a lower priority.

NUTRITIONAL THERAPY IN ACUTE RENAL FAILURE

Acute renal failure is characterized by a sudden reduction or cessation in GFR. The most common causes of acute renal failure include shock, severe infection, trauma, medications, obstruction, and certain types of glomerulonephritis. In most instances, if patients survive the underlying diseases, they will recover from acute renal failure. When patients sustain acute renal failure, they are likely to develop fluid and electrolyte disorders, uremic toxicity, and wasting. These disorders are particularly prone to develop in patients who are both oliguric and hypercatabolic, common complications of acute renal failure.

Patients with acute renal failure, and particularly those with underlying catabolic illnesses, frequently undergo metabolic changes that promote degradation of protein and amino acids and consumption of fuel substrates. Energy expenditure is often increased.[249] In vitro studies with rat muscle tissue indicate that protein degradation is enhanced and protein synthesis is reduced.[250,251] In addition, hepatic gluconeogenesis is increased. When the liver of these animals is perfused or incubated with amino acids, the elevated hepatic glucose and urea production is further enhanced.[252] As a result of these metabolic derangements, patients with acute renal failure are often unable to utilize protein, amino acids, and energy substrates efficiently. Hence it may be difficult to maintain and to improve the nutritional status of these patients by enteral or parenteral nutrition.[253,254]

GENERAL PRINCIPLES

Because available data concerning optimal nutritional therapy for acute renal failure are both limited and conflicting, one cannot strongly justify any treatment plan for such patients. The following therapeutic approach is based upon my analysis of the literature and personal experience.

Fluid and mineral balance should be carefully monitored in acute renal failure to prevent overhydration or electrolyte disorders. Water intake, in general, should equal output from urine and all other measured sources, such as nasogastric aspirate or fistula drainage, plus 400 ml per day. This regimen takes into account the contributions of endogenous water production from metabolism and the insensible water losses (from respiration, skin losses) to water balance. In general, if the patient is catabolic, weight should be allowed to decrease by 0.2 to 0.5 kg per day to avoid excessive accumulation of fluid. Sodium, potassium, phosphorus, and magnesium intake should be restricted to prevent accumulation of these minerals. Energy and, if feasible, protein intake should satisfy the patient's nutritional requirements, which may exceed normal. By controlling the water and electrolyte intake and lowering the UNA, one may be able to reduce the need for dialysis treatments.

The patient's desirable nutrient intake will depend on nutritional status, catabolic rate, residual GFR, and clinical indications for initiating dialysis therapy. For example, in a patient who is wasted, one might be more inclined to give a surfeit of nutrients and to provide dialysis as needed. A patient with acute renal failure who has a high residual GFR also may receive larger quantities of nutrients because of the lower risk of developing fluid and electrolyte disorders or accumulating potentially toxic metabolites. On the other hand, for a patient who has little or no urine flow and who is not severely catabolic or uremic, the intake of small quantities of water, minerals, and amino acids may reduce the need for dialysis. This last approach may be particularly beneficial if one anticipates that the patient will not tolerate dialysis well. Similarly, a patient who is starting to recover from acute renal failure may be given this treatment to avoid dialysis for a few days until renal function becomes adequate. In this last group of patients, high-calorie diets providing small amounts of essential amino acids or keto acids with little or no protein may be used for short periods.

Whenever feasible, patients with acute renal failure should receive oral nutrition. If the patient will not eat adequately, the use of liquid formula diets, elemental diets, and tube or enterostomy feeding should be considered. Often, parenteral nutrition is the only technique that will provide adequate nutrient intake (Table 65–4).

SPECIFIC NUTRIENT INTAKES

PROTEIN AND AMINO ACID INTAKE

The quantity of nitrogen and the composition of the amino acid formulations that are administered enterally or parenterally to patients with acute renal failure are the subject of controversy. Abel and associates carried out a series of studies that suggested benefits of parenteral nutrition for patients with acute renal failure.[255–257] The patients were infused with solutions containing hypertonic D-glucose and 12 to 30 g per day of essential amino acids but no nonessential amino acids. These authors reported that the SUN and serum potassium, phosphorus, and magnesium often stabilized or decreased, and dialysis therapy sometimes could be postponed or avoided. In a prospective, randomized, double-blind study, these investigators compared infusion of hypertonic glucose and essential amino acids to treatment with an isocaloric infusion of hypertonic glucose that contained no amino acids.[257] The patients receiving glucose and essential amino acids had significantly greater survival until renal function recovered; hospital survival was slightly but not significantly increased. Retrospective studies with nonconcurrent controls reported by other investigators suggest that parenteral nutrition providing essential and nonessential amino acids improved morbidity and mortality, particularly in patients with more complicated clinical courses.[258,259]

Leonard et al. reported that parenteral nutrition with hypertonic glucose and about 21 g per day of essential amino acids compared to isocaloric infusions with glucose alone had no advantages with regard to SUN levels, nitrogen balance, or survival in patients with acute renal failure.[260] Feinstein and co-workers carried out a randomized, prospective, double-blind study of individuals with acute renal failure who were unable to eat adequately.[253] Thirty patients were treated with 1 of 3 isocaloric parenteral nutrition formulations: hypertonic glucose with no amino acids, hypertonic glucose with 21 g of essential amino acids daily, or hypertonic glucose with 21 g of essential and 21 g of nonessential amino acids daily. The mean duration of study was 9.2 days per patient. The metabolic balance data indicated that many of these patients were severely catabolic with net rates of protein degradation, determined from the difference between nitrogen intake and the UNA, as high as 240 g per day. UNA tended to be lower with the essential amino acid regimen. Nitrogen balance and mortality rate were not different with any of these infusion regimens, but also tended to be less adverse with the essential amino acid intake.

Some investigators have argued that more than 40 g per day of a mixture of essential and nonessential amino acids may be more effective in improving nitrogen balance. Feinstein and co-workers tested this hypothesis in a randomized, prospective trial.[254] Patients received total parenteral nutrition (TPN) providing 21 g per day of essential amino acids or TPN with essential and nonessential amino acids provided in a 1.0:1.0 ratio. With the second treatment, attempts were made to infuse a quantity of nitrogen equal to the UNA. Thirteen patients with acute renal failure were randomly assigned to 1 of the 2 treatments. The results indicated that although the nitrogen intake was 5 times greater with the second regimen, the nitrogen balance, determined from the difference between intake and UNA, was not different. The UNA fell significantly only in patients receiving the essential amino acids, whereas it tended to rise in the other group.

These data suggest that high-calorie solutions providing about 21 g per day of essential amino acids may be used more effectively than isocaloric preparations containing larger quantities of essential and nonessential amino acids (e.g., 40 to 70 g per day) provided in an essential:nonessential ratio of 1.0:1.0. The essential amino acid solutions seem to reduce the UNA and total nitrogen output more than the essential and nonessential amino acids. Consequently, nitrogen balance seems to be no more negative with the former preparations, but the accumulation of nitrogenous metabolites is less. It would be of interest to examine the response to a TPN regimen that provides larger quantities of essential and nonessential amino acids but contains a larger proportion of essential amino acids.

Data from rat studies are also inconclusive. Toback and associates caused acute renal failure in rats by injection of mercuric chloride.[261,262] The rats infused with glucose and a mixture of essential and nonessential amino acids had greater regeneration of renal cortical cells, as determined by ^{14}C-choline incorporation into phospholipids, than rats infused with glucose alone. Amino acids promoted intracellular protein synthesis as determined by ^{14}C-leucine uptake.[263] The maximum serum creatinine concentration also was lower in the rats infused with glucose and amino acids, suggesting that these nutrients enhanced the recovery of renal function. However, Oken and co-workers were unable to show a consistent beneficial effect of glucose and essential amino acids or glucose and essential and nonessential amino acids as compared to glucose alone on the rate or incidence of recovery of renal function or survival in rats with acute renal failure.[264]

TABLE 65–4. TYPICAL COMPOSITION OF SOLUTIONS FOR TOTAL PARENTERAL NUTRITION IN PATIENTS WITH ACUTE RENAL FAILURE[a]

	DAILY QUANTITY OR CONCENTRATION TO BE INFUSED	
Volume	(L)	1.0
Essential and nonessential free crystalline amino acids (4.25–5.0%)[b] or	g/L	42.5–50
Essential amino acids (5%)[b]	g/L	12.5–25
Dextrose (D-glucose)[c]	g/L	350
Energy (approx.)[c]	kcal/L	1,140
Electrolytes[d]		
Sodium[e]	mmol/L	40–50
Chloride[e]	mmol/L	25–35
Potassium	mmol/day	≤35
Acetate	mmol/day	35–40
Calcium	mmol/day	5
Phosphorus	mmol/day	8
Magnesium	mmol/day	4
Iron	mg/day	2
Trace Elements		(see text)
Vitamins		
Vitamin A[f]		see text
Vitamin D		see text
Vitamin K[g]	mg/week	7.5
Vitamin E[h]	IU/day	10
Niacin	mg/day	20
Thiamin HCl (B_1)	mg/day	2
Riboflavin (B_2)	mg/day	2
Pantothenic acid (B_3)	mg/day	10
Pyridoxine HCl (B_6)	mg/day	10
Ascorbic acid (C)	mg/day	60–100
Biotin	mg/day	200
Folic acid[g]	mg/day	2
Vitamin B_{12}[g]	μg/day	3

[a]These nutrients are present in each bottle containing 500 ml of 8.5 to 10% crystalline amino acids or 250 to 500 ml of 5% essential amino acids and 500 ml of 70% dextrose. The vitamins and trace elements are an exception because they are added to only one bottle per day. The patient's fluid status and serum electrolytes and glucose must be monitored closely. The composition and volume of the infusate may need to be changed if the patient is very uremic, acidotic, or volume-overloaded, if the serum electrolyte concentrations are not normal or if they are changing, or if dialysis therapy is not readily available or is particularly hazardous to the patient (see text).

[b]For patients who are more catabolic (e.g., UNA ≥5 g/day), are undergoing regular dialysis treatments (particularly for 2 or more weeks), or who are wasted, essential and nonessential amino acids may be infused: about 1.0–1.2 g/kg/day for hemodialysis patients and 1.2–1.3 g/kg/day for intermittent or CAPD patients (see text). For patients who are less wasted, are less catabolic, are not undergoing regular dialysis therapy, and will not be receiving TPN for more than 2 or 3 weeks, 21 to 40 g/day of the nine essential amino acids may be infused. See text for discussion of the formulations of amino acids. Only solutions of crystalline amino acids should be used.

[c]To obtain an energy intake of 30 to 40 kcal/kg/day, 70% dextrose is added as necessary (see text). Lower energy intakes may be used in very obese patients. For the higher levels of energy intake (i.e., 35–40 kcal/kg/day), additional 70% dextrose may be added to the solutions. To balance the sources of calories and to prevent essential fatty acid deficiency, lipid emulsions may be used. For patients who are septic or at high risk for sepsis, about 10–20% of calories or less may be given as lipids. For more stable patients, 20–30% of calories may be given as lipids. The lipid emulsions probably should be infused over at least 12 hours, if not 24 hours, to reduce the hyperlipidemia that occurs with intravenous infusion of lipid emulsions (see text). The lipid emulsions may be infused in a separate line or mixed with the amino acid and dextrose solutions and infused soon after mixing (see text). A 20% lipid emulsion may be used to reduce the water load. The approximate calorie values are dextrose monohydrate 3.4 kcal/g; amino acids, 3.5 kcal/g; lipid emulsions 10%; 1.1 kcal/ml; 20%, 2.0 kcal/ml.

[d]When one is adding electrolytes, the amounts intrinsically present in the amino acid solution should be taken into account.

[e]Refers to the final concentrations of electrolytes after any additional 70% dextrose or other solutions have been added.

[f]Vitamin A is best avoided unless total parenteral nutrition is continued for more than 2 or 3 weeks (see text).

[g]Should be given orally or parenterally and not in the total parenteral nutrition solution because of antagonisms.

[h]May need to be increased with use of lipid emulsions.

These conflicting observations are probably the result of the following factors: (1) the clinical course of patients with acute renal failure is so complex and variable that it would be necessary to study large numbers of patients to show statistically significant benefits of nutritional therapy if they exist; (2) many of these studies were retrospective or not randomly controlled; this fact may have led to unintentional biases in the results; (3) the optimal composition of nutrients in TPN solutions has not been defined, and the use of suboptimal formulations of nutrients may reduce the clinical benefits of nutritional therapy; and (4) catabolic patients or rats with acute renal failure probably need both good nutrition and metabolic intervention to suppress catabolic processes and to promote anabolism; providing nutrients without metabolic intervention may not have a beneficial effect on nutritional status or clinical outcome, particularly in the first days after the onset of acute renal failure.

It is pertinent that the prospective studies of parenteral nutrition in patients with acute renal failure compared different regimens of nutritional therapy; that is, infusion of high-calorie solutions containing amino acids versus isocaloric infusions without amino acids and administration of isocaloric solutions with essential amino acids as compared to essential and nonessential amino acids.[253,254,257,260] No prospective, randomized study has compared the clinical course of patients receiving nutritional therapy to those receiving no nutritional support.

My current policy for amino acid or protein intake in patients with acute renal failure is as follows: Patients may be prescribed a low enteral or intravenous nitrogen intake if they have a low UNA (i.e., equal to or less than 4 to 5 g N per day), if they have no evidence of severe protein malnutrition, and if one anticipates that the patient will recover renal function within the next 1 or 2 weeks. A severely reduced GFR or the desire to avoid dialysis therapy are other factors that would suggest the use of a low nitrogen intake. Under these conditions, I may use 0.3 to 0.5 g/kg per day of primarily high-quality protein or essential amino acids with arginine. I do not give more than 0.4 g/kg per day of essential amino acids as the sole nitrogen source because larger quantities of the nine essential amino acids may cause serious amino acid imbalances.[265] Diets providing 0.10 to 0.30 g/kg per day of miscellaneous protein and 10 to 20 g per day of essential amino acids or keto acids may also be used in patients who can eat. These regimens should minimize the rate of accumulation of nitrogenous metabolites and, unless the patient is severely catabolic, will usually maintain a neutral or only mildly negative nitrogen balance. Hence the need for dialysis therapy may be minimized or avoided. If patients have substantial residual renal function (e.g., GFR of 5 to 10 ml per minute) and are not severely catabolic, I may treat them as nondialyzed patients with chronic renal failure. The individual would receive 0.55 to 0.60 g protein or amino acids/kg desirable body weight per day.

For patients who are more catabolic and have a higher UNA (more than 5 g N/day), are severely wasted, or are undergoing regular dialysis therapy and either have had or are anticipated to have acute renal failure for more than 2 weeks, I am inclined to prescribe a higher protein or amino acid intake, up to 1.0 to 1.2 g/kg desirable body weight per day. In comparison to small quantities of essential amino acids, these larger nitrogen intakes may improve nitrogen balance, particularly after the first 1 or 2 weeks of dialysis treatments. The UNA almost invariably rises, however, and the increased azotemia and, in patients receiving TPN, the larger volumes of fluid necessary to provide this amount of amino acids may increase the need for dialysis.

If acute renal failure persists for more than 2 to 3 weeks, patients undergoing regular dialysis treatment are treated as maintenance dialysis patients, with about 1.0 to 1.2 g/kg per day of protein or amino acids for patients receiving hemodialysis or 1.2 to 1.5 g/kg per day for those receiving chronic peritoneal dialysis.

Because the metabolic status of patients with acute renal failure often facilitates the catabolism of protein, amino acids, and other energy substrates,[249–252,266] there may be advantages to administering agents that promote anabolic processes or reduce catabolic pathways. Anabolic steroidal compounds, many of which are androgenic and resemble testosterone, have been used in patients with acute renal failure.[267,268] These agents can reduce UNA and increase nitrogen balance; they also have been reported to decrease the need for dialysis treatments. In vitro studies of skeletal muscle from rats with acute renal failure indicate that insulin may increase synthesis and reduce degradation of protein.[251] Studies in catabolic patients who do not have renal failure indicate that insulin may decrease the UNA.[269,270] Recombinant DNA-synthesized human growth hormone has been used to improve nitrogen balance in postoperative, acutely stressed patients without renal failure, and results have been encouraging.[271] This hormone has also improved nitrogen balance in stable, malnourished patients undergoing maintenance hemodialysis.[272] As mentioned previously, the nitrogen intake appears to be utilized more efficiently if a greater proportion of the administered amino acids is essential.[253,254] This hypothesis has not yet been tested clinically. In addition, studies in catabolic patients without renal failure suggest that intravenous infusions in which a large proportion of the amino acids comprise branched-chain acids (i.e., isoleucine, leucine, and valine) may have a specific anabolic effect.[273,274] Not all studies confirm these findings. Keto acid analogues of the branched-chain amino acids in in vitro preparations and in nonuremic individuals who are not hypercatabolic also promote anabolism.[98,99] The intravenous infusion of the salt complex of α-ketoglutarate and ornithine in postoperative patients receiving TPN is reported to reduce UNA and to increase nitrogen balance.[275] Severely stressed patients without renal failure display a rapid fall in intracellular muscle glutamine.[276] Administration of glutamine improves protein balance in these patients.[276,277] Arginine has also been reported to increase nitrogen balance.[278] The mechanism of action of this drug is not well understood. More research is clearly necessary to investigate the anabolic effects and clinical value of these agents in patients with acute renal failure.

ENERGY

Several lines of evidence suggest that patients with acute renal failure may benefit from a high energy intake. Because patients with acute renal failure are frequently in negative energy and nitrogen balance,[249,253,254,260] some investigators have argued that a greater energy intake may reduce protein wasting. Moreover, unlike nonuremic acutely ill patients who may receive large quantities of amino acids, patients with acute renal failure are usually given relatively small amounts of amino acids because of their excretory impairment. It is possible, although not proved, that higher energy intakes may improve the use of low nitrogen intakes. In two studies of patients with acute renal failure who were not randomized for energy intake, those who died were found to have a higher energy expenditure and more negative energy balance,[249] or lower energy intake,[249,253] than those who survived.

As a result of these findings, I usually administer about 30 to 40 kcal/kg desirable body weight per day (Table 65–4), except in patients who are obese (e.g., greater than 125% desirable body weight). The higher energy intakes (i.e., 40 kcal/kg per day) are used for patients who have a higher UNA, who are severely ill, and who are less obese. For example, if nitrogen balance, estimated from the difference between the patient's nitrogen intake and the nitrogen output calculated from the UNA, is negative, I try to provide an energy intake close to 40 kcal/kg per day. Alternatively, the product of the Harris Benedict equation,[279] a stress factor of 1.50,[280] may be used to estimate the patient's energy needs. Energy expenditure, measured by indirect calorimetry, can be multiplied by 1.50 to estimate the daily energy requirement. These energy intakes are higher than currently recommended for severely stressed patients without renal failure. However, because nitrogen intolerance limits the amount of amino acids or protein that can be given to the patient with renal failure and higher energy intakes tend to reduce nitrogen losses, the patient with renal failure may benefit from a larger energy load. Unfortunately, prospective studies to test this hypothesis are not available.

Larger energy intakes are not used because there appears to be little nutritional advantage to administering more calories to catabolic patients. Indeed, because high energy intakes generate more carbon dioxide from the infused carbohydrate and fat, they can promote hypercapnia if pulmonary function is impaired.[281] Carbon dioxide retention is particularly likely to occur with very high carbohydrate loads. In addition, high energy intakes may cause obesity and fatty liver,[282] and they may increase the water load to the patient.

Because most patients with acute renal failure do not tolerate large water intakes, glucose is usually administered in a 70% solution. The glucose and amino acid solutions are mixed, so the amino acids and energy are provided simultaneously (Table 65–4). Patients receiving TPN for more than 5 days should receive lipid emulsions. Patients require about 25 g per day of a lipid emulsion to prevent essential fatty acid deficiency. Some investigators have recommended giving up 30 to 40% of calories as lipid emulsions to provide sufficient fatty acids to organs that normally use lipids as their main energy source and to more closely approximate the normal American dietary intake. Some researchers have reported that infusions of large amounts of fat emulsions, such as 50 g over 8 to 12 hours, may impair the function of the reticuloendothelial system;[283] they have questioned whether infusion of lipid emulsions might lower host resistance. A prudent approach may be to infuse lipid emulsions over at least 12 hours, if not 24 hours, to prevent marked increases in plasma lipids. For patients who are septic or at high risk of severe sepsis, probably no more than 10 to 20% of total calories should be provided from fat, or fat intake may be temporarily suspended. For patients who are not septic and not at high risk of infection, about 20 to 30% of calories may be given as lipid emulsions. Intravenous lipid emulsions are available in 10% (1.1-kcal/ml) and 20% (2.0-kcal/ml) solutions. Traditionally, lipid emulsions have been infused separately from the glucose and amino acid mixtures. With careful attention to aseptic control, the lipid emulsions may be mixed with glucose and amino acids; the mixtures should be infused shortly after preparation.[284]

MINERALS

A mineral prescription for parenteral nutrition in acute renal failure is shown in Table 65–4. Any recommended intake of minerals is tentative and must be adjusted according to the clinical status of the patient. If the serum concentration of an electrolyte is increased, it may be advisable to reduce the quantity infused or to not administer it at the onset of parenteral nutrition. The patient must be monitored closely because the hormonal and metabolic changes that often occur with initiation of parenteral nutrition may cause serum electrolytes to fall rapidly. This occurrence is particularly likely for serum potassium and phosphorus. On the other hand, a low concentration of a mineral may indicate a need for greater than usual intake of that element. Again, metabolic changes and the impaired GFR can lead to a rapid rise in serum concentrations during repletion.

Trace elements are probably not necessary in parenteral nutrition solutions given to catabolic patients with acute renal failure unless this is the sole source of nutritional support for at least 2 to 3 weeks. The nutritional requirements for trace elements have not been established for uremic patients receiving TPN.

VITAMINS

The vitamin requirements have not been well defined for patients with acute renal failure. Tentative recommendations for vitamin intake for patients receiving parenteral nutrition are shown in Table 65–4. Much of the recommended intake is based on information obtained from studies in chronically uremic patients, normal individuals, or nonuremic acutely ill patients. Vitamin A is probably best avoided because, in chronic renal failure, serum vitamin A levels are elevated and small doses of vitamin A have been reported to cause toxicity to chronically uremic patients.[242,243] In addition, because most patients with acute renal failure receive parenteral nutrition for only a few days to weeks, a deficiency of this fat-soluble vitamin is unlikely.

Although vitamin D is fat-soluble and vitamin stores should not become depleted during the few days to weeks that most patients with acute renal failure receive parenteral nutrition, the turnover of its active analogue, 1,25-dihydroxycholecalciferol, is much faster. Hence this analogue may be needed in patients with acute renal failure.[246]

Although vitamin K is fat-soluble, vitamin K deficiency has been reported in nonuremic patients who are not eating and are receiving antibiotics.[244] Vitamin K therefore should be given routinely to patients receiving parenteral nutrition (Table 65–4). Ten milligrams per day of pyridoxine hydrochloride (8.2 mg/day of pyridoxine) is recommended because studies in clinically stable or sick patients undergoing maintenance hemodialysis indicate that this quantity may be necessary to prevent or to correct vitamin B_6 deficiency.[285] Patients should probably not receive more than 60 to 100 mg of ascorbic acid per day because of the risk of increased oxalate production.[240,241]

The nutrient intake of patients with acute renal failure must be carefully reevaluated each day and sometimes more frequently. This reevaluation is particularly important because these patients may undergo rapid changes in their clinical and metabolic conditions.

PERIPHERAL PARENTERAL NUTRITION

Parenteral nutrition through a peripheral vein avoids the risks of inserting a catheter into the inferior vena cava. Because the osmolality of the infusate must be restricted to reduce the risk of thrombophlebitis, it is necessary to use a larger volume of fluid and/or a lower intake of nutrients. Both approaches may have undesirable consequences for patients with acute renal failure. The financial cost of TPN administered through a peripheral vein is about the same as or greater than the cost of administration through a central vein because of the large quantities of isotonic lipid emulsions used to provide the energy needs when peripheral veins are used.

Peripheral partial parenteral nutrition may be advantageous for patients with acute renal failure who are able to ingest or be tube-fed only part of their daily nutritional requirements. The peripheral infusions may enable these patients to receive adequate nutrition without resorting to TPN through a large flow vein. In these patients, it is often most practical to infuse an 8.5 to 10% amino acid solution or a 20% lipid emulsion into a peripheral vein and to administer as much as possible of the other essential nutrients, including carbohydrates, through the enteral tract.

The peripheral vascular access used for hemodialysis can also be used for parenteral nutrition. Because of the high blood flow through the vascular access used for hemodialysis, hypertonic solutions can be used, and the water load to the patient can be reduced. This technique probably increases the risk of infection in the vascular access, however, and it should not be used in patients who will need a hemodialysis access for extended periods.

SUPPLEMENTAL PARENTERAL NUTRITION

Infusion of amino acids and glucose and/or lipids may be given as a nutritional supplement to patients with acute or chronic renal failure who eat poorly. Supplemental amino acids, glucose, and/or lipids can be infused conveniently during the hemodialysis procedure. Because most patients in need of nutritional supplements have decreased intake of both amino acids and energy, I infuse 40 to 42 g of essential and nonessential amino acids and 200 g of D-glucose (150 g of D-glucose if the hemodialysate contains glucose). This preparation is infused throughout the hemodialysis procedure at a constant rate into the blood leaving the dialyzer. Such a technique minimizes the normal fall in amino acid and glucose pools that occurs as a result of dialysis of these nutrients. Most of the infused glucose and amino acids are retained; the amino acid losses into dialysate increase by only about 4 to 5 g.[160] Lipid infusions have been substituted for glucose but are more expensive and are possibly less healthy because of the risk of hyperlipidemia and atherosclerosis in patients with chronic renal failure. Patients who have low serum phosphorus or potassium concentrations at the onset of dialysis treatment may require supplements of these electrolytes during the amino acid and glucose supplementation. To prevent reactive hypoglycemia, the infusion should not be stopped until the end of hemodialysis, and the patient should eat a carbohydrate source 20 to 30 minutes before the end of the infusion.

Whether intravenous supplements with amino acids, glucose, and/or lipids thrice weekly for about 4 hours during hemodialysis is beneficial to patients who eat poorly is controversial.[286,287] The preponderance of clinical trials do not show clear benefits of such supplements. These infusions should only be used in patients who cannot increase their intake of foods or take oral supplements. The intravenous supplements should be continued only if nutritional or clinical assessments indicate that these nourishments are beneficial.

CONTINUOUS ARTERIOVENOUS HEMOFILTRATION

Because many patients with acute renal failure are overhydrated, receive large quantities of intravenous solutions, and have impaired ability to excrete water and salt, continuous arteriovenous hemofiltration (CAVH) has been used to control salt and water balance.[288] With CAVH, catheters are placed into a large artery and vein, such as the femoral artery and vein.[288] The blood flows through a small filtering apparatus where some of the plasma water is filtered; the remaining concentrated blood is returned to the vein. Some physicians combine parenteral nutrition therapy with CAVH to provide intravenous nutrition and, at the same time, to control the water and salt balance and remove a small amount of the metabolic products that accumulate in renal failure. When CAVH is not used, patients with acute renal failure who receive parenteral nutrition may require treatment with a hemodialyzer as often as every day rather than three times weekly, which is the usual treatment for clinically stable patients receiving maintenance hemodialysis. CAVH is particularly helpful for nutritional support when patients receive the larger quantities of glucose, lipids, and amino acids.

NUTRITIONAL DIALYSIS

Some investigators have proposed adding amino acids and additional glucose to the dialysate of patients undergoing CAPD or maintenance hemodialysis.[289,290] The nutrients diffuse into the body during dialysis. At present, these techniques may provide supplemental nutrition but cannot be used for total nutritional support.

AMINO ACIDS THAT MAY PREDISPOSE TO ACUTE RENAL FAILURE

Several studies in rats suggest that amino acid or protein intake may increase the susceptibility to acute renal failure caused by ischemia or aminoglycoside nephrotoxicity.[291–294] The nutrients seem to increase both the incidence and the severity of acute renal failure induced by these agents. Although some studies have demonstrated this effect with excessively large doses of intravenous amino acids or dietary protein,[291,294] the quantities of amino acids and protein that might be prescribed for patients can also predispose them to renal failure.[292,293] D-serine, DL-ethionine, and L-lysine appear to be particularly nephrotoxic.[292,294] Whether amino acid or protein intake will predispose patients to renal failure is not known. If either one does, then patients who receive nephrotoxic medications or who are at high risk of renal ischemia might benefit from low amino acid or protein intakes. On the other hand, in vitro studies also indicate that some amino acids, particularly L-glycine and L-alanine, may protect renal tubular cells from ischemic or nephrotoxic injury.[295] Clearly, more research is needed in this area.

FUTURE DIRECTIONS FOR NUTRITIONAL SUPPORT

Several new techniques for improving nitrogen balance and host resistance could lead to major changes in nutritional support if the reported benefits are confirmed. The potential use of growth factors for patients with renal failure has been described previously.[267–272] Arginine and glutamine supplements are reported to have specific effects on enhancing nitrogen balance.[276–278] In addition, evidence indicates that supplemental arginine,[278,296] nucleotides,[297] and omega-3 fatty acids[297] may improve certain parameters of immunologic function and host resistance. The use of peptides in TPN solutions is also currently under investigation.[277]

REFERENCES

1. Kopple J.D.: Nitrogen metabolism. *In* Clinical Aspects of Uremia and Dialysis. Edited by S.G. Massry, and A.L. Sellers. Springfield, IL, Charles C Thomas, 1976, pp. 241–283.
2. Dunn, M.J.: Hormones and autacoids produced in the kidney. *In* Renal Endocrinology. Edited by M.J. Dunn. Baltimore, Williams & Wilkins, 1983.
3. Ballermann, B.J., Levenson, D.J., Brenner, B.M.: Renin, angiotensin, kinins, prostaglandins, and leukotrienes. *In* The Kidney. 3rd Ed. Edited by B.M. Brenner and F.C. Rector, Jr. Philadelphia, W.B. Saunders, 1986.
4. Audran, M., Kumar, R.: Mayo. Clin. Proc. *60:*851–866, 1985.
5. Fisher, J.W.: Kidney Hormones. Vol. 2. New York, Academic Press, 1977.
6. Caro, J., Brown, S., Miller, O., et al.: J. Lab. Clin. Med., *93:*449–458, 1979.
7. Eschbach, J.W., Egrie, J.C., Downing, M.R., et al.: N. Engl. J. Med., *316:*73–78, 1987.
8. Pullman, T.N., Alving, A.S., Dern, R.J., et al.: J. Lab. Clin. Med., *44:*320–332, 1954.

9. Klahr, S., Tripathy, K.: Arch. Intern. Med., *118:*322–325, 1966.
10. Klahr, S., Tripathy, K., Garcia, F.T., et al.: Am. J. Med., *43:*84–96, 1967.
11. Klahr, S., Tripathy, K., Lotero, H.: Am. J. Med., *48:*325–331, 1970.
12. Ichikawa, I., Purkerson, M.L., Klahr, S., et al.: J. Clin. Invest., *65:*982–988, 1980.
13. Hirschberg, R., Kopple, J.D., Blantz, R.C., Tucker, B.J.: J. Clin. Invest., *87:*1200–1206, 1991.
14. Hirschberg, R., Kopple, J.D.: J. Am. Soc. Nephrol., *1:*1034–1040, 1991.
15. Owen, O.E., Felig, P., Morgan, A.P.: J. Clin. Invest., *48:*574–583, 1969.
16. Gutman, A.B., Yu, T.-F.: Am. J. Med., *45:*756–779, 1968.
17. Bosch, J.P., Saccaggi, A., Lauer, A., et al.: Am. J. Med., *75:*943–950, 1983.
18. Bosch, J.P., Lauer, A., Glabman, S.: Am. J. Med., *77:*873–879, 1984.
19. Castellino, P., Hunt, W., DeFronzo, R.A.: Kidney Int., *32(Suppl. 22):*S15–S20, 1987.
20. Hirschberg, R., Kopple, J.D.: Kidney Int., *32:*382–387, 1987.
21. Hirschberg, R., Zipser, R.D., Slomowitz, L.A., et al.: Kidney Int., *33:*1147–1155, 1988.
22. Christiansen, J.S., Gammelgaard, J., Orskov, H.: Eur. J. Clin. Invest., *11:*487–490, 1981.
23. Hirschberg, R., Rabb, H., Bergamo, R., et al.: Kidney Int., *35:*865–870, 1989.
24. Hirschberg, R., Kopple, J.D.: J. Clin. Invest., *83:*326–336, 1989.
25. Mitch, W.E., Walser, M., Buffington, G.A., et al.: Lancet, *2:*1326–1328, 1976.
26. Rutherford, W.E., Blondin, J., Miller, J.P., et al.: Kidney Int., *11:*62–70, 1977.
27. Barsotti, G., Guiducci, A., Ciardella, F., et al.: Nephron, *27:*113–117, 1981.
28. McCormack, L.J., Beland, J.E., Schnekloth, R.E., et al.: Am. J. Pathol., *34:*1011–1022, 1958.
29. Kleinknecht, C., Grunfeld, J-P., Gomez, P.C., et al.: Kidney Int., *4:*390–400, 1973.
30. Rodriguez-Iturbe, B., Garcia, R., Rubio, L., et al.: Clin. Nephrol., *5:*198–206, 1976.
31. Torres, V.E., Velosa, J.A., Holley, K.E., et al.: Ann. Intern. Med., *92:*776–784, 1980.
32. Fishberg, A.M.: Hypertension and Nephritis. Philadelphia, Lea & Febiger, 1954.
33. Kopple, J.D., Shinaberger, J.H., Coburn, J.W., et al.: Am. J. Clin. Nutr., *21:*508–515, 1968.
34. Blatherwick, N.R., Medlar, E.M.: Arch. Intern. Med., *59:*572–596, 1937.
35. Farr, L.E., Smadel, J.E.: J. Exp. Med., *70:*615–627, 1939.
36. Addis, T.: Glomerular nephritis. *In* Diagnosis and Treatment. New York, Macmillan, Inc., 1948.
37. Ibels, L.S., Alfrey, A.C., Haut, L., et al.: N. Engl. J. Med., *298:*122–126, 1978.
38. Karlinsky, M.L., Haut, L.L., Buddington, B., et al.: Kidney Int., *17:*293–302, 1980.
39. Haut, L.L., Alfrey, A.C., Guggenheim, S., et al.: Kidney Int., *17:*722–731, 1980.
40. Laouari, D., Kleinknecht, C., Gubler, M-C., et al.: Kidney Int., *24(Suppl. 16):*S248–S253, 1983.
41. Kenner, C.H., Evan, A.P., Blomgren, P., et al.: Kidney Int., *27:*739–750, 1985.
42. French, S.W., Yamanaka, W., Ostwald, R.: Arch. Pathol., *83:*204–210, 1967.
43. Hurd, E.R., Johnston, J.M., Okita, J.R., et al.: J. Clin. Invest., *67:*476–485, 1981.
44. Howie, J.B., Helyer, B.J., Casey, T.P., et al.: Renal disease in autoimmune strains of mice. *In* Proceedings of the Third International Congress of Nephrology. Vol. 2. Basel, S. Karger, 1967, pp. 150–163.
45. Barcelli, U.O., Weiss, M., Pollack, V.E.: J. Lab. Clin. Med., *100:*786–797, 1982.
46. Zurier, R.B., Damjanov, O., Sayadoff, D.M., et al.: Arthritis Rheum., *20:*1449–1456, 1977.
47. Kelley, V.E., Winkelstein, A., Izui, S.: Lab. Invest., *41:*531–537, 1979.
48. McLeish, K.R., Gohara, A.F., Cunning, W.T., III: J. Lab. Clin. Med., *96:*470–479, 1980.
49. Deen, W.M., Maddox, D.A., Robertson, C.R., et al.: Am. J. Physiol., *227:*556–562, 1974.
50. Hostetter, T.H., Olson, J.L., Rennke, H.G., et al.: Am. J. Physiol., *241:*F85–F93, 1981.
51. Hostetter, T.H., Troy, J.L., Brenner, B.M.: Kidney Int., *19:*410–415, 1981.
52. Olson, J.L., Hostetter, T.H., Rennke, H.G., et al.: Altered charge and size selective properties of the glomerular wall: a response to reduced renal mass. *In* Proceedings of the American Society of Nephrology. Thorofare, NJ, Charles B. Slack, 1979, p. 87A.
53. Olson, J.L., Hostetter, T.H., Rennke, H.G., et al.: Kidney Int., *22:*112–126, 1982.
54. Brenner, B.M., Meyer, T.W., Hostetter, T.H.: N. Engl. J. Med., *307:*652–659, 1982.
55. Meyer, T.W., Lawrence, W.E., Brenner, B.M.: Kidney Int., *24(Suppl. 16):*S243–S247, 1983.
56. Walls, J., Williams, S.J.: Contr. Nephrol., *60:*179–187, 1988.
57. Hostetter, T.H., Meyer, T.W., Rennke, H.G., et al.: Influence of strict control of diabetes on intrarenal hemodynamics. *In* Proceedings of the American Society of Nephrology. Thorofare, NJ, Charles B. Slack, 1982, p. 122A.
58. Mogensen, C.E.: Diabetes, *25:*872–879, 1976.
59. Mogensen, C.E., Steffes, M.W., Deckert, T., et al.: Diabetologia, *21:*89–93, 1981.
60. Mogensen, C.E., Christensen, C.K., Vittinghus, E.: Diabetes, *32(Suppl. 2):*64–78, 1983.
61. Ibels, L.S., Alfrey, A.C., Huffer, W.E., et al.: Am. J. Med., *71:*33–37, 1981.
62. Alfrey, A.C., Tomford, R.C.: Phosphate and prevention of renal failure. *In* Prevention of Kidney Disease and Long-Term Survival. Edited by M.M. Avram. New York, Plenum Publishing, 1982.
63. Gimenez, L.F., Solez, K., Walker, G.W.: Kidney Int., *31:*93–99, 1987.
64. Harris, D.C.H., Hammond, W.S., Burke, T.J., et al.: Kidney Int., *31:*41–46, 1987.
65. Kasiske, B.L., O'Donnell, M.P., Schmitz, P.G., et al.: Kidney Int., *37:*880–891, 1990.
66. Wellmann, K., Wolk, B.W.: Lab. Invest., *22:*144–155, 1970.
67. Kasiske, B.L., O'Donnell, M.P., Cleary, M.P., et al.: Kidney Int., *33:*667–672, 1988.
68. Keane, W.F., O'Donnell, M.P., Kasiske, B.L., et al.: J. Am. Soc. Nephrol., *1:*S69–S74, 1990.
69. Alderson, L.M., Endemann, G., Lindsay, I., et al.: Am. J. Pathol., *123:*334–342, 1986.
70. Kaplan R., Aynedjian, H.S., Schlondorff, D., et al.: J. Clin. Invest., *86:*1707–1714, 1990.

71. Suzuki, S., Shapiro, R., Mulrow, P.J., et al.: Prostaglandins Med., *4:*377–382, 1980.
72. Purkerson, M.L., Joist, J.H., Yates, J., et al. Proc. Natl. Acad. Sci. U.S.A., *82:*193–197, 1985.
73. Dubois, E.L., Horowitz, R.E., Demopoulos, H.B., et al.: JAMA, *195:*285–289, 1966.
74. Prickett, J.D., Robinson, D.R., Steinberg, A.D.: J. Clin. Invest., *68:*556–559, 1981.
75. Rahman, M.A., Nakazawa, M., Emancipator, S.N., et al.: Kidney Int., *29:*343, 1986.
76. Badr, K.F., Brenner, B.M., Wasserman, M., et al.: Kidney Int., *29:*328, 1986.
77. Schambelan, M., Hutchinson, F.N., Kaysen, G.A., et al.: Kidney Int., *29:*344, 1986.
78. Anderson, S., Meyer, T.W., Rennke, H.G., et al.: J. Clin. Invest., *76:*612–619, 1985.
79. Beukers, J.J.B., Hoedemacker, P.J., Weening, J.J.: Kidney Int., *29:*265, 1986.
80. Taguma, Y., Kitamoto, Y., Futaki, G., et al.: N. Engl. J. Med., *313:*1617–1620, 1985.
81. Hostetter, T.H., Rosenberg, M.E.: J. Am. Soc. Nephrol., *1:*S55–S58, 1990.
82. Bauer, J.H., Reams, G.P.: J. Am. Soc. Nephrol., *1:*S80–S81, 1990.
83. Dworkin, L.D.: J. Am. Soc. Nephrol., *1:*S21–S27, 1990.
84. Anderson, S.: J. Am. Soc. Nephrol., *1:*S51–S54, 1990.
85. Purkerson, M.L., Joist, J.H., Greenberg, J.M., et al.: Thromb. Res., *26:*227–240, 1982.
86. Gimenez, L., Walker, W.G., Tew, W.P., et al.: Kidney Int., *22:*36–41, 1982.
87. Walser, M.: Clin. Nephrol., *3:*180–186, 1975.
88. Maschio, G., Oldrizzi, L., Tessitore, N., et al.: Kidney Int., *22:*371–376, 1982.
89. Alvestrand, A., Ahlberg, M., Bergstrom, J.: Kidney Int., *24(Suppl. 16):*S268–S272, 1983.
90. Barsotti, G., Morelli, E., Giannoni, A., et al.: Kidney Int., *24(Suppl. 16):*S278–S284, 1983.
91. Gretz, N., Korb, E., Strauch, M.: Kidney Int., *24(Suppl. 16):*S263–S267, 1983.
92. Mitch, W.E., Walser, M., Steinman, T.I., et al.: N. Engl. J. Med., *311:*623–629, 1984.
93. Rosman, J.B., Meijer, S., Sluiter, W.J., et al. Lancet, *2:*1291–1295, 1984.
94. Walser, M., LaFrance, N.D., Ward, L., et al.: Kidney Int., *32:*123–128, 1987.
95. Ihle, B.U., Becker, G.J., Whitworth, J.A., et al.: N. Engl. J. Med., *321:*1773–1777, 1989.
96. Zeller, J., Whittaker, E., Sullivan, L., et al.: N. Engl. J. Med., *324:*78–84, 1991.
97. Barsotti, G., Giannoni, A., Morelli, E., et al.: Clin. Nephrol., *21:*54–59, 1984.
98. Mitch, W.E., Walser, M., Sapir, D.G.: J. Clin. Invest., *67:*553–562, 1981.
99. Tischler, M.E., Desautels, M., Goldberg, A.L.: J. Biol. Chem., *257:*1613–1621, 1982.
100. Striker, G.E., Nagle, R.B., Kohnen, P.W., et al.: Arch. Pathol., *87:*439–442, 1969.
101. Lalich, J.J., Faith, G.C., Harding, G.E.: Arch. Pathol., *89:*548–559, 1970.
102. Everitt, A.V., Porter, B.D., Wyndham, J.R.: Gerontology, *28:*168–175, 1982.
103. Zucchelli, P., Cagnoli, L., Casanova, S., et al.: Kidney Int., *24:*649–655, 1983.
104. Rowe, J.W., Anres, R., Tobin, J.D., et al.: Ann. Intern. Med., *84:*567–569, 1976.
105. Kiprov, D.D., Colvin, R.B., McCluskey, R.T.: Lab. Invest., *46:*275–281, 1982.
106. Committee on Dietary Allowances, Food and Nutrition Board, National Research Council: Recommended Dietary Allowances. 10th Ed. National Academy Press, Washington, D.C., 1989.
107. Glassock, R.J., Adler, S.G., Ward, H.J., et al.: Primary glomerular diseases. *In* The Kidney. 3rd Ed. Vol. 1. Edited by B.M. Brenner, and F.C. Rector, Jr. Philadelphia, W.B. Saunders, 1986, pp. 929–1013.
108. Massry, S.G., Feinstein, E.I., Goldstein, D.A., et al.: Metabolic and endocrine complications of the nephrotic syndrome. *In* Textbook of Nephrology. Vol. 1. Edited by S.G. Massry, and R.J. Glassock. Baltimore, Williams & Wilkins, 1983, pp. 6.7–6.11.
109. Kaysen, G.A., Gambertoglio, J., Jimenez, I., et al.: Kidney Int., *29:*572–577, 1986.
110. Zeller, K.R., Raskin, P., Rosenstock, J., et al.: Kidney Int., *29:*209, 1986.
111. Kaysen, G.A., Davies, R.W.: J. Am. Soc. Nephrol., *1:*S75–S79, 1990.
112. Kopple, J.D.: Kidney Int., *14:*340–348, 1978.
113. Gonick, H.C., Maxwell, M.H., Rubini, M.E., et al.: Nephron, *3:*137–152, 1966.
114. David, D.S., Hochgelerent, E., Rubin, A.L.: Lancet, *2:*34–37, 1972.
115. Coburn, J.W., Slatopolsky, E.: Vitamin D, parathyroid hormone, and renal osteodystrophy. *In* The Kidney. 3rd Ed. Vol. 2. Edited by B.M. Brenner and F.C. Rector, Jr. Philadelphia, W.B. Saunders, 1986, pp. 1657–1729.
116. Coburn, J.W., Hartenbower, D.L., Brickman, A.S., et al.: Intestinal absorption of calcium, magnesium and phosphorus in chronic renal insufficiency. *In* Calcium Metabolism in Renal Failure and Nephrolithiasis. Edited by D.S. David. New York, John Wiley & Sons, 1977, pp. 77–109.
117. Lawson, D.H., Boddy, K., King, P.C., et al.: Clin. Sci., *41:*345, 1971.
118. Kopple, J.D., Swendseid, M.E.: Kidney Int., *7(Suppl. 2):*S79–S84, 1975.
119. Ott, S.M., Maloney, N.A., Coburn, J.W., et al.: N. Engl. J. Med., *307:*709–713, 1982.
120. Rabkin, R., Simon, N.M., Steiner, S., et al.: N. Engl. J. Med., *282:*182–187, 1970.
121. Sherwin, R.S., Bastl, C., Finkelstein, F.O., et al.: J. Clin. Invest., *57:*722–731, 1976.
122. Vajda, F.J.E., Martin, T.J., Melick, R.A.: Endocrinology, *84:*162–164, 1969.
123. Cuttelod, S., Lemarchand-Beraud, T., Magnenat, P., et al.: Metabolism, *23:*101–113, 1974.
124. Davidson, W.D., Moore, T.C., Shippey, W., et al.: Gastroenterology, *66:*522–525, 1974.
125. Samaan, N., Freeman, R.M.: Metabolism, *19:*102–113, 1970.
126. Nagel, T.C., Frenkel, N., Bell, R.H., et al.: J. Clin. Endocrinol. Metab., *36:*428–432, 1973.
127. Lim, V.S., Fang, V.S.: Am. J. Med., *58:*655–662, 1975.
128. Tourkantonis, A., Spiliopoulos, A., Pharmakioltis, A., et al.: Nephron, *27:*271–272, 1981.
129. Hershman, J.M., Krugman, L.G., Kopple, J.D., et al.: Metabolism, *27:*755–759, 1979.
130. Schiffrin, A., Guyda, H., Robitaille, P., et al.: J. Clin. Endocrinol. Metab., *46:*511–514, 1977.
131. Phillips, L.S., Kopple, J.: Metabolism, *30:*1091–1095, 1981.
132. Feldman, H.A., Singer, I.: Medicine, *54:*345–376, 1975.

133. Kopple, J.D., Fukuda, S.: Am. J. Clin. Nutr., *33:*1363–1372, 1980.
134. Tizianello, A., De Ferrari, G., Garibotto, et al.: J. Clin. Invest., *65:*1162–1173, 1980.
135. Kopple, J.D.: Nitrogen metabolism. *In* Clinical Aspects of Uremia and Dialysis. Edited by S.G. Massry and A.L. Sellers. Springfield, IL, Charles C Thomas, 1976, pp. 241–273.
136. Simenhoff, M.L., Burke, J.F., Saukkonen, J.J., et al.: Lancet, *2:*818–821, 1976.
137. Bricker, N.S.: N. Engl. J. Med., *286:*1093–1099, 1972.
138. Massry, S.G.: Semin. Nephrol., *3:*306–328, 1983.
139. Golper, T.A.: Nephron, *38:*217–225, 1984.
140. Rutsky, E.A., Rostand, S.G.: Kidney, *16:*1–8, 1983.
141. Briggs, W.A., Lazarus, J.M., Birtch, A.G., et al.: Arch. Intern. Med., *132:*21–28, 1973.
142. Bianchi, R., Mariani, G., Toni, M.G., et al.: Am. J. Clin. Nutr., *31:*1615–1626, 1978.
143. Kluthe, R., Luttgen, F.M., Capetianu, T., et al.: Am. J. Clin. Nutr., *31:*1812–1820, 1978.
144. Young, G.A., Oli, H.I., Davidson, A.M., et al.: Am. J. Clin. Nutr., *31:*1802–1807, 1978.
145. Attman, P.O., Isaksson E.J.: Am. J. Clin. Nutr., *33:*801–810, 1980.
146. Blumenkrantz, M.J., Kopple, J.D., Gutman, R.A., et al.: Am. J. Clin. Nutr., *33:*1567–1585, 1980.
147. Guarnieri, G., Faccini, L., Lipartiti, T., et al.: Am. J. Clin. Nutr., *33:*1598–1607, 1980.
148. Bansal, V.K., Popli, S., Pickering, J., et al.: Am. J. Clin. Nutr., *33:*1608–1611, 1980.
149. Thunberg, B.J., Swamy, A.P., Cestero, R.V.: Am. J. Clin. Nutr., *34:*2005–2012, 1981.
150. Heide, B., Pierratos, A., Jhanna, R., et al.: Peritoneal Dialysis Bull., *3:*138–141, 1983.
151. Young, G.A., Swanepoel, C.R., Croft, M.R., et al.: Kidney Int., *21:*492–499, 1982.
152. Salusky, I.B., Fine, R.N., Nelson, P., et al.: Am. J. Clin. Nutr., *38:*599–611, 1983.
153. Wolfson, M., Strong, C.J., Minturn, D., et al.: Am. J. Clin. Nutr., *37:*547–555, 1984.
154. Kopple, J.D.: Causes of catabolism and wasting in acute or chronic renal failure. *In* Nephrology. Vol. 2. Proceedings of the Ninth International Congress of Nephrology. Edited by R.R. Robinson. New York, Springer-Verlag, 1984, pp. 1498–1515.
155. Carlson, D.M., Duncan, D.A., Naessens, J.M., et al.: Mayo Clin. Proc., *59:*769–775, 1984.
156. Young, G.A., Kopple, J.D., et al.: Am. J. Kidney Dis., *17:*462–471, 1991.
157. Evans, R.W., Manninen, D.L., Garrison, L.P., Jr., et al.: N. Engl. J. Med., *312:*553–559, 1985.
158. Grodstein, G.P., Blumenkrantz, M.J., Kopple, J.D.: Am. J. Clin. Nutr., *33:*1411–1416, 1980.
159. Kopple, J.D., Swendseid, M.E., Shinaberger, J.H., et al.: Trans. Am. Soc. Artif. Intern. Organs, *19:*309–313, 1973.
160. Wolfson, M., Jones, M.R., Kopple, J.D.: Kidney Int., *21:*500–506, 1982.
161. Kopple, J.D., Blumenkrantz, M.J., Jones, M.R., et al.: Am. J. Clin. Nutr., *36:*395–402, 1982.
162. Blumenkrantz, M.J., Gahl, G.M., Kopple. J.D., et al.: Kidney Int., *19:*593–602, 1981.
163. Borah, M.F., Schoenfeld, P.Y., Gotch, F.A., et al.: Kidney Int., *14:*491–500, 1978.
164. Linton, A.L., Clark, W.F., Driedger, A.A., et al.: Nephron, *19:*95–98, 1977.
165. Shapiro, J.I., Argy, W.P., Rakowski, T.A., et al.: Trans. Am. Soc. Artif. Intern. Organs, *29:*129–132, 1983.
166. Acchiardo, S.R., Moore, L.W., Latour, P.A.: Kidney Int., *24(Suppl. 16):*S199–S203, 1983.
167. Lowrie, E.G., Lew, N.L.: Am. J. Kidney Dis., *15:*458–482, 1990.
168. Salusky, I.B., Fine, R.N., Nelson, P., et al.: American Society of Nephrology 15th Annual Meeting, December 1982, p. 66A. (Abstract.)
169. Calloway, D.H., Odell, A.C.F., Margen, S.: J. Nutr., *101:*775–786, 1971.
170. Kopple, J.D., Grodstein, G.: Clin. Res., *28:*597A, 1980.
171. Maroni, B.J., Steinman, T.I., Mitch, W.E.: Kidney Int., *27:*58–65, 1985.
172. Varcoe, R., Halliday, D., Carson, E.R., et al.: Clin. Sci. Mol. Med., *43:*379–390, 1975.
173. Walser, M.: J. Clin. Invest., *53:*1385–1392, 1974.
174. Sargent, J.A., Gotch, F.A.: J. Am. Diet. Assoc., *75:*547–551, 1979.
175. Kopple, J.D., Coburn, J.W.: JAMA, *227:*41–44, 1974.
176. Weigley, E.S.: J. Am. Diet. Assoc., *84:*417–423, 1984.
177. Bergstrom, J., Furst, P., Noree, L.-O.: Clin. Nephrol, *3:*187–194, 1975.
178. Noree, L.-O., Bergstrom, J.: Clin. Nephrol., *3:*195–203, 1975.
179. Furst, P., Alvestrand, A., Bergstrom, J.: Am. J. Clin. Nutr., *33:*1387–1395, 1980.
180. Kopple, J.D.: *In* Proceedings of the Eighth International Congress of Nephrology. Edited by R. Barcelo, M. Bergeron, S. Carriere, et al., Basel, S. Karger, 1978, pp. 497–507.
181. Furst, P.: Scan J. Clin. Lab. Invest., *30:*307–312, 1972.
182. Kopple, J.D., Swendseid, M.E.: J. Clin. Invest., *55:*881–891, 1975.
183. Kopple, J.D., Swendseid, M.E.: J. Nutr., *111:*931–942, 1981.
184. Jones, M.R., Kopple, J.D., Swendseid, M.E.: Am. J. Clin. Nutr., *35:*15–23, 1982.
185. Kopple, J.D., Swendseid, M.E.: Nephron, *18:*1–12, 1977.
186. Walser, M., Coulter, A.W., Dighe, S., et al.: J. Clin. Invest., *52:*678–690, 1973.
187. Kopple, J.D., Swendseid, M.E.: Am. J. Clin. Nutr., *27:*806–812, 1974.
188. Sapir, D.G., Owen, O.E., Pozefsky, T., et al.: J. Clin. Invest., *54:*974–980, 1974.
189. Freund, H., Hoover, H.C., Atamuriam, S., et al.: Ann. Surg., *190:*18–23, 1979.
190. Sherwin, R.S.: J. Clin. Invest., *61:*1471–1481, 1978.
191. Jungers, P., Chauveau, B., Lebkiri, C., et al.: Kidney Int., *32(Suppl. 22):*S67–S71, 1987.
192. Kopple, J.D., Coburn, J.W.: Medicine, *52:*583–595, 1973.
193. Blainey, J.D.: Clin. Sci., *13:*567–581, 1954.
194. Kopple, J.D., Shinaberger, J.H., Coburn, J.W., et al.: Trans. Am. Soc. Artif. Intern. Organs, *15:*302–308, 1969.
195. Blumenkrantz, M.J., Kopple, J.D., Moran, J.K., et al.: Kidney Int., *21:*849–861, 1982.
196. Kopple, J.D., Monteon, F.J., Shaib, J.K.: Kidney Int., *29:*734–742, 1986.
197. Monteon, F.J., Laidlaw, S.A., Shaib, J.K., et al.: Energy expenditure in patients with chronic renal failure. Kidney Int., *30:*741–747, 1986.
198. Cramp, D.G., Moorhead, J.F., Wills, M.R.: Lancet, *1:*672–673, 1975.
199. Chan, J.K., Varghese, Z., Moorhead, J.F.: Kidney Int., *19:*625, 1981.

200. Ciman, M., Rizzoli, V., Moracchiello, M., et al.: Am. J. Clin. Nutr., *33:*1489–1492, 1980.
201. Bellinghieri, G., Savica, V., Mallamace, A., et al.: Am. J. Clin. Nutr. *38:*523–531, 1983.
202. Sanfelippo, M.L., Swenson, R.S., Reaven, G.M.: Kidney Int., *14:*54–61, 1977.
203. Sanfelippo, M.L., Swenson, R.S., Reaven, G.M.: Kidney Int., *14:*180–186, 1978.
204. Manis, T., Deutsch, J., Feinstein, E.I., et al.: Am. J. Clin. Nutr., *33:*1485–1488, 1980.
205. Pierides, A.M., Alvarez-Ude, F., Kerr, D.N.S., et al.: Lancet, *2:*1279–1282, 1979.
206. Himizaki, T., Nakazawa, R., Tateno, S., et al.: Kidney Int., *26:*81, 1984.
207. Leaf, A., Weber, P.C.: N. Engl. J. Med., *318:*549, 1988.
208. Donadio, J.V., Jr.: *In* Renal Nutrition: Report of the Eleventh Ross Roundtable on Medical Issues. Edited by J.D. Gussler and E. Silverman. 1991, pp. 76–81.
209. Pagenkemper, J.J.: *In* Renal Nutrition: Report of the Eleventh Ross Roundtable on Medical Issues. Edited by J.D. Gussler and E. Silverman. 1991, pp. 26–33.
210. Disler, P.B.; Goldberg, R.B., Kuhn, L., et al.: Clin. Nephrol., *16:*29, 1981.
211. Shen, S.Y., Lukens, C.W., Alongi, S.V., et al.: Kidney Int., *24:*S147, 1983.
212. Pagenkemper, J.J., DiMarco, N.D., Hull, A.R., et al.: CRN Q., *13:*9, 1989.
213. Goldberg, A.P., Geltman, E.M., Hagberg, J.M., et al.: Kidney Int., *24(Suppl. 16):*S303–S309, 1983.
214. Holley, J.L., Shapiro, R., Lopatin, W.B., et al.: Transplantation, *49:*387, 1990.
215. Symposium on Role Dietary Fiber in Health. Am. J. Clin. Nutr., *31:*S1–S291, 1978.
216. Parillo, M., Riccardi, G., Pacioni, D., et al.: Diabetes Care, *8:*620, 1985.
217. Anderson, J.W., Zettwoch, N., Feldman, T., et al.: Arch. Intern. Med., *148:*292, 1988.
218. Anderson, J.W., Chen, W.L.: Am. J. Clin. Nutr., *32:*346, 1979.
219. Rampton, D.S., Cohen, S.L., Crammond, V.De.B., et al.: Clin. Nephrol., *21:*159–163, 1984.
220. Massry, S.G., Coburn, J.W.: Divalent ion metabolism and renal osteodystrophy. *In* Clinical Aspects of Uremia and Dialysis. Edited by S.G. Massry and A.L. Sellers. Springfield, IL, Charles C Thomas, 1976, pp. 304–387.
221. Tomford, R.C., Karlinsky, M.L., Buddington, B., et al.: J. Clin. Invest., *68:*655–664, 1981.
222. Cannata, J.B., Briggs, J.D., Junor, B.J.R.: Br. Med. J., *286:*1937–1938, 1983.
223. Sedman, A.B., Miller, N.L., Warady, B.A., et al.: Kidney Int., *26:*201–204, 1984.
224. Kopple, J.D., Coburn, J.W.: Medicine, *52:*597–607, 1973.
225. Pei, Y., Hercz, G., et al.: J. Am. Soc. Nephrol., *1:*572, 1990.
226. Randall, R.E., Jr., Cohen, M.D., Spray, C.C., Jr., et al.: Ann. Intern. Med., *61:*73–78, 1964.
227. Koomans, H.A., Roos, J.C., Boer, P., et al.: Hypertension, *4:*190–197, 1982.
228. Lawson, D.H., Boddy, K., King, P.C., et al.: Clin. Sci., *41:*345–351, 1971.
229. Rudolph, H., Alfrey, A.C., Smythe, W.R.: Trans. Am. Soc. Artif. Intern. Organs, *19:*456–465, 1973.
230. Atkin-Thor, E., Goddard, B.W., O'Nion, J., et al.: Am. J. Clin. Nutr., *31:*1948–1951, 1978.
231. Antoniou, L.D., Shalhoub, R.J., Sudhakar, T., et al.: Lancet, *2:*895–898, 1977.
232. Mahajan, S.K., Bowersox, G.M., Rye, D., et al.: Kidney Int., *36:*269, 1989.
233. Mahajan, S.K.: *In* Renal Nutrition: Report of the Eleventh Ross Roundtable on Medical Issues. Edited by J.D. Gussler and E. Silverman. 1991, pp. 72–75.
234. Alfrey, A.C.: Kidney Int., *29(Suppl. 18):*S53–S57, 1986.
235. Touam, M., Martinez, F., Lacour, B., et al.: Clin. Nephrol., *19:*295–298, 1983.
236. Hercz, G., Coburn, J.W.: Kidney Int., *32(Suppl.):*S215–S220, 1987.
237. Jennette, J.C., Goldman, I.D.: J. Lab. Clin. Med., *86:*834–843, 1975.
238. Spannuth, C.L., Jr., Warnock, L.G., Wagner, C., et al.: J. Lab. Clin. Med., *90:*632–637, 1977.
239. Sharman, V.L., Cunningham, J., Goodwin, F.J., et al.: Br. Med. J., *285:*96–97, 1982.
240. Balcke, P., Schmidt, P., Zazgornik, J., et al.: Ann. Intern. Med., *101:*344–345, 1984.
241. Pru, C., Eaton, J., Kjellstrand, C.: Nephron, *39:*112–116, 1985.
242. Smith, F.R., Goodman, D.S.: J. Clin. Invest., *50:*2426–2436, 1971.
243. Yatzidis, H., Digenis, P., et al.: Br. Med. J., *2:*352–353, 1975.
244. Roe, D.A.: Drug-Induced Nutritional Deficiencies. Westport, CT, AVI Publishing, 1976.
245. Kopple, J.D., Massry, S.G.: Am. J. Nephrol., *8:*437–448, 1988.
246. Slatopolsky, E., Weerts, C., Thielan, J., et al.: J. Clin. Invest., *74:*2136–2143, 1984.
247. Andress, D.L., Norris, K.C.: N. Engl. J. Med., *321:*274–279, 1989.
248. May, R.C., Kelly, R.A., Mitch, W.E.: J. Clin. Invest., *79:*1099–1103, 1987.
249. Mault, J.R., Bartlett, R.H., Dechert, R.E., et al.: Trans. Am. Soc. Artif. Intern. Organs, *29:*390–394, 1983.
250. Flugel-Link, R.M., Salusky, I.B., Jones, M.R., et al.: Am. J. Physiol. Soc., *244:*E615–E623, 1983.
251. Clark, A.S., Mitch, W.E.: J. Clin. Invest., *72:*836–845, 1983.
252. Frohlich, J., Scholmerich, J., Hoppe-Seyler, G., et al.: Eur. J. Clin. Invest., *4:*453–458, 1974.
253. Feinstein, E.I., Blumenkrantz, M.J., Healy, H., et al.: Medicine, *60:*124–137, 1981.
254. Feinstein, E.I., Kopple, J.D., Silberman, H.: Kidney Int., *26(Suppl. 16):*S319–S323, 1983.
255. Abel, R.M., Abbott, W.M., Beck, C.H., Jr., et al.: Am. J. Surg., *128:*317–323, 1974.
256. Abel, R.M., Shih, V.E., Abbott, W.M., et al.: Ann. Surg., *180:*350–355, 1974.
257. Abel, R.M., Beck, C.H., Jr., Abbott, W.M., et al.: N. Engl. J. Med., *288:*695–699, 1973.
258. Baek, S.M., Makabali, G.G., Bryan-Brown, C.W., et al.: Surg. Gynecol. Obstet., *141:*405–408, 1975.
259. McMurray, S.D., Luft, F.C., Maxwell, D.R., et al.: Arch. Intern. Med., *138:*950–955, 1978.
260. Leonard, C.D., Luke, R.G., Siegel, R.R.: Urology, *6:*154–157, 1975.
261. Toback, F.G.: Kidney Int., *12:*193–198, 1977.
262. Toback, F.G., Teegarden, D.E., Havener, L.J.: Kidney Int., *15:*542–547, 1979.
263. Toback, F.G., Dodd, R.C., Maier, E.R., et al.: Clin. Res., *27:*432A, 1979.
264. Oken, D.E., Sprinkel, F.M., Kirschbaum, B.B., et al.: Kidney Int., *17:*14–23, 1980.

265. Motil, K.J., Harmon, W.E., Grupe, W.E.: JPEN J. Parenter. Enteral Nutr., *4:*32–35, 1980.

266. Kopple, J.D., Feinstein, E.I.: Proc. EDTA, *19:*129–140, 1983.

267. McCracken, B.H., Parsons, F.M.: Lancet, *2:*885–886, 1958.

268. Gjorup, S., Thaysen, J.H.: Acta Med. Scand., *167:*227–238, 1960.

269. Hinton, P., Allison, S.P., Littlejohn, S., et al.: Lancet, *1:*767–769, 1971.

270. Woolfson, A.M.J., Healtley, R.V., Allison, S.P.: N. Engl. J. Med., *300:*14–17, 1979.

271. Ponting, G.A., Halliday, D., Teale, J.D., et al.: Lancet, *1:*438–440, 1988.

272. Kopple, J.D., Leiserowitz, M., Brunori, G., et al.: J. Am. Soc. Nephrol., *1:*364, 1990.

273. Cerra, F.B., Upson, D., Angelico, R., et al.: Surgery, *92:*192–200, 1982.

274. Daly, M., Mihranian, M.H., Kehoe, J.I., et al.: Surgery, *94:*151–159, 1983.

275. Leander, U., Furst, P., Vesterberg, K., et al.: Clin. Nutr., *4:*43–51, 1985.

276. Hammarqvist, F., Wernerman, J., Rustom, A., et al.: Ann. Surg., *209:*455–461, 1989.

277. Stehle, P., Zander, J., Mertes, N., et al.: Lancet, *1:*231–233, 1989.

278. Daly, J.M., Reynolds, J., Thom, A., et al.: Ann. Surg., *208:*512–523, 1988.

279. Harris, J.A., Benedict, F.G.: A Biometric Study of Basal Metabolism in Man. Publication No. 279. Washington, D.C., Carnegie Institute, 1919.

280. Wilmore, D.W.: *In* the Metabolic Management of the Critically Ill. New York, Plenum, 1977, p. 314.

281. Askanazi, J., Elwyn, D.H., Silverberg, B.S., et al.: Surgery, *87:*596–598, 1980.

282. Jeejeebhoy, K.N., Langer, B., Tsallas, G., et al.: Gastroenterology, *71:*943–953, 1976.

283. Seidner, D.L., Mascioli, E.A., Istfan, N.W., et al.: JPEN, J. Parenter. Enteral Nutr., *13:*614–619, 1989.

284. Driscoll, D.F., Baptista, B.J., Bistrian, B.R., et al.: Am. J. Hosp. Pharm., *43:*416–419, 1986.

285. Kopple, J.D., Mercurio, K., Blumenkrantz, M.J., et al.: Kidney Int., *19:*694–704, 1981.

286. Hecking, E., Port, F.K., Brehm, H., et al.: Kidney Int., *12:*482, 1977.

287. Ulm, A., Neuhauser, M., Leber, H.-W.: Am. J. Clin. Nutr., *31:*1827–1830, 1978.

288. Golper, T.A.: Am. J. Kidney Dis., *6:*373–386, 1985.

289. Williams, F.P., Marliss, E.B., Anderson, G.H., et al.: Peritoneal Dialysis Bull., *2:*124–130, 1982.

290. Feinstein, E.I., Collins, J.F., Blumenkrantz, M.J., et al.: Prog. Artif. Organs, *1:*421–426, 1984.

291. Zager, R.A., Johannes, G., Tuttle, S.E., et al.: J. Lab. Clin. Med., *101:*130–140, 1983.

292. Zager, R.A., Venkatachalam, M.A.: Kidney Int., *24:*620–625, 1983.

293. Malis, C.D., Racusen, C., Solez, K., et al.: J. Lab. Clin. Med., *103:*660–676, 1984.

294. Andrews, P.M., Bates, S.B.: Kidney Int., *32(Suppl. 22):*S76–S80, 1987.

295. Weinberg, J.M.: Semin. Nephrol., *10:*491–500, 1990.

296. Daly, J.M., Reynolds, J., Sigal, R.K., et al.: Crit. Care Med., *18:*S86–S93, 1990.

297. VanBuren, C.T., Rudolph, F.B., Kulkarni, A., et al.: Crit. Care Med., *18:*S114–S117, 1990.

CHAPTER 66

Nutritional Management of Infants and Children with Specific Diseases and/or Conditions

William C. Heird

The generalized deficiency of all nutrients, that is, protein-energy malnutrition, is by far the most common nutritional deficiency in the world today. Although this condition is rare in developed countries, it occurs in a number of infants and children with underlying medical problems, some of which are discussed below. Thus, it is helpful to consider the special nutrient needs and nutritional management of these children within the framework of protein-energy malnutrition as encountered in many underdeveloped parts of the world.

Protein-energy malnutrition results from a lack, in varying proportions, of protein and energy. It is seen most frequently in infants and young children and may occur in epidemic (famine-related) or endemic (disease-related) forms. Whether the cause is primary (i.e., insufficient food supply) or secondary (i.e., poor absorption, increased excretion, increased requirements), the physicochemical pattern of the tissues, the defensive capacity against environmental aggressors, and the efficiency and ability for work are affected adversely. Moreover, the condition is associated with a high mortality rate.

Protein-energy malnutrition includes two distinct syndromes, marasmus and kwashiorkor, as well as a mixed syndrome, often termed marasmic kwashiorkor. Marasmus refers to the state of chronic total undernutrition (i.e., a deficiency of both protein and energy). It results in growth failure as well as gradual emaciation and inanition. Kwashiorkor, derived from the Ga language of Ghana, was used initially to refer to the protein deficiency of weanling infants, that is, "the disease that the first child gets when the second is on the way."[1] Clinically, it is characterized by usual signs of protein deficiency, including edema and acites, as well as growth failure.

Both conditions occur in varying degrees in the groups of pediatric patients discussed below. Mild and moderate forms of both distinct syndromes are subclinical and characterized only by growth failure and possibly some retardation of mental development. Whether or not these latter consequences are permanent is a matter of debate; on balance, it appears that most can be ameliorated with appropriate treatment.[2]

CYSTIC FIBROSIS AND OTHER CHRONIC PULMONARY DISEASES

Cystic fibrosis is characterized by progressive deterioration of pulmonary and pancreatic function. The former may increase nutrient requirements somewhat but probably affects nutrition more by adversely affecting intake, particularly during acute exacerbations and in older children with severe pulmonary disease. Pancreatic insufficiency severely limits the absorption of fat, a chief energy source of most diets. Thus, the cause of malnutrition in infants and children with this disease can be both primary (i.e., inadequate nutrient intake) and secondary (i.e., fecal losses of protein and, particularly, fat). The latter cause usually can be controlled with appropriate pancreatic enzyme replacement.

Traditionally, a high-protein, low-fat diet has been advocated for patients with cystic fibrosis. However, with appropriate pancreatic enzyme replacement, most patients can maintain reasonable nutritional status with a reasonably "normal" diet. Younger patients usually have a very good appetite, but many older patients with advanced pulmonary disease have a poor appetite. In many of the latter patients, intakes of both protein and energy, especially energy, are far less than recommended. From time to time the theoretical possibility of essential fatty acid deficiency secondary to poor fat absorption is mentioned. However, unless the intake of essential fatty acids is very low, this is rarely a significant problem.

There is some concern that malnutrition may hasten deterioration of pulmonary function, but there is no definitive proof that this is the case. Nonetheless, it is clear that acute improvement of nutritional status improves muscle strength.[3] Thus, attempts either to improve nutritional status or to prevent even minimal deterioration of nutritional status are warranted.

In recent years, the advantages of a high-fat formula for patients with chronic pulmonary disease have been advocated. The rationale, supported adequately by both theory and direct observations, is that oxidation of fat produces less carbon dioxide than oxidation of carbohydrate. Thus, a high-fat intake imposes less stress on the already compromised pulmonary system. This obviously is an important consideration in patients who require mechanical ventilation or who have severely compromised pulmonary function. One product based on this principle (Pulmocare, Ross Laboratories) is available for patients with pulmonary disease. Although designed for adults, the product is used in pediatric patients; however, it should be noted that its sodium content is high.

CONGENITAL HEART DISEASE

Chronic protein-energy malnutrition, manifested chiefly by growth failure, also is a common finding in infants with congenital heart disease, particularly those with conditions associated with congestive heart failure. Although not studied extensively, the nutrient needs of patients with heart disease do not appear to be much greater, if at all, than those of similar patients without heart disease. Rather, in most patients, the cause of the accompanying malnutrition can be traced to inadequate intake. In some patients, this is a result simply of poor appetite; in others, it appears to be due to excessive tiring during feeding. In addition, fluid and sodium intakes frequently are restricted as a part of treatment, and use of diuretics is common. Either practice, of course, may limit growth even if intake of protein and energy is adequate.

The most common form of nutritional therapy for infants with congenital heart disease is use of a high-nutrient-density formula, thereby reducing the volume that must be ingested. Tube feedings via either a nasogastric tube or gastrostomy are frequently necessary, particularly in infants whose disease is sufficiently severe to cause excessive tiring during feeding. In general, if sufficient nutrients are delivered, most such patients will grow at a reasonably "normal" rate.

GASTROINTESTINAL DISORDERS

Malnutrition is endemic among infants and children with gastrointestinal disorders. The cause usually is loss of nutrients secondary to the specific derangement in gastrointestinal function, either diarrhea or vomiting. However, both diarrhea and vomiting are frequently "treated" by withholding all nutrients except water and electrolytes. This practice, of course, contributes to the development of malnutrition.

Acute Diarrhea. Acute diarrhea caused by most common organisms rarely persists for more than 4 to 5 days. During this time, the major goal of nutritional therapy is to maintain a normal state of hydration. This can be accomplished with use of oral rehydration solutions and/or special formulas (Table 66–1). Hospitalization and intravenous fluid therapy may be necessary, particularly if fever and/or vomiting accompanies the diarrhea.

What to feed and whether to feed the child with acute diarrhea have been subjects of considerable debate for many years, and both remain unresolved. In general, stool output is greater in the patient who is fed but this does not necessarily mean that feeding should be proscribed. In most patients, at least some nutrient intake is possible; however, the nature of this intake must be selected carefully, taking into account the probable cause of the diarrhea. My approach is outlined below; other approaches, of course, may be equally successful.

In general, the cause of most acute diarrhea is either bacterial or viral. Thus, a stool culture to detect the specific pathogen is indicated. In most developed countries, the recognized enteropathogenic bacteria (Salmonella, Shigella, and enteropathogenic E. coli) are infrequent causes of diarrhea. Rather, the causative organism of most acute bacterial diarrheas is one of the many toxicogenic strains of most gram-negative organisms. Thus, a routine stool culture, unless it suggests a predominant organism, usually is not helpful. On the other hand, because the pathogenesis of toxicogenic bacterial diarrhea (i.e., a secretory diarrhea resulting from stimulation of the adenylate cyclase system, as occurs in cholera[4]) is different from that of viral diarrhea (i.e., an osmotic diarrhea secondary to inhibition of glucose transport as described for Rotavirus[5]), testing the stool for pH and the presence of reducing substances

TABLE 66–1. COMPOSITION (AMOUNT/100 KCAL) OF SPECIAL FORMULAS FOR INFANTS WITH DERANGED INTESTINAL FUNCTION

COMPONENT	RCF*,†	PREGESTAMIL‡	NUTRAMIGEN‡	PORTAGEN‡	ALIMENTUM*	PEDIASURE*
Protein (g)	4.95 (soy protein isolate)	2.8 (casein hydrolysate, cystine, tyrosine, and tryptophan)	2.8 (casein hydrolysate, cystine, tyrosine, and tryptophan)	3.5 (sodium caseinate)	2.75 (casein hydrolysate, cystine, tyrosine, and tryptophan)	3.0 (low lactose whey protein and sodium caseinate)
Fat (g)	8.91 (soy and coconut oils)	5.6 (medium-chain triglycerides; corn and high-oleic safflower oils)	3.9 (corn oil)	4.8 (medium-chain triglycerides; corn oil)	5.54 (medium-chain triglycerides; safflower and soy oils)	5.0 (medium-chain triglycerides; oleic safflower oils)
Carbohydrate (g)	0	10.3 (corn syrup solids; modified corn starch; dextrose)	13.4 (corn syrup solids; sucrose)	11.5 (corn syrup solids sucrose)	10.2 (sucrose and modified tapioca starch)	11.0 (corn syrup solids and sucrose)
Calcium (mg)	173	94	94	94	105	97
Phosphorus (mg)	124	63	63	70	75	80
Magnesium (mg)	12.4	10.9	10.9	20	7.5	20
Iron (mg)	0.37	1.88	1.88	1.88	1.8	1.4
Zinc (mg)	1.2	0.94	0.78	0.94	0.75	1.2
Manganese (μg)	50	31	31	125	30	250
Copper (μg)	124	94	94	156	75	100
Iodine (μg)	25	7	7	7	15	9.7
Selenium	3.5	2.3	2.3	—	2.8	2.3
Sodium (mg)	73	39	47	55	44	38
Potassium (mg)	180	109	109	125	118	131
Chloride (mg)	103	86	86	86	80	101
Vitamin A (IU)	500	380	310	780	300	257
Vitamin D (IU)	100	75	63	78	45	51
Vitamin E (IU)	5.0	3.8	3.1	3.1	3.0	2.3
Vitamin K (IU)	25	18.8	15.6	15.6	15	3.8
Thiamine (mg)	100	78	78	156	60	270
Riboflavin B_2	150	94	94	188	90	210
Vitamin B_6	100	63	63	210	60	260
Vitamin B_{12}	0.75	0.31	0.31	0.62	0.45	0.6
Niacin (μg)	2230	1250	1250	2100	1350	1700
Folic acid (μg)	25	15.6	15.6	15.6	15	37
Pantothenic acid	1240	470	470	1050	750	1000
Vitamin C (mg)	13.6	11.7	8.1	8.1	9.0	10
Biotin (mg)	7.5	7.8	7.8	7.8	4.5	32
Choline (mg)	13	13.3	13.3	13.3	8	30
Inositol (mg)	8	4.7	4.7	4.7	5	8

*Ross Laboratories, Columbus, OH.
†Note that formula contains no carbohydrate; this accounts for the markedly different nutrient content of it compared with the others shown.
‡Mead Johnson Nutritional Division, Evansville, IN.

can be helpful. In general, a low pH (<6.0) and the presence of reducing substances suggest a viral cause. The stool must be tested, of course, following a period of adequate intake of a reducing sugar (e.g., a 5% glucose solution or a rehydration solution); in addition, the water content of the stool rather than any solid matter should be tested.

If the cause of the diarrhea appears to be viral, a carbohydrate-free formula (Table 66–1) usually is well tolerated. However, such formulas result in ketosis and sometimes hypoglycemia; thus, some carbohydrate intake is necessary. In the hospitalized child, this can be provided intravenously. Most patients who do not require hospitalization usually will tolerate at least some sugar intake by the enteral route. In general, 0.5 g of glucose (2.78 mmol) or sucrose (1.39 mmol) per ounce of formula, provided intake is adequate but not excessive, is well tolerated and prevents ketosis and/or hypoglycemia.

If this preparation is tolerated, the amount of carbohydrate can be increased daily or every other day as tolerance for carbohydrate increases. Once full carbohydrate content (i.e., approximately 2 g (11.11 mmol of glucose)/oz) is tolerated, the patient usually can be switched to a carbohydrate-containing formula.

If the cause of the diarrhea is a toxicogenic bacterium, feeding usually does not affect the volume of stool output. In many cases, in fact, a glucose-electrolyte solution appears to decrease the volume of stool output. In such patients, therefore, decisions concerning feeding must be based on clinical trial.

The tendency to avoid feedings containing lactose in all infants with diarrhea, regardless of the cause of the diarrhea, probably is unnecessary. If stool pH is normal when the child is first seen and reducing substances are not present, lactase deficiency is an unlikely contributor to the diarrhea.

Chronic Diarrhea. In a small number of patients, the acute episode of diarrhea does not resolve in the usual 4 to 5 days. In these, nutritional management becomes a much more important consideration. Although most infants can tolerate a 4- to 5-day period with little or no nutritional intake, few can tolerate a period of more than 2 weeks without becoming malnourished and developing secondary intestinal changes due to both persistent diarrhea and malnutrition. Such infants are much more likely to develop secondary deficiencies of mucosal hydrolases (e.g., lactase deficiency and, less commonly, sucrase deficiency) and monosaccharide intolerance. In these infants, management without hospitalization is much more difficult. Choice of formula, again, must be made on the basis of the suspected or culture-proven cause of the diarrhea; in addition, the much greater likelihood of secondary mucosal hydrolase deficiencies must be taken into account. If small volumes of a particular formula are reasonably well tolerated, it frequently is possible to deliver sufficient amounts to meet nutritional needs by use of a continuous infusion technique.[6] In small infants, of course, this usually requires hospitalization.

Many other congenital and/or acquired forms of chronic diarrhea (e.g., abetalipoproteinemia, coeliac disease), if not managed appropriately, frequently result in the same secondary changes in mucosal function. Nutritional management, in general, is similar to that described previously and must be coordinated with the usual medical management of these conditions. Although diet is a major aspect of the therapy of most forms of chronic diarrhea, a detailed discussion of this aspect of therapy is beyond the scope of this chapter.

Vomiting. Most acute episodes of vomiting are of short duration and present few nutritional problems. However, chronic vomiting accompanies a number of conditions. The most common of these conditions intrinsic to the gastrointestinal tract is gastroesophageal reflux, or chalasia of infancy. To some extent, this condition is physiologic in infancy; however, it assumes pathologic significance if it results in failure to thrive and/or recurrent pulmonary aspiration.

In the early stages, nutritional management of this condition includes maintaining the patient in an upright position during and immediately following feeding and reassuring the parents that the persistent vomiting is causing no harm so long as the infant is gaining weight normally and is not having respiratory symptoms. If either growth failure or a decrease in weight for height develops despite optimal medical management, remedial nutritional therapy is indicated (i.e., feedings delivered continuously into the duodenum or jejunum to minimize the risk of further reflux). In many patients, corrective surgery is necessary.

Short Bowel Syndrome. Functionally, short bowel syndrome can be considered in the same way as chronic diarrhea. In this condition, the alterations of gastrointestinal motility, secretion, digestion, and absorption are secondary to massive small intestinal loss rather than to bacterial and/or viral invasion and the secondary effects of these organisms and malnutrition. In general, the severity of the short bowel syndrome is related inversely to the length of the remaining intestinal segment; however, loss of the ileocecal valve, which acts as a physiologic sphincter to slow transit time and prevent backwash ileitis, also increases severity.[7] Specific symptoms also result from removal of specific segments of intestine. Because disaccharidase activity is greater in jejunal cells, and because cholecystokinin is secreted by jejunal sites, removal of the jejunum results in more severe carbohydrate malabsorption and probably decreased biliary and pancreatic secretions. Ileal loss, on the other hand, is associated with selective impairment of both bile salt uptake and absorption of vitamin B_{12}. In general, the ileum's potential for adaptation appears to be superior to that of the jejunum. Thus, loss of jejunum usually is better tolerated than loss of the ileum.

The early phase of the short bowel syndrome immediately after resection usually is associated with massive fluid and electrolyte losses, making effective enteral alimentation impossible. Thus, during both this phase and the intermediate phase, the majority of the nutrient requirements must be provided parenterally. As the remaining small bowel gradually adapts, enteral intake usually can be advanced, but this must proceed slowly. In general, continuous feedings via either an indwelling tube or gastrostomy are better tolerated during this phase than bolus feedings. In addition, elemental formulas (Table 66–1) generally are better tolerated than nonelemental formulas.

Eventually, maximum adaptation is achieved and more complex proteins and carbohydrates can be introduced. Even during this final phase, however, frequent small feedings may be necessary. During all phases, pharmacologic manipulations (e.g., cholestyramine to chelate bile acids; loperamide and/or paregoric to slow transit time; antibiotics to eradicate significant bacterial overgrowth) may provide symptomatic as well as physiologic improvement.

GENERAL APPROACH TO NUTRITIONAL THERAPY

Accurate determination of nutritional status obviously is the first step in all types of nutritional therapy. However, assessment of the nutritional status of infants is difficult.[8] In part, this is because there is no precise definition of malnutrition, and in part because the earliest changes of malnutrition are subtle adaptations that tend to ameliorate the effects of malnutrition. Nonetheless, some objective evaluation of nutritional status should be applied to every child who is a potential candidate for nutritional therapy. If for no other reason, this evaluation provides a baseline for monitoring the results of therapy.

Many anthropometric and biochemical assessment techniques are available; their specific advantages, disadvantages, and limitations have been discussed extensively.[8] In general, no single test or combination of tests is ideal. Indeed, clinical judgment, based on knowledge of the disease process and the status of the body's nutritional reserves, appears to be as reliable as any of the commonly used "objective" tests.[9] In my experience, assessment of weight in relation to height (length) is one of the most useful indices of nutritional status. A child who falls below the 10th percentile on this standard curve, regardless of either weight for age or height (length) for age, can be assumed to be malnourished and in need of nutritional therapy.

The situation of the child whose weight is appropriate for height (length) but whose weight and height are low for age (i.e., the stunted child) is more problematic.[10] There is no convincing evidence that such a child is malnourished and in need of aggressive nutritional intervention. On the other hand, an attempt to permit the child to achieve his or her growth potential is warranted. This usually requires both a nutritional history and a more extensive medical evaluation, including evaluation of endocrinologic status.

In general, the approach advocated for nutritional management of the low-birth-weight (LBW) infant (see Chap. 46) is equally applicable to any malnourished infant or child—indeed, for any infant or child with an underlying condition predisposing to development of malnutrition. Initially, particularly in less severely affected individuals, attempts should be made to increase nutrient intake by conventional means. If this approach is unsuccessful, one of several commercially available supplements can be used. However, these often replace usual food intake and may not achieve the desired result of increased total intake. Moreover, most of the products currently available were designed for adults and are not optimal for pediatric patients. One exception is Pediasure (Table 66–1).

If conventional foods are not tolerated, use of special formulas or supplements delivered by tube, either as a bolus or continuously, is the next step. The choice of both formula and method of delivery, of course, must be dictated by the patient's underlying condition. Tube feedings can be given throughout the day or only during part of the day (e.g., at night), depending on the patient's age, condition, and nutritional status. If the patient's condition (e.g., pulmonary disease) makes use of an indwelling nasal tube inadvisable, a gastrostomy tube, inserted percutaneously or surgically, should be considered. If gastrointestinal tolerance of even elemental formulas is severely limited, parenteral nutrients can be used, either as the sole source of nutrition or as a supplement to tolerated enteral nutrient combinations.

PARENTERAL NUTRITION

The now widespread use of parenteral nutrition usually is considered to be one of the major contributing factors to the reduction in mortality over the past several years of infants born with surgically correctable lesions of the gastrointestinal tract (e.g., omphalocele, gastroschisis, intestinal perforation) as well as infants with short bowel syndrome and intractable diarrhea.[11] Although the role of parenteral nutrient delivery in decreasing the mortality and morbidity of other groups of pediatric patients (e.g., LBW infants) is less clear, the technique is used in a wide variety of pediatric patients. Moreover, despite the many hazards of the technique,[11] most agree that the obvious anabolism usually achieved with its use is preferable to the inevitable continuation of catabolism if delivery of adequate nutrients by other routes is impossible. This is particularly true if careful attention is paid to every aspect of the technique, thereby minimizing its hazards and maximizing its benefits.

ROUTE OF ADMINISTRATION

Parenteral nutrients can be infused by either central vein or peripheral vein. An energy intake of 70 to 80 kcal/kg per day can be provided consistently and safely by the peripheral venous route but much greater intakes (100 to 120 kcal/kg per day) can be delivered by the central venous route. Acceptable intakes of all other nutrients are possible by either route.

Although the advantages and disadvantages of these two routes of delivery are frequently discussed, both are efficacious when used in the appropriate circumstances. In general, the time that parenteral nutrients are likely to be required and the nutrient needs of the patient should be the determining factors for choosing one route of administration over the other. If it is likely that parenteral nutrients will be required for more than approximately 10 days, central venous delivery usually is preferable.

In LBW infants, the infusate frequently is delivered by umbilical vessel catheters. Although this route of delivery is convenient, it cannot be recommended. The flow characteristics of the umbilical artery do not permit sufficient dilution of the nutrient infusate to circumvent vessel damage. Also, the incidence of thrombosis with umbilical arterial catheters is high. Further, malposition of either arterial or venous umbilical catheters can result in severe consequences. In addition, the incidence of sepsis appears to be greater when nutrients are delivered by umbilical vessels than when delivered by either central or peripheral vein.

NUTRIENT INFUSATE

The nutrient infusate should include a nitrogen source as well as sufficient energy (glucose and lipid), electrolytes, minerals, and vitamins. Suitable infusates for both central vein and peripheral vein delivery are shown in Table 66–2. Although these are acceptable for most infants and children, modification may be required to reflect the specific needs of individual patients.

Currently, crystalline amino acid mixtures are usually used as the nitrogen source for parenteral nutrition. Several such mixtures are available (Table 66–3); all contain most essential amino acids (exceptions are cystine and tyrosine, which are either unstable or insoluble in aqueous solution) and varying amounts of nonessential amino acids. An amino acid intake of 2.5 to 4.0 g/kg per day is recommended. Higher intakes, although tolerated by most infants, are more likely to result in elevated plasma amino acid concentrations and azotemia. Some advocate amino acid intakes of less than 2.5 g/kg per day for the LBW infant, particularly during the initial few days of therapy when nonprotein energy intake is low (because of glucose and lipid intolerance). Recent studies suggest that there is no reason to advocate this practice unless concomitant energy intake is very low.[12,13]

Glucose is the preferred nonlipid parenteral energy source; however, the ability of some infants to metabolize it is limited. Many infants, particularly during the early period of parenteral nutrition, develop hyperglycemia and osmotic diuresis with concomitant urinary loss of electrolytes when the amount of glucose infused exceeds tolerance. Collins et al. reported recently that careful, continuous administration of small doses of insulin alleviates the problem of glucose intolerance in LBW infants, thereby permitting administration of much greater glucose intakes.[14]

Most LBW infants tolerate 5 to 7% solutions of dextrose (3.5 to 5.0 mg/kg per minute or 17 to 24 kcal/kg per day), even during the first few days of life; thus, in very small and/or unstable infants, it is wise to begin parenteral nutrition with these lower glucose intakes and increase the intake as the infant's tolerance for glucose improves. In older, more stable infants, an initial glucose intake of 15 g/kg per day (about 50 kcal/kg per day) usually is well tolerated. This intake can be delivered easily by the peripheral route without exceeding a glucose concentration of 10%. With central venous delivery, much greater intakes (i.e., 25 to 30 g/kg per day or 85 to 102 kcal/kg per day) are eventually tolerated. Even in the most stable patients, however, these higher intakes should be achieved gradually with daily increments of no more than 5 g/kg. In all patients, close monitoring of glucose tolerance is necessary as glucose intake is being

TABLE 66–2. COMPOSITION OF SUITABLE PARENTERAL NUTRITION INFUSATE(S)

COMPONENT	AMOUNT IN K/G PER DAY
Amino acids	2.5 g–4.0 g
Energy	60–120 kcal
Glucose*	15–30 g
Lipid†	0.5–3.0 g
Electrolytes and minerals:	
Sodium (as chloride)	2–4 mEq
Potassium (as phosphate and chloride)‡	2–4 mEq
Calcium (as gluconate)	1.5–2.0 mmol
Magnesium (as sulfate)	0.25 mEq
Phosphorus (as potassium phosphate)‡	1.5 mmol
Trace minerals	(See Table 66–4)
Vitamins	(See Table 66–5)
Volume	100–150 ml

*For peripheral vein infusion, glucose concentration should not exceed 10–12.5%.
†Lipid must be infused separately (see text).
‡Potassium, as phosphate, should be limited to 2.5 mEq/kg per day (approximately 1.7 mmol of phosphate) unless chemical monitoring suggests need for more phosphate; if only additional potassium is required, it should be provided as the chloride salt.

TABLE 66–3. AMINO ACID CONTENT (MG/2.5 G) OF COMMERCIALLY AVAILABLE AMINO ACID MIXTURES

AMINO ACID	AMINOSYN*	AMINOSYN-PF†	TRAVASOL (B)†	NOVAMINE‡	FREAMINE III§	TROPHAMINE§
Isoleucine	180	191	120	124	175	204
Leucine	235	297	155	174	228	350
Lysine	180	170	145	198	182	204
Methionine	100	45	145	124	132	83
Phenylalanine	110	107	155	174	140	121
Threonine	130	129	105	124	100	104
Tryptophan	40	45	45	41	38	50
Valine	200	161	115	162	165	196
Histidine	75	79	109	147	71	121
Cystine	0	0	0	<12	<6	<8
Tyrosine	11	16	10	9	0	58
Taurine	0	18	0	0	0	6
Alanine	320	175	518	353	178	133
Aspartic acid	0	132	0	74	0	79
Glutamic acid	0	206	0	124	0	125
Glycine	320	96	518	174	350	92
Proline	215	204	104	147	280	171
Serine	105	124	0	100	148	96
Arginine	245	308	258	247	238	304

*Abbott Laboratories, N. Chicago, IL.
†Clintec, Deerfield, IL.
‡Kabi-Vitrum, Inc, Franklin, OH.
§McGaw Laboratories, Irvine, CA.

increased (see below). Once achieved, the higher intakes usually are well tolerated so long as infant's condition remains stable.

Electrolyte requirements vary from patient to patient; thus, the amounts suggested in Table 66–2 should not be interpreted as absolute requirements. Adjustments, which usually are necessary, should be made on the basis of close monitoring (see later).

The amounts of calcium and phosphorus required for optimal skeletal mineralization, that is, 2.5 to 3 mmol (100 to 120 mg) and 1.94 to 2.42 mmol (60 to 75 mg)/kg per day, respectively, in the "normally growing" LBW infant, often cannot be incorporated into the parenteral nutrition infusate because of the chemical incompatibility of calcium and phosphate. In general, the amounts suggested in Table 66–2 are compatible and cause no problems over the short term. However, if parenteral nutrition is required for weeks to months, skeletal mineralization may be inadequate. This is particularly true for the LBW infant.

Addition of trace minerals to the infusate is recommended if exclusive parenteral nutrition is likely to exceed 7 to 10 days. Suggested intakes[15] are given in Table 66–4. Many advocate including zinc and, perhaps, copper from the outset.

Parenteral vitamin requirements also are not known with certainty. Obviously, the usual recommended dietary allowances (RDA) may not apply when administration is by the parenteral route. Recommended intakes are given in Table 66–5.[15] Currently, however, a multivitamin preparation that provides the recommended intakes of all vitamins is not available. Intakes provided by the most commonly used pediatric multivitamin mixture are shown in Table 66–5.

TABLE 66–4. RECOMMENDED PARENTERAL INTAKES (AMOUNT PER KG PER DAY) OF TRACE MINERALS

TRACE MINERAL*	PRETERM INFANTS	TERM INFANTS AND CHILDREN†
Zinc (μg)	400	250 (5000)
Copper (μg)	20	20 (300)
Selenium (μg)	2.0	2.0 (30)
Chromium (μg)	0.2	0.2 (5)
Manganese (μg)	1.0	1.0 (50)
Molybdenum (μg)	0.25	0.25 (5)
Iodide (μg)	1.0	1.0 (1)
Iron‡		

*If parenteral nutrients are used as a supplement for tolerated enteral feeds or as sole source of nutrients for <4 weeks, only zinc is needed.
†Maximum recommended intake per day is shown in parentheses.
‡Iron dextran (1–2 mg/L) has been used safely in adults but reported experience in children, particularly infants, is limited. Estimated requirements, based on the assumption that 10% of the recommended enteral intakes is absorbed, are 100 and 200 μg/kg per day, respectively, for the term and preterm infant.
(From Greene, H.L., Hambidge, K.M., Schanler, R., et al.: Am. J. Clin. Nutr., *48:*1324–1342, 1988.)

TABLE 66–5. SUGGESTED PARENTERAL INTAKES OF VITAMINS

VITAMIN	PRETERM INFANTS* (AMOUNT/KG PER DAY)	TERM INFANTS AND CHILDREN† (AMOUNT PER DAY)
A (μg)	500	700
E (mg)	2.8	7
K (μg)	80	200
D (μg)	4 (160 IU)	10
Ascorbic acid (mg)	25	80
Thiamin (mg)	0.35	1.2
Riboflavin (mg)	0.15	1.4
Pyridoxine Cl (mg)	0.18	1.0
Niacin (mg)	6.8	17
Pantothenate (mg)	2.0	5
Biotin (μg)	6.0	20
Folate (μg)	56	140
B_{12} (μ)	0.3	1.0

*Total daily dose should not exceed that recommended for term infants and children. A dose of 2 ml of reconstituted MVI-Pediatric (Armour Pharmaceutical Co, Chicago, IL) provides the following intakes (amount/kg per day): Vitamin A, 280 mg; Vitamin E, 2.8 μg; Vitamin K, 80 μg; Vitamin D, 4 μg (160 IU); Ascorbic acid, 32 mg; Thiamin, 0.48 mg; Riboflavin, 0.56 mg; Pyridoxine, 0.4 mg; Niacin, 6.8 mg; Pantothenate, 2.0 mg; Biotin, 8.0 μg; Folate, 56 μg; Vitamin B_{12}, 0.4 μg.

†These amounts are provided by a vial of reconstituted MVI-Pediatric.

(From Greene, H.L., Hambidge, K.M., Schanler, R., et al.: Am. J. Clin. Nutro, *48:*1324–1342, 1988.)

USE OF PARENTERAL LIPID EMULSIONS

Infants who receive fat-free parenteral nutrition, particularly LBW infants and nutritionally depleted infants, develop classic essential fatty acid (EFA) deficiency, that is, an elevated triene/tetraene ratio, quickly (i.e., within days) when growth and/or regrowth is initiated.[16] Thus, use of lipid emulsions to prevent this deficiency, which becomes apparent biochemically (i.e., a ratio of eicosatrienoic to arachidonic acid of >0.25) before clinical signs appear, is desirable. Parenteral lipid emulsions also are a useful source of energy. Emulsions of either soybean oil (Intralipid, Kabi-Vitrum; Travamulsion, Travenol Laboratories; Liposyn III, Abbott Laboratories) or a mixture of safflower and soybean oils (Liposyn II, Abbott Laboratories) are available in both 10% and 20% concentrations. A dose of only 0.5 g/kg per day of soybean oil emulsion is sufficient to prevent EFA deficiency; because the linoleic acid content of the emulsion of soy and safflower oils is even greater, a smaller dose may be sufficient. However, the linolenic acid content of the latter emulsion is somewhat lower.

All infants, including LBW infants, probably can tolerate the small dose of parenteral lipid emulsion necessary to prevent EFA deficiency. However, the ability of individual infants to tolerate a larger dose varies significantly. In general, the ability to metabolize intravenous fat emulsions is related directly to maturity,[17] but the stressed and/or malnourished patient (i.e., the small-for-gestational-age LBW infant and the nutritionally depleted older child) also has difficulty metabolizing these preparations.[18,19]

Administration of doses of fat emulsion in excess of the infant's ability to metabolize it results in accumulation of triglyceride in the blood stream. This, in turn, decreases pulmonary diffusion capacity secondary, presumably, to accumulation of small lipid droplets within the pulmonary capillaries.[20] It also results in the recruitment of the reticuloendothelial system for lipid clearance and lipid accumulation in these cells, which also has been demonstrated at postmortem examination,[21] is a likely explanation of the impaired host defense mechanisms reported in patients receiving lipid emulsions.[22] Metabolism of the infused lipid results in increased serum concentrations of free fatty acids, which compete with bilirubin and other substances for binding to albumin.[23] Thus, administration of large doses of lipid emulsion may be hazardous for infants with pulmonary disease, infection, and/or hyperbilirubinemia.

Considering the difficulties of monitoring serum concentrations of both triglyceride and free fatty acids, it probably is wise to limit the dose of lipid emulsion given to patients who are likely to be intolerant to 0.5 to 1.0 g/kg per day. In most other patients, a dose of 3 g/kg per day or more usually is well tolerated; however, even in these patients, it probably is wise to use a smaller dose initially (e.g., 1 to 1.5 g/kg per day). In LBW infants, administration of lipid emulsions should be initiated with a relatively low dose and increased gradually to a maximum dose of 2 g/kg per day. In all patients, the emulsion should be infused continuously throughout the day.

The 20% soybean oil emulsion (Intralipid) appears to be cleared more rapidly than the 10% emulsion, and therefore is less likely to cause hypertriglyceridemia.[24,25] Hyperphospholipidemia and hypercholesterolemia, both of which occur routinely in patients receiving the 10% soybean emulsion, do not occur with use of the 20% emulsion.[24] The explanation, presumably, is the lower phospholipid/triglyceride ratio of the 20% versus the 10% emulsion.

Because the size of the lipid particles of the emulsions (0.4 to 0.5 μm) exceeds the pore size of an effective filter (0.22 μm), filters should not be used for the infusion of fat emulsions. Nor, in my opinion, should the emulsions be mixed directly with other components of the infusate. This practice, which appears to be relatively common, may not destroy the emulsion but it certainly inhibits detection of chemical incompatibilities within the complicated infusate (e.g., precipitation of calcium phosphate). The potential hazards of the latter possibility are compounded, of course, by the fact that filters cannot be used.

COMPLICATIONS OF TOTAL PARENTERAL NUTRITION

Despite its obvious nutritional efficacy, total parenteral nutrition (TPN) is associated with a number of complications, both catheter (or infusion)-related and metabolic.

At the time of central vein catheter insertion, pneumothorax, hemothorax, injury to an artery, and/or hematoma may occur. Thrombosis, dislodgement, perforation, infusion leaks (pericardial, pleural, mediastinal), and infections have been reported during use of central vein catheters. The most common infusion-related problem is infection. Phlebitis and soft tissue sloughs are the most frequent complications of peripheral vein infusions.

Although all of the above complications can be controlled, it is difficult to prevent them completely. Careful attention to care of the central catheter, including frequent dressing changes, is particularly important for controlling infection. Careful frequent observation of the infusion site is necessary to prevent infiltration of infusates delivered by peripheral vein as well as to ensure proper long-term function of central vein catheters.

Metabolic complications result either from the limited metabolic capacity of the patient for the various components of the nutrient infusate or from the infusate itself. The metabolic complications most commonly observed and their probable causes are listed in Table 66–6. One of the more troublesome of these is the occurrence of abnormal plasma amino acid patterns with use of many of the currently available amino acid mixtures.[26] Cyst(e)ine and tyrosine, both of which are essential amino acids for the newborn, and probably essential for all patients receiving parenteral nutrients,[27] are only sparingly soluble; hence, none of the currently marketed mixtures contains appreciable amounts of these amino

TABLE 66–6. METABOLIC COMPLICATIONS OF TOTAL PARENTERAL NUTRITION AND THEIR PROBABLE CAUSE

COMPLICATION	PROBABLE CAUSE
Disorders related to metabolic capacity of patient:	
Hyperglycemia	Excessive intake (either excessive concentration or infusion rate); change in metabolic state (e.g., infection; surgical stress)
Hypoglycemia	Sudden cessation of infusion
Azotemia	Excessive nitrogen intake
Electrolyte disorders	Excessive or inadequate intake
Mineral disorders	Excessive or inadequate intake
Vitamin disorders	Excessive or inadequate intake
Essential fatty acid deficiency	Failure to provide essential fatty acids
Hyperlipidemia	Excessive intake; change in metabolic state (e.g., stress; sepsis)
Disorders related to infusate components:	
Metabolic acidosis	Use of hydrochloride salts of cationic amino acids
Hyperammonemia	Inadequate arginine intake
Abnormal plasma aminograms	Amino acid pattern of nitrogen source
Hepatic disorders	Unknown; suggested causes include prematurity, malnutrition, sepsis, inadequate stimulation of bile flow, toxic effects of amino acids, specific amino acid deficiency, excessive amino acid and/or carbohydrate intake, and nonspecific response to lack of feeding

acids (Table 66–2) and all result in low plasma cyst(e)ine and tyrosine concentrations. Moreover, many available mixtures have large amounts of only a few nonessential amino acids (e.g., glycine) rather than a mixture of all nonessential amino acids (Table 66–3); thus, extremely high plasma concentrations of the amino acid(s) present in excess are commonly seen. Whether or not these abnormal plasma amino acid patterns are hazardous, or even undesirable is not known. However, considering the well-known relationship between abnormally high plasma amino acid concentrations and mental retardation in infants with inborn errors of metabolism (e.g., phenylketonuria) as well as the relationship between inadequate intake of a specific amino acid and a low plasma concentration of that amino acid, normalization of plasma amino acid patterns seems warranted. Some of the newer amino acid mixtures (e.g., TrophAmine, Kendall-McGaw Laboratories) accomplish this to a large extent.[28]

Although some of the metabolic complications are unavoidable, many can be controlled by careful monitoring and appropriate adjustment of the infusate. A suggested monitoring schedule is given in Table 66–7. The monitoring required to ensure safe and efficacious use of lipid emulsions is the most problematic. The most common practice (i.e., inspection of the plasma for turbidity either visually or by nephelometry) does not reliably detect elevated plasma triglyceride and free fatty acid concentrations.[29] For this purpose, actual chemical determinations are required. Because this usually is not practical, a reasonable compromise is to observe the plasma frequently (at least three times in a day), either visually or by nephelometry, for evidence of lipid accumulation (primarily triglyceride), particularly while the lipid dose is being increased, while the infant is unstable, and when a change in the infant's condition occurs. If turbidity is observed, the rate of infusion should be decreased or the infusion stopped completely until the turbidity clears. Usually, infusion can then be resumed at a lower rate. Once the desired dose of intravenous fat is achieved, serum turbidity should be checked once a day (unless the patient becomes unstable). If feasible and practical, actual determinations of serum triglyceride and free fatty acid concentrations are preferable.

WEANING INFANTS FROM TOTAL PARENTERAL NUTRITION

In most infants, administration of parenteral nutrients need not interfere with introducing enteral feedings as soon as they are tolerated. Once started, the volume of enteral feedings can be advanced as tolerated by the infant, and the volume of parenteral nutrients can be decreased. During the period of combined enteral and parenteral nutrition, care should be taken to assure both that nutrient requirements are met as nearly as possible and that tolerance for both fluids and nutrients is not exceeded. This requires careful attention to the total (parenteral *plus* enteral) intake and frequent adjustment

TABLE 66–7. SUGGESTED MONITORING SCHEDULE DURING TOTAL PARENTERAL NUTRITION (SUGGESTED FREQUENCY PER WEEK*)

VARIABLES TO BE MONITORED	INITIAL PERIOD	LATER PERIOD
Growth variables:		
Weight	7	7
Length	1	1
Head circumference	1	1
Metabolic variables:		
Plasma electrolytes	3–4	2
Plasma calcium, magnesium, phosphorus	2	1
Blood acid base status	3–4	1
Blood urea nitrogen	2	1
Plasma albumin	1	1
Liver function studies	1	1
Serum lipids†		
Hemoglobin	2	2
Urinary glucose	2–6 per day	2 per day
Variables for detection of infection:		
Clinical observations (e.g., activity, temperature)	Daily	Daily
WBC count	As indicated	As indicated
Cultures	As indicated	As indicated

*Initial period is the time during which the desired energy intake is being achieved or the time(s) of metabolic instability.
†See text.

downward of the parenteral intake as enteral intake increases.

HOME PARENTERAL NUTRITION

With increasing frequency, patients who require parenteral nutrients for a long time leave the hospital and receive this therapy at home. Considering the many difficulties of in-hospital parenteral nutrition (see above), the potential problems of TPN at home seem formidable. Nonetheless, both patients who can tolerate some enteral intake and patients who can tolerate only parenteral nutrients have been treated successfully at home for several months to years.[30] In many cases, sufficient nutrients can be administered during only a portion of the day, allowing the older patient to pursue reasonably normal daytime activities and the younger patient (as well as his or her parents) to sleep with little danger of accidental disconnection of the infusion system. Small portable infusion pumps are available such that the necessary apparatus can be enclosed in such items as vests and backpacks, allowing even the patient who requires constant infusion of parenteral nutrients to pursue a reasonably normal life. Obviously, home parenteral nutrition is more likely to be successful for the older child, adolescent, or adult. However, with careful patient selection, infants as young as 1 year of age, perhaps even less, can be managed successfully at home.

In general, the catheter used for home total parenteral nutrition is the Broviac catheter, which can be used for several months, and frequently for years. Standard nutrient infusates are obtained from the hospital pharmacy or from a number of commercial concerns and are stored in a small home refrigerator. Catheter care is managed by the patient or by a family member after careful training prior to discharge.

All the usual metabolic and catheter-related complications of parenteral nutrition can occur at home as well as in the hospital. However, patients who can be managed successfully with home parenteral nutrition usually have reached the point at which requirements are reasonably stable. Thus, less-frequent monitoring to detect metabolic problems is required. Nonetheless, successful home parenteral nutrition, particularly for the young pediatric patient, requires frequent outpatient visits as well as frequent telephone contact. Some commercial home parenteral nutrition services include frequent home visits by a visiting nurse.

On balance, administration of parenteral nutrients at home has been more successful than initially envisioned. Certainly, the practice improves the quality of life for patients who require long-term parenteral nutrition. However, the purpose of parenteral nutrition is to provide the necessary nutrients transiently while the compromised gastrointestinal function necessitating use of parenteral nutrition recovers. Some patients, of course, may never be able to survive without parenteral nutrition, but attempts to increase enteral intake must continue. In my experience, this is not always the case; rather, discharge from the hospital often is viewed as the goal of therapy and, once achieved, attempts to increase tolerance of enteral intake slow or stop. It is important that this attitude not become more common.

REFERENCES

1. Williams, C.D.: Arch. Dis. Child, *8:*423–433, 1933.
2. Grantham-McGregor, S.M., Powell, C.A., Walker, S.P., and Himes, J.H.: Lancet, *338:*1–5, 1991.
3. Mansell, A.L., Andersen, J.C., Muttart, C.R., et al.: J. Pediatr., *109:*700–705, 1984.
4. Sack, R.B.: Bacterial and parasitic agents of acute diarrhea. *In* Acute Diarrhea: Its Nutritional Consequences in Infancy. Edited by J.A. Bellanti. New York, Raven Press, 1983, pp. 53–65.
5. Hamilton, J.R.: Viral enteritis: A cause of disordered small intestinal epithelial renewal. *In* Chronic Diarrhea in Children. Edited by E. Lebenthal. New York, Raven Press, 1984, pp. 269–276.
6. Parker, P., Stroop, B.S., and Greene, H.: J. Pediatr., *99:*360–364, 1981.
7. Wilmore, D.W.: J. Pediatr., *80:*88–95, 1972.
8. Cooper, A., and Heird, W.C.: Am. J. Clin. Nutr., *35:*1132–1141, 1982.
9. Baker, J.P., et al.: N. Engl. J. Med., *306:*969–972, 1982.
10. Waterlow, J.C.: Br. Med. J., *3:*566–569, 1972.
11. Kashyap, S., and Heird, W.C.: Pediatr. Res., *27:*285A, 1990.
12. Rivera, A. Jr., Bell, E.F., Stegink, L.D., and Ziegler, E.E.: J. Pediatr., *115:*465–468, 1989.
13. Heird, W.C.: Justification of total parenteral nutrition. *In* Intravenous Feeding of the Neonate. Edited by V.Y.H. Yu and R.A. MacMahon. London, Edward Arnold, 1992.
14. Collins, J.N., Hoope, M., Brown, K., et al.: J. Pediatr., *118:*921–927, 1991.
15. Kashyap, S., Schulze, K.F., Forsyth, M., et al.: Am. J. Clin. Nutr., *52:*254–262, 1990.
16. Paulsrud, J.R., Pensler, L., Whitten, C.F., et al.: Am. J. Clin. Nutr., *25:*897–904, 1972.
17. Shennan, A.T., Bryan, M.D., and Angel, A.: J. Pediatr., *91:*134–137, 1977.
18. Park, W., Paust, H., Brösicke, H., et al.: J. Pharmacol. Exp. Ther., *10:*627–630, 1986.
19. Ricour, C., Hatemi, N., Etienne, J., and Palonovski, J.: Acta Chir. Scand., *466:*114–115, 1976.
20. Greene, H.L., Hazlett, D., and Demree, R.: Am. J. Clin. Nutr., *29:*127–135, 1976.
21. Friedman, Z., Marks, M.H., Maisels, J., et al.: Pediatrics, *61:*694–698, 1978.

22. Loo, L.S., Tang, J.P., and Kohl, S.: J. Infect. Dis., *146:*64–70, 1982.
23. Odell, G.T.B., Cukier, J.O., Ostrea, E.M. Jr., et al.: J. Lab. Clin. Med., *89:*29–307, 1977.
24. Haumont, D., Deckelbaum, R.J., Richelle, M., et al.: J. Pediatr., *115:*787–793, 1989.
25. Deckelbaum, R.J., Hamilton, J., Moser, A., et al.: Biochemistry, *29:*1136–1142, 1990.
26. Winters, R.W., Heird, W.C., Dell, R.B., et al.: Plasma amino acids in infants receiving parenteral nutrition. *In* Clinical Nutrition Update: Amino Acids. Edited by H.L. Green, M.A. Holliday, and H.N. Munro. Chicago, American Medical Association, 1977, pp. 147–154.
27. Stegink, L.D.: Am. J. Dis. Child., *137:*1008–1016, 1983.
28. Heird, W.C., Dell, R.B., Helms, R.A., et al.: Pediatrics, *80:*401–408, 1987.
29. Schreiner, R.L., Glick, M.R., Nordschow, C.W., et al.: J. Pediatr., *94:*197–200, 1979.
30. Stroebel, C.T., Byrne, W.J., Fonkalsrud, E.W., et al.: Ann. Surg., *188:*394–403, 1978.
31. Greene, H.L., Hambidge, K.M., Schanler, R., et al.: Am. J. Clin. Nutr., *48:*1324–1342, 1988.

CHAPTER 67

Nutrition Support of Inherited Metabolic Disease

Louis J. Elsas, II, and Phyllis B. Acosta

GENETIC PERSPECTIVE

Geneticists approach the general subject of nutrition and the specific requirement for nutrients with the view that the recommended daily dietary allowance for an essential nutrient is not optimum for all individuals. Rather, there is a continuum of individuals in a population with genetically determined variations in their nutrient requirements that extend over a wide range. This concept arose historically from two older scientific disciplines: human biochemical genetics and nutrition science. The former discipline originated with Sir Archibald Garrod's Croonian lectures of 1908. Garrod defined four "inborn errors of metabolism" as blocks in the normal flow of metabolic processes. Biochemical and clinical expression of these metabolic blocks demonstrated patterns of inheritance consistent with Mendel's predictions for transmission of single genes with large effect on the phenotype. Thus arose the concept that genes controlled metabolism and that disease states were created by blocks in this metabolic flow yielding accumulated precursors and deficient products.

Today, we recognize that "inborn errors" are discontinuous traits resulting from variation in the structure and function of enzymes or protein molecules. The amino acid sequences of enzymes and their quantity are dictated by genes. The control of enzyme function is predicated by molecular regulation through gene transcription, post-transcriptional processing of RNA, translation, post-translational modification, and protein turnover. Over 4900 monogenic human disorders were catalogued in 1990 and, of these, about 250 have a defined biochemical basis.[1] The extent of normal variation in genes controlling enzyme activity suggests that about 30% of our population is heterozygous for common alleles.[2] Within this continuous diversity, mutations produce discontinuous, relatively rare traits that are expressed as disease under normal environmental conditions. Mutant gene frequencies vary in populations; for example, mitochondrial branched chain α-keto acid dehydrogenase deficiency (maple syrup urine disease) occurs in one of approximately every 250,000 newborns worldwide, but occurs in 1 of 176 in an inbred Mennonite population.[3,4] The mutation produces extreme toxicity due to accumulated branched-chain α-keto acids if affected newborns are fed the recommended dietary allowance (RDA) for branched-chain amino acids. However, normal growth and development are expected if dietary leucine, isoleucine, and valine are restricted to 20 to 40% of the RDA early in life, depending on the degree of enzyme impairment.[3,5,6]

Considerable human variation occurs in the structure and activity of enzymes involved in the catabolism of essential amino acids, but only a few are so impaired that ingestion of the RDA will create severe disease. Population-based newborn screening and dietary intervention are now applied through public health programs to at least five rare inborn errors where newborn screening predicts genetic susceptibility to a normal diet.[7,8] By contrast to these relatively rare inborn errors, all humans lack the enzyme that converts L-gulono-α-lactone to ascorbic acid, but scurvy does not occur provided sufficient vitamin C is ingested and absorbed.[9] Thus, the frequency of genetic susceptibility to a "normal" diet ranges from rare to common and extends to the metabolism of amino acids, carbohydrates, lipids, pyrimidines, minerals, and vitamins.

TABLE 67–1. CRITERIA FOR NONSELECTIVE NEWBORN SCREENING

1. The disorder produces a high burden to the affected individual yet is preventable
2. Methods for screening, retrieval, diagnosis, and management must be practical and available to the population as a whole
3. Inheritance and pathogenesis of the disease should be understood
4. Benefit-to-cost ratio of the program should be greater than one
5. Patients' rights should be protected
6. False-negative laboratory screening results should not occur
7. False-positive laboratory results should be minimized

GENETIC DISORDERS BENEFITED BY NUTRITION SUPPORT

Over 250 genetic disorders have been reported in which toxic manifestations relate to accumulation, deficiency, or overproduction of normally occurring substrates and products of metabolic flow. In many of them, modifications of the dietary supply alleviate the manifestations. In a large number, however, irreversible damage has already occurred by the time symptoms appear. Optimum management of these disorders depends on identifying affected subjects while they are presymptomatic or before irreversible disease has occurred. Because the disorders are genetic in origin, markers are theoretically present from the moment of conception, and thus the genetic power of prediction and prevention is applicable. In practice, a number of disorders can be detected in the fetus in the sixteenth to eighteenth weeks of gestation by studies on amniotic fluid cells. Prenatal diagnosis has been pushed forward to the eighth to twelfth weeks of gestation through the use of chorionic villus biopsy.[10] Some intrauterine sequelae of the inborn error such as congenital cataracts in galactosemia may be prevented by removing lactose from the mother's diet. Other inherited metabolic alterations are detected postnatally in the presymptomatic infant by analysis of blood, urine, erythrocytes, leukocytes, or cultured skin fibroblasts.

A selective search for presymptomatic genetic disease is often undertaken when there is a family history of inherited disease. Selective screening for inherited disease is also initiated for relatively common symptoms such as failure to thrive in childhood. Early treatment has proved effective for many diseases such as phenylketonuria (PKU), galactosemia, isovaleric acidemia, homocystinuria, maple syrup urine disease (MSUD), argininosuccinic aciduria, and citrullinemia. Irreversible brain damage occurs if treatment is not initiated before the third week of life. To prevent this, population-wide nonselective screening of newborns has been instituted for PKU, MSUD, galactosemia, homocystinuria, and tyrosinemia. In MSUD, galactosemia, isovaleric acidemia, and disorders of the urea cycle, irreversible damage to the brain may occur within the first week of life. Thus, speed in diagnosis and treatment is of the utmost importance.

In the future, population-based presymptomatic detection will be extended to other disorders. However, before screening is initiated as a public health program, several principles should be fulfilled (Table 67–1). Note that knowledge of the pathogenesis and availability of therapy must precede the initiation of routine screening programs. Table 67–2 lists genetic disorders in which modification of nutrient intake has been employed. Effectiveness in preventing clinical sequelae is experimental in some of the therapies listed.

Although patients with many inherited disorders benefit from nutrition support, each would require a chapter for adequate discussion. Thus, this chapter emphasizes disorders for which population-based screening, retrieval, diagnosis, and nutrition support are available to prevent their irreversible, severe pathologic problems.

GENERAL PRINCIPLES OF GENETIC DISEASE MANAGEMENT

Specific enzymes produced under the direction of individual genes catalyze specific reactions as noted in the following genetic and metabolic sequences. A is converted to D through intermediates B and C using enzymes AB, BC, and CD:

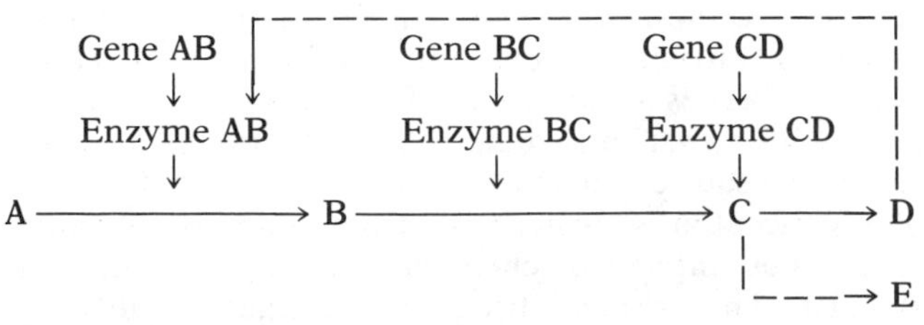

TABLE 67–2. NUTRITION TREATMENT OF GENETIC DISORDERS

DISORDER	THERAPY
Abetalipoproteinemia	Medium-chain trigylcerides; Vitamins A, D, K, and E parenterally or in excess orally
Acrodermatitis enteropathica	Zinc sulfate supplement
Adenine phosphoribosyl-transferase deficiency	Purine restriction, allopurinol; avoid alkali
Albinism	Sunscreen ointments; avoid sunlight and wear tinted lenses
Alkaptonuria (ochronosis)	Ascorbic acid supplement; phenylalanine and tyrosine restriction
Anemia, hypochromic, sideroblastic	Pyridoxine supplement
Angioneurotic edema (Hereditary C'esterase inhibitor deficiency)	Induce with Danazol
Argininemia	Protein restriction; essential amino acids supplement; ornithine supplement
Argininosuccinic aciduria	Arginine, benzoic acid, and phenylbutyrate or phenylacetate supplements; protein restriction; essential amino acids supplement
Betamethylcrotonyglycinuria	Leucine restriction
Beta-sitosterolemia	Plant sterol restriction
Biotinidase deficiency	Biotin supplement
Carbamylphosphate synthetase deficiency	Arginine, benzoic acid, and phenylbutyrate or phenylacetate supplements; protein restriction; essential amino acids supplement
Carbonic anhydrase II deficiency	Treat metabolic acidosis with bicarbonate
Chediak–Higashi syndrome	Ascorbic acid supplement
Chloride diarrhea	Sodium chloride supplement
Christmas disease (hemophilia B)	Factor IX concentrates
Citrullinemia	Protein restriction; supplement essential amino acids, arginine, phenylbutyrate, or phenylacetate and benzoic acid
Combined hyperlipidemia	Calorie, carbohydrate, saturated fatty acid restriction, nicotinic acid and mevinolin therapy, cholestyramine
Congenital adrenal hyperplasia	Cortisol, mineralocorticoid, surgery
Crigler-Najjar Syndrome (type I)	Phenobarbital induction of hepatic bilirubin UDP glucuronyl transferase
Cystathioninuria	Pyridoxine supplements
Cystic fibrosis	Enteric enzyme supplements (trypsin, lipase, chymotrypsin)
Cystinosis	Alkali, phosphate, and vitamin D supplements; cysteamine to reduce cystine
Cystinuria	Alkali, hyperhydration, D-penicillamine
Diabetes insipidus	Water, low-solute diets; vasopressin
Diabetes mellitus (type I)	Insulin, controlled diet
Dibasic aminoaciduria	Arginine supplement; protein restriction
Ehlers-Danlos Syndrome, lysyl hydroxylase defect	Ascorbic acid supplement
Folic acid reductase deficiency	N^5-formyltetrahydrofolic acid supplement
Folic acid transport defect	Parenteral folate supplement
Fructose intolerance	Fructose-free diet
Fructose-1, 6-diphosphate deficiency	Frequent glucose, folate supplement, reduced fructose intake
Galactokinase deficiency	Galactose-restricted diet
Galactosemia	Galactose-restricted diet; possible uridine supplement
Gilbert syndrome	Phenobarbital induction of UDP-glucuronyltransferase
Glucose-galactose malabsorption	Glucose, galactose restriction; fructose supplement
Glucose-6-phosphate dehydrogenase deficiency	Avoidance of fava beans and drugs that cause erythrocyte hemolysis
Glutaric acidemia type I	Restriction of lysine and tryptophan; supplement carnitine, riboflavin
Glycogen storage:	
Type I (glucose-6-phosphatase deficiency)	Frequent feeding, complex starch supplement (liver transplant)
Type III (amylo-1,6 glucosidase deficiency)	Frequent feeding, high protein
Type VI (phosphorylase deficiency)	Frequent feeding
Type VIII (phosphorylase kinase deficiency)	Avoid fasting, high protein

TABLE 67–2. *(continued)*

DISORDER	THERAPY
Glutamate-aspartate transport defect	Glutamine supplement
Gout	Purine restriction; allopurinol
Growth hormone deficiency	Growth hormone (HGH) or releasing factor (GHRF)
Hartnup disease	Nicotinamide supplement
Hemophilia A	Factor VII supplement
Hereditary methemoglobinemia	Methylene blue, ascorbate, riboflavin supplements
Hemochromatosis	Weekly phlebotomy; deferoxamine
Homocystinuria:	
Cystathionine β-synthase deficiency	Methionine restriction; cysteine supplement; pyridoxine to augment block; folate and betaine to provide alternate routes
N^5, N^{10}-methylenetetrahydrofolate reductase deficiency	Folic acid supplement
Hydroxykynureninuria	Nicotinic acid supplement
Hyperbeta-alaninemia	Pyridoxine supplement
Hypercholesterolemia	Restriction of saturated fatty acids and cholesterol; supplemental fiber, mevinolin, nicotinic acid, cholestyramine
Hyperphenylalaninemia:	
Dihydropteridine reductase deficiency	Phenylalanine restriction; carbidopa; 5-hydroxytryptophan
Biopterin biosynthetic blocks	Tetrahydrobiopterin, carbidopa; 5-OH-tryptophan
Hypertriglyceridemia	Weight reduction; carbohydrate restriction
Hypophosphatemia	Vitamin D, phosphorus supplements
Isovaleric acidemia	Leucine restriction; carnitine, glycine supplements
Ketoacidosis of infancy	Alkali, glucose supplements
Lactic acidosis, intermittent:	
(Pyruvate decarboxylase deficiency)	High-fat, low-carbohydrate diet, thiamin supplement; alkali
(Pyruvate carboxylase deficiency)	Frequent feeds; alkali, thiamin, and biotin supplements
Lactose intolerance	Lactose restriction
Lipoprotein lipase deficiency	Fat-free diet, supplement with essential fatty acids and medium-chain triglycerides
Lysine intolerance (hyperlysinemia)	Protein restriction
Maple syrup urine disease (MSUD)	Restrict leucine, isoleucine, and valine; supplement thiamin
Methionine malabsorption	Methionine restriction; cysteine supplement
Methylmalonic aciduria:	
Defective reduction or transport of cobalamin	B_{12} supplement, megadoses parenterally
Impaired cobalamin methylation	Parenteral B_{12}, megadoses
Impaired synthesis of 5′-deoxyadenosylcobalamin	Parenteral B_{12}, megadoses
Methylmalonyl-CoA mutase/racemase deficiency	Isoleucine, methionine, threonine, valine restriction
Multiple carboxylase deficiency	Biotin supplement
Nonketotic hyperglycinemia	Protein restriction, calorie supplements; strychnine; benzoic acid
Ornithine transcarbamylase deficiency	Arginine, benzoic acid and phenylacetate supplements; protein restriction; essential amino acids
Orotic aciduria	Uridine supplements
Oxalosis	Pyridoxine, magnesium, orthophosphate, water supplements (liver and kidney transplant)
Periodic paralysis:	
Hypokalemic	Carbohydrate restriction, potassium salts, sodium chloride
Hyperkalemic	Increased carbohydrates
Normokalemic	Sodium chloride
Phenylketonuria	Phenylalanine restriction, tyrosine supplement
Pseudohypoparathyroidism	Calcium and vitamin D supplements
Porphyria, acute intermittent	High glucose; hematin infusions for feedback control
Prolidase deficiency	L-proline, $MgCl_2^{++}$, vitamin C
Propionic acidemia	Isoleucine, methionine, threonine, valine restriction; biotin supplement
Pyridoxine dependency with seizures	Pyridoxine parenterally

TABLE 67–2. *(continued)*

DISORDER	THERAPY
Pyroglutamic aciduria	Alkali, protein restriction
Pyruvate dehydrogenase deficiency, partial	Thiamin supplement, carbohydrate restriction; energy supplements (lipids)
Refsum's disease	Phytanic acid restriction (diet low in dairy and ruminant fats)
Renal tubular acidosis (proximal)	Alkali supplements
Sucrose-isomaltose malabsorption	Sucrose restriction, ingestion of sucrase-isomaltase containing Streptomyces cerevesiae
Testicular feminization (XY female)	Estrogen supplement, orchiectomy
Thyroid hormone deficiency	Thyroid hormone
Tryptophanuria with dwarfism	Nicotinic acid
Tyrosinemia, type I	Phenylalanine-tyrosine restriction, high-calorie diet; hematin infusions if porphyric symptoms persist (liver transplant)
Tyrosinemia with keratosis and corneal dystrophy	Phenylalanine and tyrosine restriction
Valinemia	Valine restriction
Vitamin A defect (β-carotene 15, 15′-dioxygenase)	Vitamin A supplement
Vitamin B_{12} defect (conversion of B_{12} to precursor of 5′-deoxyadenosyl-B_{12} and methyl-B_{12}	Vitamin B_{12} supplement
Vitamin D–dependent rickets	1,25 dihydroxy D supplement
Vitamin K–dependent coagulation defects (Factors VII, IX, and X; protein C, protein S deficiency)	Vitamin K supplement
Wilson's disease	Copper restriction, D-penicillamine
Xanthinuria	Purine restriction; allopurinol, fluids, alkali supplements
Xanthurenic aciduria	Pyridoxine

If enzyme CD were genetically impaired, at least six pathophysiologic consequences might occur:

1. Deficiency of product D or some compound derived only from D. For example, in PKU, when phenylalanine is not hydroxylated to form tyrosine, not only is accumulated phenylalanine toxic, but tyrosine becomes an essential nutrient. Tyrosine must be supplemented to maintain proper infant growth in the dietary management of PKU.

2. Loss of feedback control. If product D normally functions in feedback control of enzyme AB, overproduction of an intermediate product may occur because D is not present in amounts necessary to regulate production of intermediates "B" and "C". Exemplary of this phenomenon is excessive adrenocorticotropic hormone (ACTH) and androgen production in inborn errors of hydrocortisone production such as steroid 21-hydroxylase deficiency. The consequence is overproduction of androgens and virilization of the female fetus or child.

3. Accumulation of C, the immediate precursor of the blocked reaction. In MSUD, toxic branched-chain α-keto acids accumulate because they cannot be decarboxylated and transacylated to their coenzyme A–acyl acid derivatives. The consequence in the neonate is severe central nervous system depression with apnea, stupor, coma, and death. If the neonate survives, severe mental retardation ensues if the child is not treated by diet restriction within 1–2 weeks of life.

4. Accumulation of A or B, remote precursors of the blocked reaction sequence CD. If the preceding reactions are freely reversible, a precursor, in addition to that proximal to the block, will accumulate. This process is illustrated in MSUD by increased leucine, isoleucine, and valine, which are formed by reamination of the branched-chain α-keto acids: α-ketoisocaproic, α-keto-β-methylvaleric, and α-ketoisovaleric acids, respectively.

5. Increased production of alternative products through little-used metabolic pathways. As illustrated in Fig-

ure 67–1, when phenylalanine accumulates because of impaired phenylalanine hydroxylase, phenylpyruvic, phenylacetic, and phenyllactic acids are produced in larger than normal amounts through existing pathways that normally do not function at physiologic concentrations of cellular phenylalanine.

6. Inhibition of alternate pathways by accumulated substrate (i.e., C in CD impairment). For example, neurotransmitter synthesis may be depressed in PKU owing to increased blood phenylalanine that inhibits tyrosine hydroxylase and tryptophan hydroxylase in the central nervous system. Another example is type I tyrosinemia. The accumulation of succinylacetone inhibits δ-aminolevulinic acid dehydratase (Fig. 67–2) and results in secondary accumulation of δ-aminolevulinic acid, attacks of acute porphyria with peripheral neuropathy, hypertension, and bizarre behavior.

Twelve approaches to therapy of inherited metabolic disease are discussed here. The choice of therapy depends on the mechanisms producing disease. Several therapeutic approaches may be tried sequentially or used simultaneously:

1. *Correcting the primary imbalance in metabolic relationships.* This correction involves a reduction through dietary restriction of accumulated substrate(s) that are toxic and provision of products that may be deficient. An example is phenylalanine hydroxylase deficiency in which phenylalanine is restricted and tyrosine is supplemented.

2. *Enhancing excretion of accumulated substances that are overproduced.* Treatment of gout with uricosuric agents leads to lower blood uric acid levels by blocking renal reabsorption. The tissue deposits of uric acid salts are then mobilized.

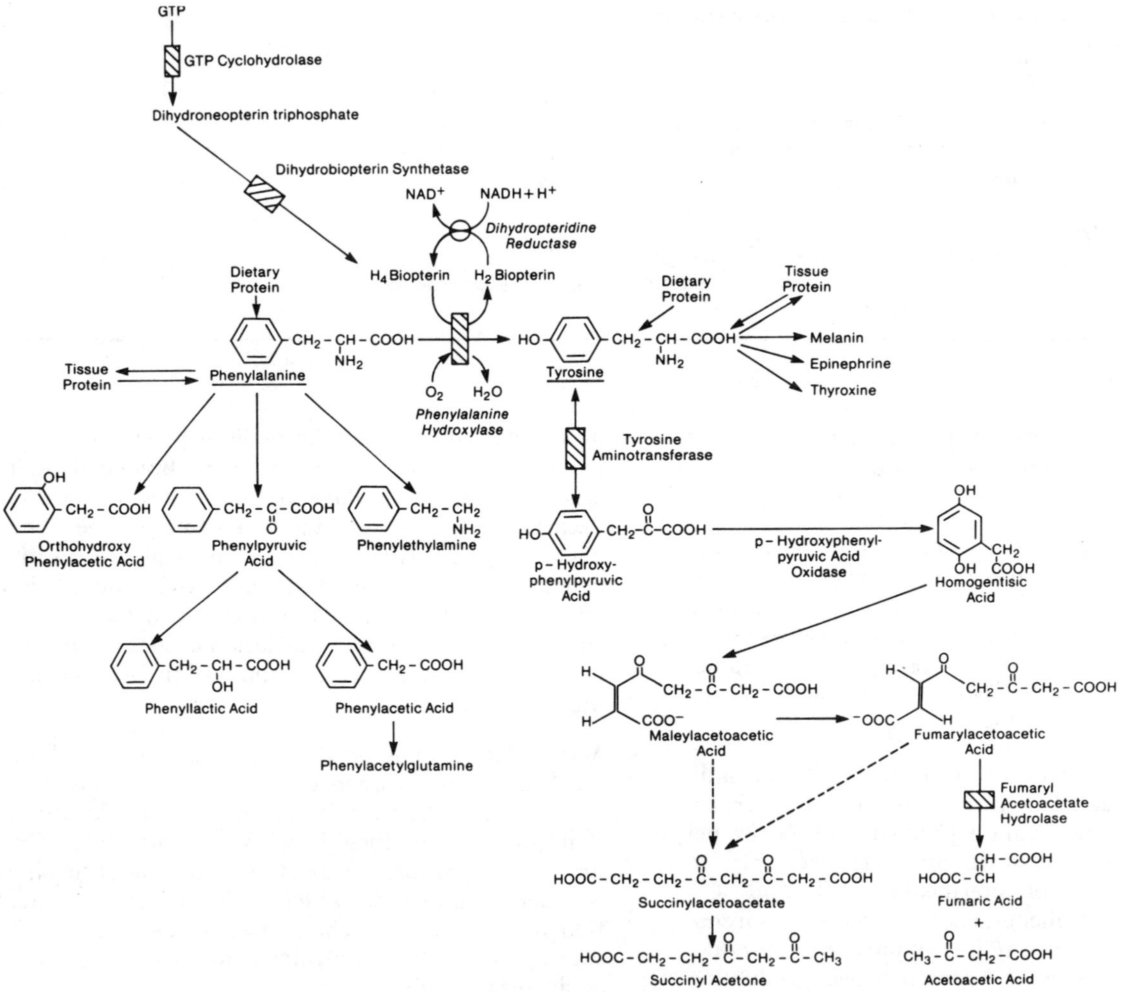

FIGURE 67–1. Metabolism of aromatic amino acids. The metabolic flow and nutrient interaction in disorders of phenylalanine and tyrosine are schematized. Crosshatched bars represent impaired enzymes involved in biopterin biosynthesis, phenylketonuria, and tyrosinemia. See text for discussion.

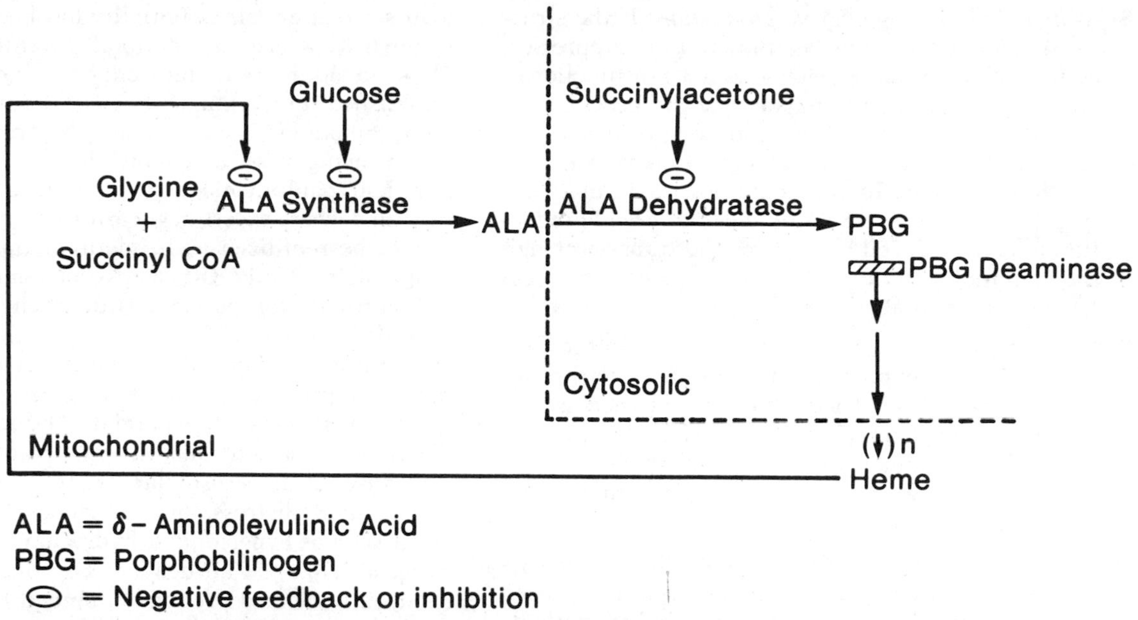

FIGURE 67–2. Inhibition site in heme biosynthesis of relevance to diagnosis and treatment of tyrosinemia type I. The hatched bar schematically represents the partial block in acute intermittent porphyria with resultant overproduction of ALA (δ-aminolevulinic acid) and PBG (porphobilinogen) with decreased heme biosynthesis. In type I tyrosinemia, succinylacetone is produced and inhibits ALA dehydratase with accumulation of ALA alone, which is neurotoxic. ALA accumulation can be reduced by the addition of excess dietary glucose (calories) and by hematin infusions that negatively control ALA synthase at levels of both enzyme and gene expression.

3. *Providing alternative metabolic pathways to decrease accumulated toxic precursors in blocked reaction sequences.* For example, the accumulated ammonia in enzyme defects of the urea cycle is reduced by removing nitrogen through administration of therapeutic amounts of phenylacetic acid to form phenylacetylglutamine from glutamine. Similarly in isovaleric acidemia, innocuous isovalerylglycine is formed from accumulating isovaleric acid if supplemental glycine is provided to drive glycine-N-transacylase. Isovalerylglycine is excreted in the urine.
4. *Using metabolic inhibitors to lower overproduced products.* Allopurinol inhibits xanthine oxidase and decreases overproduction of uric acid in gout. Lovastatin and compactin suppress hydroxymethylglutaryl coenzyme A (CoA) reductase and reduce excess cholesterol biosynthesis in familial hypercholesterolemia.
5. *Supplying products of blocked secondary pathways.* In cystic fibrosis, the exocrine pancreas does not function in a normal manner to produce and secrete digestive enzymes. Administration of these pancreatic enzymes partially corrects the digestive defect in cystic fibrosis. Similarly, supplying hematin alleviates some neurologic deficits in type I tyrosinemia in which succinylacetone has inhibited δ-aminolevulinic acid dehydratase and consequently heme biosynthesis (Fig. 67–2).
6. *Stabilizing altered enzyme proteins.* The rate of biologic synthesis and degradation of holoenzymes depends on their structural conformation. In some holoenzymes, saturation by coenzyme increases their biologic half-life and thus overall enzyme activity at the new equilibrium. This therapeutic mechanism is exemplified in homocystinuria and MSUD. Pharmacologic intake of vitamin B_6 in homocystinuria or vitamin B_1 in MSUD increases intracellular pyridoxal phosphate or thiamine pyrophosphate and will increase the specific activity of cystathionine β-synthase or branched-chain α-keto acid dehydrogenase complex, respectively.[11,12]
7. *Replacing deficient cofactors.* A variety of vitamin-dependent disorders are due to blocks in coenzyme production and are "cured" by pharmacologic intake of a specific vitamin precursor. This mechanism presumably involves overcoming a partially impaired enzyme reaction by mass action. If reactions are impaired that are required to produce methylcobalamin and/or adenosylcobalamin, homocystinuria or methylmalonic aciduria (or both) will result. Daily intakes of milligram quantities of vitamin B_{12} may cure both disorders.[13] In biotinidase deficiency the cofactor, biotin, is not released from its covalently bound state. Reviews on "vitamin dependency syndromes" have been published.[14–17]

8. *Artificially inducing enzyme production.* If the structural gene or enzyme is intact, but suppressor, enhancer, or promoter elements are not functional, abnormal amounts of enzyme may be produced. It should be possible to "turn on" or "turn off" the structural gene and enable normal enzymatic production to occur. In the acute porphyria of type I tyrosinemia, excessive δ-aminolevulinic acid production may be reduced by suppressing transcription of the δ-aminolevulinic acid synthase gene with excess glucose and hematin (Fig. 67–2).
9. *Replacing enzymes.* Many attempts to replace deficient enzymes by plasma infusions and microencapsulation have been tried with limited success. Recently the use of polyethylene glycol coating of adenosine deaminase has significantly prolonged the biologic half-life of this enzyme in treating severe combined immunodeficiency.[18]
10. *Transplanting organs.* Kidney transplant in Fabry's disease and liver transplant in type I glycogen storage disease benefit systemic metabolism with the return of organ function through replacing deficient enzyme activity.
11. *Correcting the underlying defect in DNA so that the body can manufacture its own functionally normal enzymes.* This experimental approach has great possibility for the future. The DNA for several enzymes such as phenylalanine hydroxylase, adenosine deaminase, hypoxanthine-guanine phosphoribosyl transferase, and argininosuccinic acid lyase has been cloned and retroviral constructs have been made by which gene transfer into dividing somatic cells has been accomplished. Human gene therapy is currently contemplated for these inborn errors, although several barriers to application in man must be solved first.[19]
12. *Limiting the frequency of inherited diseases through genetic counseling.* This approach might decrease the number of affected individuals from high-risk matings by developing tests for the heterozygous or carrier states, providing risks and alternatives to prospective parents and providing prenatal detection for heterozygous matings.

Nutrition management remains a principal component in treating all of these inherited disorders, and some practical considerations for nutrition control should be considered. Dietary restrictions required to correct imbalances in metabolic relationships often require the use of chemically defined or elemental foods.[20] These chemically defined products are normally accompanied by small amounts of whole natural protein that supply the restricted amino acid(s). Natural foods seldom supply more than 25%, and often supply much less, of the protein requirements of patients. Other nitrogen-free natural foods that provide energy are limited in their range of nutrients. Consequently, care must be taken to provide food constituents often considered to be contaminants because their essentiality has been demonstrated through long-term use of total parenteral nutrition.[21] Thus, in addition to nutrients for which an RDA is established, other nutrients must be supplied in adequate amounts. These include the trace metals chromium, manganese, and molybdenum, the vitamins biotin and pantothenic acid, choline and inositol and carnitine where excess acyl-carnitines are produced that cannot be reutilized as in methylmalonic acidemia or propionic acidemia. Other possible conditionally essential nutrients for patients with phenylketonuria have been described.[22]

Chemically defined diets consist of small molecules that often provide an osmolality greater than the physiologic tolerance of the patient. Abdominal cramping, diarrhea, distention, nausea, and vomiting have resulted from use of hyperosmolar feeds.[23] Aside from gastrointestinal distress, more serious consequences can occur such as hypertonic dehydration,[24] hypovolemia,[25] hypernatremia,[26] and death.[27] Osmolalities of selected chemically defined products intended for inherited diseases of amino acid metabolism have been published.[28,29]

AROMATIC AMINO ACIDS

Inborn errors of the aromatic amino acids were historically the first to respond to nutrition support. Phenylketonuria was discovered in 1933, and the prevention of its resultant mental retardation by dietary intervention is classic. By contrast, the rare disorders of tyrosine metabolism remain problematic.

BIOCHEMISTRY

The essential amino acid phenylalanine is utilized for two major purposes: tissue protein synthesis and hydroxylation to form tyrosine. The hydroxylation reaction requires phenylalanine hydroxylase, O_2, tetrahydrobiopterin, dihydropteridine reductase, and NADH + H^+ (Fig. 67–1). In the normal adult, only 10% of the RDA for phenylalanine is required for new protein synthesis, whereas approximately 90% is hydroxylated to form tyrosine. In the growing child, 60% of the phenylalanine required is used for new protein synthesis and 40% is hydroxylated to form tyrosine. Mass spectrometry and stable isotope studies of patients with phenylketonuria provide information on other pathways available for phenylalanine metabolism. These alternative pathways, outlined in Figure 67–1, are minor in the metabolism of phenylalanine at 50 μmol concentration in the plasma of normal individuals. However, byproducts become apparent when phenylalanine is not hydroxylated to tyrosine and accumulates to over 500 μmol.[30]

Tyrosine is the normal immediate product of phenylalanine and is essential to five pathways (Fig. 67–1). These include synthesis of protein, catecholamines, melanin pigment, and thyroid hormones. Tyrosine also provides energy when catabolized through parahydroxyphenyl pyruvate to fumarate and acetoacetate. Enzymes required in this latter degradative pathway include tyrosine aminotransferase, *p*-hydroxyphenylpyruvic acid oxidase, homogentisic acid oxidase, and fumarylacetoacetic acid hydrolase (see Fig. 67–1).

PHENYLKETONURIA

Phenylketonuria (PKU) is a group of inherited disorders of phenylalanine metabolism caused by impaired phenylalanine hydroxylase activity. The disease is expressed at 3 to 6 months of age and is characterized by developmental delay, microcephaly, abnormal electroencephalogram, eczema, musty odor, and hyperactivity. If not treated before 3 weeks of age, the metabolic imbalance produces irreversible mental retardation. The defect in metabolism in classic PKU is associated with less than 2% activity of normal phenylalanine hydroxylase.[31] The enzyme is expressed primarily in liver, but not in peripheral blood cells, bone marrow, or cultured cells. Considerable heterogeneity exists for mutations affecting this apoenzyme. Heterozygous parents for "classic" PKU have 50% enzyme activity but are clinically normal even though mild in vivo differences from normal are observed in semifasting phenylalanine to tyrosine plasma concentration ratios.[32] Additionally, variant forms with less severe enzymatic loss require less-stringent diet therapy.

The genetic bases for disorders of phenylalanine hydroxylase were clarified by the localization of the gene to chromosome 12q22-q24 and cloning of the gene, which has 90 kilobases (kb) and 13 exons.[33] At least eight different mutations have been identified that cause the "PKU phenotype," and these involve deletions in coding frames, missense mutations, and intron splice site mutations. Ethnic variation occurs in the type and frequency of phenylalanine hydroxylase mutations, a fact that provides clues to migration of populations in history.[33] Although the cloning of this gene and the identification of a few of many different mutations have assisted in genotyping and counseling families, the mainstay of therapy continues to be preventive newborn screening with immediate and long-term avoidance of excess phenylalanine in the diet.

Other forms of PKU may result from defects in other enzymes involved in the overall reaction. Dihydropteridine reductase is an enzyme normally present in many tissues. It reduces the quininoid form of dihydrobiopterin to tetrahydrobiopterin (see Fig. 67–1). The gene for dihydropteridine reductase is located on chromosome 4p15.3. Several other types of PKU result from defects in the synthesis of tetrahydrobiopterin[34] (see Fig. 67–1). In addition to functioning as coenzyme for phenylalanine hydroxylase, tetrahydrobiopterin is also required by tyrosine hydroxylase and tryptophan hydroxylase[35,36] (see Fig. 67–1). Because these enzymes produce essential neurotransmitters, defects in biopterin synthesis are associated with progressive neurologic disease unless tetrahydrobiopterin, L-dopa, and serotonin are replaced.[35]

Although the precise pathogenesis of mental retardation in classic PKU is not known, the accumulation of phenylalanine or its catabolic byproducts, a deficiency of tyrosine or its products, or all four circumstances will produce central nervous system damage if phenylalanine accumulates in plasma above normal values during critical periods of brain development. The pathologic consequence varies with the time in brain development at which the chemical insult occurs. Deficient myelination and abnormalities in brain proteolipids and/or proteins occur in late gestation and during the first 6 to 9 months of life.[37] During this period, oligodendroglia migration may also be impaired, resulting in irreversible brain damage later in childhood. Protein synthesis in the brain is also depressed, probably owing to competitive inhibition by high phenylalanine on blood-brain barrier transport with consequent imbalance in intraneuronal amino acid concentrations.[38] In the mature brain, neurodegeneration,[39] behavioral difficulties, and prolonged performance times may result from depressed neurotransmitter synthesis.[30,40] Impairment of these neuropsychologic functions in mature brain may be reversible when phenylalanine returns toward normal concentrations in cells and blood.[30,40]

SCREENING

The disorders of phenylalanine metabolism require identification, diagnosis, and appropriate therapy before clinical expression of the disease is apparent. Nutritional and possibly other therapy should be instituted before the third week of life. Thus a tetrapartite public health program involving screening, retrieval, diagnosis, and treatment must be coordinated and efficient to accomplish the objective of preventing mental retardation. A screening test using the bacterial inhibition assay[41] detects potential cases in the newborn population. One laboratory can effectively screen 20,000 to 200,000 samples per year using these methods. Although other methods such as fluorometry are more quantitative, the Guthrie test is used worldwide because of its ease of application. Newborns with blood phenylalanine concentrations greater than 121 μmol/L (2 mg/dl) on the screening test are restudied. The actions taken in "retrieval" depend on the concentration of blood phenylalanine, days of age, and protein intake at the time of screening. Repeat screening at 14 days of age is suggested.[42]

Newborn screening in most of the 50 states, in conjunction with aggressive approaches to retrieval and diagnosis, has led to early institution of diet therapy. To be successful, state-mandated screening programs must allow for easy collection and rapid evaluation of specimens while providing an organized, efficient retrieval system of babies whose screening tests yield positive results.[43] With the present early discharge from hospital and nursery of both mother and baby after delivery, lower phenylalanine concentrations of 121 to 242 μmol/L (2 to 4 mg/dl) are considered "positive" and follow-up is initiated.

Approximately 1 in 10,000 white newborns in the United States is affected with PKU, whereas 1 in 132,000 newborns in the black population is affected. Data in Table 67–3 detail the number of cases of PKU diagnosed since the inception of an exemplary state-wide screening program in Georgia. The mean frequency of PKU is based on a population of newborn subjects that is 63% white. Retrieval time and age at initiation of treatment for PKU cases diagnosed in 1985 are given in Table 67–4. Outcome and accountability for preventing mental retardation depend on the speed with which nutrition management is implemented. Few public health data of the type presented in Table 67–4 are available to evaluate dietary results in various programs.

DIAGNOSIS

Patients with initial blood phenylalanine concentrations of 121 μmol/L (>2 mg/dl) should have the test repeated immediately. If the initial or follow-up screening test is greater than 484 μmol/L (8 mg/dl), plasma amino acids should be quantitated by ion exchange chromatography with the infant on a known phenylalanine intake from natural protein sources. A precise diagnosis is necessary to establish the mode of therapy.

Differential diagnosis requires several laboratory methods. These include ion exchange chromatography for quantitation of plasma phenylalanine, tyrosine, and other amino acid concentrations; determination of genotype of parents and proband[32]; and assays of biopterin and dihydropteridine reductase.[34] Assessment of phenylalanine hydroxylase activity in liver biopsy material[44] has been attempted in the past but is invasive and not ethical for routine diagnosis. DNA analysis using restriction fragment length polymorphisms (RFLP) and cDNA probes for the phenylalanine hydroxylase gene will be helpful in the future.[33] For families with an affected child, prenatal diagnosis is now available using RFLP for the cDNA of phenylalanine hydroxylase.[45] Because phenylalanine hydroxylase is not expressed in cultured amniotic fluid cells, and because phenylalanine concentrations do not rise in amniotic fluid until the last trimester, prenatal monitoring was impractical in the past.

TREATMENT

Patients with plasma phenylalanine concentrations of greater than 150 μmol and plasma tyrosine concentrations below 50 μmol require prompt treatment with a phenylalanine-restricted, tyrosine-supplemented diet. The objective of nutrition support in the child with classic PKU is to maintain blood phenylalanine concentrations that will allow optimum growth and brain development by supplying adequate energy, protein, and other nutrients while restricting phenylalanine and supplementing tyrosine intake.

Although the effects of moderately elevated plasma phenylalanine are not yet known, optimum blood levels should be as close to normal as possible. This objective is met through use of a combination of proprietary, chemically defined, medical, and natural foods. Some investigators have supplemented the phenylalanine-restricted diet with isoleucine, leucine, and valine and have found improvement in behavior and decreased plasma phenyl-

TABLE 67–3. CASES DIAGNOSED SINCE INCEPTION OF COMPREHENSIVE PROGRAM: SEPTEMBER 1, 1978–DECEMBER 31, 1991

	COMPREHENSIVE TOTALS 1,286,495 LIVEBORNS)		
DISEASE	Cases Diagnosed	Incidence	Rate/100,000
PKU (Total)	73	1/17,623	5.7
Classic	47	1/27,372	3.7
Hyperphenylalaninemia	26	1/49,481	2.0
Homocystinuria			
Classic	5	1/257,299	0.4
Other Methionine abnormalities	28	1/45,946	2.2
MSUD	11	1/116,954	0.9
Tyrosinemia			
Prolonged neonatal ≥20 mg%	6	1/225,299	0.5
Transient >12 mg%	1239	1/1,038	87.5
Galactosemia* (total)	142	1/8,686	11.5
Classic	32	1/39,086	2.5
Variant	112	1/11,167	9.0

*Cases diagnosed since Feb. 1, 1979, based on 1,250,745 newborns.

TABLE 67–4. RETRIEVAL TIME FOR CASES DIAGNOSED IN 1989 (MEAN AND RANGE IN DAYS)

DISEASE	N	AGE AT FIRST ABNORMAL TEST	AGE AT START OF TREATMENT
PKU (classic)	8	2.4 (1–4)	9.8 (6–14)
Galactosemia (classic)	4	9.3 (2–28)	15.8 (1–34)

alanine.[46] This may be related to inhibition of phenylalanine transport by competition at either the intestinal or blood-brain barrier uptake steps.[38] Gene replacement therapy using recombinant viruses containing the phenylalanine hydroxylase gene may be useful in the future as one approach to management of individuals with PKU. Recombinant retroviruses may be used to introduce a functioning phenylalanine hydroxylase gene into liver or bone marrow cells and thus may enable an individual with PKU to metabolize excess phenylalanine to tyrosine.[47] However, these latter approaches are still under study, and difficulty will be encountered in coordinating dihydropteridine reductase and biopterin synthesis to accomplish the overall reaction. Thus, this approach is not yet applicable in practice.

Therapy of the child with biopterin-deficient forms of hyperphenylalaninemia requires administration of tetrahydrobiopterin and use of the phenylalanine-restricted, tyrosine-supplemented diet in combination with L-dopa and carbidopa.[35] Serotonin that is derived from tryptophan may also improve behavior if tryptophan hydroxylase is secondarily impaired by the absence of tetrahydrobiopterin.[35,36,48]

Initiation of Nutrition Support. Rapid decline of blood phenylalanine concentration at the time of diagnosis may be obtained by feeding the infant a 20 kcal/ounce (67 kcal/dl) low-phenylalanine or phenylalanine-free formula.[49] Within a mean of 4 days (SD± 3), blood phenylalanine concentration should drop to treatment range. Treatment should be initiated in hospitalized infants to enable adequate parental information transfer and to monitor blood amino acids daily. Laboratory results should be available promptly to prevent precipitation of phenylalanine deficiency and to enable rapid replacement of phenylalanine and tyrosine to optimum blood concentrations.

In the event that the infant or child is not hospitalized for initiation of nutrition support or if only weekly blood phenylalanine concentrations are obtained, a maintenance formula containing adequate phenylalanine from an appropriate source (Table 67–5) should be prescribed. Blood phenylalanine concentration will fall to treatment range within a mean of 10 days (SD 5) with this approach.[49] Choice of initial nutrition support should be predicated on producing controlled blood phenylalanine concentrations no later than the third week of life.

Chronic Care. Long-term care of the patient with classic PKU dictates that proprietary, chemically defined products (medical foods) and natural foods provide all nutrients in required amounts.

Nutrient Requirements. Table 67–6 outlines the suggested amounts of phenylalanine, tyrosine, protein, energy, and fluid to offer. A formal prescription must be written that is individualized to the specific degree of impaired enzyme activity, growth rate, and consequent needs of each patient. Weekly adjustments in the diet prescription may be necessary, particularly during the first 6 months of life, based on hunger, growth, development, and laboratory analyses of plasma phenylalanine and tyrosine concentrations. The phenylalanine provided should maintain the 3- to 4-hour postprandial blood phenylalanine concentration between 50 and 300 μmol.[50] Phenylalanine is an essential amino acid[51] and cannot be deleted from the diet without producing death.[52] Excess restriction produces growth failure, skin rashes, bone changes, and mental retardation.[52]

Phenylalanine required for growth by the infant with classic PKU is 20 to 70 mg/kg of body weight, with the younger infant requiring the larger amount.[53] Phenylalanine requirement declines rapidly between 3 and 6 months of age as growth rates plateau. Requirements for phenylalanine in the 6- to 12-month-old patient with classic PKU may fall to 15 mg/kg per day, but they vary considerably (Table 67–6). Frequent monitoring of blood phenylalanine concentration and intake is required to prevent excess intake when growth rate decelerates and to prevent inadequate intake when growth rate is at its peak.

Tyrosine is an essential amino acid for children with PKU. For this reason, plasma tyrosine values must be monitored; if they are low, L-tyrosine supplements are given. The supplement required in addition to that already present in chemically defined formula and food should be adequate to provide a total of 180 to 200 mg/kg per day for the infant and 120 to 150 mg/kg per day for the child and adult. Tyrosine supplements alone will not prevent mental retardation in classic phenylketonuria.[54]

TABLE 67–5. AMINO ACID AND PROTEIN CONTENT OF EXEMPLARY FOODS (PER 100 G EDIBLE PORTION)

FOOD	CYSTINE (MG)	ISOLEUCINE (MG)	LEUCINE (MG)	METHIONINE (MG)	PHENYLALANINE (MG)	TYROSINE (MG)	VAL. (MG)	PROTEIN (G)
Cereals								
Corn grits, cooked	32	56	215	34	73	61	47	1.4
Cream of wheat, cooked	34	67	115	28	82	48	73	1.5
Oats, cooked	64	118	197	43	141	92	151	2.6
Dairy Products								
Eggs	289	759	1,066	392	686	505	874	12.1
Cheese (cheddar)	125	1,546	2,385	652	1,311	1,202	1,663	24.9
Milk								
Cow, whole	30	199	322	83	159	159	220	3.3
Human	19	56	95	21	46	53	63	1.0
Fruits								
Apples, raw with skin	3	8	12	2	5	4	9	0.2
Apricots, raw	3	41	77	6	52	29	47	1.4
Bananas	17	33	71	11	38	24	47	1.0
Oranges, raw	10	25	23	20	31	16	40	0.9
Peaches, raw	6	20	40	17	22	18	38	0.7
Watermelon	2	19	18	6	15	12	16	0.6
Meal, Fish, Poultry								
Beef, hamburger, lean, cooked	391	1,576	2,467	748	1,240	1,081	1,673	30.1
Chicken, light meat, fried	420	1,732	2,463	908	1,303	1,108	1,828	32.8
Fish, halibut, raw	245	1,066	1,588	606	773	765	1,108	20.9
Proprietary Infant Formula								
Enfamil (per dl)	17	90	154	29	58	66	91	1.5
Similac (per dl)	13	75	145	43	75	93	84	1.5
Vegetables								
Beans, green, cooked	11	42	71	14	42	27	57	1.2
lima, cooked	83	438	535	68	336	219	425	6.8
Broccoli, cooked	21	115	139	36	90	67	136	3.0
Cabbage, raw	10	61	63	12	39	21	52	1.2
Carrots, raw	8	41	43	7	32	20	44	1.0
Peas, green, cooked	32	193	320	81	198	112	232	5.4
Potatoes, baked	29	93	138	36	102	85	130	2.3
Spinach, cooked	35	152	231	55	134	113	168	3.0
Tomatoes, raw	12	21	33	8	23	15	23	0.9

(Data from references 59 to 64.)

TABLE 67–6. APPROXIMATE DAILY REQUIREMENTS FOR SELECTED NUTRIENTS* INFANTS AND CHILDREN WITH INHERITED DISORDERS OF AMINO ACID METABOLISM

		AGE						
NUTRIENT	UNIT	0 < 6 mo.	6 < 12 mo.	1 < 4 yr.	4 < 7 yr.	7 < 11 yr.	11 < 15 yr.	15 < 19 yr.
Fluid	ml/kg	120–115	100	95	90	75	50	50
Energy	kcal/kg	145–95	135–80	—	—	—	—	—
	kcal/day (range)	—	—	1300 (900–1800)	1700 (1300–2300)	2400 (1650–3300)	2200–2700 (1500–3700)	2100–1800 (1200–3900)
Protein	g/kg	2.5–3.00	2.2–2.5	—	—	—	—	—
	g/day	—	—	25	30	35	45–50	45–55
Carbohydrate	g/day	kcal × 0.35 to 0.30 ÷ 4				← kcal × 0.50 to 0.60 ÷ 4 →		
Fat	g/day	kcal × 0.50 ÷ 9				← kcal × 0.35 ÷ 9 →		
Isoleucine	mg/kg	90–30	90–30	85–20	80–20	30–20	30–20	30–10
Leucine	mg/kg	100–60	75–40	70–40	65–35	60–30	50–30	40–15
Methionine	mg/kg	50–20	40–15	30–10	20–10	20–10	20–10	10–5
Phenylalanine	mg/kg	70–20	50–15	40–15	35–15	30–15	30–15	30–10
Tyrosine	mg/kg	80–60	60–40	60–30	50–25	40–20	30–15	30–10
Valine	mg/kg	95–40	60–30	85–30	50–30	30–25	30–20	30–15

*All known essential amino acids, essential fatty acids, minerals and vitamins must be provided in adequate amounts.

The protein content of the diet for infants with PKU has traditionally been greater than normal. Protein requirements are increased when either an L-amino acid mix or a casein hydrolysate is the primary protein source rather than natural protein.[55] Thus, recommendations for protein for nutrition support are greater than the RDA.[56,57] Recommendations for energy and fluid intake (Table 67–5) are the same as those for normal infants and children.[56,58]

Low-Phenylalanine and Phenylalanine-Free, Chemically Defined Medical Foods. Adequate protein cannot be obtained from natural foods without ingesting excess phenylalanine (natural proteins contain 2.4 to 9% by weight of phenylalanine).[59–64] Thus, special proprietary chemically defined medical foods are used to provide protein.[65–69] Sources and formulations of these products are given in Tables 67–7 and 67–8. Analog XP, designed for the infant, consists of L-amino acids, a blend of fat and carbohydrate that produces a fatty acid profile similar to breast milk, minerals, trace elements, (including chromium, molybdenum, and selenium), and vitamins. Carnitine and taurine have also been added. Analog XP is free of phenylalanine (Table 67–9). Lofenalac, formulated from a specially treated enzymatic hydrolysate of casein, is low in phenylalanine and contains fat and carbohydrate. Minerals, vitamins, and four L-amino acids are also added. The phenylalanine content of Lofenalac is between 0.06 and 0.1% and is approximately 75 mg/100 g. Lofenalac has no added chromium, molybdenum, or selenium (Table 67–9). Maxamaid XP, designed for the 1- to 8-year-old child, is an orange-flavored powder free of phenylalanine that contains L-amino acids, carbohydrate, minerals, trace elements, and vitamins. It does not contain fat, chromium, selenium, or vitamin K. Maxamum XP is formulated for children 8 years of age and older and for pregnant women. It is fat-free but has added carnitine, taurine, chromium, molybdenum, selenium, and vitamin K (Table 67–9). Phenyl-Free is an L-amino acid mix containing carbohydrate, fat, minerals, trace elements (except chromium and molybdenum), and vitamins. It is designed for children and adolescents. PKU-1, PKU-2, and PKU-3 are L-amino acid mixes that are low in carbohydrate and free of fat, chromium, and selenium. PKU-1 is designed for the infant, PKU-2 for the child, and PKU-3 for the adolescent and pregnant woman (Table 67–9).

Natural Foods. Serving lists are available to simplify the phenylalanine-restricted diet for families and professional persons guiding them (Table 67–10). The lists are similar to diabetic exchange lists in that foods of similar phenylalanine content are grouped together and can be exchanged one for another within a list to give variety to the diet.[69] Portion sizes of foods in each list may be found in reference 68.

Diet plans for children with PKU at different ages using different medical foods may be found in Tables 67–11 through 67–13. For instance, Analog XP, Lofenalac, or PKU-1 could be used to initiate a prescribed diet to a neonate at 55 mg phenylalanine/kg per day (Table 67–11). By 6 months of age the prescription would be reduced to 30 mg/kg per day, but any of the foregoing medical foods could still be used (Table 67–12). By 2 years of age a "variant" might require as much as 25 mg/kg per day. However, to allow as many natural foods as possible, Maxamaid XP or Phenyl-Free would more likely be the medical food of choice (Table 67–13).

Management Problems. Management problems described for children with PKU occur in other children with inherited disorders of metabolism. Principles described here apply to children with other disorders as well but will not be reiterated in other sections.

Maintenance of an adequate intake of protein and energy is important for the child with PKU even though phenylalanine must be restricted. Protein is obtained from chemically defined medical foods; therefore, the amount of chemically defined formula offered must be varied to provide the protein needed. Nonprotein sources of energy such as corn syrup, Moducal, Polycose, sugar, Protein Free Diet Powder (Table 67–14), and pure fats can be added to maintain energy intake and to satisfy the child's hunger without affecting blood phenylalanine concentrations. Natural foods should be prescribed in numbers of servings and introduced at the appropriate ages and in the usual textures as they would be for any child. Children should be given a variety of foods at the appropriate age so that these foods may be included in the diet later in life. In this way, increasing total phenylalanine requirements may be met.

A variety of factors may influence blood phenylalanine levels. Those that may produce an elevated blood phenylalanine concentration include acute infections with concomitant tissue catabolism, excessive or inadequate phenylalanine intake, and inadequate protein or energy intake. Infection affects plasma amino acids in normal adults.[70] Similar increases in blood phenylalanine occur in febrile, treated PKU patients. Because of this fact, any infection should be promptly diagnosed and appropriately treated. The best approach to nutrition support during short-term infections is to increase the intake of fluids and carbohydrates through the use of fruit juices, high-carbohydrate protein-free beverages, and soft drinks that do not contain caffeine.

Excess phenylalanine intake is the most common cause of elevated blood phenylalanine concentration in the older child with PKU. This condition may be due to overprescription, misunderstanding of the diet by the caretaker, or "snitching" of food by the child. Frequent evaluations of blood phenylalanine with accompanying accurate diet records for calculation of intake are used to determine the dietary phenylalanine prescription. Diet records are also useful in determining parental understanding. Misunderstanding of diet requires additional education of parents. One of the most common "misunderstandings" in older children is the total amount of an exchange group allowed. In extended families living in

TABLE 67—7. SOURCES AND INDICATIONS FOR "CHEMICALLY DEFINED" MEDICAL FOODS FOR AMINO ACID- OR NITROGEN-RESTRICTED DIETS

MANUFACTURER	PRODUCT	INDICATION(S)
Mead Johnson Nutritional Division 2404 W. Pennsylvania St. Evansville, IN 47221 (800) 457-3550	Lofenalac	PKU*
	Low Methionine Diet Powder	Hypermethioninemias Homocystinuria (cystathionine β-synthase deficiency)
	Low Phe/Tyr Diet Powder	Tyrosinemias
	Moducal	Any disorder in which amino acids or N are restricted
	MSUD Diet Powder	MSUD† IVA‡ (must add Gly, Ile and Val) Any disorder of BCAA metabolism
	Phenyl-Free	PKU
	Protein-Free Diet Powder	Any disorder in which amino acids or N are restricted
	HOM 1, HOM 2	Hypermethioninemias Homocystinuria (cystathionine β-synthase deficiency)
	MSUD 1, MSUD 2	MSUD IVA (must add Gly, Ile and Val) Any disorder of BCAA metabolism
	PKU 1, PKU 2, PKU 3	PKU
	TYR 1, TYR 2	Tyrosinemias
	UCD 1, UCD 2	Defects in urea cycle enzymes
Ross Laboratories Columbus, Ohio 43216 (800) 367-7677	Polycose Powder	Any disorder in which amino acids or N must be restricted
	Analog Range	
	MSUD	MSUD
	XLEU	Any disorder of leucine metabolism
	XMET	Hypermethioninemias Homocystinuria (cystathionine β-synthase deficiency)
	XP	PKU
	XPHEN, TYR	Tyrosinemias
	XPHEN, TYR, MET	Tyrosinemias with elevated plasma methionine
	Maxamaid Range	
	XLEU	Any disorder of leucine metabolism
	XMET	Hypermethioninemias Homocystinuria (cystathionine β-synthase deficiency)
	MSUD	MSUD
	XP	PKU
	XPHEN, TYR	Tyrosinemias
	XPHEN, TYR, MET	Tyrosinemias with elevated plasma methionine
	Maxamum Range	
	XP	PKU
	MSUD	MSUD
	XMET	Hypermethioninemias Homocystinuria (cystathionine β-synthase deficiency)

*Phenylketonuria
†Maple syrup urine disease
‡Isovaleric acidemia

TABLE 67–8. FORMULATION OF "CHEMICALLY DEFINED" MEDICAL FOODS FOR AMINO ACID- AND NITROGEN-RESTRICTED DIET

PRODUCT	PROTEIN (%)	FAT (%)	CARBOHYDRATE (%)	MINERALS (%)	VITAMINS (%)	WATER (%)
Mead Johnson Nutritional Division						
Lofenalac	14.6 casein hydrolysate; 1.07 free L-amino acids	18.0 corn oil	50.4 corn syrup solids; 9.6 modified tapioca starch	3.6	All present	3.8
Moducal	None	None	100 maltodextrin	0.4	None	5.0
MSUD Diet Powder	9.9 free L-amino acids	20.0 corn oil	52.9 corn syrup solids; 10.1 modified tapioca starch	3.5	All present	3.3
Low Methionine Diet Powder	15.5 soy protein isolate	28.0 corn oil and coconut oil	51 corn syrup solids	3.0	All present	2.1
Low Phe/Tyr Diet Powder	14.6 casein hydrolysate; 1.07 free L-amino acids	18.0 corn oil	50.4 corn syrup solids; 9.6 modified tapioca starch	3.6	All present	3.8
Phenyl-Free	20.3 L-amino acids	6.8 corn oil and coconut oil	44.2 sucrose; 14.5 corn syrup solids; 7.3 modified tapioca starch	3.8	All present	3.2
Protein-Free Diet Powder	None	22.0 corn oil	61.2 corn syrup solids; 10.8 modified tapioca starch	2.7	All present	3.0
HOM 1/ HOM 2	52/69 L-amino acids	None	18/5 sucrose	15.8/8.7	1.8/1.0	2/2
MSUD 1/ MSUD 2	41/54 L-amino acids	None	30/22 sucrose	15.8/8.7	1.8/1.0	2/2
PKU 1/PKU 2	50/67 L-amino acids	None	19/7 sucrose	15.8/8.7	1.8/1.0	2/2
PKU 3	68 L-amino acids	None	3 sucrose	11.4	1.0	2
TYR 1/TYR 2	47/63 L-amino acids	None	21/12 sucrose	15.8/8.7	1.8/1.0	2/2
UCD 1/ UCD 2	56/67 L-amino acids	None	8/6 sucrose	18.4/8.7	2.1/1.0	2/2
Ross Laboratories						
Analog Range	13.0 L-amino acids	20.9	58.0 maltodextrins 1.0 galactose	1.37	0.22	3.00
Maxamaid Range	25.0 L-amino acids	0	62.0 sucrose	3.72	0.33	3.00
Maxamum Range	39.0 L-amino acids	0	45.0 sucrose	3.49	0.53	3.00
Polycose Powder	None	None	94.0 glucose polymers	0.38	None	6.00

(Data from references 65 to 69.)

close proximity, the child may receive three to four times the allowed amount of food from different well-intentioned but uninformed relatives. "Snitching" of food by the child is the most difficult problem to handle. The child should be given sound reasons for avoiding foods not allowed on the diet, and this responsibility should be shifted to the child by 4 to 6 years of age. Appropriate disciplinary action by the parents should also be supported if the patient is unwilling to accept this responsibility. Lifetime nutrition support should be emphasized to the parents at the onset of therapy, and to both parents and child at recurring intervals.

Phenylalanine deficiency associated with inadequate phenylalanine intake has three specific stages of development.[71] The first stage is characterized biochemically by decreased blood and urine phenylalanine. Clinically, the child may appear lethargic or anorectic. Failure to gain length or weight may occur. In the older child, increases in blood alanine and mild lactic and β-hydroxybutyric acidemia occur as a consequence of muscle alanine production and β-lipolysis. In the second stage, blood phenylalanine is increased as a result of muscle protein degradation. Increased branched-chain amino acid concentrations with decreases in other plasma amino acids occur. Aminoaciduria appears as a consequence of renal tubular malabsorption.[72] In this stage, body protein stores are catabolized, energy sources are depleted, and "active" membrane functions are impaired.[72] Eczema is common. In the third stage of phenylalanine deficiency, blood phenylalanine is de-

TABLE 67–9. COMPOSITION OF "CHEMICALLY DEFINED" MEDICAL FOODS (PER 100 G OF PRODUCT) FOR PHENYLALANINE-RESTRICTED DIETS

NUTRIENTS	ANALOG XP	LOFENA-LAC	MAXAMAID XP	MAXAMUM XP	PHENYL-FREE	PKU 1	PKU 2	PKU 3
Energy (kcal)	475	460	350	340	410	280	300	290
Protein equivalent (g)	13.00	15.1	25.0	39.0	20	50	67	68
Alanine (g)	0.58	0.68	1.03	1.60	0	2.40	3.10	3.10
Arginine (g)	1.03	0.56	2.21	3.02	0.69	2.00	2.70	2.70
Aspartic acid (g)	0.96	1.40	1.85	2.81	5.30	5.70	7.60	7.60
Carnitine (g)	0.01	0.009	NA	0.02	NA	NA	NA	NA
Cystine (g)	0.38	0.06	0.71	1.11	0.35	1.40	1.80	1.80
Glutamic acid (g)	1.17	4.00	2.40	4.56	6.70	12.00	16.00	16.00
Glutamine (g)	0.11	?	0.22	0.34	NA	NA	NA	NA
Glycine (g)	0.90	0.38	1.77	2.82	3.30	1.40	1.80	1.80
Histidine (g)	0.59	0.48	1.27	1.71	0.47	1.40	1.80	1.80
Isoleucine (g)	0.90	0.87	1.70	2.66	1.10	3.40	4.50	4.50
Leucine (g)	1.55	1.66	2.91	4.56	1.73	5.70	7.60	7.60
Lysine (g)	1.06	1.65	2.22	3.49	1.89	4.00	5.40	5.40
Methionine (g)	0.25	0.54	0.48	0.73	0.63	1.40	1.80	1.80
Phenylalanine (g)	0	0.075	0	0	0	0	0	0
Proline (g)	1.10	1.42	2.05	3.23	0	5.40	7.10	7.10
Serine (g)	0.68	0.94	1.26	2.00	0	3.00	4.00	4.00
Taurine (g)	0.019	0.027	NA	0.14	NA	NA	NA	NA
Threonine (g)	0.76	0.78	1.42	2.23	0.94	2.70	3.60	3.60
Tryptophan (g)	0.30	0.20	0.57	0.89	0.28	1.00	1.40	1.40
Tyrosine (g)	1.37	0.80	2.56	4.03	0.94	3.40	4.50	6.00
Valine (g)	0.99	1.38	1.85	2.92	1.26	4.00	5.40	5.40
Carbohydrate (g)	59.0	60.0	62.0	45.0	66.0	19	7	2
Fat (g)	20.9	18.0	0	0	6.8	NA	NA	NA
Calcium (mg)	325	430	810	670	510	2,400	1,310	1,312
Chloride (mEq)	8.0	9.1	12.9	16.0	26.6	47.1	28.2	28.2
Chromium (μg)	15	?	NA	50	NA	NA	NA	NA
Copper (mg)	0.45	0.43	2.0	1.4	0.6	6.7	2.0	3.6
Iodine (μg)	47	32	134	107	45	230	120	143
Iron (mg)	7.0	8.6	12.0	23.5	12.2	34.0	15.0	21.0
Magnesium (mg)	34	50	200	285	152	520	156	540
Manganese (mg)	0.6	0.14	1.30	1.7	1.02	2.40	0.70	4.8
Molybdenum (μg)	35.00	?	60.0	110	NA	107.00	32.00	476
Phosphorus (mg)	230	320	810	670	510	1,860	1,010	1,010
Potassium (mEq)	10.7	12.1	22	18	35.1	8.9	34.1	34.1
Selenium (μg)	15	?	NA	50	6.1	NA	NA	NA
Sodium (mEq)	5.2	9.6	25	24.5	17.7	46.4	27.8	27.8
Zinc (mg)	5.0	3.6	13.0	13.6	7.1	26.0	7.8	23.8
Vitamin A (μg RE)	530	432	300	705	366	2,800	1,560	1,200
D (μg)	8.5	7.2	12.0	8.0	3.8	25.0	32.8	12.0
E (mg α-TE)	3.3	9.7	4.4	5.2	6.8	22.8	12.1	8.05
K (μg)	21	72	NA	70	102	167	167	167
Ascorbic acid (mg)	40	37	135	90	53	230	80	100
Biotin (mg)	0.026	0.036	0.12	0.140	0.030	0.100	0.300	0.179
B_6 (mg)	0.52	0.29	1.00	2.1	0.91	2.20	1.50	3.2
B_{12} (μg)	1.25	1.4	4.0	4.0	2.5	7.9	3.0	5.0
Choline (mg)	50	61	110	320	86	430	260	260
Folate (μg)	38	72	150	500	127	340	400	950
Inositol (mg)	100	22	56	86	30	500	300	300
Niacin (mg)*	4.5	5.8	12.0	13.6	8.1	54.0	24.0	18.0
Pantothenic acid (mg)	2.65	2.2	3.7	5.0	3.0	25.0	11.0	8.3
Riboflavin (mg)	0.60	0.4	1.20	1.4	1.02	4.00	2.00	1.8
Thiamin (mg)	0.50	0.4	1.1	1.4	0.61	2.70	1.40	1.8

*Preformed niacin

NA = none added

Note: Values listed, although accurate at the time of publication, are subject to change. The most current information may be obtained by referring to product labels.

(Data from references 65 to 69.)

TABLE 67–10. AVERAGE NUTRIENT CONTENT OF SERVING LISTS FOR PHENYLALANINE AND/OR TYROSINE AND PROTEIN-RESTRICTED DIETS

FOOD LIST	PHENYLALANINE (MG)	TYROSINE (MG)	METHIONINE (MG)	PROTEIN (G)	CARBOHYDRATE (G)	FAT (G)	ENERGY (KCAL)
Breads/cereals	30	20	13	0.6	7	0	30
Fats	5	4	2	0.1	0	5	60
Fruits	15	10	8	0.5	15	0	60
Vegetables	15	10	6	0.5	2	0	10
Free foods A*	5	4	2	0.1	18	0	65
Free foods B*	0	0	0	0	14	Varies	55

*Low-protein pastas and breads not included.

TABLE 67–11. DIET GUIDE FOR PHENYLKETONURIA (0 YEARS OF AGE)

NAME: PKU
AGE: 0 yrs 0 mos
WEIGHT: 3.25 kg

PRESCRIPTION:	Total	Per Kg
Phenylalanine—mg	179	55
Protein—g	9.8	3.0
Energy—kcal	390	120

FORMULA #1	PHE	TYR	PRO	KCAL	AMOUNT
Analog XP	0	630	6.0	218	46 g
Similac w/iron, concentrate	179	179	3.8	173	128 ml
Volume					600 ml
TOTALS	179	809	9.8	391	

FORMULA #2	PHE	TYR	PRO	KCAL	AMOUNT
Lofenalac	30	316	5.9	182	40 g
Enfamil w/iron, concentrate	149	172	3.8	172	127 ml
Table sugar	0	0	0	38	0.8 Tbsp
Volume					600 ml
TOTALS	179	488	9.8	392	

FORMULA #3	PHE	TYR	PRO	KCAL	AMOUNT
PKU1	0	349	5.2	28	10 g
Enfamil w/iron, concentrate	179	206	4.6	206	153 ml
Vegetable oil	0	0	0	32	4 ml
Table sugar	0	0	0	124	2.6 Tbsp
Volume					600 ml
TOTALS	179	555	9.8	390	

creased below normal, as are other amino acids. Accompanying clinical manifestations include failure to gain weight, failure to gain height, osteopenia, anemia, sparse hair, and finally death if the deficiency is not corrected by supplements of dietary phenylalanine.

Insufficient protein intake results in an inadequate supply of essential amino acids and/or nitrogen for growth. When protein synthesis is decreased, phenylalanine is no longer used for growth and accumulates in the blood. If catabolism occurs because of prolonged lack of nitrogen and/or amino acid intake, blood phenylalanine concentration increases because tissue protein contains some 5.5% phenylalanine. In case of protein insufficiency, chemically defined medical food intake should be increased to supply the required nitrogen and/or essential amino acids.

Energy, the first requirement of the body, is necessary for growth. When energy is provided as carbohydrate and fat, and if adequate nitrogen is available, nonessential amino acids may be synthesized from the keto acid

TABLE 67–12. DIET GUIDE FOR PHENYLKETONURIA (6 MONTHS OF AGE)

NAME: PKU
AGE: 0 yrs 6 mos
WEIGHT: 6.5 kg

PRESCRIPTION:	Total	Per Kg
Phenylalanine—mg	195	30
Protein—g	16.3	2.5
Energy—kcal	715	110

FORMULA #1	PHE	TYR	PRO	KCAL	AMOUNT
Analog XP	0	1247	11.8	432	91 g
Similac w/iron, concentrate	136	136	2.9	131	97 ml
Vegetable oil	0	0	0	16	2.0 ml
Polycose Powder	0	0	0	32	1.4 Tbsp
Volume					600 ml
Foods					
Breads/cereals	30	20	0.6	30	1 serving
Fruits	15	10	0.5	60	1 serving
Vegetables	15	10	0.5	15	1 serving
TOTALS	196	1423	16.3	716	

FORMULA #2	PHE	TYR	PRO	KCAL	AMOUNT
PKU1	0	756	11.2	61	22 g
Enfamil w/iron, concentrate	135	156	3.5	156	115 ml
Vegetable oil	0	0	0	171	1.4 Tbsp
Table sugar	0	0	0	222	4.6 Tbsp
Volume					720 ml
Foods					
Breads/cereals	30	20	0.6	30	1 serving
Fruits	15	10	0.5	60	1 serving
Vegetables	15	10	0.5	15	1 serving
TOTALS	195	952	16.3	715	

FORMULA #3	PHE	TYR	PRO	KCAL	AMOUNT
Lofenalac	64	648	12.8	394	86 g
Emfamil w/iron, concentrate	71	82	1.8	82	61 ml
Table sugar	0	0	0	135	2.8 Tbsp
Volume					720 ml
Foods					
Breads/cereals	30	20	0.6	30	1 serving
Fruits	15	10	0.5	60	1 serving
Vegetables	15	10	0.5	15	1 serving
TOTALS	195	806	16.3	715	

metabolites. Further, carbohydrate ingestion leads to insulin secretion, and insulin promotes amino acid transport into the cell and consequent protein synthesis.[73,74] The mechanisms by which insulin regulates amino acid uptake in muscle changes with increasing age.[74] When energy intake is inadequate, tissue catabolism occurs to meet energy needs. Such catabolism releases phenylalanine, leading to elevated blood phenylalanine concentrations. Provision of sufficient energy through generous use of nonprotein and low-protein foods is important to assure a normal growth rate.

Low blood phenylalanine concentrations (<25 μmol) may lead to depressed appetite,[75] decreased growth[76] and, if prolonged, to mental retardation.[50,52] Low blood phenylalanine concentrations are often due to inadequate prescription of phenylalanine for the affected child. In such cases, the prescription for phenylalanine can be increased by addition of measured amounts of milk and/or solid foods. In some situations, chemically defined medical food may be diluted to a volume that is too great for the child to consume in the allotted time. The volume will need to be decreased to the amount the

TABLE 67–13. DIET GUIDE FOR PHENYLKETONURIA (2 YEARS OF AGE)

NAME: PKU
AGE: 2 yrs 0 mos
WEIGHT: 13.0 kg

PRESCRIPTION:	Total	Per Kg
Phenylalanine—mg	325	25
Protein—g	25.0	1.9
Energy—kcal	1300	100

FORMULA #1	PHE	TYR	PRO	KCAL	AMOUNT
Maxamaid XP	0	1767	17.3	242	69 g
Vegetable oil	0	0	0	165	1.3 Tbsp
Polycose Powder	0	0	0	103	4.6 Tbsp
Volume					960 ml
Foods					
Breads/cereals	210	140	4.2	210	7 servings
Fats	25	20	0.5	300	5 servings
Fruits	45	30	1.5	180	3 servings
Vegetables	45	30	1.5	45	3 servings
Free Foods B	0	0	0.0	55	1 serving
TOTALS	325	1987	25.0	1300	

FORMULA #2	PHE	TYR	PRO	KCAL	AMOUNT
Phenyl-Free	0	799	17.3	345	85 g
Vegetable oil	0	0	0	113	0.9 Tbsp
Table sugar	0	0	0	52	1.1 Tbsp
Volume					960 ml
Foods					
Breads/cereals	210	140	4.2	210	7 servings
Fats	25	20	0.5	300	5 servings
Fruit	45	30	1.5	180	3 servings
Vegetables	45	30	1.5	45	3 servings
Free Foods B	0	0	0.0	55	1 serving
TOTALS	325	1019	25.0	1300	

child is able to ingest. Concentrated, chemically defined medical foods are frequently used without any untoward side effects. They may be mixed as a paste and spoon-fed, even to the young infant. The practice could begin at 3 to 4 months of age when tongue thrust is no longer evident. Extra fluid must then be offered between feedings to maintain appropriate water balance.

Assessment of Nutrition Support. Along with biweekly assessment of growth through measurement of height, weight, and head circumference and evaluation of development by appropriate developmental scales, the adequacy of phenylalanine and tyrosine intake is determined by twice-weekly quantitation of the blood phenylalanine and tyrosine concentrations. The first year is the period of most rapid growth and of greatest vulnerability to nutritional insult. Therefore, twice-weekly blood tests are suggested during the first 3 months and weekly thereafter until the child is 1 year of age. After 1 year of age, weekly blood tests are sufficient for monitoring diet. If, however, blood phenylalanine concentrations are greater than 300 μmol (5 mg/dl), more-frequent determinations should be obtained. Where indicated, the prescription for phenylalanine is decreased and frequent blood tests are obtained until blood phenylalanine concentrations are between 50 and 300 μmol. For blood tests to be of use in adjusting the prescription, laboratory methods must be both accurate and prompt. Quantitative methods of phenylalanine determination using automated ion exchange chromatography and liquid blood are preferable. This method allows evaluation of all amino acids. The microbiologic (Guthrie) method is acceptable for screening, but is nonquantitative and invalid if antibiotics are used. Fluorimetric methods are quantitative and preferred to the Guthrie test to monitor blood phenylalanine.[77] If properly instructed, parents may be given responsibility for obtaining the specimens on filter paper or in micro-capillary tubes and mailing them to a central laboratory.

A record of food ingested before and during blood sampling for blood phenylalanine measurement is essential and should be kept by the child's caregiver. The

TABLE 67–14. COMPOSITION OF NITROGEN-FREE ENERGY SOURCES (PER 100 G OF PRODUCT) FOR NITROGEN-RESTRICTED DIETS

NUTRIENT	MODUCAL	POLYCOSE POWDER	PROTEIN-FREE DIET POWDER
Energy (kcal)	380	380	490
Protein equivalent (g)	0	0	0
Carbohydrate (g)	95.0	94.0	72
Fat (g)	0	0	22
Calcium (mg)	0	30	540
Chloride (mEq)	4.2	6.3	3.9
Chromium (μg)	0	0	NA
Copper (mg)	0	0	0.54
Iodine (μg)	0	0	40
Iron (mg)	0	0	10.8
Magnesium (mg)	0	0	63
Manganese (mg)	0	0	0.18
Molybdenum (μg)	0	0	NA
Phosphorus (mg)	0	5	300
Potassium (mEq)	0.3	0.3	8.7
Selenium (μg)	0	0	NA
Sodium (mEq)	3.0	4.8	3.7
Zinc (mg)	0	0	4.5
Vitamin A (μg RE)	0	0	540
D (μg)	0	0	9.0
E (mg α-TE)	0	0	12.0
K (μg)	0	0	90
Ascorbic acid (mg)	0	0	47
Biotin (mg)	0	0	0.045
B_6 (mg)	0	0	0.36
B_{12} (μg)	0	0	1.8
Choline (mg)	0	0	76
Folate (μg)	0	0	90
Inositol (mg)	0	0	27
Niacin (mg)*	0	0	7.2
Pantothenic acid (mg)	0	0	2.7
Ribloflavin (mg)	0	0	0.54
Thiamine (mg)	0	0	0.45

*Preformed niacin
NA = none added
Note: Values listed, although accurate at the time of publication, are subject to change. The most current information may be obtained by referring to product labels.
(Data from references 65 to 69.)

correlation between the child's intake of phenylalanine, tyrosine, protein, and energy, the child's clinical status, and the blood phenylalanine and tyrosine concentrations is considered when the diet is altered.

The success of early diet management rests with the parents and depends on their understanding of the disease and their ability to cope with the diet. Later, the child's understanding of the diet and ability to assume responsibility for it are critical. These factors in turn are related to the support the parents and patient receive from various professional members of the genetic team. Roles and functions of some team members have been described.[78]

Results of Therapy. Early diagnosis and treatment of infants with PKU with a nutritionally adequate, phenylalanine-restricted, tyrosine-supplemented diet have promoted normal growth and prevented severe mental retardation. A study showed that mean height, weight, and head circumference of 111 children treated from before 120 days of age were the same as those of normal children at 4 years of age.[79] Assessment of mental development in these same children at 4 years of age yielded a mean I.Q. score of 93 on the Stanford Binet Intelligence Scale.[80] Delay in treatment and suboptimal control of blood phenylalanine concentration produced lower I.Q. than projected from parental I.Q. More recent programs with tighter control of plasma phenylalanine have improved overall outlook for normal I.Q.[50]

The semisynthetic nature of the phenylalanine-restricted diet has led to questions concerning its adequacy. Calculation of intake of major nutrients indicates that these amounts are adequate[81] when compared to the RDA. Balance studies of calcium, phosphorus, magnesium, and iron in 8 girls, 6 to 8 years of age, on Lofenalac suggested that magnesium may be inadequate to provide for optimal nutrition.[82] Our studies of plasma zinc, copper, and hair zinc in 15 treated patients 1 month to 7 years of age who were receiving Lofenalac imply that one-fourth to half the children may have subclinical zinc deficiency despite normal ingested zinc.[83,84] Studies of blood and/or plasma of children with PKU ingesting Phenyl-Free revealed low concentrations of chromium, selenium, and zinc.[85] Inadequate intake, poor absorption, or inefficient utilization may all be responsible. When Lofenalac is the protein source, the intake of vitamin E is sufficient to provide for normal plasma concentrations despite the high intake of polyunsaturated fatty acids.[86] Adequacy of niacin status in children on Lofenalac is questionable because of limited intakes of tryptophan and niacin and disturbances in tryptophan metabolism.[87]

Diet Discontinuation. Certain clinicians have suggested that the diet might be discontinued at 4, 6, or 12 years of age with no adverse effects.[88–90] Investigators have questioned this possibility because studies have shown significant differences in performance and intelligence in children who discontinued the diet at 6 years of age or older and those who remained on the diet.[30,91,92]

In studies using the same patient as his own control, elevated plasma phenylalanine concentrations prolonged the performance time on neuropsychologic tests of higher integrative function, reduced the mean power frequency of the electroencephalogram (EEG), and decreased urinary dopamine excretion and plasma L-dopa in older treated patients with PKU.[30,93] A correlation was found between high plasma phenylalanine concentration, prolonged performance time on the neuropsychologic tests, and decreased urinary dopamine in 10 patients.[30] In a study of eight additional patients, statistically significant decreases were found in the mean power frequency of the EEG and in plasma L-dopa when plasma phenylalanine increased.[93] EEG slowing occurred in PKU heterozygotes at concentration changes of blood phenylalanine that are induced by aspartame ingestion.[40] These effects were reversible and correlated in the reverse direction when plasma phenylalanine was reduced. Severe neurologic deterioration occurred in two off-diet PKU patients. Reversal of most of the symptoms was possible in the patient who returned to a strict diet.[39] Elevated plasma phenylalanine may be concentrated by the blood-brain barrier in neural cells and inhibit L-dopa and serotonin synthesis by competing for tyrosine hydroxylase and tryptophan hydroxylase.[94]

For the female with PKU, diet discontinuation poses special problems. Few women with PKU who have not been treated before and during pregnancy and who have carried the fetus to term have delivered normal infants. Congenital malformations, microcephaly, and retarded physical and mental growth are associated with in utero elevations of phenylalanine.[95] Active transport of amino acids by the placenta to the fetus leads to a fetal blood phenylalanine concentration two to three times that found in the maternal blood.[96] Such elevated fetal plasma phenylalanine concentrations may again be concentrated by the fetal blood-brain barrier. Intraneuronal phenylalanine at 600 μmol interferes with brain development by one or more of the several previously described mechanisms, including abnormal oligodendroglial migration and/or myelin and other protein synthesis.[97] Thus, it is extremely important to maintain normal plasma phenylalanine concentrations in the reproductive female before and after conception.

TYROSINEMIAS

Several known disorders of tyrosine metabolism (Table 67–15) may be amenable to nutrition support (see Fig. 67–1 and Table 67–2). Precise biochemical diagnosis is important because other disorders such as liver disease, scurvy, and prematurity may produce increases in blood tyrosine.

TABLE 67–15. INHERITED DISORDERS PRODUCING INCREASED PLASMA TYROSINE

DESIGNATION	ENZYME DEFECT	CLINICAL FEATURES
Neonatal tyrosinemia	p-OHPPA oxidase*	Prematurity (benign—?)
Tyrosinemia (type I)	Fumarylacetoacetate hydrolase	Cirrhosis, Fanconi syndrome, acute porphyria, (succinylacetone)
Tyrosinemia (type II)	Hepatic cytosol tyrosine amino transferase	Mental retardation and eye and skin disorders
Tyrosinosis (Medes)	Probably type I	Myasthenia (possibly acute prophyric attack)

*p-OHPPA oxidase is p-OH-phenylpyruvic acid oxidase. Variation in neonatal development alters the control of expression of this enzyme. Primary deficiency of p-OHPPA has not been confirmed.

Two well-recognized forms of hereditary tyrosinemia have been reported. Type I was thought to be due to a deficiency of *p*-hydroxyphenylpyruvic acid oxidase. More recently, secondary impairment in this enzyme has been attributed to a primary defect of hepatic fumarylacetoacetate hydrolyase with the production of an abnormal metabolite, succinylacetone.[98] Succinylacetoacetate and succinylacetone are formed from the accumulated substrate fumarylacetoacetate (see Fig. 67–1). Succinylacetone is extremely toxic and is associated with impaired active transport function and disordered hepatic enzymes, including *p*-OH-phenylpyruvic acid oxidase and δ-aminolevulinic acid dehydratase.[99] Decreased activity of both hepatic and erythrocyte δ-aminolevulinic acid dehydratase has been reported in these patients and is postulated as the mechanism by which acute porphyric-like episodes develop (Fig. 67–2).[100–102]

Type I tyrosinemia is characterized by generalized renal tubular impairment with failure to thrive, hypophosphatemic rickets, progressive liver failure, hypertension, episodic behavioral and peripheral nerve deficiencies, and elevated concentrations of blood phenylalanine and tyrosine.[103] This disease demonstrates an autosomal recessive mode of inheritance.

Tyrosinemia type II is characterized by greatly elevated concentrations of blood and urine tyrosine and by increases in urinary phenolic acids, N-acetyltyrosine, and tyramine. A deficiency of hepatic cytosolic tyrosine aminotransferase has been demonstrated.[103] An unusual set of symptoms is characterized by corneal erosions and plaques and bullous lesions. Persistent keratitis and hyperkeratosis occur on the fingers and palms of the hands and on the soles of the feet. These skin abnormalities respond to restriction of dietary phenylalanine and tyrosine. Intracellular crystallization of tyrosine is thought to cause these inflammatory responses. Mental retardation may occur. This disease is inherited via an autosomal recessive mode.

Neonatal tyrosinemia, associated with increased plasma and urinary concentrations of tyrosine and its metabolites, occurs in 0.2 to 10% of neonates.[103] Short-term protein restriction to 1.5 to 2.0 g/kg body weight per day has lowered plasma tyrosine concentrations in most patients within 4 weeks of life. Whether added ascorbate will stabilize and increase the activity of *p*-hydroxyphenylpyruvate oxidase in this disorder is not clear. Persistence of hypertyrosinemia in this disorder may lead to impaired mental function, and short-term diet and ascorbate therapy are indicated.[104]

DIAGNOSIS

Differential diagnosis is imperative for institution of appropriate therapy. Quantitation of plasma amino acids by ion exchange chromatography, and urinary organic acids by gas chromatography and mass spectrometry (GC/MS), are necessary approaches to diagnosis. The more severe type I tyrosinemia may not be detected by newborn screening using the bacterial inhibition assay because newborn blood tyrosine may not be above 8 mg/dl. Many newborn screening programs consider 440 μmol/L (8 mg/dl) within normal limits and do not retrieve these babies for further diagnosis. We routinely retest newborns with blood tyrosine above 220 μmol/L (4 mg/dl) if no other cause is clinically evident. If blood tyrosine is above 8 mg/dl at 14 days of age, we evaluate renal tubular and hepatic function as well as urine by organic acid analysis for the presence of parahydroxyphenyl acids and succinylacetone (Fig. 67–3). Prenatal diagnosis of type I hereditary tyrosinemia has been made by measurement of succinylacetone in amniotic fluid[105] and by measurement of fumarylacetoacetase activity in cultured amniotic fluid cells.[106]

TREATMENT

The objective of nutrition support for the hereditary tyrosinemias is to provide a biochemical environment that allows normal growth and development of intellectual potential and that prevents pathophysiologic changes. Plasma phenylalanine concentrations should be maintained between 40 and 80 μmol, and plasma tyrosine concentrations between 50 and 150 μmol. Plasma methionine should not be regulated by dietary means. Rather than restricting methionine below RDA, we follow plasma methionine as an index of S-adenosyl methionine transferase deficiency produced by liver damage.

Nutrition therapy of the hereditary tyrosinemias requires a firm diagnosis because the approaches to therapy between types I and II are different. The phenylalanine and tyrosine restriction is less severe and prognosis is excellent for type II. In type I, however, progressive liver and renal failure may occur as well as acute episodes of porphyria. Treatment of kidney impairment is also needed in type I tyrosinemia. Thus, generalized renal tubular failure may result in metabolic acidosis, hypophosphatemia, rickets, and hypokalemia unless replacement of bicarbonate, phosphate, 1,25-dihydroxycholecalciferol, and potassium is instituted. Rapid treatment of infections is required to prevent a "catastrophic" catabolic state with overproduction of succinylacetone.

Many of the "porphyric" symptoms may be due to overproduction of δ-aminolevulinic acid (ALA) secondary to the inhibitory effect of succinylacetone on ALA dehydratase and/or decreased heme biosynthesis (Fig. 67–2). Specifically, acute hypertensive crises, behavioral changes, and peripheral neuropathy abate with dietary control through high-carbohydrate feeds. Parenteral nutrition with 20 to 25% dextrose solutions may control these acute porphyric attacks.[107] Continued or progressive loss of energy-requiring functions that involve loosely bound heme to heme-proteins (plasma membrane transporters, cytochrome P-450) may be due to rapid turnover and insufficient heme biosynthesis (Fig. 67–2). Infusions of Hematin have produced transient decreases in δ-ALA and have improved acute attacks of intermittent porphyria.[108,109] We have successfully

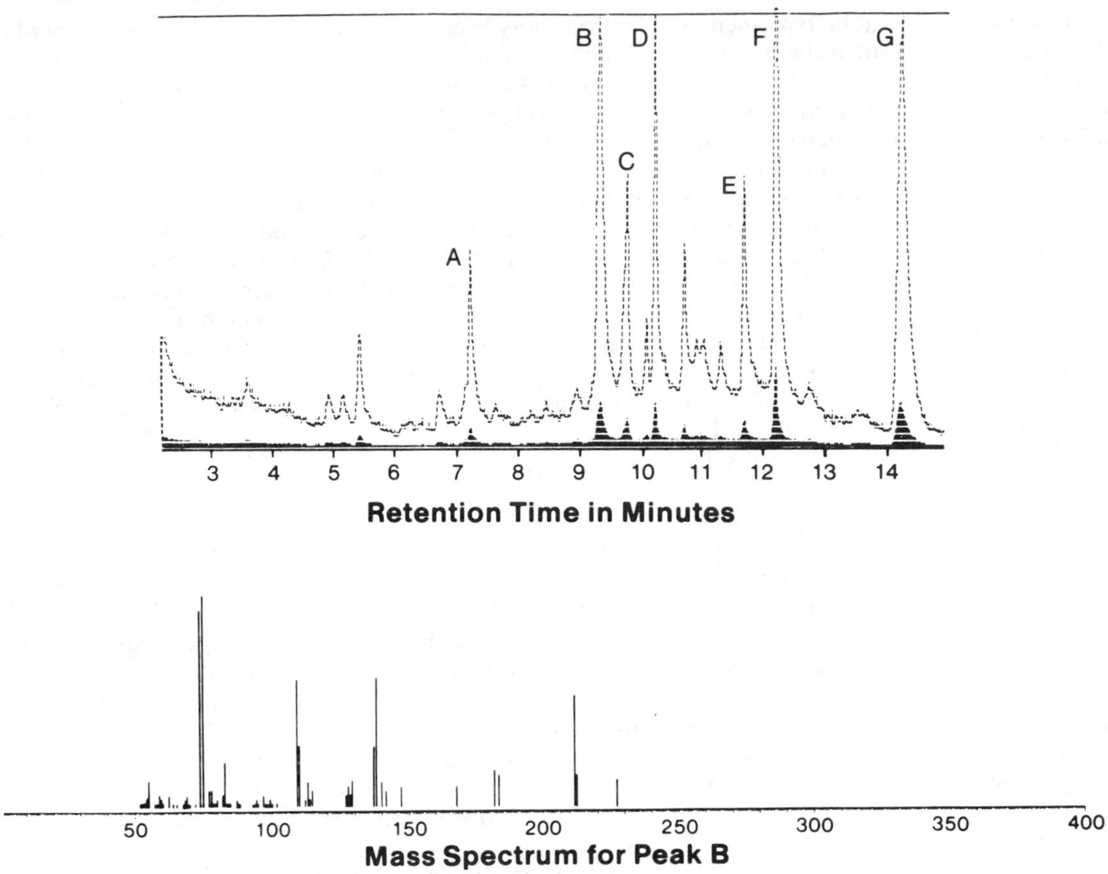

FIGURE 67–3. Chromatogram and mass spectrum of succinylacetone from urine of a patient with tyrosinemia type I. A volume of urine equivalent to 210 μg of creatinine was oximated with NaOH and hydroxyl amine hydrochloride. After acidification, organic acids were extracted, dried, and derivatized to their volatile silyl derivatives. Gas chromatography then separated organic acids by their mass (top panel). Labeled peaks were identified from the mass spectrum of their oximated o-methyl ester derivates and were: A, succinic acid; B, succinylacetone; C, α-ketoglutaric acid; D, p-OH-phenylacetic acid; E, p-OH phenyllactic acid; F, p-OH-phenylpyruvic acid; and G, tetracosane external standard. In the lower panel is the mass spectral analysis of peak B using a computer-integrated gas chromatography/mass spectroscopy system. This spectrum is identical to chemical standards for succinylacetone treated like the urine specimen with characteristic fragments of mass 227, 212, 138, 109, and 82. (Courtesy of the Division of Medical Genetics, Emory University, Atlanta, GA.)

aborted attacks and have prolonged intervals between attacks in two patients with this treatment. The efficacy of this therapy has recently been reported.[110] Long-term "cure," however, may require liver transplant not only to control metabolic homeostasis but also to prevent expected hepatoblastoma.[103,108]

Nutrition Requirements. When one is planning nutrition support for the infant or child with tyrosinemia, a formal prescription that recommends amounts of phenylalanine, tyrosine, protein, energy, and fluid for the day should be written. The prescription for phenylalanine and tyrosine is based on blood analyses correlated with intake that indicate the child's requirement and/or tolerance for each amino acid. Data in Table 67–5 describe amounts of amino acids, protein, energy, and fluid to offer as beginning therapy.

Because a large portion of phenylalanine is normally hydroxylated to form tyrosine,[111] phenylalanine must be restricted in the diet of patients with tyrosinemia. Phenylalanine requirements appear to be greater for children with tyrosinemia than for children with PKU. In general, the more distal the block is in the catabolic pathway, the more normal the amino acid requirement is. Tyrosine needs of children with tyrosinemia have been inadequately described[112] and will vary with the metabolic state of the child and the accumulation of succinylacetone.

Some investigators suggest that patients with type I tyrosinemia have decreased ability to metabolize methionine, whereas others believe that the elevated plasma methionine concentrations are secondary to liver damage.[103] Whatever the cause for hypermethioninemia, some have recommended methionine restriction when blood methionine concentrations are above 40 μmol in the absence of hepatocellular damage. Although the extent of methionine restriction to maintain normal blood methionine concentration is unknown, one recommendation is 50 mg/kg of body weight for a 15-month-old child.[113] L-Cysteine supplementation is also recommended for children with tyrosinemia type I, particularly if methionine restriction is implemented.[114]

Recommended protein intakes for infants and children with tyrosinemia are given in Table 67–5. Because the primary protein source used for the infant is either an L-amino acid mix or a casein hydrolysate, recommended intake is greater than for the normal infant.[55]

For tyrosinemia type I, high-carbohydrate feeds supplying 65 to 75% of kilocalories are recommended to suppress activity of δ-aminolevulinic acid synthase.[115–117] For the infant up to 2 years of age, 150 kcal/kg per day is a minimum need. We try to maintain greater than 100 kcal/kg per day throughout childhood.

Medical Foods Low in or Free of Phenylalanine and Tyrosine. Adequate protein cannot be obtained from natural foods without ingesting excess phenylalanine and tyrosine (proteins contain by mass 1.4 to 5.8% tyrosine). Thus, special medical foods are used in which there is little or no phenylalanine or tyrosine. Several medical foods are available to provide protein.[65–69] Sources and formulation of Analog XPHEN, TYR, Low Phe/Tyr Diet Powder, Maxamaid XPHEN, TYR and TYR 1 and TYR 2 are given in Tables 67–7 and 67–8. Their composition is given in Table 67–16. Formulation and composition of Analog XPHEN, TYR, and Maxamaid XPHEN, TYR are the same as for Analog XP and Maxamaid XP except for amino acids removed.

Low Phe/Tyr Diet Powder is an enzymatic hydrolysate of casein processed to remove most of the phenylalanine and tyrosine. Phenylalanine content is approximately 75 mg/100 g powder, and tyrosine content is less than 38 mg/100 g powder. Taurine (36 mg/100 g) has been added. Fat and carbohydrate as well as minerals and vitamins are included in appropriate amounts to meet most nutrient needs of infants. Chromium, molybdenum, and selenium are not added to Low Phe/Tyr Diet Powder.

Phenylalanine- and tyrosine-free TYR 1 and TYR 2 are formulated from L-amino acids, sucrose, minerals, and vitamins. These two products contain no fat, chromium, or selenium and only a small amount of sucrose.

The methionine content of Analog XPHEN, TYR, Low Phe/Tyr Diet Powder, Maxamaid XPHEN, TYR, TYR 1, and TYR 2 (Table 67–16) is too great for use alone if dietary methionine must be restricted. In such a situation, Analog XPHEN, TYR, MET, and Maxamaid XPHEN, TYR, MET (Table 67–16), which contain no phenylalanine, tyrosine, or methionine, could be used.

Serving Lists. Serving lists are available for the phenylalanine-tyrosine-restricted diet (Table 67–10).[68] Methionine content is given for each list in the event that methionine restriction is required for type I. Portion sizes of individual foods in each list are given in reference 68.

Initiation of Nutrition Support. The most rapid decline of blood tyrosine concentration at the time of diagnosis may be obtained by feeding a 20 kcal/ounce (67 kcal/dl) phenylalanine- and tyrosine-free formula with no added source of phenylalanine and tyrosine. Laboratory results of blood phenylalanine and tyrosine should be rapidly available or a deficiency of phenylalanine and tyrosine[118] could be precipitated. This condition is particularly undesirable in treating type I tyrosinemia because a catabolic phase with overproduction of succinylacetone will worsen the clinical state. Protein sources containing 20 to 70 mg phenylalanine and 60 to 80 mg tyrosine per kg of body weight per day are usually required after 3 to 4 days of total restriction in the newborn period.

Assessment of Nutrition Support. Frequency of assessment is dictated by the type of tyrosinemia and clinical course of the patient. In type I tyrosinemia, vital signs, height, weight, head circumference, neurologic examination, and development are documented weekly for the first 3 months, biweekly for the second 3 months, and monthly between 6 months and 1 year of life. Plasma amino acids are quantitated by ion exchange chromatography, succinylacetone and the parahydroxyphenyl organic acids by GC/MS. Additional laboratory studies include urinary δ-aminolevulinic acid, renal and liver function tests, blood and urine phosphate, potassium, and bicarbonate. Clinical status, dietary intake, and laboratory data should be monitored and correlated in managing type I tyrosinemia at intervals indicated previously.

Outcomes of Nutrition Support. Outcomes, to date, have been variable with type I tyrosinemia. Some of this "variation" is caused by the lack of clear diagnostic criteria in the past to delineate the various types of tyrosinemia. Early detection and diagnosis using GC/MS (Fig. 67–3), low-phenylalanine and -tyrosine, high-carbohydrate diets, hematin infusions, and the early replacement of renal tubular losses have brought some success in treating type I tyrosinemia. The low-phenylalanine, low-tyrosine diet has been successfully used in several patients with type II tyrosinemia with rapid resolution of clinical signs and symptoms.[103] Neonatal tyrosinemia requires early but transient protein restriction. Controlled outcome data are not yet available.

BRANCHED-CHAIN AMINO ACIDS

Disorders of branched-chain amino acid metabolism provide an interesting interface between clinical and fundamental science. Using the nutrition model of preventing mental retardation through screening and management of newborns, many rare experiments of nature have become available and have advanced our knowl-

TABLE 67–16. COMPOSITION OF "CHEMICALLY DEFINED" MEDICAL FOODS (PER 100 G OF PRODUCT) FOR TYROSINE RESTRICTED DIETS

NUTRIENT	ANALOG XPHEN, TYR	ANALOG XPHEN, TYR, MET	LOW PHE/TYR DIET POWDER	MAXAMAID XPHEN, TYR	MAXAMAID XPHEN, TYR, MET	TYR 1	TYR 2
Energy (kcal)	475	475	460	350	350	270	300
Protein equivalent (g)	13.0	13.0	15.0	25.0	25.0	47	63
Alanine (g)	0.64	0.65	0.68	1.25	1.28	2.40	3.10
Arginine (g)	1.13	1.15	0.56	2.21	2.23	2.00	2.70
Aspartic acid (g)	0.94	0.96	1.40	1.84	1.86	5.70	7.60
Carnitine (g)	0.010	0.010	0.009	NA	NA	NA	NA
Cystine (g)	0.42	0.43	0.06	0.82	0.83	1.40	1.80
Glutamic acid (g)	1.26	1.28	4.00	2.46	2.50	12.00	16.00
Glutamine (g)	0.11	0.11	NA	0.24	0.25	NA	NA
Glycine (g)	1.00	1.02	0.38	1.96	1.99	1.40	1.80
Histidine (g)	0.65	0.66	0.45	1.26	1.27	1.40	1.80
Isoleucine (g)	1.00	1.02	0.87	1.96	1.99	3.40	4.50
Leucine (g)	1.72	1.75	1.66	3.36	3.42	5.70	7.60
Lysine (g)	1.17	1.19	1.65	2.28	2.32	4.00	5.40
Methionine (g)	0.27	0	0.54	0.54	0	1.40	1.80
Phenylalanine (g)	0	0	0.075	0	0	0	0
Proline (g)	1.22	1.24	1.42	2.38	2.42	5.40	7.10
Serine (g)	0.75	0.76	0.94	1.46	1.49	3.00	4.00
Taurine (g)	0.019	0.019	0.027	NA	NA	NA	NA
Threonine (g)	0.84	0.86	0.78	1.64	1.68	2.70	3.60
Tryptophan (g)	0.34	0.34	0.20	0.66	0.67	1.00	1.40
Tyrosine (g)	0	0	<0.038	0	0	0	0
Valine (g)	1.10	1.12	1.38	2.14	2.18	4.00	5.40
Carbohydrate (g)	59.0	59.0	60.0	62.0	62.0	21	12
Fat (g)	20.9	20.9	18.0	0	0	0	0
Calcium (mg)	325	325	430	810	810	2,400	1,310
Chloride (mEq)	8.2	8.2	9.1	13	13	47.1	28.2
Chromium (μg)	15	15	NA	NA	NA	NA	NA
Copper (mg)	0.45	0.45	0.43	2.0	2.0	6.7	2.0
Iodine (μg)	47	47	32	134	134	230	120
Iron (mg)	7.0	7.0	8.6	12.0	12.0	34.0	15.0
Magnesium (mg)	34	34	50	200	200	520	156
Manganese (mg)	0.6	0.6	0.14	1.30	1.30	2.40	0.70
Molybdenum (μg)	35.0	35.0	NA	60.0	60.0	107.00	32.00
Phosphorus (mg)	230	230	320	810	810	1,860	1,010
Potassium (mEq)	10.7	10.7	12.0	22	22	59.8	34.1
Selenium (μg)	15	15	NA	NA	NA	NA	NA
Sodium (mEq)	5.2	5.2	9.6	25	25	46.4	27.8
Zinc (mg)	5.0	5.0	3.6	13.0	13.0	26.0	7.8
Vitamin A (μg RE)	530	530	432	300	300	2,790	1,560
D (μg)	8.5	8.5	7.2	12.0	12.0	25.0	32.8
E (mg α-TE)	3.3	3.3	9.7	4.4	4.4	22.8	12.1
K (μg)	21	21	72	NA	NA	167	167
Ascorbic acid (mg)	40	40	37	135	135	230	80
Biotin (mg)	0.026	0.026	0.036	0.12	0.12	0.100	0.300
B_6 (mg)	0.52	0.52	0.29	1.00	1.00	2.20	1.50
B_{12} (μg)	1.25	1.25	1.44	4.0	4.0	7.9	3.0
Choline (mg)	50	50	61	110	110	430	260
Folate (μg)	38	38	72	150	150	340	400
Inositol (mg)	100	100	22	56	56	500	300
Niacin (mg)*	4.5	4.5	5.8	12.0	12.0	54.0	24.0
Pantothenic acid (mg)	2.65	2.65	2.2	3.7	3.7	25.0	11.0
Riboflavin (mg)	0.60	0.60	0.43	1.20	1.20	4.00	2.00
Thiamin (mg)	0.50	0.50	0.36	1.1	1.1	2.70	1.40

*Preformed niacin

NA = none added

Note: Values listed, although accurate at the time of publication, are subject to change. The most current information may be obtained by referring to product labels.

edge concerning nutrition needs and metabolic utilization of leucine, isoleucine, and valine.[3]

BIOCHEMISTRY

The branched-chain amino acids isoleucine, leucine, and valine are essential nutrients. In the newborn 75% of the amounts ingested are used for protein synthesis. Those present in excess of need for synthetic purposes are degraded through many steps to provide energy (Fig. 67–4). The initial step in catabolism is reversible transamination, requiring a specific transaminase and the coenzyme, pyridoxal phosphate. The second step is irreversible oxidative decarboxylation, which uses the branched-chain α-keto acid dehydrogenase complex. This four-protein, three-enzyme complex is located on the inner mitochondrial membrane and requires the coenzymes thiamin pyrophosphate, lipoic acid, CoA, and NAD.[+119–123] Figure 67–4 schematizes this overall reaction, which is impaired in MSUD. cDNA clones for the transacylase protein (E2), E1 α and E1 β of the decarboxylase, and E3 of the multienzyme branched-chain α-keto acid dehydrogenase complex have been isolated from human cDNA expression libraries.[3,120]

Considerable progress is being made in cloning and chromosomal localization of these protein/genes. cDNA for E1 α is located on chromosome 19, E2 on chromosome 1, and E3 on chromosome 7. Although E1 β cDNA is now available, its chromosomal location is unknown.[3]

Elsas and Danner proposed a model for the role of thiamin in stabilizing the biologic turnover of the branched-chain α-keto acid dehydrogenase complex.[121] By increasing thiamin ingestion, intracellular thiamin pyrophosphate (TPP) is increased, and the TPP binding sites on the decarboxylase (E1 α) moiety of the branched-chain α-keto acid dehydrogenase complex become saturated. When these TPP binding sites are occupied, the multienzyme complex undergoes a conformational change making it more resistant to degradation. The biologic half-life of the enzyme and overall activity are increased when a new equilibrium of enzyme synthesis and degradation is reached. This model has been tested and is supported by both functional and structural studies[122–124] (Fig. 67–5).

BRANCHED-CHAIN α-KETOACIDURIA

Maple syrup urine disease (MSUD) is a group of inherited disorders of isoleucine, leucine, and valine metabolism.[3,125] These disorders result from several different mutations that impair branched-chain α-keto acid dehydrogenase (see Figs. 67–4 and 67–5). Although most mutant enzymes are immunologically present, one reported patient had absent branched-chain acyl transferase (E2) as a cause of thiamin-resistant MSUD.[119,126] An autosomal recessive mode of inheritance is defined for most of the reported cases, suggesting nuclear rather than mitochondrial genomic mutations. The cellular mechanism by which the products of these nuclear genes assemble as a multienzyme complex in mitochondria is a subject of considerable importance and current research effort.

Infants with MSUD appear normal at birth and are clinically well until after eating a protein-containing feed. The most severely impaired enzymes may produce seizures, apnea, and death within 10 days of birth. The disorder is characterized by elevated blood, urine, and cerebrospinal fluid concentrations of the branched-chain α-keto acids and their amino acid precursors. Progressive neurologic dysfunction and the production of fragrant urine with the odor of burnt sugar (caramel) or maple syrup follow. The sweet smell may only be evident in earwax, easily sensed after otoscopic examination. Neurologic impairment in the newborn is manifested by poor sucking, irregular respiration, rigidity alternating with periods of flaccidity, opisthotonos, progressive loss of Moro reflex, and seizures.

Several variants with a spectrum of impaired mitochondrial branched-chain α-keto acid dehydrogenase have been reported. Clinical manifestations are expressed intermittently upon protein loading or with febrile illness in patients with partial enzyme activity between 5 and 15% of normal.[3]

Untreated patients with classic MSUD who survive beyond early infancy have retarded physical and mental development.[5,6] Early diagnosis and therapy lead to normal growth and development. If death occurs in the first few days of life, few unique abnormalities are seen in the brain. With prolonged survival, deficient myelination is thought to be due to enzymes involved in myelin formation, inhibition of amino acid transport, and inhibition by branched-chain α-keto acids of oxidative phosphorylation.[3,5]

SCREENING

Because apnea and death may be the first clinical manifestations of the classic disorder, newborn screening, retrieval, diagnosis, and initiation of therapy are urgent, and all four processes must be completed within the first week of life. Nonselected screening of the newborn population is currently in progress (in some states) using bacterial inhibition assays for blood leucine concentrations.[43] Bedside screening in selected children uses the urinary dinitrophenylhydrazine (DNPH) reaction for branched-chain α-ketoaciduria. This reaction can also be used to monitor dietary progress. The incidence figure for MSUD based on international newborn screening appears to be about 1 in 216,000.[127] The incidence in Georgia, based on 5 years of newborn screening where 37% of newborns are black, is approximately 1 per 116,000 live births (see Table 67–3). Little information comparing frequency among ethnic groups is available, although some inbred communities have a high frequency.

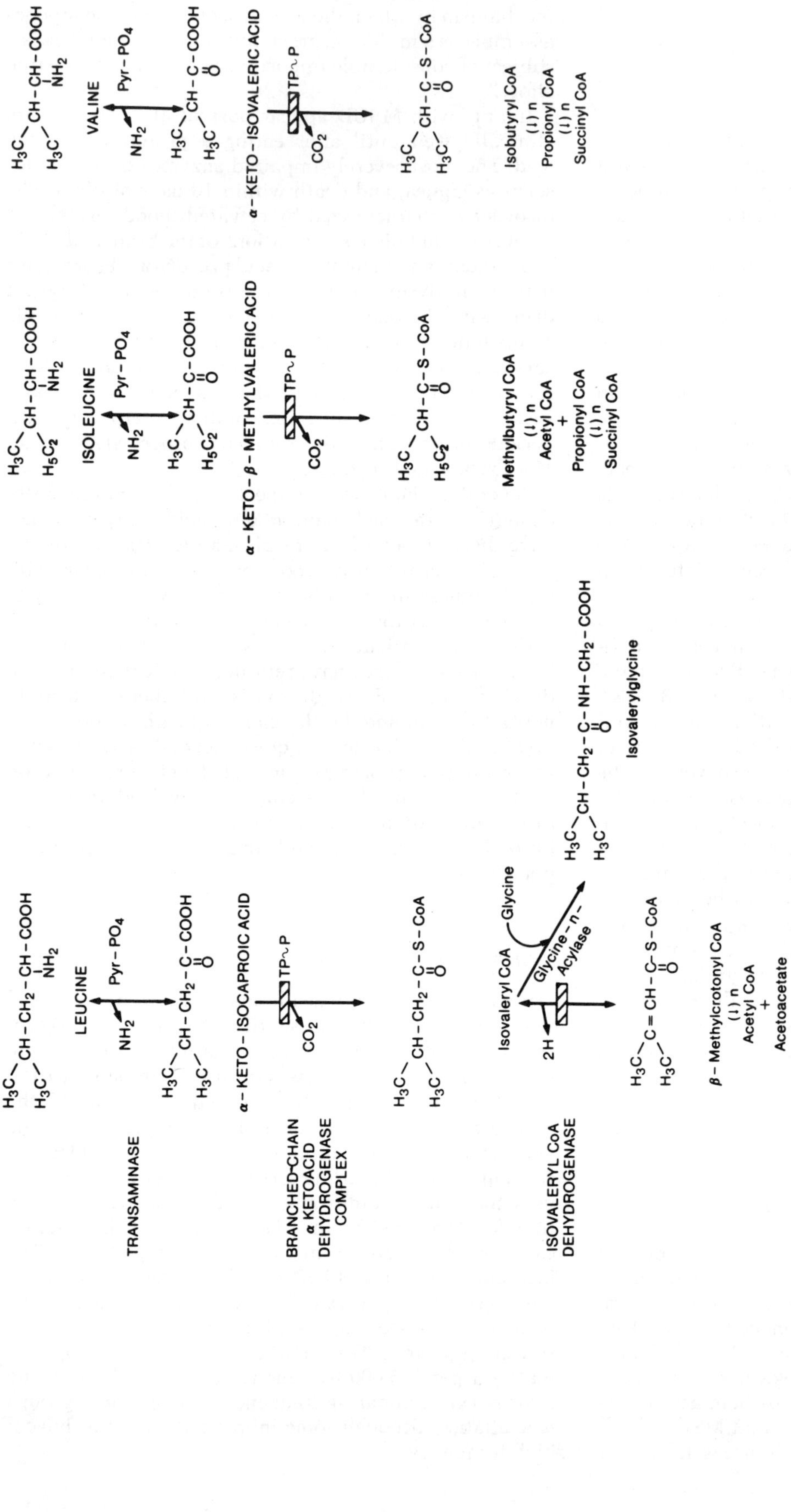

FIGURE 67–4. Catabolism of branched-chain amino acids. Crosshatch bars represent blocks in maple syrup urine disease (branched-chain α-keto acid dehydrogenase complex) and in isovaleric acidemia (isovaleryl CoA dehydrogenase). TP ~ P, the cofactor thiamin pyrophosphate; (n), several catalyzed intermediate steps.

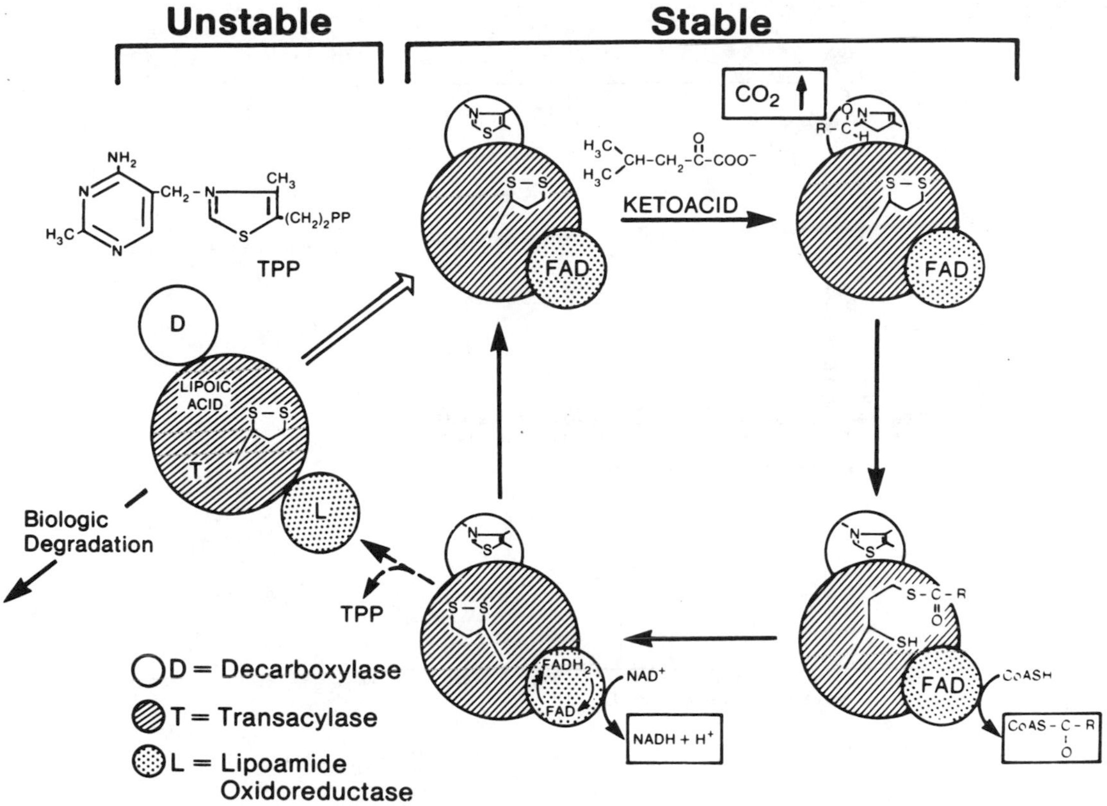

FIGURE 67–5. A model for the stabilization of the branched-chain α-keto acid dehydrogenase by thiamin pyrophosphate. The multienzyme complex branched-chain α-keto acid dehydrogenase has a configuration that is more stable to degradation when thiamin pyrophosphate (TPP) binding sites on its decarboxylase moiety are occupied. FAD and NAD, flavin and nicotinamide adenine dinucleotide.

DIAGNOSIS

Any infant with a blood leucine concentration higher than 4 mg/dl (305 μmol/L) on the newborn screening test should immediately be further evaluated. Most infants with the classic disease have greater than 8 mg/dl (610 μmol/L) leucine at 72 hours of age. Diagnosis is confirmed using ion exchange chromatography to quantitate plasma isoleucine, leucine, valine, and alloisoleucine, and GC/MS to identify urinary branched-chain α-keto acids (Fig. 67–6). The extent of enzyme impairment should be determined by rapid quantitative enzyme assay of peripheral lymphocytes, and therapy should be accordingly altered. Prenatal monitoring is available if the cellular phenotype is confirmed in fibroblasts cultured from the patient's skin.[128] In some families with severely impaired enzyme function, heterozygotes are also identifiable from enzymatic assays of cultured dermal fibroblasts.[126]

TREATMENT

Although hemodialysis with nitrogen-free dialysate[129,130] or exchange transfusion[131] may be required when diagnosis is delayed, if screening, retrieval, and diagnosis are completed within 8 to 10 days of life, this action is seldom necessary. Because hemodialysis superimposes iatrogenic risk and prolongs a catabolic phase, it is not recommended. Branched-chain amino acid-free orogastric feeding of protein and energy should be begun as soon as the diagnosis is made. The objective is to produce anabolism in the infant and thereby prevent accumulation of neurotoxic branched-chain α-keto acids. If orogastric feeding is not acceptable, gastrostomy or a central line for hyperalimentation with dextrose and lipid should be initiated for initial care of classic MSUD during the neonatal period. Except during illness, protein intake to 1.5 g/kg per day may be adequate therapy for those patients with 15% or more of enzyme activity.

Long-term therapy for MSUD is by means of diet. The objective of long-term nutrition support in the child with MSUD is to maintain plasma concentrations of branched-chain amino acids that will allow maximal development of intellect while supplying adequate energy, protein, and other nutrients for optimal growth. Plasma concentrations of branched-chain amino acids (3 to 4 hours after a meal) should be maintained between the following ranges: isoleucine, 40 to 90 μmol; leucine, 80 to 200 μmol; valine, 200 to 425 μmol.

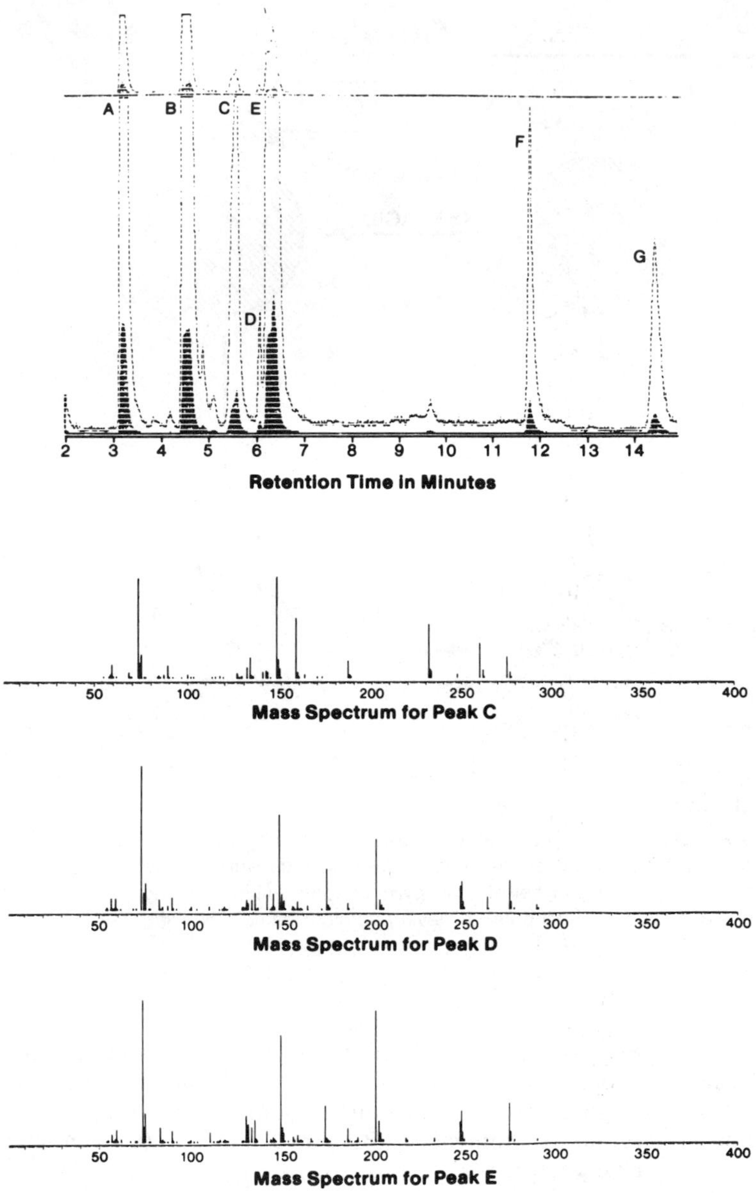

FIGURE 67–6. Chromatogram and mass spectrum of branched-chain α-keto acids in the urine of an untreated infant with maple syrup urine disease. The urine was oximated, extracted, derivatized, and chromatographed as described in Figure 67–3. Labeled peaks represent the following organic acids: A, lactic acid; B, 2-OH isovaleric acid; C, α-ketoisovaleric acid (KIC); D, α-keto-β-methylvaleric acid (KMV); E, α-ketoisocaproic acid (KK); F, is a combination of p-OH phenyllactic acid and the internal standard, pentadecanoic acid; and G, the external standard, tetracosane (C24). The mass spectra for peaks C, D, and E are in the lower half. Fragments of mass 275, 260, 232, 186, and 158 are characteristic of the trimethylsilyl derivative of KIV (C). The larger keto acids KMV and KIC differ from KIV by a larger fragment of mass 289 and a fragment of mass 246. They differ among themselves at fragments of mass 216, 143, 129, and 110 (compare spectrum for D and E). (Courtesy of the Division of Medical Genetics, Emory University, Atlanta, GA.)

The objectives of nutrition support are met through the use of a combination of medical foods (Table 67–17) and natural foods (Table 67–18). Most patients with MSUD who have the immunologic multienzyme complex will respond to oral thiamin administration of 100 to 1000 mg daily.[124,132] In classic MSUD, thiamin is only an adjunct therapy, and a diet restricted in isoleucine, leucine, and valine must also be given. Supraphysiologic amounts of oral thiamin should be added for at least a 3-month trial period because its mechanism is to stabilize the enzyme complex. Increased residual specific activity of mitochondrial membrane-bound enzymes may require this prolonged period owing to the duration of the biologic half-life of this subcellular organelle. During this period, decreased sensitivity to dietary branched-chain amino acids is usually observed, and more can be added to the diet.

Nutrient Requirements. Data in Table 67–6 outline the suggested amounts of branched-chain amino acids (BCAA), protein, energy, and fluid to offer the infant or child with MSUD. Because the BCAA are essential, they cannot be deleted from the diet without producing growth failure and death. In planning nutrition support of the infant or child with MSUD, a formal prescription should be written that includes recommended amounts of BCAA, protein, energy, and fluid for the day. Frequent adjustments in the diet prescription are necessary. Adjustments are needed daily during the first few weeks and biweekly during the first 6 months of life, based on appetite, growth, development, and laboratory analyses of plasma BCAA and α-keto acids. Because leucine residues are more prominent than isoleucine and valine in most proteins, supplemental L-isoleucine and L-valine as free amino acids may be necessary in the newborn period to prevent deficiency of these two essential amino acids. However, competition between the free BCAA at the intestinal cell can cause imbalances in plasma amino acids.[133]

Requirements for isoleucine, leucine, and valine vary considerably depending on age, growth rate, and extent of the enzyme deficit.[53] Younger infants normally have greater requirements per unit of body weight than older infants do. A rapid decline occurs in requirements for BCAA between birth and 3 to 6 months of age. Careful monitoring of plasma concentrations and intake of BCAA is required to prevent excess intake when growth rate declines.

The recommended protein intake for infants with MSUD (Table 67–6), after the initial acute period during which it is greater,[134] is slightly greater than that for normal infants and children because the primary protein source consists of L-amino acids.[55]

Recommended energy intakes, after the initial acute period, are the same as for normal infants and children but may vary considerably (see Table 67–6).[56] During the neonatal acute period, up to 170 kcal/kg per day may be required.[134]

Medical Foods Free of Branched-Chain Amino Acid. Adequate protein cannot be obtained from ordinary foods without ingesting more BCAA than are required in classic MSUD. The BCAA content of foods as a percentage of protein ranges from approximately 3.5 to 8.5%.[59–64] Because of the BCAA content of most proteins, special medical foods are used that are formulated from L-amino acids free of BCAA. In the United States, several products are available to provide protein.[65–69] Sources and formulations of these products are given in Tables 67–7 and 67–8. Composition is given in Table 67–17.

Analog MSUD, Maxamaid and Maxamum MSUD, MSUD Diet Powder, MSUD 1, and MSUD 2 are all formulated from L-amino acids. For a complete description of the Analog, Maxamaid, and Maxamum range of products see the earlier section on low-phenylalanine and phenylalanine-free chemically defined medical foods. MSUD Diet Powder contains fat, carbohydrate, minerals, and vitamins and is intended to be a complete formula except for the BCAA. However, the nitrogen-to-calorie ratio of MSUD Diet Powder is very low. This leads to inadequate nitrogen intake, especially when energy intake is low. L-Carnitine (8 mg/100 g) and taurine (36 mg/100 g) have been added to MSUD Diet Powder, but chromium, molybdenum, and selenium are not included. MSUD 1 and MSUD 2 contain, in addition to L-amino acids, a small amount of carbohydrate as well as minerals and vitamins. Fat, chromium, and selenium are not added.

Equivalent Lists. Equivalent lists of foods are available to provide variety and needed natural protein in the diet.[68] The lists are similar to diabetic exchange lists in that foods of similar content of leucine are grouped together and may be exchanged for one another within the same list. Average isoleucine, leucine, valine, protein, and energy contents of these lists are given in Table 67–18.

Initiation of Nutrition Support. A rapid decline of plasma isoleucine and valine can be achieved at the time of diagnosis by feeding formula free of BCAA. However, plasma leucine will continue to increase over the first 4 days of life even if dietary BCAA restriction is implemented at birth.[135] Most patients are not anticipated at birth, and infants whose screening results are positive are treated at 7 to 14 days of life. In our experience, branched-chain ketoacidosis can be averted by high caloric intake with no added BCAA over a 72-hour period if instituted between 8 and 11 days of age. There is an association among the degree of α-ketoisocaproic acid excretion, leucine elevations, and clinical outcome.[136] Laboratory results of plasma BCAA should be rapidly available to prevent the predicted deficiency in isoleucine and valine. When one is beginning replacement, these two amino acids may be added as free amino acids to increase their ratio to leucine in natural protein. High-energy intakes of 140 to 170 kcal/kg of body weight

TABLE 67–17. COMPOSITION OF "CHEMICALLY DEFINED" MEDICAL FOODS (PER 100 G OF PRODUCT) FOR BRANCHED-CHAIN AMINO ACID–RESTRICTED DIETS

NUTRIENTS	ANALOG MSUD	MAXAMAID MSUD	MAXAMUM MSUD	MSUD DIET POWDER	MSUD 1	MSUD 2
Energy (kcal)	475	350	340	470	280	310
Protein equivalent (g)	13.0	25.0	39.0	9.9	41	54
Alanine (g)	0.76	1.48	2.32	0.53	2.40	3.10
Arginine (g)	1.34	2.60	4.08	0.59	2.00	2.70
Aspartic acid (g)	1.12	2.17	3.40	1.38	5.70	7.60
Carnitine (g)	0.010	NA	0.019	0.009	NA	NA
Cystine (g)	0.49	0.96	1.51	0.30	1.40	1.80
Glutamic acid (g)	1.49	2.90	4.54	2.50	12.00	16.00
Glutamine (g)	0.11	0.28	0.44	NA	NA	NA
Glycine (g)	1.19	2.31	3.62	0.72	1.40	1.80
Histidine (g)	0.76	1.49	2.33	0.30	1.40	1.80
Isoleucine (g)	0	0	0	0	0	0
Leucine (g)	0	0	0	0	0	0
Lysine (g)	1.38	2.69	4.21	0.61	4.00	5.40
Methionine (g)	0.32	0.63	0.99	0.30	1.40	1.80
Phenylalanine (g)	0.90	1.75	2.74	0.66	2.40	3.20
Proline (g)	1.44	2.81	4.40	1.08	5.40	7.10
Serine (g)	0.89	1.73	2.71	0.72	3.00	4.00
Taurine (g)	0.019	NA	0.14	0.028	NA	NA
Threonine (g)	1.00	1.94	3.04	0.66	2.70	3.60
Tryptophan (g)	0.40	0.77	1.22	0.24	1.00	1.40
Tyrosine (g)	0.90	1.75	2.74	0.78	2.90	3.90
Valine (g)	0	0	0	0	0	0
Carbohydrate (g)	59.0	62.0	45.0	63	29	22.5
Fat (g)	20.9	0	0	20.0	0	0
Calcium (mg)	325	810	670	490	2,400	1,310
Choride (mEq)	8.2	13	16	10.5	47.1	28.2
Chromium (μg)	15	NA	50	NA	NA	NA
Copper (mg)	0.45	2.0	1.4	0.44	6.7	2.0
Iodine (μg)	47	134	107	33	230	120
Iron (mg)	7.0	12.0	23.5	8.9	34.0	15.0
Magnesium (mg)	34	200	285	52	520	156
Manganese (mg)	0.6	1.30	1.70	0.15	2.40	0.70
Molybdenum (μg)	35.0	60.0	110	NA	107.00	32.00
Phosphorus (mg)	230	810	670	270	1,860	1,010
Potassium (mEq)	10.7	22	18	12.5	59.8	34.1
Selenium (μg)	15	NA	50	NA	NA	NA
Sodium (mEq)	5.2	25	24	8.0	46.4	27.8
Zinc (mg)	5.0	13.0	13.6	3.7	26.0	7.8
Vitamin A (μg RE)	530	300	705	444	2,790	1,560
D (μg)	8.5	12.0	8	7.5	25.0	32.8
E (mg α-TE)	3.3	4.4	5.2	9.9	22.8	12.1
K (μg)	21	NA	70	74	167	167
Ascorbic acid (mg)	40	135	90	38	230	80
Biotin (mg)	0.026	0.12	0.14	0.037	0.100	0.300
B_6 (mg)	0.52	1.00	2.10	0.30	2.20	1.50
B_{12} (μg)	1.25	4.0	4.00	1.48	7.9	3.0
Choline (mg)	50	110	320	63	430	260
Folate (μg)	38	150	500	74	340	400
Inositol (mg)	100	56	86	22	500	300
Niacin (mg)*	4.5	12.0	13.6	5.9	54.0	24.0
Pantothenic acid (mg)	2.65	3.7	5.0	2.2	25.0	11.00
Riboflavin (mg)	0.60	1.20	1.40	0.44	4.00	2.00
Thiamin (mg)	0.50	1.1	1.40	0.37	2.70	1.40

*Preformed niacin
NA = none added
Note: Values listed, although accurate at the time of publication, are subject to change. The most current information may be obtained by referring to product labels.
(Data from references 65 to 69.)

TABLE 67–18. AVERAGE NUTRIENT CONTENT OF EQUIVALENT LISTS FOR BRANCHED-CHAIN AMINO ACID–RESTRICTED DIETS

FOOD LIST	ISOLEUCINE (MG)	LEUCINE (MG)	VALINE (MG)	PROTEIN (G)	FAT (G)	ENERGY (KCAL)
Breads/cereals	18	35	25	0.5	0	30
Fats	7	10	7	0.1	8	70
Fruits	17	25	22	0.6	0	75
Vegetables	22	30	24	0.6	0	15
Free foods A*	3	5	4	0.1	0	50
Free foods B	0	0	0	0	Varies	55

*Low-protein pastas and breads not included.

TABLE 67–19. DIET GUIDE FOR BRANCHED-CHAIN KETOACIDURIA (0 YEARS OF AGE)

NAME: MSUD
AGE: 0 yrs 0 mos
WEIGHT: 3.25 kg

PRESCRIPTION:	Total	Per Kg
Isoleucine—mg	163	50
Leucine—mg	228	70
Valine—mg	195	60
Protein—g	9.8	3.0
Energy—kcal	390	120

FORMULA #1	ILE	LEU	VAL	PRO	KCAL	AMOUNT
Analog MSUD	0	0	0	7.2	261	55 g
Isomil, concentrate	129	228	129	2.7	103	76 ml
Polycose Powder	0	0	0	0	29	1.25 ml
ILE (10 mg/ml)	34	0	0	0	0	3.4 ml
VAL (10 mg/ml)	0	0	66	0	0	6.6 ml
Volume						600 ml
TOTALS	163	228	195	9.9	393	

FORMULA #2	ILE	LEU	VAL	PRO	KCAL	AMOUNT
MSUD Diet Powder	0	0	0	7.6	362	77 g
Enfamil w/iron, concentrate	133	228	135	2.2	99	73.3 ml
ILE (10 mg/ml)	30	0	0	0	0	3 ml
VAL (10 mg/ml)	0	0	60	0	0	6 ml
Volume						600 ml
TOTALS	163	228	195	9.8	461	

should be given during this period to prevent the catabolism of body protein. If osmolality of formula permits, protein at 2.5 to 3.0 g/kg should be offered. This regimen will lower the concentrations of BCAA to near normal ranges. If deficiency of either isoleucine or valine occurs, plasma leucine concentrations will remain elevated as a function of muscle catabolism or decreased protein synthesis.

Diet guides for management of children with MSUD are listed in Tables 67–19 to 67–21. The leucine required at birth, 6 months, and 2 years may fall from 70 to 40 mg/kg per day. MSUD diet Powder and Analog MSUD can each be used, but to prevent deficiency of the essential amino acids isoleucine and valine solutions of these two BCAA are added back to the formula. As described in these sample diet guides this need persists over this 2-year developmental period.

Assessment of Nutrition Support. Frequency of assessment is dictated by the clinical course of the patient and the response of plasma amino acids. Monitoring of therapy should employ three combined approaches.

TABLE 67–20. DIET GUIDE FOR BRANCHED-CHAIN KETOACIDURIA (6 MONTHS OF AGE)

NAME: MSUD
AGE: 0 yrs 6 mos
WEIGHT: 6.5 kg

PRESCRIPTION:	Total	Per Kg
Isoleucine—mg	260	40
Leucine—mg	293	45
Valine—mg	273	42
Protein—g	16.3	2.5
Energy—kcal	715	110

FORMULA #1	ILE	LEU	VAL	PRO	KCAL	AMOUNT
Analog MSUD	0	0	0	12.4	451	95 g
Isomil, concentrate	116	203	116	2.4	92	68 ml
Polycose Powder	0	0	0	0	58	2.5 Tbsp
ILE (10 mg/ml)	87	0	0	0	0	8.7 ml
VAL (10 mg/ml)	0	0	86	0	0	8.6 ml
Volume						720 ml
Foods						
Breads/cereals	18	35	25	0.4	25	1 serving
Fruits	17	25	22	0.6	75	1 serving
Vegetables	22	30	24	0.6	15	1 serving
TOTALS	260	293	273	16.3	716	

FORMULA #2	ILE	LEU	VAL	PRO	KCAL	AMOUNT
MSUD Diet Powder	0	0	0	13.1	620	132 g
Enfamil w/iron, concentrate	154	264	156	2.6	115	85 ml
ILE (10 mg/ml)	84	0	0	0	0	8.4 ml
VAL (10 mg/ml)	0	0	93	0	0	9.3 ml
Volume						720 ml
Foods						
Vegetables	22	30	24	0.6	15	1 serving
TOTALS	260	294	273	16.3	750	

Ion exchange chromatography should be used daily to quantitate plasma amino acid concentrations for approximately 3 weeks after birth. The concentrations determine requirements for the individual BCAA.

Following establishment of requirements, quantitation of plasma amino acids is used approximately every 2 weeks to make sure the child has not "grown out" of the prescription. Samples should be obtained at midday before the noon feeding. We have found organic acid analysis of urine to be helpful (Fig. 67–6). Branched-chain α-keto acids decrease under optimum dietary conditions. If overrestriction of energy or a specific aminoacid occurs, evidence of β-lipolysis (acetoacetic acid, β-OH-butyric acid) is found.

After hospital discharge, daily testing of urine by a parent at home with dinitrophenylhydrazine (DNPH) is a rapid screen for ketoaciduria. As a rule "preventive" clinical evaluation of the child for cryptogenic infections before overt ketoacidosis occurs is more effective than trying to treat the child after a catabolic phase has produced its attendant ketoacidosis. If the urine DNPH results are positive, a blood sample should be collected on filter paper for assay of leucine and further analyzed by GC/MS. A physician should evaluate the child for infection or other causes of ketoacidosis. With a diet history, a physician's examination, and laboratory analyses, one can usually differentiate among overrestriction, intercurrent infection, or under-restriction of diet as a cause for branched-chain α-ketoaciduria. Weekly Guthrie tests and diet records are useful components in chronic management. Every effort should be made to maintain plasma BCAA in the normal range. Plasma leucine concentrations greater than 600 μmol are associated with clinically significant α-ketoacidemia and the appearance of ataxia.[5,136]

Episodes of infection bring about catabolism of tissue protein and an increase in plasma concentrations of BCAA. Clinical improvement is rapid if some BCAA are administered along with an amino acid mix that provides 150 to 200 kcal/kg per day. Parenteral amino acid

TABLE 67–21. DIET GUIDE FOR BRANCHED-CHAIN KETOACIDURIA (2 YEARS OF AGE)

NAME: MSUD
AGE: 2 yrs 0 mos
WEIGHT: 13.0 kg

PRESCRIPTION:	Total	Per Kg
Isoleucine—mg	455	35
Leucine—mg	520	40
Valine—mg	481	37
Protein—g	25.0	1.9
Energy—kcal	1300	100

FORMULA #1	ILE	LEU	VAL	PRO	KCAL	AMOUNT
Maxamaid MSUD	0	0	0	17.7	247	71 g
ILE (10 mg/ml)	149	0	0	0	0	15 ml
VAL (10 mg/ml)	0	0	93	0	0	9 ml
Volume						960 ml
Foods						
Breads/cereals	162	315	225	3.6	225	9 servings
Fats	49	70	49	0.7	490	7 servings
Fruits	51	75	66	1.8	225	3 servings
Vegetables	44	60	48	1.2	30	2 servings
Free Foods B	0	0	0	0.0	110	2 servings
TOTALS	455	520	481	25.0	1327	

FORMULA #2	ILE	LEU	VAL	PRO	KCAL	AMOUNT
MSUD Diet Powder	0	0	0	17.6	837	178 g
ILE (10 mg/ml)	162	0	0	0	0	16.2 ml
VAL (10 mg/ml)	0	0	92	0	0	9.2 ml
Volume						960 ml
Foods						
Breads/cereals	198	385	275	4.4	275	11 servings
Fruits	51	75	66	1.8	225	3 servings
Vegetables	44	60	48	1.2	30	2 servings
TOTALS	455	520	481	25.0	1367	

solutions free of BCAA have also caused a rapid decline in plasma BCAA during infection with a concomitant clinical improvement.[137]

Termination of Nutrition Support. Patients with classic MSUD are unable to terminate diet. The occurrence of death in variants with intermittent MSUD suggests the need for some form of ongoing therapy in even these relatively stable patients.[125] The branched-chain α-keto acids are relatively acute neurotoxins and probably interfere with oxygen consumption and adenosine triphosphate (ATP) production in the medullary reticular substance of the brain.[5,125]

ISOVALERIC ACIDEMIA

This disorder was first described by Tanaka in 1966 and was identified by the urinary excretion of isovaleric acid. Subsequently, a deficiency of isovaleryl-CoA dehydrogenase was defined. This enzyme is a mitochondrial flavoprotein and uses electron transfer factor (ETF). Although deficiency of ETF is also reported, mutations in the apoenzyme are specific for isovaleryl CoA as substrate. Deficiency of isovaleryl-CoA dehydrogenase results in a block in the catabolism of leucine at the next step after branched-chain α-keto acid dehydrogenase complex (see Fig. 67–4). Isovaleric acid, 3-hydroxyisovaleric acid, and the adduct isovalerylglycine accumulate in body fluids. Through gas-liquid chromatography (GC) and mass spectrometry (MS), these compounds are identified in body fluids (Fig. 67–7).

Isovaleric acid (IVA) is responsible for the sweaty-feet odor. Because IVA is a metabolite of leucine, a defect in the enzyme that was thought to oxidize the BCAA and straight-chain fatty acids with four to six carbons was suspected.[125] However, four major findings indicated the presence of an acyl-CoA dehydrogenase specific to isovaleryl-CoA, that is, isovaleryl CoA dehydrogenase: (1) an oral dose of 100 mg L-leucine per kg body weight caused

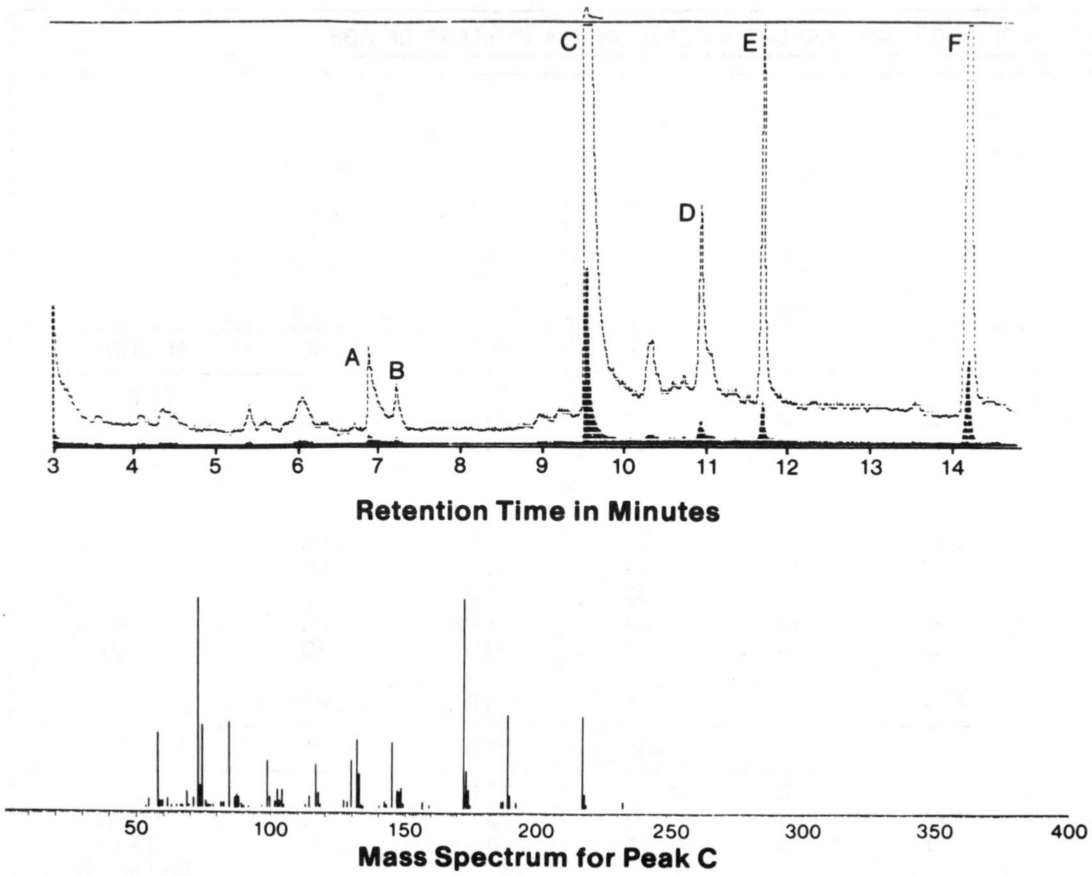

FIGURE 67–7. Chromatogram and mass spectrum of isovalerylglycine in the urine from a patient with isovaleric acidemia. This urine sample is from a stable 9-year-old girl with isovaleric acidemia who was receiving glycine supplements (see Fig. 67–8). The sample was not oximated but was extracted, dried, and derivatized with trimethylsilane as in Figures 67–3 and 67–6. A, urea; B, succinic acid; C, the monotrimethylsilyl derivative of isovalerylglycine; D, citric acid; E, the internal standard, pentadecanoic acid; F, the external standard, tetracosane. Below is the mass spectrum of C. Fragments of mass 231, 216, 189, 172, 116, 99, and 85 are characteristic of isovalerylglycine standards. (Courtesy of the Division of Medical Genetics, Emory University, Atlanta, GA.)

a 200-fold increase in serum IVA and only minimal elevations in β-methylcrotonic acid during remission; (2) similar oral loading tests with L-isoleucine and L-valine did not result in the accumulation of their corresponding short-chain fatty acid catabolites in the serum; (3) the ability of patients' leukocytes and cultured fibroblasts to oxidize [1-^{14}C] IVA to CO_2 in vitro was significantly impaired; (4) other short-chain fatty acids such as isobutyric, n-butyric, 2-methylbutyric, and n-hexanoic acids failed to increase during acidotic attacks or leucine-loading tests. Subsequently, the flavin-dependent dehydrogenase, isovaleryl-CoA dehydrogenase, was identified as the enzyme responsible for the specific oxidation of isovaleryl-CoA.[125]

Further investigation revealed the presence of N-isovalerylglycine and 3-hydroxyIVA as major metabolites in the urine of individuals with isovaleric acidemia. N-isovalerylglycine (IVG) was excreted consistently during remissions and ketotic attacks (Fig. 67–7). Unlike IVG, 3-hydroxyIVA is only present in significant amounts during ketotic attacks.[139] Several minor metabolites have also been identified in the urine of isovaleric acidemia patients including 4-hydroxyIVA, mesaconic acid, methylsuccinic acid, and 3-methylbutyrolactone.[140,141]

Analysis of numerous case reports of isovaleric acidemia has resulted in the classification of two different clinical presentations: the acute form and the chronic intermittent form.[115] Those patients with the acute form of isovaleric acidemia are generally normal full-term infants at birth. Within the first days of life, poor feeding, tachypnea, vomiting, and a characteristic "sweaty-feet" odor of the blood and urine are frequently noted. Diarrhea,[142] lethargy,[143] hypotonia, and tremors[144] may also be found. In some cases patients do not respond to treatment; they may become cyanotic or comatose, and death often results.[142–144] The exact cause of death is frequently unknown. Severe metabolic acidosis, hyperammonemia, central nervous system (CNS) hemorrhage, cardiac arrests, and sepsis are some probable causes. Those infants who respond to treatment and survive the neonatal period may develop appropriately and seem to progress into the chronic intermittent type of isovaleric acidemia.[125]

A second broad classification is the chronic intermittent form.[125] These babies generally are normal at birth. During late infancy they may develop episodes of vomiting, acidosis, stupor, and coma. A sweaty-feet odor is usually present, and a transient alopecia is occasionally seen. These episodes may begin as early as 2 weeks of age; the frequency of attacks seems to decrease with age. Urinary tract and upper respiratory infections frequently trigger these episodes, as do excessive intake of protein and aspirin. Many children affected by the intermittent form have a strong preference for fruits and vegetables over meat and milk, whereas others consume normal quantities of protein without problems. Although several patients have developed normally, some are mildly to severely retarded.

Several patients with either the acute or the chronic form of isovaleric acidemia have had moderate to severe hematologic abnormalities, including leukopenia and thrombocytopenia, with pancytopenia being the most common. This pancytopenia may be secondary to arrested maturation of hemopoietic precursors. In one instance, transfusion of packed red cells and platelets prevented further complications. Depressed hemoglobin levels were also seen in several patients. The occurrence of transient alopecia seems to be more common with the chronic intermittent form of the disease. Hyperammonemia (up to 814 μmol) has also been reported during acute attacks.

DIAGNOSIS

Because IVG is excreted during both remission and ketotic attacks, measurement of urinary IVG using GC/MS is the best method of diagnosis. Normal 3- to 5-year-old unaffected children have no detectable urinary IVG (less than 2 mg per day). Affected children of the same age excrete from 40 to 250 mg per day.[145] During ketotic episodes, urinary 3-hydroxyIVA, 4-hydroxyIVA, and methylsuccinic acids are excreted in large quantities as well.[140,141]

Diagnosis is confirmed by measuring the impaired ability of skin fibroblasts cultured from affected individuals to oxidize leucine-2-^{14}C to $^{14}CO_2$.[146] A more complicated assay using mitochondria and 1-^{14}C-isovaleric acid has also been used.[147]

Prenatal diagnosis is available by combined organic acid analysis of amniotic fluid and enzyme assay of cultured amniotic fluid cells. A heterozygote for isovaleryl-CoA dehydrogenase deficiency has been detected prenatally.[148]

The gene for isovaleryl dehydrogenase has been assigned to human chromosome 15 q12-q15.[125] To date however, specific mutations have not been identified.

TREATMENT

During acute ketotic attacks, parenteral fluid therapy and correction of the metabolic acidosis are indicated as adjuncts to high caloric intake and glycine therapy.[125] Serum IVA levels are monitored during ketotic attacks. GC/MS analysis is the most accurate means of determining serum and urinary IVA, which is an extremely volatile substance.[149] A special method of GC/MS allows separate quantitation of the two isomers, IVA and 2-methylbutyric acid.[149] Serum IVA will range from 0.1 to 84 mg/dl[148] depending on the patient's clinical status. A simple and rapid method of determining 4-hydroxyIVA levels in the plasma has recently been devised.[150] However, elevations in this metabolite lag at least 36 hours behind the maximum plasma level of IVA,[150] which limits its use clinically. Monitoring urinary IVG provides a good parameter of nutrition therapy. Titration of IVG with free glycine to a stable optimum is desirable. Excess glycine may inhibit IVG production (Fig. 67–8). When leucine restriction is optimal and the patient is stable, higher intake (300 to 600 mg/kg per day) of glycine may be necessary during infections or if dietary leucine restriction is not followed.

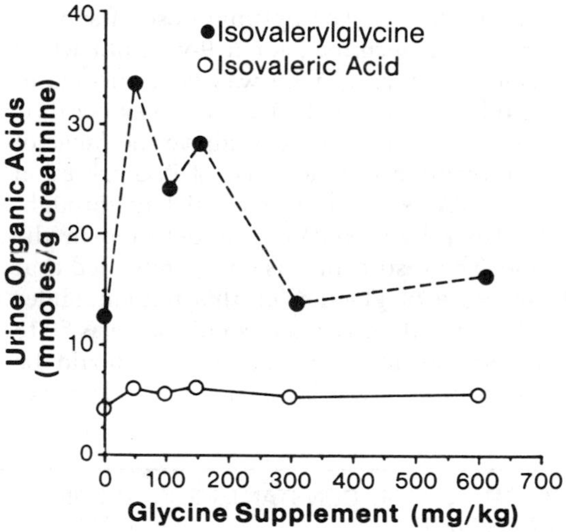

FIGURE 67–8. Effect of oral glycine supplement on isovalerylglycine production in stable isovaleric acidemia. The oral glycine supplements indicated on the abscissa were administered at weekly intervals to the patient in Figure 67–7 while she was maintained on a constant leucine-restricted diet. Isovalerylglycine (IVG) and isovaleric acid were quantitated by gas chromatography, as outlined in Figure 67–7. Symbols represent the mean of duplicate 24-hour urine samples collected over the last 2 days of each interval. Note the increase in IVG production at 50 to 150 mg/kg daily with decreased IVG production at 300 and 600 mg/kg daily of dietary glycine supplement. (Courtesy of Division of Medical Genetics, Emory University, Atlanta, GA.)

Nutrient Requirements. A low-protein diet of 1.2 to 1.5 g/kg per day in children less than 1 year of age improves clinical symptoms, and many patients restrict protein by choice.[125] This represents only 60% of the RDA. Total protein restriction is therefore not the best mode of therapy because over-restriction of essential branched chain aminoacids (Ile, Val) is inevitable if leucine is adequately restricted in natural food.

Leucine restriction and the use of pharmacologic doses of glycine have been reported. In six patients with isovaleric acidemia, glycine therapy resulted in decreased IVA in plasma and urine.[125] Urinary IVG simultaneously increased, often two to three times (see Figs. 67–5 and 67–8). Clinical improvement occurred that was characterized by increased growth, control of acidosis, and resolution of pancytopenia on glycine supplement and protein restriction over a 2-week period.

Glycine used to remove isovaleric acid through an alternative pathway is a prototype for nutritional detoxification of accumulated substrates in inborn errors of metabolism (see Fig. 67–5).[151,152] The ubiquitous enzyme glycine-N-acylase has a broad range of substrates (Table 67–22) that accumulate in other inborn errors of metabolism and might also be amenable to this approach. The relative amounts of glycine required to optimize removal of isovaleric acid (or other substrates for the glycine-N-acylase reaction) need careful evaluation and will change with the clinical condition of the patient.[152]

Some evidence exists for substrate inhibition of the reaction when excess glycine is added under stable conditions (see Fig. 67–7). The optimal dose of supplemental glycine was determined for a 9-year-old white girl with isovaleric acidemia who was well and maintained on an intake of leucine of 54 ± 3.6 mg/kg per day. Supplementation of glycine below or above the range of 50 to 150 mg/kg resulted in a decrease of IVG excretion by 50%. Urinary IVA excretion was consistent throughout the study. No β-hydroxylIVA was detected in the plasma or urine. The results of this study indicated that (1) the optimal dose of glycine for this patient under these stable clinical and nutritional conditions was 50 to 150 mg/kg, (2) an optimal dose of glycine should be quantitated for specific ages, clinical states, the degree of enzyme activity, and levels of leucine intake in the treatment of isovaleric acidemia, and (3) glycine supplements above 300 mg/kg per day increased plasma and urine concentrations of glycine, but resulted in decreased IVG excretion as if this substrate were inhibiting glycine-N-acylase when concentrations of its cosubstrate, isovaleryl CoA, were controlled.[152]

Systemic carnitine deficiency has been demonstrated in several patients with isovaleric acidemia.[153] Although plasma levels of carnitine were low in these patients, the acylcarnitine ester—that is, isovalerylcarnitine (IVC)—was increased, especially during illness.[153,154] Relative deficiency of muscle carnitine and use of carnitine as an adduct for isovaleric acid are two reasons for treating with extra L-carnitine. The relative therapeutic value of L-carnitine has been compared with that of glycine in the treatment of isovaleric acidemia in a 4 1/2-year-old black boy.[154] Administration of glycine plus leucine resulted in the excretion of more isovaleric acid as isovalerylglycine than when leucine was administered alone. Leucine plus L-carnitine increased isovalerylcarnitine excretion from a pretreatment level of 7 μmol per 24 hours to a post-treatment level of 1470 μmol per 24 hours. Large doses of carnitine are needed in the range of 100 to 200 mg/kg per day to accomplish this therapeutic excretion, whereas 100 to 150 mg/kg per day of glycine will suffice. Smaller doses of carnitine supplements are recommended to prevent "deficiency."

SULFUR-CONTAINING AMINO ACIDS

The biochemistry and nutrition requirements for sulfur-containing amino acids have been largely elucidated in humans by studies of inherited blocks in their metabolic pathways.

BIOCHEMISTRY

Natural protein contains approximately 0.3 to 5.0% methionine. Some dietary methionine is used by the body for tissue protein synthesis but the majority is

TABLE 67–22. KINETIC CONSTANTS FOR GLYCINE-N-ACYLASE FROM BOVINE LIVER

SUBSTRATE	K_M (10^{-4} M)	V_{MAX} (μmol/minute/mg protein)
Tiglyl-CoA	1.1	33.3
Isovaleryl-CoA	1.8	12.3
Benzoyl-CoA	0.09	10.4
2-Methylbutyryl-CoA	1.1	8.3
3-Methylcrotonyl-CoA	0.14	5.7
Propionyl-CoA	1.8	4.4
Acetyl-CoA	2.1	1.6

(From Barlett, K., Gompertz, D.: Biochem. Med., *10*:15, 1974, by permission.)

utilized through the trans-sulfuration pathway to form adenosylmethionine, adenosylhomocysteine, homocysteine, cystathionine, α-ketobutyrate, cysteine, and their derivatives (Fig. 67–9). The first step in the trans-sulfuration pathway is the synthesis of S-adenosylmethionine (SAM), a reaction catalyzed by methionine adenosyltransferase. In this reaction, the adenosyl portion of ATP is transferred to methionine. Biologically important compounds that obtain their methyl group from SAM include creatine, choline and phosphatidylcholines, methylated DNA and RNA, and epinephrine. Decarboxylated SAM is the source of the three carbon moieties of spermidine and spermine. S-adenosylhomocysteine is formed as an intermediary product in this pathway. S-adenosylhomocysteine is hydrolyzed to homocysteine. Homocysteine then has four possible pathways open to it. Homocysteine reacts with serine in the presence of cystathionine β-synthase, found in liver and brain, to form cystathionine (Fig. 67–9). Cystathionine β-synthase requires pyridoxal phosphate as a coenzyme.

Homocysteine can also be remethylated to form methionine through two different enzymatic reactions. In one reaction, the methyl group is derived from betaine

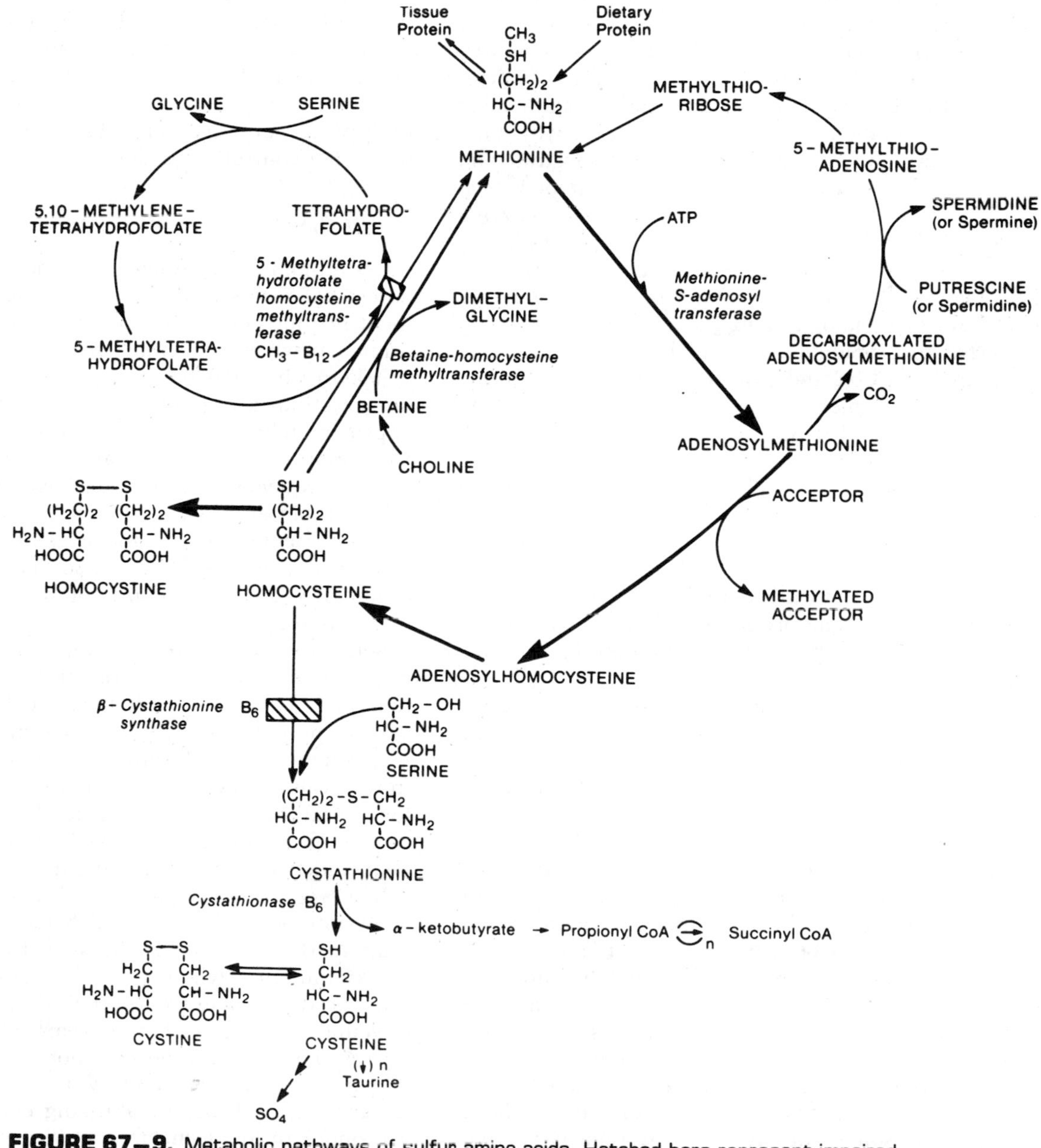

FIGURE 67–9. Metabolic pathways of sulfur amino acids. Hatched bars represent impaired reactions in two inherited metabolic disorders resulting in homocystinuria.

and is catalyzed by betaine-homocysteine methyltransferase. The second reaction requires N^5-methyltetrahydrofolate as a methyl donor and methylcobalamin (CH_3-B_{12}) as coenzyme (Fig. 67–9). The enzyme catalyzing this reaction is 5-methyltetrahydrofolate-homocysteine methyltransferase. Finkelstein and Martin used an in vitro system that approximated in vivo conditions in rat liver to measure the simultaneous product formation by the three enzymes that utilize homocysteine.[155] In this control system, 5-methyltetrahydrofolate homocysteine methyltransferase, betaine homocysteine methyltransferase, and cystathioniné β-synthase accounted for 27%, 27% , and 46%, respectively, of the homocysteine consumed.

The fourth pathway open to homocysteine is spontaneous oxidation to homocystine (Fig. 67–9). This reaction occurs only when homocysteine is present in tissue in abnormal amounts. It is essentially irreversible because the disulfide bond of homocystine is covalent. Homocystine is not further metabolized. Cystathionine β-synthase metabolizes most homocysteine with high affinity to cystathionine using serine as cosubstrate and pyridoxal phosphate as coenzyme. Cystathionine is then hydrolyzed to cysteine and α-ketobutyrate. The enzyme cystathionase, which also utilizes pyridoxal phosphate as coenzyme, is required for this reaction (Fig. 67–9). A deficiency of cystathionase results in cystathioninuria, which has no pathologic consequence. α-Ketobutyrate is converted to propionyl CoA, which is carboxylated to methylmalonyl CoA and isomerized to succinyl CoA, a Krebs-cycle intermediate. L-Cysteine is catabolized to pyruvate, NH_3, and H_2S.

HOMOCYSTINURIA

One of several genetically determined errors of methionine metabolism that produces defects in function of cystathionine β-synthase or 5-methlytetrahydrofolate-homocysteine methyltransferase may result in homocystinuria. Impaired activity of the latter enzyme may be caused by failure to synthesize methylcobalamin from vitamin B_{12} or by a deficiency in 5, 10 methylenetetrahydrofolate reductase. Several different defects impair the uptake, transfer, and conversion of dietary vitamin B_{12} to methylcobalamin.[15,16,156]

The most common form of homocystinuria is caused by a deficiency of cystathionine β-synthase. The mutant enzymes are now being chemically characterized, and one deletion of 60 amino acid residues has been reported.[157] Severely impaired enzyme function produces accumulation of plasma homocyst(e)ine and methionine and decreased cyst(e)ine in cells and physiologic fluids. If this biochemical circumstance is not treated early in life, skeletal changes, dislocated lenses, intravascular thromboses, osteoporosis, malar flushing, and, in some patients, mental retardation will occur.

The skeletal changes and dislocated lenses are presumably due to a structural defect in collagen formation produced by α-homocystine interaction with aldose groups on collagen.[156] Intravascular thromboses may occur at any age and have been found in coronary, renal, carotid, and intracranial arteries. Fifty percent of untreated patients die before 20 years of age, and 95% before 50 years of age.[158] The natural history of homocystinuria due to cystathionine β-synthase deficiency has been clarified in a large series of patients.[159] Heterozygosity for homocystinuria may predispose patients to the development of premature occlusive arterial disease.[160]

It is not known to what degree the mental retardation seen in homocystinuria is due to a metabolic sequela, such as deficient cystathionine in myelin formation, or is a result of multiple small cerebrovascular thromboses. In a series of 84 patients, half were of average intelligence, several were university graduates, and one held a Ph.D.[158] Mental deficiency may occur with severely impaired cystathionine β-synthase as a consequence of multiple cerebral-arteriolar obstructions if homocystinemia is not controlled by diet.

SCREENING

Cystathionine β-synthase deficiency is inherited as an autosomal recessive disease. Accurate estimates of the incidence for homocystinuria are not available, but in limited newborn screening, figures varying from 1 in 36,000 to 1 in 330,000 have been found.[156] Screening for homocystinuria in Georgia has yielded an incidence of approximately 1 per 257,299 live births (see Table 67–3). Homocystinuria occurs in many ethnic groups, but has a higher frequency in persons of Irish extraction than in other ethnic groups.[156] This finding may be a bias of ascertainment because of the original description of and continued screening for this disorder in the Irish population. Worldwide screening for homocystinuria is not yet available.

Selective screening uses the inexpensive urinary nitroprusside reaction. In this reaction, reduced homocysteine and cysteine form a stable red color with nitroprusside if present in excessive amounts. This selective screening test for sulfur amino acids should be included in the evaluation of any patient with an unknown cause for arterial thrombosis, dislocated lens, or mental retardation. The test is also positive in cystinuria and should be included as a screen for patients with nephrolithiasis.

In a large survey of patients with homocystinuria due to cystathionine β-synthase deficiency, only 13% were vitamin B_6 responsive.[159] Most of these patients were "leaky mutants" who had residual cystathionine β-synthase activity and expressed their disease in adolescence or young adulthood rather than early childhood. Vitamin B_6 responsivity may be common to all mutations in which some enzyme activity is present because the mechanism is through stabilizing enzyme turnover.[156] The more residual enzyme activity present, the more dramatic the response to vitamin B_6. Hypermethioninemia may not be present in the newborn if the activity of cystathionine β-synthase is greater than 15%.

DIAGNOSIS

Positive results to a screen by bacterial inhibition assay for methionine or urinary nitroprusside reaction should be followed by assay of plasma amino acids using ion exchange chromatography. With a cystathionine β-synthase defect, homocystine, cysteine-homocysteine, and methionine are all elevated in plasma. Normal or low plasma methionine concentrations are associated with homocystinuria due to decreased remethylation pathways (Fig. 67–9). Demonstration of significantly decreased cystathionine β-synthase, CH_3-B_{12}, or homocysteine methyltransferases is necessary to confirm the diagnosis and to implement appropriate therapy. Methionine may be elevated in the absence of homocystinemia in liver disease and in specific impairment of S-adenosylmethionine methyltransferase. By contrast, in defects of homocysteine remethylation to methionine, methionine is low whereas homocysteine concentrations are elevated. Thus, disorders of cobalamin methylation to CH_3-B_{12} or the two homocysteine methyltransferases will not be detected by nonselective newborn screening that only discriminates elevated blood methionine.

Management of these rare forms of homocystinuria does not include methionine-restricted diets. Rather, pharmacologic amounts of vitamin B_{12}, folate, or choline are added depending on the primary defect. Liver biopsy specimens, transformed lymphoblasts, or cultured skin fibroblasts express cystathionine β-synthase and are used to confirm the most common cause of homocystinuria. Prenatal diagnosis has been accomplished.[156,159] "Leaky mutants" should be suspected later in life when unexplained arterial thrombosis, mental retardation, or dislocated lens is encountered.

TREATMENT

Objectives of nutrition support in homocystinuria vary according to the age at which diagnosis is made and the type and degree of enzymatic impairment. If homocystinuria is due to cystathionine β-synthase deficiency expressed in the newborn, the clinical objectives are (1) to prevent the development of skeletal and ocular abnormalities, (2) to prevent intravascular thromboses, and (3) to assure normal intellectual development.

Pharmacologic doses of pyridoxine should be tried in all patients with hypermethioninemia and homocystinemia.[17,159] Trials of 1 g of oral pyridoxine daily should be given to determine its effects on plasma methionine and homocysteine levels. Because enzyme stabilization is the most common mechanism of vitamin responsivity, weeks may be required for a biochemical response to occur. If the plasma methionine and homocysteine concentrations are reduced, the amount of pyridoxine should be gradually lowered until the minimum dose required to maintain biochemical normality is reached. Doses of 25 to 750 mg per day have been required for some patients.[17] Excess vitamin B_6 for prolonged periods may cause peripheral neuropathy[161] and liver injury[162]; consequently, if vitamin B_6 is not helpful, it should be discontinued. Betaine supplements (6 g daily) will assist in maintaining postprandial plasma homocysteine concentrations in the near-normal range in vitamin B_6–responsive individuals.[163]

Patients who do not respond to pyridoxine will require a methionine-restricted diet supplemented with L-cysteine. L-cysteine becomes an essential amino acid in homocystinuria (Fig. 67–9). If plasma folate concentrations are below normal owing to excess use in remethylating homocysteine to methionine, folate should be added as a supplement.

Nutrient Requirements. In prescribing and implementing nutrition care plans for infants and children with homocystinuria due to cystathionine β-synthase deficiency, one must consider energy, protein, methionine, cysteine, folate, vitamins B_6 and B_{12}, betaine, and fluid needs. Younger infants have a greater methionine requirement per kilogram of body weight than older infants. Suggested daily methionine intakes range from 50 mg/kg in the young infant to 5 mg/kg in the 15- to 19-year-old. Suggested beginning energy, protein, methionine, and fluid intakes for infants and children of different ages are given in Table 67–6. If the medical food provides more than 20 kcal/ounce, extra fluid should be offered between feedings to prevent dehydration.[20]

Calcium cystinate, a soluble form of L-cysteine, should supplement the methionine-restricted diet at all ages. The young infant should be offered 300 mg/kg body weight. This amount may be decreased to 200 mg/kg at 6 months of age and 100 mg/kg at 3 years of age and thereafter. The calcium cystinate should be mixed with the chemically defined low-methionine or methionine-free formula to provide even distribution throughout the day.

Low-Methionine and Methionine-Free Chemically Defined Medical Foods. Several medical foods have been developed as protein sources for patients with homocystinuria.[65–69] These include Analog XMET, Low Methionine Diet Powder, Maxamaid and Maxamum XMET, HOM 1, and HOM 2. For a complete description of the Analog, Maxamaid, and Maxamum range of products, see the section on low-phenylalanine and phenylalanine-free chemically defined medical foods. Sources and formulation of these products are given in Tables 67–7 and 67–8. Composition is given in Table 67–23. Low Methionine Diet Powder, a soy protein isolate that contains carbohydrate, fat, minerals, and vitamins, is relatively high in methionine: 138 mg/100 g powder. Taurine (31 mg/100 g) is added. HOM 1 and HOM 2 are formulated from L-amino acids, minerals, and vitamins and are free of methionine, fat, chromium, and selenium.

TABLE 67–23. COMPOSITION OF "CHEMICALLY DEFINED" MEDICAL FOODS (PER 100 G OF PRODUCT) FOR METHIONINE-RESTRICTED DIETS

NUTRIENTS	ANALOG XMET	HOM 1	HOM 2	LOW METHIONINE DIET POWDER	MAXAMAID XMET	MAXAMUM XMET
Energy (kcal)	475	280	300	520	350	340
Protein equivalent (g)	13.0	52	69	15.5	25.0	39.0
Alanine (g)	0.59	2.40	3.10	0.60	1.16	1.81
Arginine (g)	1.04	2.00	2.70	0.99	2.04	3.16
Aspartic acid (g)	0.87	5.70	7.60	1.74	1.70	2.64
Carnitine (g)	0.01	NA	NA	0.01	NA	0.02
Cystine (g)	0.39	2.50	3.40	0.14	0.75	1.18
Glutamic acid (g)	1.16	12.00	16.00	3.00	2.27	3.54
Glutamine (g)	0.11	NA	NA	NA	0.22	0.32
Glycine (g)	0.93	1.40	1.80	0.62	1.81	2.82
Histidine (g)	0.60	1.40	1.80	0.36	1.16	1.81
Isoleucine (g)	0.93	3.40	4.50	0.71	1.81	2.82
Leucine (g)	1.59	5.70	7.60	1.18	3.10	4.85
Lysine (g)	1.08	4.00	5.40	0.93	2.10	3.30
Methionine (g)	0	0	0	0.16	0	0
Phenylalanine (g)	0.70	2.40	3.20	0.76	1.37	2.14
Proline (g)	1.12	5.40	7.10	0.76	2.19	3.43
Serine (g)	0.69	3.00	4.00	0.68	1.35	2.12
Taurine (g)	0.019	NA	NA	0.31	NA	0.14
Threonine (g)	0.78	2.70	3.60	0.50	1.52	2.38
Tryptophan (g)	0.31	1.00	1.40	0.19	0.61	0.95
Tyrosine (g)	0.70	2.90	3.90	0.53	1.37	2.14
Valine (g)	1.01	4.00	5.40	0.71	1.97	3.09
Carbohydrate (g)	59.0	18	5	51.0	62.0	45.0
Fat (g)	20.9	0	0	28.0	0	0
Calcium (mg)	325	2,400	1,310	480	810	670
Chloride (mEq)	8.2	47.1	28.2	12.2	13	16
Chromium (μg)	15	NA	NA	NA	NA	50
Copper (mg)	0.45	6.7	2.0	0.48	2.0	1.4
Iodine (μg)	47	230	120	52	134	107
Iron (mg)	7.0	34.0	15.0	9.7	12.0	23.5
Maganesium (mg)	34	520	156	56	200	285
Manganese (mg)	0.6	2.40	0.70	0.13	1.30	1.70
Molybdenum (μg)	35.0	107.00	32.00	NA	60.0	110
Phosphorus (mg)	230	1,860	1,010	380	810	670
Potassium (mEq)	10.7	59.8	34.1	16.1	22	18
Selenium (μg)	15	NA	NA	NA	NA	50
Sodium (mEq)	5.2	46.4	27.8	8.0	25	24
Zinc (mg)	5.0	26.0	7.8	4	13.0	13.6
Vitamin A (μg RE)	530	2,790	1,560	483	300	705
D (μg)	8.5	25.0	32.8	8	12.0	8
E (mg α-TE)	3.3	22.8	12.1	10.8	4.4	5.2
K (μg)	21	167	167	81	NA	70
Ascorbic acid (mg)	40	230	80	42	135	90
Biotin (mg)	0.026	0.100	0.300	0.04	0.12	0.14
B_6 (mg)	0.52	2.20	1.50	0.32	1.00	2.10
B_{12} (μg)	1.25	7.9	3.0	1.61	4.0	4.00
Choline (mg)	50	430	260	40	110	320
Folate (	38	340	400	80	150	500
Inositol (mg)	100	500	300	24	56	86
Niacin (mg)*	4.5	54.0	24.0	6.5	12.0	13.6
Pantothenic acid (mg)	2.65	25.0	11.0	2.4	3.7	5.0
Riboflavin (mg)	0.60	4.00	2.00	0.48	1.20	1.4
Thiamin (mg)	0.50	2.70	1.40	0.40	1.10	1.4

*Preformed niacin

NA = none added

Note: Values listed, although accurate at the time of publication, are subject to change. The most current information may be obtained by referring to product labels.

(Data from references 65 to 69.)

Serving Lists. Methionine may be provided for the young infant through the addition of specified amounts of evaporated milk or proprietary infant formula to the low-methionine or methionine-free medical foods. As growth and development proceed, solid foods should be added at the usual ages. Methionine requirement is small, and most foods contain moderate amounts in relation to requirement.[65–69] Because of this, the amount of solid food that can be ingested is small. To provide variety to the methionine-restricted diet, serving lists have been prepared.[68] Average methionine, cystine, protein, and energy contents of these lists are given in Table 67–24.

Diet guides for children aged 0 to 2 years apply these principles in Tables 67–25 through 67–27. Prescriptions for methionine in a patient nonresponsive to vitamin B_6 will fall from 35 mg/kg per day in the newborn period to 10 mg/kg per day. Newborn requirements are met by either Analog XMET with added proprietary infant formula or Low-Methionine Diet Powder. Both require L-cysteine supplement. One-year-olds and older will use Maxamaid XMET, but additional L-cysteine will still be needed.

Assessment of Nutrition Support. Following introduction of diet and stabilization, plasma methionine and cysteine concentrations should be monitored twice weekly until 3 months of age. Weekly monitoring is suggested until 6 months of age and twice monthly thereafter if blood methionine levels are stable. Following a diet change, plasma methionine and cysteine should be measured after 3 days have elapsed. A 3-day record prior to each blood sample is necessary to evaluate plasma methionine and cysteine. Plasma methionine should be maintained between 15 and 30 μmol in fasting plasma.[112] Little or no homocystine should be present in blood and urine. Growth and development as well as clinical evaluation of the pulses, skeletal growth and development, and ocular lenses are routinely assessed clinically.

Results of Nutrition Support. In a retrospective study of 629 patients with cystathionine β-synthase deficiency, methionine restriction initiated neonatally prevented mental retardation, slowed the rate of lens dislocation, and reduced the incidence of seizures.[159] Pyridoxine treatment of late-detected vitamin B_6–responsive patients decreased the rate of thromboembolic events.

Termination of Nutrition Support. Most clinicians who treat individuals with homocystinuria believe that patients should be kept on the diet indefinitely. Termination of diet after growth is achieved may lead to thromboembolisms and ciliary muscle laxity with lens dislocation. Where initiation or maintenance of nutrition support is not possible, acetylsalicylic acid (1 g daily) and dipyridamole (100 mg daily) increase platelet survival time and decrease thrombotic events.[164]

REPRODUCTIVE PERFORMANCE

For both men and women, fewer conceptions are reported for patients who do not respond to vitamin B_6 than for patients who do. Offspring of male patients do not suffer excess losses and are generally reported to be normal. A study showed that higher rates of fetal loss occurred in presumptive heterozygous fetuses carried by cystathionine β-synthase–deficient mothers than occurred in normal women.[159] Whether hypermethioninemia, homocysteinemia, or other metabolic variations in methionine metabolism are teratogenic is as yet unclear, but a teratogenic mechanism as defined for "maternal PKU" is possible.

AMMONIA

Nutrition management of disorders involving ammonia fixation and urea production use all the traditional rules for treating inborn errors of metabolism; restricting toxic precursor, adding deficient product, and encouraging alternative pathways for nitrogen excretion are three essential rules to follow. Additionally, the biologic variation imparted on ammonia fixation and the urea cycle by heritable mutations has greatly increased our understanding of the normal physiology, biochemistry, and molecular biology of these complex functions.

TABLE 67–24. AVERAGE NUTRIENT CONTENT OF SERVING LISTS FOR METHIONINE-RESTRICTED DIETS

FOOD LIST	METHIONINE (MG)	CYSTINE (MG)	PROTEIN (G)	FAT (G)	ENERGY (KCAL)
Breads/cereals	20	20	1.2	0	55
Fats	2	0	0.1	2	25
Fruits	5	5	0.5	0	60
Vegetables	10	8	1.0	0	20
Free foods A*	1	1	0.2	0	50
Free foods B	0	0	0	Varies	55

*Low-protein pastas and breads not included.

TABLE 67–25. DIET GUIDE FOR HOMOCYSTINURIA (0 YEARS OF AGE)

NAME: Homocystinuria
AGE: 0 yrs 0 mos
WEIGHT: 3.3 kg

PRESCRIPTION:	Total	Per Kg
Methionine—mg	115	35
Cystine—mg	975	300
Protein—g	9.9	3.0
Energy—kcal	390	120

FORMULA #1	MET	CYS	PRO	KCAL	AMOUNT
Analog XMET	0	164	5.5	200	42 g
Similac w/iron, concentrate	114	28	4.3	194	142 mL
L-Cys (10 mg/mL)	—	780	—	—	78 mL
Volume					600 mL
TOTALS	114	972	9.8	394	

FORMULA #2	MET	CYS	PRO	KCAL	AMOUNT
Low Methionine Diet Powder	115	104	11.5	385	74 g
L-Cys (10 mg/mL)	0	200	0	0	20 mL
Polycose Powder	0	0	0	8	1 tsp
Volume					600 mL
TOTALS	115	304	11.5	393	

TABLE 67–26. DIET GUIDE FOR HOMOCYSTINURIA (6 MONTHS OF AGE)

NAME: Homocystinuria
AGE: 0 yrs 6 mos
WEIGHT: 6.5 kg

PRESCRIPTION:	Total	Per Kg
Methionine—mg	98	15
Cystine—mg	1300	200
Protein—g	16.2	2.5
Energy—kcal	715	110

FORMULA #1	MET	CYS	PRO	KCAL	AMOUNT
Analog XMET	0	359	12.0	437	93 g
Similac w/iron, concentrate	63	16	2.4	107	79 ml
Polycose Powder	0	0	0	35	1.5 Tbsp
L-Cys (10 mg/ml)	0	890	0	0	89 ml
Volume					720 ml
Foods					
Breads/cereals	20	20	1.2	55	1 serving
Fruits	5	5	0.5	60	1 serving
Vegetables	10	8	0.1	20	1 serving
TOTALS	98	1298	16.2	714	

BIOCHEMISTRY

Normally, ammonia is converted to urea in the liver through the Krebs-Henseleit cycle (Fig. 67–10). The first two enzymes of the cycle and N-acetylglutamate synthetase are mitochondrial. N-acetylglutamate synthetase catalyzes the conversion of acetyl-CoA plus glutamate to N-acetylglutamate, an essential cofactor for carbamylphosphate synthesis. Carbamylphosphate synthetase I catalyzes the conversion of ammonia, ATP, and bicarbonate to carbamylphosphate. Ornithine transcarbamylase carboxylates ornithine, forming citrulline. Citrulline

TABLE 67–27. DIET GUIDE FOR HOMOCYSTINURIA (2 YEARS OF AGE)

NAME: Homocystinuria
AGE: 2 yrs 0 mos
WEIGHT: 13 kg

PRESCRIPTION:	Total	Per Kg
Methionine—mg	139	10
Cystine—mg	1950	150
Protein—g	25.0	1.9
Energy—kcal	1300	100

FORMULA #1	MET	CYS	PRO	KCAL	AMOUNT
Maxamaid XMET	0	472	15.8	220	63 g
L-Cys (10 mg/ml)	0	1360	0	0	136 ml
Sugar	0	0	0	288	6 Tbsp
Volume					960 ml
Foods					
Breads/cereals	80	80	4.8	220	4 servings
Fats	10	0	0.5	125	5 servings
Fruits	20	20	2.0	240	4 servings
Vegetables	20	16	2.0	40	2 servings
Free Foods B	0	0	0	165	3 servings
TOTALS	130	1948	25.1	1298	

is exported from mitochondria to the cytoplasm where it combines with aspartate to form argininosuccinic acid, a reaction catalyzed by argininosuccinic acid synthetase. Fumarate is cleaved from argininosuccinic acid by argininosuccinic acid lyase, yielding arginine. Urea is then formed by the action of arginase, regenerating ornithine, which is transported back into the mitochondria.

UREA CYCLE ENZYME DEFICIENCIES

Disorders of the urea cycle are a heterogeneous group of inherited defects in ureagenesis.[165] These disorders may result from impairment of one of six enzymes, three of which occur in the mitochondria and three of which occur in the cytosol (hatched bars in Fig. 67–10). With the exception of ornithine transcarbamylase (OTC) deficiency, all have an autosomal recessive mode of inheritance. OTC deficiency is inherited as an X-linked dominant trait that is usually lethal in males.[165]

Hyperammonemia is a biochemical manifestation characteristic of all disorders of the urea cycle. Other biochemical characteristics of each defect follow: Carbamylphosphate synthetase I defect causes decreased plasma citrulline; OTC deficiency results in orotic aciduria and X-linked patterns of transmission; argininosuccinate synthetase deficiency is associated with increased plasma citrulline accompanied by orotic aciduria; argininosuccinate lyase deficiency causes increased argininosuccinate in plasma and urine; and arginase deficiency has increased arginine in plasma and urine. Clinical features in the newborn suggestive of urea cycle defects occur with protein ingestion. In increasing order of severity, these defects include poor feeding, vomiting, lethargy, hypotonia or spasticity, irritability, respiratory distress, convulsions, and coma. Mental retardation occurs in survivors, but successful control of hyperammonemia in the newborn may prevent this sequela.

VARIABILITY OF EXPRESSION

Hyperammonemia and its clinical sequelae of vomiting, lethargy, and coma relate to excessive protein intake or catabolism and are observed in all the defects. However, the biochemical and phenotypic manifestations differ in the individual enzyme deficiencies. In argininosuccinate lyase deficiency a specific hair abnormality, trichorrhexis nodosa, is evident (Fig. 67–11). This condition is related to arginine deficiency and the relatively high arginine content of normal hair protein. Hair reverts to normal with arginine supplementation (Fig. 67–11). In patients with defects of the first four enzymes, arginine deficiency has also been associated with progressive degeneration of the central nervous system, with control of hyperammonemia through protein restriction alone.[166]

Within each enzyme defect there is a spectrum of clinical manifestations ranging from death in the newborn period to cyclical vomiting and migraine in adolescence. For example, the typical male with OTC deficiency has less than 5% activity and dies in the neonatal period. A surviving male child with a variant form of OTC deficiency shows decreased affinity for ornithine, a shift of pH optimum, and 25% of normal activity under physiologic conditions.[167]

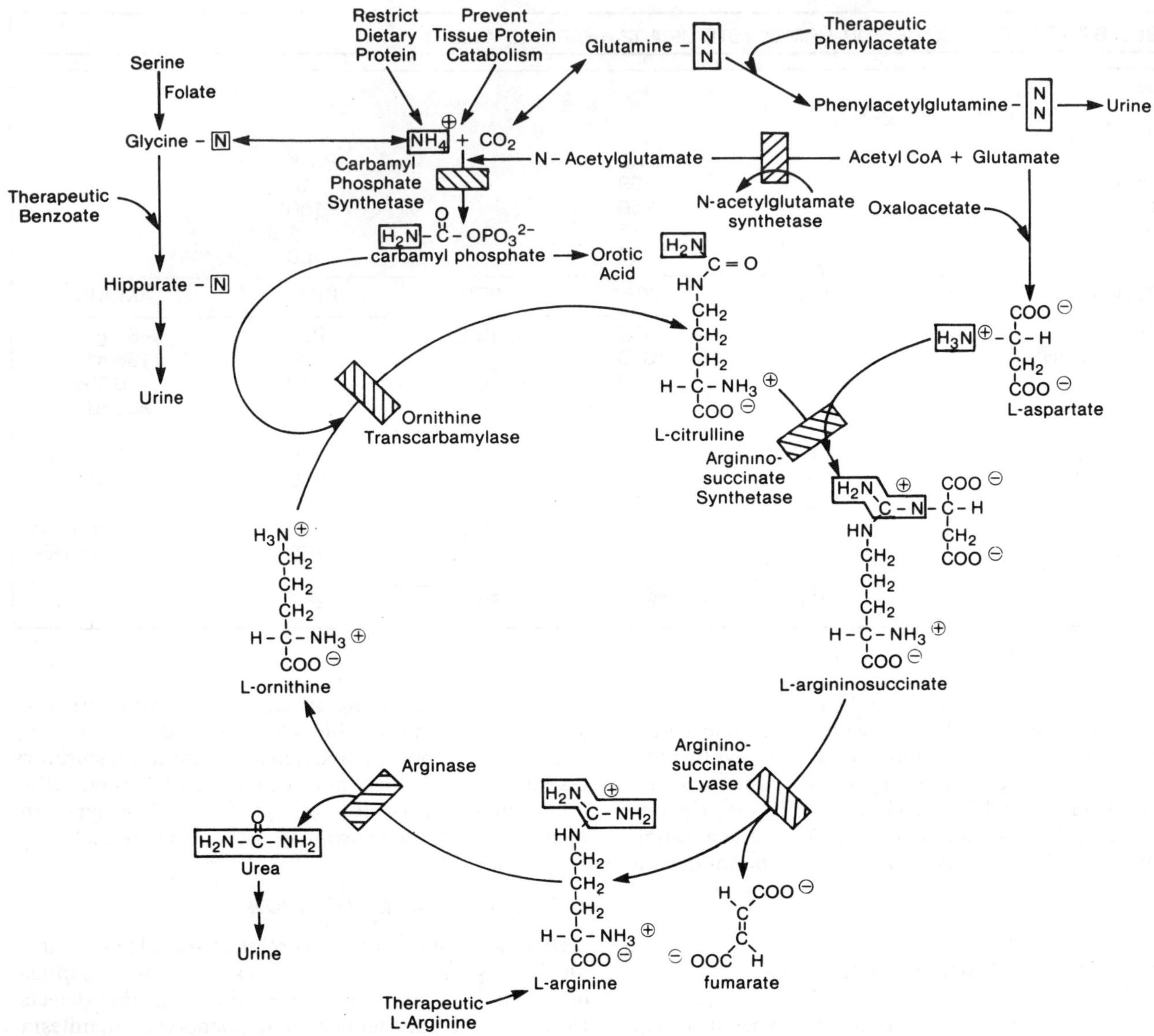

FIGURE 67–10. Inborn errors in the urea cycle and nutrition approaches to their management. Ammonia fixation and urea production are metabolically cycled with inherited blocks producing hyperammonemia indicated by hatched bars. Important nitrogen molecules and their biochemical origins are outlined in boxes. Mitochondrial enzymes in urea synthesis are carbamylphosphate synthetase, N-acetylglutamate synthetase, and ornithine transcarbamylase. The use of benzoate and phenylacetate is indicated to provide alternate pathways for nitrogen excretion. The addition of dietary arginine is to provide urea cycle substrate distal to genetically impaired reactions. Restriction of dietary protein and addition of dietary energy to prevent protein catabolism are also indicated.

Enzymatic evidence for genetic heterogeneity comes from kinetic studies in fibroblasts of patients with argininosuccinic acid synthetase deficiency. A study showed that enzymes from patients all showed decreased binding of citrulline and/or aspartate, but the residual argininosuccinic acid synthetase had a distinct and different curve of activity in each patient.[168] In a case of argininosuccinic acid lyase deficiency, the enzyme was defective in the liver but not in the brain and kidney, suggesting that more than one gene may be responsible for the activity of this enzyme.[169]

The genes for all six urea cycle enzymes have been cloned, and specific mutations have been identified for many.[165,170] The cytosolic enzyme argininosuccinate synthetase has multiple pseudogenes, requiring that mRNA be used from patients in northern blots to

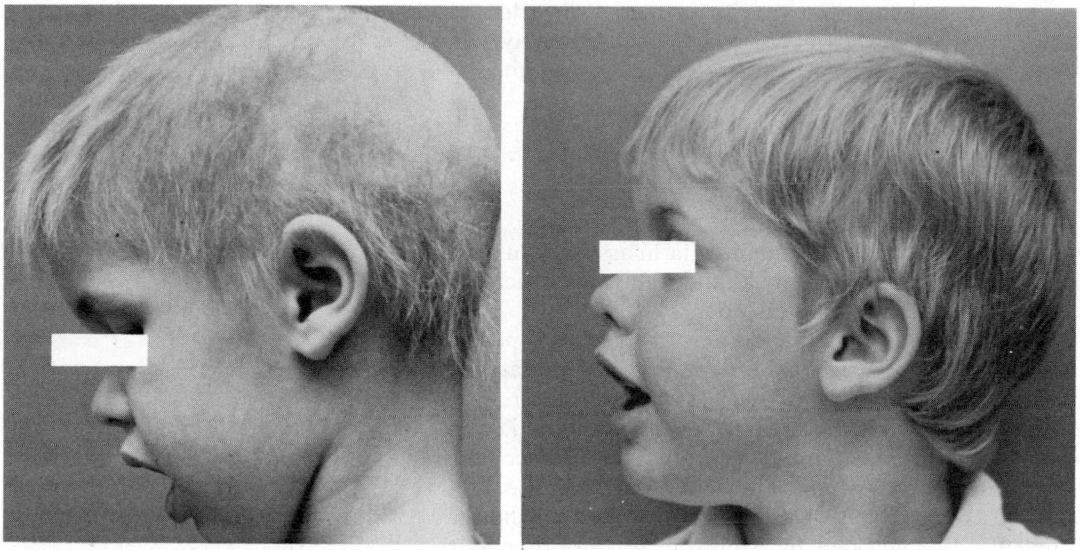

FIGURE 67–11. Effect of arginine on hair growth in argininosuccinic aciduria. A 6-year-old boy with hyperammonemia, trichorrhexis nodosa, and developmental delay was diagnosed with argininosuccinic aciduria. *A*, Before diet therapy he had diffuse, brittle hair. *B*, Six months later, while receiving 350 mg/kg per day arginine, he had luxuriant blond hair and his first haircut. (Courtesy of P. Fernhoff, Division of Medical Genetics, Emory University, Atlanta, GA.)

evaluate mutations leading to citrullinemia. This technique identifies the expressed transcripts by hybridization with the cDNA probe and digestion with S1 nuclease.[171,172] Several different types of abnormal mRNA have been defined in citrullinemia.[172] In OTC deficiency, mutations are found that produce immunologically absent mitochondrial protein in addition to variation in enzyme function. Regulation of the mechanisms involved in mitochondrial import of this nuclear-coded X-linked protein is under current intensive study.[173,174] Arginase may have differing genetic origins in kidney, liver, and brain.[175] Molecular analysis of this autosomal gene (or genes) is also under investigation. A syndrome known as HHH, for hyperammonemia, homocitrullinemia, and hyperornithinemia, may be caused by defective ornithine transport by mitochondria.[176]

EXPRESSION OF THE HETEROZYGOUS STATE FOR OTC DEFICIENCY

The heterozygous state of OTC deficiency may be characterized by mild protein intolerance manifested clinically by migraine in adults and by cyclic vomiting in children.[177] A grandmother and a mother of two children with OTC deficiency suffered from migrainous attacks and voluntarily avoided high-protein foods. Ammonium chloride tolerance tests were done, and within 4 hours both women developed nausea and headache, and their plasma ammonium levels rose to three times normal.

When protein or ammonium chloride loads were administered to 15 children with migraine and cyclic vomiting, 9 had abnormally high baseline plasma ammonium levels. The tests produced marked hyperammonemia in 8; 6 developed migraine symptoms. Of 7 girls with cyclical vomiting subjected to enzyme assay, 3 had deficient activity of ornithine transcarbamylase.[177] Heterozygous females with OTC deficiency may be asymptomatic or as severely affected as hemizygous males.[178]

SCREENING

Nonselected screening of all newborns for urea cycle disorders is routinely conducted only in Massachusetts.[179] A report shows that with the use of a bacterial auxotroph that required arginine, nine of 700,000 newborn tests were found to be homozygous-affected or heterozygous for argininosuccinate lyase deficiency.[179] Selective screening tests for disorders of the urea cycle are available.[180–184] One method for selective screening for hyperammonemia in the newborn nursery requires only one drop of blood, can be performed at the bedside, and gives results in 15 minutes.[183] This method can be readily adopted in offices and hospitals for selective screening.

The incidence of hyperammonemia in an institutionalized mentally retarded population was studied.[184] Thirty female patients with a history of protein intolerance out of a population of 6000 were evaluated; of 21 for whom ammonia level was reported, 17 were abnormally high. Unfortunately, enzyme diagnoses were not completed and artifactual elevation of blood ammonia due to contamination with feces, nail polish, and tobacco smoke was not considered. The true incidence of disorders of ureagenesis is not known, but genetic variation may well remain undiagnosed as causes of idiopathic mental retardation.

DIAGNOSIS

The presence of hyperammonemia in association with other appropriate biochemical and clinical characteristics suggests a urea cycle disorder.[165,185]

The enzyme defect can be inferred from the specific metabolite in addition to ammonia that accumulates in blood and urine: orotic acid in the urine in OTC deficiency; and citrulline, argininosuccinic acid, and arginine in the plasma and urine in argininosuccinate synthetase, argininosuccinate lyase, and arginase deficiencies, respectively. Carbamylphosphate synthetase deficiency is suggested by exclusion of the other four enzymopathies. Hyperammonemia can also be caused by acute or chronic liver diseases, Reye's syndrome, asparaginase treatment, propionic acidemia, hyperlysinemia, hyperornithinemia, isovaleric acidemia and methylmalonic aciduria, and FreAmine II solution exposure in infants. Definitive diagnosis depends on biochemical and enzymatic assays in addition to adequate clinical history.[185]

TREATMENT

The treatment of inherited urea cycle enzymopathies can be divided into short- and long-term therapy.[186]

Short-Term Therapy. Hemodialysis may be useful in the presence of coma in reducing plasm ammonium levels.[187] Peritoneal dialysis for 7 days in a male neonate with OTC deficiency removed 50 times more ammonia than a single exchange transfusion did.[188] However, peritoneal dialysis includes risks such as Candida peritonitis and continued catabolism. If dialysis is used, parenteral L-arginine and Ucephan should begin as well. We prefer to begin orogastric perfusion with high caloric intake (150 kcal/kg per day) but no protein. Protein-Free Diet Powder is useful for this approach (see Tables 67–7, 67–8, and 67–14). L-Arginine (350 to 500 mg/kg per day) should be added to this formulation. Sodium benzoate (300 mg/kg per day) can successfully reduce acute hyperammonemia in the neonatal period. Phenylbutyric acid or phenylacetic acid (550 mg/kg per day) is also given to form phenylacetylglutamine, which is excreted in the urine, eliminating from the body two nitrogen atoms per molecule (see Fig. 67–10).[189] Addresses and telephone numbers of suppliers of these compounds are given in Table 67–28. Urine potassium loss is enhanced by the excretion of hippurate and phenylacetylglutamine. Consequently, plasma potassium levels should be monitored and supplements should be given if needed. A priority of newborn therapy is to "force" the neonate into an anabolic phase with high-calorie feeds. Peripheral venous hyperalimentation with 10 to 20% glucose and lipid (2 to 4 g/kg) may be necessary if gavage is tolerated. As gavage feeds are increased, peripheral alimentation should be decreased. After 4 days of "no-protein," high-calorie, arginine- and benzoate-supplemented feeds, blood ammonia should revert to near normal. Cautious addition of 1.0 to 1.5 g/kg per day of protein is then necessary.

Long-Term Therapy. The objectives of therapy in a child with a defect of the urea cycle are to maintain plasma concentrations of ammonia as near normal as possible, and to supply protein and other essential amino acids and nutrients that will allow maximal development of intellect and optimal growth. Four major approaches are used in treatment of individuals with urea cycle defects (see Fig. 67–10). These include (1) reducing precursors of ammonia, (2) correcting arginine deficiency, (3) enhancing alternate mechanisms of waste nitrogen loss, and (4) accelerating renal excretion of accumulated intermediates.[186,189]

Methods used to reduce ammonia precursors include protein restriction, prevention of body protein catabolism and use of essential and semiessential amino acids.[186] In any situation in which intake of protein or essential amino acids is severely restricted, precursors for synthesis of carnitine (lysine, methionine), glutathione (cysteine, glutamate), and taurine (cysteine) may be limiting. Restricted methionine intake may result in a decrease in the available pool of labile methyl groups required for synthesis of important metabolic compounds.

L-Arginine supplementation is required in all of the urea cycle defects except arginase deficiency. To maintain normal or slightly elevated plasma arginine concentrations, 350 to 500 mg/kg of body weight daily are used.[190] L-Arginine can then produce ornithine for ammonia fixation and drive the "cycle" to citrulline and argininosuccinate (see Fig. 67–10). These two amino acids are poorly absorbed by kidney and allow nitrogen loss.

Acceleration of renal excretion of accumulated intermediates in the impaired cycle is sought. Arginine supplementation increases citrulline and argininosuccinic acid excretion in argininosuccinic acid synthetase and argininosuccinic acid lyase deficiency, respectively.[186,190]

Waste nitrogen urinary loss can be enhanced by the use of sodium benzoate, phenylacetate, or phenylbutyrate[191] (see Fig. 67–10). Glycine conjugates with benzoate using glycine-N-acylase and leads to the excretion of a nearly stoichiometric quantity of nitrogen as hippurate (see Fig. 67–10). Toxicity is low on 200 to 500 mg/kg

TABLE 67–28. SUPPLIERS OF MEDICATIONS AND NUTRITION SUPPLEMENTS REQUIRED FOR TREATMENT OF UREA CYCLE DISORDERS

PRODUCT	SUPPLIER
Medications	
Sodium benzoate plus sodium phenylacetate (intravenous); an investigational new drug	Saul Brusilow, MD The Johns Hopkins Hospital 600 N. Wolfe Street Baltimore, MD 21205 (301) 955-0885
Sodium phenylbutyrate powder and tablets; an investigational new drug	Saul Bruisilow, MD The Johns Hopkins Hospital 600 N. Wolfe Street Baltimore, MD 21205 (301) 955-0885
Ucephan: a 10% solution of sodium benzoate plus sodium phenylacetate (oral)	Kendall McGaw Laboratories, Inc. 2525 McGaw Avenue Irvine, CA 92714 (800) 854-6851
Nutrition Supplements	
L-Arginine powder* (free base) L-Citrulline powder*	Ajinomoto USA, Inc. 500 Frank W. Burr Boulevard Teaneck, NJ 07666-6894 (201) 488-1212 Tanabe USA, Inc. 7071 Convoy Court San Diego, CA 93138 (619) 571-8410
L-Arginine powder* and Capsules (free base)	Tyson and Associates, Inc. 1661 Lincoln Boulevard Santa Monica, CA 90494 (800) 367-7744
L-Arginine HCL† (10% pyrogen-free solution; 10% sterile solution for intravenous use)	KabiVitrum, Inc. 1311 Harbor Bay Parkway Alameda, CA 94501 (800) 227-1518
L-Citrulline powder*	Seybridge Pharmacy 37 New Haven Road Seymour, CT 06483 (203) 888-0073 Ask for Peter Przybylski Tyson and Associates, Inc. 1661 Lincoln Boulevard Santa Monica, CA 90494 (800) 367-7744

*Amino acid powders have different densities. Consequently, they should be measured on a scale that reads in grams. A 1-week supply may be weighed and placed in a vial. The week's supply may then be mixed to a known volume in boiled water, capped, and stored in the refrigerator. The daily amount required may be measured in a disposable syringe or volumetric flask.

†Hypochloremic acidosis may occur with high-dose L-arginine HCL. Consequently, plasma concentrations of chloride and bicarbonate should be monitored and bicarbonate administered if needed.

per day. Folate must be administered to provide a source of one-carbon fragments for synthesis of glycine from serine in order to prevent glycine depletion.[192] Pyridoxine is necessary for transamination.

Phenylbutyrate and phenylacetate increase urinary nitrogen excretion as phenylacetylglutamine[189–192] (see Fig. 67–10). The suggested dose is 550 mg/kg of body weight. This efficient alternative pathway removes two molecules of nitrogen per molecule of phenylacetylglutamine and requires monitoring of protein intake to prevent deficiency.

Catabolism during a febrile illness may lead to life-threatening elevations in blood ammonia. In addition to prompt diagnosis and treatment of the infection, decreased protein intake (to 0 g for 1 to 2 days), increased energy intake, and peritoneal dialysis may all be required.

In planning nutrition support of the infant or child with a defect of a urea cycle enzyme, a formal prescription should be written that includes recommended amounts of protein, energy, fluid, L-arginine, and benzoic acid for the day. The prescription for protein should be based on blood ammonia concentrations and correlated with growth.

Protein intakes suggested in Table 67–29 are based on amounts required to cover obligatory losses and growth needs[193] of infants and children fed an excellent protein source such as egg or milk. Intakes may need to be increased if the child fails to grow adequately on the recommended intake or if sodium benzoate, phenylacetate, or phenylbutyrate is administered.

Energy intakes recommended in Table 67–29 are somewhat greater than those for normal infants and children in order to provide ketoacid precursors from carbohydrate for synthesis of nonessential amino acids and to prevent protein degradation. Carbohydrate should not provide more than 50% of the energy because of frequently elevated plasma triglyceride concentrations.

In any situation in which protein-restricted diets are fed, carnitine supplements may be necessary. If carnitine deficiency occurs, recommended amounts of supplemental L-carnitine are 50 to 100 mg/kg per day.

L-Cysteine or L-methionine may be required with protein-restricted diets to provide precursors for synthesis of sulfur amino acids and taurine. If UCD 1 is used as the protein source (see next section), adequate cysteine and methionine are included. Monitoring plasma amino acids helps to prevent this type of iatrogenic deficiency.

Iafolla and co-workers have reported citrate deficiency in patients with argininosuccinate lyase deficiency and have recommended supplementation.[194]

TABLE 67–29. RECOMMENDED PROTEIN AND ENERGY INTAKES FOR INFANTS AND CHILDREN WITH DISORDERS OF THE UREA CYCLE

AGE	PROTEIN*	ENERGY
	(g/kg)	(kcal/kg)
<3 mo.	1.6–1.4	130–145
3<6 mo.	1.4–1.3	125–145
6<9 mo.	1.3–1.2	120–125
9<12 mo.	1.2–1.0	115–135
1<4 yr.	1.0–0.9	110–120
4<7 yr.	0.9–0.8	100–110
7<11 yr.	0.8–0.7	80–90
11<19 yr.	0.7–0.6	55–65
≥19 yr.	0.6–0.5	35–50

*Amount of protein required may be greater than indicated if sodium benzoate, sodium phenylacetate, and sodium phenylbutyrate are administered.

Medical Foods for Urea Cycle Disorders. Nutrition support of urea cycle disorders requires restriction of nitrogen intake. This restriction is best accomplished by providing about half the prescribed protein in the form of essential amino acids only. UCD 1, intended for the infant, is formulated from essential L-amino acids, L-cystine, L-tyrosine, sucrose, minerals, and vitamins. UCD 2 is formulated in a similar fashion, but it is free of L-cystine and L-tyrosine (Tables 67–7, 67–8, and 67–30). UCD 1 contains 55 mg L-cystine per gram of protein. These two products contain no fat, chromium, magnesium, or selenium.

Serving Lists. Serving lists of natural foods are available to simplify the protein-restricted diets for professionals and for families (Table 67–10).

Assessment of Nutrition Support. Frequency of assessment is, in part, dictated by the clinical course of the patient. Blood ammonia concentrations should be monitored routinely and maintained below 50 μmol. Plasma concentrations of amino acids should be monitored and maintained in the normal range. Plasma albumin and globulin concentrations are indices of protein status and should be evaluated frequently. Plasma prealbumin and retinol-binding protein have shorter half-lives than albumin and can provide information on protein status at an earlier stage in deficiency than albumin can. Caretakers should provide diet diaries and records of health status in tandem with blood for ammonia and plasma amino acids. Growth and development should be routinely assessed. If evidence of protein deficiency occurs or growth is not maintained, increased protein intake is necessary.[165,193]

Results of Nutrition Support. Results of therapy in infants with complete or near-complete enzyme deficiencies have been less than optimal, with delayed death and below-normal development. If the serious brain swelling and coma are prevented in the neonatal period or if onset of disease expression is delayed, physical growth and mental development are more nearly normal with nutrition and pharmacologic support.[165,185,190] If diagnosis is anticipated and treatment is begun in early infancy in affected siblings with citrullinemia or argininosuccinic acidemia, relatively normal outcome is observed even in the severe enzyme defects.

TABLE 67–30. COMPOSITION OF "CHEMICALLY DEFINED" MEDICAL FOODS FOR NITROGEN-RESTRICTED DIETS (PER 100 G OF PRODUCT)

NUTRIENT	UCD 1	UCD 2
Energy (kcal)	260	290
Protein equivalent (g)	56	66
Alanine (g)	0	0
Arginine (g)	0	0
Aspartic acid (g)	0	0
Carnitine (g)	0	0
Cystine (g)	3.10	0
Glutamic acid (g)	0	0
Glutamine (g)	0	0
Glycine (g)	0	0
Histidine (g)	3.10	3.60
Isoleucine (g)	7.60	8.90
Leucine (g)	12.80	15.00
Lysine (g)	9.00	10.70
Methionine (g)	3.10	7.10
Phenylalanine (g)	5.30	14.10
Proline (g)	0	0
Serine (g)	0	0
Taurine (g)	0	0
Threonine (g)	6.00	7.10
Tryptophan (g)	2.20	2.80
Tyrosine (g)	6.50	0
Valine (g)	9.0	10.70
Carbohydrate (g)	8.0	6.0
Fat (g)	0	0
Calcium (mg)	2,800	1,310
Chloride (mEq)	55.4	28.2
Chromium (μg)	NA	NA
Copper (mg)	8.0	2.0
Iodine (μg)	270	120
Iron (mg)	40.0	15.0
Magnesium (mg)	0	0
Manganese (mg)	2.8	0.7
Molybdenum (μg)	128	32
Phosphorus (mg)	2,200	1,010
Potassium (mEq)	71.8	34.1
Selenium (μg)	NA	NA
Sodium (mEq)	54.7	27.8
Zinc (mg)	31.0	7.8
Vitamin A (μg RE)	3,360	1,560
D (μg)	30	33
Vitamin E (mg α-TE)	27.5	12.1
K (μg)	200	167
Ascorbic acid (mg)	280	80
Biotin (mg)	0.12	0.30
B_6 (mg)	2.6	1.5
B_{12} (μg)	8	3
Choline (mg)	510	260
Folate (μg)	400	400
Inositol (mg)	590	300
Niacin (mg)*	65	24
Pantothenic acid (mg)	30	11
Ribloflavin (mg)	4.8	2.0
Thiamin (mg)	3.2	1.4

*Preformed niacin

NA = none added

Note: Values listed, although accurate at the time of publication, are subject to change. The most current information may be obtained by referring to product labels.

(Data from references 65 to 69.)

GALACTOSE

BIOCHEMISTRY

Because lactose is the principal carbohydrate and energy source for infants and young children, galactose maintains a central metabolic role in human nutrition. Lactose is hydrolyzed in the intestine by lactase to glucose and galactose (Fig. 67–12). Prior to utilization, galactose must be converted to glucose. This occurs primarily in the liver where galactose becomes glucose through three enzymatic steps. First, galactose is phosphorylated to galactose-1-phosphate by galactokinase. Then the phosphorylated hexose is interchanged with the glucose moiety of uridyldiphosphoglucose by galactose-1-phosphate uridyl transferase. Finally, galactose is rearranged to glucose by uridine diphosphate (UDP) galactose-4-epimerase (Fig. 67–12). The glucose thus formed can be used for glycogen synthesis or phosphorylated to glucose-1-phosphate for further utilization.

GALACTOSEMIA

Galactosemia may occur because of deficient functioning of any of three enzymes: galactokinase, galactose-1-phosphate uridyl transferase (gal-1-P transferase), or UDP galactose-4-epimerase[195] (Fig. 67–12). Patients with galactokinase deficiency have only cataracts. Galac-

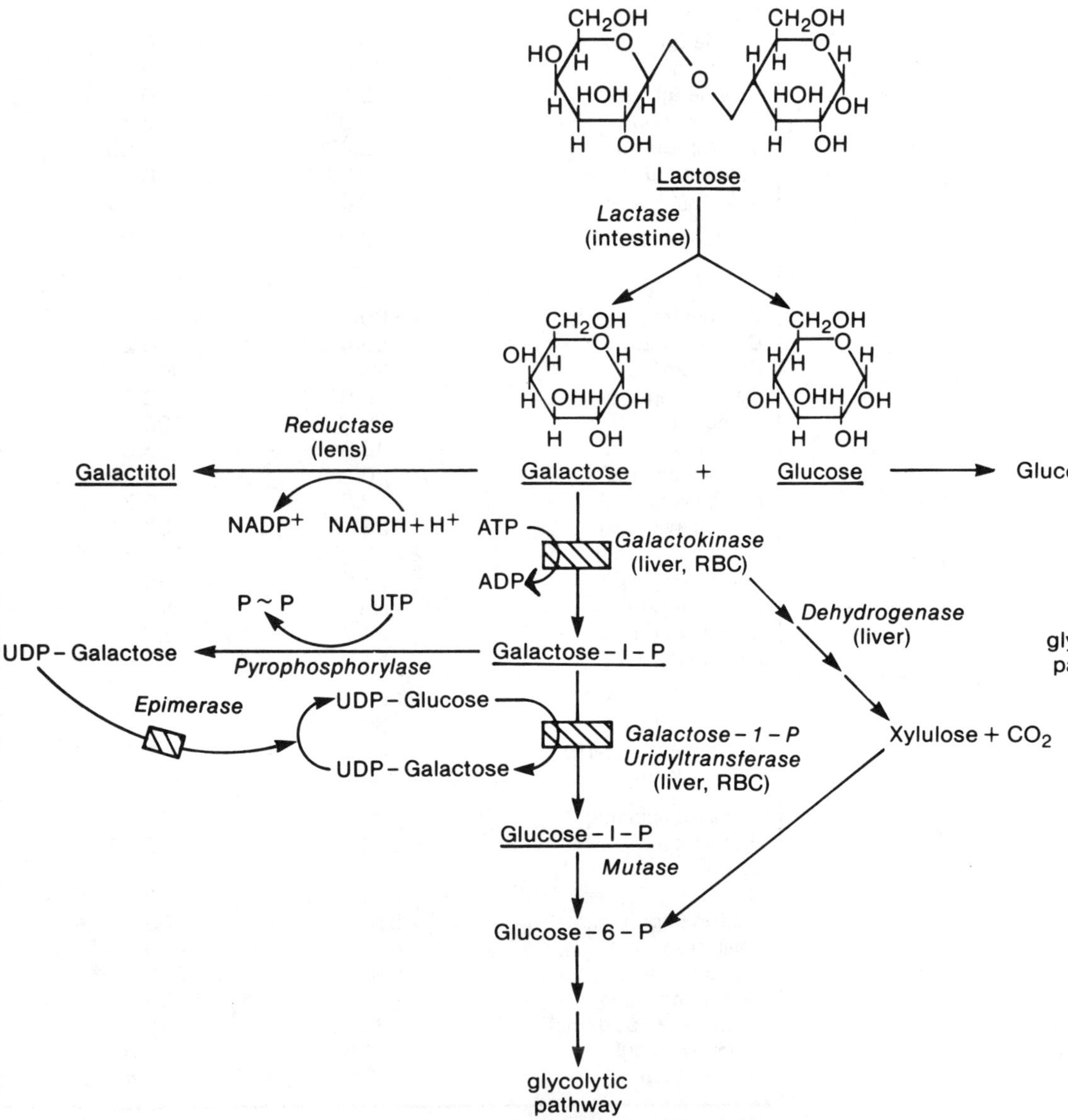

FIGURE 67–12. Metabolic blocks in galactose metabolism that lead to galactosemia. Genetic disorders of catalyzed reactions are indicated by hatched bars.

tokinase deficiency does not produce severe clinical manifestations or the accumulation of galactose-1-phosphate seen with gal-1-P transferase deficiency. At least nine variants with different degrees of function and structure have been described for mutant gal-1-P transferase.[195] This gene locus is on chromosome 9p.[196,197] The cDNA for gal-1-p transferase has been accurately sequenced, and many different mutations within the traditional "classic" category now called G/G are being identified.[197] New classifications based on both mutation and enzyme function are imminent.

Galactosemia due to deficiency of gal-1-P transferase leads to accumulation of galactose-1-phosphate, which acts as a phosphate sink–reducing intracellular phosphate for high-energy phosphate bonds. Thus, ATP, GTP (guanosine triphosphate), and CTP (cytidine triphosphate) are reduced. An alternative hypothesis suggests a deficiency of UDPgal with consequently impaired glycolipid synthesis.[195] Progressive damage to the central nervous system, liver, and renal tubule results if galactose restriction is not instituted in the first few days of life.

Clinical symptoms of the gal-1-P transferase defect appear early in infancy. Some infants are born with cataracts and cirrhosis, which may be due to maternal lactose ingestion. Symptoms generally appear with the onset of milk feedings. Prolonged neonatal jaundice at 4 to 10 days of age is common. Hyperbilirubinemia is secondary to toxic injury to liver cells by gal-1-P, delayed maturation of glucuronyl transferase,[198] mild hemolysis, and bleeding. Bleeding diatheses, Escherichia coli sepsis, and shock are catastrophic events that occur during the neonatal period. Therefore, rapid screening, retrieval, diagnosis, and treatment are essential for population-based newborn screening programs if the clinical sequelae of galactosemia are to be prevented. Other relatively minor symptoms occur. Anemia from various causes is present in about 40% of untreated patients. Lethargy, hypotonia, food refusal, vomiting, and diarrhea are also common symptoms.

Retarded mental and physical growth occur in most of the untreated patients who survive. The pathophysiology of galactosemia remains unclear, but early diet clearly prevents neonatal sepsis, shock, and bleeding. However, even well-treated patients may have some specific speech defects or disorders and infertility. Whether intrauterine effects of accumulated galactose or gal-1-P or whether deficiency of UDPgal cause the pathology remains for further study. Additional nutritional causes such as food refusal, vomiting, diarrhea, renal failure, loss of galactose-derived energy, and depressed protein synthesis are also possible.

Cataracts occur in about 45% of untreated individuals. They are thought to result from the formation and accumulation of galactitol in the lens of the eye, which is impermeable to efflux. Galactitol creates an osmotic gradient that allows glutathionine to efflux with consequent decreased concentrations of lens glutathione. When glutathione concentrations are decreased, glutathione peroxidase is inactivated and hydrogen peroxide accumulates to toxic levels. Hydrogen peroxide denatures lens protein, causing production of lenticular cataracts.[195,198]

Hepatomegaly occurs in nearly all cases of gal-1-P transferase deficiency, and cirrhosis develops in untreated patients. The hepatomegaly is associated with abnormally large amounts of gal-1-P, UDP galactose, and glycogen in the liver. Liver damage results in decreased synthesis of prothrombin and albumin.

Because of decreased albumin synthesis and proteinuria, ascites and generalized edema occur in about 36% of untreated patients.[195] The albumin synthesized by untreated galactosemic patients contains large amounts of galactose, whereas albumin of normal individuals is free of galactose.[199] Untreated or poorly controlled patients are extremely susceptible to infection with gram-negative organisms. Immunoincompetence is probably a direct result of inhibition by gal-1-P of immune protein synthesis by lymphocytes and inactivation of leukocyte phagocytosis.

Galactose and its accumulated metabolites are toxic to the glomeruli and tubules of the kidney. Additionally, active tubular transport is impaired because of deficient ATP. Aminoaciduria is generalized.

On rare occasions, hypoglycemia occurs. Causes include defective hepatic gluconeogenesis, the inability to convert glycogen to glucose because of inhibition of phosphorylase kinase by gal-1-P, and hyperinsulinemia that may result from galactose stimulation of pancreatic β cells and decreased hepatic extraction of insulin.[198]

SCREENING

Gal-1-P transferase deficiency is inherited via an autosomal recessive mode. Estimates of the frequency of the gal-1-P transferase defect have increased with the improvement of screening and diagnostic procedures. Ten years of experience with screening of over 1,000,000, infants for galactosemia in Georgia have yielded an incidence of 2.5 in 100,000 patients with classic galactosemia and 9.0 in 100,000 patients with variant forms (see Table 67–3). Other authors have reported variable frequencies in United States populations between 1 in 18,000 and 1 in 70,000.[195]

The most common screening method is the Beutler fluorescent test for galactosemia.[200] This procedure consists of incubating dried blood on filter paper disks with a mixture of uridine diphosphoglucose (UDPG), phosphoglucomutase, glucose-6-phosphate dehydrogenase, and NADP. Erythrocytes from normal individuals contain the enzyme gal-1-P uridyl transferase and will produce glucose-1-phosphate as follows (items preceded by an asterisk are added to produce enzyme-linked NADPH for ultraviolet fluorescent assay):

Galactose-1-P + UDP glucose

↓ galactose-1-P uridyl transferase

UDP galactose + Glucose-1-P

↓ *Phosphoglucomutase

Glucose-6-P + *NADP

↓ *Glucose-6-P dehydrogenase

6-P-gluconate + NADPH

Glucose-1-phosphate is converted to glucose-6-phosphate which, in the presence of glucose-6-dehydrogenase, reduces NADP to NADPH. Blood from patients with classic galactosemia has impaired gal-1-P uridyl transferase activity. This enzyme-linked reaction is determined by the presence or absence of produced NADPH, which is fluorescent when viewed under shortwave ultraviolet light.

Positive screening results occur if variants of gal-1-P uridyl transferase are inactivated by exposure of the blood disks to heat, as in the summer. The Duarte/galactosemia compound heterozygote is more sensitive to heat than the homozygous normal is. Confirmation of positive Beutler screening test results requires the use of erythrocyte hemolysates for quantitative enzyme activity. Quantitation of intact erythrocyte gal-1-P content in the erythrocytes of the proband and isoenzymal analysis of parental gal-1-P uridyl transferase is necessary for final diagnosis and genetic counseling.

An alternative screening test to determine the presence of excess galactose concentrations has been developed.[7] This test depends on the fact that lysis of certain strains of E. coli by bacteriophage is inhibited by galactose or gal-1-P. Climatic changes should not affect this screening procedure.

DIAGNOSIS

Patients with positive Beutler and/or positive E. coli bacteriophage test results should have all lactose removed from their diets immediately while enzyme diagnosis and family work-up proceed. Fresh, sterile heparinized blood should be sent to a central laboratory experienced in enzyme analysis. Both patient and family should be evaluated by the center for genotype and form of impaired enzyme.

Diagnosis of galactosemia is accomplished through measurement of activity of gal-1-P transferase in erythrocytes. No activity occurs in individuals homozygous for the classic disease (G/G), whereas heterozygotes (G/N) have approximately one-half normal activity (Table 67–31). Several types of gal-1-P transferase deficiency have been described that are based on the percentage of activity in the erythrocyte and on isozyme patterns on starch gel electrophoresis. The need for therapy in patients with an activity of 25% or less of gal-1-P transferase, as in compound heterozygotes for Duarte/galactosemia alleles, has not been established. However, galactose should be restricted in early life for patients with any mutant genotype if erythrocyte gal-1-P is elevated above 2 mg/dl.

Gal-1-P transferase is expressed in cultured amniotic fluid cells from the normal fetus. Thus, prenatal detection of gal-1-P transferase deficiency is possible. Amniotic fluid of a fetus with galactosemia has recently been found to have an elevated concentration of galactitol. Assessment of the galactitol content of amniotic fluid by GC/MS provides a rapid ancillary method for prenatal diagnosis of galactosemia.[201]

TREATMENT

Objectives of therapy in galactosemia are to ameliorate or to prevent symptoms while providing adequate energy and nutrients for normal growth and development. Treatment should begin as early in the first week

TABLE 67–31. SOME ALLELIC DISORDERS OF GALACTOSE-1-PHOSPHATE URIDYL TRANSFERASE

TYPE	GENOTYPE	ERYTHROCYTE UDP-GAL-1-P TRANSFERASE (% OF CONTROL)
Classic	G/G	0
Chicago	C/N	75
	D/N	75
Duarte	D/D	50
	G/N	50
Durate/Gal	D/G	25
Indiana	I/N	0–45
Negro	gt/gt (mosaic)	0 (normal hepatic activity)
Rennes	R/N	7

of life as possible and consists of removal of all sources of lactose and galactose from the diet.

Nutrient Requirements. Energy and nutrient requirements of infants and children with well-controlled galactosemia are the same as those for normal individuals of the same age, gender, and physical activity level. Whether greater-than-normal energy and protein intakes will prevent the linear growth retardation seen in poorly controlled children is not known.

Formulas. Human milk contains 6 to 8% lactose, cow's milk 3 to 4% lactose, and many proprietary infant formulas 7% lactose. These milks must be replaced by a formula low in galactose (Isomil or Prosobee).

Formulas containing soy protein isolate have about 14 mg galactose/L in the form of raffinose and stacchyose, oligosaccharides that contain galactose. At one time it was thought that these oligosaccharides yielded free galactose on hydrolysis in the intestine. It is now believed that the human intestine has no enzymes to hydrolyze these oligosaccharides.[202] Thus, they may be safely used for feeding infants and children with galactosemia. Casein hydrolysates such as Nutramigen and Pregestimil have been treated to remove lactose but contain about 160 mg galactose/L.[203]

Solid Foods. When solid foods (Table 67–32) are added at appropriate ages, careful reading of labels is required to ensure that neither galactose nor lactose has been added in food processing. Lactose is added to baked goods, dry mixes, ice cream, sherbets, confections, and batter mixes, among other items, to improve flavor, texture, body, viscosity, and mouth feel.[204] Standards of identity for "standard name" foods that do not require ingredient lists on the label should be obtained from the Food and Drug Administration. Examples of such foods are imitation milk, white bread, and mayonnaise. Foods such as peas and organ meats that naturally contain galactose must also be excluded from the diet. Certain artificial sweeteners contain lactose as an extender. These artificial sweeteners and any products prepared with these sugar substitutes must be avoided.

Some clinical centers treating patients with galactosemia have allowed fermented dairy products and aged cheese under the mistaken impression that all lactose has been converted to lactic acid. This is not the case,[205–208] however, and these products should be excluded from the diet. Vegetable gums such as agar, acacia (gum arabic), carrageenen, locust bean (carob), and guar are complex galactosides or galactomannans that contain mostly β-D-1—>3, 1—>4, and 1—>6 linkages that are not digested by humans. Thus, foods containing these gums may be used in galactose-restricted diets. Only tragacanthic acid, which has a main chain of 1—>4-β-D-galacturonopyranosyl units, may need to be excluded from the diet. One report suggested that all legumes, textured vegetable protein, spinach, and vegetable gums be excluded from the galactose-restricted diet.[209] However, no scientific data were presented to justify this recommendation.

Drugs. Drugs often contain lactose for a variety of purposes. Neocalglucon, often used to supplement calcium, is high in galactose. Lists of sugar-free drug preparations are published that should be updated frequently and scrutinized when galactosemic children require drug therapy.

Results of Nutrition Support. Treatment, although lifesaving, may not result in complete freedom from the sequelae of accumulated gal-1-P. Those infants diagnosed and treated early who maintain excellent dietary control have better intellectual function than those who have poor control or are diagnosed late.[210,211] Control is defined on the basis of erythrocyte gal-1-P levels and is considered excellent if consistently below 2 mg/dl.[212] However, even with excellent nutrition control, children frequently have a higher RBC Gal-1-P and a lower I.Q. than their normal siblings.[213] They may have difficulty with language,[214] abstract thinking, and visual perception. Females may have ovarian failure. These clinical deficits may be related to intrauterine damage from maternal blood galactose crossing the placenta into the vulnerable fetus,[215] from galactose synthesis, or from UDPgal deficiency. Membranes are constantly being synthesized and degraded, requiring and producing galactose. Many fruits and vegetables contain free galactose. Prevention of all gal-1-P accumulation by restriction of exogenous galactose is thus impossible. Early-onset cataracts and infertility in affected females are reported despite "good" dietary control. Galactose (i.e., milk) restriction in at-risk pregnant females is generally advised.[216]

The recent observation that UDPgal is partially deficient in erythrocytes of galactosemic patients offers another potential reason for chronicity of disease despite adequate lactose restriction. These findings have not as yet been confirmed by other laboratories. Whether uridine supplements will help is speculative.[195]

Assessment of Nutrition Support. Frequent evaluation of growth, development, and erythrocyte gal-1-P concentrations is necessary to determine if the diet is being followed. Use of galactosylated hemoglobin A1 as an index of dietary control has also been suggested, but is less sensitive and is an indirect test.[217]

Diet Termination. Although some investigators have recommended liberalization of the galactose-restricted diet at 12 to 13 years of age, this is not warranted because the damaging effects of accumulated galactitol in the lens and gal-1-P in the liver and kidney remain. Galactosemic females must continue treatment with galactose exclusion to prevent gonadal atrophy and in utero damage to the fetus.[218] Hypogonadism has been reported

TABLE 67–32. GALACTOSE-RESTRICTED DIET

FOODS ALLOWED	FOODS EXCLUDED
<u>Beverages</u>	
Isomil*; ProSobee;† RCF*; carbonated drinks; fruit drinks free of apple, grape, pear, and papaya; lactose-free products	All untreated milk of any species and all products containing milk, whether whole, skim, dried, evaporated, or condensed; yogurt, cheese, aged cheese, ice cream, sherbet; malted milk; Ovaltine, hot chocolate; some cocoas and instant coffees (read labels); powdered soft drinks with lactose; curds; whey and casein; milk treated with lactobacillus acidophilus culture or lactase; imitation or filled milks; calcium caseinate or sodium caseinate
<u>Breads and Cereals</u>	
Breads, crackers, and rolls made without milk; Italian bread, some cooked and prepared cereals (read labels), soda crackers, pasta; contact bakeries in each geographic area for milk-free breads	Prepared mixes, such as muffins, biscuits, waffles, pancakes; some dry cereals (read labels carefully); instant Cream of Wheat; cereals, breads, crackers, zwieback, French toast made with milk
<u>Cheeses</u>	
None	All excluded
<u>Desserts</u>	
Water and fruit ices; gelatin, angel food cake; homemade cakes, pies, cookies made from allowed ingredients; puddings made with water, Isomil, ProSobee, or RCF; sorbets	Commercial cakes, cookies and mixes; custard, puddings, sherbets, and ice cream made with milk; any containing chocolate; pie crust made with butter or margine
<u>Eggs</u>	
All	Omelets and soufflés containing milk
<u>Fats</u>	
Margarines and dressings that do not contain milk or milk products, oils, shortening, bacon, some nondairy creamers (read labels), nut butters, nuts, lard	Margarines and dressings containing milk or milk products; butter, cream, cream cheese, peanut butter with milk solid fillers, salad dressings containing lactose, nondairy creamers containing sodium or calcium caseinate
<u>Fruits</u>	
Canned, fresh, or frozen fruits that do not contain galactose and are not processed with lactose	Any canned or frozen fruits processed with lactose; apples, applesauce, apple juice, banana, dates, figs, grapes, kiwi fruit, papaya, pears, persimmon, watermelon

*Ross Laboratories, Columbus, Ohio 43216.
†Mead Johnson Nutritional Division, Evansville, IN 47221.
‡Gross, K.C., Sams, C.E.: Changes in cell wall neutral sugar composition during fruit ripening: A species survey. Phytochemistry, *23*:2457–2461, 1984.
§Gross, K.C.: Correspondence with P.B. Acosta, March, 1990.
‖Matthews, R.H., Pehrsson, R., Farhat-Sabet, M.: Sugar content of selected foods; individual and total sugars. USDA Home Economics Research Report No. 48. Washington, D.C., U.S. Government Printing Office, 1987.

in female patients with gal-1-P transferase deficiency in whom nutrition support was delayed.[219–222] Examined males have had normal gonadal function. Offspring of pregnant rats fed a 50% galactose diet have had a striking reduction in oocyte number. The most prominent effects have been noted after exposure to galactose during the premeiotic stages of oogenesis.[223,224]

REFERENCES

1. McKusick, V.A.: Mendelian Inheritance in Man: Catalog of Autosomal Dominant, Recessive, and X-Linked Phenotypes. 9th Ed. Baltimore, Johns Hopkins University Press, 1990.
2. Harris, H.: The Principles of Human Biochemical Genetics. 3rd Ed. Amsterdam, North-Holland Publishing, 1980.
3. Danner, D.J., Elsas, L.J.: Disorders of branched chain aminoacid and ketoacid metabolism. *In* The Metabolic Basis of Inherited Disease. 6th Ed. Edited by C. Scriver, A. Beaudet, W. Sly, et al. New York, McGraw-Hill, 1989.
4. Marshall, L., DiGeorge, A.: Am. J. Hum. Genet., *33*:138A, 1981.

TABLE 67–32. CONTINUED

FOODS ALLOWED	FOODS EXCLUDED
Legumes, Nuts, Seeds[‖]	
Exclude all legumes; nuts and seeds except those excluded	All legumes; fermented soybean products such as miso, natto, tempeh, or fermented soy sauce in which enzyme processing has been used; hazelnuts, safflower seed kernels
Meat, Fish, Poultry	
Plain beef, chicken, fish, ham, lamb, pork, veal, strained or junior meats that do not contain milk or milk products, kosher frankfurters	Creamed or breaded meat, fish, or fowl; sausage products, such as weiners, liver sausage, cold cuts containing nonfat milk solids; brains, liver, kidney, pancreas, sweetbreads
Soups	
Clear soups, consommés, cream soups made with nondairy creamers free of caseinate, vegetable soups made with allowed vegetables	Cream soups; vegetable soups unless made with allowed ingredients; chowders, commercially prepared soups containing lactose
Vegetables[‡§]	
Fresh, canned, or frozen vegetables; artichokes, asparagus, beets, cabbage, cauliflower, celery, chard, corn, cucumbers, eggplant, kale, lettuce, mustard, okra, parsley, parsnips, potatoes, rutabagas, spinach, and yams; all vegetables not containing galactose if prepared without lactose	Any vegetable to which lactose is added during processing; creamed, breaded, or buttered vegetables; instant potatoes, corn curls, and frozen French fries if processed with lactose; bell peppers, broccoli, brussels sprouts, carrots, onions, peas, pumpkin, sweet potatoes, tomatoes
Miscellaneous	
Carob powder, popcorn, olives, pure sugar candy, jelly or marmalade, sugar, corn syrup, gravy made with water, baker's cocoa, pickles, pure seasoning and spices, molasses, beet sugar, pure monosodium glutamate, honey	Chewing gum; milk chocolate; neocalglucon; some cocoas; toffee, peppermint; butterscotch, caramels; dietetic preparations (read labels); certain drugs and vitamin and mineral preparations; spice blends if they contain lactose; monosodium glutamate extender; artificial sweeteners containing lactose

*Ross Laboratories, Columbus, Ohio 43216.
†Mead Johnson Nutritional Division, Evansville, IN 47221.
‡Gross, K.C., Sams, C.E.: Changes in cell wall neutral sugar composition during fruit ripening: A species survey. Phytochemistry, *23*:2457–2461, 1984.
§Gross, K.C.: Correspondence with P.B. Acosta, March, 1990.
‖Matthews, R.H., Pehrsson, R., Farhat-Sabet, M.: Sugar content of selected foods; individual and total sugars. USDA Home Economics Research Report No. 48. Washington, D.C., U.S. Government Printing Office, 1987.

5. Elsas, L.J., et al.: Metabolic consequences of inherited defects in branched chain a-ketoacid dehydrogenase: Mechanisms of thiamine action. *In* Metabolism and Clinical Implications of Branched Chain Amino Acids and Ketoacids. Edited by M. Walser and G.R. Williamson. New York, Elsevier, 1981.
6. Snyderman, E.: Maple syrup urine disease. *In* Congenital Metabolic Disease: Diagnosis and Treatment. Edited by L.A. Wapnir. New York, Marcel Dekker, 1985.
7. Elsas, L.J.: Newborn Screening. *In* Pediatrics. 19th Ed. Edited by A.M. Rudolph. New York, Appleton-Century-Crofts, 1990.
8. Elsas, L., Brown, A., Fernhoff, P.: Newborn screening. *In* Neonatal Screening. Edited by H. Naruse and M. Irie. Amsterdam, Excerpta Medica, 1983.
9. Burns, J.J.: Am. J. Med., *26:*740, 1959.
10. Jackson: Hosp. Pract., *15:*39, 1985.
11. Lipson, M.H., et al.: J. Clin. Invest., *66:*188, 1980.
12. Elsas, L.J., Danner, D.J.: Ann. N. Y. Acad. Sci., *378:*404, 1982.
13. Baumgartner, E.R., et al.: Helv. Paediatr. Acta, *34:*483, 1979.
14. Elsas, L.J., McCormick, D.B.: *In* Vitamins and Hormones. Vol. 43. New York, Academic Press, 1987, pp. 103–144.
15. Elsas, L., McCormick, D.: Vitamins and Hormones. Vol. 44. New York, Academic Press, 1987.
16. Rosenberg, L.E.: *In* Advances in Human Genetics. Vol. 6. Edited by Harris Hirschorn. New York, Plenum Press, 1976, pp. 1–69.
17. Fernhoff, P.M., et al.: Vitamin-responsive disorders. *In* Human Nutrition: Clinical and Biochemical Aspects. Edited by P. Garry. Washington, D.C., American Association of Clinical Chemistry, 1980.
18. Hershfield, M.S., et al.: N. Engl. J. Med., *316:*589, 1987.
19. Thompson, M.W., McKinnes, R.R., Willard, H.F. (eds.): Thompson and Thompson Genetics in Medicine. 5th Ed. Philadelphia, W.B. Saunders, 1991.
20. Acosta, P.B.: *In* Practice of Pediatrics. Edited by V. Kelly. Philadelphia, J.B. Lippincott, 1983.
21. Chipponi, J.X., et al.: Am. J. Clin. Nutr., *35:*1112, 1982.
22. Acosta, P.B., Stepnick-Gropper, S.: J. Inherited Metab. Dis., *9(Suppl. 2):*1983, 1986.
23. Cashel, K.M., et al.: J. Hum. Nutr., *32:*264, 1978.
24. Abrams, C.A.L., et al.: JAMA, *232:*1136, 1975.

25. Coodin, F.J., et al.: Pediatrics, *47:*438, 1971.
26. Seegar, W.E., Chesney, R.W.: Am. J. Dis. Child., *131:*137, 1977.
27. Endres, W., et al.: J. Inherited Metab. Dis., *7:*8, 1984.
28. Anderson, K., et al.: J. Inherited Metab. Dis., *9:*39, 1986.
29. Martin, S., Acosta, P.B.: J. Am. Diet. Assoc., *87:*48, 1987.
30. Krause, W., et al.: J. Clin. Invest., *75:*40, 1985.
31. Friedman, et al.: Proc. Natl. Acad. Sci. U.S.A., *70:*552, 1973.
32. Griffin, R.F., Elsas, L.J.: J. Pediatr., *86:*572, 1975.
33. Scriver, C.R., Kaufman, S., Woo, S.L.L.: The hyperphenylalaninemias. *In* The Metabolic Basis of Inherited Disease. 6th Ed. Edited by C. Scriver, A. Beaudet, W. Sly, and D. Valle. New York, McGraw-Hill, 1989.
34. Niederwieser, A., et al.: J. Inherited Metab. Dis., *8(Suppl. 1):*34, 1985.
35. Kaufman, S.: J. Inherited Metab. Dis., *8(Suppl. 1):*20, 1985.
36. Curtius, H.C. et al.: J. Inherited Metab. Dis., *8(Suppl. 1):*28, 1985.
37. Dobbing, J.: The later development of the brain and its vulnerability. *In* Scientific Foundations of Paediatrics. Edited by J.A. Davis and J. Dobbing. London, Heinemann, 1981.
38. Pardridge, W.M., Choi, T.B.: Fed. Proc., *45:*2073, 1986.
39. Villasana, D., Butler, I.J., Williams, J.C., Roongta, S.M.: J. Inherited Metab. Dis., *12:*451–457, 1989.
40. Epstein, C.M., et al.: Electroencephalogr. Clin. Neurophysiol., *72:*133, 1989.
41. Guthrie, R.A., Susi, A.: Pediatrics, *32:*338, 1963.
42. Genetic Screening: Programs, Principles, and Research. Washington, D.C., National Academy of Sciences, 1975.
43. Fernhoff, P.M., et al.: South. Med. J., *75:*529, 1982.
44. Berry, H., et al.: Am. J. Dis. Child., *136:*111, 1982.
45. Daiger, S.P., et al.: Lancet, *1:*229, 1986.
46. Jordan, M.K., et al.: Dev. Med. Child Neurol., *27:*33, 1985.
47. Cournoyen, D., Caskey, C.T.: N. Engl. J. Med., *323:*601–602, 1990.
48. Reichle, F.A. et al.: JAMA, *178:*939, 1961.
49. Acosta, P.B., et al.: J. Am. Diet. Assoc., *72:*164, 1978.
50. Smith, I., Beasley, M.G., Ades, A.E.: Arch. Dis. Child., *65:*472–478, 1990.
51. Rose: Nutr. Abstr. Rev., *27:*631, 1957.
52. Hanley, W.B., et al.: Pediatr. Res., *4:*318, 1970.
53. Acosta, P.B.: The contribution of therapy of inherited amino acid disorders to knowledge of amino acid requirements. *In* Congenital Metabolic Disease: Diagnosis and Treatment. Edited by R.A. Wapnir. New York, Marcel Dekker, 1985.
54. Batshaw, M.L., et al.: J. Pediatr., *99:*159, 1981.
55. Holt, L.E., et al.: Protein and Amino Acid Requirements in Early Infancy. New York, New York University Press, 1960.
56. Food and Nutrition Board, National Research Council: Recommended Dietary Allowances. 10th Ed. Washington, D.C., National Academy Press, 1989.
57. Kindt, E., et al.: Am. J. Clin. Nutr., *37:*778, 1983.
58. Barness, L.: Nutrition and nutritional disorders. *In* Nelson's Textbook of Pediatrics. 12th Ed. Edited by Behrman and Vaughan. Philadelphia, W.B. Saunders, 1983.
59. Douglass, J.S., et al.: Composition of Foods: Breakfast Cereals: Raw, Processed, Prepared. Agricultural Handbook 8-8. Washington, D.C., U.S. Government Printing Office, 1982.
60. Gebhardt, J.E., et al.: Composition of Foods: Fruits and Juices: Raw, Processed, Prepared. Agricultural Handbook 8-9. Washington, D.C., U.S. Government Printing Office, 1982.
61. Haytowitz, D.B., Matthews, R.H.: Composition of Foods: Vegetables and Vegetable Products: Raw, Processed, Prepared. Agricultural Handbook 8-11. Washington, D.C., U.S. Government Printing Office, 1984.
62. Pennington, J.A.T., Church, H.N.: Bowes and Church's Food Values of Portions Commonly Used. 14th Ed. New York, Harper & Row, 1985.
63. Posati, L.P.: Composition of Foods: Poultry Products: Raw, Processed, Prepared. Agricultural Handbook 8-5. Washington, D.C., U.S. Government Printing Office, 1979.
64. Posati, L.P., Orr, M.L.: Composition of Foods: Dairy and Egg Products: Raw, Processed, Prepared. Agricultural Handbook 8-1. Washington, D.C., U.S. Government Printing Office, 1976.
65. Mead Johnson Nutritional Division: Pediatric Products Handbook. Evansville, IN, Mead Johnson, 1988.
66. Mead Johnson Nutritional Division: Products for Dietary Management of Inborn Errors of Metabolism and Other Special Feeding Problems. Evansville, IN, Mead Johnson, 1989.
67. Polycose. Glucose Polymers. Columbus, OH, Ross Laboratories, 1984.
68. Acosta, P.B.: Nutrition Support Protocols. Columbus, OH, Ross Laboratories, 1989.
69. Acosta, P.B.: Nutrition Support of Inborn Errors of Metabolism. Rockville, MD, Aspen Publishers, 1990.
70. Wannemacher, R.W.: Am. J. Clin. Nutr., *30:*1269, 1977.
71. Umbarger, B., et al.: JAMA, *193:*128, 1965.
72. Ingall, G.B., et al.: J. Pediatr., *65:*1073A, 1964.
73. Elsas, L.J., et al.: J. Biol. Chem., *243:*1846, 1968.
74. Elsas, L.J., et al.: J. Biol. Chem., *246:*6452, 1971.
75. Nakagawa, I., et al.: J. Nutr., *77:*61, 1962.
76. Sibinga, M.S., et al.: Dev. Med. Child. Neurol., *13:*63, 1971.
77. McCaman, R.E., Robins, A.J.: J. Lab. Clin. Med., *59:*885, 1962.
78. Acosta, P.B., et al.: PKU—A Guide to Management. Berkeley, CA, California State Department of Health, 1972.
79. Holm, V.A., et al.: Pediatrics, *63:*700, 1979.
80. Dobson, J.C., et al.: Pediatrics, *60:*822, 1977.
81. Acosta, P.B., et al.: Am. J. Clin. Nutr., *30:*198, 1977.
82. Wong, R., et al.: J. Am. Diet. Assoc., *57:*229, 1970.
83. Acosta, P.B., et al.: J. Parent. Ent. Nutr., *5:*406, 1981.
84. Acosta, P.B., et al.: J. Inherited Metab. Dis., *5:*107, 1982.
85. Acosta, P.B., et al.: J. Parent. Ent. Nutr., *11:*287, 1987.
86. Lewis, J.S., et al.: Am. J. Clin. Nutr., *26:*136, 1973.
87. Lewis, J.S., et al.: Fed. Proc., *33:*666A, 1974.
88. Hudson, F.P.: Arch. Dis. Child., *42:*198, 1967.
89. Holtzman, N.A., et al.: N. Engl. J. Med., *293:*1121, 1975.
90. Horner, F.A., et al.: N. Engl. J. Med., *266:*79, 1962.
91. Seashore, M.R., et al.: Pediatrics, *75:*226, 1985.
92. Holtzman, N.A., et al.: N. Engl. J. Med., *314:*593, 1986.
93. Krause, W., et al.: Pediatr. Res., *20:*1112–1116, 1986.
94. Elsas, L.J., Trotter, J.F.: Changes in physiological concentrations of blood phenylalanine produce changes in sensitive parameters of human brain function. *In* Dietary Phenylalanine and Brain Function. Boston, Birkhauser Publishing, 1987, pp. 187–195.
95. Lenke, R.R., Levy, H.L.: N. Engl. J. Med., *303:*1202, 1980.
96. Ghadimi, H., Pecora, P.: Pediatrics, *33:*500, 1964.
97. Okano, Y., et al.: J. Inherited Metab. Dis., *9:*15, 1986.
98. Lindblad, B., et al.: Proc. Natl. Acad. Sci. U.S.A., *74:*4641, 1971.
99. Sassa, S., Kappas, A.: J. Clin. Invest., *71:*625, 1983.
100. Christensen, E., et al.: Clin. Chim. Acta, *116:*331, 1981.
101. Kvittingen, E.A., et al.: Pediatr. Res., *14:*541, 1983.

102. Furukawa, N., et al.: Pediatr. Res., *18:*409, 1984.
103. Goldsmith, L.A., Laberge, C.: Tyrosinemia and related disorders. *In* The Metabolic Basis of Inherited Disease. 6th Ed. Edited by C. Scriver, A. Beaudet, W. Sly, et al. New York, McGraw-Hill, 1989.
104. Mamunes, P., et al.: Pediatrics, *57:*675, 1976.
105. Gagne, R., et al.: Prenat. Diagn., *2:*185, 1982.
106. Kvittingen, E.A., et al.: Pediatr. Res., *19:*334, 1985.
107. Elsas, L.J.: Personal experience.
108. Sassa, S., Granick, S.: Proc. Natl. Acad. Sci. U.S.A., *67:*517, 1970.
109. Goetsch, C.A., Bissell, D.M.: N. Engl. J. Med., *315:*235, 1986.
110. Rank, J.M., et al.: J. Pediatr., *118:*136, 1991.
111. Tolbert, B.M., Watts, D.T.: J. Nutr., *80:*111, 1963.
112. Acosta, P.B., Elsas, L.J.: Dietary Management of Inherited Metabolic Diseases: Phenylketonuria, Galactosemia, Tyrosinemia, Homocystinuria and Maple Syrup Urine Disease. Atlanta, ACELMU Publishers, 1976.
113. Michals, K., et al.: J. Am. Diet. Assoc., *73:*507, 1978.
114. Soirdahl, S., et al.: Pediatr. Res., *13:*74, 1979.
115. Bonkowsky, H.L., et al.: Metabolism, *25:*405, 1976.
116. Tschudy, D.P., et al.: Metabolism, *13:*396, 1964.
117. Welland, F.H., et al.: Metabolism, *13:*232, 1964.
118. Cohn, R.M., et al.: Am. J. Clin. Nutr., *30:*209, 1977.
119. Danner, D.J., et al.: J. Clin. Invest., *75:*858, 1985.
120. Litwer, S., Danner, D.J.: Biochem. Biophys. Res. Commun., *131:*961, 1985.
121. Elsas, L.J., Danner, D.J.: Ann. N.Y. Acad. Sci., *378:*404, 1982.
122. Danner, D.J., Elsas, L.J.: Biochem. Med., *13:*7, 1975.
123. Heffelfinger, S., et al.: Am. J. Hum. Genet., *36:*802, 1984.
124. Fernhoff, P.M., et al.: Pediatr. Res., *19:*1011, 1985.
125. Sweetman, L.: Branched chain organic acidurias. *In* The Metabolic Basis of Inherited Disease. 6th Ed. Edited by C. Scriver, A. Beaudet, W. Sly, et al. New York, McGraw-Hill, 1989.
126. Elsas, L.J., et al.: Metabolism, *21:*929, 1972.
127. Naylor, E.W., Guthrie, R.: Pediatrics, *61:*262, 1978.
128. Elsas, L.J., et al.: Metabolism, *23:*569, 1974.
129. Wendel, L.L., et al.: Eur. J. Pediatr., *138:*293, 1982.
130. Clow, C.L., et al.: Pediatrics, *68:*856, 1981.
131. Wendel, U., et al.: Eur. J. Pediatr., *138:*293, 1982.
132. Duran, M., Wadman, S.K.: J. Inherited Metab. Dis., *8(Suppl. 1):*70, 1985.
133. Szmelcman, S., Guggenheim, K.: Biochem. J., *100:*7, 1966.
134. Hammerson, G., et al.: Monogr. Hum. Genet., *9:*84, 1978.
135. DiGeorge, A.M., et al.: N. Engl. J. Med., *307:*1492, 1982.
136. Snyderman, J.E., et al.: Pediatr. Res., *18:*851, 1984.
137. Berry, G.T., et al.: N. Engl. J. Med., *324:*175, 1991.
138. Tanaka, K., et al.: Proc. Natl. Acad. Sci. U.S.A., *56:*236, 1966.
139. Shigamatsu, Y., et al.: Pediatr. Res., *16:*771, 1982.
140. Truscott, R.T.W., et al.: Clin. Chim. Acta, *110:*187, 1981.
141. Lehnert, W., Niederhoff, H.: Eur. J. Pediatr., *136:*281, 1981.
142. Mendiola, J., et al.: Tex. Med., *80:*52, 1984.
143. Wysocki, S.J., et al.: Clin. Chem., *29:*1002, 1983.
144. Yoshino, M., et al.: Adv. Exp. Biol. Med., *153:*141, 1982.
145. Yudkoff, M., et al.: J. Pediatr., *92:*813, 1978.
146. Dubiel, B., et al.: J. Clin. Invest., *72:*1543, 1983.
147. Ikeda, T., et al.: Purification and characterization of isovaleryl 1-CoA dehydrogenases from a liver mitochondria. *In* Metabolism and Clinical Implications of Branched Chain Amino Acids and Ketoacids. Edited by M. Walser and G.R. Williamson. New York, Elsevier, 1981.
148. Blascovics, M., Donnell, G.: J. Inherited Metab. Dis., *1:*9, 1978.
149. Tanaka, K., Yu: Clin. Chim. Acta, *138:*333, 1984.
150. Shigematsu, Y., et al.: Clin. Chim. Acta, *138:*333, 1984.
151. Bartlett, K., Gompertz, D. Biochem. Med., *10:*15, 1974.
152. Naglak, M, Elsas, L.J.: Pediatr. Res., *24:*9, 1988.
153. Stanley, C.A., et al.: Pediatr. Res., *17:*296A, 1983.
154. Roe, C.R., et al.: J. Clin. Invest., *74:*2290, 1984.
155. Finkelstein, J.D., Martin, J.J.: J. Biol. Chem., *259:*9508, 1984.
156. Mudd, S.H., Levy, H.L., Skorby, F.: Disorders of transsulfuration. *In* The Metabolic Basis of Inherited Disease. 6th Ed. Edited by C. Scriver, A. Beaudet, W. Sly, et al. New York, McGraw-Hill, 1989.
157. Skovby, F., et al.: Am. J. Hum. Genet., *36:*452, 1984.
158. McCusick, V.A. et al.: The clinical and genetic characteristics of homocystinuria. *In* Inherited Disorders of the Sulfur Metabolism. Edited by N. Carson and N. Raine. London, Churchill Livingstone, 1971.
159. Mudd, J.H., et al.: Am. J. Hum. Genet., *37:*1, 1985.
160. Boers, G.H.J., et al.: N. Engl. J. Med., *313:*709, 1985.
161. Schaumburg, H., et al.: N. Engl. J. Med., *309:*445, 1983.
162. Yoshida, I., et al.: J. Inherited Metab. Dis., *8:*91, 1985.
163. Wilcken, D.E.L., et al.: Metabolism, *34:*1115, 1985.
164. Marcus, A.J.: N. Engl. J. Med., *309:*1515, 1983.
165. Brusilow, S., Horwich, A.: Urea cycle enzymes. *In* The Metabolic Basis of Inherited Disease. 6th Ed. Edited by C. Scriver, A. Beaudet, W. Sly, et al. New York, McGraw-Hill, 1989.
166. Cederbaum, S., et al.: J. Pediatr., *90:*5–69, 1977.
167. Levin, B., et al.: Arch. Dis. Child., *44:*152, 1969.
168. Kennaway, N., et al.: Pediatr. Res., *9:*554, 1975.
169. Glick, N.R., et al.: Am. J. Hum. Genet., *28:*22, 1976.
170. Beaudet, A.: Am. J. Hum. Genet., *37:*386, 1985.
171. Su, T.S., et al.: J. Biol. Chem., *256:*11826, 1981.
172. Beaudet, A., et al.: Adv. Hum. Genet., *15:*161, 1986.
173. Horwich, et al.: Science, *224:*1068, 1984.
174. Kraus, et al.: Nucleic Acids Res., *13:*943, 1985.
175. Spector, E.B., et al.: Pediatr. Res., *17:*941, 1983.
176. Valle, D., Simell, O.: The hyperornithinemias. *In* The Metabolic Basis of Inherited Disease. 5th Ed. Edited by J.B. Stanbury. New York, McGraw-Hill, 1983.
177. Russell, A.: Mt. Sinai J. Med., *40:*723, 1973.
178. Rowe, P.C., et al.: N. Engl. J. Med., *314:*541, 1986.
179. Levy, H., et al.: The New England experience. *In* Neonatal Screening for Inborn Errors of Metabolism. Edited by H. Bickel et al. Berlin, Springer-Verlag, 1980.
180. Naylor, E.W., et al.: J. Lab. Clin. Med., *89:*987, 1977.
181. Naylor, E.W.: Pediatrics, *68:*453, 1981.
182. Talbot, H.W., et al.: Pediatrics, *70:*526, 1982.
183. Tada, K., et al.: Eur. J. Pediatr., *130:*105, 1979.
184. Rett, A.: Wien. Med. Wochenschr., *118:*311, 1968.
185. Symposium on Disorders of the Urea Cycle. Pediatrics, *68:*271, 1981.
186. Brusilow, S., Horwich, A.: Urea cycle enzymes. *In* Metabolic Basis of Inherited Disease. 6th Ed. Edited by C. Scriver, A. Beaudet, W. Sly, et al. New York, McGraw-Hill, 1989.
187. Batshaw, M.L., et al.: Pediatr. Res., *13:*472, 1979.
188. Snyderman, S.E., et al.: Pediatrics, *56:*65, 1975.
189. Bachmann, C.: Enzyme, *32:*56, 1984.
190. Batshaw, M.L., et al.: Pediatrics, *68:*290, 1981.
191. Brusilow, S.W.: Pediatr. Res., *29:*147, 1991.
192. Msall, M., et al.: N. Engl. J. Med., *310:*1500, 1984.

193. Ad Hoc Expert Committee: Energy and Protein Requirements. Rome, Food and Agriculture Organization of the United Nations, 1973.
194. Iafolla, A.K., et al.: J. Pediatr., *117:*102, 1990.
195. Segal, S.: Disorders of galactose metabolism. *In* The Metabolic Basis of Inherited Disease. 6th Ed. Edited by C. Scriver, A. Beaudet, W. Sly, et al. New York, McGraw-Hill, 1989.
196. Sparkes, R.C., et al.: Am. Hum. Genet. (London), *43:*343, 1980.
197. Flach, J.E., Reichardt, J., Elsas, L.: Mol. Biol. Med., *7:*365–369, 1990.
198. Sidbury, J.B., Jr: Investigations and speculations on the pathogenesis of galactosemia. *In* Galactosemia. Edited by D. Hsia. Springfield, IL, Charles C Thomas, 1969.
199. Urbanowski, J.C., et al.: N. Engl. J. Med., *306:*84, 1982.
200. Beutler, B.: J. Lab. Clin. Med., *68:*137, 1966.
201. Jakobs, C., et al.: Pediatr. Res., *18:*714, 1984.
202. Gitzelman, R., Auricchio, S.: Pediatrics, *36:*231, 1965.
203. Galactosemia in Infancy. Evansville, IN, Mead Johnson, 1976.
204. Nickerson, T.A.: Food Tech., *32:*40, 1978.
205. Hettinga, D.H.: J. Dairy Sci., *53:*1377, 1970.
206. Gallagher, C.R.: J. Am. Diet. Assoc., *65:*418, 1974.
207. Lee, P.E., Lillibridge, C.B.: Am. J. Clin. Nutr., *29:*428, 1976.
208. Fagen, J.H.: J. Dairy Sci., *35:*779, 1952.
209. Clothier, C.M., Davidson, D.C.: Hum. Nutr. Appl. Nutr., *37A:*483, 1983.
210. Fishler, K., et al.: Pediatrics, *50:*412, 1972.
211. Lee, D.H.: J. Ment. Def. Res., *16:*173, 1972.
212. Donnell, G., et al.: Pediatrics, *31:*802, 1963.
213. Gitzelman, R., Steinmann, B.: Enzyme, *32:*37, 1984.
214. Waisbren, S.E., et al.: J. Pediatr., *102:*75, 1983.
215. Irons, M., et al.: J. Pediatr., *107:*261, 1985.
216. Fensom, A.H., et al.: Br. Med. J., *4:*386, 1974.
217. Howard, N.J., et al.: Acta Paediatr. Scand., *70:*695, 1981.
218. Komrower, G.M.: J. Inherited Metab. Dis., *5(Suppl. 2):*96, 1982.
219. Anon: Lancet, *2:*1379, 1982.
220. Komrower, G.M.: Lancet, *1:*190, 1983.
221. Kaufman, F.R., et al.: N. Engl. J. Med., *30:*994, 1981.
222. Kaufman, F.R., et al.: J. Inherited Metab. Dis., *9:*140, 1986.
223. Chen, Y.T., et al.: Science, *214:*1145, 1981.
224. Chen, Y.T., et al.: Pediatr. Res., *18:*345, 1984.

SELECTED READINGS

Desnick, R.J. (Ed.): Treatment of Genetic Diseases. New York, Churchill Livingstone, 1991, p. 350.
Fernandes, J., Saudubray, J.M., Tada, K. (Eds.): Inborn Metabolic Diseases. Diagnosis and Treatment. New York, Springer-Verlag, 1990, p. 730.
Scriver, C.S., Beaudet, A., Sly, W., et al. (Eds.): The Metabolic Basis of Inherited Disease. 6th ed. Vol. 1. New York, McGraw-Hill, 1989, p. 3006.
Tada, K., Colombo, J.P., Desnick, R.J., (Eds.): Recent Advances in Inborn Errors of Metabolism. New York, Karger, 1987, p. 332.

CHAPTER 68

Diet and Nutrition in the Care of the Patient with Surgery, Trauma, and Sepsis

Wiley W. Souba, Jr., and Douglas W. Wilmore

Surgeons care for patients who undergo major operative procedures, sustain severe injuries, and develop life-threatening infections such as sepsis. Such individuals exhibit marked changes in metabolism and often require nutritional support. No discipline in medicine has benefited more from the current advances in nutritional support of hospitalized patients than has surgery. As recently as two decades ago, many surgical patients died of malnutrition, sepsis, and multiple-system organ failure because sophisticated techniques of enteral and parenteral feedings were not available. Such patients now routinely survive complex surgical procedures, major trauma, debilitating gastrointestinal disease, and complications such as sepsis and enterocutaneous fistulas. Today, virtually all hospitalized patients can be fed safely and effectively because of three developments: (1) the technique of central venous cannulation and infusion of hypertonic nutrient solutions into the superior vena cava;[1] (2) the development of specific enteral formula diets, usually delivered by a feeding tube;[2] and (3) the availability of fat emulsion for safe intravenous administration.[3]

Investigators in the mid-1970s suggested that 20 to 50% of patients in major hospitals were malnourished. It was proposed that much of this undernutrition was iatrogenic, resulting from the provision of sophisticated medical care without concern for satisfying nutritional requirements.[4] Indeed, many patients lose weight during hospitalization, as the result of withholding of meals for diagnostic tests or other periods of inadequate nutrient intake associated with acute illness, major operation, or medical therapy. These patients can now be fed; however, controlled trials in patients with normal body composition who undergo elective operations show that such nutritional support produces little improvement in outcome. Therefore, limited weight loss in selected hospitalized patients is acceptable because short-term undernutrition does not prolong a life-limiting illness, nor does it complicate convalescence following major operation or other therapy.

Not all hospitalized patients are malnourished because of diagnostic and therapeutic measures, however; the disease process is often the major culprit. Critically ill patients are frequently anorexic secondary to illness and confinement. Patients who have multiple injuries, with or without complications such as sepsis, rarely take adequate calories spontaneously from a food tray.[5] Others often initially have some degree of gastrointestinal ileus and hence cannot or should not eat. Patients with inflammatory bowel disease or those who are critically ill frequently cannot tolerate adequate feedings; enteral feedings result in pain, fever, bloating, or diarrhea. Cancer patients have a diminished appetite secondary to the tumor burden or concomitant treatment regimens, and weight loss is a sign of disease progression.

This chapter reviews the metabolic alterations that occur in patients undergoing elective operations, in patients with accidental injury, and in patients with sepsis. Methods of nutritional assessment of individuals in each of these general groups are provided, along with current knowledge of the nutritional requirements of patients with these illnesses. The basis for selecting the safest and most effective route of nutrient administration is discussed, and a review of newer methods of modifying the catabolic response to critical illness is provided.

ELECTIVE OPERATIVE PROCEDURES

PHYSIOLOGIC RESPONSES TO SURGERY

Although cytokines clearly play an important role in regulating the body's response to stress, their role appears to be more significant in patients with major injury and infection. Therefore, the importance of cytokines in the cellular response to injury and infection is discussed in the section of this chapter on trauma.

ENDOCRINE CHANGES AND THEIR METABOLIC CONSEQUENCES

One of the earliest consequences of a surgical procedure is the rise in levels of circulating cortisol that occurs in response to a sudden outpouring of adrenocorticotropic hormone (ACTH) from the anterior pituitary gland. Activation of the pituitary gland occurs when afferent nervous signals from the operative site reach the hypothalamus to initiate the stress response. The rise in ACTH stimulates the adrenal cortex to elaborate cortisol. This hormone remains at two to five times normal levels for approximately 24 hours after a major operation.[6] Cortisol has generalized effects on tissue catabolism and mobilizes amino acids from skeletal muscle that provide substrates for wound healing and serve as precursors for the hepatic synthesis of acute-phase proteins or new glucose. Associated with the activation of the adrenal cortex is stimulation of the adrenal medulla through the sympathetic nervous system, with elaboration of epinephrine. This circulating neurotransmitter plays an important role in circulatory adjustment, but it may also elicit metabolic responses if the augmented secretion rate continues over a prolonged period of time.

In addition to increased circulating levels of epinephrine, norepinephrine levels rise during and following elective operative procedures.[7] The excitement, pain, fear, and hypovolemia that may accompany the surgical procedure are potent stimulators of the sympathetic nervous system. Urinary catecholamines may be elevated for 24 to 48 hours after operation any may then return to normal. The major catabolic role of this regulatory system may be the stimulation of hepatic glycogenolysis and gluconeogenesis in concert with glucagon and glucocorticoids.

The neuroendocrine responses to operation also modify the various mechanisms that regulate salt and water excretion. Alterations in serum osmolarity and tonicity of body fluids secondary to anesthesia and operative stress stimulate the secretion of aldosterone and antidiuretic hormone (ADH).[7,8] Aldosterone is a potent stimulator of renal sodium retention, whereas ADH stimulates renal tubular water reabsorption. Although the neutral and humoral mediators that result from tissue trauma may stimulate aldosterone release, afferent signals from volume receptors appear to be the major stimuli for these hormonal adjustments.

The ability to excrete a water load after elective surgical procedures is restricted.[9] The usual postoperative patient concentrates urine to 1 to 2 ml water/mOsm solute excreted, corresponding to a urine osmolarity of 500 to 1000 mOsm/L, even in the presence of adequate hydration. Hence weight gain secondary to salt and water retention is usual following operation. Edema occurs to a varying extent in all surgical wounds, and this accumulation is proportional to the extent of tissue dissection and local trauma. Administration of sodium-containing solutions during operation replaces this functional volume loss as extracellular fluid redistributes in the body. This "third-spaced" fluid eventually returns to the circulation as the wound edema subsides, and diuresis commences 2 to 4 days following the operation.

Alterations occur in the response of the endocrine pancreas following elective operation. In general, insulin elaboration is diminished, and glucagon concentrations rise.[10] This response may be related to increased sympathetic activity or to the rise in levels of circulating epinephrine, which is known to suppress insulin release.[11] The increased elaboration of glucagon may be related to increased sympathetic nervous system stimulation or to alterations in circulating mediators. The rise in glucagon and the corresponding fall in insulin are a potent signal to accelerate hepatic glucose production, and, with other hormones (epinephrine and glucocorticoids), gluconeogenesis is maintained.

The postoperative hormonal responses are thought to orchestrate physiologic and biochemical changes that benefit the host. Salt and water conservation support the circulating blood volume. Augmented hepatic glucose production provides adequate essential fuel for the nervous system, red and white blood cells, and the healing wound. Skeletal muscle proteolysis provides amino acid precursors for gluconeogenesis and hepatic protein synthesis. Postoperative lipolysis provides abundant quantities of free fatty acid, as an additional energy source. Current techniques of postoperative care minimize, but do not reverse, these responses.

STAGE OF SURGICAL CONVALESCENCE

The period of catabolism initiated by operation, a combination of inadequate nutrition and alteration of the hormonal environment, has been termed the "adrenergic-corticoid phase." This period is followed by the onset of anabolism, which occurs at a variable time in the patient's convalescence. In general, in the absence of postoperative complications, this phase starts 3 to 6 days after an abdominal operation of the magnitude of a colectomy or gastrectomy, often concomitant with the commencement of oral feedings. This "turning point" from catabolism to anabolism is referred to as the "corticoid-withdrawal phase" because it is characterized by a spontaneous sodium and free-water diuresis, a positive potassium balance, and a reduction in nitrogen excretion. This transitional phase usually lasts only 1 to 2 days.

The patient then enters a prolonged period of early anabolism characterized by positive nitrogen balance and weight gain. Protein synthesis is increased as a result of sustained enteral feedings, and this change is related to the return of lean body mass and muscular strength. The positive nitrogen balance is usually in the range of 2 to 4 g of nitrogen per day in the average adult, a range representing a daily gain of 60 to 120 g lean tissue. The total amount of nitrogen ultimately gained equals the amount lost, but the rate of gain is much slower than the rate of initial loss.

The fourth and final phase of surgical convalescence is late anabolism, the hallmark of which is much slower weight gain. During this period, the patient is in nitrogen equilibrium but in positive carbon balance, which results from the deposition of body fat.

EFFECTS OF NUTRITIONAL SUPPORT ON POSTOPERATIVE METABOLISM

Most patients undergoing elective operations are adequately nourished. Following an operation of the magnitude of cholecystectomy with common duct exploration, aneurysmectomy, or colectomy, oral feedings are generally not tolerated for 2 to 6 days. In a patient without postoperative complications, the duration of postoperative ileus depends on the extent of manipulation of the abdominal viscera and the length of the operation. Nasogastric decompression is frequently required, and the patient is routinely supported by 2 to 4 L intravenous fluids, usually containing 5% dextrose and appropriate electrolytes. Unless the patient has suffered significant preoperative malnutrition, characterized by a weight loss >10%, or has had a major intraoperative or postoperative complication, solutions containing 5% dextrose may be administered for 5 to 7 days before the initiation of enteral nutrition, with no detrimental effect on outcome. With no dietary nitrogen and with insufficient calories, negative nitrogen balance occurs, in which urinary nitrogen excretion averages 10 to 15 g per day for 2 to 3 days and then gradually diminishes. This nitrogen excretion is associated with a loss of potassium and phosphorus and indicates a loss of lean body mass.

Early investigators who studied the catabolic responses to operation concluded that the negative nitrogen balance was "obligatory" and an irreversible consequence of the metabolic response to injury. This view was challenged by data from two studies in postoperative patients. Riegel and associates fed patients who had undergone gastrectomy and neurosurgical procedures with tube-feeding techniques and showed that nitrogen equilibrium could be achieved when 0.30 g nitrogen and 125 kJ/kg (30 kcal/kg)* were provided daily.[12] Subsequently, Holden and colleagues nutritionally supported patients who had undergone gastrectomy in the early postoperative period with intravenous nutrients and noted that body weight was maintained and near nitrogen balance was achieved when adequate calories and nitrogen were administered.[13] These investigators concluded that the catabolic response to operation is due in large part to inadequate food intake and is not an obligatory consequence of operative stress.

In general, if the patient is well nourished preoperatively and is expected to eat by the fifth to seventh postoperative day, 5% dextrose solutions will provide adequate calories to prevent detrimental losses of endogenous body protein. Although a balanced nutrient intake administered in the postoperative period reduces the brief negative nitrogen balance associated with elective surgery and may maintain body weight, such as approach appears to be unwarranted in most patients undergoing elective operations. Such feedings have not accelerated recovery or decreased hospital stays in this group of patients. Therefore, the increased cost of feedings and the potential complications associated with intravenous nutrition cannot be justified. On the other hand, jejunal feedings may be useful in the postoperative period in some patients, especially those undergoing extensive upper gastrointestinal operations. Such feedings are considerably less expensive than total parenteral nutrition (TPN) and can be administered safely. Studies evaluating the effectiveness of postoperative nutrition are reviewed in this chapter.

NUTRITIONAL SUPPORT OF ELECTIVE SURGICAL PATIENTS

NUTRITIONAL ASSESSMENT

The two major objectives of nutritional assessment are: (1) to determine the patient's nutritional status; and (2) to determine energy, protein, and macro- and micronutrient requirements. The nutritional status of a patient is determined by a careful history and physical examination, followed by additional tests to confirm the

*4.18 kJ = 1 kcal.

clinical impression. The medical history should include inquiries about associated disease processes, medication, and history of weight loss and dietary habits. The physical examination may establish the diagnosis of cachexia, protein-energy malnutrition, or specific nutrient deficiencies. Weight loss of more than 10% of the patient's weight before illness may compromise the patient's ability to combat infection or to heal wounds.

Anthropometric measurements include measurement of body weight and height. The features are compared with population norms.[14] Measurements of skinfold thickness are helpful to determine fat mass, and a 24-hour urine collection with measurement of creatine allows determination of the creatine-height index (CHI), a factor proportional to the size of muscle mass.[15] More sophisticated techniques to determine body composition include isotopic dilution methods, underwater weighing, total-body computed tomography, and γ-neutron activation; these methods are not generally practical in routine screening of most elective surgical patients. A detailed evaluation of assessment procedures is given in Chapters 49 to 51 (see also Appendix Tables A–11 to A–15).

Immunologic status has been used to evaluate nutritional status; total peripheral lymphocyte count, delayed hypersensitivity using a skin-test response to common antigens, and lymphocyte transformation have all been used as indicators of immunocompetence in the critically ill patient.[16] Depressed immune function often returns to normal with nutritional repletion, but altered immunologic responses are not specific for nutritional deficiencies and are observed in patients with advanced malignant disease or in those who have had a severe injury. Moreover, delayed hypersensitivity may return on resolution of the disease process, despite inadequate nutrient intake.

Laboratory tests are useful to confirm the clinical suspicion of malnutrition. Serum albumin and transferrin are the most common serum proteins measured, and they correlate well with body protein deficiency in isolated cases of malnutrition. Most nutritional deficits in surgical patients are secondary to a disease process, however, and the presence of disease may alter these indicators. Other laboratory studies that may be useful in nutritional assessment include red blood cell indices to determine iron and micronutrient deficiencies, plasma glucose to assess insulin resistance, blood urea nitrogen (BUN) to determine renal status, and liver function tests to evaluate hepatic function.

DETERMINING NUTRITIONAL REQUIREMENTS

Nutritional therapy should be directed to a specific goal; depending on the patient's nutritional status, this goal should be: (1) to diminish the rate of weight loss and body protein breakdown; (2) to maintain body weight and protein stores; and (3) to achieve weight gain and anabolism. In general, patients with abnormal body composition (no major nutritional deficiencies) and who are not hypercatabolic do not develop significant nutritional deficits during 5 to 7 days of undernutrition. For example, the patient with an uncomplicated postoperative course may receive intravenous infusions of 5% dextrose in water or inadequate oral intake for this period of time without any detrimental effect on recovery or ultimate health. The malnourished patient who has lost more than 10% of normal preillness weight requires vigorous nutritional support, however. The immediate goal in such an individual is nutritional maintenance, whereas the ultimate goal is restoration of body mass, which generally occurs in the later phases of surgical convalescence.

Total energy requirements are based on several factors: (1) the basal metabolic rate (BMR); (2) the degree of stress imposed by the disease process; and (3) the amount of energy expended with activity. Available nomograms relate normal metabolic requirements to a person's age, sex, height, and weight.[14] Once basal metabolic requirements of the nonstressed individual have been determined, additional factors such as the stress of the disease and hospital activity should be considered. These relationships are expressed in Table 68–1.

The principal influences on nitrogen balance in surgical patients are total energy intake, nitrogen intake, and the metabolic state of the patient. Energy and nitrogen relationships are altered in nutritionally depleted and hypermetabolic patients. Persons with nutritional deficits have intact protein-conserving mechanisms that allow nitrogen equilibrium when 7 to 8% of the total caloric needs are provided as protein. This translates into a calorie-to-nitrogen ratio of approximately 350:1. Hypermetabolic, catabolic patients, on the other hand, have a diminished protein economy and require much more protein. For example, Duke and associates showed that, in injured patients, protein contributes 15 to 20% of the total energy expenditure, such that the optimal calorie-to-nitrogen ratio is approximately 150:1.[17]

ROUTES OF FEEDING

Enteral or intravenous feedings are prescribed, depending on the patient's conditions.

Enteral Feedings. For patients who can eat and who have a functional gastrointestinal tract, adequate nutrition can best be provided by the regular hospital diet. This diet may be supplemented with between-meal snacks if necessary. Daily calorie counts and body weight determinations are necessary to monitor intake and the response to therapy.

Some patients with a functional intestinal tract will not or cannot eat. Such patients include neurosurgical patients, those with oropharyngeal or esophageal obstruction, the elderly, and small children. In these patients, nasogastric or nasojejunal feedings may be indicated. Gastric feedings can be delivered 5 to 6 times daily by bolus feedings. Jejunal feedings require continuous administration. When permanent feedings are an-

TABLE 68–1. FORMULAS FOR DETERMINATIONS OF TOTAL ENERGY REQUIREMENTS

Daily Energy Requirement for Weight Maintenance =
Normal BMR[a] × Stress Factor[b] × 1.25[c]

Daily Energy Requirement for Weight Gain =
Maintenance Energy + 1,000 kcal[d,e]

[a]Normal BMR (basal metabolic rate, usually 1,500 to 1,800 kcal/day) can be determined using standard nomograms or formulas. The approximate values of the basal metabolic rate for adults of average size are given below:

Body Weight (kg)	50	55	60	65	70	75	80
Normal BMR (kcal/day)	1,316	1,411	1,509	1,602	1,694	1,784	1,872

[b]Stress factor is the term used to correct the normal BMR for the effects of a disease process:

Condition	Stress Factor
Mild starvation	0.85–1.00
Postoperative recovery (no complications)	1.00–1.05
Cancer*	1.10–1.45
Long-bone fracture	1.25–1.30
Peritonitis	1.05–1.25
Severe infection of multiple trauma*	1.30–1.55
Burns >40% body surface area	2.0

*Proportional to the extent of the disease.
[c]The basal caloric requirements of the stressed patient are adjusted upward an additional 20 to 25% for hospital activity and the stress associated with treatment. This adjustment is unnecessary for patients receiving artificial ventilation who are paralyzed or are heavily sedated.
[d]If anabolism and weight gain are the goals, an additional 1,000 kcal/day may be added to maintenance requirements to provide for a weight gain of approximately 1 kg (2 lb)/week. Weight maintenance, not weight gain, should be the primary objective in most critically ill patients.
[e]1 kilocaloric (kcal) = 4.18 kilojoules, (kJ)

ticipated, a gastrostomy or feeding jejunostomy should be considered.[18] A variety of nutrient formulas are now available for enteral feedings. In general, intact or partially hydrolyzed nutrients are most appropriate. These diets should be nutritionally complete and free of lactose (see Chap. 79).

Intravenous Feedings. Frequently, surgical patients require nutritional support, but have a diseased or nonfunctional gastrointestinal tract. These persons are candidates for parenteral nutrition, which can be infused through a peripheral or central vein. Peripheral venous feedings provide dilute nutrients in a large fluid volume and rely on fat emulsions as a principal calorie source. Central venous feedings consist of hypertonic glucose and amino acid solutions infused through a catheter placed in the superior vena cava. Adequate calories can be administered in a small fluid volume, but this method of feeding requires placement and care of a central venous catheter (see Chap. 80).

FORMULATING A NUTRITION SUPPORT PLAN

Most patients undergoing elective operative procedures recover quickly, resume oral feeding early in the postoperative period, and require no specialized nutritional support. Other surgical patients do not fit this description and require formal nutritional care. This group includes patients with preoperative malnutrition, those with dysfunctional gastrointestinal tracts (prolonged ileus, inflammatory bowel disease), or those with specific diseases associated with a catabolic course (severe infection, major injury). These patients generally fall into one of these categories. In normally nourished patients, the nutritional goal is to maintain body weight and protein stores. In malnourished patients and nonstressed patients, weight gain and repletion of lean body tissue are indicated and are usually accomplished by providing an extra 4180 kJ (1000 kcal) per day. Anabolism is difficult to achieve in stressed catabolic patients, but body mass is generally restored simultaneously on resolution of the disease process. Hence the nutritional goal in these patients is weight maintenance and treatment of the underlying disease process.

PERIOPERATIVE NUTRITIONAL SUPPORT—IS IT BENEFICIAL?

In general, one cannot justify the use of perioperative nutrition, particularly parenteral feedings, unless a clear benefit to the patient can be demonstrated. Unfortunately, many of the studies undertaken to evaluate the effectiveness of perioperative nutritional support have design flaws that make their interpretation difficult. However, several clear-cut indications for preoperative and postoperative nutrition have emerged because of these trials, and all surgeons should be familiar with these indications and how to monitor during feedings (Fig. 68–1).

PREOPERATIVE NUTRITIONAL SUPPORT

Total Parenteral Nutrition (TPN). Retrospective studies in the 1970s suggested that preoperative nutritional repletion with TPN was of benefit to the malnourished cancer patient. Copeland and Dudrick studied cancer patients undergoing major surgical procedures and suggested that malnourished patients who were not fed preoperatively often developed complications such as prolonged ileus, wound infection and dehiscence, and anastomotic disruption that required prolonged periods of postoperative TPN for resolution.[19] Rombeau and colleagues suggested, from a retrospective analysis, that preoperative parenteral nutrition was beneficial in patients requiring operation for inflammatory bowel disease.[20] Patients who received preoperative parenteral nutrition for at least 5 days had fewer postoperative complications than patients who received TPN for fewer than 5 days. Mullen et al. retrospectively applied the Prognostic Nutritional Index (PNI) to surgical patients to evaluate the effectiveness of at least 7 days of preoperative TPN.[21,22] In the high-risk group of patients (PNI >50%), the incidence of postoperative septic complications and mortality were decreased five-fold in the group receiving TPN.

Although these aforementioned studies suggest that preoperative TPN may benefit certain patients, retrospective studies are fraught with pitfalls and assumptions that often make them invalid. In this regard, prospective trials are more reliable. Holter and Fischer prospectively studied the effects of preoperative TPN in patients with gastrointestinal malignant disorders who had lost 10 lb of body weight over the prior 2 to 3 months.[23] The TPN group received TPN for 72 hours preoperatively surgery and were continued on this form of nutritional support for 10 days postoperatively or until 6300 kJ (1500 kcal) per day was taken orally. This group was compared to a group of patients with weight loss who did not receive TPN and a group of patients without significant weight loss who did not receive TPN. Patients in the TPN group demonstrated increases in serum albumin and body weight, but no difference was found in the incidence of major or minor complications among the groups. In a similar study, Thompson et al. randomized patients with weight loss from malignant

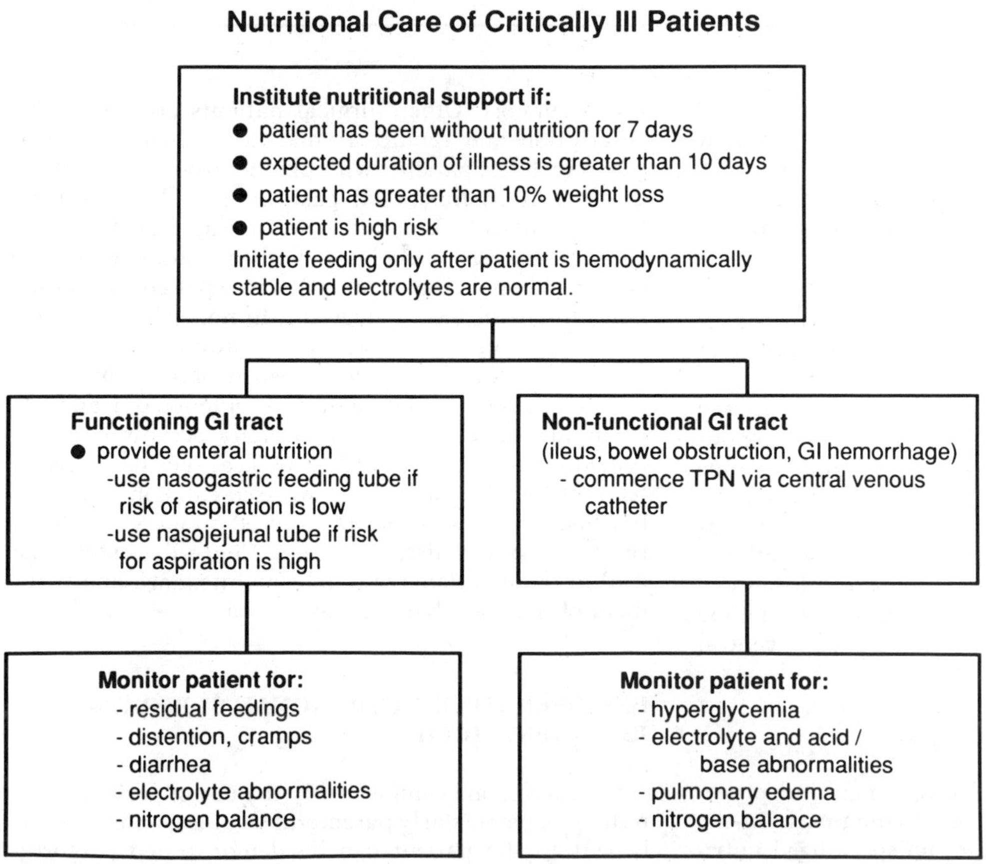
Nutritional Care of Critically Ill Patients
Institute nutritional support if:
patient has been without nutrition for 7 days
expected duration of illness is greater than 10 days
patient has greater than 10% weight loss
patient is high risk
Initiate feeding only after patient is hemodynamically stable and electrolytes are normal.
Functioning GI tract
provide enteral nutrition
-use nasogastric feeding tube if risk of aspiration is low
-use nasojejunal tube if risk for aspiration is high
Non-functional GI tract
(ileus, bowel obstruction, GI hemorrhage)
- commence TPN via central venous catheter
Monitor patient for:
- residual feedings
- distention, cramps
- diarrhea
- electrolyte abnormalities
- nitrogen balance
Monitor patient for:
- hyperglycemia
- electrolyte and acid / base abnormalities
- pulmonary edema
- nitrogen balance

FIGURE 68–1. Nutritional management of the critically ill patient.

gastrointestinal diseases to receive either preoperative and postoperative TPN or no TPN.[24] A third group, serving as controls, had weight loss less than 4.5 kg and did not receive TPN. The patients in the TPN group received adequate calories and nitrogen for a mean of 8 days preoperatively and 10 days postoperatively. Although the TPN group was better able to maintain body weight, postoperative complications were equal among the groups. A prospective, randomized study from the National Cancer Institute compared the use of preoperative (12 days) and postoperative TPN (13 days) to an ad libitum oral diet in patients with upper gastrointestinal tract cancers and weight loss.[25] This study terminated after accruing only 26 patients because early analysis showed a trend toward an increase in the complication rate in the TPN group. The TPN patients received 75 to 101% of their estimated caloric requirements. The increase in complications was largely attributed to infections.

Contrary to the foregoing studies, several prospective reports support the use of preoperative TPN in certain circumstances. In a frequently cited publication, Müller et al. studied 125 surgical patients with gastrointestinal tract cancers.[26] Patients were randomized to receive either TPN or no TPN (control) preoperatively. The control group received a hospital diet (the amount consumed was not recorded). Patients received TPN for 10 days preoperatively and postoperatively until they resumed oral intake. Of the 66 patients in the TPN group, only 41% were considered malnourished. A similar percentage of patients in the control group were malnourished. The incidence of major complications was 30% in the control group and 20% in the TPN group. Mortality in the control group was 18.6%, whereas mortality in the TPN group was only 4.5%. This study is biased against TPN because many of the patients were well nourished. Nevertheless, TPN resulted in an overall reduction of morbidity and mortality. This prospective trial provides the best evidence for the use of a 10-day preoperative course of TPN in the malnourished patient.

In a more recent study, Bellatone et al. prospectively studied 100 patients undergoing major surgical procedures for gastrointestinal disease.[27] Forty-nine of these patients received preoperative TPN for at least 7 days, whereas the control group of 51 patients did not receive preoperative nutritional support. The TPN regimen consisted of 125 kJ (30 kcal)/kg per day (30% of total calories supplied as lipid) and 200 mg nitrogen/kg per day. The overall septic complication rate was not significantly different between groups. However, in those patients who were malnourished (serum albumin level less than 3.5 g/dl and/or total lymphocyte count less than 1500 cells/mm^3), a statistically significant difference was observed in the incidence of sepsis between the TPN group and the control group (21% versus 53%, respectively). This was most dramatic in the group undergoing gastrectomy for gastric cancer. In a more recent publication, Bellatone and colleagues studied only those patients who were malnourished.[28] Significantly fewer total complications were noted in the group randomized to preoperative TPN, including a decrease in the incidence of serious septic complications.

In 1981, the Cooperative Studies Program of the Veterans Administration Medical Research Service appropriated funds to initiate planning of a multi-institutional clinical study to evaluate the efficacy and cost effectiveness of preoperative TPN in surgical patients. The study is now published and demonstrates that preoperative TPN reduces the noninfectious complication rate but increases the infectious complication rate.[29] Overall, the severely malnourished patient appears to benefit most from preoperative TPN, with the decrease in serious noninfectious complications outweighing the slight increase in infectious complications. Meta-analyses of prospective, randomized trials have also shown a marginal benefit of preoperative TPN.[30] The authors of this analysis of 11 separate trials concluded that the use of preoperative TPN in well-nourished patients is not justified and that its routine use in malnourished patients requires further study to define which groups of patients are most likely to benefit from preoperative TPN.

Enteral Nutrition. Beneficial effects of preoperative nutrition have been observed in two trials. The first of these studies demonstrated that 10 days of a preoperative polymeric diet decreased the complication rate, death rate, and length of hospital stay in patients undergoing surgical procedures for a variety of diseases.[31] More recently, an Italian study by Foschi et al. indicated that preoperative enteral alimentation following percutaneous transhepatic biliary drainage for obstructive jaundice was beneficial.[32] Patients in this study received an average of 20 days of enteral feedings by feeding tube or were allowed ad libitum intake of a regular hospital diet. The patients receiving the enteral diet had a reduced incidence of complications (anastamotic disruptions and organ failure) and a decrease in mortality rate. In a noncontrolled trial, Flynn and Leighty were able to show a reduction in postoperative morbidity and in length of hospital stay in patients with head and neck cancer who were given aggressive enteral nutritional supplements preoperatively.[33]

POSTOPERATIVE NUTRITIONAL SUPPORT

Indications for Postoperative Feedings. Indications include postoperative complications and certain risk factors.

Complications Following Operation in the Well-Nourished Patient. One common complication is prolonged postoperative ileus. Despite enemas and ambulation, the absence of peristalisis persists, and nasogastric tube losses occur. If the ileus continues for more than 5 to 7 days, intravenous feedings should be initiated. More frequently, ileus is the hallmark of an intra-abdominal inflammatory process, be it secondary to infection, pancreatitis, or active inflammatory bowel disease. Unlike the unstressed postoperative patient with simple ileus, these individuals are often febrile and hypermetabolic. In conjunction with appropriate treatment of the intra-abdominal process, nutritional support should be instituted; the nutritional goal is maintenance of body weight and protein stores and provision of adequate quantities of vitamins and micronutrients. The insertion of a central venous catheter for the delivery of hypertonic nutrient solutions provides 9200 to 10,500 kJ (2200 to 2500 kcal) and 14 to 17 g nitrogen per day with a calorie-to-nutrition ratio of approximately 150:1. When an abscess is associated with a gastrointestinal anastomosis, an enterocutaneous fistula may form. Adequate nutritional care, coupled with prompt surgical care (drainage) and appropriate antibiotics, has reduced the mortality rate from this complication from 40 to 60% to as low as 6%.[34]

High-Risk Surgical Patients. Only an occasional previously healthy patient undergoing elective operation develops complications and subsequently requires nutritional support. The majority of surgical patients requiring nutritional support are individuals at increased operative risk. Many of these patients are malnourished; preoperative nutritional support should be a major objective. Other high-risk patients are these with diabetes, cirrhosis, heart disease, renal failure, marked obesity, or known abuse of drugs or alcohol. In addition, immunocompromised patients should be carefully evaluated, and their nutritional deficits should be restored before operation.

A major complication of the high-risk patient is wound dehiscence. This separation of the wound is most impressive when it occurs following laparotomy. When abdominal evisceration occurs, the patient should be taken to the operating room, and the wound should be debrided and approximated. Because wound disruption is frequently associated with infection and results in a massive inflammatory reaction, calorie and nitrogen demands increase and should be provided by intravenous feedings.

Hepatic failure occurs most commonly in the alcoholic cirrhotic patient who has a major gastrointestinal hemorrhage that requires operative intervention. Although the origin of hepatic encephalopathy is unknown, central nervous system function may be influenced by circulating levels of amino acids.[35] The branched-chain amino acids (leucine, isoleucine, and valine) circulate at unusually low levels in patients with liver failure, whereas levels of the aromatic amino acids (phenylalanine, tyrosine, and tryptophan) are elevated. The hypothesis states that branched-chain amino acids compete with neutral amino acids for uptake across the blood-brain barrier. Because of the low blood levels of the branched-chain amino acids, brain uptake of several of the amino acids that serve as precursors for the synthesis of false neurotransmitters may increase.[36] This therapeutic effect has not consistently been observed,[37] and appropriate nutritional therapy for encephalopathic patients is currently under investigation (see also Chaps. 63 and 80).

When acute renal failure follows a major operation, the kidneys are unable to excrete waste solute (nitrogen) or solvent, although occasionally polyuric renal failure occurs. Provision of the usual amounts of amino acids in the diet exacerbates the already elevated level of blood urea nitrogen. In these patients, adequate calories should be provided to minimize protein breakdown, and nitrogen intake should be restricted if the patient does not require hemodialysis.[38] Potassium, magnesium, and zinc are administered with caution.

A special solution of essential amino acids (Nephramine) may improve protein synthesis and may reduce urea generation.[36] These amino acids are mixed with a 50 to 70% dextrose solution, to minimize fluid intake. This mixture is administered through central venous catheters. This renal failure formula has been evaluated in patients with postoperative acute renal failure. Abel and associates reported that such parenteral nutrition improved survival rates and diminished renal dysfunction in patients with acute renal failure following aortic aneurysmectomy.[39] In this prospective, randomized, double-blind trial, patients given glucose and essential amino acids had a better chance of surviving acute renal failure than those receiving only glucose (75 versus 44%; $p=0.02$). Because patients were carefully selected for entry into this study, these results may only be applicable to a select group of individuals with postoperative acute renal failure. Other studies generally support the conclusions of Abel and colleagues, however[38] (see also Chap. 65).

Postoperative TPN. Few studies have examined the effects of postoperative TPN as a sole means of perioperative nutritional support. Copeland and Dudrick, in a retrospective analysis of malnourished cancer patients, suggested that the advantage of TPN is primarily from preoperative administration.[19] Preshaw et al. randomized patients undergoing elective colon resection to receive 5 days of postoperative TPN or no TPN.[40] Forty-seven patients were radiographically studied 10 to 14 days postoperatively, and 8 anastamotic leaks in the TPN group and 4 leaks in the control group were found. Ordinarily, such patients would not have been provided nutritional support postoperatively, so the meaning of such data is unclear.

Yamada et al. prospectively studied the effects of TPN with adjunctive chemotherapy in 57 patients immediately after gastrectomy for advanced stomach cancer.[41] Postoperative TPN restored cell-mediated immunocompetence, increased body weight, enhanced serum protein and albumin levels, and increased the total lymphocyte count. In the TPN group, chemotherapy was better tolerated and a higher dose of 5-fluorouracil could be administered. Postoperative complications were significantly decreased in the TPN group, as were disease-free survival and overall survival. Askanazi et al. retrospectively reviewed patients who were randomized to receive TPN or 5% dextrose in water after radical cystectomy.[42] TPN was administered for 1 week postoperatively. Although patients entering the study were not malnourished, the median duration of hospitalization was significantly shorter in the TPN group.

Postoperative Enteral Nutrition. Benefits of postoperative enteral nutrition have been observed in at least six controlled trials: 3 for gastrointestinal diseases requiring operation,[43,44,45] one for hip fractures, and two for abdominal trauma necessitating laparotomy.[46,47] The benefits of enteral nutrition observed in these trials included a decrease in the duration of intravenous feedings, a decrease in septic complications, and a reduction in length of hospital stay and rehabilitation. These trials were prompted by animal studies indicating that delivery of nutrients through the gastrointestinal tract is superior to TPN in maintaining gut structure, metabolism, and immunologic function. In the first of these studies, Hoover and colleagues randomized 51 patients undergoing extensive upper gastrointestinal operations to receive either standard intravenous fluids or an elemental diet via needle-catheter jejunostomy (NCJ) in the immediate postoperative period.[44] Increases in weight gain, nitrogen balance, and total serum protein levels were noted in the enterally fed group. The duration of intravenous fluid therapy in the enteral group was 2.1 days, compared to 8.4 days in the control group. NCJ-related complications were not reported. In a subsequent study, Daly et al. prospectively studied the effects of immediate postoperative jejunostomy feedings in patients undergoing cystectomy and ileal conduit for bladder cancer.[43] Twenty patients were randomized to receive an enteral diet via NCJ or the standard postoperative 5% dextrose solution. Improved nitrogen balance was noted in the patients nourished by NCJ, but half the patients in the NCJ group suffered some type of gastrointestinal complication, compared to 36% in the control group. The length of hospital stay was not different between groups and infectious complications were not reported. In a 1979 study, Sagar and associates randomized 30 patients undergoing major gastrointestinal operations to receive an elemental diet (beginning on postoperative day 1 through a nasojejunal tube) or standard intravenous fluids and a "light diet" started on the sixth postoperative day.[45] Control patients lost more weight, had a more pronounced negative nitrogen balance, and had a longer hospital stay than the group fed an elemental diet. However, wound infection rates were similar.

TRAUMA

USUAL RESPONSE TO INJURY

GENERAL OVERVIEW AND TIME COURSE

Accidental injury is followed by a well-described pattern of physiologic responses. The events are generally related to the severity of injury; that is, the greater the insult, the more pronounced the specific response (Fig. 68–2). Although alterations following injury were first described in the 1860s, not until the 1930s were changes in injured humans carefully studied and an integrated response pattern described. David Patton Cuthbertson studied patients with long-bone fractures. He noticed that these patients lost large quantities of nitrogen, potassium, and phosphorus in their urine following injury, and this accelerated excretion rate could not be reversed by vigorous oral feedings.[46] Cuthbertson noted that the injured patient's oxygen consumption gradually rose, with simultaneous elevation in body temperature. Because no apparent site of infection was identified, this febrile response was referred to as "post-traumatic fever". Cuthbertson described the time course for many of the post-traumatic responses, and two distinct periods were identified, an early "ebb" or shock phase was usually brief (12 to 24 hours) and occurred immediately following injury. Blood pressure, cardiac output, body temperature, and oxygen consumption were reduced. These events were often associated with hemorrhage and resulted in hypoperfusion and lactic acidosis. With restoration of blood volume, ebb-phase alterations gave way to more accelerated responses. The flow phase was then characterized by hypermetabolism, increased cardiac output, increased urinary nitrogen losses, altered glucose metabolism, and accelerated tissue catabolism (Table 68–2).

The flow-phase responses to accidental injury are similar to those seen following elective operation. The response to injury is usually much more intensive and extends over a long period of time, however. For example, following soft tissue injury, patients often have an impaired ability to excrete a water load because of the heightened elaboration of aldosterone and ADH. The retention of large quantities of sodium and water that may occur during fluid resuscitation results in a dramatic increase in body weight, which may rise 10 to 20% over the patient's weight before injury. During recovery, the edema fluid reenters the vascular compartment, and the salt and water load is gradually excreted by the kidneys. Although sodium and water retention may occur following elective operation, the magnitude is much less great, and subsequent events (fluid mobilization followed by volume expansion and diuresis) are much less dramatic than in injured patients.

CHARACTERISTICS OF THE FLOW PHASE OF THE INJURY RESPONSE

This phase is characterized by hypermetabolism and by alterations in the metabolism of glucose, protein, and fat.

Hypermetabolism. Hypermetabolism is defined as an increase in BMR above that predicted on the basis of age, sex, and body size. Metabolic rate is usually determined by measuring the exchange of respiratory gases and by calculating heat production from oxygen consumption

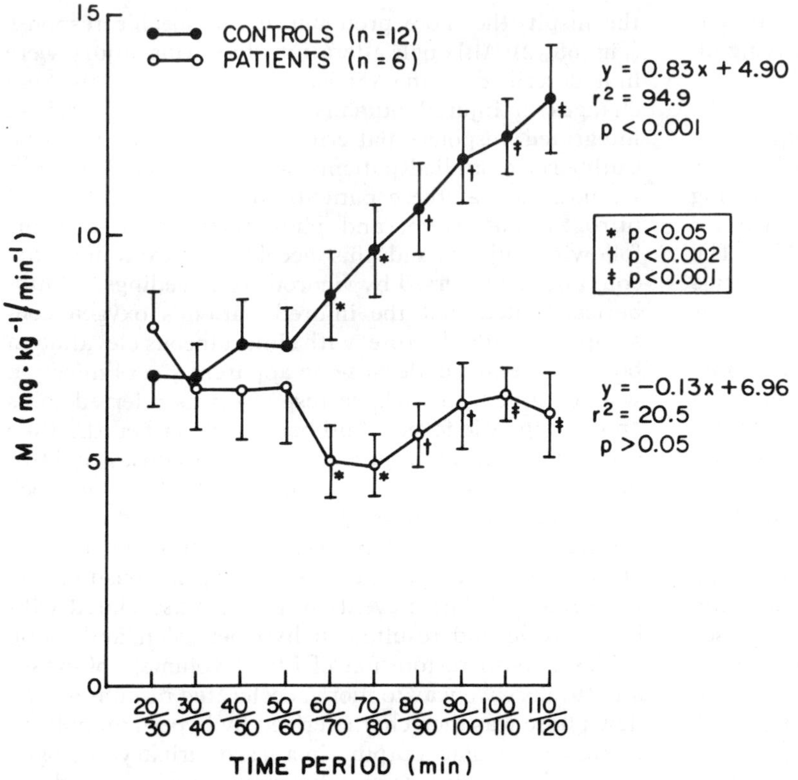

FIGURE 68–2. With time, the rate of glucose disposal (M) progressively increases in the control subjects during the hyperglycemic glucose clamp. In contrast, glucose removal was constant in these patients over the 2 hours of study and averaged approximately 7 mg/kg per minute. (From Black, P.R., Brooks, D.C., Bessey, P.Q., et al.: Ann. Surg., *196*:420–433, 1982.)

TABLE 68–2. METABOLIC ALTERATIONS FOLLOWING INJURY

EBB PHASE	FLOW PHASE
Blood glucose elevated	Glucose normal or slightly elevated
Glucose production normal	Glucose production increased
Free fatty acids elevated	Free fatty acids normal or slightly elevated; flux increased
Insulin concentration low	Insulin concentration normal or elevated
Catecholamines and glucagon elevated	Catecholamines high normal or elevated; glucagon elevated
Blood lactate elevated	Blood lactate normal
Oxygen consumption depressed	Oxygen consumption elevated
Cardiac output below normal	Cardiac output increased
Core temperature below normal	Core temperature elevated

and carbon dioxide production (see Chap. 5). The degree of hypermetabolism (increased oxygen production) is generally related to the severity of the injury. Patients with long-bone fractures have a 15 to 25% increase in metabolic rate, whereas the metabolic needs of patients with multiple injuries increase by 50%. Patients with severe burn injury, greater than 50% of body surface area (BSA), have resting metabolic rates that may reach twice basal levels.[14] These rates of heat production in trauma patients are contrasted with those in postoperative patients, who rarely increase their BMR by more than 10 to 15% following operation.

Concomitant with the development of hypermetabolism, the trauma patient usually develops a 1 to 2° C elevation in body temperature. This post-traumatic fever is a well-recognized component of the injury response and represents an upward shift in the thermoregulatory set point of the brain.[47] In general, if the patient is asymptomatic, the fever will rarely be treated.

Altered Glucose Metabolism. Hyperglycemia commonly occurs following injury, and the elevation of fasting blood sugar levels generally parallels the severity of stress in the ebb phase. At that time, insulin levels are low, and glucose production is only slightly elevated.[48] Later, during the flow phase, insulin concentrations are normal or elevated; yet hyperglycemia persists. This phenomenon suggests an alteration in the relationship between insulin sensitivity and glucose disposal. Hepatic glucose production is increased,[49] and the accelerated gluconeogenesis is generally related to the extent of the injury. Studies in injured patients show that much of the new glucose generated by the liver arises from 3-carbon precursors (lactate, pyruvate, amino acids, and glycerol) released from peripheral tissues.[49]

To determine which peripheral tissues use the large quantity of glucose produced by the liver, investigators measured substrate exchange across injured and uninjured extremities of severely burned patients matched for age, weight, and extent of total-body-surface burn.[50] That net glucose flux across uninjured extremities was low suggests that fat, not glucose, is the primary fuel for resting skeletal muscle in the postabsorptive state. Similar observations have been made in a study of normal volunteers; however, glucose uptake was increased across the burned extremity. In addition, the injured extremity released large quantities of lactate, which accounted for as much as 80% of the glucose consumed. This finding is consistent with our knowledge of the biochemistry of the specialized cells of the wound and inflammatory tissue (fibroblasts, macrophages, leukocytes), which undergo anaerobic metabolism and have a large capacity for lactate production. Additional measurements of blood flow and substrate concentration differences across the kidney to the brain further characterize the glucose disposal in stable trauma patients.[50,51] The glucose consumed by the central nervous system in the injured patient is approximately normal (120 g per day), whereas that consumed by kidney is approximately twice normal (75 g per day). Only a small fraction of the glucose is taken up by the resting skeletal muscle, and the remainder is consumed by the wound. The wound converts most of the glucose to lactate, which is recycled to the liver in the Cori cycle.

These alterations in glucose metabolism have a profound impact on the handling of exogenously administered glucose contained in enteral or parenteral feedings. To characterize glucose disposal during the flow phase of injury, 6 traumatized patients who did not have sepsis were studied by means of the hyperglycemic glucose "clamp" technique for 5 to 10 days after injury.[52] The results were compared with 11 age-matched control subjects. After an overnight fast, a 20% glucose solution was infused intravenously to elevate plasma glucose concentrations suddenly 125 mg/dl above basal levels. This elevation was maintained for 2 hours with bedside glucose monitoring and negative feedback servocontrol. The results showed a progressive increase in glucose disposal with time in normal control subjects, whereas the injured patients maintained a constant glucose disposal throughout the study (Fig. 68–2). Moreover, the quantity of insulin elaborated by the patients was greater than in control subjects; nonetheless, these rising insulin concentrations failed to increase glucose clearance in these patients.

Other studies have demonstrated a failure to suppress hepatic glucose production in trauma patients during glucose loading or insulin infusion.[53] Either of these perturbations usually inhibits hepatic glucose production in normal subjects. Wolfe and colleagues, using tracer methods, found that endogenous suppression comprised only 73% of the infused glucose load in burn patients (2.6 mg/kg per minute).[54] This rate of glucose infusion completely suppresses glucose production in normal subjects. When investigators used the hyperglycemic glucose "clamp" technique combined with tracer methods, endogenous glucose production was only partially reduced in trauma patients, in spite of high concentrations of both glucose and insulin.[52]

To quantitate the extent of insulin resistance in peripheral tissues, Brooks and associates measured glucose uptake across the uninjured forearm in conjunction with hyperinsulinemic-euglycemic clamp studies in 11 normal subjects and in 5 patients with multiple trauma.[55] Glucose uptake by uninjured forearm skeletal muscle of trauma patients was much less than that observed in control subjects.

Thus, profound insulin insensitivity occurs in injured patients. Direct measurements show that liver and skeletal muscle are resistant tissues, and studies by Carpentier and associates suggest that lipolysis is not attenuated in trauma patients after glucose administration.[56] The cause of this marked insensitivity to insulin is unknown; however, similar effects are observed following alterations in the hormonal environment. For example, insulin-mediated forearm glucose uptake is diminished in normal subjects following 2 hours of epinephrine infusion.[57] Similarly, 3 days of glucocorticoid administration will decrease glucose consumption.[58]

Alterations in Protein Metabolism. Extensive urinary nitrogen loss occurs following major injury. Because of the magnitude of these losses and the progressive wasting of skeletal muscle mass and associated muscle weakness, it was originally hypothesized that the nitrogen loss represented a generalized and accelerated breakdown of muscle protein. Like other responses, the loss of nitrogen following injury is related to the extent of the trauma, but it also depends on the previous nutritional status, as well as the age and sex, of the patient, because these factors determine, in part, the size of the muscle mass.

Although nitrogen balance studies demonstrate marked negative nitrogen balance following injury, these studies reflect only net nitrogen catabolism, not the absolute rate of nitrogen breakdown. In normal subjects, nitrogen equilibrium is maintained by a careful balance between rates of protein synthesis and rates of degradation. Negative nitrogen balance will occur if the breakdown rate increases and protein synthesis remains the same, or if the breakdown rate of synthesis decreases. The use of isotopically labeled, nonradioactive amino acids allows quantification of the alterations in synthesis and breakdown rates associated with many disease processes (Table 68–3).

Herrmann and associates administered ^{15}N glycine to achieve a steady state and measured ^{15}N urea nitrogen enrichment using the two-pool model of Picou and Taylor-Roberts.[59,60] Turnover rates of protein were measured, and rates of synthesis and catabolism were calculated in fed and fasted states in normal subjects. During feeding, synthesis and catabolism were equal. Restriction of food intake caused a marked reduction in synthesis, with minimal impact on rates of protein catabolism.

Birkhahn and associates described protein kinetics in four patients following multisystemic injury, including long-bone fractures.[61] In contrast to patients undergoing elective orthopedic operations, these patients had a marked increase in catabolic rate and a slight increase in synthesis; because catabolism exceeded synthesis, these patients were in marked negative nitrogen balance while receiving standard infusions of 5% dextrose and water.

Thus, trauma accelerates nitrogen turnover. In unfed patients, breakdown rates exceed synthesis, and negative balance results. Providing exogenous calories and nitrogen increases synthesis, and, when adequate nutrients are provided, the two rates are matched and nitrogen balance is maintained (Fig. 68–3).

That muscle is the origin of the nitrogen lost in the urine following extensive injury was initially suggested by Cuthbertson.[62] In his patients with long-bone fractures, he suggested that this reaction was a uniform response of the entire muscle mass, and nitrogen was not lost solely from damaged muscle at the site of injury. This concept has been supported by a variety of studies that measured important markers of muscle catabolism, such as creatinine, creatine, zinc, and 3-methylhistidine. Further evidence of net skeletal muscle breakdown has been demonstrated by quantification of the loss of amino acids from extremities of severely injured patients. Aulick and Wilmore used plethysmographic techniques to measure leg blood flow and simultaneously to determine arterial and femoral venous amino acid concentrations in traumatized patients.[63] These investigators found a three- to fourfold increase in amino acid flux from the extremities of injured patients compared to normal subjects. Alanine efflux was the most highly elevated of the amino acids measured, but glutamine was not measured. The increase in alanine release from the legs of the severely traumatized patients was generally related to the extent of injury and the oxygen consumption of the patient, but it was not related to the size of the limb injury or to blood flow in the leg. The accelerated rate of α-amino nitrogen release from the limbs of these patients appeared to be a generalized catabolic effect of injury, rather than a response to local inflammatory or metabolic events in the injured extremities. This response may be the result of chronic hypercortisolism, which occurs in injury.

Using dogs catheterized on a long-term basis to study hindquarter amino acid metabolism, Muhlbacher and colleagues observed that the long-term administration of dexamethasone (a potent glucocorticoid) resulted in a fourfold increase in glutamine and alanine release from skeletal muscle.[64] Although glutamine stores in muscle were reduced by 50% within 10 to 14 days, the accelerated glutamine release was exceeded by an accelerated consumption of this amino acid, and plasma glutamine levels fell by 30%.

It is now recognized that amino acids are released by muscle in increased quantities following injury and that the composition of amino acid efflux does not reflect the composition of muscle protein. Alanine and glutamine comprise 50 to 60% of amino acids released, whereas each makes up only about 6% of muscle protein. The branched-chain amino acids (valine, leucine, and isoleucine), on the other hand, make up approximately 6% of the released amino acids, but constitute nearly 15% of muscle protein. To explain these observations, Goldberg and Chang proposed that the branched-chain amino acids serve as amino donors for α-ketoglutarate, yielding the corresponding branched-chain keto acids and glutamate.[65] The keto acids can be converted to tricarboxylic-cycle intermediates in skeletal muscle, or they can be exported through the circulation. Glutamate may be a precursor for glutamine synthesis or an amino donor for alanine synthesis. These coupled reactions could explain the synthesis and increased release of alanine and glutamine as well as the diminished release of branched-

TABLE 68–3. ALTERATIONS IN RATES OF PROTEIN SYNTHESIS AND CATABOLISM THAT MAY AFFECT HOSPITALIZED PATIENTS

	SYNTHESIS	CATABOLISM*
Normal: patient starved	↓	o
Normal: patient fed, during bedrest	↓	o
Elective surgical procedure	↓	o
Injury/sepsis: patient receiving Intravenous dextrose	↑ ↑	↑ ↑ ↑
Injury/sepsis: patient fed	↑ ↑ ↑	↑ ↑ ↑

* ↓ = decrease; o = no change; ↑ = increase.

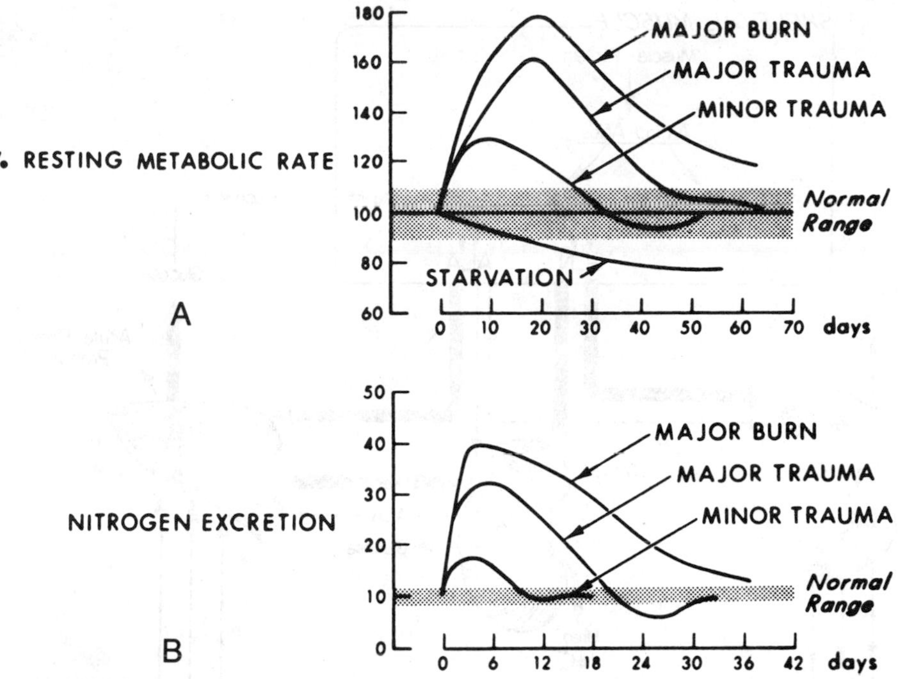

FIGURE 68–3. Metabolic rate (*A*) and nitrogen excretion (*B*) are related to the extent of injury. The two responses generally parallel each other. Patients received 12 g nitrogen daily. (From Wilmore, D.W.: The Metabolic Management of the Critically Ill. New York, Plenum Medical Book, 1977.)

chain amino acids (Fig. 68–4). Oxidation of branched-chain amino acids by skeletal muscle is accelerated following injury,[66] and skeletal muscle release of glutamine and alanine is increased.

Glutamine is also extracted by the kidney, where it contributes ammonium groups for ammonia generation, a process that excretes acid loads.[67] This effect can be augmented in the dog by the administration of glucocorticoids. Glutamine is taken up by the gastrointestinal tract and serves as an oxidative fuel.[68] The gut enterocytes convert glutamine primarily to ammonia and alanine, and these two substances are released into the portal venous blood. This ammonia is then removed by the liver and is converted to urea; the alanine may also be removed by the liver and may serve as a gluconeogenic precursor. Following elective surgical stress, glutamine consumption by the bowel and the kidney is accelerated,[69] a reaction that appears to be regulated by the increased elaboration of the glucocorticoids.[70] Although skeletal muscle releases alanine at an accelerated rate, the gastrointestinal tract and kidney also release increased amounts of alanine. This amino acid is extracted by the liver and is used in the synthesis of glucose and acute-phase proteins. Hence glutamine and alanine are important participants in the transfer of nitrogen from skeletal muscle to visceral organs; however, their metabolic pathways favor the production of urea and ammonia, both of which are lost from the body (Fig. 68–5).

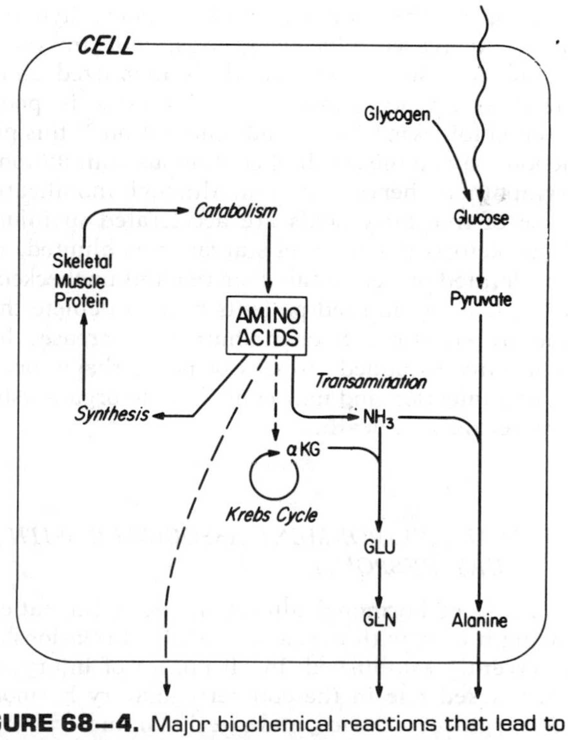

FIGURE 68–4. Major biochemical reactions that lead to the synthesis of glutamine (GLN) and alanine in skeletal muscle.

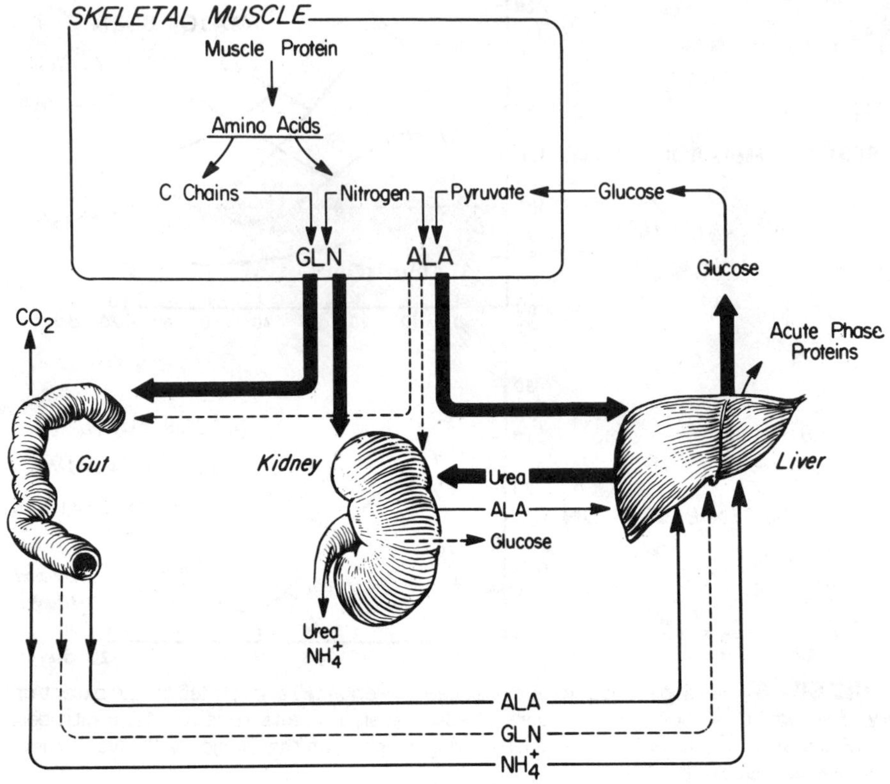

FIGURE 68–5. Major pathways of "obligatory" loss of nitrogen from the body. ALA, Alanine; GLN, glutamine.

Alterations in Fat Metabolism. To support hypermetabolism, increased gluconeogenesis, and interorgan substrate flux, stored triglyceride is mobilized and is oxidized at an accelerated rate. Lipolysis is poorly attenuated following glucose administration,[56] this phenomenon may be the result of continuous stimulation of the sympathetic nervous system. Although mobilization and use of free fatty acids are accelerated in injured subjects, ketosis during brief starvation is blunted, and the accelerated protein catabolism remains unchecked.[71] If unfed, severely injured patients rapidly deplete their fat and protein stores. Such malnutrition increases their susceptibility to added stresses of hemorrhage, operations, and infection and may contribute to organ-system failure, sepsis, and death.

HORMONAL ENVIRONMENT ASSOCIATED WITH THE INJURY RESPONSE

A variety of hormonal alterations occur in patients following injury, with the cause-and-effect relationships more recently established. In all phases of injury, one sees a marked rise in the counterregulatory hormones glucagon, glucocorticoids, and catecholamines.[72] During the ebb phase of injury, the sympathoadrenal axis primarily maintains the pressure-flow relationships necessary for an intact cardiovascular system. With the onset of hypermetabolism, characteristic of the flow phase, these and other hormones exert a variety of metabolic effects. Glucagon has potent glycogenolytic and gluconeogenic effects on the liver, and these effects signal the liver to make new glucose from hepatic glycogen stores and gluconeogenic precursors. Cortisol mobilizes amino acid from skeletal muscle, increases hepatic gluconeogenesis, and maintains body fat stores. The catecholamines stimulate hepatic gluconeogenesis and glycolysis and increase lactate production from peripheral tissues (skeletal muscle). Catecholamines also increase metabolic rate and stimulate lipolysis. The level of growth hormone is elevated, even in the presence of hyperglycemia, and thyroid levels are reduced to low-normal concentrations.

CYTOKINES AND THE METABOLIC RESPONSE TO INJURY

Although the classic counterregulatory hormones of stress (cortisol, catecholamines, glucagon) play an important role in mediating the body's response to injury and infection, they exert their influence largely by endocrine mechanisms. Other mediators, peptide compounds known collectively as cytokines, which are produced both at the site of injury by endothelial cells and by diverse immune cells throughout the body, also occupy a pivotal position in the stress response.[73] Those cytokines that have been studied most extensively and appear to play the most important role in the injury response are tumor necrosis factor-α (TNF, cachectin), interleukin-1 (Il-1), interleukin-2 (Il-2), interleukin-6 (Il-6), and interferon γ (IFN).

Originally, it was thought that the cytokines' primary influence was on immune cell function. It is now clear that cytokines are key regulators of the metabolic response to injury and infection (Fig. 68–6). These polypeptide signals, produced by the organism in response to bacteremia or endotoxemia, induce many of the adverse responses seen following severe infection.[74,75] Many of these reticuloendothelial cell products have now been described and summarized in Chapters 40 and 41. Circulating TNF and IL-1 and IL-6 have been convincingly demonstrated in the circulation of humans following administration of endotoxin.[73,76]

TNF is believed to be the primary signal that initiates many of the metabolic responses to injury and infection. The host response to endotoxin includes a rapid increase in circulating TNF levels, which are no longer detectable after several hours. Although infusion of TNF to patients results in fever, malaise, tachycardia, and chills, indicating an acute phase response, the potent effects of TNF on body metabolism may in concert be beneficial for the host because they promote mobilization of nitrogen and carbon from the periphery to the splanchnic circulation. TNF has no effect on skeletal muscle protein balance or amino acid efflux when it is administered to healthy animals or incubated with skeletal muscle. However, TNF stimulates glutamine uptake by the liver (Souba et al., unpublished data) and by endothelial cells.[77]

Il-1 is a protein with a molecular weight of about 17 kd. Previously called lymphocyte-activating factor or endogenous pyrogen, this peptide plays a central role in the acute-phase protein response, including an increase in myofibrillar protein breakdown, and in the release of amino acids from skeletal muscle, in particular glutamine. Like TNF, Il-1 stimulates glutamine transport by endothelial cells,[77] as well as by the liver. Its effects on intestinal glutamine metabolism are similar to those of endotoxin and include a decrease in glutamine extraction from the blood and a fall in mucosal glutaminase activity.[78]

The pattern of appearance of various cytokines in the circulation has been examined in animals receiving intravenous infusions of bacteria.[79] TNF levels peaked at about 90 minutes, whereas IL-1 peaked at 3 hours. Il-6 levels continued to rise for up to 8 hours. Thus, the pattern of cytokinemia appears to be monophasic and probably explains the failure to always detect these mediators in the blood of infected patients. In addition, many of the biologic responses to cytokines may be due to tissue levels of cytokines rather than circulating levels. Clearly, cytokines may exert their effects in a paracrine, autocrine, or endocrine fashion.[80,81] They also appear to work in synergy to produce the metabolic derangements that occur in traumatized and septic patients.

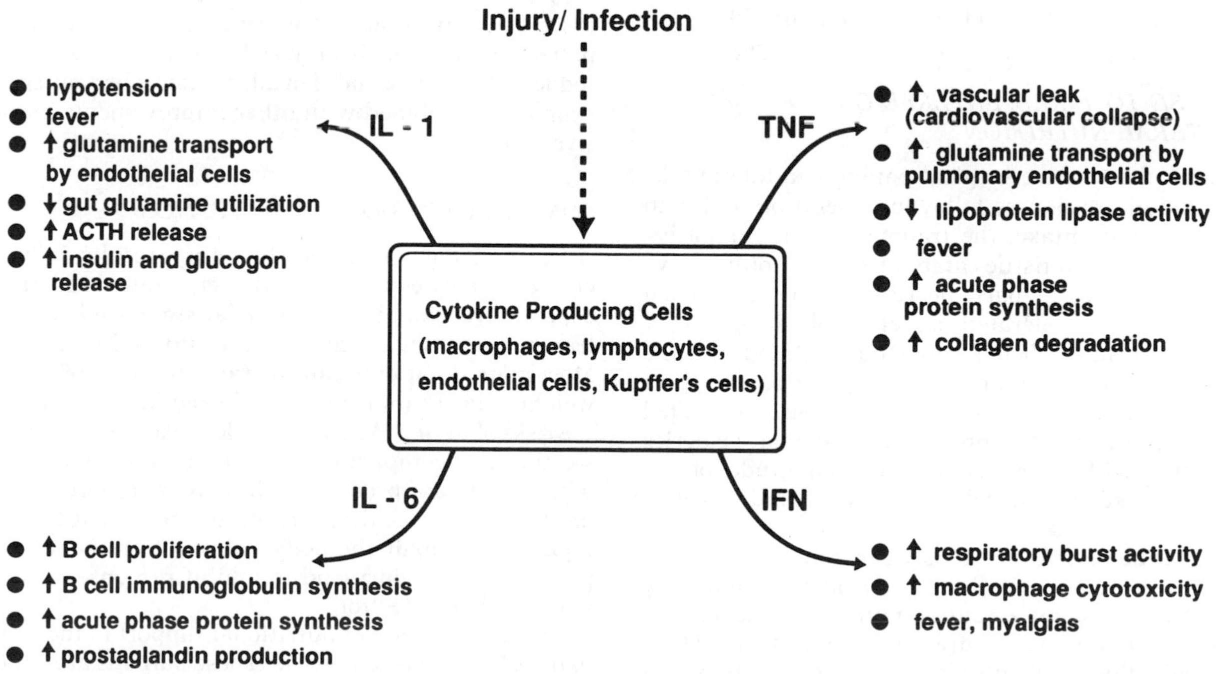

FIGURE 68–6. Some metabolic activities of selected cytokines as they relate to the body's response to injury and infection.

NUTRITIONAL SUPPORT OF THE INJURED PATIENT

USUAL COURSE: CASE EXAMPLE

A 28-year-old, nonobese male (183 cm tall; 77 kg (6′, 170 lb), body surface area (BSA), 2.0 m^2) is admitted to the hospital with a pelvic fracture and soft tissue injury following a motor vehicle accident. He has always been in good health prior to this accident. He is resuscitated without incident with intravenous fluids and blood products. The patient is admitted to the trauma intensive care unit of the hospital, and a nasogastric tube is placed. Over the next 24 hours, his blood volume is restored, and he is given maintenance solutions with 5% dextrose and appropriate electrolytes at the rate of 125 ml per hour (3 L per day). His urine output on his first hospital day is 1500 ml, and he gains 5 kg following fluid resuscitation. Because of prolonged ileus, the patient is not fed, and he continues to receive intravenous fluids. On the seventh day of the injury, the ileus resolves and a spontaneous diuresis of 3000 ml ensues. On the eighth day following the accident, the patient starts taking clear liquids and is gradually advanced to regular diet over the next 4 days. He is discharged from the hospital 4 weeks later, when his fractures have stabilized.

Nitrogen balance studies from hospital day 1 through day 7 reveal a cumulative 7-day nitrogen loss of 108 g. During this 7-day period, the patient had 0 nitrogen intake and 2500 kJ (600 kcal) glucose per day. By the eighth day of hospitalization, the patient lost 5 kg. Approximately half the weight represented loss of lean body mass,* and the remainder the loss of fat. On discharge from the hospital a month later, the patient had regained his initial body weight (Fig. 68–7).

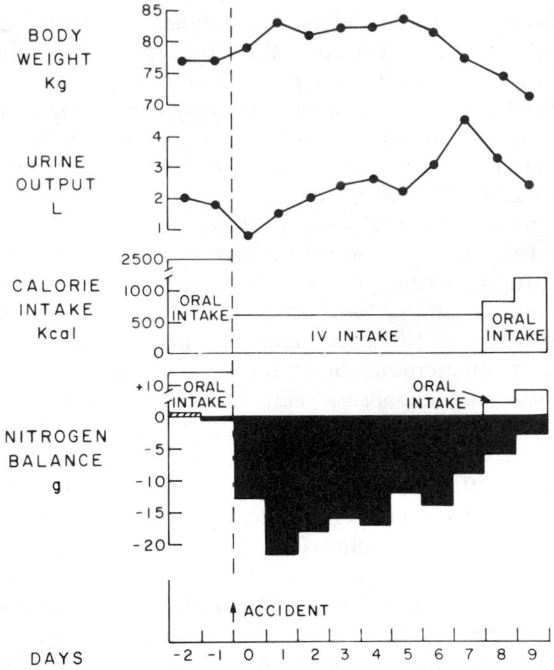

FIGURE 68–7. The metabolic response of a previously healthy individual to an injury of moderate severity.

RESPONSE TO FIXED ENTERAL OR PARENTERAL NUTRITION

Whereas the elective surgical patient can tolerate the mild catabolic responses following operation and with inadequate food intake, the trauma patient cannot because of accelerated tissue catabolism. This "obligatory" nitrogen loss can, in part, be reversed by nutritional means, but the accelerated excretion of nitrogen only returns to normal when the wound is closed and the fracture is stabilized and is healing. Nutritional support does not affect the hypermetabolic response associated with severe trauma, but provision of adequate calories and amino acids does reduce the magnitude of net lipogenesis, skeletal muscle proteolysis, and negative nitrogen balance.

Suppose the patient previously described sustains the same injury, but his postinjury period is modified by administration of all essential nutrients. The patient receives 3 L parenteral solution that delivers 11,700 kJ (2800 kcal) plus 15 g nitrogen per day as a balanced amino acid mixture (Fig. 68–8). This caloric intake is judged to be adequate to maintain body weight. Nitrogen balance studies show cumulative losses of 140 g from hospital day 1 through hospital day 7, so the patient's net loss for the 7 days equals 35 g. The patient lost 1 kg during this time, primarily lean body tissue. In this patient, the administration of nutrients is designed to combat the negative nitrogen balance and weight loss associated with injury. The benefits of such feedings in patients with extensive injury have been translated into reduced morbidity and mortality rates when nutritional support is combined with other improvements in intensive care.

*108 g nitrogen = 675 g protein = 2.5 kg lean body mass

CONSEQUENCES OF MALNUTRITION

The metabolic response to injury results in an increased energy expenditure. If energy intake is less than expenditure, oxidation of body fat stores and erosion of lean body mass will occur, with resultant loss of weight. Most injured patients can tolerate a loss of 10% of their weight prior to injury without a significant increase in the risks of injury. When weight loss exceeds 10% of body weight, the complications of undernutrition interact with the disease process, with increased morbidity and mortality rates. Undernutrition to this extent following injury may impair the body's ability to respond appropriately to the injury and to inhibit responses to added stress such as infection.

The major impact of nutritional support in the trauma patient is to aid host defense. These patients are exposed to a variety of infectious agents in the hospital, and their injuries and requirements of care increase the risk of

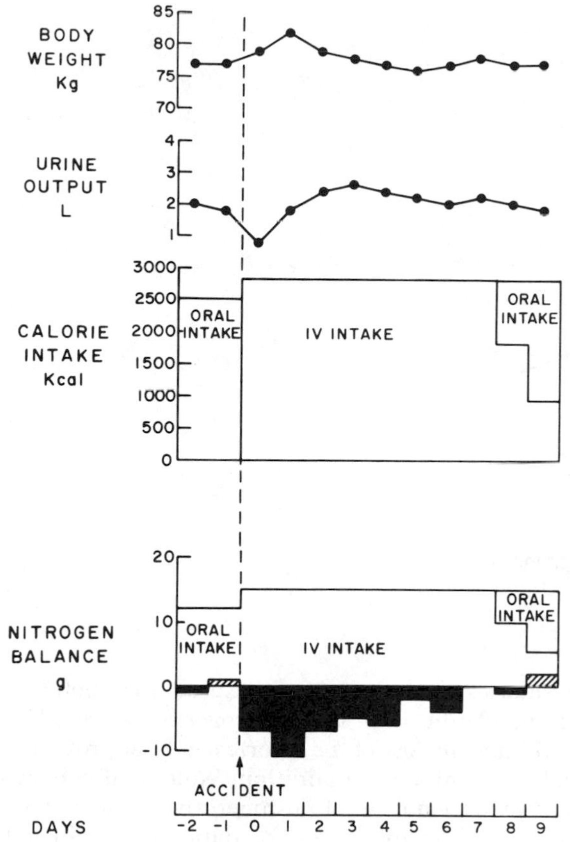

FIGURE 68–8. The injury response with nutrition provided by central vein infusions.

infection. The normal barrier defense mechanisms are disrupted by multiple indwelling catheters, nasotracheal and nasogastric tubes, and breakdown of skin and mucous membrane. Undernutrition may compromise the available host defense mechanism and may thus increase the likelihood of invasive sepsis, multiple organ-system failure, and death. Additional consequences of malnutrition include poor wound healing, decreased mobility and activity, the occurrence of pressure sores and decubitus ulcers, altered gastrointestinal function, and the occurrence of edema secondary to reduced colloid osmotic pressure. Whereas these complications are most frequently observed in patients with severe malnutrition (>15% body weight loss), adequate nutritional support helps to prevent them.

PRIORITIES OF CARE

Nutrition should be integrated into the overall care of the critically ill patient to maximize the benefits of nutritional support, yet minimize complications in a complex intensive care setting. Priorities in care should be established at various points following injury. Resuscitation, oxygenation, and arrest of hemorrhage are immediate priorities for survival. Wounds should then be repaired or stabilized as expeditiously as possible. During wound repair, a patient's intensive metabolic demands abate, and nutrients become more effective in achieving anabolism. Early excision and grafting of burns and internal fixation of fractures are examples of early definitive wound care; yet even these procedures may be followed by several weeks of post-traumatic hypermetabolism. While the wound is treated, care should be taken to minimize other potential stresses that heighten metabolic demands in addition to those imposed by the injury alone. Such factors include pain, fever, mild cold exposure, acidosis, and hypovolemia. The greatest acceleration of catabolism occurs with infection, however, and every effort should be made to prevent sepsis.

Nutritional support is an essential part of the metabolic care of the critically ill trauma patient. Adequate nutrition allows normal responses that optimize wound healing and recovery. Nutritional support should be instituted before significant weight loss occurs. The development of techniques for intravenous administration of hypertonic nutrient solutions, the use of peripheral venous feedings with fat emulsions, and the availability of specific enteral diets have made it possible for virtually all injured patients to receive safe and effective nutritional support.

GOALS OF NUTRITIONAL SUPPORT

The majority of injured persons are not malnourished at the time of injury. The increased metabolic demands following injury will quickly lead to a malnourished state if the patient is not nutritionally supported (Fig. 68–9). Thus, nutritional support should be considered in all injured patients. The provision of full nutritional support early after injury may be fraught with metabolic complications, however. Hyperglycemia, hyperosmolarity, and electrolyte disorders are frequently observed. Therefore, intravenous feedings are not usually begun immediately following the admission of the patient to the hospital. On stabilization of the patient's condition and development of a care plan, nutritional support can be gradually initiated. The goal of nutritional support is the maintenance of body cell mass and the limitation of weight loss to less than 10% of preinjury weight.

FEEDING THE PATIENT

Considerations include nutritional evaluation, requirements, monitoring, routes of administration, and specific formulas.

Nutritional Assessment and Requirements. Nutritional assessment of the trauma patient helps to determine energy and protein requirements. A careful medical history and physical examination are essential, but the usual indicators of malnutrition are frequently misleading in the trauma patient. For example, body weight is increased in these patients because of edema, and serum albumin and transferrin decrease in concentration be-

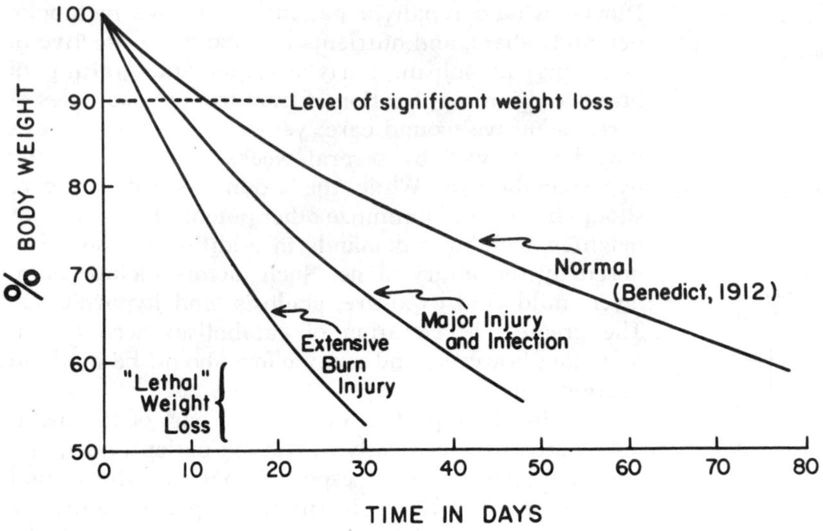

FIGURE 68–9. Weight loss with starvation is accelerated after major injury and infection.

cause of an enlarged distribution space. Hence nutritional support should be considered for all injured patients, with the goal to maintain usual (preinjury) body weight and body tissue mass.

Basal energy requirements are determined from standard tables based on age, sex, and BSA.[14] These requirements are adjusted for the increase in metabolic rate due to the injury or disease process by multiplication of a stress factor based on the severity of injury (see Table 68–1). An additional 25% is added to account for the energy expenditure associated with treatment and activity, but this addition is not required in inactive patients, such as those sedated or paralyzed while receiving artificial ventilation. The product of the factors (BMR times stress factors times 1.25, if needed) is an estimate of the patient's energy requirements.

The next step is to calculate nitrogen requirements. In normal subjects, the ratio of nitrogen to nonprotein calorie intake is usually 1:1250 to 1450; that is, for every 1250 to 1450 kJ (300 to 350 kcal), 1 g nitrogen is provided. Because of the heightened protein catabolism associated with the post-traumatic response, more dietary protein is required to achieve nitrogen balance. For critically ill patients, the optimal nitrogen-to-joule ratio is thought to range between 1:400 and 1:800. This ratio indicates that approximately twice the quantity of protein is required to achieve "balance" in the injured patient than in healthy persons. Approximately 15 to 20% of calorie intake should be protein.

Once energy and nitrogen requirements have been determined, the proportions of fat and carbohydrate need to be estimated, to maximize nitrogen retention. Long and associates studied the nitrogen-sparing effects of different isocaloric mixtures of glucose and fat in patients receiving 11.7 g nitrogen/m^2 per day.[82] They found no additional nitrogen-sparing effects when glucose calories exceeded the measured metabolic rate. Nitrogen equilibrium was approached when glucose comprised 60 to 70% of the caloric needs, approximately 7 mg/kg per minute. In addition, Wolfe and colleagues studied oxidation rates of postoperative patients receiving glucose.[83] No increase in oxidation of administered glucose was observed when patients received glucose infusions above 7 mg/kg per minute. Black and colleagues, using the glucose clamp technique, demonstrated that injured patients had an upper limit to glucose disposal of approximately 6 to 7 mg/kg per minute, a value that represented 60 to 70% of the estimated caloric needs.[52] In contrast, normal subjects could dispose of increasing quantities of glucose and approached an upper limit of 15 to 17 mg/kg per minute. The results of these three independent studies using different techniques point to the same conclusion: no clear-cut gain is made in providing glucose calories in excess of 60 to 70% of daily metabolic requirements to injured patients. The administration of larger glucose loads, however, has been associated with an increasing incidence of complications such as hyperglycemia, hyperosmotic states, hepatic dysfunction, and respiratory insufficiency.[84] For patients who are tolerant of large caloric loads, the provision of 60% of caloric needs as glucose and the rest as fat should minimize complications and should maximize protein synthesis.

Multivitamins are administered daily, along with supplemental vitamin C, which is believed by some to be required in increased amounts following injury[85] (see Chap. 80). Electrolytes are present in standard diets or tube feedings; trace elements are variably present; they must be added to parenteral infusions. Potassium, magnesium, and phosphate supplements, in addition to those in tube formulas, may be required to maintain normal serum concentrations of these electrolytes. They must be added to parenteral fluids to meet needs, except when present in amino acid-electrolyte combinations. Although the need for zinc has been demonstrated experimentally, clinical reports of zinc-replacement therapy in burn patients provide no definitive answers on the benefit of this supplement following injury.[86] Zinc supplements should be administered to severely malnourished individuals or to those with a history of poor nutrient intake, such as alcoholic patients, who have a major injury or major intestinal fluid losses. (See Chap. 80 concerning other trace elements.)

In summary, the nutritional requirements of the trauma patient can be determined as follows:

1. Determine BMR for age, sex, and BSA from the tables of Fleisch or the Harris-Benedict equation (BMR in kcal per day).[14]
2. Determine the percentage of increase in metabolism rate due to the injury (see Table 68–1), multiply by BMR, and add to 1 (% × BMR + BMR).
3. Add 25% × BMR for hospital activity (walking, physical therapy, sitting, treatment).
4. The sum of steps 1 to 3 is an estimated daily caloric requirement for maintenance of body weight.
5. Divide step 4 by 150 to determine nitrogen requirements (protein = 6.25 × nitrogen).
6. Give approximately 60% of caloric requirement (determined in step 4) as glucose.
7. Give remaining caloric requirement as fat (glucose can be used if tolerated by the patient). Glucose is much less expensive, and a central venous catheter will be necessary to administer the glucose solution. If glucose is used as the remaining caloric source, insulin may need to be given to avoid hyperglycemia. Fat emulsion should then be given 2 to 3 times per week to provide essential fatty acid requirements.
8. Reassess energy and nitrogen needs at least twice weekly. Weigh the patient daily.
9. If nutritional support seems unsatisfactory because of progressive weight loss, consider direct measurement of oxygen consumption or measurement of nitrogen loss and calculation of nitrogen balance.

Nutritional Monitoring. Once the trauma patient is nutritionally assessed, feedings can be gradually commenced. Protein and calorie intake should be measured and recorded daily. If nutritional requirements are not met by current therapy, then other feeding techniques should be used. Combined nutritional support techniques may be necessary during the convalescence of a severely injured patient (Fig. 68–10).

If the patient continues to lose more weight than can be attributed to a postresuscitation diuresis, then additional nutritional assessment techniques, such as indirect calorimetry or nitrogen balance testing, should be performed. Plasma glucose levels should be determined regularly, especially when one is beginning or increasing nutritional support. Insulin should be administered to maintain a plasma glucose level of 100 to 150 mg/dl. Urine sugar content should be evaluated by the hospital nursing staff every 6 to 8 hours. Levels of serum electrolytes, BUN, and creatinine and liver function should be determined regularly, as consistent with proper care. Serum potassium concentrations may need to be followed more closely because of increased potassium losses after injury and a tendency toward metabolic alkalosis.

Additional Nutritional Assessment Techniques. Energy requirements may be estimated with reasonable accuracy in 85% of hospital patients. If estimated requirements are delivered by current nutritional support, but therapy seems inadequate because of persistent weight loss in excess of estimated net fluid losses or an unsatisfactory clinical course, energy requirements may be measured by indirect calorimetry. Oxygen consumption ($\dot{V}O_2$) and carbon dioxide production ($\dot{V}CO_2$) are deter-

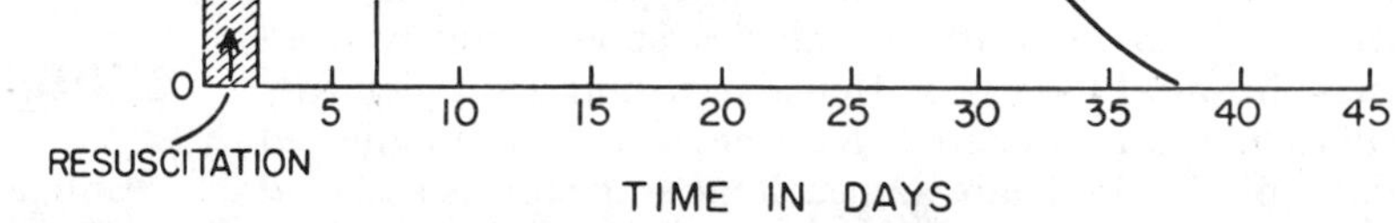

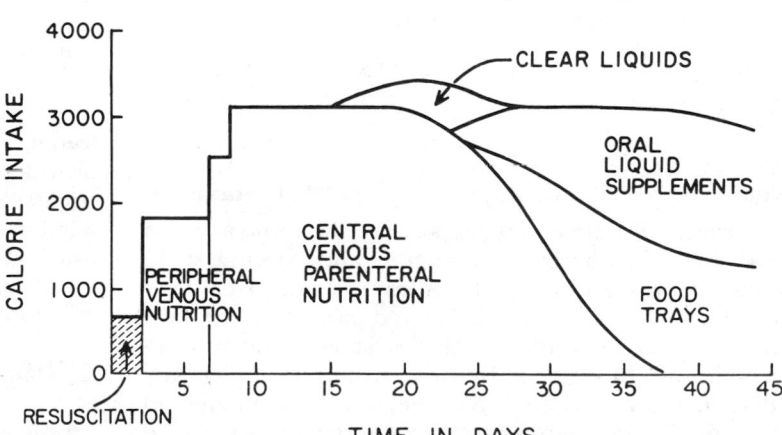

FIGURE 68–10. In subjects with moderate-to-severe injury, various techniques are necessary to provide safe and efficient nutrition.

mined under resting, unstressed, basal conditions. These respiratory parameters are interrelated to energy expenditure by the following relationships:

$$\text{Metabolic rate (kcal/hour)} = 3.9 \times \dot{V}o_2 \text{ (L/hour)} + 1.1 \times \dot{V}co_2 \text{ (L/hour) or}$$

$$\text{Metabolic rate (kJ/hour)} = 16.3 \times \dot{V}o_2 \text{ (L/hour)} + 1.1 \times \dot{V}co_2 \text{ (L/hour)}$$

This value is the resting energy expenditure of the patient and should be increased 20 to 30% to account for minimal daily activity when used to determine energy requirements.

Nitrogen balance studies help to define the effectiveness of nutritional support. These should be performed in patients whose clinical course is unsatisfactory or in whom nutritional efficacy cannot be estimated on clinical grounds alone. Nitrogen balance is the quantity of nitrogen taken in or administered to the patient minus the quantity of nitrogen lost:

$$N_{bal} \text{ (g/day)} = N_{in} - N_{out}$$

Most nitrogen is lost in the urine, mainly as urea. The urine is collected for 24-hour periods and is stored in acidified containers. Urinary urea nitrogen (UUN) is measured. This represents approximately 80% of urinary nitrogen. Additionally, about 2 g per day are lost in the feces and from the skin. If the BUN changes during the 24-hour period, the whole-body changes in urea nitrogen (ΔBUN) should be estimated as follows:

$$\Delta\text{BUN g/day} = (\text{BUN day 2 in mg/dl} - \text{BUN day 1 in mg/dl}^{a}) \times 0.6 \times \text{body weight kg}^{b} \div 1{,}000$$

where a = Change in concentration and
b = Estimated quantity of total body water

$$N_{out} \text{ (g/day)} = \frac{\text{UUN}}{0.8} \text{ g/day} + 2 \text{ g/day}^{c} + \Delta\text{BUN g/day}^{d}$$

where c = Estimate for stool and skin and
d = Other loss from wounds or drains, as measured or estimated

Nitrogen is conventionally taken to be 16% of the total protein intake; that is, N_{in}/day = protein intake g/day × 0.16.

Routes of Nutritional Support and Nutrient Formulas. The routes of nutritional support are the same as those described elsewhere: oral, enteral, and parenteral. In general, oral and enteral routes are preferred over intravenous administration. Injured patients rarely take the required quantity of calories spontaneously from their hospital food tray. Hence oral liquid supplements should be administered. Nutrient intake is monitored daily by the dietician, and each nursing shift is assigned a quantity of supplement to be provided. Free water or low-calorie drinks are not offered. All liquid is a calorie-dense nutrient supplement.

The patient's injuries may, however, preclude the use of oral feedings; for example, patients with facial trauma may have their jaws wired together. Children, older adults, patients with head injuries, and those receiving artificial ventilation are all potential candidates for tube feedings. Retro- or intraperitoneal hematomas, intra-abdominal sepsis, severe gastrointestinal injury and extensive repair, or other factors may lead to reduction in intestinal motility (ileus) or intolerance to enteral feedings. Jejunal or duodenal tube feedings are often successful even if the stomach must be continuously decompressed. Thus, for all patients who have undergone abdominal operations, feeding jejunostomy placement should be considered.[18] Alternatively, the jejunum or duodenum can be intubated perorally with special tubes, with or without the aid of fluoroscopy. The development of diarrhea in a patient receiving enteral feedings may limit the caloric load given by these routes. When the nutritional needs of the patient cannot be met by oral and enteral feedings, intravenous techniques can be used.

Enteral formulas are usually balanced mixtures of fat, carbohydrate, and protein. Several recently developed formulas are particularly rich in calories and protein, yet have low osmolarity. In light of the injured patient's nutritional requirements, these formulas would seem to be particularly advantageous; however, a variety of formulas are available and may be preferred in selected cases.

Intravenous feedings may be necessary to supplement enteral feedings, or they may be required to provide adequate nutritional intake if enteral feedings cannot be tolerated or are inadequate. Peripheral nutrient solution can be given to supplement enteral feedings. These dilute solutions of glucose and amino acids should be minimized, and fat infusion should be maximized, while high-carbohydrate tube feeding is provided. Such an approach ensures adequate carbohydrate loads in a minimal fluid volume. Trauma patients, and particularly burn patients, are usually young adults without cardiovascular disease and with large daily fluid requirements. Thus, these patients are ideal candidates for peripheral-vein nutrient infusion. Unfortunately, however, adequate carbohydrate calories can rarely be provided solely by this route, and when parenteral nutrition is required, central venous feedings are usually indicated. The hypertonic solution provides glucose, amino acids, and other essential nutrients. Fat emulsion and supplemental fluids are easily administered through a second intravenous access site, usually a peripheral vein.

SEPSIS

Unlike in elective operations and uncomplicated trauma, the response patterns following major infection are often unpredictable. The variability in the metabolic and physiologic responses is related in part to the patient's age, previous state of health, preexisting disease, previous stresses, site of infection, and specific pathogens. Moreover, organ-system failure, such as septic shock or pulmonary insufficiency, may mask the more subtle manifestations of systemic infection. In spite of numerous advances in the treatment of infection and a better understanding of its mediators and pathophysiologic features, the mortality and morbidity rates for septicemia remain high.

In general, two physiologic response patterns have been described, based on cardiac output.[87] The first is characterized by an increased cardiac output and heightened systemic perfusion. This state varies, depending on the patient's physiologic compensation and administered fluid volume. The second response pattern is characterized by cardiac decompensation, inadequate tissue perfusion, and profound acidosis. This pattern is described as "low-flow sepsis." Both these responses reflect the body's reaction to systemic infection. These patterns are also modified by the underlying disease process and the physiologic reserve of the particular patient. In this section, we review the metabolic responses to sepsis and the priorities for safe nutritional support. Sepsis is defined as the presence of infection resulting in systemic signs and symptoms and diagnosed by bacteremia. Low-flow sepsis is difficult to reverse and usually results in death. Most of this discussion focuses on the metabolic responses that occur during the hyperdynamic high-flow state.

USUAL PHYSIOLOGIC RESPONSE TO SYSTEMIC INFECTION

GENERAL OVERVIEW AND TIME COURSE

The invasion of the body by microorganisms initiates many host responses. Local penetration of tissues stimulates mobilization of phagocytes, initiates an inflammatory response at the local site, and may activate additional host immunologic mechanisms. If the infection progresses, fever, tachycardia, and other systemic responses occur; these more generalized reactions may reflect direct or indirect effects of the inflammatory response. Systemic events during the hyperdynamic phase of sepsis can be categorized into two general types of responses: (1) those related to the host's immunologic defenses; and (2) those related to the body's general metabolic and circulatory adjustments to the infection. The predominant alterations in host defense mechanisms include fever, leukocytosis, changes in acute-phase protein synthesis, and activation of a variety of immunologic reactions. The changes in metabolism relate to alterations in glucose, nitrogen, and fat metabolism, as well as those related to the redistribution of trace metals. These events are initiated by invasion of the microorganism and evolve as the infectious disease progresses through its period of incubation, through the initiation of metabolic responses and fever, and into early convalescence and recovery.

Several general characteristics describe the systemic events that occur after infection, as follows:

1. These responses appear stereotyped and can be produced after administering many microorganisms or their toxins. The systemic responses to infection are similar in many respects to events that follow injury, but these processes are not the same.
2. The magnitude of the responses varies with the extent and duration of the infection.
3. The complex sequence of systemic events that follows infection appears to change in time, and hence sequential studies must be performed to locate the responses precisely within that time.
4. Although the systemic responses to infection are stereotyped, these processes are modulated by the physiologic reserves of the individual. The magnitude of the responses to infection depends on the patient's age and sex, previous nutritional state, function of vital organs, immunologic memory, and associated disease processes. The classic response to infection has been observed in young, previously healthy, well-nourished, active adults with no other medical problems. These patients are rarely admitted to surgical services, however. Surgeons usually see patients at extremes of life or those who are hospitalized because of disease processes and who have additional stress, usually an operation or injury, that limits physiologic, biochemical, or immunologic responses to infection. Thus, infection complicating the recuperative course of a surgical patient may not evoke standard systemic responses. Limitations in the patient's capacity to respond to infection may affect recovery or survival.
5. As infection progresses, additional functional limitations may be imposed on one or more specific organs and may further impair the host systemic response. These limitations can be observed in patients with severe pneumonia and marked pulmonary dysfunction causing hypoxemia, associated with circulatory failure and hypotension related to severe gram-negative sepsis.

In spite of the complexities of unraveling and understanding the systemic responses to infection in critically ill surgical patients, a large body of investigative and clinical data is available to aid our understanding of these host defense mechanisms.

Beisel has described the time course of metabolic and immunologic responses during a typical febrile illness.[88] Phagocytic activity is an early response that occurs shortly after the moment of exposure to the pathogen. The febrile period is the hallmark of systemic effects. With the onset of fever, negative nitrogen balance, accelerated losses of potassium, phosphate, and magnesium, and retention of salt water all occur. On resolution of the sepsis, one sees spontaneous diuresis and a return to positive nitrogen balance. Associated with the losses of elements from the body is an internal redistribution of substances, particularly iron and zinc, which are sequestered in the body, presumably to make them unavailable to the invading organisms (Fig. 68–11).

SYSTEMIC METABOLIC RESPONSES

Many of the metabolic responses to infection are similar to those observed following injury. Hence investigators have speculated that a final common pathway may apply to all catabolic states. Severe infection is characterized by prolonged fever, hypermetabolism, diminished protein economy, altered glucose dynamics, and accelerated lipolysis. Anorexia is commonly associated with systemic infection and contributes to the loss of body tissue. These effects are compounded in the patient with sepsis by multiorgan-system failure, which includes the gastrointestinal tract, liver, heart, and lungs.

Hypermetabolism. Oxygen consumption is usually elevated in the infected patient. The extent of this increase is related to the severity of infection, with peak elevations reaching 50 to 60% above normal.[14] Such responses often occur in the postoperative and postinjury periods secondary to severe pneumonia, intra-abdominal infection, or wound invasion. If the patient's metabolic rate is already elevated to a maximal extent because of severe injury, no further increase will be observed.[49] In patients with only slightly accelerated rates of oxygen consumption, the presence of infection causes a rise in metabolic rate that appears additive to the preexisting state. A portion of the increase in metabolism may be ascribed to the increase in reaction rate associated with fever (Q10 effect). Calculations suggest that the metabolic rate increases 10 to 13% for each elevation of 1° C in central temperature. On resolution of the infection, the metabolic rate returns to normal.

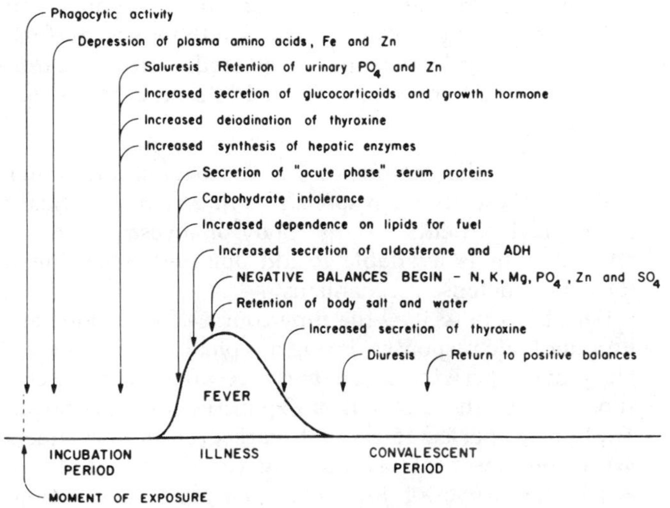

FIGURE 68–11. Nutritional responses that evolve following a generalized febrile, infectious illness. (From Beisel, W.R.: Am. J. Clin. Nutr., *30*:1, 236, 1977.)

Altered Glucose Dynamics. Blood glucose levels are generally elevated in the infected patient, but the descriptive term "diabetes of infection" is inappropriate because plasma insulin concentrations are generally normal or elevated in previously healthy individuals who develop infection.[89] That glucose production is increased in infected patients appears to be additive to the augmented gluconeogenesis that occurs following injury.[49] For example, uninfected burn patients have a glucose production rate approximately 50% above normal; with the onset of bacteremia in similar individuals, hepatic glucose production increases to twice basal levels. Glucose dynamics following infection are complex, and profound hypoglycemia and diminished hepatic glucose production have also been described in both animals and human patients.[90,91] The best clinical example of the imbalance in hepatic glucose production and tissue glucose consumption is found in neonatal hypoglycemia associated with gram-negative septicemia.[92] Studies in animals and in human patients show that deterioration in glucogenesis is associated with more progressive stages of infection and may be related to alterations in splanchnic blood flow.[49] Hepatic dysfunction this profound is usually associated with other complications of sepsis, such as respiratory insufficiency and renal failure, and usually heralds impending cardiovascular instability and death.

Alterations in Protein Metabolism. Accelerated proteolysis, increased nitrogen excretion, and prolonged negative nitrogen balance occur following infection, and the response pattern is similar to that described for injury. Long and associates noted that the protein catabolic rate in infected patients was accelerated,[93] and Herrmann and colleagues showed that protein synthesis could be augmented in the infected patient by vigorous feeding.[59] Amino acid flux from skeletal muscle is accelerated in patients with sepsis,[94] and this flux is matched by accelerated visceral amino acid uptake. In infected burn patients, splanchnic uptake of amino acids is increased 50% above rates in uninfected burn patients with injuries of comparable size.[49] These amino acids serve as glucose precursors and are used for synthesis of acute-phase proteins. In addition, acidosis frequently occurs in the patient with sepsis, and this stimulus serves as a signal for accelerated glutamine uptake by the kidney. Glutamine liberates an ammonia ion that combines with a hydrogen ion and is excreted in the urine, thus participating in acid-base homeostasis.[67] Because the glutamine arises from skeletal muscle proteolysis, this complication of sepsis is yet another stimulus of heightened skeletal muscle breakdown.

Although operative stress is characterized by abnormal gut glutamine metabolism, these abnormalities are generally inconsequential because most patients recover and their glutamine metabolism returns to normal. During sepsis or endotoxemia, however, the altered interorgan glutamine metabolism that occurs is more significant (Fig. 68–12). Severe infection is often associated with a hypercatabolic state that initiates marked changes in glutamine metabolism. Bacteria and their endotoxins stimulate macrophages to release cytokines, which activate the pituitary/adrenal axis. The release of cortisol accelerates muscle proteolysis and net skeletal

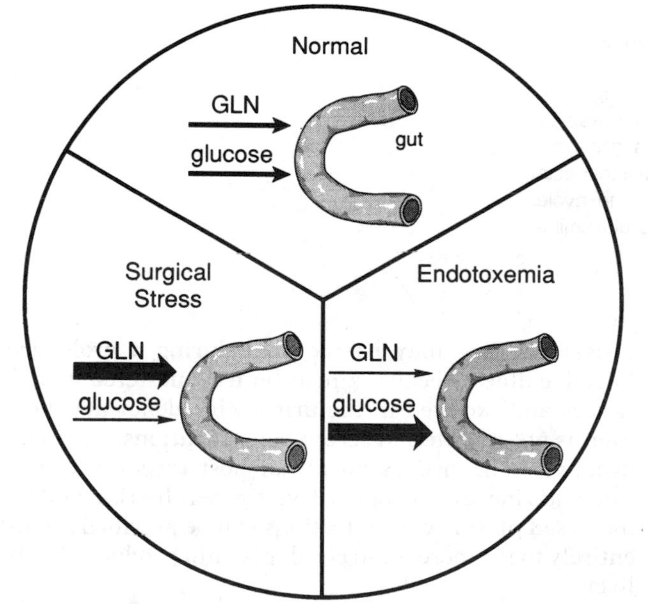

FIGURE 68–12. Fuel use by the gut in normal and stress states. Under normal circumstances the gastrointestinal tract extracts large amounts of circulating glutamine. Following surgical stress gut glutamine utilization is increased, an event mediated by the glucocorticoid hormones and glucagon. This accelerated utilization of glutamine following operative stress may help support mucosal metabolism and function at a time when food intake is often interrupted. During sepsis and endotoxemia, intestinal glutamine extraction is diminished and may be associated with an injured gut mucosal barrier.

muscle glutamine release. Recent studies indicate that the lung is also a key organ of glutamine metabolism. Studies in surgical patients with indwelling pulmonary artery catheters demonstrate that the lungs release large amounts of glutamine into the systemic circulation during hyperdynamic sepsis.[95] The regulator of these events is unknown, but animal studies demonstrate that the glucocorticoid hormones accelerate pulmonary glutamine release.[96] The lungs may work together with skeletal muscle to help maintain circulating glutamine levels (Fig. 68–13).

The effects of sepsis on glutamine metabolism by the gastrointestinal tract have been studied in rodents and in man.[97] Endotoxin or saline was administered to adult rats 15 hours prior to cannulation of the carotid artery and portal vein. Despite a slight elevation of arterial glutamine in endotoxic animals, the gut glutamine uptake, extraction, and glutaminase activity were significantly depressed ($p<0.01$). Patients with sepsis who were undergoing laparotomy for their primary disease had a 70% reduction in gut glutamine extraction and a 50% reduction in gut oxygen extraction. Mucosal transport of glutamine and several other amino acids and glucose was also diminished during sepsis.[98] The decreased transport of glucose from the lumen that occurs during endotoxemia is in contrast to the increased uptake from the circulation. It appears that sepsis and endotoxemia impair gut metabolism of glutamine, an effect that may be related to the breakdown of the gut mucosal barrier and the development of bacterial translocation (see Fig. 68–12).

Alterations in Fat Metabolism. Fat is a major fuel oxidized in infected patients, and the increased metabolism of lipids from peripheral fat stores is especially prominent during a period of inadequate nutritional support. Lipolysis is most probably mediated by the heightened sympathetic activity that is a potent stimulus for fat mobilization and accelerated oxidation. Serum triglyceride levels reflect the balance between rates of triglyceride production by the liver and use and storage by peripheral tissues. Marked hypertriglyceridemia has been associated with gram-negative infection,[99] but plasma triglyceride concentrations are usually normal or low. The use of free fatty acids is coupled with increased hepatic fat clearance. During starvation, hepatic uptake of free fatty acids is associated with ketosis, and concentrations of β-hydroxybutyrate and acetoacetate rise. This change does not occur in infected patients, and investigators have hypothesized that the accelerated proteolysis seen during infection is a consequence of this hypoketonemic state. This hypothesis was tested by the infusion of β-hydroxybutyrate into infected animals, however.[100] Following this infusion, the accelerated gluconeogenesis and proteolysis were not diminished; this finding suggests that these factors are governed by regulators other than the simple regulation of the oxidation of fat and carbohydrate. Other investigators have suggested that the hypoketonemic state of infection may be a conse-

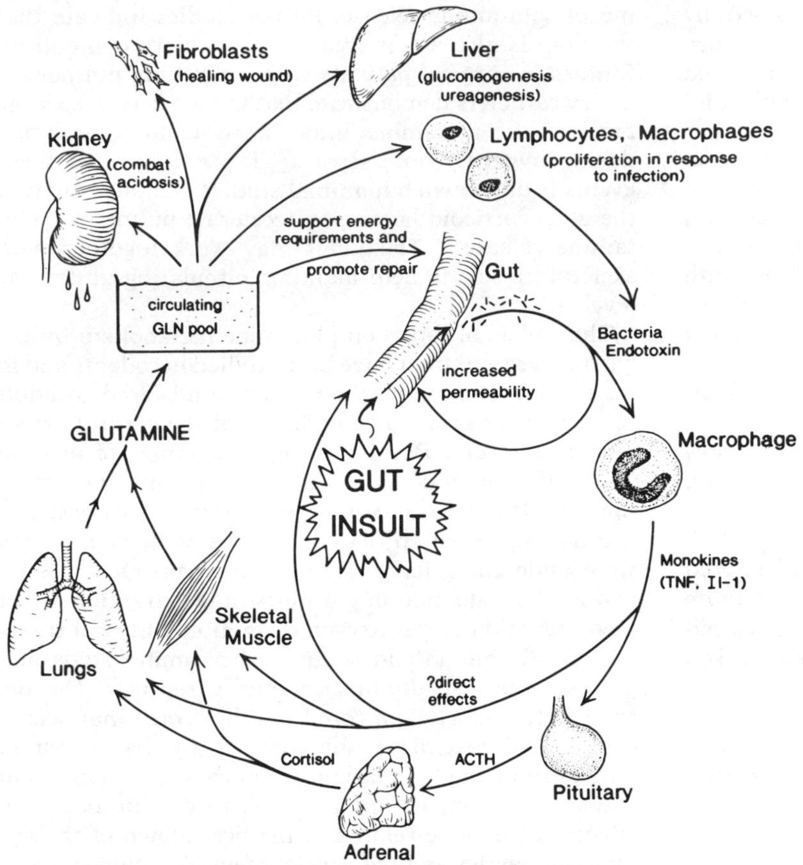

FIGURE 68–13. The interorgan glutamine cycle can be initiated by local and/or systemic gut insults that cause an increase in bowel permeability and bacterial translocation. Bacteria and endotoxins stimulate macrophages to release cytokines, which activate the pituitary/adrenal axis. The release of cortisol accelerates muscle and lung glutamine release and enhances intestinal glutamine uptake. Simultaneously, glutamine supports renal ammoniagenesis and lymphocyte proliferation in response to bacterial invasion. If the cycle persists, or if the patient is unable to take oral feedings or remains glutamine deficient, a prolonged catabolic state will develop.

quence of the hyperinsulinemia associated with catabolic states.[101] Studies in rats and in human patients lend credence to this argument.[102]

Changes in Trace Mineral Metabolism. Changes in balance of magnesium, inorganic phosphate, zinc, and potassium generally follow alterations in nitrogen balance. Although the iron-binding capacity of transferrin is usually unchanged in early infection, iron disappears from the plasma, especially during severe pyrogenic infections; similar alterations are observed with serum zinc levels. These decreases cannot be totally accounted for by losses of the minerals from the body. Rather, both iron and zinc accumulate within the liver, and this accumulation appears to be another host defense mechanism. The administration of iron to the infected host, especially early in the disease, is contraindicated because increased serum iron concentrations may impair resistance. Zinc may be required during a prolonged, infective illness because zinc is both sequestered in body tissues and excreted in the urine. Zinc deficiency, however, is not reflected in serum concentrations, which are usually diminished as an initial host response. Unlike iron and zinc levels, copper levels generally rise, and the increased plasma concentrations can be ascribed almost entirely to the increase in ceruloplasmin produced by the liver.

MEDIATORS OF THE CATABOLIC RESPONSE

HORMONES AND CYTOKINES

The hormonal and cytokine responses that occur during the hypermetabolic phase of infection are similar to those described following injury. Serum cortisol levels are elevated and lose their usual circadian rhythm.[103]

Glucagon levels are increased, but the insulin-to-glucagon ratio, a hormonal relationship considered to indicate hepatic stimulation of gluconeogenesis, remains below normal. Levels of catecholamines, growth hormone, ADH, and aldosterone are all elevated. The growth hormone level persists into convalescence, presumably to promote anabolism. These hormonal and cytokine responses to infection are the subjects several reviews.[73-75]

GUT MUCOSAL BARRIER FUNCTION AND GUT-ORIGIN SEPSIS

Although the intestinal tract is generally viewed as an organ of digestion and absorption, it also protects the host from intraluminal bacteria and their toxins. The maintenance of an intact brush border and the presence of intercellular tight junctions prevent the movement of toxic substances into the intestinal lymphatics and circulation. Those bacteria that do translocate appear to do so in small numbers and the mesenteric lymph nodes effectively dispose of them without deleterious systemic effects. Bacterial endotoxins absorbed into the portal venous blood are rapidly detoxified by Kupffer's cells of the liver.

Gut immune function is the term applied to the structural and functional characteristics of the gastrointestinal tract that make it resistant to the entry of infectious or toxic agents into the systemic circulation.[104] This function is a combination of nonimmunologic processes (physical factors, intestinal flora) and the local mucosal immune system function. Immune factors include the secretion of secretory IgA (S-IgA) and the function of macrophages and lymphocytes in Peyer's patches, mesenteric lymph nodes, and lamina propria of the intestinal mucosa.[104] These collections of cells of the immune system within the gastrointestinal tract are known collectively as the gut-associated lymphoid tissue (GALT). Maintenance of a gut mucosal barrier that effectively excludes luminal bacteria and toxins requires an intact epithelium and normal mucosal immune mechanisms.

A particularly important component of gastrointestinal immune function is S-IgA.[105] The stimulation of gut S-IgA secretion begins in Peyer's patches of the small intestine. Enteric antigens are presented to immunocompetent cells through M cells, which are specialized epithelial cells overlying Peyer's patches. The antigens are processed by macrophages and are presented to T and B lymphoblasts. The B cells are then committed to the production of antigen-specific S-IgA. These cells are released from Peyer's patch, pass through mesenteric lymph nodes, and eventually enter the systemic circulation through the thoracic duct. The B cells then home to the intestinal lamina propria where they mature and secrete specific S-IgA in response to enteric antigen presentation. B cells are also distributed to other tissues such as the liver, and thus S-IgA is found in bile as well as intestinal succus. In the gastrointestinal tract, the bile appears to contribute about 90% of the S-IgA present in the intestinal lumen. S-IgA works by preventing the binding of enteric pathogens to the cells of the intestinal mucosa and acts in conjunction with the indigenous intestinal microflora to control enteric pathogenic bacteria.

Bacterial translocation is the process by which microorganisms migrate across the mucosal barrier and invade the host.[106] The most extensive work on bacterial translocation has been done in animal models, where the number and pathogenicity of the endogenous flora can be precisely controlled and the microorganisms that invade the host carefully quantified. Three principal mechanisms generally promote bacterial translocation: (1) altered permeability of the intestinal mucosa, as caused by hemorrhagic shock, sepsis, distant injury, or administration of cell toxins; (2) decreased host defense secondary to glucocorticoid administration, immunosuppression, or protein depletion; and (3) an increased number of bacteria within the intestine, as caused by bacterial overgrowth, intestinal stasis, or the feeding of bacteria to experimental animals. Several retrospective and epidemiologic studies have associated infection in specific patient populations with bacterial invasion from the gut.[107-109] These reports suggest that bacterial invasion occurs in patients after injury, multiorgan-system failure, or severe burns and in persons with cancer after undergoing chemotherapy or bone marrow transplantation. Nonmetabolizable markers of known size, such as lactulose or mannitol, have also been used to determine permeability. These studies have demonstrated an increase in mucosal permeability in normal volunteers receiving endotoxin and in infected burn patients. Because many of the factors that facilitate bacterial translocation occur simultaneously in surgical patients, and because their effects may be additive or cumulative, patients in an intensive care unit may be extremely vulnerable to the invasion of enteric bacteria or to the absorption of their toxins (Fig. 68–14). Such patients do not generally receive enteral feedings, current parenteral therapy results in gut atrophy, and methods used to support critically ill patients neither facilitate repair of the intestinal mucosa nor maintain gut barrier function.

NUTRITIONAL ASSESSMENT AND REQUIREMENTS

As with accidental injury, the onset of sepsis is generally sudden and unplanned. On the other hand, in contrast to trauma victims who are well nourished and healthy prior to their injury, infected patients are often nutritionally depleted when bacteremia develops. Malnutrition is inseparable from the occurrence and effects of infectious diseases, and their interaction is synergistic.

As with all patients, the primary objectives of nutritional assessment are to evaluate the patient's present nutritional status and to determine energy, protein, and macro- and micronutrient requirements. Assessment of

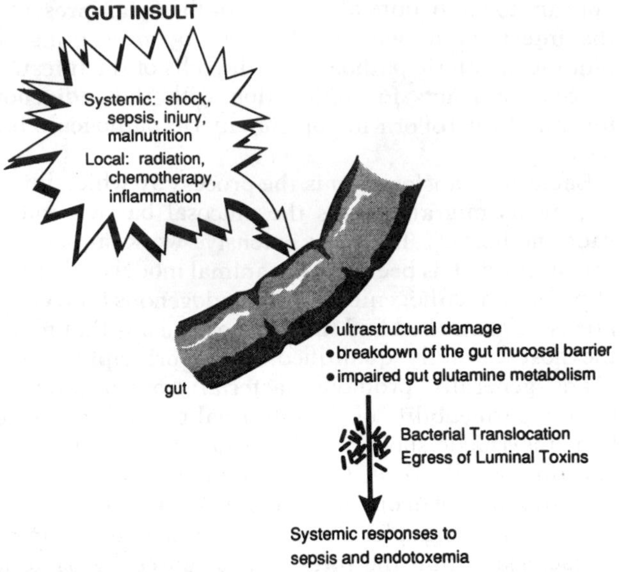

FIGURE 68–14. The gut hypothesis proposes that local and systemic insults can damage the gut epithelium and allow egress of luminal bacteria and toxins. If the systemic responses such as hypermetabolism and persistent catabolism are self-perpetuating, multiple organ failure can develop.

patients with sepsis should start with a medical history and physical examination, which are frequently difficult to obtain and perform because of the severity of the patient's illness. Use of anthropometric measurements is helpful, but weight may be an inaccurate reflection of nutritional status because of fluid retention. Serum protein concentrations (albumin and transferrin) are low because of redistribution secondary to the infection; hence these values are not useful indicators of malnutrition.

The immediate goal of nutritional therapy is weight maintenance. Weight gain and anabolism are generally difficult to achieve during the septic process, but they do occur once the disease process has abated. Total energy requirements can be calculated using the stress equation; mild-to-moderate infections increase energy requirements 20 to 30%, and severe infection increases caloric needs ≃ 50% above basal levels. The optimal calorie-to-nitrogen ratio is approximately 150:1, although providing more nitrogen has been proposed.

USUAL COURSE: CASE EXAMPLE

The usual response pattern following infection is difficult to outline because of the many possible variations. The following case example illustrates the value of nutritional support in the overall integrated care of a patient with prolonged sepsis.

A 65-year old man (183 cm tall, 80 kg (6', 175 lb) BSA, 2.0 m^2) appeared in the hospital emergency ward with right-upper-quadrant pain, a temperature of 103° F, and mild jaundice. A recent ultrasonic study had shown the presence of gallstones, but the patient was otherwise well nourished and in good health. Initial laboratory studies showed a white blood cell count of 17,000, with a left shift, total bilirubin level of 5 mg/dl, and an alkaline phosphatase level of 550 Bodansky units. Shortly after hospital admission, the patient became confused, and his blood pressure fell to 70 mm Hg systolic. His skin was warm and pink, and a diagnosis of ascending cholangitis and septic shock was made. Intravenous fluid was administered, and the patient's blood pressure returned to normal. Antibiotics were started, and shortly thereafter the patient was taken into the operating suite, where he was found to have an impacted gallstone in the common bile duct. A cholecystectomy and common duct exploration were performed, and the impacted stone was removed. Pus was present in the gallbladder and the biliary tract.

Postoperatively, the patient required ventilatory support. On postoperative day 1, he was no longer dependent on cardiotonic agents to maintain normal blood pressure. He had a marked ileus and remained febrile. He received 5% dextrose solutions containing appropriate electrolytes. He gradually became alert, but remained dependent on the ventilator. On postoperative day 5, the patient's fever increased to 103.6° F, and he had marked leukocytosis. Diagnostic studies showed an intra-abdominal abscess, and the patient returned to the operating room for surgical drainage. Postoperatively, the patient received large doses of antibiotics, and 3 days after the second operation, he was weaned from the ventilator. Results of liver function tests gradually returned to normal, and the patient's ileus resolved. During this postoperative period, routine intravenous fluids with glucose were given. On postoperative day 15, the patient started a clear-liquid diet, and he was discharged from the hospital on postoperative day 22. Nitrogen balance studies from postoperative day 1 to day 16 showed a cumulative 15-day negative balance of 225 g (Fig. 68–15). The patient had lost 11 lb by postoperative day 15, half of which was lean tissue and the remainder fat. By day 15, the patient had started oral intake, and by discharge day (day 22), he was clearly afebrile and anabolic, taking adequate quantities of nutrients.

RESPONSE TO FIXED NUTRIENT INTAKE

To evaluate the effect of fixed nutrient intake in sepsis, let us suppose that the foregoing patient with ascending cholangitis is supported vigorously throughout his course with adequate parenteral nutrition. A combination of sepsis, anesthesia, and tissue trauma in this patient increased the metabolic rate by 50%, so the energy needs were approximately 12,100 kJ (2900 kcal) per day. The patient received 3 L central venous nutrition, which provided 21 g nitrogen and 12,540 kJ (3000 kcal) per day. Nitrogen balance studies from postoperative day 1 to 16 showed a cumulative loss of 375 g, and cumulative nitrogen balance for this 15-day period was −60g. On postoperative day 16, the patient had lost only

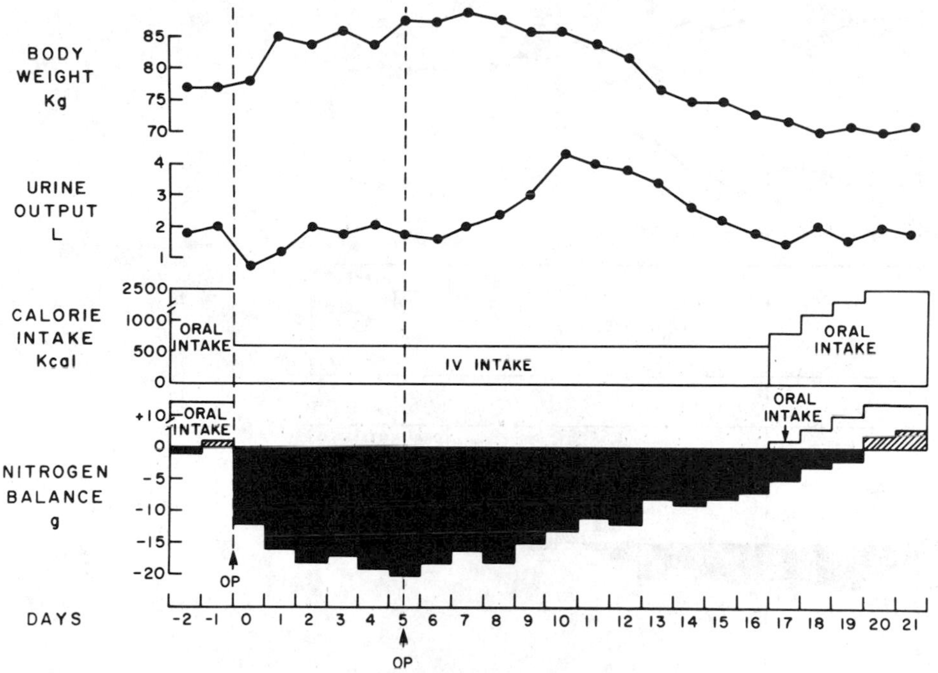

FIGURE 68–15. Metabolic responses to sepsis.

4 lb, half of which was body fat and the remainder lean body mass (Fig. 68–16).

Prompt initiation of nutritional support in patients with sepsis who cannot eat enough or should not eat is mandatory. On the other hand, provision of nutrients requires integration into the patients' management and support plan. The patient in the case example, after about 5 weeks on routine intravenous infusions, was started gradually on nutritional feedings, to avoid untoward complications of hyperglycemia, and the infusion was diminished during the second septic interval. Adequate parenteral nutrition in this case should include fat in a moderate proportion of the infused energy, to avoid the complications of hyperglycemia and to diminish the possibilities of increased carbon dioxide production complicating hypercaloric glucose infusions. Nutritional support helps to diminish the severe erosion of lean body mass possible in such a patient. This provision of calories and nitrogen cannot attenuate the hypermetabolism characteristic of sepsis, but it does reduce accelerated catabolism.

ROUTES OF FEEDING

The routes of nutrient administration are similar to those for the elective surgical patient and the trauma victim. The enteral route should always be used when possible, but patients with sepsis usually have an ileus and therefore require parenteral nutrition. In general, this condition requires central venous nutrition because peripheral nutritional support cannot provide adequate calories in a moderately restrictive fluid volume. The risks of catheter sepsis are minimized by dedicating the central line solely to the infusion of the hypertonic nutrient solutions and maintenance of strict asepsis at the catheter entrance site. In addition, the catheter may be changed over a guidewire using a strict aseptic technique, and the catheter tip may be cultured.[110] This culturing is done at intervals of 3 to 5 days and ensures that the catheter has not become the focus of the septic process.

COMPLICATIONS, ORGAN FAILURE, AND SPECIAL FEEDING PROBLEMS

The most severe complication of sepsis is the failure of essential organs, which may result in death. Current treatment of systemic infection consists of: (1) bacteriologic control by removal and drainage or containment of the source; (2) use of appropriate antibiotics; (3) support of cardiovascular and respiratory function; (4) supportive therapy of specific organ failure, whether cardiac, pulmonary, hepatic, renal, or gastrointestinal; and (5) vigorous support of the host through nutritional means.

RESPIRATORY INSUFFICIENCY

A common problem associated with systemic infection is oxygenation and elimination of carbon dioxide. A variety of endotoxins and vasoactive factors mediated by the infectious process can alter pulmonary vascular permeability and may lead to pulmonary insufficiency. Patients often require intubation and vigorous ventila-

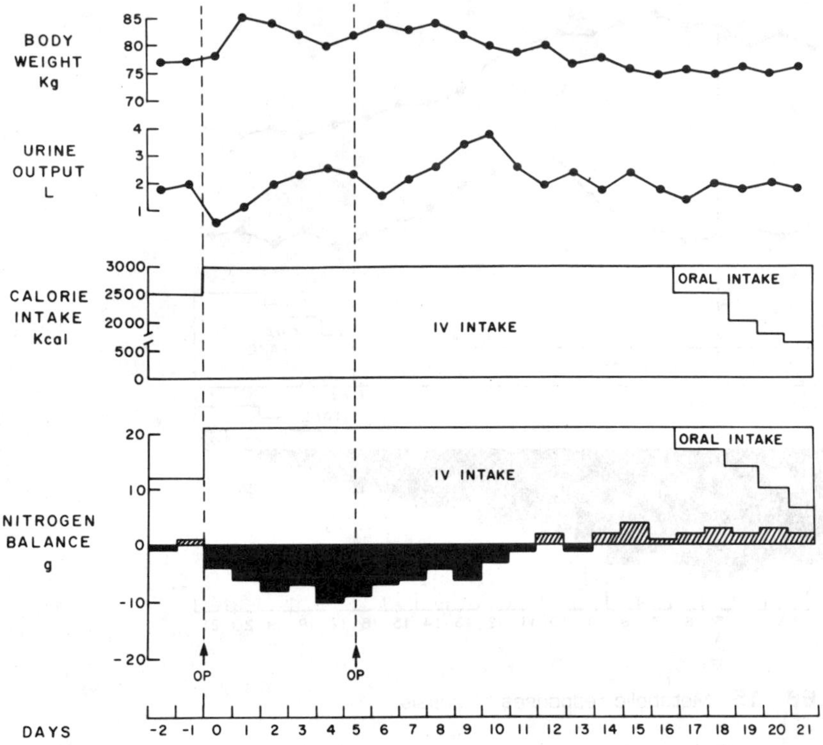

FIGURE 68–16. Metabolic responses to sepsis with constant intravenous nutrition.

tory support with volume cycle ventilation and positive expiratory pressure. Ongoing problems include the development of pneumonia and pulmonary insufficiency secondary to increased capillary permeability. Most of the central and parenteral formulas used to provide nutritional support for critically ill patients contain large amounts of carbohydrate, which generate large quantities of carbon dioxide following oxidation. Such a large carbon dioxide load may worsen pulmonary function or may delay weaning from the ventilator.[84] If this factor becomes a problem, the carbohydrate load should be reduced to 50% of metabolic requirements and fat emulsion should be administered to provide additional calories.

RENAL FAILURE

The origin of renal failure associated with sepsis is unclear. Circulating factors are associated with increasing blood flow to the kidney. If cardiac output is inadequate, however, such a response will not be possible, and this failure, coupled with redistribution blood flow, may cause progressive deficiency of the cortical portion of the kidney. In addition, the use of aminoglycoside antibiotics, which are nephrotoxic, may also cause progressive impairment and malfunction. When renal failure becomes progressive, the early use of hemodialysis, with or without filtration, minimizes the effects of uremia superimposed on the metabolism of sepsis. Adequate caloric support limits ureagenesis and normalizes alterations in serum electrolyte levels. Because uremia itself is a potent catabolic signal,[111] this condition further impairs the hypercatabolic infected host. Metabolic studies in patients with acute and chronic renal failure have limited the intake of nonessential amino acids, in an attempt to lower urea production. Proteins of high biologic value, but in much smaller quantities (<0.5 g/kg per day) than usually given, are administered along with adequate calories, usually in the form of glucose. When enteral feedings are not feasible, a central venous infusion of an essential amino acid solution and hypertonic dextrose provides calories and a small quantity of nitrogen, to reduce protein catabolism while simultaneously controlling the rise in BUN. Whether such nutritional therapy reduces mortality rates for renal failure associated with sepsis remains controversial. During dialysis, protein intake is liberalized, but the BUN is maintained below 100 mg/dl.

GUT DYSFUNCTION

Sepsis causes marked changes in gastrointestinal function. The most common abnormality is ileus, which can result from intra-abdominal disease or from the effects of bacteria elsewhere. Stress ulcers lead to upper gastrointestinal bleeding, which may require operative treatment. Factors that promote breakdown of the gut mucosal barrier and lead to translocation of luminal bacteria and their toxins have been discussed.

HEPATIC FAILURE

Hepatic dysfunction is a common manifestation of septicemia. The degree of dysfunction is variable and may appear early as a slight elevation of liver enzymes, or it may cause severe jaundice and hyperbilirubinemia. Specific bacteria overwhelm the reticuloendothelial system of the liver and result in fulminant hepatic failure. Localized infections, such as hepatic abscesses, pylephlebitis, and hepatitis, may cause profound liver dysfunction because of the direct effect of infection on this organ. Occasionally, hypoglycemia accompanies ascending cholecystitis because of the direct effect of hepatic inflammation. Fulminant hepatic failure in the patient with sepsis has a high mortality rate, especially when hepatic encephalopathy occurs. As discussed in the section of this chapter on trauma, the effects of normalization of amino acid concentration and reversal of hepatic coma remain controversial. More common, however, are alterations on liver function studies, such as elevations in levels of alkaline phosphatase, hepatic enzymes, and serum bilirubin, which appear secondary to the septic event, but may worsen with intravenous feedings.[112] Hepatic dysfunction generally resolves on resolution of the sepsis, but if the inflammatory process persists, adjustments in the feeding formulation will be necessary. The carbohydrate load is usually reduced to consist of no more than 50% of metabolic requirements, and the additional calories should be provided as fat emulsion. If the patient's serum bilirubin level becomes elevated (generally above 12 mg/dl), the patient should be observed for the presence of encephalopathy. If this complication occurs, then the protein load should also be reduced.

CARDIAC DYSFUNCTION

The myocardial dysfunction that occurs in sepsis may be secondary to the elaboration of cytokines or to heart failure secondary to pulmonary insufficiency. Malnourished patients with sepsis may be sensitive to volume overload, and use of a concentrated solution of hypertonic dextrose (D-70%) mixed with amino acids may be indicated to maximize calories and to minimize volume. In addition, a 20% fat emulsion can be administered to provide additional energy.

CHOICE OF NUTRITION IN CRITICALLY ILL PATIENTS

ENTERAL OR PARENTERAL?

Although the physiologic advantage of enteral nutrition is apparent, preoperative nutritional repletion by the enteral route has not been as extensively studied as preoperative TPN. Although it can be associated with the development of nausea, diarrhea, and distention, we recommend the use of enteral nutrition (by a feeding tube or as in-between-meal supplements) in malnourished patients who need an elective operation. Candidates must have a functional gastrointestinal tract and must be able to receive adequate amounts of calories and nitrogen. In general, we limit such preoperative nutritional support to 10 to 14 days.

Studies in elective surgical patients comparing the efficacy of parenteral and enteral nutrition in the postoperative setting have failed to show significant differences. However, significant benefits of enteral feedings have been shown in trauma patients. Moore and colleagues demonstrated that septic complications were significantly reduced in trauma patients fed immediately after emergency celiotomy.[113] In a later study, these authors suggested that early postoperative feeding supported hepatic protein synthesis.

Magnússon and colleagues randomized 20 patients undergoing resection for colorectal cancer to receive identical amounts of glucose either enterally or parenterally.[114] Glucose tolerance and the hypoglycemic response to insulin were superior in the enterally fed group. The group receiving enteral glucose had less subjective postoperative distress and required fewer doses of analgesics. Muggia-Sullam et al. compared the effects of immediate postoperative enteral nutrition (by NCJ) to TPN in patients undergoing major gastrointestinal surgical procedures with regard to subjective tolerance.[46] Both treatment methods maintained body weight and serum protein levels and afforded a positive nitrogen balance. These authors reported that the enterally fed group had a higher incidence of gastrointestinal complaints related to the tube feedings. In our experience, the incidence of postoperative tube feeding intolerance is approximately 20% and is generally manifested as distention or diarrhea. This appears to be due, in most cases, to increasing the rate of the tube feedings too rapidly. Decreasing the rate of feedings usually corrects these complaints. Luminal nutrition is beneficial even when relatively small amounts of the formula, below caloric requirements, are provided.

In an effort to evaluate the cost effectiveness and metabolic consequences of nutritional support, investigators have compared postoperative TPN and enteral nutrition. The cost of enteral nutrition is considerably less than the cost of TPN and home administration is easier in patients who are nourished enterally. Bower et al. randomized 20 patients undergoing major upper gastrointestinal or pancreaticobiliary operations to receive either postoperative TPN or an elemental diet via NCJ.[115] Early nitrogen balance was improved in the TPN group, but late nitrogen balance was similar between groups. Complications were minimal, and differences in serum albumin concentration and transaminase levels were insignificant. The major difference between groups was the estimated cost of nutritional support: $2313 in the TPN group, compared to $849 in the NCJ group for an average of 5 days of feeding after surgery.

NUTRITION AND THE GASTROINTESTINAL TRACT

The intestinal tract has long been considered an organ of inactivity following operation or injury. Ileus is generally present, nasogastric decompression is often necessary, and the gut is usually unused in the immediate postoperative period. In the past, digestion and absorption were thought to be the only physiologic roles of the gut. However, more recent studies have shown that the gut functions as a central organ of amino acid metabolism, a role that may become more pronounced during critical illness.[116,117] Disuse of the gastrointestinal tract, either by starvation or through nutritional support by TPN, may lead to numerous physiologic derangements as well as changes in gut microflora, impaired gut immune function, and disruption of the integrity of the mucosal barrier. Thus, maintaining gut function in the perioperative period may be essential to minimize septic complications and organ failure.

Treatment strategies designed to support the gut during critical illness should be directed toward providing appropriate nutrition and maintenance of mucosal structure and function. Presumably, such efforts will assist the gut in its role as a metabolic processing station and as a barrier.

NUTRITIONAL SUPPORT: ENTERAL FEEDINGS

Enteral feedings are probably the best single method of maintaining mucosal structure and function (Table 68–4).The trophic effects of luminal nutrition are key and the beneficial effects are well documented even if relatively small amounts of nutrients are provided. Elegant studies utilizing Thiry-Vella loops to study the effects of excluding a segment of small intestine from the nutrient stream demonstrated the superiority of enteral stimulation.[118] On the other hand, the detrimental effects of TPN may include mucosal atrophy characterized by a fall in mucosal mass and brush border activity.[119,120] Elemental diets provided to rats promote translocation, but the incidence is significantly lower than that observed when an identical solution is administered intravenously for 2 weeks. In rats subjected to an intraperitoneal injection of hemoglobin and Escherichia coli, the survival rate was clearly enhanced when the same nutrient solution was given enterally rather than parenterally.[121] Mochizuki and colleagues studied endocrine and gut responses to burn injury in guinea pigs and demonstrated that early enteral nutrition blunted the catabolic response and helped to preserve mucosal integrity.[122]

TABLE 68–4. PROPOSED EFFECTS OF LACK OF ENTERAL STIMULATION ON THE GUT

Decreased villous height
Decreased cellular mass
Decreased brush border enzyme activities
Increased gut permeability
Changes in gut microflora
Decreased gut immunity

NUTRITIONAL SUPPORT: GUT-SPECIFIC NUTRIENTS

It is now clear that the composition of the diet and the route of delivery play important roles in maintaining gut structure and function. Several gut-specific nutrients have been studied, but glutamine has received the most attention.[116] Glutamine has several unique properties that suggest an important role in health and during critical illness. It is the most important substrate for renal ammoniagenesis, an essential precursor for the synthesis of nucleotides, and a regulator of protein synthesis. Glutamine is avidly consumed by replicating cells such as gut mucosa cells, lymphocytes, and fibroblasts.

Glutamine has been classified as a nonessential or nutritionally dispensable amino acid. Because this categorization implies that glutamine can be synthesized in adequate quantities from other amino acids and precursors, it has not been considered necessary to include glutamine in nutritional formulas. It has been eliminated from TPN solutions because of its relative instability and short shelf-life compared to other amino acids. With few exceptions, glutamine is present in oral and enteral diets only at the relatively low levels characteristic of its concentration in most animal and plant proteins (about 7% of total amino acids).[117] This view of glutamine as a dispensable nutrient belies its qualitative and quantitative importance in mammalian metabolic pathways. This may be of central importance in critically ill patients because researchers recognized several years ago that glutamine concentrations in the body are not only high, but also labile. Its concentrations in whole blood and tissues decrease significantly during critical illness, leading to a start of marked glutamine depletion. The decrease in glutamine concentrations is greater than for any other amino acid, correlates in general to the severity of the underlying insult, and is reversed only late in the course of recovery.

Several studies demonstrate that glutamine plays an important role in the maintenance of intestinal metabolism, structure, and function. Shive et al. demonstrated its use in the treatment of peptic ulcers 35 years ago.[123] Okabe et al. demonstrated that glutamine protects against aspirin-induced gastric ulceration.[124] Baskerville et al. infused glutaminase to lower blood glutamine levels and noted the development of diarrhea, mild villous atrophy, mucosal ulcerations, and intestinal necrosis in several animal species.[125] Hwang et al. demonstrated that glutamine supplementation of TPN solutions resulted in an increase in jejunal mucosal weight and DNA content and significantly decreased villous atrophy.[126] Jacobs et al. demonstrated that the combination of glutamine supplementation and epidermal growth factor had a synergistic effect on the thickness of the small intestine.[127] Grant also demonstrated that glutamine supplementation of TPN solutions increase villous height and nitrogen content.[128] Subsequent studies by Burke and Alverdy and their associates showed that glutamine-enriched TPN results in decreased bacterial translocation when compared to standard formulas.[129] Salloum et al. demonstrated the ability of glutamine-supplemented elemental diets to stimulate intestinal mucosal growth following starvation.[130]

Other studies have shown that provision of glutamine-supplemented nutrition may be an important adjunct to the therapy of patients with an intestinal mucosal injury secondary to chemotherapy and radiation therapy. Fox and colleagues showed that the addition of glutamine to an elemental, enteral diet resulted in a significant reduction in the severity of methotrexate-induced enterocolitis, as reflected by improved morphometric parameters in the jejunum and colon.[131] In addition, these investigators demonstrated that provision of glutamine reduced endotoxin transmigration from the gut lumen. Similar benefits were reported by Jacobs and associates, who demonstrated that a glutamine-enriched intravenous diet accelerated healing of the gut mucosa in rats receiving 5-fluorouracil.[132] O'Dwyer et al. also showed that after 5-fluorouracil, rats maintained on glutamine-enriched TPN demonstrated greater mean jejunal villous height and increased mucosal DNA content.[133] Similarly, administration of glutamine-enriched oral diets prior to abdominal radiation affords small bowel mucosal protection.[134] Additional studies have shown that the provision of oral glutamine following abdominal irradiation supports gut glutamine metabolism and decreases the morbidity and mortality associated with this entity.[135]

Gut glutamine extraction by the human gastrointestinal tract is about 12%, whereas consumption is approximately 1000 to 1500 nmol/kg per minute. Two European studies suggest that glutamine-supplemented TPN is safe and potentially useful. Hammargvist et al. studied patients following cholecystectomy and demonstrated the ability of glutamine-enriched TPN to improve nitrogen balance.[136] Provision of approximately 20 g of free glutamine as a TPN additive significantly diminished the fall in muscle glutamine content and intracellular ribosomal concentration that characterizes operative stress. Similar benefits were reported by Stehle et al., who used a stable dipeptide, l-alanyl-L-glutamine to supplement standard TPN.[137] Wilmore and colleagues have noted significant benefits of glutamine-enriched TPN in bone marrow transplant patients. Specifically, provision of glutamine-enriched TPN improves water balance in this group of catabolic patients.[138]

Studies to date have failed to demonstrate any toxicity associated with glutamine-supplemented parenteral nutrition. Concern exists about infusing glutamine because of its biochemical relation to ammonia, but elevated circulating levels of ammonia or glutamine have not been reported. Glutamine in solution undergoes hydrolysis in a relatively short time, but this process can be slowed by adjusting the pH and temperature of the solution. Therefore, it appears that breakdown is negligible when the glutamine is added to the TPN mixture at the time the pharmacist prepares the final solution. Nevertheless, it may be more practical to use much more stable and soluble glutamine dipeptides.

USE OF GROWTH FACTORS TO SUPPORT THE GUT MUCOSA

Specific growth factors that may promote intestinal mucosal growth have been implicated in certain physiologic processes including growth, tissue repair, and regeneration. Among these is epidermal growth factor, a polypeptide secreted by submaxillary glands and by Brunner's glands of the small intestine. The most widespread effect of this growth factor on the gastointestinal mucosa is the overall stimulation of DNA synthesis as evidenced by thymidine incorporation. Provision of epidermal growth factor subcutaneously to rats receiving TPN decreases the degree of villous atrophy that otherwise occurs.[127]

OTHER METHODS OF MODIFYING THE CATABOLIC RESPONSE TO SURGERY AND CRITICAL ILLNESS

Besides nutritional intervention, several other methods of modifying the physiologic and biochemical responses to an elective operative procedure have been studied in an effort to reduce the magnitude of the stress of operations and to provide insight into mechanisms in these responses. A variety of human studies have shown that many postoperative responses can be ablated following denervation of the wound.[139,140] These studies suggest that regional anesthetic techniques block afferent signals from the wound and interrupt sympathetic nervous efferent signals to the adrenal gland and possibly the liver. The effect of sympathetic blockade is a reduction in the apparent magnitude of the stress response. These techniques have also been used during the postoperative period. Bromage and colleagues suppressed hyperglycemia and hypercortisolism with maintenance of an epidural anesthetic for the first 24 hours after operation.[141] Brandt and associates reported an improved 5-day cumulative nitrogen balance in patients undergoing elective abdominal hysterectomy with epidural anesthesia, as compared to a similar group receiving general anesthesia.[142]

Several investigators have studied stress responses in animals that have undergone sympathectomy by blocking the efferent limb of the neuroendocrine reflex response. Propranalol has been shown to improve postoperative nitrogen balance and decrease muscle protein breakdown. Herndon and associates reported that the adminsitration of propranalol to burned children decreased cardiac work without affecting wound healing or mortality.[143] Brandt and colleagues reported that large doses of morphine (4 mg/kg) given prior to skin incision diminished the normal rise in plasma ACTH, cortisol, growth hormone, and glucose in patients undergoing aortic valve replacement.[144] These reports indicate that central nervous system blockade interrupts afferent signals stimulated by operative procedures.

Studies in the 1960s and 1970s demonstrated that short courses of growth hormone promoted nitrogen retention following thermal injury. More recent studies have documented the safety and efficacy of long-term exogenous recombinant growth hormone administration.[145] Growth hormone stimulates protein synthesis during hypocaloric feedings and increases retention of sodium and potassium by the kidney. The potential synergistic effects of specialized nutrition in combination with growth hormone require further study.

Cyclooxygenase inhibitors such as aspirin and ibuprofen attenuate the symptoms and endocrine responses that occur during critical illness without altering cytokine elaboration. For example, pretreatment with ibuprofen may attenuate the undesirable symptoms associated with the inflammatory response.[146] It is anticipated that researchers will eventually be able to block selectively the deleterious effects of excessive cytokines and preserve their beneficial effects. Specific antibodies are already used in the clinical setting to block the TNF and Il-1 receptor. Clearly, the type of nutrition used in critically ill patients can influence the metabolic alterations seen with infection.[147] No doubt patient-care strategies in the future will use combination therapies designed to minimize the undesirable consequences of the body's response to critical illness and simultaneously accelerate wound healing, immune function, and recovery.[148]

REFERENCES

1. Dudrick, S.J., Wilmore, D.W., Vars, H.M., et al.: Surgery, *64:*134–142, 1968.
2. Stephens, R.V., Randall, H.T.: Ann. Surg., *170:*642–667, 1969.
3. Wretlind, A.: Nutr. Metab., *14(Suppl):*1–57, 1972.
4. Butterworth, C.E., Blackburn, G.L.: Nutr. Today, *10:*8–18, 1975.
5. Wilmore, D.W., McDougal, W.S., Peterson, J.P.: Am. J. Clin. Nutr., *30:*1498–1505, 1977.
6. Burke, G., Francsson, C., Plaintin, C.O.: Acta Endocrinol., *18:*201–209, 1955.
7. Traynor, C., Hall, G.M.: Br. J. Anaesth., *53:*153–160, 1981.
8. Deutsch, S.: Surg. Clin. North Am., *55:*775–786, 1975.
9. Philbin, D.M., Coggins, C.H.: Anesthesiology, *49:*95–98, 1978.
10. Russell, R.C., Walker, C.J., Bloom, S.R.: Br. Med. J., *1:*10–12, 1975.
11. Porte, D., Graber, A.L., Kuzuwa, T., et al.: J. Clin. Invest., *45:*228–236, 1966.
12. Riegel, C., Koop, C.E., Drew, J., et al.: J. Clin. Invest., *26:*18–23, 1947.
13. Holden, W.D., Krieger, H., Levey, S., et al.: Ann. Surg., *146:*563–579, 1957.
14. Wilmore, D.W.: The Metabolic Management of the Critically Ill. New York, Plenum Medical Book, 1977.
15. Rombeau, J.L., Rolandelli, R.H., Wilmore, D.W.: Nutritional Support. *In* Care of the Surgical Patient. Vol. 1. Critical Care: Care in the I.C.U. New York, Scientific American, 1988, pp. 1–40.
16. Meakins, J.H., McLean, A.P.H., Kelly, R., et al.: J. Trauma, *18:*240–247, 1978.
17. Duke, J.H., Jorgensen, S.B., Broell, J.R., et al.: Surgery, *68:*168–174, 1970.
18. Page, C.P., Ryan, J.A., Haff, R.C.: Surg. Gynecol. Obstet., *142:*184–188, 1976.
19. Copeland, E.M., III, Dudrick, S.J.: Curr. Probl. Cancer, *1:*1–51, 1976.
20. Rombeau, J.L., Barot, L.R., Williamson, C.E., et al.: Am. J. Surg. *143:*139–143, 1982.
21. Mullen, J.L., Buzby, G.P., Waldman, M.T., et al.: Surg. Forum, *30:*80–82, 1979.
22. Mullen, J.L., Buzby, G.P., Matthews, D.C., et al.: Ann. Surg., *192:*604–613, 1980.
23. Holter, A.R., Fischer, J.E.: J. Surg. Res., *23:*31–34, 1977.
24. Thompson, B.R., Julian, R.B., Stremble, J.F.: J. Surg. Res., *30:*497–500, 1981.
25. Cromack, D.C., Moley, J.F., Pass, H.I., et al.: A perspective randomized trial of parenteral nutrition compared to ad lib oral nutrition in patients with upper gastrointestinal carcinoma and significant weight loss undergoing surgical treatment. Presented at the 22nd Annual Meeting of the Association for Academic Surgery, 1988, p. 96.
26. Müller, J., Dienst, C., Brenner, U., et al.: Lancet, *1:*68–71, 1982.
27. Bellantone, R., Doglietto, G.B., Bossola, M., et al.: JPEN J. Parenter. Enteral Nutr., *12:*195–197, 1988.
28. Bellatone, R., Doglietto, G.B., Bossa, M., et al.: Nutrition, *6:*168–170, 1990.
29. Buzby, G.P., and The Veterans Affairs Total Parenteral Nutrition Cooperative Study Group: N. Engl. J. Med., *325:*525, 1991.
30. Detsky, J.M., Baker, J.P., O'Rourke, K., et al.: Ann. Intern. Med., *107:*195–203, 1987.
31. Shukla, H.S., Rao, R.R., Banu, N., et al.: Indian J. Med. Res., *80:*339–344, 1984.
32. Foschi, D., Cavagna, G., Callioni, F., et al.: Br. J. Surg., *73:*716–719, 1986.
33. Flynn, M.B., Leighty, F.: Am. J. Surg., *154:*359–362, 1987.
34. McFadyen, B.V., Dudrick, S.J., Ruberg, R.L.: Surgery, *74:*100–105, 1973.
35. Fischer, J.E., Rosen, H.M., Ebeid, A.M., et al.: Surgery, *80:*77–91, 1976.
36. Cerra, F.B., McMillen, M., Angelico, R., et al.: Surgery, *94:*612–619, 1983.

37. Wahren, J., Denis, J., Desurmont, P., et al.: Intravenous administration of branched-chain amino acids in the treatment of hepatic encephalopathy. *In* Amino Acids: Metabolism and Medical Applications. Edited by G.L. Blackburn et al. Boston, John Wright, 1983.
38. Wesson, D.E., Mitch, W.E., Wilmore, D.W.: Nutritional support. *In* Acute Renal Failure. Edited by B. Brenner and J.M. Lazarus. Philadelphia, W.B. Saunders, 1983.
39. Abel, R.M., Beck, C.H., Abbott, W.M., et al.: N. Engl. J. Med., *288:*695–699, 1973.
40. Preshaw, R.M., Attisha, R.P., Hollingsworth, W.J., et al.: Can. J. Surg. *22:*437–439, 1979.
41. Yamada, N., Koyama, H., Kioki, K, et al.: Br. J. Surg., *70:*267–274, 1983.
42. Askanazi, J., Hensle, T.W., Starker, P.M., et al.: Ann. Surg., *203:*236–239, 1986.
43. Daly, J.M., Bonau, R., Stofberg, P., et al.: Am. J. Surg., *153:*198–206, 1987.
44. Hoover, H.C., Ryan, J.A., Anderson, E.J., et al.: Am. J. Surg., *139:*153–159, 1980.
45. Sagar, S., Harland, P., Shields, R.: Br. Med. J., *1:*293–295, 1979.
46. Muggia-Sullam, M., Bower, R.H., Murphy, R.F., et al.: Am. J. Surg., *149:*106–112, 1985.
47. Wilmore, D.W., Orcutt, T.W., Mason, A.D., et al.: J. Trauma, *15:*697–703, 1975.
48. Wilmore, D.W.: *In* Clinics in Endocrinology and Metabolism. Vol. 5. Edited by K.G.M.M. Alberti. Philadelphia, W.B. Saunders, 1976, pp. 731–745.
49. Wilmore, D.W., Goodwin, C.W., Aulick, L.H., et al.: Ann. Surg., *192:*491–504, 1980.
50. Wilmore, D.W., Aulick, L.H., Mason, A.D., et al.: Ann. Surg., *186:*444–458, 1977.
51. Goodwin, C.W., Aulick, L.H., Powanda, M.C., et al.: Eur. J. Surg. Res., *12(Suppl. 126):*126–127, 1980.
52. Black, P.R., Brooks, D.C., Bessey, P.Q., et al.: Ann. Surg., *196:*420–433, 1982.
53. Wilmore, D.W., Aulick, L.H., Goodwin, C.W., et al.: Acta Chir. Scand., *498(Suppl.):*43–47, 1980.
54. Wolfe, R.R., Durkot, M.J., Allsop, J.R., et al.: Metabolism, *28:*1031–1039, 1979.
55. Brooks, D.C., Bessey, P.Q., Black, P.R., et al.: J. Surg. Res., *34:*100–107, 1984.
56. Carpentier, Y.A., Askanazi, J., Elwyn, D.H., et al.: J. Trauma, *19:*649–654, 1979.
57. Bessey, P.Q., Brooks, D.C., Black, P.R., et al.: Surgery, *94:*172–179, 1983.
58. Bessey, P.Q., Watters, J.M., Aoki, T.T., et al.: Ann. Surg., *200:*264–281, 1984.
59. Herrmann, V.M., Clark, D., Wilmore, D.W., et al.: Surg. Forum, *31:*92–94, 1980.
60. Picou, D., Taylor-Roberts, T.: Clin. Sci., *36:*283–296, 1969.
61. Birkhahn, R.H., Long, C.L., Fitkin, D., et al.: Am. J. Physiol., *241:*E64–E71, 1981.
62. Cuthbertson, D.P.: Q.J. Med., *1:*233–246, 1932.
63. Aulick, L.H., Wilmore, D.W.: Surgery, *85:*560–565, 1979.
64. Muhlbacher, F., Kapadia, C.R., Colpoys, M.F., et al.: Am. J. Physiol., *247:*E75–E83, 1974.
65. Goldberg, A.L., Chang, T.W.: Fed. Proc., *37:*2301–2307, 1978.
66. Moldawer, L.L., Echenique, M.M., Bistrian, B.R., et al.: *In* Advances in Clinical Nutrition. Edited by I.D.A. Johnson. Boston, MTP Press, 1983.
67. Pitts, R.F.: Am. J. Med., *36:*720–742, 1964.
68. Windmueller, H.G., Spaeth, A.E.: J. Biol. Chem., *249:*5070–5079, 1974.
69. Souba, W.W., Wilmore, D.W.: Surgery, *94:*342–350, 1983.
70. Souba, W.W., Kapadia, C.R., Smith, R.J., et al.: Surg. Forum, *34:*74–78, 1983.
71. Birkhahn, R.H., Long, C.L., Fitkin, D.L., et al.: J. Trauma, *21:*513–519, 1981.
72. Wilmore, D.W., Aulick, L.H., Becker, R.A.: Hormones and the control of metabolism. *In* Surgical Nutrition. Edited by J.E. Fischer. Boston, Little, Brown, 1983, pp. 65–96.
73. Michie, H.R., Wilmore, D.W.: Arch. Surg., *125:*531–536, 1990.
74. Akira, S., Hirano, T., Taga, T., et al.: FASEB J., *4:*2860–2867, 1990.
75. Arai, K., Lee, F., Miyajima, A., et al.: Annu. Rev. Biochem., *59:*783–836, 1990.
76. Michie, H.R., Manogue, K.R., Spriggs, D.R.: N. Engl. J. Med., *318:*1481–1486, 1988.
77. Souba, W.W., Salloum, R.M., Bode, B.P., et al.: Surgery. *110:*295–302, 1991.
78. Austgen, T.R., Chen, M.K., Flynn, T.C., et al.: J. Trauma. *31:*742–752, 1991.
79. Fong, Y., Tracey, K.J., Moldawer, L.L., et al.: J. Exp. Med., *170:*1627–1631, 1989.
80. Fong, Y., Moldawer, L.L., Marano, M., et al.: J. Immunol., *142:*2321–2327, 1989.
81. Fong, Y., Marano, M.A., Moldawer, L.L., et al.: J. Clin. Invest., *85:*1896–1903, 1990.
82. Long, J.M., III, Wilmore, D.W., Mason, A.D., et al.: Ann. Surg., *185:*417–422, 1977.
83. Wolfe, R.R., Allsop, J.R., Burke, J.F.: Metabolism, *28:*210–220, 1979.
84. Askanazi, J., Rosenbaum, S.H., Hyman, A.I., et al.: JAMA, *243:*1444–1447, 1980.
85. Levenson, S.W., Green, R.W., Taylor, F.H.L., et al.: Ann. Surg., *124:*840–856, 1946.
86. Brodribb, A.J.M., Ricketts, C.R.: Injury, *3:*25–29, 1971.
87. Clowes, G.H.A., Vucinic, M., Weidner, M.G.: Ann. Surg., *163:*866–885, 1966.
88. Beisel, W.R.: Annu. Rev. Med., *26:*9–20, 1975.
89. Gump, F.E., Long, C., Killian, P., et al.: J. Trauma, *14:*378–388, 1974.
90. LaNoue, K.F., Mason, A.D., Daniels, J.P.: Metabolism, *17:*606–611, 1968.
91. McFadzean, A.J.S., Yeung, R.T.T.: Trans. R. Soc. Trop. Med. Hyg., *59:*179–185, 1965.
92. Yeung, C.Y.: J. Pediatr., *77:*812–817, 1970.
93. Long, C.L., Jeevanandam, M., Kim, B.M., et al.: Am. J. Clin. Nutr., *30:*1340–1344, 1977.
94. Duff, J.H., Viidik, T., Marchuk, J.B., et al.: Surgery, *85:*344–348, 1979.
95. Plumley, D.A., Souba, W.W., Hautamaki, R.D., et al.: Arch. Surg., *125:*57–61, 1990.
96. Souba, W.W., Plumley, D.A., Salloum, R.M., et al.: Surgery, *108:*213–219, 1990.
97. Souba, W.W., Herskowitz, K., Klimberg, V.S., et al.: Ann. Surg., *211:*543–551, 1990.
98. Salloum, R.M., Copeland, E.M., III, Souba, W.W.: Ann. Surg., *213:*401–410, 1991.
99. Gallin, J.I., Kaye, D., O'Leary, W.M.: N. Engl. J. Med., *281:*1081–1086, 1969.
100. Radcliffe, A.G., Wolfe, R.R., Colpoys, M.F., et al.: Am. J. Physiol., *244:*R667–R675, 1983.
101. Neufeld, H.A., Kaminski, M.V., Wannemacher, R.W.: Am. J. Clin. Nutr., *30:*1357–1358, 1977.

102. Watters, J.M., Wilmore, D.W.: Br. J. Surg., *73:*108–110, 1986.
103. Egdahl, R.H.: J. Clin. Invest., *38:*1120–1125, 1959.
104. Maddaus, M.A., Wells, C.L., Platt, J.L., et al.: Ann. Surg., *207:*387–398, 1988.
105. Alverdy, J.C.: JPEN J. Parenter. Enteral Nutr., *14(Suppl.):*109S–113S, 1990.
106. Deitch, E.A.: Arch. Surg., *125:*403–404, 1990.
107. Hollander, D., Vadheim, C.M., Brettholz, E., et al.: Ann. Intern. Med., *105:*883–885, 1986.
108. Border, J.R., Hassett, J., LaDuca, J., et al.: Ann. Surg., *206:*427–445, 1987.
109. Jarrett, F., Balish, E., Moylan, J.A., et al.: Surgery, *83:*523–527, 1978.
110. Graeve, A.H., Carpenter, C.M., Schiller, W.R.: Am. J. Surg., *142:*752–755, 1981.
111. Garber, A.J.: J. Clin. Invest., *62:*623–632, 1978.
112. Kaminski, D.L., Adams, A., Jellinek, M.: Surgery, *88:*93–100, 1980.
113. Moore, F.A., Moore, E.E., Jones, T.N., et al.: J. Trauma, *29:*916–923, 1989.
114. Magnússon, J., Trenberg, K.G., Jeppsson, B., et al.: Scand. J. Gastroenterol., *24:*539–549, 1989.
115. Bower, R.H., Talaman, M.A., Sax, H.C., et al.: Arch. Surg., *121:*1040–1045, 1986.
116. Souba, W.W., Klimberg, V.S., Plumley, D.A., et al.: J. Surg. Res., *48:*383–391, 1990.
117. Lacey, J., Wilmore, D.W.: Nutr. Rev., *48:*297–313, 1990.
118. Gleeson, M.H., Dowling, R.H., Peters, T.J.: Clin. Sci., *43:*743–757, 1982.
119. Johnson, L.R., Copeland, E.M., Dudrick, S.J., et al.: Gastroenterology, *68:*1177–1183, 1975.
120. Levine, G.M., Deren, J.J., Steiger, E., et al.: Gastroenterology, *67:*975–982, 1974.
121. Kudsk, K.A., Carpenter, G., Petersen, S., et al.: J. Surg. Res., *31:*105–110, 1981.
122. Mochizuki, H., Trocki, O., Dominioni, L., et al.: Ann. Surg., *200:*297–310, 1984.
123. Shive, W., Snider, R.N., DeBillar, B., et al.: Tex. State J. Med., *Nov.:*840–843, 1957.
124. Okabe, S., Honda, K., Takeuchi, K., et al.: Dig. Dis., *20:*626–632, 1975.
125. Baskerville, A., Hambleton, P., Benbough, J.E.: Br. J. Exp. Pathol., *61:*132, 1980.
126. Hwang, T.L., O'Dwyer, S.T., Smith, R.J., et al.: Surg. Forum, *38:*56, 1987.
127. Jacobs, D.O., Evans, D.A., Mealy, K., et al.: Surgery, *104:*358–364, 1988.
128. Grant, J.: J. Surg. Res., *44:*506–513, 1988.
129. Burke, D., Alverdy, J.C., Aoys, E., et al.: Arch. Surg., *124:*1396–1399, 1989.
130. Salloum, R.M., Souba, W.W., Klimberg, V.S., et al.: Surg. Forum, *40:*6, 1989.
131. Fox, A.D., Kripke, S.A., DePaula, J., et al.: JPEN J. Parenter. Enteral Nutr., *12:*325–331, 1988.
132. Jacobs, D.O., Evans, A., O'Dwyer, S.T., et al.: Surg. Forum, *38:*45–49, 1987.
133. O'Dwyer, S.T., Scott, T., Smith, R.J., et al.: Clin. Res., *35:*369a, 1987.
134. Klimberg, V.S., Souba, W.W., Dolson, D.J., et al.: Cancer, *66:*62–68, 1990.
135. Klimberg, V.S., Souba, W.W., Hautamaki, R.D., et al.: Arch. Surg., *125:*1040–1045, 1990.
136. Hammargvist, F., Wernerman, J., Ali, R., et al.: Ann. Surg., *209:*455–461, 1989.
137. Stehle, P., Zander, J., Mertes, N., et al.: Lancet, *1:*231, 1989.
138. Scheltinga, M., Young, L.S., Benfell, K., et al.: Ann. Surg., *214:*385–395, 1991.
139. Kehlet, H., Brandt, R.M., Rem, J.: JPEN J. Parenter. Enteral Nutr., *4:*152–155, 1980.
140. Engquist, A., Brandt, M.R., Fernandes, A., et al.: Acta Anaesthesiol. Scand., *21:*330–335, 1977.
141. Bromage, P.R., Shibata, H.R., Willoughby, H.W.: Surg. Gynecol. Obstet., *132:*1051–1056, 1971.
142. Brandt, M.R., Fernandes, A., Mordhorst, R., et al.: Br. Med. J., *1:*1106–1108, 1978.
143. Herndon, D.N., Barrow, R.E., Rectan, T.C., et al.: Ann. Surg., *208:*484–490, 1988.
144. Brandt, M.R., Korshin, J., Prange Hansen, A., et al.: Acta Anaesthesiol. Scand., *22:*400–412, 1978.
145. Ziegler, T.R., Lorraine, S., Young, R.D., et al.: JPEN J. Parenter. Enteral Nutr., *14:*574–581, 1990.
146. Revhaug, A., Michie, H.R., Manson, J. McK., et al.: Arch. Surg., *123:*162–170, 1988.
147. Fong, Y., Marano, M.A., Barber, A., et al.: Am. Surg., *210:*449–457, 1990.
148. Wilmore, D.W.: N. Engl. J. Med., *325:*695–702, 1991.

CHAPTER **69**

Nutrition and Infection

Gerald T. Keusch

The temporal relationship between nutrition and infection has long been appreciated and there are many historical references to the concurrence of pestilence and famine.[1] Even the catabolic response to infection was well known, as indicated by the popular designation of tuberculosis as "consumption." A more recent example of the obvious nature of the interaction of nutrition and infection is acquired immune deficiency syndrome (AIDS), which was first recognized in East Africa by the lay term "slim disease," because of the dramatic wasting that occurred in these patients.[2]

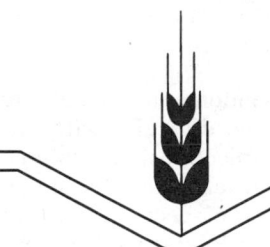

What has been slower to develop has been an understanding of the mechanisms involved, and an appreciation of the intricate coupling of the altered host metabolism, which underlies catabolic responses, to activation and amplification of host defenses. In the course of intensive studies over the past 25 years, however, new information has been obtained. At the same time, extrapolation and application of this information to clinical settings has been less than satisfactory, especially to the critical assessment of the impact of specific nutrient deficiencies on immunologic host defense mechanisms. In this chapter, these issues are explored, and the multifaceted relationship between nutrition, immune responses, and infection is described. To provide the background needed to understand the complexities involved, certain aspects of host defense mechanisms are reviewed first (see also Chap. 41).

HOST DEFENSE MECHANISMS

The immune system is highly organized; its function in the host response to infection represents an extraordinary integration of multiple functional components.[3] Host defense is not synonymous with immunity because both immunologic and nonimmunologic based defense mechanisms are involved. An example of the latter is thc ability of gastric acid to protect against infection with certain enteric pathogens that are acid intolerant; for example, *Vibrio cholerae*, the causative agent of cholera, or nontyphoidal salmonella, common causes of food or water-borne diarrhea. Individuals with defects in gastric acid production for any reason, whether because of previous ulcer surgery or current use of H-2 blockers, are therefore at increased risk if exposed to the pathogens. During the 1970s, clinical cholera in Europe was observed primarily among individuals with hypochlorhydria.[4] Although protection based on creating a hostile environment (such as low pH) is "nonspecific" in that no stereospecific recognition events are involved, not all pathogens are affected by the gastric acid barrier (for example, no relation has been found between hypochlorhydria and shigella infection), which creates the appearance of "specificity."

In contrast, immunologic mechanisms are truly specific in the sense that they depend on stringent receptor-ligand recognition mechanisms. Similar specific recognition also underlies the typical species, organ, and cellular selectivity of infectious agents. On the host side of the equation, immune responses are mediated by effector cells such as T lymphocytes, macrophages, and granulocytes, or soluble molecules such as antibodies, complement-derived peptides, and cytokines (see Chap. 41). Given this organization of the immune system, and the basic specificity principle inherent to both infection and immune responses, it is not surprising that immune defenses exhibit selectivity as well, that is, individual responses are specialized for certain classes of infecting agents and not for others. Convincing clinical evidence of this level of specialization comes from observations of patients with genetically mediated immunodeficiency states that predispose to some, but not all, types of infection (Table 69–1).[5] In general, humoral defects of antibody or complement predispose to pyogenic systemic bacterial infections; defects of T cells and cell-mediated immunity (CMI) commonly predispose to viral, fungal, and intracellular bacterial infections; and defects of phagocytes increase the prevalence and severity of pyogenic bacterial and certain fungal infections.

X-linked agammaglobulinemic males develop recurrent pyogenic infections of the respiratory tract, middle ear, and skin, beginning in the second year of life after maternally acquired immunity wanes. The most common pathogen is Haemophilus influenzae; however, significant problems with Streptococcus pneumoniae, Streptococcus pyogenes, and Pseudomonas spp. also are found. Yet these children have no difficulty with diarrheal diseases, urinary tract infections, or common childhood viral illnesses. Congenital deficiency of complement components also results in specific heightened susceptibility to encapsulated bacterial organisms, even though complement activation products are critical to the orderly and effective activation of the entire inflammatory response. Deficiencies of the early components of the classical pathway, C1, C2, or C4, are not ordinarily accompanied by increased systemic infections, but when these do occur they are commonly due to S. pneumoniae or another encapsulated bacteria. No doubt the ability to activate complement through the alternative pathway serves an important protective function in these patients. When C3 is deficient, however, neither pathway can be effectively activated, and encapsulated bacteria such as S. pneumoniae, H. influenzae, and Neisseria meningitidis cause severe and recurrent infections. Deficiency of either late components or properdin of the alternative pathway frequently leads to invasive infection, particularly with N. meningitidis.

Severe combined immunodeficiency is a syndrome with different genetic causes, but all are characterized by reduction in T cells and a decrease of cell-mediated immune competence. Affected children experience AIDS-like opportunistic infections with Candida albicans and

TABLE 69–1. INFECTIONS IN CONGENITAL IMMUNODEFICIENCY SYNDROMES

	COMMONLY ASSOCIATED PATHOGENS			
NATURE OF DEFECT	Bacteria	Viruses	Protozoa	Fungi
Agammaglobulinemia	Hib, Sp, Sa, Ps	Echo	Gl, ?Pc	—
IgA deficiency	—	—	—	—
IgE deficiency	OM, S, CSP			
HyperIgE syndromes*	Sa, Hib, Sp	RSV, Pi		
IgG1 deficiency	CSP			
IgG2, 4 deficiency	Hib, Sp, CSP			
DiGeorges syndrome†	CSP, DD		Pc	Ca
SCID‡	CSP, BCG	VZ, A, HSV, CMV	Pc	Ca
Bare lymphocytes§	DD		Pc	Ca
Wiscott-Aldrich‖	OM, CSP	VZ, HSV, CMV	Pc	Ca
HAT#	CSP	CMV		
CGD**	Sa, Psc, Lp, Nc			As
MPO deficiency††	—	—	—	—
C3 deficiency	Sp, Hib, Nm, GNB			

Abbreviations: Hib, Haemophilus influenzae type b; Sp, Streptococcus pneumoniae; Sa, Staphylococcus aureus; Psc, Pseudomonas cepacia; Lp, Legionella pneumophila; Nc, Nocardia spp; Mc, Neissernia meningiditis; GNB, gram-negative bacilli; Echo, echovirus meningoencephalitis; RSV, respiratory syncytial virus; Pi, parainfluenza virus; VZ, varicella-zoster virus; A, adenovirus; H, herpesvirus; Gl, Giardia lamblia; Pc, Pnemocystis carinii; Ca, Candida albicans; As, Aspergillus spp; OM, otitis media; S, sinusitis; CSP, chronic suppurative pneumonia; RSP, recurrent suppurative pneumonia; DD, diarrheal disease; BCG, bacillus Calmette-Guérin; Ps, Pseudomona species; HSV, Herpes simplex virus; CMV, cytomegalo virus.

*Associated with various lymphocyte defects.

†Pure T cell defect.

‡Severe combined immunodeficiency, combined T and B cell defect.

‖Associated with T cell defects, hyper IgE, poor antipolysaccharide antibody responses.

#Hereditary ataxia telangiectasia–IgA deficiency, poor CMI.

**Chronic granulomatous disease, defective neutrophil oxidative response.

††Myeloperoxidase deficiency.

other skin pathogens, chronic diarrhea, and interstitial pneumonia commonly attributed to Pneumocystis carinii; if BCG was given as a routine childhood immunization at birth, progressive systemic BCG infection may occur. Whereas varicella, herpesvirus, or adenoviruses often cause disseminated and severe infections in these patients, the pyogenic bacteria are not especially troublesome.

Defects of phagocytic cell function such as chronic granulomatous disease (CGD), in which neutrophils cannot generate normal oxidative bactericidal products, result in excess susceptibility to catalase-positive organisms. Catalase-negative organisms, such as S. pneumoniae or S. pyogenes, are not a problem because they lack the catalase activity needed to detoxify and resist their own bacteria-derived hydrogen peroxide; hence, these organisms are quickly eliminated. Patients with CGD typically develop serious infections with S. aureus, gram-negative bacilli such as Pseudomonas aeruginosa and Serratia marcescens, and fungi such as aspergillis, but not with routine upper respiratory bacterial pathogens or usual childhood viral pathogens.

Some caution is required in extrapolating evidence of defective host defenses to clinical susceptibility to infection. Thus, specific defects in host responses may be measurable by in vitro functional tests but still fail to be associated with increased clinical infections because alternative defense mechanisms are available to the host. Congenital IgA deficiency is an example in which production of IgM and IgG antibodies appears to compensate for diminished mucosal immunity related to lack of IgA. Similarly, patients with congenital absence of myeloperoxidase, a neutrophil enzyme involved in the generation of bactericidal oxygen radicals, usually do not experience recurrent or unusually severe infections because other bactericidal products are still produced. Based on the general correlations between particular immune mechanisms and susceptibility to specific types of organisms, it should be possible to predict the effects of nutritional immunodeficiencies on clinical susceptibility to infection (Table 69–2). These predictions hold rather well, presumably because the breadth of the acquired defects in the malnourished host is sufficient to overcome the redundancy and capacity for adaptation in the immune system, resulting in susceptibility to a broad range of infections in the severely malnourished individual.

FUNCTIONAL ORGANIZATION OF THE IMMUNE SYSTEM

This organization was detailed in Chapter 41; this section addresses interactions between components of the immune system and various infectious agents. Activation of these host responses may involve simply the triggering of biochemical reactions or proteolytic cascades such as the complement system, or may involve the clonal proliferation of specific antigen-reactive T and/or B lymphocyte subsets or bone marrow granulocyte precursors. The latter events are probably the most important aspect of effective immune responses, and therefore it is reasonable to predict that any nutritional deficit that impairs the ability of a host to sustain cellular proliferation can have an adverse effect on host defense. Because it is often the speed with which these host responses are called into play that determines the difference between harmless and fatal infections, a reduced capacity to support growth and expansion of immunologically capable cells because of nutrient deficiencies (or in some situations, even nutrient excess) can tip the balance toward more dire outcomes as well.

Once set in motion, however, host defense responses generate products able to damage normal structures, and the host must be able to dampen and control these reactions. For this reason, elaborate mechanisms involving regulatory cells and proteins have evolved for all classes of immune reactions in order to modulate responses and ultimately prevent such an "immunologic runaway." Also, in well-characterized situations, it is the host response that results in clinical pathologic change. These abnormal responses can be amplified in the presence of nutritional deficits that alter immunoregulation and lead to more extensive immunopathology. There are also contrary examples of nutritionally induced immunodeficiency that may diminish immunopa-

TABLE 69–2. IMMUNE DEFECTS AND INFECTIONS IN PROTEIN-ENERGY MALNUTRITION

IMMUNE DEFECT	ASSOCIATED MICROORGANISMS
T cell functions (cell-mediated immunity)	Facultative intracellular bacteria, measles virus, Pneumocystis carinii, Candida albicans
Antibody abnormalities (↓ s-IgA, ↓ affinity)	Mucosal infections, pyogenic and encapsulated bacteria, fungi
Neutrophil function (↓ microbial killing)	Pyogenic bacteria, gram-negative bacilli
Complement (↑ use, ↓ synthesis)	Gram-negative bacilli, encapsulated bacteria

thology, such as occurs in infection with Schistosoma mansoni. In this case, nutritional deficiencies resulting in a reduced ability to mount CMI reactions can decrease the size of the granuloma formed in response to schistosome eggs deposited in the liver. This nutritional modulation of granuloma size can favorably influence organ damage and dysfunction, at least as documented in experimental murine infection.

Separating the immune system into its cellular (including T lymphocyte and phagocytic cell responses) and humoral compartments (including complement, antibody, and cytokines), although convenient, obscures the extent of the interactions among these elements. For example, B lymphocytes are essential but not sufficient for antibody formation, which requires antigen-presenting macrophages and T cells; normal phagocytes cannot function without complement and antibody for opsonization; and various cytokines produced by either lymphocytes or monocyte-macrophages interact with all of these cells to up- or down-regulate their function. The term *immune system* should be interpreted literally to suggest that the various "compartments" really do function as an interactive "system" in which communication among the individual parts is critical.

VIRUSES

Viruses are obligate intracellular pathogens because the number of viral genes is insufficient to encode their necessary life support "housekeeping" functions. Therefore, a virus must usurp the host cell to carry out its life cycle. Yet, it is remarkable how intricate this simple life form is, and how diverse their habitats can be, as well as the pathologic processes they induce, ranging from acute to chronic to latent infections of particular organ systems, to the induction of tumors and autoimmune diseases, to the infection and destruction of CD4+ helper T lymphocytes, the distinctive feature of HIV infection that leads to the dramatic immunosuppression of AIDS.

Viruses can enter the host across the skin or mucous membranes, by inhalation, or by inoculation from infected blood or tissues. Viremia or replication within specific organs or cell types, or both, can result in almost any combination of cellular dysfunction, inflammatory responses, or damage and destruction. All of these features determine the nature of the subsequent disease a viral infection will cause. Species specificity and both tissue and cell tropism also can differ significantly among isolates of the same virus.

As a general rule, soluble antigens produce good humoral immunity but poor lymphocyte-mediated cytotoxic cellular immunity, whereas antigens synthesized within cells and presented as a complex with the major histocompatibility (MHC) glycoproteins generally induce cytotoxic cellular immunity. Viruses are capable of stimulating both kinds of response. The MHC antigens in humans are called HLA, for human leukocyte antigen, and they comprise several distinct groups of molecules. Class I MHC determinants are transplantation antigens, and include three loci in humans (HLA-A, B, and C) present on the surface of virtually all nucleated cells. Class I molecules act as antigen-presenting sites for molecules from intracellular pathogens and are recognized by CD8+ cytotoxic lymphocytes (CTL). In this way, virus-infected cells are killed by the CTL response, virus replication is interrupted, and the disease process is controlled. This process is accomplished largely by the production of a membrane attack protein similar to the complement C7, 8, 9 complex that punches holes in the infected target cell surface. Some viruses also induce suppressor lymphocyte responses among CD8+ cells, thus down-regulating both virus-specific CMI and antibody mechanisms, and in a nonspecific manner altering the response for unrelated infectious agents as well.

In contrast, class II molecules are more restricted in their distribution to macrophages and T and B lymphocytes, and are used to present extrinsic soluble antigens to the humoral immune system. Thus, soluble antigens encountered by macrophages are internalized, processed, and placed on the surface of the antigen-presenting cell together with the class II molecule. The complex is recognized by T cell receptors on CD4+ helper cells, which in turn interact with B cells capable of antibody responses. Certain viruses such as poliovirus are effectively neutralized by antibody present in secretions or in plasma. Live oral polio vaccine, like natural infection, induces a local immune response in the gut, including neutralizing secretory IgA, which inactivates orally ingested virus before it can invade through the intestinal mucosa and systemically spread to the central nervous system. Killed polio vaccine induces only systemic antibodies that must interact with the virus in the circulation before it reaches target neurons in the spinal cord if the vaccine is to be effective. Both vaccine approaches work.

Some antiviral effects are mediated or conditioned by soluble host products such as interferons (IFN), a family of immunoregulatory proteins with direct or, more likely, indirect antiviral properties. Three related IFN classes include α (leukocyte derived), β (fibroblast derived), and τ or "immune" interferon (produced by antigen or mitogen-activated lymphocytes). These IFN have diverse biologic effects but all regulate the expression of normally repressed cellular genes. Surprisingly, several clinical trials of the antiviral effects of recombinant IFN have shown that α-IFN and not τ-IFN is of greatest efficacy, although the underlying mechanism remains uncertain.

Complement can also contribute to antiviral effects by binding to the agent and preventing attachment to receptors, by opsonizing virus-antibody complexes for phagocytosis and later degradation, or by mediating direct lysis of lipid enveloped viruses. Typical complement-antibody lysis of virus-infected cells is demonstrable in vitro as well. Viruses can also cause immunologically mediated pathology, and a variety of mechanisms are known. With persistent infections such as hepatitis B, measles, or cytomegalovirus, even normal antibody responses can lead to deposition of circulating antigen-antibody complexes in tissues with fenestrated vessels, e.g., the renal glomerulus, resulting in acute glomerulonephritis. Recent data indicate that IgE virus-specific antibodies to parainfluenza or respiratory syncytial virus cause local mast cell degranulation in the lung, leading to the severe respiratory symptoms sometimes associated with these agents, especially in children with hyper-IgE responses. Viruses are also suspected as an inciting cause of autoimmune phenomena, as in postinfection encephalitis after common viral infections such as measles, mumps, and varicella-zoster.

BACTERIA

Bacteria, like viruses, are exceedingly diverse life forms, ranging from strict anaerobes, to facultative anaerobes able to survive in the presence or absence of oxygen, to organisms that require oxygen. Some are able to grow at high temperature (in hot springs) whereas others prefer cool temperatures; most rapidly divide but some are slow growing; certain organisms possess polysaccharide capsules, others have a proteinaceous coat; many are motile and many are not; a few make lethal toxins and some others produce required nutrients for the host.

A major host defense against bacteria resides in the ability of phagocytic cells to ingest the organisms, leading to the activation of bacterial killing mechanisms, including those related to alterations in host cell metabolism of oxygen. Ingestion usually requires the presence of immunoglobulin or complement-derived opsonins, particularly when the infecting microorganism makes antiphagocytic carbohydrate capsules, as is the case with S. pneumoniae or gram-negative organisms such as Klebsiella pneumoniae. Unless the ingested organism is capable of inhibiting the subsequent activation of antibacterial mechanisms within the phagolysosome, as Legionella pneumophila can, neutrophil ingestion of a microorganism triggers the release of bactericidal oxidative and nonoxidative metabolic products. However, the success of this response depends in part on sufficient numbers of host cells able to produce these bactericidal substances (500 neutrophils/mm^3 is a threshold below which infection is highly likely to occur), and the cells must also be able to migrate to the site of infection and respond to external stimuli in appropriate fashion.

Some bacterial pathogens are capable of surviving and multiplying within phagocytic cells, using a variety of strategies. Organisms that survive briefly in the intracellular niche in neutrophils, or chronically within macrophages, may be sensing unique signals in the phagolysosome in which they reside, such as low pH or Ca^{++} concentration, that regulate bacterial genes controlling the ability to resist phagocyte antibacterial mechanisms. How to activate the latent bactericidal mechanisms for such "facultative intracellular" organisms is a frontier question in microbiology. For many of this sort of pathogen, later immunologic engagement of T lymphocytes leads to macrophage activation and the production of interferons and other cytokines that induce acquired microbicidal capability.

Specific immunoglobulins (Ig) serve many functions in the immune response. Those Ig that recognize and bind to bacterial surface structures via their antibody combining site (Fab region) can opsonize and facilitate the attachment of the organism to phagocyte receptors for the other end of the Ig molecule, the Fc portion. Binding of opsonized organisms to Fc receptors also initiates phagocytic uptake. Ig on the bacterial surface can also lead to complement activation and assembly of the terminal complex of C7, 8, 9, directly resulting in bacterial lysis and microbial death. Thus, it is not surprising that bacteria recovered from the blood of septic patients usually are resistant to this complement-mediated lysis. In many instances, complement resistance is not related either to the failure of complement activation or its assembly on the bacterial cell surface, but rather to a more fundamental failure of microbial response to complement deposition.

Antibody directed to specific virulence attributes of a bacterium can interfere with disease pathogenesis. For example, anticolonization factor antibodies may prevent the initial establishment of infections on mucosal surfaces, and such colonization antigens are targets for vaccine development for mucosal pathogens of the oral, respiratory, intestinal, and genitourinary tracts. A variation of the same theme is the strategy to induce antibody to the invasins mediating epithelial cell penetration by invasive bacteria. These antibodies should restrict systemic infection by organisms such as salmonella, including the typhoid bacillus, Listeria monocytogenes, and many others.

When disease results from the action of specific bacterial products, such as toxins, pre-existing antitoxins can prevent symptoms even if the same antibodies arising during infection have no impact on its course. In fact, this strategy was the first success of applied microbiology almost a century ago, when vaccines were developed for tetanus and diphtheria based on inactivated toxin antigens. Much contemporary research on microbial pathogenesis is therefore designed to identify molecular targets for immunization, although few infections have turned out to be as simple to deal with as tetanus or diphtheria. Protective antibody-mediated immunity can be induced by a proper vaccine even when antibody may play no role in recovery from natural infection. For example, an unimmunized patient surviving clinical tetanus remains susceptible to the disease unless immunized with toxoid, because so little antigen is produced during the natural infection that no effective immune response results. Similarly, it is possible to protect against Salmonella typhi by immunizing with the Vi polysaccharide antigen of the organism, where Vi antibodies arising during the course of established typhoid fever have no impact on recovery. Pre-existing anti-Vi is bactericidal during the initial bacteremia of S. typhi infection, and by preventing initial invasion of macrophages by the organism, it prevents the disease. But the same antibody has little impact on the later course of the intramacrophage phase of the infection.

Complement activation is essential for efficient initiation of the inflammatory response and phagocytic cell antimicrobial functions, especially for bacterial infections. Products of complement activation are potent chemotactic factors for neutrophils, they increase vascular permeability and facilitate movement of phagocytic cells from the intravascular to the tissue compartment, and they serve as opsonins or mediate bacteriolysis. However, the complement cascade can be activated by two different pathways, the classical pathway (for which the presence of specific antibody is needed to form a complex with the first, second, and fourth components of complement that can cleave C3 and activate the rest of the cascade) or the alternative pathway (which does not require specific antibody and uses a set of distinctive initial proteins, including factors B and D, to form a C3 cleavage product). Once either system gets going, the biologic results are the same, and because specific antibody is not needed for activation through the alternative pathway, this system is of particular importance early in infection before antibody develops.

FUNGI

Humans are rather resistant to systemic fungal invasion, although mucosal yeast infections are common, and often are severe in patients with defects in CMI such as AIDS. In the presence of severe neutropenia, however, invasive candidiasis becomes prominent. Risk of fungal infection is increased as well in the presence of debilitating illness, especially when patients have tracheal tubes, catheters, and/or multiple indwelling intravenous lines in place, including those for intravenous nutrition support.

PARASITES

Relatively little is known about immune defenses against protozoa and worms. Many of the disease-causing parasites have evolved strategies to fool the host by turning off immune responses. They can masquerade as "self" by expressing host self antigens on their surface, or evade recognition by continuously shedding surface antigens recognized by the host immune system or by rapidly changing their exposed antigens. Some parasites may be able to directly subvert killing mechanisms within phagocytic cells. For example, they may be polyclonal B cell activators, stimulating production of a large array of irrelevant instead of protective antibodies, or they may induce selective immunosuppression. In general, however, defects in CMI responses, but not antibody, complement, or phagocytic cell abnormalities, increase risk of parasitic infection.

EFFECTS OF PROTEIN-ENERGY MALNUTRITION ON HOST DEFENSE MECHANISMS

The development of laboratory methods to study immune responses of relevance to host defense have permitted studies in patients with protein-energy malnutrition (PEM) (see Chap. 57). A broad range of abnormalities have been identified, including both cellular and humoral immune defects, suggesting that an immunodeficiency state may be responsible for the high frequency of severe infections in these patients (see Table 69–2). However, many subjects have been infected at the time of study, making it difficult to determine cause and effect of immunologic deficits (infection can be immunosuppresive), and few studies have been longitudinal, which would permit determination of the temporal impact of the defect on clinical responses.

PEM has been described as a mosaic of nutrient deficits resulting from diverse dietary inadequacies, complicated by infection-induced anorexia and catabolism.[6] It is best understood as a syndrome associated with variable losses of protein, carbohydrate, and fat stores, along with changes in micronutrients such as minerals and vitamins. However, in practice, the physical and biochemical markers of protein and energy depletion are most obvious and most likely to be recorded. The clinical definitions of PEM are broad and cover a range of physiologic abnormalities within limited categories. Because PEM patients are not metabolically homogeneous, it is surely perilous to describe any associated immunologic abnormalities in general terms. Nevertheless, a common finding in these patients is depletion of lymphocytes from the central and peripheral lymphoid tissues, particularly in T cell regions of thymus, spleen, and lymph nodes.[7]

Based on current understanding of normal T lymphocyte development and the role of thymic peptide hormones, the limited assay data indicating reduced circulating thymic factor levels in PEM patients suggests that the T cell defect in PEM may represent maturational arrest related to an abnormal thymic microenvironment.[8] The impact is a relative reduction in circulating mature T lymphocytes so that blood samples obtained for study are enriched in immature and functionally defective cells. The reduction in mature T helper cells and to a lesser and more variable extent of T suppressor cells results in impaired delayed-type skin hypersensitivity responses in vivo and inhibited mitogen and antigen-driven lymphocyte proliferation in vitro. The clinical consequence of this finding is a reduction in the efficacy of host defenses that depend on T cell function, including macrophage microbicidal mechanisms for intracellular pathogens and T cell-mediated cytotoxic responses to viruses.

Antibody production to most protein antigens is T cell dependent and requires signals from primed antigen-specific T lymphocytes. T cells are also involved in switching antibody production from the first response of low-affinity IgM antibody to the second response, high-affinity IgG antibody. Because serum Ig levels usually are normal or elevated in PEM, the ability of malnourished hosts to make Ig is unaffected, and in fact, in developing countries, high serum levels of IgE frequently are detected.[7] This finding probably reflects both the effect of helminths as stimulators of IgE production as well as the loss of T cell suppression of IgE, a normal control mechanism for this immunoglobulin.[9]

In contrast to the simple measurement of Ig levels, the effect of PEM on formation of specific functional antibody in humans has not been studied systematically. Available data are derived principally from observing the response to vaccines. These studies are crude because no titration of antigen dose is possible and limited sampling precludes assessing the kinetics of the response. However, the results suggest that antibody responses to protein antigens often are relatively preserved in PEM, whereas the response to polysaccharide antigens is often subpar. A recent study showed that breast-fed Swedish infants receiving "low" protein cow milk formula (1.6 g/kg per day) produce similar levels of serum, salivary, and fecal antibodies to oral poliovirus vaccine or parenteral diphtheria or tetanus toxoids as infants fed a conventional protein isocaloric formula (2.2 g/kg per day), but that both groups are significantly less responsive than comparable breast-fed infants.[10] The authors conclude that breast milk promotes antibody responses. However, no mechanism is suggested and the relevance of the observation to the malnourished child is uncertain. In most studies investigators have neither looked at very young infants nor compared breast with formula-fed babies under controlled conditions.

Antipolysaccharide antibodies are present mostly in IgG2 and IgG4 subclasses that are either locally produced in the lungs or transported into respiratory secretions.[11] If the difficulty in making antibody to polysaccharide antigens results from a special defect in synthesis of these Ig subclasses in PEM, it could contribute to the frequency and severity of infection by encapsulated bacteria in PEM patients. In addition, when levels and activity of secretory IgA have been evaluated, they typically are depressed in PEM patients. This defect could also be a factor in the frequency of mucosal infections of the gut and urinary tract in these individuals.

The complement system is a typical proteolytic cascade resulting in formation of biologically active products during sequential activation of complement components; when the cascade is activated, complement proteins are consumed. To sustain the response, enhanced production is required, and the normal host does indeed increase complement synthesis as a part of the acute-phase response to inflammatory stimuli. In PEM patients, however, active complement levels are depressed, often in the presence of breakdown products of activation, suggesting consumption and inadequate replacement.[12] The deficit is more profound for the less efficient alternative pathway, suggesting that early responses to infection are particularly impaired. This deficiency may be a significant factor predisposing to gram-negative sepsis, a well-described complication during the course of PEM. It is not clear whether the complement deficit is secondary to consumption induced by infection and/or impaired acute-phase response (thus increasing the severity of the process) or whether it preceeds and thus predisposes to infection, or possibly both.

When phagocytic cells from PEM patients are studied in vitro, impaired chemotaxis and reduced oxidative metabolic response are often found, whereas the initial and subsequent events in phagocytosis, including microbial ingestion, fusion of the phagocytic vesicles with lysosomes, and degranulation, are preserved. In the presence of normal opsonins, the intracellular killing of organisms by neutrophils from PEM patients in vitro remains intact or only mildly impaired. However, because these patients have reduced complement and they may not make high-affinity antibody, serum opsonic activity should be depressed in vivo. This finding has been reported,[12,13] and therefore, phagocytic host-defense mechanisms are likely to be more impaired in vivo than they appear to be in vitro.

The summation of these data indicates that PEM patients have the potential for problems in CMI and phagocytosis, as well as in antibody and complement-mediated defenses. As such, PEM patients should exhibit increased frequency and/or severity of certain bacterial, viral, fungal, and parasitic infections, which is generally consistent with clinical observations.

IRON

Phlebotomy was once a traditional remedy used for a diverse range of maladies, including some infectious diseases.[14] It has been suggested that the apparent benefits of phlebotomy may have been related to the removal of enough iron from the host to create a state of iron deficiency.[15] In its more modern form, exchange transfusion, blood letting does provide a significant beneficial effect in a few specific infections, such as severe falciparum malaria or babesiosis, presumably because the procedure results in rapid and major reduction in the number of circulating parasitized erythrocytes. Whether or not actual removal of iron from the host is beneficial to the response to these or other infectious agents remains controversial. The controversy has even spread to public health decision making. Concerns have been raised about implementing iron supplementation programs to combat nutritional anemia in areas with a high burden of infection.[16] The suggestion that low iron levels are helpful is based on limited in vivo observations; these include the well-described reduction in circulating iron levels during acute infection and inflammation because of iron uptake into tissue stores, and the susceptibility of patients with iron overload to certain infections. In addition, in vitro data show that removing iron from media reduces microorganism growth.[17] Protective responses based on nutrient alterations in the host have been termed "nutritional immunity."[18] In the case of iron, the benefits should theoretically be reversed by the administration of iron, and clinical data have been advanced to support this thesis.[19]

However, the basic concept has come into question as other studies have demonstrated just the opposite, i.e., impaired in vitro immune function and increased infection morbidity in vivo in iron deficiency states.[20] These data have fueled the controversy over the impact of iron on susceptibility to infection. This section considers two opposing questions: does iron deficiency impair immune responses, increase susceptibility to infection, and consequently should be corrected by iron administration, and conversely, does iron deficiency impede infection by withholding a required nutrient from pathogens, so that iron replacement favors microbial virulence.[21]

PHYSIOLOGY IN VIVO

Iron is a highly reactive transition metal that readily catalyzes oxidative/peroxidative processes and interacts with oxygen to form unstable reactive intermediates able to damage cell membranes or degrade DNA. To prevent such destructive events and still safely deliver oxygen in mammals, virtually all iron is maintained tightly bound to metalloproteins and enzymes involved in oxygen transport and use, energy metabolism, and DNA synthesis; the bound metal is required for their activity. Excess free iron is precluded by the normal excess high-affinity iron-binding capacity present in transferrin, lactoferrin, and ferritin. The best characterization of normal iron balance in all mammalian hosts, including humans, is that they represent a highly iron-restricted environment.

Because mammalian pathogens encounter a "low-iron" compartment in the host, they must compete for this tightly bound iron in order to survive and grow. They accomplish this goal primarily by making iron chelator proteins (siderophores) with extremely high affinity for iron, which are able to strip bound iron from host proteins and have receptors to bind the metal chelate and transport proteins to bring it into the cell.[22] A few microorganisms are even known to synthesize receptors for transferrin that resemble the natural receptors of the host, enabling them to acquire iron directly from transferrin.[23]

In conditions of iron sufficiency in the environment, microbes do not need to make these siderophores, microbial outer membrane protein (OMP) siderophore receptors, or transport proteins. However, human pathogens have evolved mechanisms to turn on the synthesis of these same iron-regulated OMP (or IROMP) under conditions of limited iron. IROMP are made by bacteria growing in vivo in mammalian hosts, just as occurs in vitro in experimental conditions of iron deprivation.[24] Pathogens should therefore be seen as constitutively adapted to respond to low iron levels. This ability to use low iron concentration as a critical signal to transcriptionally regulate the proteins pathogens need to obtain iron when supply is limited certainly raises the question of whether the additional iron restriction imposed by clinical iron deficiency states or the hypoferremia of infection (nutritional immunity) can have an impact on microbial growth in vivo.

REGULATION OF MICROBIAL GENES

Many successful pathogens regulate production of virulence factors so that these are made only when needed in the host, and they have evolved mechanisms to monitor environmental signals such as temperature, cyclic nucleotides, or divalent cations such as calcium or iron[25] to determine their presence in a potential host. Only when detection of the signal triggers gene transcription are the needed virulence proteins made. One of the best known of these environmental regulators is an iron-responsive gene called *fur*, (ferric uptake regulator).[26] In an iron-dependent manner, fur exerts control over other genes, many of which are involved in disease causation.[25] Thus, low iron states are used by disease-causing microorganisms to increase pathogenic potential, overcoming the putative protection of the host attributable to iron deficiency predicted by the nutritional immunity hypothesis.

IRON, IRON-BINDING PROTEINS, AND THE IMMUNE SYSTEM

Because transferrin-iron is continuously required for all DNA synthesis,[27] lymphocytes undergoing clonal expansion in immune responses must take up iron to synthesize ribonucleotide reductase, the rate-limiting iron-metalloenzyme for DNA synthesis. For this reason, receptors for transferrin receptors appear on lymphocytes responding to interleukin 2 (IL-2) during the period of activation. Therefore, at some point during the development of iron deficiency states, cellular proliferation may be impaired.

Immune responses in iron-deficient humans have been studied primarily by testing skin test reactivity to recall antigens in vivo or by assessing in vitro incorporation of ^{3}H-thymidine by mitogen-stimulated cells. Reported results are somewhat variable, although a common theme is reduced skin test reactivity in iron-deficient hosts, with enhanced reactivity after iron therapy.[28–30] In vitro proliferation data are even more variable, more often than not showing decreased mitogen responses.[31–34] It is at least possible that enough iron can be present in the media to sometimes correct defects in cells obtained from iron-deficient subjects. Thus, iron deficiency most likely impedes rapid proliferation during lymphocyte activation, and in this way may adversely affect the course of an infection.

A more constant finding in iron deficiency is diminished activity of the neutrophil iron metalloenzyme, myeloperoxidase.[35–37] This enzyme generates reactive bactericidal halide radicals during the oxidative burst of phagocytosis. However, this defect alone is not likely to be of clinical significance, because congenital absence of myeloperoxidase does not increase the risk of infection. However, iron is also required to produce oxygen radicals used in phagocyte bactericidal reactions.[38] Therefore, the effects of iron deficiency on neutrophil function may be more pervasive than just a reduction in myeloperoxidase activity. As evidence of this possibility, the reduction of nitroblue tetrazolium by peroxide released from activated neutrophils is abnormal in iron-deficient subjects.[39,40] This deficit predicts abnormal bactericidal activity, and a modest diminution in bacterial killing capacity has been shown by some investigators,[41–43] although contradictory data also exist.[44,45] Other neutrophil functions, such as chemotaxis, phagocytosis, and degranulation are consistently reported to be normal in iron deficiency, as might be expected if the effects of iron deficiency on neutrophils are specific and related to the biologic functions of the metal.

The amount of human data on iron deficiency and macrophage function is small. Animal studies have shown reduced clearance of polyvinyl pyrrolidone and impaired generation of oxygen radicals in iron-deficient mice,[46,47] and diminished IL-1 responses in iron-deficient rat leukocytes.[48] If these findings mean that iron deficiency can adversely affect macrophage presentation of antigens, then one consequence may be a negative effect on antibody production. Limited data in animals support this possibility.[49]

EFFECTS OF EXCESS IRON

The evidence for nutritional immunity includes the finding of enhanced microbial growth in vitro or increased infections in vivo in conditions of iron excess.[50,51] Impaired growth of bacteria in the presence of iron-binding proteins in vitro is reversed when excess iron is added back. Hemochromatosis serum supports the growth of Vibrio vulnificus, which fails to survive in normal human serum. It also has been suggested that clinical iron overload states (such as β-thalassemia, sickle cell anemia with multiple transfusions, idiopathic hemochromatosis, or so-called Bantu hemosiderosis resulting from grossly excessive oral iron loads) are associated with increased infection morbidity.[52] In these patients, transferrin is fully iron saturated, and iron is readily available to pathogens from circulating low molecular weight loose complexes of iron and albumin.[53] However, more careful analysis puts these clinical findings into question, as it is difficult to separate the effects of excess iron itself from the associated hepatic or splenic dysfunction or effects of secondary diabetes.

Review of infection deaths in thalassemia patients shows that nearly all events occur in splenectomized patients, long before significant transfusion siderosis could develop. When experimental iron overload states in animals are examined, susceptibility is increased, but only to certain organisms that do not produce their own siderophores and depend instead on available environmental iron sources.[54,55] This finding is consistent with the clinical association of human iron excess with severe yersinia infections in both chronic iron overload patients[56–60] and in patients after acute oral ingestion of iron.[61,62] Many yersinia strains are of low virulence and growth restricted in the normal host,[63] except when transport proteins are iron saturated and free iron becomes available. These strains can also obtain iron from iron-desferoxamine chelates, and an association between desferoxamine therapy and yersinia sepsis has been reported.[64,65] Organisms with analogous mechanisms of iron acquisition, including Vibrio vulnificus,[66] and possibly listeria,[67] mucor, rhizopus, and cunninghamella species,[68–70] seem to be associated with iron excess states.

Immune function is probably impaired as well because of tissue-damaging oxidative and peroxidative reactions associated with iron excess. This decreased function would explain why neutrophils, which use iron-catalyzed reactions to produce bactericidal oxygen radicals, are less able to kill microorganisms when obtained from patients with iron excess. Thus, superoxide and hydrogen peroxide production and NBT dye reduction are reduced in cells from β-thalassemia or dialysis patients with transfusion siderosis.[71–75] Chemotactic responses and random migration are also said to be reduced in thalassemic cells,[76] and peripheral blood monocytes from subjects with β-thalassemia show diminished capacity to kill Candida pseudotropicalis[77] or S. aureus.[78,79]

CLINICAL DATA IN EXCESS STATES

Malaria is an interesting example to consider, because the parasite spends most of its lifetime within red blood cells, in close association with an enormous pool of iron in the form of hemoglobin, and because the infection is so often associated with anemia. Several investigators report an increase in malaria parasitemia in individuals given parenteral or oral iron,[80–82] however, these studies have been criticized because of the lack of simultaneous placebo controls, failure to control for the presence of PEM and associated reduced transferrin levels, and lack of proper blinding of investigators. An association of parenteral iron with increased rates of smear-positive malaria has been confirmed in a carefully designed, properly conducted double-blind study in Papua, New Guinea;[83] a 64% increase in parasitemia rate in infants given iron supplements was observed, although the parasite density was no different from that in the control group. A significant increase in malaria-related hospital admissions, measles-associated admissions, and otitis media and pneumonia was found in the iron group as well.[84]

Another careful study of total dose iron-dextran infusion in pregnant women in Papua, New Guinea also found increased risk of malaria parasitemia in treated compared to untreated women.[85] Because the parasites use the globin portion of hemoglobin for nutrition, relative depletion of hemoglobin in red cells from iron-deficient subjects may be a key limiting factor for parasite growth, whether or not heme iron is used by the parasite to meet its iron requirements.[86] When iron is given to deficient subjects, synthesis of hemoglobin and uptake of iron is stimulated, providing both protein and iron for parasite development, because it too requires iron for essential metalloenzymes.[87,88]

Hemolysis is a known risk factor for bacterial infection, particularly salmonellosis, regardless of the cause,[89–91] presumably because of macrophage defects in phagocytosis and/or killing of salmonella secondary to the uptake of iron-hemoglobin by macrophages rather than increased circulating iron for the pathogen. Consistent with this concept, hemolysis induced by the mouse malaria parasite Plasmodium berghei or phenylhydrazine administration dramatically increased the virulence of Salmonella typhimurium, whereas simple iron deficiency induced by bleeding did not.[92]

CLINICAL DATA IN DEFICIENCY STATES

These examples indicate clearly that the relationship between iron and infection depends in part on the causative organism, the metabolism of the pathogen, and its ability and mechanisms used to acquire the iron it needs. Although iron deficiency has an adverse impact on certain host defenses, and most pathogens appear to be well equipped to compete for available iron stores, clinical examples do exist of iron deficiency apparently protecting the host.[82,93–97] However, some negative results have been reported,[98,99] with no difference being found in iron-supplemented or unsupplemented groups, whereas other investigators have found increased prevalence and severity of infections in treated subjects.[100] Unfortunately, interpretation is difficult because published studies on iron deficiency and susceptibility to infection often are flawed in design, sometimes lack sufficient numbers of subjects to permit statistical analysis, or fail to control for the numerous confounders liable to be encountered in a field study. Thus, differences in the age of subjects, route and form of the iron administered, failure to include simultaneous controls or to demonstrate the comparability of the control group except for iron status, the presence of other nutritional deficiencies such as PEM, the lack of laboratory confirmation of infection, use of imprecise criteria to characterize iron nutrition state of the host, and a lack of correlation of infectious episodes with the severity of the nutrient deficiency or the effect of the supplement, all complicate the final interpretation.[101,102]

Although conclusive proof is lacking, the impression from these various reports is that iron deficiency is likely associated with some increased incidence of common infections in children. Also, iron supplementation by the parenteral route in very young infants, or use of iron chelators in disease states with iron excess, probably increases the incidence of some specific infections. There is, however, no justifiable rationale for the use of parenteral iron in very young infants. Newborns normally have an excess of iron and highly saturated serum iron-binding proteins, they are immunologically immature and susceptible to invasive bacterial infections under any circumstances, and they are the group most likely to experience an adverse effect of the therapy. In addition, because severe PEM is known to result in reduced transferrin levels, it is unwise to administer iron in any form while the iron-binding capacity is low. An association between low transferrin and severe systemic infection in PEM has been inferred,[103] although such patients have multiple defects in all limbs of host defense. For these reasons, nutritional rehabilitation of PEM patients usually does not include iron supplements during the first week. This supplementation commonly is delayed until the second week of treatment, when new protein synthesis is actively occurring and the circulating levels of export proteins, such as transferrin, are increasing.[104]

ZINC

Like iron, alterations in the distribution of zinc is part of the acute-phase response in infections, with the ion being rapidly removed from circulation to an intracellular locus primarily in liver, thymus, and bone marrow. This effect is related to increased synthesis of the intracellular zinc-binding protein, metallothionein,[105] which is transcriptionally regulated by a central player in inflammation, IL-1.[106]

Zinc plays a critical role in the function of some enzymes involved in DNA transcription and RNA translation (see Chapter 10).[107,108] Thus, the shift of zinc to the intracellular compartment of lymphocytes may prime the proliferation of lymphoid cells involved in immune responses and host defense. A potential unfortunate corollary is that zinc deficiency can restrict rapid multiplication and clonal expansion of critical cell populations.

Zinc-binding finger loop domains, known as "zinc fingers," are also involved in conformational stabilization of transcription factor proteins, permitting sequence-specific DNA recognition and gene expression.[109] Zinc deficiency of a magnitude sufficient to impede these regulatory signals further impairs the host response by limiting the translation of proteins encoded by genes turned on during the acute-phase response to infection.

Finally, certain thymus-derived peptides, postulated to function as thymic hormones in the differentiation of T cells, are zinc metalloproteins.[110,111] These proteins may be the normal regulators of T cell maturation, and the T cell maturational arrest in PEM, which is almost always accompanied by zinc deficiency, as well as the depletion of mature T cells observed in other zinc depletion or deficiency situations, may be traceable to this defect. Zinc deficiency is also often manifested by lesions of skin and mucous membrane, which break their mechanical barrier functions, providing a route for both high and low virulence microorganisms to invade and initiate infection.[112] Thus, in a number of ways, abnormal zinc nutrition can be related to heightened infection susceptibility and/or severity.

EFFECTS ON IMMUNE FUNCTION (SEE ALSO CHAP. 41)

It has been noted that IL-1 induces metallothionein and shifts zinc from plasma to tissues. At the same time, production and/or membrane binding of certain cytokines that regulate the immune system may depend on zinc, including IL-1, IL-2, and IFN.[113–115] However, careful systematic studies of zinc status, cytokines, and immune function have not yet been reported. What seems clear is that zinc deprivation in animals has an effect on the thymus, which undergoes involution, associated with splenic atrophy and lymphopenia.[116–118] In the early stages of deficiency, a preferential loss of cells occurs from the cortical regions normally populated by glucocorticoid-sensitive immature thymocytes. This change is actually independent of any glucocorticoid effect, because it occurs even when the adrenal glands are removed.[119] Similar thymic involution occurs in a breed of cattle with a genetic defect that impairs zinc absorption and results in severe zinc deficiency.[120]

Despite an unresolved controversy over whether zinc deficiency affects particular T cell subpopulations,[121] little doubt remains that the proliferative response to both T-dependent and T-independent mitogens is reduced.[122,123] This may happen in several ways, such as indirectly by altered cytokine metabolism[124] or directly by effecting lymphocyte DNA replication. As a consequence of impaired T cell function, delayed-type hypersensitivity responses are diminished in zinc deficiency,[125] although if this is related to lymphocyte abnormalities alone or to additional changes in macrophage function that are demonstrable in zinc-deficient cells is not clear.[126]

Consistent with these diverse abnormalities in the immune system, increased susceptibility to infection has been reported in animals experimentally infected with a wide variety of pathogens, including bacteria (Francisella tularensis), protozoa (Trypanosoma cruzi), and fungi (Candida albicans).[127] Consistent with these observations, Fresian cattle with the equivalent of human acrodermatitis enteropathica are also hypersusceptible to infection, which often is fatal.[128]

IMMUNITY AND SUSCEPTIBILITY TO INFECTION IN HUMANS

The data in humans concerning zinc and infection are limited. Several situations associating zinc deficiency, immune defects, and hypersusceptibility to infection have been reported. In one of the earliest reports in humans, zinc deficiency associated with geophagia in Iranian children was found to result in growth retardation, hypogonadism, and frequent infections.[129] Subsequently, recognition of zinc deficiency in a series of clinical situations associated with immunologic deficits and infections, namely, acrodermatitis enteropathica, in patients receiving total parenteral nutrition without added zinc, in malabsorption states, in Down's syndrome, and in sickle cell disease, and correction by zinc administration, has supported the notion that increased infections are associated with the lack of this mineral.[129]

The development of a diet-induced zinc deficiency model in humans has helped to establish this relationship.[130] Dietary restriction of zinc results in negative zinc balance of around 1 mg per day, with a cumulative loss approaching 180 to 200 mg over a 6-month period. Because most zinc is present in bone and muscle, only 200 to 400 mg are in a mobile exchangeable pool in the liver and the circulation. Because zinc is not stored in quantity, the diet rapidly leads to a deficiency mostly affecting tissues with high turnover rates such as liver and leukocytes. In some instances, abnormalities in zinc deficiency can be reversed by providing this ion. For example, the reduced serum thymulin activity in zinc-deficient subjects was related to circulation of inactive thymulin protein, and the addition of zinc restored biologic activity.[131] Similarly, the increase in immature T cells and the decrease in the T4 to T8 ratio, IL-2 production,[131] and natural killer cell (NK) activity[132] are also reversed by correcting the zinc deficiency, as are the abnormalities in patients with acrodermatitis enteropathica.

These findings are consistent with the observations in humans with genetic diseases associated with zinc deficiency, in whom thymic atrophy, lymphopenia, diminished NK activity and IL-2 production, decreased serum thymulin levels, and alterations in lymphocyte subpopulations are reported.[131,133–135] Alterations in the zinc-dependent enzyme, nucleoside phosphorylase, may result in accumulation of toxic levels of nucleotides leading to impaired cell division or to cell death.[136] In addition to these deficits, zinc-reversible chemotaxis and motility abnormalities of granulocytes from zinc-deficient uremic patients have been described.[137] Data attributing immunologic defects in PEM to zinc deficiency are thin at present, but the concept is plausible. These data include enlarging thymic shadows on radiographs in PEM children after zinc therapy or increased skin delayed-type hypersensitivity reactions when topical zinc is applied directly to the test site.[138,139] It is unclear whether correcting a zinc deficit without altering protein or energy will lead to any improvement in immunologic function, or especially an improvement in the excess susceptibility of these patients to infectious diseases. Considerable work remains to be done.

VITAMIN A

A high degree of interest has focused on the relationship of mild vitamin A deficiency and high morbidity and mortality owing to infectious diseases and the potential benefit that improved vitamin A nutriture might provide. This interest is based primarily on the results of a limited number of field trials in children with evidence of mild vitamin A deficiency in developing countries in which reduced morbidity and mortality have been observed. There is a theoretic as well as an experimental basis (see Chap. 16) to postulate that vitamin A might influence host susceptibility to infection by alterations in both nonspecific and specific defense mechanisms. First, vitamin A deficiency is known to be associated with metaplasia of mucosal epithelium and the replacement of ciliated cells with keratinized cells, reducing the efficacy of the ciliary ladder in clearance of bacteria on mucosal surfaces as a result. This increase in keratinized cells occurs, at least in part, because of the negative transcriptional regulation of keratin synthesis by retinoids. Second, because of the known sugar acceptor and donor capacity of retinyl phosphate in glycoprotein biosynthesis, vitamin A deficiency alters the production of mucous glycoconjugates. Thus, in vitamin A deficiency states, mucus-secreting cells are either reduced in number or replaced by multilayered keratinized cells. This change is likely to be associated with a loss of the nonspecific barrier function of mucus, as its ability to bind to microorganisms through specific carbohydrate recognition events can modify microbial adherence to epithelial cells and subsequent colonization or systemic invasion. In addition, because cell surface glycoconjugates often serve as receptors for pathogens or their virulence products, or in the activation of host immune cells, vitamin A deficiency may alter surface-expressed host cell glycoconjugates, with additional and unforseen effects on the host-pathogen interaction.

Therefore, the lack of vitamin A presumably impairs the mucosal barrier function for infectious agents. In fact, animals maintained on low vitamin A diets are more susceptible to infection than those fed adequate diets.[140,141] As a result, vitamin A came to be known as the "anti-infective vitamin" soon after its discovery.[142]

Third, abnormal immunologic functions develop in experimental vitamin A deficiency in animals, including reduced mitogen-induced lymphocyte proliferation, cytotoxic lymphocyte responses, delayed-type skin hypersensitivity reactions, and impaired antibody production.[143–145] However, when the possibility was tested in humans in a large field study in Bangladesh, no effect was noted when vitamin A was given together with tetanus toxoid on the vaccine response in children, although perhaps testing the booster response as in this study is not as important as assessing the impact of vitamin A on primary immunization.[146] In addition, the levels of lysozyme, a bactericidal enzyme present in mucosal secretions that hydrolyzes the peptidoglycan layer of certain gram-positive bacteria, is reduced in vitamin A deficiency.[147]

It is difficult to draw conclusions on the effect of vitamin A deficiency on human host defenses because of the paucity of available information. It also appears that low circulating concentrations of retinol and retinol-binding protein (RBP) are a part of the acute-phase response to infection and inflammation, similar to the hypoferremia that rapidly develops at the onset of infection,[148,149] and therefore biochemical evidence of vitamin A deficiency may be unusually difficult to interpret during the course of infections. One suggestion is that vitamin A functions as an antioxidant, which is essential for maintaining tissue integrity, particularly in protection from reactive oxygen species generated in the host response to infection and inflammation.[150] Hence, reduction of circulating retinoids and their distribution into extravascular fluids and tissues may be an adaptive host response to minimize oxidative damage during inflammation. The concept that reduced circulating vitamin A is part of the programmed host response to infection will certainly stimulate debate on the possible protective effects of this response and on the possible harmful effects of interventions to replete the host with exogenous retinoids. Thurnham suggests that both possibilities may be true, with protective effects seen in hosts with normal vitamin A nutriture,[148] but when initial levels of vitamin A are low, the acute-phase response is more likely to impair recovery and increase mortality.

DEFICIENCY AND INFECTION MORTALITY

The suggestion that administration of vitamin A by itself can reduce morbidity and mortality has come from an initial set of field studies in Indonesia by one group of workers. The proposition is attractive, a magic bullet to target the malnutrition/infection complex in developing countries. In these studies, mild vitamin A deficiency was detected by eye signs such as night blindness or the presence of Bitot's spots. Children with these findings experienced an unexpected increase in mortality and morbidity from respiratory and diarrheal disease.[151,152] Almost 5000 children were evaluated every 3 months for 18 months. Children with severe xerophthalmia were treated immediately, and the remaining children were followed. The prevalence of mild xerophthalmia increased during the first 3 years of life to a plateau of 7%, and was associated with a fourfold increase in risk of death. Survivors with mild eye signs had a relative risk of 2 and 2.8 for respiratory and diarrheal diseases, respectively, compared to those without eye signs. One problem in these and other field studies attempting to evaluate the clinical role of vitamin A as a determinant of susceptibility or response to infection is the current difficulty in assessing vitamin A nutriture.[153] Although new methods such as the relative dose response test or conjunctival impression cytology promise better sensitivity, specificity, and simplicity, these techniques have yet to be applied.

On the basis of these data, several interventional trials were implemented (Table 69–3). The first trial, conducted by the same group of workers in Indonesia, revealed a 34% reduction in mortality among children in the treatment group, assigned to receive 200,000 IU of vitamin A every 6 months.[154] When the analysis was carried out on those children documented to have received their doses, the results were even more impressive, with a 75% reduction in mortality in the vitamin A recipients. However, a number of methodologic issues have been raised and the results questioned because the study design did not permit randomization of treatment in individuals, baseline mortality data in the control and experimental villages were lacking, and potentially important differences were observed in the baseline nutritional status between control and experimental villages. In another trial in Indonesia, constant vitamin A supplementation through use of vitamin A-fortified monosodium glutamate (MSG) led to a nearly twofold decrease in risk of death among children.[155]

Four subsequent intervention trials have been published. In one, a small dose of vitamin A (8333 IU = 2.5 mg all trans retinol = 0.72 mmol) plus vitamin E or vitamin E alone was given weekly by community health workers to more than 7500 South Indian children in each group.[156] The dose was placed directly in each child's mouth, and nearly 90% were seen at each weekly contact. During 1 year of observation, there was a striking 54% reduction in non-accident-related deaths in those individuals receiving vitamin A in addition to vitamin E, most prominently in the under 3-year-old children. In a second study in Nepal, a randomized, double-masked, placebo-controlled community trial, 60,000 retinol equivalents (= 17.2 mmol all trans retinol) or identical placebo capsules were given every 4 months to children from 6 to 72 months of age.[157] After 1 year, a 30% reduction in mortality among the treated children was detected, independent of overall nutritional status assessed by arm circumference. By standardized retrospective and objective assignment of cause of death derived from verbal information from parents (verbal autopsies), the effect of vitamin A was associated with diarrhea or dysentery, wasting malnutrition, and measles. The positive results led to interruption of the trial midway through the planned 2-year investigation.

In the third study (in South India), villages with almost 16,000 children were assigned to receive either 200,000 IU (= 17.3 mmol) of vitamin A or placebo.[158] Morbidity and mortality were recorded every 3 months by trained field workers and clinical examinations were carried out at 6-month intervals by physicians, all of whom were blinded as to the treatment given in each village. As in the Indonesian trial, corneal lesions were treated immediately, but children with less severe eye signs were followed. No significant difference was noted in mortality comparing children receiving one, two, or three doses of vitamin A with similarly treated placebo controls. The authors' interpretation is that confounding factors associated with vitamin A deficiency, including PEM and infections, independently contribute to mortality. The explanation for the differences observed in this study are not apparent, although it may relate to an impact of the study itself, because seriously ill children were referred for care and may, as a result, have survived. The frequent contacts between field workers and villagers in control villages would certainly lead to the transmittal of health advice that may be heeded, as reflected by the higher mortality rate among children who did not participate in the trial compared to those who did. It may also be explained by basic differences in

TABLE 69–3. MORTALITY IN FIELD TRIALS OF VITAMIN A SUPPLEMENTATION*

AUTHOR	VITAMIN A DOSE	COUNTRY (AGE RANGE)	OBSERVATION PERIOD	CHANGE IN MORTALITY
Sommer et al.[154]	200,000 IU 6 monthly × 2	Indonesia (0–5 years)	1 year	−34%
Ramathullah et al.[156]	8,333 IU weekly	India (6–60 months)	1 year	−54%
West et al.[157]	60,000 RE 4 monthly × 3	Nepal (6–72 months)	1 year	−30%
Vijayaraghavan et al.[158]	200,000 IU 6 monthly × 2	India (1–5 years)	1 year	Nil
Daulaire et al.[159]	50–200,000 IU by age, once	Nepal (1–59 months)	6 months	−26%

*1 μg cell-*trans* retinol = 1 retinol equivalent (RE) = 3.3. IU_a = 3.49 nmol of all-*trans* retinol.

health-related behavior between those who elect to join a clinical trial compared to those who opt not to join.

The possible role of Hawthorne effects has been addressed in another field trial of vitamin A supplementation in a population of children 5 years old and younger with evidence of severe vitamin A deficiency in the highlands of western Nepal.[159] Surveys in the study area revealed high prevalence of eye signs of vitamin A deficiency, with 13% of children in the under 5-year-old group showing signs of active xerophthalmia, including a high rate of 1.5% among infants. In this study, a single dose of vitamin A was administered to 88% of 8786 children under 5 years of age (50,000 to 200,000 IU, = 4.33 to 17.3 mmol, increasing according to age) in 8 districts who were enrolled in a pneumonia therapeutic interventional study involving 2 weekly home surveillance visits. Except for the visit to give the dose, no other changes in the provision of health care or home visits were instituted. The control group consisted of 3411 children of similar age and health characteristics in 8 adjacent districts. Mortality and disease-specific mortality rates (based on verbal postmortem reports) were ascertained over the subsequent 5 months by 2 weekly visits in all 16 districts. A 26% reduction in overall mortality was noted in the supplemented children. No beneficial effect was present in the 0 to 5-month-old infants, but in those 6 to 11 months of age, the reduction in mortality was 49%. This change was accounted for by a reduction in diarrheal disease mortality, decreasing from 97.5/1000 child years at risk to 63.5/1000 child years at risk (RR = 0.65; 95% CL = 0.44 to 0.95). No convincing reduction was observed in mortality attributed to pneumonia, measles, or "other" causes.

An important aspect of this study was an evaluation of the cost and feasibility of implementing vitamin A supplementation. The extra cost for supplementation, including supplies, personnel, and management time, was estimated to be less than $0.20 per dose, leading to a total marginal cost of approximately $11.00 per death averted, a highly cost-effective measure. The authors acknowledge that this highly favorable benefit ratio is largely attributable to the high underlying under age 5 years mortality, the prevalence of severe clinical vitamin A deficiency eye signs, and the presence of a logistical delivery system to which the vitamin A supplementation could be engrafted. The cost-benefit is likely to be less favorable when these factors do not exist.

DEFICIENCY AND INFECTION MORBIDITY

Since the initial Indonesian studies, other groups have examined the relationship between vitamin A status and morbidity. An increase in respiratory but not diarrheal disease morbidity was reported in Indian patients with mild vitamin A deficiency,[160] whereas diarrheal but not respiratory disease rates were increased in Thai children with xerophthalmia.[161] Interestingly, the number of deaths was too small in either study to be able to analyze the association of vitamin A deficiency with mortality. The effects of vitamin A on morbidity have since been analyzed in two of the four vitamin A intervention trials discussed previously; results showed a decrease in respiratory and diarrhea-related morbidity in one[154] and no difference in either respiratory or diarrheal disease rates in the other.[162]

DEFICIENCY AND MEASLES MORTALITY AND MORBIDITY

In some of these studies, investigators also attempted to examine the effect of vitamin A on the specific mortality associated with measles; other trials of vitamin A interventions for measles have been reported. Two reports from Africa demonstrate that administration of a large bolus of vitamin A to measles patients on admission significantly reduces the associated in-hospital mortality. In one study from Tanzania,[163] 12 of 96 controls compared to 6 of 88 treated children died; the difference was significant when the group under 2 years of age was analyzed separately. In another report from South Africa,[164] serum retinol levels, assessed before the administration of vitamin A, were low in over 90% of both treatment and control groups. Patients with measles seen within 5 days of the onset of the rash and with pneumonia, diarrhea, or croup were randomly assigned to receive an oral dose of 400,000 IU (34.6 mmol) of retinyl palmitate or placebo. Baseline data were similar in the two groups except for a slightly lower serum albumin value in the vitamin A recipients. Twelve (6.3%) children died, nearly all from associated pneumonia. The majority of deaths (10 of 12) were in the control group, and vitamin A administration was associated with a significantly reduced risk of death (RR = 0.21). In addition, the recovery from pneumonia as well as from diarrhea was significantly more rapid in the treated patients.

These results are supported by data from another center in South Africa.[165] Sixty children 2 years old and younger with measles rash documented for 5 or fewer days and no history of vitamin A administration in the past month were randomly assigned to receive 54.5 to 109 mg of retinyl palmitate drops or placebo syrup by mouth when admitted to the center. The baseline data, including the high (more than 90%) prevalence of reduced serum vitamin A levels, were comparable in the two groups. Subjects were seen in follow-up at 6 weeks, when another dose of vitamin A or placebo was given, and again 6 months after discharge. A total integrated morbidity score was calculated for each visit, based on cumulative episodes and severity of diarrhea, upper respiratory infections, laryngotracheobronchitis, and pneumonia. Initial in-hospital recovery from pneumonia, diarrhea, and fever was more rapid in the treated group, and the morbidity score was 82% lower than in the controls. Eighty percent of subjects were seen at the 6-week follow-up, and the morbidity score was 61% lower in the vitamin A group. The follow-up at 6 months was only 60%, but again the morbidity score was significantly lower (85%) in the vitamin A group.

When assigned cause of death was evaluated in interventional community trials in India and Nepal, measles mortality was significantly reduced in one study,[157] and a trend in the same direction was noted in a second study.[156]

These studies spawned editorials in the *New England Journal of Medicine* and the *Lancet.* The authors of the article entitled "Vitamin A supplements—too good not to be true," recommended both continued study and immediate implementation of vitamin A interventions wherever vitamin A deficiency is clinically evident in the population, wherever PEM is common, and wherever an excess of measles deaths is detected.[166] Authors of the second editorial, although acknowledging the evidence that vitamin A interventions can have a "striking impact" on child mortality, concluded that it was "unlikely that global approaches for vitamin A are indicated" because the need for vitamin A would likely differ from one country to another.[167] They also recommended that further studies be designed and carried out to provide the needed guidance for those nations, "who may come under pressure from international agencies to launch 'vitamin A capsules for all' programmes."

These statements do not imply the lack of a consensus for reducing the global prevalence of vitamin A deficiency.[166,167] Most public health nutrition experts agree that the best long-term measure to improve vitamin A status in developing countries is to ensure dietary adequacy of vitamin A; it is the suggestion that supplementation or food fortification be used as immediate stop-gap measures that is in question, because of cost and logistics. Current evidence would suggest giving a bolus of vitamin A to all measles patients at risk, especially if the disease is severe enough to warrant admission to the hospital. Methods to fortify MSG or sugar have been developed (see Chap. 91); the debate continues on whether to implement these measures in developing countries. The cost, feasibility, and sustainability of periodic vitamin A distribution schemes remain as questions limiting commitment to implementation now, and it may be necessary to approach the answer by cost-benefit analysis to determine how to spend the restricted health care budgets of national and international bodies concerned with global health. Such data are not yet available.

REFERENCES

1. Keusch, G.T., Scrimshaw, N.S.: Rev. Infect. Dis., *8:*349–353, 1986.
2. Serwadda, D., Sewankambo, N.K., Carswell, J.W., et al.: Lancet, *2:*849–852, 1985.
3. Keusch, G.T.: Immunologic mechanisms in infectious diseases. *In* Immunologic Disorders in Infants and Children. 3rd Ed. Edited by E.R. Stiehm. Philadelphia, W.B. Saunders, 1989.
4. Gitelson, S.: Isr. J. Med. Sci., *7:*663–667, 1971.
5. Rosen, F.S.: Semin. Hematol., *27:*333–341, 1990.
6. Keusch, G.T.: Semin. Infect. Dis., *2:*265–303, 1979.
7. Keusch, G.T., Wilson, C.S., Waksal, S.D. Nutrition, host defenses, and the lymphoid system. *In* Advances in Host Defense Mechanisms. Edited by J.D. Gallin, A.S. Fauci. New York, Raven Press, 1983.
8. Keusch, G.T.: Malnutrition and the thymus gland. *In* Nutritional Modulation of Immune Response. Edited by S. Cunningham-Rundles. New York, Marcel Dekker, 1992.
9. Purtilo, D.T., Riggs, R.S., Evans, R., et al.: Am. J. Trop. Med. Hyg., *25:*229–232, 1976.
10. Hahn-zoric, M., Fulconis, F. Minoli, I., et al.: Acta Paediatr. Scand., *79:*1137–1142, 1990.
11. Reynolds, H.Y.: Mayo Clin. Proc., *63:*161–174, 1988.
12. Keusch, G.T., Torun, B., Johnston, R.B. Jr, et al.: J. Pediatr., *105:*434–436, 1984.
13. Keusch, G.T., Urrutia, J.J., Guerrero, O., et al.: Bull. WHO, *59:*923–929, 1981.
14. Brain, P.: S. Afr. Med. J., *56:*149–154, 1979.
15. Weinberg, R.J., Weinberg, E.D.: Med. Hypotheses, *21:*441–443, 1986.
16. deMaeyer, E.M.: Preventing and controlling iron deficiency anemia through primary health care. A guide for health administrators and programme managers. Geneva, WHO, 1989.
17. Weinberg, E.D.: Physiol. Rev., *64:*65–102, 1984.
18. Kochan, I.: Curr. Top. Microbiol. Immunol., *60:*1–30, 1973.
19. Murray, A.M., Murray, A.B., Murray, M.B., et al.: Br. Med. J., *2:*1113–1115, 1978.
20. Hershko, C., Peto, T.E.A., Weatherall, D.A.: Br. Med. J., *296:*660–664, 1988.
21. Keusch, G.T.: Ann. N.Y. Acad. Sci., *587:*181–188, 1990.
22. Griffiths, E.: The iron-uptake systems of pathogenic bacteria. *In* Iron and Infection. Edited by J.J. Bullen, E. Griffiths. New York, John Wiley & Sons, 1987.
23. Martinez, J.L., Delgado-Iribarren, A., Baquero, F.: FEMS Microbiol. Lett., *6:*45–56, 1990.
24. Chart, H., Stevenson, P., Griffiths, E.: J. Gen. Microbiol., *134:*1549–1559, 1988.
25. DiRita, V.J., Mekalanos, J.J.: Annu. Rev. Genet., *23:*455–482, 1989.
26. DeLorenzo, V., Wee, S., Herrero, M., et al.: J. Bacteriol., *169:*2624–2630, 1987.
27. Kay, J.E., Benzie, C.R.: Immunol. Lett., *12:*55–58, 1986.
28. Joynson, D.H.M., Jacobs, A., Walker, D.M., et al.: Lancet, *2:*1058–1059, 1972.
29. Macdougall, L.G., Anderson, R., McNab, G.M., et al.: J. Pediatr., *86:*833–843, 1975.
30. Krantman, H.J., Young, S.R., Ank, B.J., et al.: Am. J. Dis. Child., *136:*840–844, 1982.

31. Fletcher, J., Mather, J., Lewis, M.J., et al.: J. Infect. Dis., *131*:44–50, 1975.
32. Sawitsky, B., Kanter, R., Sawitsky, A.: Am. J. Med. Sci., *272*:153–160, 1976.
33. Gupta, K.K., Dhatt, P.S., Singh, H.: Indian J. Pediatr., *49*:507–510, 1982.
34. Grosch-Warner, I., Grosse-Wilde, H., Bender-Gotze, et al.: Klin. Wochenschr., *62*:1091–1093, 1984.
35. Prasad, J.S.: Am. J. Clin. Nutr., *32*:550–552, 1979.
36. Yetgin, S., Altay, C., Ciliv, G., et al.: Acta Haematol. (Basel), *61*:10–14, 1979.
37. Turgeon-O'Brien, H., Amiot, J., Lemieux, L., et al.: Acta Haematol. (Basel), *74*:151–154, 1985.
38. Fridovich, I.: Science, *201*:875–880, 1978.
39. Chandra, R.K.: J. Pediatr., *86*:899–902, 1975.
40. Celada, A., Herreros, V., Pugin, P., et al.: Br. J. Haematol., *43*:457–463, 1979.
41. Chandra, R.K.: Arch. Dis. Child., *48*:864–866, 1973.
42. Moore, L.L., Humbert, J.R.: Pediatr. Res., *18*:684–689, 1984.
43. Walter, T., Arredondo, S. Arevalo, M., et al.: Am. J. Clin. Nutr., *44*:877–882, 1986.
44. Kulapongs, P., Vithayasai, V., Suskind, R., et al.: Lancet, *2*:689–691, 1974.
45. Van Heerden, C., Oosthuizen, R., Van Wyk, H., et al.: S. Afr. Med. J., *24*:111–113, 1981.
46. Kuvibidila, S., Wade, S.: J. Nutr., *117*:170–176, 1987.
47. Thompson, H.L., Brock, J.H.: FEBS Lett., *200*:283–286, 1986.
48. Helyar, L., Sherman, A.R.: Am. J. Clin. Nutr., *46*:346–352, 1987.
49. Kochanowski, B.A., Sherman, A.R.: Am. J. Clin. Nutr., *41*:278–284, 1985.
50. Chart, H., Griffiths, E.: FEMS Microbiol. Lett., *26*:227–231, 1985.
51. Bullen, J.J., Ward, C.G., Wallis, S.N.: Infect. Immun., *10*:443–450, 1978.
52. Barrett-Connor, E.: Medicine, *50*:97–112, 1971.
53. Hershko, C., Peto, T.E.A.: Br. J. Haematol., *66*:149–151, 1987.
54. Robins-Browne, R.M., Pripc, J.K.: Infect. Immun., *47*:774–779, 1985.
55. Fletcher, J., Goldstein, E.: Br. J. Exp. Pathol., *51*:280–285, 1970.
56. Chiu, H., Flynn, D.M., Hoffbrand, A.V., et al.: Br. Med. J., *292*:97, 1986.
57. Marlon, A., Gentry, L., Merigan, T.C.: Arch. Intern. Med., *27*:947–949, 1971.
58. Rabson, A.R., Hallett, A.F., Koornhof, H.J.: J. Infect. Dis., *131*:447–451, 1975.
59. Kelly, D.A., Price, E., Wright, V., et al.: J. Pediatr. Gastroenterol. Nutr., *6*:643–645, 1987.
60. Capron, J.P., Capron-Chivrac, D., Tossou, H., et al.: Gastroenterology, *87*:1372–1375, 1984.
61. Melby, K., Slordahl, S., Guttenberg, T.J., et al.: Br. Med. J., *285*:467–468, 1982.
62. Mofenson, H.C., Caraccio, T.R., Sharieff, N.: N. Engl. J. Med., *316*:1092–1093, 1988.
63. Carniel, E., Mercereau-Puijalon, O., Bonnefoy, S.: Infect. Immun., *57*:1211–1217, 1989.
64. Hadjiminas, J.M.: J. Antimicrob. Chemother., *21*:680–681, 1988.
65. Gallant, T., Freedman, M.H., Vellend, H., et al.: N. Engl., J. Med., *314*:1643, 1986.
66. Wright, A.C., Simpson, L.M., Oliver, J.D.: Infect. Immun., *34*:503–507, 1981.
67. Mossey, R.T., Sondheimer, J.: Am. J. Med., *79*:397–399, 1985.
68. Goodili, J.J., Abuelo, J.G.: N. Engl. J. Med., *317*:54, 1987.
69. Abe, F., Inaba, H., Katoh, T., et al.: Mycopathologia, *110*:87–91, 1990.
70. Daly, A.L., Velazquez, L.A., Bradley, S.F., et al.: Am. J. Med., *87*:468–471, 1989.
71. Martino, M., Rossi, M.E., Resti, M., et al.: Acta Haematol. (Basel), *71*:289–298, 1984.
72. Waterlot, Y., Cantinieaux, B., Hariga-Mulier, C., et al.: Br. Med. J., *291*:501–504, 1985.
73. Flament, J., Goldman, M., Waterlot, Y., et al.: Clin. Nephrol., *25*:227–230, 1986.
74. Tavo, T.A., Minlero, R., Ponsono, A.: J. Pediatr., *90*:666, 1977.
75. Cantinieaux, B., Hariga, C., Ferster, A., et al.: Eur. J. Haematol., *389*:28–34, 1987.
76. Khan, A.J., Lee, C., Wolff, J.A., et al.: Pediatrics, *60*:349–351, 1983.
77. Ballart, I.J., Estevez, M.E., Sen. L., et al.: Blood, *67*:105–109, 1986.
78. Van Asbeck, B.S., Marx, J.J.M., Struyvenberg, A., et al.: J. Immunol., *132*:851–856, 1984.
79. Van Asbeck, B.S., Marx, J.J.M., Struyvenberg, A., et al.: J. Infect., *85*:232–240, 1984.
80. Byles, A.B., D'Sa, A.: Br. Med. J., *3*:625–627, 1970.
81. Masawe, A.E.J., Muindi, J.M., Swai, G.B.R.: Lancet, *2*:314–317, 1974.
82. Murray, M.J., Murray, A.B., Murray, M.B., et al.: Br. Med. J., *2*:113–115, 1978.
83. Oppenheimer, S.J., Gibson, F.D., Macfarlane, S.B., et al.: Trans. R. Soc. Trop. Med. Hyg., *80*:603–612, 1986.
84. Oppenheimer, S.J., Macfarlane, S.B.J., Moody, J.B., et al.: Trans. Soc. Trop. Med. Hyg., *80*:596–602, 1986.
85. Oppenheimer, S.J., Macfarlane, S.B.J., Moody, J.B., et al.: Trans. Soc. Trop. Med. Hyg., *80*:818–822, 1986.
86. Hershko, C., Peto, T.E.A.: J. Exp. Med., *168*:375–387, 1988.
87. Scheibel, L.W., Sherman, I.W. Metabolism and organellar function during various stages of the life cycle: Proteins, lipids, nucleic acids and vitamins. *In* Malaria: Principles and Practice of Malariology. Edited by W. Wernsdorfer and I. McGregor. Edinburgh, Churchill Livingstone, 1988.
88. Scheibel, L.W.: Plasmodial parasite biology: Carbohydrate metabolism and related organellar function during various stages of the life cycle. *In* Malaria: Principles and Practice of Malariology. Edited by W. Wernsdorfer and I. McGregor. Edinburgh, Churchill Livingstone, 1988.
89. Black, P.H., Kunz, L.J., Swartz, M.N.: N. Engl. J. Med., *262*:811–817, 921–927, 1960.
90. Cuadra, M.: Tex. Rep. Biol. Med., *14*:96–113, 1956.
91. Bennett, I.L., Hook, E.W.: Annu. Rev. Med., *10*:1–20, 1959.
92. Kaye, D., Gill, F.A., Hook, E.W.: Am. J. Med. Sci., *254*:205–215, 1967.
93. Murray, M.J., Murray, A.B., Murray, M.B., et al.: Lancet, *1*:653–654, 1975.
94. Keusch, G.T., Farthing, M.J.G.: Annu. Rev. Nutr., *6*:131–154, 1986.
95. MacKay, H.M.: Arch. Dis. Child., *3*:117–147, 1928.
96. Andelman, M.B., Sered, B.R.: Am. J. Dis. Child., *111*:45–55, 1966.
97. Basta, S.S., Soekirman, M.S., Karyadi, D., et al.: Am. J. Clin. Nutr., *32*:916–925, 1979.

98. James, J.A., Combes, M.: Pediatrics, *26:*368–373, 1960.
99. Damsdaran, M., Naidu, A.N., Sarma, K.V.R.: Indian J. Med. Res., *69:*448–456, 1979.
100. Oppenheimer, S.J., Hendrickse, R.: Nutr., Abstr. Rev., *53:*585–598, 1983.
101. Strauss, R.G.: Am. J. Clin. Nutr., *31:*660–666, 1978.
102. Dhur, A., Galan, P., Hercberg, S.: Comp. Biochem. Physiol., *94A:*11–19, 1989.
103. McFarlane, H., Reddy, S., Adcock, K.J., et al.: Br. Med. J., *4:*268–270, 1970.
104. Torun, B., Viteri, F.E. Protein-energy malnutrition. *In* Tropical and Geographical Medicine. 2nd Ed. Edited by K.S. Warren, A.A.F. Mahmoud, New York, McGraw-Hill, 1990.
105. Sobocinski, P.A. Canterbury, W.J. Jr., Mapes, C.A. et al.: Am. J. Physiol., *234:*E399–E406, 1978.
106. Cousins, R.J., Leinart, A.S.: FASEB J., *2:*2884–2890, 1988.
107. Lieberman, I., Abrams, R., Hunt, N., et al.: J. Biol. Chem., *238:*3955–3962, 1963.
108. Beisel, W.R.: Am. J. Clin. Nutr., *35:*417–468, 1982.
109. Schwabe, J.W.R., Rhodes, D.: TIBS, *16:*291–296, 1991.
110. Dardenne, M., Pleau, J.M., Nabarra, P., et al.: Immunol. Today, *2:*225–227, 1981.
111. Prasad, A.S., Meftah, S., Abdallah, H., et al.: J. Clin. Invest., *82:*1202–1210, 1988.
112. Hambridge, K.M., Casey, C.E., Krebs, N.F.: Zinc. *In* Trace Elements in Human Health and Animal Nutrition. Edited by W. Mertz. New York, Academic Press, 1986.
113. Flynn, A., Loftus, M.A., Finke, J.H.: Nutr. Res., *4:*673–679, 1984.
114. Salas, M., Kirchner, H.: Clin. Immunol. Immunopathol., *45:*139–142, 1987.
115. Winchurch, R.A., Togo, J., Adler, W.H.: Clin. Immunol. Immunopathol., *49:*215–222, 1988.
116. Beach, R.S., Gershwin, M.E., Hurley, L.S.: Dev. Comp. Immunol., *3:*725–738, 1979.
117. Dowd, P.S., Kelleher, J., Guillou, P.J.: Br. J. Nutr., *55:*59–69, 1986.
118. Mercalli, M.E., Seri, S., Aquilio, E., et al.: Nutr. Res., *4:*665–671, 1984.
119. DePasquale-Jardieu, R., Fraker, P.J.: J. Immunol., *124:*2650–2655, 1980.
120. Brummerstedt, E., Basse, A., Flagstad, T.: Am. J. Pathol., *87:*725–728, 1977.
121. Keen, C.L., Gershwin, M.E.: Annu. Rev. Nutr., *10:*415–431, 1990.
122. Gross, R.L., Osdin, N., Fong, L., et al.: Am. J. Clin. Nutr., *32:*1260–1265, 1979.
123. Zanzonica, P., Fernandes, G., Good, R.A.: Cell Immunol., *60:*203–211, 1981.
124. Winchurch, R.A.: Clin. Immunol. Immunopathol., *47:*174–180, 1988.
125. Fraker, P.J., Zwicki, C.M., Luecke, R.W.: J. Nutr., *112:*309–313, 1982.
126. Chvapil, M., Stankova, L., Weldy, P., et al.: The role of zinc in the function of some inflammatory cells. *In* Zinc Metabolism: Current Aspects in Health and Disease. Edited by G.J. Brewer and A.S. Prasad. New York, Alan Liss, 1977.
127. Salvin, S.B., Rabin, B.S.: Cell Immunol., *87:*546–552, 1984.
128. Miller, W.J.: J. Dairy Sci., *53:*1123–1135, 1970.
129. Prasad, A.S.: Am. J. Clin. Nutr., *53:*403–412, 1991.
130. Prasad, A.S., Rabbani, P., Abbasi, A., et al.: Ann. Intern. Med., *89:*483–490, 1978.
131. Prasad, A.S., Meftah, S., Abdallah, J., et al.: J. Clin. Invest., *82:*1202–1210, 1988.
132. Tapazoglou, E., Prasad, A.S., Hill, G., et al.: J. Lab. Clin. Med., *105:*19–22, 1985.
133. Moynahan, E.J.: Immunodermatology, *30:*437–447, 1981.
134. Fraker, P.J., Gershwin, M.E., Good, R.A., et al.: Fed. Proc., *45:*1474–1479, 1986.
135. Ballester, O.F., Prasad, A.S.: Ann. Intern. Med., *98:*180–182, 1983.
136. Meftah, S., Prasad, A.S.: J. Lab. Clin. Med., *114:*114–119, 1989.
137. Briggs, W.A., Pedersen, M., Mahajan, S.: Kidney Int., *21:*827–832, 1982.
138. Golden, M.H.N., Golden, B.E., Jackson, A.A.: Lancet, *2:*1057–1059, 1977.
139. Golden, M.H.N., Golden, B.E., Harland, P.S.E.G., et al.: Lancet, *1:*1226–1228, 1978.
140. Cohen, B.E., Elin, R.J.: J. Infect. Dis., *129:*597–600, 1974.
141. Bang, F.B., Bang B.G., Foard, M.: Am. J. Pathol., *78:*417–426, 1975.
142. Green, H.N., Mellanby, E.: Br. Med. J., *2:*691–696, 1928.
143. Nauss, K.M., Mark, D.A., Suskind, R.M.: J. Nutr., *109:*1815–1823, 1979.
144. Bhaskaram, C., Reddy, V.: Br. Med. J., *3:*522, 1975.
145. Soppi, E., Lehtonen, O-P.: J. Immunopharmacol., *8:*91–96, 1984.
146. Brown, K.H., Rajan, M.M., Chakraborty, J., et al.: Am. J. Clin. Nutr., *33:*212–217, 1980.
147. Neumann, C.: Non-specific host factors and infection in malnutrition — a review. *In* Malnutrition and the Immune Response. Edited by R.M. Suskind. New York, Academic Press, 1977.
148. Thurnham, D.I.: Trans. R. Coll. Trop. Med. Hyg., *83:*721–723, 1989.
149. Thurnham, D.I., Ratree, S.: Trans. R. Soc. Trop. Med. Hyg., *85:*194–199, 1991.
150. Thurnham, D.I.: Proc. Nutr. Soc., *49:*247–259, 1990.
151. Sommer, A., Tarwotjo, I., Hussaini, G., et al.: Lancet, *2:*585–588, 1983.
152. Sommer, A., Katz, J., Tarwotjo, I.: Am. J. Clin. Nutr., *40:*1090–1095, 1984.
153. Underwood, B.A.: J. Nutr., *120:*1459–1463, 1990.
154. Sommer, A., Tarwotjo, I., Djunaedi, E., et al.: Lancet, *1:*1169–1173, 1986.
155. Muhilal, Permeisih, D., Idradinata, Y.R., et al.: Am. J. Clin. Nutr., *48:*1271–1278, 1988.
156. Rahmathullah, L., Underwood, B.A., Thulasiraj, R.D., et al.: N. Engl. J. Med., *323:*929–935, 1990.
157. West. K.P., Jr., Pokhrel, R.P., Katz, J., et al.: Lancet, *338:*67–71, 1991.
158. Vijayaraghavan, K., Radhaiah, G., Prakasam, B.S., et al.: Lancet, *336:*1342–1345, 1990.
159. Daulaire, N.M.P., Starbuck, E.S., Houston, R.M., et al.: Br. Med. J., *304:*207–210, 1992.
160. Milton, R.C., Reddy, V., Naidu, A.N.: Am. J. Clin. Nutr., *46:*827–829, 1987.
161. Bloem, M.W., Wedel, M., Egger, R.J., et al.: Am. J. Epidemiol., *131:*332–339, 1990.
162. Rahmathulla, L., Underwood, B.A., Thulasiraj, R.D., et al.: Am. J. Clin. Nutr., *54:*568–577, 1991.

163. Barclay, A.J.G., Foster, A., Sommer, A.: Br. Med. J., *294:*294–296, 1987.
164. Hussey, G.D., Klein, M.: N. Engl. J. Med., *323:*160–164, 1990.
165. Coutsoudis, A., Broughton, M., Coovadia, H.M.: Am. J. Clin. Nutr., *54:*890–895, 1991.
166. Keusch, G.T.: N. Engl. J. Med., *323:*985–987, 1990.
167. Anon.: Lancet, *336:*1349–1351, 1990.

SELECTED READINGS

Bendich, A., Chandra, R.K.: Ann. N.Y. Acad. Sci., *587:*5–350, 1990.
Bullen, J.J., Griffiths, E.: Iron and Infection. New York, John Wiley and Sons, 1987.
Burkholder, W.J., Swecker, W.S. Jr.: Semin. Vet. Med. Surg. (Small Anim.), *5:*154–165, 1990.
Gershwin, M.E., Beach, R.S., Hurley, L.S.: Nutrition and Immunity. Academic Press, San Diego, 1985.
Keusch, G.T., Scrimshaw, N.S.: Rev. Infect. Dis., *8:*349–353, 1986.
Keusch, G.T., *In* The Malnourished Child. Edited by R.M. Suskind, L.L. Suskind. New York, Raven Press, 1990.

CHAPTER 70

Nutritional Management of Diabetes Mellitus

James W. Anderson and Patti Bazel Geil

Diabetes mellitus is a major health problem. In the United States, an estimated 11 to 15 million persons have diagnosed and undiagnosed diabetes.[1] Diabetes is not a benign disease. It causes 50% of all amputations of the lower extremities in adults, 25% of all kidney failure, and is the leading cause of blindness in adults in the United States.[2] Diabetes ranks sixth as a primary cause of death in the United States, and when its complications are considered, it ranks third. The estimated economic impact of diabetes exceeds 20 billion dollars annually in the United States.[3] Proper care of diabetes is essential because no known cure exists and good management reduces the frequency of complications.[4] Diabetes management requires education and communication; the patient's knowledge is vital because diabetes health care is primarily self-care.

The nutrition plan is the foundation for successful diabetes management. This chronic disease necessitates a strategy with short-term and long-term goals. Short-term goals include health and freedom from disability, whereas long-term goals include freedom from diabetic complications and atherosclerosis. Diabetic individuals and health-care teams jointly create comprehensive plans to foster an optimal life style while maintaining desirable blood glucose and lipid concentrations.

HISTORIC OVERVIEW

Ancient civilizations in Egypt, Greece, Rome, and India recognized diabetes and recommended dietary modifications. Early medical writers reported weight loss, excessive urination, and the sweet taste of urine. The Roman Aretaeus (A.D. 70) noted polydipsia and polyuria and named the condition *diabetes*, meaning "to flow through." Thomas Willis, a London physician, described the sweet taste of urine and introduced the term *mellitus*, meaning "honeylike," in 1675. Most early physicians recommended carbohydrate replacement.[5]

During previous centuries, recommendations about dietary carbohydrate for diabetic individuals were based on theory rather than on scientific fact. Proponents of carbohydrate replacement debated proponents of carbohydrate restriction. Believers in low-carbohydrate, high-fat diets argued that diabetic individuals have excess sugar in blood and urine and should eat less sugar and carbohydrate. Believers in high-carbohydrate diets argued that dietary carbohydrate should replace sugar lost in urine. One important feature, still relevant today, was almost universally endorsed—diabetes is best treated by energy-restricted diets.

John Rollo, a British Army Surgeon-General, launched modern diabetes nutrition therapy in 1797 by recommending a low-carbohydrate, high-fat diet.[6] He advised complete avoidance of dietary carbohydrate and abstinence from all vegetables. Therapy was directed to minimizing glycosuria. He noted that small amounts of bread allowed "saccharine matter" to return to urine. When his patients improved, he allowed them to resume a cautious intake of vegetables. In 1860, Charles Henry Pike of Philadelphia reiterated the "strict use of animal foods alone."[5]

In 1865, the French clinician Apollinaire Bouchardat developed a more palatable low-carbohydrate, high-fat diet by eliminating milk and allowing some boiled vegetables. He observed that limited food supplies during wartime were accompanied by less glycosuria for diabetic patients. In addition to limiting carbohydrate intake, he emphasized a major nutrition principle, the restriction of energy intake. He also initiated intermittent fasting to control glycosuria. His reports galvanized the widely accepted practice of using a low-carbohydrate, energy-restricted diet for diabetic individuals in the preinsulin era.[5]

The German physician and investigator Bernhard Naunyn introduced carefully measured diets in 1906. He noted that dietary protein increased glycosuria and recommended restriction of protein and carbohydrate. He also reported that intermittent 24-hour fasts reduced glycosuria for less severely affected individuals. Frederick M. Allen of New York developed the famous "Allen Starvation Treatment" of diabetes in 1912. Using 1000-kcal diets containing 10 g carbohydrate, he sustained the lives of a few young men until insulin became available.[7] Thus, just prior to the discovery of insulin, diabetes was treated with low-carbohydrate, semistarvation regimens.[5]

High-carbohydrate, energy-restricted diets were advanced by Thomas Willis. He developed the milk diet that became standard treatment until the time of Bouchardat. In 1875, Plorry of Paris also argued that sugar lost in urine should be replaced with dietary carbohydrate. Donkin recommended skim milk in 1869; others developed "cures" using various carbohydrate sources. Van During in 1875 used rice, whereas Dujardin-Beaumetz in 1889 and Mosse in 1898 used potatoes. Carl Harko von Noorden developed an "oatmeal cure" for diabetes in 1906. His report sustained the minority view that high-carbohydrate, energy-restricted diets were the treatment of choice for diabetes.[5]

Even after insulin was discovered in 1921, most Western diabetes specialists used low-carbohydrate, high-fat diets to treat lean diabetic individuals. The few clinicians to report that high-carbohydrate, low-fat diets benefited diabetic individuals included Geyelin in 1935,[8] Sansum in 1926,[9] Rabinowitch in 1935,[10] and Kempner in 1958.[11] Table 70–1 outlines changes in nutrition recommendations over 50 years. Recent clinical and experimental data support recommendations of national diabetes associations for a generous-carbohydrate, fat-restricted diet.

CLASSIFICATION

Diabetes mellitus is a chronic metabolic condition characterized by major derangements in metabolism of glucose and abnormalities in metabolism of fat, protein,

TABLE 70–1. CHANGES IN NUTRITION RECOMMENDATIONS FOR PERSONS WITH DIABETES (VALUES ARE FOR 2000-KCAL INTAKE)

	1930	1955	1970	1990
Carbohydrate, total, g/d	70	176	225	290
Percentage of energy (%)	(14)	(35)	(45)	(58)
Simple (g/d)	40	71	112	130
Complex (g/d)	30	105	113	160
Fat, total (g/d)	153	99	82	60
Percentage of energy (%)	(69)	(45)	(37)	(27)
Saturated (g/d)	87	46	35	14
Monounsaturated (g/d)	50	37	31	26
Polyunsaturated (g/d)	9	11	13	17
Cholesterol (mg/d)	1060	690	550	150
Protein (g/d)	85	101	90	75
Dietary fiber (g/d)	8	15	20	40

and other substances. Hyperglycemia is the hallmark. Pathologic changes of small blood vessels of eyes, kidneys, and other tissues and degeneration of peripheral nerves develop with time. This condition, usually inherited, results from an absolute or relative deficiency of insulin, the hormone secreted by the pancreatic beta cells. Diabetes can be primary or secondary (Table 70–2). Spontaneous diabetes is the major form in the West, whereas malnutrition-related diabetes is a major form in Africa and Asia.[12] Malnutrition-related diabetes, also called pancreatic diabetes, usually develops in young people and is characterized by moderate-to-severe hyperglycemia without ketonemia. The chronic calcifying pancreatitis generally develops in children as a result of protein-calorie malnutrition.

Ten percent of patients have type I diabetes, which usually develops during childhood, but can develop after age 20.[13] One of every 700 school children in North America develops type I diabetes. Characterized by a proneness to ketoacidosis, these individuals have virtually no capacity to secrete insulin after their diabetes is entrenched. The presentation of diabetes is often acute because of a reduction in insulin secretion usually related to autoimmune damage to pancreatic beta cells in a genetically susceptible individual.[14] Viral destruction of the beta cells is a rare cause of type I diabetes. Some individuals with type I diabetes have strong family histories of autoimmune conditions such as autoimmune thyroid or adrenal disease.

Type II diabetes usually develops insidiously because of gradual reduction of insulin secretion. This genetic disorder is associated with resistance of skeletal muscle to insulin action. Obesity is a major cause of insulin resistance, although some lean individuals are insulin resistant. Even in insulin-resistant individuals, impaired insulin secretory capacity appears to be responsible for the diabetic state.[15,16] In type II diabetes, the pancreatic beta cells act like an aging factory whose production steadily declines. The only satisfactory response to limited output is to reduce requirements. Individuals susceptible to type II diabetes can increase insulin sensitivity by weight loss, diet, and exercise.

In North America, 90% of diabetic individuals have type II disease.[17] This form usually develops after age 30. Diabetes is 10% more prevalent in men than women and twofold higher in black than in white individuals, especially black women. Lower income or education is accompanied by twice the rate of diabetes than higher income or education.

Secondary factors account for diabetes development in 10% of cases in the West and 25% of cases in Eastern countries such as India.[17] Total pancreatectomy leads to insulin-dependent diabetes; other secondary causes may produce either insulin-dependent or noninsulin-dependent forms. Hormonal disorders or drug therapy may trigger diabetes in genetically susceptible individuals.

DIAGNOSIS

Classic symptoms such as polydipsia, polyuria, and rapid weight loss associated with gross and unequivocal elevation of blood glucose (over 11.1 mmol/L or 200 mg/dl) make the diagnosis of diabetes mellitus. A fasting plasma glucose level exceeding 7.8 mmol/L (140 mg/dl) on two occasions is diagnostic. An oral glucose tolerance

TABLE 70–2. CLASSIFICATION OF DIABETES MELLITUS

Spontaneous Diabetes Mellitus (DM)
Insulin-dependent (IDDM or type I)
Noninsulin-dependent (NIDDM or type II)
Nonobese NIDDM
Obese NIDDM
Maturity-onset diabetes of young people
Secondary Diabetes
Malnutrition-related diabetes
Pancreatic disease (pancreatitis, pancreatitic insufficiency, or surgical pancreatectomy)
Hormonal: excess of counterregulatory hormones (growth hormone, as with acromegaly, glucocorticoids as with Cushing's syndrome, catecholamines as with pheochromocytoma, or thyroid hormones as with thyrotoxicosis)
Drug- or chemical-induced (as with potassium-wasting diuretics, β-blocking agents, or phenytoin)
Insulin-receptor abnormalities
Structurally abnormal insulin
Certain genetic disorders (such as myotonic dystrophy)
Impaired Glucose Tolerance
Gestational Diabetes
Glucose intolerance discovered during pregnancy

test (OGTT) is indicated for borderline fasting plasma glucose (6.4 to 7.8 mmol/L, 115 to 140 mg/dl), when 2-hour postprandial plasma glucose exceeds 7.8 mmol/L (140 mg/dl), or for individuals at high risk of diabetes.[12]

The OGTT identifies individuals with diabetes, impaired glucose tolerance, and gestational diabetes. For proper interpretation the individual must be ambulatory, otherwise healthy, and taking no medications that impair glucose tolerance.[13,18] For at least 3 days before the test, individuals use a weight-maintaining diet providing at least 150 g of carbohydrate daily. After an overnight fast of 10 to 16 hours, an oral glucose load of 50 to 100 g (or 40 g/M^2) is given. The subject remains seated during the test. Water is permitted but smoking is not. Blood is taken before glucose administration and 1/2, 1, 1 1/2, and 2 hours later for plasma glucose.

Nondiabetic adults have fasting plasma glucose levels lower than 7.8 mmol/L (140 mg/dl) and values during the OGTT of less than 7.8 mmol/L (140 mg/dl) at 2 hours and less than 11.0 mmol/L (200 mg/dl) at 1/2, 1, and 2 hours. Diabetes mellitus is present in nonpregnant adults when two OGTT results are abnormal with plasma glucose levels exceeding 11.0 mmol/L (200 mg/dl) at 2 hours and one other time (1/2, 1, 1 1/2 hours).[18]

Glycosylated hemoglobins are convenient screening tests for diabetes. When the glycosylated hemoglobin is more than three standard deviations about the "normal" mean, this indicates the presence of diabetes, but glycosylated hemoglobins are much less sensitive than the OGTT.[13,19]

BODY FUEL REGULATION

ROLE OF HORMONES

Insulin, the major hormonal regulator of fuel storage and release, is synthesized and secreted in response to specific stimuli. After synthesis, proinsulin splits, producing the connecting peptide (C-peptide) and insulin (51 amino acids).

Healthy lean adults secrete approximately 31 U insulin daily. Because of peripheral insulin resistance, obese nondiabetic adults secrete about 114 U daily. Type I diabetic individuals release only 0 to 4 U insulin daily, on average, whereas lean type II diabetic individuals produce about 14 U daily. These estimates of insulin secretion support other evidence that diabetes usually results from an absolute or relative deficiency of insulin.[15,16,20]

Insulin is the main signal to the body for the "fed" or "fasting" states. After a large meal, high serum insulin levels stimulate fuel and energy storage. After an overnight fast, low serum insulin levels permit mobilization of fuel and energy from storage depots. Glucagon, the pancreatic alpha cell hormone, facilitates fuel and energy release with low blood insulin levels (Fig. 70–1). Under stressful circumstances, hypoglycemia, or trauma, glucagon and other "counterregulatory" hormones, which oppose or counter insulin action, are released. These hormones—glucagon, catecholamines, glucocorticoids, and growth hormone—act specifically to decrease glucose use, to promote glucose production, and to mobilize fatty acids. During fasting, exercise, and stress, fatty acids emerge as major sources of energy.

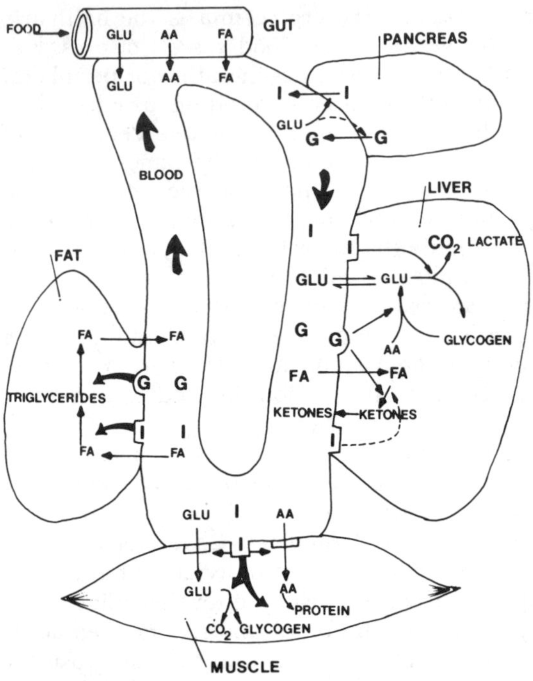

FIGURE 70–1. Action of insulin and glucagon shown schematically. GLU, Glucose; AA, amino acids; FA, fatty acids; I, insulin; and G, glucagon.

ENERGY STORES

A healthy 70-kg man stores approximately 70 g liver glycogen, 200 g muscle glycogen, and 30 g glucose in body fluids to total 300 g glucose or 5023 kJ (1200 kcal) of energy. Available glucose stores can meet energy needs for only 12 to 18 hours. However, adipose tissue triglycerides typically represent energy depots of 502,320 kJ (120,000 kcal), 100 times the glucose energy reserves. During starvation or stress, fatty acids are released for energy. Body proteins, skeletal and visceral structures, and other vital components are unavailable for energy except under dire conditions of prolonged starvation or severe stress.

FED STATE

After meals, gastrointestinal enzymes hydrolyze carbohydrates and proteins to component monosaccharides and amino acids. After absorption, these nutrients enter the portal vein and stimulate insulin secretion. Sugars and amino acids enter liver cells with high ambient insulin. Insulin stimulates glycogen synthesis, aerobic and anaerobic glycolysis, protein synthesis, and fatty acid syntheses in liver. Insulin inhibits glycogenolytic, gluconeogenic, proteolytic, and lipolytic processes. After activation by phosphorylation, glucose enters glycogen depots, generates energy in glycolytic and Krebs cycle pathways, and yields precursors for fatty acid and protein synthesis. Other simple sugars enter the glycogen pool, generate energy, or become precursors for synthetic processes. Amino acids enter precursor pools for protein synthesis.

Muscles and adipose tissue receive a large percentage of glucose and amino acids released after large meals. High serum insulin concentrations specifically stimulate the transport of glucose and amino acids into muscle cells and glucose into adipose tissue. In muscle cells, under the influence of insulin, glucose enters glycogen depots and generates energy while amino acids serve as precursors for protein synthesis. Insulin also facilitates the conversion of glucose products to fatty acids for storage as triglycerides in fat cells. Most other tissues are freely permeable to glucose as well as amino acids and use the nutrients for glycogen formation, energy, and protein synthesis.

Gut, liver, and other tissues handle ingested fat differently from glucose and amino acids. Gut hydrolyzes fats to fatty acids, glycerol, cholesterol, phospholipids, and other constituents. Short- and medium-chain fatty acids are absorbed and enter the portal vein for use in the liver. Long-chain fatty acids, cholesterol, and phospholipids are repackaged by gut mucosa and enter lymphatics as chylomicrons, which enter the superior vena cava through the thoracic duct. In the systemic circulation, chylomicrons release fatty acids for use by liver, muscle, fat, and other cells.

High serum insulin levels affect lipid metabolism in several ways. Insulin stimulates synthesis of lipoprotein lipases, which are secreted onto capillary membranes. These lipases extract fatty acids from triglyceride-rich circulating lipoproteins and facilitate entry of fatty acids into various tissues. In the fed state, a large proportion of these fatty acids are extracted by adipose tissue and are incorporated into triglyceride storage. Liver cells exposed to generous amounts of insulin extract fatty acids from chylomicrons and repackage them as very low-density lipoprotein (VLDL) particles, which are secreted into the systemic circulation. VLDL also deliver fatty acids to adipose tissue for deposition.

FASTING STATE

The transition from fed to fasted states is accompanied by a gradual fall in serum insulin and a rise in serum glucagon. The falling ratio of insulin to glucagon slowly switches the liver enzyme machinery from glucose use to glucose production. After 12 or more hours of fasting, half the liver glycogen is depleted. During longer starvation, hepatic glycolytic rates and activities of key glycolytic enzymes decline over 48 to 96 hours and then stabilize, whereas hepatic gluconeogenesis rates and key gluconeogenic enzyme activity increase. After 72 hours of fasting, the liver has low glycolytic rates and has retooled for maximal gluconeogenesis.

Brain, other nervous tissues, red blood cells, and renal medulla have ongoing requirements for glucose for energy, whereas other tissues begin using fatty acids and ketones for energy. Low serum insulin levels stimulate lipolysis in adipose tissue; fatty acids are released at rates required for energy by various tissues. Lipolysis is further stimulated by high serum concentrations of glucagon and catecholamines. Liver burns fatty acids to meet energy needs and to fuel gluconeogenesis. Ketones are hepatic byproducts of fatty acid oxidation. Glucogenic amino acids released by muscles and other tissues are major substrates for active gluconeogenesis. When glycogen reserves of liver and muscle are exhausted, most tissues are dependent on fatty acids and ketones to meet their energy needs.

High levels of free fatty acids decrease the number of insulin receptors on various tissues and act in other ways to block insulin action. Because of low serum insulin and high serum free fatty acids, glucose and other amino acids are not transported into muscle cells. Protein synthesis stops and proteolysis is activated with amino acids released into circulation. Glucocorticoids also foster release of amino acids to support gluconeogenesis in liver.

During a short-term fast, serum insulin and glucagon orchestrate changes in fuel homeostasis resulting in a steady supply of glucose to brain and other glucose-dependent tissues while mobilizing free fatty acids to meet energy needs of other tissues. After a 7- to 10-day fast, brain develops the capacity to use ketones for fuel and the need to convert amino acids to glucose abates, allowing adjustment to long-term fasting with sparing of skeletal and visceral proteins.

METABOLIC DERANGEMENTS

Diabetes resembles fasting, especially in responses of liver, muscle cells, and adipose tissues. With low ratios of insulin to glucagon and the high levels of fatty acids, liver produces glucose while other tissues use fatty acids and ketones instead of glucose. Muscle cells and adipose tissue respond by using ketones and fatty acids. Although these resemblances between fasting and diabetes are striking, pathologically low serum insulin levels disrupt the efficiency seen during fasting.

With low insulin, key glycolytic enzyme activities decrease. Glucose use falls to levels far below those seen during fasting. Concurrently, hepatic gluconeogenic enzyme activities increase and gluconeogenic rates rise. Bombarded with free fatty acids, the liver increases gluconeogenesis, secreting large amounts of VLDL, and accumulates fatty acids in droplet form. A long-term toxic effect of diabetes is the accumulation of 25% more lipid than normal. In the diabetic state, the liver oxidizes these fatty acids and produces acetone, acetoacetate, and β-hydroxybutyrate.

Muscle cells and adipose tissue also show major metabolic changes in diabetes. Muscle glycogen almost disappears and muscle protein is broken down to support gluconeogenesis. Cardiac and skeletal muscles meet their energy needs from ketones and fatty acids. Fat cells actively release fatty acids under the lipolytic stimuli of glucagon, catacholamines, and insulin deficiency.

Noninsulin-dependent tissues respond to diabetes totally differently. Hexokinase, the key stimulus of glucose use, is increased in jejunal mucosa, renal cortex, and peripheral nerves of diabetic animals. In hyperglycemia, glucose use increases and sugars accumulate.

Excess glucose accumulation leads to tissue damage. Diabetic rats have 30% more total body glycogen than nondiabetic rats. Glycogen accumulates in renal tubules to values 50 times higher than in nondiabetic rats. Glycogen accumulation may contribute to tubular dysfunction and susceptibility to damage from x-ray dyes. Unimpeded entry of glucose into many tissues increases cellular glucose, producing linkage of glucose to tissue proteins (glycosylation). The diabetic state damages noninsulin-dependent tissues, including glomeruli, retinal vessels, nerves, and circulating blood cells.[21]

DIABETIC COMPLICATIONS

ACUTE PROBLEMS

Diabetes can first become manifest with either symptomatic hyperglycemia or a medical emergency caused by severe hyperglycemia, ketoacidosis, or severe hyperlipidemia. Most symptoms of diabetes are related to hyperglycemia or accumulation of glucose in various tissues. As hyperglycemia develops, individuals have increased polyuria, thirst, lack of energy, irritability, blurred vision, and weight loss. Adults usually develop these symptoms over weeks to months, whereas children may develop them in hours or days. If hyperglycemia goes undetected or if stress or illness intervenes, the individual will develop stupor or coma (Table 70–3).

Adults with type II diabetes are likely to develop the hyperglycemic nonketotic state characterized by plasma glucose values exceeding 750 mg/dl without significant ketonemia.[22] These individuals may be protected from ketoacidosis by circulating insulin in spite of low-normal or low levels. The hyperglycemic nonketotic condition can be precipitated by excessive sugar intake, dehydration, heat exposure, illness, or drug therapy.

Individuals with type I diabetes are vulnerable to diabetic ketoacidosis characterized by hyperglycemia and ketonemia, which occurs either in insulin deficiency or from stress.[23] Either hyperglycemic nonketotic state or ketoacidosis can be fatal. Vigorous therapy includes insulin, fluids, and electrolytes.

Severe hypertriglyceridemia can be a serious medical emergency. Serum triglycerides exceed 22.6 mmol/L (2000 mg/dl) and may be accompanied by neurologic symptoms, skin lesions, or abdominal symptoms from pancreatitis. Treatment includes intravenous fluids or a clear liquid diet to lower serum triglycerides, insulin to control hyperglycemia, and appropriate therapy for other medical problems.[24]

SHORT-TERM COMPLICATIONS

Sustained hyperglycemia alters glucose metabolism in virtually every tissue. Cells that are noninsulin dependent are particularly vulnerable because sugar alcohols (polyols) accumulate and proteins are glycosylated. Most tissues gradually convert glucose to polyols, which are used slowly (Fig. 70–2). Hyperglycemia causes high intracellular glucose leading to rapid formation of polyols, which accumulate rapidly but are degraded slowly. Sorbitol and fructose, the major polyols, accumulate and cause cell distention and toxicity. Blurred vision, for example, is caused by distention of the lens. Polyol accumulation can alter the function of peripheral nerves.[25]

Excess glucose affects production of glycoproteins, proteins containing sugar side chains (Fig. 70–3). The condensation reaction between glucose and an amino acid component of protein has two stages: (1) the aldehyde group of glucose links to the amino group of an amino acid forming an aldimine (Schiff base); and (2) the unstable aldimine releases glucose or undergoes an Amadori rearrangement to form the stable ketoamine linkage. This process, occurring spontaneously without enzyme action, is termed nonenzymatic glycosylation. Hemoglobin, serum albumin, and many other proteins are glycosylated. In diabetes, glycosylation is related to the magnitude and duration of hyperglycemia.[26]

The sugar content of hemoglobin, the best-characterized glycoprotein, is normally less than 6%. In diabetes, the percentage of glycosylated hemoglobin can exceed 25% of total hemoglobin. When erythrocytes are incubated with glucose, glycohemoglobin doubles within hours. Most glucose is attached by the unstable aldimine linkage, which can be dissociated if erythrocytes are incubated in low glucose solutions. Long-term exposure to high glucose levels causes the formation of irreversible ketoamine linkages that persists until the cell is degraded. Thus, glycohemoglobin measurements reflect glycemic control over the previous 6 to 8 weeks. In patients with excellent glycemic control, glycohemoglobin concentrations are normal. Poor diabetic control yields glycohemoglobin values exceeding 9%. The degree of glycosylation of circulating proteins, hormones, lipoproteins, plasma membranes of cells, basement membranes, and other proteins in diabetes has not been determined. This may contribute to basement membrane thickening, vascular permeability, microcircula-

TABLE 70–3. DIABETIC COMPLICATIONS AND PATHOPHYSIOLOGIC CONSIDERATIONS

COMPLICATION	PATHOPHYSIOLOGIC CONSIDERATION
	Acute
Moderate hyperglycemia	Polydipsia, polyuria, weight loss, fatigue, blurred vision
Severe hyperglycemia	Hyperglycemic nonketotic state
Severe ketosis	Diabetic ketoacidosis
Hyperlipidemia	Chylomicronemic syndrome with neurologic skin and/or pancreatitis symptoms
	Short-term
Protein glycosylation	Premature aging of collagen, lens, and other tissue proteins; functional abnormalities of hormones, lipoproteins and membrane proteins
Polyol accumulation	Nerve and lens dysfunction
Mucopolysaccharide abnormalities	Alterations in arterial walls
Glycogen accumulation	Renal tubular lesions
Lipoprotein abnormalities	Accelerated atherosclerosis
Vascular permeability abnormalities	Protein leakage from capillaries
Microcirculation defects	Abnormal renal and muscle blood flow
White blood cell abnormalities	Altered response to infection and immune challenges
Platelet abnormalities	Contribution to micro- and macrovascular abnormalities
Erythrocyte abnormalities	Stiffness and altered oxygen transport
Nerve dysfunction	Decreased nerve conduction velocity
	Long-term
Renal glomeruli	Nodular or diffuse thickening
Retinal vessels	Hemorrhage, ischemia, new vessel proliferation
Neurologic disorders	Peripheral and autonomic neuropathies
Capillary disorders	Basement membrane thickening and microcirculation abnormalities
Arterial disorders	Generalized and accelerated atherosclerosis

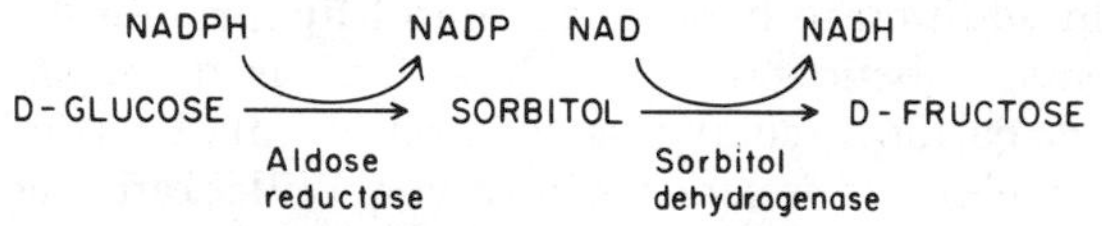

FIGURE 70–2. Polyol pathway.

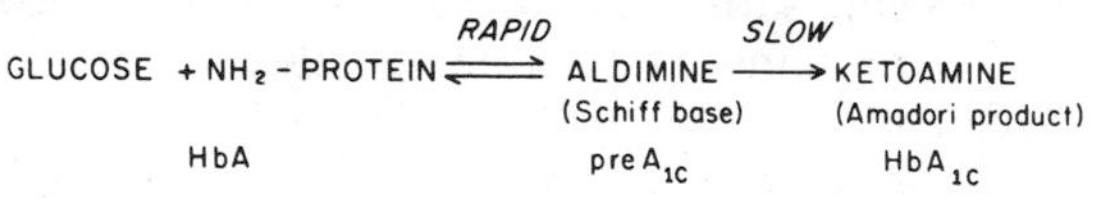

FIGURE 70–3. Pathway for nonenzymatic glycosylation.

tion defects, and functional abnormalities of erythrocytes, leukocytes, and platelets.[27]

Hyperglycemia induces a host of other metabolic derangements. Glycogen accumulates in noninsulin-dependent tissues. Increased flux of glucose through insulin-insensitive pathways such as mucopolysaccharide synthesis leads to abnormalities of mucopolysaccharides, possibly contributing to atherosclerosis. Hyperglycemia alters the orderly formation of glycoproteins in the kidney and other tissues, contributing to diabetic glomerulosclerosis. Many short-term problems of hyperglycemia can be avoided by maintaining satisfactory plasma glucose concentrations, and in some cases, derangements can be reversed by good glycemic control.[27]

LONG-TERM COMPLICATIONS

The pathogenesis of the long-term manifestations of diabetes remains controversial (Table 70–3). Metabolic, genetic, and other factors affect major diabetic complications: retinopathy, nephropathy, and neuropathy.[28] Most authorities believe that chronic hyperglycemia accelerates the development of these complications. Pirart carefully documented the prevalence of diabetic complications among 4400 diabetic patients (Fig. 70–4).[29] After 25 years, most patients had complications of some type; however, complications were less frequent in patients who maintained fairly good glycemic control than in those who had maintained poor diabetic control. Individual genetic tendencies toward complications also affect their frequency. Some diabetic individuals develop complications at an accelerated rate despite reasonable glycemic control, whereas others show little tendency toward these complications. The most prudent course is to achieve the best glycemic control possible without undue hypoglycemic episodes or severe limitations of the patient's life style.

ATHEROSCLEROSIS

Atherosclerosis is the most common complication of diabetes. Diabetic men have a two- to threefold higher risk of coronary heart disease, stroke, and peripheral vascular disease, whereas diabetic women have a three- to fivefold higher risk than matched nondiabetic individuals.[30,31] Mechanisms responsible for accelerated atherosclerosis are not understood, and many interacting factors contribute. Figure 70–5 illustrates major risk factors for atherosclerosis in diabetes and indicates the influence of nutrition. Reducing risk of vascular disease requires improved glycemic control, avoidance of cigarette smoking, normal blood pressure, and desirable serum lipoprotein levels. Hypertension is the major risk factor for coronary heart disease in type I diabetes.[32] Diabetic individuals, particularly women, develop hypertension more frequently than the general population.[33] Hypertension-related factors may act synergistically with arterial wall abnormalities, cellular dysfunction, lipoprotein abnormalities, and platelet derangements to accelerate atherosclerosis.

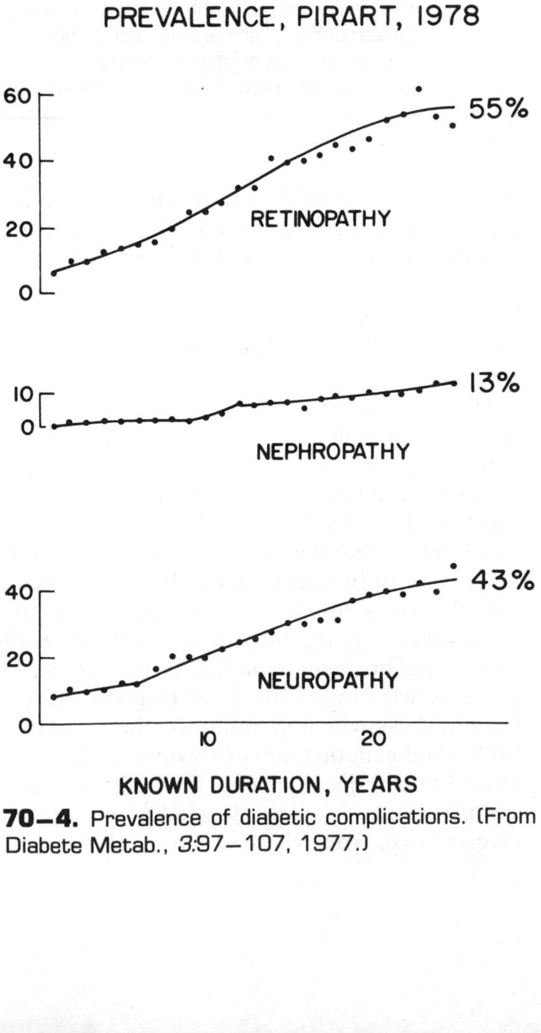

FIGURE 70–4. Prevalence of diabetic complications. (From Pirart, J.: Diabete Metab., *3*:97–107, 1977.)

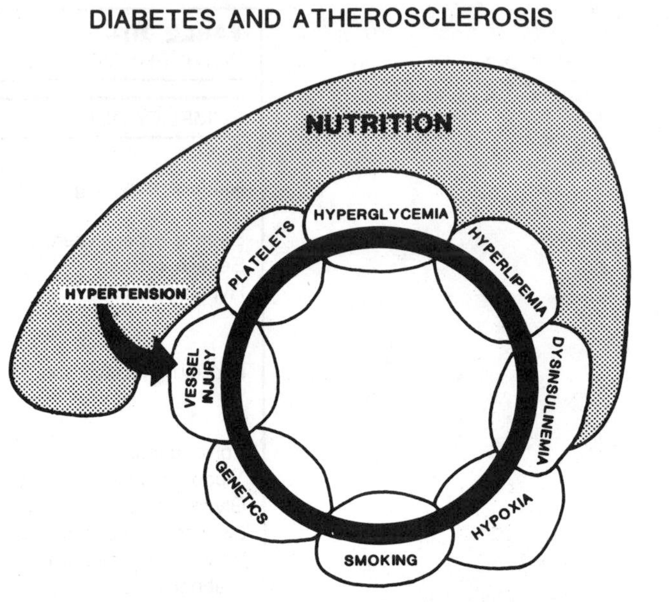

FIGURE 70–5. Relationship of diabetes, nutrition, and atherosclerosis.

Lipoprotein abnormalities play a major role in atherosclerosis. Serum low-density lipoprotein (LDL) abnormalities, decreased serum high-density lipoproteins (HDL), and increased serum triglycerides contribute to accelerated atherosclerosis in diabetes. LDL may be glycosylated or altered in other ways to enhance atherogenicity in diabetes.[34] Many lipoprotein alterations in diabetes increase the risk of atherosclerosis.

In addition to hypertension and lipoprotein derangements, diabetic individuals have increased prevalence of other cardiovascular risk factors: elevated serum insulin,[35] elevated fibrinogen and von Willebrand factor,[36] platelet function abnormalities,[37] and obesity. The nutrition plan focuses on reducing the risk of atherosclerosis by reducing saturated fat intake, achieving desirable serum lipoproteins, and reducing other cardiovascular risk factors.

GOALS FOR NUTRITIONAL THERAPY

The ultimate goal of nutritional intervention is a healthy individual with a complete life style and normal longevity. The diabetes nutrition plan attempts to diminish the effects of the disease by maintaining a normal metabolic state. Table 70–4 lists specific and general goals of nutrition therapy. While maintaining desirable blood glucose values over the short range, one must consider intermediate psychologic effects. Because the long-term effects of specific diabetic diets are not known, one should use diets that have the

TABLE 70–4. GOALS FOR NUTRITIONAL THERAPY OF DIABETES

SPECIFIC
Achieve physiologic blood glucose levels
Maintain desirable plasma lipids
Reduce likelihood of specific diabetic complications
Retard development of atherosclerosis
GENERAL
Provide optimal selection of nutrients
Attain and maintain desirable body weight
Meet energy needs in a timely manner
Individualize to preferences and food available
Address special requirements (such as pregnancy)
Tailor for therapeutic needs (such as renal failure)

greatest potential for sustaining life with a minimum of complications.

Specifically, the primary goal of nutritional therapy is to achieve normal blood glucose levels by optimizing glucose use, normalizing glucose production, and enhancing insulin sensitivity. This therapy will maintain normal blood levels of other fuels such as fatty acids, ketones, and amino acids. Undue hyperglycemia, as well as consequential hypoglycemia, is hazardous and should be minimized by diet. Second in priority is maintaining desirable plasma lipid levels. The third goal of nutritional therapy is reducing the frequency of specific diabetic complications such as retinopathy, nephropathy, and neuropathy. Although their pathogenesis is not fully understood, success with the first goal should reduce the development of these complications. The last goal addresses the causes of atherosclerosis. Appropriate nutrition reduces the risk of hypertension, hypercholesterolemia, hypertriglyceridemia, and hyperinsulinemia. Theoretically, measures that normalize platelet aggregation, restore desirable serum lipids, and avoid hyperinsulinemia will retard atherosclerotic processes.

Regarding general goals, the diabetes nutrition plan first provides adequate amounts and varieties of nutrients for optimal nutrition. As a guide, daily Recommended Dietary Allowances (RDAs) are presented in the Appendix (Appendix Table A–16). Second, it provides appropriate energy intake to achieve desirable body weights. The lean adult should maintain a healthy weight, whereas the obese individual should lose weight. Third, it provides three reasonable meals and snacks as required to meet energy needs. Fourth, it is as consistent as possible with the established eating patterns of the individual, although changes in eating patterns should be recommended for good cause. Breakfast, for example, is a must; other habits such as excessive intake of fat, sugar, or alcohol should be changed. Diet modifications can be achieved when the diabetic individual and the family work with the health-care team. Through education, patients learn the purpose of recommended changes and adopt these goals as their own. Fifth, special requirements for growth, pregnancy, or lactation are considered in the nutrition plan. Finally, the plan incorporates modifications for problems such as hypertension, congestive heart failure, osteopenia, or renal disease. The diabetes nutrition plan focuses not only on diabetes, but also on overall health and well-being.

NUTRITION PLAN

After generations of controversy, consensus recommendations have emerged regarding the diet for diabetes. National diabetes associations recommend a nutrition plan with generous amounts of complex carbohydrate and fiber and restrictions of fat and cholesterol.[38] Table 70–5 summarizes these recommendations, compared with components of a high-fiber maintenance approach to the diabetes nutrition plan. Dietary guidance for a healthy American population centers on increasing complex carbohydrate and fiber intake and reducing total fat, saturated fat, and cholesterol to decrease the risk of atherosclerosis and certain forms of cancer, especially colon, breast, and prostate cancer.[39] Current nutritional recommendations for persons with diabetes include all nutritional principles of a health-promoting diet.

Carbohydrate should provide 55 to 60% of energy for diabetic persons, but up to 70% is well tolerated. Complex carbohydrate should provide approximately two thirds of total carbohydrate. Unrefined carbohydrates in their natural fiber packages have advantages over highly refined carbohydrates.

According to American Diabetes Association (ADA) recommendations, protein should provide 12 to 20% of energy intake, although the adult RDA of 0.8 g/kg body weight more closely matches actual protein needs. High levels of protein intake may contribute to diabetic nephropathy.[40] To accommodate usual eating patterns including red meat and poultry and to meet the need for vegetables, grains, and beans, we recommend diets providing 12 to 16% of energy as protein.

Fat intake should not exceed 30% of energy; intakes of less than 20 to 25% are more desirable. Saturated fat intake should not exceed 10% of energy intake, and cholesterol intake should not exceed 200 to 300 mg per day. Polyunsaturated fats such as vegetable oil are preferred to saturated fats such as butter, but intake of polyunsaturated fats should also be less than 10% of energy intake. The remainder of fat should be monounsaturated. These recommendations are consistent with those of the American Heart Association and other groups.[39]

Generous intakes of fiber improve glycemic control and lower the lipid values of diabetic individuals.[41] Fiber intakes of 30 to 50 g per day are safe and well tolerated; the measurable benefits outweigh the potential side effects.

TABLE 70–5. COMPARISON OF NUTRITIONAL RECOMMENDATIONS FOR PERSONS WITH DIABETES

COMPONENT	RECOMMENDATIONS OF DIABETES ASSOCIATIONS	HIGH-FIBER MAINTENANCE DIET
Carbohydrate (CHO)	55–60% Unrefined CHO emphasized Modest amounts of refined sugars may be acceptable	55–60% 60–70% complex CHO 30–40% simple CHO
Protein	12–20% Adult RDA: 0.8 g/kg	12–16% Minimum of 45 g/day
Fat	<30%	20–25% or less 10% or less as saturated fat
Cholesterol	<300 mg/day	<200 mg/day 100 mg/1000 calories
Fiber	<25 g/1000 calories Maximum of 50 g/day	25 g/1000 calories 40–50 g/day total 10–15 g/day soluble

TABLE 70–6. GENEROUS CARBOHYDRATE INTAKES: ADVANTAGES AND DISADVANTAGES

ADVANTAGES
- Improved tissue insulin sensitivity
- Increased number of insulin receptors
- Enhanced intracellular glucose metabolism
- Higher rate of glycogenesis and glycolysis
- Lower rates of liver gluconeogenesis
- Lower postprandial and average serum lipids

DISADVANTAGES
- Temporary worsening of glycemic control
- Increased postprandial blood glucose and fasting serum triglycerides, unless accompanied by increased intake of dietary fiber

CARBOHYDRATE

AMOUNT

Recommendations on the carbohydrate content of the diabetes diet are controversial. The long-term use of high-carbohydrate diets for diabetic individuals is well documented. Early studies showed improved blood lipids and glucose tolerance with use of a high-carbohydrate diet.[42–44] More recent research documents the beneficial effects of diets high in carbohydrate and fiber for diabetic individuals; these diets also lower serum cholesterol concentrations.[41,45]

The advantages of higher carbohydrate intake outweigh the disadvantages (Table 70–6). Individuals are more sensitive to insulin when consuming high-carbohydrate as opposed to high-fat diets because they have increased numbers of insulin receptors.[41] Of greater importance is the enhanced intracellular glucose metabolism associated with high-carbohydrate diets. Most of these findings have been documented in experimental animals, but selected measurements in humans are confirmatory. Rates of glycogen synthesis and glycogen accumulation in liver, skeletal muscle, and jejunal mucosa are higher with high- rather than low-carbohydrate diets. Rates of glycolysis and activities of key glycolytic enzymes are higher in several tissues with high-carbohydrate diets. These diets are associated with lower rates of gluconeogenesis in liver and lower activities of rate-limiting gluconeogenic enzymes. Many metabolic changes that facilitate glucose use accompany high-carbohydrate, low-fat diets.[45]

Concerns about high-carbohydrate diets include higher postprandial blood glucose, temporary worsening of glycemic control, and increases in fasting serum triglycerides.[46] Including fiber in a high-carbohydrate diet ameliorates the rise in blood glucose and triglycerides.[41,47] Postprandial plasma glucose values are lower in diabetic individuals who are on high-carbohydrate (70% of energy), high-fiber (70 g), low-fat (12%) diets than in those who are on control (43% carbohydrate, 20 g fiber, and 38% fat) diets.[45] Although temporary worsening of glycemic control can occur when changing high-fat diets to high-carbohydrate, low-fat diets, this effect is of short duration. For diabetic individuals, no scientific evidence indicates that the long-term use of high-carbohydrate diets adversely affects glycemic control.[45]

High-carbohydrate, low-fiber diets induce increased fasting serum triglycerides in nondiabetic and diabetic subjects; however, high-fiber, high-carbohydrate diets lower fasting and postprandial triglyceride levels in diabetic or hypertriglyceridemic patients over short and long periods.[45] Figure 70–6 illustrates our experience using high-carbohydrate (70%), high-fiber (70 g per day) diets on a short-term basis and generous-carbohydrate (55 to 58 %), high-fiber (50 g per day) maintenance diets on a long-term basis in diabetic patients.[48] High-fiber, high-carbohydrate diets decrease triglycerides and do not jeopardize the triglyceride metabolism of most individuals with diabetes.

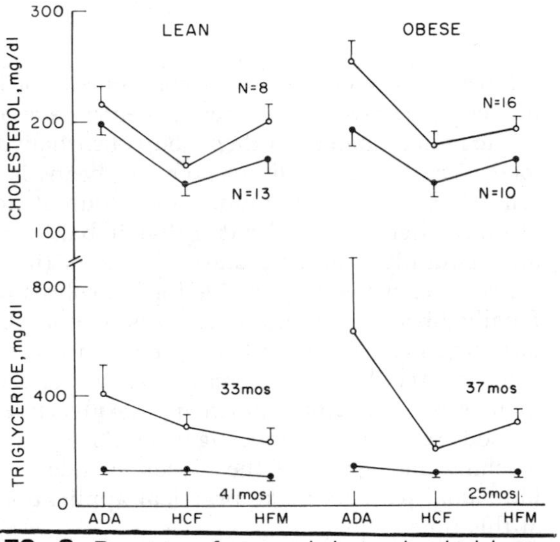

FIGURE 70–6. Response of serum cholesterol and triglyceride concentration to high-carbohydrate, high-fiber (HCF) and high-fiber maintenance (HFM) diets in lean and obese diabetic individuals. Open circles represent individuals with elevated serum triglyceride concentration on an American Diabetes Association (ADA) diet. Duration of follow-up is indicated in months.

GLYCEMIC RESPONSE

Carbohydrates in foods have traditionally been classified as either "simple" (sugars) or "complex" (starches). Simple carbohydrates from commonly used foods raise blood glucose more than complex carbohydrates from starchy foods. The glycemic response to 50 g glucose is much greater than the response to a variety of foods providing 50 g starch. Whereas glucose, maltose, and sucrose produce large increases in the blood glucose level, fructose does not (Fig. 70–7). Fructose, metabolized without insulin, evokes little increase in serum insulin in nondiabetic individuals; it produces only minimal increases in blood glucose levels in nondiabetic and diabetic persons with reasonable glycemic control. Fructose may play a role as a sweetener for selected individuals with diabetes.[49] Although simple carbohydrate worsens glycemic control and promotes weight gain,[50] the American Diabetes Association has suggested that "modest amounts of sucrose and other refined sugars may be acceptable, contingent on metabolic control and body weight."[51]

Complex carbohydrates in different forms also evoke different glycemic responses. Bread and potatoes raise blood glucose levels much more than beans (Fig. 70–7). Many investigators have compared the glycemic response of foods rich in complex carbohydrate.[52–54] Jenkins and colleagues introduced the term "glycemic index" to describe these responses comparing test foods to the glycemic response from a reference food such as bread or glucose.[53] Table 70–7 compares the glycemic response to selected foods (see also Appendix Table A–24a for more quantitative data).

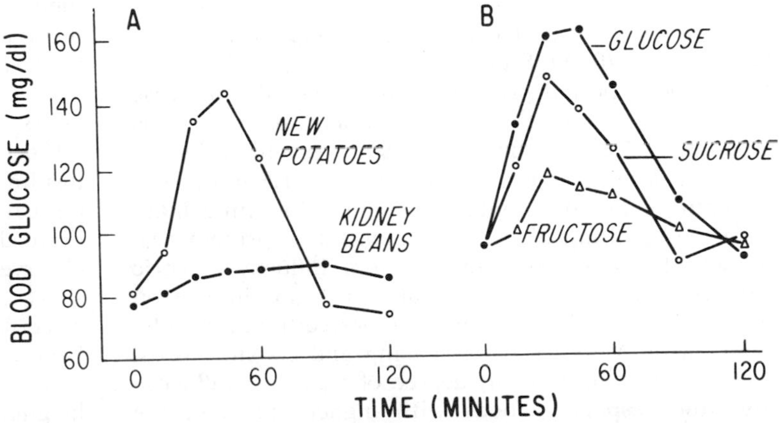

FIGURE 70–7. A, Glycemic response of healthy individuals to 50 g carbohydrate from new potatoes or kidney beans. B, Glycemic response of healthy individuals to 50 g glucose, sucrose, or fructose.

TABLE 70–7. GLYCEMIC INDEX (GI) RANKING OF SELECTED STARCHY FOODS

CLASS I (HIGHER: GI >90)	CLASS II (INTERMEDIATE: GI 70–90)	CLASS III (LOWER: GI <70)
Most breads	All bran	Pumpernickle bread
Plain crackers	Oatmeal	Most pasta
Most breakfast cereals	Most cookies or biscuits	Parboiled rice
Most potatoes	Polished rice	Most dried legumes
Millet	Buckwheat	Nuts
Corn chips	Sweet corn	Barley
	Boiled new potatoes	Bulgar (cracked wheat)
	Yams	
	Sweet potatoes	

(Adapted from Wolever, T.M.S., Jenkins,D.J.A.: Diet and diabetes. *In* Diet, Nutrition and Health. Edited by K.K. Carroll. Montreal, McGill-Queen's University Press, 1989.)

TABLE 70–8. FACTORS AFFECTING THE GLYCEMIC RESPONSE TO FOOD

- Rate of ingestion
- Food form
- Food components
  - Fat content
  - Fiber content
  - Protein content
  - Starch characteristics
  - Food ingredients
- Methods of cooking and processing food
- Physiologic effects
  - Pregastric hydrolysis
  - Gastric hydrolysis
  - Gastric emptying rate
  - Intestinal response
  - Intestinal hydrolysis and absorption
  - Pancreatic and gut hormone responses
  - Colonic effects

Many factors influence the glycemic response to foods (Table 70–8). Sipping 50 g glucose slowly over a several-hour period produces a much smaller increase in blood glucose than rapid intake of the same amount.[55] Eating three apples takes 15 minutes, whereas their juice can be consumed in 1.5 minutes.[56] Differences in fiber content and ingestion time influence the resultant glycemic response. Fat, protein, water-soluble fiber, and other factors influence gastric emptying time. Food form makes a major impact on digestion time; bread can be digested more rapidly than pasta. Methods of processing and cooking foods, and in the case of fruit, degree of ripeness, influence glycemic response. Foods with higher ratios of the amylopectin to the amylose form of starch are digested more rapidly than those with low ratios.[57]

Fiber is only one of many components of food that influence the glycemic response. Beans have lower glycemic indices than any other group of carbohydrate-rich foods. The low glycemic response to beans is probably related to their high soluble fiber content, food form (usually eaten as cooked rather than in bakery products), and naturally occurring starch blockers (inhibitors of digestive enzymes responsible for hydrolysis of starch). Finally, fiber fermentation products such as short-chain fatty acids are absorbed from the colon into the portal vein; in the liver they may directly affect glucose metabolism.[58] Factors influencing the glycemic response to foods require more investigation. The complexities of teaching and applying the glycemic index concept to individual patients make practical application difficult at this time.

FAT

AMOUNT

Traditionally, carbohydrate restriction led to high-fat diets (see Table 70–1). These diets may provide short-term advantages, but longer-term consequences are unclear. Substituting fat for carbohydrate in a meal lowers the postprandial glycemic response. Over 24 hours, replacing most of the dietary carbohydrate with fat decreases apparent insulin requirements.[59] When insulin-dependent diabetic subjects change from generous-carbohydrate, low-fat diets to high-fat, low-carbohydrate diets, no changes in insulin requirements were observed over a longer period.[60] High-fat diets offer short-term benefits for glycemic control and have no discernable adverse effects on insulin requirements over 2- or 3-week periods.

Dr. Elliott P. Joslin expressed concern about the long-term consequences of high-fat diets in 1928, suggesting "with an excess of fat diabetes begins and from an excess of fat diabetics die."[61] Limited epidemiologic evidence indicates that high-fat diets contribute to the atherosclerosis so common in diabetic persons.[62,63] However, almost all risk factors for atherosclerosis occur more frequently in persons with diabetes. Hyperlipidemia, glycosylated lipoproteins, platelet dysfunction, arterial wall changes, hyperinsulinemia, hypertension, and obesity all combine in diabetes to accelerate atherosclerosis. Maintenance of desirable serum lipid levels is a primary management goal.[38]

High-fat diets have metabolic disadvantages. They cause insulin resistance and impair intracellular glucose metabolism. Animal studies show that dietary fat not only antagonizes the use of glucose, but also stimulates inappropriate glucose production. High-fat diets decrease the number of insulin receptors in several tissues, decreasing glucose transport into muscle and adipose tissue and decreasing activities of insulin-stimulated processes. Rates of glycolysis and activities of key glycolytic enzymes are lower in a variety of tissues with high-fat versus high-carbohydrate diets. Glycogen synthesis rates, glycogen accumulation, and glucose oxidation are also lower with high-fat diets. High-fat diets stimulate rates of gluconeogenesis and increase activities of rate-limiting gluconeogenic enzymes.[45]

High serum levels of free fatty acids may mediate some of the adverse effects of high-fat diets on glucose metabolism.[64] High free fatty acid levels may act directly to reduce the number of insulin receptors for certain tissues. The intracellular metabolism of free fatty acids inhibits the essential glycolytic enzyme phosphofructokinase and further acts to stimulate gluconeogenesis. The two- to threefold rise in serum free fatty acids associated with high-fat diets antagonizes the diabetic state.

TYPE

The long-term effects of altering the type of fat in the diabetic diet are not well documented. In one long-term (30-week) study, diets rich in polyunsaturated fat were compared with diets rich in saturated fat in patients with noninsulin-dependent diabetes. The polyunsaturated-fat diet significantly lowered cholesterol and LDL cholesterol without affecting triglycerides, HDL cholesterol, or apoproteins when compared with the saturated-fat diet.[65] When a high-carbohydrate diet was compared with a diet high in monounsaturated fat in patients with noninsulin-dependent diabetes, after 4 weeks the monounsaturated-fat diet significantly decreased insulin dose, glucose, triglycerides, and VLDL cholesterol while significantly increasing HDL cholesterol and apolipoprotein A-I.[66] Although increased intake of fat usually leads to decreased insulin sensitivity, this preliminary short-term study suggests that this may not occur with monounsaturated fat intake.

OMEGA-3 FATTY ACIDS

Certain essential fatty acids of the omega-3 class lower serum cholesterol moderately and serum triglyceride levels markedly.[67] These omega-3 fatty acids, popularly known as fish oils, may also decrease platelet aggregation,[68] which may potentially reduce the cardiovascular disease risk in diabetes. Initially, fish oil supplementation in individuals with noninsulin-dependent diabetes appeared to improve their insulin sensitivity.[69] More recent research suggests that such supplementation worsens diabetic control, increasing blood glucose and glycohemoglobin levels by increasing hepatic glucose production. This outweighs the potentially beneficial effects of increased insulin sensitivity.[70,71]

FAT SUBSTITUTES

New fat substitutes, developed to lower dietary fat content, are being tested for safety and efficacy. Olestra, or sucrose polyester, is a nondigestible fat made from sucrose bonded with eight long-chain fatty acids into a molecule too large to be hydrolyzed in the small intestine.[72] Olestra provides no calories or cholesterol and may bind to cholesterol molecules from other foods in the digestive tract to remove their cholesterol and calories. In two studies of patients with noninsulin-dependent diabetes, Olestra appeared to offer substantial metabolic benefits when used as part of a hypocaloric, low-fat diet.[73,74] Olestra is targeted for use in oils, cooking, frying, fast foods, and snack foods. Another product in the same category is Simplesse, a fat substitute made using a microparticulation process to convert protein from egg whites and milk into particles less than 3 mm in diameter, which the tongue perceives as the creamy sensation of fat. Because this product is derived from protein, it contains 1.5 calories/g versus 9 calories/g of fat, which must be considered in the calculation of a diabetic meal plan. Simplesse has been approved for use in frozen desserts and cheese foods; projected uses include dairy products and oil-based products such as salad dressings. Additional fat substitutes in development include combinations of water and surface-active lipids or nonlipids having emulsifying or gelling properties. Few controlled studies of fat substitutes have been conducted in patients with diabetes. The potential usefulness of products such as these lies in their effectiveness in assisting diabetic individuals in staging dietary changes to reach realistic nutritional goals.

FIBER

Dietary fiber has emerged as a major dietary component in the management of diabetes. It has therapeutic value and may reduce the prevalence of diabetes. In 1960, Trowell reported diabetes to be rare among African hospital patients.[75] Walker then postulated that increased cereal fiber intake might prevent development of diabetes.[76] Walker and colleagues documented that healthy Bantu school children in South Africa had lower glycemic responses than urban children, and these differences were related to dietary fiber intake.[77] Trowell speculated that prolonged intake of fiber-depleted starch

TABLE 70–9. EFFECTS OF HIGH-CARBOHYDRATE, HIGH-FIBER, HIGH-FAT, AND LOW-FAT DIETS ON BLOOD GLUCOSE AND LIPID LEVELS OF TEN TYPE II DIABETIC MEN (ISOCALORIC DIETS WERE FED FOR 2 WEEKS WITH WASHOUT PERIODS OF 6 TO 14 WEEKS)

	HIGH-CARBOHYDRATE, HIGH-FIBER	HIGH-CARBOHYDRATE, LOW-FIBER	LOW-CARBOHYDRATE, HIGH-FAT	LOW-CARBOHYDRATE LOW-FAT
Carbohydrate (% of energy)	65	63	27	23
Protein (% of energy)	24	25	18	62
Fat (% of energy)	10	12	55	15
Dietary fiber (g/d)	45	20	14	13
Fasting plasma glucose (mmol/L)	−17*	+1	+27*	−30*
Oral glucose tolerance test (change in mean glucose (mmol/L)	−2.6	−0.9	+2.5	−1.8
Serum cholesterol (% change)	−16*	−2	+6	−9*
LDL cholesterol (% change)	−22	+1	+7	−14
Serum triglycerides (% change)	−17	−11	+4	−30

*p vs. initial <.05

(Data from O'Dea, K., Traianedes, K., Ireland, P., et al.: J. Am. Diet. Assoc., *89*:1076, 1989.)

TABLE 70–10. HIGH FIBER INTAKES: ADVANTAGES AND DISADVANTAGES

ADVANTAGES

- Slow nutrient digestion and absorption
- Decrease postprandial plasma glucose
- Increase tissue insulin sensitivity
- Increase insulin receptor number
- Stimulate glucose use
- Attenuate hepatic glucose output
- Decrease counterregulatory hormone release (such as glucagon)
- Lower serum cholesterol
- Lower fasting and postprandial serum triglycerides
- May attenuate hepatic cholesterol synthesis
- May increase satiety between meals

DISADVANTAGES

- Increase intestinal gas
- Temporarily may cause abdominal discomfort or gastrointestinal distress
- May alter pharmocokinetics of certain drugs

promoted the development of diabetes and formulated the dietary fiber hypothesis of the etiology of diabetes.[78] Epidemiologic data indicate that low fiber intake correlates with a higher prevalence of diabetes.[79]

The therapeutic value of fiber in diabetes emerged in 1976 when the Oxford group reported that fiber supplements reduced postprandial glycemic responses,[80] whereas we reported that high-fiber diets decreased the insulin requirements of lean diabetic individuals.[81] Many others confirmed that either fiber-supplemented diets or high-fiber diets benefit diabetic individuals.[41,82,83]

O'Dea and colleagues compared the impact of different diets for 2 weeks on blood glucose and lipid values in type II diabetic individuals (Table 70–9).[84] The detrimental effects of high fat intakes on blood glucose and lipid values and the beneficial effects of a high-carbohydrate, high-fiber, low-fat diet were illustrated. Although a low-carbohydrate, low-fat, high-protein intake providing 221 g of protein daily was used to test the effects of low carbohydrate and low fat intake, this diet is impractical and contraindicated in diabetic individuals at risk of diabetic nephropathy. This study demonstrates the clear superiority of a high-carbohydrate, high-fiber diet to either a high-carbohydrate, low-fiber diet or a low-carbohydrate, high-fat diet.

Table 70–10 outlines the pros and cons of recommending increased dietary fiber intake in diabetic individuals. For many individuals, the advantages outweigh the disadvantages. In addition to its effects on the gastrointestinal tract, fiber enhances peripheral sensitivity to insulin.[85–87] Increasing dietary fiber intake offers these major advantages: improved glucose control with decreased swings in blood glucose resulting in less hyperglycemia and less hypoglycemia; decreased requirements for insulin or sulfonylureas; lower atherogenic lipoproteins; and other health benefits such as lower blood pressure,[39] reduced risk of coronary heart disease,[39] enhanced weight management,[48] and reduced risk of colorectal cancer.[88] A generous intake of dietary fiber from fruits, vegetables, legumes, whole-grain cereals, and breads also fosters intake of many nutrients such as vitamins and minerals.

Different types of fiber are distinguished by their physiologic properties and systemic effects. Water-insoluble fiber, found primarily in wheat, vegetables, and most grain products, alters gastrointestinal function by decreasing intestinal transit time and increasing fecal bulk. Insoluble fiber generally does not lower blood glucose or cholesterol levels. Soluble fiber becomes viscous or gummy when mixed with water, increasing intestinal transit time, delaying gastric emptying, and slowing glucose absorption. These actions lower postprandial blood glucose concentrations and decrease blood cholesterol, both important goals for individuals with diabetes. Food sources of soluble fiber include fruits, oats, barley, and legumes. Research into fiber supplements such as pectin, guar, and psyllium has documented the beneficial effects of these substances in diabetes control,[41] but fiber supplements are not commonly used in clinical practice. Newly developed, safe, and palatable fiber supplements may assist patients in reaching recommended levels of fiber intake and in improving metabolic control.

The major disadvantages of increased fiber intake relate to gastrointestinal symptoms. Theoretic concerns about detrimental effects on vitamin or mineral availability have not been documented.[89,90] Some individuals note mild abdominal discomfort while increasing fiber intake; this usually can be avoided by gradually increasing fiber intake, and it usually disappears after a few days. Most individuals have more flatulence with increased fiber intake; this usually persists but is better tolerated in time. Increased fiber intake increases fecal bulk and usually increases frequency of bowel movements. Individuals with irritable bowel syndrome often do not tolerate an abrupt increase in fiber intake well and should increase fiber intake slowly to avoid gastrointestinal symptoms. Individuals with autonomic neuropathy of the gastrointestinal tract need special consideration. Increased soluble fiber may aggravate delayed gastric emptying. Increased fiber intake may benefit diabetic diarrhea and also promotes laxation for individuals with constipation. In our experience, dietary fiber has a beneficial effect in most diabetic individuals with autonomic neuropathy. Most diabetic individuals who gradually increase fiber consumption have net beneficial effects.

Many national health organizations recommend that healthy adults should increase their dietary fiber intake by 50 to 100%. Because the average fiber intake of American adults is approximately 13 g per day for women and 18 g per day for men, this recommendation suggests that an intake of 20 to 35 g per day would be healthy and desirable.[39] The ADA recommends that diabetic adults consume approximately 40 g of dietary fiber per day or 15 to 25 g per 4186 kJ (1000 kcal).[51] These recommendations are appropriate for diabetic individuals because of the fiber-related benefits such as increased insulin sensitivity, better glycemic control, and lower atherogenic serum lipids. This level of fiber intake can easily be achieved using high-carbohydrate, high-fiber (HCF) exchanges (Table 70–11) or ADA exchanges (Table 70–12), with an emphasis on higher-fiber choices such as whole-grain breads, high-fiber cereals, generous intakes of fruits and vegetables, and regular use of legumes.[91]

SWEETENERS

Most people consume sweetened foods and beverages. To avoid aggravating hyperglycemia, individuals with diabetes are advised to limit foods that worsen glycemic control or foster weight gain; however, they should enjoy foods that are safe and compatible with their nutrition plan. Diabetic individuals cannot entirely avoid foods containing glucose, sucrose, or fructose, and the ADA has suggested that modest amounts of sucrose and other refined sugars may be acceptable in the diet, contingent on individual metabolic control and body weight.[51] Foods containing large amounts of these sugars may produce hyperglycemia and weight gain. In addition, these foods often have a high fat and energy content that contributes to poor metabolic control. Alternative sweeteners are acceptable in the management of diabetes. If sweeteners are used, a multiple-sweetener approach is recommended, so only small amounts of any one type are consumed. Each sweetener has its own advantages and risks. The two basic categories of sweeteners are nutritive (calorie containing) and nonnutritive (noncalorie containing).

The use of modest amounts of nutritive sweeteners, such as fructose or the polyols (sorbitol, mannitol, or xylitol) probably poses no risk to diabetic or nondiabetic individuals,[92] as long as their caloric contribution is

TABLE 70–11. NUTRIENT VALUES PER SERVING: 1987 HIGH-CARBOHYDRATE, HIGH-FIBER (HCF) EXCHANGE LIST

FOOD GROUP	ENERGY (KCAL)	CARBOHYDRATE (G)	PROTEIN (G)	FAT (G)	FIBER (G)
Starches	70	15	2	—	2
Cereals	90	20	3	—	4
Proteins	50	—	8	2	—
Beans	95	17	7	—	5
Vegetables	25	5	1	—	2
Fruits	60	15	—	—	2.5
Skim milk	85	12	8	0.5	—
Fats	45	—	—	5	—

TABLE 70–12. NUTRIENT VALUES PER SERVING: 1986 AMERICAN DIABETES ASSOCIATION (ADA) EXCHANGE LIST*

FOOD GROUP	ENERGY (KCAL)	CARBOHYDRATE (G)	PROTEIN (G)	FAT (G)
Starch/bread	80	15	3	trace
Meat and substitutes				
Lean	55	—	7	3
Medium-fat	75	—	7	5
High-fat	100	—	7	8
Vegetables	25	5	2	
Fruit	60	15	—	—
Milk				
Skim	90	12	8	trace
Low-fat	120	12	8	5
Whole	150	12	8	8
Fat	45	—	—	5

*Multiplying the grams of carbohydrate and protein by 4 in the starch/bread and skim milk lists will not yield the total number of calories given for these two lists. These exchanges contain less than a gram of fat per serving and the term "trace" is used to make teaching easier. Dietitians may wish to use 1 gram fat in their calculations to achieve the total caloric value for the exchange group.

counted in the meal plan. Fructose offers advantages over sucrose because it tastes sweeter, is metabolized without insulin, and produces less hyperglycemia. Although fructose may increase blood glucose levels in poorly controlled diabetes, it is otherwise well metabolized. It produces only 20% of the glycemic response of glucose and 33% of the response of sucrose in well or fairly well controlled insulin- or noninsulin-dependent diabetes. Substituting fructose for glucose and sucrose in the diet lowers average blood glucose values in diabetic individuals. When fructose displaces fat from the diet, improved sensitivity to insulin results. However, the long-term safety of fructose for persons with diabetes is not established. We incorporated 50 to 60 g of fructose daily into a prudent diet for 14 diabetic men.[49] Over a 24-week period, no adverse effects were observed in plasma glucose, glycohemoglobin, cholesterol, triglycerides, lactate, or urate. Studies such as this indicate that diabetic individuals can consume moderate amounts of fructose with reasonable safety, provided they do not gain weight.

Nonnutritive sweeteners are widely used in beverages and other products. Saccharin, discovered in 1879, is a petroleum derivative that may be associated with an increased risk of bladder cancer when the substance is ingested in large amounts. At present, we recommend that pregnant women avoid saccharin, children not exceed two cans of saccharin-sweetened soft drinks daily, and nonpregnant adults exercise moderation in its use. Although not available in the United States, cyclamate, a chemical-based artificial sweetener, has limited sweetening power and is most effective when used synergistically with other high-intensity sweeteners. Aspartame, a dipeptide containing aspartic acid and phenylalanine, appears reasonably safe for individuals without phenylketonuria.[93] This sweetener has negligible caloric value, but is unable to withstand heat exposure and has limited use in baking. Acesulfame potassium (ACE-K), discovered in 1967, is a derivative of acetoacetic acid approved for broad product applications. Limited research has indicated that ACE-K can induce insulin secretion in rats.[94] Excessive intake of any sweetener requires nutritional counseling and should be limited to the established safe level. Practical resources are available to assist in counseling patients with diabetes in regard to sweeteners.[95,96]

ALCOHOL

The same precautions regarding alcohol use apply to both the general public and people with diabetes. To reduce the risk of chronic disease in healthy adults, alcohol should be consumed only in moderation (no more than two drinks per day), if at all.[97] The ADA advises no more than two equivalents of an alcoholic beverage once or twice a week.[51] One equivalent or 1 ounce of liquor equals the amount of alcohol in a 1.5-ounce shot of distilled spirits (i.e., whiskey, scotch, vodka, gin, rum), a 4-ounce glass of wine, or 12 ounces of beer.

Alcohol is absorbed across the gastrointestinal mucosa of the stomach, duodenum, and jejunum. The liver is the major organ for alcohol metabolism and the site of its oxidation; alcohol does not require insulin to be metabolized. Excessive alcohol enters the general circulation, where it becomes part of all body fluids and cells, exerting effects on the central nervous system. In diabetes, alcohol has detrimental effects, particularly alcohol-induced fasting hypoglycemia caused by inhibition of gluconeogenesis and hypoglycemia caused by the alalcohol-enhanced hypoglycemic effects of insulin, oral hypoglycemic agents, and exercise.[17] Additional alcohol-specific concerns include aggravation of hypertriglyceridemia, interaction with concurrent medications (particularly the disulfiram reaction of flushing, nausea, and dizziness that may occur when alcohol and chlorpropamide are used), and impaired judgment that may result in disruption of usual eating patterns, excessive energy intake, or errors in insulin dose.

Alcoholic beverages are "empty calories," providing 7 cal/g and no other nutritional value. For individuals with insulin-dependent diabetes, the caloric value of an alcoholic beverage should be calculated in addition to the regular meal plan. For those with noninsulin-dependent diabetes, alcohol is best substituted for fat exchanges in the meal plan (1 ounce = 2 fat exchanges), because it is high in calories and metabolized like fat. "Light" beer and dry wine are better choices than regular beer or wine and sugary, sweetened drinks because they contain less carbohydrate.

Diabetic individuals who wish to use alcohol should be provided with the following practical guidelines: (1) the use of alcohol should be discussed with the physician and nutrition counselor; (2) pregnant women should abstain from alcohol, as should anyone with poorly controlled diabetes; (3) alcohol should be consumed slowly and with food to prevent hypoglycemia; (4) one should use moderation and never drink to the extent that judgment is impaired, nor should one drive after drinking; and (5) one should wear medical identification indicating diabetes because the symptoms of insulin reaction are similar to those of intoxication.

ADDITIONAL CONSIDERATIONS

CHILDREN

Children with diabetes cannot be treated as small adults; they have unique needs and should not be immersed in an adult-oriented therapeutic program. Health-care teams need special skills and interests to communicate effectively with both the child and the parents during each stage of childhood.

Immediate treatment alleviates symptoms and restores a sense of "feeling good." Short-term objectives include: eliminating polydipsia, polyuria, and polyphagia; preventing ketonuria, ketonemia, and ketoacidosis; avoiding hypoglycemia and hyperglycemia; and minimizing energy losses associated with heavy glycosuria. After medical treatment, the child should resume usual activities.

Intermediate objectives include: satisfactory glycemic control; normal blood lipid values; and normal growth and development. Growth data should be obtained several times yearly and plotted on standardized height, weight, and velocity charts. Other aims are the incorporation of a prudent nutrition plan and a high level of physical fitness into the child's life style. Both child and parents are educated about diabetes so they can participate intelligently in its management. Gradually, the child assumes increased responsibilities for daily care and management. The child should develop increasing self-reliance while parents avoid overprotectiveness. The diabetic child should function as a normal family member and should not be singled out for special attention at school.

The ultimate goal in the management of the diabetic child is the development of a well-adjusted, healthy adult without physical or psychosocial limitations. Long-term objectives include: maturing to adulthood with appropriate intellectual, emotional, and physical capabilities; preventing diabetic complications; and minimizing the likelihood of atherosclerotic disease.

To achieve these goals, the nutrition plan must be individualized and flexible. Based on the guidelines outlined earlier, it must evolve to meet changing requirements with growth and be reassessed on an ongoing basis. The nutrition plan promotes acceptable glycemic control and normal lipid levels. A generous carbohydrate and fiber intake coupled with restricted fat provides the same advantages for children as for adults with diabetes.[98] During periods of rapid growth or increased energy requirements, more carbohydrates (starches and, to a limited extent, sugars) can be added to meet energy needs. Carbohydrate need not be distributed evenly throughout the day. Children with insulin-dependent diabetes need a consistent level of food intake, with three meals and usually three snacks per day. Generally, each meal provides at least 20% of daily energy requirements. The dietitian develops meal plans according to the food preferences of the child, and insulin doses are adjusted to achieve suitable glycemic control. The child receives guidelines for increasing or decreasing energy intake with snacks in anticipation of variable physical activity. Insulin doses are also adjusted for unusually active or sedentary days. Self-monitoring of blood glucose is a valuable tool for demonstrating food and exercise effects on glucose levels, allowing the child to learn from supervised "trial and error."[99]

ELDERLY PATIENTS

Diabetes is a major chronic problem for a growing elderly population. The prevalence of diabetes is almost 10% for Americans over age 60 and approximately 20% for those over 80 years old. Diabetic individuals over age 65 have a relative risk of mortality that is approximately 1.5 fold higher than nondiabetic individuals.[100] Factors that contribute to glucose intolerance and development of diabetes in the elderly include decreased physical activity, intake of less complex carbohydrate and a higher percentage of energy from fat, and increased adiposity with decreased lean body mass. Other illnesses or medications may contribute to the development of diabetes in the elderly.[101]

Because the elderly have multiple defects including impaired insulin secretion, decreased action of insulin to suppress hepatic glucose output, and peripheral insulin resistance, treatment should first focus on increasing sensitivity to insulin through nutrition and physical activity. When required, second-generation sulfonylureas (glipizide or glyburide) should be initiated. If insulin is necessary, a single injection of NPH or of a premixture of NPH and regular (e.g., 70/30 insulin) will usually supplement endogenous insulin secretion adequately. Commonly, the sulfonylurea agent is continued after insulin is instituted to minimize the amount of insulin required. The goals for blood glucose control are tailored to each individual's circumstances.[102]

Eating a nutritious diet providing adequate energy from a variety of foods is extremely important. Fat intake should be less than 30% of energy, with limits in saturated fat and cholesterol. The generous carbohydrate intake can include simple and complex carbohydrates rich in dietary fiber. Fruits, juices, and sweeteners usually do not need to be limited if fat guidelines are followed. The sulfonylurea or insulin regimen can usually be adjusted to allow individuals to follow meal plans that suit their preferences or circumstances. Special teaching skills and involvement of the patient are required to optimize learning for elderly diabetic individuals. Nutrition counselors need a positive attitude, patience, and use of praise to enable elderly individuals to change lifelong dietary and exercise habits successfully.[103]

PREGNANCY

Pregnancy changes eating habits, exercise patterns, emotional state, insulin sensitivity, and hormone secretions. These changes alter glucose control and insulin requirements. In the nondiabetic woman, as placental and ovarian hormones decrease insulin sensitivity, more insulin is secreted to maintain satisfactory glucose levels. Two to 13% of women lack the pancreatic reserve to meet this challenge and develop gestational diabetes.[104] This condition usually abates after delivery, but these women are much more likely to develop diabetes during subsequent pregnancies or later in life, particularly if they are obese. For all diabetic women, the reduction of maternal, fetal, and perinatal risks requires excellent glucose control.

Insulin requirements change dramatically during pregnancy. To sustain a healthy fetus, the diabetic woman must adjust her nutrient intake and insulin dose to control glucose levels and avoid ketosis. During the first half of pregnancy, insulin requirements drop by 20 to 30% because of decreased food intake and increased glucose uptake by the fetus and placenta. During the second half of pregnancy, insulin requirements rise by 60 to 100% above prepregnancy levels because of placental hormone production and insulin resistance related to other factors. After delivery and removal of the placenta, insulin requirements drop precipitously; much smaller doses are required the week after delivery, but insulin requirements gradually increase to prepregnancy levels by 6 weeks after delivery. Proper adjustment of insulin therapy during pregnancy and post partum requires careful blood glucose monitoring.

Pregnant women have lower fasting glucose levels than nonpregnant women; normal fasting blood glucose is 55 to 65 mg/dl. This level normally peaks at 140 mg/dl 1 hour after a meal; the 24-hour average level is 80 to 85 mg/dl. To ensure the best possible outcome, normal glucose levels are the goal for diabetic pregnant women.[105] Goals during pregnancy include meeting the nutrition needs of both mother and fetus while maintaining excellent blood glucose control. Specifically, these goals are: to achieve glucose control before gestation and during the early weeks of pregnancy to reduce the risks of congenital malformations; to provide energy intake for appropriate weight gain (a range of 6.8 to 18.1 kg (15 to 40 lb), based on prepregnancy Body Mass Index (BMI)[106]), to meet increased protein needs; to provide carbohydrate to minimize ketosis, meeting the needs of the fetus and placenta; to optimize tissue sensitivity to insulin; and, during the critical 3 to 4 weeks prior to delivery, to maintain excellent glucose control to reduce neonatal risk and fetal macrosomia.

Requirements for most nutrients increase with pregnancy and are similar for diabetic and nondiabetic women. During the first trimester, most women should gain 0.9 to 1.8 kg (2 to 4 lb); this can be achieved by increasing energy intake by 419 kJ (100 kcal) per day. During the second and third trimesters, a gain of about 1 lb per week depending on prepregnancy BMI is the goal. This is achieved by increasing energy intake by 15%, or 1256 kJ (300 kcal) per day. To meet increased needs, intake of high-quality protein is increased by 30 g per day to at least 1.3 g of protein per kg of body weight. Carbohydrate should provide at least 50% of the energy intake; some individuals benefit from higher intakes of complex carbohydrate and fiber.[107] Fat provides the remaining energy intake. Most women require supplemental iron and folic acid; a multiple vitamin and mineral supplement including these is usually prescribed if evidence indicates that usual intake is low enough to produce adverse effects on maternal or fetal health or on the outcome of the pregnancy.

Gestational Diabetes. Gestational diabetes presents a special challenge. Because affected individuals usually remain unaware that they have diabetes until it is discovered during pregnancy, they need intensive education. These women are often obese, requiring a diet permitting a steady weight gain of 9.1 to 11.4 kg (20 to 25 lb), although pregnancy is not the time for weight reduction. Good glucose control must be maintained and, if necessary, insulin prescribed to reduce risks of fetal macrosomia, neonatal hypoglycemia, and perinatal mortality. Glucose tolerance tests are important in identifying high-risk individuals because early control of hyperglycemia decreases the risks to the fetus.

Pregnancy in Overt Diabetes. A successful diabetic pregnancy requires planning and a commitment of time and money. Because poorly controlled diabetes threatens the health of the mother and safety of the fetus and newborn, most women make these commitments. To reduce the risks of congenital malformations, excellent glycemic control prior to conception and during early pregnancy is necessary. Maintaining excellent glycemic control throughout pregnancy demands careful attention to diet, exercise, and insulin adjustments. Health professionals educate women about special needs during pregnancy, with the patient, physician, dietitian, and nurse educator working as a team to accomplish goals.

Nutrition management plans for pregnant and nonpregnant women with overt diabetes are similar, but pregnancy necessitates greater attention to the day-to-day nutrition plan. Guidance during early pregnancy includes a special consideration of food cravings or nausea. An individualized nutrition plan that evolves throughout pregnancy is essential to meet changing nutritional needs and insulin requirements. Three meals and three snacks supply energy requirements in the timely fashion necessary to prevent hypoglycemia.

The pregnant diabetic woman requires intensive management to achieve a successful outcome. Frequent office visits and vigorous nutrition therapy are important. Using frequent home blood glucose measurements, the individual strives to maintain normal fasting and postprandial glucose values while avoiding frequent or severe hypoglycemic reactions. The health-care team monitors the fetus and assesses fetal maturity to select the optimal time for and mode of delivery. Hospitalization may be necessary to reestablish blood glucose control; early hospitalization for glycemic control prior to delivery is advisable. Finally, intensive neonatal management is essential. The use of these principles can reduce maternal risk to near that of nondiabetic women and their offspring.

Diabetic women should be encouraged to breast-feed their infants, while paying special attention to changing insulin and food requirements. A caloric intake of 31 kcal/kg maternal body weight is associated with the ability of mothers with insulin-dependent diabetes to sustain lactation.[108]

RENAL DISEASE

Renal disease is a major complication that affects 30 to 50% of type I and over 20% of type II diabetic individuals. Diabetic nephropathy is accompanied by proteinuria, decreased glomerular filtration rate, and hypertension. Development of *microalbuminuria,* urine protein of 40 to 300 mg per 24 hours, is the forerunner of overt nephropathy.[109] Hypertension accelerates the development and progression of renal disease, whereas poor glycemic control and high protein intakes may contribute to the development and progression of nephropathy.[110]

Protein restriction in management of chronic renal failure is discussed elsewhere (see Chap. 65). High protein intakes are proposed to lead to renal damage in diabetic individuals by various mechanisms. Extensive protein feeding increases glomerular filtration rate, renal blood flow, single nephron glomerular filtration rate, and transcapillary hydraulic pressure in laboratory animals.[111,112]

Unlimited protein intake is inappropriate in patients with diabetic nephropathy. Protein restriction decreases the progression of chronic renal failure in nondiabetic individuals and perhaps in diabetic nephropathy.[113] At present, it appears prudent to restrict protein intake to 0.6 g/kg body weight for individuals with established diabetic nephropathy with appropriate adjustments for proteinuria and careful clinical monitoring. Carbohydrate should provide at least 50% of energy intake, and saturated fat and cholesterol intake should be restricted.

HYPERLIPIDEMIA

Most diabetic individuals have lipoprotein abnormalities. There are multiple abnormalities of VLDL and HDL metabolism and to a smaller extent of LDL metabolism. Hypertriglyceridemia and low HDL cholesterol values are seen more commonly in diabetic than nondiabetic individuals.[34] Hypertriglyceridemia appears to confer a higher risk of atherosclerotic cardiovascular disease on diabetic than on nondiabetic individuals, whereas low HDL cholesterol values are a major risk factor.[34]

Serum lipid and lipoprotein goals for diabetic individuals are still being actively discussed.[114] To minimize the risk of atherosclerotic cardiovascular disease, the following desirable or goal fasting values for diabetic individuals are recommended: total cholesterol <200 mg/dl (<5.2 mmol/L); LDL cholesterol <130 mg/dl (<3.4 mmol/L); triglycerides <150 mg/dl (<1.7 mmol/L); and HDL cholesterol for males >45 mg/dl (>1.2 mmol/L) and for females >55 mg/dl (>1.4 mmol/L). Because abnormally low HDL cholesterol levels are difficult to increase by dietary or pharmacologic measures, LDL cholesterol should be decreased to achieve ratios of LDL to HDL cholesterol of <2.9 for males and <2.4 for females.

The diabetes nutrition plan outlined in this chapter and elsewhere is the basic approach for most hyperlipidemic individuals.[115,116] Good glycemic control, attaining and maintaining a desirable body weight, regular exercise, and moderation in alcohol intake—practices recommended for all diabetic individuals—reduce hyperlipidemia. Approach to hyperlipidemia can focus on management of elevated LDL cholesterol, elevated triglycerides, decreased HDL cholesterol, or combinations of these disorders.

Elevations of LDL cholesterol occur with the same frequency in diabetic as in nondiabetic individuals;

treatment is similar. A high-carbohydrate (55 to 60% of energy), high-fiber (25 g/4186 kJ (1000 kcal)), low-fat (about 25% of energy with less than 10% saturated), low-cholesterol (<200 mg per day) diabetes diet is the first step. This diet should include generous amounts of soluble dietary fiber from oat and bean products. Increasing soluble fiber intake by 6 g per day without other changes in diet can decrease LDL cholesterol by 10 to 20%.[117–119] The second step is daily inclusion of 4 to 12 g of psyllium, a well-tolerated concentrated source of soluble fiber.[120] When desirable LDL cholesterol levels are not achieved, a bile acid sequestrant is added. Bile acid sequestrants and psyllium can be mixed together in 8 to 12 oz of fluid and taken two or three times daily. Hydroxymethylglutaryl coenzyme A (HMG CoA) reductase inhibitors are the second pharmacologic agent of choice.[114]

Hypertriglyceridemia is more common in diabetic individuals, especially in type II diabetes, than in nondiabetic individuals and carries a greater risk of atherosclerosis. Almost all individuals can be managed effectively with a high-fiber, high-carbohydrate diet if they decrease their fat intake to a satisfactorily low level.[121,122] Persistently elevated triglyceride levels usually are due to excessive dietary fat intake because triglyceride levels plummet when individuals are hospitalized and receive a low-fat diet. Sometimes excessive alcohol or simple sugar intake aggravates hypertriglyceridemia. Fibric acid derivatives are the pharmacologic agent of choice for individuals not responding to diet.

Type II diabetic individuals commonly have decreased HDL cholesterol levels. Taking regular physical exercise such as walking 2 to 3 miles daily and not smoking are important life-style practices to increase HDL cholesterol. Dietary measures to decrease serum triglycerides and the regular use of oat products may increase HDL cholesterol by 10 to 20%.[117] HDL cholesterol usually decreases when intensive nutritional measures are used. Decreases in HDL cholesterol may parallel decreases in LDL cholesterol levels for several months before HDL cholesterol levels begin to increase. The increase in HDL cholesterol with exercise and diet occurs slowly over 3 to 6 months. However, most individuals cannot increase HDL cholesterol levels by more than 0.13 to 0.26 mmol/L (5 to 10 mg/dl) by these life-style measures. Often, LDL cholesterol levels must be decreased to below goal levels to achieve desirable LDL-to-HDL ratios of <2.9 for males or <2.4 for females. Pharmacologic agents that increase the HDL cholesterol somewhat are fibric acid derivatives and HMG CoA reductase inhibitors. These agents are introduced when LDL cholesterol or triglyceride concentrations do not reach goal levels with dietary measures.

The hyperlipidemia of most diabetic individuals responds well to nutritional measures. Most individuals with LDL cholesterol of 5.23 mmol/L (<200 mg/dl) can be managed effectively with high-fiber diets including generous amounts of soluble fiber. Most hypertriglyceridemic individuals respond to a high-fiber diet moderately or severely restricted in saturated and total fat. Regular exercise such as walking 2 to 3 miles daily and achieving and maintaining a desirable body weight also enhance the lipoprotein response to nutritional measures.

OBESITY

PREVALENCE

About 75% of type II diabetic individuals in the United States are obese; obesity is a major contributor to the development and maintenance of the diabetic state. Achieving and maintaining a desirable body weight through diet and exercise comprise the treatment of choice. Oral sulfonylureas and insulin are important adjunctive measures, but they cannot be substituted for exercise and a diet appropriate in energy, fat, and complex carbohydrate.

WEIGHT-LOSS PROGRAMS

The health-care team sets the stage for effective weight loss by being empathetic and supportive while continuing to emphasize the detrimental effects of overeating on diabetes and health. However, the obese individual must make a commitment to losing weight before nutrition counseling will be effective. Our team offers a variety of weight-loss programs, including: instruction in a hypocaloric diet; referral to a community program; an intensive high-fiber, weight-reduction diet with frequent medical and dietetic follow-up; and medically supervised low-calorie or very low-calorie diet programs. Diabetic individuals who have BMI above 30 kg/m^2 or have more than 22.7 kg (50 lb) to lose should have medical supervision during the weight-loss phase and should not enroll in medically unsupervised programs.

WEIGHT MAINTENANCE

Weight loss is not the cure for obesity. This chronic condition requires a long-term maintenance program and access to lifelong counseling about life-style changes important in weight maintenance. After nonsurgical weight-loss programs, long-term weight maintenance, as a percentage of initial weight loss, is reported to be about 36% at 2 years and about 5% at 5 years. Most obese individuals who complete community weight-loss programs, behavioral modification programs, and very low-calorie programs regain all the weight they lost within 2 to 5 years.[123] Newer very low-calorie diet programs that stress physical activity, use the best available behavioral techniques, and facilitate achievement of desirable body weights are obtaining better long-term weight maintenance. Obese individuals completing the HMR Fasting Program at the University of Kentucky are maintaining about 63% of their initial weight loss at 2 years after completing the weight-loss phase.[123] The best predictors of good weight maintenance are low fat intakes and good levels of physical activity such as walking 20 miles per week. Much further development is required to enable formerly obese individuals to maintain desirable weights for long periods.

HIGH-FIBER WEIGHT-LOSS PROGRAMS

High-carbohydrate, high-fiber, weight-reducing diets are excellent choices for diabetic individuals with BMIs ranging from 28 to 35 kg/m^2.[38] The diet is individualized to provide 5 to 7 kcal/lb actual weight so many women receive 4186 to 5023-kJ (1000- to 1200-kcal) diets and many men receive 5023- to 6698-kJ (1200- to 1600-kcal) diets. These diets provide 55 to 60% of energy from carbohydrate, 50 to 70 g protein, the remainder of energy from fat, and about 15 to 25 g fiber per 4186 kJ (1000 kcal). Patients also are encouraged to walk 2 to 3 miles per day and keep records of food intake, exercise, and blood glucose values. Initially, patients are seen every 2 weeks, then every 3 to 6 weeks during the weight-loss phase, and then every 4 to 8 weeks during the first year after completing the weight-loss phase.[124,125]

LOW-CALORIE AND VERY LOW-CALORIE WEIGHT-LOSS PROGRAMS

Intensive low- or very low-calorie diet programs are the treatment of choice for obese diabetic individuals with BMIs exceeding 35 kg/m^2. Responsible very low-calorie diets programs provide: careful medical evaluation and ongoing medical supervision by trained physicians; a high-quality supplement adequate in protein, carbohydrate, vitamins, and minerals; a weekly program providing the most current behavioral and life-style education; an emphasis on physical activity that enables average participants to achieve and maintain the expenditure of 8372 kJ (2000 kcal) per week in physical activity such as walking; and a maintenance program of 18 or more months.[123,126]

MEDICATION ADJUSTMENT WITH LOW-CALORIE DIETS

Because high energy intakes sustain hyperglycemia and requirements for insulin or sulfonylureas, energy-restricted diets reduce requirements for these medications. Figure 70–8 shows insulin dose reductions over 12 weeks when 20 insulin-treated type II diabetic individuals were given low- or very low-calorie diets providing 2093 to 3349 kJ (500 to 800 kcal) per day. Insulin doses

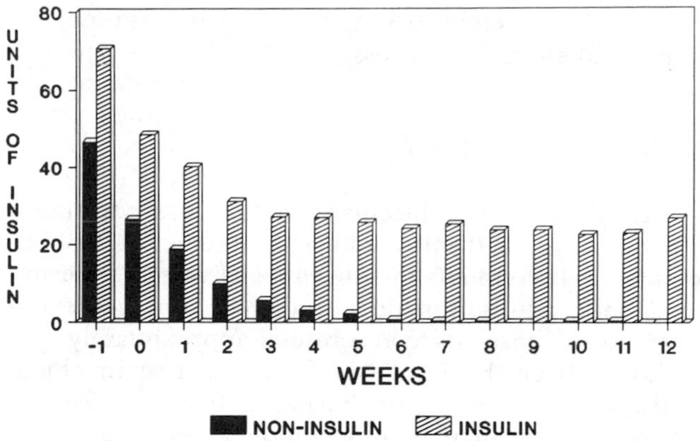

FIGURE 70–8. Reduction of insulin dose for type II individuals treated for 12 weeks with low-calorie diets. Subjects designated "noninsulin" were able to discontinue insulin during the 12-week study.

decreased about 50% during the first week. We routinely decrease insulin doses by 50% when we initiate low- or very low-calorie diets. With less severe degrees of energy restriction, we reduce insulin doses by 10 to 30%, based on prior glycemic control and degree of energy restriction. Subsequent doses are decreased as required based on home glucose monitoring. Similarly, sulfonylurea doses must be reduced when diabetic individuals initiate energy-restricted diets. Usually, we reduce sulfonylurea doses by 50% when initiating low- or very low-calorie diets. Individuals treated with either insulin or sulfonylureas must monitor their glucose when initiating energy-restricted diets to avoid serious hypoglycemia.

EXERCISE

Regular exercise has an important role in weight loss and long-term weight maintenance. Exercise regimens are individualized, but walking is the best exercise for most obese individuals. They can usually begin walking 10 to 20 minutes once or twice daily and increase this gradually over a few weeks to walking 30 minutes twice daily. A treadmill is a good alternative to walking. Swimming and the use of an exercise bicycle or rowing machine are satisfactory alternatives if arthritis or other problems do not favor walking. After agreeing with the patient about an exercise goal, we give each patient a written reminder of this goal. For most individuals, even 75-year-old women with severe degenerative disease of both knees, we can find some way to allow them to increase physical activity by at least 2930 kJ (700 kcal) per week. Exercise not only enhances weight loss, but also lowers blood pressure, improves glycemic control, and improves cardiovascular fitness. Keeping written records of physical activity, blood glucose, and food intake while on weight-loss programs facilitates problem solving and enhances success.

INSULIN THERAPY

Although insulin replacement therapy has been used for about 70 years, the physiologic replacement of insulin for diabetic individuals remains an elusive goal. In lean, nondiabetic adults, insulin is secreted into the portal system in the basal state at a rate of approximately 1 U per hour. After the intake of food, the rise in blood glucose and gastrointestinal hormones triggers a five- to tenfold increase in insulin secretion rates. Basal plus food-related insulin secretion totals approximately 40 U per day for lean, nondiabetic adults. Even though human insulin is available, this physiologic response cannot be mimicked.[127]

Both diet and exercise have major effects on insulin sensitivity in type I and type II diabetic individuals. High-carbohydrate, high-fiber diets increase insulin sensitivity and decrease insulin requirements, whereas high-fat diets have opposite effects.[41,86] For example, a slender 38-year-old farmer required 57 U of insulin per day for good glycemic control on a conventional high-fat (37% of energy), low-carbohydrate (43% of energy), low-fiber diet in 1974.[128] After 16 years of good adherence to a high-carbohydrate (about 60% of energy), high-fiber (about 45 g per day), low-fat (less than 25% of energy) diet, he takes 36 U of insulin daily to maintain fairly good control as an outpatient. Regular physical activity appears to act in a similar manner by increasing skeletal muscle sensitivity to insulin. For example, when a family-practice physician trains for marathons by running over 60 miles per week, he requires only 20 U of insulin daily, but when not in training he requires about 50 U daily. Physiologic considerations, risks, and benefits of exercise are reviewed elsewhere.[129]

The insulin regimen is usually tailored to the nutrition plan and the physical activity of the individual. Some nutritional guidelines for insulin-treated type II diabetic individuals, type I diabetic individuals receiving conventional insulin therapy, and type I diabetic individuals receiving intensive insulin therapy are presented. Table 70–13 compares insulin preparations widely used in the United States.

More than 2 million type II diabetic individuals receive insulin therapy in the United States. Many receive sulfonylurea therapy as well as insulin because this combination decreases the amount of insulin required.[130] About 75% of these insulin-treated type II individuals are obese. When diabetes and obesity occur together, "diabesity," overeating is the major cause of hyperglycemia. Any reduction in energy intake promptly reduces insulin requirements. When starting any weight-reduction diet, reductions in insulin needs should be anticipated.

Insulin therapy in type II diabetes usually supplements endogenous insulin and often is given as a single injection before breakfast or at bedtime. When doses exceed 50 U per day, usually injections are given twice daily before breakfast and the evening meal. Some patients mix NPH insulin and regular insulin for these injections or use premixed combinations of 70% NPH insulin and 30% regular insulin. Most insulin-treated type II diabetic individuals can be managed with three meals and a bedtime snack. The major adverse effects of insulin therapy in type II diabetes are hypoglycemic attacks and weight gain. Because overeating is the major contributor to hyperglycemia, undereating predictably produces hypoglycemia in the insulin-treated, obese type II diabetic individual. Avoiding hypoglycemia and weight gain in these individuals challenges both the physician who counsels the patient on insulin dosage and the dietitian who counsels on diet.

TABLE 70–13. USUAL TIMING OF ACTION OF HUMAN INSULINS

TYPE	ONSET (H)	PEAK (H)	MAXIMUM DURATION (H)
Regular	0.5–1	2–3	4–6
NPH	2–4	4–10	14–18
Lente	3–4	4–12	16–20
Ultralente	6–10	?	20–30

(Modified from American Diabetes Association: Physician's Guide to Insulin-Dependent (Type I) Diabetes: Diagnosis and Treatment. Alexandria, VA, American Diabetes Association, 1988.)

Conventional insulin management in type I diabetes usually involves two daily injections of a mixture of NPH and regular insulin and a meal plan including three meals and two to three snacks. Many individuals can achieve fairly good glycemic control if they self-monitor the blood glucose (SMBG) and make appropriate adjustments in food intake, physical activity, and insulin doses based on their blood glucose level.[131] Because most type I diabetic individuals do not adjust their own insulin doses based on twice-daily SMBG, the energy intakes at meals and snacks need to be consistent from day to day. Most of these individuals benefit from using a meal plan based on exchanges.

Intensive insulin therapy is now used more widely by type I diabetic individuals and is the treatment of choice for a majority of these individuals. The elements of an intensive therapy program include: multiple daily injections of insulin or use of an insulin infusion pump; multiple SMBG daily; careful balance of food intake, physical activity, and insulin dose through self-monitoring and self-adjustment of these parameters; careful and frequent coaching and support by the health-care team.[131] The diet plan for these individuals is highly tailored to their needs, and patients need to have the skills to make daily adjustments in food intake in response to blood glucose values and physical activity.

ORAL HYPOGLYCEMIC AGENTS

Currently, sulfonylureas are the only oral hypoglycemic agents available in the United States. The sulfonylureas lower blood glucose principally by stimulating insulin secretion from the pancreatic beta cells. These agents also may enhance peripheral sensitivity to insulin by unknown mechanisms. Persons of normal weight and obese individuals who develop diabetes after age 40, those who have had diabetes for less than 5 years, or those whose diabetes is well controlled on 20 U of insulin for lean persons or 40 U for obese persons are likely to respond well to sulfonylurea agents.

Nearly 40% of type II diabetic individuals take sulfonylureas; cholorpropamide, glipizide, and glyburide account for 75% of the market.[1] The two second-generation sulfonylureas are the preferred agents for initiating therapy. All sulfonylureas have the same mechanism of action, but they differ in potency, duration of action, and metabolic fate. The second-generation agents, glipizide and glyburide, are more potent than the first-generation agents, have fewer side effects, and may have other advantages.[1] A significant disadvantage of sulfonylureas is the tendency for individuals to gain weight as they achieve good glycemic control.

The combination of insulin and sulfonylureas is widely used for type II diabetes because it lower insulin requirements and frequently improves glycemic control. Theoretically, the sulfonylureas increase peripheral sensitivity to insulin and reduce hyperinsulinemia.[132] When insulin doses exceed 70 to 100 U per day for obese type II diabetic individuals, we incorporate sulfonylureas into the regimen.

Diet and exercise retain central importance in the management of type II diabetes. Our experience indicates that approximately three fourths of type II individuals treated with insulin, sulfonylureas, or the combination can be managed with diet and exercise alone. Whether insulin or sulfonylureas are used or not, overeating is the major cause of hyperglycemia in type II diabetes; a mildly energy-restricted diet generous in complex carbohydrate and fiber and restricted in fat almost universally improves glycemic control as it facilitates weight loss.

EDUCATION AND COUNSELING

Nutrition education and counseling are central to the control of diabetes. Both are ongoing processes with the ultimate goal of positive behavioral change.[133] Unfortunately, many diabetic individuals do not follow their prescribed diet plan because they have not received adequate education or they lack the required skills. This low success rate has led to a degree of therapeutic nihilism. Some physicians believe that nutrition counseling is a waste of time, and many dietitians are frustrated because of the patient's poor dietary adherence, attitudes that often undermine the program's effectiveness. When the entire health-care team is enthusiastic and supportive of a nutrition plan, diabetic individuals can change their eating patterns and closely adhere to a diet plan. Approximately 70% of a group of diabetic individuals adhered in a good or excellent manner to a high-fiber maintenance diet for almost 2 years; only 5% demonstrated poor adherence.[91]

The team approach to diabetes management enhances effectiveness. Successful control of diabetes requires a partnership between the patient and the health-care team. The core health-care team includes a physician, dietitian, or nutritionist, and nurse educator; a pharmacist, social worker, psychologist, physical therapist, podiatrist, and exercise physiologist may complement the core team. The core team acts as coaches who train and assist the patient. Multiple sessions with different team members are required. The physician and nurse must reinforce the message of the dietitian, just as each team member must reinforce any aspect of the diabetes-care program when the opportunity occurs. Education and management of diabetes have become oriented more toward prevention and less toward crisis intervention. Realizing that teaching is not synonymous with education, more professionals are interacting with patients to transmit knowledge that leads to behavioral changes. A successful educational approach presents basic "survival" skills initially, followed by ongoing in-depth continuing education. Diabetes education, though time consuming, is cost effective in achieving the long-term goals of diabetes management.

The individualized nutrition plan is a key element of the diabetes education program. Usually, the physician introduces the plan by discussing the role of diet in diabetes management and by outlining its critical features. The dietitian then collects information to tailor the diet to the patient. Whereas group sessions strengthen learning, the dietitian must provide individual instruction for each patient and others involved in meal preparation. A minimum of two sessions is necessary to initiate diet instruction, and follow-up visits are critical. Ideally, the patient with newly diagnosed diabetes should receive 6 to 12 hours of nutritional education. Instruction sessions should be short but frequent, allowing the patient to assimilate new information, ask questions, and test this information.

Many hospitals and group practices channel the expertise of health-care team members from different disciplines into diabetes classes. Table 70–14 lists some important topics for diabetes nutrition education programs. The American Association of Diabetes Educators also serves as an excellent resource. High-priority items for discussion in a diabetes class include: (1) a description of diabetes, its inheritance, pathogenesis, and aggravating factors such as obesity; (2) meal planning to achieve optimal glucose and lipid levels; (3) the role of exercise in diabetes control and good health; (4) medications, including insulin and oral hypoglycemic agents; (5) the importance of monitoring blood glucose and/or

TABLE 70–14. DIABETES NUTRITION EDUCATION TOPICS

SURVIVAL SKILLS
Relation of food to insulin and activity
Importance of good nutrition in the control of blood glucose and lipid levels
Necessity of maintaining normal weight
Types and amounts of food in meal plan
Modification of food intake during brief illnesses
IN-DEPTH COUNSELING
Meal planning
Types of nutrients, their functions, relation to insulin, and effect on blood glucose and lipid levels
Calorie level of meal plan and percentages of carbohydrate, protein, and fat
Food sources of fiber
Importance of reducing total fat, saturated fat, and cholesterol in the diet
Relation of sodium to hypertension
Proper serving sizes
Changes in food intake based on activity level
Eating out and special occasions
Label reading and grocery shopping
Use of sweeteners, alcohol, and "dietetic" foods
Food modifications for other disorders
Incorporation of favorite recipes

(Adapted from Franz, M., Krosnick, A., Maschak-Carey, B.J., et al.: Goals for Diabetes Education. Chicago, American Diabetes Association, 1986.)

urine glucose and ketones; (6) acute complications such as hyperglycemia and hypoglycemia; (7) psychosocial adjustments; (8) health habits including foot care and smoking cessation; (9) guidelines to delay or prevent long-term complications; (10) community resources; and (11) benefits and use of health-care systems.[131] Effective diabetes education involves communication between experienced and empathetic health professionals and diabetic individuals.

INDIVIDUALIZATION

To be effective in the long term, the health-care team must individually tailor the nutrition plan. Readily available, preprinted diet sheets provide clues to changes in eating habits, but they allow no flexibility and are doomed to eventual failure. Although the effects of diet components such as carbohydrate and fat have been extensively studied, implementing the diet has received much less attention. The best nutrition plans will not work if they are not followed.

Initially, team members must realistically assess the motivation and capabilities of each patient and the family or support group. An optimistic approach is imperative; previous failures do not necessarily predict failure with a nutrition plan at this point. The individual may be unable to learn an exchange system and should be taught a "no-added-sugar" plan. Shortly after the diagnosis of diabetes, some individuals are best taught a simplified "survival" diet, with more detailed nutritional education provided when they are better able to cope with their condition.

After initial evaluation, the dietitian assesses exercise habits, work schedule, socioeconomic level, living situation, and past eating habits. Diet recalls, food records, or food-frequency checklists provide useful information. A history of food eaten in the past 24 hours is a practical way to estimate energy intake and percentage contribution of carbohydrate, protein, and fat. A 7-day food-frequency survey offers a better overview of food intake. To obtain accurate information, the interviewer should ask nonjudgmental questions. Finally, food preferences are elicited. Information about prior food habits forms the foundation for building a solid nutrition plan.

Desirable body weight estimations are made during the initial nutrition assessment. After obtaining a weight history (lightest and heaviest adult weights, recent weight changes, prior use of weight-reducing regimens), we often ask individuals how much they would like to weigh. Ideally, the individuals identify "good" weight goals, and we avoid designating a weight they consider unrealistic. Desirable body weight estimations from tables or formulas provide guidance in setting weight goals. The diabetic individual and dietitian work together to develop targets for short- and long-term weight. The simple process of establishing an estimate of desirable body weight signals to diabetic individuals that the management of their condition is a partnership venture.

Developing the specific nutrition plan is the next step. Based on the available information, the dietitian and physician decide which nutrition strategy best suits the individual. For some, a plan avoiding sucrose and foods rich in sugars works best. Simplified educational materials have been developed for this purpose.[134] For others, a plan using food exchanges is more appropriate. Some individuals are good candidates for high-fiber diets. Once the team establishes a basic plan, it must be modified for other conditions such as hyperlipidemia, congestive heart failure, or weight loss.

Tailoring the diet to the specific individual is probably the most difficult task in the management of nutrition in diabetes. In doing so, the dietitian considers the treatment regimen (frequency and type of insulin injections or use of oral hypoglycemic agents), as well as other factors. The individualized nutrition plan should be as compatible as possible with the food habits and life style of the patient. However, an effective nutrition plan usually requires change. The dietitian's goal is to develop the most therapeutically effective plan and to train the diabetic individual and support group to put this plan into practice.

FOOD EXCHANGES

Flexibility has slowly emerged as an integral part of the diabetes nutrition plan. The American Diabetes Association and American Dietetic Association Exchange Lists for Meal Planning were first released in 1950 and have remained the most acceptable, universal method of meal planning. To better reflect current nutrition recommendations for people with diabetes, these exchanges were revised in 1986.[135] Other specialized exchange plans have been developed based upon the same principles.[136] Exchange-based nutrition plans provide flexibility and choice while maintaining consistency from day to day.

Exchange groups include foods of similar nutrient composition; all serving sizes or portions in one exchange provide similar amounts of energy, carbohydrate, protein, and fat. Using an exchange diet, an individual chooses a certain number of items from each food group daily. Because each exchange group includes many different foods, the diet can be quite varied.

Although several methods of diet instruction are available, exchange nutrition plans are widely used by health professionals. When individuals change health-care providers, use of a universally understood nutrition plan facilitates communication and continuity of care.

STEP-BY-STEP GUIDE TO EXCHANGE DIET CALCULATIONS

1. Estimate energy requirements. For weight maintenance, tables or diet histories provide guidance. As a rough approximation, allow 10 to 12 kcal per pound (current weight) for sedentary adults, 13 to 15 kcal per pound for moderately active adults, and 16 to 20 kcal per pound for very active adults.[41] This estimation may be revised at a following visit. For weight reduction, eliminate approximately 500 kcal daily for a weight loss of roughly 1 lb per week. Weight loss can be enhanced by exercise.
2. Distribute energy intake between carbohydrate, protein and fat. Carbohydrate usually contributes 55 to 60% of energy intake, protein contributes 12 to 20% and fat provides the balance (less than 30%).
3. Convert energy to grams by dividing calories by conversion factors: 4 cal/g protein and carbohydrate, 9 cal/g fat. For example, a 2000-kcal diet to provide 58% carbohydrate, 15% protein, and 27% fat would have:

$$58\% \text{ carbohydrate} = 1160 \text{ kcal or } 290 \text{ g} \quad (1160 \div 4 = 290)$$

$$15\% \text{ protein} = 300 \text{ kcal or } 75 \text{ g} \quad (300 \div 4 = 75)$$

$$27\% \text{ fat} = 540 \text{ kcal or } 60 \text{ g} \quad (540 \div 9 = 60)$$

4. Set the number of servings from each exchange group to provide the desired grams of carbohydrate, protein, and fat. With experience, it becomes easy to estimate the number of exchanges required to approximate the target amounts. Food preferences are also incorporated at this stage. Table 70–15 illustrates a worksheet used to develop an exchange meal plan for the foregoing sample 2000-kcal diet, based on lean meat and skim milk. On the bottom line, list the target grams of carbohydrate, protein, and fat. Estimate the number of exchanges needed to meet the target amounts by assigning servings of starch/bread, vegetables, fruits, and milk to meet the carbohydrate target. Add the meat and substitutes required to meet the protein target. Finally, add fat. Many alternative meal plans can be developed, including those without milk for the lactose intolerant and those without meat for vegetarians.
5. Assign exchanges to meals and snacks. We routinely develop meal plans to include three meals and an evening snack. For most persons taking insulin, midmorning and midafternoon snacks are needed. Distribute energy intake according to these guidelines:

TABLE 70–15. WORKSHEET FOR DEVELOPING 2000-KCAL EXCHANGE MEAL PLAN

EXCHANGE	SERVINGS	ENERGY (KCAL)	CARBOHYDRATE (G)	PROTEIN (G)	FAT (G)
Starch/Bread	8	640	120	24	trace
Meat and substitutes	3	165	—	21	9
Vegetables	7	175	35	14	—
Fruit	7	420	105	—	—
Milk	2	180	24	16	trace
Fat	10	450	—	—	50
TOTAL	—	2030	284	75	59
TARGET	—	2000	290	75	60

the three main meals should provide at least 65% of energy intake, whereas snacks provide up to 35%. Breakfast has 20 to 30%, the noon meal 20 to 35%, and the evening meal 25 to 40% of energy intake. Snacks provide 0 to 15% at midmorning, 0 to 15% at midafternoon, and 0 to 15% in the evening. Insulin-treated individuals should be taught methods of increasing their food intake in response to exercise or hypoglycemia.

6. As an optional sixth step, compute the fiber content of the diet. Based on fiber values developed for the high-carbohydrate high-fiber (HCF) exchange list,[137] the diet example provides 18 g of fiber from starches and breads, at least 12 g from vegetables and 15 g from fruits for a total of at least 45 g. This is a generous-fiber diet; higher fiber intakes can be attained using the HCF exchanges.

In conclusion, an individualized nutrition plan is vital to the successful management of diabetes. The diabetic individual and the health-care team integrate the nutrition plan into the daily schedule of activities to match the available insulin. The diet, physical activities, levels of stress, and available insulin (endogenous or exogenous) change daily. The diabetic individual needs information, education, motivation, and experience to respond to these changes. The health-care team should provide education, encouragement, and coaching in an empathetic manner to help the diabetic individual integrate diet, exercise, and medication to achieve blood glucose goals from day to day. Both short-term and long-term considerations affect the nutrition plan. Feeling good and avoiding trouble, while desirable attributes, should not lull the diabetic individual or the health-care team into accepting undesirable nutrition practices. Achieving good glycemic control, having desirable serum lipoprotein levels, and reducing risks for metabolic, microvascular, and atherosclerotic complications are the key goals of the diabetes nutrition plan.

REFERENCES

1. Gerich, J.E.: N. Engl. J. Med., *321:*1231–1245, 1989.
2. National Diabetes Advisory Board: Sixth Annual Report. NIH Publication No. 84–1587. Bethesda, MD, United States Department of Health and Human Services, 1984.
3. Anonymous: JDF Int. Countdown, *9:*9, 1988.
4. Raskin, P., Pietri, A.O., Unger, R., et al.: N. Engl. J. Med., *309:*1546–1550, 1983.
5. Wood, F.C., Jr., Bierman, E.L.: Nutr. Today, *7:*4–12, 1972.
6. Rollo, J.: A General View of this History, Nature and Appropriate Treatment of Diabetes Mellitus. London, T. Gillet for C. Dilly, 1798.
7. Allen, F.M.: JAMA, *63:*639–643, 1914.
8. Geyelin, H.R.: JAMA, *104:*1203–1208, 1935.
9. Sansum, W.D., Blatherwick, N.R., Bowden, R.: JAMA, *86:*178–181, 1926.
10. Rabinowitch, I.M.: Can. Med. Assoc. J., *33:*136–140, 1935.
11. Kempner, W., Peschel, R.L., Schlayer, C.: Postgrad. Med. J., *24:*359–371, 1958.
12. Fajans, S.S., Rifkin, H., Porte, D., Jr.: Diabetes Mellitus. 4th Ed. New York, Elsevier, 1990.
13. American Diabetes Association: Physician's Guide to Insulin-dependent (Type I) Diabetes: Diagnosis and Treatment. Alexandria, VA, American Diabetes Association, 1988.
14. Eisenbarth, G.S.: N. Engl. J. Med., *314:*1360–1368, 1986.
15. DeFronzo, R.A., Ferrannini, E., Koivisto, V.: Am. J. Med., *74(Suppl. 1):*52–81, 1983.
16. Reaven, G.M. (Ed.): Am. J. Med., *74(Suppl. 1):*1–112, 1983.
17. American Diabetes Association: Physician's Guide to Non-insulin-Dependent (Type II) Diabetes: Diagnosis and Treatment. 2nd Ed. Alexandria, VA, American Diabetes Association, 1988.
18. National Diabetes Data Group: Diabetes, *28:*1039–1057, 1979.
19. Singer, D.E., Coley, C.M., Samet, J.H., et al.: Ann. Intern. Med., *110:*125–137, 1989.
20. Genuth, S.M.: Quoted by Cahill, G.F., Jr. *In* Harrison's Principles of Internal Medicine. 9th Ed. New York, McGraw-Hill, 1980.
21. Anderson, J.W.: Nutrition management of diabetes mellitus. *In* Modern Nutrition in Health and Disease. 7th Ed. Edited by M.E. Shils and V.R. Young. Philadelphia, Lea & Febiger, 1988.
22. Khardori, R., Soler, N.G.: Am. J. Med., *77:*889–904, 1984.
23. Gerich, J.E., Cryer, P., Rizza, R.A.: Metabolism, *29:*1165–1175, 1980.
24. Anderson, J.W. Hyperlipidemia and diabetes: nutrition considerations. *In* Nutrition and Diabetes. Edited by C. Peterson and L. Jovanovic. New York, Alan R. Liss, 1985.
25. Greene, D.A., Lattimer, S.A., Sima, A.A.F.: N. Engl. J. Med., *316:*599–606, 1987.
26. Brownlee, M., Cerami, A., Vlassara, H.: N. Engl. J. Med., *318:*1315–1322, 1988.
27. Camerini-Davalos, R.A., Velasco, C., Glasser, M., et al.: N. Engl. J. Med., *309:*1551–1556, 1983.
28. Harate, Y.: Ann. Intern. Med., *107:*546–59, 1987.
29. Pirart, J.: Diabete Metab., *3:*97–107, 1977.
30. Kannel, W.B.: Am. Heart J., *110:*1100–1107, 1985.
31. Brand, F.N., Abbott, R.D., Kannel, W.B.: Diabetes, *38:*504–509, 1989.
32. Christlieb, A.R., Warram, J.H., Krolewski, A.S., et al.: Diabetes, *30(Suppl.2):*90–96, 1981.
33. Working Group on Hypertension in Diabetes: Arch. Intern. Med., *147:*830–842, 1987.
34. Howard, B.V.: J. Lipid Res., *28:*613–628, 1987.
35. Stout, R.W.: Diabetes Care, *13:*631–654, 1990.
36. Colwell, J.A., Winocour, P.D., Lopes-Virella, M., et al.: Am. J. Med., *75:*67–79, 1983.
37. Colwell, J.A., Winocour, P.D., Holushka, P.V.: Diabetes, *32(Suppl.2):*14–19, 1983.

38. Anderson, J.W., Geil, P.B.: Am. J. Med., *85(Suppl. 5A)*:159–165, 1988.
39. Anderson, J.W., Deakins, D.A., Floore, T.L., et al.: Crit. Rev. Food Sci. Nutr., *29*:95–147, 1990.
40. Zeller, K., Whittaker, E., Sullivan, L., et al.: N. Engl. J. Med., *324*:78–84, 1990.
41. Anderson, J.W., Gustafson, N.J., Bryant, C.A., et al.: J. Am. Diet. Assoc., *87*:1189–1197, 1987.
42. Stone, D.B., Connor, W.E.: Diabetes, *12*:127–135, 1963.
43. Weinsier, R.L., Seeman, A., Herrera, G.: Ann. Intern. Med., *80*:332–341, 1974.
44. Brunzell, J.D., Lerner, R.L., Hazzard, W.R., et al.: N. Engl. J. Med., *284*:521–524, 1971.
45. Anderson, J.W.: High-carbohydrate diet effects on glucose and triglyceride metabolism of normal and diabetic men. *In* Metabolic Effects of Utilizable Carbohydrates. Edited by S. Reiser. New York, Marcel Dekker, 1982.
46. Coulston, A.M., Hollenbeck, C.B., Swislocki, A.C.M., et al.: Diabetes Care, *12*:94–101, 1989.
47. Anderson, J.W., Chen, W.L.: Am. J. Clin. Nutr., *32*:346–363, 1979.
48. Anderson, J.W., Bryant, C.A.: Am. J. Gastroenterol., *81*:898–906, 1986.
49. Anderson, J.W., Story, L.J., Zettwoch, N.C., et al.: Diabetes Care, *12*:337–344, 1989.
50. Crapo, P.A., Kolterman, O.G., Olefsky, J.M.: Diabetes Care, *3*:575–581, 1980.
51. American Diabetes Association: Diabetes Care, *10*:126–132, 1987.
52. Crapo, P.A., Reaven, G.M., Olefsky, J.: Diabetes, *25*:741–747, 1976.
53. Jenkins, D.J.A., Wolever, T.M.S., Taylor, R.H., et al.: Am. J. Clin. Nutr., *34*:362–366, 1981.
54. Jenkins, D.J.A., Wolever, T.M.S., Jenkins, A.L.: Diabetes Care, *11*:149–159, 1988.
55. Jenkins, D.J.A., Wolever, T.M.S., Jenkins, A.L., et al.: Diabetologia, *24*:257–264, 1983.
56. Haber, G.B., Heaton, K.W., Murphy, D., et al.: Lancet, *2*:679–682, 1977.
57. Anderson, J.W.: Clin. Nutr., *3*:59–64, 1984.
58. Anderson, J.W., Bridges, S.R.: Proc. Soc. Exp. Biol. Med., *177*:372–376, 1984.
59. Nuttall, F.Q.: Diabetes Care, *6*:197–207, 1983.
60. Anderson, J.W.: J. Am. Coll. Nutr., *8*:615–675, 1989.
61. Joslin, E.P.: The Treatment of Diabetes Mellitus. 4th Ed. Philadelphia, Lea & Febiger, 1928.
62. Paisey, R.B., Arredondo, L.N., Villalobos, A., et al.: Diabetes Care, *7*:421–427, 1984.
63. West, K.M., Ahuja, M.M.S., Bennett, P.H., et al.: Diabetes Care, *6*:361–369, 1983.
64. Randle, P.J., Garland, P.B., Hales, C.N., et al.: Lancet, *1*:785–789, 1963.
65. Heine, R.J., Mulder, C., Popp-Snijders, C., et al.: Am. J. Clin. Nutr., *49*:448–456, 1989.
66. Garg, A., Bonanome, G., Grundy, S.M., et al.: N. Engl. J. Med., *319*:829–834, 1988.
67. Phillipson, B.E., Rothrock, D.W., Connor, W.E., et al.: N. Engl. J. Med., *312*:1210–1216, 1985.
68. von Schacky, C., Fischer, S., Weber, P.C.: J. Clin. Invest., *76*:1626–1631, 1985.
69. Popp-Snijders, C., Schouten, J.A., Heine, R.J., et al.: Diabetes Res., *4*:141–147, 1987.
70. Glauber, H., Wallace, P., Griver, K., et al.: Ann. Intern. Med., *108*:663–668, 1988.
71. Sorisky, A., Robbins, D.C.: Diabetes Care, *12*:302–304, 1989.
72. Crouse, J.W., Grundy, S.M.: Metabolism, *28*:994–1000, 1979.
73. Geil, P.B., Lawrence, S.R., Anderson, J.W.: J. Am. Diet. Assoc., *89*:A-9, 1989.
74. Grundy, S.M., Anastasia, J.V., Kesaniemi, Y.A., et al.: Am. J. Clin. Nutr., *44*:620–629, 1986.
75. Trowell, H.C.: Non-infective disease. *In* Disease of Africa. London, Edward Arnold. 1960.
76. Walker, A.R.P.: S. Afr. Med. J., *35*:114–115, 1961.
77. Walker, A.R.P., Walker, B.F., Richardson, B.D.: Lancet, *2*:51–52, 1970.
78. Trowell, H.C.: Diabetes, *24*:762–766, 1975.
79. Trowell, H.: Am. J. Clin. Nutr., *31*:1489–1490, 1978.
80. Jenkins, D.J.A., Leeds, A.R., Gassull, M.A., et al.: Lancet, *2*:172–174, 1976.
81. Kiehm, T.G., Anderson, J.W., Ward, K.: Am. J. Clin. Nutr., *29*:895–899, 1976.
82. Ebeling, P., Yki-Jarvinen, H., Aro, A., et al.: Am. J. Clin. Nutr., *48*:98–103, 1988.
83. Hagander, B., Asp, N.-G., Efendic, S., et al.: Am. J. Clin. Nutr., *47*:852–858, 1988.
84. O'Dea, K., Traianedes, K., Ireland, P., et al.: J. Am. Diet. Assoc., *89*:1076–1086, 1989.
85. Tagliaferro, V., Cassader, M., Bozzo, C., et al.: Diabete Metabol., *11*:380–385, 1985.
86. Fukagawa, N.K., Anderson, J.W., Hageman, G., et al.: Am. J. Clin. Nutr., *52*:524–528, 1990.
87. Anderson, J.W., Zeigler, J.A., Deakins, D.A., et al.: Am. J. Clin. Nutr., *54*:936–943, 1991.
88. DeCosse, J.J., Miller, H., Lesser, M.L.: J. Natl. Cancer Inst., *81*:1290–1297, 1989.
89. Behall, K.M., Scholfield, D.J., McIvor, M.E., et al.: Diabetes Care, *12*:357–364, 1989.
90. Rattan, J., Levin, N., Graff, E., et al.: J. Clin. Gastroenterol., *3*:389–393, 1981.
91. Anderson, J.W., Gustafson, N.J.: Diabetes Educator, *15*:429–34, 1989.
92. Talbot, J.M., Fisher, K.D.: Diabetes Care, *1*:231–240, 1978.
93. Butchko, H., Kotsonis, F.N.: Comment. Toxicol., *3*:253–278, 1989.
94. Liang, Y., Steinbach, G., Maier, V., et al.: Horm. Metab. Res., *19*:285–289, 1987.
95. American Diabetes Association: Diabetes Care, *13*:26–27, 1990.
96. American Dietetic Association: J. Am. Diet. Assoc., *87*:1690–1694, 1987.
97. United States Department of Health and Human Services, Public Health Services: The Surgeon General's Report on Nutrition and Health. DHHS (PHS) Publication No. 88-50210. Washington, D.C., U.S. Government Printing Office, 1988.
98. Kinmonth, A.L., Angus, R.M., Jenkins, P.A., et al.: Arch. Dis. Child., *57*:187–194, 1982.
99. Brink, S.J.: Diabetes Care, *11*:192–200, 1988.
100. Morley, J.E., Mooradian, A.D., Rosenthal, M.J., et al.: Am. J. Med., *83*:533, 1987.
101. Wilson, P.W.F., Anderson, K.M., Kannel, W.B.: Am. J. Med., *80(Suppl. 5A)*:3–9, 1986.
102. Lipson, L.G.: Am. J. Med., *80(Suppl. 5A)*:10–21, 1986.
103. Heins, J.M.: Diabetes Care Educ. Newslett., *11*:1–19, 1990.
104. Jovanovic, L., Peterson, C.M.: Diabetes, *34(Suppl.2)*:21–23, 1985.

105. Jovanovic, L., Peterson, C.M.: Acta Endocrinol., *277:*77–80, 1986.
106. Institute of Medicine: Nutrition During Pregnancy. Part I: Weight Gain. Part II: Nutrient Supplements. Washington, D.C., National Academy Press, 1990.
107. Ney, D., Hollingsworth, D.R., Counsins, L.: Diabetes Care, *5:*529–533, 1981.
108. Ferris, A.M., Dalidowitz, C.K., Ingardia, C.M., et al.: J. Am. Diet. Assoc., *88:*317–322, 1988.
109. Mogensen, C.E., Christensen, C.K.: N. Engl. J. Med., *311:*89–93, 1984.
110. Wiseman, M., Bognetti, E., Dodds, R., et al.: Diabetologia, *30:*154–159, 1987.
111. Hostetter, T.H., Meyer, T.W., Renneke, H.G., et al.: Kidney Int., *30:*509–517, 1986.
112. Collins, D.M., Coffman, T.M., Ruiz, P., et al.: J. Lab. Clin. Med., *114:*545–553, 1989.
113. Ihle, B.U., Becker, G.J., Whitworth, J.A., et al.: N. Engl. J. Med., *321:*1773–1777, 1989.
114. Garg, A., Grundy, S.M.: Diabetes Care, *13:*153–169, 1990.
115. Anderson, J.W., Smith, B.M., Geil, P.B.: Postgrad. Med., *88:*157–168, 1990.
116. Anderson, J.W., Gustafson, N.J.: Postgrad. Med., *82:*40–50, 1987.
117. Anderson, J.W., Gustafson, N.J.: Am. J. Clin. Nutr., *48:*749–753, 1988.
118. Anderson, J.W., Gustafson, N.J., Spencer, D.B., et al.: Am. J. Clin. Nutr., *51:*1013–1019, 1990.
119. Anderson, J.W., Spencer, D.B., Hamilton, C.C., et al.: Am. J. Clin. Nutr., *52:*495–499, 1990.
120. Anderson, J.W., Zettwoch, N., Feldman, T., et al.: Arch. Intern. Med., *148:*292–296, 1988.
121. Anderson, J.W.: Can. Med. Assoc. J., *123:*975–979, 1980.
122. Anderson, J.W., Tietyen-Clark, J.: Am. J. Gastroenterol., *81:*907–919, 1986.
123. Anderson, J.W., Brinkman, V., Hamilton, C.C.: Am. J. Clin. Nutr. In press.
124. Anderson, J.W.: High-fiber diets for obese diabetic men on insulin therapy: short-term and long-term effects. *In* Dietary Fiber and Obesity. Edited by G.V. Vahouny. New York, Alan R. Liss, 1985.
125. Anderson, J.W., Gustafson, N.J.: Int. Med. Specialist, *7:*100–117, 1986.
126. Anderson, J.W., Hamilton, C.C., Crown-Weber, E., et al.: J. Am. Diet. Assoc., *91:*1582–1584, 1991.
127. Zinman, B.: N. Engl. J. Med., *321:*363–370, 1989.
128. Anderson, J.W., Ward, K.: Am. J. Clin. Nutr., *32:*2312–2321, 1979.
129. Vranic, M., Wasserman, D., Bukowiecki, L.: *In* Diabetes Mellitus. Edited by H. Rifkin and D. Porte, Jr. New York, Elsevier, 1990.
130. Genuth, S.: Diabetes Care, *13:*1240–1264, 1990.
131. Hirsch, I.B., Farkas-Hirsch, R., Skyler, J.S.: Diabetes Care, *13:*1265–1283, 1990.
132. Leibovitz, H.E., Pasmantier, R.M.: Diabetes Care, *13:*667–675, 1990.
133. Franz, M., Krosnick, A., Maschak-Carey, B.J., et al.: Goals for Diabetes Education. Chicago, American Diabetes Association, 1986.
134. American Diabetic Association and American Dietetic Association: Healthy Food Choices. Chicago, 1986.
135. American Diabetes Association and American Dietetic Association: Exchange Lists for Meal Planning. Chicago, 1986.
136. HCF Diabetes Foundation: The HCF Exchanges: The High-Carbohydrate High-Fiber (HCF) Nutrition Plan. Lexington, KY, 1987.
137. Anderson, J.W.: Plant Fiber in Foods. Lexington, KY, HCF Nutrition Research Foundation, 1990.

CHAPTER 71

Nutrition, Diet, and Hypertension

Theodore A. Kotchen and Jane Morley Kotchen

Hypertension is a major risk factor for the development of cardiovascular disease, and as many as 58 million people in the United States have elevated blood pressure or are taking antihypertensive medications.[1] In more than 90% of hypertensive individuals, there is no specific identifiable cause for the elevation of arterial pressure; these individuals are considered to have primary or essential hypertension. A variety of renal, endocrine/metabolic, and vascular disorders accounts for the blood pressure elevation in approximately 10% of hypertensives.

In both normotensive and hypertensive individuals, cardiovascular disease risk is related to the height of both the systolic and diastolic blood pressures.[2,3] A pragmatic definition of hypertension is that level of blood pressure at which a therapeutic intervention will reduce the risk of subsequent cardiovascular disease. It was clearly demonstrated over 20 years ago that antihypertensive drug therapy decreases the risk of cardiovascular disease morbidity and mortality in individuals with diastolic blood pressures greater than 104 mm Hg.[4] However, approximately two-thirds of hypertensive Americans have "mild" hypertension, arbitrarily defined as a diastolic blood pressure in the range of 90 to 104 mm Hg. Mild hypertension carries double the baseline risk of cardiovascular disease over that of normotension. In general, results of clinical trials document that drug therapy of mild hypertension results in a statistically significant decrease of cardiovascular morbidity and mortality. However, only a relatively small percentage of individuals with mild hypertension develop clinically apparent cardiovascular disease over a relatively prolonged period; particularly in these patients, there are concerns about potential adverse consequences versus benefits of long-term antihypertensive drug therapy.

An understanding of the relationship between diet and blood pressure has important implications for the prevention and treatment of hypertension. With appropriate dietary modifications, it may be possible to treat hypertensive patients with fewer drugs and with lower doses; in a significant percentage of hypertensives, particularly patients with mild hypertension, dietary modifications may totally obviate the need for drug therapy. In hypertensives whose blood pressures have been controlled with medications, weight loss or NaCl restriction more than doubles the likelihood of maintaining normal blood pressure after withdrawal of drug therapy.[5] Additionally, in individuals with normal and "high-normal" blood pressures, diet modifications may decrease the long-term risk of developing cardiovascular disease and hypertension.

The purpose of this chapter is to describe the relationships between diet and blood pressure and to review the physiologic mechanisms by which alterations in nutrient intake affect blood pressure. Dietary recommendations for the primary prevention and treatment of hypertension will also be reviewed.

OBESITY AND HYPERTENSION

An association between obesity and hypertension has been amply documented. Data from cross-sectional studies indicate a direct, linear correlation between body weight (or body mass index) and blood pressure.[6–12] Centrally located body fat is a more important determinant of blood pressure elevation than peripherally located body fat. In longitudinal studies, there is a direct correlation between change in weight and change in blood pressure over time, even when dietary salt intake is held constant.[12–15] The proportion of the prevalence of hypertension attributable to obesity is an important public health question. It has been estimated that 60% of hypertensives are more than 20% overweight.[12] In the National Heart Foundation of Australia Risk Factor Prevalence Survey., approximately one-third of the cases of hypertension was potentially attributable to obesity in men and women aged 25 to 64 years; in men between the ages of 25 and 44 years, two-thirds of hypertension cases were attributable to obesity.[16]

A beneficial impact of weight reduction on blood pressure in hypertensive individuals has clearly been documented in short-term trials. Based on pooling results of controlled dietary intervention trials, it has been estimated that a mean change in body weight of 9.2 kg is associated with 6.3-mm Hg change in systolic blood pressure and a 3.1-mm Hg change in diastolic blood pressure.[12]

Obesity-related hypertension has been variously ascribed to hypervolemia and an increased cardiac output without an appropriate reduction of peripheral resistance, and to increased sympathetic nervous system activity.[17–24]

In the experimental animal and in man, obesity is also associated with resistance to insulin-stimulated glucose uptake, hyperinsulinemia, and hypertriglyceridemia, and it has been suggested that elevated insulin concentrations in some way contribute to obesity-related hypertension.[25–31] Weight loss or exercise training without weight loss enhances insulin sensitivity, decreases plasma insulin concentrations, and lowers blood pressure in obesity-related hypertension.[32–35] Recent reports suggest that nonobese patients with essential hypertension are also resistant to insulin-stimulated glucose uptake, hyperinsulinemic, and relatively hypertriglyceridemic.[36–40] Although its effect may be nonspecific, somatostatin has been reported to lower both plasma insulin and blood pressure in patients with essential hypertension.[41]

Insulin has an antinatriuretic effect due to increased renal tubular reabsorption of sodium in the proximal tubule and increased aldosterone responsiveness to angiotensin II.[42–46] In the dog fed a high-fat diet, increases of blood pressure associated with weight gain are related to sodium retention, which in turn is related to increases of plasma insulin and aldosterone concentrations.[47] Resistance to insulin-stimulated glucose uptake is accompanied by resistance to the antinatriuretic effect of insulin.[31,48]

In both the experimental animal and in man, insulin may increase sympathetic nervous system activity. Acute intravenous infusions of insulin increase cardiac contractility, vascular responses to norepinephrine, plasma catecholamine concentrations, and total peripheral resistance in the absence of hypoglycemia.[49–54] However, the inotropic effect of insulin may or may not depend on adrenergic mechanisms and may be related to pharmacologic rather than to physiologic increases of serum insulin concentrations.[55] In the dog, euglycemic hyperinsulinemia enhances the pressor and aldosterone responses to angiotensin II.[46] In the rat, sucrose and fructose feeding cause a defect in insulin-stimulated glucose utilization and hyperinsulinemia, as well as elevation of arterial pressure.[56–61] Sucrose feeding is also associated with increased sympathetic nervous system activity.[20,57,62–65] Again, resistance to insulin-stimulated glucose uptake is accompanied by resistance to insulin-induced neural stimulation.[66]

TABLE 71–1. PUTATIVE MECHANISMS BY WHICH INSULIN MAY INCREASE ARTERIAL PRESSURE

1. Sodium retention
2. Increased sympathetic nervous system activity
3. Alteration of ion transport in vascular smooth muscle cells
4. Mitogenic effect on vascular smooth muscle cells

Considerable evidence links insulin with ion transport and growth of cells, including cardiovascular cells,[67–72] and these alterations could also contribute to insulin-induced elevations of arterial pressure. Insulin may affect intracellular sodium and calcium concentrations by stimulating Na^+K^+ ATPase activity, by activating the Na^+H^+ antiporter and thus increasing intracellular pH, and by inhibiting sarcolemmal $Ca^{++}Mg^{++}$ ATPase.[73–81] The net effect of these insulin-induced transport alterations would be an elevation of intracellular calcium concentrations.[74,82] Increased intracellular calcium in vascular smooth muscle has been related to increased peripheral resistance,[83] and elevated intracellular calcium has been observed in platelets, erythrocytes and adipocytes of patients with essential hypertension, obese individuals, and both normotensive and hypertensive patients with type II diabetes.[84–88] Additionally, if cell sodium rises, $Ca^{++}Na^+$ antiport activity would decrease, and this would also increase intracellular calcium.[89] Insulin may also increase Ca^{++} influx via voltage-dependent calcium channels, an effect that is potentiated by higher ambient glucose concentrations.[90] In the obese Zucker rat, elevations of arterial pressure are associated with impaired calcium efflux from vascular smooth muscle cells and decreased Ca-ATPase activity and increased intracellular calcium in erythrocytes.[91,92] Increased cytosolic free calcium may also be a factor in inducing insulin resistance associated with hyperinsulinism and/or obesity.[91]

There is unambiguous evidence for increased growth of vascular smooth muscle in small-resistance arteries and arterioles in hypertension,[93,94] and insulin promotes growth of cells, including vascular smooth muscle cells.[95,96] This would increase peripheral resistance. Resistance to insulin-mediated glucose uptake is not accompanied by resistance to the mitogenic effects of insulin.[97,98] The growth-promoting effects of insulin may be linked to increased intracellular cytosolic free calcium.[99] Additionally, activation of the Na^+H^+ antiporter participates in the initiation of cell growth and proliferation and also in the agonist-induced vasoconstriction of vascular smooth muscle cells and glomerular mesangial cells.[100–105] Decreased intracellular pH and activation of the Na^+H^+ antiporter have been observed in human and rat models of hypertensive disease, including obesity-associated hypertension.[106–110]

Alternatively, increased plasma insulin concentrations may not be causally related to hypertension. In obese humans, there is no correlation between plasma insulin and blood pressure.[111] In acute experiments, insulin may reduce vascular resistance despite increases of peripheral sympathetic nerve activity.[112] In the absence of a compensatory increase of plasma catecholamines, insulin has been reported to induce frank hypotension.[113] Insulin may also antagonize the cardiovascular actions of circulating catecholamines.[114] In the euglycemic, normotensive dog with reduced renal mass, infusion of insulin for 7 to 28 days has been reported to cause only a transient retention of sodium, without increases of arterial pressure, plasma catecholamine concentrations, or vascular responsiveness to norepinephrine.[115] These responses to short-term infusions of pharmacologic doses of infused insulin may not reflect the long-term responses to physiologic increases of plasma insulin.

DIETARY SODIUM CHLORIDE AND BLOOD PRESSURE

Evidence for an association between sodium chloride (NaCl) intake and blood pressure is provided by both observational and intervention studies. Among populations, the prevalence of hypertension is related to NaCl intake, although the strength of this association depends on the extremes of salt intake.[116] A recently completed study, Intersalt, describes the relationship between blood pressure and 24-hour urine sodium excretion in over 10,000 individuals at 52 centers around the world.[117] Two principal findings of this study are (1) a difference of 100 mmol (100 mEq) per day in sodium intake is associated with a 2.2 mm Hg difference of systolic blood pressure, and (2) a 100 mmol (100 mEq) per day lower sodium intake attenuates the rise of systolic blood pressure between the ages of 25 and 55 years by 9 mm Hg. Within single populations, correlations of blood pressure with NaCl intake are modest or nonexistent.

Based on results of acute NaCl depletion or acute NaCl loading protocols, it has been estimated that approximately 30 to 50% of hypertensives and a smaller percentage of normotensives are NaCl-sensitive—that is, arterial pressure is decreased by NaCl depletion and/or increased by NaCl loading.[118,119] In relatively short-term intervention trials of the effects of moderate NaCl restriction on blood pressure, the overall reduction of blood pressure is small. Cutler et al. recently summarized the results of 23 published randomized clinical trials of the effect of moderate NaCl restriction on blood pressure[120]; in aggregate, based on a total of 1536 subjects, NaCl restriction resulted in a 4.9 ±1.3 (95% confidence level) mm Hg reduction of systolic blood pressure and a 2.6 ±0.8 mm Hg reduction of diastolic blood pressure in hypertensives and a 1.7 ±1.0 mm Hg reduction of systolic blood pressure and a 1.0 ±0.7 mm Hg reduction of diastolic blood pressure in normotensives. These changes were associated with mean reductions of urine sodium excretion ranging from 16 to 171 mmol per 24 hours for individual trials. A dose-response relationship across trials was found in both normotensives and hypertensives. A dose-response relationship between NaCl restriction and blood pressure has also been observed in a single double-blind, crossover study using three levels of NaCl intake in patients with essential hypertension.[121]

These overall responses mask individual variability of blood pressure responses to NaCl restriction. In clinical trials, NaCl sensitivity of blood pressure is associated with a number of demographic variables, including black race, obesity, older age, and higher levels of blood pressure.[118,119,122] In addition, experimental models provide convincing evidence for a genetic susceptibility and a genetic resistance to the effects of dietary NaCl on arterial pressure. In man, there may also be a genetic susceptibility to NaCl. A familial resemblance of the change of blood pressure in response to salt restriction has been described,[123] and it has recently been suggested that a phenotype of haptoglobin is a marker of NaCl sensitivity.[124]

Several mechanisms for salt sensitivity of blood pressure have been proposed. A decreased capacity of the kidney to excrete sodium may contribute to NaCl-induced elevations of arterial pressure in the susceptible host. The Dahl salt-sensitive (Dahl-S) rat is a well-characterized genetic model of NaCl-sensitive hypertension.[125] In this model, the pressure natriuresis curve (inflow pressure versus sodium excretion) from the isolated kidney is shifted to the right—that is, the kidney of the NaCl-sensitive animal requires a greater pressure to excrete sodium than the kidney from the salt-resistant (Dahl-R) animal does. The development of hypertension in this model appears to be related to the diminished capacity to excrete sodium and fluid retention.[126–129] Similarly, several but not all investigators have reported that NaCl-sensitive hypertensive humans retain more sodium in response to a NaCl load than NaCl-resistant patients do.[130,131]

The sympathetic nervous system and alterations of baroreflex function also contribute to the NaCl-induced elevation of arterial pressure. Sympathetic nervous system activity is increased in several models of NaCl-sensitive hypertension,[132–136] and surgical or chemical sympathectomy protects against the development of hypertension.[137–139] Further, in the Dahl-S rat, dietary NaCl loading potentiates the increment of vascular resistance in response to neural stimulation and increases the rate of basal firing of the splanchnic nerve.[140,141] A high NaCl intake also increases vascular reactivity to norepinephrine in the prehypertensive Dahl-S rat.[142] Impaired baroreflex control of heart rate and peripheral vascular resistance in response to acute alterations of arterial pressure has also been described in the prehypertensive Dahl-S rat.[143–146] Cardiopulmonary baroreflex activity is also impaired in the Dahl-S rat.[147–150] A high-NaCl diet exacerbates impairment of baroreceptor reflex control of heart rate in the Dahl-S rat,[151,152] whereas in the Dahl-R rat, a high-NaCl diet enhances afferent discharge of aortic baroreceptors and augments sympathoinhibitory responses to volume expansion.[153] In the normotensive rat, dog, and rabbit, impaired baroreflex function renders the animal susceptible to NaCl-induced elevations of blood pressure.[154,155]

Increased sympathetic nervous system activity and impaired baroreflex function may also contribute to NaCl sensitivity of blood pressure in man. In NaCl-sensitive normotensives and hypertensives, forearm vascular resistance is inappropriately increased by NaCl loading and plasma and/or urine norepinephrine is not normally suppressed.[150,156–158] In patients with essential hypertension, it has recently been reported that baroreflex function, estimated from the slope of the line relating change in heart rate to change in blood pressure in response to tilt, is enhanced by a high NaCl intake in NaCl-insensitive but not in NaCl-sensitive subjects.[159]

Alterations of ion transport in vascular smooth muscle may also contribute to NaCl sensitivity of blood pressure. Based primarily on studies in circulating blood cells, most but not all evidence suggests that active membrane Na^+ transport is suppressed by a high NaCl intake, and that suppression of sodium transport by a high-NaCl diet may be less prominent in circulating cells of hypertensives than of normotensives.[160–172] Hypertension is also associated with increased red blood cell Li^+Na^+ countertransport and decreased $Na^+K^+/2Cl^-$ cotransport[162,169,170]; increased red cell Li^+Na^+ countertransport may be a marker for NaCl sensitivity of blood pressure.[173] In the Dahl-S rat, there is an acceleration of ouabain-sensitive and ouabain-resistant Rb^+ uptake in vascular smooth muscle,[174] although it has recently been reported that Na^+K^+ pump rates are not altered in red cells of the mature Dahl-S rat.[175] Dietary NaCl loading has been reported to increase intracellular calcium in lymphocytes of NaCl-sensitive humans.[176] Similar to the case in obesity-related hypertension, decreased intracellular pH and activation of the Na^+H^+ antiporter have been observed in the Dahl-S rat.[115–119]

INTERACTION OF DIETARY SALT AND INSULIN RESISTANCE

Similar physiologic mechanisms may account for NaCl sensitivity of blood pressure and for hypertension related to insulin resistance, and insulin resistance/hyperinsulinemia may lead to the development of NaCl sensitivity. Blood pressure of obese individuals tends to be NaCl-sensitive, and insulin resistance may be a predictor of NaCl sensitivity of blood pressure in both obese and nonobese humans.[177]

High-sucrose feeding increases arterial pressure in several normotensive strains of rats and in man.[56,57] Although a high sucrose intake is not associated with increased weight gain in the rat, sucrose feeding causes a defect in insulin-stimulated glucose utilization and hyperinsulinemia.[58] A high sucrose intake potentiates the effect of a high NaCl intake on blood pressure in normotensive and hypertensive rats.[62,178–182] Further, it has recently been reported that a 4-week insulin infusion decreases sodium excretion and increases blood pressure in the NaCl-sensitive spontaneously hypertensive rat (SHR), but not in the NaCl-resistant SHR.[183]

CHLORIDE

The effect of dietary NaCl on blood pressure has generally been attributed to the sodium ion. However, recent evidence indicates that the anion accompanying sodium plays an important role in determining the magnitude of the blood pressure increase in response to a high dietary intake of NaCl.[184] The full expression of NaCl-sensitive hypertension depends on the concomitant administration of both sodium and chloride. In both experimental models of NaCl-sensitive hypertension and in man, blood pressure is not increased by a high dietary sodium intake provided with anions other than chloride, and high chloride intakes without sodium have less effect on blood pressure than NaCl does. The failure of nonchloride sodium salts to produce hypertension may be related to their failure to expand plasma volume.

Although sodium in the diet is generally present as the chloride salt, certain processed foods may contain considerable quantities of nonchloride salts of sodium such as sodium bicarbonate and monosodium glutamate.

POTASSIUM

In societies with high potassium intakes, both mean blood pressure and the prevalence of hypertension tend to be lower than in societies with low potassium intakes.[185–187] Several large surveys have also demonstrated a significant inverse correlation between potassium intake and blood pressure among individuals[117,185]; this inverse association may be particularly prominent in the presence of a high-NaCl diet. However, not all surveys have documented an association between potassium intake and either hypertension prevalence or level of blood pressure. Failure to observe this association may be related to insufficient sample sizes.

More than 50 years ago, Addison reported that a high potassium intake has an antihypertensive effect in humans.[188] More recently, several relatively small clinical trials have shown that an increased potassium intake decreases blood pressure in patients with hypertension.[185–187] Conversely, potassium depletion induced either by diuretics or by a low-potassium diet is associated with an elevation of blood pressure, possibly due to volume expansion.[189,190] The effect of a high potassium intake on blood pressure is more pronounced in blacks than in whites, in individuals consuming a high NaCl intake, and in hypertensives rather than normotensives.[185–191] An increased intake of potassium appears not to effect blood pressure in individuals on a low-NaCl diet,[192] and the blood pressure lowering effect of dietary potassium may be related to its natriuretic capacity. The urine sodium/potassium ratio may be a stronger correlate of blood pressure than either sodium or potassium alone[117,185–187]; in children, the rise of blood pressure with age is directly related to the urine sodium/potassium ratio.[193]

Potassium loading also prevents or ameliorates the development of hypertension in several animal models of genetic and sodium chloride–induced hypertension.[185] In addition to its natriuretic effect, other proposed mechanisms by which a high dietary intake of potassium may lower blood pressure include inhibition of renin release, antagonism of the pressor response to angiotensin II, direct vasodilation, decreased production of the vasoconstrictor thromboxane, and increased production of the vasodilator kallidin.

Recent data suggest that dietary potassium may effect morbidity and mortality, independent of its effect on blood pressure. Unrelated to an effect on blood pressure, a high-potassium diet has been reported to decrease stroke mortality in the stroke-prone SHR and to decrease renal damage in the Dahl-S rat.[194,195] Similarly, in a prospective study in man, the 12-year risk of stroke death was negatively associated with potassium intake, independent of blood pressure.[196]

CALCIUM

Interest in calcium and magnesium was initially provoked by epidemiologic studies suggesting a protective effect of "hard water" on the development of cardiovascular disease. Similar to the case with potassium, within and among populations there is an inverse association between dietary calcium intake and blood pressure, and calcium deficiency is associated with an increased prevalence of hypertension.[197–201]

Most clinical trials evaluating the effect of increased dietary calcium on blood pressure have supplemented the diets of subjects with 25 to 37 mmol (1000 to 1500 mg) of elemental calcium per day. Reductions of blood pressure by an increased calcium intake have been modest and inconsistent, and no gradient of calcium effect or threshold intake level has been identified.[200–204] A low calcium intake may amplify the effects of a high NaCl intake on blood pressure in susceptible individuals, and calcium supplementation has been reported to blunt the effect of a high NaCl intake on blood pressure.[204–206] Hypertensives appear to be more responsive to calcium supplementation than normotensives, particularly patients with low renin hypertension and NaCl-sensitive hypertension. High dietary calcium also preferentially lowers blood pressure or attenuates the development of hypertension in NaCl-sensitive experimental models. In contrast, calcium supplementation may increase blood pressure in patients with high renin or with renin-dependent hypertension, and in experimental models of renin-dependent hypertension.[207]

This interaction of NaCl sensitivity of blood pressure and responsiveness to dietary calcium may provide clues about the mechanism by which dietary calcium affects blood pressure. In both man and the intact normotensive rat, NaCl loading produces hypercalcuria and increases serum concentrations of both parathyroid hormone (PTH) and 1,25-dihydroxy vitamin D. Hypercalcuria, decreased plasma ionized calcium concentrations, and increased PTH concentrations have also been observed in experimental models of NaCl-sensitive hypertension and in patients with low renin hypertension.[207,208] Serum concentrations of 1,25-dihydroxy vitamin D are also increased in the prehypertensive Dahl-S rat and in patients with low-renin essential hypertension. In contrast, vitamin D concentrations are either normal or decreased in the hypertensive SHR, in DOCA-salt hypertension, and in patients with primary aldosteronism.[207]

There is considerable speculation about mechanisms by which these alterations of calcium and calcium-regulating hormones may contribute to hypertension.[207] The following effects of calcium supplementation may contribute to the putative effect of calcium on blood pressure: a diuretic effect, a membrane-stabilizing effect, effects on sympathetic tone, and elevation of circulating levels of the potent vasodilator, calcitonin-gene-related peptide (CGRP). Some studies have focused on a role for elevated PTH in the hypertensive process. PTH may influence neural activity and/or vasoactive hormones either directly or indirectly via changes in serum calcium. PTH may also act as a calcium ionophore and hence provide calcium to the contractile apparatus of vascular smooth muscle. Other studies have emphasized a potential role for vitamin D, especially in NaCl-related hypertension. For example, dietary NaCl loading in essential hypertension increases blood pressure to the extent that it suppresses serum ionized calcium and stimulates serum 1,25-dihydroxy vitamin D. Furthermore, calcium supplementation has been reported to blunt NaCl-induced hypertension and to suppress endogenous 1,25-dihydroxy vitamin D levels. The ability of dietary calcium to lower blood pressure in elderly hypertensive patients is best correlated with initial 1,25-dihydroxy vitamin D levels.

Thus, NaCl-sensitive hypertension may be a calcium-losing state, resulting in secondary hyperparathyroidism. Calcium supplementation may reduce blood pressure by correcting this calcium deficiency and the associated secondary hyperparathyroidism. Alternatively, alterations of calcium metabolism and calcium-regulating hormones may be epiphenomena of NaCl loading that are not causally related to the development of hypertension, and the blood pressure lowering effect of high dietary calcium may be secondary to calcium-induced natriuresis rather than to a specific effect of calcium or calcium-regulating hormones on vascular smooth muscle.

MAGNESIUM

Relatively little information is available concerning dietary magnesium and blood pressure (see also Chap. 8). Although magnesium is found in a variety of foods, it is not as easily identified and quantified as calcium is. Nevertheless, as with calcium, there is suggestive evidence for an association between lower magnesium in the diet and higher blood pressures.[207] Over the past century, the availability of magnesium-rich foods has declined, and processed foods that have lost magnesium have increased. It has been proposed that subclinical magnesium deficiency has developed in industrialized countries[209,210] and that this has paralleled the increased prevalence of hypertension. Conversely, persons consuming vegetarian diets, which are usually high in magnesium, tend to have lower blood pressures than nonvegetarians, raising the possibility that dietary magnesium is inversely related to blood pressure. Limited evidence suggests that dietary intake of magnesium is lower in hypertensives than in normotensives; in one prospective study, lower calcium and magnesium intakes predicted risk of subsequent hypertension.[199] Limited information is available about the effects of magnesium supplementation on blood pressure in hypertensives, and the results are inconsistent.

There is a satisfactory physiologic rationale for an effect of magnesium on blood pressure. Magnesium decreases vascular tone and contractility, possibly by decreasing cellular uptake of calcium and thereby decreasing cytosolic calcium. Conversely, magnesium deficiency enhances vascular contractility.[207]

ALCOHOL

Alcohol intake has recently become recognized as an important independent correlate of blood pressure, unrelated to potentially confounding variables such as age and body mass.[211–213] In comparison to nondrinkers, there is a small but significant elevation of blood pressure in individuals consuming three or more drinks per day (a standard drink contains approximately 14 g of ethanol and is defined as a 12-ounce glass of beer, a 6-ounce glass of table wine, or 1.5 ounces of distilled spirits). The contribution to the prevalence of hypertension of alcohol consumption greater than two drinks per day has been estimated to be 5 to 7%; the contribution in men is greater than in women, although in women the risk of hypertension increases progressively with alcohol intakes in excess of 20 g per day. Several short-term studies suggest a therapeutic benefit of decreasing alcohol consumption in hypertensives. In controlled studies, reduction of alcohol consumption has been associated with a 4 to 8 mm Hg reduction of systolic blood pressure and a lesser reduction of diastolic pressure. Blood pressure of normotensives may also decrease in response to a reduction of alcohol consumption. The mechanism(s) by which alcohol may affect blood pressure has not been established.

DIETARY LIPIDS

Limited epidemiologic evidence suggests a direct association between diets high in saturated fats and blood pressure, and many populations that have low mean blood pressure levels eat a diet low in total fat and saturated fatty acids.[214] Conversely, diets high in ω-3 fatty acid content may be associated with lower blood pressures.[215] Several trials have failed to show a significant blood pressure effect by varying the dietary content of fat or by exchanging polyunsaturated fatty acids for saturated fatty acids, and there is ongoing debate as to whether the reduction of saturated fat and/or the increase of polyunsaturated fat in the diet results in a decrease of blood pressure.[216] Linoleic acid–enriched diets have been shown to reduce blood pressure in the rat and in normotensive and hypertensive humans. Further, it has recently been reported that high doses of fish oil lower blood pressure in men with essential hypertension.[217] Whether these putative changes in blood pressure are related to alterations of prostaglandin metabolism is unclear.

VEGETARIAN DIET

In general, vegetarian diets reduce both systolic and diastolic blood pressures, although the specific nutrient(s) responsible for this reduction has not been defined.[218] In general, vegetarians have lower intakes of total fat, saturated fat, cholesterol, and protein than omnivores have. Dietary intakes of carbohydrate, fiber, polyunsaturated fats, potassium, magnesium, and calcium tend to be increased in vegetarian diets. In addition, the type of protein eaten by vegetarians is markedly different. The effect of dietary fiber on blood pressure remains an unresolved issue;[219] there is a need for carefully controlled studies with different types of fiber. Although there is little evidence for an effect of dietary protein on blood pressure, studies in animal models raise the possibility that the type and level of protein in the diet may effect cardiovascular responses to elevated arterial pressure.

HYPERTENSION PREVENTION

Evidence for the preventability of hypertension through altered dietary intake comes from prevention studies in adults and longitudinal studies that have followed blood pressures in children over time.

Two recent trials have tested the efficacy of preventing the onset of diastolic hypertension in adults through altered dietary intake. Both of these studies suggest that primary prevention of hypertension is feasible through beneficial life-style changes. In the first trial, approximately 200 subjects with diastolic blood pressures in the high-normal ranges (80 to 89 mm Hg) were assigned to either a control group or a combined intervention consisting of weight loss, sodium restriction, moderate alcohol restriction, and moderate isotonic physical activity.[220] Subjects were followed over a 5-year period. Nine percent of intervention subjects developed hypertension, compared to 19% of control subjects ($p < 0.027$).

In the second prevention trial, 841 men and women between the ages of 25 and 49 years with diastolic blood pressures ranges between 78 and 89 mm Hg were assigned to one of five groups: (1) control, (2) reduced calories, (3) reduced sodium, (4) reduced calories and sodium, and (5) reduced sodium and increased potassium.[221] Calorie counseling reduced mean diastolic and systolic blood pressures at 6 months (2.8 and 5.1 mm Hg, respectively) and 3 years (1.8 and 2.4 mm Hg). Somewhat unexpectedly, the combination of calorie and sodium counseling was less effective than calorie counseling alone. The other interventions did not significantly affect blood pressure.*

Studies evaluating the association between dietary NaCl and blood pressure in infants, children, and adolescents have found either no association or weak associations.[222] However, in children, there is a strong correlation between obesity and blood pressure, and a direct association between changes in body weight and blood pressure.[223] In addition, blood pressures in the young tend to track over time, and a large proportion of obese children become obese adults. Prevention of obesity, beginning in childhood, would seem to be an important strategy for the primary prevention of hypertension and cardiovascular disease.

*Phase I of an additional trial of hypertension prevention has recently been completed in men and women with diastolic blood pressures ranging from 80 to 89 mm Hg. Different groups of subjects were exposed to different interventions. Compared to controls, stress management or dietary supplementation with calcium, magnesium, potassium, or fish oil did not significantly reduce systolic or diastolic blood pressure; however, blood pressure was reduced by weight reduction and to a lesser extent by modest salt restriction.[229]

PUBLIC HEALTH IMPLICATIONS AND THERAPEUTIC RECOMMENDATIONS

Dietary recommendations for the prevention and treatment of hypertension should address overall cardiovascular disease risk, not simply elevated blood pressure, and should be incorporated into a comprehensive program that also addresses other cardiovascular disease risk factors such as cigarette smoking and a sedentary life style. In developing recommendations, the potential impact of changing the intake of a single nutrient on the dietary content and/or bioavailability of a wide range of nutrients should also be considered.

Based on the strength of the association between body weight and blood pressure, and between change in weight and change in blood pressure over time, it is apparent that avoidance of obesity or weight reduction in overweight individuals should be key strategies for both the prevention and the treatment of hypertension.[224–226] A potentially favorable impact on other cardiovascular disease risk factors is another advantage of avoidance of obesity or weight reduction.

Currently, there is no clear method for identifying those hypertensive patients who are most apt to benefit from NaCl restriction. It is generally recommended that hypertensive individuals be advised to restrict dietary NaCl to 68 to 102 mmol (4 to 6 g) per day.

Opinion is divided concerning a recommendation on NaCl restriction for the entire population.[117,224–227] Arguments for this recommendation include the following: current NaCl intake is in excess of the physiologic need; the tendency for blood pressure to increase with a high NaCl intake occurs over the entire population; although relatively large differences of dietary NaCl have a relatively small impact on blood pressure within and across populations, these blood pressure differences may significantly affect the overall incidence of cardiovascular disease; within a population, a certain percentage of individuals may be particularly susceptible to the effect of dietary NaCl on blood pressure; and identification of NaCl sensitive individuals is not practical. Arguments against the recommendation for NaCl restriction for the entire population include the following: limited or no proven benefit for a large segment of the population; potential benefit restricted to NaCl-sensitive hypertensives; and potential adverse health consequences of NaCl restriction. Despite these reservations, it is generally recommended that excessively high intakes of dietary NaCl be avoided; as an example of a specific guideline, the American Heart Association recommends that dietary NaCl be restricted to no more than 128 mmol (7.5 g) per day.[228]

Recommendations about other nutrients should also be considered.[224–226] Because of the association of alcohol intake with blood pressure, a recommendation to restrict alcohol intake to two drinks per day would seem reasonable, particularly in individuals with hypertension. Although data are currently inadequate to recommend high intakes of potassium, calcium, or magnesium to prevent or treat hypertension, deficient intakes of these ions are associated with hypertension, and the effects of a high NaCl intake on blood pressure may be amplified by dietary deficiencies of both potassium and calcium. Furthermore, dietary deficiencies of these ions may be associated with other disorders such as calcium deficiency and osteoporosis. Consequently dietary deficiencies of these ions should be avoided. Although serum cholesterol and hence cardiovascular disease risk may be modified by dietary fat intake, there is currently insufficient information to make recommendations about dietary intakes of lipids or carbohydrates for the prevention or treatment of hypertension.

REFERENCES

1. Subcommittee on Definition and Prevalence of the Joint National Committee on Detection, Evaluation, and Treatment of High Blood pressure: Hypertension, *7:*457–468, 1985.
2. Castelli, W.P.: Am. J. Med., *76:*4–12, 1984.
3. Stamler, J., Neaton, J.D., Wentworth, D.N.: Hypertension, *13(Suppl. I):*2–12, 1989.
4. Collins, R., Peto, R., MacMahon, S., et al.: Lancet, *335:*827–838, 1990.
5. Langford, H.G., Blaufox, D., Oberman, A., et al.: JAMA, *253:*657–664, 1985.
6. Kannell, W., Brand, N., Skinner, J., et al.: Ann. Intern. Med., *67:*48–59, 1967.
7. Chiang, B.N., Perlman, L.V., Epstein, R.H.: Circulation, *39:*403–421, 1969.
8. Epstein, F.H.: Am. J. Epidemiol., *81:*307–322, 1965.
9. Stamler, R., Stamler, J., Riedlinger, W.E., et al.: JAMA, *240:*1607–1610, 1978.
10. Mann, G.V.: N. Engl. J. Med., *291:*178–185, 1974.
11. National Institutes of Health Consensus Development Panel on the Health Implications of Obesity: Ann. Intern. Med., *103:*1073–1077, 1985.
12. MacMahon, S.W., Cutler, J., Brittan, E., et al.: Eur. Heart. J., *8(Suppl. B):*57–70, 1987.
13. Fagerberg, B., Andersson, O.K., Isaksson, B., et al.: Br. Med. J., *288:*11–14, 1984.
14. Reisin, E., Frohlich, E.D., Messerli, F.H., et al.: Ann. Intern. Med., *98:*315–319, 1983.
15. Dornfield, L.P., Maxwell, M.H., Waks, A.U., et al.: Int. J. Obes., *9:*381–389, 1985.
17. Sims, E.A.H.: Hypertension, *4:*43–49, 1982.
18. Dustan, H.P.: Ann. Intern. Med., *98:*860–864, 1983.
19. Messerli, F.H., Ventura, H.O., Reisin, E., et al.: Circulation, *66:*55–60, 1982.
20. Landsberg, L., Young, J.B.: N. Engl. J. Med., *298:*1295–1301, 1978.
21. Frohlich, E.D., Reisin, E.: Hemodynamics in patients with overweight and hypertension. *In* The Heart in Hypertension. Edited by M.E. Safar. Amsterdam, Martinus Nijhoff, 1989, pp. 117–125.
22. Landsberg, L., Krieger, D.R.: Am. J. Hypertens., *2:*125S-132S, 1989.
23. Rocchini, A.D., Moorehead, C.P., DeRemer, S., et al.: Hypertension, *13:*922–928, 1989.
24. Tuck, M.L., Sowers, J.R., Dornfeld, L., et al.: Acta Endocrinol., *102:*252–257, 1983.
25. Sims, E.A.H., Berchtold, P.: JAMA, *247:*49–52, 1982.
26. Modan, M., Halkin, H., Almog, S., et al.: J. Clin. Invest., *75:*809–817, 1985.
27. Christlieb, A.R., Krolewski, A.S., Warram, J.H., et al.: Hypertension, *7:*54–57, 1985.
28. Reaven, G.M., Hoffman, B.B.: Am. J. Med., *87(Suppl. A):*2S–6S, 1989.
29. Rocchini, A.P., Katch, V., Schork, A., et al.: Hypertension, *10:*267–273, 1987.
30. Glass, A.R.: Med. Clin. North Am., *73:*139–160, 1989.
31. Rocchini, A.P., Katch, V., Kveselis, D., et al.: Hypertension, *14:*367–374, 1989.
32. Rocchini, A.P., Key, J., Bondie, D., et al.: N. Engl. J. Med., *321:*580–585, 1989.
33. Krotkiewski, M., Mandroukas, K., Sjostrom, L., et al.: Metabolism, *68:*650–658, 1979.
34. Reisin, E., Abel, R., Modan, M., et al.: N. Engl. J. Med., *298:*1–6, 1978.
35. Rosenthal, M., Haskell, W.L., Solomon, R., et al.: Diabetes, *32:*408–411, 1983.
36. Singer, P., Gadick, W., Voigt, S., et al.: Hypertension, *7:*182–186, 1985.
37. Ferrannini, E., Buzzigoli, G., Bonadona, R.: N. Engl. J. Med., *317:*350–357, 1987.
38. Shen, D.-C., Shieh, S.-M., Fuh, M.-J., et al.: J. Clin. Endocrinol. Metab., *66:*580–583, 1988.
39. Swislocki, A.L.M., Hoffman, B.B., Reaven, G.M.: Am. J. Hypertens., *2:*419–423, 1989.
40. Manolio, T.A., Savage, P.J., Burke, G.L., et al.: Arteriosclerosis, *10:*420–426, 1990.
41. Izumi, Y., Honda, M., Tsuchiya, M., et al.: Endocrinol. Jpn., *27:*505–511, 1980.
42. DeFronzo, R.A., Cooke, C., Andres, R., et al.: J. Clin. Invest., *55:*845–855, 1975.
43. Baum, M.: J. Clin. Invest., *79:*1104–1109, 1987.
44. DeFronzo, R., Goldberg, M., Agus, Z.: J. Clin. Invest., *58:*83–90, 1971.
45. Krichner, K.: Am. J. Physiol., *255:*F1206–F1213, 1988.
46. Rocchini, A.P., Moorehead, C., DeRemer, S., et al.: Hypertension, *15:*861–866, 1990.
47. Rocchini, A.P., Moorehead, C.P., DeRemer, S., et al.: Hypertension, *13:*922–928, 1989.
48. Finch, D., Davis, G., Bower, J., et al: Hypertension, *15:*514–518, 1990.
49. Alexander, W.D., Oake, R.J.: Diabetes, *26:*611–614, 1977.
50. Rowe, J.W., Young, J.B., Minaker, K.L., et al.: Diabetes, *30:*219–225, 1981.
51. Christensen, N.J., Gundersen, H.J.G., Hegedus, L., et al.: Metabolism, *29:*1138–1145, 1980.
52. Kreiger, D.R., Landsberg, L.: Am. J. Hypertens., *1:*84–90, 1988.

53. Liang, C.S., Doherty, J.V., Faillace, R., et al.: J. Clin. Invest., *69:*1321–1336, 1982.
54. Pereda, S.A., Eckstein, J.W., Abboud, J.E.: Am. J. Physiol., *202:*249–252, 1962.
55. Fitzovtich, D.E., Randall, D.C.: Am. J. Physiol., *258:*R624–R633, 1990.
56. Presuss, H.G., Fournier, R.D.: Life Sci., *30:*879–886, 1982.
57. Bunag, R.D., Tomita, T., Sasaki, S.: Hypertension, *5:*218–225, 1983.
58. Wright, D.W., Hansen, R.I., Mondon, C.E., et al.: Am. J. Clin. Nutr., *38:*879–883, 1983.
59. Zavaroni, I., Sander, S., Scott, S., et al.: Metabolism, *29:*970–973, 1980.
60. Hwang, I.-S., Ho, H., Hoffman, B.B., et al.: Hypertension, *10:*512–516, 1987.
61. Reaven, G.M., Ho, H., Hoffman, B.B.: Hypertension, *12:*129–132, 1988.
62. Young, J.B., Landsberg, L.: Metab. Clin. Exp., *30:*421–424, 1981.
63. Gradin, K., Nissbrand, H., Ehrenstom, F., et al.: Arch. Pharmacol., *337:*47–52, 1988.
64. Young, J.B., Landsberg, L.: Nature, *269:*615–617, 1977.
65. Berne, C., Farius, J., Miklasson, F.: J. Clin. Invest., *84:*1403–1409, 1989.
66. O'Hare, J.A., Minaker, K., Young, J.B.: Clin. Res., *33:*441A, 1985.
67. Ku, D.D., Sellers, B.M.: J. Pharmacol. Exp. Ther., *222:*395–400, 1982.
68. Moore, R.D., Rabovsky, J.L.: Am. J. Physiol., *236:*C249–C254, 1979.
69. Hougen, T.J., Hopkins, B.E., Smith, T.W.: Am. J. Physiol., *234:*C59–C63, 1978.
70. Stout, R.W., Bierman, E.L., Ross, R.: Circ. Res., *36:*319–327, 1975.
71. Koschinsky, T., Bunting, C.E., Schwippert, B., et al.: Atherosclerosis, *33:*245–252, 1979.
72. Pfeifle, B., Ditschuneit, H.H., Ditschuneit, H.: Horm. Metab. Res., *12:*381–385, 1980.
73. Mir, M.A., Charalambous, B.M., Morgan, K., et al.: N. Engl. J. Med., *305:*1264–1268, 1981.
74. Pershadsingh, H.A., McDonald, J.M.: Cell Calcium, *5:*111–130, 1984.
75. Chimori, K., Miyazaki, S., Kosaka, J., et al.: Clin. Exp. Hypertens., *8:*185–199, 1986.
76. Clausen, T., Kohn, P.G.: J. Physiol. (Lond.), *265:*19–42, 1977.
77. Gavryck, W.A., Moore, R.D., Thompson, R.C.: J. Physiol. (Lond.), *252:*43–58, 1975.
78. Moore, R.D., Fidelman, M.L., Seeholzer, S.H.: Biochem. Biophys. Res. Commun., *91:*905–910, 1979.
79. Fidelman, M.L., Seeholzer, S.H., Walsh, K.B., et al.: Am. J. Physiol., *242:*C87–C93, 1982.
80. McDonald, J.M., Bruns, D.E., Jarett, L.: Biochem. Biophys. Res. Commun., *71:*114–121, 1976.
81. Schudt, C., Gaertner, U., Pette, D.: Eur. J. Biochem., *68:*103–111, 1976.
82. Ferrari, P., Weidmann, P.: J. Hypertens., *8:*491–500, 1990.
83. Postnov, Y.V., Orlov, S.N.: Physiol. Rev., *65:*904–945, 1985.
84. Postnov, Y.V., Orlov, S.N.: J. Hypertens., *2:*1–6, 1984.
85. Erne, P., Bolli, P., Burgisser, E., et al.: N. Engl. J. Med., *310:*1084–1088, 1981.
86. Lindner, A., Kenny, M., Meacham, A.J.: N. Engl. J. Med., *316:*509–513, 1987.
87. Resnick, L.M.: Am. J. Med., *87(Suppl. A):*175–225, 1987.
88. Cooper, R.S., Sham, N., Katz, S.: Hypertension, *9:*234–239, 1987.
89. Blaustein, M.P.: Am. J. Physiol., *232:*C165–C173, 1977.
90. Draznin, B., Sussman, K.E., Kao, M., et al.: J. Biol. Chem., *262:*14385–14388, 1987.
91. Draznin, B., Sussman, K.E., Eckel, R.H., et al.: J. Clin. Invest., *82:*1848–1852, 1988.
92. Zemel, M.B., Sowers, J.R., Shehin, S., et al.: Metabolism, *39:*704–708, 1990.
93. Folkow, B.: Physiol. Rev., *62:*347–504, 1982.
94. Liu, J., Bishop, S.P., Overbeck, H.W.: Circ. Res., *62:*1001–1010, 1988.
95. Nakao, J., Ito, H., Kanayasu, T., et al.: Diabetes, *34:*185–191, 1985.
96. Ewton, D.Z., Florini, J.R.: Proc. Soc. Exp. Biol. Med., *194:*76–80, 1990.
97. Kwok, C.F., Goldstein, B., Muller-Wieland, D., et al.: J. Clin. Invest., *83:*127–136, 1989.
98. King, G., Kahn, C.R., Rechler, M., et al.: J. Clin. Invest., *66:*130–140, 1980.
99. Marban, E., Koretsune, Y.: Hypertension, *15:*652–658, 1990.
100. Moolenaar, W.H., Tsien, R.Y., Van Der Saag, P.I., et al.: Nature, *304:*645–648, 1983.
101. Ganz, M.B., Boyarsky, B., Sterzel, R.B., et al.: Nature, *337:*648–651, 1989.
102. Huang, C.I., Cogan, M.G., Cragoe, E.J. Jr., et al.: J. Biol. Chem., *262:*14134–14140, 1987.
103. Mitsuhashi, T., Ives, H.E.: J. Biol. Chem., *263:*8790–8796, 1988.
104. Hatori, N., Fine, B.P., Nakamura, E., et al.: J. Biol. chem., *262:*5073–5078, 1987.
105. Berk, B.C., Vallega, G., Muslin, A.J., et al.: J. Clin. Invest., *83:*822–829, 1989.
106. Resnick, L.M., Gupta, R.K., Sosa, R.E., et al.: Proc. Natl. Acad. Sci. U.S.A., *84:*7663–7667, 1987.
107. Feig, P.U., D'Occhio, M.A., Boylan, J.W.: Hypertension, *9:*282–288, 1987.
108. Livne, A., Balfe, J.W., Veitch, R., et al.: Lancet, *1:*533–536, 1987.
109. Batlie, D.C., Saleh, A., Rombola, G.: Hypertension, *15:*97–103, 1990.
110. Saleh, A., Batlie, D.C.: J. Clin. Invest., *85:*1734–1739, 1990.
111. Grugni, G., Ardizzi, A., Dubini, A., et al.: Horm. Metab. Res., *22:*124–125, 1990.
112. Liang, C.S., Doherty, J., Faillace, R.: J. Clin. Invest., *69:*1321–1336, 1982.
113. Mathias, C.J., daCosta, D.F., Fosbraey, P., et al.: Br. Med. J., *295:*161–163, 1987.
114. Alexander, W.D., Oake, R.J.: Diabetes, *26:*611–614, 1977.
115. Hall, J.E., Brands, M.W., Kivlighn, S.D., et al.: Hypertension, *15:*519–527, 1990.
116. Dahl, L.K.: Am. J. Clin. Nutr., *25:*231–244, 1972.
117. Intersalt Cooperative Research Group: Br. Med. J., *297:*319–328, 1988.
118. Weinberger, M.H., Miller, J.H., Luft, F.C., et al.: Hypertension, *8(Suppl. II):*127–134, 1986.
119. Sullivan, J.M., Prewitt, R.L., Ratts, T.E.: Am. J. Med. Sci., *295:*370–377, 1988.
120. Cutler, J.A., Follmann, D., Elliott, P., et al.: Hypertension, *27(Suppl. I):*27–33, 1991.
121. MacGregor, G.A., Markandu, N.D., Sagnella, G., et al.: Lancet, *2:*1244–1247, 1989.

122. Grobbee, D.E., Hofman, A.: Br. Med. J., *293:*27–29, 1986.
123. Miller, J.Z., Weinberger, M.H., Christian, J.C., et al.: Am. J. Epidemiol., *126:*822–830, 1987.
124. Weinberger, M.H., Miller, J.Z., Fineberg, N.S., et al.: Hypertension, *10:*443–446, 1987.
125. Rapp, J.P.: Hypertension, *4:*753–763, 1982.
126. Roman, R.J.: Am. J. Physiol., *251:*F57–F65, 1986.
127. Tobian, L., Lange, J., Azar, S., et al.: Circ. Res., *43(Suppl. I):*I-92–I-97, 1978.
128. Roman, R.J., Osborn, J.L.: Am. J. Physiol., *252:*R833–R841, 1987.
129. Greene, A.S., Yu, Z.Y., Roman, R.J., et al.: Am. J. Physiol., *258:*H508–H514, 1990.
130. Fujiata, T., Henry, W.L., Bartter, F.C., et al.: Am. J. Med., *69:*334–344, 1980.
131. Gill, J.R., Gullner, H.G., Lake, C.R., et al.: Hypertension, *11:*312–319, 1988.
132. Genain, C., Reddy, S.R., Ott, C.E., et al.: Hypertension, *12:*568–573, 1988.
133. Takeshita, A., Mark, A.L., Brody, M.J.: Am. J. Physiol., *236:*H48–H52, 1979.
134. Winternitz, S.R., Oparil, S.: Clin. Exp. Hypertens., *4:*751–760, 1982.
135. Iwai, J.: Am. J. Physiol., *245:*H762–H766, 1983.
136. Chen, Y.F., Meng, Q., Wyss, J.M., et al.: Hypertension, *11:*55–62, 1988.
137. Goto, A., Ikeda, I., Tobian, L., et al.: Clin. Sci., *61:*53s–55s, 1981.
138. Haywood, J.R., Brennan, T.J., Hinojosa, C.: Fed. Proc., *44:*2393–2399, 1981.
139. Friedman, R., Tassinari, I.M., Heine, M., et al.: Clin. Exp. Hypertens., *1:*779–799, 1979.
140. Takeshita, A., Mark, A.L.: Circ. Res., *43(Suppl. I):*86–91, 1978.
141. Bunag, R.D., Butterfield, J., Sasaki, S.: Hypertension, *5:*460–467, 1983.
142. Friedman, S.M.: *In* Hypertension. 2nd Ed. Edited by J. Genest, O. Kuchel, P. Hamet, et al. New York, McGraw-Hill, 1983, pp. 457–473.
143. Miyajima, E., Bunag, R.D.: Clin. Exp. Hypertens., *8:*1049–1061, 1986.
144. Whitescarver, S.A., Ott, C.E., Kotchen, T.A.: Am. J. Physiol., *259:*R76–R83, 1990.
145. Andresen, M.C.: Circ. Res., *64:*695–702, 1989.
146. Gordon, F.J., Mark, A.L.: Circ. Res., *54:*378–387, 1984.
147. Thornton, R.M., Wyss, J.M., Oparil, S.: Hypertension, *14:*518–523, 1989.
148. VeelKen, R., Swain, L.L., DiBona, G.F.: Hypertension, *13:*822–827, 1989.
149. Thoren, P., Morgan, D.A., Mark, A.L.: Am. J. Physiol., *253:*H133–H137, 1987.
150. Reddy, S., Baylis, C., Kotchen, T.A.: Am. J. Physiol., *260:*R32–R38, 1991.
151. Miyajima, E., Bunag, R.D.: Am. J. Physiol., *252:*H402–H409, 1987.
152. Bunag, R.D., Miyajima, E.: J. Clin. Invest., *74:*2065–2073, 1984.
153. Ferrari, A.U., Mark, A.L.: Hypertension, *10:*55–60, 1987.
154. Howe, P.R., Rogers, P.F., Minson, J.B.: J. Hypertens., *3:*457–460, 1985.
155. Weinstock, M., Schorer-Apelbaum, D.: Clin. Sci., *68:*489–493, 1985.
156. Campese, V.M., Romoff, M.S., Levitan, D., et al.: Kidney Int., *21:*371–378, 1982.
157. Sullivan, J.M., Prewitt, R.L., Ratts, T.E., et al.: Hypertension, *9:*398–406, 1987.
158. Koolen, M., Van Brumnelen, P.: Hypertension, *6:*820–825, 1984.
159. Sakaguchi, A., Saito, T., Yamamoto, Y.: J. Hypertens., *6(Suppl. 4):*209–212, 1988.
160. Ambrosioni, E., Costa, F.V., Borhgi, C., et al.: Hypertension, *4:*789–794, 1982.
161. Poston, L., Johnson, V.E., Gray, H.H., et al.: Klin. Wochenschr., *63(Suppl. III):*136–138, 1985.
162. Krzesinski, J.M., Rorive, G.L.: Klin. Wochenschr., *63(Suppl. III):*45–58, 1985.
163. Weissberg, P.L., West, M.L., Kendall, M.J., et al.: J. Hypertens., *3:*475–480, 1985.
164. Saito, K., Furuta, Y., Sano, H., et al.: Clin. Exp. Hypertens., *A7:*1217–1232, 1985.
165. Stokes, G.S., Monaghan, J.C., Middleton, A.T., et al.: J. Hypertens., *4:*35–38, 1986.
166. Zidek, W., Karoff, C., Losse, H., et al.: Klin. Wochenschr., *64:*1183–1185, 1986.
167. Zemel, M.B., Kraniak, J., Standley, P.R., et al.: Am. J. Hypertens., *1:*386–392, 1988.
168. Quintanilla, A.P., Weffer, M.I., Koh, H., et al.: Clin. Sci., *75:*167–170, 1988.
169. Cooper, R., Trevisan, M., Van Horn, L., et al.: Hypertension, *6:*731–735, 1984.
170. Gudmundsson, O., Herlitz, H., Jonsson, O., et al.: Clin. Sci., *66:*427–433, 1984.
171. Canessa, M., Redgrave, J., Laski, C., et al.: Am. J. Hypertens., *2:*515–523, 1989.
172. Swales, J.D., Bing, R.F., Bradlaugh, R., et al.: J. Cardiovasc. Pharmacol., *6:*S42–S48, 1984.
173. Redgrave, J., Canessa, M., Gleason, R., et al.: Hypertension, *13:*721–726, 1980.
174. Overbeck, H.W., Ku, D.D., Rapp, J.P.: Hypertension, *3:*306–312, 1981.
175. Zicha, J., Duhm, J.: Hypertension, *15:*612–627, 1990.
176. Oshima, T., Matsuura, H., Matsumoto, K., et al.: Hypertension, *11:*703–707, 1988.
177. Rocchini, A.P., Moorehead, C., London, M., et al.: Abstracts of 1990 Annual Meeting of the American Heart Association, Abstract No. 2624.
178. Hall, C.E., Hall, O.: Exp. Biol. Med., *123:*370–374, 1966.
179. Hall, C.E., Hall, O.: Tex. Rep. Biol. Med., *23:*435–444, 1965.
180. Beebe, C., Schemmel, R., Mickelsen, O.: Proc. Soc. Exp. Biol. Med., *151:*395–399, 1976.
181. Presuss, M.B., Presuss, H.B.: Lab. Invest., *43:*101–105, 1980.
182. Smith-Barbaro, P.A., Quinn, M.R., Fisher, H., et al.: Proc. Soc. Exp. Biol. Med., *165:*283–290, 1980.
183. Tomiyama, H., Kushiro, T., Abeta, H., et al.: Abstracts of 44th Annual Fall Conference of Council for High Blood Pressure Research, Abstract No. 15. Baltimore, American Heart Association, 1990.
184. Boegehold, M.A., Kotchen, T.A.: Hypertension, *14:*579–583, 1989.
185. Svetkey, L.P., Klotman, P.E.: Blood pressure and potassium intake. *In* Hypertension: Pathophysiology, Diagnosis, and Management. Edited by J.H. Laragh and B.M. Brenner. New York, Raven Press, 1990.
186. Khaw, K.T., Barrett-Conner, E.: Circulation, *77:*53–61, 1985.

187. Veterans Administration Cooperative Study Group on Antihypertensive Agents: J. Chronic Dis., *40:*839–847, 1987.
188. Addison, W.: Can. Med. Assoc. J., *18:*281–285, 1928.
189. Lawton, W.J., Fita, A.E., Anderson, E.A., et al.: Circulation, *81:*173–184, 1990.
190. Krishna, G.C., Miller, E., Kapoor, S.: N. Engl. J. Med., *320:*1177–1182, 1989.
191. Barden, A.E., Vandongen, R., Beilin, L.J.: J. Hypertens., *4:*339–343, 1986.
192. Grimm, R.H., Neaton, J.D., Elmer, P.J., et al.: N. Engl. J. Med., *322:*569–574, 1990.
193. Geleijnse, J.M., Grobbee, D.E., Hofman, A.: Br. Med. J., *300:*899–902, 1990.
194. Tobian, L., Lange, J.M., Ulm, K.M., et al.: J. Hypertens., *2(Suppl. 3):*363–366, 1984.
195. Tobian, L., MacNeill, D., Johnson, M.A., et al.: Hypertension, *6(Suppl. I):*170–176, 1984.
196. Kwaw, D.T., Barrett-Connor, E.: N. Engl. J. Med., *316:*235–240, 1987.
197. McCarron, D.A., Morris, C.D., Henry, H.J., et al.: Science, *224:*1392–1398, 1984.
198. Cutler, J.A., Brittain, E.: Am. J. Hypertens., *3:*137s–146s, 1990.
199. Witteman, J.C.M., Willett, W.C., Stampfer, M.J., et al.: Circulation, *80:*1320–1327, 1989.
200. Grobbee, D.E., Waal-Manning, H.J.: Drugs, *29:*7–18, 1990.
201. Harlan, W.R., Harlan, L.C.: Blood pressure and calcium and magnesium intake. *In* Hypertension: Pathophysiology, Diagnosis, and Management. Edited by J.H. Laragh and B.M. Brenner. New York, Raven Press, 1990.
202. Resnick, L.M., Difabio, B., Marion, R.M., et al.: J. Hypertens., *4(Suppl. 6):*679–681, 1986.
203. Resnick, L.M., Sealey, J.E., Laragh, J.H.: Fed. Proc., *42:*300, 1983.
204. Zemel, M.B., Gualdoni, S.M., Sowers, J.R.: J. Hypertens., *4*(Suppl. 6):343–345, 1986.
205. Langford, H.G., Watson, R.L.: Clin. Sci. Molec. Med., *45:*111S–113S, 1978.
206. Saito, K., Sano, H., Furuta, Y., et al.: Hypertension, *13:*219–226, 1989.
207. Resnick, L.M.: The role of dietary calcium and magnesium in the therapy of hypertension. *In* Hypertension: Pathophysiology, Diagnosis, and Management. Edited by J.D. Laragh and B.M. Brenner. New York, Raven Press, 1990.
208. Kotchen. T.A., Ott, C.E., Whitescarver, S.: Am. J. Hypertens., *2:*749–753, 1989.
209. Marier, J.R.: Magnesium, *1:*3–15, 1982.
210. Durlach, J., Bara, M., Guiet-Bara, A.: Magnesium, *4:*5–15, 1985.
211. MacMahon, S.: Hypertension, *9:*111–121, 1987.
212. Witteman, J.C.M., Willett, W.C., Stampfer, M.J., et al.: Am. J. Cardiol., *65:*633–637, 1990.
213. Klatsky, A.L.: Blood pressure and alcohol intake. *In* Hypertension: Pathophysiology, Diagnosis, and Management. Edited by J.D. Laragh and B.M. Brenner. New York, Raven Press, 1990.
214. Sacks, F.M.: Nutr. Rev., *47:*291–300, 1989.
215. Knapp, H.R.: Nutr. Rev., *47:*301–313, 1989.
216. Iacono, J.M., Dougherty, R.M.: Blood pressure and fat intake. *In* Hypertension: Pathophysiology, Diagnosis, and Management. Edited by J.D. Laragh and B.M. Brenner. New York, Raven Press, 1990.
217. Knapp, H.R., Fitzgerald, G.A.: N. Engl. J. Med., *320:*1037–1043, 1989.
218. Rouse, I.L., Beilin, L.J.: Hypertensive disease and kidney structure. *In* Hypertension: Pathophysiology, Diagnosis, and Management. Edited by J.D. Laragh and B.M. Brenner. New York, Raven Press, 1990.
219. Swain, J.F., Rouse, I.L., Curley, C.B.: N. Engl. J. Med., *322:*147–152, 1990.
220. Stamler, R., Stamler, J., Gosch, F.C., et al.: JAMA, *262:*1801–1807, 1989.
221. Hypertension Prevention Trial Research Group: Arch. Intern. Med., *150:*153–162, 1990.
222. Kotchen, T.A., Kotchen, J.M., Boegehold, M.: Hypertension, *18(Suppl. I):*115–120, 1991.
223. Kotchen, J.M., Holley, J., Kotchen, T.A.: Semin. Nephrol., *9:*296–303, 1989.
224. The Surgeon General's Report on Nutrition and Health. Washington, D.C., U.S. Dept. of Health and Human Services, 1988.
225. The 1988 Report of the Joint National Committee on Detection, Evaluation, and Treatment of High Blood Pressure: Arch. Intern. Med., *148:*1023–1038, 1988.
226. Kaplan, N.M.: Ann. Intern. Med., *102:*359–373, 1985.
227. Swales, J.D.: Br. Med. J., *297:*307–308, 1988.
228. Grundy, S.M., Bilheimer, D., Blackburn, H., et al.: Circulation, *65:*839A–854A, 1982.
229. Trials of Hypertension Prevention Collaborative Research Group: JAMA, *267:*1213–1220, 1992.

CHAPTER **72**

Nutrition and Diet in The Management of Hyperlipidemia and Atherosclerosis

Elaine B. Feldman

LIPID HYPOTHESIS OF ATHEROSCLEROSIS

That the fat content and fatty acid composition of the diet were important factors in the pathogenesis of atherosclerosis was inferred from the decline in mortality from coronary heart disease that occurred during periods of food deprivation in the United States during the Depression and in the Western countries involved in World War II. During those times consumption of milk, butter, cheese, and eggs declined. Epidemiologic studies were designed and implemented that examined the dietary fat-heart hypothesis and specifically examined the relationship between the intake of saturated fatty acids and coronary heart disease (see Keys in the selected readings list at the end of this chapter). The wide differences in prevalence of coronary heart disease could be related in part to consumption of fat; severe atherosclerosis was common and the serum cholesterol increased sharply with age when the diet provided about 40% of energy as fat. Cholesterol intake also correlated with death rates from coronary heart disease.

The results of some primary and secondary intervention trials relating blood lipids and coronary heart disease (CHD) risk are discussed in Chapter 87. These data formed the bases for the guidelines to diagnose and manage hyperlipidemias.[1]

BLOOD LIPIDS AND LIPOPROTEINS

The blood lipids include free cholesterol and cholesterol esterified with long-chain fatty acids, triglycerides (triacylglycerols), phospholipids (lecithin or phosphatidylcholine, phosphatidylethanolamine, sphingomyelin, phosphatidylserine, and phosphatidylinositol), and unesterified or free fatty acids (see Chap. 3). The lipids are transported in plasma incorporated into lipoprotein particles that vary in atherogenicity.[2–4] The plasma lipoproteins are classified according to their physical and chemical properties (Table 72–1) and include the following:

Chylomicrons

Very low-density lipoproteins (VLDL)

Intermediate-density lipoproteins (IDL, or β-VLDL)

TABLE 72–1. PLASMA LIPOPROTEINS IN HUMANS

					CHEMICAL COMPOSITION, %				
					Surface			Core	
Class	Particle Diameter (nm)	Flotation Density	Electro-phoretic Mobility	Major Apoproteins	Proteins	Phospho-lipids	Choles-terol	Cholesterol Esters	Triglyc-erides
Chylo-microns	80–500	<0.95	α 2	B, E, A-I, A-IV, C	2	7	2	3	86
VLDL	30–80	0.93–1.006	pre-β	B, E, C	8	18	7	12	55
IDL	25–35	1.006–1.019	slow pre-β	B, E	19	19	9	29	23
LDL	18–28	1.019–1.063	β	B	22	22	8	42	6
HDL_2	9–12	1.063–1.125	α 1	A-I, A-II	40	33	5	17	5
HDL_3	5–9	1.125–1.210	α 1	A-I, A-II	55	25	4	13	3

VLDL, Very low-density lipoprotein; IDL, intermediate-density lipoprotein; LDL, low-density lipoprotein; HDL, high-density lipoprotein.
(Modified from Feldman, E.B.: Essentials of Clinical Nutrition. Philadelphia, F.A. Davis, 1988, p. 433.)

Low-density lipoproteins (LDL)
High-density lipoproteins (HDL)

CIRCULATING LIPIDS

CHOLESTEROL

Cholesterol is a sterol that is synthesized in the body and ingested in the animal products of the diet. Levels of cholesterol in plasma vary with age; in men cholesterol increases from puberty to about the fifth decade of life and in women until the seventh decade of life (Table 72–2).[5] Values exceeding the 75th percentile are associated with moderate risk of atherosclerosis; those above the 90th percentile convey high risk (Table 72–3). Plasma cholesterol levels in women generally are lower than those of men until middle age. Plasma cholesterol levels among adults in the United States range (5th to 95th percentile) from 3.2 to 7.1 mmol/L (125 to 275 mg/dl), with averages between 4.2 and 6.0 mmol/L (160 and 230 mg/dl) depending on age and gender. Mean serum cholesterol levels in adults have declined recently by 0.05 to 0.5 mmol/L (2 to 20 mg/dl), depending on age and gender.

About two-thirds of the plasma cholesterol is transported as LDL; levels of LDL cholesterol parallel those of total cholesterol. HDL transports about 25% of the plasma cholesterol with levels averaging about 1.17 mmol/L (45 mg/dl) in men and are 0.23 to 0.44 mmol/L (9 to 17 mg/dl) higher in women. In patients with diseases such as diabetes mellitus, hypothyroidism, the nephrotic syndrome, renal failure, pancreatitis, and obstructive liver disease—as well as ingestion of some drugs and hormones, especially adrenal and gonadal hormones—plasma cholesterol levels are increased, resulting in secondary hypercholesterolemia. These elevated levels will decline with appropriate treatment of the underlying disease or change in the type or dose of medication.[6] Thus patient evaluation must include screening for these diseases, especially checking thyroid function and obtaining a complete history of medications.

TRIGLYCERIDES

Circulating triglyceride levels average about 1.13 mmol/L (100 mg/dl) in fasting young adults; triglycerides are lower in women. Triglycerides increase by 50 to 75% with age (Table 72–2). Median triglyceride levels range from 0.90 to 1.47 mmol/L (80 to 130 mg/dl); levels in the population (5th to 95th percentile) range from 0.45 to 3.61 mmol/L (40 to 320 mg/dl) depending on age and gender. Triglyceride levels are increased by genetic and dietary factors (calories, fat, carbohydrate, alcohol) as well as diseases such as diabetes mellitus, pancreatitis, and the nephrotic syndrome and some antihypertensive medications and thyroid and gonadal hormones. Triglyceride levels are labile and may vary by up to 50% daily depending on the recent diet.

APOPROTEINS

The apolipoproteins, or apoproteins, are the primary determinants of the metabolic fate of the individual lipoprotein particles (see Chap. 3) and maintain the solubility of lipoprotein lipids in the plasma.[7,8] Apoproteins include A-I, A-II and A-IV, B (big or B-100 and little/small B-48), C-I, C-II, and C-III, D, and three isoforms of E (2, 3, and 4), as well as F, G and H and apo(a). Their distribution in lipoproteins and the average levels in plasma are shown in Tables 72–1 and 72–4. Apoprotein measurements, together with lipid levels, may aid in diagnosing disorders of lipoprotein transport—the dyslipoproteinemias[9–11]—and may be useful in predicting the risk of developing coronary heart disease or other cardiovascular disease.[12] Survivors of

TABLE 72–2. AVERAGE LEVELS OF CIRCULATING LIPIDS (50TH PERCENTILE)

	TOTAL C		LDL C		HDL C		TG	
Age, Yr	mmol/L	mg/dl	mmol/L	mg/dl	mmol/L	mg/dl	mmol/L	mg/dl
White men								
15–19	3.95	152	2.42	93	1.20	46	0.77	68
20–24	4.13	159	2.63	101	1.17	45	0.88	78
25–29	4.58	176	3.02	116	1.14	44	0.99	88
30–34	4.94	190	3.22	124	1.17	45	1.15	102
35–39	5.04	194	3.41	131	1.12	43	1.23	109
40–44	5.30	204	3.51	135	1.12	43	1.39	123
45–49	5.46	210	3.67	141	1.17	45	1.34	119
50–54	5.49	211	3.72	143	1.14	44	1.45	128
55–59	5.56	214	3.77	145	1.20	46	1.32	117
60–64	5.59	215	3.72	143	1.27	49	1.25	111
65–69	5.54	213	3.80	146	1.27	49	1.22	108
70+	5.56	214	3.69	142	1.25	48	1.30	115
White women								
15–19	4.08	157	2.42	93	1.33	51	0.72	64
20–24	4.29	165	2.65	102	1.33	51	0.90	80
25–29	4.63	178	2.81	108	1.43	55	0.86	76
30–34	4.63	178	2.83	109	1.43	55	0.82	73
35–39	4.84	186	3.02	116	1.38	53	0.94	83
40–44	5.02	193	3.17	122	1.46	56	0.77	68
45–49	5.30	204	3.30	127	1.51	58	1.06	94
50–54	5.56	214	3.48	134	1.61	62	1.16	103
55–59	5.95	229	3.77	145	1.56	60	1.25	111
60–64	5.88	226	3.87	149	1.59	61	1.18	105
65–69	6.06	233	3.93	151	1.61	62	1.33	118
70+	5.88	226	3.82	147	1.56	60	1.24	110

C = cholesterol, TG = triglycerides (see Table 72–1 for other abbreviations)
(Adapted from Lipid Research Clinics Program: JAMA, *251*:351–374, 1984.)

myocardial infarction, for example, have low levels of apo-A-I and increased levels of apo-B. Apoprotein levels or changes in size or amino acid composition may be better predictors of coronary heart disease than lipid levels, and may correlate with the severity of the disease.[7,12] The apoprotein level indicates the number of lipoprotein particles in plasma (i.e., concentration) compared to the lipoprotein cholesterol level that reflects changes in lipoprotein composition.

LIPOPROTEINS, LIPID TRANSPORT, AND METABOLISM

Each lipoprotein contains specific amounts of the various lipid components and apoproteins (Table 72–1). Their transport and metabolism are described in detail in Chapter 3.

CHYLOMICRONS

Chylomicron particles form in the intestine when triacylglycerol esters of long-chain fatty acids are ingested and are present in plasma only after a fatty meal. Chylomicrons in plasma that is kept refrigerated in a test tube may be seen as a creamy layer on top of the plasma. Chylomicrons are present in the blood when triglyceride levels exceed 7.90 mmol/L (700 mg/dl) and approach 11.3 mmol/L (1000 mg/dl).

Chylomicrons are absorbed from the small intestine into the lymphatics and then into the blood. They are removed from the circulation by the action of lipoprotein lipase, an enzyme that is induced by heparin and regulated by insulin. The remnant particle produced is taken up by the liver via receptors that specifically recognize the apoprotein constituents.[13]

VLDL

VLDL is produced by the liver and is the main transporter of endogenous triglyceride produced from carbohydrate precursors in the diet. Excess VLDL particles in plasma make the plasma diffusely cloudy. Plasma appears cloudy when triglyceride levels exceed 2.25 mmol/L or 200 mg/dl. Lipoprotein lipase activity generates VLDL remnants or intermediate-density lipoproteins (IDL) that are removed from the circulation by the

TABLE 72–3. LEVELS OF CIRCULATING LIPIDS WARRANTING ATTENTION

	LDL C* 75TH PERCENTILE		HDL C 25TH PERCENTILE		TG 90TH PERCENTILE	
Age, yr	mmol/L	mg/dl	mmol/L	mg/dl	mmol/L	mg/dl
White men						
15–19	2.83	109	1.01	39	1.41	125
20–24	3.07	118	0.99	38	1.64	146
25–29	3.59	138	0.96	37	1.92	171
30–34	3.74	144	0.99	38	2.41	214
35–39	4.00	154	0.94	36	2.81	250
40–44	4.08	157	0.94	36	2.84	252
45–49	4.24	163	0.99	38	2.84	252
50–54	4.21	162	0.94	36	2.74	244
55–59	4.37	168	0.99	38	2.36	210
60–64	4.29	165	1.07	41	2.17	193
65–69	4.42	170	1.01	39	2.55	227
70+	4.26	164	1.04	40	2.27	202
White women						
15–19	2.89	111	1.12	43	1.26	112
20–24	3.07	118	1.14	44	1.52	135
25–29	3.28	126	1.22	47	1.54	137
30–34	3.33	128	1.20	46	1.58	140
35–39	3.61	139	1.14	44	1.91	170
40–44	3.80	146	1.25	48	1.81	161
45–49	3.90	150	1.22	47	2.02	180
50–54	4.16	160	1.30	50	2.14	190
55–59	4.37	168	1.30	50	2.60	229
60–64	4.37	168	1.33	51	2.36	210
65–69	4.78	184	1.27	49	2.49	221
70+	4.42	170	1.25	48	2.13	189

*See Tables 72–1 and 72–2 for abbreviations.

TABLE 72–4. AVERAGE LEVELS OF APOPROTEINS IN PLASMA (MG/L)

APOPROTEIN	MEAN ± SD
A-I	1200 ± 200 (men)
	1350 ± 250 (women)
A-II	330 ± 50 (men)
	360 ± 60 (women)
B	1000 ± 200
C-I	70 ± 20
C-II	40 ± 20
C-III	130 ± 50
D	60 ± 10
E	50 ± 20

(From Albers, J.J.: The determination of apoproteins and their diagnostic value in clinical chemistry. *In* Eleventh International Congress of Clinical Chemistry. Edited by E. Kaiser, F. Gabal, M.M. Muller, et al. Berlin, Walter de Gruyter, 1982.)

liver and receptor pathway. The VLDL remnants remaining in the circulation generate most of the LDL in plasma.

IDL

IDL is enriched in the proportion of cholesterol relative to triglyceride, compared with VLDL (Table 72–1). Atherogenic diets may give rise to the related β-VLDL particle that is cholesterol-rich, contains apo-B and apo-E, and interacts with both the LDL receptor and the chylomicron (and VLDL) remnant receptor.[10]

LDL

LDL is taken up by the specific cell surface lipoprotein receptor (see Brown and Goldstein, Selected Readings) in the liver and (to a lesser extent) in peripheral tissues. The LDL is the most atherogenic of the lipoproteins because of mechanisms that remain unclear. LDL particles may be large and buoyant or small and dense. The latter are associated with a three-fold increased risk of myocardial infarction. Peroxidation of LDL also contributes to its atherogenicity.[14] A variant of LDL, Lp(a), normally present in small amounts in blood, is highly atherogenic. Lp(a) levels range from virtually undetectable to 1000 mg/L and may be increased in patients with cerebrovascular disease as well as in patients with coronary disease.[15] Levels are under genetic control and not easily modified by diet or lipid-lowering drugs other than niacin. Lp(a) levels greater than 300 mg/L are associated with significantly increased risk of vascular disease.

HDL

The HDL particle is produced when lipoprotein lipase transfers surface lipids from other triglyceride-rich lipoprotein particles (Fig. 72–1). Lipoprotein lipase activity generates HDL_2 and hepatic lipase converts HDL_2 to HDL_3. Feeding cholesterol results in the production of specific HDL particles that are larger, float at a lower density, and are enriched in cholesterol esters and apo-E. The HDL particle content of apo-A-I or apo-A-II may affect its antiatherogenic potential. High levels of HDL cholesterol are associated with decreased risk of atherosclerosis in both men and women and up to age 80. The protective effect of HDL may result from enhancing cholesterol removal from the body (reverse cholesterol transport)[16] or stabilizing vascular prostacyclin. The Framingham study showed a strong inverse correlation between levels of HDL cholesterol and coronary heart disease in both men and women, independent of the total cholesterol level. This has led to the development of various ratios to predict cardiovascular risk, such as total to HDL cholesterol, LDL to HDL cholesterol, or HDL to total HDL cholesterol. Very low HDL cholesterol in women results in high risk of CHD equivalent to that of men with similar HDL cholesterol. HDL cholesterol is decreased in smokers and increases within 1 year of stopping smoking. Most correlations are best with the HDL_2 subfraction.

DIETS AND SERUM LIPIDS AND LIPOPROTEINS

FATS, CHOLESTEROL, AND STEROLS

Diets high in total fat—especially saturated fat—are atherogenic for many animal species, particularly when cholesterol intake also is high.[2] Dietary saturated long-chain fatty acids raise plasma cholesterol levels and decrease LDL receptor activity.[17–19] Eicosapentaenoic acid and the other ω-3 (n-3) fatty acids found in fish and fish oils may have a hypocholesterolemic effect in normal

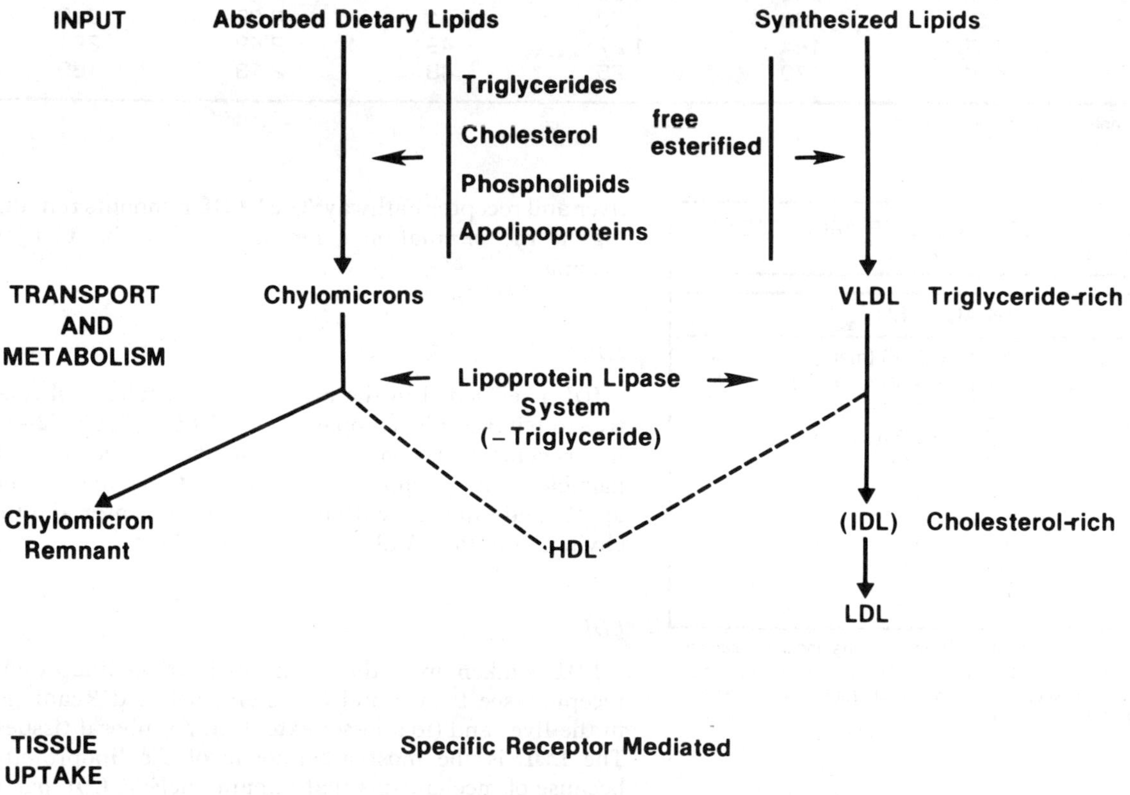

FIGURE 72–1. Diagram for the origin and removal of lipids and lipoproteins in the body. HDL, High-density lipoprotein; VLDL, very low-density lipoprotein; IDL, intermediate-density lipoprotein; LDL, low-density lipoprotein. (From Kuske, T.T., Feldman, E.B.: Arch. Intern. Med., *147*:357–360, 1987.)

subjects or raise LDL and HDL cholesterol in hyperlipidemic subjects and have significant hypotriglyceridemic effects in normal and hyperlipidemic subjects.[20–22] Rather than consuming fish oil capsules, however, eating more deep water ocean fatty fish such as herring, mackerel, tuna, halibut, and salmon is recommended because these foods do not contain the potentially toxic levels of vitamins A and D that may be present in fish liver oils. Monounsaturated liquid vegetable oils have a cholesterol-lowering effect, perhaps by replacing saturated fat.[23] Polyunsaturated fats of the ω-6 series in liquid vegetable oils such as corn, safflower, and sunflower oils result in decreased levels of LDL cholesterol and at high intake may decrease HDL cholesterol. Saturated fats are about twice as potent in raising serum cholesterol levels as polyunsaturated fats are in lowering them[2] (see also Chap. 87).

DIET COMPARISONS

Quantitative effects on serum or plasma levels of total, LDL, and HDL cholesterol and triglyceride of various diets using different amounts of total fats (high, moderate, low) with various modifications of levels and proportions of saturated, monounsaturated and polyunsaturated fats (n-3 and n-6) are provided in Table 72–5. Data are derived from recent published studies feeding healthy subjects (mostly young men) diets using foods in meals in an ambulatory setting.[21,24–28]

These studies conclude that with a low-fat diet (27% energy) HDL cholesterol may decrease, but the LDL-to-HDL ratio improves.[24] Although a diet high in fat with a high MFA content was "better" than a very low-fat (22% energy) diet, the exact compositions of the diets were not provided.[25] Others[26] showed that at less extreme P-to-S ratios there was no advantage in using MFA rather than PUFA in a low-fat diet in terms of plasma HDL cholesterol, and that HDL cholesterol does not necessarily fall with either a low-fat diet or a diet with a higher P-to-S ratio, nor does it increase with MFA.[27] When the saturated fat in a high-fat diet was replaced by MFA or PUFA there was no difference between them other than a greater fall in LDL cholesterol with the PUFA-enriched diet; neither diet affected HDL cholesterol.[28]

Thus, it seems that there are no special benefits of MFA, nor are there special adverse effects of PUFA or

TABLE 72–5. EFFECTS OF TYPICAL, CONTROLLED, AND MODIFIED FAT DIETS ON BLOOD LIPIDS*

		LIPID AND LIPOPROTEIN LEVELS				
Type of Diet	Specific Fat Concentration and Composition	Total Cholesterol	LDL Cholesterol	HDL Cholesterol	LDL/HDL Ratio	Triglycerides
A. Typical American diet ↑F, ↑SFA[25,27-29]	37–43% F; P:S = 0.2–0.6	↑	↑	↑	No report —[29]	±[27,29] (?) ↑[28] ↑ (if calories ↑)
B. Low-fat diet ↓F, ↓SFA, ↑CHO[24-26,27,29]	<30% F (20–29); P:S = 1	↓	↓	↓[24,29] —[27]	↓[24] —[29]	—[24,29] ↑[25] (some subjects)
C. Typical American diet + ↑MFA[25,27,28]	40–41% F; P:S = 0.7–1.0	↓	↓	—	↓	↓
D. Typical American diet + ↑PFA[28]	36–42% F; P:S = 2–3	↓	↓	—[28] ↓	↓	↓
E. Mod F, ↓SFA, Mod CHO[26]	32% F (29–35); P:S = 0.7–1.0	↓	↓	—	No report	—
F. Mod F, + ω-3 FA, Mod CHO[20-22,26]	5 g (2–10 g) ω-3 FA	—[21] ↓[22]	—[21] ↑[22] ↓[22]	±[21] ↑[22]	No report	↓
G. Mod F, ↑PFA, Mod CHO[26]	32% F (28–35); P:S = 1.25–1.5	↓	↓	—	No report	↓

Abbreviations and Symbols:
↓ = low level in the diet; ↓ = decrease in the blood lipid or lipoprotein level with the diet; ↑ = high level in the diet; ↑ = increase in the blood lipid or lipoprotein level with the diet; ± = variable response of lipids and lipoproteins to the diet; — = no effect of the diet on the blood lipid level; Mod = moderate concentration in the diet; F = fat; SFA = saturated fatty acids; MFA = monounsaturated fatty acids; PFA = polyunsaturated fatty acids; CHO = carbohydrate.

*The effect of any one type of diet on circulating lipids may differ among the investigators' studies cited. This is indicated for the respective lipid parameters by citation of the appropriate reference for each effect. Where only one effect is tabulated for a diet the studies cited are in agreement.

low-fat–high-carbohydrate diets if extremes are avoided (i.e., very low fat/very high carbohydrate, very high absolute PUFA, or extreme reduction in dietary cholesterol).[27] Incidentally, a diet low in fat and saturated fat has been estimated by the American Medical Association to cost $230 per year less than the typical American diet. In compliant free-living hypercholesterolemic subjects, about half will reduce LDL cholesterol by 16% on average with a low-fat, low-saturated-fat diet, whereas 10% may be diet-unresponsive. The remaining 40% show less than a 10% reduction in LDL cholesterol.[29] Overall, the step 2 NCEP diet (Appendix Table A–28) can be predicted to lower LDL cholesterol about 10% in hypercholesterolemic subjects.

Significantly different effects of dietary fats on plasma lipids and lipoproteins may be obtained when similar diets are provided to healthy normolipidemic subjects compared to hyperlipidemic patients (1) when studies are compared among similar subjects in metabolic units, free-living and provided meals, or free-living and diet counseled and monitored, (2) when formula diets are provided compared to meals, and (3) when the duration varies from a few weeks to the long term (years).

The usual daily diet in the United States for men contains about 450 mg cholesterol. Reducing the cholesterol intake to 300 mg or less (80 to 100 mg per 1000 kcal) will decrease plasma cholesterol levels (see the *Report of the National Cholesterol Education Program* listed in the selected readings at the end of this chapter). Cholesterol, synthesized by all animal cells, therefore is present in all animal products (see Appendix Table A–19) and is not present in any plant products, including all vegetable oils. Cholesterol intake increases LDL synthesis and decreases LDL catabolism via the LDL receptor.

Large doses of plant sterols (sitosterol, campesterol) produce a hypocholesterolemic effect when given at or before mealtime. Marine sterols from clams or oysters also may be hypocholesterolemic. These sterols presumably inhibit intestinal absorption of cholesterol.

CARBOHYDRATE AND FIBER

High-fiber, low-fat diets have been proposed as protective against atherosclerosis; addition of some forms of fiber to diets may lower cholesterol levels and reduce hyperglycemia in diabetics.[30] Partially digestible noncellulose pectin (in the "zest" of fruit) and gums and mucilages and lignin may have a specific lipid-lowering effect. For example, most wheat bran varieties do not lower cholesterol, but oat bran and some barleys do. Intake of refined carbohydrates may exacerbate hypertriglyceridemia.[4]

CALORIES, PROTEIN, AND ALCOHOL

Restriction of calories in the obese patient will reduce serum lipid levels; diet modifications are indicated in such subjects at least up to age 70. Lower levels of HDL cholesterol in the obese will increase with weight reduction. Excess calories increase VLDL production and decrease VLDL removal, resulting in increased triglyceride levels. LDL overproduction can ensue along with increased cholesterol levels. Impaired glucose tolerance with obesity will contribute to the lipid metabolic defects, especially to hypertriglyceridemia.

Some types of animal protein (e.g., casein or meat) may be hypercholesterolemic, and some kinds of vegetable protein (e.g., soy) lower cholesterol.[4]

Consumption of alcohol increases VLDL production by the liver. Chylomicron synthesis increases when alcohol is consumed with a fatty meal. These effects of alcohol can induce hypertriglyceridemia and convert a patient with endogenous hypertriglyceridemia (type 4) to a mixed hyperlipidemia (chylomicronemia syndrome, type 5).

TABLE 72–6. FACTORS AFFECTING HDL CHOLESTEROL LEVELS

INCREASED LEVELS	DECREASED LEVELS
Saturated fats	Simple sugars/high carbohydrate diet (short period)
Dietary cholesterol	Polyunsaturated fat, high
Alcohol (≤2 drinks daily)	Androgens
Long-term aerobic exercise program	Anabolic steroids
Estrogens	Progestogens
Female gender	Some antihypertensive drugs
	Obesity
	Diabetes mellitus
	Cigarette smoking
	Physical inactivity
	Male gender

DIET AND HDL

Diets that decrease HDL cholesterol include high-carbohydrate diets or diets very high in polyunsaturated fat and diets decreased in saturated fat or very low in fat. HDL increases with modest intake of alcohol (Table 72–6).

HYPERLIPIDEMIAS

The hyperlipidemias may occur from increased levels of cholesterol and/or triglycerides in a variety of lipoproteins (Table 72–7). These disorders may be inherited or of dietary origin. Responses to diet modifications vary with the disorder and among individuals.

CLASSIFICATION

Hypercholesterolemia may be inherited as a single gene abnormality or may develop from the effects of multiple genes (polygenic hypercholesterolemia). Ele-

TABLE 72–7. HYPERLIPIDEMIAS

TYPE	DESIGNATION AND LIPOPROTEIN ABNORMALITY
1	Increased exogenous triglycerides in the form of chylomicrons
2a	Hypercholesterolemia (increase in LDL) with normal triglyceride levels
2b	Hypercholesterolemia combined with mild hypertriglyceridemia (increase in LDL and VLDL, overproduction of apo-B)
3	Hypercholesterolemia with hypertriglyceridemia and increase in IDL
4	Mild to moderate endogenous hypertriglyceridemia (2.8–7.9 mmol/L, or 250–700 mg/dl) with increased VLDL
5	Moderate to severe hypertriglyceridemia (11.3 mmol/L or 1000 mg/l) with mixed VLDL and chylomicrons

vated cholesterol levels in plasma usually involve LDL and result from the increased production and/or delayed or defective removal of LDL cholesterol. Hypercholesterolemia can occur without (type 2a) or combined with (type 2b, familial combined hyperlipidemia) mild hypertriglyceridemia. Elevated triglyceride levels in association with hypercholesterolemia result from genetic defects or diet or both. Primary hypertriglyceridemia may result from overproduction of VLDL alone (type 4), or with chylomicrons (type 5), or from defective removal via lipoprotein lipase (type 1). A defect in removal of IDL results in hypercholesterolemia and hypertriglyceridemia (type 3 hyperlipoproteinemia). Thus, the primary hyperlipoproteinemias are metabolic disorders characterized by an excess of one or more lipoproteins in the circulation.[31]

Hyperlipoproteinemias may be diagnosed after at least three measurements of plasma lipids after the patient has fasted overnight for 12 to 14 hours. The lipoproteins are fractionated to determine the type of hyperlipoproteinemia. A preliminary lipid profile can be provided by measurement in a blood sample of total cholesterol, triglycerides, and HDL cholesterol and calculating the LDL cholesterol using the equation LDL cholesterol (mg) = total cholesterol − HDL cholesterol − triglyceride ÷ 5. The latter factor approximates VLDL cholesterol and is only valid when triglyceride values are less than 350 to 400 mg/dl. The presence of diseases causing secondary hyperlipidemia should be ruled out. Hypercholesterolemia per se is asymptomatic in most of the population. Its detection is possible only by measurement of circulating lipids. Family members, especially first-degree relatives, also should be screened. This may provide clues to inheritance and detect new patients.

GENETICS

Genetic hyperlipidemias have been associated with mutations underlying lipoprotein lipase deficiency, apo-B gene variants, and variations in the apo AI-CIII-AIV gene[32–34] (Table 72–8). New insights into genetic disorders of lipoprotein metabolism will result from the application of molecular biologic techniques. Nutrition may be an important factor controlling gene expression.

TABLE 72–8. GENETIC BASIS OF FAMILIAL HYPERLIPOPROTEINEMIAS

Type 1	Familial lipoprotein lipase deficiency	Missense and nonsense mutations of gene encoding enzyme
	Familial lipoprotein lipase inhibitor	?
	Familial apo-C-II deficiency	Four variant genes
	Familial hepatic lipase deficiency	?
Type 2	Familial hypercholesterolemia	45 mutations in four classes of the LDL receptor gene
	Familial defective apo-B_{100}	Defective apo-B gene impairs binding
	Polygenic hypercholesterolemia	Apo-A-I/C-III/A-IV gene clusters
Type 2b	Familial combined hyperlipidemia	?
Type 3	Type III	Apo-E gene polymorphism affects amino acid coding
Type 4	Familial hypertriglyceridemia—Type IV	Apo-A-I/C-III/A-IV
Type 5	Type V	Apo-A-I/C-II/A-IV; apo-A-II

Gene-gene interactions may explain some differences in susceptibility to atherosclerosis.

A family history of premature coronary disease is found in almost half of CHD patients. More than half of the variability in serum cholesterol between individuals is attributable to genetic variation, presumably largely polygenic. Many genes are possible causes of the hyperlipidemias (Table 72–8). About 7% of the variation in cholesterol between individuals is attributable to the effect of apo-E polymorphism on LDL cholesterol levels, and approximately 3.5% of the variance is explained by apo-B gene polymorphism. Other genes may influence LDL receptor activity and apo-B synthesis and may interact with nongenetic factors such as the diet and physical activity.

About 30% of all survivors of premature myocardial infarction (under 55 years of age) have some form of familial hyperlipidemia.

TYPES OF HYPERLIPOPROTEINEMIAS

CHYLOMICRONEMIA (TYPE 1 HYPERLIPOPROTEINEMIA)

Exogenous triglycerides transported as chylomicrons are increased in type 1 hyperlipoproteinemia. The condition is rare and results from a defect in the removal of chylomicrons from the blood. The disorder is due to a recessive gene that results in a deficiency of lipoprotein lipase, the absence of or an abnormality of its apoprotein-C-II activator, or the presence of a circulating inhibitor. Type 1 hyperlipoproteinemia may be observed in infants and children and does not necessarily predispose to vascular disease. Patients are at risk of recurrent severe pancreatitis. They may exhibit lipemia retinalis (Fig. 72–2*A*), eruptive xanthomas (Fig. 72–2*B*), and hepatoplenomegaly. The plasma shows a chylomicron layer over a clear infranatant. Plasma triglyceride levels usually exceed 17 mmol/L (1500 mg/dl).

HYPERCHOLESTEROLEMIA (TYPE 2A AND TYPE 2B HYPERLIPOPROTEINEMIA)

Hypercholesterolemia characterizes type 2a and type 2b hyperlipoproteinemia. In type 2a, the level of plasma triglycerides is normal; the levels of cholesterol and its lipoprotein transporter LDL are increased. Type 2b combines hypercholesterolemia and hypertriglyceridemia, with increases in LDL and VLDL, and overproduction of apo-B. The most common hyperlipidemic syndrome in families with early coronary disease (by age 55) is familial combined hyperlipidemia (FCH), occurring in 15% of such families.

Familial Combined Hyperlipidemia (FCH). Dense LDL with increased apo-B levels is a marker of this disorder. These heterogeneous particles have great atherogenic potential. Apo-B levels exceeding 1300 mg/L are diagnostic of the hyper apo-B variant of FCH. There is a strong family history of premature coronary disease.

Familial Hypercholesterolemia. Familial hypercholesterolemia (FH) is a single gene defect in the cell surface receptor that binds or internalizes circulating LDL (see Brown and Goldstein, and Scriver, Beaudet, and Sly in the selected readings list at the end of this chapter). One in 500 individuals is heterozygous for the FH gene; the homozygous state occurs in 1 in 1,000,000. More than 40 mutations have been characterized involving the synthesis, processing, binding, and clustering of the cell surface receptor. The homozygous phenotype also may be the result of a compound heterozygote with two genetic defects.

Mechanism. The specific cell surface receptor delivers cholesterol to cells. Cholesterol is freed from the lipoprotein within the cell and regulates endogenous cholesterol synthesis by suppressing the activity of hydroxymethylglutaryl coenzyme (HMG CoA) reductase, the rate-limiting step in cholesterol synthesis. Cholesterol is re-esterified and stored as cholesteryl ester within the cell. This suppresses the synthesis of the LDL receptor. In the FH heterozygote, the number of LDL receptors is about half normal; the LDL cholesterol level doubles in the circulation, and the fractional catabolic rate of LDL is halved. With no receptors (the FH homozygote), LDL synthesis is greatly enhanced and its removal is decreased, with a marked decrease in the fractional catabolic rate of LDL.

Clinical Manifestations. Hypercholesterolemia is present from birth in the FH patient. Cholesterol levels average 9.0 mmol/L (350 mg/dl) in heterozygotes and 19 mmol/L (740 mg/dl) in homozygotes. Corneal arcus (Fig.

FIGURE 72–2. *A*, Funduscopic photograph of the retinal blood vessels from a patient with severe type 5 hyperlipoproteinemia (chylomicronemia syndrome). *B*, Eruptive xanthomas of the skin of the arm in a patient with severe type 5 hyperlipoproteinemia (chylomicronemia syndrome). *C*, Premature and extensive corneal arcus in a patient with heterozygous familial hypercholesterolemia. *D*, Achilles tendon xanthomas from a patient with type 2b hyperlipoproteinemia, heterozygous familial hypercholesterolemia (case). *E*, Xanthomas of the extensor tendons of the hands in a patient with heterozygous familial hypercholesterolemia. *F*, Tuberous xanthomas of the skin over the elbows of a teenager with heterozygous familial hypercholesterolemia, type 2a. *G*, Eyelid xanthelasma from a patient with type 2 hyperlipoproteinemia. *H*, Extensive planar xanthomas of the palms, typical of a patient with type 3 hyperlipoproteinemia.

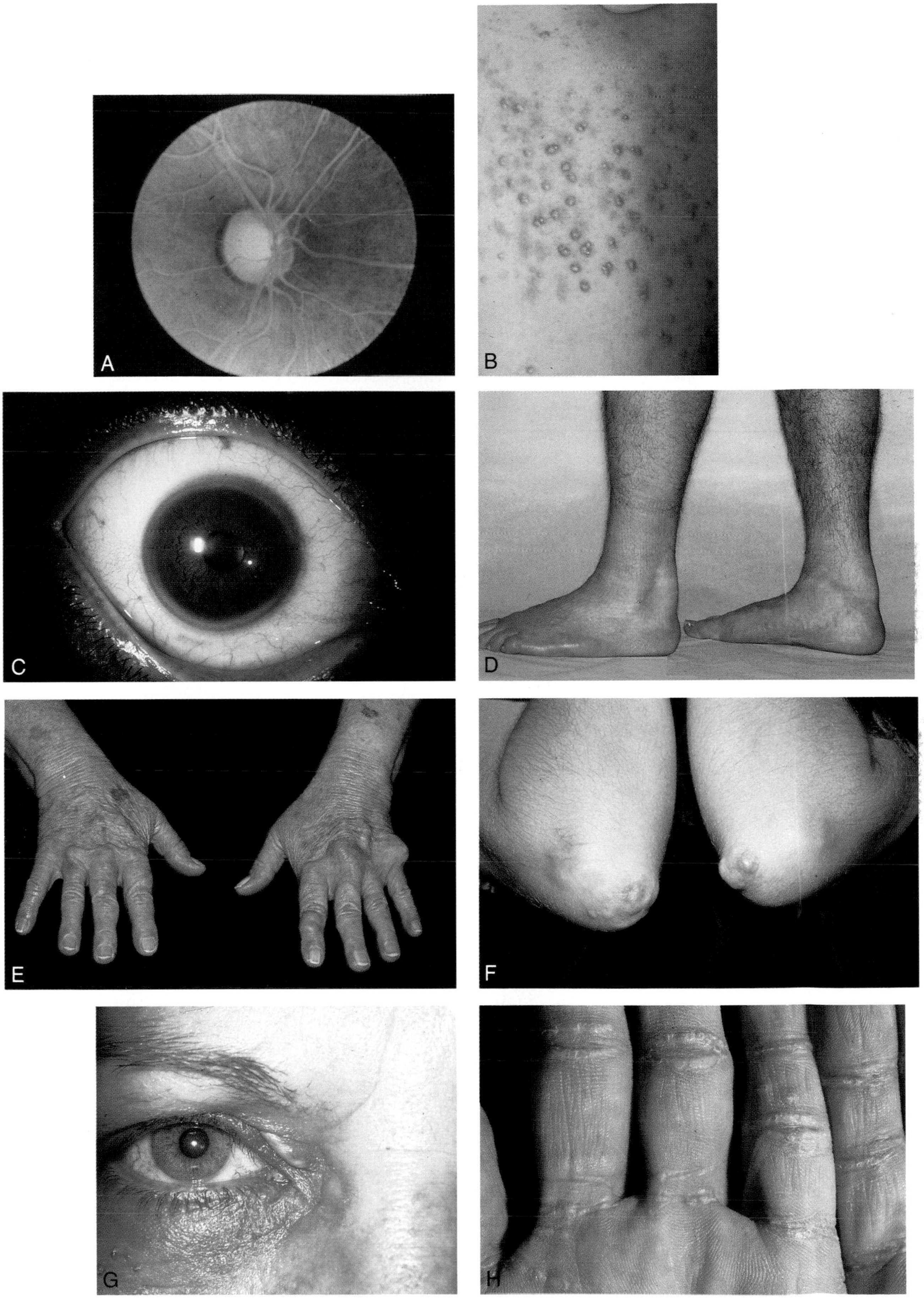
A
B
C
D
E
F
G
H

72–2*C*) and tendon xanthomas (Fig. 72–2*D* and *E*) and/or tuberous xanthomas (Fig. 72–2*F*) may be seen in heterozygotes by the latter half of the second decade of life; by the third decade these signs appear in more than half of these patients. Tendon xanthomas typically involve extensor tendons (e.g., Achilles, digits); up to 80% of FH patients have them sometime in life. By age 4 homozygotes have unique cutaneous xanthomas on the buttocks, the creases of the hands, and over the kneecaps. Eyelid xanthelasma (Fig. 72–2*G*) comprises planar xanthomas observed in patients with hypercholesterolemia. Cholesterol levels are normal in about half of patients with xanthelasma; recent studies have indicated that these patients have abnormal isoforms of apo-E (E phenotypes).

The incidence of coronary heart disease in FH patients is 25 times that of persons not carrying the gene and occurs at a mean age that is 15 to 20 years younger than in the general population. The first heart attack occurs in 51% of men with heterozygous FH by age 50 and in 85% by age 60. Over 70% have triple-vessel disease. In women with FH 12% will have a heart attack by age 50 and 58% by age 60. The mean age of death of patients with homozygous FH is 21 years, with heart attacks occurring in infancy and early childhood.

Case History: Familial Type 2b Hyperlipidemia. A 55-year-old physician had known hyperlipidemia for 32 years. His plasma cholesterol was 33.8 mmol/L (1300 mg/dl), and total lipid levels of 37.3 mmol/L (3300 mg/dl) were reported at the onset. With a diet low in fat, saturated fat, and cholesterol and an exercise program, his plasma cholesterol ranged from 13 to 15 mmol/L (500 to 600 mg/dl) with triglycerides of 6 to 14 mmol/L (600 to 1200 mg/dl). His tendon and tuberous xanthomas of hands, feet, elbows, and knees increased in size. Angina developed at age 40. Cardiac catheterization at age 48 showed an obstructed right coronary artery. Several siblings died in their forties of coronary heart disease.

When seen his HDL cholesterol was 1.4 mmol/L (55 mg/dl), and LDL cholesterol was 7.1 mmol/L (275 mg/dl). He had a corneal arcus, tendon xanthomas of hands and ankles, skin xanthomas over knees, and prominent tibial tubercles (Fig. 72–2*C* to *E*). A 15-lb weight-loss goal was set, and a stringent diet was prescribed. In view of prior treatment failures using clofibrate, niacin, and colestipol, he was treated with an HMG CoA reductase inhibitor. Addition of cholestyramine to the drug regimen resulted in increases in triglycerides and cholesterol and was stopped. At routine ultrasonography of the gallbladder an abdominal aortic aneurysm was found, and surgery was performed. With niacin (3 g per day) added to lovastatin (40 mg bid), lipid values were as follows: total cholesterol 5.3 mmol/L (203 mg/dl), triglycerides 1.0 mmol/L (88 mg/dl), HDL cholesterol 2.2 mmol/L (83 mg/dl), LDL cholesterol 2.8 mmol/L (109 mg/dl). The tendon xanthomas decreased in size and the tuberous xanthomas disappeared.

Adverse effects, attributed to niacin, that normalized with decrease in drug dose or discontinuance included increased liver enzymes (alkaline phosphatase and transaminases), nausea, vomiting, and itching.

This patient is a classic example of the disorder of heterozygous familial hypercholesterolemia. Typical are the clinical stigmata of hypercholesterolemia and premature atherosclerosis and the resistance of the elevated levels of LDL cholesterol to a prudent diet, even combined with one or more cholesterol-lowering medications. Family screening and early and aggressive therapy are mandatory preventive measures.

For adults with FH the use of the new class of drugs that inhibit cholesterol synthesis offers the possibility of normalizing lipid levels and preventing the severe premature atherosclerosis that develops in untreated or inadequately managed patients.

TYPE 3 HYPERLIPOPROTEINEMIA

Type 3 hyperlipoproteinemia also is termed dysbetalipoproteinemia, or broad beta or floating beta disease. Hypercholesterolemia combined with hypertriglyceridemia is due to increased IDL (VLDL remnants), at times mixed with chylomicrons. Type 3 hyperlipoproteinemia may be suspected when the levels of cholesterol and triglycerides in plasma are increased proportionally. Type 3 hyperlipoproteinemia is relatively uncommon and is characterized by planar xanthomas in the creases of the palms of the hands and fingers (Fig. 72–2*H*). Tuberous xanthomas also may appear over the elbows and the knees (Fig. 72–2*F*). The disorder usually appears in the third decade of life; it may be secondary to and precipitated by an endocrine abnormality such as hypothyroidism or hypopituitarism, which should be treated. Over half of the type 3 hyperlipoproteinemia patients have premature peripheral vascular disease and coronary heart disease.

This disorder is diagnosed by preparative ultracentrifugation of lipoproteins to demonstrate the increased amounts of cholesterol relative to triglycerides in the lipoprotein fraction floating at $d < 1.006$ (VLDL). A mass ratio of cholesterol to triglyceride exceeding 0.42 is diagnostic. Electrophoresis of this fraction shows β-migrating lipoprotein, β-VLDL. This accounts for another name for type 3 hyperlipoproteinemia, "floating beta disease." Type 3 disease is characterized by a genetic defect with abnormal E isoforms (one or two E-2 rather than E-3, or E-4 isoforms with defective receptor binding—see Scriver, Beaudet, Sly, et al., Selected Readings). The apo-E phenotype should be determined to establish the diagnosis. For the clinical expression of this disorder as hyperlipidemia, a second genetic lipoprotein disorder or other metabolic abnormalities also may need to be present. The abnormal apo-E–containing IDL binds less avidly to the LDL (apo-B, E) receptor than normal VLDL remnants do, and its lesser rate of removal results in increased circulating levels of IDL.

Case History: Type 3 Hyperlipoproteinemia. A 38-year-old hospital employee was referred for cardiac catheterization. He had a history of intermittent claudication and angina for 2 years and had sustained a myocardial infarction 3 months earlier. He was a heavy smoker with a history of alcohol abuse and a family history of myocardial infarction (father at age 60 and uncle at age 46). Physical examination showed decreased arterial pulses in the lower extremities. Yellowish streaks (2 × 10 mm linear plaques) were visible in the creases of the palms of his hands (Fig. 72–2*H*). His pulses were diminished in both popliteal regions. Plasma lipid values were as follows: total cholesterol 13.6 mmol/L (526 mg/dl), triglycerides 13.2 mmol/L (1173 mg/dl). Ultracentrifugation of plasma obtained after the patient had received diet counseling yielded the following values: total cholesterol 10.66 mmol/L (410 mg/dl), VLDL cholesterol 7.2 mmol/L (279 mg/dl), LDL cholesterol 2.8 mmol/L (106 mg/dl), and HDL cholesterol 0.6 mmol/L (25 mg/dl), with triglycerides at 6.5 mmol/L (573 mg/dl). Electrophoresis showed a broad beta pattern in whole plasma and a "floating beta" band in the VLDL fraction, confirming the diagnosis of type 3 hyperlipoproteinemia.

This patient illustrates that blood lipids may not be measured even when symptomatic premature coronary heart disease is present. His type 3 disorder showed the classic manifestations of peripheral vascular disease and planar xanthomas of the hands along with elevated levels of cholesterol with similar levels of triglycerides. The patient died 2 years later; he had not reported for follow-up treatment.

TYPE 4 AND TYPE 5 HYPERLIPOPROTEINEMIA

Mild-to-moderate increase in triglyceride values (3 to 8 mmol/L, or 250 to 700 mg/dl) with increased VLDL characterize type 4 hyperlipoproteinemia (endogenous hypertriglyceridemia). The defect may involve both overproduction and decreased removal of VLDL triglycerides (see Schaefer and Levy in the selected readings list at the end of this chapter). LDL cholesterol levels are within the normal range. This type of hyperlipoproteinemia is associated with an increased risk of atherosclerosis, perhaps because of the usual association of elevated VLDL and triglycerides with decreased HDL cholesterol. Hypertriglyceridemia per se may be an independent risk factor for atherosclerosis. Moderate to severe increases in triglyceride values (exceeding 11.3 mmol/L, or 1000 mg/dl) occur in type 5 hyperlipoproteinemia. Triglyceride levels may rise, though rarely, to 225 mmol/L (20,000 mg/dl). In type 5 hyperlipoproteinemia, chylomicrons appear along with the increased levels of VLDL.

The chylomicronemia syndrome is characterized by eruptive xanthomas correlated with increased triglyceride levels (Fig. 72–2*B*). The xanthomas often are observed earliest involving the skin over the back of the neck or the buttocks. When the triglyceride level exceeds 34 mmol/L (3000 mg/dl), lipemia retinalis will be observed on funduscopic examination (Fig. 72–2*A*). These patients with chylomicronemia are at increased risk to develop recurrent acute pancreatitis and may develop pancreatic insufficiency. They may have recurrent abdominal pain without elevated amylase levels. Type 5 hyperlipoproteinemia patients are at increased risk for atherosclerosis, especially with low HDL. More than half of these patients have diabetes mellitus that must be controlled to lower triglycerides effectively. Alcohol intake sometimes will convert a type 4 hyperlipoproteinemia patient to type 5 disease and may precipitate pancreatitis. Administration of corticosteroids or estrogens also may aggravate the hypertriglyceridemia and precipitate pancreatitis. The underlying mechanisms and genetic defects in these disorders are unknown.

Case History: Type 5 Hyperlipoproteinemia. A 60-year-old college professor had known of increased levels of circulating triglycerides for more than 15 years, with levels exceeding 22 mmol/L (2000 mg/dl). He had been treated unsuccessfully with a cholesterol-lowering diet and clofibrate, cholestyramine, probucol, and lovastatin in turn. The triglyceride value on referral was 9 mmol/L (832 mg/dl) with total cholesterol at 6.12 mmol/L (237 mg/dl), HDL cholesterol at 0.36 mmol/L (14 mg/dl), and LDL cholesterol at 1.3 mmol/L (50 mg/dl). The patient was advised to decrease intakes of alcohol, fat (peanut butter), and sweets with an increase in fish, seafood, pasta, soluble fiber, and complex carbohydrates. Because there was no sustained improvement in triglycerides after 4 months of compliance with the diet, the patient was started on treatment with gemfibrozil. The triglyceride value was 3.6 mmol/L (320 mg/dl), LDL cholesterol increased to 4.19 mmol/L (161 mg/dl), and HDL cholesterol was 0.57 mmol/L (22 mg/dl). Niacin (500 mg bid) was added, and values were as follows: triglycerides 2.79 mmol/L (248 mg/dl), total cholesterol 4.86 mmol/L (187 mg/dl), LDL cholesterol 3.10 mmol/L (120 mg/dl), and HDL cholesterol 0.67 mmol/L (26 mg/dl).

This patient illustrates the need to prescribe an appropriate triglyceride-lowering diet and triglyceride-lowering medicines for the type 4 or type 5 hyperlipoproteinemia patient. He was fortunate not to have experienced recurrent abdominal pain and acute pancreatitis.

Other recently described lipid atherogenic syndromes include: familial dyslipoproteinemic hypertension with hyperlipidemia, glucose intolerance, and hypertension; and abnormal lipoprotein phenotypes with increased atherogenicity such as hypertriglyceridemia, dense LDL, and reduced HDL cholesterol with insulin resistance and abdominal obesity.

EVALUATION OF THE HYPERLIPIDEMIC PATIENT

The hyperlipidemic patient is evaluated by the usual tools of the history, the clinical examination, and laboratory tests. Are there xanthomas, symptoms of vascular insufficiency, abdominal pain? Were lipids measured previously? Has the patient had a myocardial infarction, bypass surgery, angioplasty? Is the gallbladder present? A history of diabetes, thyroid, hepatic, or renal disease or gout is relevant. The family history of coronary heart disease, hyperlipidemia, hypertension, diabetes, and gout should be sought. Have the children been tested for hyperlipidemia? The diet history includes alcohol and use of supplements. Smoking habits, exercise, and medications should be asked about.

The physical examination looks for corneal arcus, xanthelasma, xanthomas; one should pay attention to the palms, elbows, knees, buttocks, dorsum of hands and feet, tibial tuberosities, and Achilles tendons. Are there aortic murmurs, reduced pulses, bruits, or retinopathy (or lipemia retinalis)? Liver and spleen size should be assessed. Is skin dry or hair lost, and is there delayed relaxation of deep tendon reflexes? The blood pressure should be measured along with the height and weight.

Plasma should be obtained after an overnight fast of 12 to 14 hours. Total cholesterol, triglycerides, and HDL cholesterol should be measured with calculation of LDL cholesterol (and HDL ratio). Apo-B, apo-A-I, and Lp(a) should be measured, if available. The plasma should be examined after standing overnight at 4° C. Lipoprotein ultracentrifugation, electrophoresis, and E phenotyping will differentiate type 3 from type 2b or type 5 hyperlipoproteinemia. Measurements of post-heparin lipolytic activity and agarose gel electrophoresis of C-apoproteins will aid in evaluation of type 1 and type 5 hyperlipoproteinemia patients. The latter tests are usually available only in university and research laboratories.

Tests of renal, hepatic, and thyroid function should be included, with measurement of blood glucose. A resting electrocardiogram should be routine.

The dietitian's assessment should include the patient's intake of energy, protein, carbohydrate, and sucrose, the amount and type of fat, and cholesterol content.

MANAGEMENT OF HYPERLIPIDEMIAS BY DIET

Goals of treatment are as follows: for the hypertriglyceridemic patient, to prevent pancreatitis; for the patient with coronary disease, to lower lipids and prevent progression of atherosclerosis and occurrence of new and other clinical events; and for the asymptomatic patient, to prevent symptomatic coronary disease, especially if the patient is at high risk. Treatment is by diet, with medication added if target lipid and lipoprotein levels are not reached.

CHOLESTEROL LOWERING

To reduce hypercholesterolemia to levels below the 75th percentile (Table 72–3) and for levels that warrant treatment (Table 72–9), the dietary intake of calories, total fat, saturated fat, cholesterol, and animal protein are restricted, and increases in consumption of complex carbohydrates and fiber, the proportion of polyunsaturated or monounsaturated fats, and vegetable protein are ordered.[34,35] Diet counseling should be continued for several months in the treatment of hypercholesterolemia to enhance compliance, with measurements of plasma lipids made at 6- to 8-week intervals to monitor the response (see Report of the National Cholesterol Education Program, Selected Reading).

Calories are regulated to achieve desirable weight. An exercise regimen will aid in weight loss and in raising HDL cholesterol. Total fat initially should be decreased to 30% or less of calories, with saturated fat reduced to less than 10% of calories, polyunsaturates (including about 2% as n-3 fatty acids) increased up to 10% of calories, and the remainder given as monounsaturates. The cholesterol intake should be less than 100 mg/1000 kcal. Dietary changes include limiting visible fats and oils, especially solid fat, by trimming meats; using low-fat dairy products and lean meats in moderation, substituting fish and poultry (white meat, no skin) for red meats; avoiding "invisible" fats hidden in snacks and desserts; limiting egg yolks and substituting egg whites or egg substitutes; and using whole grains, pastas, fruits, and vegetables (raw or lightly cooked). The diet of the United States should be modified to resemble that of Mediterranean or Asian populations.

Compliance with and response to these changes may lower total cholesterol and LDL cholesterol by 10 to 20%; the greatest effect will come from the elimination of

TABLE 72–9. BLOOD LIPID AND LIPOPROTEIN CHOLESTEROL LEVELS WARRANTING TREATMENT

	RECOMMENDED	BORDERLINE	NEEDING TREATMENT
Cholesterol	<5.20 (<200)*	5.20–6.24 (200–240)	6.24+ (240+)
LDL cholesterol	<3.38 (<130)	3.38–4.16 (130–160)	4.16+ (160+)
HDL cholesterol			<0.91 (<35)
Triglycerides		>2.82 (>250)	>5.65 (>500)

(Adapted from the Report of the National Cholesterol Education Program expert panel on detection, evaluation, and treatment of high blood cholesterol in adults: Arch. Intern. Med., *48:* 36-69, 1988.)

*Values are given in mmol/L; values in parentheses are in mg/dl.

saturated fat (each 1% decrease in saturated fat = −2.7 mg, or 0.07 mmol, cholesterol). Patients with more-severe forms of hypercholesterolemia, with very high levels of total and LDL cholesterol, should be prescribed a more rigorous diet that further reduces total fat, with saturated fat decreased to less than 7% of calories and cholesterol limited to less than 70 mg/1000 kcal.

TRIGLYCERIDE LOWERING

Triglycerides in VLDL (endogenous hypertriglyceridemia) are increased by excess calories, especially the proportion of calories from refined carbohydrates, and by alcohol. Triglycerides are decreased by n-3 fatty acids in fish oils.[20,21] Chylomicron triglycerides (exogenous hypertriglyceridemia) are sensitive to fat and alcohol intake and are lowered by limiting fat intake severely to 50 g or less daily, or to less than 20% of calories. Alcohol also should be restricted. Weight control with caloric restriction and exercise especially is helpful.[36] The immediate and long-term goals are to decrease triglycerides in the type 5 hyperlipoproteinemia patient to less than 5.65 mmol/L (500 mg/dl) to avoid drug treatment and lessen the risk of acute pancreatitis. The risk of atherosclerosis may be decreased when triglyceride levels are reduced by diet to less than 2.26 mmol/L (200 mg/dl).

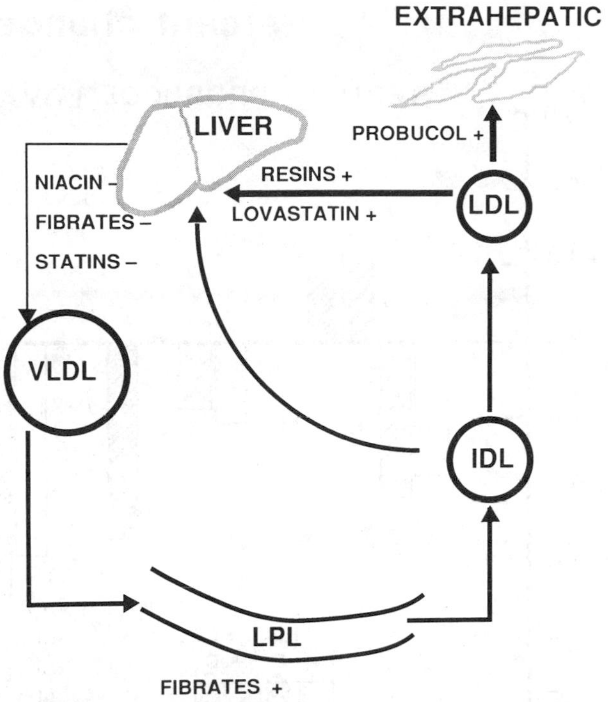

FIGURE 72–3. Interrelation of apo-B-containing lipoprotein production and removal in blood and tissues of normolipidemic subjects. The sites of action of the lipid-lowering drugs are indicated. LPL, Lipoprotein lipase; see Figure 72–1 for other abbreviations.

MANAGEMENT OF HYPERLIPIDEMIAS BY DRUGS

If the appropriate lipid-lowering diet does not control blood lipid levels adequately within 3 to 6 months (Table 72–9), then appropriate medication should be added to (not substituted for) the diet (see *Report of the National Cholesterol Education Program* in the selected readings list at the end of this chapter). Patients with severe familial hypercholesterolemia should be started on medication sooner because they are unlikely to be controlled with diet alone. Drug treatment should be monitored for efficacy and safety and must be considered life-long therapy.

CHOLESTEROL LOWERING

Drugs that lower total and LDL cholesterol significantly include the bile acid binding resins (cholestyramine, colestipol), niacin, HMG CoA reductase inhibitors (lovastatin, pravastatin, simvastatin), fibric acid derivatives (gemfibrozil), and probucol.[18,37] Their efficacy, side effects, and mechanisms of action are described in Figures 72–3 and 72–4 and in Table 72–10. Drugs may need to be used in combinations of two or three in the management of severe hypercholesterolemia (Fig. 72–4). Average cost to the pharmacist in 1990 for 1 month's treatment of hypercholesterolemia with usual dosages of medications ranged from $7 for generic niacin to $80 for cholestyramine. Gemfibrozil, lovastatin, and probucol costs were $50, $52, and $54, respectively.

TRIGLYCERIDE LOWERING

Fibric acid derivatives and niacin are potent triglyceride-lowering drugs that also increase HDL cholesterol.[18] Either drug should be added to the diet early on in patients with severe hypertriglyceridemia (type 5) to prevent pancreatitis. If LDL levels increase when VLDL and chylomicrons decrease, a cholesterol-lowering drug may need to be combined with the initial agent. Metabolic diseases such as diabetes mellitus and hypothyroidism must be controlled. There are no effective drugs for the treatment of chylomicronemia (type 1); this disorder must be controlled by diet.

INTERFERING MEDICATIONS

Some medications used to treat hypertension or angina may have adverse effects, increasing total and LDL cholesterol and/or triglycerides and lowering HDL cholesterol. Lipids should be evaluated and monitored in patients receiving some diuretics or β-blockers for treatment of hypertension or coronary heart disease as well as

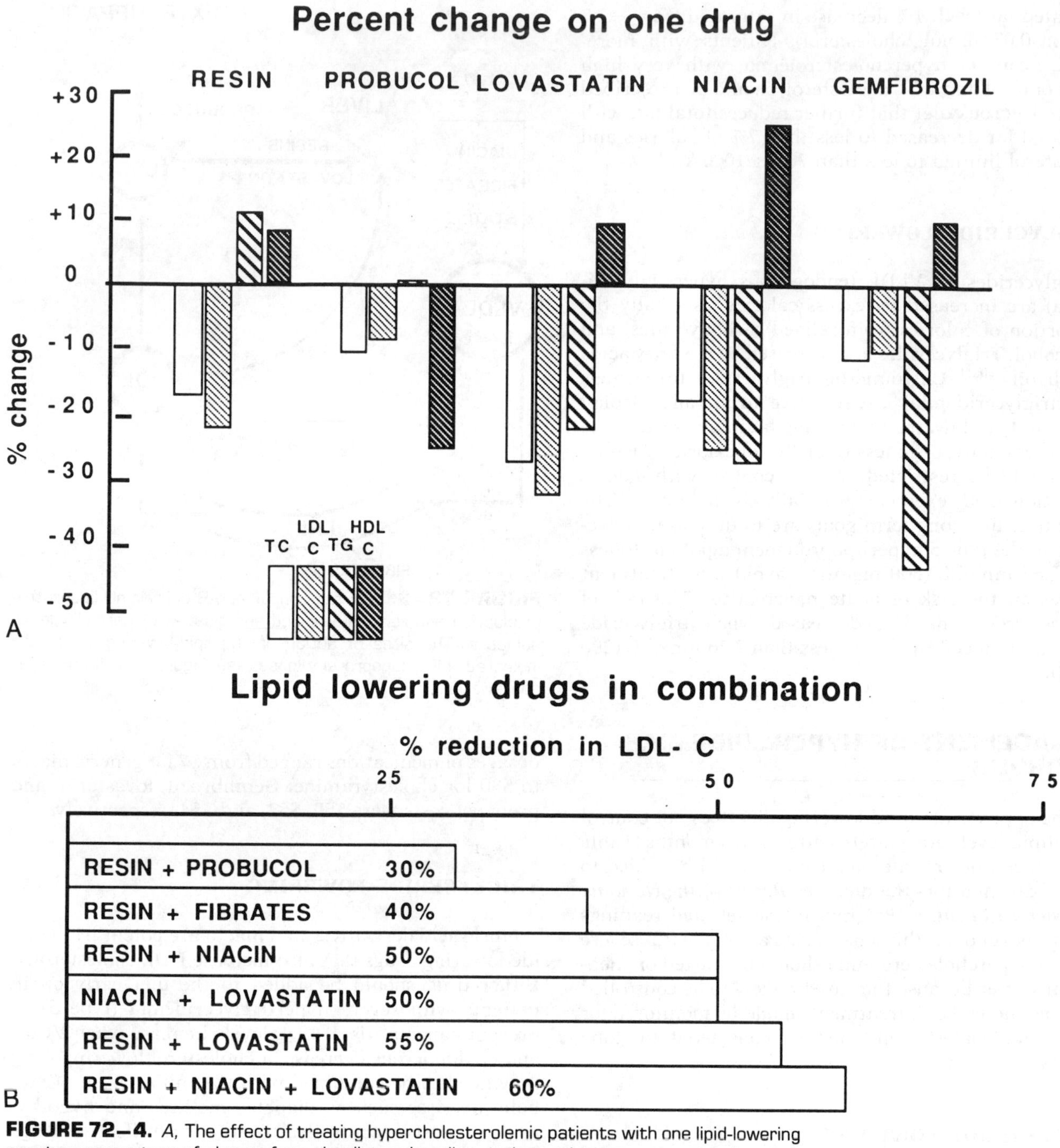

FIGURE 72–4. *A*, The effect of treating hypercholesterolemic patients with one lipid-lowering agent as percentage of change from the dietary baseline; patients also are eating a cholesterol-lowering diet. Total cholesterol is represented by clear bars, low-density lipoprotein cholesterol by stippled bars, triglyceride by hatched bars, and high-density lipoprotein by dotted bars. *B*, The effect on levels of LDL-C (low-density lipoprotein cholesterol) of treating hypercholesterolemia with various combinations of lipid-lowering medications in patients already ingesting a cholesterol-lowering diet. (From Feldman, E.B., Kuske, T.T.: Mod. Med., *56*:60–71, 1988.)

TABLE 72–10. LIPID-LOWERING DRUGS

DRUG	TOLERANCE/COMPLIANCE	SIDE EFFECTS
Resin	Compliance poor; side effects frequent (5–34%)	Constipation, heartburn Belching, nausea ↑ Enzymes, binds other drugs ↑ Triglycerides
Niacin	Compliance poor or fair; rarely tolerated by older patients and menopausal women not on estrogen	Flushing (80%) Peptic ulcer disease, gastritis Hepatitis, glucose intolerance Gout, ichthyosis (20% dry skin)
HMG CoA reducatase inhibitors	Well tolerated; 1–4% report dose-related side effects	Acute myositis-rhabdomyolysis (rare) Cataract (beagles) ↑ Transaminase (0.5–1.5%) Flatulence, diarrhea
Fibric acid derivatives	Well tolerated	Lithogenic bile Nausea, abdominal pain ↓ Libido, weight gain Myositis, drowsiness
Probucol	Well tolerated; 2–5% report side effects	Diarrhea, abdominal pain Flatulence, nausea

in hyperlipidemic women prescribed oral contraceptives or gonadal or corticosteroid hormones.[18]

ATHEROSCLEROSIS—CURRENT STATE OF THE DISEASE AND ITS PREVENTION

The death rates of coronary heart disease in males in 24 countries (1984) ranged from 64 (Japan) to 436 (Scotland) per 100,000. The United States ranks tenth-highest (348), with England seventh (360) and Canada twelfth (325). Rates also are high in New Zealand, Australia, Scandinavia, West Germany, and the Netherlands compared to eastern European and Mediterranean countries. Death rates in women are more consistent among countries and were lowest in Japan (~50/100,000) and highest in Czechoslovakia (~250/100,000) in 1978.

The risk of developing coronary heart disease is continuous over the range of serum cholesterol screening results, rising appreciably with levels above 6.5 mmol/L (12 per 1000) and even more steeply above 7.8 mmol/L (16 per 1000), with the lowest rates occurring at cholesterol levels below 5.2 mmol/L (3 per 1000). The correlation between LDL cholesterol and coronary heart disease is present in both men and women, although death rates of women are lower. Coronary heart disease in women occurs a decade or so later than in men, but morbidity and mortality rates of women are similar to those of men after age 75, and the protective effect of being female is lessened after menopause. Coronary heart disease is the leading cause of death in both men (31%) and women (24%).

The absolute risk of CHD increases 2 to 10 times with age at all serum cholesterol levels, but the relative risk increases with increasing serum cholesterol more steeply in males at age 35 (5 times greater) than at age 65 (20% higher risk). For women at comparable age and serum cholesterol levels, the relative risk of CHD is one third to one sixth that of men except when HDL cholesterol levels are less than 0.92 mmol/L (35 mg/dl). In the United States (1987) approximately 7 million people (4 million men, 3 million women) had symptomatic CHD. Half the men were under 65 years of age, and two thirds of the women were over 65.

About 20% of men in Britain who are 50 to 60 years old have CHD. Their mortality rate is about 1% per year, so about 15% will die prematurely (i.e., before age 65). 75% of the 300,000 deaths per year in men from coronary disease occur in the 50% with serum cholesterol levels between 5.7 and 8 mmol/L (225 and 300 mg/dl). Fifteen percent of deaths occur in the 5% of men with cholesterol levels over 8 mmol/L (300 mg/dl). Only 10% of deaths occur in men with serum cholesterol levels lower than 5.7 mmol/L (225 mg/dl) (45% of total).

Atherosclerosis occurs in relation to increased serum cholesterol (LDL, apo-B), blood pressure, and age, and decreased HDL.[38–40] LDL particles deliver cholesterol to the arterial wall. Endothelial injury initiating proliferation of vascular smooth muscle cells and fibroblasts can result from hemodynamic stress, cigarette smoking, immune complexes, viruses, and homocysteine as well as from increased levels of LDL per se. The early lesion (fatty streak) foam cell is a cholesterol ester–laden macrophage transformed from a monocyte by action of growth factors. Oxidized LDL may accelerate foam cell formation and subsequent atheroma development with a fibrous plaque. The accumulation of LDL at the site of internal damage depends on the plasma LDL level and the efficiency of reverse cholesterol transport.

REGRESSION STUDIES

Presumably, regression can result from mobilization of the cholesterol that makes up 25 to 35% of atheromatous plaques by creating a reverse concentration gradient between the arterial wall and plasma. Crystalline, unesterified cholesterol deep in the plaque turns over much more slowly than esterified cholesterol in the more superficial layers that is more susceptible to mobilization.

The severity of coronary artery disease as judged by angiography relates to hyperlipidemia (namely, hypercholesterolemia), increase in LDL cholesterol, and decrease in HDL cholesterol, especially HDL_2.[39] Progression is inversely related to the ratio of HDL cholesterol or HDL_2 to LDL cholesterol. Similar data are observed in grafts after bypass surgery. Effective lipid-lowering therapy can slow the rate of progression or induce regression.[41–45] Double-blind controlled trials showed that moderate reduction of LDL cholesterol (from 5.7 to 4.6 mmol/L; 220 to 180 mg/dl) and increase in the HDL-to-LDL ratio (from 0.2 to 0.26) reduced the percentage of lesions that progressed.[46] More marked reduction in LDL cholesterol (4.1 to 2.5 mmol/L; 160 to 95 mg/dl) and increase in the HDL-to-LDL ratio (0.59 to 2.7) resulted in significant increase in regression of lesions.[41–43] Recent trials show that with conventional treatment 46% of patients progressed, whereas with aggressive treatment with lipid-lowering drugs lovastatin and colestipol, or niacin and colestipol, 21 to 25% showed *progression;* 32 to 39% showed *regression* with these drugs, compared to an 11% regression rate with conventional treatment. Improvement was associated with 46 and 32% reduction in LDL, 15 to 43% increase in HDL, and 9 and 29% decrease in triglycerides.[44]

MANAGEMENT OF THE ATHEROSCLEROTIC PATIENT

The goal set in patients with atherosclerosis to achieve arrest or regression of disease is to reduce total cholesterol to less than 6.24 mmol/L (240 mg/dl), preferably to less than 5.2 mmol/L (200 mg/dl), and optimally to less than 4.6 mmol/L (180 mg/dl). Levels of LDL cholesterol achieved with treatment that are associated with arrest of progression of atherosclerosis or regression are less than 3.4 mmol/L (130 mg/dl), perhaps optimally to less than 2.6 mmol/L (100 mg/dl).[41–45] Levels of HDL cholesterol less than 0.90 mmol/L (35 mg/dl) and levels of triglycerides exceeding 2.28 mmol/L (200 mg/dl) also increase the risk of secondary myocardial infarction and warrant intervention.

Although the hyperlipidemias markedly increase the risk of atherosclerosis, most patients with myocardial infarction have total and LDL cholesterol levels between the 50th and 75th percentiles (see Table 72–2) rather than the higher values associated with the primary hyperlipoproteinemias. For atherosclerotic patients, diet modification is always warranted to prevent recurrent events. After 3 to 6 months, drug intervention is recommended for patients with LDL cholesterol levels exceeding 4.1 mmol/L (160 mg/dl). The goal is to lower these levels to less than 2.6 mmol/L (100 mg/dl). Increase in HDL cholesterol to levels exceeding 1.5 mmol/L (60 mg/dl) may be protective. Results of a multitude of primary and secondary intervention trials using diet or both diet and drugs with myocardial infarction as the end point indicate that coronary events are reduced by 2 to 3% for every 1% decrease in LDL cholesterol and by 3% for every 1% increase in HDL cholesterol[46–48] (see Chap. 87).

This chapter is based on the principles of the National Cholesterol Education Program (NCEP) for high-risk patients. Other approaches have been developed, for example, in Canada, the United Kingdom, Europe, and Norway. At times the policy recommendations differ among different groups within the country, which is the case in Canada. Also, strategies differ for a population approach (see Chap. 87) versus the recommendations in this chapter for treatment of hyperlipidemic patients or patients who already have CHD (secondary prevention). The diet recommended is the same among these countries, however.

The policy statement of the European Atherosclerosis Society is similar to the NCEP guidelines and deals with the recognition and management of hyperlipidemia in adults. The LDL goal is 3.5 mmol/L (135 mg/dl). The Society categorizes five treatment groups according to lipid levels, rather than the three groups in the United States. Their action limits differ slightly (6.5 mmol/L, or 250 mg/dl, for moderate increases in total cholesterol from the U.S. target of 240 mg/dl (6.24 mmol/L) for cholesterol. Desirable total cholesterol is the same as in the United States, namely 5.2 mmol/L (200 mg/dl). The recommendation to add drugs is delayed somewhat compared to the United States: the usual is 6 months, or 3 months in more severe or serious situations.[49]

The Canadian Consensus Conference report also is similar to that of the NCEP.[50] The report recommends a mean population value for cholesterol of 4.9 mmol/L (190 mg/dl) as a feasible long-term goal. The desirable goal for patients with hypercholesterolemia is 5.2 mmol/L (200 mg/dl), the same as in the United States. The limits set by the Canadian Consensus Conference for moderate risk for cholesterol, LDL cholesterol, and HDL cholesterol are the same as those set by the NCEP. The Canadian

Consensus Conference level of triglyceride for diet counseling is the same as the European level, which is above 2.3 mmol/L (200 mg/dl). The Toronto Working Group on Cholesterol Policy addresses the early detection and management of asymptomatic hypercholesterolemia.[51] The treatment guidelines from five expert panels (NCEP, two Canadian, European, and British) are detailed in their review. The more conservative approach of the Canadian Task Force on the Periodic Health Examination recommends diet and drug therapy at total cholesterol levels exceeding 6.85 mmol/L (265 mg/dl) and drug therapy alone when LDL exceeds 4.53 mmol/L (175 mg/dl).

The population strategy in Norway promotes diet therapy for those with total cholesterol levels of 6.0 to 7.9 mmol/L (230 to 300 mg/dl), adding drug therapy at serum cholesterol concentrations of 8.0 mmol/L (310 mg/dl) or higher.[52]

REFERENCES

1. NIH Consensus Development Conference Summary: Arteriosclcrosis, *4:*443A–468A, 1984.
2. Dupont, J., White, P.D., Feldman, E.B.: J. Am. Coll. Nutr., *10:*577–592, 1991.
3. Dawber, T.R.: The Framingham Study: The Epidemiology of Atherosclerotic Disease. Cambridge, MA., Harvard University Press, 1980.
4. Feldman, E.B.: Diet and plasma lipids and lipoproteins. *In* Nutrition and Heart Disease, Vol. 6: Contemporary Issues in Clinical Nutrition. Edited by E.B. Feldman. New York, Churchill Livingstone, 1983.
5. Lipid Research Clinics Program: JAMA, *251:*351–374, 1984.
6. Feldman, E.B.: Essentials of Clinical Nutrition. Philadelphia, F.A. Davis, 1988.
7. Levy, R.I.: Clin. Chem., *27:*653–662, 1981.
8. Brewer, H.B., Gregg, R.E., Hoeg, J.M., et al.: Clin. Chem., *34:*B4–B8, 1988.
9. Albers, J.J.: The determination of apoproteins and their diagnostic value in clinical chemistry. *In* Eleventh International Congress of Clinical Chemistry. Edited by E. Kaiser, F. Gabal, M.M. Muller, et al. Berlin, Walter de Gruyter, 1982.
10. Mahley, R.W.: Med. Clin. North Am., *66:*375–402, 1982.
11. Ghiselli, G., Schaefer, E.J., Gascon, P., et al.: Science, *214:*1239–1241, 1981.
12. Barber, M., Wile, D., Trayner, I., et al.: Br. Heart J., *60:*397–403, 1988.
13. Kuske, T.T., Feldman, E.B.: Arch. Intern. Med., *147:*357–360, 1987.
14. Steinberg, D., Parthasarathy, S., Carew, T.E., et al.: N. Engl. J. Med., *320:*915–924, 1989.
15. Utermann, G.: Science, *246:*904–910, 1989.
16. Reichl, D., Miller, N.E.: Arteriosclerosis, *9:*785–797, 1989.
17. Feldman, E.B., Kuske, T.T.: J. Am. Coll. Nutr., *6:*475–484, 1987.
18. Feldman, E.B., Kuske, T.T.: Mod. Med., *56:*60–71, 1988.
19. Dupont, J.: Lipids. *In* Present Knowledge in Nutrition. 6th Ed. Edited by M. Brown. Washington, D.C., International Life Sciences Institute, Nutrition Foundation, 1990.
20. Harris, W.S., Connor, W.E., Inkeles, S.B.: Metabolism, *33:*1016–1019, 1984.
21. Harris, W.S.: J. Lipid Res., *30:*785–807, 1989.
22. Simopoulos, A.P.: Am. J. Clin. Nutr., *54:*438–463, 1991.
23. Mattson, F.H., Grundy, S.M.: J. Lipid Res., *26:*194–202, 1985.
24. Sacks, F.M., Handysides, G.H., Marais, G.E., et al.: Arch. Intern. Med., *146:*1573–1577, 1986.
25. Mensink, R.P., diGroot, M.J.M., Vanden Broeke, L.T., et al.: Metabolism, *38:*172–178, 1989.
26. Dreon, D.M., Vranizen, K.M., Krauss, R.M., et al.: JAMA, *263:*2462–2466, 1990.
27. Ginsberg, H.N., Barr, S.L., Gilbert, A., et al.: N. Engl. J. Med., *322:*574–579, 1990.
28. Wardlaw, G.M., Anook, J.T.: Am. J. Clin. Nutr., *57:*815–821, 1990.
29. Hunninghake, D.B., Stein, E.A., Dujovne, C.A., et al.: N. Engl. J. Med., *328:*1213–1219, 1993.
30. Anderson, J.W., Story, L., Sieling, B., et al.: Am. J. Clin. Nutr., *40:*1146–1155, 1984.
31. Patsch, W., Patsch, J.R., Gotto, A.M. Jr.: Med. Clin. North Am., *73:*859–893, 1989.
32. Lusis, A.J.: J. Lipid Res., *29:*397–429, 1988.
33. Breslow, J.L.: J. Clin. Invest., *84:*373–380, 1989.
34. Mahley, R.M., Weisgraber, K.H., Innerarity, T.L., et al.: JAMA, *265:*78–83, 1991.
35. Recommendations for the Treatment of Hyperlipidemia in Adults. Arteriosclerosis, *4:*443A–468A, 1984.
36. Greene, J.M., Feldman, E.B.: J. Am. Coll. Nutr., *10:*443–452, 1991.
37. The Lovastatin Study Group III: JAMA, *260:*359–366, 1988.
38. Pekkanen, J., Linn, S., Heiss, G., et al.: N. Engl. J. Med., *322:*1700–1707, 1990.
39. Nikkila, M., Kiuula, T., Niemela, K., et al.: Br. Heart J., *63:*78–81, 1990.
40. PDAY Research Group: JAMA, *264:*3018–3024, 1990.
41. Blankenhorn, D.H., Nessum, S.A., Johnson, R.L., et al.: JAMA, *257:*3233–3240, 1987.
42. Blankenhorn, D., Johnson, R.L., Mack, W.J., et al.: JAMA, *263:*1646–1652, 1990.
43. Cashin-Hemphill, L., Mack, W.J., Pagoda, J.M., et al.: JAMA, *264:*3013–3017, 1990.
44. Brown, G., Albers, J.J., Fisher, L.D., et al.: N. Engl. J. Med., *323:*1289–1298, 1990.
45. Kane, J.P., Mulloy, M.J., Ports, T.A., et al.: JAMA, *264:*3007–3012, 1990.
46. Levy, R.I., Brensike, J.F., Epstein, S.E., et al.: Circulation, *69:*2325–2336, 1984.
47. Canner, P.L., Berg, K.G., Wenger, N.K., et al.: J. Am. Coll. Cardiol., *8:*1245–1255, 1986.
48. Frick, M.H., Elo, O., Haapa, K.K., et al.: N. Engl. J. Med., *317:*1237–1245, 1987.
49. Study Group, European Atherosclerosis Society: Eur. Heart J., *9:*571–600, 1988.

50. Canadian Consensus Conference on Cholesterol: Final Report: Can. Med. Assoc. J., *139(Suppl.)*:1–8, 1988.
51. Toronto Working Group on Cholesterol Policy: J. Clin. Epidemiol., *43*:1028–1121, 1990.
52. Kristiansen, I.S., Eggen, A.E., Thelle, D.S.: Br. Med. J., *302*:1119–1122, 1991.

SELECTED READINGS

Brown, M.S., Goldstein, J.L.: A receptor-mediated pathway for cholesterol homeostasis. Science, *232*:34–47, 1986.

Keys, A.: Seven Countries. Cambridge, MA, Harvard University Press, 1980.

Report of the National Cholesterol Education Program Expert Panel on Detection, Evaluation and Treatment of High Blood Cholesterol in Adults: Arch. Intern. Med., *48*:36–69, 1988.

Schaefer, E.J., Levy, R.I.: Pathogenesis and management of lipoprotein disorders. N. Engl. J. Med., *312*:1300–1310, 1985.

Scriver, C.R., Beaudet, A.L., Sly, W.S., et al. (Eds.): The Metabolic Basis of Inherited Disease. 6th Ed. Part 7. Lipoprotein and Lipid Metabolism Disorders. New York, McGraw-Hill, 1989, pp. 1129–1302.

Second report of the National Cholesterol Education Program (NCEP) Expert Panel on Detection, Evaluation and Treatment of High Blood Cholesterol in Adults (Adult Treatment Panel II). JAMA *269*:3015–3023, 1993.

CHAPTER **73**

Nutrition and Diet in Cancer Management

Maurice E. Shils

HEALTH BURDEN OF CANCER

The designation of cancer includes many disease conditions characterized by growth of cells that have lost their usual growth restraints and thus multiply and spread. The localized and/or distant spread interferes with the function of adjacent organs and often has undesirable systemic effects.

In 1991, the estimated number of deaths from cancer in the United States was about 514,000. Total death rates in the United States from cancer at each of the 9 most common anatomic sites at intervals from 1930 to 1987 are shown in Figure 73–1. The striking changes over the years have been the dramatic rise in death from lung cancer and the marked decline in mortality from gastric and uterine (predominantly cervical) malignancies.

Although deaths from cancer are appreciably less than those from cardiovascular diseases, the gap between the percentage of all deaths and the probability of dying from these two causes is narrowing for men and for women[1] (Table 73–1). This trend is attributable to the continuing decline in deaths from ischemic heart disease and stroke with little or no change in overall cancer mortality and to the increased likelihood of dying from cancer, particularly from lung cancer.

Mortality rates from cancer in the United States in persons younger than age 45 years have decreased markedly for both men and women, especially for those below the age of 20 years.[2] In the same period (1970 to 1987), cancer mortality rates have increased for men and women aged 65 years and older.[2] Other reports claim that all forms of cancer, except lung and stomach, are increasing in persons over the age of 54 years (mortality rate from lung cancer is beginning to decline in men under 45 years in the United States.)[3] Some authors suggest that these rate increases are not attributable solely to diagnostic artifacts or to increased access to health care, i.e., there may well be a true increase.[3]

The *incidence** of cancer increased for men of all ages between 1973 to 1977 to 1983 to 1987 and for women younger than 20 years and older than 65 years.[2] For men aged 20 to 44 years, the recorded incidence increased significantly in this period for testicular cancer, melanoma and nonmelanoma of the skin, and nonHodgkin's

*Incidence and patient survival data on various sites of cancer have been collected since 1973 in the United States by the National Cancer Institute through their Surveillance, Epidemiology, and End Results (SEER) program. These data are collected from 9 population-based cancer registries covering about 10% of the population.

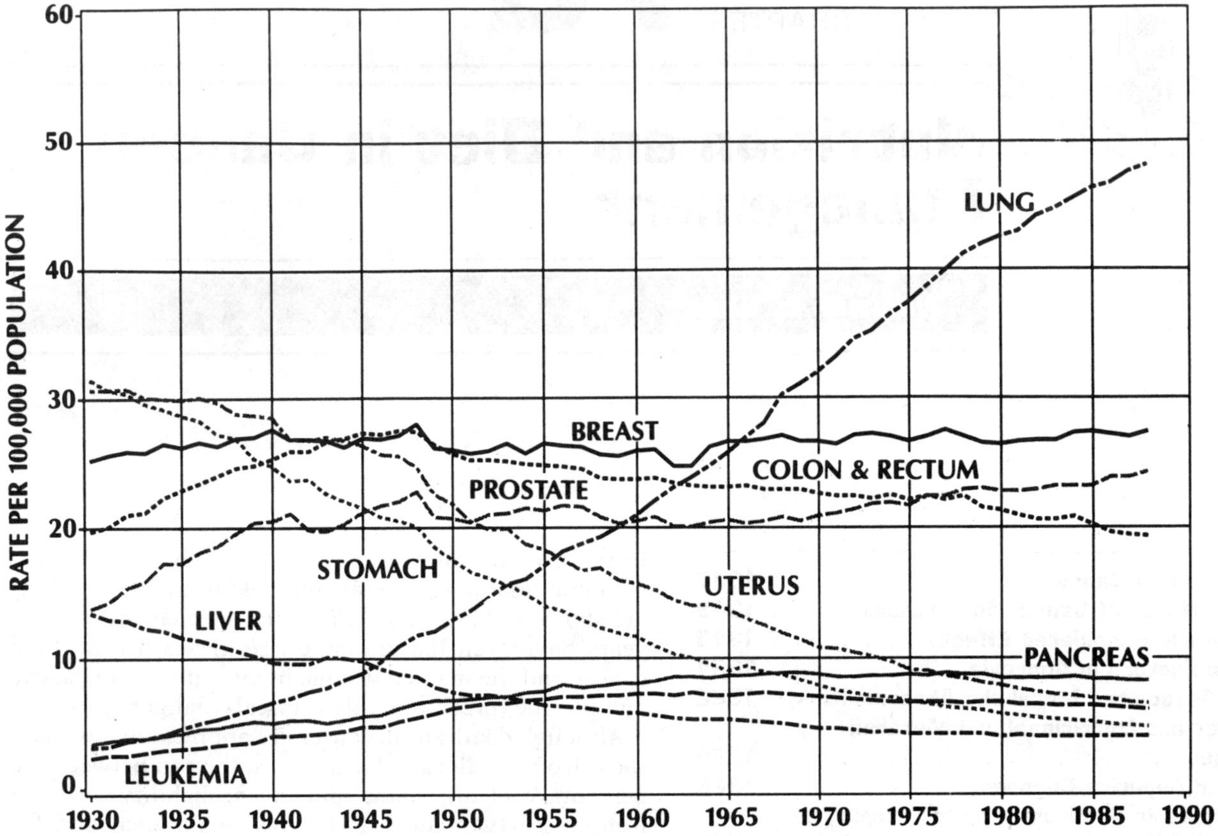

FIGURE 73–1. Cancer death rates by site, United States, 1930 to 1988. Rates are adjusted to the age distribution of the 1970 census population. Rates are both sexes combined, except breast and uterus (female population only) and prostate (male population only). Data are from the National Center for Health Statistics and United States Bureau of the Census. (From Cancer Facts and Figures, 1992. Atlanta, American Cancer Society, 1992.)

TABLE 73–1. COMPARATIVE MORTALITY IN THE UNITED STATES FROM CANCER, ISCHEMIC HEART DISEASE (IHD), AND STROKE IN 1955 AND 1986

		MEN		WOMEN	
CAUSE	YEAR	Percentage of all Deaths	Probability of Dying from Cause (%)	Percentage of all Deaths	Probability of Dying from Cause (%)
Cancer	1955	14.5	14.6	17.5	15.5
	1986	22.7	22.5	21.9	19.5
IHD	1955	33.1	35.8	27.9	32.3
	1986	24.8	26.4	24.6	26.5
Stroke	1955	9.6	11.1	13.7	15.7
	1986	5.4	6.0	9.0	9.9

(Data from Lopez, A.D.: Ann. N.Y. Acad. Sci., *609*:70, 72 (Tables 1 and 2), 1990.)

lymphoma; in women of this age group, the incidence of melanoma and nonmelanoma of the skin and of non-Hodgkin's lymphoma also increased.[2] Because the validity of data for incidence is less reliable than that for mortality for various reasons, some controversy exists on whether true increases have occurred.[4,5] Whatever the outcome of this debate, the type of data indicated in Table 73–1 foretells an increasing proportion of patients with cancer in our population unless widespread applications are made of new and major improvements in the preventive and curative treatments of the major malignant disorders.

SYSTEMIC EFFECTS OF CANCER ON NUTRITION

Cancer and the various antitumor treatments in use can have adverse effects on the nutritional status of the affected patient. An understanding of the various nutritional, metabolic, and physiologic changes that can occur provides the basis for evaluating the need for nutritional support in various clinical situations and for planning and providing such support when indicated.

Even a localized cancer may exert various systemic (i.e., generalized) effects in the patient. As the tumor grows and metastasizes, these influences often become more obvious as a result of the bulk of the tumor and of its local and distant invasion. In addition, malignant tumors can produce signs and symptoms at a distance from the original tumor or its metastases. These remote effects, termed "paraneoplastic syndromes," are reviewed in this section (Table 73–2).

ANOREXIA AND ASSOCIATED EFFECTS

Loss of appetite (anorexia) can occur in patients with various cancers or as a consequence of such treatments as surgery, radiation, chemotherapy, and other drug treatments. In addition, anorexia can be a systemic effect of the malignant tumor per se, however, anorexia often is intensified by fear, depression, sepsis, and treatment effects. When persistent and severe, the anorexia, in association with or as the result of various metabolic and physiologic changes, can eventually lead to severe undernutrition and the wasting of body tissues commonly termed cancer cachexia. This condition is advanced protein-energy malnutrition.

Although anorexia is not unique to cancer, its high incidence in certain types of cancers and its severity and persistence in a significant number of patients cause special concern. In his 1932 paper reporting the major prevalence of cachexia as a cause of death in individuals with carcinoma at various primary sites, Warren noted that cachexia was associated most frequently with carcinoma of the stomach (45%), breast (33.1%), and large bowel (22%); bladder and prostate cancers were associ-

TABLE 73–2. NUTRITIONAL PROBLEMS ASSOCIATED WITH THE PRESENCE OF NEOPLASTIC DISEASE

1. Anorexia with progressive weight loss and undernutrition
2. Taste changes causing depressed or altered food intake
3. Alterations in protein, carbohydrate, and fat metabolism
4. Increased energy expenditure despite weight loss
5. Impaired food intake and malnutrition secondary to
   - A. Mechanical bowel obstruction at any level
   - B. Intestinal dysmotility induced by various tumors, particularly lung cancer
6. Malabsorption associated with
   - A. Deficiency or inactivation of pancreatic enzymes
   - B. Deficiency or inactivation of bile salts
   - C. Failure of food to mix with digestive enzymes (e.g., enzyme dilution, pancreaticocibal asynchrony)
   - D. Fistulous bypass of small bowel
   - E. Infiltration of small bowel wall or lymphatics and mesentery by malignant cells
   - F. Blind loop syndrome occurring with depressed gastric secretion or partial upper small bowel obstruction leading to bacterial overgrowth
   - G. Malnutrition-induced villous hypoplasia in the small intestine
7. Protein-losing enteropathy
8. Metabolic abnormalities induced by tumor-derived eutopic hormones
   - A. Hypercalcemia induced by parathyroid hormone–like polypeptides, osteolytic processes, increased calcitriol
   - B. Osteomalacia with hypophosphatemia often associated with depressed serum calcitriol
   - C. Hypoglycemia induced by insulin-secreting tumors
   - D. Hyperglycemia, e.g., with islet glucagonoma or somatostatinoma
9. Anemia of chronic blood loss and bone marrow suppression.
10. Electrolyte and fluid problems with
    - A. Persistent vomiting with intestinal obstruction or intracranial tumors
    - B. Intestinal fluid losses through fistulas or diarrhea
    - C. Intestinal secretory abnormalities with hormone-secreting tumors (e.g., carcinoid syndrome, Zollinger-Ellison syndrome [gastrinoma], Verner-Morrison syndrome [ViPoma], increased calcitonin, villous adenoma)
    - D. Inappropriate antidiuretic hormone secretion associated with certain tumors (e.g., lung carcinomas)
    - E. Hyperadrenalism with tumors producing corticotropin or corticosteroids
11. Miscellaneous organ dysfunction with nutritional implications, e.g., intractable gastric ulcers with gastrinomas, Fanconi's syndrome with light-chain disease, coma with brain tumors
12. Tumor products stimulating monocyte production of various interleukins (see Table 73–7)

ated with the least incidence.[6] Lymphomas, leukemias, and sarcomas were not included in that study. The subjects with breast cancer in Warren's study revealed extensive lung involvement (76%) and/or liver insufficiency (30%) at postmortem examination. These factors presumably contributed to the high prevalence of cachexia. More recent studies indicate that tumors of nonvisceral organs, such as those of the breast and sarcomas, are not usually associated with significant weight loss in contrast to the significant weight loss associated with tumors of the upper gastrointestinal tract and to the intermediate effects of tumors of the lung and colon.[7]

Breast cancer, even with bone involvement, is usually associated with relatively little or no weight loss.[7] In a recent study of 923 women diagnosed as having breast cancer without distant metastases, weight evaluation (in relation to height and build) prior to mastectomy and axillary dissection revealed that 13% were underweight, 42.4% were at their desired weight, 22.1% were overweight, and another 22.4% were obese.[8] Obesity at this stage was associated with a significantly increased risk for recurrence compared to that for nonobese patients.

Various reports since 1980 have indicated that 40 to 80% of cancer patients develop some clinically detectable malnutrition.[9,10] In different types of cancer, weight loss was associated with a shorter median survival as compared to the median survival of patients with no weight loss (Table 73–3).[7] Anorexia may be regarded as the primary event for the onset of undesired weight loss in patients with malignant disease.[10]

The effects of serious weight loss and of nutrient deficiencies on metabolic and immune functions with resulting increased morbidity and mortality have been reviewed in various chapters of this book (see Chaps. 41, 50, 56, 57, and 69). Weight loss greater than 10% may be present in as many as 45% of hospitalized adult cancer patients,[11] and this degree of loss is an independent risk factor for survival (Table 73–3).[7,12] In quantitative terms, the minimum range of corrected arm muscle area compatible with survival of cancer patients is 9 to 11 cm.[13]

Onset of anorexia may be insidious and may not be accompanied by obvious manifestations of disease other than the progressive weight loss. A dictum of medicine states that the patient with an unexplained weight loss should undergo a search for an occult neoplasm. Detailed initial medical evaluation usually reveals the cause.[14]

The anorexia of malignancy appears to be a general phenomenon exhibited by several other tumor-bearing species. Anorexia in these species, as in humans, is not necessarily induced by all tumor types. A comparison of the reactions of rats to transplanted tumor types is instructive.[15] A Leydig's cell–derived tumor (LTW) caused early anorexia and failure of growth when transplanted in young rats. A breast carcinosarcoma, however, was not associated with significant anorexia; tumor and host grew almost until death. Parabiotic studies were performed in which two rats were subcutaneously attached so that a small persistent blood exchange occurred. In each paired group, one of the pair

TABLE 73–3. WEIGHT LOSS IN ADULT CANCER PATIENTS: INCIDENCE AND EFFECT ON SURVIVAL

		PATIENTS WITH WEIGHT LOSS IN PREVIOUS 6 MONTHS (%)			MEDIAN SURVIVAL (WEEKS)		
TUMOR TYPE/LOCATION	TOTAL NO. PATIENTS	No Loss	Some Loss	>10% Loss	No Weight Loss	Any Weight Loss	p*
Pancreas	111	17	83	26	14	12	N.S.
Gastric							
Nonmeasurable	179	17	83	30	41	27	.05
Measurable	138	13	87	38	18	16	N.S.
Colon	307	46	54	14	43	21	.01
Breast	289	64	36	6	70	45	.01
Prostate	78	44	56	10	46	24	.05
Sarcoma	189	60	40	7	46	25	.01
Lung							
Non-small cell	590	39	61	15	20	14	.01
Small cell	436	43	57	14	34	27	.05
Hodgkin's disease							
Favorable	290	69	31	10	—	138	.01
Unfavorable	311	52	48	15	107	55	.01
Acute nonlymphocytic leukemia	129	61	39	4	8	4	N.S.

*N.S. = no significant difference.

(Adapted from DeWys, W.D., Begg, C., Lavin, P.T., et al.: Prognostic effect of weight loss prior to chemotherapy in cancer patients. Am. J. Med., *68*:683–690, 1980.)

had either the LTW or the breast tumor type and the other had no tumor. Two attached sham-operated rats served as controls. Over a period of time, none of the rats bearing breast cancer lost weight (as expected), and neither did their parabiotic nontumor-bearing partners. In contrast, the rats with the Leydig's cell–derived tumor lost weight (as expected), and their parabiotic nontumor-bearing partners also lost significant weight. Such general results have been observed by others.[16]

Anorexia developed in rats bearing a Walker 256 tumor that previously had been made hyperphagic by lesions in the ventromedial hypothalamus, thus indicating that anorexia in the presence of a tumor is not mediated by this mechanism.[17]

ETIOLOGIC FACTORS IN ANOREXIA

The usual regulation of total food intake obviously fails in this syndrome (see Chap. 35). The parabiotic rat studies just mentioned suggest that one or more anorexigenic agents derived from anorexia-inducing tumors are transmitted via the lymphatic or vascular systems to influence food intake of nontumor-bearing animals. Various hormones, neurotransmitters, cytokines, and other factors may be involved.

HORMONES AND NEUROTRANSMITTERS

Hormones, such as cholecystokinin, and neurotransmitters, such as serotonin, norepinephrine, and the opiates, normally operate to influence food intake and choice (see Chap. 35). Efforts to delineate a specific role for cholecystokinin in tumor-induced anorexia in various experimental models have been unsuccessful. On injection, cholecystokinin was no more effective in inducing hypophagia in tumor-bearing rats than it was in nontumor-bearing controls.[18] Injection of several antiserotonin drugs did not modify the anorectic response to the rat Walker 256 tumor despite significant reductions of brain serotonin and hydroxyindoleacetic acid.[19]

Insulin was used to overcome anorexia in nondiabetic malnourished individuals in the early days of its commercial availability. The effect of this hormone has been studied in anorectic rats bearing various tumors at differing stages of tumor growth. In early stages, food intake and carcass weights were greater in those given insulin as compared to those of untreated tumor-bearing controls, but survival was slightly reduced.[20] When given during the cachectic period, insulin increased food intake and weight gain but did not increase survival.[20] In longer experiments, food intake was increased with insulin, but only for 6 days; thereafter, appetite decreased and the animals died despite continued administration of insulin.[21]

In attempts to overcome the decreased insulin/glucagon ratio and to increase hepatic gluconeogenic enzyme activities associated with tumor weight gain and host carcass loss, researchers tested a somatostatin analogue, octreotide (which inhibits pancreatic glucagon and insulin secretion), and exogenous insulin in mammary tumor-bearing and nontumor-bearing rats. Although insulin alone increased the serum insulin/glucagon ratio many times over that attained with saline treatment in tumor-bearing rats, carcass weight loss and tumor weight gain were unchanged. Octreotide and insulin together further increased insulin/glucagon ratios and significantly decreased both carcass weight loss and tumor weight gain.[22]

Growth hormone given to rats with transplanted methylcholanthrene-induced sarcoma and supported by total parenteral nutrition (TPN) resulted in weight gain of the host similar to that of nontumor-bearing rats given either saline or growth hormone. Insulin-like growth factor essentially stopped weight gain in the host without affecting tumor burden.[23] Acivin, a glutamine antimetabolite, reduced tumor growth in tumor-bearing (sarcoma) rats given TPN, but did not improve protein content of muscle or of serum albumin.[24] Acivin did improve survival with TPN feedings, but not with chow feedings.[25] When given subcutaneously every other day, acivin markedly depressed oral intake on the day of injection; the resulting anorexia led to marked hypoglycemia when insulin was added to the regimen.[25]

Clenbuterol, a selective β_2 agonist, plus acivin decreased tumor mass and increased lean body mass in rats on TPN.[26] The recent research on clenbuterol and similar β-agonists has been reviewed with respect to their protein anabolic properties.[27]

The cyclo-oxygenase inhibitor indomethacin given orally or subcutaneously to tumor-bearing mice at 1 μg/g prolonged survival by about 50%. This increase was associated with inhibition of tumor growth, decreased anorexia, and improved lean body mass compared to that of untreated tumor-bearing animals.[28]

The progestational agent megestrol acetate (Megace) has been noted to stimulate appetite and food intake in a significant proportion of women with documented advanced breast cancer and weight loss, but it has glucocorticoid side effects.[29,30] Megace has proved to be a potent dose-dependent stimulator of a fibroblast cell line differentiation into adipocytes, whereas tumor necrosis factor blocks this differentiation.[29]

Whether any of these antianorexia agents has significant value in the management of serious anorexia in cancer patients remains to be seen. At present, the biochemical basis of anorexia in cancer is unknown. Further insight into anorexia has been gained through advances in the understanding of the roles of interleukins (cytokines), which are reviewed in a subsequent section of this chapter.

CANCER-ASSOCIATED METABOLIC ABNORMALITIES

The presence of malignant growth in human subjects and laboratory animals clearly is associated with numerous metabolic abnormalities. When transplanted tumors begin to grow rapidly and anorexia becomes apparent with decreased growth rate, forced tube feeding initially helps to maintain host weight. Continuation of this feeding and the absence of either effective antitumor therapy or surgical removal of the tumor, however, cause undesirable metabolic reactions, and a more rapid death ensues.[31] This result was well exemplified in experiments when energy in the form of TPN was varied in groups of tumor-bearing and nontumor-bearing animals. Weights of the host and the tumor increased in relation to the energy provision. Above 133% of energy need, significantly more fat was in the liver of the tumor-bearing rats than in the liver of nontumorous controls, and at 167%, all tumor-bearing animals died (cause undetermined) while the control population survived.[32] In paired feeding experiments in which carcass weights of tumor-bearing animals were compared to those of nontumor-bearing animals, decreased food intake alone did not explain all the tissue depletion in the tumor-bearing animals.[33]

ENERGY EXPENDITURE IN PATIENTS WITH CANCER

Because patients with advanced cancer tend to lose weight, measurements of resting energy expenditure (REE) have been performed frequently to determine whether increased REE is a possible causative factor.

When the daily REE of cancer patients was compared to predicted values by the Harris-Benedict equation, some investigators noted a hypermetabolic rate (i.e., > 10% above the predicted value) in varying degree[34,35]; others found that patients with gastrointestinal cancers were variable, with some patients hypometabolic, some normometabolic, and some hypermetabolic[36,37]; and Merrick and colleagues found no difference in patients with colon and rectal cancer.[38]

In the last 12 years, many reports have been issued on this subject with increasing attention to adequacy of patient data, procedures, and relevant controls. Comparisons have been made more frequently between cancer patients with different degrees of weight loss and either healthy subjects or those with nonmalignant diseases. Warmold and associates used heart rate to determine REE and reported that cancer patients had a mean REE 29% above the mean of patients with no cancer.[39] One group of investigators reported that a small absolute increase in REE was observed in patients with gastrointestinal cancer who were losing weight as compared to that in patients without malignant disease ($p < 0.05$).[40] These results, however, were not found by another group studying different cancer patients.[41] In patients with bony and soft tissue sarcoma, those with localized tumor and a 7.2% average weight loss had a total daily REE similar to that of age- and sex-matched controls; however, the REE/kg per day was significantly higher, whereas the REE/kg$^{0.75}$ per day was not different.[42] Of these patients with sarcoma, 4 had diffuse disease and a 15.4% mean weight loss; their total REE per day was the same as that of the other 2 groups, but their REE/kg per day and REE/kg$^{0.75}$ per day were increased. Resection of the tumor led to a postoperative fall in REE.[42]

Patients with gastrointestinal cancers who had lost weight (average 17%) had a REE per day significantly greater than that of patients with benign disease who had lost a similar percentage of weight. This relationship held true when REE was expressed per kg per day or per mmol total body potassium.[43] The cancer patients who either had lost weight or had not lost weight had similar daily REE and REE/kg, but the REE in relation to total body potassium was higher in those who had lost weight.[43]

When REE was expressed in kg per day or kg$^{0.75}$ per day or kg lean body mass (LBM)/day, no significant difference existed between patients with gastric and colorectal cancer who had lost an average of 18% body weight and patients with benign gastrointestinal diseases who had lost an average of 16% body weight.[44] When a relatively large group of patients with colon and nonsmall cell lung cancer who had experienced some weight loss were compared to malnourished patients without cancer and to healthy volunteers, no difference appeared in their REE/kg LBM.[45] No significant difference existed among weight-losing or weight-stable patients with gastric and colon cancer, or among weight-losing patients with benign gastrointestinal disease when their energy expenditure was expressed as daily REE, REE/kg body weight, or REE/kg fat-free mass (FFM).[46] Weight-stable patients with cancer and healthy volunteers had a total daily REE significantly greater ($p < 0.001$) than that of weight-losing patients with cancer or gastrointestinal disease, but no difference existed among any groups per kg body weight or per kg FFM.[47] Patients who were in a semistarving condition with localized resectable esophageal cancer had a REE/kg body weight similar to that of better-nourished controls admitted for minor surgery.[48]

Even though some of the controlled studies indicate some increased REE in patients with cancer, especially in those with weight loss, the differences among patients with and without cancer are not marked; some studies, in fact, have found no differences. Furthermore, data expressed per unit weight or LBM tend to eliminate or decrease any differences. The presence of liver metastases or more extensive disease did not increase REE in some studies,[38,44,47] but other studies reported a positive relation.[40] Several groups noted that the Harris-Benedict equation tended to underestimate the REE/day for weight-losing cancer patients.[43,44] On the other hand, Fredrix and associates concluded that this equation overestimated energy expenditure in all groups studied, whether with or without cancer and whether weight losing or weight stable.[47] They found that the current FAO/WHO/UNU prediction equation reduced the predicted number of "hypermetabolic" patients.[49]

The evidence presented supports the concept that increased REE contributes relatively little to the development of cancer cachexia; on the other hand, weight-losing cancer patients often *maintain* their energy expenditure in contrast to otherwise healthy semistarving weight-losing individuals who *decrease* their energy expenditure.[50]

ABNORMALITIES IN CARBOHYDRATE METABOLISM (TABLE 73–4)

Glucose intolerance has been noted frequently in patients with cancer;[9] it may be mild in early stages and increase with tumor burden. This glucose intolerance results from increased insulin resistance and perhaps from inadequate insulin release. In addition to these peripheral tissue changes, evidence shows that nontumor factors, e.g., extent of weight loss, bedrest, and sepsis, may play a role.[51]

An example of insulin resistance and its associated changes in glucose turnover in cancer patients was demonstrated in a small group of patients with untreated gastrointestinal malignant tumors and serious weight loss. The euglycemic clamp technique was used to infuse graded doses of insulin in the group with cancer and in a group of healthy volunteers.[52] Although the patients with cancer had normal fasting glucose levels, their mean postabsorptive rate of glucose appearance (i.e., gluconeogenesis rate) was significantly greater than that of the control group, and their glucose disappearance lessened with increasing insulin infusion rates. At high physiologic insulin doses, endogenous glucose production was completely suppressed. The impaired insulin action on peripheral glucose use was associated with an increase in peripheral lactate release in the patients with cancer.

Gluconeogenesis and Glucose Turnover and Disappearance. The reports of an increased rate of endogenous glucose production in cancer patients are numerous. Tumor type, stage, and histology influence the rate. This increased production, combined with other carbohydrate changes, is associated with weight loss.[9,50–57]

Patients with more extensive colon cancer (Dukes' C and D) had significantly increased glucose turnover rates compared to those observed in patients whose cancer had a more limited spread (Dukes's B). No relation to pre-illness weight loss existed.[53] Rates of glucose and urea turnover and glucose oxidation have been determined in normal volunteers, in a group of patients with early gastrointestinal (colon) cancer, and in those with advanced gastrointestinal (esophagus, stomach, pancreas) cancer.[54] Basal rates of glucose turnover were similar in the normal and early cancer groups (13.9 and 13.3 μmol/kg per minute), but were significantly higher in the advanced cancer group (17.6 μmol/kg per minute). The glucose oxidation rate increased progressively in proportion to tumor burden (23.9% for controls, 32.8% for early tumors, and 43.0% for advanced tumors). After curative resection in the early tumor groups, glucose utilization decreased significantly. Urea turnover was significantly higher in the advanced tumor group (8.4 μmol/kg per minute) as compared to that in the control group (5.9 μmol/kg per minute); glucose infusion significantly suppressed urea turnover in the healthy control group but did not induce a significant decrease in the advanced tumor group.[54] Glucose turnover rates in patients with sarcoma and leukemia have been either 2 or nearly 3 times those of normal volunteers[55,56]; on the other hand, no difference from the normal rate was observed in patients with lymphoma.[56]

Glucose infusion into patients with sarcoma and leukemia suppressed hepatic glucose production by somewhat less than one third.[55,56] In those with early and advanced gastrointestinal cancer, glucose production was suppressed with glucose by 76% and 69% respectively, whereas in normal volunteers, glucose production was almost completely suppressed (94%).[54] Glucose production rates in weight-stable cancer patients were similar to those of normal volunteers, but the weight-losing cancer patient had markedly elevated rates.[57] Weight loss caused by uncomplicated starvation *reduced* glucose turnover.[58] Glucose turnover rates in cachectic patients with cancer have been estimated to account for up to 42% of spontaneous glucose intake, a result of increased recycling of glucose through lactate.[58]

Cori Cycling. An increased rate of Cori cycling has been reported to occur in cancer patients. In this cycle, glucose released by peripheral tissues is metabolized to lactate, which is then resynthesized to glucose in the liver.[57–61] The process is energy consuming because six adenosine triphosphates (ATP) are required for the glucose resynthesis, and only two are produced in the glycolytic cycle; hence, the term "futile cycle." If anaerobic glycolysis by tumor cells with release of lactate is quantitatively large, the small energy release from glucose would be exacerbated by the Cori cycling of lactate in the liver. Hence, the Cori cycle could be a significant factor in the development of weight loss.

TABLE 73–4. ABNORMALITIES IN CARBOHYDRATE METABOLISM ASSOCIATED WITH ADVANCED CANCER

Glucose intolerance
Insulin resistance
Abnormal insulin secretion
Delayed glucose clearance
Increased glucose production
Increased glucose turnover
Variably increased Cori cycle activity

Holyroyde and colleagues noted increased cycle activity in patients with metastatic disease and progressive weight loss but no increase in patients with cancer and stable weight.[57] Cori cycling was significantly higher in patients with cancer who either were fasting or were in the fed state than in patients without cancer but who experienced a similar degree of weight loss.[60] In contrast, an association has not been noted between the rate of Cori cycle activity and the extent of colon cancer or a weight loss of more than 10%.[53] Although increased Cori cycling would appear likely to play some role in energy balance problems of certain cancer patients, its quantitative significance in inducing cachexia is uncertain.[60,61]

The source of recycled lactate that accompanies accelerated Cori cycling in human cancer cachexia has not been completely elucidated.[52] Earlier work focused on glucose consumption by the tumor with lactate formation, because glucose utilization by the tumor can be substantial. A massive tumor, however, would be required to consume the amount of glucose estimated to occur. Such a size is unusual for most human tumors of the type often associated with cancer cachexia;[52] more recent reports have emphasized the release of lactate from glucose recycling in peripheral tissues.[52]

Of interest in relation to the possible association of lactate production and weight loss is a comparison between two experimental colonic tumors, one (Mac 16) that induces cachexia when transplanted into the animal host and one (Mac 13) that does not induce cachexia.[62] Mac 13 utilizes glucose to a much greater extent than does Mac 16; however, both tumors are the largest glucose consumers after the brain. Irrespective of cachexia, a marked decrease in glucose utilization, particularly by the brain, but also by fat cells, testes, colon, spleen, and kidney, occurs in the presence of these tumors. Brain metabolism from these tumor-bearing animals was maintained in vitro by an increased use of lactate and hydroxybutyrate; presumably this characteristic was true of the various organs in vivo. Hence, in this model at least, increased glucose oxidation and lactate production by the tumor are divorced from cachexia and from glucose utilization by normal tissues.

TABLE 73–5. ABNORMALITIES IN FAT METABOLISM ASSOCIATED WITH ADVANCED CANCER

Excess body fat depletion relative to protein loss
Increased lipolysis, free fatty acids, and glycerol turnover
Decreased lipogenesis
Hyperlipidemia
Failure of glucose to suppress oxidation of free fatty acids
Decreased serum lipoprotein lipase activity despite normal insulin

ABNORMALITIES IN LIPID METABOLISM (TABLE 73–5)

Many reports have stated that the major portion of weight loss in many cancer patients is attributable to fat depletion.[9,53,63,64]

Fat Mobilization. Fat from adipose tissue is mobilized in the fasting state by the action of specific lipases that eventually complete the lipolytic conversion of triglycerides to free fatty acids and glycerol. The lipase that releases the first fatty acid, triglyceride lipase, is regulated by various circulating hormones, some of which, especially catecholamines, are stimulatory, whereas insulin is antilipolytic. In the nonfasting state, fatty acids are derived from chylomicrons and very low-density lipoprotein (VLDL) under the influence of lipoprotein lipase.

Klein and Wolfe have noted four possible mechanisms that may increase lipolytic rates in cancer patients: (a) increased lipolytic rates caused by decreased food intake and malnutrition; (b) increased lipolysis when expressed per kilogram of body weight caused by body weight loss and an increased percentage of body weight as lean body mass; (c) stimulation of lipolysis caused by the stress response to illness with adrenal medullary stimulation, increased circulating catecholamines, and insulin resistance, and (d) the release of lipolytic factors produced by the tumor itself or by myeloid tissue cells.[65] Hence, these mechanisms must be controlled insofar as possible to delineate the role of the tumor per se.

Stable isotopic tracers have revealed that weight-losing patients with gastrointestinal malignant disease had significantly elevated rates of release of both glycerol and free fatty acids into the plasma. Significant differences in whole body glycerol and fatty acid kinetics were not evident between weight-stable cancer patients and normal volunteers.[66] A later study from the same laboratory, however, controlled the factor of weight loss by including a group of cachetic patients without cancer.[65] The results of this study showed that weight loss per se was associated with increased lipolytic rate. Other reports concerning whole body lipolytic rates in patients with cancer are contradictory; the rates were normal in two reports and increased in two reports.[65]

Loss of body fat occurs when both lipolysis *and* fatty acid oxidation are increased. Increased lipolysis without an equal increase in fatty acid oxidation causes an increase in triglyceride-fatty acid cycling, i.e., released fatty acids are subsequently re-esterified to triglyceride. Although this cycle does not increase net flux of reactants, the reaction does require energy. Beta-adrenergic activity has been noted to stimulate both lipolysis and triglyceride-fatty acid recycling in burn patients[67]; serious undernutrition may be such a stimulus also.[65]

In laboratory animal models with transplanted tumors, including those in the genetically abnormal nude mouse, carcass lipid depletion occurs with varying degrees of tumor burden.[68] Urine and plasma from mice and human subjects with cancer cachexia were found by assay to contain higher levels of lipid metabolizing activity than did the urine and plasma from either normal controls or volunteers after a period of acute starvation.[69]

Hyperlipidemia. Elevated lipid levels usually are not marked in cancer patients but do occur in association with certain tumors. One mechanism for this elevation is decreased lipoprotein lipase (LPL) activity, which has been noted, for example, in patients with lung cancer. The lowest levels of LPL activity are associated with the greatest weight loss. Patients with breast cancer had normal LPL and minimal weight loss.[70]

Fat Oxidation. The considerable literature reporting that fat is oxidized at an increased rate in patients with cancer was summarized.[9,53] Fat oxidation rates were higher and carbohydrate oxidation rates were lower in those patients with cancer (colorectal and gastric) who had lost significant weight than in patients with cancer who had not lost weight or in patients with benign disease who had lost weight.[44]

ABNORMALITIES IN PROTEIN METABOLISM (TABLE 73–6)

The rates of whole-body protein turnover and the synthetic and catabolic rates of muscle protein increase with advancing stage of disease and its clinical expression of weight loss.[53,71–73] Whole-body protein turnover may be consistently increased to about 50% or more in patients with small cell sarcoma.[72] Increases of 50 to 70% in whole-body protein turnover rate have been noted in large groups of patients with lung and colorectal cancer.[46] Turnover studies in a diverse group of cancer patients found, however, one subpopulation with increased turnover whereas another was normal. These data indicate that an increased rate of protein mobilization can occur even in the presence of malnutrition and that supplying nutrition by the intravenous route in such individuals did not depress the turnover.[74] Kinetic studies further delineated metabolic abnormalities in malnourished untreated patients with cancer (with no liver metastases) (group 1) from those in malnourished patients with benign disease (group 2) and from those in healthy subjects on a starvation regimen for 10 days (group 3).[75] Whole-body protein turnover was 32% higher in group 1 than in group 2 and 35% higher in group 1 than in group 3. In this study, patients with cancer and weight loss had *increased* protein turnover, synthesis, and proteolysis in contrast to reduced rates, which are the normal adaptive response to acute malnutrition.

TABLE 73–6. ABNORMALITIES IN PROTEIN METABOLISM ASSOCIATED WITH ADVANCED CANCER

Increased whole-body protein turnover
Increased protein fractional synthetic rates in liver
Reduced fractional synthetic rates in muscle
Increased hepatic protein synthesis
Persistent muscle protein breakdown
Decreased plasma branched-chain amino acids

In another kinetics study using labeled leucine during intraoperative periods, no significant differences were noted in whole-body protein synthesis (WBPS), whole-body protein catabolism (WBPC), net protein catabolism (NPC), or albumin fractional synthesis rates between patients with benign disease who had maintained weight (group 1) and patients with cancer who had not lost weight (group 2).[76] In contrast, patients with cancer cachexia ($\geqq$ 15% weight loss, group 3) had a significant ($p < 0.005$) elevation in WBPC. WBPS was also elevated, but to a lesser extent, and the NPC rate was also increased ($p < .05$). Group 3 patients also had significantly higher fractional synthetic rates (FSR) in skeletal muscle ($p < .05$), liver ($p < .05$), and albumin ($p < .01$). The study concluded that patients with cancer cachexia were actively losing protein as a result of an increase in WBPC that was only partially compensated for by an increase in WBPS. Protein FSR in the primary tumors of patients in groups 2 and 3 were not significantly different; however, the values for protein FSR in the nodal and systemic metastases were higher than those for the primary tumor.[76]

Is the inability of many undernourished patients with cancer to reduce protein turnover (the normal adaptation to undernutrition) a causative factor in the development of cancer cachexia? As previously noted, studies of numerous cancer patients and normal subjects have confirmed the significantly increased protein turnover in the cancer patients. Fearon et al., in a comparative study of patients with colon and lung cancer and controls, found no correlation, however, between individual turnover rates, energy expenditure, and weight loss in the patients with cancer.[46]

Cancer patients who have lost significant weight often have protein kinetics similar to those of traumatized or infected individuals. As previously indicated, when the whole-body catabolic rate exceeds that of the synthetic rate of normal tissues plus that of the malignancy, depletion of body protein occurs.

Liver Protein Metabolism. Laboratory animal tumor models have demonstrated that the synthetic rate of total cellular hepatic protein is increased, unlike that of muscle.[77] An increase has been noted also in liver biopsy specimens from cancer patients[78] and in the fractional synthetic rate in vivo in the liver tissue of cachectic cancer patients.[76] These findings have been supported by organ imaging in a small sample of patients with cancer cachexia that indicates that liver size has been spared,[79] presumably as the result of transfer of nitrogen to the liver. Body composition data of Cohn et al. indicated that, although patients with cancer and serious weight loss had a significant decrease in the percentage of lean body mass, the percentage of nonmuscle lean body mass (i.e., visceral protein) rose markedly.[64] Their patients who had lost weight over a 6-month period had an average total weight loss of 15.29 kg, which was accounted for by the loss of 7.4 kg of body water, 6.2 kg of fat, and 1.63 kg of protein.[80]

Hypoalbuminemia and Albumin Synthesis. Albumin is the principal secretory protein of the liver; its depletion is common in cancer and results in hypoalbuminemia. The relatively few reports on albumin kinetics in cancer patients are contradictory with respect to synthetic rates,[76] and several studies report normal degradation rates.[53] These studies are in contrast to recent reports comparing rates in tumor-bearing and nontumor-bearing mice that indicate depressed synthesis secondary to malnutrition and an increased degradation by tumor liposomes.[81]

CYTOKINES AND NUTRITIONAL AND METABOLIC CHANGES

Many of the metabolic changes induced by cancer are seen also in patients with infections and trauma. These changes are believed to be endogenous host responses rather than the direct action of a pathogen or a tumor and to be attributable to the release of mediators derived from cells of the immune system. These mediators are termed cytokines.

Many cytokines are now known (see Chaps. 41, 68, and 69). They are polypeptide products of activated cells that, in most instances, provide short-range communication between cells by influencing their proliferation, differentiation, metabolism, and activation. Individual cytokines have the capacity to induce other cytokines in activated blood cells.

Three areas in cancer have special relations to these peptide regulatory factors. One, which we now mention only in passing but will undoubtedly become of major importance, relates to the interactions of stimulating and growth-inhibiting cytokines with activated oncogenes, loss of tumor suppressor genes, emergence of drug resistance, and loss of intimate cell-cell contacts.[82] Another area concerns the use of certain cytokines in antitumor therapy; this area is reviewed later. The third area concerns the roles of these regulatory factors in intermediary metabolism, in tumor growth, and in the development of various cancer metabolic abnormalities.

In studies that resulted in the isolation of the protein designated cachectin, Cerami and his colleagues originally noted that rabbits infected with Trypanosoma brucei had wasting of body protein and fat, severe anorexia, cachexia, hypertriglyceridemia associated with VLDL, and a suppression of lipoprotein lipase.[83] Cachectin and tumor necrosis factor (TNF) proved to be identical chemically and biologically.[84]

Additional reports indicate that, in the absence of sepsis or acute parasitic infections, serum TNF is not increased in patients with cancer,[85–87] chronic infection, or AIDS. Failure to find elevated TNF levels in anorectic and cachectic patients does not necessarily imply that TNF and/or one or more of the interrelated cytokines are not operating at some level. First, when TNF production in healthy volunteers is stimulated acutely by endotoxin, the TNF concentration in plasma peaks in about 2 hours and is back to normal in another 2 hours.[88] In addition, the plasma half-life in humans is 15 to 17 minutes. Hence, TNF may be difficult to detect. Second, the paracrine activity (action on nearby cells) of these factors may mean that systemic distribution and plasma level increases may not occur (see the following).

Dietary supplementation of healthy subjects with n-3 fish oils induced a depressed production by mononuclear blood cells, of the cytokines interleukin-1 (IL-1) α and β, and of TNF when the cells were stimulated by endotoxin or by phytohemagglutinin.[89] Infusion of recombinant (r) TNF over 5 days into cancer patients was associated with a negative nitrogen balance attributed to TNF-induced anorexia rather than to a specific effect on protein metabolism.[90]

Observations on interrelations between various cytokines and transplanted tumor models in mice indicate that numerous regulatory agents are involved with weight loss and other metabolic abnormalities. (The reader interested in learning more about the complexity of these relationships and intriguing aspects of tumor-monocyte interleukin interactions may wish to read references 91 to 96.)

Striking similarities and some discrepancies exist among the metabolic changes observed in cachetic cancer patients and those observed with AIDS patients with secondary infection and with septic patients. All have reactions in obvious contrast to those of patients with simple starvation and to those of the nonanorectic cancer patient maintaining weight.

TASTE AND APPETITE CHANGES

TASTE

Many patients ascribe diminished appetite to unpleasant and unacceptable alterations in the tastes of foods. The anatomic, physiologic, and other factors affecting taste and smell are complex (see Chap. 36).

Most studies of altered taste in patients with cancer have used the method of detecting the lowest perceptible solution concentration of sodium chloride (for salt), hydrochloric or citric acid (for sour), urea (for bitter), and sucrose (for sweet). This method has been criticized, and forced-choice methods, although more time consuming, have been recommended to eliminate some response biases.[97]

An early paper in this field noted that 25 of 50 patients with metastatic carcinoma of various primary sites had less pleasurable taste of food.[98] This change was associated with an elevated taste threshold for sweetness (i.e., food tasted less sweet) and a lowered taste threshold for bitterness. The likelihood of the presence of a taste abnormality increased with the increasing extent of disease but not with histologic type of neoplasm. Subsequent papers have challenged the concept of a consistent pattern of altered taste and have differed from each other. No threshold taste differences were noted between matched controls and patients with esophageal cancer.[99] Other studies have reported a higher threshold for sour and sweetness,[100] a higher threshold for salt in patients with breast cancer, and a higher threshold for sweets in patients with colon cancer.[101] Responses of patients with upper gastrointestinal cancers to five suprathreshold concentrations of the four basic tastes were graded on the basis of the range of intensity and hedonic reactions.[102] Intensity scores indicated no abnormalities of taste perception among patients on the basis of tumor site, type of therapy, or appetite. Hedonic reactions differed among individuals and groups.

Thus, findings on taste are inconsistent or variable both within patient groups and among reports. Such inconsistencies should not be regarded as an indication that taste changes do not occur; usually, such changes are frequent. When they cause rejection of nutritious foods, they are contributory factors to anorexia and appear to be influenced to a variable degree by psychosomatic factors, fear, pain, and side effects of medications. Physicians and dietitians should ascertain the preferences and dislikes for foods of their individual patients and thereby develop appropriate diet patterns based on their specific responses.

LEARNED FOOD AVERSIONS

Psychologic factors undoubtedly play a role in appetite. The fear and uncertainty engendered by the diagnosis of cancer and its uncertain outcome and the stress of diagnostic procedures are exacerbated by the physiologic and metabolic effects of various antitumor interventions. One aspect of these stresses is so-called learned food aversion. This behavior is the unconscious association (by person or animal) of the consumption of a particular food with a concurrent or subsequent unpleasant reaction, such as nausea or vomiting. The result is subsequent avoidance of that food. In cancer patients, the unpleasant reactions may occur in association with antitumor therapy, such as a chemotherapeutic drug or ionizing radiation. Children who were given anticancer drugs that induced nausea or vomiting were tested for learned food aversion by offering the experimental group of children with cancer an unusually flavored ice cream shortly before drug administration. Controls were not given this flavored ice cream. When tested later for aversion to the same ice cream, controls chose it three times more frequently than did the experimental groups.[103] Such studies were extended to include adult patients. Contradictory evidence exists, however, because patients undergoing chemotherapy did not have a significantly greater aversion, decrease in appetite, earlier satiety, or weight loss than did patients not receiving chemotherapy.[104]

The possible role of learned food aversions in tumor-bearing animals was based on the hypothesis that tumor-bearing rats would avoid foods associated with aversive physiologic effects of the tumor itself without any relation to treatment. The results have been variable and have depended, in part, on the tumor and diets tested.[105,106] Reservations have been expressed that this reaction is a physiologic expression of tumor effects rather than a conditioned response.[107]

PARANEOPLASTIC SYNDROMES AND "ECTOPIC" OR "EUTOPIC" PEPTIDES

Secretion of polypeptide hormones by certain malignant tumors has been known for many decades to cause distinct paraneoplastic syndromes. Many new active peptides recently have been discovered within the central nervous system and the gastrointestinal tract and also are expressed by human tumors. In addition to these true endocrines, various interleukins, including growth factors, are expressed by tumors. As previously noted, transplanted animal tumors derived from human tumor cell lines can produce soluble substances that, in turn, stimulate monocytes elsewhere to produce peptides, such as TNF-α.

Every known naturally occurring hormone is produced by one or more human tumor types. Unlike the firmly regulated feedback controls of the normal endocrine systems, such hormone production is more autonomous. Hence, unregulated production can have a powerful influence on adjacent and distant organs. These tumor-produced hormones had been believed to be abnormal with respect to source[108]; however, many normal cells not previously considered to be hormone producers are now known to have the capability of making small amounts of hormones. For example, chorionic gonadotropin made by colonic adenocarcinoma can also be produced in normal colonic mucosa; ACTH and calcitonin made "ectopically" by bronchiogenic cancer can be produced in small amounts by normal bronchial epithelial cells. Hence, the tumor-derived peptide production is more appropriately designated as "eutopic;" i.e., the production is abnormal with respect to quantity but not with respect to source.

Metabolic, nutritional, electrolyte, and other clinical problems can result from increased production. Hormones with such implications include gastrin, vasoactive intestinal peptide (VIP), serotonin, glucagon, insulin, vasopressin, parathyroid hormone and its analogues, growth hormone, somatostatin, and the vitamin D derivative, calcitriol. Cushing's syndrome is related to the production of ACTH by lung cancer of all types, pancreatic islet cells, carcinoid, and adenocarcinoma. The syndrome of inappropriate antidiuretic hormone (SIADH) has been associated with lung and colon cancers. When insulin from insulinomas is added to that produced by its normal cells of production, severe hypoglycemia results. Gastrin from pancreatic tumor cells (also produced by gastric cells normally capable of its production) can induce the Zollinger-Ellison syndrome. Somatomedins, which are believed to account for the development of hypoglycemia in instances of hepatic carcinomas, are normally produced in the liver and act like insulin. Of the types of neoplasms that produce hypoglycemia, 21% were found to be hepatic in origin, and a few were adenocarcinomas of the stomach and colon.[108]

Some polypeptide hormones produced by tumors may have activities of other hormones because of common peptide sequences in their molecules. Many neuroendocrine tumors that produce hormones contain opioid peptides. Secretion of opioid peptides has been postulated to contribute to psychiatric disturbances, such as depression, mood swings, and psychosis.[109] Severe diarrhea can result from tumors secreting serotonin (carcinoid syndrome), calcitonin, gastrin (Zollinger-Ellison syndrome), and VIP (Verner-Morrison syndrome). Zollinger-Ellison syndrome can be associated with steatorrhea induced by the inhibitory effects of decreased intestinal pH on pancreatic lipase function, as well as by epithelial damage.[110] Potassium and fluid losses in the diarrhea of Verner-Morrison syndrome may be severe.[111]

Several recently available drugs have proved useful in the management of some of these gut-derived endocrine tumors when resection is not feasible. Omeprazole, which inhibits acid secretion by the gastric mucosa, can eliminate or greatly reduce the gastrin effects in the Zollinger-Ellison syndrome. The analogue of somatostatin, octreotide, has proved beneficial when administered in several daily subcutaneous injections in suppressing endocrine secretions associated with the Verner-Morrison syndrome (VIPomas) and the carcinoid syndrome. Benefit from octreotide has also been reported with insulinomas and glucagonomas.[112]

HYPERCALCEMIA

Hypercalcemia is one of the most common metabolic complications of cancer. Approximately 20 to 40% of patients with breast, squamous, bladder, and renal carcinomas, multiple myeloma, and lymphomas develop hypercalcemia at some point in their disease. It is steadily progressive unless treated and may be symptomatic at relatively lower calcium concentrations than is the case with hyperparathyroidism. The more common symptoms are nausea, muscle weakness, excess urine, elevated blood pressure, anorexia, lethargy, confusion, and stupor progressing to coma.

Major mechanisms of hypercalcemia include[113]:

1. Local osteolytic hypercalcemia. This mechanism is involved in 20 to 40% of malignancy-associated cases of hypercalcemia, primarily in breast cancer, multiple myeloma, lymphomas, and leukemias. Of interest is the finding that plasma cells in multiple myeloma liberate into their culture media a factor or factors that stimulate bone resorption. The main osteoclast activating factor appears to be TNF-β (lymphotoxin). Other malignant tumors stimulate production of the bone-resorbing cytokines TNF-α and IL-1 and of transforming growth factor.

2. Osteoclastic bone resorption with discrete lytic lesions caused by bone-metastasizing solid tumors (breast, lung, pancreatic tumors).

3. Parathyroid hormone–like peptides (PTHLP) induced by a gene produced by nonmetastatic breast, lung, renal and pancreatic tumors and by lymphoma.[114] These peptides are homologous in some regions with parathyroid hormone (PTH) and they act on PTH receptors. The response of bone and kidney to PTHLP, however, differs in certain respects from that to regular PTH in that calcium reabsorption by the kidney is enhanced, a tendency to alkylosis is apparent, plasma calcitriol is decreased, and circulating iPTH is decreased. Hypercalcemia in patients with breast cancer usually is the result of this PTHLP mechanism. The kidney also plays a role in producing hypercalcemia, depending on the tumor involved.[113]

Seven reported cases of hypercalcemia in patients with lymphoma have been associated with increased circulating calcitriol.[115]

OSTEOMALACIA

Certain tumors reduce plasma calcitriol concentration in conjunction with hypophosphatemia, thereby inducing an oncogenic osteomalacia. Approximately 50 such cases were reported as of 1986; undoubtedly many more have occurred. Most reported cases have usually involved benign nonendocrine tumors of mesenchymal origin (e.g., hemangiopericytoma or giant cell tumor).[116] In addition, hypophosphatemic osteomalacia has been noted with prostatic carcinoma.[117] Muscle weakness of varying degree and variable back pain have been frequent complaints with findings of hypophosphatemia, renal phosphate wasting, and decreased calcitriol, PTH, and calcium; serum calcidiol has been normal. Histologically, osteoclast activity has been markedly enhanced. Gastrointestinal malabsorption of calcium and phosphate has been observed. Where resection of the tumor has been possible, serum calcitriol and phosphate levels rose within 36 hours, with subsequent correction of the bone disease.[117]

VILLOUS CHANGES

Creamer suggested that malignant tumors external to the gastrointestinal tract induced an abnormal small-intestinal mucosa with resultant malabsorption to which he attributed some of the ill health and loss of weight characteristic of malignant disease.[118] In a more definitive study, Barry showed that malnourished patients with extra-alimentary tract malignant tumors often displayed abnormalities of mucosal cell structure, loss of epithelial cells, and decreased xylose absorption. Because he found similar changes in seriously malnourished patients without cancer, he suggested that the mucosal changes were the *result* of malnutrition rather than a direct effect of nongastrointestinal tract malignant tumors.[119] Once present, impaired mucosal function can contribute further to malnutrition by depressing the efficiency of absorption.

LOCALIZED TUMOR EFFECTS

In addition to the systemic effects of cancer, numerous more localized effects of various neoplasms may lead to nutritional problems (see Table 73–2).

OBSTRUCTION OF THE ALIMENTARY TRACT

The most common direct effect of alimentary tract neoplasms on nutritional status relates to partial or complete obstruction at one or more sites. Approximately 20% of surgical hospital admissions for acute abdominal conditions are associated with intestinal obstruction; the second most common cause of obstruction is neoplasm of the alimentary tract.[120] Esophageal, gastric, and colorectal carcinomas are important etiologic factors in the older age group. Obstructive symptoms can occur from peritoneal tumor seeding; intestinal dysfunction without mechanical obstruction may develop secondary to abdominal metastases. When obstruction occurs acutely, the patient seeks medical attention immediately. Most neoplasms, however, obstruct slowly and progressively; consequently, a significant number of patients defer seeking medical care until one or more of their symptoms (anorexia, dysphagia, nausea, vomiting, pain, diarrhea, or anemia from chronic blood loss) have resulted in weight loss and/or weakness. In addition to weight loss secondary to poor intake of food, problems of fluid, electrolyte, and acid-base balance result from persistent vomiting or diarrhea or as a consequence of dehydration and/or malnutrition.

MALABSORPTION

Malabsorption occurs for numerous reasons.

BLIND LOOP SYNDROME

This syndrome occurs with partial obstruction in the upper small bowel, the presence of jejunal diverticuli, or lack of motility in an intestinal loop. The associated overgrowth of bacteria in the upper small bowel may result in steatorrhea and vitamin B_{12} deficiency. Not only is there direct interaction of bacteria with certain nutrients, but resulting abnormalities of the intestinal epithelium also cause malabsorption.[121]

FISTULA

Bypass of a significant portion of the bowel can occur as the result of fistula formation between widely separated portions of the gastrointestinal tract. The resulting degree of malabsorption depends on the site and the completeness and extent of the bypass. Severe malabsorption occurs with a fistula between stomach and large bowel (gastrocolic type) or between small bowel and large bowel (enterocolic type) or between small bowel and small bowel (entero-entero fistula) or from small bowel to skin (enterocutaneous fistula).

MALIGNANCIES OF THE SMALL INTESTINE

These are uncommon in the duodenum and small intestine and account for only about 1% of all malignancies of the gastrointestinal tract. They may be associated with pain and bleeding (often occult, resulting in microcytic anemia), weight loss, partial obstruction, and diarrhea or steatorrhea, especially with lymphomas of the upper intestine. An association exists between celiac disease and an increased incidence of intestinal lymphoma and carcinoma.[122] (See also Chap. 62D.) A type of intestinal lymphoma in individuals in the Middle East involves the mesentary lymph nodes with resultant malabsorption.[123]

CARCINOID TUMORS

Carcinoid tumors derived from argentaffin cells may produce serotonin (with an associated increase in urinary excretion of 5-hydroxyindoleacetic acid), histamines, catecholamines, and kinins. When the tumor is metastatic to the liver, these substances can be synthesized in sufficient quantities to cause flushing, episodic watery diarrhea, and dyspnea or asthma.[124]

PROTEIN-LOSING ENTEROPATHY

Infiltration of the lamina propria and draining lymph nodes by tumor cells can lead to obstruction and dilation of the lymphatics within the intestinal villi, which, in turn, can lead to development of protein-losing enteropathy with hypoalbuminemia, hypoglobulinemia, and lymphocytopenia.[125] This condition was described originally with intestinal lymphoma and gastric carcinoma, but now is known to occur with tumors arising outside the alimentary tract, e.g., malignant melanoma, ovarian carcinoma, and metastatic lung carcinoma.

NUTRITION SUPPORT RECOMMENDATIONS

Reversal of the undesirable clinical, metabolic, and nutritional changes secondary to systemic and localized effects of cancer depends primarily on elimination of the malignant condition by complete eradication or by major palliation. The physician frequently must correct significant malnutrition and fluid and electrolyte imbalances in patients who require surgical intervention or in those who need prolonged maintenance in therapeutic trials of radiation and/or chemotherapy. As with all chronic wasting diseases, one cannot and should not expect to restore significant amounts of tissue in a short period of time. Urgent treatments cannot and should not be postponed until the goal of nutritional rehabilitation can be achieved. In such a situation, correction of acute or chronic vitamin and mineral deficiencies, blood loss, and electrolyte and fluid imbalances can often be accomplished rapidly, thus decreasing the risk.

When surgery, radiation, and/or chemotherapy are indicated for the debilitated patient who faces a further significant period of little or no oral intake of food as a consequence of such treatment, efforts to improve nutritional and metabolic status by adequate parenteral or enteral feeding may be an aid to survival or to decreased morbidity and shorter period of convalescence. These issues are reviewed later. The nutrition support methods of enteral and parenteral feedings are discussed in Chapters 79 and 80, respectively.

CANCER THERAPIES: RESULTANT NUTRITION PROBLEMS AND THEIR MANAGEMENT (TABLE 73–7)

Significant nutritional problems may arise not only from the systemic effects of the malignant condition, but also from specific treatments undertaken to control the neoplastic process. These treatment methods are reviewed in the following sections. More general issues in nutrition support are reviewed later.

SURGICAL INTERVENTION

Surgery is the primary therapeutic method available to patients with gastrointestinal malignancies in whom eradication of the tumor or significant palliation is deemed reasonably certain. Significant nutritional problems may arise and nutrition support may be helpful, depending on the type and extent of resection. Because radiation therapy and chemotherapy may also be utilized pre- and postoperatively, their effects also are noted.

HEAD AND NECK TUMORS

In addition to impaired food intake as a result of the obstructing tumor, male patients, especially, often have a history of chronic heavy alcohol intake and smoking. Such patients may be in a nutritionally depleted state prior to therapy. Treatment often involves combined surgery and radiation, with chemotherapy also used in some cases (Table 73–7). Radiation can induce loss of taste ("mouth blindness"), xerostomia (dry mouth) as the result of salivary gland damage, and trismus and some nerve damage, depending on the site radiated. Injury to teeth may also occur, but this outcome can be minimized by adequate dental care before treatment. Radiation effects may be long term. Of 13 patients studied 1 to 7 years after radiotherapy, 9 had measurable taste losses, especially for salt and bitter; 12 had reduced salivary flow and secretion rates, with no saliva being collected in 7; and 9 complained of dry mouth.[126] Surgery may include partial or total glossectomy and mandibulectomy, and resection of portions of the hard or soft palate and of soft tissues of the lower face and neck. These procedures add to the difficulties in chewing and swallowing. The likelihood of chronic aspiration on swallowing may be serious enough to require tube feeding or, alternatively, laryngectomy with its physical separation of the respiratory and alimentary tracts and resultant loss of normal voice.

Nutrition Support Recommendation. For the patient who is seriously malnourished on admission, early nutritional intervention should be considered. Feeding tubes usually can be placed despite the tumor. If tube feeding is not possible, parenteral nutrition through a peripheral vein or through a long anecubital line into a central vein can be given if placement of a neck or subclavian central catheter is contraindicated. Post-treatment attention is directed to providing attractive foods with pleasant aroma that are lubricated by gravies and salad dressings and are of high caloric nutrition content to encourage better food intake. Nutritious liquid formulas can be administered by mouth if they can be swallowed or, alternatively for the short term, by intermittent nasoesophageal tube feeding. Gastrostomy tubes should be inserted for long-term maintenance of patients requiring such support (see Chap. 79). For patients who are at serious risk of aspiration of regurgitated food (tendency to vomit, absent gag reflex, significant pulmonary disease), bolus feeding through a tube with its tip in the stomach or duodenum increases the risk. This danger is reduced by placing the tip of the tube in the small bowel and infusing the formula by slow drip over several hours using a pump to assure regular flow rate.

TABLE 73–7. CONSEQUENCES OF CANCER TREATMENT PREDISPOSING TO NUTRITION PROBLEMS

I. Radiation treatment
- **A.** Radiation of oropharyngeal area
  - **1.** Destruction of sense of taste; xerostomia and odynophagia; loss of teeth
- **B.** Radiation to lower neck and mediastinum
  - **1.** Esophagitis with dysphagia
  - **2.** Fibrosis with esophageal stricture
- **C.** Radiation of abdomen and pelvis
  - **1.** Bowel damage, acute and chronic, with diarrhea, malabsorption, stenosis and obstruction, fistulization

II. Surgical treatment
- **A.** Radical resection of oropharyngeal area
  - **1.** Chewing and swallowing difficulties
- **B.** Esophagectomy
  - **1.** Gastric stasis and hypochlorhydria secondary to vagotomy
  - **2.** Steatorrhea secondary to vagotomy
  - **3.** Diarrhea secondary to vagotomy
  - **4.** Early satiety
  - **5.** Regurgitation
- **C.** Gastrectomy (high subtotal or total)
  - **1.** Dumping syndrome
  - **2.** Malabsorption
  - **3.** Achlorhydria and lack of intrinsic factor and R protein
  - **4.** Hypoglycemia
  - **5.** Early satiety
- **D.** Intestinal resection
  - **1.** Jejunum
    - **a.** Decreased efficiency of absorption of many nutrients
  - **2.** Ileum
    - **a.** Vitamin B_{12} deficiency
    - **b.** Bile salt losses with diarrhea or steatorrhea
    - **c.** Hyperoxaluria and renal stone
    - **d.** Calcium and magnesium depletion
    - **e.** Fat and fat-soluble vitamin malabsorption
  - **3.** Massive bowel resection
    - **a.** Life-threatening malabsorption
    - **b.** Malnutrition
    - **c.** Metabolic acidosis
    - **d.** Dehydration

Discharged patients who require long-term liquid feedings at home should be given information to assure that the purchased or home-made formulas used are nutritionally adequate in all respects, are of the "prudent diet" type, are as inexpensive as possible, and have sufficient bulk-forming materials to prevent constipation.

ESOPHAGEAL CARCINOMA

Antitumor management of patients with esophageal cancer often employs surgery, radiation, and combination chemotherapy.

Radiation to the lower neck and mediastinum can induce esophagitis; although this condition usually disappears following cessation of therapy, some patients may develop fibrosis with resultant esophageal stricture. Fistulas and hemorrhage may also occur and commonly are related to regrowth of the cancer. Chemotherapy may induce nausea, anorexia, sore mouth, and odynophagia, thus further inhibiting food intake and decreasing the acceptance of tube feeding.

Surgical treatment usually involves total or distal esophagectomy requiring bilateral vagotomy, proximal gastrectomy, and anastomosis of the retained portion of the esophagus to the remaining stomach, which is placed into the chest. Esophageal anastomotic leakage may occur (see the following). Easy regurgitation, rapid satiety, decreased rate of gastric emptying of solid food despite pyloroplasty, diarrhea (intermittent or continuous), and steatorrhea (mild to moderate) are common results of this surgery (Table 73–7).[127] The causes of diarrhea and steatorrhea are unknown, but are related to the vagotomy.

TABLE 73–7. *(continued)*

- **4.** Ileostomy and colostomy
  - **a.** Complications of salt and water balance
- **E.** Blind loop syndrome
  - **1.** Vitamin B_{12} malabsorption
- **F.** Pancreatectomy
  - **1.** Malabsorption
  - **2.** Diabetes mellitus

III. Drug treatment
- **A.** Corticosteroids
  - **1.** Fluid and electrolyte problems
  - **2.** Nitrogen and calcium losses
  - **3.** Hyperglycemia
- **B.** Sex hormone analogues
  - **1.** Fluid retention
  - **2.** Nausea
  - **3.** Megesterol acetate—glucocorticoid effects
- **C.** Immunotherapy
  - **1.** Tumor necrosis factor (TNF)
    - **a.** Fluid retention
    - **b.** Hypotension
    - **c.** Nausea, vomiting
    - **d.** Diarrhea
  - **2.** Interleukin-2
    - **a.** Hypotension
    - **b.** Fluid retention
    - **c.** Azotemia
  - **3.** Interferons
    - **a.** Anorexia
    - **b.** Nausea/vomiting
    - **c.** Diarrhea
    - **d.** Azotemia
- **D.** Cytotoxic chemotherapy (see Table 73–8)

Nutrition Support Recommendations. A significant number of these patients already have lost weight as a result of decreased food intake secondary to progressive dysphagia. In addition, a significant number of men have a history of chronic ethanol use. Weight loss of greater than 10% is a negative prognostic factor.[128] When obstruction is partial and regurgitation is not a problem, ingestion of adequate amounts of complete liquid formulas is often beneficial in preventing or ameliorating malnutrition. When serious anorexia is also present, passage of a feeding tube is possible. Oral or tube feeding is often inadequate to meet the need in the period of radiation and chemotherapy because of interference with the feeding program, nausea, pain, or combinations thereof. In such instances, preoperative parenteral feeding is indicated to improve nutritional status. Postoperative complications in patients who received at least 5 days of preoperative TPN support were noted to be reduced significantly over those in patients who did not receive such support; fewer complications were also reported in the preoperative TPN group as compared to those in patients given TPN only postoperatively.[129] Either enteral or parenteral nutrition supports normalized glucose turnover, suppressed gluconeogenesis, and increased protein synthesis in patients with esophageal cancer.[130]

In their review of 16 cases of esophageal anastomotic leakages after tumor resection, Riboli et al. noted that, in the period from 1978 to 1980, 8 patients with such leakage underwent immediate reoperation to create a new anastomosis; 7 died postoperatively. In the period from 1980 to 1982, 8 other patients with leakage were treated with TPN and complete fasting; 6 survived with spontaneous healing of the leaks, and 2 died of septic mediastinitis and respiratory failure.[131]

Following resumption of oral intake by the patient who has undergone esophagectomy, the dietary prescription should provide for frequent small meals (to overcome easy satiety and the tendency to regurgitation) high in carbohydrate and adequate in protein and fat. If steatorrhea occurs with increased frequency and foul-smelling stools and abdominal discomfort ensue, partial substitution of long-chain fats (LCT) by medium-chain triglycerides (MCT) can be tested and may be helpful.[127] True "dumping" does not occur in such patients eating solid food because the gastric-duodenal continuity is normal and gastric emptying is usually delayed despite pyloroplasty. Postoperative stricture may occur and requires dilation; the patient may temporarily require oral or tube-fed liquid formulas to assure adequate intake until the stricture is overcome.

Carcinoma of the esophagogastric junction creates pre- and postoperative physiologic and nutritional problems similar to those just described. Because an appreciably larger portion of the proximal stomach may be resected, early satiety may be more marked and production of gastric juice may be reduced, thereby resulting in decreased B_{12} absorption.

GASTRIC CANCER

Surgical treatment for gastric cancer involves either a radical subtotal gastrectomy (80 to 85%) with a gastrojejunal anastomosis or a total gastrectomy with an esophagojejunal anastomosis with or without some type of reservoir in the upper jejunum. Long-term survival following curative surgery is reasonably good; reported outcome is better in Japan than in the United States. The 5- and 10-year survival rates after curative total gastrectomy with lymphadenectomy in 292 patients in Japan were 48.6 and 23.2%, respectively, for patients older than 70 years of age and 49.4 and 33.6%, respectively, for younger patients.[132] For the treatment of the patient with resected but residual localized disease, radiation and/or chemotherapy are utilized.

Removal of most or all of the stomach reduces or deletes its reservoir, digestive, secretory, diluting, and metering functions. These modifications from the normal have both physiologic and nutritional consequences that may vary from mild to severe, depending on the extent of resection, the individual patient response, the appropriateness of the intervention, and the postoperative care. The physiologic and nutritional problems of patients with high subtotal or total gastrectomy are different from those of patients with esophagogastrectomy (Table 73–7).

Depending on the types and amounts of foods ingested postoperatively and on the response of the patient, various signs and symptoms, which have been termed the "dumping syndrome," can occur. This syndrome develops with varying severity (depending in part on the composition of the meal) in approximately one half of patients with gastrojejunal or esophagojejunal anastamoses. Usually the signs and symptoms occur within 15 to 30 minutes following ingestion of a meal. Vasomotor manifestation includes diaphoresis, palpitations, weakness, and faintness; in addition, gastrointestinal signs and symptoms include abdominal bloating, cramping, and diarrhea, which may become pronounced shortly after the meal. Another set of symptoms, which may occur in conjunction with those just mentioned, but usually occurs approximately 2 hours after eating, is also characterized by sweating, tachycardia, and faintness; mental confusion also may occur. This set of symptoms is related to catecholamine discharge mediated by hypoglycemia induced by the insulin response to the rapid entry of the meal into the upper small bowel.

Malabsorption of fat occurs especially in those who have undergone total or near total gastrectomy.[133] Deficiencies of iron, calcium, and fat-soluble vitamins may occur.

Numerous reports have described the beneficial effect of somatostatin and especially of its analogue, octreotide, in the treatment of the dumping syndrome. In dumping provocation tests induced by diet, the drug reduced or abolished the early and late signs and symptoms associated with hypovolemia and hypoglycemia, respectively.[112,134] Some patients benefited from long-term use, but many others were unable to tolerate the drug because of diarrhea.[112] The use of octreotide has provided important information on the possible cause of the dumping syndrome. Geer et al. found that the plasma levels of pancreatic polypeptide, neurotensin, and glucagon were markedly elevated during the "dump" treated with placebo, but each was suppressed with octreotide pretreatment. On the basis of specific findings and other data, the authors postulate that neurotensin is most likely the mediator peptide.[134]

Nutrition Support Recommendations. Because octreotide must be given parenterally and chronic use may be associated with diarrhea, diet therapy still remains a useful and practical approach. The dumping syndrome can be greatly minimized or prevented by provision of and adherence to an antidumping diet (see Appendix Table A–33). In general, such a diet is high in protein, has adequate fat, is quite low in soluble carbohydrates, somewhat decreased in total carbohydrates, restricted in fluids at meal time, and served approximately six times per day. An additional measure for those who continue to be somewhat symptomatic includes reclining for a period immediately after eating. The use of a pectin derivative has been reported to prolong gastric emptying; to decrease dumping, blood volume changes, and serum insulin; and to minimize the fall in blood sugar (see Chap. 39).[135]

Steatorrhea can be significant (i.e., 20 to 25% fat malabsorption) in some patients and can be reduced by progressive replacement of a portion of LCT with MCT as tolerated. A trial of pancreatic extract in this situation is indicated to rule out luminal pancreatic enzyme insufficiency resulting from dilution of pancreatic enzymes by rapid food and fluid entry into the upper small bowel or from a pancreatic secretory defect or from both.

Deficiencies of vitamins and minerals can be prevented or treated by adequate oral administration of iron with ascorbic acid and by supplementary vitamins containing both water-soluble and fat-soluble vitamins (high-potency vitamin formulations are usually not necessary). Monthly injections of 100 μg of vitamin B_{12} are required because the extensive gastric resection will eventually result in B_{12} deficiency because of lack of gastric juice, intrinsic factor, and R protein.

Symptoms of milk intolerance, which are common in these patients, can be prevented and adequate calcium obtained by instructing the patient to drink milk in small amounts frequently over the day, or preferably to drink a lactase-treated milk or to use yogurt as tolerated. If these approaches are unsatisfactory, the more soluble calcium salts should be taken in divided doses over the day to provide at least 1 g of this ion.

The weight loss seen so often in patients who have undergone gastrectomy is not primarily the result of malabsorption, but is usually attributable to poor food intake. In addition to the food antipathy related to the recurrence of the unpleasant dumping syndrome with meals, discomfort associated with eating may result from the afferent loop syndrome, esophagitis secondary to bile regurgitation, anorexia associated with depression, or the side effects of drugs and/or radiation. Hence, a careful diet history, adequate explanation of the basis for dietary modifications, and periodic review to manage problems as they arise are important.

When the most careful dietary advice and the adherence to an antidumping diet do not prevent the dumping syndrome or assure an adequate food intake to maintain or gain weight, testing of intermittent slow-drip tube feedings of a complete formula is recommended. Because of the slow entry of food into the upper intestine by this technique, dumping is not likely to occur. Such feedings may need to be given only during the period of chemotherapy, following which appetite may improve. When patients remain seriously anorectic following cessation of chemotherapy, nightly tube feedings are helpful.

PANCREATIC CARCINOMA

The adverse impacts on nutritional status of this type of tumor and of its treatments are listed in Table 73–7. Pancreatic carcinoma is a malignant condition often associated with abdominal pain, anorexia, nausea and vomiting, and weight loss as presenting complaints; some of the nausea and vomiting are associated with duodenal obstruction. Eating may aggravate pain. Carcinoma of the pancreas may cause digestive enzyme deficiency when the duct of Wirsung is obstructed. The resulting malabsorption, combined with anorexia, contributes to progressive weight loss. Bile insufficiency can occur as a result of obstruction, such as the obstruction that occurs with involvement by tumor of the ampulla of Vater, of the common bile duct behind the pancreatic head, or at the porta hepatis. Bile insufficiency reduces intestinal absorption of vitamin K and leads to reduction in plasma levels of the vitamin K-dependent coagulation factors. Pancreatic carcinoma is an aggressive disease, and by the time of diagnosis, most patients are at a stage in which curative treatment is not feasible.

Surgical resection offers the only possible chance of cure at present. Pancreaticoduodenectomy was described by Whipple et al. in 1935 for the surgical treatment of carcinoma of the ampulla of Vater. The procedure is utilized for surgical management of cancer of the head of the pancreas, distal common bile duct, and the duodenum. In the usual operative procedure, the distal portion of the stomach is removed, the pancreas is transected (usually at its neck, but varying amounts or even the entire organ may be removed), and the entire duodenum and a few inches of jejunum distal to the ligament of Treitz are resected. The postoperative complication rate of this procedure is still significant and may result in prolonged hospitalization with numerous problems interfering with normal food intake. Five-year survival rates have been uncommon after surgery, but appear to be increasing with reported rates of as high as 18 to 36%.[136]

The decision concerning management of the remaining pancreas has nutrition implications. Ligation of the pancreatic duct with oversewing of the transected end of the pancreas (a procedure that is occasionally done) leads to complete exocrine pancreatic insufficiency.[137] Even when the remainder of the duct in the pancreatic stump was anastomosed into the stomach or duodenum in an effort to utilize exocrine secretions, fat malabsorption occurred in 27%[137] and 50%[138,139] of patients.

Approximately 10 to 12% of patients who appear with carcinoma of the pancreas are overtly diabetic,[138] and depending on the site of the tumor, 10 to 35% have asymptomatic glycosuria or hyperglycemia.[140] Another aspect of this surgical procedure concerns the endocrine function of the postoperative remnant of the pancreas. Decreased glucose tolerance has been noted in patients who have undergone pancreaticoduodenectomy (in whom fasting blood sugar levels were within normal limits) with an insufficient insulin response to a glucose load.[141] Hemipancreatectomy performed on healthy donors for the purpose of obtaining pancreatic tissue for transplantation into recipients with type I diabetes resulted in deterioration of insulin secretion and glucose tolerance in the donors 1 year later.[142]

Debate continues about total pancreatectomy as a preferred procedure over more limited resections. This procedure results in a difficult metabolic situation because of the dual exocrine and endocrine insufficiencies with "brittle" diabetes mellitus. In a series of 48 patients who underwent total pancreatectomy and were followed with respect to their control of diabetes, 50% were easily managed, 8% were managed with difficulty only when a concomitant illness existed, 19% had occasional hypoglycemic reactions managed with oral carbohydrate, 4% did poorly with persistent glycosuria, and 20% were managed with great difficulty, with ketoacidosis or hyperglycemic episodes requiring hospitalization.[143] Efforts continue to develop to prove that resections more radical than pancreaticoduodenectomy with or without adjuvant radiotherapy have better 5-year survival rates.[136]

Regional pancreatectomy as developed by Fortner involved en bloc removal of all or most of the pancreas, adjacent tissues, and primary lymph drainage and portions of involved vessels, soft tissues, distal stomach, duodenum, spleen, gallbladder, and common bile duct with skeletonizing of the porta hepatis, celiac axis, and superior mesenteric artery, vena cava, and aorta.[144] Anorexia, marked diarrhea, and severe malabsorption usually occurred together. This procedure is no longer used.

Nutrition Support Recommendations. When pancreaticoduodenectomy is associated with evidence of deficiency of exocrine pancreatic secretions, adequate amounts of pancreatic extract are helpful and should be administered with all meals and snacks, particularly when moderate to severe fat malabsorption exists.[145] MCT are more efficiently absorbed in the absence of pancreatic enzymes and decreased bile salts than are the usual LCT. Glucose oligosaccharides may also help to increase the caloric intake and absorption of patients with pancreatic insufficiency, because these relatively short-chain glucose polymers can be hydrolyzed to glucose by the brush-border enzyme sucrase-α-dextrinase. This white powdery material is not sweet and may be used in a variety of ways to supplement intake.

OTHER SURGICAL INTERVENTIONS

Ileal Resection. Major resection of the small bowel because of primary gastrointestinal malignant tumors is relatively uncommon, as is resection of only the jejunum. The ileum is damaged, bypassed, or removed to varying extent in cancer patients because of involvement with metastatic disease, fistula development, or radiation enteritis. Resection of the ileum leads to certain physiologic and nutritional problems that are reviewed in Chapter 62A and listed in Table 73–7.

Colectomy (Partial, Total, and Diverting). Resection of the right colon with the ileocecal valve and a portion of the distal ileum may be associated with watery diarrhea in large part caused by entry of increased amounts of bile salts into the colon, as well as by functional loss of the valve.[146] Only a small segment of distal ileum usually is sacrificed; therefore, vitamin B_{12} deficiency is not likely to occur.

Total proctocolectomy is performed for ulcerative colitis, which carries with it a significant risk of colorectal cancer, and for familial polyposis of the colon, which, if unresected, also has a high risk for occurrence of this malignant disease. An ileostomy with stool collected in an external pouch over the stoma is the oldest procedure and is still used for older patients. Even though the distal ileum is functionally intact, losses of water and sodium through the ileostomy may be significant over the first 7 to 10 postoperative days. Thereafter, most patients adapt, and the fluid and electrolyte losses decrease. These patients usually lose 300 to 600 ml of water daily with 40 to 100 mEq of sodium and 2.5 to 10 mEq of potassium. When sodium intake is restricted, a "low sodium" diuresis tends to result; this diuresis together with an obligatory ileal sodium loss predisposes the patient to severe salt and water depletion. Some authors have reported that the "low sodium" diuresis can be prevented by intramuscular injections of desmopressin, a synthetic antidiuretic vasopressin agonist that conserves water.[147] Patients can be managed in most instances with increased fluids and salt, however. Even patients who adapt well may experience an episode of gastroenteritis, partial intestinal obstruction, or prolonged excessive sweating that causes additional losses and may cause dehydration. Various procedures have been designed to provide a continent ileostomy with an internal (e.g., Koch) pouch and an ileorectal continuity without or with ileoanal reservoir.[148] Eating patterns and dietary recommendations to minimize stool frequency have been published.[149]

When a significant segment of the large bowel is taken out of continuity by a diverting procedure that leaves only the distal rectoanal area in continuity, an inflammatory process termed diversion colitis can occur in this residual area. Diversion colitis occurs at a variable time after the completion of the bypass and is characterized by persistent histologic features resembling those of ulcerative colitis, i.e., absent or variably symptomatic abdominal cramping with mucoid or bloody discharge and with stricture. Resolution occurred in the past only with reanastomosis.[150] Studies have shown more recently that infusion of a salt solution containing short-chain fatty acids (SCFA) into the rectal remnant results in healing.[151] The role of colonic bacteria in metabolizing unabsorbed carbohydrate and fiber to acetic n-propionic and n-butyric acids, as well as to their alcohols and various gases, is discussed in Chapters 4 and 39. Diversion colitis is a deficiency state in colon mucosa deprived of SCFA.

RADIATION THERAPY

This subject has been reviewed in Chapter 62C.

CYTOTOXIC CHEMOTHERAPY

Multiple combinations administered cyclically in maximum tolerated dosages are given because of the frequent development of resistance of malignant cells to a single agent and the need to kill all the malignant cells to obtain a "cure." The therapeutic effectiveness of available agents against certain malignant cells has been significant, with high percentages of cures particularly of acute leukemias, certain lymphomas, testicular tumors, Wilms' tumor, osteogenic sarcoma, and rhabdomyosarcoma. On the other hand, the most common cancers have, on the whole, responded poorly to chemotherapy and adjuvant chemotherapy. These malignant conditions include those of the head and neck, lung, stomach, pancreas, liver, cervix, colon-rectum, melanoma, and soft tissue sarcoma.[152] Major efforts continue to develop and test new agents and to vary the combinations of new and approved drugs and their dosages to obtain better responses.[153]

Because these drug activities are not specific to cancer cells, side effects on host cells are common. The severity and manifestation of these side effects are related to the specific agent, dosage, duration of treatment, accompanying drugs, and individual susceptibility. Because the epithelial cells of the alimentary tract have a relatively rapid turnover, many of the drugs affecting cell division have adverse effects in this area, as well as more pronounced effects on cells in the bone marrow. In some instances, major effects occur on renal tubules, as well as on hepatic, cardiac, pulmonary, and nerve cells.

Nausea and vomiting may occur acutely with chemotherapy, or may occur in some patients with previous chemotherapy exposure who are again exposed to treatment-related associations (anticipatory emesis), or may be delayed for 24 hours or more after receiving chemotherapy. Factors influencing emesis include patient sensitivity, emetic potential of a drug and its combinations, dosage and frequency, and route of administration.

A summary is given in Table 73–8 of some of the more commonly used chemotherapeutic agents, their mechanisms of action, and potential side effects that influence nutritional status. Marked nausea and vomiting tend to result from dosages usually given of dactinomycin, dacarbazine, bleomycin, doxorubicin, cisplatin, pentostatin, cyclophosphamide, and hexamethylmelamine. Mucositis and stomatitis may be severe with bleomycin, dactinomycin, fluorouracil, methotrexate, and amsacrine (AMSA). Diarrhea may be marked with dactinomycin, azacytidine, fluorouracil, methotrexate, gallium nitrate, and amsacrine. Combinations of drugs may exacerbate symptoms. Vincristine may cause neurologic damage leading to severe ileus. Abdominal pain occurs with dactinomycin, cyclophosphamide, methotrexate, and vincristine. Hepatotoxicity occurs with busulfan (in high doses, as used in bone marrow transplantation treatments), pentostatin, and asparaginase. Nephrotoxicity is frequent with asparaginase, cisplatin, gallium nitrate pentostatin, methotrexate, and, to a lesser extent, with some others. Cisplatin leads to renal wasting of magnesium with resultant hypokalemia and hypocalcemia if magnesium in adequate supplementary dosages is not given.[154] Some hormonal agents, such as diethylstilbestrol and tamoxifen citrate, may induce some nausea and vomiting. Corticosteroids cause sodium and water retention and nitrogen and calcium loss (Table 73–7). Daunorubicin and doxorubicin are cardiotoxic. Bleomycin and busulfan may induce pulmonary toxicity. The dose-limiting toxicity of many chemotherapeutic agents is leukopenia and thrombocytopenia.[153]

Plasma levels of taurine fell markedly in patients who had received intensive chemotherapy (and in some cases, total-body irradiation) in preparation for bone marrow transplantation.[155] The mechanism of the decline in taurine is caused by, in part, urinary loss. The nutritional significance, if any, of this decrease is unclear.

Other data indicate negative effects of single or combined chemotherapeutic agents on nutritional and metabolic parameters. This effect is illustrated in a report in which protein kinetic studies were performed before and in conjunction with chemotherapy (vinblastine, cisplatin, and bleomycin) in patients with stage III testicular carcinoma. The nitrogen equilibrium present before chemotherapy changed to negative nitrogen balance; protein turnover, synthesis, and catabolism (initially similar to those of normal controls) decreased with the drug therapy by 23%, 34%, and 30%, respectively, despite continuing intravenous nutrition support.[156]

BLOOD-STIMULATING FACTORS

Permanent bone marrow injury caused by high-dose chemotherapy can be overcome in most patients by the use of autologous bone marrow or peripheral stem cell rescue. Even with these procedures, a finite period of absolute neutropenia remains and can contribute to the occurrence of life-threatening bacterial and fungal infections. Granulocyte-macrophage colony stimulating factor (GM-CSF) is being used to shorten the period of neutropenia.[157,158] Recombinant GM-CSF has been reported to cause hypomagnesemia, hypocalcemia, and hypokalemia,[159] as well as hypoalbuminemia.[160]

ANTIEMETICS

Advances have been made over the years in managing chemotherapy-induced nausea and vomiting. Phenothiazines, cannabinoids, and metoclopramide have now been buttressed by the selective serotonin antagonists, the first being ondansetron. Ondansetron, when given with dexamethasone, is currently the most effective antiemetic regimen for minimizing or preventing acute and delayed emesis.[161] Decreased nausea and vomiting improve the quality of life of the patients, allow better adherence to therapeutic programs, and help to achieve better oral intake of food and fluid.

DIETARY INFLUENCES ON TOXICITY AND EFFICACY

Toxicity. Numerous studies have reviewed the effects of different types of diets on toxicity of certain chemotherapeutic compounds. Early studies claimed that the feeding of an "elemental" diet (hydrolyzed protein with a major percentage of its amino acids in free form) reduced 5-fluorouracil toxicity in humans[162] and in rats.[163] On the other hand, rats fed a chemically defined liquid diet and injected intraperitoneally with methotrexate had increased mortality from severe enterocolitis compared to mortality of rats on a chow diet. This increase was a result of delayed clearance of the drug from serum and intestinal tissue.[164] The enhanced toxicity was reversible by feeding the chow diet within 24 hours before drug injection. A protein-depleted diet markedly increased the incidence of hemorrhagic cystitis in rats with Morris hepatoma given cyclophosphamide; protein-repleted rats were free of this complication.[165] The morbidity and mortality resulting from methotrexate administered to rats were reduced by enteral administration of glutamine.[166] A purified diet containing intact protein was

TABLE 73–8. ACTIONS AND POTENTIAL ADVERSE NUTRITIONAL EFFECTS OF CYTOTOXIC CHEMOTHERAPEUTIC AGENTS

ACTIONS	EXAMPLES	POTENTIAL FOR ADVERSE NUTRITIONAL EFFECTS *
I. Inhibition of a stage of DNA synthesis		
A. Single carbon transfer blocking purine synthesis		
1. Inhibits H_2 folate reductase	Methotrexate†	$A^{+}, N^{+}, P, M^{2+}, U, D^{2+}$
2. Blocks thymidylate and inosinic acid synthesis	Methotrexate†	$A^{+}, N^{+}, P, M^{2+}, U, D^{2+}$
B. Inhibits purine synthesis or interconversion	6-Mercaptopurine	$A, N^{2+}, M+, D^{+}$
	Pentostatin	A, N^{3+}
C. Blocks interconversion of pyrimidines (thymidylate synthase inhibition)	5-Fluorouracil	A, N^{+}, M^{2+}, D^{2+}
D. Inhibits pyrimidine metabolism	Streptozocin	A, N^{3+}, U, CT
E. DNA polymerase inhibition; also inhibits DNA strand growth	Cytarabine†	$A+, N^{2+}, M^{+}$
F. Incorporates into RNA and inhibits protein synthesis	Azacitidine	A^{2+}, N^{2+}, D^{3+}
	Fluorouracil	A, N^{2}, M^{+}, D^{+}
G. Inhibits ribonucleotide reductase	Hydroxyurea†	A, N^{+}, M^{+}
II. Inhibition of DNA replication and transcription		
A. Alkylating agents react with susceptible DNA sites	Hexamethylmelamine	A, N^{3+}
	Chlorambucil	A, N^{+}
	Cyclophosphamide	A, N^{3+}
	Dacarbazine	A, N^{3+}, D
	Cisplatin	A, N^{3+}, Mg
	Carmustine (BCNU)	A, N^{3+}
B. Inhibiting DNA synthesis and DNA-dependent RNA synthesis by intercalating between DNA base pairs		
1. Antibiotic anthracycline glycosides	Doxorubicin	A, N^{+}, M^{+}
	Idarubicin	$A, N^{+}, M+$
2. Streptomyces antibiotic	Dactinomycin	A, N^{3+}, M, D
C. Causes scission of single- and double-stranded DNA, free radical formation, and inhibition of DNA ligase	Bleomycin‡	M^{3+}, D, N^{+}
D. Degrades DNA by forming hydroxy radicals and inhibits DNA, RNA, and protein synthesis	Procarbazine	A, N^{2+}
E. Causes DNA strand breakage	Etoposide‡	N^{+}, M, D
	Amsacrine#‡	A^{2+}, M^{2+}, CT
III. Enzyme inhibiting protein synthesis and delaying DNA and RNA synthesis		
A. Hydrolysis of asparagine to aspartic acid in cells lacking asparagine synthase	Asparaginase§	A^{2+}, N^{2+}
IV. Inhibition of mitosis		
A. Binds tubulin preventing microtubule assembly	Vinblastine	C,M,N,D
	Vincristine‖	C^{3+}, P
B. Interferes with microtubule network	Taxol	A,M,N,D,O
C. Causes G2 phase arrest	Etoposide‡	N^{+}, M, D
D. Causes metaphase arrest	Teniposide‡	N^{+}, M, D

* A = anorexia; C = constipation/ileus; CT = cardiac toxicity; D = diarrhea; M = mucositis/stomatitis; Mg = renal magnesium loss; N = nausea/vomiting; O = odynophagia; P = abdominal pain; U = intestinal ulceration. Letter without + = occurs uncommonly; letter with + = low potential; letter with 2+ = moderate potential; letter with 3+ = high potential.

† = S phase specific.

‡ = causes G2 phase arrest or delay.

‖ = M phase specific.

§ = G1 phase specific.

as effective as a chow diet in permitting rats to survive a toxic dose of methotrexate; both of these diets were much more effective than a highly purified diet with amino acids rather than protein. The amino acid diet resulted in some survival when supplemented with glutamine, but not when supplemented with glycine. The purified protein diet, like the chow diet, allowed better mucosal histology and decreased the cecal gram-negative anaerobes.[167] This decrease in anaerobes suggests that when amino acids replace protein or when a protein-deficient diet is given, resistance to enterocolitis of bacterial origin is decreased.

Efficacy. Tumor-bearing rats on a glutamine-containing elemental type of diet treated with methotrexate had smaller tumors than did controls that received glycine. The rats that received glutamine also experienced reduced bacteremia and improved survival.[168] Enhanced tumor responsiveness occurred following methotrexate administration when protein-depleted rats were repleted with protein.[169] When methotrexate was administered to rats with transplanted mammary tumors 2 hours after initiating various nutritional regimens, significant reduction in tumor volume occurred in those animals given TPN or parenteral amino acids or chow as compared to the tumor volume in those on a protein-depleted diet.[170–172] Adjuvant short-term TPN enhanced tumor responsiveness to the cell cycle–specific chemotherapeutic agents methotrexate or doxorubicin, but not to the cell cycle–nonspecific agent Cytoxan (cyclophosphamide).[171] As noted later, this effect may be related to stimulation of the S phase of the cell by more adequate diets following a protein-deficient diet.

DIFFERENTIATION THERAPY

This relatively new strategy uses chemical compounds to induce differentiation of human cancer cells rather than destroying them. This therapy has achieved striking success with the retinoids all-*trans*-retinoic acid (tretinoin) and 13-*cis*-retinoic acid (isotretinoin). Isotretinoin has caused regression of premalignant leukoplakia of the buccal mucosa and has prevented secondary primary tumors in patients with squamous cell carcinoma of the head and neck. In a series of reports, tretinoin has caused an aggregate rate of complete remission of approximately 80% in acute promyelocytic leukemia; however, because of relapses despite continued therapy, the follow-up use of cytotoxic chemotherapy is being studied.[173,174] The genetic mechanism of this retinoid response[173] has been reviewed also in Chapter 16. Highly objective response rates have been observed in patients with squamous cell carcinoma of the skin and cervix treated with isotretinoin and α-interferon.[174]

Side effects of tretinoin observed in patients with acute promyelocytic leukemia have been termed the "retinoic acid syndrome." This syndrome consists of fever, respiratory distress, edema, pleural or pericardial effusions, and episodic hypotension.[175] Early treatment with high-dose dexamethasone resulted in prompt improvement and recovery.

Calcitriol (1,25-dihydroxycholecalciferol) promotes tissue differentiation, inhibits cellular proliferation in cell culture, affects cellular oncogene transcription and growth factor receptor expression in vivo, and inhibits proliferation of several breast cancer cell lines.[176] Because calcitriol tends to cause hypercalcemia, analogues are being developed that retain its cell differentiation effect but reduce the effect on calcium metabolism. One such analogue, calcipotriol, when applied topically to cutaneous metastatic breast cancer caused some reduction in size of such deposits in some of the patients.[176]

ADOPTIVE IMMUNOTHERAPY

This term has been given to various biologic strategies designed to destroy cancer cells by utilizing cells and cell products of the natural defense mechanisms of the immune system.[177] They are mentioned here because they may either influence nutritional state or be influenced by some dietary modification.

MONOCLONAL ANTIBODIES

Tumor cells often bear surface molecules that are immunogenic in the natural host or in other animal species. By immunizing animals with tumor cell preparations, antisera can be prepared that recognize the various antigens found on the surface of the tumor cell. Each clone of cells produces a single type of antibody, called a "monoclonal antibody," that has a single type of antigen binding site. These cells can be grown in large numbers with manufacture of the monoclonal antibody in a highly purified state and in essentially unlimited amounts. In addition to their use in radiolocalization of tumors, monoclonal antibodies can be used as antitumor cancer therapy as carriers of cytotoxic substances in vivo; to purge bone marrow in vitro of either T-lymphocytes to prevent graft-versus-host disease; or to purge tumor cells before autologous transplantation in conjunction with high-dose system chemotherapy. These potential applications and existing problems have been discussed.[178]

IMMUNOTHERAPY USING INTERLEUKIN-2 ALONE OR WITH CELLS

Approximately 12 years ago it was noted that lymphocytes exposed to interleukin-2 (IL-2) developed the ability to kill fresh tumor cells but not normal cells. The availability of large amounts of purified recombinant IL-2 made possible phase I and II studies in patients with advanced cancer combining lymphokine-activated killer (LAK) cells plus IL-2 or IL-2 alone. Numerous studies have been reported on the toxicity and clinical evaluation of IL-2.[177,179]

One nutritionally interesting side effect of both interferon and IL-2 is their ability to induce the enzymes indoleamine 2,3 dioxygenase, thereby resulting in tryptophan degradation to kynurenine as the result of opening of the indole ring. Decrements in plasma tryptophan were dose related to IL-2. At high doses of IL-2, the decline in this essential amino acid was so marked that the IL-2 had to be discontinued.[183]

GENE THERAPY

The objectives of this approach are either to deliver concentration of cytotoxic agents, such as TNF, directly to the tumor site or to modify the genetic characteristics of tumor cells (e.g., by inserting cytokine-producing genes) to increase their immunogenicity, thereby leading to the production by the host of cytolytic cells that are not produced in response to the parental unmodified tumor. The genetic immunologic and historical backgrounds have been recently summarized,[184] as have the current efforts by Rosenberg and colleagues in this therapeutic approach.[177,185]

NUTRITION INTERVENTION AND TUMOR GROWTH

RAT STUDIES

Many reports have compared the effects of intravenous feeding to various oral diets on host and tumor weights and other parameters following transplantation of various tumors. In general, complete TPN formulas resulted in tumor and carcass weights that were about the same as or somewhat greater than those resulting from ad libitum chow or semisynthetic diets. The tumor and carcass weights were appreciably greater in those with intravenous feeding than in animals that were starved or given only some carbohydrate or amino acids. Reports have been contradictory, however, on the key issue relating the type of nutrition support to the growth of tumor in proportion to host carcass weight. Some have found that the weight ratio of tumor to host carcass did not change with TPN, i.e., growth was proportionate, whereas others have found that tumor growth exceeded that of increased carcass weight on lean body mass.[32,186]

A TPN formula including amino acids, dextrose, and LCT resulted in larger primary tumor volume and weight and in the presence of many more tumor metastases than were observed with the formula devoid of lipid but with proportionate increases in glucose.[186] This finding implies, at least for the rat strain utilized, a tumor growth stimulus with LCT either directly or perhaps through a prostaglandin or membrane effect. When LCT alone was compared to a 75% MCT/25% LCT mixture, the mixed lipid was found to inhibit the number of lung metastases.[187]

As has been mentioned previously, tumor responsiveness to cell cycle–specific chemotherapy improved in rats that were nutritionally repleted either orally or intravenously.[171] Tumor cytokinetic analysis by flow cytometry revealed that the percentage of tumors in the S phase was significantly increased in previously protein-deficient rats after only 2 hours of infusion of a complete TPN solution as compared to the percentage of such tumors after use of a saline infusion containing minerals and micronutrients.[188]

HUMAN STUDIES

How do such rat data compare with human tumor responses to provision of nutrition? One approach to this question has been to measure the rates of protein synthesis or the enzyme and cytokinetic responses in patients with gastrointestinal malignant disease to TPN administered just before surgery in comparison to those in nonTPN controls. In one study, presurgical nutrition with TPN was more adequate than the presurgical oral diets of the voluntary control group. The fractional protein synthesis (FPS) rates (measured by ^{15}N-glycine) were essentially the same in the tumors from both groups and no difference appeared among the FPS rates in the tissues from which the tumors arose.[189] When human tumors and normal muscle and liver in cachectic patients were sampled after ^{14}C-leucine infusion at the onset of and again during surgery, TPN promoted whole-body protein synthesis and FPS rates in muscle, but no significant change occurred in the FPS rate in the tumors. In other patients, infusion of lipid emulsion only did not significantly change muscle or tumor FRS rates.[76] On the other hand, in patients with localized colorectal cancer who were randomly chosen either to receive TPN or to fast for 24 hours before surgery, tumor FPS was 89% higher in the TPN group than in the fasted group.[190]

Malnourished patients with various untreated malignant tumors of the head and neck participated in a series of studies performed on biopsy specimens of their tumors taken while fasting and after 5 to 7 days of continuous TPN.[191] Unlike the rat study previously noted,[188] tumor cytokinetics in these patients were not changed with TPN, nor did any upregulation occur in the activity of ornithine decarboxylase (increases of which precede induction of DNA synthesis) nor any change in the growth fraction of tumor cells as measured by a proliferation-associated nuclear antigen. With these varied tumors tested under different circumstances in varying numbers of patients the evidence remains equivocal as to whether TPN stimulates human tumor cell replication.

EVALUATION OF THE EFFICACY OF NUTRITION SUPPORT

Two major and apparently contradictory themes present themselves in this review of the relation of cancer and nutrition. One theme documents the numerous mechanisms by which the systemic and localized effect of malignant disorders and their various treatments can impact negatively on the nutritional status of affected patients (see Tables 73–2 and 73–7). The other theme relates to accumulating evidence that, with progressive weight loss and debility (cachexia) in cancer patients, a series of alterations from normal occur in energy expenditure and carbohydrate, fat, and protein metabolism. These alterations appear to be associated with tumor-mediated metabolically potent interleukins. The themes converge in the general proposition that, for most patients with aggressive tumors and weight loss, current nutritional efforts at reversal become increasingly futile unless the underlying malignant condition can be eradicated or significantly palliated by antitumor treatment methods. Before some related issues can be explored, a brief review of patient outcome data with nutritional support is indicated.

Much of these data are derived from studies utilizing TPN because TPN has been a primary method of assuring continued administration of nutrients in surgical and other seriously ill patients undergoing antitumor treatments. Early retrospective and uncontrolled reports suggested that undernourished cancer patients were more responsive to radiation therapy and/or chemotherapy and had fewer side effects from treatment when nutrition support was provided.[192,193] These reports were followed by additional studies that were better controlled and were conducted with randomization of patients and treatments. A series of detailed tabular summaries and several meta-analyses published between 1986 and 1991 are reviewed here briefly.[194–200] Their data are derived from individual studies that varied in the numbers, ages, and sexes of patients entered, as well as in the types and stages of malignant disease, the nature and duration of treatment methods, and the duration and frequency of nutritional support.

A meta-analysis of 28 preoperative randomized studies of cancer patients on TPN concluded that (1) when used preoperatively in patients with gastrointestinal cancer, TPN helped to reduce major surgical complications ($p = .01$) and operative mortality ($p = .02$) and (2) no statistically significant benefit was derived from TPN on survival, treatment tolerance, toxicity, or tumor response in patients given chemotherapy and TPN ($p < .00001$).[194]

Subsequent summaries repeated and added some new data. A 1986 survey analyzing results separately for patients receiving radiation therapy and chemotherapy and for patients undergoing major surgery concluded that "the routine use of preoperative IVF (intravenous feeding) should be confined to patients unable to sustain lean body mass by enteral or oral feeding."[195] The authors state that " . . IVF has not been documented . . . to affect favorably either responses to therapy or survival in patients receiving radiation therapy or chemotherapy." Selecting patients for TPN remains a matter of clinical judgment; however, the authors state that "when therapy response rates and nutritional morbidity are high, IVF should be instituted until the host can recover from the effects of antitumor therapy. . . . The utilization of prolonged periods of parenteral nutrition, particularly in the outpatient setting, cannot be *routinely* (authors' emphasis) justified in the anticipation of restoring patients to a 'treatable' status." Thus, ". . . prolonged and/or home parenteral nutrition is indicated in those patients for whom enteral nutrition is not feasible *and* in whom antitumor therapy has clearly been successful." The authors conclude that ". . . there is clear evidence that in *individual* patients with cancer, IVF can prevent death from starvation and decrease the morbidity of treatment" but "only those patients undergoing surgery for gastrointestinal neoplasia have benefited significantly from the addition of adjuvant IVF."[195]

Another meta-analysis was based on a pool of 12 randomized studies of cancer patients receiving chemotherapy and given TPN. The American College of Physicians report concluded in part, "that for tumor response rates the best estimate was that nutritionally supported patients were only 68% as likely to achieve complete partial responses ($p = 0.12$) . . . We are 95% confident that total parenteral nutrition does not result in any improvement in overall survival . . . that total parenteral nutrition does not result in a 30% or greater improvement in short term survival or that total parenteral nutrition does not result in a 10% or greater improvement in response to chemotherapy."[196,197] The report deemed the effect of TPN on chemotherapy toxicity as small and reported TPN to be associated with four times the increased risk of significant infection ($p = 0.0001$). A systematic search to reveal any conditions for which TPN could be shown to be beneficial resulted in the conclusions that "no such condition could be found although there was a trend of borderline significance toward such support being less detrimental in patients who were malnourished."[196] With respect to infection rates, a meta-analysis of the same data by another group revealed that the infection rate for TPN patients who received no intravenous lipid was not different from that of controls, whereas those receiving lipid 1 to 3 times per week had an odds ratio of infection rates with controls of 2.3 ($p < .02$) and those given lipid daily had an odds ratio of infection rates with controls of 6.3 ($p < .01$).[198] This type of study needs confirmation.

A 1989 review used the same treatment division as that used in the 1986 review,[195] but with updated information.[199] The authors concluded that chronically malnourished patients given nutrition support often have restoration of a sense of well-being and become more physically functional; however, "whether this support results in long-term clinical benefits is difficult to evaluate."[199] Despite their reservation concerning many deficiencies in the reviewed studies, the authors stated that "it appears that routine application of nutritional support to all patients undergoing treatment for malignancy is not justified" and "that the primary indication for nutritional support is for the malnourished patients undergoing a major operation for upper GI malignancy and for the chemotherapy patient with severe gastrointestinal dysfunction. These issues will not be resolved without a large-scale clinical trial."[199]

Analysis of 18 trials in which adults were given only chemotherapy and of 5 trials in which children were treated with chemotherapy in all and with additional radiation in some was undertaken by Lipman.[200] The author concluded that, although weight gain or decreased weight loss can often be achieved with nutritional support, "early weight gain with nutritional support usually results from accumulation of water and fat" and that "this is of questionable benefit."[200] "Consistent improvement in other nutritional parameters has not been found in the trials here. . . This reviewer would argue that changes in nutritional parameters without concomitant improvement in clinical outcome are of no clinical utility. . . . Based upon prospective, randomized, controlled clinical trials *with the exception of bone marrow transplantation* (author's emphasis), there appears to be little support for the routine aggressive nutritional support in the nonsurgical oncology patient."[200] Nevertheless, the author recognized circumstances in which aggressive nutrition by any route can be provided. These circumstances include prolonged inability to eat, especially when malnutrition is secondary to poor intake, a nutrition support team to decrease complications, and the presence of a tumor deemed likely to respond to treatment.

Numerous pertinent issues were not discussed in these reviews. One issue involves the adequacy of the TPN solutions given during the trials. Because more than one half of the individual trial publication dates were 1981 or earlier, one can conclude that most of the subjects in the studies were given TPN in the late 1970s and in 1980. Analyses of trial outcomes with TPN support must take this possibility into account. Careful attention to the micronutrient and other nutrient composition of the TPN formulations of the 1970s resulted in adequate nutrition over long periods for patients with a short bowel syndrome who did not have cancer. Cancer patients with serious weight loss and widespread disease, however, might have benefited from an altered formulation.

The Food and Drug Administration (FDA) did not approve the use of Intralipid in the United States until 1977, although it was used experimentally in some hospitals in the United States earlier. Its utilization in many hospitals was delayed because of its novelty, its high cost, and some initial concern about its safety. Accordingly, if the report of Desai et al. is corroborated,[198] one must include an analysis of infection rates before and during the rise of intravenous lipid use and its frequency before attributing infections to TPN and catheters generally.

Another factor that changed in the early 1980s was the introduction of a new and more complete parenteral multivitamin solution for TPN. This new solution had been approved by the FDA in July 1979 and became generally available in 1981.[201] Until that time, the multivitamin solution primarily used in TPN was MVI or MVI concentrate, which were deficient in folate, B_{12}, biotin, and vitamin K and provided high levels of vitamins A and D. The AMA-FDA complete pediatric multivitamin formula was not approved by the FDA until 1984. Unless the physician directing the clinical trial, or the TPN pharmacist preparing the solutions, was aware of the inadequacies of MVI and took steps to modify that formula by adding the individual missing vitamins, the TPN solution administered before 1981 was inadequate in its vitamin content.

The same point would hold true for trace elements. Sterile solutions of zinc, copper, chromium, and manganese were not commercially available until approximately 1980. The presence of selenium in TPN did not become recognized as a potential clinical problem until 1981 to 1983, when case reports of cardiomyopathy appeared in medical journals in the United States. Selenite solutions did not become commercially available until approximately 1983. How many of the solutions used in 1977 to 1980 were adequate in their trace elements?

Are other substances essential for the patient with advanced cancer? The question of taurine has been noted.[155] Choline has been noted recently to maintain more normal liver function tests when present.[202] Of perhaps greater significance are two recent reports on the benefits of glutamine supplementation in TPN solutions in randomized double-blind controlled clinical trials in cancer patients. Adult patients who had undergone resection of the colon or rectum and who were given a TPN solution with an alanyl-glutamine peptide had less negative nitrogen balances than did controls on TPN solutions containing equivalent nitrogen in the form of extra alanine and glycine. The patients who received glutamine supplementation maintained intramuscular glutamine concentration near to the preoperative level, whereas the controls had a decline of about 40%.[203] Parenteral nutrition either with or without glutamine was given to adults the day after allogeneic bone marrow transplantation for hematologic malignant disease following high-dose radiation plus chemotherapy or chemotherapy alone. Those receiving glutamine-supplemented TPN had improved nitrogen balance, less clinical infection, lower rates of microbial colonization, and shortened hospital stays compared to those of patients receiving standard TPN.[204] Whether any of these additives has a consistently positive effect on muscle protein kinetics and improved nutritional status in the hypermetabolic cancer patient remains to be seen.

In addition, none of these reviews remarked on the fact that, in long-term antitumor treatment trials (i.e., when, after initial workup and treatment, patients were hospitalized only for chemotherapy or for terminal management), TPN was often given only for relatively short periods. One such trial involving patients with advanced colorectal cancer received much attention because one of its conclusions stated that "overall median survival was significantly decreased in TPN patients (79 vs. 305 days, $p = 0.03$)."[205] Analysis of the protocol reveals that patients who entered the trial were randomly chosen to receive either an ad libitum diet or TPN. TPN was given for 14 days prior to chemotherapy (5-fluorouracil plus methyl CCNU) and continued during *the first course only*, which lasted an average of 12 days. TPN was then stopped, although this group continued to receive chemotherapy every 4 weeks while eating ad libitum. The study included 20 TPN patients and 25 controls. The data indicate the following: female patients (9 TPN vs. 17 controls) had a slightly higher but not significantly different survival; only those patients with prior weight loss of 0 to 6% had significantly decreased survival, and of these, 7 of 8 in the TPN group had liver metastases compared to 5 of 10 in the control group; and those patients, male and female, who had a pretrial weight loss of 6% or greater had no diminution in survival with TPN. This trial was actually a test to determine the possible adjuvant effect of a relatively short-term initial period of TPN. The results on survival as stated were complex and involved sex and tumor extension differences.

Some of the surveys on effectiveness vs. noneffectiveness of nutrition support have made survival an important criterion. Several points on this score are worth considering. First, most of the surveys did not include survival data, thus leaving only a relatively small number in this category. Second, if such malignancies as metastatic colon, lung, stomach, and esophageal cancers do not respond well to any known antitumor treatments, why should a nutrition support method be expected to assist such patients beyond perhaps slowing death and perhaps improving the quality of life in some patients in whom starvation existed in varying degree? Finally, the reader interested in this subject of efficacy of nutrition support is advised to review the meta-analyses and also to read the original trial reports and other reviews that provide evidence of the value in many cases of improved nutrition for appropriate patients.[206,207] Much more must be learned about the metabolism of cancer patients with progressive disease. Such knowledge will, hopefully, provide the basis for improvements in nutritional support when more effective antitumor therapies are discovered.[208]

GUIDELINES FOR NUTRITION SUPPORT

Recognizing the metabolic problems, complications, and uncertainties that have been briefly mentioned, the physician frequently must reach a decision concerning initiation of some form of nutritional support for the cancer patient. The multiple reasons for undernutrition in such patients have been reviewed in some detail. Subjective and objective responses to nutrition support can and do occur with improved feeling of well-being, strength, and activity. Individual responses to such support vary; unfortunately, no simple objective tests enable the physician to predict who will and who will not improve. Hence, nutrition support is worth considering as part of the overall patient care program as indicated in the following guidelines.

1. Early evaluation is indicated for patients who have developed or who are at risk of developing significant and persistent nutritional deficits as a consequence of prior surgery and/or radiation that induces primarily alimentary tract dysfunction but also dysfunction of liver or kidney. These procedures should be followed where indicated by appropriate nutritional intervention and periodic evaluation to assure adequate therapy.
2. For the patient with mild to moderate anorexia and taste changes who may require a prolonged period of treatment, careful evaluation of food likes and dislikes and provision of attractive solid and liquid foods and supplements, properly timed, may make the difference between weight maintenance and loss.
3. Another criterion for instituting nutrition support is progressive weight loss or the high risk of significant weight loss in the patient deemed to have a good probability of responding to therapy. The specific period of active support depends on the nature and duration of the antitumor therapy or therapies and on patient responsiveness.
4. Factors affecting the decision for enteral vs. parenteral routes are reviewed in Chapters 79 and 80. In general, the seriously ill leukopenic and thrombocytopenic patient with seriously impaired gastrointestinal function is a candidate for parenteral nutrition through a central vein. If the gastrointestinal route can be safely used without significant distress to the patient, however, oral and tube feeding should be tried.
5. Enteral and parenteral nutrition formulations for the cancer patient are basically the same as those for the mildly to moderately ill patient without cancer. Due consideration must be given, however, to special problems related to organ failure and the effects of the various antitumor or other therapies being used. The decision as to which method to use depends on functional capabilities of the alimentary tract in a given situation. In general, if the gut works, use it.
6. For the patient requiring major surgery who has lost little (< 5%) or no weight, routine fluid and electrolyte support in the postoperative period is indicated unless serious complications that postpone enteral intake for at least 7 to 10 postoperative days occur. In such an instance, either peripheral or central TPN is indicated unless gastrostomy or jejunostomy tube feedings are appropriate and feasible.
7. For the patient requiring major surgery who has become progressively and seriously underweight (15 to 20% body weight loss) and who cannot be fed enterally by gastrostomy or jejunostomy tube, perioperative peripheral or central nutrition support is indicated because of the likelihood of increased risk secondary to malnutrition.
8. For the seriously anorectic patient who is no longer a candidate for further antitumor therapy, who has a functioning alimentary tract, and whose quality of life is reasonably acceptable and likely to be maintained or improved by enteral supplementary feeding at home, this method should be utilized if desired by the patient.

9. The patient with active cancer who has persistent intestinal obstruction or other severe intestinal dysfunction and who has failed all therapy and cannot be sustained on enteral feeding will experience a rapid downhill course as an inpatient or outpatient without intravenous feeding. This situation presents difficult emotional problems, especially for the family when the patient is to be discharged home without TPN, particularly if prior use of parenteral nutrition had improved strength and weight. The physician frequently is pressured to continue this method at home despite the clear statement that TPN has no antitumor benefit and may have its own potential complications, particularly in a patient with obstruction. The attending physician, preferably with the assistance of other health professionals, must present to the patient and/or family the options and drawbacks of home parenteral nutrition (including financial costs); the mentally competent patient or the family of the incompetent patient then must make the decision. Personal experience and more recent data[209,210] indicate poor survival (i.e., mean survival of 3 months or less) for most of these patients.
10. Experience has also indicated that the cancer patient with a severely dysfunctional alimentary tract (as the result of radiation, surgery, chemotherapy, or their combinations) but who is free of residual malignant disease has an entirely different outlook from that of the cancer patient just mentioned. Proper management of such patients by oral, enteral, and/or parenteral feedings can lead to prolonged life of good quality. (See Chaps. 62A and 62C, 79, and 80.)

UNPROVEN DIET AND NUTRITION CLAIMS

Historically, diseases with major morbidity and mortality associated with a relatively poor response rate to conventional medical practice of the time have attracted various therapeutic "innovations" with little or no evidence of proof of efficacy. Cancer is no exception. The reasons are not hard to find. (1) Cancer is second on the list of diseases in terms of mortality, and its major types at the disseminated stage have relatively low "cure" rates by conventional medical practice. (2) Expensive conventional therapies for cancer often have serious, if often transient, side effects with no certainty of "cure." (3) Such therapies are often provided impersonally in a multidisciplinary setting. This chapter began with evidence of controversy on the question of whether the incidence of cancer is becoming more frequent despite great effort at its control.[3,4] Many patients and family members are aware of statements in recognized medical publications such as that which concluded that "35 years of intense effort focused largely on improving treatment must be judged a qualified failure."[211]

Exact numbers of cancer patients in the United States and elsewhere who are under treatments that are not accepted by the medical profession are unknown. Although probably a relatively small percentage of all cancer patients, they are a "visible minority."[212] The terms for these types of treatment range from "fraud," "quackery," "unproven," or "disproved" (e.g., Laetrile) by those mainly in scientific medicine, to "unconventional" or "unorthodox" by those in the middle ground, to "alternative" by those favorable to unproven methods. The demand for such treatment exists, and the financial cost to the patients and families and, in some instances, the public is quite large.[212,213]

The nature of some of these unproven treatments, their claims for efficacy, and attempts to rationally evaluate some of them have been reviewed periodically. One of the most recent and detailed analyses is that from the Office of Technology of the United States Congress,[212] but many others have appeared about treatments in the United States[214–216] and in Europe.[217] Many of these unconventional treatment programs have special dietary and nutritional components in addition to using herbal and gland extracts, purgatives, Laetrile administration, and spiritual guidance in various combinations to form one or another "system" of management. Some of these appear innocuous, whereas others raise a concern for safety. Vigorous use of coffee enemas has been associated with deaths[218]; high doses of Laetrile by mouth provided potentially toxic doses of cyanide[212]; and persistent use of diets deficient or excessive in one or more essential nutrients may create problems if taken chronically as the primary food source.[212,214–219]

Physicians, dietitians, and nurses who care for cancer patients must be aware of the extent of this problem, know the details of some of the more common components of unproven systems of care, and be willing to discuss frankly this area with patients who ask questions about such methods. The need for an informed and understanding approach to patients on this issue is underscored by data collected on cancer patients by Cassileth et al.[219] Interviews were conducted of 304 cancer center inpatients and of 356 cancer patients (primarily outpatients) under the care of "unorthodox" practitioners; 31% of the total were treated with conventional (i.e., medically accepted) therapy only; 49% were treated with both conventional and unorthodox therapy; and 8% were treated with unorthodox therapy only.

In addition to the 171 patients treated with both types of therapies who received chemotherapy and/or radiation and/or surgery, 10% of the remaining patients had refused recommended chemotherapy, 9% had refused recommended radiation therapy, and 2% had refused recommended surgery. Of the patients treated with unorthodox therapy only, 28% had refused recommended chemotherapy, 26% had refused recommended radiation therapy, and 28% had refused recommended surgery. Of the total of 325 patients treated with the two types of therapies, 64% had sought conventional treatment first and then added alternative treatment an average of 24 months later; although 60% continued both systems of treatment, 40% had discontinued conventional care entirely after an average of 8 months.

This study revealed that physicians constituted 60% of unorthodox practitioners; they played an active role in prescribing unorthodox treatments for the 378 patients receiving such therapies, particularly "metabolic," megavitamin, and "immune" treatments. Of patients treated with dual systems, 75% had informed their regular physicians of their adoption of alternative care. Of these physicians, 39% reacted with disapproval to this information, whereas 30% were supportive and 12% were neutral. Disapproval resulted in 4% of patients being denied further treatment by their physicians. No data were provided on the nature of the unorthodox treatments that led to rejection, disapproval, or approval by physicians.

One of the arguments advanced by proponents of unproven therapies has been superior patient support offered by the therapists, thereby leading to improved quality of life. This characteristic has been widely claimed, although the proponents' position is weak because of the lack of scientific documentation supportive of their claim that their remedies are effective against cancer. Both aspects have been examined in a prospective randomized study of patients with advanced malignant disease and an expected median survival time of not more than 1 year. One group received care at an academic cancer center and the other at a cancer clinic that provided its "autogenous immune enhancing vaccine" plus the conventional care of the academic center.[213] Survival times were the same in these two settings. Of considerable interest was the finding that the quality of life scores were consistently better among those treated at the academic center beginning from the time of enrollment.

A continuing and urgent need exists for adequately informed health professionals to advise the public, the media, and legislatures about the personal and societal costs of health frauds. The failures of the health professions, the media, and legislators are made clear in a review of the debacle with Laetrile.[220] At least 21 legislatures passed and almost all the governors involved approved legislation decriminalizing this fraudulent agent; the legislation may still be law in most of these states. Such legislation fundamentally attacked the integrity of the Food, Drug, and Cosmetic Act and the powers of the Food and Drug Administration by giving state appointees power to approve a federally unapproved substance, thus opening the door to legalized charlatanism. It misled the public by giving the false impression that Laetrile was safe. It derogated the role of physicians as patient advocates by misstating health facts to the public and introducing the potential for mistrust between physician and patient by unwarranted state actions.

The failure of the health professions to exert significant educational influence on Congress is underscored again by a recent Congressional directive to the National Institutes of Health to create a new Office on Unconventional Medical Practices to evaluate a broad range of unorthodox therapies, with cancer as the initial focus.[221] In Germany, approximately 7 of 10 general practitioners practice "alternative" medicine, which is reimbursible by insurance. The German government has established a research program on alternative medicine for cancer in response to "public demand" and a movement is underway to integrate alternative with conventional medicine in medical schools.[222]

REFERENCES

1. Lopez, A.D.: Ann. N.Y. Acad. Sci., *609:*58–74, 1990.
2. Doll, R.: Am. J. Epidemiol., *134:*675–688, 1991.
3. Davis, D.L., Hoel, D., Fox, J., et al.: Lancet, *336:*474–481, 1990.
4. Marshall, E.: News and Comment. Science, *250:*900–902, 1990.
5. Editorial: The cancer epidemic: fact or misinterpretation. Lancet, *340:*399–400, 1992.
6. Warren, S.: Am. J. Med. Sci., *184:*610–615, 1932.
7. DeWys, W.D., Begg, D., Lavin, P.T., et al.: Am. J. Med., *69:*491–497, 1980.
8. Serrie, R., Rosen, P.P., Rhodes, P., et al.: Ann. Intern. Med., *116:*26–32, 1992.
9. Kern, K.A., Norton, J.A.: JPEN J. Parenter. Enteral Nutr., *12:*286–298, 1988.
10. Ollenschläger, G., Viell, B., Thomas, W., et al.: Recent Results Cancer Res., *121:*249–259, 1991.
11. Shils, M.E.: Cancer, *43:*2093–2102, 1979.
12. Costa, G.: Cancer Res., *37:*2327–2335, 1977.
13. Heymsfield, S.B., McManus, C., Smith, J., et al.: Am. J. Clin. Nutr., *36:*680–690, 1982.
14. Morton, K.I., Sox, H.C., Krupp, J.R.: Ann. Intern. Med., *95:*568–574, 1981.
15. Mordes, J.P., Rossini, A.A.: Science, *213:*565–567, 1981.
16. Norton, J.A., Moley, J.F., Green, M.V., et al.: Cancer Res., *45:*5547–5552, 1985.
17. Baille, P., Millar, F.K., Pratt, A.W.: Am. J. Physiol., *209:*293–300, 1965.
18. Van Lammeren, F.M., Chance, W.T., Fischer, J.E.: Peptides, *5:*97–101, 1984.
19. Chance, W.T., von Myenfeldt, M., Fischer, J.E.: Pharmacol. Biochem. Behav., *18:*115–121, 1983.
20. Peacock, J.L., Norton, J.A.: JPEN J. Parenter. Enteral Nutr., *12:*260–264, 1988.
21. Chance, W.T., Muggia-Sullam, M., Chen, M-H., et al.: J. Natl. Cancer Inst., *77:*497–503, 1986.
22. Bartlett, D.L., Charland, S.L., Torosian, M.H.: Surg. Forum, *42:*14–16, 1991.

23. Ng, E.H., Rock, C.S., Hawes, A.S., et al.: Surg. Forum, *42:*444–446, 1991.
24. Chance, W.T., Cao, L., Fischer, J.E.: JPEN J. Parenter. Enteral Nutr., *14:*122–128, 1990.
25. Fischer, J.F., Chance, W.T.: JPEN J. Parenter. Enteral Nutr., *14 (4-S):*86S–89S, 1990.
26. Chance, W.T., Lequn, C., Zhang, F., et al.: Am. J. Surg., *161:*51–56, 1991.
27. Editorial: Muscling in on clenbuterol. Lancet, *340:*403, 1992.
28. Gelin, G., Andersson, C., Lundholm, K.: Cancer Res., *51:*880–885, 1991.
29. Aisner, J., Paines, H., Tait, N., et al.: Semin. Oncol., *17:*2–7, 1990.
30. Loprinzi, C.L., Ellison, N.M., Goldberg, R.M., et al.: Semin. Oncol., *17:*8–12, 1990.
31. Mider, G.B.: Annu. Rev. Med., *4:*187–198, 1953.
32. Popp, M.B., Wagner, S.C., Brito, O.J.: Surgery, *94:*300–308, 1983.
33. Lundholm, K., Edström, S., Karlberg, I., et al.: Cancer Res., *40:*2516–2522, 1980.
34. Bozzetti, F., Pagnoni, A., DelVecchio, M.: Surg. Gynecol. Obstet., *150:*229–234, 1980.
35. Russell, D. McR., Shike, M., Marliss, E.B., et al.: Cancer Res., *44:*1706–1711, 1984.
36. Knox, C.S., Crosby, L.O., Feuer, I.B., et al.: Ann. Surg., *197:*152–162, 1983.
37. Dempsey, D.T., Feuer, I.D., Knox, L.S., et al.: Cancer, *53:*1265–1273, 1984.
38. Merrick, H.W., Long, C.L., Grecos, G.P., et al.: JPEN J. Parenter. Enteral Nutr., *12:*8–14, 1988.
39. Warmold, I., Lundholm, K., Schersten, T.: Cancer Res., *38:*1801–1807, 1978.
40. Macfie, J., Burkenshaw, L., Oxby, C., et al.: Br. J. Surg., *69:*443–446, 1982.
41. Edström, S., Bennegåard, K., Eden, E., et al.: Arch. Otolaryngol., *108:*697–699, 1982.
42. Arbeit, J.M., Lees, D.E., Corsey, R., et al.: Ann. Surg., *199:*292–298, 1984.
43. Lindmark, L., Bennegård, K., Eden, E., et al.: Gastroenterology, *87:*402–408, 1984.
44. Hansell, D.T., Davies, J.W.L., Born, H.J.G.: Ann. Surg., *203:*240–245, 1986.
45. Nixon, D.W., Kutner, M., Heymsfield, S., et al.: Metabolism, *37:*1059–1064, 1988.
46. Fearon, K.C.H., Hansell, D.T., Preston, T., et al.: Cancer Res., *48:*2590–2595, 1988.
47. Fredrix, E.W.H.M., Soeters, P.B., Rouflart, M.J.J., et al.: Am. J. Clin. Nutr., *53:*1318–1322, 1991.
48. Thomson, S.R., Hirschberg, A., Haffejee, A.A., et al.: JPEN J. Parenter. Enteral Nutr., *14:*119–121, 1990.
49. FAO/WHO/UNU: Energy and protein requirements. Report of a joint expert consultation. WHO Technical Report Series No. 724. Genera, World Health Organization, 1985.
50. Douglas, R.G., Shaw, J.H.F.: Br. J. Surg., *77:*246–254, 1990.
51. Chlebowski, R.T., Heber, D.: Surg. Clin. North Am., *66:*957–968, 1986.
52. Cerosimo, E., Pisters, P.W.T., Pesola, G., et al.: Surgery, *109:*459–467, 1991.
53. Kokal, W.A., McCullough, A., Wright, P.O., et al.: Ann. Surg., *198:*146–150, 1983.
54. Shaw, J.H.F., Wolfe, R.R.: Surgery, *101:*181–191, 1987.
55. Shaw, J.H.F., Humberstone, D.M., Wolfe, R.R.: Ann. Surg., *207:*283–289, 1988.
56. Humberstone, D.M., Shaw, J.H.F.: Cancer, *62:*1619–1624, 1988.
57. Holyroyde, C.P., Gabuzda, T.G., Putnam, R.C., et al.: Cancer Res., *35:*3710–3714, 1975.
58. Holyroyde, C.P., Reichard, G.A.: Cancer Treat. Rep., *65(Suppl. 5):*55–59, 1981.
59. Waterhouse, C.: Cancer, *33:*66–71, 1974.
60. Eden, E., Edström, S., Bennegård, K., et al.: Cancer Res., *44:*1717–1724, 1984.
61. Young, V.R.: Cancer Res., *37:*2336–2347, 1977.
62. Mulligan, H.D., Tisdale, M.J.: Biochem. J., *277:*321–326, 1991.
63. Lundholm, K.: Surg. Clin. North Am., *66:*1013–1024, 1986.
64. Cohn, S., Gartenhaus, W., Sawitsky, A., et al.: Metabolism, *30:*222–229, 1980.
65. Klein, S., Wolfe, R.R.: J. Clin. Invest., *86:*1403–1408, 1990.
66. Shaw, J.H.F., Wolfe, R.R.: Ann. Surg., *205:*368–376, 1987.
67. Wolfe, R.R., Herndon, D.N., Jahoor, F., et al.: N. Engl. J. Med., *317:*403–408, 1987.
68. Hollander, D.M., Ebert, E.C., Roberts, A.I., et al.: Surgery, *100:*292–297, 1986.
69. Beck, S.A., Tisdale, M.J.: Br. J. Cancer, *63:*846–850, 1991.
70. Vlassara, H., Spiegel, R.J., Doval, D.S., et al.: Horm. Metab. Res., *18:*698–703, 1986.
71. Carmichael, M.J., Clague, M.B., Kier, M.J., et al.: Br. J. Surg., *67:*736–739, 1980.
72. Heber, D., Chlebowski, R.T., Ishibashi, D.E., et al.: Cancer Res., *42:*4815–4819, 1982.
73. Eden, E., Ekman, L., Lindmark, L., et al.: Metabolism, *33:*1020–1027, 1984.
74. Norton, J.A., Stein, T.P., Brennan, M.F.: Ann. Surg., *194:*123–128, 1981.
75. Jeevanandam, M., Horowitz, G.D., Lowry, S.F., et al.: Lancet, *1:*1423–1426, 1984.
76. Shaw, J.H.F., Humberstone, D.A., Douglas, R.G., et al.: Surgery, *109:*37–50, 1991.
77. Warren, R.S., Jeevanandam, M., Brennan, M.F.: J. Surg. Res., *42:*43–50, 1987.
78. Lundholm, K., Edström, S., Ekman, L.A.: Cancer, *42:*453–461, 1978.
79. Heymsfield, S.B., McManus, C.B.: Cancer, *55:*238–249, 1985.
80. Cohn, S.H., Gartenhaus, W., Vartsky, D., et al.: Am. J. Clin. Nutr., *34:*1997–2004, 1981.
81. Andersson, C.E., Lönnroth, I.C., Gelin, J.L., et al.: Gastroenterology, *100:*938–945, 1991.
82. Steel, C.M.: Lancet, *2:*30–34, 1989.
83. Moldawer, L.L., Lowry, S.F., Cerami, A.: Annu. Rev. Nutr., *8:*585–609, 1988.
84. Old, L.J.: Science, *230:*630–632, 1985.
85. Philip, S., Lam, S.L., Ryan, K.J., et al.: Lancet, *2:*1364–1365, 1986.
86. Waage, A., Espivak, T., Lamvik, J.: Scand. J. Immunol., *24:*739–743, 1986.
87. Socher, S.H., Martinez, D., Craig, J.B., et al.: J. Natl. Cancer Inst., *80:*595–598, 1988.
88. Michie, H.R., Kirk, R.M., Spriggs, D.R., et al.: N. Engl. J. Med., *318:*1481–1486, 1988.
89. Endres, S., Ghorbani, R., Kelley, V.E., et al.: N. Engl. J. Med., *320:*265–271, 1989.
90. Michie, H.R., Sherman, M.L., Spriggs, D.R., et al.: Ann. Surg., *209:*19–24, 1989.
91. Gelin, J., Moldawer, L.L., Lönnroth, C., et al.: Cancer Res., *51:*415–421, 1991.

92. Yoneda, T., Alsina, M.A., Chavez, J.B., et al.: J. Clin. Invest., *87:*977–985, 1991.
93. Black, K., Garrett, I.R., Mundy, G.R.: Endocrinology, *128:*2657–2659, 1991.
94. Strassman, G., Fong, M., Kenney, J.S., et al.: J. Clin. Invest., *89:*1681–1684, 1992.
95. Van Snick, J.: Annu. Rev. Immunol., *8:*253–278, 1990.
96. Beck, S.H., Smith, K.L., Tisdale, M.J.: Br. J. Cancer, *62:*816–821, 1990.
97. Bartoshuk, L.M.: Am. J. Clin. Nutr., *31:*1068–1077, 1978.
98. DeWys, W.D., Walters, K.: Cancer, *36:*1888–1896, 1975.
99. Kamath, S., Booth, P., Lad, T.E., et al.: Cancer, *52:*386–389, 1983.
100. Williams, L.A., Cohen, M.H.: Am. J. Clin. Nutr., *31:*122–125, 1978.
101. Carson, J.A.S., Gormican, A.: J. Am. Diet Assoc., *70:*361–365, 1977.
102. Trant, A.S., Serin, J., Douglass, H.O.: Am. J. Clin. Nutr., *36:*46–58, 1982.
103. Bernstein, I.L.: Cancer Res., *42(Suppl.):*715S–720S, 1982.
104. Nielsen, S.S., Theologides, A., Vickers, Z.M.: Am. J. Clin. Nutr., *33:*2253–2261, 1980.
105. Bernstein, I.L., Fenner, D.P.: Appetite J. Intake Res., *4:*79–86, 1983.
106. Levine, J.A., Emering, P.W.: Br. J. Cancer, *56:*73–78, 1987.
107. Morrison, S.D.: Cancer Res., *42(Suppl.):*720S, 1982.
108. Odell, W.D., Wolfsen, A.R.: Annu. Rev. Med., *29:*379–406, 1978.
109. Bostwick, D.G., Null, W.E., Holmes, D., et al.: N. Engl. J. Med., *317:*1439–1443, 1987.
110. Shimoda, S.S., Saunders, D.R., Rubin, C.E.: Gastroenterology, *55:*705–723, 1968.
111. Fahrenkrug, J.: Clin. Gastroenterol., *9:*633–643, 1980.
112. O'Donnell, L.D.J., Farthing, M.G.J.: Gut, *30:*1165–1172, 1989.
113. Mundy, G.R.: J. Clin. Invest., *82:*1–6, 1988.
114. Broadus, A.E., Mangin, M., Ikeda, K., et al.: N. Engl. J. Med., *319:*556–563, 1988.
115. Rosenthal, N., Insogna, K.L., Godsall, J.W., et al.: J. Clin. Endocrinol. Metab., *60:*29–33, 1985.
116. Siris, E.S., Clemens, T.L., Dempster, D.W., et al.: Am. J. Med., *82:*307–312, 1987.
117. Case records of the Massachusetts General Hospital Case 52-1989:N. Engl. J. Med., *321:*1812–1821, 1989.
118. Creamer, B.: Br. Med. J., *2:*1435–1436, 1964.
119. Barry R.E.: Gut, *15:*562–565, 1974.
120. Schwartz, S.I.: Manifestations of gastrointestinal disease. *In* Principles of Surgery. 5th Ed. Edited by S.I. Schwartz, G.T. Shires, and F.C. Spencer. New York, McGraw Hill, 1989.
121. Mathias, J.R., Clench, M.H.: Am. J. Med. Sci., *289:*243–248, 1985.
122. Herbsman, H., Wetstein, L., Rosen, Y., et al.: Curr. Probl. Surg., *17:*121–184, 1980.
123. Novis, B.H., Banks, S., Marks, S.W., et al.: Q. J. Med., *40:*521–540, 1971.
124. Tilson, M.D.: Surg. Clin. North Am., *54:*409–423, 1974.
125. Waldman, T.A., Broder, S., Strober, W.: Ann. N.Y. Acad. Sci., *230:*306–317, 1974.
126. Mossman, K., Schatzman, A., Chencharick, J.: Int. J. Radiat. Oncol. Biol. Phys., *8:*991–997, 1982.
127. Shils, M.E.: Surg. Gynecol. Obstet., *132:*709–715, 1971.
128. Pedersen, H., Hansen, H.S., Cederqvist, C., et al.: Acta Clin. Scand., *148:*363–366, 1982.
129. Daly, J.M., Massar, E., Gracco, G., et al.: Ann. Surg., *196:*203–208, 1982.
130. Burt, M.E., Stein, T.P., Schwade, J.G., et al.: Cancer, *53:*1246–1254, 1984.
131. Riboli, E.B., Bertoglio, S., Arnulfo, G., et al.: J. Parenter. Enteral Nutr., *10:*82–85, 1986.
132. Bandoli, T., Isoyama, T., Toyoshima, H.: Surgery, *109:*136–142, 1991.
133. Lawrence, W.: Cancer Res., *37:*2379–2388, 1977.
134. Geer, R.J., Richards, W.O., O'Dorisio, T.M., et al.: Ann. Surg., *212:*678–687, 1990.
135. Leeds, A.R., Ralphs, D.N.C., Ebeid, F., et al.: Lancet, *1:*1075–1078, 1981.
136. Ratner, D.W.: Mayo Clin. Proc. (editorial), *67:*907–909, 1992.
137. Goldsmith, H.S., Ghosh, B.G., Huvos, A.G.: Surg. Gynecol. Obstet., *132:*87–92, 1971.
138. Wallaeger, E.E., Comfort, M.W., Clagett, O.T., et al.: J.A.M.A., *137:*838–848, 1948.
139. Brooks, J.R., Culebras, J.M.: Am. J. Surg., *131:*516–520, 1976.
140. Warren, K.W., Veidenheimer, M.C., Pratt, H.S.: Surg. Clin. North Am., *47:*639–645, 1967.
141. Miyata, M., Takao, T., Uozumi, T., et al.: Ann. Surg., *179:*494–498, 1974.
142. Kendall, D.M., Sutherland, D.E.R., Najjarian, J.S., et al.: N. Engl. J. Med., *322:*898–903, 1990.
143. Pliam, M.N., ReMine, W.H.: Arch. Surg., *110:*506–511, 1975.
144. Fortner, J.G.: Cancer, *47:*1712–1718, 1981.
145. Perez, M.M., Newcomer, A.D., Moertel, C.G., et al.: Cancer, *52:*346–352, 1983.
146. Weser, E., Fletcher, J.T., Urban, E.: Gastroenterology, *77:*572–579, 1979.
147. Sutters, M., Carmichael, D.J.S., Unwin, R.J., et al.: Gut, *32:*649–653, 1991.
148. Wong, W.D., Rotherberger, D.A., Goldbert, S.M.: Curr. Probl. Surg., *22:*1–78, 1985.
149. Tyus, F.J., Austhof, S.I., Chima, C.S., et al.: J. Am. Diet Assoc., *92:*861–863, 1992.
150. Cummings, J.H.: Gut, *22:*763–779, 1981.
151. Haing, J.M., Soergel, K.N., Komorowski, R.A., et al.: N. Engl. J. Med., *320:*23–28, 1987.
152. Krakoff, I.H.: CA. (Am. Cancer Soc. J. Clin.), *37:*93–105, 1987.
153. Wittes, R.E., Hubbard, S.M.: Chemotherapy: the properties and uses of single agents. Chap. 22. *In* Manual of Oncologic Therapeutics 1991/1992. Edited by R.E. Wittes. Philadelphia, J.B. Lippincott, 1991.
154. Schilsky, R.L., Anderson, T.: Ann. Intern. Med., *90:*929–931, 1979.
155. Desai, T.K., Maliakkal, J., Kinzie, J.L., et al.: Am. J. Clin. Nutr., *55:*708–711, 1992.
156. Herrmann, V.M., Garnick, M.B., Moore, F.D., et al.: Surgery, *90:*381–387, 1984.
157. Editorial: Lancet, *338:*217–218, 1991.
158. Editorial: Ann. Intern. Med., *117:*261–262, 1992.
159. Potter, M.N., Mott, M.G., Oakhill, A.: Ann. Intern. Med., *112:*715, 1990.
160. Kaczmarski, R.S., Mufti, G.J.: Br. Med. J., *301:*1312–1313, 1990.
161. Gralla, R.M.: Treatment of Emesis. Chap. 58. *In* Manual of Oncologic Therapeutics 1991/1992. Edited by R.E. Wittes. Philadelphia, J.B. Lippincott, 1991.

162. Bounous, G., Gentile, J.M., Hugon, J.: Can. J. Surg., *14*:312–324, 1971.
163. Bounous, G., Hugon, J., Gentile, J.M.: Can. J. Surg., *14*:298–311, 1971.
164. Harvey, L.P., McAnena, O.J., Mehta, B.M., et al.: JPEN J. Parenter. Enteral Nutr., *11*:119–123, 1987.
165. Daising, M.C., Grosfeld, J.L., Remley, K., et al.: J. Pediatr. Surg., *17*:721–727, 1982.
166. Fox, A.D., Kripke, S.A., DePaula, J.: JPEN J. Parenter. Enteral Nutr., *12*:325–331, 1988.
167. Shou, J., Lieberman, M.D., Hofmann, K., et al.: JPEN J. Parenter. Enteral Nutr., *15*:307–312, 1991.
168. Klimberg, V.S., Nwokedi, E., Hutchins, C.F., et al.: Surg. Forum, *41*:16–18, 1991.
169. Reynolds, H.M., Daly, J.M., Rowlands, B.J., et al.: Cancer, *45*:3069–3074, 1980.
170. Torosian, M.H., Mullen, J.L., Miller, E.E., et al.: JPEN J. Parenter. Enteral Nutr., *7*:337–345, 1983.
171. Torosian, M.H., Mullen, J.L., Miller, E.E., et al.: Surgery, *94*:291–299, 1983.
172. Torosian, M.H., Mullen, J.L., Stein, T.P., et al.: J. Surg. Res., *39*:103–113, 1988.
173. Cheson, B.D. (editorial): N. Engl. J. Med., *327*:422–423, 1992.
174. Parkinson, D.R., Smith, M.A. (editorial): Ann. Intern. Med., *117*:338–340, 1992.
175. Frankel, S.R., Eardley, A., Lauwers, G., et al.: Ann. Intern. Med., *117*:292–296, 1992.
176. Bower, M., Colston, K.W., Stein, R.C., et al.: Lancet, *337*:701–702, 1991.
177. Rosenberg, S.A.: Cancer Res., *51(Suppl.)*:5074S–5079S, 1991.
178. Dillman, R.O.: Ann. Intern. Med., *111*:592–603, 1989.
179. Rosenberg, S.A., Lotze, M.T., Mule, J.J.: Ann. Intern. Med., *108*:853–864, 1988.
180. Kradin, R.L., Lazarus, D., Dubrinett, S.M., et al.: Lancet, *1*:577–580, 1989.
181. Atzpodien, J., Korfer, A., Franks, C., et al.: Lancet, *335*:1509–1512, 1990.
182. Webb, D.E., Austin, H.A., Belldegrum, A., et al.: Clin. Nephrol., *30*:141–145, 1988.
183. Brown, R.R., Lee, C.M., Kohler, P.C., et al.: Cancer Res., *49*:4941–4944, 1989.
184. Gutierrez, A.A., Lemoine, N.R., Sikora, K.: Lancet, *339*:715–721, 1992.
185. Culliton, B.J.: Science (News and Comments), *249*:974–976, 1990.
186. Torosian, M.H., Donaway, R.B.: Surgery, *109*:597–601, 1991.
187. Bartlett, D., Charland, S., Torosian, M.: JPEN J. Parenter. Enteral Nutr., *16*:275, 1992 (abstract).
188. Torosian, M.H., Tsou, K.C., Daly, J.M., et al.: Cancer, *53*:1409–1415, 1984.
189. Mullen, J.L., Busby, G.P., Gertner, M.H., et al.: Surgery, *87*:331–338, 1980.
190. Heys, S.D., Park, K.G.M., McNurlan, M.A., et al.: Br. J. Surg., *78*:483–487, 1991.
191. Westin, T., Stein, H., Niedobritek, G., et al.: Am. J. Clin. Nutr., *53*:764–768, 1991.
192. Copeland, E.M., MacFayden, B.V., Lanzotti, V.J., et al.: Am. J. Surg., *129*:167–173, 1975.
193. Copeland, E.M., Souchon, E.A., MacFayden, B.V., et al.: Cancer, *36*:609–616, 1977.
194. Klein, S.M., Simes, J., Blackburn, G.L.: Cancer, *58*:1378–1386, 1986.
195. Lowry, S.F., Brennan, M.F.: Intravenous feeding of the cancer patient. *In* Parenteral Nutrition. Edited by J.L. Rombeau and M.D. Caldwell. Philadelphia, W.B. Saunders, 1986.
196. Am. College Physicians: Position Paper. Parenteral Nutrition in Patients Receiving Cancer Chemotherapy. Ann. Intern. Med., *110*:734–736, 1989.
197. McGeer, A.J., Detsky, A.S., O'Rourke, K.: Nutrition, *6*:478–483, 1990.
198. Desai, T.K., Kinzie, J.: JPEN J. Parenter. Enteral Nutr., *14(Suppl)*:7S, 1990 (abstract).
199. Shike, M., Brennan, M.F.: Supportive care of the cancer patient. Chap. 59. *In* Cancer Principles and Practice of Oncology. 3rd Ed. Edited by V.T. DeVita Jr., S. Hellman, and S.A. Rosenberg. Philadelphia, J.B. Lippincott, 1989.
200. Lipman, T.O.: Hemotol./Oncol. Clin. North Am., *5*:91–102, 1991.
201. Shils, M.E., Baker, H., Frank, O.: JPEN J. Parenter. Enteral Nutr., *9*:179–188, 1985.
202. Zeisel, S.H., DaCosta, K.A., Franklin, P.D., et al.: FASEB J., *5*:2093–2098, 1991.
203. Stehle, P., Zander, J., Mertes, N., et al.: Lancet, *1*:231–233, 1989.
204. Ziegler, T.R., Young, L.S., Benfell, K., et al.: Ann. Intern. Med., *116*:821–828, 1992.
205. Nixon, D.W., Moffitt, S., Lawson, D.H., et al.: Cancer Treat. Rep., *65(Suppl. 5)*:121–128, 1981.
206. Bozetti, F.: JPEN J. Parenter. Enteral Nutr., *13*:406–420, 1989.
207. Chen, M.K., Souba, W.W., Copeland, E.M.: Hematol./Oncol. Clin. North Am., *5*:125–145, 1991.
208. Ng, E.H., Lowry, S.F.: Hematol./Oncol. Clin. North Am., *5*:161–184, 1991.
209. Howard, L., Heaphey, L., Fleming, C.R., et al.: JPEN J. Parenter. Enteral Nutr., *15*:384–393, 1991.
210. August, D.A., Thorn, D., Fisher, R.L., et al.: JPEN J. Parenter. Enteral Nutr., *15*:323–327, 1991.
211. Bailar, J.C., Smith, E.M.: N. Engl. J. Med., *314*:1226–1232, 1986.
212. U.S. Congress, Office of Technology Assessment: Unconventional Cancer Treatments. OTA-H-405. Washington, D.C., U.S. Government Printing Office, 1990.
213. Cassileth, B.R., Lusk, E.J., Guerrey, DuP., et al.: N. Engl. J. Med., *324*:1180–1185, 1991.
214. Am. Soc. Clin. Oncol.: Ineffective Cancer Therapy: A Guide for the Lay Person. J. Clin. Oncol., *1*:154–163, 1983.
215. Herbert, V.: Cancer, *58*:1930–1941, 1986.
216. Cancer: Questionable Nutritional Therapies in the Treatment of Cancer. Atlanta, American Cancer Society, 1991.
217. Schraub, S., Bernheim, J.: Quackery in the quest of quality. Reflections on the impact of unproven methods in the treatment of cancer. *In* The Quality of Life of Cancer Patients. Edited by N.K. Aaronson and J. Beckmann. New York, Raven Press, 1987.
218. Eisele, J.W., Reay, D.T.: JAMA, *244*:1608–1609, 1980.
219. Cassileth, B.R., Lusk, E.J., Strouse, T.B., et al.: Ann. Intern. Med., *101*:105–112, 1984.
220. Lerner, I.J.: Cancer, *53*:815–819, 1984.
221. Nelson, H.: Lancet, *340*:106–107, 1992.
222. Tuffs, A.: Lancet, *340*:107, 1992.

SELECTED READINGS

Bloch, A.S. (Ed.): Nutrition Management of the Cancer Patient. Rockville, MD, Aspen, 1990.

Mertelsmann, R., Rosenthal, F.M., Lindemann, A., et al.: Cytokines and hematopoietins: physiology, pathophysiology, and potential as therapeutic agents. Recent Results Cancer Res., *121*:121–140, 1991.

Ng, E-H., Lowry, S.F.: Nutritional support and cancer cachexia, evolving concepts of mechanisms and adjunctive therapies. Hematol./Oncol. Clin. North Am., *5*:161–184, 1991.

Wittes, R.E. (Ed.): Manual of Oncologic Therapeutics 1991/1992. Philadelphia, J.B. Lippincott, 1991.

CHAPTER **74**

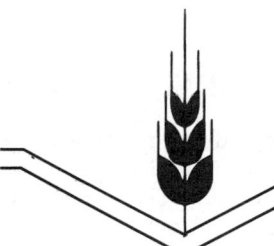

Diet and Nutrition in Neurologic Disorders

Pierre M. Dreyfus and Masud Seyal

Improper and inadequate nutrition that is allowed to persist over weeks and months can lead to neurologic diseases that affect either or both the central or the peripheral nervous system. Nutritional diseases of the nervous system have been documented carefully from a clinical, pathologic, and biochemical point of view since their etiology was first identified a century ago. In fact, the study of some of these diseases has been responsible in large part for several advances in the field of modern nutrition. More specifically, the discoveries of the pathogenesis of beriberi,[1] a disease that affects the heart and the peripheral nervous system, and pellagra,[2] an affliction of the central nervous system, led to the eventual discovery of vitamins and active cofactors and an understanding of their function in metabolism. The successful nutritional management of beriberi antedated by some 29 years the discovery of the specific cause of the disease and the description of the deficient nutrient: thiamin. Before 1882, when a drastic change in the diet of the Japanese navy virtually eliminated beriberi among Japanese sailors, beriberi had occurred in epidemic proportions throughout the world. Although the disease continues to be seen in underprivileged, severely malnourished, and chronically alcoholic individuals, it no longer constitutes a major public health problem.

Nutritional disorders of the nervous system are seen most commonly as a consequence of chronic alcoholism, debilitating diseases that affect the gastrointestinal tract, starvation resulting from unavailability of nutrients (e.g., poverty or drought), and malnutrition caused by individual ignorance about diet and nutrition. Among the more privileged populations of the world, nutrition-related neurologic diseases most often affect patients seeking to shed excess weight by dietary, pharmacologic, or surgical means, as well as in food cultists and individuals with peculiar dietary habits. In this type of population, nutritional deficiency sufficiently severe to lead to neurologic dysfunction can also occur as the result of stress, although the dietary intake is considered adequate. Examples of such stressful conditions are chronic infection, endocrine imbalance, overwhelming psychiatric disease, and pernicious vomiting; occasionally, pregnancy is a culprit.

The various nutritional syndromes that affect the nervous system, all of which are described in this chapter, may manifest separately in relatively pure form or together in varying combinations. Some are more common than others. Basic constitutional and genetic factors undoubtedly underlie individual responses to altered nutrition. Some individuals have no clinical manifestations; others experience an array of symptoms and signs referable to the central, peripheral, or autonomic nervous system. All nutritional disorders of the nervous system share certain characteristic etiologic and pathologic attributes. The known biochemical lesions that can be demonstrated in these diseases invariably antedate the appearance of clinical manifestations and pathologic changes, which affect areas of the nervous system in a predictable, reproducible, selective, and symmetric fashion. Most of these diseases are eminently preventable or, when they occur, can be treated by a simple dietary approach.

Some neurologic diseases and syndromes are engendered by metabolic disturbances. In some instances, the metabolic defect may be well defined, whereas in others it is as yet unknown. The prevention and successful treatment of some of these disorders frequently involve nutritional manipulation consisting of the addition, elimination, or substitution of some basic nutrient or nutrients. Various chronic afflictions of the nervous system are attended by severe, life-threatening malnutrition that can be reversed with relative ease, leading to increased comfort on the part of the patient, although the course of the underlying disease remains unaltered.

The adverse consequences of diet or dietary elements on behavior, the potential neurotoxicity of certain vitamins, and the interrelationship of antiepileptic drugs and vitamins also are considered in this chapter.

Finally, the rationale behind the use of diet and vitamins as therapy for neurologic disorders that do not have a nutritional correlation, such as headache, neuralgia, and dementia, is also discussed.

NEUROLOGIC DISORDERS CAUSED BY MALNUTRITION

The chronic ingestion of alcohol, when it is accompanied by undernutrition (in some instances, malnutrition), can lead to several clearly defined neurologic disorders. During periods of heavy drinking, the absorption of vitamins, their intestinal transport, tissue storage, use, and conversion to metabolically active forms are sharply curtailed, while the need for vitamins and essential nutrients increases. In addition, chronic alcoholism affects mineral, carbohydrate, protein, and lipid metabolism adversely. Nutritional disorders of the nervous system, although most commonly associated with chronic alcoholism, can affect malnourished, debilitated, nonalcoholic individuals who suffer from such illnesses as malabsorption syndromes, carcinomatosis, thyroid, renal disease, and acquired immunodeficiency syndrome (AIDS). Considering the ever-increasing size of the chronic alcoholic population throughout the world and the magnitude of the consequent general medical problems, alcohol-induced nutritional diseases of the nervous system are relatively rare. Nutritional disorders constitute only 1 to 3% of all alcohol-related problems affecting the nervous system that come to the attention of physicians.[3]

WERNICKE-KORSAKOFF SYNDROME

Wernicke-Korsakoff syndrome, although relatively rare, constitutes the most common alcoholic-nutritional affliction of the central nervous system.[4,5] This syndrome is not restricted to the alcoholic population; it can affect patients in whom nutritional depletion is unrelated to the abusive intake of alcohol. Wernicke's encephalopathy is characterized by the acute onset of ophthalmoplegia, nystagmus, and ataxia of stance and gait. Mental symptoms, which evolve during the course of the illness, affect more than 90% of patients. At the onset of the illness, global confusion, profound disorientation, apathy, indifference, inattentiveness, drowsiness, and decreased spontaneity of speech are the characteristic presenting symptoms. On rare occasions, stupor and coma are the initial symptoms. The clinical picture of Wernicke's disease may include such superimposed symptoms of alcohol withdrawal as delirium tremens or clinical evidence of hepatic decompensation.

With improved nutrition, the clinical picture improves and patients can be tested more easily. It is then possible to demonstrate the presence of ocular palsies, nystagmus, ataxia, and peripheral neuropathy—the classic hallmarks of Wernicke's disease. These clinical signs are frequently accompanied or followed by obvious Korsakoff's psychosis, otherwise referred to as amnestic-confabulatory syndrome. This condition is characterized by spotty loss of memory, the inability to learn and form new memories, impaired conceptual or perceptual functions, and confabulation, which usually vanishes during the more chronic stage of the illness. On rare occasions, Korsakoff's psychosis may be present without the ocular signs and ataxia of Wernicke's encephalopathy.

Wernicke-Korsakoff syndrome is caused by severe thiamin deficiency.[5] The requirements for thiamin are greatest when large amounts of glucose or alcohol are being metabolized and when metabolic demands are high. A sudden increase in brain glucose levels in a patient with marginal thiamin reserves may precipitate symptoms and signs of Wernicke-Korsakoff's syndrome.[6] Therefore, whenever glucose is being administered rapidly to a chronically malnourished and/or metabolically stressed individual, the parenteral fluids should always include a mixture of B vitamins. Because Korsakoff's psychosis, whether associated with or subsequent to the onset of Wernicke's encephalopathy, is essentially irreversible, urgent therapeutic intervention is essential. A delay of a few hours in a patient with ataxia and ocular signs may result in the development of irreversible changes of Korsakoff's psychosis. Small doses of thiamin may correct the ocular disturbances seen in Wernicke's encephalopathy. However, larger doses are needed to replenish thiamin stores and to stimulate the transketolase reaction optimally. The dosage is 50 mg thiamine intravenously followed by 50 mg daily intramuscularly until the patient can resume adequate oral feedings. The improvement of the acute neurologic signs and symptoms of Wernicke-Korsakoff disease correlates well with erythrocyte transketolase activity, a sensitive test of the adequacy of thiamin nutriture.[7] Reduced erythrocyte transketolase activity reverts toward normal levels as thiamin is administered and the patient improves. Genetic abnormalities in red cell transketolase may underlie a predisposition to Wernicke-Korsakoff syndrome.[8] Wernicke-Korsakoff syndrome and acute beriberi with metabolic acidosis may be precipitated by iatrogenic factors such as total parenteral nutrition.[6,9] For additional discussion on this syndrome, see Chapter 65.

NUTRITIONAL NEUROPATHY

Nutritional neuropathy is probably the most frequently-encountered nutritional disorder of the peripheral nervous system. In common with all nutritional disorders of the nervous system, the disease occurs in a variety of clinical settings. The characteristic clinical features of nutritional polyneuropathy,[10] as is the case with most polyneuropathies, consist in the early stages of the disease of symmetric impairment of motor and sensory function accompanied by reduced or absent reflex activity affecting the legs to a greater extent than the arms. The distal segments of the extremities usually are more affected than are the proximal ones, and autonomic dysfunction occasionally, accompanies the classic symptoms and signs of polyneuropathy. Also in the early stages of the disease, sensory symptoms tend to be more prominent than motor dysfunction. Patients frequently complain of paresthesias, dysesthesias, and a burning sensation. In the more advanced stages of the disease, motor impairment, such as foot drop, wrist drop, or complete paralysis of the legs, may be elicited. No specific clinical manifestations distinguish polyneuropathies caused by nutritional deficiency from those that occur by other causes.

One of the various clinical entities that have been attributed to nutritional factors is beriberi neuropathy ("dry beriberi"), which stems from a primary deficiency of thiamin. Another entity, alcoholic or nutritional neuropathy, seen predominantly in developed countries, is likely associated with severe thiamin deficiency caused by abnormal vitamin metabolism, or with inadequate intake of the vitamin in the face of a high energy intake (derived mainly from alcohol).[10] It has been demonstrated that alcohol alone may have a direct effect on neuronal metabolism. Consequently, alcoholic neuropathy is perhaps a prime example of what may be called a "toxonutritional" polyneuropathy.[11] Deficiencies of thiamin, pyridoxine, niacin, pantothenic acid, biotin, vitamin B_{12}, and possibly folate are associated with disease of the peripheral nervous system. Rarely is deficiency of a single vitamin (with the exception of B_{12}) identified as the sole cause of polyneuropathy. Usually, the deficiency state is multifactorial, involving the lack of several vitamins and other nutrients. Whereas the peripheral nervous system may be the most susceptible to nutritional depletion, other parts of the nervous system, such as the spinal cord, optic nerve, and cerebellum, may be affected coincidentally, but to a lesser degree. In such instances, the symptoms and signs of neuropathy tend to mask those of myelopathy or cerebellar involvement. In most cases of nutritional polyneuropathy, the presence of such systemic manifestations as weight loss, seborrheic dermatitis, follicular hypokeratosis, glossitis, cheilosis, angular stomatitis, changes in the color and texture of hair, anemia, and circulatory disturbances helps in establishing the nutritional etiology of the disease.

Attempts to investigate clinically the specific etiologic factors of nutritional polyneuropathies have encountered difficulties. The disease process is slow, with both onset and recovery measured in terms of weeks or even months. The underlying biochemical lesion or metabolic insult usually antedates the advent of clinical signs and symptoms, abnormal physiologic parameters, and pathologic changes. By the time a patient seeks the care of a physician, the underlying biochemical defect may already have been corrected, yet the disease continues to evolve. Patients frequently complain of severe weakness, sensory loss, or troublesome dysesthesia at the same time that electrical studies and pathologic changes suggest improvement of the underlying disease. Although electrical studies may ascertain the stage of the disease and provide some clues whether the underlying pathologic process involves primarily the axon or the myelin sheath, they cannot possibly elucidate etiologic factors.

The treatment of nutritional polyneuropathies is straightforward: provision of improved nutrition and supplemental vitamins, preferably administered by the parenteral route, and removal of noxious substances. Nutritional neuropathy may persist indefinitely in spite of improved nutrition.[12] Alcohol-induced neuropathy may worsen after bouts of heavy drinking and malnutrition.[13]

NUTRITIONAL AMBLYOPIA

This remarkably uniform and stereotyped disorder of vision occurs infrequently and affects only persons who are chronically undernourished.[14] Characteristically, the disease evolves slowly and subacutely, with the mode of onset of symptoms being much the same in all patients. Visual impairment usually has an insidious beginning and reaches its maximum in several weeks to months. Common presenting complaints are blurred or dim vision, difficulty in reading, photophobia, and discomfort in the retrobulbar region on moving the eyes. On examination, the patient has bilateral asymmetric scotomata of varying sizes. Ophthalmoscopic changes are at first restricted to slight redness of the temporal margins of the optic discs. At a later stage of the illness, minimal pallor may be observed, but frequently no abnormality is visible. Peripheral vision is intact. Although the syndrome most frequently afflicts patients who neglect their nutrition and who are habituated to alcohol or occasionally to tobacco, it has been encountered during periods of famine in undernourished populations all over the world and among civilian and military prisoners of war who have had no access to either alcohol or tobacco. The disease has been observed in patients afflicted with Crohn's disease and as a complication of jejunoileal bypass surgery for morbid obesity.[15,16] On occasion, a similar syndrome may present as one of the complications of pernicious anemia as well as of other deficiency states caused by a lack of vitamin B_{12}.[17]

The metabolic aberration or specific vitamin deficiency responsible for the development of nutritional amblyopia has not as yet been defined; deficiency of vitamin B_{12}, thiamin, riboflavin, and pyridoxine and a failure in the detoxification of the cyanide present in tobacco smoke have both been implicated. In isolated cases, reduced serum vitamin B_{12} levels, the abnormal urinary excretion of methylmalonic acid, and low levels of blood transketolase activity have been detected; none of these abnormalities is specific and to date no others have been demonstrated.[14]

Treatment with oral or parenteral B vitamins and improved nutrition is usually followed by clinical amelioration. Improvement depends on the duration of the visual syndrome and its severity at the time that therapy is instituted.[14]

CEREBELLAR DEGENERATION

Cerebellar cortical degeneration, sometimes referred to as alcoholic cerebellar degeneration, is a syndrome characterized primarily by progressive unsteadiness of stance and gait, with relative sparing of arms and cranial nerves. The disease can be set apart from all other known forms of cerebellar degeneration because of the uniformity of the clinical and pathologic manifestations.[18]

A substantial body of evidence implicates nutritional factors as the most likely causes of the disease. Although the disease is encountered most frequently in chronic alcoholic patients, it has also occurred in malnourished individuals who allegedly did not drink. Many patients with cortical cerebellar degeneration have a history of progressive weight loss before the onset of their symptoms. Signs of malnutrition are common, and the cerebellar syndrome frequently occurs in conjunction with cirrhosis and other nutritional complications of alcoholism. Nonalcoholic patients may develop cortical cerebellar degeneration in the setting of other diseases associated with nutritional depletion, such as pellagra, gastrointestinal cancer, and protracted vomiting.[19]

Improved nutrition and the administration of B vitamins may result in some degree of improvement of ataxia. On occasion, abstinence alone may be effective. It has been postulated that alcohol and/or some of its metabolites superimposed on malnutrition may be responsible for the damage caused to the cerebellum.[18]

VITAMIN B_{12} DEFICIENCY

Malabsorption of vitamin B_{12} from the gastrointestinal tract, such as that caused by pernicious anemia, can result in subacute degeneration of the spinal cord, optic nerves, cerebral white matter, and peripheral nerves. Most often, the neurologic manifestations of vitamin B_{12} deficiency are associated with the typical macrocytic anemia of pernicious anemia. In patients afflicted with dementia, the neuropsychiatric manifestations may precede the hematologic abnormality by months to years.[20] The neurologic symptoms and signs of the deficiency state may occur independently of the megaloblastic anemia.[21] Neurologic symptoms rarely occur as a result of vitamin B_{12} deficiency related to fish tapeworm infestation, sprue, gastrointestinal surgery, or vegetarianism.

Progressive symmetric paresthesia of hands and feet, weakness, spasticity and ataxia of legs, occasional confusion and dementia, and sometimes bilateral failing vision constitute the main neurologic symptoms of vitamin B_{12} deficiency. The main physical findings consist of diminution or loss of position and vibratory senses (blunting of pain, temperature, and tactile sensations over the distal parts of the legs), hyperactive knee jerks, and the absence of ankle jerks and extensor plantar responses. Psychologic symptoms may range from apathy, irritability, and depression to confusion and frank dementia.

Why a deficiency of vitamin B_{12} results in neurologic complications remains unknown. Treating patients afflicted with vitamin B_{12} deficiency with folic acid or conversely a folate-deficient patient with vitamin B_{12} may exacerbate the neuropsychiatric symptoms of either deficiency state.[20] Neurologic symptoms and signs may appear when the anemia has been corrected by folic acid. The biochemical lesion responsible for the neurologic manifestations of vitamin B_{12} deficiency appears to involve the enzyme methylmalonyl-CoA-isomerase that normally converts methylmalonyl-CoA to succinyl-CoA, a metabolic step in the utilization of propionic acid.[22,23] The excessive urinary excretion of methylmalonic acid that results as a consequence of the deficiency state has been demonstrated in patients with vitamin B_{12} deficiency and neurologic complications. Detection of this substance in the urine constitutes a sensitive index of vitamin B_{12} deficiency. More recently, the assay of methylmalonic acid and total homocysteine levels in the serum has proven to be useful as an indicator of vitamin B_{12} deficiency in patients with a hematologic picture, Schilling test, and serum vitamin B_{12} level that are normal or borderline.[15] The isomerase that converts methylmalonyl-CoA to succinyl-CoA may be essential to the maintenance of the myelin sheath. Sural nerve specimens obtained from patients with pernicious anemia show abnormal fatty acid metabolism, i.e., they accumulate branched-chain and odd-chain fatty acids that are derived from labeled propionate. The presence of these abnormal fatty acids may explain, in part, the structural changes observed in central and peripheral myelin of patients.[24]

The early neurologic manifestations of vitamin B_{12} deficiency are rapidly and completely reversible. Therefore, prompt initiation of therapy is of the utmost importance. The greatest degree of improvement is achieved when treatment takes place within 3 months of the onset of symptoms. However, variable degrees of amelioration can be obtained even 6 to 12 months after the onset of symptoms. Daily intramuscular injections of 1000 μg of cyanocobalamin should be given during the first 2 weeks. Subsequently, 1000 μg of cyanocobalamin should be given intramuscularly twice a week for 2 months, after which the patient should receive a minimum of 100 μg intramuscularly every month for life to prevent relapse.

PELLAGRA

Pellagra, characterized by dementia, dermatitis, and diarrhea, is becoming increasingly rare in the Western world as a consequence of improved nutrition, the enrichment of flour, and the increasingly common practice of vitamin supplementation. When the disease was prevalent in the United States, a large proportion of cases occurred in chronic alcoholic individuals, among whom it can still be encountered, particularly among those who, in addition to their chronic imbibition, have a combination of impaired gastrointestinal absorption and faulty nutrition. The neurologic manifestations of pellagra resemble those of an encephalopathy, occasionally accompanied by signs of peripheral nerve and spinal cord involvement. The psychologic symptoms often precede the skin changes, which characteristically develop on exposure to sunlight. In the early stages of the disease, the patient may be depressed, apathetic, fearful, and apprehensive. Insomnia, dizziness, and headache are common. As the disease progresses, a florid psychosis characterized by confusion, delusion, disorientation, and hallucinations may develop. Later, the patient may lapse into coma. Some patients exhibit spasticity of the legs and ataxic gait.[25] The neurologic symptoms and signs are promptly reversed by the administration of niacin. Niacin, 10 to 20 mg per day in the presence of adequate amounts of dietary tryptophan is sufficient to treat endemic pellegra. Larger amounts of niacin are required in Hartnup disease (an inherited disorder in which several amino acids, including tryptophan, are poorly absorbed). Larger amounts of niacin are also required in the carcinoid syndrome, in which a large percentage of tryptophan is catabolized by alternate, normally minor, pathways.

VITAMIN E DEFICIENCY

Severe deficiency of vitamin E in children and adults results in neurologic afflictions.[26–29] The salient clinical features consist of a motor-sensory polyneuropathy, truncal and limb ataxia, ophthalmoplegia, retinal degeneration, and myopathy. In its most advanced stage, vitamin E deficiency results in neuroaxonal degeneration[30] and destruction of muscle fibers. The deficiency state occurs as the result of abnormal lipid metabolism and consequent malabsorption of the vitamin. The neurologic dysfunction has been described in association with various congenital pediatric, and acquired adult disorders including primary biliary congenital cholestatic hepatobiliary diseases, cystic fibrosis, abetalipoproteinemia (Bassen-Kornzweig disease),[31] primary biliary cirrhosis,[32] exocrine pancreatic failure, intestinal lymphangiectasia, and short gut syndrome.[27] On rare occasions, vitamin E deficiency may occur as the result of a selective defect of vitamin E absorption.[33] The retinal lesions seen in children afflicted with vitamin E deficiency may occur because of deficiencies of both vitamins A and E.[27]

In patients afflicted with the various disorders, the serum level of D, 1, α-tocopherol is reduced. The tissue tocopherol levels, including those of the nervous system, are reduced before histologic changes become apparent.[34] The neurologic symptoms and signs can often be prevented by the early detection of the state of deficiency and by the administration of large doses of the vitamin. In children afflicted with chronic cholestasis, the early administration of α-tocopherol (120 mg/kg/day orally or 0.8 to 2.0 mg/kg/day intramuscularly), can prevent the advent of neuromuscular symptoms.[27] A beneficial effect may follow vitamin E therapy in cystic fibrosis associated with spinocerebellar degeneration with replacement therapy. Clinical improvement may also occur in vitamin E deficiency states resulting from malnutrition and from chronic fat malabsorption.

NEUROLOGIC DISORDERS AFFECTED BY DIET OR DIETARY ELEMENTS

In several genetically determined metabolic neurologic diseases, a part of the treatment consists of either the elimination of certain foods that contain nutrients known to be damaging to the nervous system and other organs or, in vitamin-dependent diseases, the supplementation of a specific vitamin because of a demonstrated enzymatic defect that can be overcome in part by pharmacologic rather than nutritional doses of the vitamin (Table 74–1). Examples of such disorders will be discussed briefly.[43]

WILSON'S DISEASE

A classic example of a disease affected by the elimination of a nutrient is Wilson's disease (hepatolenticular degeneration),[39,40] a progressive familial illness inherited through an autosomal recessive gene. This condition is characterized by cirrhosis of the liver, neurologic signs and symptoms related to damage of the basal ganglia of the brain, and a rust, pigmented ring of the cornea of the eye near the scleral junction (Kayser-Fleischer ring) in all patients with neurologic impairment. The salient symptoms and signs include progressive tremors, rigidity, dysarthria, dysphasia, drooling, dementia, and psychosis. The basic underlying biochemical defect consists of a deficiency of the copper-carrying protein ceruloplasmin in the blood. This genetic defect causes the increased accumulation of copper in various organs, including the liver, the nervous system, and the cornea (hence the Kayser-Fleischer ring), and the elimination of large quantities of copper in the urine. Treatment of this disease is best achieved by the exclusion from the diet of foods high in copper content, such as broccoli, liver, mushrooms, shellfish, cocoa, nuts, and beans. Agents that either chelate copper, such as penicillamine and triethylenetetramine (trientine),[44] or prevent its absorption from the gastrointestinal tract, such as zinc acetate,[45] are used in conjunction with a low copper diet. The combined dietary and pharmacologic treatment leads to significant amelioration of hepatic dysfunction and of neurologic symptoms and signs.[40,46]

REFSUM'S DISEASE (HEREDOPATHIA ATACTICA POLYNEURITIFORMIS)

This relatively rare autosomal recessive disease of the peripheral nervous system was first described by Refsum in 1944.[41] The illness is characterized by the onset in either late childhood or early adolescence of signs and symptoms suggestive of motor, sensory, symmetric, areflexic neuropathy, sometimes accompanied by cerebellar ataxia, cataracts, retinitis pigmentosa, diminished hearing or deafness, cardiomyopathy, and cutaneous changes (ichthyosis). Phytanic acid accumulates in the liver and kidneys because of a lack of phytanic acid α-hydroxylase, which converts phytanic acid to α-hydroxyphytanic acid. The metabolic block causes the accumulation of a branched-chain fatty acid, phytanic acid, in the blood, with increased excretion of the acid in the urine and the accumulation of abnormal lipids in peripheral nerves. Phytanic acid is derived from phytol, which is contained in a large variety of foods, such as nuts, spinach, and coffee. Elimination from the diet of dairy products, ruminant fat, and chlorophyll-containing foods leads to decreased phytanic acid levels in the blood, followed over the course of many months by slow but steady improvement of the neurologic disorder.[42] In individuals in whom the peripheral nerve disorder is

TABLE 74.1 INBORN ERRORS OF METABOLISM WITH NEUROLOGIC MANIFESTATIONS

DISEASE	DEFECT	DIETARY TREATMENT	REF.
Phenylketonuria	Phenylalanine hydroxylase	Restrict phenylalanine	35, 36
Maple syrup urine disease	Branched-chain ketoacid decarboxylase	1. Restrict leucine, isoleucine, valine 2. Thiamin	35, 32
Urea cycle defects			
Argininosuccinicaciduria	Argininosuccinase		
Citrullinemia	Argininosuccinic synthetase		
Hyperammonemia	Ornithine transcarbamylase Carbamyl phosphate synthetase	Restrict protein	
Lysine intolerance	Interference with arginase		
Homocystinuria	Cystathionine synthetase	1. Restrict methionine 2. Pyridoxine 3. Folic acid, vitamin B_{12}	
Galactosemia	Galactose-1-phosphate uridyl transferase	Lactose-free diet Low-galactose diet	37,38
Wilson's disease	Low serum ceruloplasmin	Low-copper diet	39, 40
Refsum's disease	Alpha oxidation of phytanic acid to pristanic acid	Phytol-free diet	41, 42

(Adapted from Menkes, J.H.: Textbook of Child Neurology. 3rd Ed. Philadelphia, Lea & Febiger, 1985.)

either partial or intermittent, the strict adherence to a phytol-free diet, although important, may not be crucial.

VITAMIN-RESPONSIVE DISEASES

Vitamin-responsive, or vitamin-dependent, diseases are a group of genetically determined metabolic disorders in which either a vitamin-dependent enzymatic step or a reaction involving the conversion of a vitamin to its active cofactor form is defective, causing the abnormal accumulation of metabolites, or substrates, in the blood.[43,47–49] In these diseases, blood vitamin levels are normal. The basic metabolic defect involves the structure of the apoenzyme, its coenzyme binding sites, or some aspect of coenzyme synthesis. The neurologic manifestations observed in vitamin-responsive diseases tend to be protean, ranging from mental retardation, psychiatric symptoms, and convulsive seizures to ophthalmologic signs, ataxia, spasticity, and peripheral neuropathy (Table 74–2). The degree of response of these disorders to the appropriate vitamin varies considerably. In some patients, neurologic symptoms and signs improve dramatically after therapy with amounts exceeding nutritional or physiologic doses. In pyridoxine dependency, a disorder of neonates characterized by generalized seizures and most likely resulting from abnormal glutamic acid decarboxylase coenzyme binding sites, convulsions can be controlled with daily doses of pyridoxine that are 5 to 20 times greater than the recommended daily requirement.[43,47,48] Because no specific diagnostic test for pyridoxine dependency is known, a child with persistent seizures should be given 50 mg of pyridoxine intravenously. If the seizures cease within minutes, dependency should be suspected. Rapid normalization of the electroencephalogram (EEG) results and cessation of seizures confirm the diagnosis.[50]

ACQUIRED AND HEREDITARY HYPERAMMONEMIC DISORDERS

Acute and chronic liver disease caused by either a primary hepatic pathologic process or portacaval shunting may lead to a metabolic encephalopathy that evolves over a period of days and weeks and proceeds to progressive mental confusion and drowsiness followed by stupor, coma, and sometimes death. On occasion, these symptoms are preceded by generalized or focal seizures and asterixis (liver flap). The encephalopathy can be reversible by appropriate treatment, including dietary measures, but the outcome frequently is fatal. Recurring bouts of hepatic encephalopathy may cause episodic stupor and coma or persistent extrapyramidal movement disorder, ataxia, myelopathy, and irreversible dementia. The EEG of a patient with hepatic encephalopathy assumes a characteristic triphasic delta wave pattern that is also observed in association with other metabolic encephalopathies. The abnormal EEG pattern correlates with high serum ammonia levels detected in well-established cases.[51] The nutritional support of patients afflicted with acute and chronic liver disease, the prevention of hepatic encephalopathy, and the successful treatment of this devastating disorder are discussed in Chapters 63 and 64.

Several genetically determined disorders caused by hyperammonemia that results from the failure of removal of blood urea have been recognized. In these diseases, which are inherited in an autosomal recessive manner, a deficiency of urea cycle enzymes has been detected (see Table 74–1 and Chap. 67). The clinical features of these genetic hyperammonemic disorders vary according to the degree of enzymatic defect. Symptoms may consist of mental retardation, generalized seizures, ataxia, intermittent stupor and coma, rigidity, and opisthotonos. However, some patients merely dis

TABLE 74–2. VITAMIN-RESPONSIVE DISEASES WITH NEUROLOGIC MANIFESTATIONS

VITAMIN	DISEASE
Thiamin (vitamin B_1)	Maple syrup urine disease
	Pyruvate decarboxylase deficiency
	Leigh's disease*
Pyridoxine (vitamin B_6)	Neonatal convulsions
	Homocystinuria
	Cystathioninuria
Cobalamin (vitamin B_{12})	Methylmalonuria
	Homocystinuria
Folic acid	Homocystinuria
Nicotinamide	Hartnup disease†
Biotin	Propionicacidemia
	Methylcrotonylglycinuria

*Defective regulation of thiamin-dependent pyruvate dehydrogenase complex; cytochrome C oxidase deficiency.

†Defective intestinal and renal tubular transport of tryptophan and other neutral amino acids.

(Adapted from Mudd, S.H.: Adv. Nutr. Res., *4*:1–34, 1982.)

play learning disability and are otherwise normal. In general, the patient improves when the diet is restricted in protein. Of interest, some afflicted children display a natural distaste for meat.[49]

SPINA BIFIDA

Because of previous contradictory evidence, a large prospective randomized clinical trial was conducted in Europe, Australia, Canada, and Israel.[52] Women at high risk of having a pregnancy with a neural tube defect, because of a previous pregnancy, were randomized to receive folic acid, or other vitamins or both or neither. Folic acid supplementation, but not other vitamins, had a 72% protective effect (relative risk 0.28, 95% CI 0.12 to 0.71). The U.S.P.H.S. now recommends 0.4 mg for all women capable of becoming pregnant.[94]

CHRONIC NEUROLOGIC DISEASES

Acute and chronic neurologic diseases of non-nutritional origin that impair consciousness or motor functions essential to adequate nutritional intake, such as paralysis or weakness or the facial muscles, the tongue, the pharynx, and the muscles of deglutition, frequently require the temporary or permanent use of a nasogastric tube or a gastrostomy. These measures make proper enteral nutrition possible and may, in fact, prove to be lifesaving. In most of these disorders, nutritional support does not affect the basic pathogenesis of the disease. The use of B-complex vitamin preparations for a variety of acute and chronic neurologic diseases of cryptic origin continues to be common medical practice. To date, however, no objective evidence exists that this practice has any effect on the speed of recovery of the afflicted nervous tissue.

Specific nutritional therapy has been advocated for several neurologic diseases of undetermined origin. For instance, a lowfat diet has been recommended as an effective means of reducing the incidence of exacerbations in patients with multiple sclerosis. However, objective evaluation of the efficacy of this treatment has not yet been possible. Epidemiologic studies relating multiple sclerosis to nutritional factors have revealed a possible correlation between the incidence of the disease, the total fat intake, and the percentage of calories of animal origin consumed.[53] Multiple sclerosis tends to be more prevalent in countries in which the use of animal fat is high. It has also been suggested that the administration of unsaturated fatty acids, such as linoleic or arachidonic acid, may reduce the number and severity of multiple sclerosis attacks. This idea is based on the observation that brain and spinal cord gleaned from patients who have died of multiple sclerosis are deficient in unsaturated fatty acids and that linoleic and arachidonic acid tend to inhibit the lymphocyte-antigen interaction, the cellular mechanism that may enhance demyelination. Sensitized lymphocytes probably interact with myelin components in the affected parts of the nervous system during an attack. That the ingestion of unsaturated fatty acids, such as linoleic acid, affects the course of multiple sclerosis remains unproved.[53]

Although Parkinson's disease is not caused by altered nutrition, it responds favorably to a combination of specific therapy and dietary manipulation. The administration of the amino acid levodopa (L-dihydroxyphenylalanine) is known to improve the symptoms of Parkinson's disease, i.e., rigidity, bradykinesia, and tremor. On entry into the appropriate nerve cells of the affected parts of the brain, levodopa is converted to the deficient catecholamine dopamine. Most of the ingested levodopa is converted to dopamine in nerve cells located in peripheral ganglia, and only 1% of the amino acid is made available to the brain. The enzymatic reaction that converts levodopa to dopamine, a vitamin B_6-dependent decarboxylase, can be stimulated by excessive amounts of the vitamin, shunting even more levodopa to the periphery. As a result, the beneficial effects of levodopa may be drastically reduced when supplemental vitamin preparations containing pyridoxine are added to the daily dose of levodopa. Therefore, use of such preparations should be avoided. Because the amino acids contained in the standard diet tend to compete with the gastrointestinal absorption of levodopa, the daily protein intake of parkinsonian patients receiving levodopa should be kept in the vicinity of 0.5 g protein/kg/day. In addition, the medication should not be ingested with foods rich in amino acids, such as meat and dairy products.[54]

Anticonvulsant Effect of Ketogenic Diet. Ketosis and acidosis resulting from minimal caloric intake or starvation have an anticonvulsant effect. This knowledge had led to the successful clinical use of a diet high in fat and low in carbohydrate, the ketogenic diet, as therapy for seizure disorders in which all other forms of treatment have failed. The mechanism of action of the ketogenic diet on seizures remains unknown, but the anticonvulsant effect of the diet is maintained as long as blood levels of ketone bodies remain elevated. Because the diet has such an impressive effect on certain seizure types (absence and myoclonic), it deserves consideration as a mode of therapy. The diet appears to be most effective in children under the age of 10 years. To ensure success, the diet must be followed rigidly, which presents problems in terms of acceptance and compliance. A more recently developed ketogenic diet including medium-chain triglycerides has permitted liberalization of carbohydrate and protein intake, making the diet more acceptable to the patient.[55]

HEADACHE

A link between the consumption of certain foods and the occurrence of headaches, particularly of the migraine type, has been suspected since Hippocratic days.[56] Such foods as chocolate, cheese, citrus fruit, and alcoholic beverages are most frequently associated with migraine headaches.[57] It is postulated that tyramine, a monoamine contained in relatively high concentrations in these foods, triggers the symptoms.[56] Tyramine is found mainly in foods and beverages that have undergone bacterial decomposition, such as cheddar and blue cheese and certain wines.[56] Theoretically, tyramine, by virtue of sympathomimetic properties, acts either directly or indirectly through the release of norepinephrine, a powerful vasoconstrictor, on sensitive blood vessels that in turn provoke a migraine attack. Biochemical studies on the platelets of some patients with migraine headaches have revealed a deficiency of phenosulfotransferase, an enzyme that detoxifies the phenol groups contained in certain foods by the addition of a sulfate radical.[58,59] Tyramine ingestion may result in intense throbbing headache sometimes associated with hypertension in patients receiving monoamine oxidase inhibitors for depression. Dietary phenylethylamine, contained in such foods as chocolate, cheese, and alcoholic beverages, may also precipitate migraine attacks in some individuals, presumably by virtue of defective phenylethylamine oxidation. Certain food additives, notably sodium nitrite and nitrate (meat preservatives used in processed meats), sodium glutamate (a flavor enhancer and a food preservative), and tartrazine (a coloring agent), have also been associated with headaches. Sodium glutamate, frequently used in certain Chinese dishes, when consumed in large quantities, may precipitate a generalized vasomotor reaction consisting of perioral numbness, flushing of the face, dizziness, and headache (Chinese restaurant syndrome) in sensitive individuals.[60,61] Whereas nitrates and nitrites contained in such processed meats as hot dogs have been blamed for migraine attacks, one clinical study suggests that the headaches are in fact provoked by the amount of pork contained in these products, rather than by the preservatives.[62]

In general, the results of clinical investigations of the association of foods and their constituents and headaches remain controversial. Results of some studies seem to confirm the connection whereas others deny it, attributing "diet-induced" headaches to psychologic factors. Until a consensus has been established, migraine sufferers should be advised to abstain whenever possible from foods thought to provoke an attack.

NEUROPATHY, NEURALGIA, AND DEMENTIA

Nutritional therapy consisting of vitamins and other nutrients continues to be used to treat neurologic disorders of unknown cause, in spite of a total lack of scientific rationale. The popularity of administering large doses of B vitamins as therapy for peripheral neuropathies, neuralgias, and dementias of uncertain origin stems from the fact that experimentally induced deficiencies of these vitamins in animals frequently result in symptoms caused by reversible lesions of the peripheral and central nervous system. In most instances, the far-advanced lesions show demyelination and destruction of nerve fibers as well as damage to nerve cells, a frequent finding in many human neurologic diseases. These observations have led to the erroneous belief that diseases in human beings with similar clinical and pathologic attributes will improve more rapidly and more completely after the administration of vitamins in doses that frequently exceed those used to maintain adequate nutrition. In most instances, lack of knowledge, frustration on the part of the patient and the physician, and the desire to try any type of "shotgun" therapy have led to the irrational and medically unsound use of vitamins and special diets in the treatment of such neurologic disorders as neuropathies, neuralgias, and dementias.

Thiamin, in huge doses, is used frequently to treat peripheral neuropathy of undetermined cause. To date, no scientific evidence shows that the vitamin either protects peripheral nerve fibers from further damage or enhances regeneration or remyelination, except when severe thiamin deficiency has been demonstrated by appropriate laboratory tests. The same can be said for the use of large doses of vitamin B_{12} in trigeminal or postherapeutic neuralgia. The neuropathy, subacute degeneration of the spinal cord, degeneration of the optic nerve, and dementia associated with vitamin B_{12} deficiency respond dramatically to appropriate doses of the vitamin, as does the rare case of dementia caused by folate or niacin deficiency. Treatment with large doses of B-vitamin complex has no effect on toxic, metabolic, familial, or traumatic neuropathies. Similarly, dementias, such as Alzheimer's and Pick's diseases, do not respond to megavitamin therapy.

VITAMIN TOXICITY AND NEUROLOGIC DEFECTS

Recent decades have witnessed the misuse of vitamins in doses that far exceed the accepted daily requirements. Along with an emphasis on weight-reduction diets, better nutrition, and improved physical and mental health, a belief has developed that vitamins will increase athletic stamina and performance and that if a small dose of a vitamin is good, a megadose must, by necessity, be better. This concept has been responsible for the overcommercialization and indiscriminate use of vitamins.[63] However, considering the large doses of vitamins consumed daily, for a variety of reasons, by an ever-increasing number of people, vitamin toxicity affecting the nervous system is relatively rare. Of all the vitamins, both water- and fat-soluble, only two—vitamin A and pyridoxine (vitamin B_6)—are known to produce adverse neurologic reactions when ingested in pharmacologic rather than recommended nutritional doses.

Vitamin A. This vitamin has been used to excess by patients suffering from acne and health food addicts.

Although susceptibility to vitamin A toxicity tends to be highly variable, a dose in excess of 25,000 IU per day (10 times the recommended daily allowance) ingested over a period of months can lead to toxic symptoms. Infants and children tend to be more susceptible,[64,65] as are those with renal insufficiency. The abusive intake of alcohol further enhances the toxicity of this vitamin.[65]

Toxicity occurs when the capacity of the retinol binding system in the plasma and cells is exceeded. The excessive vitamin A is then presented to cell membranes and organelles in unbound form. It is presumed that an excess of the vitamin leads to increased permeability of the choroid plexus in the brain and a consequent increase in the formation of cerebrospinal fluid. The result is a clinical condition known as pseudotumor cerebri, or benign increased intracranial pressure. Patients complain of headache, drowsiness, blurred vision, and diplopia. They may exhibit nuchal rigidity, papilledema, and bilateral abducens weakness, all caused by increased intracranial pressure. Once the vitamin has been withheld, recovery from toxicity occurs in 2 to 3 days. In some instances, resolution of symptoms and signs of toxicity may take several weeks.[66,67]

Vitamin A ingested in excessive amounts during the first trimester of pregnancy may be responsible for cleft palate, harelip, macroglossia, defective eye development, or hydrocephalus in the fetus.

Vitamin B_6. Excessive doses of vitamin B_6 have been used for general health purposes, premenstrual syndrome, carpal tunnel syndrome, schizophrenia, and childhood autism. Until recently, it was assumed that high doses of the vitamin were generally harmless. One group of authors has shown that when pyridoxine is ingested in gram quantities per day (6 g per day) for 5 to 40 months, a severe, slowly reversible, symmetric, distal, areflexic, sensory neuropathy may ensue.[68] Even smaller doses (500 mg per day) may result in neuropathy.[69] Patients complain of progressive ataxia, particularly in the dark (loss of visual cues), accompanied by numbness of the feet and severe sensory dysfunction characterized by a decrease in joint position and vibratory sense, a decrease in the sense of touch in a distal symmetric distribution, and a decrease in the sensation of the lips and tongue. Results of spinal fluid examination tend to be normal. Standard electrical studies performed after the illness is well established reflect degeneration of large axons and small myelinated fibers that in turn reflect pathologic changes in the dorsal root and gasserian ganglia.[68]

ANTICONVULSANT-INDUCED VITAMIN INSUFFICIENCY

Folate. Patients taking anticonvulsant drugs for seizure disorders may incur a significant degree of folic acid deficiency.[70,71] Although phenytoin appears to be the drug implicated most frequently, phenobarbital and primidone may also be involved, but to a lesser degree and frequency. These drugs are thought to affect the metabolism of folate or its metabolites because of similarities in chemical structure, because of a drug-induced impairment of absorption or of tissue transport, or because of competitive inhibition of vitamin coenzyme formation.[72] After the long-term administration of these drugs, a decrease in the serum, cerebrospinal fluid, and red blood cell folate levels can be detected, and a megaloblastic anemia and/or neuropsychiatric complications characterized by apathy, depression, and, eventually, dementia may occur.

Reports on the effects of folic acid on seizure control are conflicting. It has been suggested that in some patients, the administration of folic acid may increase the frequency of seizures and that folic acid and its derivatives may have significant convulsive properties.[73] Results of experiments in animals suggest a possible blockade of inhibitory γ-aminobutyric acid receptors by folic acid, reducing seizure thresholds.[74]

Carefully controlled clinical studies are needed before the relationship among anticonvulsants, folate, and seizure control can be confirmed and fully understood.[75] It seems reasonable to screen the serum folate levels of patients who have received phenytoin for recurrent seizures over a prolonged period, particularly in patients who demonstrate such unusual neuropsychiatric problems as dementia.

Vitamin D. The prolonged administration of anticonvulsant drugs, such as phenytoin, may lead to a decrease in bone mineral content. The severity of demineralization appears to be related to the dose of the drug, a deficiency of physical activity, and a lack of exposure to sunlight. However, pathologic fractures as a result of demineralization are rare. The drugs interact with the vitamin, decreasing intestinal calcium absorption and redistribution. The problem in the United States does not appear to be of sufficient clinical importance to warrant the routine vitamin D supplementation of patients treated with antiepileptic drugs; however, the possibility should be borne in mind, and vitamin D metabolites should be estimated periodically in patients on longterm phenytoin therapy with poor intake or malabsorption.

Vitamin K. The use of antiepileptic drugs phenytoin, phenobarbital, and primidone, individually or in combination, to treat epileptic pregnant women can cause bleeding in the neonate by depressing the production or the release of the vitamin K-dependent clotting factors prothrombin and factors V and VII. Vitamin K should be administered in the late stages of pregnancy to the neonate and the mother under treatment for epilepsy.[76]

Valproic Acid and Hyperammonemia. Valproic acid, a widely used and effective anticonvulsant drug, can cause hepatic failure and hyperammonemia. The latter has been reported in the absence of laboratory evidence of hepatic dysfunction in children receiving multiple anticonvulsant drugs.[77–81] In this group of patients, hyperammonemia appears to be dose related and may occur after several years of therapy. Hyperammonemia may underlie unexplained episodes of stupor, coma, and increased seizure activity, weight loss, nausea, anorexia, and vomiting. According to some investigators, the biochemical mechanism responsible for the hyperammonemia consists of the accumulation of propionate, one of the metabolites of valproic acid, and the inhibition of carbamyl phosphate synthetase, one of the enzymes involved in the conversion of ammonia to urea.[77] A partial inborn error of ammonia metabolism in certain children may render them more vulnerable to hyperammonemia when they are treated with valproic acid. Valproic acid therapy may cause asymptomatic hepatic dysfunction and hyperammonemia. Therefore, liver function tests, including ammonia blood levels, are indicated at periodic intervals in patients receiving this drug, and its use should be discontinued in the presence of abnormal liver function tests and/or hyperammonemia. In patients in whom valproic acid has proved to be the most effective anticonvulsant agent, the drug can be continued cautiously, provided the dietary intake of protein is sharply curtailed. This regimen may result in the reversal of abnormal liver function test results, including hyperammonemia.[82]

FOOD ADDITIVES

The idea that food additives, such as synthetic food dyes and certain naturally occurring ingredients, adversely affect the behavior and learning of children has attracted considerable attention since it was first suggested several decades ago. Clinical data gathered to date have been extremely controversial. Feingold has claimed that strict adherence to his **diet,** a diet totally devoid of additives, including dyes and antioxidants, leads to improvement or complete remission of hyperkinetic behavior and learning disability in 50 to 70% of afflicted children.[83] Furthermore, in 75% of such children, the diet has been claimed to be as effective as such stimulants as methylphenidate hydrochloride (Ritalin) and dextroamphetamine. The beneficial effect of the diet, sometimes referred to as "the Feingold effect," has been reported to occur in a matter of days to weeks, provided there is 100% adherence to the diet. The younger the child, the more rapid and complete the degree of improvement. The published accounts of the dramatic effects of the diet are either anecdotal or based mainly on essentially uncontrolled clinical trials.[83,84]

In 1982, a Consensus Development Conference was convened at the National Institutes of Health to evaluate the available information on the subject.[85] Anderson has summarized some of the conference findings as follows:[86]

Some significant and well-controlled studies have verified the following impressions:

1. The Feingold type of diet may be helpful in some children with the attention deficit disorder with hyperkinesis (not 50% as Feingold stated).[87,88*]
2. The diet seemed most helpful in younger children.
3. Challenge with higher doses of food colors in children might produce a pharmacologic-like effect to depress learning in a specific test situation.[89]
4. Allergic (hypersensitivity) as well as other reactions to foods or food additives probably have nothing to do with the effects of the diet on behavior.

Significant biochemical and neurobehavioral effects of artificial food colors have been reported by a number of research laboratories. The best-studied example is erythrosin B (FDC Red #3). This artificial coloring agent, when added in vitro, alters membrane conductance, changing the movement of the cations sodium and potassium across the membrane. The dye has the unique property of acting only on the sodium and potassium ATPase of brain; it is not active on the enzyme found in other tissues, such as liver and red blood cells. It is a potent noncompetitive inhibitor of dopamine uptake by nerve endings prepared from rat brain exposed to the dye for 5 minutes. Other authors have shown that the compound inhibits the uptake of many other neurotransmitters and precursors, an effect diluted by increasing amounts of tissue in the biochemical assay. Whether these neurochemical properties of this particular food dye can be extrapolated to hyperactive behavior and learning disorders in children remains to be shown.[90–93]

Well-designed clinical studies that take into consideration genetic predisposition, variability and heterogeneity, dosage, time of administration, and easily measured objective and significant clinical end points seem essential before it is possible to establish beyond doubt that food additives have an adverse effect on behavior.

In summary, neurologic diseases and their relationship to nutritional and dietary factors have been discussed. In some of the disorders, improper or inadequate nutrition is implicated; therefore, dietary manipulation constitutes the main mode of therapy. In others, a combination of genetic and metabolic factors, as well as dietary factors, underlies the symptoms and signs of neurologic dysfunction that can be ameliorated by changes in the diet and/or vitamin supplementation. In some disorders, such as migraine headache and hyperactivity in children, the beneficial effects of altered nutrition remain controversial. In such neurologic diseases as dementia, in which no obvious nutritional cause has been established, dietary treatment has not been successful.

Despite significant advances over the past decades in the field of nutrition, large gaps remain in our understanding of the role of nutrition in the normal and

*Reference numbers in this quotation are those of this chapter.

abnormal metabolic activity of the nervous system. More sensitive and critical methods for the assessment of the nutritional status of the nervous system and for the valuation of the dietary management of neuropsychiatric disorders are essential before more rational and effective therapeutic manipulations can be developed.

REFERENCES

1. Williams, R.R.: Toward the Conquest of Beriberi. Cambridge, MA, Harvard University Press, 1970.
2. Terris, M.: Goldberger on Pellagra. Baton Rouge, Louisiana State University Press, 1964.
3. Victor, M., Adams, R.D.: Am. J. Clin. Nutr., *9:*379–397, 1961.
4. Victor, M., Adams, R.D., Collins, G.H.: The Wernicke-Korsakoff's Syndrome. 2nd Ed. Philadelphia, F.A. Davis, 1989.
5. Charness, M.E., Simon, R.P., Greenberg, D.A.: N. Engl. J. Med., *321:*442–453, 1989.
6. Watson, A.J.S., Walker, G.H., Tomkin, M.M.R., et al.: Ir. J. Med. Sci., *150:*301–303, 1981.
7. Dreyfus, P.M.: N. Engl. J. Med., *267:*596–598, 1962.
8. Pratt, O.E., Jayosingham, M., Shaw, G.K., et al.: Transketolose variant enzymes and brain damage. Alcohol Alcohol., *20:*223–232, 1985.
9. Velez, R.J., Myers, B., Guber, M.S. Severe acute metabolic acidosis (acute beriberi): An avoidable complication of total parenteral nutrition. JPEN J. Parenter. Enteral Nutr., *9:*216–219, 1985.
10. Victor, M.: Polyneuropathy due to nutritional deficiency and alcoholism. *In* Peripheral Neuropathy. Edited by P.J. Dyck. Philadelphia, W.B. Saunders, 1975.
11. Mayer, R.F., Garcia-Mullin, R.: Peripheral nerve and muscle disorders associated with alcoholism. *In* Biology of Alcoholism. Edited by B. Kissin and H. Begleiter. New York, Plenum Publishing, 1972.
12. Gill, G.V., Bell, D.R.: J. Neurol. Neurosurg. Psychiatry, *45:*861–865, 1982.
13. Hawley, R.J., Kurtzke, J.F., Armbrustmacher, J.W., et al.: Acta Neurol. Scand., *66:*582–589, 1982.
14. Dreyfus, P.M.: Amblyopia and other neurological disorders associated with chronic alcoholism. *In* Handbook of Clinical Neurology. Edited by P.J. Vinken and G.W. Bruyn. Amsterdam, North Holland Publishing, 1976.
15. Iansek, R., Edge, C.J.: J. Neurol. Neurosurg. Psychiatry, *48:*1307–1308, 1985.
16. Thompson, R.E., Felton, J.L.: Ann. Ophthalmol., *14:*848–850, 1982.
17. Lerman, S., Feldman, A.L.: Arch. Ophthalmol., *65:*381–385, 1961.
18. Victor, M., Adams, R.D., Mancall, E.L.: Arch. Neurol., *1:*479–688, 1959.
19. Mancall, E., McEntee, W.J.: Neurology, *15:*303–313, 1965.
20. Martin, D.C.: Clin. Geriatr. Med., *4:*841–842, 1988.
21. Lindenbaum, J., Healton, E.B., Savage, D.G., et al.: N. Engl. J. Med., *318:*1720–1728, 1988.
22. Frenkel, E.P.: J. Clin. Invest., *52:*1237–1245, 1973.
23. Frenkel, E.P., Kitchens, R.L., Johnston, J.M.: J. Biol. Chem., *248:*7540–7546, 1973.
24. Dreyfus, P.M., Dube, V.: Clin. Chim. Acta, *15:*525–528, 1967.
25. Jolliffe, N., Bowman, K.M., Rosenblum, L.A., et al.: JAMA, *114:*307–312, 1940.
26. Muller, D.P.: Lancet, *1:*225–228, 1983.
27. Sokol, R.J., Guggenheim, M., Iannaccone, S.T., et al.: N. Engl. J. Med., *313:*1580–1586, 1985.
28. Gutmann, L., Shockor, W., Guttman, L., et al.: Neurology, *36:*554–556, 1986.
29. Muller, D.P., Lloyd, J.K., Wolff, O.H.: Ciba Found. Symp., *101:*106–121, 1983.
30. Landrieu, P., Selva, J., Alvarez, F., et al.: Neuropediatrics, *16:*194–201, 1985.
31. MacGilchrist, A.J., Mills, P.R., Noble, M., et al.: J. Inherited Metab. Dis., *11:*184–190, 1988.
32. Jeffrey, G.P., Muller, D.P., Burroughs, A.K., et al.: J. Hepatol., *4:*307–317, 1987.
33. Harding, A.E., Matthews, A.I.M.L.S., Jones, S., et al.: N. Eng. J. Med., *313:*32–35, 1985.
34. Traber, M.G., Sokol, R.H., Ringel, S.P., et al.: N. Engl. J. Med., *317:*262–265, 1987.
35. Centerwall, W.R., Centerwall, A.S., Armon, V., et al.: Pediatrics, *59:*93–101, 1961.
36. Holliday, M.A., Anderson, A.S., Barness, L.A., et al.: Pediatrics, *57:*783–792, 1976.
37. Cornblath, M., Schwartz, R.: Disorders of Carbohydrate Metabolism in Infancy. 2nd Ed. Philadelphia, W.B. Saunders, 1976.
38. Fischler, K.: Pediatrics, *50:*412–419, 1972.
39. Scheinberg, I.H.: Wilson's Disease. Philadelphia, W.B. Saunders, 1984.
40. Sternleib, I., Scheinberg, I.H.: JAMA, *189:*748–754, 1964.
41. Refsum, S.: Acta Psychiatr. Scand., *(Suppl. 38):*1, 1946.
42. Steinberg, D., Mize, C.E., Herndon, J.H., Jr., et al.: Arch. Intern. Med., *125:*75–87, 1970.
43. Mudd, S.H.: Adv. Nutr. Res., *4:*1–34, 1982.
44. Scheinberg, I.H., Jaffe, M.E., Sternlieb, I.: N. Engl. J. Med., *317:*209–213, 1987.
45. Bremer, G.J., Hill, G.M., Prasad, A.S., et al.: Oral zinc therapy for Wilson's disease. Ann. Intern. Med., *99:*314–320, 1983.
46. Strickland, G.T., Blackwell, R.A., Walten, R.H.: Am. J. Med., *51:*31–40, 1971.
47. Rosenberg, L.E.: Curr. Concepts Nutr., *8:*55–64, 1979.
48. Dodge, P.R., Prensky, A.L., Feigin, R.D., et al.: Nutrition and the Developing Nervous System. St. Louis, C.V. Mosby, 1975.
49. Menkes, J.H.: Textbook of Child Neurology. 3rd Ed. Philadelphia, Lea & Febiger, 1985.
50. Freeman, J.M. Neonatal seizures. *In* Pediatric Epileptology. Edited by F.E. Dreifuss. John Wright. Littleton, MA, PSG, 1983.
51. Conn, H.O.: Hosp. Pract., *8:*65–72, 1973.
52. MRC Vitamin Study Research Group: Lancet, *338:*131–137, 1991.
53. Fields, E.J.: J.R. Soc. Med., *72:*487–488, 1979.
54. Mena, I., Cotzias, G.C.: N. Engl. J. Med., *292:*181–184, 1975.

55. Withrow, C.D.: The Ketogenic Diet: Mechanism of anticonvulsant action. *In* Antiepileptic Drugs. Edited by D.M. Woodbury, J.K. Penry, and R.P. Schmidt. New York, Raven Press, 1972.
56. Kohlenberg, R.J.: Headache, *22:*30–34, 1982.
57. Wilson, C.W.M., Kirker, J.G., Warnes, H., et al.: Postgrad. Med. J., *56:*617–621, 1980.
58. Littlewood, J., Glover, V., Sandler, M., et al.: Lancet, *1:*983–985, 1982.
59. Glover, V., Littlewood, J., Sandler, M., et al.: Headache, *23:*53–58, 1983.
60. Medina, J.L., Diamond, S.: Headache, *18:*31–34, 1978.
61. Hanington, E.: J. Hum. Nutr., *34:*175–180, 1980.
62. Bernstein, A.: Personal communication, 1986.
63. Rudman, D., Williams, P.J.: N. Engl. J. Med., *309:*488–489, 1983.
64. Farris, W.A., Erdman, J.W., Jr.: JAMA, *247:*1317–1318, 1982.
65. Herbert, V.: Am. J. Clin. Nutr., *36:*185–186, 1982.
66. Leo, M.A., Arai, M., Sato, M., et al.: Gastroenterology, *82:*194–205, 1982.
67. Bauernfeind, J.C.: *In* The Safe Use of Vitamin A. Edited by G. Arroyare, et al. New York, Nutrition Foundation, 1980.
68. Schaumburg, H., Kaplan, J., Windebank, A., et al.: N. Engl. J. Med., *309:*445–448, 1983.
69. Berger, A., Schaumburg, H.H.: N. Engl. J. Med., *311:*986–987, 1984.
70. Reynolds, E.H., Mattson, R.H., Gallagher, B.B.: Neurology, *22:*841–844, 1972.
71. Smith, D.B., Obbens, E.A.M.T.: Antifolate-antiepileptic relationships in folic acid. *In* Neurology, Psychiatry, and Internal Medicine. Edited by M.I. Botez and E.H. Reynolds. New York, Raven Press, 1979.
72. Pisciotta, A.V.: Phenytoin, hematological toxicity. *In* Antiepileptic Drugs. Edited by D.M. Woodbury, J.K. Penry, and C.E. Pippenger. New York, Raven Press, 1982.
73. Baylis, E.M., Crowley, J.M., Preece, J.M., et al.: Lancet, *1:*62–64, 1971.
74. Roberts, P.J.: Nature, *250:*429–430, 1974.
75. Mattson, R.H., Gallagher, B.B., Reynolds, E.H., et al.: Arch. Neurol., *29:*78–81, 1973.
76. Kutt, H., Solomon, G.E.: Antiepileptic drugs. Phenytoin: Relevant side effects. *In* Antiepiieptic Drugs. Edited by D.M. Woodbury, J.K. Penry, and R.P. Schmidt. New York, Raven Press, 1972.
77. Coulter, D.L., Allen, R.J.: Lancet, *1:*1310–1311, 1980.
78. Rawat, S., Borkowski, W.J., Swick, H.M.: Neurology, *31:*1173–1174, 1981.
79. Murphy, J.V., Marquardt, K.: Arch. Neurol., *39:*591–592, 1982.
80. Cotariu, D., Zaidman, J.L.: Clin. Chem., *34:*890–897, 1988.
81. Iinuma, K., Hayasaka, K., Narisawa, K., et al.: Eur. J. Pediatr., *148:*267–269, 1988.
82. Dreyfus, P.M.: Personal observation, 1985.
83. Feingold, B.F.: Dietary management of behavior and learning disabilities. *In* Nutrition and Behavior. Edited by S.A. Miller. Philadelphia, Franklin Institute Press, 1981.
84. Feingold, B.F.: Why Your Child is Hyperactive. New York, Random House, 1975.
85. National Institutes of Health Consensus Development Conference: Defined Diets in Childhood Hyperactivity. Office for Medical Applications of Research, Bethesda, Maryland. Washington, D.C., National Institutes of Health, January, 1982.
86. Anderson, J.A.: Nutr. Rev., *42:*112, 1984.
87. Harley, J.P., Ray, R.S., Tomasi, L., et al.: Pediatrics, *61:*818–828, 1978.
88. Weiss, B., Williams, J.H., Margen, S.: Science, *207:*1487–1488, 1980.
89. Swanson, J.M., Kinsbourne, M.: Science, *207:*1485–1487, 1980.
90. Silbergeld, E.K., Anderson, S.M.: Bull. N.Y. Acad. Med., *58:*275–295, 1982.
91. Rose, T.L.: J. Appl. Behav. Anal., *11:*439–446, 1978.
92. Mailman, R.B., Ferris, R.M., Tang, F.L.M., et al.: Science, *207:*535–537, 1980.
93. Dickerson, J.W., Pepler, F.: J. Hum. Nutr., *34:*167–174, 1980.
94. Centers for Disease Control: MMWR, *41:*81–85, 1982.

CHAPTER **75**

Nutrition and Diet in Rheumatic Diseases

Alfred Jay Bollet

The field of rheumatic diseases encompasses a wide range of diseases and pathologic processes, most of which affect joint tissues and thus cause symptoms of arthritis. The basic structure affected by these diseases is the connective tissue, and these disorders are also known as connective tissue diseases, or "collagen diseases," the latter term arising when collagen meant all connective tissue. Because collagen now refers to a group of specific fibrillar proteins in that tissue, the name collagen disease is obsolete.

The connective tissues usually affected in rheumatic diseases include synovial membrane lining joint surfaces, cartilage, bone, tendons, ligaments, interstitial tissues in all organs, and blood vessels. Vasculitis occurs commonly, particularly affecting arterioles and venules, but in some instances, large arteries, including the aorta, are affected. By convention, arteriosclerotic vascular lesions and inflammation of large veins (phlebitis) are not considered connective tissue diseases.

Because connective tissues are found in every organ, manifestations of rheumatic diseases can vary, but joint tissues are affected most commonly and arthritis is a frequent manifestation of these diseases. There are over 100 different rheumatic diseases, with a wide variety of pathologic processes, including local or widespread inflammation, immune mechanisms, physical wear, and inherited metabolic abnormalities. Muscle diseases and vaguely defined painful syndromes such as "fibrositis" are common rheumatic diseases, along with many temporary but annoying focal connective tissue syndromes, including traumatic sprains and strains, focal myositis, tendinitis, and tendon-sheath abnormalities. The most frequent serious rheumatic diseases are rheumatoid arthritis (RA), osteoarthritis (OA), gout, and systemic lupus erythematosus (SLE). The focus of this chapter is primarily on nutritional considerations in those diseases.

Pain is the most frequent manifestation of rheumatic disease. Although spontaneous improvement eventually occurs in most instances, therapy for many forms of arthritis is not curative. Therefore, most connective tissue diseases become chronic and patients are always seeking more satisfactory treatment. Food faddists prey on patients with rheumatic diseases because of the attractiveness of nonpharmacologic therapy; the lay literature abounds in dietary "cures" for arthritis. When spontaneous improvement occurs, patients usually attribute it to the last therapy tried; favorable testimonials result, providing quotes for lay articles and books, which rarely identify the nature of the arthritis in the patients quoted. Because the causes and underlying pathologic processes of the diseases that cause arthritis are extremely varied, any publication that fails to identify the nature of the disease treated, lumping all "arthritis" as if it is one disease, is valueless.

Nutritional deficiency syndromes may result from limiting intake to what have been referred to as "miracle foods." Growth retardation is a possible consequence of bizarre diets in children with juvenile chronic arthritis.[1]

Fasting, experimental diets, use of or elimination of specific foods or types of food, and studies of food allergy have been the subject of numerous papers concerning human disease or experimentally induced arthritis in animal models. A list of articles of this type can be found elsewhere.[2]

NUTRITIONAL INFLUENCES ON THE STRUCTURE AND METABOLISM OF CONNECTIVE TISSUE

Mature connective tissues are varied in structure and function. Articular cartilage is easily compressed, making it energy absorbing; it is self-lubricating, its high water content making it weep like a sponge when a load is applied, keeping friction during joint motion extremely low. Ligaments, tendons, and bone provide support and strong attachments for muscles. Loose areolar interstitial tissue and capillary walls control diffusion of large molecules, allowing rapid movement of nutrients and wastes between cells and plasma. The cells synthesize the basic constituents of each of these forms of connective tissue, and are named according to the physical characteristics of the mature tissue they form (osteocytes, fibrocytes, chondrocytes, etc.) When the tissue is immature, with active synthesis of its extracellular constituents, the cells usually are referred to as "blasts" (chondroblasts, fibroblasts, etc.)

The main fibrillar components of the connective tissues are the proteins elastin, reticulin, and the various types of collagen. Interspersed among the fibers are the constituents of the "ground substance," including the proteoglycans, which are high-molecular weight substances containing large, complex polysaccharides (the glycosaminoglycans). The proteoglycans can bind large amounts of water and electrolytes. Space does not permit a thorough description of the chemistry and metabolism of these compounds; it is worthy of emphasis, however, that the polysaccharide components are synthesized from glucose and the rates of synthesis can be affected by the availability of this sugar or its metabolic derivatives, such as uridine diphosphoglucose (UDPG).

The protein components of connective tissue, including the collagens and the protein moieties of the proteoglycans, are affected by nutritional influences in a fashion similar to those that affect other structural proteins. The first true connective tissue disease described was scurvy; ascorbic acid is essential for synthesis of collagen. Scurvy, then, is actually a "collagen disease;" weakness of the collagenous structure of small blood vessels leads to the multiple, small, interstitial hemorrhages that occur in this disease (see subsequent discussion). Collagen serves in part as a reservoir protein, providing a source of amino acids in times of negative nitrogen balance,[3] although not as readily as muscle protein. Mobilization of collagen does occur during starvation or protein deficiency, or in states of protein catabolism, such as occurs when corticosteroids are administered.

Loss of collagen becomes evident in the structures with the most collagen; namely, the bone and the skin, with 50 and 25% of the collagen, respectively. The rest of the connective tissues contain the remaining 25% of the collagen. Diminution of bone collagen content, resulting in thinning of the bone owing to the decrease in bone matrix (osteoporosis) occurs in starvation or other states of prolonged negative nitrogen balance.

NUTRITION, INFLAMMATION, AND IMMUNE PHENOMENA

The most frequent pathologic process affecting the connective tissues in the rheumatic diseases is inflammation. In the past, it was not realized that inflammation was susceptible to nutritional influences, but now, it is clear that fatty acid derivatives, the prostaglandins, play a key role in the pathogenesis of the inflammatory process, and experimental data (see subsequent section) have shown that dietary changes can modify the production of prostaglandins during inflammation. In many rheumatic diseases, antibodies are formed that react with tissue components, so-called autoantibodies, and these diseases are often referred to as "autoimmune" diseases. A variety of immune mechanisms occur in these diseases; we are beginning to recognize and understand nutritional influences on these immune phenomena,[4] which may become more important in the near future.

The most common and serious forms of chronic arthritis are rheumatoid arthritis (RA) and osteoarthritis (OA). The former is a widespread inflammation affecting small and large joints resulting from immune-mediated tissue damage; it can begin at any age, and varies greatly in severity and manifestations. Osteoarthritis, on the other hand, is a wear-and-tear process, characterized by degeneration of articular cartilage with secondary changes in underlying bone and surrounding tissues. It usually occurs in older people, primarily affecting joints that have endured excessive wear, and often it is limited to one or a few joints. Genetic factors play a role in certain forms of familial OA, but most patients have no major metabolic abnormality.

Muscle wasting is a common manifestation of chronic joint disease, because muscle inflammation occurs commonly as part of all types of arthritis, and joint immobility because of pain also leads to focal muscle atrophy around affected joints. Some patients with RA have fever and other systemic manifestations, leading to anorexia, weight loss, and even inanition in severe cases. In such instances, the negative nitrogen balance can contribute to the muscle wasting, and nutritional influences are of importance in these patients.

Inflammation is a complicated process that includes activation of cascade systems of plasma proteins and attraction of proinflammatory cells, resulting in release or activation of enzymes, cytokines, and other factors that play a role in mobilization of responsive cells and in tissue destruction. These phenomena include formation of active products of the kinin and complement systems, release of endogenous pyrogen and other mediators from cells, release of lysosomal enzymes, and appearance in the plasma of "acute phase reactants" formed in the liver.

In chronic inflammatory states, mononuclear phagocytes release agents with phlogistic activity, including interleukin 1 (IL-1), the leukocyte pyrogen, which affects the hypothalamus and produces fever and a hypermetabolic state, and tumor necrosis factor (TNF). These agents cause lipolysis and gluconeogenesis, secondarily causing hyperglycemia, hyperinsulinemia, elevated free fatty acid levels, and glucocorticoid release. Another finding is increased proteolysis of muscle protein mediated by prostaglandin E_2 (PGE_2), which causes muscle wasting and release of free amino acids, some of which are used in the synthesis of acute phase proteins. Thus, chronic inflammation leads to a hypermetabolic state with protein wasting, a condition that can impair immune function.[4]

ROLE OF ESSENTIAL FATTY ACIDS AND EICOSANOIDS

The process of inflammation includes the generation of biologically active fatty acids, the prostaglandins and leukotrienes, from arachidonic acid. The nature of these active products can be influenced by dietary fatty acids (see also Chap. 3).

Prostaglandins and leukotrienes are synthesized by a wide variety of cells, including leukocytes, platelets, and endothelial cells of blood vessels. Arachidonic acid, a constituent of the phospholipids that form mammalian cell membranes, is substrate for cyclooxygenase and lipoxygenase; the former enzyme leads to formation of prostaglandins and thromboxanes, which are proinflammatory and promote platelet adhesion, whereas the latter leads to synthesis of hydroperoxy fatty acids and leukotrienes, which are less potent mediators of inflammation.

Prostaglandins modulate the actions of many tissues and organs, particularly those containing smooth muscle. The prostaglandins of the E series cause vasodilatation, hyperemia, exudation, and increased sensitivity to painful stimuli (tenderness). Prostaglandins also mediate the interrelationships of antibody-producing cells, inhibiting the action of suppressor T cells, leading to increased antibody production, at least in vitro.[5]

Arachidonic acid is the main precursor of prostaglandins, resulting in the formation of compounds of the E series; in cells, this essential fatty acid is located mainly in membrane phospholipids. Dietary arachidonic acid is incorporated preferentially into the phospholipids of activated lymphocytes; this fatty acid constitutes over 20% of the total phospholipid fatty acid content of macrophages.[6]

The fatty acid composition of membrane phospholipids can be altered by diet. Polyunsaturated n-3 fatty acids including eicosopentaenoic acid (EPA, C20:5) and docosahexaenoic acid (DHA, C22:6), which are found in certain marine foods (see Appendix Table A–19b), differ from arachidonic acid in that they contain an extra double bond at the third carbon atom from the methyl terminal. EPA and DHA decrease production of prostaglandins and thromboxanes from arachidonic acid; this is probably the explanation of the prolonged bleeding time of Greenland eskimos whose diet is rich in marine lipids and whose tissues contain large amounts of EPA and DHA. This phenomenon has been linked to the lower incidence of thromboembolic disease and myocardial infarction in this population compared to populations ingesting diets richer in animal fats.[7,8] EPA and DHA also are substrates for lipoxygenase, leading to the formation of leukotriene B_5 (LTB_5), which has less proinflammatory and platelet aggregating effect than leukotriene B_4 (LTB_4), the product derived from arachidonic acid.[9,10]

Polymorphonuclear leukocytes of patients with RA treated with fish oil concentrates produce less LTB_4, resulting in less platelet aggregation.[11] It has also been shown that less IL-1 and TNF are produced by mononuclear cells of volunteers fed 18 g of fish oil concentrate daily for 6 weeks.[12]

Modest beneficial effects of diets supplementated with fish oil fatty acids have been noted in patients with RA in a nonrandomized double-blind trial.[13] A decrease was noted in the number of tender joints and fatigue time in the EPA-treated group, correlating with decreased levels of neutrophil LTB_4. A longer double-blind randomized trial showed similar improvement in the number of tender and swollen joints.[14]

Experimental forms of inflammation in rats have also shown improvement with diets supplemented with γ-linolenic acid (C18:3, n-6), a precursor of monoenoic prostaglandins such as PGE_1. γ-Linolenic acid competes with arachidonic acid for the active site of the cyclooxygenase and lipoxygenase does not act on it, thus curtailing the production of inflammatory leukotrienes.[15] In a study involving the use of a diet containing borage oil, prostaglandin synthesis was shifted toward PGE_1 from PGE_2. Evening primrose oil has been reported to contain 72% linoleic acid and 10% γ-linoleic acid.[16] Borage seed oil, referred to by Tate et al., is stated to contain 47.2% linoleic acid and 23.1% γ-linoleic acid.[15] The chemotactic response of polymorphonuclear leukocytes of rats on this diet was significantly impaired.[17]

Diets deficient in essential fatty acids can modify the response of laboratory animals to inflammatory stimuli. For example, mice on a diet deficient in essential fatty acids showed a significant reduction in both primary and secondary immune responses.[18] Responses to both T cell-dependent and T cell-independent antigens were blunted.[19]

Evidence for diminution in immune response on a diet deficient in essential fatty acid was reported in F1 hybrids of New Zealand Black and New Zealand White mice (NZB/NZW), who develop a form of glomerulonephritis accompanied by antinuclear antibodies; pathologically, this disease resembles the renal disease seen in association with SLE in humans. These rats uniformly die before 1 year of age, but littermates kept on a diet deficient in essential fatty acids have a lower incidence of renal disease, and a considerably longer survival.[20] A similar observation has been made in another strain of mice that develop autoimmune lupus.[21] The rats on a diet deficient in essential fatty acids showed a decreased incidence of glomerulonephritis, decreased subepidermal deposition of immunoglobulins, and decreased development of antibodies to double-stranded DNA.[22]

On the other hand, skin-graft rejection in rats deficient in polyunsaturated fatty acids is potentiated, and the incidence of induced tumors is reduced, suggesting that cell-mediated immune responses are augmented.[6,18,23] Rats on a diet deficient in essential fatty acids show reduced experimentally induced chronic inflammation.[17,24] Adjuvant arthritis, an experimental form of inflammation that has many similarities to human RA and is used widely for screening potential antirheumatic drugs, is suppressed in rats fed such a diet.[24] Inflammatory exudate induced experimentally in these animals is decreased in quantity, and has a lower concentration of prostaglandins that in controls fed a normal diet.[24]

Many of the drugs used in the treatment of the rheumatic diseases affect synthesis of prostaglandins; these agents, called nonsteroidal anti-inflammatory drugs (NSAID), inhibit a key enzyme that catalyzes an early step in the synthesis of these compounds, the cyclooxygenase.[25] Phospholipase A_2 activity, which releases arachidonic acid from membrane lipids, is decreased by treatment with corticosteroids. These pharmacologic approaches diminish prostaglandin formation and are more useful than dietary modifications at present, but the latter may prove to be a safe and effective means of altering the responsiveness of the cells involved in the inflammatory process.

OTHER CLINICAL FINDINGS IN RHEUMATIC DISEASES

The renal involvement that occurs in some patients with systemic connective tissue disease, such as SLE, can lead to the nephrotic syndrome. Loss of protein and various nutrients may be severe and can lead to hypoproteinemia, edema, and other forms of malnutrition, as occurs in other causes of nephrotic syndrome.

Some patients with arthritis have leg edema, in part because of salt and water retention from the effect of NSAID on renal handling of sodium and water through their effect on renal prostaglandin synthesis,[25] but the immobility caused by joint pain is also a contributory factor. Whatever the mechanism of the edema in these patients, salt restriction is helpful, and diuretics are often valuable as well.

Gastrointestinal abnormalities occur in association with some connective tissue diseases, particularly in scleroderma (progressive systemic sclerosis). Widespread gastrointestinal tract involvement in this disease can result in atrophy of the intestinal mucosa and loss of secretory activity and absorptive surface.[26] Malabsorption, with severe nutritional consequences, may occur. Elemental diets or parenteral nutrition may be necessary. These problems do not differ fundamentally from those seen in other causes of malabsorption, but the prognosis is usually poor because of progression of the underlying disease.

Restriction of the ability to open the mouth to eat and chew can occur in patients with scleroderma as a result of tightness of the skin around the mouth or contracture of the capsules of the temporomandibular joints, and involvement of those joints can occur in RA. Such problems can interfere with food consumption; a liquid diet may be needed, and teeth may have to be removed in order to feed a patient through a straw.

OBESITY

Because the spine and lower extremities are weight-bearing, body weight plays a role in the strain on these joints and can contribute to the development or progression of arthritis. Osteoarthritis (OA) is the form of arthritis most likely to be affected by obesity, because it is a wear-and-tear process characterized by breakdown of cartilage and bone with secondary proliferative changes. Mechanical factors that put an extra strain on joint tissues can accelerate the development or rate of progression of this disease. Studies of dietary intake and body weight in OA, however, have not clearly established obesity as a factor in the pathogenesis of this disease process.[27] Engel reported a higher incidence of OA in both weight-bearing and nonweight-bearing joints in obese patients,[28] but several other authors found the effect in weight-bearing joints but not in nonweight-bearing joints, such as the distal interphalangeal joints.[29,30] In a population survey in New Haven, CT, the weight-to-height ratio was found to correlate with the incidence of OA.[31]

A strikingly high frequency of OA occurs in a strain of obese mice,[32] but a genetic factor was identified that did not correlate with body weight.[33]

The hip joint, which is commonly affected by both OA and RA, has been well studied from the standpoint of the influence of body weight on the progression of established arthritis. For example, a group of 89 patients who had total hip replacement for OA or RA showed a striking correlation between body weight and the degree of loss of substance of the femoral head.[34] Another study of 25 grossly obese patients, who averaged 91 kg above their ideal weights, failed to show an increase in the frequency of OA above that expected, but the mean age of these patients was only 44.7 years, which is relatively young for a study of OA.[35]

Obesity has been shown to correlate with the finding of hyperuricemia and the development of gout;[36] weight loss caused lowering of the plasma uric acid level in these people.[37]

In a more recent report, the author noted that the relationship between risk factors and OA may differ across joints. For knees, obesity and knee injury either from acute events or repetitive impact loading may be the most important preventable causes of disease. Hand OA is probably also caused by repetitive use, but its association with other risk factors is unknown. Hip OA is probably different from OA in other joints, in that many cases are associated with congenital and developmental abnormalities.[38]

ARTHRITIS AFTER SURGICAL TREATMENT OF OBESITY

Some patients with particularly severe obesity were subjected to a surgical procedure to limit the intestinal surface available for absorption, the so-called "intestinal bypass." This operation (which is no longer performed) created a bypassed loop of jejunum and ileum that was not involved in transport or absorption of food. Such patients commonly developed arthritis, perhaps because of bacterial overgrowth in such loops leading to absorption of bacterial antigens and formation of immune complexes that reach the joints. The arthritis in these cases had a predilection for small joints of the upper and lower extremities.[39]

METABOLIC DISEASES AFFECTING CONNECTIVE TISSUE

Gout is the most common metabolic disorder associated with arthritis. Hyperuricemia, whatever the cause, can lead to formation of uric acid crystals in joint tissues, producing a severe inflammatory reaction. This form of "crystal synovitis" occurs most often on a familial basis, especially in men. Usually, no underlying disease is present, although patients with gout have a higher frequency of obesity, and some of the correlates of obesity such as diabetes, hypertension, and ischemic heart disease occur with higher frequency in people with gout than in the general population.[36]

Some patients with gout are in positive urate balance, excreting less uric acid each day than they form from endogenous and exogenous precursors. The accumulation of urate leads to deposition of insoluble masses of crystals, particularly in cartilage, and a foreign-body granulomatous reaction develops around these depositions. These deposits, called tophi, can cause destruction of joint tissues, leading to chronic arthritis.

Studies of patients with gout have not revealed any significant differences in diet from control groups, with the exception of ethanolic beverages; patients with gout had a greater intake of beer.[40] A clear association exists, however, between alcoholic intake, especially in the form of binges, and gout.

Dietary therapy in the management of gout is useful in some patients. About 15% of the urate formed each day comes from dietary sources; the remainder is an obligatory end product of tissue nucleic acid turnover. A diet restricted in purine content can reduce the urinary excretion of uric acid by 200 to 400 mg per day and lower the serum uric acid level by about 59.5 μmol/dl (1 mg/dl).[41] Such a diet is relatively unpalatable, and compliance is difficult. Fortunately, it is not necessary, because drugs are effective in controlling the manifestations of the disease, but control of obesity, reduction in alcohol intake, and, when necessary, control of hypertriglyceridemia, remain important aspects of the nutritional management of gout. However, all patients with gout should avoid foods particularly high in purine content, such as sweetbreads, fish roe, anchovies, sardines, liver, and kidney, and to restrain intake of foods moderately high in purines, such as animal meats, seafood, beans, lentils, spinach, and peas.[41]

Hyperlipidemias can be associated with joint symptoms, particularly the type IIa and type IV hyperlipoproteinemias. Patients with type IA disease often have polyarthritis, Achilles tendinitis, and tenosynovitis, and thus seem to have a rheumatic disease. Usually, the patients have xanthelasma and numerous xanthomas, especially in tendons, and thus the diagnosis is evident (see Chap. 72). Patients with type IV hyperlipoproteinemia commonly have mild joint pains, usually involving one or a few joints, with periodic exacerbations. The episodic nature of the symptoms provides a diagnostically helpful clue, but false-positive serologic tests for rheumatoid factor in these patients may lead to confusion. Diagnosis must be made by lipoprotein electrophoresis, demonstrating elevated levels of β-lipoproteins and serum triglycerides. Dietary therapy, including restriction of intake of carbohydrates, alcohol, and total calories, with consequent reduction in triglyceride levels, is often helpful in relieving the joint symptoms; drug therapy is being evaluated.[42]

Ochronosis is an inherited metabolic disorder characterized by urine that darkens on standing because of the presence of excessive quantities of homogentisic acid. Also called alkaptonuria, the disease is associated with an inherited deficiency of the enzyme homogentisic acid oxidase. As a result, homogentisic acid increases in quantity in body fluids, and is excreted in the urine. Polymers of homogentisic acid form in cartilaginous structures, especially joint cartilage, darken with time, and the resulting black pigment in cartilage is a characteristic finding. Degeneration of chondrocytes results, leading to breakdown of the cartilage matrix, a form of OA. The abnormal cartilage becomes calcified, and thus the disease can be diagnosed radiographically as well as by the dark urine and the pigmentation visible in cartilaginous structures, such as the ear lobes. At present, no dietary therapy is useful in management of this disorder.

METABOLIC PHENOMENA IN CONNECTIVE TISSUE DISEASES

HISTIDINE AND SULFHYDRYL GROUPS

The plasma of patients with RA has a lower level of free sulfhydryl groups [43] and decreased levels of histidine compared to normal individuals,[44,45] whereas levels of other amino acids are in the same range as in normal subjects. The decreased level of histidine correlates with the degree of clinical activity of the RA, as measured by various parameters that reflect disease activity, such as the erythrocyte sedimentation rate, duration of morning stiffness, and titer of rheumatoid factor. The subnormal level of this amino acid in the plasma is not explained by poor absorption.[46] In view of these biochemical findings, treatment with 4.5 g per day of histidine was evaluated in the treatment of RA in a double-blind study. Although no significant improvement was noted in the group as a whole, patients with more active and more prolonged disease did show some suggestion of benefit, compared to their status on placebo therapy.[47]

Drugs used in the therapy of RA that give significant improvement in patients with the disease do not alter the abnormal plasma level of histidine, with one exception; penicillamine raises the levels of histidine and total serum sulfhydryl levels and lowers the plasma viscosity and C-reactive protein content.[48] Because penicillamine itself has free sulfhydryl groups, it has been suggested that its mechanism of action involves those groups. This subject is controversial, however, because gold, which is given as a complex with a sulfhydryl compound, is clearly of value in the treatment of RA. Gold is believed to be the therapeutic substance, but the possibility exists that the sulfhydryl compounds accompanying the gold constitute the true therapeutic agent.[48] The amount of sulfhydryl in these gold salts is not sufficient to affect total level of these compounds in the serum, however. Chloroquin, another drug that has a disease suppressive effect in RA, albeit a weak one, does not affect plasma levels of histidine, nor do other useful agents such as the NSAID, corticosteroids, and immunosuppressants.

Rheumatoid factor is present in the plasma of most patients with RA; it is an antibody to γ globulin that has become antigenic. In vitro, low levels of histidine allow aggregation of γ globulin molecules to form more readily by formation of disulfide bonds, a process that can augment its antigenicity. Maintenance of free sulfhydryl groups in plasma is a possible protective mechanism, minimizing the tendency of the γ globulin to become antigenic.[44] This concept is not generally accepted, however.

TYROSINE AND TRYPTOPHAN METABOLISM IN RHEUMATOID ARTHRITIS

Abnormal quantities of metabolites of tyrosine and tryptophan have been found in the urine of patients with RA and other forms of inflammatory arthritis. Degradation of tryptophan results in excretion of 3-hydroxykynurenine, xanthurenic acid, 3-hydroxyanthranilic acid, and N-methylnicotinamide. Increased urinary excretion of these metabolites of tryptophan has been reported in patients with RA and scleroderma, but not in a pattern that would suggest a defect at a specific enzymatic step; the reason for these abnormalities has not been elucidated.[49] Deficiencies of vitamins involved in the metabolism of these amino acids have not been found in patients with these connective tissue diseases, and administration of pyridoxine neither is clinically beneficial nor does it correct the abnormalities in urinary excretion (except in one study in which pyridoxine administration caused a reversal of the increased urinary excretory of these metabolites after administration of tryptophan.[50]

Several authors report aggravation of RA and other systemic connective tissue diseases after oral administration of L-tyrosine, and improvement of patients on diets low in phenylalanine and tyrosine. Several patients with RA on diets low in tryptophan showed some clinical improvement with a drop in sedimentation rate; notably, these diets are low in total protein (20 g per day).[41] In a study of the glomerulonephritis that develops in hybrid New Zealand Black mice (NZB/NZW), a diet low in phenylalanine and tyrosine reduced the frequency and severity of development of the renal lesions.[6]

EOSINOPHILIA-MYALGIA SYNDROME (EMS)

A syndrome with features of scleroderma has been observed in patients who had ingested tryptophan as a dietary supplement. The syndrome included the accumulation of eosinophils in connective tissues, muscle and joint pains, neurologic manifestations including cognitive changes, as well as skin changes including proliferation of fibroblasts with excessive collagen deposition. The disease process caused long-term sequelae including skin tightening, arthralgias, muscle aches and weakness, anxiety, depression, and decreased cognitive function.[51] Disability and death occurred in many patients, even after discontinuing the tryptophan. A variety of patho logic mechanisms must have been involved, including chemotaxis of eosinophils, production of cytokines, and stimulation of fibroblasts.[52]

It was originally unclear whether the disease was produced by the tryptophan itself or by an accompanying toxin formed during the fermentation process used in production of the tryptophan.[52,53] Results of later studies have identified a dimer of tryptophan in the lots associated with EMS that may have been the responsible toxin.[54] Serotonin, a product of tryptophan metabolism, can induce dermal fibrosis[55] and a serotonin analogue, methsergide, which has been used therapeutically for relief of chronic pain, has been shown to cause retroperitoneal fibrosis.[56] The reports of abnormal tryptophan metabolism in scleroderma mentioned previously may be relevant; increased levels of kynenurine in the blood and urine in patients with scleroderma was also found in patients with eosinophilic fasciitis (a rare, benign, localized process) and those with EMS.[52,57,58]

CANAVANINE AND SYSTEMIC LUPUS ERYTHEMATOSUS

During a study of the cholesterol-lowering effect of alfalfa, a syndrome resembling human SLE, including hemolytic anemia, pluerisy, and antinuclear antibodies, was observed in mice, monkeys, and one human. Two patients with SLE were observed to have flareups of their disease after ingesting alfalfa tablets. Alfalfa contains large amounts of canavanine, one of about 200 nonprotein amino acid occurring in higher plants; it has toxic properties, protecting some plants from insects. Canavanine is present in alfalfa seeds and sprouts, as well as in several food crops, including onions and soybeans and in forage crops, including clover,[59] but it usually is destroyed by heating or cooking.[60]

When large amounts of canavanine were fed to mice, their lymphocytes showed impaired DNA synthesis in response to mitogens. A similar decrease in mitogenic response of human B cells has been observed.[61] Mice that spontaneously develop a syndrome closely resembling human SLE were shown to have a decreased life span when fed that amino acid.[62] Canavanine appeared to interfere with the interaction between B and T cells, resulting in B cell dysfunction and autoantibody production; suppressor cell function seems to be impaired, increasing antibody production.[59]

Canavanine is chemically similar to arginine, and can be incorporated into protein in place of that amino acid.[59,60] Because histone, the main protein of nucleoproteins, is particularly rich in arginine, it is possible that large amounts of canavanine in the diet could result in nucleoproteins changing their antigenicity in relation to antinuclear antibody production, or, in the case of lymphocytes, changing their immunoregulatory function.

SPECIFIC NUTRIENTS

TRACE MINERALS

Iron. Anemia is a frequent finding in severe, uncontrolled RA, and occasionally is seen in other forms of chronic inflammatory joint disease. True iron deficiency can occur in RA, but in the usual form of anemia with low iron in the plasma and hypochromic normocytic cells, the total iron-binding capacity of the plasma is not increased and the bone marrow usually shows normal or increased iron stores. Thus, the findings in RA are typical of the anemia of chronic disease rather than of true iron deficiency.[63] Serum[64] and red cell ferritin concentrations are normal; the red cell ferritin concentration provides a reliable index of true iron deficiency in RA and thus is predictive of the response to iron therapy.[65]

A study of the role of iron, vitamin B_{12}, and folic acid deficiency, erythropoietin responsiveness, and iron absorption in the anemia of patients with RA revealed that more than one type of anemia may be present. The clinical findings of the different types of anemia may be masked by changes of another type, disease activity, and, possibly, erythropoietin unresponsiveness.[66]

The anemia in RA and other chronic inflammatory states probably represents a defect in reutilization of iron after red blood cell destruction, the exact cause of which is still obscure. The process is not specific for RA, and is not critical to the pathogenesis of the disease. Only rarely does the anemia itself require treatment, and usually another contributory factor is involved, such as significant gastrointestinal blood loss (which can result from drug toxicity) or a superimposed, acquired, immunologically mediated hemolytic process.[67]

Although iron absorption was thought to be normal in patients with RA, findings of recent studies revealed that iron retention was considerably decreased in patients with RA. Analysis of the two sequential steps in iron absorption showed that mucosal uptake was normal in iron-replete patients with RA but was significantly decreased in patients with RA who had depleted iron stores, compared with iron-deficient controls. Mucosal transfer of iron was considerably decreased in patients with RA with normal iron stores.[68,69]

Increased amounts of iron have been demonstrated in synovial tissues of patients with RA,[70–72] suggesting recurrent intra-articular microhemorrhages. This small amount of iron accumulation probably has no effect on the stores of iron available for marrow function. The amount of free iron was significantly higher in the synovial fluid of patients with RA compared with those with OA, and, although iron-binding proteins were increased, the ferritin saturation index, transferrin saturation index, and bound iron were lower in RA. These findings suggest sufficient amounts of free iron are present in rheumatoid synovial fluid to allow formation of toxic hydroxyl radicals, which contribute to the production of inflammation.[73]

Copper. Plasma levels of both free copper and ceruloplasm are elevated in patients with RA. Levels of both total copper and ultrafilterable copper are elevated.[74] The plasma copper levels correlate with the degree of joint inflammation. These findings have been interpreted to mean that both copper and ceruloplasmin behave as acute phase reactants in a nonspecific fashion; they are elevated in patients with a variety of inflammatory diseases.[74,75] The levels of copper decrease with control of the RA with therapy, as do levels of other acute phase reactants.[74]

In rats with experimental adjuvant arthritis, a large increase in the concentrations of copper, zinc, and iron was found in the liver and pancreas; these changes in metal concentrations showed a strong correlation with the degree of inflammation.[76]

Copper and ceruloplasmin levels are particularly elevated in female patients with RA receiving oral contraceptives containing estrogen, whereas normal levels were found in men and women not receiving estrogen;[74,77] oral contraceptives raise titers of antinuclear antibodies and rheumatoid factor.[74] The levels of total serum copper correlate inversely with the serum iron level in patients with RA,[74,75] but ultrafilterable copper levels do not correlate with anything.[74]

A strong direct correlation exists between ceruloplasmin levels and antioxidant activity of the serum.[75] This phenomenon suggests a potential protective role for the increased ceruloplasmin levels in inflammatory states, because toxic oxygen radicals are formed during inflammation; scavengers of these radicals decrease the severity of inflammation in experimental models. Ceruloplasmin may act to minimize the toxicity of such radicals.[74,75] In this context, it is notable that the wearing of copper bracelets is a folk remedy for arthritis. These bracelets or bangles usually cause some discoloration of the underlying skin, suggesting absorption of copper from the jewelry.[74]

The serum concentrations of zinc, copper, and selenium were abnormal in 125 patients with juvenile chronic arthritis (JCA) as compared with those of a large group of healthy children. Serum zinc and selenium concentrations were lower and those of copper higher in children with arthritis, especially in those with polyarthritis. Serum zinc levels showed a direct correlation with hemoglobin and an inverse correlation with values for the erythrocyte sedimentation rate, whereas copper correlated directly with sedimentation rate. Selenium values did not correlate with the activity of the disease, but were low in the patients with arthritis of long duration.[78] Similar changes were observed in experimental adjuvant arthritis in rats.[79]

Zinc. Patients with RA have lower serum levels of zinc than normal individuals or patients with other rheumatic diseases. Niedermeier and Griggs found a zinc level averaging 11.2 μmol/dl (73 μg/dl) in patients with RA, compared to a mean in controls of 115;[80] in a study with atomic absorption spectrophotometry, plasma zinc levels averaged 13.2 μmol/dl (86 μg/dl) in patients with RA in contrast to 15.1 μmol/dl (99 μg/dl) in controls. Zinc levels correlated directly with the level of serum albumin, and inversely with the erythrocyte sedimentation rate but do not correlate with the degree of joint tenderness.[81,82]

Low zinc levels have also been reported in patients receiving corticosteroid therapy, and in people who have had severe burns.[82] Zinc could be of importance in the genesis of manifestations of RA because it has been shown to stabilize lysosomal membranes, inhibit prostaglandin synthesis, interfere with complement action, and impair macrophage function.[83]

In a double-blind controlled study of therapy with oral zinc sulfate in 24 patients with chronic, refractory RA, significant improvement was noted in the amount of joint swelling, the duration of morning stiffness, the time it took to walk a set distance, and the overall evaluation of their status by the patients. Several other clinical trials have failed to show a beneficial effect of zinc.[84–86]

Enzymes involved in the synthesis of collagen require zinc; in zinc-deficient animals, wound healing is impaired, implying a defect in collagen synthesis. Failure of collagen synthesis is not a feature of the rheumatic diseases, however.

Most of the direct reacting zinc in the plasma is bound to histidine, and the low levels of serum histidine may be the cause or the effect of the low levels of zinc.[83]

At least one therapeutic agent used in patients with RA can alter zinc metabolism; penicillamine increases both zinc absorption and urinary excretion, but a positive balance results. Gold therapy may decrease plasma levels of zinc.[48]

Selenium. A deficiency of this element has been reported in a patient in New Zealand receiving parenteral hyperalimentation who developed muscle pain and tenderness and was unable to walk. Findings in this case resemble those in patients with myositis, the so-called "fibrositis syndrome," and also as a component of other rheumatic diseases, such as RA. Surgical stress and lack of selenium in the i.v. fluid contributed to the negative balance of this element in addition to previous low intake in the patient who lived in an area with low selenium content in the soil.[87] This observation pointed to a need for further investigation of possible trace metal deficiencies that might contribute to symptoms of patients with rheumatic diseases. A controlled trial of a compound containing selenium failed to demonstrate any significant efficacy for the compound over placebo at 3 or 6 months in patients with OA.[88] It should be noted that in most clinical reports of severe selenium depletion, focal cardiac necrosis is an associated finding (see Chap. 12).

Manganese. This cofactor is critical to the activity of some enzymes involved in glycosaminoglycan synthesis. Manganese deficiency in laboratory animals results in defective synthesis of these compounds, which are key components of the extracellular material in connective tissue.[89] These findings may be relevant to disease affecting connective tissues, but no clinical studies have been performed.

VITAMINS

Among the other dietary claims made regarding treatment of arthritis, "megavitamin therapy," especially large doses of vitamins C and D, have been advocated. Vitamin D was used therapeutically for RA in the 1930s and early 1940s, in uncontrolled trials. Although many physicians thought it was of benefit, and little else was available to treat these patients at that time, a great deal of toxicity occurred. Huge doses were given, often parenterally, with resulting hypercalcemia, renal calculi, and pathologic calcifications. Objective signs of improvement were few and unconvincing.[90]

Vitamin C was used as treatment for RA in the 1940s, at a time when vitamin deficiency diseases were more common, and therapeutic use of vitamins was popular. Numerous studies showed low levels of ascorbic acid in the plasma and blood cells of patients with RA, findings that have been confirmed with improved methods of assay. The reason for the low levels has never been clarified; it is possible that therapy, particularly aspirin, may increase the rate of clearance of ascorbic acid, lowering plasma levels secondarily. Because of these observations, therapeutic doses of ascorbic acid were prescribed, but they were without clinical benefit.[91] Large doses of vitamin C were used for a variety of problems, but there are no reports of controlled studies showing clinical benefit in any form of arthritis.

Ascorbic acid is essential for the synthesis of collagen, the main extracellular protein of connective tissue, and vitamin C deficiency is characterized by failure of synthesis of adequate quantities of collagen, accounting for the impaired wound healing and capillary fragility seen in patients with scurvy. Decreased synthesis of collagen is not a feature of any of the rheumatic diseases. Thus, there is no reason to expect this form of therapy to be of benefit. On the other hand, the synthesis of collagen requires only the small amounts of ascorbic acid in the recommended daily allowance, and so benefit from intake of larger amounts should not be expected. In fact, deleterious effects seem more likely if collagen synthesis could be accelerated, because fibroblast proliferation and excessive collagen formation occurs in many forms of arthritis. However, such harmful effects have not been reported.

EFFECTS OF THERAPY ON NUTRITIONAL STATUS

GOLD AND ZINC

The mechanism of action of gold compounds in RA is unclear; most research is focusing on a controlling influence on immunologic processes, through an effect on either macrophages or lymphocytes. Some investigators are looking into possible effects of gold on heavy metal nutrition. In patients with RA, a response to gold correlates with a decrease in the elevated plasma copper levels that occur in patients with active disease, the copper behaving as an acute phase reactant. A slower rise in plasma zinc levels occurs as the arthritis comes under control.[48]

CORTICOSTEROIDS

Among the therapeutic agents used in the treatment of rheumatic diseases, corticosteroids have the most metabolic effects. Although rarely used in the treatment of RA, except in small doses, corticosteroids are used in relatively large amounts in the treatment of SLE and other serious systemic connective tissue diseases, especially those that are the result of immune mechanisms. The antianabolic effect of corticosteroids is well known and only the effect on vitamin D metabolism and bone is discussed here.

Inhibition of the synthetic activity of connective tissue cells by corticosteroids is well established, with the most important clinical manifestations seen in skin and bone, the two organs with the most abundant collagen. Osteoporosis and thin skin are thus major side effects of corticosteroid therapy, especially when the drugs are used for long periods in moderate doses. Women, who constitute a majority of the patients with rheumatic diseases, are more susceptible to these side effects of corticosteroids.

The mechanisms responsible for the altered bone metabolism when corticosteroids are administered include a direct effect on the bones, inhibiting synthesis of bone matrix, and an effect on calcium absorption in the intestine, resulting from modification of the effects of vitamin D. Osteoporosis results, and collapse of vertebral bodies and increased susceptibility to femoral fractures are the most important clinical sequelae. Corticosteroids inhibit synthesis of the carrier protein involved in calcium absorption; the resulting decrease in calcium entering the plasma leads to secondary stimulation of parathyroid function, contributing to the skeletal thinning.[92]

NONSTEROIDAL ANTI-INFLAMMATORY AGENTS

The therapeutic agents used most frequently in the treatment of patients with rheumatic diseases are the nonsteroidal anti-inflammatory agents (NSAID). Aspirin was the most widely used drug in this category and it is a mainstay of therapy for arthritis. Other NSAID introduced more recently are occasionally more effective, generally have fewer gastrointestinal side effects than aspirin, and are now widely available in over-the-counter preparations. These drugs are analgesic, anti-inflammatory, and antipyretic. A major aspect of the action of the entire group of drugs is inhibition of synthesis of prostaglandins. A consequence of the inhibition of prostaglandin synthesis in the kidney is retention of salt and water by some patients because the vasodilating effect of increased prostaglandin synthesis maintains glomerular filtration when renal perfusion is decreased. This form of adaptation occurs when hypovolemia exists, such as in patients receiving diuretics. In susceptible individuals, azotemia can result, but retention of salt and water rarely has serious consequences.

Methotrexate, an antagonist of folic acid, causes manifestations of deficiency of that amino acid; most patients getting benefit from the drug show evidence of macrocytosis (a high mean corpuscular volume) while some get distressing ulcerations of the buccal mucosa and a few develop cytopenia. It has been suggested that all patients receiving this drug be given 1/mg of folate each day;[93] this amount does not seem to prevent the drug from being clinically effective.[94]

Sulfasalazine, a combination of a sulfonamide chemotherapeutic agent with a salicylate, is also used to treat RA and the arthritis of inflammatory bowel disease. This drug inhibits the absorption of folate,[95] and the addition of 1/mg of folate to the diet daily is recommended when patients are receiving this drug.

Most of the drugs used in treating rheumatic diseases have gastric toxicity; abdominal pain is the most frequent manifestation, but nausea and vomiting may develop. Nutritional consequences can occur.

UNPROVEN DIETS FOR TREATMENT OF ARTHRITIS

The lay literature abounds with suggestions of diets that cause or cure arthritis.[96,97] Although published as nonfiction, some reaching bestseller lists in that category, these books should be classified as fiction. A hallmark of the group is a claim that the proposed diet is good for "arthritis" without making any distinction among the 100 or so causes of arthritis. Clearly, in view of the diversity of the diseases in this field, no treatment can be expected to cure all forms of arthritis. A second feature of this group of publications is the use of testimonials, without mention of controlled trials. Many rheumatic diseases spontaneously fluctuate in severity or improve spontaneously; descriptions of improvement without controlling for the frequency of these spontaneous variations makes such claims impossible to evaluate and scientifically worthless. Such occurrences probably account for the bulk of the testimonials.

In 1935, Walter Bauer, one of the founders of American rheumatology, reviewed six diets that had been advocated as treatment for arthritis, including omission of acid fruits and vegetables, limiting content of any meal to only one type of food, alterations in the acid-base balance, omission of foods suspected of causing hypersensitivity, and low-protein, low-carbohydrate, and low-calorie regimens. None were thought to be efficacious. A "well-balanced diet" containing abundant fruits and vegetables was recommended.[98]

A controlled study of diet was performed on 11 patients with RA who, after a period of fasting, spent 10 weeks on a regimen limited in preservatives, additives, herbs, milk products, fruit, and red meat, following suggestions made in a popular book (the "Dong diet"). Fifteen patients with RA who remained on their regular diet served as controls. Six patients on the placebo diet improved, as did 5 on the experimental diet. Although no effect of this elimination diet was shown, 2 patients elected to remain on the diet because they were convinced that it helped them.[97] Thus, dietary manipulation can help individual patients, but no regimen clearly deserves widespread adoption or the immodest claims made in lay media.

Joint pain can be a manifestation of food allergy.[99,100] Rheumatic complaints have been induced in patients with established allergic reactions to foods, including soy extracts, coffee, eggs, milk, potatoes, apples, lettuce, oranges, ethanol, beef, and pork.[100] Also, in individual case reports, authors describe patients with RA who have demonstrated definite adverse reactions to specific items of food, and benefit from an elimination diet. In one well-studied case, the specific food item was cheese, and evidence for circulating immune complexes was found; the patient benefited from withdrawal of dairy products from the diet.[101] Reactions to milk,[102] English walnuts,[103] nitrates,[104] gluten,[105] and an amino acid in alfalfa sprouts[106] have also been associated with rheumatic complaints relieved by eliminating the offending agent from the diet.

Classic tests for allergies, using skin reactions and in vitro tests, are not dependable, giving a high frequency of both false-negative and false-positive results. Allergy can be established in patients by elimination diets followed by challenge with the suspected offending antigen in hidden form (e.g., freeze-dried samples in opaque capsules). Once established, specific elimination diets can be helpful.[107]

Although digestive processes would be expected to destroy antigenicity of food components, a variety of mechanisms have been proposed by which antigens could be absorbed, enter the circulation, and lead to immunologically mediated disease.[108]

When food is responsible for joint complaints, or aggravation of underlying joint disease, improvement can be expected from dietary manipulation. These in stances may account for some of the testimonials claiming improvement on certain diets, such as the "no nightshades diet," which eliminates potatoes, tomatoes, peppers, and related vegetables.

Dietary manipulation may be of benefit to some patients, at least in the inflammatory forms of arthritis, but care is necessary to obtain this benefit without inducing significant nutritional deficiencies.

REFERENCES

1. Henderson, C.J., Lovell, D.J.: Rheum. Dis. Clin. North Am., *17:*403–413, 1991.
2. Panush, R.S.: Rheum. Dis. Clin. North Am., *17:*259–272, 1991.
3. Bollet, A.J.: Mt. Sinai J. Med., *37:*445–449, 1970.
4. Pike, M.C.: J. Rheumatol., *161:*718–720, 1989.
5. Goodwin, J.S., Webb, D.R.: Clinical Immunol. Immunopathol., *15:*106–122, 1980.
6. Hurd, E.R., Johnston, J.M., Okita, J.R., et al.: J. Clin. Invest., *67:*467–485, 1981.
7. Dyerberg, J., Bang, H.O., Stoffersen, E., et al.: Lancet, *II:*117–119, 1978.
8. Kromann, N., Green, A.: Acta Med. Scand., *208:*401–406, 1980.
9. Robinson, D.R.: Rheum. Dis. Clin. North Am., *17:*213–222, 1991.
10. Lee, T.H., Hoover, R.L., Williams, J.D., et al.: N. Engl. J. Med., *312:*1205–1209, 1985.
11. Sperling, R.I., Weinblatt, M., Robin, J.-L., et al.: Arthritis Rheum., *30:*988–997, 1987.
12. Endres, S., Ghorbani, R. Kelley, V.E. et al.: N. Engl. J. Med., *320:*265–272, 1989.
13. Kremer, J.M., Jubiz, W., Michalek, K., et al.: Ann. Intern. Med., *106:*497–503, 1987.
14. Kremer, J.M., Lawrence, D., Jubiz, W., et al.: Arthritis Rheum., *33:*810–820, 1990.
15. Tate, G., Mandell, B.F., Laposata, M., et al.: J. Rheumatol., *16:*729–734, 1989.
16. Fisher, J.M., Donnegan, D.R., Leon, H., et al.: Prog. Lipid Res., *20:*799–805, 1982.
17. Kunkel, S.L., Ogawa, H., Ward, P.A.: Prog. Lipid Res., *20:*885–888, 1981.
18. Ziff, M.: Arthritis Rheum., *26:*457–481, 1983.
19. DeWille, J.W., Fraker, P.J., Romsos, D.R.: J. Nutr., *109:*1018–1027, 1979.
20. Prickett, J.D., Robinson, D.R., Steinberg, A.D.: J. Clin. Invest., *68:*556–559, 1981.
21. Kelley, V.E., Ferreti, A., Izu, S., et al.: J. Immunol., *134:*1914–1919, 1985.
22. Hurd, E., Gilliam, J.N.: J. Invest. Dermatol., *77:*381–384, 1981.
23. Mertin, J., Hunt, R.: Proc. Natl. Acad. Sci. USA, *73:*928–931, 1973.
24. Denko, C.W.: Agents Actions, *6:*636–641, 1976.
25. Bollet, A.J.: Nonsteroidal anti-inflammatory drugs. *In* Textbook of Rheumatology. Edited by W.N. Kelly, E.D. Harris, Jr., S. Ruddy, et al. Philadelphia, W.B. Saunders, 1985.
26. Rodnan, G.P.: Progressive systemic sclerosis (scleroderma). *In* Arthritis and Allied Conditions. 9th Ed. Edited by D.J. McCarty. Philadelphia, Lea & Febiger, 1979.
27. Elsin, L.: J. Bone Joint Surg., *45:*69–81, 1963.
28. Engel, A.: Publication 1000:29. Washington, U. S. Public Health Service, 1968.
29. Kellgren, J.H., Lawrence, J.S.: Ann. Rheum. Dis., *17:*370–387, 1975.
30. Stecher, R.M.: Ann. Rheum. Dis., *14:*1–10, 1955.
31. Acheson, R.M., Collart, A.B.: Ann. Rheum. Dis., *34:*379–387, 1975.
32. Silberberg, M., Jarrett, S.F., Silberberg, R.: Arch. Pathol. Lab. Med., *61:*117–123, 1956.
33. Sokoloff, L., Michelson, O.: J. Nutr., *85:*117–121, 1965.
34. Watson, M.: Rheumatol. Rehab., *15:*264–269, 1976.
35. Goldin, R.J., McAdam, L., Louie, J.S., et al: Ann. Rheum. Dis., *35:*349–353, 1976.
36. Hall, A.P., Barry, P.E., Dawber, R.R., et al.: Am. J. Med., *42:*27–37, 1967.
37. Nicholls, A., Scott, J.T.: Lancet, *2:*1223–1224, 1972.
38. Felson, D.T.: Rheum. Dis. Clin. North Am., *16:*499–512, 1990.
39. Utsinger, P.D., Farber, N., Shapiro, N., et al.: Arthritis Rheum., *21:*599, 1978.
40. Gibson, T., Highton, J., Potter, C.: Ann. Rheum. Dis., *39:*417–423, 1980.
41. Kelly, W.N.: Gout and related disorders of purine metabolis. *In* Textbook of Rheumatology. Edited by W.N. Kelly, E.D., Harris, Jr., S. Ruddy, et al. Philadelphia, W.B. Saunders, 1981.
42. Fishel, B., Rosenbach, T.O., Yaron, M., et al.: Clin. Rheumatol., *5:*75–79, 1986.
43. Lorber, A., Bovy, R.A., Chang, C.C.: Metabolism, *20:*446–455, 1971.
44. Gerber, D.J.: J. Rheumatol., *2:*384–392, 1975.
45. Gerber, D.J.: J. Clin. Invest., *55:*1164–1173, 1975.
46. Gerber, D.J., Tannebaum, L., Ahrens, M.: Metabolism, *25:*655–657, 1976.
47. Pinals, R.S., Harris, E., Burnett, J.B., et al.: J. Rheumatol., *4:*414–419, 1977.
48. Bird, H.A.: Ann. Rheum. Dis., *42:*474–475, 1983.
49. Houpt, J.R., Ogryzlo, M.A., Hunt, M.: Semin. Arthritis Rheum., *2:*333–353, 1973.
50. Robinson, W.: Nutrition in the Rheumatic Diseases. *In* Textbook of Rheumatology. Edited by W.N. Kelly, E.D. Harris, Jr., S. Ruddy, et al. Philadelphia, W.B. Saunders, 1981.
51. Centers for Disease Control: MMWR, *40:*401–403, 1991.
52. Kaufman, L.D., Seidman, R.J.: Rheum. Dis. Clin. North Am., *17:*427–441, 1991.
53. Centers for Disease Control: MMWR, *39:*14–15, 1990.
54. Mayeno, A.N., Lin, F., Foote, C.S., et al.: Science, *250:*1707–1708, 1990.
55. MacDonald, R.A., Robbins, S.L., Mallory, G.K.: Proc. Soc. Exp. Biol. Med., *97:*334–337, 1956.

56. Utz, D.C., Rooke, E.D., Spittel, J.A., et al.: JAMA, *191:*983–985, 1965.
57. De Antoni, A., Muggeo, M., Costa, C., et al.: Acta Vitamin. Enzymol., *30:*134–139, 1976.
58. Houpt, J.B., Ogryzlo, M.A., Hunt, M.: Semin. Arthritis Rheum., *2:*333–353, 1973.
59. Montanaro, A., Bardana, E.J. Jr.: Rheum. Dis. Clin. North Am., *17:*323–332, 1991.
60. Rosenthal, G.A.: Q. Rev. Biol., *52:*155–178, 1977.
61. Alocer-Valera, J., Iglesias, A., Llorente, L., et al.: Arthritis Rheum., *28:*52–57, 1985.
62. Prete, P.E.: Can. J. Physiol. Pharmacol., *64:*1189–1196, 1986.
63. Mowat, A.G.: Semin. Arthritis Rheum., *1:*195–219, 1971.
64. Harju, E.: Clin. Pharmacokinet., *17:*69–89, 1989.
65. Das, K.C., Sattar, M.A.: Scand. J. Rheumatol., *18:*399–405, 1989.
66. Vreugdenhil, G., Wognum, A.W., van Eijk, H.G., et al.: Ann. Rheum. Dis., *49:*93–98, 1990.
67. Owen, E.T., Lawson, A.A.H.: Ann. Rheum. Dis., *25:*547–552, 1966.
68. Weber, J., Werre, J.M., Julius, H.W., et al.: Ann. Rheum. Dis., *47:*404–409, 1988.
69. Benn, H.P., Drews, J., Randzio, G., et al.: Ann. Rheum. Dis., *47:*144–149, 1988.
70. Muirden, K.D., Senator, G.B.: Ann. Rheum. Dis., *27:*38, 1968.
71. Senator, G.B., Muirden, K.D., Balazs, N.: Ann. Rheum. Dis., *27:*49, 1968.
72. Bennett, R.M., Williams, E.D., Lewis, S.M., et al.: Arthritis Rheum., *16:*298, 1973.
73. Ahmadzadeh, N., Shingu, M., Nobunaga, M.: Clin. Rheumatol., *8:*345–351, 1989.
74. Brown, D.H., Buxhn, W.W., El-Ghobery, A.F., et al.: Ann. Rheum. Dis., *38:*174–176, 1979.
75. Scudder, R., Al-Timini, D., McMurray, W., et al.: Ann. Rheum. Dis., *37:*67–70, 1978.
76. Kishore, V.: Res. Commun. Chem. Pathol. Pharmacol., *63:*153–156, 1989.
77. Bajpayee, D.P.: Ann. Rheum. Dis., *34:*162–165, 1975.
78. Honkanen, V., Pelkonen, P., Mussalo-Rauhamaa, H., et al.: Clin. Rheum., *8:*64–70, 1989.
79. Neve, J., Fontaine, J., Peretz, A., Famaey, J.P.: Agents Actions, *25:*146–155, 1988.
80. Niedermeier, W., Griggs, J.H.: J. Chronic Dis., *23:*527–536, 1971.
81. Balogh, Z., El-Ghobarey, A.F., Fell, G.S., et al.: Ann. Rheum. Dis., *39:*329–332, 1980.
82. Kennedy, A.C., Fell, G.S., Rooney, P.J., et al.: Scand. J. Rheumatol., *4:*243–245, 1975.
83. Simkin, P.A.: Lancet, *2:*539–542, 1976.
84. Job, C., Menkes, C.J., Delbarre, F.: Arthritis Rheum., *23:*1408–1409, 1980.
85. Mattingly, P.C., Mowat, A.G.: Ann. Rheum. Dis., *41:*456–457, 1982.
86. Mascioli, E.A., Blackburn, G.L.: Nutrition and the rheumatic diseases. *In* Textbook of Rheumatology. Edited by W.N. Kelly, E.D. Harris, Jr., S. Ruddy, et al. Philadelphia, W.B. Saunders, 1981.
87. Young, V.R.: N. Engl. J. Med., *304:*1228, 1982.
88. Hill, J., Bird, H.A.: Br. J. Rheumatol., *29:*211–213, 1990.
89. Cotzias, G.C., Papavasiliou, P.S., Hughes, E.R., et al.: J. Clin. Invest., *47:*992, 1968.
90. Ellman, P.: Br. J. Rheumatol., *1:*263–277, 1939.
91. Hall, M.G., Darling, R.C., Taylor, F.H.: Ann. Intern. Med., *13:*415–423, 1939.
92. Hahn, T.J., Hahn, B.H.: Arthritis Rheum., *6:*165–188, 1976.
93. Med. Lett. Drugs Ther., *33:*65–70, 1991.
94. Morgan, S.L., Baggott, J.E., Vaughn, W.H., et al.: Arthritis Rheum., *33:*9–18, 1990.
95. Franklin, J.L., Rosenberg, H.H.: Gastroenterology, *64:*517–525, 1973.
96. Panush, R.S., Carter, R.L., Katz, P., et al.: Arthritis Rheum., *26:*462–471, 1983.
97. Darlington, L.G.: Rheum. Dis. Clin. North Am., *17:*273–285, 1991.
98. Bauer, W.: JAMA, *104:*1–6, 1935.
99. Bock, S.A.: Medical Times, Sept. 1983, pp. 27–43.
100. Mandell, M.: Medical World News, *31:*16–17, 1980.
101. Parke, A.L., Hughes, G.V.H.: Br. Med. J., *282:*2027–2029, 1981.
102. Panush, R.S., Stroud, R.M., Webster, E.M.: Arthritis Rheum., *29:*220–226, 1986.
103. Marquart, J.L., Snyderman, R., Oppenheim, J.J.: Cell. Immunol., *9:*263–272, 1973.
104. Epstein, S.: Ann. Allergy, *27:*343–348, 1969.
105. O'Farrelly, C., Melcher, D., Price, R., et al.: Lancet, *2:*819–822, 1988.
106. Malinow, M.R., Bardona, E.J.: Science, *216:*415–417, 1982.
107. Bahua, S.L., Katzanga, J.: Rheum. Dis. Clin. North Am., *17:*243–250, 1991.
108. Cunnigham-Rundles, C.: Rheum. Dis. Clin. North Am., *17:*287–308, 1991.

CHAPTER 76

Nutrition, Respiratory Function, and Disease

Robert Chin, Jr., and Edward F. Haponik

Cellular respiration is essential for the normal function of all tissues. Oxygen is required for the efficient use of the nutrients, and carbon dioxide is produced as a by-product. The respiratory system provides for these essential functions of gas exchange by taking up oxygen and removing carbon dioxide for the entire organism. This system responds to the dynamic metabolic needs of the organism, increasing oxygen uptake and carbon dioxide elimination when oxygen consumption and carbon dioxide production are increased. Such immediate adjustments are integrally related to overall substrate use. Moreover, compromise of nutritional status imposes major limits on respiratory function in health and disease. This chapter includes an overview of the components of the respiratory system, their relationships to nutritional status, and how these interactions are altered by acute and chronic illnesses. In addition, potential strategies to nutritional replenishment and their benefits and risks in patients with pulmonary disease are presented.

THE RESPIRATORY SYSTEM

The respiratory system consists of (1) the lungs, including alveoli, blood vessels, the supporting structure, and the conducting airways; (2) the thoracic cage housing the lungs; (3) the respiratory muscles; (4) the nervous system; and (5) the cellular constituents that provide for the host defense mechanism and the metabolic activity of the lungs (Table 76–1). Defects in any of these individual components can lead to clinical disease. Selected components of the respiratory system (central control of breathing, respiratory muscles, and the lung itself) are particularly affected by nutritional deficiency.

CONTROL OF BREATHING

The respiratory system is modulated by the nervous system. The brain stem governs automatic respiration, but voluntary breathing is controlled by the cerebral cortex. However, before the final message is delivered to the respiratory muscles (e.g., the respiratory "pump"), complex interactions occur in the spinal cord between the descending impulses from the central nervous system (CNS) and afferent modifying impulses from the periphery. These interactions are key to the rapid response of the respiratory system to changing metabolic demands.

Rhythmic automatic respiration arises from neural input originating in the pontomedullary portion of the brain stem and sets the resting breathing pattern.

TABLE 76–1. THE RESPIRATORY SYSTEM

Central and peripheral nervous system
Control of breathing
Respiratory muscles
The "pump"
Thoracic cage
Lungs
Conducting airways
Terminal respiratory unit and alveoli
Pulmonary vasculature
Supporting structures
Trafficking cells
Host defense cells

Deviant respiratory patterns can reflect a specific anatomic problem at one of the brain stem loci of respiratory neurons. Input from the higher voluntary center, the cerebral cortex, can modify the rate, rhythm, and depth of respiration or interrupt the automaticity to permit behavior-related patterns of respiration (i.e., breathholding, cough, tachypnea, and bradypnea). Rapid adjustments in the pattern of breathing are required to adapt to the changing environment of the organism. Feedback from the periphery allows integration of peripheral needs of the organism with the central output. Such adjustments maintain the acid-base and respirable gas (oxygen and carbon dioxide) balance within a narrow range. Thus, although higher centers set the automaticity of the respiratory system, peripheral receptors modify this pattern to accomodate the metabolic needs.

The peripheral chemoreceptors (carotid and aortic bodies) respond to changes in the arterial Po_2 (Pao_2), $Paco_2$, and arterial pH. Reduced Pao_2 and pH and elevated $Paco_2$ result in increased chemoreceptor activity and respiratory stimulation. Reduced blood flow to these bodies also stimulates chemoreceptor activity. The carotid bodies assume more importance in humans in regard to these responses than the aortic bodies.[1]

Central chemoreceptors located in the medulla also respond to changes in $Paco_2$ and pH, but not to the Pao_2. Like the peripheral chemoreceptors, they lead to an increase in minute ventilation (respiratory rate times tidal volume) in the presence of acidemia or hypercapnia, but are slower to react to the changes in the arterial blood. The central chemoreceptors respond to changes in cerebral interstitial fluid $Paco_2$ and pH, which reflect the arterial changes and not the acid-base changes in the bathing cerebrospinal fluid.

Other sensors are located in the lungs, upper airways, and respiratory muscles and influence breathing in diverse ways. For the most part, the receptors in the lungs and upper airways respond to focal conformational changes and irritant stimuli. They are important in the origination of the cough reflex, coordination of the upper and lower airway caliber, control of inspiration and expiration, and the production of mucous secretion. The role of the respiratory muscles sensors is unclear, but they may contribute to the balance between agonist and antagonist muscle groups, posture, and the sensation of dyspnea. Final integretation of the afferent and efferent information takes place in the spinal cord, from which segmental motor neurons destined for the respiratory muscles carry the fully integrated message.

RESPIRATORY MUSCLES

Normally at rest, inspiration is active and expiration occurs passively with relaxation of the inspiratory muscles. With increased ventilatory demands, however, expiration may become active. Contraction of the inspiratory muscles leads to expansion of the thoracic cage, resulting in negative intrathoracic pressure. The resulting pressure gradient between the opening of the respiratory system (the mouth), which is at atmospheric pressure, and the alveoli, the pressures of which become subatmospheric with inspiration, initiates airflow. Inspiratory flow ceases when these pressures attain equilibrium. The return of the thoracic cage to its resting position increases intra-alveolar pressure, reversing the pressure gradient, and leads to exhalation.

The muscles of the respiratory pump are the diaphragm, the intercostal and accessory muscles, and the abdominal muscles. The diaphragm is the major inspiratory muscle and, anatomically, separates the thoracic cavity from the abdominal cavity. It is composed of striated skeletal muscle with a central tendon and has a rich vascular supply. Diaphragmatic contraction flattens its resting dome shape, enlarging the intrathoracic cavity. Although this muscle contracts rhythmically throughout a lifetime, it does not have intrinsic automaticity like the smooth muscle of the heart. The intercostal and accessory muscles consist of the internal and external intercostal muscles group, and the scalene, chest wall, and the sternocleidomastoid muscles. These groups have primarily inspiratory functions, lifting the rib cage and increasing its anterior-posterior dimension; however, part of the internal intercostal muscle group (the interosseous portion) may become expiratory as the lungs reach full inspiratory volume. The chest wall muscles, including the pectoralis, latissimus dorsi, serratus anterior, and trapezius, assist in inspiration. The abdominal muscles are recruited principally during active exhalation associated with vigorous breathing maneuvers such as exercise, but can also augment the inspiratory function of the diaphragm of an individual in the upright or sitting position.

Like other skeletal muscle groups, the respiratory muscles are subject to fatigue from an imbalance between supply and demand. Roussos defined muscle fatigue as the inability of a muscle to continue to generate prior attainable force,[2] whereas respiratory muscle weakness is the chronic inability of the muscle to attain adequate force. Respiratory muscle fatigue results in the failure of the muscles to produce sufficient force to support continuous gas exchange in and out of the lung. Clinically, hypercapnic respiratory failure and, subsequently, hypercapnic and hypoxemic respiratory failure occur as the result of the incapacity of the respiratory system to meet metabolic demands. Respiratory muscle fatigue may be central (resulting from loss of appropriate central neural drive) or peripheral (resulting from primary failure of muscle performance).

Both fatigue and weakness have obvious relationships to nutritional status. The diaphragm and the other respiratory muscles are composed of type I and type II muscle fibers. Type I fibers are slow-twitch fibers requiring more time to reach peak tension after stimulation than the type II, fast-twitch fibers. Type I fibers also have higher levels of oxidative enzymes, are more resistant to fatigue, and are recruited earlier than type II fibers, which have relatively higher levels of glycolytic enzymatic activity. Type II fibers can be characterized further on the basis of the level of oxidative enzymes that relate to fatigue resistance: the more oxidative enzyme, the less fatiguable. Functionally, type II muscle fibers are able to generate a greater peak force than the type I fibers.

The effect of malnutrition on these two fiber types has been well studied. In rats subjected to 6 weeks of undernutrition (reduction of body weight to 50% of expected body weight), a significant reduction in the cross-sectional area was found in both types of fibers of the diaphragm, but the fast-twitch fibers were quantitatively more affected.[3] Greater atrophy of the fast-twitch fibers compared to the slow-twitch fibers in animal skeletal muscle preparations was reported with malnutrition and protein-deficient nutrition.[4,5] The fast-twitch fibers, lower in oxidative enzymes, were more affected than the higher oxidative enzyme-containing fast-twitch fibers. Fatigue resistance was actually improved in an in vitro nerve muscle strip preparation from the diaphragms of nutritionally deprived rats (daily food access restricted to one third of estimated daily consumption until body weight was approximately 50% of the controls), despite a significant reduction in the cross-sectional area of both fibers.[6] Type II fibers showed more atrophy than type I fibers when compared to controls; no change was noted in the oxidative capacity of the muscle fibers.[6] The increase in fatigue resistance was believed to be related to the selective atrophy of the more fatiguable type II fibers.[6] These observations suggest that a clinical sequela of malnutrition is a diminished peak pressure generation of the respiratory muscles with little or no effect on endurance.

In physiologic terms, inspiratory muscle fatigue can be predicted by the length of time of the respiratory cycle that the muscles are in active contraction and the ratio of tension developed to peak tension. Bellemare and Grassino described the relationship between the product of the ratio of inspiratory time to the total respiratory cycle (T_I/T_{TOT}) and the ratio of diaphragmatic pressure generation to peak pressure (Pdi/Pdimax) as the tension time index ($TTdi = Pdi/Pdimax \times T_I/T_{TOT}$).[7] A TTdi in normal subjects and patients with chronic airflow obstruction exceeding 0.15 is associated with electromyographic evidence of diaphragmatic fatigue.[7,8] If the peak pressure that can be generated is reduced, then any given pressure produced during the inspiratory cycle represents a greater percent of the reduced peak pressure than of a normal peak pressure. Thus, if malnutrition contributes to a decline in peak pressure, the pressure required for a normal tidal breath represents a larger proportion of the "lower" peak pressure and can result in inspiratory muscle fatigue.

Although diseases affecting primarily the respiratory muscles are less common than those affecting the lung itself, the respiratory muscles are important as a compensating mechanism. Despite major alterations in the lung parenchyma or communicating airways, gas exchange at the capillary level may still occur as long as increased bulk air exchange can offset the deficiencies. In fibrotic lung diseases, the elastic load to respiratory muscles is increased, whereas in obstructive airway diseases, the resistive load is increased. If the respiratory muscles are able to overcome such increased loads without fatigue, even though the work of breathing is increased, function is preserved, but respiratory reserve is diminished.

THE LUNGS

The lungs comprise the conducting airways, the gas exchange organ (alveoli and pulmonary capillary bed), the supporting structural elements, the pulmonary and bronchial vasculature, and trafficking immune effector cells.

THE TRACHEOBRONCHIAL TREE

The conducting airways are a series of dichotomously branching structures extending from the proximal main airway (the trachea) to the periphery (alveoli). They consist of two major types; the bronchi or cartilaginous airways and the bronchioles, noncartilaginous or membranous airways. As the bronchioles further divide toward the periphery, they are subdivided into nonrespiratory and respiratory bronchioles. The latter contain alveoli and participate in gas exchange as well as conduct the gas stream to more distal gas exchange units (alveolar ducts and alveoli).

The airways not only conduct the gas to the alveoli, but also further condition it (humidifying, warming, and filtering) through specialized bronchial epithelial cells and bronchial submucosal glands. The bronchial epithelium consists mostly of ciliated columnar cells that sweep inhaled particles, by the coordinated beating of the cilia, proximally for removal ("mucociliary elevator"). Other cell types include mucous and serous cells that are responsible in part for the production of the mucus that helps entrap particles for the ciliary elevator; basal and intermediate cells that migrate toward the surface to replace the luminal epithelial cells; argyrophil cells that may have endocrinologic properties; and Clara cells found in the distal respiratory bronchioles that may contribute to the luminal liquid lining.[1] The submucosal bronchial glands contribute to the bronchial mucous layer and are of greatest number in the medium-sized bronchi.[1] In response to chronic irritation, as seen in chronic bronchitis, they can increase their output and size and contribute to airway lumen narrowing.

Smooth muscle is found throughout the walls of the tracheobronchial tree. Muscle contraction imparts rigidity to the airways[1] as well as reduces the caliber of the airway lumen. Innervation is primarily through the parasympathetic and the nonadrenergic nervous pathways, but receptors are present for other neurotransmitters. Gas flows through the tracheobronchial tree down a pressure gradient. Airflow is inversely related to the airway resistance, which, in turn, is inversely related to the radius of the tracheobronchial tube.

THE TERMINAL RESPIRATORY UNIT

This unit consists of respiratory bronchioles, alveolar ducts, and alveoli. The total surface area of the alveoli in a normal human adult is estimated to be 140 m^2.[1] Gas exchange occurs at the alveolar-capillary membrane, which consists of the alveolar and capillary epithelium and their basement membranes, the tissue and cellular components of the contiguous interstitial space, and the surfactant lining.[1] Oxygen diffuses down a concentration gradient across this membrane into the capillary red blood cells, with carbon dioxide moving in the opposite direction. Surfactant, a complex phospholipid and protein mixture produced by the alveolar epithelium (type II pneumocyte), lines the alveolar airspace. Surfactant reduces the surface tension of the alveolus at the air interface, thus decreasing its tendency to collapse and maintaining alveolar stability at low lung volumes.

PULMONARY PHYSIOLOGY

The right side of the heart returns oxygen-poor blood to the lungs for oxygenation and carbon dioxide removal. At the alveolar-capillary level, oxygen diffuses down a concentration gradient from the alveoli to the capillary blood to combine with the hemoglobulin of the red blood cell, with a minor amount dissolving in the plasma; simultaneously, carbon dioxide leaves the blood and enters into the alveoli across a concentration gradient in the opposite direction. Inspired air, at sea level, has a partial pressure of oxygen of 160 torr and a partial pressure of carbon dioxide of 0 torr. After hydration and mixing with the resident gas in the alveoli, the normal partial pressures of oxygen and carbon dioxide in the terminal respiratory units alveoli are 100 torr and 40 torr, respectively. The partial pressure of oxygen and carbon dioxide in the capillary blood entering into the gas exchange area is 40 torr and 46 torr, respectively; therefore, the driving pressure for oxygen normally is 60 torr and that for carbon dioxide normally is 6 torr. Equilibrium between alveoli gas and entering capillary blood is accomplished within 0.25 seconds with a capillary transit time of 0.75 seconds at rest.[1]

Implied in this system is the rapid replenishment of fresh gas to alveoli to match the arrival of desaturated, carbon dioxide-loaded blood to the alveolar-capillary unit. Impairment of the fresh supply of gas to match perfusion of alveoli translates into a pathophysiologic state. The gas supply can be impaired by obstruction to airflow (increased airway resistance) or limited expansion of the lungs (decreased compliance). These obstacles lead to ventilation and perfusion mismatch. When perfused alveoli are not ventilated, deoxygenated blood mixes with oxygen saturated blood, reducing the total oxygen content of the blood. This results in arterial hypoxemia and represents shunt physiology. On the other end of the spectrum, ventilated but not perfused alveoli lead to wasted ventilation and do not contribute to carbon dioxide elimination. This phenomenon is termed dead space ventilation. The ventilation/perfusion mismatches caused by airflow obstruction or decreased compliance can range anywhere between these two extremes with a variable impact on gas exchange. Altered respiratory physiology increases the work of breathing, not only from the need to overcome the increased airway resistance or decreased lung compliance, but also from the compensatory mechanisms (usually increased minute ventilation) required to meet the continuing metabolic demands of the individual. Eventually, when metabolic demand exceeds the respiratory reserve, gas exchange abnormalities appear.

In addition to its gas exchange functions, the lung acts as a "filter" for the blood and has a surprising number of metabolic functions. The latter include synthesis of surfactant, various proteins (both structural and enzymatic), and humoral substances (arachidonic acid metabolites, histamine, substance P, and vasoactive intestinal protein), and the transformation of biochemical substances.[1] Relatively little is known about the effects of altered nutrition in these areas.

In a broad sense, pulmonary diseases can be categorized as obstructive airflow diseases and restrictive diseases; both can be acute or chronic (Fig. 76–1). With obstructive airflow disease, maintaining adequate alveolar ventilation (respiratory rate times alveolar tidal volume) to match perfusion and allow for adequate gas exchange in the setting of increased airflow resistance is the primary problem. The resulting ventilation/ perfusion mismatch leads to hypoxemia. As minute alveolar ventilation falls, CO_2 excretion falls and $Pa{CO_2}$ rises. In disease processes marked by decreased lung compliance (e.g., pulmonary fibrosis, pneumonia, and pulmonary edema), destruction of functioning alveolar-capillary units as well as ventilation/perfusion mismatches from regional changes in compliance lead to hypoxemia. Compensation occurs with an increased respiratory rate to replenish alveolar oxygen stores, but the tidal volume falls because of the increased work to inflate stiffer lungs; a greater pressure change must be generated to achieve a given change of lung volume. If the process progresses or the respiratory reserve decreases (e.g., respiratory muscle fatigue), CO_2 elimination suffers and $Pa{CO_2}$ rises, leading to hypercapnic, hypoxemic respiratory failure.

The importance of adequate respiratory muscle energy supply and central drive to compensate for altered gas exchange becomes apparent. Interference with these two critical compensatory mechanisms, as seen with malnutrition, limits the reserve (supply) of this system and leads to premature clinical deterioration. Nutritional supplementation usually does not primarily affect the underlying lung disease. However, it plays a major secondary role in supporting the respiratory muscles that are essential in overcoming the increased work of breathing imposed by disease conditions, maintaining

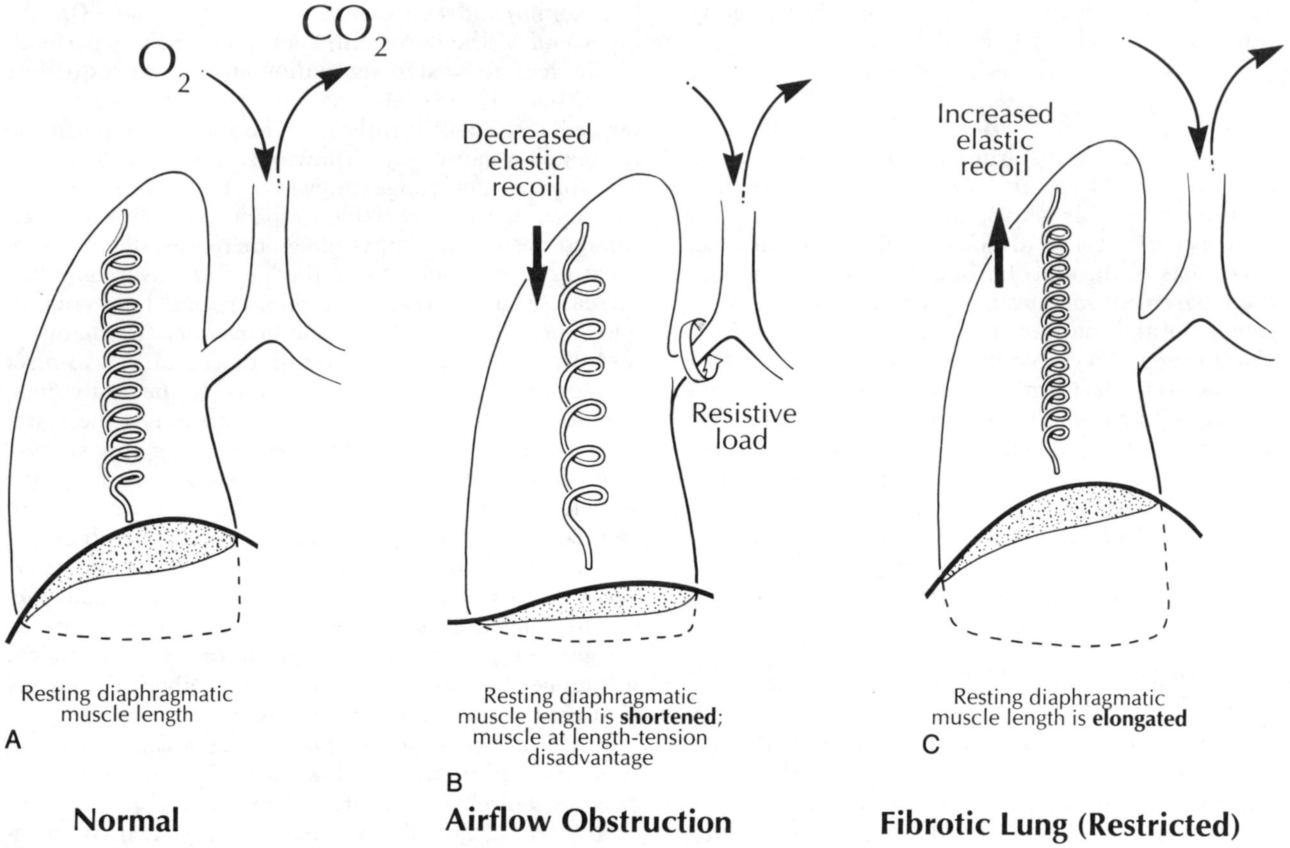

FIGURE 76–1: Normal *(A)*, obstructive *(B)*, and fibrotic *(C)* lungs. *B*, Airflow obstruction leads to an increased resistive load for the respiratory muscles to overcome. In emphysema elastic recoil is lost because of destruction of multiple alveolar-capillary units. As expiratory flow is limited, the lungs become hyperinflated and flatten the normal curvature of the diaphragm. This places the diaphragm at a mechanical disadvantage by the shortened resting length of the diaphragm. The work of breathing is increased because of the increased resistive load and the relative inefficiency of the respiratory muscles because of the shortened resting length. *C*, In the fibrotic lung elastic recoil is increased (decreased compliance of the lung), placing an elastic load on the respiratory muscles that increases the work of breathing.

the ventilatory drive, and reducing damage from possible infection.

NUTRITION AND THE RESPIRATORY SYSTEM: GENERAL CONSIDERATIONS

Results of both laboratory investigations and clinical studies suggest that the major adverse effects of malnutrition on the respiratory system are in respiratory muscle structure and function, ventilatory drive, and host immune defenses (Table 76–2). Although adverse effects on lung architecture, its repair after injury, and surfactant production and other metabolic functions probably also occur, these events are less clear.

Studies based on animal models have shown a linear correlation between diaphragm weight and body weight.[9,10] One investigation of the effects of a short-term fast in young rats leading to a 28% loss of body weight demonstrated a proportional loss in diaphragmatic weight.[11] Similar correlation exists between body weight and diaphragm weight in normal humans[12] and persons with emphysema.[12] Arora and Rochester showed

TABLE 76–2. RESPIRATORY COMPLICATIONS OF MALNUTRITION

Established
Decrease in respiratory muscle structure and function
Decrease in ventilatory drive
Decrease in pulmonary host immune defenses
Proposed
Altered lung architecture especially in immature animals
Decreased ability for repair after injury
Decreased surfactant production

that poorly nourished (body weights were 71 ± 6% of ideal body weight based on height and sex from Metropolitan Life Insurance tables) patients had diminished respiratory muscle strength manifested by reductions in both peak inspiratory and expiratory pressures.[14] The extent of muscle mass loss could not fully account for the disproportionately severe decline in respiratory muscle strength; it was suggested that poor nutritional status could also result in possible myopathy of the remaining muscles.[14] Although the effects of underlying disease (such as malignancy) cannot be excluded as a contributing factor in this study, it does suggest a clinical correlate to the anatomic findings.

Normal subjects limited to a 500-kcal carbohydrate diet have been found to experience a decrease in both the hypoxic ventilatory drive and metabolic rate.[15] These abnormalities proved reversible after refeeding.[15] In another study, normal male volunteers given only a daily infusion of 3 liters of a 5% amino acid solution (550 kcal [2300 kJ] daily) to maintain nitrogen balance for 10 days showed a depression in the hypoxic ventilatory drive compared to a control group given a daily infusion of 3 liters of 5% amino acid solution supplemented with 500 ml of 10% safflower oil emulsion (1100 kcal per day).[17] The latter study suggests that reasonably adequate calorie intake is necessary to preserve the normal ventilatory drive in semistarvation.[17] However, neither study demonstrated a significant alteration in the hypercapnic response in semistarvation. Conversely, after an overnight fast in normal volunteers, enteral protein feedings (100 kcal of egg albumin) caused the normal ventilatory response slope to CO_2 to rise compared to that of a carbohydrate meal (1000 kcal of a glucose solution); both feedings caused an increase in the resting metabolism as well as an increase in the hypoxic ventilatory response.[16]

Along with a general susceptibility to infections, malnourished (both protein and calorie-deficient) individuals are likely to develop alterations in pulmonary defense mechanisms. In infant rats, protein calorie malnutrition has reduced T lymphocyte-dependent alveolar macrophage function, although neutrophil-dependent alveolar macrophage function was preserved.[18] In adult rats, effects of malnutrition on alveolar macrophage function are conflicting. One study showed a reduction in alveolar macrophages recovered by bronchoalveolar lavage but normal phagocytic function in protein-restricted adult rats.[19] In another investigation, more severe starvation resulted in reduction in alveolar macrophage phagocytosis and bactericidal activity.[20] In a clinical study, Niederman and associates demonstrated a positive correlation between gram-negative bacterial adherence and colonization of the lower respiratory mucosa and nutritional status in tracheostomized patients.[21] Fuenzalida et al. measured reactivity to skin antigens and absolute lymphocyte counts in patients with chronic obstructive lung disease and mild malnutrition.[22] Absolute lymphocyte count and reactivity to common skin test antigens improved with refeeding and weight gain, suggesting a link between these parameters in this patient population.[22] Existing animal studies also suggest that adequate nutrition may be important in maintaining normal lung repair and structure and in pulmonary surfactant production,[23] but the clinical relevance of these observations is unclear.

DISEASES OF THE LUNGS

Diseases of the pulmonary system can be categorized into those that cause acute alterations in normal function and those that cause chronic changes. The potential benefits, hazards, and clinical priorities of nutritional care differ with these settings. In acute lung injury, the general goal of nutritional support is to provide for the expanded requirements of a hypercatabolic state to prevent protein breakdown. In chronic obstructive lung disease, the emphasis is on maintaining respiratory muscle strength, mass, and function in an effort to optimize the patient's overall performance status.

ACUTE LUNG INJURY

Acute lung injury can range from a simple localized lung infection (pneumonia) to diffuse alveolar damage as seen with the the adult respiratory distress syndrome (ARDS). Most respiratory illnesses are associated with the systemic symptoms of anorexia, fatigue, and malaise. When these symptoms are combined with cough, shortness of breath, and/or dyspnea, oral intake generally is poor. If the patient requires endotracheal intubation and assisted ventilation, oral intake becomes essentially nil. If the illness is thought to be brief (less than 3 days), then the question of supplemental nutrition may be moot. However, it is often difficult to estimate presumptively the length of decreased oral intake. If negative nitrogen balance ensues, decreased respiratory muscle strength because of protein catabolism, diminished ventilatory drive, and altered immune function can result and compromise recovery.[24] Thus, nutritional status has assumed a priority during the earliest phase of treatment.

METABOLIC REQUIREMENTS

The metabolic response and requirements of severe lung injury (e.g., ARDS) are similar to those associated with sepsis, trauma, major injury, or burns, and differ from the normal fasting state. In ARDS, the degree of metabolic alteration depends more on the underlying insult than on the degree of lung injury as ARDS may represent only the pulmonary response to an underlying local or distant injury. In the phase characterized by hypercatabolism, negative nitrogen balance generally occurs. Carbohydrate metabolism is altered. Hyperglycemia results from increased glucose turnover caused by relative insulin "resistance" with expanded hepatic gluconeogenesis and an excess of counter-regulatory hormones (glucagon, epinephrine, and cortisol).[25] Fat oxidation appears to be preferred and may be the main caloric source in the stressed patient.[26] However, in shock states and multisystem organ failure (MSOF), fat may be used poorly, leading to fat accumulation.[26] Muscle proteolysis develops to maintain a steady glucose supply to the brain, and other glucose dependent tissues leading to negative nitrogen balance.[27]

In this complex setting, the energy requirements can be measured practically by indirect calorimetry at the bedside or estimated by using the Harris-Benedict equation (Table 76–3). Oxygen consumption ($\dot{V}O_2$), an estimate of caloric use, can be calculated using the Fick equation: [$\dot{V}O_2 = CO \times (CaO_2\text{-}CvO_2)$, in which CO is the cardiac output, CaO_2 is oxygen content of arterial blood, and CvO_2 is the mixed oxygen venous content of blood]. The disadvantages of this approach are the requirements of a pulmonary artery catheter to sample mixed venous blood, a relatively stable patient, the inherent inaccuracies of using multiple measurements with their own standards of error to calculate a final product, and the intermittent timing of measurements. Despite these limitations, Liggett et al. found an excellent correlation ($r = 0.90$) between the calculated resting energy expenditure (REE = $\dot{V}O_2$ multiplied by 4.86 kcal/L) using the Fick method and the results of the gas exchange method of calorimetry in 19 stable patients.[28] Alternatively, VO_2 can be assessed more directly by means of a metabolic cart (the gas exchange method). This method requires the technical ability to measure directly exhaled gases and is not universally available. Problems related to its use include the need for skilled technicians trained to operate the analyzer, a leak-free system, a stable FIO_2 (fraction of inspired oxygen), and expensive instrumentation. In addition, at high FIO_2 (greater than or equal to 0.80), the assumptions made in the derivation of the $\dot{V}O_2$ by this method begin to fail.[29] Nevertheless, if it can be preformed accurately, this approach has the advantage that it can be used continuously and represents more of a "direct" measurement. The $\dot{V}O_2$ (ml/min) obtained by either method is converted to kcal kilocalories per day by simply using the caloric value of oxygen (4.69 to 5.05 kcal/L of O_2 per day based on a nonprotein respiratory quotient [RQ])[18] or by using the modified Weir equation if the $\dot{V}CO_2$ is also known: energy expenditure (EE) = $(3.9\ \dot{V}O_2 + 1.1\ \dot{V}CO_2) \times 1.44$[29] (see Table 76–3).

TABLE 76–3. ESTIMATES OF ENERGY REQUIREMENTS

1. EE = $\dot{V}O_2 \times 4.7$ kcal/L $\times$ 1440 min/day
   or
   EE = $(3.9 \times \dot{V}O_2 + 1.1 \times \dot{V}CO_2) \times 1.44$
2. Harris-Benedict Equation
   Females:
   REE = $655 + [4.3 \times \text{Wt(lbs.)}] + [4.3 \times \text{Ht(in.)}] - [4.7 \times \text{age}]$
   Males:
   REE = $65 + [6.2 \times \text{Wt(lbs.)}] + [12.7 \times \text{Ht(in.)}] - [6.8 \times \text{age}]$

Another estimate of the resting energy requirement can be derived from standard regression formulas based on various population studies. The most common formula used is the Harris-Benedict equation (see Table 76–3).[30] This regression equation was derived from studies on normal subjects at rest and was not designed to address the stress and hypercatabolism seen in association with many disease states, especially those encountered in the critical care setting. Therefore, "stress factors" have been developed for certain common clinical scenarios. These range from 1.2 times the calculated REE for elective surgery[29] to 1.5 or greater times the REE for burn patients.[31] However, the correlation between the measured REE by indirect calorimetry and that predicted from the Harris-Benedict equation has been found to be only moderate in postoperative, hemodynamically stable, noncomatose, but critically ill patients requiring mechanical ventilation (Fig. 76–2).[32] More recently, Ligget and Renfro showed that in nonseptic, mechanically ventilated medical intensive care unit patients, the Harris-Benedict equation satisfactorily predicted EE using the Fick method of determining $\dot{V}O_2$ (EE = $\dot{V}O_2 \times 4.86$ kcal/L) without modification or "stress factors."[33] In patients with sepsis, an increase of 20% over that predicted from the Harris-Benedict equation approximated the energy requirements of this group.[33]

Proper estimation of caloric requirements is particularly important in this group with acute lung injury. Overfeeding can lead to fluid overload, glucose intolerance, fatty infiltration of the liver with either parenteral or enteral feedings, diarrhea with enteral feedings, net lipogenesis increasing the minute ventilation demand secondary to increases in the net $\dot{V}CO_2$ (CO_2 production), and an increase in the baseline REE because of diet-induced thermogenesis. Underestimation of caloric needs can lead to underfeeding and negative nitrogen balance with muscle proteolysis. As indicated previously, clinical evidence shows that malnutrition has detrimental effects on pulmonary mechanics by impairing ventilatory drive, respiratory muscle function, and normal lung defense mechanisms,[24] thereby increasing the need for mechanical assistance. Nutritional supplementation may aid in weaning patients with respiratory failure from mechanical ventilation.[34,35] Despite anecdotal experience and the hypothetical benefits of nutritional support in this population, no prospective, randomized, controlled investigations have as yet demonstrated clearly the efficacy of nutritional support in pulmonary disease.[36] Although early enteral feedings can blunt the hypermetabolism and catabolism in severe burn patients,[37] nutritional support does not totally reverse the changes in intermediary metabolism (rela-

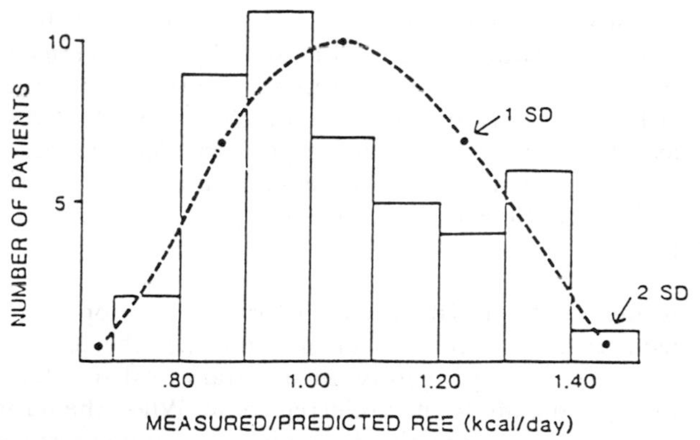

FIGURE 76–2. The distribution of the ratio of measured resting energy expenditure (REE) by indirect calorimetry to the predicted energy requirement using the Harris-Benedict equation in mechanically ventilated, postoperative, critically ill patients who were hemodynamically stable and noncomatose. Perfect correlation would have a value of 1.00. (From Weissman, C., Kemper, M., Askanazi, J., et al.: Anesthesiology, *64*:673–679, 1986.)

tive increase in nitrogen excretion for a given nitrogen intake, increased gluconeogenesis, and increased fat use) in the catabolic state.[25] Balance should be the goal of nutritional sustenance rather than net gain or replenishment in the acute setting.

ENTERAL AND PARENTERAL NUTRITIONAL SUPPORT

Despite clinical uncertainties, several strategies for nutritional support of patients with acute lung failure have evolved. Selection of substrates appropriate for the patient's clinical circumstances and an optimum route of administration are major management issues.

Substrate Supplementation. Nutritional supplementation can be in the form of various mixtures of protein, carbohydrate, or fat. The nutritional characteristics of these substrates are detailed in Chapters 1 to 3 and clinical aspects of formulations in Chapters 79 and 80. In this chapter, we discuss the relative merits of these substrates as they relate to pulmonary diseases.

Most patients with acute respiratory failure that require mechanical ventilation are in a hypercatabolic state and catabolize their protein stores in order to meet their immediate metabolic needs. In addition, glucose-dependent tissue (brain, red blood cells, and healing wounds) requirements are met through gluconeogenesis from amino acids if glucose supplies are limited. Inhibition of glucose neosynthesis with protein sparing can be accomplished in normal fasting patients by the administration of 100 g of glucose per day. Injured or septic patients may require 600 g or more.[38] Intravenous fat emulsions can also be protein sparing if administered with at least 500 kcal per day of carbohydrate calories (either glycerol or glucose).[39] Exogenous protein administration can also replace endogenous protein stores as a substrate for gluconeogenesis and limit proteolysis.[39] Protein supplementation, although, may increase oxygen consumption (thermic effect of protein),[40] minute ventilation,[40] and the ventilatory response to hypercarbia and hypoxemia.[16] Clinically, a high-protein diet could result in increased dyspnea in patients with an already augmented respiratory drive and/or those with borderline respiratory reserve. Because of the integral role of protein in normal physiologic and cellular function (structural support, enzyme activity, transport, and receptor activity and messager activity), protein sparing is essential to recovery from any insult.

Most of the prepared alimentation products provide or can be supplemented to provide the recommended dietary allowances for the micronutrients (vitamins, minerals, and trace elements). These formulas can also be adjusted for fluid and electrolyte deficiencies or excesses and/or other clinical states (hepatic, renal, intestinal, cardiac, or pulmonary failure).

The appropriate mix of substrate (protein, carbohydrate, or fat) delivered depends on the clinical state and the goals to be achieved. In patients with acute or chronic respiratory failure in whom respiratory reserve is limited, carbohydrates impose a greater demand on the respiratory system than the other substrates because of the relative greater carbon dioxide production during its oxidation. For every molecule of glucose oxidized, one molecule of carbon dioxide is produced, giving a respiratory quotient (RQ = molecule of O_2 used/molecule of CO_2 produced) of 1. On the other hand, the RQ of fat is 0.7 (less CO_2 produced for every molecule of O_2 consumed) and the RQ of protein is 0.8. Therefore, more CO_2 is produced in oxidizing carbohydrate than fat or protein for the lung to eliminate (Fig. 76–3).[41]

The partial pressure of arterial CO_2 is determined by the relationship:

$$Pa_{CO_2} = K(\dot{V}_{CO_2}/\dot{V}_A)$$

in which $\dot{V}_{CO_2}$ is CO_2 production, $\dot{V}_A$ is alveolar minute ventilation ($\dot{V}_A = RR \times V_T(1 - V_D/V_T)$ in which RR is the respiratory rate, V_T is the tidal volume, and V_D/V_T is the fraction of wasted or dead space ventilation), and K is a constant. It is apparent from this relationship that if the $\dot{V}_{CO_2}$ increases, alveolar ventilation must also increase to keep the Pa_{CO_2} normal. The increase in alveolar ventilation can be accomplished by increasing the respiratory rate or tidal volume, which in turn increases the work of breathing. Reducing the physiologic dead space (that which is ventilated but not perfused) will also improve alveolar ventilation, but such a reduction usually is not easily accomplished. If the patient has little or no respiratory reserve to meet the augmented ventilatory demand of increased CO_2 production, further exacerbation of respiratory failure may ensue and complicate weaning from artificial ventilatory support.

Respiratory failure may be precipitated or aggravated by administration of high glucose loads to respiratory

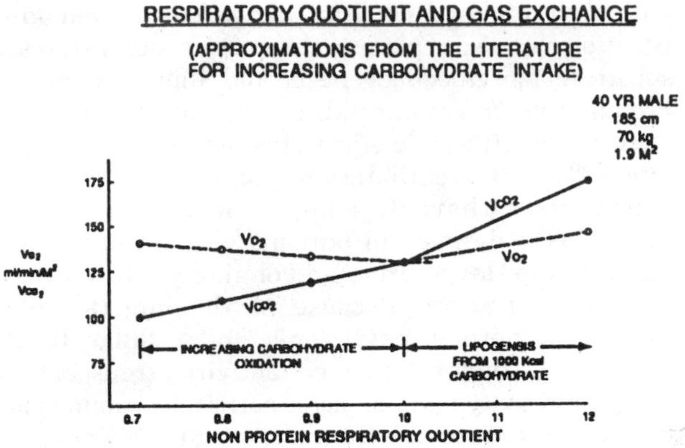

FIGURE 76–3. Effects of increasing carbohydrate intake on CO_2 production and O_2 consumption and respiratory quotient in a normal subject. As the carbohydrate intake increases, CO_2 production and, eventually, O_2 consumption increase. (From Elwyn, D.H., Askanazi, J., Kinney, J.M.: Acta Chir. Scand., *507 (Suppl.)*:209–219, 1981.)

function-compromised patients.[42–44] In chronic nutritionally depleted patients and acutely ill patients with injury or infection,[42] Askanazi et al. studied the effect of total parenteral nutrition (TPN) supplementation at 1.5 times their REE with either glucose or fat emulsions making up to 50% of the nonprotein calories. Neither of two groups required assisted ventilation or were noted to have respiratory impairment. In the chronically nutritionally depleted group, however, CO_2 production rose by 20% and minute ventilation (mostly because of an increase of the V_T) rose by 26% after conversion from a high-fat to a high-glucose source.[41] In the acutely ill individuals, CO_2 production also rose significantly by 21%. Changes in minute ventilation in the acutely ill were not characterized in this report, but in an earlier investigation of high-glucose TPN (1.2 to 2.25 times REE), minute ventilation increased by 71% in the hypermetabolic patients and by 121% in those with mild or moderate injury.[44] Respiratory deterioration was not reported in either study. In stable medical patients with chronic illness, the $\dot{V}co_2$ difference between a high-fat versus high-carbohydrate infusion was exaggerated once supplementation was increased from a maintenance rate to a replenishment rate.[45] This result may be explained by the amount of CO_2 liberated in the production of trigylceride from glucose, which is 30 times greater than the amount of CO_2 produced with dietary fat conversion into triglyceride.[45]

Although some authors suggest that weaning patients from assisted mechanical ventilation may be facilitated by switching from a high-carbohydrate formulation to a high-fat, low-carbohydrate composition,[43,46,47] no compelling evidence exists that this change alters acute management in most of these patients or influences their ultimate outcome. It is certainly prudent, however, to use a high-fat design (greater than 50% of the nonprotein calories from a fat source) rather than a high-carbohydrate diet and to abstain from overfeeding in those patients with marginal respiratory reserve at risk for respiratory failure. In this way, one might avoid precipitating acute respiratory decompensation or, when weaning these patients from assisted mechanical ventilation, ease the transition to ventilator independence.

Route of Administration. The route of supplemental feeding may be parenteral or enteral. If the patient is able to eat independently, then dietary oral supplementation is definitely the preferred route. When the patient is unable to eat the choice lies between the enteral and parenteral routes. At our institution, we prefer the enteral route if at all possible.

Enteral Feeding. This type of supplemental feeding can be accomplished by a gastric feeding tube or by a small caliber duodenal feeding tube. Gastric tubes are easier to place but are also more likely to be complicated by aspiration and/or nosocomial pneumonia, despite intubation with a cuffed endotracheal tube. Gastric paresis is common in critically ill patients, especially those using ventilators. The presence of a tube traversing the lower esophageal sphincter can allow passage of regurgitated gastric material into the hypopharynx and lead to pulmonary aspiration. In addition, the neutralization of the gastric acid pH by enteral supplements is conducive to bacterial overgrowth in the stomach and subsequent colonization in the oropharynx.[48] Although raising the pH in the stomach may reduce stress gastritis/ulceration, factors that increase the gastric pH may increase the risk of nosocomial pneumonia in patients requiring mechanical ventilation.[49] Continuous intragastric feedings are more effective in elevating gastric pH than intraduodenal feedings.[50] To minimize either bolus or micro aspiration, patients should have the head of the bed elevated at least 45° and feedings held when residuals exceed 100 ml. Unfortunately, it is difficult to maintain this posture in the intubated patient because frequent turning and moving are indicated to reduce decubitus ulcers and to promote pulmonary toilet. Moreover, residuals often exceed ideal limits because of gastric paresis. These factors have led to the introduction of various feeding tubes designed to enter the duodenum.

Duodenal tubes generally are small-caliber flexible tubes made of nonreactive materials with a weighted distal tip designed to help the tube migrate distally into the small intestine. The smaller size and flexibility usually make placement into the stomach better tolerated by the patient than the stiffer nasogastric tubes, but a guide wire may be required to pass the tube through the upper pharynx and esophagus. Unless the tube passes through the pylorus into the duodenum, it offers little advantage over stiffer nasogastric tubes other than increased patient comfort and, perhaps, less nasopharyngeal irritation and sinus ostia blockage. In a limited study, a 30% incidence of aspiration was detected by tracheal glucose strips from tube tips in the stomach as compared to no occurrences with tubes documented to be in the duodenum.[51] Spontaneous or metaclopramide-aided passage accounts for only a relatively small percentage of tubes left in the stomach transversing the pylorus into the duodenum. Direct placement into the duodenum by bedside manipulation can be accomplished in approximately one half the cases in our experience. The use of fluoroscopic guidance results in a higher success rate, but may require transportation to the radiology suite, which is not always easily accomplished with a ventilated patient. Guided placement under direct visualization using a fiberoptic endoscope has the highest success rate but increases the cost. Manual placement should probably be attempted first. Appropriate tube position is confirmed by abdominal radiographs. Bedside techniques to confirm placement (e.g., auscultation of air insufflation through the tube in the right upper quadrant or aspiration of bile) are helpful, but not definitive. Needle catheter jejunostomies placed at the time of intra-abdominal surgery can afford immediate postoperative nutritional support as well as maintenance fluid and electrolyte replacement. Formal operative jejunostomy or gastrostomy can also provide access to the intestinal tract but usually are reserved for those patients who require long-term nutritional replacement.

Mechanical problems associated with nasoenteric tubes include improper insertion, clogging of the tube, and pulmonary aspiration. Tubes have been placed in the tracheobronchial tree beyond cuffed endotracheal tubes, occasionally with perforation into the pleural space, leading to catastrophic complications.[52] These problems underscore the need to confirm proper placement before use. In addition epistaxis, sinusitis, esophagitis, tracheoesophageal fistula, and ruptured esophageal varices can complicate the use of nasoenteral tubes.[53] Because of the thin caliber of the duodenal feeding tubes, obstruction with inspissated feedings and viscous solutions do occur. Continuous feedings, flushing with water or saline when the feedings are discontinued, and the avoidance of administering thick viscous material (especially medications and protein supplements)through the tube reduce the incidence of clogging that necessitate tube replacement. The use of duodenal feeding tubes theoretically should reduce the incidence of aspiration by bypassing the problem of delayed emptying secondary to gastric paresis and adding the pylorus as a barrier to regurgitation. The prevalence reported in the literature of aspiration with naso-oroenteral tube feedings (not specifically duodenal tubes) ranges from 1 to 44%.[54]

Other difficulties that can be encountered with enteral feeding, including diarrhea, nausea with vomiting, fluid and electrolyte abnormalities, and hyperglycemia, are addressed in Chapter 79.

Total Parenteral Nutrition. Total parenteral nutrition (TPN) can be accomplished through a central vein, allowing for more concentrated and hypertonic solutions, or peripherally (see Chap. 80). The peripheral route, however, may require a greater obligate fluid load to meet similar caloric needs compared to the central route (Table 76–4). Impaired fluid handling is common in patients with acute lung injury and limited fluid intake is preferred.

Access to the central venous circulation is obtained through percutaneous catheterization of one of the central veins (most commonly the subclavian and jugular veins). Technical difficulties with insertion can lead to ipsilateral pneumothorax, arterial puncture, thoracic duct disruption, catheter misdirection, catheter fracture, thrombosis, catheter or air embolism, infection at the local site with subsequent bloodstream seeding, and local bleeding and hematoma formation.

In cardiac patients, fluid and sodium restriction is important; therefore, a high-fat, dextrose, amino acid, and low-sodium mixture can be used to minimize fluid and sodium load. A high-lipid portion of the nonprotein calories resulting in an overall RQ (CO_2 produced/O_2 consumed) of 0.8 can also be beneficial in the respiration-limited patient. If the ventilatory reserve is limited, the formula that produces the least CO_2 during metabolism will impose the least demand on the ventilatory system. This balance is especially important when attempting to wean a patient from mechanical ventilation.

TABLE 76–4. STANDARD CONSTITUENTS OF PARENTERAL NUTRITION BASE SOLUTIONS (PER LITER)*

Standard central parenteral nutrition	Dextrose 21%	Fat 3%	Amino acids 5%	1.2 kcal/ml
Standard peripheral parenteral nutrition	Dextrose 5%	Fat 3%	Amino acids 5%	0.67 kcal/ml

*Peripheral solutions have approximately one half the caloric content per milliliter of fluid and require double the volume load for equivalent calorie supplementation.

Intralipid (soybean oil; 50% linoleic acid and 9% linolenic acid) and Liposyn II (safflower and soybean oil) are two of the most common lipid emulsions approved by the Food and Drug Administration (FDA) in the United States. Studies from several centers have shown alterations in lung function (decreased oxygen saturation and diffusing capacity of carbon dioxide) in both humans and animal models.[55] These changes appear to be caused principally by an increase in ventilation/perfusion inequalities induced by the lipid infusions, but their clinical relevance even in the severely compromised patient is not clear and usually of little practical significance. However, the conversion of linoleic acid, an essential fatty acid, into arachidonic acid, the precursor to eicosanoids (both prostaglandins and leukotrienes), may have important effects on the cytokine regulation of an immune response.[56] Linolenic acid, an ω-3 fatty acid, can, conversely, decrease eicosanoid production and therefore may attenuate an inflammatory response.[56] Despite being an excellent compact calorie source, the potential effects of the lipid emulsions on the immune regulating system may prove to be more important in critically ill, respiratory function-compromised, and usually infected patients and could affect their usefulness in this population.

Enteral versus parenteral alimentation. Because of the cost of TPN, which is greater than that of enteral feedings, the attendant complications of central venous catheterization, and the more physiologic approach achieved with enteral feedings, we favor the enteral approach when appropriate. In our intensive care unit, we strive to have an enteral tube placed in the duodenum or beyond and feedings started by the third day. We attempt a bedside approach first and then resort to endoscopy if that fails. Because of the difficulty in transporting critically ill patients, fluoroscopy is seldom used. If the gut cannot be used, TPN is instituted for caloric needs; however, we still try to support intestinal integrity by providing at least minimal calories by using an enteral route and formula. Based on results of studies in severely burned patients that early enteral nutrition can blunt postburn hypermetabolism and catabolism[37] and decrease the duration of care in these patients,[57] we stress the early initiation of enteral feeding when possible.

CHRONIC LUNG DISEASE

Most chronic lung diseases present pathophysiologically with either a fixed obstructive or restrictive defect, singly or in combination, in lung mechanics. The most common chronic lung disease is chronic obstructive pulmonary disease (COPD). It is the best studied in regard to the effects of malnutrition and nutritional support on the disease process. Studies of the effects of nutrition on other chronic lung diseases (except for cystic fibrosis, which is not discussed in detail here) have been relatively lacking. However, because most of these conditions place an inspiratory load on ventilatory mechanics, interventions designed to improve respiratory muscle function in COPD should prove helpful in these diseases. The other beneficial effects of nutrition on lung function should also be advantageous in other specific lung diseases.

A subject of particular interest is dietary composition manipulation to reduce the incidence of lung cancer. Some authorities have shown a protective benefit from lung cancer from β-carotene or perhaps other factors in green leafy vegetables, but an increased risk from dietary cholesterol and possibly animal fat.[58] However, the relative benefit and risk are far less than that associated with nonsmoking or smoking cessation and cigarette smoking, respectively.

Cystic fibrosis, physiologically, resembles COPD, although a restrictive defect may also be present. However, in addition to lung involvement, the underlying defect in ion transport also affects other organs. Pancreatic deficiency resulting in malabsorption, glucose intolerance, intestinal obstruction, salt depletion, fatty liver, and gallbladder disease are common nonpulmonary complications of cystic fibrosis and contribute to the problem of maintaining an adequate nutritional status. Weight gain or loss correlates to the overall general health of the patient and is an important monitor and predictor of prognosis. Although considerable advances have been made in the genetic defect of cystic fibrosis, treatment is still largely supportive. The use of a high-calorie, high-protein diet with supplemental pancreatic enzymes and multivitamin fortification is recommended to maintain weight.

CHRONIC OBSTRUCTIVE PULMONARY DISEASE

This generic term encompasses emphysema, bronchitis, and chronic asthma. The hallmark of the disease is airflow obstruction during expiration caused by airway smooth muscle contraction, bronchial inflammation and edema, bronchial gland hypertrophy with mucous plugging, loss of elastic recoil, or accentuated dynamic collapse of airways as the lung volume decreases; most commonly, it is a combination of these events. These changes result in hyperinflation and airtrapping, elevating the residual volume, and flattening the diaphragms (see Fig. 76–1). The diaphragms are then at a mechanical disadvantage by the shortening of their resting length prior to inspiratory contraction (e.g., Starling's law relating length to tension). Patients, thereby, become inspiration limited as well as expiration limited.

In 1984, COPD was the fifth leading cause of death in the United States.[59] In the Tecumseh Community Health Study, the prevalence rate for obstructive airways disease, chronic bronchitis, or both was approximately 14% of the adult males and 8% of the adult females.[60]

Nutritional depletion is exceedingly common in the COPD population: 24% of 779 men with COPD enrolled in the IPPB (Intermittent Positive Pressure Breathing) study group were malnourished, defined as a weight less than 90% of ideal body weight.[61] Braun found that 48% of 60 outpatients with COPD presenting to a pulmonary rehabilitation program proved to be nutritionally depleted based on the criteria of weight loss of greater than 5% during the preceding year or abnormal anthropometrics (triceps skin fold of less than 60% of standard) at presentation.[62] Schols and colleagues, using a nutritional index composed of the percentage of ideal body weight, serum albumin level, serum prealbumin level, and total lymphocyte count found 19% of 153 patients with COPD admitted to a rehabilitation center were nutritionally compromised.[63] Other investigators using different criteria of undernutrition have found similar ranges for nutritional depletion in their subgroups of COPD patients.[64–66]

After the onset of progressive weight loss in patients with COPD, mortality has been found to be 30% at 3 years and 49% at 5 years, compared to 25% at 5 years for those without weight loss.[67] Several other epidemiologic surveys have also shown that a poor prognosis is associated with a compromised nutritional status in this group of patients.[68–70] In retrospectively analyzed patients enrolled in the IPPB trial, it was found that individuals who were less than 90% of ideal body weight on entry into the study had a greater overall 5-year mortality rate even after normalization for the severity of their lung dysfunction (Fig. 76–4).[61] This effect was seen in patients with mild obstruction (forced expiratory volume [FEV_1] greater than 46% predicted) as well as in those with severe obstruction (FEV_1 less than 35% predicted), and therefore was independent of lung function.[61] The 3-year mortality rate (30 to 40%) in the patients with lowest percentage of ideal body weight regardless of degree of airflow obstruction was remarkably similar to the rate Vanderbergh reported in 1966.[61,67] This similarity suggests that 20 years of medical advances in the treatment of COPD have not changed the adverse prognosis associated with a poor nutritional status in this group.

The possible pathophysiologic mechanisms for this weight loss in patients with chronic lung disease have been summarized.[23] Impaired gastrointestinal function, inadequate dietary intake, an adaptive mechanism to lower oxygen consumption to theoretically lower the work of breathing, altered pulmonary and cardiovascular hemodynamics limiting nutrient supply to other tissues, and a hypermetabolic state could all contribute to the malnutrition seen in this group of patients.[23] In their review, Wilson et al. concluded that an increase in daily energy expenditure led to weight loss in patients with chronic lung disease because of an increased resistive load and decreased respiratory muscle efficiency.[23] Coupled with this increase in resting energy requirement, they postulated that decreases in caloric intake could occur when energy requirements are further increased by stresses such as intervening illness, surgery, or infection. In this way, a stepwise decline in pulmonary function and nutritional status can occur.

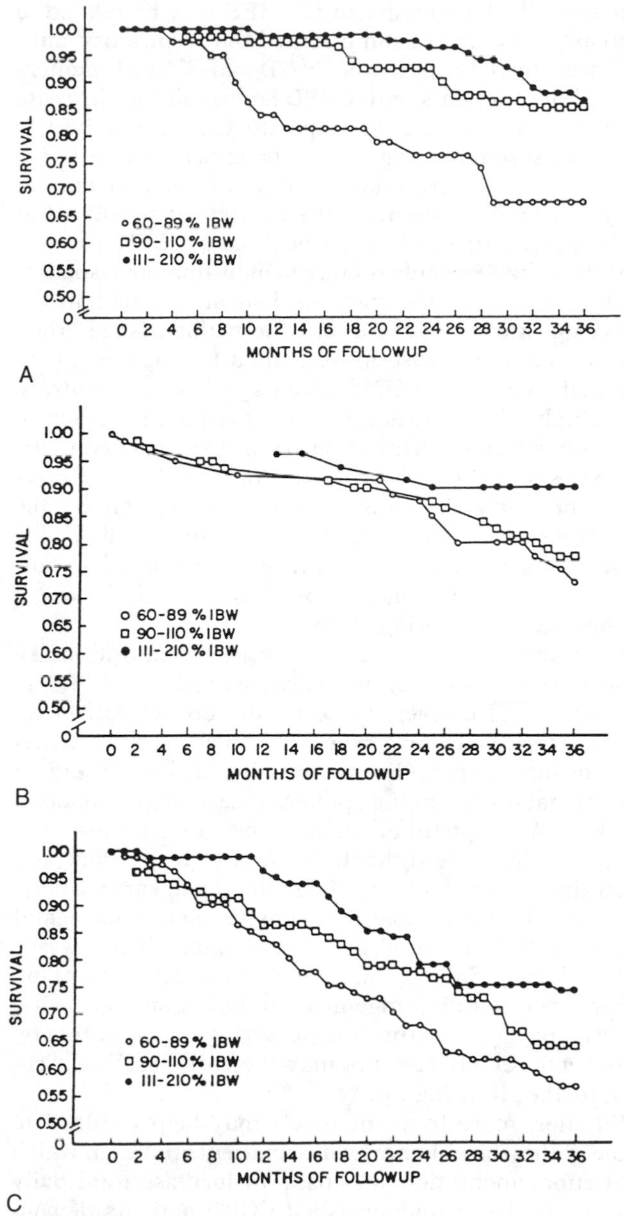

FIGURE 76–4. Survival curves for patients with chronic obstructive pulmonary disease who were enrolled in the National Institutes of Health Intermittent Positive-Pressure Breathing Trial. *A*, Survival of patients with a forced expiratory volume in 1 second (FEV_1) higher than 47% predicted by percentage of ideal body weight (%IBW) category. *B*, Survival of patients with FEV_1 of 35 to 47% predicted by %IBW category. *C*, Survival of patients with a FEV_1 lower than 35% predicted by %IBW. (From Wilson, D.O., Rogers, R.M., Wright, R.C., et al.: Am. Rev. Respir. Dis., *139*:1435–1438, 1989.)

Several investigators have shown that the measured REE in patients with COPD with and without weight loss significantly exceed the calculated REE from the Harris-Benedict equation.[62,71,72] Although the patients are hypermetabolic, they do not seem to be hypercatabolic, as would be seen in stress states with preferential fat oxidation.[71] The increase in the REE may be related to increased oxygen consumption of the respiratory muscles seen in these patients.[72,73] Donahoe et al. demonstrated that patients with COPD had significant increase in energy expenditure for respiratory muscle activity.[72] They measured the oxygen cost of augmented ventilation with dead-space stimulation of ventilation in normal subjects, COPD patients with greater than 90% ideal body weight (normal nourished), and COPD patients with less than 90% ideal body weight (malnourished).[72] Both groups of COPD patients had an increase in the oxygen cost of ventilation, but the malnourished group had a notable increase in oxygen cost compared to the normally nourished COPD patients and normal controls. Presumbly, this elevation in energy requirements for an increase in minute ventilation can be extrapolated to the increases seen in daily activities of normal life. Therefore, the higher level of energy consumption by the respiratory muscles to meet the demands of daily life could induce a hypermetabolic state compared to normal subjects, and lead to progressive weight loss if output exceeds caloric intake.

Most studies show adequate or better caloric intake than that predicted or measured at rest in COPD patients.[62,64,74] However, these results do not satisfactorily address the caloric expenditure necessary for activity[62] or intercurrent illness, and also tend to depend on nutritional inventory (i.e., patient recall) to assess caloric intake.[75] Attempts to augment caloric intake over baseline levels may be difficult because of respiratory and gastrointestinal symptoms (e.g., anorexia, early satiety, dyspnea, fatigue, bloating, constipation, and dental problems).[75,76] Some of these symptoms (bloating, satiety, and anorexia) may be related to the flattening of the diaphragms with impingement on the abdominal cavity. Arterial oxygen desaturation occurring during eating by hypoxemic COPD patients may increase baseline dyspnea, further limiting intake.[77,78]

Smaller, more frequent meals may help to alleviate some of these problems. Two outpatient studies in which oral supplementation was used to increase total daily caloric intake in malnourished COPD patients demonstrated difficulty in maintaining significant caloric intake over baseline on entry into the study.[79,80] In one of the studies, increased enteral formula intake was associated with a tendency to decrease usual food intake.[79] Schols et al. found that COPD patients with weight loss had similar REE as COPD patients without weight loss, but the former group had a lower caloric intake in relation to the measured REE.[81]

Nutritional Supplementation. Wilson et al. studied six malnourished (less than 90% ideal body weight) patients with emphysema admitted to an inpatient clinical research unit with a target caloric ingestion of 150% of the basal metabolic rate calculated daily by indirect calorimetry.[74] Within 3 weeks, all patients had been able to ingest sufficient calories to exceed both their calculated resting energy requirements from indirect calorimetry and the Harris-Benedict equation (some even prior to nutritional intervention). All patients gained weight and increased their percentage ideal body weight. Maximal inspiratory mouth and transdiaphragmatic pressures (measures of respiratory muscle function) increased as did peripheral skeletal muscle strength (handgrip). Spirometry, lung volumes, and the diffusion capacity of carbon monoxide (physiologic lung function measurements) did not change significantly. In another study of short-term nutritional support of inpatients with COPD, Whittaker et al. showed that caloric supplementation over 16 days led to significant weight gain and improvement of the maximal inspiratory pressure compared to a control group.[82]

Lewis et al. evaluated the effect of an 8-week outpatient nutritional supplementation on 21 malnourished COPD patients randomized to a control and "fed" group.[79] The mean caloric intake was increased in the "fed" group but not sufficiently enough to obtain a significant increase in their weight. A trend toward weight gain was noted, but no changes in anthropometric measurements, pulmonary function studies, or respiratory muscle strength occurred. A greater increase in daily caloric intake over baseline (approximately 1.5 times basal energy expenditure calculated using the Harris-Benedict equation) was difficult to obtain because the patients tended to decrease their own food intake while drinking the enteral study formula. The investigators then compared respiratory muscle function (maximal inspiratory pressure, maximal expiratory pressure, and maximal sustained ventilatory capacity) of poorly nourished patients with COPD (less than 90% ideal body weight) and well-nourished COPD patients and found no difference.[79]

In another outpatient study of dietary supplementation in patients with COPD, Knowles et al. also could not demonstrate a difference in respiratory muscle function (maximal inspiratory pressure, maximal expiratory pressure, and sustainable inspiratory pressure) in the nutritionally supplemented group versus controls.[80] This study was a randomized observer-blinded crossover trial in which each group was supplemented for 8 weeks and then held as a control without supplementation for 8 weeks or in reverse order. Any improvement in respiratory muscle function during the 16-week study was thought to be due to learning rather than resulting from improved nutritional status, as improvement occurred during both the supplement phase and the control period. Although small increases in body weight were noted after 8 weeks of nutritional supplementation, the patients tended to lose weight within 1 month of stopping the supplements. This study included patients with body weights greater than 90% of ideal body weight at entry, but 13 of 25 were less than 85% of ideal body weight.

Efthimiou et al. undertook a longer, 3-month outpatient oral nutritional support trial in COPD patients, and noted an increase in body weight and other anthropometric measurements after 3 months of dietary supplementation.[83] Along with this gain, improvement in respiratory muscle strength as well as peripheral strength was demonstrated, but these changes were not accompanied by improvements of pulmonary function or arterial blood gases. Nevertheless, patients' feeling of general well-being, breathlessness scores, and 6-minute walking distances improved significantly.

In comparing these observations, the three studies[74,82,83] in which significant weight gain was achieved with nutritional supplementation were those that demonstrated improvements in respiratory muscle function (Table 76–5). The other two studies noted in this table showed a tendency toward weight gain, but the lack of improvement in respiratory muscle function might have been related to the shorter duration of nutritional supplementation. Interestingly, the degree of airflow obstruction in the patients was similar in all five studies, but the average baseline maximal inspiratory pressure was lower in Wilson's patients compared to those in the three outpatient trials.[73,74,79,83] The average baseline caloric intake before supplementation was lower in Efthimiou's and Whittaker's patients (who showed significant weight gain) as opposed to the two other outpatient study without significant weight gain, but total supplemented calories were similar in all four studies.[79,80,82,83] It may be that those patients with weight loss and the lowest caloric intake derive greater benefit from nutritional supplementation, especially if supplementation is continued for 3 months or longer and significant weight gain occurs. The likelihood of improvement of respiratory muscle function, therefore, may be linked to the degree of weight gain and, possibly, the severity of initial deficits. Further information is needed in this area.

Both Lewis et al.[79] and Knowles et al.[80] commented about the difficulty these patients have in ingesting and maintaining sufficient caloric intake to gain weight. This problem may relate to diet-induced thermogenesis (an energy requiring process to biochemically convert dietary substances into usable fuel for consumption and storage). Goldstein et al. demonstrated that malnourished COPD patients had a greater increase in resting oxygen consumption after a meal than malnourished patients without COPD.[84] Suchner et al. used growth hormone in a preliminary study to determine whether they could promote positive nitrogen balance in malnourished COPD patients with an eucaloric intake that alone achieved equilibrium.[85] They were able to achieve significant positive nitrogen balance with 60 μg/kg daily of growth hormone compared to TPN alone.[85] Pape et al. administered recombinant growth hormone (0.05 mg/kg daily subcutaneously) to malnourished COPD patients (less than 90% ideal body weight) together with a balanced diet of 35 kcal/kg for 3 weeks of monitoring in their clinical research center.[86] While receiving growth hormone, these patients showed improved nitrogen balance, weight gain, and an increase in maximal inspiratory pressure compared to 1 week receiving the balanced diet alone. Rudman et al. gave biosynthetic growth hormone to a group of healthy elderly males to test the hypothesis that declining activity of growth hormone as indicated by low insulin growth factor I (IGF-I) levels may contribute to the decrease in lean body mass and an increase in fatty tissue associated with aging.[87] The group receiving the biosynthetic growth hormone (0.03 mg/kg subcutaneously three times per week for 6 months) had a significant increase in lean body mass and a decrease in adipose tissue mass compared to a control group with similar caloric intake (25 to 30 kcal/kg). This approach of using exogenous growth hormone may allow replenishment and protein synthesis while minimizing the thermogenic effect of nutritional replacement by reducing the total amount calories needed for anabolism.[85]

A body weight of less than ideal body weight is used as an index of a poor nutritional state and respiratory muscle function as assessment of an improved pulmonary status in most studies. Although there are other

TABLE 76–5. NUTRITIONAL INTERVENTION IN MALNOURISHED CHRONIC OBSTRUCTIVE PULMONARY DISEASE PATIENTS

AUTHORS	NUMBER FED	STUDY TYPE	RMS*	WEIGHT GAIN
Wilson et al.[74]	6	Inpatient, 3 weeks	MIP improved Mean: 143%	Yes
Whittaker et al.[82]	6	Inpatient, 2.3 weeks	MIP improved Mean: 119%	Yes
Lewis et al.[79]	10	Outpatient, 8 weeks	MIP no change Mean: 89%	No
Knowles et al.[80]	25	Outpatient, 8 weeks	MIP no change† Mean: 105–115%	No
Efthimiou et al.[83]	7	Outpatient, 12 weeks	MIP improved Mean: 116%	Yes

*RMS, respiratory muscle strength; MIP, maximal inspiratory pressure; mean, mean percent of baseline after supplementation.

†No significant change in MIP between fed and control patients.

methods of nutritional assessment (other anthropometrics, measurements of body compartments, and parameters of functional status), weight loss has been most clearly associated with a poor outcome in these patients.[67–70] Respiratory muscle function tests are relatively easy to perform and reproduce and would be expected to change with nutritional status. Other pulmonary function tests (spirometry, static lung volumes, and diffusion capacity of the carbon monoxide) should not be expected to improve and relate to the underlying cause of airflow obstruction, which nutritional support would not be anticipated to change directly. However, there are other determinants of respiratory muscle strength independent of nutrition. Important in the COPD population is the initial length of muscle fibers in the diaphragm when inspiratory and expiratory force are measured. If the fibers are shortened because of hyperinflation and airtrapping (increased residual volume), it can be expected that maximal inspiratory force would be reduced (see Fig. 76–1). In chronic overinflated states, respiratory muscle adaptation may occur, overcoming some of the mechanical disadvantage altering the normal length-tension relationship.[79,88] In addition, short-term caloric replenishment may have a greater impact on improving electrolyte-related respiratory muscle function than protein anabolism and muscle reconstitution.[79,89]

No long-term studies examining nutritional support in this population and improvement in overall prognosis are available. If survival is linked to decreased body weight and is an independent variable, and nutritional support can improve and maintain body weight, it would be expected that survival should improve with optimizing nutritional support. It is not clear which potential effects of nutritional support on respiratory muscle function, immunocompetence, control of ventilation, lung repair, or surfactant production might lead to improved clinical outcomes. Despite the mixed results from the short-term studies and the difficulties in maintaining satisfactory long-term nutritional intake, appropriate dietary supplementation is of greater potential benefit than of clinical toxicity.

Nutrient Composition and Administration. Because COPD patients have a limited ventilatory reserve, it may be expected that a high-carbohydrate diet that produces more CO_2 for each mole of O_2 consumed for energy requirements would stress the respiratory system. A high-fat diet, on the other hand, would be expected to produce less CO_2 per mole of oxygen consumed and perhaps be beneficial. Angelillo et al. performed a randomized double-blinded study of COPD patients with hypercarbia and found that a 5-day, low-carbohydrate diet (28% carbohydrate calories, 55% fat calories) resulted in a significantly lower CO_2 production and arterial $Paco_2$ than a 5-day, high-carbohydrate diet (74% carbohydrate calories, 9.4% fat calories).[90] Kwan and Mir also noted a benefit (reduced $Paco_2$) from a low-carbohydrate diet in COPD patients with hypercapnia (chronic hypoventilatory respiratory failure).[91] In addition, Pao_2 and mouth pressure at 100 msec (a measure of respiratory center output) also increased with the carbohydrate restriction.[91] Brown et al. assessed a meaningful functional parameter, the 12-minute walk, and found that a large carbohydrate load reduced the walking distance compared to placebo in patients with COPD.[92] Sue et al. examined in normal subjects the exercise gas exchange response to altering dietary fat and carbohydrate proportions.[93] The mean CO_2 production, respiratory gas exchange ratio, and minute ventilation at rest were higher (the latter not significantly higher) on a high-carbohydrate diet versus a low-carbohydrate diet; with exercise, however, mean minute ventilation was not significantly different between the two diets.[93] The authors concluded that if these changes can be extrapolated to COPD patients, then exertional dyspnea is unlikely to be related to acute changes in dietary composition. These studies did not specifically address underweight individuals or whether long-term benefits of changes in dietary composition in COPD patients might occur.

As mentioned in a previous section, protein supplementation can increase oxygen consumption from its thermic effect,[40] increase minute ventilation,[40] and increase the ventilatory response to hypoxemia and hypercarbia.[16] These effects could result in dyspnea in patients with limited respiratory function.

Electrolyte deficiencies such as hypophosphatemia, hypokalemia, and hypocalcemia can also adversely effect respiratory muscle function. Aubier et al. have shown improvement in diaphragmatic contractility after phosphorus replacement in hypophosphatemic patients with acute respiratory failure.[94] This observation is particularly relevant to patients with COPD who rely on mechanical ventilation; intracellular shifts after correction of respiratory acidosis commonly occur in these individuals.[95] An acute drop in serum phosphorus levels in asthmatic individuals may occur after intensive bronchodilator therapy, which probably relates to intracellular shifts and parallels improvement in the arterial pH and $Paco_2$.[96,97] The clinical consequences of the acute hypophosphatemia were not clear in these reports. The clinical manifestations of hypophosphatemia generally result from intracellular phosphorus depletion, which is associated more often with chronic hypophosphatemia. Aubier et al. also reported that lowering the serum calcium level acutely with a chelating agent (EGTA) can also reduce diaphragmatic maximal contraction.[98] Dorin and Crapo reported a case of hypokalemic respiratory arrest that occurred in association with diabetic ketoacidosis that was thought to be secondary to hypokalemic respiratory muscle paralysis.[99] Electrolyte replenishment may ultimately prove to be more important than protein anabolism in accounting for acute improvements of respiratory muscle strength by restoring normal intracellular concentrations of these ions in short-term replenishment.

The relationships between micronutrients and respiratory illness have also received increasing attention. In an epidemiologic study from the Second National Health and Nutrition Examination Survey (NHANES II), the authors developed a comprehensive nutrient-specific logistic regression analysis.[100] Controlling for other variables, they found a negative association of respiratory symptoms of bronchitis with serum vitamin C and the serum zinc to copper ratio and a negative association between wheezing and serum vitamin C, niacin, and the serum zinc to copper ratio. Vitamin C is an antioxidant and copper is an important cofactor for the enzyme lysyl-oxidase, which catalyzes the cross-linking of collagen and elastin; severe copper deficiency can lead to weakened collagen.[100] Lung injuries, both acute (e.g., ARDS) and chronic (emphysema, in particular), may be related to free radical oxidant damage when the lung's natural antioxidant defense system is overwhelmed (cigarette smoking) or deficient (α1-antitrypsin deficiency). Dietary deficiencies in micronutrients could lead to increased susceptibility to oxidant damage and/or respiratory symptoms, but more information is needed.[100]

In summary, nutritional intervention in lung disease is a relatively new frontier. Clinical investigations as well as anecdotal observations have shown that malnutrition is common in both acute and chronic lung diseases. Current research supports nutritional intervention in these cohorts of patients, but the optimum method, type, and duration of nutritional support and/or impact on the prognosis of these diseases is not distinct.

Modification of nutritional factors may not reverse the underlying disease processes affecting the lungs, but it might help in lung injury by supporting repair and providing an energy source for normal and compensatory function until the lung insult is removed. What is apparent, however, is that nutritional intervention is and will continue to be important in the management of acute and chronic lung diseases. The rational use of dietary components and micronutrients may further refine nutritional supplementation for specific diseases.

REFERENCES

1. Murray, J.F.: The Normal Lung. 2nd Ed. Philadelphia, W.B. Saunders, 1986.
2. Roussos, C., Macklem, P.T.: N. Engl. J. Med. *307*:786–797, 1982.
3. Lewis, M.I., Sieck, H.C., Founier, M., et al.: J. Appl. Physiol., *60*:596–603, 1986.
4. Goldspink, G., Ward, P.S.: J. Physiol. (Lond), *296*:453–469, 1979.
5. Oldfor, A., Mairk, W.G.P., Sourander, P.: Neurol. Sci., *59*:291–302, 1983.
6. Sieck, G.C., Lewis, M.I., Blanco, C.E.: J. Appl. Physiol., *66*:2196–2205, 1989.
7. Bellemare, F., Grassino, A.: J. Appl. Physiol., *53*:1190–1195, 1982.
8. Bellemare, F., Grassino, A.: J. Appl. Physiol., *55*:8–13, 1983.
9. Davidson, M.B.: Growth, *32*:221–223, 1968.
10. Rochester, D.F., Pradel-Guena, M.: J. Appl. Physiol., *34*:68–74, 1973.
11. Goldberg, A.L., Odessey, R.: Am. J. Physiol., *223*:1384–1391, 1972.
12. Thurlbeck, W.M.: Thorax, *33*:483–487, 1978.
13. Arora, N.S., Rochester, D.F.: J. Appl. Physiol., *56*:64–70, 1982.
14. Arora, N.S., Rochester, D.F.: Am. Rev. Respir. Dis., *126*:5–8, 1982.
15. Doekel, R.C., Zwillich, A.V., Scoggins, C.H., et al.: N. Engl. J. Med., *295*:358–361, 1976.
16. Zwillich, C.W., Sahn, S.A., Weill, J.A.: J. Clin. Invest., *60*:900–906, 1977.
17. Baier, H., Somani, P.: Chest, *85*:222–225, 1984.
18. Martin, T.R., Altman, L.C., Alvares, O.F.: Am. Rev. Respir. Dis., *128*:1013–1019, 1983.
19. Moriguchi, S., Sine, S., Kishina, Y.: J. Nutr., *113*:40–46, 1983.
20. Shennib, H., Chin, R.C., Mulder, D.S., et al.: Surg. Gynecol. Obstet., *158*:535–540, 1984.
21. Niederman, M.S., Merrill, W.W., Feranti, R.D., et al.: Ann. Intern. Med., *100*:795–800, 1984.
22. Fuenzalida, C.E., Petty, T.L., Jones, M.L., et al.: Am. Rev. Respir. Dis., *142*:49–56, 1990.
23. Wilson, D.O., Rogers, R.M., Hoffman, R.M.: Am. Rev. Respir. Dis., *132*:1347–1367, 1985.
24. Pingleton, S.K.: Am. Rev. Respir. Dis., *137*:1463–1493, 1988.
25. Kinney, J.M.: Critical Care Clinics 3:1–10, 1987.
26. Wiener M., Rothkopf M.M., Rothkopf G., et al. Crit. Care Clin., *3*:25–56, 1987.
27. Elwyn, D.H.: Crit. Care Clin., *3*:57–69, 1987.
28. Liggett, S.B., John, R.E., Lefrak, S.S.: Chest, *91*:562–566, 1987.
29. Damask, M.C., Schwarz, Y., Weissman, C.: Crit. Care Clin., *3*:71–96, 1987.
30. Harris, J.A., Benedict, F.G.: Standard Basal Metabolism Constants for Physiologists and Clinicians; A Biometric Study of Basal Metabolism in Man. Philadelphia, J.B. Lippincott, 1919.
31. Saffle, J.R., Medina, E., Raymond, J., et al.: J. Trauma, *25*:32–39, 1985.
32. Weissman, C., Kemper, M., Askanazi, J., et al.: Anesthesiology, *64*:673–679, 1986.
33. Liggett, S.B., Renfro, A.D.: Chest, *98*:682–686, 1990.
34. Bassili, H.R., Deital, M.: J. Parenter. Enter. Nutr., *5*:161–163, 1981.
35. Laaban, J.P., Lemaire, F., Baron, J.R., et al.: Chest, *87*:67–72, 1985.

36. Koretz, R.L.: Chest, *98:*524–526, 1990.
37. Mochizuke, H., Trocki, O., Dominioni, L.: Ann. Surg., *200:*297–310, 1984.
38. Elwyn, D.H., Kinney, J.M., Jeevanandam, M., et al.: Ann. Surg., *190:*117, 1979.
39. Edens, N.K., Gil, K.M., Elywyn, D.H.: Clin. Chest Med., *7:*3–17, 1986.
40. Weissman, C., Askanazi, J., Rosenbaum, S.H., et al.: Ann. Intern. Med., *98:*41–44, 1983.
41. Elwyn, D.H., Askanazi, J., Kinney, J.M.: Acta Chir. Scand. *507(Suppl.):*209–219, 1981.
42. Askanazi, J., Elwyn, D.H., Silverbery, P.A., et al.: Surgery, *8:*596–599, 1980.
43. Al-Saady, N.M., Blackmore, C.M., Bennett, E.D.: Intensive Care Med., *15:*290–295, 1989.
44. Herve, L., Simonneau-Girard, P., Cerrina, J., et al.: Crit. Care Med., *13:*537–540, 1988.
45. Heymsfield, S.B., Erbland, M., Casper, K., et al.: Clin. Chest Med., *7:*41–67, 1986.
46. Covelli, H.D., Black, J.W., Olsen, M.: Ann. Intern. Med., *95:*579, 1981.
47. Dark, D.S., Pingleton, S.K., Kerby, G.R.: Chest, *88:*141–143, 1988.
48. Pingleton, S.K., Hinthorn, D.R., Liu, C.: Am. J. Med., *80:*827–832, 1986.
49. Driks, M.R., Craven, D.E., Celli, B.R., et al.: N. Engl. J. Med., *318:*1376–1382, 1987.
50. Valentine, R.J., Turner, W.W., Bowman, K.R., et al.: Crit. Care Med., *14:*599–600, 1986.
51. Zaloga, G.P.: Chest, *100:*1643–1646, 1991.
52. Miller, K.S., Tomlinson, J.R., Sahn, S.A.: Chest, *88:*230–233, 1985.
53. Berger, R., Adams, L.: Chest, *96:*372–378, 1989.
54. Koruda, M.J., Guenter, R.N., Rombeau, J.L.: Crit. Care Clin., *3:*133–153, 1987.
55. Hageman, J.R., Hunt, C.E.: Clin. Chest Med., *7:*69–72, 1986.
56. Zaloga, G.P.: Nutrition and Prevention of Systemic Infection. Critical Care State of the Art. Edited by R.W. Taylor and W.C. Shoemaker. Fullerton, CA, Society of Critical Care Medicine, 1991.
57. Garrel, D.R., Davignon, I., Lopez, D.: J. Burn Care Rehabil., *12:*85–90, 1991.
58. Miller, A.B., Risch, H.A.: Chest, *96:*8S–9S, 1989.
59. Higgins, M., Thom, T.: Curr. Pulmonol., *9:*1–24, 1988.
60. Higgins, M.W., Keller, J.B., Bedar, M., et al.: Am. Rev. Respir. Dis., *125:*144–151, 1982.
61. Wilson, D.O., Rogers, R.M., Wright, R.C., et al.: Am. Rev. Respir. Dis., *139:*1435–1438, 1989.
62. Braun, S.R., Keim, N.L., Dixon, R.M., et al.: Chest, *86:*558–563, 1984.
63. Schols, A., Moslert, R., Soetters, P., et al.: Chest, *96:*247–249, 1989.
64. Hunter, A.M.B., Carey, M.A., Larsh, H.W.: Am. Rev. Respir. Dis., *124:*376–381, 1981.
65. Fiaccadori, E., Canale, S.F., Coffrini, E., et al.: Am. J. Clin. Nutr., *48:*680–685, 1988.
66. Gray, D.K., Gibbons, L., Shupin, S.H., et al.: Am. Rev. Respir. Dis., *140:*1544–1548, 1989.
67. Vandenbergh, E., Van de Woestijne, K.P., Gyselen, A.: Am. Rev. Respir. Dis., *95:*556–566, 1967.
68. Boushy, S.F., Adhikari, P.K., Sakamoto, A., et al.: Dis. Chest, *45:*402–410, 1964.
69. Burrows, B.A., Nidon, A.H., Barclay, W.R., et al.: Am. Rev. Respir. Dis., *91:*665–678, 1964.
70. Renzetti, A.D., McClement, J.H., Litt, B.D.: Am. J. Med., *41:*115–129, 1966.
71. Goldstein, S.A., Thomashaw, B.M., Kvetan, V., et al.: Am. Rev. Respir. Dis., *138:*636–644, 1988.
72. Donahoe, M., Rogers, R.M., Wilson, D.O., et al.: Am. Rev. Respir. Dis., *140:*385–391, 1989.
73. Cherniack, R.M.: J. Clin. Invest., *38:*494–499, 1959.
74. Wilson, D.O., Rogers, R.M., Sanders, M.H., et al.: Am. Rev. Respir. Dis., *134:*672–677, 1986.
75. Donahoe, M., Rogers, R.M.: Clin. Chest Med., *11:*487–504, 1990.
76. Browning, R.J., Olsen, A.M.: Mayo Clin. Proc., *36:*537–543, 1961.
77. Brown, S.E., Castari, R.J., Light, R.W.: South. Med. J., *76:*194–198, 1983.
78. Schols, A., Mostert, R., Cobben, N.: Chest, *100:*1287–1292, 1991.
79. Lewis, M.I., Belman, M.J., Dorr-Uyemura, L.: Am. Rev. Respir. Dis., *135:*1062–1068, 1987.
80. Knowles, J.B., Fairburn, M.S., Wiggs, B.J., et al.: Chest, *93:*977–983, 1988.
81. Schols, A., Soeters, P.B., Mostert, R., et al.: Am. Rev. Respir. Dis., *143:*1248–1252, 1991.
82. Whittaker, J.S., Ryan, C.E., Buckley, P.A., et al.: Am. Rev. Respir. Dis., *142:*283–288, 1990.
83. Efthimiou, J., Fleming, J., Gomes, C., et al.: Am. Rev. Respir. Dis., *137:*1075–1082, 1988.
84. Goldstein, S.A., Askanazi, J., Weismann, C., et al.: Chest, *91:*22–224, 1987.
85. Sucher, U., Rothkopf, M.M., Stanilaus, G., et al.: Arch. Intern. Med., *150:*1225–1230, 1990.
86. Pape, G.S., Friedman, M., Underwood, L.E., et al.: Chest, *99:*1495–1499, 1991.
87. Rudman, D., Fellor, A.G., Nagraj, H.S.: N. Engl. J. Med., *323:*1–6, 1991.
88. Marks, J., Pasterkamp, H., Tal, A., et al.: Am. Rev. Respir. Dis., *133:*414–417, 1986.
89. Rochester, D.F.: Am. Rev. Respir. Dis., *134:*646–648, 1986.
90. Angelillo, V.A., Sukhdarshan, B., Durfee, D., et al.: Ann. Intern. Med., *103:*883–885, 1985.
91. Kwan, R., Mir, M.A.: Am. J. Med., *82:*751–758, 1987.
92. Brown, S.E., Nagendran, R.C., McHugh, J.W., et al.: Am. Rev. Respir. Dis., *132:*960–962, 1985.
93. Sue, D.Y., Chung, M.M., Grosvenor, M., et al.: Am. Rev. Respir. Dis., *139:*1430–1434, 1989.
94. Aubier, M., Murcianeo, D., Lecocquic, Y., et al.: N. Engl. J. Med., *313:*420–424, 1985.
95. Laaban, J.P., Grateau, G., Psychoyos, I., et al.: Crit. Care Med., *17:*1115–1120, 1989.
96. Laaban, J.P., Waked, M., Laromiguiere, M., et al.: Ann. Intern. Med., *112:*68–69, 1990.
97. Brady, H.R., Ryan, F., Cunningham, J., et al.: Arch. Intern. Med., *149:*2367–2368, 1989.
98. Aubier, M., Viires, N., Piquet, J., et al.: J. Appl. Physiol. *58:*2054, 1985.
99. Dorin, R.I., Crapo, L.: JAMA, *257:*1517–1518, 1987.
100. Schwartz, J., Weiss, S.T.: Am. J. Epidemiol., *130:*67–76, 1990.

CHAPTER **77**

Food Allergy

Hugh A. Sampson

BACKGROUND AND DEFINITIONS

Hippocrates was among the first to record an adverse reaction to food over 2000 years ago. However, not until the turn of the century did scattered reports of food allergic reactions appear in the medical literature. Most accounts of food allergic reactions were based simply on the history of the patient until 1950, when Loveless reported the first blinded, placebo-controlled food challenges; one study involving 8 patients for milk allergy[1] and one involving 25 patients for cornstarch sensitivity.[2] Subsequently, Goldman et al. published a series of articles describing their studies in 89 children suspected of milk allergy.[3,4] These authors considered the diagnosis of food allergy established only when the patient had resolution of symptoms after withdrawal of milk from the diet and duplication of presenting symptoms on three successive challenges with milk. Although the "Goldman criteria" firmly established the diagnosis of food allergy, most investigators were reluctant to subject highly allergic patients to three challenges. In 1976, May introduced the use of double-blind, placebo-controlled oral food challenges (DBPCFC) to diagnose food allergy, ushering in the recent era of scientific investigation into food allergic disorders.[5]

To facilitate research in this area, a joint American Academy of Allergy and Immunology —National Institute of Allergy and Infectious Disease (NIH) publication proposed a standardized nomenclature[6]: *adverse food reaction* is a generic term referring to any untoward reaction after the ingestion of a food. Adverse food reactions can be categorized into two types: *food allergy* (food hypersensitivity) or *food intolerance*. A food allergic reaction is an abnormal immunologic response, whereas food intolerance is the result of nonimmunologic mechanisms. Food intolerances constitute the majority of adverse reactions to foods and may result from toxic contaminants (e.g., histamine in scombroid fish poisoning, toxins secreted by Salmonella, Shigella, and Campylobacter), pharmacologic properties of the food (e.g., caffeine in coffee and soft drinks), metabolic disturbances (e.g., lactase deficiency), or idiosyncratic reactions of the host. Most well-characterized food allergic reactions are IgE-mediated (type I) hypersensitivity. However, a variety of gastrointestinal disorders are believed to occur on the basis of non-IgE mediated immune mechanisms (e.g., delayed cell-mediated (type IV) hypersensitivity).

PREVALENCE

No satisfactory epidemiologic studies have been conducted to determine the prevalence of food allergic reactions in adults, although the figure of less than 1% is quoted frequently. A recent household survey indicated that about one third of women believed at least one family member suffered from a food allergy.[7] In a prospective study of 480 children 3 years of age or younger, parents reported that 28% of their children experienced adverse food reactions.[8] However, the investigator was able to confirm adverse food reactions by blinded or open challenge in only 8% of the population studied. Eighty percent of adverse food reactions were acquired in the first year of life. Overall, 2 to 4% of the pediatric population are believed to have food allergies. However, the prevalence of food allergy may be as high as 30% in some groups, such as children with atopic dermatitis.[9]

PATHOPHYSIOLOGY

Foods and beverages ingested in everyday life constitute the largest exogenous antigenic load to which human beings are subjected, estimated by some to be in excess of several tons over a lifetime. The gastrointestinal tract uses a variety of immunologic and nonimmunologic mechanisms to prevent the entry of foreign proteins from entering the body. Nonimmunologic barriers include gastric acid secretion, proteolysis by various intestinal and pancreatic enzymes, peristalsis, the mucous coat, and the microvillous membrane. The gut enterocyte selectively absorbs small peptides and amino acids, and lysosomal activity further breaks down small peptides into nonantigenic fragments. The main immunologic barrier to foreign proteins is the secretion of secretory-IgA molecules into the gut lumen, that complex with foreign proteins and block their absorption. In addition, immune complexes promote both mucus release from goblet cells and mucosal surface proteolysis. Serum IgG and IgA antibodies may bind foreign proteins that gain access to the circulation, and lead to their clearing by the reticuloendothelial system.[10]

Despite the intricate barrier network evolved to prevent the entry of foreign protein into the body, Walzer and colleagues established unequivocally that food proteins readily gain access to the circulation and are transported to distal target organs. Using normal volunteers in a series of experiments using Prausnitz-Küstner (P-K) tests with serum from highly food allergic individuals, Walzer demonstrated that food antigens gain access to the body at all levels of the gastrointestinal tract.[11] In addition, other investigators have presented evidence to suggest that antigen permeability is increased after gastroenteritis, and in young infants. The increased susceptibility of young infants to various antigens appears to be the result of relatively low secretory IgA in intestinal secretions and immature, submaximal nonimmunologic mechanisms.

The development of food allergy is the result of an abnormal interaction between food allergens and the immune system and/or the gastrointestinal tract. The glycoprotein fractions of the foods are implicated in allergic responses. The predominant allergenic glycoproteins are water soluble, largely heat resistant, and acid stable, and are commonly in the range of 14,000 to 40,000 d. Only a few foods have been documented to cause the majority of allergic reactions: milk, eggs, peanuts, soy, and wheat in children and fish, shellfish, tree nuts, and peanuts in adults.

Normal individuals generate IgA, IgM, and IgG antibodies to the minute quantities of food antigens that pass the intestinal barrier or are selectively absorbed by M cells that overlie intestinal Peyer's patches and present antigens to resident lymphocytes. After a meal, circulating food antigen-antibody complexes often are found in normal individuals.[12] In subjects developing food allergic reactions, food antigen-specific IgE antibodies and/or abnormal T cell responses develop, for reasons not fully understood.

IgE-Mediated Reactions. Food allergic reactions involving IgE antibodies are the most well characterized. IgE antibodies bind to high affinity Fc_ϵ receptors on mast cells and basophils. Perivascular mast cells are prominent in all surfaces that confront the environment, such as the skin, respiratory tract, and gastrointestinal tract. When allergens react with IgE antibodies bound to mast cells, mediators such as histamine, prostaglandins, and leukotrienes are released. These mediators cause vasodilatation, smooth muscle contraction, and secretion of mucus, resulting in symptoms of immediate hypersensitivity. The activated mast cells also release a variety of cytokines, including interleukins, platelet-activating factor, and other mediators that promote the IgE-mediated late-phase response. Neutrophils, eosinophils, and to a lesser extent, lymphocytes infiltrate the area during the first 6 to 8 hours. These cells are activated and release a variety of mediators including platelet-activating factor, peroxidases, eosinophil major basic protein, and eosinophil cationic protein. In the subsequent 24 to 48 hours, lymphocytes and monocytes infiltrate the area and establish a more chronic inflammatory picture. With repeated ingestion of a food allergen, mononuclear cells are stimulated to secrete "histamine-releasing factor" (HRF), a cytokine that interacts with IgE molecules bound to the surface of mast cells and basophils and increases their releasability.[13] HRF production has been associated with bronchial hyperreactivity in patients with asthma,[14] and may be related to cutaneous irritability in children with atopic dermatitis.[13] IgE-mediated allergic reactions may provoke urticaria/angioedema, eczematous rashes, rhinoconjunctivitis, asthma, vomiting, and diarrhea.

Non-IgE-Mediated Reactions. Non-IgE-mediated reactions may consist of antibody-mediated (type II) hypersensitivity, immune complex reactions (type III), or cell-mediated (type IV) hypersensitivity. In contrast to the IgE-mediated reactions, the non-IgE reactions may involve IgA, IgM, and IgG antibodies. No reports are available describing any type II food allergic responses. The complexes formed by the interaction of non-IgE antibodies with antigen may or may not result in adverse reactions, but to date, support is minimal for type III, food antigen-immune complex mediated disease.[12] Studies in animal models revealed that cell-mediated (type IV) reactions can cause intestinal damage, including villus atrophy. It is believed that abnormal cell-mediated immune responses may be responsible for some of the allergic gastrointestinal syndromes in humans, but data to support this theory are not convincing. In both food allergic and nonallergic individuals, stimulation of peripheral blood lymphocytes with food antigens in vitro may result in blastogenesis, interleukin 2 (IL-2) production, and/or leukocyte inhibitory factor (LIF) production.

CLINICAL SIGNS AND SYMPTOMS

The symptoms attributed to food allergy are legion. However, only a few specific symptoms have been documented as related to food hypersensitivity reactions. The majority are the result of IgE-mediated reactions (Table 77–1).

IgE-Mediated Mechanisms. Acute urticaria/angioedema after the ingestion or contact with a food is relatively common, although the actual prevalence is unknown. Most individuals with this disorder are aware of the association between the ingestion of a specific food and the development of symptoms and therefore simply avoid the food. Chronic urticaria/angioedema related to food allergy is believed to be rare. The development of atopic dermatitis has been associated with food allergy in children. During blinded food challenges, a pruritic, erythematous morbilliform rash develops within 10 to 90 minutes of allergen ingestion.[15] Repeated ingestion of the offending allergen leads to activation of cutaneous mast cells and induction of the late-phase IgE inflammatory response, both of which result in pruritus, consequent scratching, and the development of eczematous lesions.[16]

Both upper and lower respiratory symptoms have been demonstrated as a result of food allergy by DBPCFC.[15,17] In one study of 300 patients attending a pulmonary clinic, 6 patients (2%) had significant food allergy by DBPCFC.[18] In a second study of children with asthma, 5% of patients had food allergies contributing to their asthmatic symptoms.[19]

Symptoms involving the oropharynx and gastrointestinal tract may occur within minutes of ingesting a food allergen. Pruritus and swelling of the lips, tongue, and soft palate, as well as nausea, abdominal pain, vomiting, and diarrhea have all been demonstrated secondary to food allergy. The "oral allergy syndrome" consists of symptoms confined almost exclusively to the oropharynx and is most commonly reported in association with a variety of fresh fruits and vegetables.[20] Interestingly, patients with respiratory allergy to birch pollen may develop oral symptoms after ingestion of potatoes, carrots, celery, hazelnuts, and apples, whereas patients allergic to ragweed may develop oral symptoms after eating melons and bananas.

Systemic anaphylaxis owing to food allergy does occur, but because of a lack of a formal reporting mechanism for such reactions, the prevalence of food-induced anaphylaxis is unknown. In a report of fatal

TABLE 77–1. FOOD ALLERGIC REACTIONS SUBSTANTIATED BY BLINDED CHALLENGES AND APPROPRIATE LABORATORY STUDIES

IgE Mediated	
Skin	Urticaria/angioedema*
	Atopic dermatitis
Respiratory	Rhinoconjunctivitis
	Laryngeal edema
	Asthma
Gastrointestinal	Nausea and abdominal cramps
	Vomiting and diarrhea
	"Oral allergy syndrome"
	Infantile colic?
General	Anaphylactic shock*
Non-IgE Mediated	
Skin	Dermatitis herpetiformis
Respiratory	Heiner's syndrome
Gastrointestinal	Food-induced enterocolitis
	Food-induced colitis
	Malabsorption syndromes (celiac disease)
	Allergic eosinophilic gastroenteritis
	Infantile colic?
Other	Migraine headaches
	Seizures in children with epilepsy and migraine
	Iron deficiency anemia associated with gastrointestinal blood loss
	Arthritis (one case)

*Symptoms also may be provoked by the combination of ingesting specific food(s) in conjunction with exercising, but not by ingestion of the food alone or exercise alone.

anaphylactic reactions in 7 individuals, the authors expressed concern that 6 of 7 subjects had ingested the food allergen unknowingly, that all patients tended to minimize the symptoms initially, and that the initiation of emergency medical management was delayed.[21] Anaphylactic shock after the ingestion of certain foods in association with exercise also has been reported in some individuals.

Non-IgE-Mediated Immune Reactions. A variety of disorders have been associated with the ingestion of food and are believed to be the result of an immunologic mechanism(s). Although cell-mediated mechanisms often are implied, insufficient information is available to determine the pathogenic process involved.

Heiner's Syndrome (a form of pulmonary hemosiderosis) is a chronic or recurrent pulmonary disease characterized by chronic rhinitis, pulmonary infiltrates and hemosiderosis, gastrointestinal blood loss, iron deficiency anemia, and failure to thrive. It is associated most often with a hypersensitivity to cow's milk, but reactivity to egg and pork have also been reported.[22] Although peripheral blood eosinophilia and multiple serum precipitins to cow's milk are relatively constant features, the immunologic mechanisms responsible for this disorder are not known. Avoidance of the precipitating allergen leads to resolution of symptoms.

Given the presence of food antigen-immune complexes in many individuals after meals, several claims have been made for the use of fasting or hypoallergenic diets in the treatment of rheumatoid arthritis. However, exacerbation of arthritis has been established in only two patients associated with ingestion of a specific food by DBPCFC.[23]

A variety of gastrointestinal disorders believed to have an immunologic basis have been described. Infants with cow's milk- or soy protein-induced enterocolitis generally present between 1 week and 3 months of age with protracted diarrhea and projectile vomiting, often severe enough to produce dehydration.[24] Stools generally contain occult blood, polymorphonuclear neutrophils (PMN), and eosinophils, and are generally positive for carbohydrate (reducing substances). The syndrome is associated most commonly with ingestion of cow's milk and soy in infants, but also is reported in association with eggs in older individuals. Some patients present only with bloody diarrhea (gross or occult) or hematochezia with lesions confined to the distal bowel, i.e., food-induced colitis. Both disorders resolve clinically within 72 hours of allergen elimination.

Malabsorption syndromes include a spectrum of disorders that generally require medical attention because of protracted diarrhea, vomiting in up to two thirds of patients, failure to thrive, and carbohydrate malabsorption, demonstrated by the presence of reducing substances in the stools. Increased fecal fat and abnormal D-xylose absorption generally are present. Cow's milk sensitivity is the most frequent cause of this syndrome, but it also has been associated with soy, egg, and wheat hypersensitivity. Patchy villous atrophy with cellular infiltrate on biopsy is characteristic of this disorder.[25] A more extensive enteropathy with total villous atrophy and extensive cellular infiltrate is associated with sensitivity to gliadin, a component of gluten (celiac disease). Patients often present with diarrhea or frank steatorrhea, abdominal distention and flatulence, weight loss, and occasionally nausea and vomiting. Dermatitis herpetiformis is a highly pruritic skin rash (sometimes mistaken for atopic dermatitis) associated with gluten-sensitive enteropathy.[26] Biopsy of the skin rash reveals an infiltration of PMN and deposits of IgA at the dermal-epidermal junction. Administration of dapsone or other sulfones often relieves the skin itching within 24 hours.[27] Elimination of the responsible allergen for 3 to 4 months may be required to normalize intestinal biopsy findings in the malabsorption syndromes.

Allergic eosinophilic gastroenteritis often presents as postprandial nausea with vomiting, abdominal pain, diarrhea, occasionally steatorrhea, and weight loss in the adult, and failure to thrive in the infant.[28] In the mucosal form, patients often have atopic disease, elevated serum IgE levels, positive immediate skin tests to a variety of foods and aeroallergens, peripheral eosinophilia, iron deficiency anemia, and hypoalbuminemia. In some patients, symptoms are associated with specific foods. The protein-losing enteropathy syndrome in infants is a form of eosinophilic gastroenteritis that has been described in association with ingestion of cow's milk.[29] Gastrointestinal symptoms are minimal (occasional diarrhea and vomiting) and children have edema related to hypoalbuminemia. Eosinophilic gastroenteritis rarely presents as pyloric stenosis with outlet obstruction.[30] Removal of the suspect allergen for up to 12 weeks may be required to bring about resolution of symptoms and intestinal histologic changes.

Infantile colic is an ill-defined syndrome of paroxysmal fussiness characterized by inconsolable crying, abdominal distention, excessive gas, and drawing up of the legs. It generally develops in the first 2 to 4 weeks of life and resolves in the third to fourth month, and has been associated with the ingestion of foreign food proteins (most frequently cow's milk) in some breast-fed and formula-fed infants.[31] A review of current studies suggests that approximately 10 to 15% of infantile colic is related to food allergy.[32]

Non-IgE-Mediated Reactions; Mechanism Unknown. In several disorders, symptoms have been associated with reactivity to ingested foods, but an associated immune response is unclear. Reports since the turn of the century have suggested that oligoantigenic diets also may be useful in the treatment of certain neurologic disorders. In one study, 15% of 80 adult patients with frequent migraine headaches had clearing of their headache while on a specific food elimination diet, and exacerbation of their symptoms during double-blind challenge with a

TABLE 77–2. UNSUBSTANTIATED SYMPTOMS ASCRIBED TO FOOD ALLERGY

General	Fatigue (tension-fatigue syndrome)
	Nervousness
	Weakness
	Sleep disturbances (other than infantile colic)
	Learning disorders
	Hyperactivity
	Schizophrenia
	Neuroses
	Depression
	Obesity
Gastrointestinal	Crohn's disease
	Ulcerative colitis
	Irritable bowel syndrome
Genitourinary	Enuresis
	Dysmenorrhea
Cardiovascular	Vasculitis
	Recurrent phlebitis
	Cardiac arrhythmias

single food.[33] In another study, 16 children with epilepsy and migraine developed seizures only while receiving a specific food during DBPCFC.[34]

The feeding of pasteurized, whole cow's milk to infants, especially less than 6 months of age, frequently leads to occult blood loss from the gastrointestinal tract,[35] and occasionally to iron deficiency anemia.[36] Substitution of infant formula (including cow's milk-derived formulas that have been subjected to more extensive heating) for whole cow's milk generally normalizes fecal blood loss within 3 days. Considerable interest has resurfaced on the possible role of food allergy in inflammatory bowel disease (Crohn's disease and ulcerative colitis). Although considerable circumstantial evidence makes such hypotheses attractive, convincing proof remains to be established.

Table 77–2 is a list of a variety of other symptoms reported to be related to food allergy. Convincing proof that any of these disorders manifest as isolated findings in association with food allergy is lacking. However, subjects experiencing a typical allergic reaction to a food may become irritable or lethargic after an IgE-mediated reaction, and whether this response is attributable to the discomfort of the allergic symptoms or the release of various cytokines, such as IL-1, IL-6, and/or tumor necrosis factor, remains to be established.

DIAGNOSTIC TESTS

Much of the confusion surrounding food allergy has resulted from the lack of a sensitive, specific laboratory test to confirm the diagnosis. Confirmation of the diagnosis usually depends on a clinical test, the DBPCFC, which is the current "gold standard" for diagnosing food allergy.[37,38] The initial evaluation of a patient with suspected food allergy should focus on a careful history and physical examination. The history should emphasize the following points: food suspected and the approximate quantity ingested, time between the ingestion and development of symptoms, description of the symptoms, frequency and reproducibility of symptoms, the most recent occurrence, and whether other factors (i.e., exercise) are necessary for reaction to occur. The physical examination should note any atopic features, which frequently are present in individuals with IgE-mediated food allergy.

Several laboratory tests have evolved for use in the diagnosis of IgE-mediated food hypersensitivity reactions and that may be used in the initial screening of food allergic complaints. Skin tests with food extracts are used to demonstrate the presence of food antigen-specific IgE antibodies on the surface of cutaneous mast cells, which are presumed to reflect the IgE present on mast cells in the gastrointestinal and respiratory tracts. When compared to DBPCFC, the negative puncture or prick skin test is extremely useful for excluding IgE-mediated food allergy, but inadequate for predicting the presence of clinical reactivity, i.e., low positive predictive accuracies.[39] Intradermal skin tests are even less specific than prick skin tests, and therefore are not recommended in the evaluation of IgE-mediated food allergy. Radioallergosorbent tests (RAST) or similar in vitro tests measure food antigen-specific IgE antibodies in the blood. RAST performed in a reliable laboratory provide predictive information that is not significantly different from prick skin tests. Once suspected foods are identified by history and skin testing (or RAST), they are eliminated from the diet for 1 to 2 weeks. Because DBPCFC are so time-consuming, single-blind challenges often are performed to eliminate foods considered unlikely to provoke an allergic reaction. DBPCFC are then used to establish a diagnosis of food allergy.[38] All challenges suspected of provoking an IgE-mediated response must be conducted in a physician's office or a hospital setting because of the risk of a generalized anaphylactic reaction. Although a DBPCFC is rarely equivocal when investigating typical IgE-mediated symptoms, a variety of laboratory measurements are used sometimes to quantitate the response: plasma histamine, serum tryptase, pulmonary function, and/or nasal lavage histamine concentration.

No satisfactory laboratory tests have emerged to assist in the diagnosis of non-IgE-mediated food allergic disorders. For ailments in which cell-mediated reactions are considered important, stimulation of peripheral blood mononuclear cells in vitro with specific food antigens has been investigated for blastogenesis, e.g., ^{3}H-thymidine uptake, leukocyte inhibitory factor production, and IL-2 generation. Although many patients with presumed food allergy have increased activity compared to normal controls, these tests are not discriminatory. In addition, no evidence exists that measurement of food antigen-specific IgG or IgG subclass antibodies, or of food antigen-antibody complexes, is of any diagnostic value. Other tests (e.g., cytotoxic tests, sublingual and intradermal provocation tests) have been suggested for use in diagnosing food allergy, but their diagnostic efficiencies have never been validated.

Food-induced enterocolitis may be diagnosed by a single food allergen challenge, preferably blinded, after a brief period of allergen exclusion. Up to 0.6 g of the implicated protein per kilogram of body weight is administered in a physician's office or hospital setting, because of the risk of protracted vomiting and hypotension. A positive challenge generally provokes vomiting and diarrhea, with occult or grossly apparent blood in the stools, an increase in stool PMN and eosinophils over baseline, and an increase in the total peripheral blood PMN count of 3500 cells/mm^3 over baseline at 6 to 8 hours postchallenge.[40]

Food-induced colitis often has a characteristic appearance on sigmoidoscopy. The bowel wall is edematous, erythematous, and friable with scattered ulcerations. Biopsy reveals an inflammatory infiltrate and prominent eosinophilia.[41] Cultures of the stools for bacteria, virus, and parasites are necessary to rule out infection. Examination of the stools reveals significant numbers of leukocytes, and examination of the blood may demonstrate a mild elevation in the number of peripheral blood eosinophils. Exclusion of the responsible allergen generally leads to resolution of symptoms within 72 hours, and re-feeding the allergen provokes a recurrence of hematochezia within 24 to 48 hours.

Both the malabsorption syndromes and allergic eosinophilic gastroenteritis require endoscopy and intestinal biopsy while the patient is ingesting the suspected allergen, after being placed on an allergen exclusion diet for up to 3 months, and after re-instituting the food allergen into the diet. Endoscopy and biopsy before challenge should reveal normal intestinal mucosa. Reintroduction of the responsible allergen to patients with the malabsorption syndromes leads to villous atrophy, which may be partial or complete, and often is patchy. In allergic eosinophilic gastroenteritis, the characteristic eosinophilic infiltrate may also be patchy. Consequently, multiple biopsies are required to exclude this diagnosis, especially in young children. Breath hydrogen and D-xylose absorption may be abnormal because of secondary disaccharidase deficiency. In celiac disease and dermatitis herpetiformis, both forms of malabsorption syndrome, IgA antigliadin and IgA antiendomysial antibodies are present in over 90% of patients with untreated disease. In addition, the presence of IgA deposits in the dermal-epidermal junction is characteristic of patients with dermatitis herpetiformis.

Confirmation of infantile colic resulting from food allergy requires at least two double-blind, placebo-controlled cross-over trials of the suspected food allergen. To be considered positive, symptoms should be prominent during the allergen challenges and absent during the placebo challenges.

Many structural and enzymatic abnormalities in both children and adults can result in gastrointestinal symptoms that closely mimic food allergic reactions. The differential must be considered carefully in all patients undergoing evaluation, because many of these other disorders can also be life-threatening.[42] Foods may contain a variety of preservatives, dyes, and other chemicals that occasionally have been implicated in adverse reactions to foods. Many foods also have endogenous pharmacologic agents that can trigger symptoms in highly susceptible individuals. Occasionally, improper handling of food (scombroid poisoning) or ingestion of a toxin by an animal (ciguatera poisoning) results in symptoms that mimic an allergic reaction.

THERAPY

Once the diagnosis of food allergy has been established, the only proven form of therapy is strict elimination of the offending food. This action requires considerable time and effort (ideally with the help of a dietitian) to educate the patient (or parent). Teaching patients to read food labels is necessary to guarantee exclusion of many "hidden forms" of common foods.[43] For example, most individuals are unaware that casein (milk protein) is found in canned tuna fish; M&M's (plain) contain peanut; most nondairy creamers contain caseinate, etc. In addition, the importance of a nutritionally sound diet must be stressed.

In food-induced enterocolitis, a short course of corticosteroids may be lifesaving in the initial acute stages. However, long-term management involves identification and removal of the responsible food. Allergic eosinophilic gastroenteropathy syndrome often requires treatment with corticosteroids, especially when no food is clearly implicated. Although several other methods have been suggested for the treatment of food allergies (e.g., oral sodium cromolyn, desensitization), they have not been effective in controlled trials in which the diagnosis of food allergy has been established unequivocally.

NATURAL HISTORY

Results of follow-up studies on food allergic individuals indicate that food allergies may resolve after several years. A loss of symptomatic, IgE-mediated food allergy occurred in approximately 40% of children and adults adhering to an allergen exclusion diet for 1 to 3 years, even though results of skin tests and RAST did not change (i.e., food allergen-specific IgE was still present).[44,45] The probability of symptomatic resolution appeared to depend on compliance with the exclusion diet and the specific food provoking the symptoms; allergies to peanuts, tree nuts, fish, and other seafood were more long lasting. In a cohort of 100 children with various forms of cow's milk allergy, only 22% remained clinically allergic after 6 years.[46] Consequently, it is recommended that allergic individuals be rechallenged to most foods every 1 to 2 years and to peanuts, tree nuts, and seafood every 4 to 8 years to determine whether their clinical allergy persists. No evidence exists that individuals who lose a food allergy will redevelop symptomatic reactivity after reintroducing the food into the diet. In addition to the longevity of clinical allergy to peanuts, tree nuts, fish, and shellfish, patients with these allergies must be warned about the greater risk of a generalized anaphylactic reaction compared to other foods.

It is generally accepted that infants with milk-induced enterocolitis and colitis syndromes "outgrow" their sensitivity in 1 to 2 years. Although this notion may be true, no formal studies have been performed to support it and follow-up of a few patients for 3 to 5 years indicates persistent sensitivity in at least some patients. No information is available on the natural history of allergic eosinophilic gastroenteritis.

A similar presumption is that many infants with milk-induced malabsorption syndrome "outgrow" their sensitivity. Again, no studies address this issue. Most clinicians agree that patients with celiac disease must exclude gluten-containing grains for life. Some patients with celiac disease can tolerate gluten-containing products with little gastrointestinal discomfort, especially after avoiding it for a time. However, the risk of malignancy of the mouth, pharynx, and esophagus, and non-Hodgkins lymphoma is significantly increased in patients with celiac disease ingesting gluten, regardless of the presence of clinical symptoms.[47]

PROPHYLAXIS

The role of breast feeding and food allergen avoidance in the prevention of atopy and food allergy remains highly controversial. Findings of recent studies suggest that breast feeding (especially with maternal avoidance of such major allergens as milk, egg, peanut, and fish during lactation) can postpone atopic disease in high-risk infants. An infant is considered at "high risk" when both parents have atopic disease (i.e., atopic dermatitis, asthma, and/or allergic rhinitis), one parent and one sibling have atopic disease, or one parent or one sibling has atopic disease and the infant has an elevated cord blood IgE level (greater than 0.9 IU/ml). In a large controlled trial, maternal and infant avoidance of allergenic foods (egg, milk, peanut, and fish) lowered the prevalence of atopic dermatitis, urticaria, and/or gastrointestinal disorders at 12 and 24 months, but had no effect on the prevalence of asthma, allergic rhinitis, or positive skin tests to inhalant allergens.[48] Because of the difficulty in maintaining a prophylactic regimen, many investigators recommend prophylactic measures only in "high-risk" infants with highly motivated families, until our understanding of immunologic sensitization to food allergens is more complete. This plan includes exclusive breast feeding, maternal avoidance of major food allergens, and supplementation with hypoallergenic formula (Alimentum, Nutramigen, Pregestimil) if necessary for the first 6 months of life. Highly allergenic foods (i.e., milk, egg, peanut, peanut butter, and fish) should then be excluded from the child's diet for the first 2 to 3 years.

In summary, food allergy probably affects 2 to 4% of the pediatric population and 1 to 2% of the adult population. It has been implicated in all forms of atopic diseases, including anaphylactic shock and death, and a variety of gastrointestinal disorders. IgE-mediated food allergic reactions have been best characterized, but several other immunologic mechanisms are believed responsible for some adverse food reactions. Appropriate diagnosis of these disorders requires a provocative food challenge, preferably blinded, and in several gastrointestinal syndromes, endoscopy and intestinal biopsy. Rechallenges should be done at set intervals to determine whether clinical sensitivity has been lost, because most food allergies are not lifelong. At present, strict allergen avoidance remains the only documented form of therapy that is universally successful.

REFERENCES

1. Loveless, M.H.: J. Allergy Clin. Immunol., *21:*489–499, 1950.
2. Loveless, M.H.: J. Allergy Clin. Immunol., *21:*500–509, 1950.
3. Goldman, A.S., Anderson, D.W., Sellers, W.A., et al.: Pediatrics, *32:*425–443, 1963.
4. Goldman, A.S., Sellers, W.A., Halpern, S.R., et al.: Pediatrics, *32:*572–579, 1963.
5. May, C.D.: J. Allergy Clin. Immunol., *58:*500–515, 1976.
6. American Academy of Allergy & Immunology-/NIAID: Adverse Reactions to Foods. Edited by J.A. Anderson, D.D. Sogn. NIH Publication 84-2442. Washington, D.C., National Institutes of Health, 1984, pp. 1–6.
7. Sloan, A.E., Powers, M.E.: J. Allergy Clin. Immunol., *78:*127–132, 1986.
8. Bock, S.A.: Pediatrics, *79:*683–688, 1987.
9. Burks, A.W., Mallory, S.B., Williams, L.W., et al.: Pediatrics, *113:*447–451, 1988.
10. Walker, W.A.: Transmucosal passage of antigens. *In* Food Allergy. Edited by D. Reinhardt, E. Schmidt. New York, Raven Press, 1988, pp. 15–34.
11. Walzer, M.: J. Allergy Clin. Immunol., *13:*554–562, 1942.
12. Paganelli, R., Quinti, I., D'Offizi, G.P., et al.: Ann. Allergy, *59:*157–161, 1987.
13. Sampson, H.A.: N. Engl. J. Med., *321:*228–232, 1989.
14. Alam, R., Kuna, P., Rozniecki, J., et al.: J. Allergy Clin. Immunol., *79:*103–108, 1987.
15. Sampson, H.A., McCaskill, C.M.: J. Pediatr., *107:*669–675, 1985.
16. Sampson, H.A.: J. Allergy Clin. Immunol., *81:*635–645, 1988.
17. Bock, S.A., Atkins, F.M.: J. Pediatr., *117:*561–567, 1990.
18. Onorato, J., Merland, N., Terral, C., et al.: J. Allergy Clin. Immunol., *78:*1139–1146, 1986.
19. Novembre, E., Martino, M., Vierucci, A.: J. Allergy Clin. Immunol., *81:*1059–1065, 1988.
20. Ortoloni, C., Ispano, M., Pastorello, E.A., et al.: J. Allergy Clin. Immunol., *83:*683–690, 1989.
21. Yunginger, J.W., Sweeney, K.G., Sturner, W.Q., et al.: JAMA, *260:*1450–1452, 1988.
22. Lee, S.K., Kniker, W.T., Cook, C.D., et al.: Adv. Pediatr., *25:*39–57, 1978.
23. Panush, R.S., Stroud, R.M., Webster, E.M.: Arthritis Rheum., *29:*220–226, 1986.
24. Powell, G.K.: J. Pediatr., *93:*553–560, 1978.
25. Kuitunen, P., Visakorpi, J.K., Savilahti, E., et al.: Arch. Dis. Child., *50:*351–356, 1975.
26. Hall, R.P.: J. Am. Acad. Dermatol., *16:*1129–1144, 1987.
27. Katz, S.I.: Ann. Intern. Med., *93:*857–874, 1980.
28. Kettelhut, B.V., Metcalfe, D.D.: Adverse reactions to foods. *In* Allergy: Principle and Practice. 3rd Ed. Edited by E. Middleton, C.E. Reed, E.F. Ellis, et al.: St. Louis, C.V. Mosby, 1988, pp. 1481–1502.
29. Waldman, T.A., Wochner, R.D., Laster, R.D., et al.: N. Engl. J. Med., *276:*761–769, 1967.
30. Snyder, J.D., Rosenblum, N., Wershil, B., et al.: J. Pediatr. Gastroenterol. Nutr., *6:*543–547, 1987.
31. Loethe, L., Lindberg, T.: Pediatrics, *83:*262–266, 1989.
32. Sampson, H.A.: J. Pediatr., *115:*583–584, 1989.
33. Vaughn, R.T.: Medical/Scientific Update, National Jewish Center for Immunology and Respiratory Disease, *7:*4–5, 1988.
34. Egger, J., Carter, C.M., Soothill, J.F., et al.: J. Pediatr., *114:*51–58, 1989.
35. Ziegler, R.E., Fomon, S.J., Nelson, S.E., et al.: J. Pediatr., *116:*11–18, 1990.
36. Wilson, J.F., Heiner, D.C., Lahey, M.E.: JAMA, *189:*568–572, 1964.
37. Sampson, H.A.: Ann. Allergy, *60:*262–269, 1988.
38. Bock, S.A., Sampson, H.A., Atkins, F.M., et al.: J. Allergy Clin. Immunol., *82:*986–997, 1988.
39. Sampson, H.A., Albergo, R.: J. Allergy Clin. Immunol., *74:*26–33, 1984.
40. Powell, G.K.: J. Pediatr., *93:*553–560, 1976.
41. Goldman, H., Proujansky, R.: Am. J. Surg. Pathol., *10:*75–86, 1986.
42. Sampson, H.A.: J. Allergy Clin. Immunol., *78:*212–219, 1986.
43. Leihnas, J.L., McCaskill, C., Sampson, H.A.: J. Am. Diet. Assoc., *87:*604–608, 1987.
44. Sampson, H.A., Scanlon, S.M.: J. Pediatr., *115:*23–27, 1989.
45. Pastorello, E.A., Stocchi, L., Pravettoni, V., et al.: J. Allergy Clin. Immunol., *84:*475–483, 1989.
46. Bishop, J.M., Hill, D.J., Hosking, C.S.: J. Pediatr., *116:*862–867, 1990.
47. Holmes, G.K.T., Prior, P., Lane, M.R., et al.: Gut, *30:*333–338, 1989.
48. Zeiger, R.S., Heller, S., Mellon, M.H., et al.: J. Allergy Clin. Immunol., *84:*72–89, 1989.

CHAPTER **78**

Diet, Nutrition, and Drug Reactions

Daphne A. Roe

The gulf that formerly separated nutrition and pharmacology has closed, particularly since it has been realized that nutrients can behave as drugs, and drugs may have some of the properties of nutrients. An interscience of drug-nutrient interactions has been created. The concerns of this newer discipline must include nutrients as drugs. However, to the clinical pharmacologist, drug effects on food intake and dietary factors influencing the disposition of drugs are of primary importance. The toxicologist is concerned with nutritional factors in teratogenesis, as well as dietary and nutritional influences on the initiation and promotional phases of carcinogenesis. Pharmacologic problems related to change in body composition, drug-food and drug-nutrient incompatibilities, and alcohol-drug and alcohol-food interactions are of particular concern to the physician, whereas adverse or positive effects of drugs on nutrient absorption, transport, metabolism, cellular uptake, and excretion are of special importance to the nutritionist. The aims of this review are to both describe and classify drug-nutrient interactions and to discuss adverse outcomes.

DRUG AND NUTRIENT INTERACTIONS

The umbrella terms "drug and nutrient interactions" and "diet, nutrition, and drug interactions" are used to mean either the interactions themselves or the outcomes of these interactions. Interactions between diet and drugs can be physicochemical, physiologic, or pathophysiologic. Physicochemical interactions between diet ingredients and drug ingredients include absorption, complexation, precipitation, and effects of one interactant on another whereby stability of one or both is altered. Physiologic interactions include all those in which diet variables affect the disposition of drugs in the body or vice versa. Pathophysiologic interactions are those in which the toxic effects of drugs result in impairment of nutrient absorption or use.

Outcomes of these different types of interaction differ. Most commonly, physicochemical interactions result in reduced absorption of the drug and nutrient interaction. The result may be either reduced absorption of the drug or nutrient interaction or both reactants may be poorly absorbed. This occurs, for example, when tetracycline is taken within 2 hours of a calcium-containing food or supplement.[1] Physiologic interactions on the other hand are more likely to change the rate of absorption of a drug or nutrient in either direction. Such effects of diet on drug disposition or drug on nutrient disposition are reversible and often transient. However, they may result in an important change in the time taken for a drug to take effect, acute drug toxicity, or massive loss of a

TABLE 78–1. CLASSIFICATION OF DRUG AND NUTRIENT INTERACTIONS BY CAUSAL MECHANISMS INTO GALAXIES

GALAXY 1 PHYSICOCHEMICAL	GALAXY 2 PHYSIOLOGIC	GALAXY 3 PATHOPHYSIOLOGIC
Adsorption	GI functional change	Enterotoxicity
Solubilization	Vasodilatation	Hepatotoxicity
Precipitation	Hyperphagia	Nephrotoxicity
Chelation	Hypophagia	Neurotoxicity
Gel formation	Electrolyte imbalance	Embryotoxicity
Ion exchange		Hemolysis
Photoactivation		

TABLE 78–2. OUTCOMES OF DRUG-NUTRIENT INTERACTIONS

GALAXY 1 PHYSICOCHEMICAL	GALAXY 2 PHYSIOLOGIC	GALAXY 3 PATHOPHYSIOLOGIC
Nasogastric tube block or reduced absorption of drug or nutrient owing to pH-dependent component interaction and gel formation	Functional change in GI motility, diet or drug-induced, affecting rate of drug or nutrient absorption	Reversible or irreversible pathologic change that is drug related and cause of drug-induced malnutrition

nutrient that can be life-threatening. From the point of view of reducing side effects of drugs that are unpleasant to patients, slowed drug uptake may be desirable. On the other hand, rapid absorption of a high dose of a drug can cause acute signs of drug toxicity.

Examples of physiologic interactions that cause slowed drug uptake include the effect of dietary fiber of the hemicellulose type on the absorption of digoxin.[2] This result has been explained as being related to the effect of the fiber in slowing gastric emptying time. Slowed uptake of the calcium channel blocker nifedipine occurs if the drug is taken with a lowfat meal or snack; this reduces drug-related flushing and may bring relief to those taking the drug.[3] However, rapid uptake of sustained release preparations of theophylline associated with concurrent intake of a high-fat meal frequently produces signs of drug toxicity with headache, tachycardia, and agitation.[4] The most important example of a life-threatening event in which acute nutrient depletion is associated with a drug-induced change in gut motility is hypokalemia resulting from diarrhea brought on by laxative abuse.[5]

Pathophysiologic interactions include those in which drugs by their toxicologic effects block biosynthetic pathways or cause cellular damage so that nutrients cannot be activated, used, or retained by the body. Examples of such effects include the antifolic acid effects of methotrexate, trimetrexate, and sulfasalazine.[6]

Thus, physicochemical interactions most likely occur because of errors in the timing of food intake with drug intake. On the other hand, the most important risk factors for physiologic reactions are dietary changes imposed without concurrent adjustment of drug dose or formulation. Finally, major risk factors for pathophysiologic reactions are antinutrient properties of the drug and prior impairment of organ function. Classification of drug and nutrient interactions into these three categories is best conceptualized as galaxies or domains that indicate causes, outcomes, and risk factors for these problems (Tables 78–1 to 78–3).

DISEASE DETERMINATION OF DRUG-NUTRIENT INTERACTIONS AND OUTCOMES

The clusters of drugs that are prescribed are determined by the primary diagnosis and the spectrum of diseases present. Prediction of risk of drug and nutrient interactions is determined by patient group. Thus, risk is determined on the basis of whether the individual is, for example, a cardiac, hypertensive, or diabetic patient. Furthermore, these disease groups are what determine not only the therapeutic drugs prescribed but also the types of drugs the patients take for symptom relief, including over-the-counter drugs. For example, the drug and nutrient interactions encountered in diabetic patients are either related to the antidiabetic drugs they take, or to the effects of drugs they take for complications of their primary disease.[7] The complexity of the influences imposed by comorbidity and age on risk of drug-nutrient interaction risk is exemplified by the risk of severe iron deficiency anemia in an elderly diabetic patient with an autonomic neuropathy of the colon.[8] If

TABLE 78–3. RISKS OF DRUG AND NUTRIENT INTERACTIONS

Galaxy 1 (Physicochemical)	
	Chemistry of the drug
	Formulation of the drug
	Composition of the diet
	Timing errors
	Ultraviolet exposure
Galaxy 2 (Physiologic)	
	Pharmacologic action of drug on the gut
	Physiologic action of food on GI motility
	Food and nutrient effect on splanchnic circulation
	Competitive absorption of drug and nutrient
	Intake of alcohol
	Central effect of drug or nutrient on satiety center
	Drug or nutrient effect on renal function
Galaxy 3 (Pathophysiologic)	
	Drug toxicity
	Previous organ damage
	Drug dose
	Drug frequency
	Drug duration
	Drug as antinutrient
	Reversibility of drug toxicity
	Protein-energy malnutrition
	Functional immaturity
	Pregnancy
	Lactation
	Aging
	Current diet
	Fasting
	Diet-related disease

this patient has pain related to osteoarthritis, it is likely a nonsteroidal anti-inflammatory drug (NSAID) will be prescribed or taken as an over-the-counter preparation. This patient is at risk for colonic ulceration and secondary drug-induced bleeding, which causes the anemia.[9] The risks of anemia owing to NSAID-induced bleeding also include concurrent use of anticoagulant drugs.

On the other hand, chronic iron deficiency anemia in arthritic patients is most commonly the result of NSAID-induced bleeding from a peptic ulcer. The risk of bleeding in such patients receiving these drugs is increased in the elderly, and in those persons with a history of recurrent peptic ulcer. Bleeding is also more frequent in patients receiving NSAID who are also taking coumarin anticoagulants and in alcohol abusers.[10]

The association of drug and nutrient interactions with particular patient groups and risk factors related to comorbidity is shown in Table 78–4.

NUTRIENTS AS DRUGS

Vitamins and their analogues may have both pharmacologic and nutritional properties. The pharmacologic effect of vitamins has long been appreciated and has been used for therapeutic purposes. The inhibitory effects of massive doses of vitamin A on keratinization were described by Miescher in 1954.[11] In patients given daily doses of 200,000 to 400,000 IU (209.5 to 419 μmol or 60,000 to 120,000 μg) of vitamin A, ichthyosis disappeared more or less completely within 2 to 3 months but recurred when treatment was discontinued. It was claimed that no side effects were encountered.

About the same time, however, the toxic effects of vitamin A overload were reported in children to include skeletal abnormalities and hemorrhages.[12] These side effects were observed to follow doses of vitamin A in the order of 500,000 IU daily. Sulzberger and Lazar reported signs of vitamin A intoxication in a woman of 44 years who took 600,000 IU daily for 18 months.[13]

Vitamin D_3 (calciferol) was advocated by Dowling and co-workers in England,[14] Michelson in the United States,[15] and Charpy in France[16] for the treatment of tuberculosis of the skin (lupus vulgaris). Dosage ranges were equivalent to between 6.5 to 40 mmol (2500 to 15,000 μg) vitamin D_3 daily. The clinical experience of these investigators was critically reviewed by Goldsmith and Hellier in 1954.[12] Toxic reactions, including fatalities, were observed frequently. Anning et al. reported that in a group of 200 patients with lupus vulgaris receiving vitamin D_3, 19% developed toxic symptoms including anorexia, vomiting, tiredness, malaise, nausea, headache, constipation, abdominal pain, and polyuria.[17] Laboratory tests revealed hypercalcemia and evidence of impaired renal function.

Three years after the isolation of niacin and its effective use at physiologic doses in the treatment of pellagra, studies were carried out by Bean and Spies to examine the vasodilator effect of niacin and several analogues.[18] Pyridine compounds, which produced vasodilatation, included nicotinic acid (niacin), sodium nicotinate, ammonium nicotinate, and ethyl nicotinate. Nicotinamide did not have vasodilator potency. Ruffin and Smith observed that vasodilatation and headache occurred in normal subjects who took 250 mg niacin four times a day. Vasodilator effects of niacin were subsequently used therapeutically in the treatment of Raynaud's phenomenon.[19]

The vasodilatory effect of niacin has been considered as justification for administration to elderly patients with cerebrovascular disease. However, although authors claim that the vitamin could cause dilatation of cerebral vessels and thereby improve memory and brain function. No scientific evidence supports such a claim.

Niacin has been and is still used in megadosages (≧ 1 g per day) for the treatment of familial hypercholesterolemia and other disorders of lipoprotein metabolism. The hypocholesterolemic effects of large doses of niacin were first reported by Altschul et al. in 1955.[20] Since that time, niacin has been in use as a hypocholesterolemic agent, and although its use for this function declined after the mid-1960s for several years, niacin is again used as an adjunct drug with coadministration with a bile acid sequestrant. It has been demonstrated that niacin decreases total plasma triglycerides and very

TABLE 78–4. EFFECTS OF PRIMARY DIAGNOSIS AND COMORBIDITY ON THE RISK OF DRUG AND NUTRIENT INTERACTIONS

PRIMARY DIAGNOSIS	OTHER DISEASE PRESENT	DRUG PRESCRIBED	DRUG-NUTRIENT INTERACTION
Diabetes	Arthritis Peptic ulcer	NSAID*	Bleeding →anemia
	Hypertension	Thiazide	Hyperglycemia
	Peripheral vascular disease	Niacin	Flush

*NSAID, nonsteroidal anti-inflammatory drugs.

low density lipoprotein triglyceride. It also decreases plasma cholesterol and increases the hepatic secretion of biliary cholesterol.

Reported side effects occurring in patients receiving niacin therapy at dosages ≧300 mg per day include flushing, dryness of the skin, nausea and diarrhea, and, rarely, the skin changes of acanthosis nigricans. Some patients have developed impaired hepatic function, hyperglycemia, and hyperuricemia. Hepatotoxicity with elevation of plasma transaminases and alkakine phosphatase levels is dose-dependent, occurring with greater frequency when the niacin dose exceeds 2.5 g per day. Glucose intolerance is usually moderate: hyperuricemia occurs in about one third of the patients receiving pharmacologic doses of niacin, but is not usually associated with gout. Arrythmia has been described.[21-23]

Niacin is still used extensively as a lipid-lowering agent. The prescribed dose of the vitamin, when it is used for this purpose, is 1000 to 4000 mg per day. While short-acting crystalline preparations are available in 250-mg tablets, timed-release formulations frequently are prescribed because they are available as capsules in a larger unit dose (500 mg) and also because the vasodilator effects of the large niacin dose are thereby lessened. Hepatotoxicity of the timed-release products has been reported.[24] Elevated transaminase levels, together with weakness and nausea, believed to be related to toxic hepatitis, occurred in a man who was taking niacin in the form of a Nature's Plus Niacin-500 product (Nature's Plus, Farmingdale, NY) (4.5 g/day) concurrently with cholestyramine.[25] Their use is highly inadvisable. To lessen the severity of niacin-induced flushing, the total daily dose is divided and taken at the three mealtimes, and each dose of niacin is taken with aspirin.

The vasodilator effects of niacin, including the flushing and infrequently associated tachycardia, tinnitus, and pruritus, may be partially or completely inhibited by aspirin (0.3 g), but the hepatotoxic and other metabolic effects of niacin can be reversed only when the "drug" is discontinued.[26]

Limitations on the use of vitamins as drugs stem from toxic effects and limited therapeutic effectiveness. The availability of vitamin analogues has reactivated interest in the use of vitamin-like substances as drugs. 13-*cis*-retinoic acid (isotretinoin) is being used in the treatment of acne vulgaris, particularly cystic and inflammatory forms of acne.[27] This "drug" is an oral synthetic vitamin A derivative, which actually is effective in controlling a wide variety of dermatoses characterized by defective keratinization. Long-term use (15 to 20 weeks) produces sustained remission of severe refractory cystic acne. However, higher doses and long-term administration of 13-*cis*-retinoic acid have been used to control such keratinizing dermatoses as lamellar ichthyosis.[28] 13-*cis*-retinoic acid, at a dose of 1 to 2 mg/kg, has also been recommended as a treatment for oral leukoplakia. Because relapse of the leukoplakia has been found to occur 2 to 3 months after discontinuing treatment, the risk of retinoid toxicity with continued use seems likely.[29]

Adverse side effects of 13-*cis*-retinoic acid at dosages of 1 to 2 mg/kg/day, as used in acne, include dry skin, fissuring of the lips, headache, dryness of the conjunctiva, and in some patients, moderate elevation of plasma cholesterol and triglyceride levels. At daily dosages of 3 to 4 mg/kg/day taken over a prolonged period (1 to 2 years), this drug has caused hyperostoses with multiple bony outgrowths of the vertebral column.[30] Both 13-*cis*-retinoic acid and the related retinoid, etretinate, which has been shown to be of therapeutic benefit in psoriasis, can induce severe birth defects when women take these drugs in the first trimester of pregnancy.[31]

Patients with acute promyelocytic leukemia have a characteristic translocation with a break on chromosome 17 in the region of the retinoid receptor. Because it has been shown that this receptor is involved in growth and differentiation of myeloid cells, a successful therapeutic trial of all-trans-retinoic acid has been carried out. This agent induces complete disease remission. Also, clinical response to this agent is associated with leukemic cell differentiation and expression of the aberrant RAR-α nuclear receptor. On the basis of these intervention studies, it has been suggested that molecular detection of the aberrant receptor may serve as a marker for residual leukemia.[32]

The ingestion of tryptophan products containing a contaminant has been associated with an epidemic of the eosinophilia-myalgia syndrome in the United States. Cases have also been reported from Europe. Other previously diagnosed cases of eosinophilic fasciitis have been attributed to this cause.[33]

DRUGS AS CALORIC SOURCES AND NUTRIENTS

Whereas vitamins administered in high dosages can exert pharmacologic effects, drugs may have nutritional functions. Alcohol, now the most widely used social drug, was formerly a therapeutic drug used in the treatment of fevers and of diabetes mellitus.[34,35] By ancient tradition, beer and wine were given to acutely ill patients as sources of nourishment when solid food could not be tolerated. Atwater and co-workers, who carried out the first fundamental studies on the metabolism of alcohol, cited cases in which alcohol was used as the only means of nutritional support.[36] One of the cases cited was a girl in the Massachusetts General Hospital with pneumonia who received more than a gallon of brandy over 7 days and no other form of food. Atwater and Benedict's human studies, carried out in the years 1898 to 1900, were the first to provide information that alcohol is oxidized and serves as a fuel.[37] They found that alcohol spares protein, fat, and also possibly carbohydrates. The viewpoint held at the beginning of the twentieth century was that alcohol resembles food with respect to its oxidation, but that it differs from foods in that it is not retained in the body for any considerable period.[38]

Today, alcohol is seldom used as a therapeutic drug because better drugs are available and also because of its toxic properties. Becker et al. summarized the history and current position of alcohol as a therapeutic drug as follows:[39] "Alcohol has been used clinically as an appetite stimulant, as a sedative-hypnotic drug, and as a caloric source for intravenous alimentation. Such medicinal uses of alcohol have never been subjected to controlled evaluation. Health tonics contain substantial quantities of alcohol and may as a consequence be abused."

Alcohol is absorbed as a drug and is metabolized both as a macronutrient and as a drug. In high dosages, it behaves as an antinutrient in that alcohol abuse can be associated with malabsorption and impaired use of a number of nutrients, particularly fat and water-soluble vitamins.[40] Today, we use alternate synthetic food-energy sources that are free of the toxicity of alcohol; for example, glucose polymers, which are used as caloric sources in enteral formulas for acutely ill or chronically sick patients. In contrast to alcohol, these alternate energy sources can promote micronutrient absorption of riboflavin and the rate of folic acid absorption.[41]

At present, when concern is high about obesity and fat-related chronic disease, caloric dilution of the United States diet by the use of a noncaloric fat replacement agent, Olestra (Proctor and Gamble) has been proposed. However, this agent, a sucrose polyester, has been shown to reduce the absorption of fat-soluble vitamins and certain drugs.[42]

DIETARY FACTORS INFLUENCING THE DISPOSITION OF DRUGS

Absorption of most drugs occurs by diffusion through the mucosa of the gastrointestinal tract. Although absorption of drugs can occur through any portion of the tract, absorption of most orally administered drugs is maximal at the level of the proximal part of the small intestine. Absorption across the mucosa of this part of the intestine is enhanced by the large surface area provided by the folds of Kerckring, the villi, and the microvilli. However, before absorption can occur, solid formulations of drugs must first be disintegrated and dissolved in the stomach by the gastric juice. The drug solution then leaves the stomach at a rate that depends on the gastric emptying time.[43]

Food components have been shown to affect drug absorption and bioavailability.[44] Three general mechanisms explain these effects: gastric emptying time, interactions with the gut lumen, and competitive inhibition.

Gastric Emptying Time. Absorption of drugs may be increased or decreased by physiologic changes in the gastrointestinal tract in the fed versus the fasted state. Gastric emptying time influences the rate of drug absorption. In the fasted state, or when little food is in the stomach, drugs leave the stomach rapidly and therefore soon reach the small intestine where they are optimally absorbed. Conversely, if a drug is formulated as a solid preparation—such that disintegration of drug particles as well as dissolution of the drug in stomach fluid must precede absorption—then rapid stomach emptying time militates against efficient drug absorption. In this case, the drug may be better absorbed after food intake, particularly after intake of foods or forms of foods that delay stomach emptying. Slow stomach emptying time occurs after heavy meals, meals containing fat, and after hot meals.[44]

The volume of a beverage taken with a drug and the characteristics of such a beverage can also influence drug absorption. Drugs are absorbed more efficiently when they are in dilute solution and therefore when the drug is taken with a beverage.[45]

Postprandial conditions that delay gastric emptying may also enhance drug absorption because the drug is metered out more slowly and efficiently to its intestinal absorption site. This effect is believed to explain the enhanced absorption of the thiazide diuretic chlorothiazide after food intake, as well as the enhanced absorption of pharmacologic doses of riboflavin after food intake.[46,47] Dietary factors that enhance the absorption of pharmacologic doses of riboflavin include food as such dietary fiber, cola beverages, and intake of a glucose polymer.[48]

Interactions Within the Gut Lumen. A physical or chemical interaction of the food and drug may occur within the gut lumen. For example, tetracycline is less well absorbed when taken with foods containing calcium, magnesium, iron, or zinc. The drug forms chelates with these minerals, which then are not absorbed.[49] Drugs can also interact with the components of enteral feeding formulas so that a gel or precipitate is formed, which can reduce drug or nutrient absorption and clog feeding tubes. In 1982, Bauer reported that when neurosurgical patients were given phenytoin during continuous nasogastric feeding, the plasma levels of the drug were reduced and there was escape from the desired anticonvulsant effects of the drug.[50] These effects were explained by direct interaction of formula constituents and this anticonvulsant within the gut lumen.

Competitive Inhibition. Food-induced increases in splanchnic blood flow may also increase the bioavailability of certain drugs after food. This effect is seen with some of the beta blocker drugs such as propranolol and metoprolol.[51] The absorption of drugs can also be influenced by individual nutrients. For example, absorption of L-dopa is reduced when this drug is taken with a high protein meal or with an amino acid mixture. Competitive inhibition of L-dopa absorption occurs when other amino acids absorbed from the same transport system are presented.[52] A similar protein or amino acid effect has been reported with methyldopa.[53]

A significant reduction of particular drug formulations by food has been reported in patients (Table 78–5). Slowing of drug absorption by food occurs with the drug formulations listed in Table 78–6. On the other hand, significant enhancement of the drugs listed in Table 78–7 occurs when the drug is taken with food. However, a report of different effects of food on different slow-release preparations of theophylline[54] indicates a need to explore food effects on drug absorption further so that we may be better able to predict the direction of the food effect. The lipid-lowering agent lovastatin and related drugs are better absorbed if given after a main meal. Further adherence to a lowfat diet increases the effectiveness of these drugs.[55]

TABLE 78–5. COMPOUNDS WHOSE ABSORPTION MAY BE REDUCED BY FOOD OR FOOD SUPPLEMENTS

COMPOUND	DOSAGE FORM
Amoxycillin	Capsules
Ampicillin	Capsules
Aspirin	Tablets
Aspirin, calcium	Tablets
Atenolol	Tablets
Captopril	Tablets
Cephalexin	Capsules, suspension
Demeclocycline (demethylchlortetracycline)	Capsules
Doxycycline	Capsules
Ethanol	Solution
Folic acid	Tablets*
Hydrochlorothiazide	Tablets
Iron	Solution, tablets
Isoniazid	Tablets
Ketoconazole	Tablets
Levodopa	Tablets
Lincomycin	Capsules
Methacycline	
Nafcillin	Tablets
Oxytetracycline	
Penicillamine	Tablets
Penicillin G	Tablets, suspension
Penicillin V (K)	Capsules, suspension, tablets
Penicillin V (Ca)	Tablets
Penicillin V (acid)	Tablets
Phenacetin	Suspension
Phenazone (antipyrine)	Syrup
Phenethicillin	Capsules, tablets
Phenylmercaptomethylpenicillin	Capsules
Phenytoin	Capsules†
Pivampicillin	Capsules
Propantheline	Tablets
Rifampicin	
Sotalol	Tablets
Tetracycline	Capsules
Theophylline	Capsules, controlled release‡

*Absorption reduced by calcium carbonate.
†Absorption reduced by folic acid and by enteral formula.
‡Absorption reduced by controlled release preparation of theophylline (Theo-Dur Sprinkle, Key Pharmaceuticals).
(Adapted from Welling, P.: Nutrient effects on drug metabolism and action in the elderly. Drug-Nutrient Interac., *4:*183, 1985.)

DIETARY FACTORS INFLUENCING DRUG METABOLISM

Rates of drug metabolism in the intestine, as well as in the liver, are influenced by dietary composition. High protein diets enhance drug metabolism, and protein-deficient diets slow drug metabolism. Effects of protein restriction on the drug-metabolizing activity of the liver have been reported in both in vitro and in vivo studies.[56,57]

Dietary factors that influence drug oxidation or conjugation reactions include protein quality, indolic compounds in vegetables of the *Brassica* family (cabbage and brussel sprouts), methylxanthine-containing beverages (coffee, tea, cocoa, chocolate), dietary fiber, and cooking method. Charcoal broiling of meats promotes drug metabolism in human subjects. Rapid effects of non-nutrient dietary components such as flavones on drug metabolism occur when a drug is taken concurrently or in close temporal proximity to food.[58]

Whereas relatively few dietary factors have been examined in human subjects for their effects on drug metabolism, a wide range of macro- and micronutrients, such as vitamins and trace elements, as well as other minerals, have been investigated in laboratory animals with regard to this effect. In a 1981 review of the subject, McLean emphasized the major nutrient influences on the rate and direction of drug metabolism that are superimposed on the genetic determinants of drug metabolism.[59]

TABLE 78–6. COMPOUNDS WHOSE ABSORPTION MAY BE DELAYED BY FOOD

COMPOUND	DOSAGE FORM
Alclofenac	Suspension
Amoxycillin	Tablets
Aspirin	EC tablets
	Effervescent tablets
Cefaclor	Capsules, suspension
Cephalexin	Capsules
Cephradine	Capsules
Cimetidine	Tablets
Cinoxacin	Capsules
Diclofenac	EC tablet
Digoxin	Tablets
Furosemide	Tablets, solution
Glipizide	Tablets
Indoprofen	Capsules
Metronidazole	Tablets
Paracetamol (acetaminophen)	Tablets
Phenytoin	Capsule, powder or suspension*
Piroxicam	Capsules
Potassium ion	Tablets and solution
Quinidine	
Sulfadiazine	Suspension
Sulfadiazine, sodium	Solution
Sulfadimethoxine	Tablets
Sulfafurazole (sufisoxazole)	Tablets
Sulfanilamide	Suspension
Sulfamethoxypyridazine	Tablets
Sulfasymasine	Tablets
Theophylline	Solution, sustained release tablet
	Sustained release tablets
	Sustained release tablets and capsules, enteric-coated tablets
	Tablets
Valproic acid	Syrup, capsules

*Absorption delayed by protein solution or enteral formula.

(Adapted from Welling, P.: Nutrient effects on drug metabolism and action in the elderly. Drug-Nutrient Interact., *4*:187, 1985.)

McLean also pointed out that weaker nutritional influences may have significant effects on the response to foreign compounds in the natural environment.

Animal experiments have shown that not only the level but also the quality of dietary protein affect drug metabolism. When the level of dietary protein is reduced so that it is limiting for growth, the basal rate of the cytochrome P-450-linked drug metabolism, as well as the response to inducers of drug metabolism such as phenobarbital, is diminished. When animals are fed a low-protein diet that is adequate in energy content, glucuronidation increases. Diets low in the sulfur-containing amino acids methionine and cystine cause a reduction in sulfate conjugation rates.[60,61]

Outcomes of protein restriction on drug or xenobiotic toxicity depend on whether the parent substance or the metabolite is more toxic. If the parent substance is more toxic, then protein restriction will increase toxicity, whereas if the metabolite is more toxic, then protein restriction may diminish toxicity. Reduction in toxicity by protein restriction has been dramatically demonstrated with respect to the pesticide heptachlor.[62] Previously, it was considered that reduction in the metabolic activation of carcinogens (initiators of the carcinogenic process) by protein restriction explained the lessening of tumor development in animals on a low protein diet; it has now been shown that protein restriction has its major influence on the promotional phase of carcinogenesis.[63,64]

The level of dietary fat also influences drug metabolism, as does the quality of fats administered. When fat-free diets are fed to laboratory animals, a reduction is noted in the cytochrome P-450 levels and in the activity of drug-metabolizing enzymes.[65,66]

In guinea pigs, it has been shown that diets deficient in ascorbic acid cause a reduction in the level of hepatic cytochrome P-450 and also in the activity of drug-metabolizing enzymes.[67]

Numerous animal studies have shown large effects of diet composition on drug metabolism and drug toxicity, but relatively few of these effects have been demonstrated in human populations or in subjects enrolled in drug trials. Indeed, the need to carry out epidemiologic

TABLE 78–7. COMPOUNDS WHOSE ABSORPTION MAY BE INCREASED BY FOOD OR FORMULA

COMPOUND	DOSAGE FORM
Alafostalin	Capsules
Canrenone	Tablets
Carbamazepine	Tablets
Chlorothiazide	Tablets
Dextropropoxyphene	Capsules
Diazepam	Tablets
Dicoumarol	Tablets
Diftalone	Capsules
Griseofulvin	Tablets or capsule
Hydralazine	Tablets
Hydrocholorothiazide	Tablets
Labetalol	Tablets
Lithium citrate	Tablets
Mebendazole	Tablets
Methoxsalen	Coated tablets
Metoprolol	Tablets
Nitrofurantoin	Capsules, tablets
Phenytoin	Capsules
Pivampicillin	Capsules
Propranolol	Capsules
Riboflavin*	Tablets, solution
Riboflavin-5′-phosphate*	Tablets, solution
Sulfamethoxydiazine	Tablets
α-Tocopherol nicotinate	Capsules

*Absorption is slowed by increased by food by specific dietary fiber sources including bran and by a glucose polymer solution (Polycose.Ross).

(Adapted from Welling, P.: Nutrient effects on drug metabolism and action in the elderly. Drug-Nutrient Interact., *4*:193, 1985.)

and metabolic studies of effects of diet composition on drug toxicity has been highlighted as a much needed area for research, particularly in aging populations and in elderly individuals in whom it is not clear whether the high prevalence of drug reactions can be explained by drug overuse or misuse, by the effects of aging on drug disposition, or by diet-related factors.[68]

EFFECTS OF DIET ON DRUG EXCRETION

Low-protein diets that decrease renal plasma flow and creatinine clearance can also reduce the renal clearance of certain drugs. For example, restriction of dietary protein decreases the clearance of the antigout drug allopurinol. Such diets also promote the renal tubular reabsorption of the chief metabolite of allopurinol, oxypurinol.[69–71] Practical implications of these findings are that elderly patients with gout should not follow prescribed low-protein conventional or formula diets when they are receiving allopurinol, unless the drug dosage is reduced sufficiently to avoid the risk of toxicity, which is related to persistence of the parent drug and its metabolite in the body. This precaution is particularly important in elderly patients with compromised renal function. Indeed, it is well known that in such patients, the risk of allopurinol toxicity is increased. This toxicity is manifested by fever, rash, peeling skin, hepatitis, and worsening of renal function.[72]

A low-protein diet can also lessen the rate of excretion of basic drugs such as the antibiotic gentamicin or the antiarrhythmic drug procainamide. This result is explained by the alkalinizing effect of the diet, which leads to less of the ionized form of these drugs presented in the renal tubule and therefore more of the drug being reabsorbed. A similar effect is produced by intake of antacids that are commonly taken by elderly patients. In patients receiving basic drugs, the urinary pH should be monitored, and if the pH is increasing, the physician should reduce the drug dose or consider an alternative drug.[73]

Competition between drugs or between drugs and nutrients for a common renal secretory pathway can also change the rate of drug excretion. For example, the renal clearance of the antifolate drug methotrexate is reduced significantly by administration of aspirin.

INFLUENCE OF FOOD AND NUTRIENTS ON PRESYSTEMIC CLEARANCE OF DRUGS

Melander and McLean pointed out that drugs can have a low degree of oral bioavailability in spite of the fact that gastrointestinal absorption is complete.[74] They explained that some drugs undergo extensive presystemic metabolism during their first passage through the gut mucosa and the liver. The intake of specific nutrients has been found to influence the bioavailability of certain drugs that are known to undergo presystemic metabolic clearance. These drugs are lipophilic bases including propranolol, metoprolol, labetalol, and hydralazine, which are metabolized presystemically by hydroxylation, glucuronidation, and acetylation. Marley et al. reported that food-induced increases in the bioavailability of propranolol are related to the amount of protein in a meal,[75] probably by the effect of the protein in the meal on splanchnic blood flow. It is not clear, however, from published studies whether this protein effect is of clinical significance when the drug is given in several doses per day and on a long-term basis.

Erratic responses to these drugs can be explained by administration in a haphazard way in relation to meal times, so that the food sometimes has an effect on their bioavailability and at other times does not. It is recommended, therefore, that these drugs always be given with a meal and preferably always with a meal of similar composition.

EFFECTS OF DIET ON MICROBIAL METABOLISM OF XENOBIOTICS

The gut microflora are capable of metabolizing foreign compounds as well as endogenous metabolites. Most of the studies that have demonstrated metabolism of drugs by the gut microflora have been carried out in vitro. Prins pointed out, however, that in vitro demonstration that the intestinal microflora metabolize a drug does not actually mean that this process takes place in vivo.[76] For in vivo metabolism of drugs to take place, the drug or its metabolites must actually be in contact with the bacteria within the lumen of the intestine. Criteria have been developed to indicate whether a drug is metabolized by the gut microflora in vivo. These criteria can be summarized as follows: (1) the reaction should occur more extensively after oral rather than parenteral administration of the drug; (2) the microbial drug metabolism should be decreased when antibiotics are given; and (3) the reaction should not occur in germ-free animals. Most metabolic activities of the gut microflora with respect to therapeutic drugs and other xenobiotics are degradative. In rodents, microbial metabolism of foreign compounds and endogenous metabolites is more extensive than in man, because the upper gastrointestinal tract is colonized with bacteria capable of these activities and the animals practice coprophagy so that drugs and their primary metabolites may be returned to the tract several times. In the human, as in other animals, most of the microbial metabolism of foreign compounds occurs after initial absorption of the parent drug and its conversion by the microsomal drug-metabolizing system to primary metabolites. These metabolites are absorbed into the enterohepatic circulation and are then excreted via the bile into the gut lumen. In human subjects, the microbial metabolism of drugs presumably occurs in the large intestine, because the major colonization of the gut by bacteria is in the large intestine, except under conditions of disease when the small intestine may be colonized.

EFFECTS OF OBESITY ON DRUG PHARMACOKINETICS

Differences in body composition may influence drug disposition. The disposition of gentamicin and tobramycin have been studied in mildly obese subjects, and the mean relative volume of distribution is similar to that in normal-weight subjects when normalized body mass is used in the calculation.[77] Following this study, these and other investigators recommended that dosing schedules for tobramycin and for other aminoglycosides should be based on ideal body weight.[78,79]

Tobramycin pharmacokinetics was studied by Blouin et al. in subjects who were 124.9 ± 36% S.D. overweight.[79] The volume of distribution of the drug (v_{area}) related to ideal body weight was approximately 1.7 times as high as in published reports on normal subjects. Specifically, Blouin et al. recommended that the loading dose of tobramycin in morbidly obese subjects should be based on a v_{area} of 0.26 L/kg × (IBW + 58% adipose mass).[79] However, there is still a need to determine whether multiple doses or the duration of multiple doses would alter the volume of distribution of aminoglycosides at the steady state.

DRUG EFFECTS ON FOOD INTAKE, BODY WEIGHT, NUTRIENT REQUIREMENTS, AND GROWTH

Drugs can reduce food intake because they cause a perversion or loss of appetite, induce sedation, or evoke an adverse response when food is taken. Drugs affecting appetite may do so by central or peripheral effect. Appetite-reducing drugs acting centrally include unsubstituted and substituted amphetamines, as well as related compounds. Although this class of drugs has not shown outstanding effectiveness in the treatment or control of obesity, it has been shown that, when children are given a similar drug, such as dextroamphetamine, for the control of hyperactivity, growth may be retarded while the drug therapy is maintained. Fortunately, rebound growth occurs when the drug is discontinued. Ethoxzolamide (Ethamide) has a similar effect to that of dextroamphetamine with respect to inhibition of growth.

Intentional or unintentional modulation of appetite by drugs has been a subject of much research and of several major reviews.[80,81] Whereas all reviews on appetitive control by drugs stress drugs that have been and are used in the treatment of obesity, our present concern is with other therapeutic drugs for which change in appetite and, hence, change in food intake are unwanted side effects. Any drug that induces nausea is likely to reduce food intake and hence contribute to weight loss. Digitalis, which usually is administered for long periods, if also prescribed at a high dosage level, can cause severe wasting (digitalis cachexia) because associated nausea diminishes the desire for food.[82]

Among all drug groups that reduce appetite, the cancer chemotherapeutic drugs are most important. At effective therapeutic dosages, these drugs commonly have an acute anorectic effect, which is an integral part of the systemic toxicity. However, intake of food may be reduced after administration of cancer chemotherapeutic drugs because of either oral or intestinal ulceration. A reduction in food intake is related to gastroenterologic toxicity. It is largely explained by the reluctance to eat, because food causes unpleasant symptoms, which may include pain and diarrhea.[83]

A wide range of environmental chemicals that have significant systemic toxicity induce a reduction in food intake. For example, experience has shown that in the Yusho disease that occurred in Fukuoka, Japan, as a result of exposure to polychlorinated biphenyls, poor appetite was a consistent symptom of intoxication.[84]

Risks from the effects of drug-induced anorexia depend on both the primary toxicity of the substance and the secondary effects of the anorexia or loss of desire to consume food. The latter includes not only weight loss, but also specific nutrient deficiencies that may ensue because of diminished intake of nutrients. A classification of anorectic drugs is given in Table 78–8.

Drugs that increase appetite include the phenothiazine and benzodiazepine tranquilizers and lithium carbonate, which is used as a psychotherapeutic agent in patients with manic depressive psychoses. Effects of these drugs, which increase appetite and food intake in psychotic

TABLE 78–8. CLASSIFICATION OF ANORECTIC DRUGS

A. Primary → appetite suppression
  1. *Centrally acting*
    a) Catecholaminergic, e.g., dextroamphetamine
    b) Dopaminergic, e.g., levodopa
    c) Serotoninergic, e.g., fenfluramine
    d) Endorphin modulators, e.g., naloxone
  2. *Peripherally acting*
    a) Agents that inhibit gastric emptying, e.g., levodopa
    b) Bulking agents, e.g., methyl cellulose

B. Secondary → Adverse response to food → Loss of appetite
  a) Drugs causing nausea and vomiting, e.g., digoxin-toxin dose
  b) Drugs causing loss of taste, e.g., penicillamine
  c) Drugs causing stomatitis, e.g., fluorouracil
  d) Hepatotoxic agents, e.g., alcohol

(Based on Pawan, G.L.S.: Proc. Nutr. Soc., *33*:239–244, 1974.)

patients, are related to both direct pharmacologic effects and the fact that administration of the drug reduces mental agitation. Cyproheptadine is another drug that can increase appetite. It is used as an antihistamine and serotonin antagonist. The hyperphagic effect of this drug has been used in the nutritional management of the debilitated individual whose appetite is precarious.[85]

DRUG EFFECTS ON NUTRIENT REQUIREMENTS

In human subjects, as in laboratory animals, microbial nutrient synthesis occurs in the intestine. Contribution of this synthesis to the nutrition of the host has been considered modest in the human, whereas in rodents, the nutrient synthesis in the small and large intestine is important in contributing to vitamin needs. However, in certain circumstances, microbial synthesis of specific nutrients becomes critical, particularly when intake of said nutrients is inadequate. For example, the synthesis of biotin in the intestine may supply needs for this vitamin in patients who are totally fed with a biotin-free enteral formula. A case report illustrates the development of biotin deficiency in an adult that was induced by lack of biotin intake as well as by suppression of the normal colonic bacterial flora by long-term antibiotic therapy. The patient who had inflammatory bowel disease of long standing may also have had gastrointestinal losses of biotin through fistulae. Food-energy and nutrient intake of this man was supplied by parenteral alimentation using a formula that did not contain biotin.[86]

Broad-spectrum antibiotics, such as tetracycline, can also depress vitamin K synthesis in the intestine. The impact of this nutrient effect of the antibiotic with respect to vitamin K status is not important unless concurrently the patient is vitamin K-deficient because of liver disease or a warfarin anticoagulant that is a vitamin K antagonist is also being administered.[87,88]

DRUG-INDUCED MALDIGESTION AND MALABSORPTION

Drugs that may cause nutrient malabsorption include antacids, laxatives, antibacterial agents such as sulfasalazine, and also isoniazid (isonicotinic acid hydrazide, INH). Absorption induced by antacids is multifactorial. When the pH of the upper part of the jejunum is increased after ingestion of sodium bicarbonate, folate absorption is reduced. However, our own studies of peptic ulcer patients taking antacids suggest that folate deficiency is not common and that when it does occur, it is more often associated with inadequate intake of the vitamin, rather than intake of sodium bicarbonate. A risk does exist, nevertheless, that if large doses of sodium bicarbonate are taken concurrently with food sources of folate, significant malabsorption could lead to folate depletion and deficiency.

A phosphate depletion syndrome is known to occur in elderly people taking heavy doses of antacids containing aluminum or magnesium hydroxide or mixtures of these substances. Dietary phosphate combines with aluminum and magnesium hydroxide to form insoluble aluminum and magnesium phosphates, which are excreted through the gastrointestinal tract. The risk of phosphate depletion is greatest when there is an interactive effect with a low-phosphate diet. Some effects of phosphate depletion are muscle weakness, which may be limited to the proximal limb muscles, malaise, parasthesias in the limbs, anorexia, hemolytic anemia, and convulsions. Congestive heart failure may also occur. In a few patients with phosphate depletion, low-phosphate osteomalacia has developed.[89,90]

It has been proposed that folate malabsorption associated with intake of sulfasalazine occurs because of inhibition of folate enzymes in the gastrointestinal tract. Sulfasalazine is a competitive inhibitor of folate transport by the intestine.[91] Folate malabsorption in patients with inflammatory bowel disease who are receiving this drug depends not only on drug intake but also on whether they obtain a sufficiency or otherwise of dietary folate.[92]

Two drugs used in the treatment of tuberculosis, rifampicin and isoniazid, interfere with the normal metabolism of vitamin D and, hence, may impair calcium absorption. Isoniazid inhibits both the hepatic 25-hydroxylase and the renal 1 α-hydroxylase. Rifampicin is a microsomal enzyme inducer that stimulates metabolism of 25-hydroxycholecalciferol with a resultant decrease in circulating levels of this vitamin D metabolite. Whether or not hypocalcemia and metabolic bone disease (osteomalacia) occur as a result of ingestion of these drugs depends on the age of the patient, physiologic stress (pregnancy or lactation), ultraviolet exposure, vitamin D or calcium intake, presence of alcoholic liver disease, administration of both isoniazid and rifampicin, and a previous partial gastrectomy.[93,94]

Malabsorption of protein-bound vitamin B_{12} has been reported with intake of the H_2 receptor blocking drugs, cimetidine and ranitidine. Cimetidine, in a dosage of 1,000 mg per day (200 mg 3 times daily + 400 mg at night), has been shown to reduce the absorption of protein-bound cobalamin by peptic ulcer patients and also by normal subjects. When cimetidine was administered in a dosage of 400 mg per night, it had no significant effect on the absorption of the vitamin.[95] Ranitidine can also cause protein-bound vitamin B_{12} malabsorption, but these effects are rapidly reversible when the drug is discontinued.[96]

The anticonvulsant drugs phenytoin and phenobarbital can cause hypocalcemia and rickets or osteomalacia in epileptic children and adults who receive these anticonvulsant drugs. The mechanisms responsible for the adverse effects of these drugs on calcium absorption are not entirely clear. The drugs may have a direct effect on bone growth, but also both drugs inhibit the synthesis of calcium-binding protein and thereby inhibit calcium absorption. It has been further proposed that these drugs stimulate the catabolism of 25-hydroxycholecalciferol to vitamin D metabolites, which are inactive in promoting calcium absorption.[97–99]

Mechanisms responsible for drug-induced maldigestion and malabsorption include interaction of the drug and nutrient in the gastrointestinal tract, change in gastrointestinal function, and drug-induced enteropathy with damage to the brush border of the intestinal villi, causing interference with active transport mechanisms for nutrients. Drug-induced maldigestion and malabsorption are classified in Table 78–9 together with mechanisms.

VITAMIN ANTAGONISTS

Vitamin antagonists are those therapeutic drugs and environmental chemicals that have antinutrient function by virtue of the fact that they interfere with the metabolism and physiologic function of vitamins. The antivitamin effects of drugs may be used intentionally in the treatment of disease, or these effects may be an unwanted side effect of drug therapy.[100]

Drugs for which the therapeutic effect is related to vitamin antagonism include methotrexate, which is used in the treatment of choriocarcinoma, head and neck cancer, and acute lymphoblastic leukemia, and pyrimethamine, which is used in the prevention and treatment of malaria. Another class of therapeutic compounds that are vitamin antagonists are the coumarin anticoagulants. Methotrexate has several antifolate effects. In the tissues, this drug binds tightly to the dihydrofolate reductase enzyme. Folate from dietary sources is thereby displaced from the dihydrofolate reductase enzyme by the drug and is thereafter excreted in the urine. Methotrexate polyglutamates are formed, and synthesis of folate polyglutamates is diminished. Thymidylate synthetase is inhibited. The synthesis of DNA, RNA, and protein are thereby also inhibited. Methotrexate reduces the incorporation of deoxyuridine (dU) into DNA and favors incorporation of thymidine into DNA by the alternate pathway. The dU suppression test is abnormal in people who are receiving methotrexate.[101] Methotrexate is being used at low dosages for the treatment of rheumatoid arthritis. In this regimen, the risk of antifolate effects of the drug are reduced. It has also been found that folic acid supplements can further reduce the risk of these side effects.[102]

Methotrexate has a greater affinity for folate-binding protein at the pH optimum for the radiometric assay for plasma folate. It has therefore been proposed that this assay, which involves competitive protein binding in plasma and erythrocytes, should not be used to measure this vitamin in the plasma or erythrocytes of patients receiving the drug.[103]

Sulfasalazine is also a folate antagonist. Inhibitory actions of sulfasalazine include inhibition of three enzymes in vitro, including dihydrofolate reductase, methyltetrahydrofolate reductase, and serine transhydroxymethylase, which each catalyze a different reaction involving folate coenzymes. Sulfasalazine has been shown to act as a folate antagonist in intact lymphocytes.[104] Another folate antagonist, pentamidine, is currently the drug of choice for the control of Pneumocystis carinii pneumonia in AIDS patients.[105]

Nitrous oxide, long used as an anesthetic and more recently used in the management of patients after cardiac bypass surgery, has been shown to be a vitamin B_{12} antagonist. Megaloblastic erythropoiesis and neurologic disorders have been reported both in man and in

TABLE 78–9. DRUG-INDUCED MALDIGESTION AND MALABSORPTION

MECHANISM	EXAMPLE OF INDUCING DRUG(S)	EFFECT ON NUTRIENT ABSORPTION
Intraluminal interaction of drug and nutrient	Mineral oil	↓ Absorption fat-soluble vitamins: ∵ solubilization and ↓ micelle formation
	Cholestyramine	↓ Absorption of folic acid ∵ absorption onto drug
Change in milieu of GI tract or GI function	Sodium bicarbonate	↓ Absorption of folic acid ∵ ↑ pH*
	Cimetidine	↓ Absorption of vitamin B_{12} ∵ ↓ gastric digestion
	Alcohol	↓ Absorption of fat ∵ ↓ exocrine pancreatic function
Drug-induced enteropathy	Neomycin Colchicine	Disaccharide intolerance and fat malabsorption ∵ damage to brush border

*∵ = "due to . . ."

laboratory animals after exposures to high concentrations of this gas. Nitrous oxide causes multiple metabolic defects. It oxidizes vitamin B_{12} and causes an inhibition of methionine synthetase. When inactivation of methionine synthetase is produced by nitrous oxide, cobalamin is displaced from the enzyme. Further, there is an increased formation of inactive cobalamin analogues.[106-109]

Vitamin antagonism is a significant side effect of a number of therapeutic drugs, including isoniazid and hydralazine. Both of these drugs are vitamin B_6 antagonists. Isoniazid can also induce a secondary niacin deficiency with development of pellagra. Such secondary niacin deficiency is rare, but it has been reported in tuberculous patients who have been on a marginal intake of niacin. It is thought that the deficiency in these patients results from an inhibition of the enzyme kynureninase in the pathway of nicotinamide nucleotide synthesis from tryptophan as a result of complex formation between isoniazid and pyridoxal phosphate (Schiff base formation).[110,111]

Vitamin K antagonists include coumarin drugs such as warfarin, dicoumarol, and phenprocoumon, as well as coumarins in plants, which sometimes are used in making herbal teas. These coumarin derivatives inhibit the hepatic reductase, which converts the storage form of vitamin K (vitamin K 2.3-epoxide) to the active form of the vitamin.[112] High doses of vitamin K decrease the anticoagulant effect of coumarin drugs and lessen their clinical effectiveness in the prevention of thromboses.[113]

Moxalactam, which is a β-lactam cephalosporin antibiotic as well as a β-lactam antibiotic, can decrease vitamin K-dependent clotting factors, including prothrombin. Hemorrhagic events after use of these antibiotics are most frequent with moxalactam. This drug can interfere with blood clotting through three different mechanisms: production of hypoprothrombinemia, platelet dysfunction, and occasionally thrombocytopenia. Only hemorrhage that is associated with hypoprothrombinemia can be reversed or prevented by administration of vitamin K.[114,115]

The cancer chemotherapy drug doxorubicin (Adriamycin) produces a dose-dependent cardiomyopathy when the total cumulative dose is greater than 500 mg/m.[2] In laboratory animals, the histopathologic aspects of the cardiac lesion are similar to those of vitamin E deficiency. The lesions seen in vitamin E deficiency, and apparently in doxorubicin toxicity, are the result of free radical reactions that cause lipid peroxidation of membrane lipids. The incidence and severity of the doxorubicin-induced cardiac damage has been reduced by administration of vitamin E to laboratory animals, but this vitamin has not been effective in preventing doxorubicin cardiotoxicity in man.[116]

Adverse effects of alcohol excess on nutritional status include an impairment in the utilization of B vitamins.[117] For example, the Wernicke-Korsakoff syndrome is a thiamin dependency disease that occurs mainly in alcoholics. The acute phase of this disease (Wernicke's encephalopathy) responds to intravenous administration of high doses of thiamin.[118]

Wernicke's encephalopathy has also been reported in a diabetic patient after administration of the oral hypoglycemic agent tolazamide. Signs were reversed by administration of thiamin given as combined intramuscular and oral therapy. It was suggested that administration of this hypoglycemic agent to diabetic patients may increase the demand for thiamin because of a sudden increase in use of glucose in an individual who previously is thiamin-depleted.[119] Drugs that have significant effects as vitamin antagonists are classified in Table 78–10.

DRUG-INDUCED FETAL MALNUTRITION

All drugs given to a pregnant woman can be considered potentially harmful to the fetus because they cross the placental membrane. The highest risk for disruption in fetal development is during the period of embryogenesis.[120] The most important toxic effect of drug administration during the period of embryogenesis is the development of fetal malformations (teratogenic effect).

TABLE 78–10. THERAPEUTIC DRUGS THAT ARE VITAMIN ANTAGONISTS

ANTAGONISTS	DRUG	USAGE
Folacin	Methotrexate	Cancer chemotherapy
	Pyrimethamine	Antimalarial
	Triamterene	Diuretic
	Trimethoprim	Antibacterial
	Sulfasalazine	Anti-inflammatory
Vitamin B_6	Isoniazid	Antituberculosis agent
	Hydralazine	Antihypertensive agent
Vitamin B_{12}	Nitrous oxide	Anesthetic
Vitamin K	Warfarin	Anticoagulant
	Moxalactam	Antibiotic

The teratogenic potential of drugs is related to drug properties, including drug metabolism; to the time of administration during gestation; to dosage and maternofetal transfer; to the species, strain, and genetic susceptibility of the animal or individual; and to nutritional status. Drugs that are vitamin antagonists impose a high risk for teratogenic effects.

Specific associations between the change in nutritional status and the fetal malformations have been identified as follows: (1) A disturbance in DNA synthesis, such as that imposed by folacin deficiency, causes multiple malformations. Interference with DNA synthesis can be brought about by drugs such as methotrexate or pyrimethamine, which are folate antagonists. (2) Impaired glycosaminoglycan synthesis or sulfation can result in malformations related to the skeleton. Sulfation of the glycosaminoglycans in the fetal skeleton depends on substrate availability. When drugs that require sulfoconjugation, such as salicylamide, are administered during pregnancy, competitive use of sulfate for sulfoconjugation and sulfation of the skeletal elements occurs.[121] (3) Riboflavin deficiency induced by administration of the flavin antagonist, galactoflavin, can induce congenital anomalies in the fetus because of impairment of the electron transport system. Depressed function of the electron transport system during the critical period of development usually results in malformations.[122]

Epidemiologic studies have been carried out to determine whether the vitamin folic acid can reduce the risk of neural tube defects. Observations in the United Kingdom indicated a protective effect of folic acid, but in subsequent studies, it was shown that the risk of neural tube defects is determined by both genetic and environmental factors. Women who take folic acid or multivitamins containing folic acid are less likely to bear infants with neural tube defects, but it is not clear whether it is their vitamin-taking practices or other health or nutritional practices that have the protective effect.[123]

DRUG EFFECTS ON MINERAL STATUS

Drug effects on mineral status include overload and depletion. Sodium overload with development of congestive heart failure can result from intake of antacids containing sodium bicarbonate. The risk is most severe in elderly people with pre-existing heart disease who are also consuming high-sodium diets. Intake of other high-sodium drugs can also cause sodium overload, particularly in cardiac patients. The antihypertensive agent diazoxide, which increases the proximal tubular reabsorption of sodium, can also cause sodium overload.[100,124] Angiotensin-converting enzyme inhibitor drugs such as captopril are also under current trial for control of nephropathy in insulin-dependent diabetes. These drugs reduce blood pressure and reduce decline of glomerular filtration rates.[125]

Potassium Overload. A number of drugs are known to produce hyperkalemia. Administration of succinylcholine can produce significant increases in serum potassium levels that may result in arrhythmia and cardiac arrest.[126] Hyperkalemia with development of metabolic acidosis can result from administration of a biguanide such as phenformin when this drug is given to a diabetic patient with impaired renal function.[127]

Hyperkalemia can follow use of potassium-sparing diuretics. Hyperkalemia resulting from administration of spironolactone, an aldosterone antagonist, is caused by blocking of the distal tubular sodium-potassium exchange. Hyperkalemia owing to the use of spironolactone is more severe in patients with impaired renal function.[128] Triamterene, which is also a potassium-sparing diuretic, can cause hyperkalemia.[129] Increases in serum potassium levels have been reported with use of beta-blocking drugs.[130,131]

Hypercalcemia. Hypercalcemia may be drug-related, but usually this metabolic disorder is multifactorial. Hypercalcemia can occur with administration of thiazide diuretics; however, this side effect of thiazide therapy is relatively uncommon and may only be temporary.[132]

Thiazide diuretics cause calcium retention, and the actual effect of these drugs on the mineral content of bone has been measured. Thiazide users have a greater bone mineral content than nonusers who have been matched. It has been suggested that thiazide drugs might have a therapeutic role in the management of osteoporosis.[133]

Editronate is another drug that is known to be of benefit in osteoporosis. This biphosphonate compound, when given as intermittent cyclic treatment, increases spinal bone mass and reduces the incidence of new vertebral fractures in women with postmenopausal osteoporosis.[134]

Pharmacologic doses of vitamin D and its metabolites cause hypercalcemia. In vitamin D intoxication, hypercalcemia is associated with polyuric renal failure and also soft tissue calcification. When high doses of vitamin D are taken, the hypercalcemic effect is potentiated by concurrent intake of calcium salts.[135,136]

The milk-alkali syndrome occurs as a complication of excessive ingestion of soluble alkali and milk. It is characterized by hypercalcemia with hypercalciuria. Renal insufficiency with azotemia can develop with alkalosis. Signs include band keratitis owing to deposition of calcium in the cornea. The milk-alkali syndrome has been reported in people taking large amounts of sodium bicarbonate or calcium carbonate. Persons at particular risk are those with pre-existent renal insufficiency.[137]

When malignant tumors metastasize to bone, they may induce hypercalcemia, and it has been shown that when androgenic steroids are used in the treatment of metastases from breast tumors, hypercalcemia may thereby be increased.[138]

Another concern is that chronically supplementing dietary calcium with calcium salts, as a means to delay age-related bone loss or to prevent hypertension, could also cause the milk-alkali syndrome.[139] Previous estimates of the amount of ingested calcium and alkali necessary to produce the syndrome were 4 to 5 g up to 60 g of calcium carbonate daily.[140] The current extensive use of calcium carbonate tablets for osteoporosis and hypertension prevention may therefore lead to an increased prevalence of the syndrome such as was encountered in peptic ulcer patients when the Sippy diet and antacid treatment were in vogue.

Magnesium Overload. Magnesium intoxication has been reported in patients with chronic renal failure who have been taking magnesium-containing antacids. Signs include nausea, vomiting, flushing, impaired respiratory function, and partial or complete heart block. Lithium carbonate, used in the management of manic-depressive psychosis, may induce hypermagnesemia.[141,142]

Drug-Induced Mineral Depletion. Drug-induced mineral depletion is commonly multifactorial. For example, in the elderly, it may be the outcome of concurrent use of several drugs that have this side effect, as well as intake of the mineral. Such common drugs causing potassium deficiency, for example, are diuretics, including both thiazide and loop-type diuretics, and elderly individuals who are taking one of these drugs while using laxatives, which also cause potassium depletion, may also have an inadequate potassium intake. Factors contributing to mineral depletion in such individuals include prolonged drug intake and renal disorder. Crooks and Stevenson drew attention to the relationship between an age-related decline in renal function and the potential for mineral depletion by nephrotoxic drugs.[143] Related diseases that potentiate drug-related mineral depletion include renal disease and catabolic diseases, including metastatic cancer. Drugs that cause potassium depletion may damage the renal tubule and thereby cause secondary depletion of magnesium and zinc.[100] Drug causes of mineral depletion as well as the sequelae of such depletion are classified in Table 78–11.

DRUG-FOOD AND DRUG-ALCOHOL INCOMPATIBILITIES

Food and drug incompatibilities usually arise as outcomes of the drug-induced inhibition of enzymes acquired in the catabolism of potentially toxic endogenous metabolites. Many of the incompatibilities result in flush reactions. "Histamine poisoning" has been reported in individuals receiving isoniazid as an antituberculous drug during intake of certain kinds of fish, including tuna and skipjack. Signs include redness of the face, itching of the eyes, face, and palms, and severe headache. It is known that isoniazid is a potent histaminase inhibitor and it has therefore been suggested that eating fish that is not fresh and contains high levels of histamine may produce these side effects.[144]

Chlorpropamide-alcohol flushing (CPAF) has been found in many patients with noninsulin-dependent diabetes. This type of flushing can be blocked by administration of prostaglandin inhibitor drugs such as aspirin and indomethacin. These findings have indicated an etiologic association between prostaglandins and the flush reaction.[145–147]

Tyramine reactions have occurred when fermented foods such as cheese have been consumed by people receiving monamine oxidase inhibitor drugs. These drugs include certain antidepressants such as phenelzine, the cancer chemotherapeutic drug procarbazine, and isoniazid. In these patients, absorption of tyramine, because of inhibition of its metabolism in the intestine, triggers release of catecholamines with resultant acute elevation in blood pressure. Attacks of hypertension of short duration are associated with headaches, palpitations, nausea, and vomiting. In some cases, major cerebrovascular accidents have occurred. Severity of each attack is related both to the current drug dosage and also to the level of tryamine in the particular food ingested. Foods high in tyramine documented in these incompatibility reactions include not only aged cheese but also Chianti wine and chicken livers.[148–152] The amino acid dopa or its amine derivative, dopamine, present in broad beans may trigger the tyramine reaction in patients on monamine oxidase inhibitor drugs.[148]

The disulfiram reaction occurs when people receiving the drug disulfiram (Antabuse) either drink alcoholic beverages or consume foods containing alcohol, or apply alcohol-containing lotions or other solutions to the skin. The reaction is associated with flushing and headache followed by nausea, vomiting, and a variable degree of chest and/or abdominal pain. Because these symptoms are unpleasant, the drug has come to be used as an alcohol deterrent for alcoholics. Disulfiram-like reactions are caused by all drugs that are aldehyde dehydrogenase inhibitors. Disulfiram is such a drug. Other drugs in this category are: metronidazole, furazolidone, griseofulvin, quinacrine, tolazoline, and procarbazine. Inkycap mushroom *(Coprinus atramentarius)* contains an aldehyde dehydrogenase inhibitor such that consumption of these mushrooms with or following an alcoholic beverage, including beer, causes a disulfiram reaction.[117,153–156]

Hypoglycemic reactions may occur when diabetic patients receiving hypoglycemic agents ingest alcohol. Symptoms are characterized by weakness, mental confusion, irrational behavior, and, if untreated, loss of consciousness. Hypoglycemic attacks have occurred when sweet or semisweet drinks containing alcohol are ingested on an empty stomach.[157]

TABLE 78–11. DRUG CAUSES, SIGNS, AND SEQUELAE OF MINERAL DEPLETION

MINERAL DEPLETION	DRUGS CAUSING	SIGNS AND SEQUELAE
Sodium	Chlorpropamide	Hyponatremia, anorexia
	Tolbutamide	Nausea
	Vincristine	Vomiting
	Amitryptyline	Muscle weakness, seizures
	Mannitol	Loss of consciousness
	Thiazides	
	Spironolactone	
	Captopril	
Potassium	Thiazides	Hypokalemia, anorexia
	Furosemide	Muscle weakness
	Ethacrynic acid	Renal tubular damage
	Laxatives, e.g., phenolphthalein	Arrhythmias, hyperglycemia
	Nephrotoxic antibiotics, e.g., gentamicin	Magnesium and zinc depletion
Calcium	Aluminum hydroxide	Hypocalcemia, tetany, osteomalacia
	Phenytoin	
	Phenobarbital	
	Corticosteroids	Osteoporosis
Magnesium	Thiazides	Muscle weakness
	Furosemide	Tremors
	Ethacrynic acid	Seizures
	Gentamicin	Tetany
	Cisplatin	Psychotic behavior
	Neomycin	
	Colchicine	
Iron	Aspirin	Anemia
	Indomethacin	
Zinc	Penicillamine	Loss of taste
		Dermatitis
		Impaired wound healing

PREDICTING AND DIAGNOSING DIET, NUTRITION, AND DRUG INTERACTIONS

Predictions of the risk of drug and nutrient interaction can be made if the primary and secondary diagnoses are known, if organ function is known from laboratory tests, if the characteristics of prescribed drugs and diet are known, and if the regimen is known. Diagnosis of a clinical problem as an adverse outcome of a drug and nutrient interaction rests initially on the knowledge that for this association to be correct the problem must have appeared after the drug has been prescribed and/or after a change in diet or drug regimen has occurred. In addition, changes in laboratory tests occurring in temporal relationship to the event will help to clarify the diagnosis. For example, if plasma glucose levels are elevated in a diabetic patient within 2 days of corticosteroid administration, the likelihood that this drug has induced the hyperglycemia is strong. Situations in which prediction and diagnosis are critical are in relation to drugs for which the therapeutic window is narrow,[158] because otherwise, a toxic reaction will occur, or conversely, the drug will be ineffective.

In summary, the emphasis of this account of drug-nutrient interactions has been on the impact on human health. Whereas drug-nutrient interactions can be defined as events and outcomes that ensue as a result of physical, chemical, physiologic, or pathophysiologic relationships between drugs and nutrients, the significance of drug-nutrient interactions is in their adverse or unwanted outcomes. Unwanted outcomes include reduction in the intended or expected response to a therapeutic drug because of diet-induced changes in drug bioavailability or metabolism, drug-induced nutritional deficiencies or overload, drug-induced fetal malnutrition, and drug-food and drug-nutrient incompatibility reactions. Risk of drug-nutrient interactions and their outcomes depends most on the characteristics of the exposed individual, including age, physiologic status, multiple drug exposure, hepatic and renal function, and diet. However, as emphasized in this account, whether or not a drug-nutrient interaction occurs depends largely on the concurrent use or exposure to drug and nutrients at the critical period. Avoidance of drug-nutrient interactions depends on a knowledge of the risk and also avoidance of temporal proximity of drug-nutrient, drug-alcohol, or drug-food intake that imposes a high risk situation.

REFERENCES

1. Hansten, P.D.: Drug Interactions. 5th Ed. Philadelphia, Lea & Febiger, 1985, p. 241.
2. Nordstrom, M., Melander, A., Robertson, E. et al.: Drug-Nutrient Interact., *5:*67–69, 1987.
3. Reitberg, D.P., Love, S.J., Quercia, G.T. et al.: Clin. Pharmacol. Ther., *42:*72–75, 1987.
4. Vaughan, L., Milavetz, G., Hil, M., et al.: Drug Intell. Clin. Pharm., *18:*510–513, 1984.
5. Fleming, B.J., Genuth, S.M., Gould, A.B., et al.: Ann. Intern. Med., *83:*60–62, 1975.
6. Roe, D.A.: Drug-folate interrelationships: Historical aspects and current concerns. *In* Folic Acid Metabolism in Health and Disease. Edited by M.F. Picciano, E.L.R. Stokstad, J.F. Gregory. New York, Wiley-Liss, 1990, pp. 277–287.
7. Roe, D.A.: Handbook on Drug Nutrient Interactions: A Problem-Oriented Reference Guide for Dietitians. Chicago, American Dietetic Association, 1989, pp. 41–43.
8. Lamy, P.P.: Adverse drug effects. *In* Clinics in Geriatric Medicine. Edited by P.P. Lamy. Philadelphia, W.B. Saunders, 1990, pp. 293–307.
9. Brown, C.B.: Handbook of Drug Therapy Monitoring. Baltimore, Williams & Wilkins, 1990, pp. 165–166.
10. Carson, J.L., Strom, B.L., Taragin, M.I., et al.: Arch. Intern. Med., *147:*85–88, 1987.
11. Miescher, G.: Dermatologica, *108:*300–303, 1954.
12. Goldsmith, W.N., Hellier, F.F.: Recent Advances in Dermatology. 2nd. Ed. New York, Blakiston, 1954.
13. Sulzberger, M.B., Lazar, M.P.: JAMA, *146:*788–793, 1951.
14. Dowling, G.B., Gauvain, S., Macrae, D.E.: Br. Med. J., *1:*430–435, 1948.
15. Michelson, H.E.: Arch. Dermatol. Syphol., *58:*680–695, 1948.
16. Charpy, M.J.: Ann. Dermatol. Syphol. (Paris), *6:*310–346, 1946.
17. Anning, S.T., Dawson, J., Dolby, D.E., et al.: Q.J. Med., *17:*203–228, 1948.
18. Bean, W.B., Spies, T.D.: Am. Heart J., *20:*62–75, 1940.
19. Ruffin, J.M., Smith, D.T.: South. Med. J., *32:*40–47, 1939.
20. Altschul, R., Hoffer, A., Stephen, D.: Arch. Biochem. Biophys., *54:*558–559, 1955.
21. Cook, P., James, I.: N. Engl. J. Med., *305:*1560–1564, 1981.
22. Grundie, S.M., Mok, H.Y.I., Zec, L., et al.: J. Lipid Res., *22:*24–36, 1981.
23. Illingworth, D.R., Phillipson, B.E., Rapp, J.H., et al.: Lancet, *1:*296–298, 1981.
24. Henkin, Y., Johnson, K.C., Segrest, J.P.: JAMA, *264:*241–243, 1990.
25. Frost, P.H.: Ann. Intern. Med., *114:*1065, 1991.
26. Havel, R.J., Kane, J.P.: Annu. Rev. Med., *33:*417–433, 1982.
27. Peck, G.L., Olsen, T.G., Yoder, F.W., et al.: N. Engl. J. Med., *300:*329–333, 1979.
28. Peck, G.L., Gross, E.G., Butkus, D.: *In* Retinoids: Advances in Basic Research and Therapy. Edited by C.E. Orfanos. New York, Springer, V. 1981, pp. 279–286.
29. Hong, W.K., Endicott, J., Itri, L.M., et al.: N. Engl. J. Med., *315:*1501–1505, 1986.
30. Pittsley, R.A., Yoder, F.W.: N. Engl. J. Med., *308:*1012–1014, 1983.
31. Morison, W.L.: Arch. Dermatol., *122:*133–134, 1986.
32. Warrell, R.P., Frankel, S.R., Miller, W.H., et al.: N. Engl. J. Med., *324:*1385–1393, 1991.
33. Gordon, M.L., Lebwohl, M.G., Phelps, R.G., et al.: Arch. Dermatol., *127:*217–220, 1991.
34. Anstie, F.E. On the Uses of Wines in Health and Disease. London. Macmillan, 1977.
35. Hutchison, R.: Food and the Principles of Dietetics. New York, W. Wood. Co., 1905, pp. 335, 464–466.
36. Atwater, W.O., Woods, C.D., Benedict, F.G.: Bull. 44, Office of Experiment Stations, Washington, D.C., USDA, 1903.
37. Atwater, W., Benedict, F.B.: Bull. 69, 109, Washington, D.C., USDA, 1900.
38. Billings, J.S. (Ed.): The Nutritive Value of Alcohol. *In* Psychological Aspects of the Alcohol Problem. Vol. 2, Boston, Houghton-Mifflin, 1903, pp. 174–343.
39. Becker, C.E., Roe, R.L., Scott, R.A.: Alcohol as a Drug: A Curriculum on Pharmacology, Neurology and Toxicity. Baltimore, Williams & Wilkins, 1974.
40. Roe, D.A.: Alcohol and the Diet. Westport, CT., AVI Publishing, 1979.
41. Belko, A., Rotter, M., Roe, D.A.: J. Am. Coll. Nutr., *1:*413, 1982.
42. Jones, D.Y., Miller, K.W., Koonsvitsky, B.P., et al.: Am. J. Clin. Nutr., *53:*1281–1287, 1991.
43. Gibaldi, M.: Biopharmaceutics and Clinical Pharmacokinetics, 2nd Ed. Philadelphia, Lea & Febiger, 1977, pp. 15–41.
44. Welling, P.G.: J. Pharmacokinet. Biopharm., *5:*291–331, 1977.
45. Borowitz, J.L., Moore, P.F., Yim, G.K.W., et al.: Toxicol. Appl. Pharmacol., *19:*164–168, 1971.
46. Welling, P.G., Barbhaiya, R.H.: J. Pharm. Sci., *71:*32–35, 1982.
47. Jusko, W.J., Levy, G.: J. Pharm. Sci., *56:*56–58, 1967.
48. Roe, D.A.: *In* Nutrition and Drugs. Edited M. Winick. New York, John Wiley & Sons, 1983, pp. 129–138.
49. Neovonen, P., Gothoni, G., Hackman, R.: Br. Med. J., *4:*532–534, 1970.
50. Bauer, L.A.: Neurology, *32:*570–572, 1982.
51. Melander, A., Danielson, K., Schersten, B., et al.: Clin. Pharmacol. Ther., *22:*108–122, 1977.
52. Goldin, B.R., Goldman, P. Fed. Proc., *32:*798, 1973, (Abstract)

53. Sved, A.F., Goldberg, I.M., Fernstrom, J.D.: J. Pharm. Exp. Ther., *214:*147–151, 1980.

54. Karim, A., Burns, T., Wearley, L., et al.: Clin. Pharmacol. Ther., *38:*77–83, 1985.

55. Lovastatin Study Group III: JAMA, *260:*359–366, 1988.

56. Anderson, K.E., Conney, A.H., Kappas, A.: Clin. Pharmacol. Ther., *26:*493–501, 1979.

57. Kato, R., Oshima, T., Tomizawa, S.: J. Pharmacol., *18:*356–366, 1968.

58. Conney, A.H., Pantuck, E.J., Pantuck, C.B., et al.: *In* Proceedings First World Conference Clinical Pharmacology and Therapeutics. London, Aug. 3–9, 1980. Macmillan, 1980.

59. McLean, A.E.M.: *In* Nutrition in Health and Disease and International Development. Symposium 12th International Congress Nutrition. New York, Alan R. Liss, 1981, pp. 729–737.

60. Woodcock, B.G., Wood, G.C.: Biochem. Pharmacol., *20:*2703, 1971.

61. Krijgsheld, K.R., Scholtens, E., Mulder, G.J.: Biochem. Pharmacol., *30:*1973–1981, 1981.

62. Campell, T.C., Hayes, J.R.: Pharm. Rev., *26:*181–197, 1974.

63. Weatherholtz, W.M., Campbell, T.C., Webb, R.E.: J. Nutr., *98:*90–94, 1969.

64. Campbell, T.C.: *In* Nutrition and Drug Interrelations. Edited by J.N. Hathcock, J. Coon, New York, Academic Press, 1978, pp. 409–422.

65. Marshall, W.J., McLean, A.E.M.: Biochem. J., *122:*569–573, 1971.

66. Nored, W.P., Wade, A.E.: Biochem. Pharmacol., *21:*2887–2897, 1972.

67. Sato, P.H., Zannoni, V.G.: J. Pharmacol. Exp. Ther., *198:*295–307, 1976.

68. Conclusions and Perspectives of the International Conference on Nutrients, Medicine and Aging. Bellagio, Italy. Drug-Nutrient Interact., *4:*251–263, 1985.

69. Berlinger, W.A., Park, G.D., Spector, R.: N. Engl. J. Med., *313:*771–776, 1985.

70. Elion, G.B., Kovensky, A., Hitchings, G.H., et al.: Biochem. Pharmacol., *15:*863–880, 1966.

71. Hande, K.R., Noone, R.M., Stone, W.J.: Am. J. Med., *76:*47–56, 1984.

72. Hande, K., Reed, E., Chabner, B.: Clin. Pharmacol. Ther., *23:*598–605, 1978.

73. Reidenberg, M.M.: N. Engl. J. Med., *313:*816–818, 1985.

74. Melander, A., McLean, A.E.M.: Clin. Pharmacokinet., *8:*286–296, 1983.

75. Marley, T., Fagan, T.C., Wiley, K., et al.: Clin. Pharmacol. Ther., *30:*790–795, 1981.

76. Prins, R.A.: *In* Nutrition and Drug Interactions. Edited by J.N. Hathcock, J. Coon. New York, Academic Press, 1978.

77. Schwartz, S.N., Pazin, G.J., Lion, J.A., et al.: J. Infect. Dis., *138:*499–505, 1978.

78. Sarubbi, F.A., Jr., Hull, J.H.: Ann. Intern. Med., *89:*612–618, 1978.

79. Blouin, R.A., Mann, H.J., Griffen, W.O., et al.: Clin. Pharmacol. Ther., *26:*508–512, 1979.

80. Sullivan, A.C., Cheng, L.: *In* Nutrition and Drug Interrelations. Edited by J.N. Hathcock. J. Coon. New York, Academic Press, 1978, pp. 21–65.

81. Sullivan, A.C., Triscari, J., Cheng, L.: *In* Nutrition and Drugs. Edited by M. Winick. New York, John Wiley & Sons, 1983, pp. 139–167.

82. Pawan, G.L.S.: Proc. Nutr. Soc., *33:*239–244, 1974.

83. Pratt, W.B., Ruddon, R.W.: The Anticancer Drugs. New York, Oxford University Press, 1979.

84. Lindsey, D.G., Sherlock, J.C.: *In* Adverse Effects of Foods. F.P. Jelliffe, D.B. Jelliffe. New York, Plenum Press, 1982, p. 95.

85. Pawan, G.L.S.: Proc. Nutr. Soc., *33:*239–244, 1974.

86. McClain, C.J., Baker, H., Onstad, G.R.: JAMA, *247:*3116–3117, 1982.

87. Gabuzda, G.J., Gocke, T.M., Jackson, G.G., et al.: Arch. Intern. Med., *101:*476–513, 1958.

88. Mezey, E.: Gastroenterology, *74:*770–783, 1978.

89. MacKenzie, J.F., Russell, R.I.: Clin. Sci., *51:*363–368, 1976.

90. Russell, R.I., Dahr, G.J., Dutta, S.K., et al.: J. Lab. Clin. Med., *93:*428–436, 1979.

91. Selhub, J., Dahr, G.J., Rosenberg, I.H.: J. Clin. Invest., *61:*221–114, 1978.

92. Halstead, C.H.: Annu. Rev. Med., *31:*79–87, 1980.

93. Brodie, M.J., Boobis, A.R., Hillvard, C.J., et al.: Clin. Pharmacol. Ther., *30:*363–367, 1981.

94. Brodie, M.J., Boobis, A.R., Hillvard, C.J., et al.: Clin. Pharmacol. Ther., *32:*525–530, 1981.

95. Streeter, A.M., Goulston, K.J., Bathur, F.A., et al.: Dig. Dis. Sci., *27:*13–16, 1982.

96. Belaiche, J., Cattan, D., Zittoun, J., et al.: Dig. Dis. Sci., *28:*667–668, 1983.

97. Sotaniemi, E.A., Hakkarainen, H.K., Puranen, J.A., et al.: Ann. Intern. Med., *77:*389, 1972.

98. Dent, C.E., Richens, A., Rowe, D.J., et al.: Br. Med. J., *1:*69–72, 1970.

99. Hunter, J., Maxwell, J.D., Stewart, D.A., et al.: Br. Med. Jr., *4:*202, 1971.

100. Roe, D.A.: Clin. Lab. Med., *1:*647–664, 1981.

101. Wickramasinghe, S.N., Saunders, J.E.: Acta Haematol. (Basel), *58:*193–206, 1977.

102. Morgan, S.L., Baggott, J.E., Vaughn, W.H., et al.: Arthrit. Rheumat., *33:*9–18, 1990.

103. Waxman, S.: *In* Folic Acid in Neurology, Psychology, and Internal Medicine. Edited by M.I. Boter, E.H. Reynolds. New York, Raven Press, 1979, p. 47.

104. Baum, C.L., Selhub, J., Rosenberg, I.H.: J. Lab. Clin. Med., *97:*778–784, 1981.

105. Weston, K.A., Perera, D.R., and Schulz, M.G.: Ann. Intern. Med., *73:*695–702, 1970.

106. Amess, J.A.L., Burman, J.F., Reese, G.M., et al.: Lancet, *2:*339–342, 1978.

107. Deacon, R., Lumb, M., Perry, J., et al.: Lancet, *2:*1023–1024, 1978.

108. Agamolis, D., Chester, M., Victor, M., et al.: Neurology, *26:*905–914, 1976.

109. Kondo, H., Osborn, M.L., Kolhouse, J.F., et al.: J. Clin. Invest., *67:*1270–1283, 1981.

110. Biehl, J.P., Vilter, R.W.: Proc. Soc. Exp. Biol. Med., *85:*389–395, 1954.

111. Bender, D.A., Russell-Jones, R.: Lancet, *2:*1125–1126, 1979.

112. O'Reilly, R.A.: Pharmacology, *7:*149, 1972.

113. Koch-Weser, J., Sellers, E.M.: N. Engl. J. Med., *285:*487–498, 1971.

114. Bang, U., Tessler, S.S., et al.: Rev. Infect. Dis., Suppl., *4:*S546–S554, 1982.

115. Bruch, K.: Lancet, *1:*535–536, 1983.

116. Legha, S.S., Wang, Y-M., MacKay, B., et al.: Ann. N.Y. Acad. Sci., *393:*411–418, 1982.

117. Roe, D.A. Alcohol and the Diet. Westport, CT., AVI Publishing Co., 1979, pp. 119–130.
118. Victor, M., Adams, R.D., Collins, G.H.: The Wernicke-Korsakoff Syndrome. A Clinical and Pathological Study of 245 Patients, 82 with Post Mortem Examination. Philadelphia, F.A. Davis, 1971.
119. Kwee, I.L., Nakada, T.: N. Engl. J. Med., *309:*599–600, 1983.
120. Krauer, B., Krauer, F.: Clin. Pharmacokinet., *2:*157–181, 1977.
121. Knight, E., Roe, D.A.: Teratology, *18:*17–22, 1978.
122. Landauer, W.: J. Exp. Zool., *120:*469, 1952.
123. NAS. Nutrition during Pregnancy, Part II: Nutrient Supplements. National Academy of Sciences, Washington, D.C., 1990, pp. 412–419.
124. Bartorelli, C., Gargano, N., Leonnetti, G., et al.: Circulation, *27:*895–903, 1963.
125. Bjork, S., Nyberg, G., Mulec, H., et al.: Br. Med. J., *293:*471–474, 1986.
126. Gronert, G.A.: JAMA, *211:*300, 1970 (Letter).
127. Mestman, J.H., Pocock, D.S., Kirchner, A.: Calif. Med., *111:*181–185, 1969.
128. Herman, E., Rado, J.P.: Arch. Neurol., *15:*4–77, 1966.
129. Dorph, S., Olgaard, A.: Nord. Med., *79:*516–518, 1968.
130. Pederson, E.B., Kornerup, H.G.: Acta Med. Scand., *200:*263–267, 1976.
131. Pederson, O.L., Mikkelsen, E.: Clin. Pharmacol. Ther., *26:*339–343, 1979.
132. Duarte, C.G., Winnaker, J.L., Becker, K.L., et al.: N. Engl. J. Med., *284:*828–830, 1971.
133. Wasnich, R.D., Benfante, R.J., Yano, K., et al.: N. Engl. J. Med., *309:*344–347, 1983.
134. Watts, N.B., Harris, S.T., Genant, H.K., et al.: N. Engl. J. Med., *323:*73–79, 1990.
135. Milne, M.D.: *In* Clinical Effects of Interaction Between Drugs. Edited by L.E. Cluff, J.C. Petrie. New York, Elsevier Publishing Inc., 1974, p. 193.
136. Stewart, V.L.: Herling, P., Dalinka, M.K.: JAMA, *250:*78–81, 1983.
137. Randall, R.E. Jr., Strauss, M.B., McNeeley, W.: Arch. Intern. Med., *107:*163–181, 1961.
138. Spencer, H., Lewin, I.: J. Chronic Dis., *16:*713–726, 1963.
139. Editorial: Ann. Intern. Med., *103:*946–947, 1985.
140. Orwoll, E.S.: Ann. Intern. Med., *97:*242–248, 1982.
141. Wacker, W.E.C., Parisi, F.: N. Engl. J. Med., *278:*658–663, 712–717, 771–776, 1968.
142. Nielson, J.: Acta Psychiatr. Scand., *40:*190–196, 1964.
143. Crooks, J., Stevenson, I.H.: Age Ageing, *10:*73–80, 1981.
144. Uragoda. C.G.: Am. Rev. Respir. Dis., *121:*157–159, 1980.
145. Pike, D.A., Leslie, R.D.G.: Br. Med. J., *2:*1521–1522, 1978.
146. Strakosch, C.R., Jefferys, D.B., Keen, H.: Lancet, *2:*394–396, 1980.
147. Barnett, A.H., Spiliopoulos, A.J., Pike, D.A.: Lancet, *2:*164–166, 1980.
148. Blomley, B.J.: Lancet, *2:*1181–1182, 1964.
149. Blackwell, B., Mabbit, L.A.: Lancet, *1:*938–940, 1965.
150. Marley, E., Blackwell, B.: Adv. Pharmacol. Chemother., *8:*185–239, 1970.
151. Kent-Smith, C., Durack, D.T.: Ann. Intern. Med., *88:*520–521, 1978.
152. Spivack, S.D.: Ann. Intern. Med., *81:*795–800, 1974.
153. Seixas, F.A.: Ann. Intern. Med., *83:*86–92, 1975.
154. Penick, S.B., Carrier, R.N., Sheldon, J.B.: Am. J. Psychiatr., *125:*1063–1066, 1969.
155. Bruck, R.W.: N. Engl. J. Med., *265:*681–686, 1961.
156. Reynolds, W.A., Lowe, S.H.: N. Engl. J. Med., *272:*630–631, 1965.
157. O'Keefe, S.J.D., Marx, V.: Lancet, *1:*1286–1287, 1977.
158. Roe, D.A.: Diet and Drug Interactions. New York, Van Nostrand Reinhold, 1988, pp. 61–176.

CHAPTER 79

Enteral Feeding

Moshe Shike

Enteral feeding is a method of provision of nutrient solutions into the gastrointestinal (GI) tract through a tube. This method is increasingly utilized for nutritional support in patients who cannot ingest or digest sufficient amounts of food. The increasing popularity of enteral feeding in various clinical states can be attributed mostly to two factors: (1) the development of simple and low-risk procedures for placement of tubes in the GI tract, particularly percutaneous endoscopic gastrostomies and jejunostomies, and (2) the availability of a wide variety of commercial enteral feeding formulas with diverse nutrient components that allow for a choice of suitable formulas for patients with limitations in GI function or for those who require special nutrition.

Advantages of enteral feeding over the alternative of parenteral feeding include preservation of the structure and function of the GI tract (absence of nutrients in the intestines is associated with atrophy of the intestinal mucosa and decreased function of the pancreatic-biliary system), more efficient nutrient utilization, fewer infectious and metabolic complications, greater ease of administration, and lower cost.

HISTORY

The history of enteral feeding has been reviewed by Randall.[1] The practice of placing nutrients into the GI tract while bypassing the mouth originated in ancient times with the Egyptians, who used nutrient enemas for preservation of general health. Greek physicians used enemas containing wine, whey, milk, and barley broth for the treatment of diarrhea and for provision of nutrients. In the nineteenth century, European physicians installed various foods and liquids in patients' rectums. These nutrient enemas included beef extracts, milk, and whiskey. Rectal feeding was widely used until the beginning of the twentieth century, when Einhorn pointed out its inadequacies.[2] Capivacceus, a Venetian physician, is considered to have been the first (in 1598) to use a hollow tube attached to an animal's bladder for feeding into the esophagus. The use of a small silver tube passed from the nose to the esophagus was reported in 1617 for feeding patients suffering from tetanus. A major development in provision of nutrition through tubes occurred at the end of the eighteenth century, when John Hunter, a famous surgeon at the time, proposed that a nasogastric tube be made from eel skin to feed a patient suffering from neurogenic dysphagia. The tube was made and used successfully for 5 weeks, after which the patient resumed his ability to swallow. The use of nasogastric tubes both for feeding and for emptying the stomach became widespread in the nineteenth century.

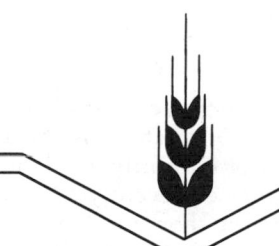

The concept of early postoperative enteral feeding was introduced by Andresen in 1918 when he started jejunal feeding in a patient following a gastrojejunostomy.[3] This practice gained increasing popularity because of the realization that, following an operation, the small bowel peristalsis is preserved although the stomach remains nonmotile for a few days. Regular foodstuffs were mixed and ground or blenderized into a fine solution, which was instilled into the stomach through a tube. As many as 2000 kcal per day were provided. In 1959, Barron reported on enteral feeding in the postoperative period in a few hundred patients who had undergone various surgical procedures.[4] He used natural juices and foods broken into fine solutions, and interestingly, he also infused GI secretions collected from drainage from biliary, pancreatic, gastric, and intestinal fistulas. The solutions were introduced through polyethylene tubes passed through the nose.

Specialized enteral feeding formulas appeared in the 1930s with the introduction of casein hydrolysate for use in both enteral and parenteral feeding. Subsequently, crystalline amino acids were used in combination with various amounts of carbohydrates, fats, minerals, and vitamins. The first commercial enteral feeding formula was Nutramigen, introduced to the market in 1942 for treatment of children with intestinal diseases and allergies. A major advance in knowledge and utilization of chemically defined formulas was achieved through studies that were sponsored by the National Aeronautics and Space Administration.[5] These studies demonstrated that normal volunteers could be maintained during a 6-month period, in a normal nutritional and physical status while being fed solely with chemically defined solutions. Based on the results of these studies, Randall and colleagues started a series of studies using commercial chemically defined diets.[1] They demonstrated the usefulness of these diets given to patients with a variety of GI diseases.

FEEDING TUBES

Enteral feeding requires administration of the nutrient solutions through a tube into the upper GI tract. (The ancient practice of feeding through the rectum has been abandoned.) At present, enteral feeding devices can be divided into two major categories—those entering the GI tract through the nose (nasogastric or nasoenteral tubes) and those entering through the abdominal wall (gastrostomies, duodenostomies, or jejunostomies). Occasionally feedings are given through a pharyngostomy or an esophagostomy.

NASOGASTRIC AND NASOENTERAL TUBES

Numerous types of nasogastric tubes are available commercially. Most are made of silicone or polyurethane. Tubes used in adults vary in length between 30 and 43 inches with diameters from 5 to 16 French. The shorter tubes are used for nasogastric feeding and the longer tubes are used for nasoduodenal or nasojejunal feeding, usually in patients who are at an increased risk from aspiration.

The tip of the tube contains tungsten or silicone to facilitate passage through the GI tract. Mercury is no longer used because of its toxicity.

The tubes come with a stylet, which facilitates insertion through the nose and into the GI tract. A historical review and a comprehensive list of currently available nasogastric tubes have been published recently.[6] Nasogastric tubes are usually utilized for short-term enteral feeding, mostly in the hospital. They are placed by health professionals, and verification of the location of the tip of the tube in the stomach or the small intestines is required. This verification can be made by obtaining a radiograph of the abdomen. (Listening for airflow over the upper abdomen can also be done; however, this procedure must be performed cautiously because flow of air can also be heard when the tip of the tube is in the esophagus).

In the past, when long-term enteral feeding in the home was required, patients were trained to place a nasogastric tube so that they could pass it prior to beginning feeding and remove it at the end of the feeding. This practice is rarely utilized now, however, because percutaneous endoscopic gastrostomies and button gastrostomies are currently used for long-term enteral feeding.

Complications related to nasogastric and nasoenteral tubes can be divided into two categories: (1) those resulting from the insertion of the tube and (2) those arising thereafter. Insertion-related complications include trauma and bleeding from the nose and upper GI tract, perforation, misplacement of the tube (mostly into the respiratory tract), respiratory compromise caused by coiling of the tube in the nasopharynx, aspiration pneumonia, and vomiting of gastric contents as a result of pharyngeal irritation. Postinsertion complications include migration of the tube (especially into the esophagus), aspiration of infused solutions, erosion of the GI tract mucosa by the tip of the tube, and ear and nose infections.

Malfunction of the nasogastric and nasoenteral tube can occur because of clogging of the tube with nutrition solutions or medications, kinking, or bursting (secondary to forceful injection of solutions). These malfunctions can be avoided with appropriate care of the tube. Complication rates of feeding tubes vary, depending on the experience of the person inserting the tube and on the care of the tube after it is inserted. The reported complication rate varies between 7.6 and 19%.[7,8]

GASTROSTOMY AND JEJUNOSTOMY TUBES

For long-term enteral feeding, gastrostomy or jejunostomy tubes are advantageous for the following reasons.

1. They have a larger diameter (16 to 24 French) and thus do not tend to clog. The wider tubes also allow for a quicker and easier administration of feeding solution and medications.
2. Because they are fixed in the stomach or upper intestines and do not migrate into the esophagus (as

may happen with nasogastric tubes), the risk of aspiration is considerably decreased.

3. They are more convenient and aesthetically acceptable to the patient.

Gastrostomy and jejunostomy tubes can be placed either surgically or endoscopically. For many years only the surgical technique was used. Although the operation is relatively minor, it requires a laparotomy, which has a complication rate of 2.5 to 16% and a mortality rate of 1 to 6%.[9-12] In recent years, the percutaneous endoscopic gastrostomy (PEG), originally described by Ponsky et al.,[13] has become increasingly popular because of the ease of the procedure, its safety, and the ability to perform the procedure on an outpatient basis. The technical aspects of the procedure have been reported widely in the last decade.[13,14] In patients with gastric resection and in those with increased risk for aspiration, jejunal tubes can be placed using a modification of the technique of endoscopic gastrostomy tube placement.[15] Such tubes can be placed endoscopically directly into a jejunal loop. This technique is difficult and requires a high level of expertise because of the small diameter of the jejunum compared to that of the stomach. A technically easier alternative is to place a wide PEG tube (28 French) through which a small-diameter (usually 8 French) jejunal tube is passed into the stomach and carried into the jejunum by forceps passed through the endoscope. This apparatus can also be used for simultaneous jejunal feeding and gastric decompression in patients with gastric outlet obstruction. The endoscopic placement of PEG and percutaneous endoscopic jejunostomy (PEJ) tubes is associated with a morbidity rate of 5 to 15% and a mortality rate of 0.3 to 1%.[13-15] The tubes function well in the long term with few complications.[14] Active patients who require long-term enteral feeding can benefit from a skin-level button gastrostomy,[16] which is less obtrusive and more convenient compared to the regular tube gastrostomy.

ENTERAL FEEDING SOLUTIONS*

More than 100 commercial solutions are available for enteral feeding. The names and types of various enteral feeding products and the companies that produce them are listed in the Appendix (Table A–37).

The composition of the different solutions varies greatly, with some intended for general nutrition and others designed for specific metabolic or clinical conditions. In addition to, or instead of, using commercial products, patients can blenderize regular foods and use them for enteral feeding. Such foods can be easily administered through PEGs and PEJs because of the relatively wide diameter of the tubes. When given through small-diameter nasogastric tubes, however, such ground foods can quickly clog the tubes. Therefore, blenderized foods should be strained prior to administration through nasogastric tubes.

Solutions used for enteral feeding have been classified according to various criteria. The names given to different classes of solutions have not always been consistent and often overlap, thus leading to lack of clarity and confusion. The general term "medical foods" has been used since 1989 by the United States Food and Drug Administration (FDA) to define enteral nutrition products as follows[17]:

Medical foods (MF) are distinguished from other foods for special dietary purposes or foods which make health claims (e.g., fiber in relation to cancer) by the requirement that they (MF) be used under medical supervision. In addition, single ingredient nutrient products that are promoted for the treatment of specific disease states will continue to be regulated under existing drug law (e.g., zinc sulfate for the treatment of acrodermatitis enteropathica), as with all injectable nutrient formulations. In general, in order to be considered a MF a product must, at a minimum, meet the following criteria:

- The product is a food for oral or tube feeding.
- The product is labeled for the dietary management of a medical disorder, disease or condition.
- The product is labeled to be used under medical supervision.

This is a general definition which includes all products for enteral feedings.

The definitions and regulatory aspects of enteral feeding products have been summarized in a recent report by Talbot,[18] which was also presented to the FDA as possible guidelines for evaluating studies designed to demonstrate the safety and suitability of enteral products for their proposed purposes.

The term "defined formula diets" was suggested as a general term to indicate that the ingredients (including nutrients processed from foods and/or relatively purified compounds, simple or complex) are prepared commercially by designated procedures so that their composition is established fairly well, although not necessarily with chemical precision.[19]

The term "elemental" has been used mostly to indicate formulas containing predigested protein. Most of the so-called "elemental solutions," however, are not elemental in the chemical sense (see the following).

Solutions for enteral feeding can be classified in different ways. The following classification is based on practical considerations according to the clinical indications for the solution.

1. Natural foods: blenderized foods that can be used for the provision of adequate nutrition by the oral route or through a tube.
2. Polymeric solutions: contain macronutrients in the form of isolates of intact protein, triglycerides, and carbohydrate polymers; can be used orally or through a tube and provide complete nutrition.

*The term solutions is used here more broadly than in its strict physiochemical meaning, and it includes homogenates, suspensions, and powders mixed with water.-

3. Monomeric solutions: contain protein as peptides and/or amino acids, fat as long-chain triglycerides (LCT) or a mixture of LCT and medium-chain triglycerides (MCT), and carbohydrates as partially hydrolyzed starch maltodextrins and glucose oligosaccharides; often used for patients with impaired digestion or absorption; it is questionable whether they are necessary or more advantageous than polymeric solutions.
4. Solutions for specific metabolic needs: intended for patients who have unique metabolic requirements, i.e., inborn errors of metabolism, renal failure.
5. Modular solutions: consist of nutritional components that can be given by themselves or can be mixed to provide solutions that meet the special needs of a given patient, i.e., increased calories, increased minerals.
6. Hydration solutions: provide minerals, water, and small amounts of carbohydrates.

NATURAL FOODS

Natural blenderized foods are available commercially or can be prepared by the patient at home. The commercial blenderized food solutions are prepared from milk, beef, fruits, vegetables, and fiber; hence their nutrient content is not determined precisely. Although they have the advantage of being "natural foods," they are prepared from a limited number of food items, and thus, their nutritional completeness is not assured. Commercial blenderized food products are usually more expensive than others. Currently the use of blenderized products is limited. The ranges of the nutrient contents are listed in Table 79–1.

Patients who use enteral feeding in the home can prepare blenderized foods from regular foods in the household. If this practice is used, the nutritional adequacy of the blenderized foods must be ensured.

POLYMERIC SOLUTIONS

The term "polymeric formulas" refers to those that contain macronutrients in the form of isolates of intact protein, triglycerides, and carbohydrate polymers. A wide variety of polymeric commercial enteral feeding solutions is available. In most of these solutions, protein constitutes 12 to 18% of total calories, carbohydrates 40 to 60%, and fats 30 to 40%. In the standard formulas, the ratio of nonprotein calories to nitrogen is about 150 kcal/1 g nitrogen. In the high-nitrogen polymeric solutions, this ratio is much lower, about 75 kcal/1 g nitrogen.

Polymeric solutions contain whole proteins isolated from casein, lactalbumin, whey, egg white, or a combination of these. The carbohydrates are usually glucose polymers in the form of starch and its hydrolysates. The fats are of vegetable origin, such as corn oil, safflower oil, sunflower oil, and others. Vitamins and essential trace elements are present in adequate quantities so that a daily intake of 1500 to 2000 kcal provides the necessary recommended daily allowance (RDA) of these nutrients. The amounts of such minerals as sodium and potassium vary considerably among the various solutions, thus allowing a choice when restriction of the intake of these minerals is necessary. Polymeric solutions are lactose free. The osmolality varies between 300 and 450 mOsm/kg in solutions that contain 1 kcal/ml. In solutions that contain more than 1 kcal/ml, however, the osmolality is higher and may reach 650 mOsm/kg. Some polymeric solutions contain fiber in the form of complex nondigestible carbohydrates. The amounts of fiber range between 6 and 14 g/1000 kcal. The caloric density is between 1 and 2 kcal/ml. The high-caloric formulas allow provision of large amounts of calories in a smaller volume and are particularly suitable for patients who require fluid restriction. Administration of these formulas requires close follow-up, however, because they can be associated with dehydration and electrolyte abnormalities. The ranges of the nutrient contents of polymeric solutions are listed in Table 79–1.

Polymeric solutions can be infused through a tube in patients with a functioning GI tract. In those with intact stomachs, the daily volume can be administered in 3 to 5 bolus feedings of 300 to 500 ml, thereby making the feeding process easier and less cumbersome than that with continuous infusion.[14] In patients fed through a jejunostomy, the daily volume of solution can be given in a pump-controlled continuous drip at a rate of 75 to 250 ml per hour.

MONOMERIC SOLUTIONS

The main feature of monomeric solutions is that they require less digestion than do regular foods or polymeric solutions. The protein in these solutions is in the form of peptides and/or free amino acids and is derived from hydrolysis of casein, whey, and other proteins. The net absorption of dipeptides and tripeptides, and the amino acids generated from their digestion, is more rapid and efficient than the absorption of equivalent amounts of free amino acids.[20] In addition, tripeptides and dipeptidase create less of an osmotic load than do the corresponding amounts of amino acids. Therefore, monomeric solutions containing partially digested protein have physiologic advantages over those containing only free amino acids.

The carbohydrates are in the form of partially hydrolyzed starch (maltidextrins and glucose oligosaccharides). The fat is frequently a mixture of MCT and LCT of plant origin. The majority of the calories are present as carbohydrates (as much as 80%), whereas only 1 to 5% are in the form of fat. Protein contributes 12 to 20% of the

TABLE 79–1. RANGES OF NUTRIENT CONTENT OF ENTERAL FEEDING PRODUCTS

NUTRIENTS	BLENDERIZED FOODS OR MILK-BASE FORMULAS: COMPLETE	POLYMERIC FORMULAS: COMPLETE	POLYMERIC FORMULAS WITH FIBER: COMPLETE	MONOMERIC FORMULAS	DISEASE-SPECIFIC FORMULATIONS
Kcal/ml	0.7–1.0	0.5–2.0	1.0–1.2	1.0–1.33	1.0–2.0
Protein					
Intact g/L	42.0–84.0	17.5–83.7	39.7–53.0	0	30.0–83.0
Hydrolyzed g/L	0	0	0	31.5–58.1	0
Amino acids g/L	0	0	0	20.6–38.2	19.4–69.7
Carbohydrate g/L	82.8–192.0	68.0–250.0	123.0–162.0	127.0–226.3	93.7–365.6
Fat g/L	20.0–42.8	17.5–106.0	35.0–46.0	1.45–52.0	7.4–96.0
MCT/LCT ratio	NA	20:80–73:27*	NA	40:60–70:30*	25:75–70:30*
Fiber g/L	4.24	NA	5.9–14.4	NA	NA
Osmolality	300–450	120–710	303–480	270–650	320–910
Volume to meet 100% RDA	—	750–2,000	1,250–1,800	1,500–2,250	947–3,000
Nonprotein calorie/ nitrogen ratio	131/1	75/1–167/1	116/1–148/1	125/1–284/1	NA
Vitamin A (I.U.)	3,332–9,000	1,250–10,000	3,300–5,000	2,500–5,000	735–6,700*
Vitamin D (I.U.)	266.8–800.0	100.0–560.0	267.0–420.0	140.0–280.0	84.5–423.0*
Vitamin E (I.U.)	24–42	15–75	21–64	15–40	10–60*
Vitamin K (μg)	66.8–80.0	38.0–320.0	48.0–160.0	22.3–160.0	35.0–160.0*
Vitamin C (mg)	60.0–120.0	56.0–317.0	120.0–254.0	33.3–200.0	30.0–317*
Thiamin (mg)	1.48–2.12	0.75–4.0	1.2–3.22	0.83–2.00	0.69–3.17*
Riboflavin (mg)	1.68–4.76	0.85–4.8	1.36–3.64	0.94–2.4	0.7–3.59*
Niacin (mg)	16.0–28.0	10.0–56.0	16.0–42.4	11.1–28.0	8.82–42.0*
Vitamin B_6 (mg)	2.0–2.8	1.0–8.0	1.6–4.24	1.11–4.0	1.07–8.61*
Folate (μg)	266.8–560.0	200.0–1,080.0	270.0–540.0	210.0–540.0	47.6–1056.0*
Pantothenic acid (mg)	6.68–14.0	5.0–28.0	8.0–21.2	5.00–14.0	2.62–21.1*
Vitamin B_{12} (μg)	4.8–12.0	3.0–16.0	4.8–12.7	2.0–8.0	2.94–12.7*
Biotin (μg)	49.2–440.0	150.0–800.0	240.0–400.0	100.0–400.0	142.5–634.0*
Sodium (mg)	760–1,320	350–1,184	500–930	460–1,000	235–1,310*
Potassium (mg)	1,400–3,640	600–2,500	1,250–1,800	782–1,661	882–1,902*
Chloride (mg)	1,132–3,600	500–2,000	1,000–1,440	819–2,501	677–1,691*
Calcium (mg)	668–2,320	250–1,400	667–910	451–800	491–1,284*
Phosphorus (mg)	868–2,000	250–1,400	667–850	499–700	491–1,056*
Magnesium (mg)	240–560	100–680	267–340	200–400	192–423*
Iron (mg)	12.0–25.2	4.5–24.0	12.0–15.0	9.0–13.3	8.82–19.0*
Iodine (μg)	100.0–212.0	37.5–200.0	100.0–127.0	74.7–101.3	73.5–158.4*
Copper (mg)	1.32–2.8	0.5–3.0	1.3–1.7	1.0–1.6	0.96–2.11*
Zinc (mg)	12.0–21.2	3.75–30.0	12.0–20.0	8.33–15.0	7.35–23.8*
Manganese (mg)	0.16–4.0	1.0–5.4	1.77–3.8	0.94–3.33	1.23–5.3*

NA, Not available
*Information available only on some of the solutions.

total calories. The caloric density of monomeric formulas varies between 1 and 1.5 kcal/ml. Because the solutions contain sufficient minerals, trace elements, and vitamins, a daily administration of 2000 kcal provides the RDA of these nutrients. Some of the micronutrients, however, may be inadequate for a patient with increased needs.

Monomeric formulas are lactose free and do not contain fiber. The partially digested macronutrients in monomeric solutions contribute to the higher osmolality in comparison to that of the polymeric solutions. The osmolality of monomeric solutions ranges between 400 and 700 mOsm/kg (See Table 79–1).

Based on physiologic considerations, these solutions might be regarded as suitable for patients with impaired digestion, such as those with pancreatic insufficiency or short bowel syndrome (in which case time for digestion and absorption is insufficient because of the shortened bowel). Clinical trials to demonstrate such an advantage, however, have not been adequate.

The high osmolality of monomeric solutions is a disadvantage because it tends to induce shift of free water into the intestinal space and thus induce rapid transit and diarrhea. Some polymeric solutions have a high osmolality; however, these are the more concentrated solutions that contain more than 1.5 kcal/ml. The osmolality of monomeric solutions is higher than that of polymeric solutions with the same caloric density.

SOLUTIONS FOR SPECIFIC METABOLIC NEEDS

These are mostly complete nutritional solutions in which specific nutrients are added or removed to meet special metabolic requirements. Specific metabolic solutions can be divided into two categories.

1. Those designed for use in patients with inherited metabolic disorders (see Chap. 67). They are low in or devoid of specific nutrients, e.g., phenylalanine or other amino acids, that cannot be properly metabolized because of enzymatic defects or deficiencies.
2. Those designed for use in patients with specific medical conditions, such as liver failure, renal failure, or critical illness with multiple organ failure. The feeding solutions in this category are designed to lessen the metabolic burden on the failing organ or to correct metabolic abnormalities that result from the organ dysfunction.

BRANCHED-CHAIN AMINO ACID (BCAA) SOLUTIONS

These solutions contain about 40 to 50% of the amino acids as leucine, isoleucine, and valine. The concentration of the aromatic amino acids (AAA) tryptophan, tyrosine, and phenylalanine is low.

Solutions high in branched-chain amino acid have been designed for use in two conditions: (1) liver failure and hepatic encephalopathy and (2) severe illness and stress with multiple organ failure, such as sepsis and major injury.

Patients with hepatic encephalopathy tend to have decreased levels of BCAA and increased levels of AAA in blood and in cerebrospinal fluid. The AAA were originally postulated to act as false neurotransmitters in the central nervous system and to contribute to hepatic encephalopathy. Thus, the provision of a nutrition solution containing high levels of BCAA and low levels of AAA was postulated to act to reverse or improve the hepatic encephalopathy induced by the AAA false neurotransmitters. Randomized studies examining the use of solutions high in BCAA in patients with hepatic encephalopathy, however, have not shown a clear benefit, and their role in these patients is controversial[21,22] (see Chap. 63).

Major acute illnesses with severe metabolic stress, such as sepsis, severe trauma, major operations, and burns, are associated with accelerated muscle catabolism. Because BCAA are used mostly by muscles, provision of solutions high in BCAA has been proposed to be beneficial for muscle preservation in severely ill and catabolic patients. Some clinical trials have shown improved nitrogen balance with enteral or parenteral solutions high in BCAA in critically ill patients[23,24]; however, other studies have not shown such benefit or any clinically relevant benefit in decreasing morbidity or mortality.[25,26] At present, no decisive information supports the routine use of solutions high in BCAA in patients who either are suffering from liver failure or are critically ill. Recommendations for adequate testing of enteral feeding solutions to demonstrate efficiency have been made to the FDA.[18]

ESSENTIAL AMINO ACID SOLUTIONS

These solutions are intended for the feeding of patients with renal failure (see Chap. 65). The failing kidneys have a decreased ability to handle protein and have a reduced capacity for clearance of various metabolites (urea, creatinine, uric acid) and minerals (potassium, phosphate, magnesium). The serum levels of some nonessential amino acids are elevated and the levels of essential amino acids, such as leucine, isoleucine, and valine, are decreased. The objectives of nutritional support in patients with renal failure are to provide optimal nutrition and to minimize the load of metabolites presented for handling by the compromised kidneys. The renal enteral feeding solutions contain essential amino acids, histidine, small amounts of fat, and electrolytes. They do not contain vitamins or trace elements, which must be supplemented as needed. The low content of electrolytes allows flexibility in their utilization because the patient with kidney failure has difficulties in handling electrolytes. The necessary amounts of electrolytes can be added on an individual basis. Randomized trials that show a clear advantage of these solutions over other enteral feeding solutions have not been conducted. Physiologically, such an advantage would be expected, but still must be demonstrated.

HIGH-FAT/LOW-CARBOHYDRATE SOLUTIONS

In these formulas, the fat content is increased to between 50 to 55% of the total calories, with a corresponding decrease in the carbohydrate content. The rationale for these solutions is based on the observation that feeding carbohydrates presents a larger respiratory burden, with increase in oxygen utilization and carbon dioxide production, in comparison to the burden from feeding fat (see Chap. 76). In most patients, the difference is not clinically significant; however, in those with borderline pulmonary function, the difference may be important, especially when excess calories are supplied.[27,28]

IMMUNE-MODULATING SOLUTIONS

Specific nutrients can have a profound effect on the immune response (see Chaps. 41 and 69). The immune-enhancing role of zinc and the immune-inhibiting effect of certain fatty acids have long been known. Recent experimental studies suggest that substances that have not been considered essential nutrients for adults, such as ω-3 polyunsaturated fat,[29] ribonucleic acid (RNA),[30] and arginine,[31] may also have beneficial effects on the immune response. These developments prompted the formulation of a new enteral feeding solution (Impact) that contains these nutrients in addition to the regular other nutrients. In a recent randomized study in surgical cancer patients, the effects of Impact were compared to those of a standard enteral feeding solution (Osmolite) when started on the first postoperative day. Feeding with Impact resulted in better immunologic and metabolic outcomes, with a decrease in infectious and wound complications and a decrease in postoperative hospitalization.[32] More clinical studies will have to be performed to confirm these results and to determine whether immune-modulating solutions can benefit nonsurgical patients as well.

MODULAR SOLUTIONS

Modular solutions provide each of the macronutrients or micronutrients in suitable combinations or singly and can be used to prepare specialized formulas or to augment regular enteral or oral feeding.

The protein modular products are usually available as powder, which is mixed with water prior to administration. Carbohydrates are available in the form of glucose polymers; fat is supplied as triglycerides of long-chain polyunsaturated or medium-chain fatty acids. These nutrients can be added when extra calories or protein are needed. They are particularly useful when the patient cannot receive the required macronutrient by increasing the amount of enteral feeding formula because of limited tolerance to fluids or to other components present in the regular feeding solution. The use of these solutions to modify commercial solutions or to prepare a special solution is limited by the difficulty they present and the lack of specific indication for their use. For instance, fat emulsions require an emulsifier to keep them dispersed in solutions after they have been mixed with other enteral solutions. Glucose polymers added to solutions can increase the osmolality and induce diarrhea once they are digested to glucose. Protein powder is hard to mix and tends to clump, thereby creating mechanical difficulties when administered.

When requirements increase for certain micronutrient solutions, those available for oral intake and parenteral use can also be used for enteral feeding; thus, in patients needing additional potassium, an oral potassium solution can be added to regular enteral feeding to increase potassium intake. Caution must be exercised, however, when adding nutrients to enteral feedings to prevent precipitation that will decrease absorption. For instance, phosphate added to enteral feedings may cause precipitation of calcium, which can clog small-diameter tubes and may not be absorbed in the intestines. Such problems can be avoided, preferably by administering additives separately from the enteral feeding solutions, unless advance testing has been adequate.

HYDRATION SOLUTIONS

Hydration solutions have been designed mostly to provide fluid and minerals to children and adults with acute diarrhea to prevent dehydration. They have been used successfully in underdeveloped countries during epidemics of infectious diarrhea. These solutions can be used for administration through tubes to patients with excessive fluid and mineral requirements, such as patients with certain types of the short bowel syndrome. (For a detailed discussion of these solutions, see Chap. 37.)

INDICATIONS

Enteral feeding is indicated in patients who cannot ingest adequate amounts of food, but have enough GI function to allow digestion and absorption of feeding solutions delivered into the GI tract through tubes. This broad functional indication covers the various clinical situations in which enteral feeding is used. Knowledge of the physiology and pathophysiology of the GI tract (Chap. 37) and choice of appropriate feeding solutions are essential to maximize the digestion and absorption of enteral feeding in the compromised GI tract. Specific indications include:

1. Severe dysphagia from obstruction or dysfunction of the oropharynx or esophagus.[14]
2. Coma or delirious state.
3. Persistent anorexia.
4. Nausea or vomiting. Patients who suffer from nausea and vomiting that arise from a gastric disorder (gastroparesis, gastritis, gastric outlet obstruction) can be safely fed enterally into the jejunum. If these symptoms are the result of intestinal obstruction, however, enteral feeding should be avoided.
5. Partial obstruction of the stomach or small bowel.
6. Fistulas of the distal small bowel or colon.
7. Severe malabsorption secondary to decreased absorption capacity of the GI tract, such as a short bowel or inflammatory disease of the bowel. In these conditions, a pump-controlled slow drip of enteral feeding solution can maximize utilization of the limited absorption capacity, which may be overwhelmed by the large volume of food and fluids delivered to the intestines in oral feeding.
8. Recurrent aspiration. In this condition, feeding solutions should be delivered through a jejunostomy. Feeding into the stomach must be avoided.
9. Diseases or disorders that require administration of specific solutions (see Chap. 67).
10. Increased nutritional requirements that cannot be met by oral intake. This indication applies mostly to burn patients who have high nutritional requirements.

The clinical efficacy of enteral feeding in specific clinical conditions is reviewed in the various chapters dealing with these conditions.

Enteral feeding is contraindicated in patients with complete intestinal obstruction, paralytic ileus, severe pseudointestinal obstruction, severe diarrhea, or extreme malabsorption. In patients with a proximal intestinal fistula, enteral feeding can be attempted only if the tip of the feeding tube is distal to the fistula. In these conditions, however, enteral feeding may still aggravate the fistula by increasing the amounts of fluids secreted into the GI tract (from stomach, pancreas, and bile). Enhanced secretion can occur even if the enteral feedings enter the GI tract distal to the duodenum.

A general indication for enteral feeding relates to maintaining the GI tract mucosa in a healthy state and preventing its atrophy, particularly in patients with trauma, postsurgical patients, or those for whom prolonged fasting is associated with a lengthy illness. Atrophy of the intestinal mucosa can occur rapidly after trauma and major illness.[33] In an experimental setting, these disorders may lead to bacterial translocation from the gut.[33] The presence of nutrients in the GI tract can serve as trophic factors both in the short bowel syndrome (Chap. 62A) and in the presence of severe trauma. Thus, oral or enteral feeding early in the course of trauma or severe illness has been suggested not only to provide nutrition, but also to maintain a healthy GI mucosa and prevent bacterial translocation and sepsis.[33] Whether such a benefit can be achieved in humans remains to be seen.

METHODS OF INFUSION

Enteral feedings can be administered either by a bolus[14] or a continuous drip.[15] When possible, the bolus method is preferable because it takes less time, gives the patient more freedom, and is easier to use. It does not require pump control. The bolus of the feeding solution can be given by an administration of as many as 500 ml over 5 to 10 minutes. The solution can be administered through a syringe with a slow push or by a gravity-driven drip from a bag.

Bolus feeding is suitable when the tip of the feeding tube is in the stomach. The bolus of the feeding solution is delivered into the stomach, and the outflow of the solution into the duodenum is regulated by the stomach and the pyloric sphincter (see Chap. 37). Thus, a bolus containing one third of the daily volume can be delivered without dumping in a patient with a normal stomach.[14] When the tip of the feeding tube is in the duodenum or the jejunum, the feeding solution must be delivered in a continuous drip (preferably pump controlled) to avoid intestinal distention and dumping. Feeding into the small bowel usually can be tolerated at a rate of as many as 150 ml/hour, although some patients can tolerate higher rates.

When bolus feeding is used, such as in patients with dysphagia who are fed with gastrostomy tubes, the daily intake of about 2000 ml can be given in 3 to 5 boluses administered every 3 to 5 hours.[14] The bolus must be administered with the patient sitting or reclining in 45° to prevent aspiration. When feeding into the stomach, iso-osmolar and hyperosmolar solutions can be used because the pylorus prevents passage of a large volume of solution into the duodenum. When feeding into the small bowel, iso-osmolar solutions usually are preferable to avoid passage of free water from the intestinal wall into the lumen.

COMPONENTS AND ABSORPTION

PROTEIN

Protein is absorbed through the intestinal mucosa in the form of dipeptides, tripeptides, or as single amino acids.[20,34] Therefore, one must establish whether provision of protein in the form of dipeptides and tripeptides offers an absorptive advantage over provision of whole proteins or free amino acids, particularly in patients with malabsorption. Based on physiologic considerations, such an advantage may be expected for the following reasons.

1. Dipeptides and tripeptides are only one half or one third as active osmotically as the same amount of amino acids in free form. Ordinarily, osmolality is not a problem; however, in the compromised intestinal tract, high osmolality may decrease tolerance to enteral feeding, particularly when solutions are infused directly into the jejunum.
2. Pancreatic proteolytic enzymes are not required for hydrolysis of small oligopeptides because this hydrolysis occurs by mucosal peptide hydrolysis. Hence, the small peptides would be absorbed in pancreatic insufficiency, whereas intact protein hydrolysis would be less efficient.
3. In patients with rapid transit through the GI tract, the time required for proteolytic enzymes to break down whole protein may be lacking. Dipeptides and tripeptides may be advantageous because their absorption can proceed at once.

In spite of these seemingly physiologic advantages of dipeptides and tripeptides, a clear clinical advantage has to be demonstrated before a claim of their superiority can be made.[18]

In perfusion studies in persons with a normal GI tract, administration into the jejunum of lactalbumin in the form of low molecular hydrolysates (dipeptides to pentapeptides) resulted in better absorption in comparison with administration of the corresponding large proteins or free amino acids.[35] Another study showed that hydrolysates prepared from ovalbumin that contained mostly dipeptides and tripeptides were absorbed better than those that contained mainly larger proteins (tetrapeptides and pentapeptides).[36] Other observations have not confirmed these results, however.[37]

The question of whether the administration of peptides or free amino acids as part of an enteral feeding solution rather than as a single nutrient offers an advantage has been addressed in numerous studies comparing the nitrogen availability from solutions containing intact protein, protein hydrolysates of various manufactures, and free amino acids. In undernourished patients with no malabsorption who were fed by a tube positioned in the proximal jejunum, nitrogen absorption was as effective from a solution with intact protein (Isocal) as from an isocaloric isonitrogenous solution containing protein hydrolysates (Criticare HN).[38] Better nitrogen retention was observed in subjects given Criticare HN than in those given a free amino acid formula (Vivonex).[39,40] Jones et al. showed that only small differences existed between a solution containing free amino acids (Vivonex) and an intact protein diet (Clinifeed 400) when infused by tube over 24 hours in a randomized fashion in 70 malnourished patients needing nutrition support after a period of inadequate intake.[41] With similar nitrogen and caloric intakes, nutritional parameters were about the same, but the intact protein formula allowed somewhat better nitrogen balance. Other studies have shown that feeding a peptide-based formula (Reabilan) resulted in levels of serum transferrin and prealbumin that were higher than those attained by feeding a solution with intact protein.[42,43]

Of more interest is the question of whether a peptide-based formula offers any advantages in patients with a compromised absorptive and digestive capacity. A randomized crossover study in patients with short bowel syndrome compared the nutritional and metabolic effects of an enteral solution containing a free amino acid mixture to a solution containing equivalent hydrolyzed whey protein. Nitrogen balance and protein turnover estimated by leucine kinetics showed no difference between the two enteral feeding solutions.[44] Another study compared enteral feeding using Reabilan HN to total parenteral nutrition (TPN) in postoperative patients. Feedings in both arms of the study started 6 hours postoperatively. The authors reported good tolerance of the enteral solutions with a positive nitrogen and caloric balance in both groups. Although the study demonstrated feasibility of enteral feeding with a peptide-based formula in the immediate postoperative period, it did not show a clear clinical benefit from such feeding nor did it have an arm with enteral feeding with an intact protein-based solution.[45] A crossover study in patients with the short bowel syndrome (less than 150 cm of residual jejunum ending in a stoma) examined the absorption from a defined-formula diet with a protein isolate, a defined-formula diet with a protein hydrolysate (15 to 20% free amino acids, 80 to 85% 2 to 6 amino acid peptides), and 3 solid diets.[46] The diets varied in fat, fiber, and carbohydrate. Although the variations in absorption among patients were marked, almost all had similar percentages of caloric and nitrogen absorption when on the two defined-formula diets; however, caloric and nitrogen absorption were generally better with the defined-formula diets than with the solid diets. The investigators concluded that a liquid diet consisting of peptides, oligosaccharides, and MCT is not more beneficial than a polymeric diet in a patient with the short bowel syndrome. The various enteral feeding solutions differ not only in their sources and amounts of amino acids, but also in their content of carbohydrates, fats, and other nutrients. This point should be remembered in the evaluation of results of comparative experiments because these variables are essentially uncontrolled. Furthermore, in most of the comparison experiments that have been reported, the amino acid composition of the free amino acid formulation was different from that of the protein hydrolysate or protein in the respective formulations.[47,48]

At present, no clear consistent clinical data support the use of solutions in which the protein is in the form of hydrolysates or free amino acids. One reason for the lack of clear superiority of these forms of protein is the great reserve and adaptive capacity of the absorptive mucosa of the small bowel (see Chap. 62A). Even when a large percentage of the small bowel mucosa is injured or resected, the remaining parts can still process adequate amounts of nutrients. Although some patients with malabsorption might benefit from a peptide enteral feeding solution, this possibility must be clearly demonstrated in clinical trials.[18] Because of the high cost of enteral solutions with free amino acids or peptides, their routine use cannot be supported at present.

The amino acid glutamine is present in only minute nonsignificant amounts in enteral feedings (except for Alitraq and Vivonex Standard Diet, which contain added glutamine). Glutamine is unstable in aqueous solutions and spontaneously breaks down to ammonia and pyroglutamic acid; thus, inclusion of glutamine in nutritional solutions poses a manufacturing hurdle. Glutamine is the most abundant free amino acid in the body (see Chaps. 1, 68, and 80). It is synthesized mostly in muscle and is used as the primary fuel in the intestines. In recent years, glutamine has become increasingly recognized as important for maintenance of healthy intestinal mucosa,[49] and may protect the mucosa from injury induced by chemotherapy, radiation, and other injurious factors.[50,51] In rats with the short bowel syndrome, the addition of glutamine (25% of total amino acids) to a defined-formula diet resulted in a trophic effect on the mucosa of the remaining small bowel with increased villous height and a greater degree of hyperplasia.[52]

In catabolic states, release of glutamine from muscle and utilization of glutamine by the GI mucosa seem to increase.[53,54] This increase may result in severe loss of muscle tissue.

During prolonged periods of catabolism, glutamine synthesis and release from muscle decrease and may not be adequate to meet the increased utilization by various tissues, especially the GI mucosa. Thus, glutamine deficiency may ensue. Glutamine consequently has been suggested as an essential nutrient for the intestinal mucosa and for other organs of patients in catabolic states and thus may need to be added to nutritional regimens given to patients with catabolic illnesses.[55] The provision of adequate glutamine in nutritional regimens results in better immune response in the GI mucosa and in maintenance of mucosal mass and of its barrier function against bacteria.[56] Such maintenance may provide protection against bacterial translocation and sepsis. Before glutamine is added in large amounts to enteral feedings, however, studies must be performed regarding its safety and efficacy. Some investigators are concerned that glutamine, being a primary nutrient in some tumors, may act as a tumor stimulator,[57] and therefore, a careful evaluation must be performed regarding any potential adverse effects of glutamine, particularly in cancer patients.

CARBOHYDRATES

The various starches put in commercial enteral feeding solutions are eventually hydrolyzed to glucose in the small intestine. Starches vary in glucose units from 400 to many thousands. Hydrolysis forms polymers with decreasing numbers of glucose units. The osmolality of a formula is influenced to a major extent by the sources and amounts of glucose, sucrose, and the shorter-chain glucose units and to a lesser extent by free amino acids and electrolyte concentrations.

The initial rapid infusion into the stomach or jejunum of large volumes of high osmolality should be avoided in patients with vagotomy (which also occurs with esophagectomy), gastrectomy, and intestinal dysfunction, because this infusion can induce rapid transit, glucose malabsorption, abdominal discomfort, and diarrhea. Hyperosmolar nonketotic coma can occur with high-carbohydrate feedings; coma is most likely to develop in the diabetic patient who is infected and dehydrated. Excess carbohydrate calories in enteral feeding can result in hypercarbia in patients with respiratory insufficiency and in a rise in metabolic rate.

In the individual with normal GI function, hydrolysis of starch and long-chain glucose polymers is rapid. In patients with marked pancreatic insufficiency, oligosaccharides may be useful because they are hydrolyzed to glucose by the intestinal brush-border enzyme α-dextrinase.

LIPIDS

The concentration of fat in enteral feeding solutions varies from less than 2% to 45% of the total calories (Table 79–1). The lipids, usually corn oil or soy oil, have a large amount of polyunsaturated fatty acids; some have lecithin added (presumably as an emulsifier). Others have MCT in small or large proportions. The rationale for adding MCT is based on the observation that they are easily hydrolyzed and absorbed in various states of malabsorption (see Chap. 3);[58,59] however, the absorption of enteral feeding solutions containing MCT has not been proved superior to that of LCT-based solutions. Because MCT are ketogenic, they should be avoided in patients with diabetes, ketosis, or acidosis.[59] The relatively large amounts of polyunsaturated fat in most formulas provide more than an adequate amount of essential fatty acids, the need for which is approximately 3 to 4.5% of the total calories (see Chap. 3). Recently, an enteral feeding solution (Impact) has been introduced in which part of the fat is in the form of fish oil. Fish oil, which has a high content of ω-3 fatty acids, has been reported to be superior to vegetable oil in its effect on the immune response.[29]

As for other nutrients, the efficiency of absorption of lipids depends on the rate of infusion, the concentration of the nutrient, and the digestive and absorptive capacities of the GI tract. (Lipid characteristics and other factors affecting digestion, absorption, and metabolism are reviewed in detail in Chap. 3). Patients with exocrine pancreatic insufficiency may absorb more than 50% of dietary fat despite the absence of measurable pancreatic lipase activity. This absorption appears to be related to roles of lingual and gastric lipases.[60] Nevertheless, administration of pancreatic extracts is useful in patients with pancreatic insufficiency. Patients with the short bowel syndrome have been reported to absorb 54% of the fat from a diet containing 46% of the calories as fat.[61] Fat did not have an adverse effect on absorption of magnesium, calcium, and zinc. This finding dispels the notion that patients with the short bowel syndrome must be on a low-fat diet and has an important implication regarding the use of enteral feeding in such patients. A high-fat enteral feeding solution administered through a continuous drip can provide a large amount of calories and thus ensure absorption of adequate calories in spite of the malabsorption. A report compared the effectiveness of 5 different levels of fat (from 10 to 50% of nonprotein calories) in enteral feeding solutions given to guinea pigs with 30% total-body-surface full-thickness burns.[62] Lipid levels between 5 and 15% of nonprotein calories were deemed optimal for nutritional support.

VITAMINS AND TRACE ELEMENTS

Enteral feeding solutions were designed to provide the RDA of vitamins and trace elements with an intake of 1500 to 2000 calories. Complete enteral nutrition solutions contain the full range of vitamins. Patients maintained on enteral feeding for periods exceeding 6 months were shown to have normal or high blood levels of the various vitamins.[63]

The stability of vitamins in commercial enteral feeding solutions has been determined only to a limited extent. Short- and long-term studies demonstrated stability of vitamins A and E and riboflavin for as long as 3 months.

Specific data regarding absorption of vitamins from enteral feeding solutions are lacking. The adequate or high levels of vitamins in the blood of patients who received long-term enteral feeding suggest that both stability and absorption are adequate and, consequently, that current enteral feeding solutions contain adequate vitamins.[63]

Most enteral feeding formulas contain sufficient amounts of trace elements, including iron, zinc, copper, and iodine, so that intake of 1500 to 2000 calories per day provides adequate amounts of these nutrients. Zinc and other micronutrient deficiencies, however, can occur when the caloric intake from enteral feeding is low, or when GI losses of zinc persistently exceed intake, as can happen in patients with active Crohn's disease.

FIBER

Enteral feeding formulas initially had been fiber free, except for those that were prepared by blenderizing natural foods. With the increasing recognition that dietary fiber offers numerous physiologic and metabolic benefits (see Chap. 4), the tendency now is toward including fibers in enteral feeding.[64]

Most Americans ingest 8 to 12 g of dietary fiber a day.[65] The recommended amounts for healthy Americans are 10 to 13 g of dietary fiber per 1000 calories.[66] Blenderized enteral feeding solutions contain 1.9 to 3.3 g of dietary fiber per 250 ml.[67] To date, the only fiber added to enteral feeding solutions has been soy polysaccharide (except for one product that also contains oat fiber). Soy polysaccharide is a tasteless and odorless material and physically can be added easily to enteral feeding solutions. Only about 6% of soy polysaccharide is water soluble. It can improve lipid metabolism and diabetic control in hyperlipidemic patients.[68] The amounts of soy polysaccharide added to enteral feeding solutions vary between 2.5 and 5.9 g per 250 ml.[67]

Various dietary fibers have divergent physiologic effects (see Chap. 4). Thus, fiber derived from oats may have a cholesterol-lowering effect when added to enteral feeding solutions, whereas most insoluble fibers, such as cellulose and hemicellulose, would serve mostly as laxatives. The main reason for adding fiber to enteral feeding solutions is to facilitate bowel movements. If a formula without fiber is used, however, fiber can be administered separately in other forms, such as natural bran and Metamucil.

In addition to its direct effect on bowel function, fiber may have important trophic effects on the mucosa of the large bowel, because short-chain fatty acids derived from fiber metabolism by colonic bacteria constitute the primary fuel source of the colonic mucosa (see Chaps. 4 and 39).

In a study of healthy young male subjects, the effects of adding 0, 30, or 60 g per day of soy fiber to a feeding solution (Ensure) were determined and compared. The results showed that dietary fiber increased daily fecal weights and frequency of bowel movements. All dosages of fiber resulted in decreased transit time in the GI tract.[69]

The effects on bowel function of a fiber-containing enteral feeding solution (Enrich, 12.8 g fiber/1000 kcal) were compared in a crossover randomized study to the effects of a solution without fiber (Ensure).[70] Mean daily fecal weight and frequency of bowel movements were similar during administration of the two solutions; however, patients who were fed Ensure required more laxatives and had more diarrhea. Constipation was similar in both groups. The authors reported that the fiber-containing solution was associated with improved GI function. Because the patients fed Ensure received more laxatives, it cannot be ruled out that their worsened GI function (i.e., more diarrhea) was caused by the laxative use. Most of the patients in this study were comatose, and therefore, the results are of limited clinical application in other groups of patients.

Some authors have expressed concern that fiber in enteral feeding solutions would result in a decrease in absorption of minerals and vitamins.[71] The addition of 120 g per day of soy polysaccharides to an elemental solution did reduce the overall absorption rate of magnesium, zinc and phosphorus, but did not affect potassium and calcium absorption. The balance for all 5 minerals was still positive, however.[72] In another study, the effect of adding 20, 30, and 40 gs of soy polysaccharides was studied. The 40 gs of fiber caused a negative balance for copper and iron, whereas zinc, calcium, and magnesium were in a positive balance.[73]

The administration of enteral feeding solutions that contain soy polysaccharide apparently does not result in malabsorption and deficiency of major minerals and vitamins in the short term. The effects, however, in patients receiving long-term enteral feeding with fiber as the primary or sole diet are unclear. Appropriate monitoring for these nutrients is recommended.

COMPLICATIONS

Enteral feeding can be a safe and effective nutritional support method. Its safety depends on (1) the choice of the appropriate formula and infusion method, (2) the delivery of the formulas into the appropriate part of the GI tract, and (3) the clinical and metabolic evaluation of the patient prior to and during enteral feeding.

The most severe potential complication of enteral feeding is aspiration. This complication is most likely to occur when patients suffer from impaired gastric emptying, when the tip of the tube is misplaced in the upper stomach or in the esophagus, or when the patient receives the feeding in a supine position. This potential complication can be avoided by appropriate positioning of the feeding tube, elevating the upper body to 30 to 45°, and avoiding enteral feeding when contraindicated. In the presence of impaired gastric emptying or in the absence of gag reflex, the feeding solution is best delivered into the jejunum. The incidence of aspiration depends on how vigorously it is looked for and on the type of patient. Severe aspiration was reported in 1% of patients receiving an average of 10 days of enteral feeding.[74] In a prospective study, the incidence of aspiration was 2.4 per 1000 enteral feeding days. Little morbidity and no mortality resulted from aspiration.[75]

Bacterial contamination of enteral feeding formulas can occur easily because the solutions are an ideal growth medium for bacteria. Such contamination apparently does not cause clinical problems, although occasional case reports of sepsis associated with feeding of contaminated enteral feeding solutions have surfaced.

Nausea and vomiting have been reported to occur in as many as 20% of patients.[41] Nonspecific symptoms of abdominal cramps, distention, and bloating can occur and are usually caused by too rapid an infusion or by an underlying intestinal disorder.

Diarrhea has been reported in 5 to 30% of patients receiving enteral feeding.[76] Defining and determining diarrhea in patients receiving enteral feeding presents a great difficulty, however, and the method of reporting may significantly alter the reported incidence of this complication.[77] Tolerance to enteral feeding depends on several factors, including the functional capacity of the GI tract, the rate of infusion, the type of formula, and concomitant medications. The healthy GI tract can easily handle bolus feedings of as many as 500 ml given over 10 to 15 minutes. This feeding method has been used successfully in patients with dysphagia secondary to cancer of the head and neck.[14]

Patients with GI diseases may require a slow rate of infusion. Those with a short bowel or with small bowel mucosal disease, such as radiation enteritis or Crohn's disease, may require a pump-controlled continuous feeding over 10 to 15 hours with a rate not exceeding 100 ml per hour. Iso-osmolar solutions are better tolerated in patients prone to diarrhea because hyperosmolar solutions tend to draw fluids into the upper intestines, thereby increasing the load that must be absorbed distally. When using solutions with an osmolality of approximately 300 m0sm/kg, the solutions do not require dilution as a means of enhancing tolerance and decreasing diarrhea.

One of the most important factors in causing diarrhea during enteral feeding is concomitant use of medications, particularly antibiotics and magnesium-containing antacids. In some reports, as many as half of the patients on enteral feeding and receiving antibiotics developed diarrhea; these two factors seem to work synergistically to induce diarrhea.[78]

Constipation occurs in as many as 15% of patients receiving long-term enteral feedings. As mentioned earlier, no clear evidence from clinical trials shows that fiber-containing enteral feeding solutions alleviate this problem.

Metabolic abnormalities can occur in patients receiving enteral feeding. Their frequency and severity depend mostly on the general medical condition of the patient. Thus, patients with renal failure are at risk for developing increased azotemia, hyperkalemia, hypermagnesemia, and hyperphosphatemia, whereas the diabetic patient is at risk for hyperglycemia. These potential complications are not inherent to enteral feeding and can be avoided by careful attention to the medical condition of the patient.

Dehydration is a potential complication in patients given high-osmolality enteral feeding solutions, such as those used in the past. Current solutions with osmolality in the range of 300 to 700 m0sm/kg do not pose this risk.

REFERENCES

1. Randall, H.T.: JPEN J. Parenter. Enteral Nutr., *8:*113–136, 1984.
2. Einhorn, M.: Med. Rec., *78:*92–95, 1910.
3. Andresen, A.F.R.: Ann. Surg., *67:*565–566, 1918.
4. Barron, J.: Surg. Clin. North Am., *39:*1481–1491, 1959.
5. Winitz, M., Seedman, D.A., Graff, J.: Am. J. Clin. Nutr., *23:*525–545, 1970.
6. Fagerman, K.E.: Nutr. Supp. Services, *7:*10–14, 1987.
7. Benya, R., Langer, S., Mobrahan, S.: JPEN J. Parenter. Enteral Nutr., *14:*108–109, 1990.
8. Ghahremani, G.G.: Dig. Dis. Sci., *31:*574–578, 1981.
9. Shellito, M.: Ann. Surg., *201:*763–767, 1985.
10. Gallagher, M.W., Tyson, K.R.T., Ashcraft, K.W.: Surgery, *74:*536–539, 1973.
11. Holder, T.M., Leape, L.L., Ashcraft, K.W.: N. Engl. J. Med., *286:*1345–1347, 1972.
12. Campbell, J.R., Sasaki, T.M.: Am. Surg., *40:*505–508, 1974.
13. Ponsky, J.L., Gauderer, M.W.L., Stellato, T.A.: Arch. Surg., *118:*913–914, 1983.
14. Shike, M., Berner, Y.N., Gerdes, H.: Otolaryngol. Head Neck Surg., *101:*549–554, 1989.
15. Shike, M., Wallach, C., Likier, H.: Gastrointest. Endosc., *37:*62–65, 1991.
16. Shike, M., Wallach, C., Herman-Zaidins, M.: JPEN J. Parenter. Enteral Nutr., *13:*648–650, 1989.
17. U.S. Food and Drug Administration. Compliance Program Guidance Manual. Chap. 21. Program No. 7321.002. Washington, D.C., 1989–1991.
18. Talbot, J.M.: Guidelines for the Scientific Review of Enteral Food Products for Medicinal Purposes. Bethesda, MD, Life Sciences Research Office, Federation of American Societies for Experimental Biology, 1990.
19. Shils, M.E. (Ed.): Introduction to Proceedings of Conference: Defined-Formula Diets for Medical Purposes. Chicago, American Medical Association, 1977.
20. Grimble, G.K., Silk, D.B.A.: Nutr. Clin. Practice, *5:*227–230, 1990.
21. Eciksson, L.S., Conn, H.O.: Hepatology, *10:*228–246, 1989.

22. Naylor, C.D., O'Rourke, K., Detsky, A.S., et al.: Gastroenterology, *97:*1033–1042, 1990.
23. Cerra, F.B., Mazuki, J., Teasley, K., et al.: Crit. Care Med., *11:*775–778, 1983.
24. Cerra, F.B., Shronts, E.P., Raup, S., et al.: Crit. Care Med., *17:*619–622, 1989.
25. Yu, Y.M., Wagner, D.A., Walesrewski, J.C., et al.: Ann. Surg., *207:*421–429, 1988.
26. Von Meyenfeldt, M.F., Socters, P.B., Vente, J.P., et al.: Br. J. Surg., *77:*924–929, 1990.
27. Goldstein, S.A., Thomashow, B.M., Kvetan, V., et al.: Am. Rev. Respir. Dis., *138:*636, 1988.
28. Brandstetter, R.D., Zakky, Y., Gutherz, P., et al.: Heart Lung, *17:*170, 1988.
29. Alexander, J.W., Saito, H., Ogle, C.K., et al.: Ann. Surg., *204:*1–8, 1986.
30. Kulkarnic, A.D., Fanslow, W.C., Drath, D.B., et al.: Arch. Surg., *121:*169–172, 1986.
31. Kirk, S.J., Barbul, A.: J. Parenter. Enteral Nutr., *14:*226S–229S, 1990.
32. Daly, J.M., Lieberman, M.D., Goldfine, J., et al., Surgery, *112:*56–67, 1992.
33. Alexander, J.W.: JPEN J. Parenter. Enteral Nutr., *14:*170S–174S, 1990.
34. Adibi, S.A., Fogel, M.P., Agrawal, R.M.: Gastroenterology, *67:*586–591, 1974.
35. Grimble, G.K., Keohane, P.P., Higgins, B.E., et al.: Clin. Sci., *71:*65–69, 1986.
36. Grimble, G.K., Silk, D.B.A.: Nutr. Res. Rev., *2:*87–108, 1989.
37. Moriarty, K.J., Hegarty, J.E., Fairclough, P.D., et al.: Gastroenterology, *26:*694–699, 1985.
38. Heymsfield, S.B., Bloir, J., Whitmir, L., et al.: Am. J. Clin. Nutr., *39:*234–250, 1984.
39. Smith, J.L., Arteago, C., Heymsfield, S.B.: N. Engl. J. Med., *306:*1013–1018, 1982.
40. Beer, W.H., Halsted, C.H.: Am. J. Clin. Nutr., (Abstr.) *39:*689, 1984.
41. Jones, B.J.M., Lees, R., Andrews, J., et al.: Gut, *24:*78–84, 1983.
42. Meridith, J.W., Ditesheim, J.A., Zeluga, G.P.: J. Trauma, *30:*825–829, 1990.
43. Heimburger, D.C.: Nutr. Clin. Practice, *5:*225–226, 1990.
44. Rees, R.G., Grimble, G.K., Halliday, D.: Gut, *28:*A1397, 1988.
45. Hamaoui, E., Lefkowitz, R., Olender, L., et al.: JPEN J. Parenter. Enteral Nutr., *14:*501–507, 1990.
46. McIntyre, P.B., Fitchew, M., Lennard-Jones, J.E.: Gastroenterology, *91:*25–33, 1986.
47. Trocki, O., Mochizuki, H., Dominion, L.: JPEN J. Parenter. Enteral Nutr., *10:*139–145, 1986.
48. Moriarty, K.J., Hegarty, J.E., Fairclough, P.D., et al.: Gut, *6:*694–696, 1985.
49. Souba, W.W., Herskowitz, K., Salloum, R.M.: JPEN J. Parenter. Enteral Nutr., *14:*45S–50S, 1990.
50. Klimberg, V.S., Sauba, W.W., Dolson, D.J., et al.: Cancer, *66:*62–68, 1990.
51. Fox, A.D., Kriple, S.A., Depauler, J.A., et al.: JPEN J. Parenter. Enteral Nutr., *12:*324–331, 1988.
52. Smith, R.J., O'Dwyer, T., Wang, X.O.: Report of the 8th Conference on Medical Research. Columbus, OH, Ross Laboratories, 1988.
53. Souba, W.W., Smith, R.J., Wilmore, D.W.: JPEN J. Parenter. Enteral Nutr., *9:*608–617, 1985.
54. Stehle, P., Zonder, J., Merters, N.: Lancet, *1:*231–235, 1989.
55. Smith, F.R.: JPEN J. Parenter. Enteral Nutr., *14:*40S–44S, 1990.
56. Alverdy, J.C.: JPEN J. Parenter. Enteral Nutr., *14:*109S–113S, 1990.
57. Fischer, J., Chance, W.T.: JPEN J. Parenter. Enteral Nutr., *14:*86S–89S,
58. Jandacek, R.J., Whiteside, J.A., Holcombs, B.N., et al.: Am. J. Clin. Nutr., *45:*940–945, 1987.
59. Bach, A.C., Babeyan, V.K.: Am. J. Clin. Nutr., *36:*950–962, 1982.
60. Abrams, C.K., Hamosh, M., Dutta, S.K., et al.: Gastroenterology, *92:*125–129, 1987.
61. Woolf, G.M., Miller, C., Kurian, R., et al.: Dig. Dis. Sci., *32:*8–15, 1987.
62. Mochizuki, H., Trocki, O., Dominioni, L., et al.: JPEN J. Parenter. Enteral Nutr., *8:*638–646, 1984.
63. Berner, Y.N., Morse, R., Frank, O., et al.: JPEN J. Parenter. Enteral Nutr., *13:*525–528, 1989.
64. Slavin, J.: Nutr. Clin. Practice, *5:*247–249, 1990.
65. Lanza, E., Jones, Y., Block, G., et al.: Am. J. Clin. Nutr., *46:*790–797, 1987.
66. Pilch, S.M. (Ed.): Physiological Effects and Healthy Consequences of Dietary Fiber. Washington, D.C., U.S. Food & Drug Administration, Federation of American Societies of Experimental Biology, 1987.
67. Fredstron, S.B., Baglien, K.S., Lampe, J.W., et al.: JPEN J. Parenter. Enteral Nutr., *15:*450–453, 1991.
68. Lo, G.S., Goldberg, A.P., Lim, A., et al.: Atherosclerosis, *622:*239–244, 1986.
69. Slavin, J.L., Nelson, N.L., McNamara, E.A., et al.: JPEN J. Parenter. Enteral Nutr., *9:*317–321, 1985.
70. Shankardass, K., Chuchmach, S., Chelswick, K., ét al.: JPEN J. Parenter. Enteral Nutr., *14:*508–512, 1990.
71. Scheppach, W., Burghardt, W., Bartram, P., et al.: JPEN J. Parenter. Enteral Nutr., *14:*204–209, 1990.
72. Heymsfield, S.B., Roongspisuthipong, C., Evert, M., et al.: JPEN J. Parenter. Enteral Nutr., *12:*265–273, 1988.
73. Taper, L.J., Milam, R.S., McCallister, M.S., et al.: Am. J. Clin. Nutr., *48:*305–311, 1988.
74. Kohane, P.P., Attecill, H., Silk, D.B.A.: J. Clin. Nutr. Gastroenterol., *1:*189–193, 1986.
75. Mullen, H., Roubenoff, R.A., Roubenoff, R.J.: JPEN J. Parenter. Enteral Nutr., *16:*160–164, 1992.
76. Keohane, P.P., Attcill, H., Love, M.: Br. Med. J., *288:*678–681, 1984.
77. Bliss, D.Z., Guenter, P.A., Settle, R.G.: Am. J. Clin. Nutr., *55:*753–759, 1992.
78. Silk, D.B.A.: Clin. Nutr., *6:*61–74, 1987.

CHAPTER 80

Parenteral Nutrition

Maurice E. Shils

HISTORY

The long and interesting efforts to introduce fluid, salt, and food intravenously that began with Sir Christopher Wren in 1658 have been summarized.[1–3] The scientific groundwork resulting in successful parenteral nutrition was laid in the third to fifth decades of this century. Such developments included (1) the ability to provide pyrogen-free fluids as a result of Seibert's work,[4] (2) elucidation by many investigators of the chemical nature of essential nutrients and their eventual availability in safe intravenous forms, (3) increased understanding of fluid electrolyte needs and acid-base balance aided by advances in analytic instrumentation, and (4) recognition of the metabolic and nutritional changes associated with disease.[5,6]

World War II stimulated further research into the metabolic changes induced by trauma and infection, led to wider recognition of the importance of nutrition in these and other clinical states,[1,7] and furthered the use of parenteral nutrition in the seriously ill.[8,9]

Peripheral (and occasionally central) parenteral feedings utilizing 5 or 10% glucose, protein hydrolysates, intravenous fat (Lipomul), electrolytes, and multivitamins were utilized from 1955 to 1965 by various clinicians for limited periods.[3] Serious side effects led to withdrawal of intravenous Lipomul from the United States market in the early 1960s. This created a serious problem requiring that glucose be given either in large, relatively isotonic volumes for peripheral vein infusion or else in hyperosmolar form requiring infusion into a major vein. Although central catheters threaded into veins had been used as early as 1944,[3] these were uncommon. A safe and effective intravenous lipid preparation (Intralipid) had been developed by Wretlind, tested by 1961 in Sweden,[10] and approved for use in most European countries by 1963; it was not approved for use in Canada or in the United States until 1977. Intralipid availability in Europe in the early 1960s led to the increased use of parenteral nutrition through peripheral veins.

Widespread interest and utilization of parenteral nutrition occurred after publication of reports by Dudrick, Wilmore, Vars, and Rhoads.[11] Utilizing percutaneous central catheters as the route for nutrient solutions, with glucose as the source of nonprotein calories, these investigators demonstrated convincingly in malnourished infants and adults that parenteral nutrition as the sole source of nutrients resulted in good growth in infants and positive nitrogen balance and nutritional and clinical improvement in adults over periods of many weeks.

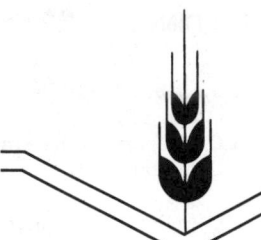

The development of parenteral nutrition has been marked by the replacement of hydrolyzed casein or blood fibrin by free amino acid mixtures and by the advent of safe lipid formulations and the availability of improved formulations of parenteral vitamins and trace elements.[3,10,12,13] Sophisticated pumps with programmed metering controls have increased safety and have simplified the care of these patients.

All parenteral solutions and emulsions are classified as drugs and must meet the standards of the United States Food and Drug Administration (FDA) for sterility, safety, and efficacy. Accordingly, these agents are appreciably more expensive than enteral products, with consequent limitations on development of new items or modifications of older ones. Nutrients of poor solubility or stability in aqueous solutions still present problems in formulations.

The major physiologic difference between parenteral and enteral products is the direct entry of parenteral solutions into the systemic circulation, bypassing the alimentary tract or the first circulatory pass through the liver. Related problems are those of venous access, sterile technique in administration, nutritional adequacy, and the problems related to the presence of an indwelling catheter in the vascular system.

NOMENCLATURE

The issue of ensuring adequate nutrition is presented forcibly to the physician confronted by the patient who cannot eat or be tube fed or who, for various reasons, cannot digest or absorb sufficient amounts of oral or tube fed nutrients. The solution to each of these problems is the use of what has been described as parenteral feeding.

The objective is to provide nutrients in amounts that meet the needs of the individual patient, needs that may be high in the hypercatabolic patient or relatively low in the obese patient on a weight-reduction diet. The term "hyperalimentation" entered into the clinical nutrition lexicon in various ways to indicate the need for large amounts of calories and certain other nutrients. Co Tui et al. used the term in 1944 and 1945 in describing "hyperalimentation" with large amounts of casein hydrolysate and carbohydrates given postoperatively by tube to patients who had undergone gastrectomy[14] and orally or by tube to patients with peptic ulcer.[15] In 1965, the term was used by others to describe supplementary intravenous (IV) lipid feeding given to cancer patients.[16] The term was reintroduced by the University of Pennsylvania group,[11] and it was widely used to designate the procedure later known as total parenteral nutrition (TPN). It became widely used in the context of high-calorie formulation and was often shortened to "hyperal." It was applied also to tube feeding, and so "IV hyperalimentation" and "enteral hyperalimentation" have appeared in the literature.

From both historical and etymologic aspects, the term has implied the need for and provision of relatively large amounts of energy and protein. With more information, it has become apparent that used in this way, the term "hyperalimentation" has a misleading connotation. As noted later in this chapter, the excess provision of energy and of certain nutrients is often undesirable. In my view, the term "IV hyperalimentation" should be abandoned in favor of a more precise term such as parenteral nutrition with the qualifiers of total or supplementary, central or peripheral to designate amount and route.

INDICATIONS

The primary objective of parenteral nutrition is the maintenance or improvement of the nutritional and metabolic status of patients who, for a critical period of time, cannot be adequately nourished by oral or tube feeding (Table 80–1). The value and use of this treatment method in the management of patients are discussed in this book in chapters concerned with obstetric problems (see Chap. 44[17]), short bowel syndromes (see Chap. 62A), other types of bowel dysfunction (see Chap. 62B and C), pediatric problems (see Chap. 66), cancer (see Chap. 73), neurologic injuries,[18–20] and in surgical problems (see Chap. 68). The use of parenteral nutrition in the perioperative period in patients undergoing surgery has been evaluated and is discussed further in Chapter 68 and in many publications.[21–23]

For those individuals who are well nourished or minimally malnourished before undergoing elective surgery and who are likely to be eating again in 5 to 7 days, postoperative nutritional support is usually considered sufficient as hypocaloric glucose, electrolytes, and micronutrients. Preexisting serious undernutrition, however,

TABLE 80–1. CLINICAL STATES OF PATIENTS LIKELY TO BENEFIT FROM PARENTERAL NUTRITION

Severe malabsorption with electrolyte and fluid abnormalities not adequately responsive to oral and/or tube feeding
Massive bowel resection (see Chap. 62A)
Severe chronic radiation enteritis with obstructive symptoms (see Chap. 62C)
Severe inflammatory bowel disease (see Chap. 62B)
Small bowel fistula that cannot be bypassed by tube feedings
Immune diseases with intestinal villous atrophy
Prolonged postoperative ileus
Inability to ingest food
Persistent vomiting (e.g., secondary to obstruction, increased intracranial pressure, or medications)
Intestinal motility disorders (e.g., severe pseudointestinal obstruction)
Support for the underweight premature infant (see Chaps. 46 and 66)
Persistent hypermetabolic states where enteral feeding is contraindicated or inadequate (e.g., severe burns with trauma or sepsis; see Chap. 68)

increases the likelihood of postoperative complications, especially with major surgery (see Chaps. 50, 57, and 68).[21–23]

The decision to undertake parenteral nutrition requires the weighing of several factors and due consideration for the patient's diagnosis and prognosis as discussed in appropriate chapters. In general, parenteral nutrition is indicated to improve serious undernutrition or to avoid the risk of serious undernutrition when more routine parenteral support (fluids, glucose, and minerals) is deemed inadequate, and oral and/or tube feeding is contraindicated. It is not a defensible substitute for oral or tube feeding when either of these methods is feasible. Issues related to its use in the hopelessly ill are reviewed in Chapters 73 and 81.

VENOUS ACCESS: PERIPHERAL AND CENTRAL

Infusion of the nutrient solution directly into a small peripheral vein has an advantage over central vein infusion by avoiding the insertion and maintenance of a central catheter. Peripheral parenteral nutrition (PPN) reduces peripheral vein damage by the use of isotonic lipid emulsions with their large caloric content together with 5 or 10% glucose, 5% or less amino acids, electrolytes, and micronutrients.[24,25] It is feasible, for example, to provide 2500 kcal in 3 L of relatively isotonic solutions with 75% of the energy as lipid. PPN may be useful (although the restricted carbohydrate may on occasion present some problems) for the patient who needs parenteral nutrition and who has a goodly supply of patent peripheral vessels. Many patients requiring IV nutrition, however, have had numerous prior peripheral infusions and venesections with consequent vessel sclerosis. The critically ill patients whose condition is unstable must have reliable venous access at all times; a central catheter in such a patient is a necessity.

To provide adequate energy without providing a large percentage as lipid, central parenteral nutrition requires the infusion of hypertonic glucose solutions. Consequently, the catheter tip should be in a vessel with high blood flow causing rapid dilution; this minimizes the occurrence of phlebitis and thrombosis. Numerous routes for such vascular access have been used (Table 80–2). Popularized by Dudrick et al., the percutaneous subclavian vein approach in adults and the jugular vein approach in infants were widely adopted.[10,11,26] Percutaneous peripheral vein placement of a long catheter threaded into the superior vena cava has also been used. Arteriovenous fistulas of the internal type have been prepared, usually with a bovine graft, and external fistulas have been used; some of the early patients discharged home on TPN had one or another of these fistulas. Other vascular approaches have been adopted in situations where the usual vessels have not been patent or otherwise available.

TABLE 80–2. VASCULAR ACCESS ROUTES FOR PARENTERAL NUTRITION

ROUTE	REFERENCE
Peripheral vein: percutaneous approach	25
Jugular vein (internal or external): percutaneous approach	26
Jugular vein (internal or external): surgical approach*	27
Subclavian vein or tributary: percutaneous approach	26
Subclavian vein or tributary: surgical approach*,†	28
Portal vein	29
Arteriovenous fistulas	
Internal	30, 31
External	32
Femoral or iliac vein	
Azygos vein (via right thoracotomy)	33
Common facial vein	27
Inferior epigastric vein	34
Saphenous vein	35
Right atrium	36

*Used in placement of tunneled catheter.
†Used in placement of tunneled catheter or subcutaneous port.

In an effort to reduce the incidence of infection, tunneled central catheters were introduced in 1973; these are usually placed surgically within the subclavian or jugular vein with the tip in the superior vena cava. The extravascular portion of the catheter is tunneled under the skin for a variable distance before being taken through the skin. The catheter is often anchored at the skin exit with a Dacron cuff to eliminate the need for sutures in the skin. More recently, subcutaneously placed chambers, termed *ports,* of silicone or other elastomer have been developed; the chamber is connected by a catheter usually placed into the subclavian vein with its tip in the superior vena cava.[37] The nutrient solution is infused into the chamber through special needles inserted through the skin. Such chambers are a development from an earlier concept using an Omaya shunt.[38]

The insertion and use of an indwelling central venous catheter impose the possibility of various risks to the patient; these include pneumothorax, hemothorax, aneurysms, venous or nerve injury, and microbial contamination with colonization of the catheter. Thrombogenicity varies with the catheter material; the earlier and stiffer polyvinyl and polyethylene catheters were associated with more thrombus formation than silicone or polyurethane elastomers. Multilumen catheters have increased in use to provide additional access for infusing medications and blood and for blood sampling without interfering with TPN administration. Their use has been associated with a significant increase in catheter-related sepsis, however.[39,40]

Complications tend to occur less frequently when experienced surgical and other personnel, preferably members of a clinical nutrition team, exercise necessary precautions, including aseptic technique in catheter insertion and maintenance, assurance of proper placement (checked by x-ray study before use), and adequate care of the insertion site. Recommendations for infection control in association with parenteral nutrition have been published.[41]

In general, a diagnosis of bacteremia or fungemia with the possibility of catheter colonization should be seriously considered when the patient experiences sudden spiking fever and/or shaking chills. A sustained fever is more likely to be related to an abscess somewhere, often without catheter colonization. With the onset of fever, sources of infection should be sought, and appropriate cultures should be taken both from a peripheral vein and through the catheter. Appropriate antibiotic treatment should be instituted as indicated.

When bacterial or fungal colonization is suspected in a percutaneously placed catheter, a modified Seldinger technique may be useful because this involves rapid replacement of a central catheter over a flexible wire using appropriate sterile technique without another venipuncture.[42,43] This technique greatly reduces the need for further venipunctures and possible complications and is particularly valuable for the patient who is deemed a candidate for long-term TPN, for which continued vascular access is critical.

My experience and that of many others indicate that, with good technique in placement and solution preparation and with proper maintenance indwelling catheters of the percutaneous or tunneled type may remain safely in place for months and years without infection or disruption.[44–46] Evidence indicates that the use of tunneled catheters is associated with less infection and fewer technical problems (e.g., dislodgment).

The use of subcutaneously placed ports has been increasing, presumably on the assumption that the risk of infection is reduced during the 8 to 16 hours of infusion by having a fine needle as the only external vascular access. No controlled comparative data are available to allow an objective appraisal of the value of this technique against that of other types of catheters. Such devices are expensive and are not free of the occurrence of infection and maintenance problems.

DELIVERY SYSTEMS

The nutrient solutions for PPN are delivered from bottles or plastic bags by gravity flow with or without drop counters. Central parenteral nutrition solutions are generally delivered using propulsion pumps of various types. These have become increasingly sophisticated and automated but increasingly expensive, in part because of the need for special tubing. They ensure even flow rates, overcome the increased resistance of filters of small porosity (especially with continued use), minimize the likelihood of clotting at the catheter tip, and reduce need for frequent nursing surveillance. In-line membrane filters (usually 0.22 μm) have been used in an effort to provide greater assurance of sterile delivery of parenteral fluids and to prevent introduction of particulate matter; however, these filters are rarely used now. Such fine-bore filters cannot be used with "triple-mix" lipid-containing infusions (see later in this chapter for a discussion of filter use in this situation).

The use of pliable plastic bags of various sizes eliminates the danger of breakage, simplifies transportation and storage, and reduces storage space requirements before and after filling, as compared to glass or formed-plastic bottles. The usual water solutions of nutrient formulations do not extract measurable amounts of phthalate plasticizer used in the manufacture of polyvinyl chloride (PVC) bags; albumin, lipids, and blood take up the plasticizer.[47] The amount of plasticizer eluted from PVC administration sets by lipid emulsions is relatively small compared to that from the bags. Plasticizer-free tubing and bags are available in the form of ethylene vinyl acetate (EVA). Another elastomer contains the plasticizer trioctyl trimellitate (TOTM), which is not extracted by lipid. These are useful with certain lipid formulas.

Insulin adsorption varies appreciably, depending on the binding characteristics of the nutrients present, the type of plastic in the delivery system, the presence of filters, and the concentration of insulin added.[48] When insulin is added to parenteral solutions in diabetic patients, the dosage must be tested with close monitoring until properly adjusted.[48,49]

PARENTERAL COMPONENTS AND REQUIREMENTS

These are reviewed with a brief general summary and a more detailed review of specific nutrient requirements and metabolic issues.

GENERAL REQUIREMENTS

Approximately 30 kcal (7.2 kJ) per kg of body weight per day should be sufficient to maintain weight for the relatively unstressed middle-aged patient in an acceptable weight range whose activity is restricted and who has no fever or other hypermetabolic condition. The formula content of the ratio of grams of nitrogen to kilocalories (N/kcal) of approximately 1:250 to 1:300 (1:60 to 1:72 N/kJ) is appropriate for such a patient. Malnourished nonhypercatabolic adults can be placed into positive nitrogen balance on a caloric intake approximately equal to 1.3 times resting energy expenditure (REE) or 29 kcal/kg while receiving parenteral solutions supplying 1.13 g of amino acids/kg (= 180 mg N/kg) per day.[50] When twice this amount of amino acids per kilogram were given, nitrogen retention was better. Such patients appear to behave like growing children in this respect. To allow for weight gain, more calories are required depending on the weight gain desired. Shaw et al. have developed a graphic presentation of the effects of nitrogen and energy intakes on nitrogen and fat balance in depleted patients.[50] To minimize or help regain loss of lean body mass in adult patients acutely stressed by trauma, burns, or infection, the N/kcal ratio is generally increased (1:150) (see Chap. 68). Caloric provision to such adult patients may be as high as 40 to 45 kcal/kg or occasionally higher. Care must be taken not to exceed caloric expenditure consistently. The goals for infants and children are reviewed in Chapter 66, and those for adolescents are given in Chapter 47.

All essential and sufficient nonessential amino acids should be provided in amounts needed for adequate protein synthesis. Essential fatty acids should be supplied regularly. Macrominerals, trace elements, and vitamin intakes should meet individual requirements without excessive wastage or toxicity. A key point to remember in all nutrition support is that a deficiency of any essential nutrient—no matter how adequate the formula is in other respects—may lead to negative balance of nitrogen and other nutrients. Rudman et al. found that a single deficiency of either potassium, sodium, phosphate, or nitrogen impaired or abolished retention of other elements,[51] whereas Wolman et al. found that depletion of zinc caused negative nitrogen balance.[52]

WATER

The fluid component must be sufficient to meet individual needs and to avoid the twin dangers of over- and underhydration in patients who may have difficulty in excreting or retaining needed water. The close interrelationships of water, electrolytes, and hormonal factors are considered in Chapter 6. The water derived from the metabolism of energy substrates is sodium-free water; the volumes may be a significant addition to that infused (Table 80–3).

Expansion of extracellular fluid (ECF) is a common finding in hospitalized patients with malnutrition, and this influences body weight and serum albumin levels. Starker et al. have described different patterns of changes of body weight and serum albumin in various clinical situations during the first week of TPN.[53,54] Severe malnutrition and inflammatory processes are associated with sodium and fluid retention in the early period of nutritional rehabilitation.

CARBOHYDRATES

Glucose is the commonly used carbohydrate for caloric replacement in TPN and is usually the major source of energy. Parenteral glucose is in the form of the monohydrate, with 1 g providing about 3.4 kcal. It is readily available in various concentrations in liquid form, is relatively inexpensive, and is rapidly metabolized by most patients. A large glucose contribution to energy needs within a tolerable fluid volume requires an extremely hypertonic solution (Table 80–4).

Other carbohydrates given intravenously are metabolized whole or in part. Fructose is converted to glucose in the liver and requires insulin for utilization of the formed glucose. The utilization of even small amounts of exogenous fructose is seriously impaired in hypoinsulinemic

TABLE 80–3. WATER FORMED IN THE METABOLISM OF TISSUE AND CALORIC SOURCES

SOURCE	AMOUNT
Muscle	1 g yields 0.85 ml (0.1 ml from protein + 0.75 ml cellular water)
Mixed tissue	100 kcal yields 10 ml
Fat	1 g yields 1.0 ml
Protein	1 g yields 0.4 ml
Glucose	1 g yields 0.64 ml
Glucose · H_2O	1 g yields 0.60 ml
Mixed diet	100 kcal yields 20 ml
Example: High-glucose TPN solution	
750 ml 10% amino acids	= 300 kcal yields 30 ml H_2O
1175 ml 50% glucose/water	= 2,000 kcal yields 353 ml H_2O
143 ml 10% lipid	= 157 kcal yields 14 ml H_2O
Total: 2068 ml	= 2,457 kcal yields 397 ml H_2O
Example: Glucose-lipid TPN solution	
750 ml 10% amino acids	= 300 kcal yields 30 ml H_2O
750 ml 50% glucose/water	= 1,275 kcal yields 225 ml H_2O
500 ml 20% lipid	= 1,000 kcal yields 100 ml H_2O
Total: 2,000 ml	= 2,575 kcal yields 355 ml H_2O

TABLE 80–4. OSMOLALITIES AND ENERGY VALUES OF INTRAVENOUS GLUCOSE AND LIPID PREPARATIONS

SOLUTION	PERCENTAGE (%)	mOsm/kg H_2O*	kcal/L
Glucose†	5	278	170
Glucose	10	523	340
Glucose	20	1250	680
Glucose	50	3800	1700
Lipid	10	280	1100
Lipid	20	330	2000

*Plasma, 290; 0.9% NaCl, 308 mOsm/kg H_2O.
†Monohydrate form.

conditions.[55] When fructose is given in large quantities, it increases serum lactate, urate, and bilirubin and depresses hepatic adenosine triphosphate (ATP) and serum phosphate concentrations.[56] It has a low renal threshold with resultant urinary loss when given in high concentration. Sorbitol, a hexose hydroxyalcohol, is used in some countries other than the United States; it is converted to fructose. Xylitol is a pentose hydroxyalcohol that bypasses insulin-dependent glucose pathways;[57] like sorbitol, it is not available in the United States. Neither intravenous maltose[58] nor oligosaccharide[59] is hydrolyzed sufficiently to be useful as a source of carbohydrate energy in TPN. A solution containing 3% glycerol, amino acids (3%), and electrolytes (Procalamine, McGaw) is available for use in PPN. The glycerol is well utilized as an energy source in traumatized patients when it is given with 10% lipid.[60] In comparison with glucose, glycerol required only about half the amount of insulin to maintain the glycemia of diabetics in the range of 150 to 200 mg/dl.[61]

GLUCOSE METABOLISM AND HORMONAL CHANGES

Byrne et al. studied the adaptation to increasing loads of parenteral glucose and other nutrients as the duration of infusion was decreased in relatively stable patients who were being prepared for or were already receiving home TPN (HPN).[62] After adaptation to successive periods of 24, 17, and 12 hour infusions of the same TPN formulas and volumes, glucose and various hormone concentrations were measured in the course of each infusion and during the postinfusion period (Fig. 80–1). With the 24- and 17-hour infusions, subjects responded well; the major response to abrupt initiation of the infusion was brisk insulin secretion. Tapering resulted in a fall of glucose to fasting levels and a rapid decline in insulin. No significant changes in glucagon, cortisol, or growth hormone were noted. With the 12-hour infusion, one of the five patients developed marked hyperglycemia, hyperinsulinemia, hyperglucagonemia, and increased growth hormone and cortisol levels, and the elevated hormone levels persisted into and beyond the tapering period. Because such patients are not uncommon, it is necessary to check tolerance to glucose before infusing large amounts in cyclic fashion.

ALTERED SUBSTRATE METABOLISM IN HYPERCATABOLIC PATIENTS

The metabolism of glucose is markedly different from that of normal individuals in patients with trauma, injury, and sepsis or advanced cancer that induces weight loss. This subject is discussed in Chapters 68 and 73 and elsewhere.[63–66] Some aspects that relate directly to TPN formulation follow.

The reasonably stable patient can oxidize infused glucose to CO_2 efficiently up to approximately 14 mg/kg per minute, whereas the critically ill patient has a capacity of only about half or less of that figure; that is, 5 mg/kg per minute in burn patients and 6 to 7 mg/kg per minute in postoperative patients.[63] Infusion above the limiting rate results in the conversion of glucose to fat, with a rise in energy expenditure and a rise above 1.0 of the respiratory quotient (RQ). The conversion of excess glucose to fat is energy dependent; after the oxidation of the resultant fat, energy as ATP sources is derived that is 30% of that which would theoretically have been obtained if direct oxidation of the amount of converted glucose had occurred.[67]

Other potentially detrimental effects of providing glucose in excess exist. Wolfe et al. have calculated that, at an infusion rate of 9 mg/kg per minute into the stressed patient, 206 g per day of triglyceride were synthesized in the liver. Only a small fraction of newly synthesized fat would have to remain in the liver to account for the development of fatty liver.[65] Other undesirable effects of excess glucose relate to the risk of hyperglycemia and glycosuria, with resultant water and sodium losses and, particularly in the dehydrated and infected diabetic patient, the danger of hyperosmolar nonketotic coma.

Elwyn et al. demonstrated that malnourished individuals had no increase in REE with increasing glucose intake in amounts below those needed for energy equilibrium; however, with excess glucose, REE increased by

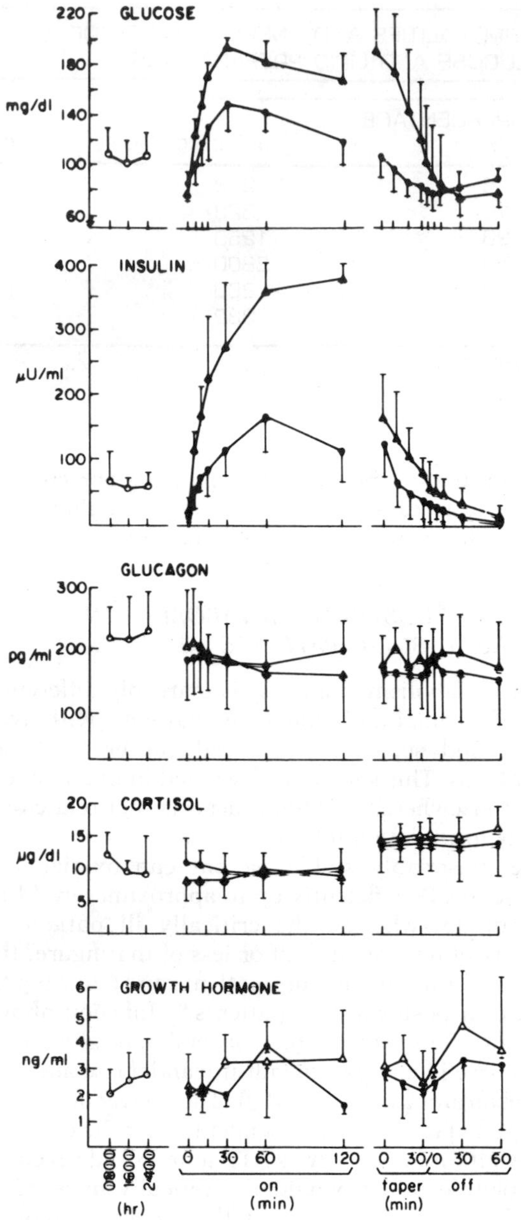

FIGURE 80–1. The responses of glucose, insulin, glucagon, cortisol, and growth hormone to infusions of TPN solution in the same five adapted patients over 24 hours (○—○), 17 hours (●—●) and 12 hours (△—△), and over a 30-min period during which the infusions were tapered and stopped and over the first 60 min following cessation of infusion. Mean ± SEM is depicted for all 5 patients at 24 and 17 hours and for 4 patients at 12 hours. (Reprinted with permission from Byrne, W.J., et al., Gastroenterology, Vol. 80, pp. 947–956. Copyright 1981 by The American Gastroenterological Association.)

1 kcal for each 5 kcal of intake in association with fat deposition and rise in RQ above 1.0.[68] In contrast, the injured and/or septic patient given a large amount of glucose with lipid-free TPN exhibited major increases in both resting CO_2 production and O_2 consumption; however, the nonprotein RQ remained below 1.0.[69] This finding is compatible with other evidence indicating that some fat oxidation persists despite a glucose intake that normally abolishes fat oxidation.[65,70]

Differences in energy expenditure were apparent when surgical patients receiving a high-glucose TPN formula were compared with those receiving an isocaloric glucose-fat formula with 69% of non-nitrogen calories as fat. When the high-glucose formula was given at an infusion rate to provide the carbohydrate at 4 mg/kg per minute, the energy increase was 11% of the mean daily energy intake and 21% of the mean REE; those receiving the glucose-fat formula had an increase of 3 and 7%, respectively.[71]

VENTILATORY RESPONSE TO GLUCOSE

When glucose infusion was given in amounts greater than the REE to malnourished individuals with resultant lipogenesis, minute ventilation at rest was found to increase by about 32%; it was increased appreciably more in hypermetabolic patients who had an elevated resting ventilation before TPN.[72] In patients with a decreased sensitivity to CO_2 or in those with compromised lung function or who are already hyperventilating, the added ventilatory stimulus of high-glucose TPN may aggravate preexisting pulmonary dysfunction (see Chap. 76).

TPN solutions with glucose as the non-nitrogen energy source have been associated with low serum cholesterol and triglyceride levels, a 26% increase in the fractional catabolic rate of low-density lipoprotein (LDL), and an associated reduction of plasma cholesterol levels through changes in both LDL and high-density lipoprotein (HDL).[73]

LIPIDS

These substances consist of tiny droplets (0.5 μm or less) with triglyceride as the core and with the cholesterol derived from the egg yolk phosphatides surrounded by a solubilizing and stabilizing surface layer of the emulsifying phospholipids. Both 10 and 20% concentrations of several lipid preparations are available and serve as a source of calories and essential fatty acids (EFA).

The cholesterol content per liter of Intralipid is appreciably higher than that of Liposyn II and III, presumably because of the preparation of the phosphatide (Table 80–5). Per kilocalorie, the 20% emulsion has only half as much cholesterol as the 10% preparation. The rise in serum cholesterol after a single infusion of lipid emulsion is transient and usually reverts to near preinfusion levels within 4 to 6 hours. As noted later in this discussion however, persistent use of lipid infusions such as Intralipid is associated with an elevation of plasma phospholipid and free cholesterol.

Glycerin (glycerol) serves to make the emulsions isotonic and is also a carbohydrate source. The isotonicity

TABLE 80–5. COMPARISON OF PARENTERAL LIPID EMULSION FAT SOURCE

	SOYBEAN OIL				SOYBEAN PLUS SAFFLOWER OIL (EQUAL PARTS)	
	Intralipid*		Liposyn III†		Liposyn II†	
Total fat (%)	10	20	10	20	10	20
kcal/ml	1.1	2.0	1.1	2.0	1.1	2.2
Glycerin (%)	2.25		2.5		2.5	
Egg phosphatides (%)	1.2		1.2		1.2	
Linoleic acid (%)‡	49§		55		66	
Oleic acid (%)	21§				18	
Palmitic acid (%)	11§				9	
Linolenic acid (%)	6.5§		8.3		4	
Cholesterol (mg/L)	250–300		19–21		13–22	
Phosphorus (mg/L)	150–200		267–500		267–500	
mOsm/L	300		284–292		260–280	
pH	8.0		8.3		8.3	8.0
vitamin E activity‖	18#	18#	18	36	19	46

*Clintec Nutrition, Deerfield, IL.
†Abbott Laboratories, Abbott Park, IL. Data on Liposyn II and III courtesy of Paul D. Rosen.
‡As percentage of total fatty acid.
§Data from Ito, Y., Hudgens, L.C., Hirsch, J., et al.: Am. J. Clin. Nutr., *53*:1487–1492, 1991.
‖Activity in milligrams per milliliter.
#Tocopherol isomers in Intralipid in mg/L (and E activity): α, 7.7 (7.7); δ, 383 (0.38); β and α, 51.1 (10.2); total, 97.1 (18.3). Data from Gutscher, G.R., Lax, A.M., Farrell, P.M.: J. Parenter. Enteral Nutr., *8*:269–273, 1984.

and tolerance of the endothelium of small vessels for the IV lipid preparation permit the peripheral infusion of a large amount of calories. The equivalent of 2000 kcal in 1 L of 20% lipid emulsion is 1 L of 59% glucose solution, an extremely hypertonic solution.

As noted in Table 80–5, Intralipid and Liposyn III contain more linolenic acid (C18:3,n-3) than Liposyn II, whereas Liposyn II has more linoleic acid (C18:2,n-6) because of the incorporation of safflower oil. The role of these essential fatty acids in nutrition and their metabolism and requirements are discussed in Chapter 3 and in other chapters of this book. EFA deficiency is prevented by average daily provision of about 3.2% of total calories as IV fat in adults.[74] The requirements for infants and children are noted later in this discussion and are reviewed in Chapter 66.

METABOLISM

Although the particle size of these lipid emulsions is within the range of chylomicrons, significant differences exist between these two types of particles. Whereas no lipoprotein is present on the surface of emulsion particles prior to infusion, coating with lipoproteins occurs in the circulation.[75] Their phospholipid content is higher than that of chylomicrons, especially in the 10% emulsions. With ultracentrifugation of an emulsion, two particle populations are noted: one consists of triglyceride-rich particles and the other of phospholipids.[76] As with circulating chylomicrons, lipoprotein lipase (LPL) on the surface of capillary endothelial cells is activated by apolipoprotein C (Apo C) on the lipid droplet and hydrolyzes the triglyceride in the core, releasing free fatty acids (FFA) and glycerol. This is the rate-limiting step in clearance. FFA bind to albumin and circulate as metabolic fuel to heart, liver, and skeletal muscle, and in liver they are converted to very low density lipoproteins, which are secreted into plasma.[77] The released FFA enter various tissues; in adipose tissues, they are re-esterified to triglycerides and are stored; in muscle they are oxidized. In liver, they are converted to very low-density lipoproteins (VLDL), which are secreted into plasma.[77]

Lipoprotein X. As noted previously, Intralipid particles differ from chylomicrons in their elevated phospholipid content (10% Intralipid >20% Intralipid). Early studies with infusion of 10% Intralipid at 83% of non-nitrogen calories indicated a sixfold increase in plasma phospholipid content in a period of 4 weeks, a similar rise in free cholesterol, only a 2.5-fold rise in cholesterol esters, and only a modest rise in triglycerides.[78] Ultracentrifugation of plasma of patients infused with Intralipid revealed a marked elevation of an abnormal lipoprotein associated with an LDL fraction high in free cholesterol and phospholipid. Its composition approximated that of lipoprotein X (LpX), which is characteristic of cholestasis.[79] In several studies, LpX has been associated with Intralipid administration in varying concentrations and durations of infusions both in children and adults.[80–83] It seemingly occurs by an intravascular physicochemical union of phospholipid with free cholesterol.[80] The level of LpX is appreciably higher in the plasma of patients receiving 10% Intralipid than in those receiving 20% Intralipid, presumably because of the higher phospholipid content per kcalories infused in the 10% preparation. The half-life of LpX appears to be 2 to 4 days, with small amounts still present 7 days after termination of the lipid infusion.[80] Apolipoproteins CIII and E are reportedly the main components of LpX. Infusion of Intralipid 10% is associated with an increase in Apo B, which indicates an accompanying rise of normal LDL.[82]

Tolerance. When the concentration of lipid increases to the level where binding sites on LPL are saturated, a maximum elimination capacity has been reached. In normal adults, this maximum rate is about 3.8 g of fat/kg per 24 hours, corresponding to about 35 kcal/kg per 24 hours. It is increased in starvation (approximately 50%) and even more in trauma.[77]

Daily infusion of the fat emulsion over a period of a week or more is associated with increased tolerance, as indicated by decreased preinfusion serum triglycerides. Serum FFA are cleared more rapidly with simultaneously administered carbohydrate. Clearance rate from plasma is not equivalent to the oxidative rate of lipid.

Effect of Lipid Infusion with TPN. When lipid (supplying one third the calories) is infused for approximately 8 hours, together with a glucose-based TPN formula given over 24 hours, fat oxidation is approximately 6 kcal/kg per minute; thus, it falls to about 3 kcal/kg per minute after cessation of lipid. A TPN formula with glucose and no lipid is associated with a fat oxidation rate of about 2 kcal/kg per minute, decreasing to approximately 0 by end of 24 hours.[83]

Hypermetabolic patients with sepsis and/or trauma in the basal state have increased rates of lipolysis, as indicated by elevation in glycerol flux and fat oxidation as compared with normal individuals (e.g., 5.3 versus 2.2 μmol/kg per minute and 2 versus 1 mg/kg per minute, respectively).[66,84] In a study of patients with sepsis who were given TPN with lipid, most of the fat oxidized was from endogenous fat stores, rather than from infused cleared lipid.[84]

In postoperative patients, comparisons have been made of two parenteral solutions providing equal calories (38 kcal/kg per day); one provided 70% of nonprotein calories as lipid and 30% as glucose, and the other provided 100% as glucose. No differences in nitrogen balance, plasma liver enzymes, urea, albumin, and prealbumin were noted; however, the lipid formulation was associated with continuing gluconeogenesis of alanine and delayed recovery of plasma transferrin after surgery.[85] In such patients, more glucose may be needed to suppress gluconeogenesis given either at a faster infusion rate or with an increased glucose percentage.

Non-Nitrogen Caloric Sources and Nitrogen Retention. Solid evidence exists for the nitrogen-sparing effect of carbohydrate (including glycerol) in the absence of and with amino acids. In the absence of amino acids, fat appears not to spare nitrogen beyond its glycerol content released on hydrolysis and its metabolism as a carbohydrate precursor. At low energy intakes, the effects of carbohydrate on nitrogen balance are much greater than those of fat. Increasing amounts of carbohydrate from 0 up to about 100 to 150 g intake (400 to 600 kcal) increase nitrogen balance by approximately 7.5 mg/N per added kcal (1.8 mg N/kJ). This effect is not shared by fat. Above this amount, however, the effect of added carbohydrate on increased nitrogen balance is only about 1.5 mg N per added kcal; this effect is thought to be shared by fat.[86]

Some investigators have disagreed on the nitrogen-sparing effect of fat in the presence of amino acids in hypercatabolic subjects. Long et al. were unable to achieve nitrogen equilibrium or positive balance when fat was supplied as the non-nitrogen energy source in burn or trauma patients. Calories from carbohydrate were required in an amount equal to the resting metabolic rate to achieve maximum nitrogen retention.[87] A review of nitrogen balance studies in patients with various inflammatory diseases, however, indicates that fat and carbohydrate are comparable in promoting nitrogen balance,[88] presumably after the minimum of 100 g glucose has been met.[86]

TOTAL NUTRIENT ADMIXTURE

Intravenous lipids have been infused in most instances by piggybacking the tubing from the emulsion into the tubing carrying a water-based TPN or PPN solution. Admixtures in a single container with amino acids, dextrose, minerals, vitamins, and a fat emulsion are used and are designated total nutrient admixture (TNA) or "triple mix." The admixture system is potentially unstable. Davis reviewed the relevant aspects of the properties of the phosphatide emulsifiers and various factors influencing the stability of the fat emulsions in the presence of various additives in the admixture.[89] The cumulative effects on aggregation of various cations of different charge can be predicted from an equation termed the critical aggregation number (CAN) at and above which neutralization of anionic surface groups results in lipid particle aggregation. Theoretically, CAN should be less than 130 to avoid aggregation;[89] however, considerable experience indicates that certain emulsions are stable above 130 and some even above 200.[90] Emulsion stability for 3 days has been noted with newer pediatric complete TNA formulations containing taurine, cystine, and tyrosine,[91] and with storage for 1 month of a TPN formula including heparin, ranitidine, and iron.[92] For solutions with larger amounts of either electrolytes or lipid, storage time is a matter of days.

Decreased microbial growth over 24 hours occurs in TNA, as compared to fat emulsions per se.[91] This finding led the Centers for Disease Control of the United States Public Health Service to recommend a 12-hour maximal infusion time for fat emulsions not in TNA.[93] The use of TNA over 24 hours increases tolerance to IV lipids in neonates. The major advantages and disadvantages of the TNA system are listed in Table 80–6. Reduction in the cost of lipid emulsions has facilitated the daily use of lipids.

Various investigators have reported blockage of catheters in patients receiving TNA for periods of 37 to 206 days, with deposition of a soft, creamy material on the internal catheter surface.[94] Analysis was made of material obtained after filtration (5-μm filter) of a specific TNA formulation stored for 7 days at 4° C in four different commercial EVA bags.[94] The small amount of material collected averaged 99.4% as fat and <0.5% as mineral salts. Of concern was the finding of plasticizer particles (numbers ranging from means of 2890 to 16,204 from different bags) with a size range of 1.4 to 43.8 μm that had been flushed out of the bags with saline before adding the TNA solution. The use of appropriate filters was suggested as a means of minimizing catheter occlusion and entry of plasticizer particles.[94]

TABLE 80–6. ADVANTAGES AND DISADVANTAGES OF THE TOTAL NUTRIENT ADMIXTURE (TNA) SYSTEM

ADVANTAGES
1. Decrease in nursing personnel time and subsequent cost savings resulting from simplification of administration
2. Increased compliance in home patients resulting from ease of administration
3. Decrease in training time for home patients requiring daily lipid emulsion
4. Potential decrease in rate of extrinsic contamination because of a reduced number of manipulations of IV delivery system by nursing personnel
5. Less likelihood of lipid toxicity by increased dilution and duration of lipid infusion
DISADVANTAGES
1. Apparent support of the growth of a variety of microorganisms that is significantly better than that of the conventional dextrose/amino acid solutions, but less than that of fat emulsions per se
2. Undesired effects (i.e., oiling out) resulting when base solutions ratios and/or additives exceed the amounts tested under stipulated controlled conditions
3. Inability of TNA systems to be filtered with a 0.22-μm bacterial retention filter
4. Inability to use total membrane sampling on TNA systems for a pharmacy quality assurance sterility testing program
5. Unknown consequences of long-term administration of larger particle size (larger than 0.4 μm) in TNA systems

COMPLICATIONS OF LIPID INFUSIONS

Because the ability to metabolize these emulsions is related directly to infant maturity, the risk of lipid accumulation in blood and its sequelae are greatest in the premature infant, the small-for-age gestational low birth weight (LBW) infant, and the nutritionally depleted older child (see Chap. 66).

Possible Altered Pulmonary Function. Lipid accumulation in the hepatic reticuloendothelial system with the likelihood of depressed immune responses and its competition with bilirubin and other substances for albumin binding have been described (see Chap. 66). Cases have been reported, primarily in young children, of bleeding dyscrasia in association with high plasma lipid levels and with platelets engorged with lipid.[95] Reports of altered pulmonary function during acute hyperlipidemia have varied; whereas decreased preliminary diffusion capacity has been noted,[96] other investigators have found no change in lung dynamics, but rather, a decrease in arterial oxygenation,[97] and still others have not found oxygen impairment in neonates with hyperlipidemia,[77] or in healthy men.[98] Impaired oxygenation has been noted when patients with adult respiratory distress syndrome were given IV lipid, however.[99] Infusion of lipid at a rate (0.15 g/kg per hour) that did not produce hypoxemia in healthy sheep produced hypoxemia after endotoxin pretreatment.[100] While recognizing the toxic potential of lipid infusions in infants, one must note that biochemical evidence of EFA deficiency has been present in more than half of premature infants at 7 days of age.[101] A progressive program of lipid infusion for such infants has been described.[101]

Fat Overload Syndrome. The fat overload syndrome, a rare complication of IV administration of fat, is characterized by sudden elevation of serum triglycerides in association with fever, hepatosplenomegaly, coagulopathy, and variable end-organ dysfunction. Fat sludging occurs within the microvasculature in spleen, liver, kidney, lungs, and brain. The use of plasma exchange was beneficial in one patient who did not respond to conservative medical therapy.[102]

Various fat emulsions given intravenously are known to result in the presence of lipid particles and deposition of a "ceroid" pigment in the reticuloendothelial system (RES) of the bone marrow, lymph nodes, spleen, and in the Kupffer cells and hepatocytes of the liver of adults, children, and laboratory animals.[103,104] To date, no effect of these histologic changes on hepatic function has been discovered.

LIPIDS AND IMMUNITY

The increased uptake of long-chain lipids by the RES in patients with hepatosplenomegaly and decreased clearance of lipid have led to concern of possible depression of immune responses with such infusions and increased susceptibility to infection. Mice injected with streptococci demonstrated higher mortality rates and incidence of bacteremia and decreased neutrophil chemotaxis when Intralipid was given.[103] In healthy and in burned guinea pigs, IV long-chain triglyceride (LCT) infusion at 75% or more of total nonprotein calories resulted in RES overload and an altered pattern of IV administered pseudomonas.[105] In vitro studies of neutrophil chemotaxis have given variable results reflecting different dosages and conditions.

What has been observed with respect to infection rates in patients receiving TPN? Various immune functions have been studied in malnourished cancer patients who are maintained on either a glucose TPN formula or one with both glucose and lipid; depressed cell-mediated immunity was noted before starting TPN, and no alteration in these parameters was observed with fat infusion.[106] In a randomized trial of preoperative TPN, patients receiving 50% of their caloric intake as lipid experienced more major complications and deaths than control subjects and, although the numbers of patients were small, more deaths than in the group receiving lipid-free TPN.[107] A meta-analysis of randomized studies of cancer patients receiving chemotherapy and TPN reported that TPN was associated with four times the increased risk of significant infection than in control subjects who did not receive TPN.[108] A meta-analysis of the same data by another group revealed that the infection rate for those patients receiving TPN who did not receive IV lipid was not different from that of the control subjects, and those receiving lipid one to three times per week had a 2.3-times increased risk of infection of ($p<.02$) compared to controls, whereas those given lipid daily had a 6.3-times increased risk ($p<.01$).[109] Freeman et al. analyzed risk factors associated with bacteremia due to coagulase-negative staphlococci in neonatal intensive care units; this organism is now the most common blood-culture isolate in this situation.[110] Infants with this type of bacteremia were 5.8 times as likely as control subjects to have received IV lipid emulsion before the onset of bacteremia; because lipid infusions were common, 56.6% of all cases of nosocomial infections were attributed to lipid administration.

NEWER INTRAVENOUS LIPID SOURCES

Beyond providing the small basic needs for linoleic and linolenic acids, are there lipids suitable for intravenous use that are metabolically and nutritionally more efficacious than the present vegetable oil-derived LCT?

Medium-Chain Triglycerides (MCT). MCT (see Chap. 3) have an established role when given enterally and parenterally in the management of malabsorptive disorders (see Chaps. 62 and 63). Experimental laboratory animal studies have indicated that MCT is cleared and oxidized more rapidly than LCT and is an equivalent in providing energy and in supporting protein synthesis; MCT increases energy expenditure appreciably more than does LCT.[111,112]

MCT (with octanoic acid as the main fatty acid) has been tested experimentally in laboratory animals as physical mixtures of MCT and LCT and as chemically structured triglycerides.[111] The latter has triglycerides with their fatty acids in various combinations of medium-chain and long-chain fatty acids (MCFA and LCFA) or other fatty acids from butter, depending on the starting proportion of the types of fatty acids.[112] Data obtained with laboratory animals indicate their ability to induce weight gain in trauma and to have effects superior to that of MCT on nitrogen balance and liver protein fraction synthetic rates.[111]

Physical mixtures of MCT and LCT as soybean oil in equal amounts have been given intravenously to patients in Europe,[76,111] and clinical investigations have been conducted in the United States with 75/25 physical mixtures of MCT and LCT.[111] Rapid hydrolysis and uptake of the MCT and a thermogenic effect of the latter have been found with no increase in body temperature. Long-term studies were conducted in Belgium in patients with inflammatory bowel disease with 20% LCT or a 20% MCT-LCT mixture (equal amounts), with glucose providing equal proportion of energy; each emulsion was infused for 3 months, followed by the other in random order.[76] None of the patients receiving an MCT-LCT mixture developed abnormal liver function tests; three of eight patients receiving LCT developed abnormal liver function tests that regressed to normal when LCT was replaced by an MCT-LCT mixture. MCFA released in high amounts during MCT-LCT infusion were oxidized in greater proportions than LCFA and produced ketone bodies in higher amounts. LCT infusion led to a significant increase in the LDL/HDL cholesteryl ester ratio, whereas MCT-LCT infusion did not; LCT infusion caused an imbalance in the fatty acid pattern of erythrocyte phospholipids, which were corrected by MCT-LCT infusion.[76]

Ultrasonic comparison of liver size and gray-scale value (which relates to liver density and incorporation of fat and connective tissue) was made before and after patients were given TPN with either 10% Intralipid or a 10% mixture of MCT and LCT in equal amounts; no changes were noted in either parameter with the MCT-LCT infusion, whereas both rose significantly with the LCT.[113] Although the rates and amounts of MCT infused in these and other studies[114] appear to be safe, infusion of octanoate as the salt or as MCT in various laboratory species at higher doses can produce lactic acidosis and encephalopathy.[115]

One of the stated reasons for favoring MCT over LCT has been the belief that, unlike with LCFA, carnitine is not required for MCFA transport into the mitochondria.[112,116] Measurements of the levels of the various plasma carnitine fractions in healthy subjects before and during infusion of glucose or amino acids, LCT, and 50% MCT-50% LCT revealed significant differences in the fractions between LCT and MCT infusions, however; such data support the hypothesis that metabolism of MCFA involves carnitine in some manner and suggest more study of these interactions.[116]

ω-3 (n-3) Fatty Acids. Important physiologic differences among the prostanoids and leukotrienes, derived from linoleic and linolenic acids (see Chap. 3), have directed attention to the possible advantages of including n-3 fatty acids and/or γ-linolenic acid as triglycerides or phospholipids in intravenous fat emulsions.[117–119] Eicosanoid synthesis must be carefully regulated, to provide their various mediators in appropriate quantities in response to appropriate stimuli and at the same time to avoid harmful excesses of these potent compounds. To produce clinically significant alterations in various clinical conditions, relatively large amounts of n-3 fatty acids may be necessary.[119] Much careful experimental work in laboratory animals followed by studies in human subjects will be necessary before a clear-cut decision can be made on the usefulness and safety of IV lipid emulsions containing n-3 fatty acids or compounds such as γ-linolenic acid.

AMINO ACIDS

Intravenous amino acid solutions have evolved from the original hydrolysates of casein or blood fibrin to those of formulations of crystalline L-amino acids of different compositions and varying concentrations based in part on the amino acid composition of hydrolysates of modifications of high-quality dietary proteins on the basis of aminogram data. This history has been reviewed.[3,12] Variations continue to appear on the market.[120] Formulations of crystalline L-amino acids for specific clinical problems have been developed, with claims for superiority over general formulas in renal and hepatic failure, in trauma, and for growth of infants. The compositions of some commercially available solutions are given in Table 80–3, Chapter 66, and reference 120. Such commercial formulations differ between and within manufacturers in amino acid composition and concentrations per liter depending on clinical purpose; in addition, they may have added electrolytes and/or glucose.[120]

The eight amino acids essential for normal adults are present in all formulas, as are histidine and arginine, which are needed for young children. Glycine, alanine, and proline are present in moderately large concentration in the general adult formulations as sources of nonessential amino nitrogen. Some manufacturers add serine, tyrosine, glutamic acid, and aspartic acid in variable amounts, and a few have taurine in small amounts. The ratio by weight of essential to total amino acids in the pediatric and standard adult solutions varies between 0.41 and 0.54; higher ratios are present in formulas designed for patients with renal or hepatic failure.

Achievement of nitrogen equilibrium or positive nitrogen balance requires sufficient essential amino acids and sufficient nonessential amino nitrogen, adequate nonnitrogen energy, and other nutrients (such as potassium and phosphorus) essential for nitrogen utilization. Recent research on amino acids or their derivatives of current interest is summarized in the next few sections of this chapter.

BRANCHED-CHAIN AMINO ACIDS

The muscle uptake and the metabolism of the essential amino acids isoleucine, leucine and valine are reviewed in Chapter 1, and the role of these branched-chain amino acids (BCAA) as amino group donors in accelerated protein catabolism in muscle of hypermetabolic patients is noted in Chapter 66. Is the need for BCAA increased in injured and/or septic patients? Claims have been contradictory concerning beneficial effects (e.g., improved nitrogen balance with levels of BCAA higher than the 19 to 25% in standard United States amino acid formulations). An expert panel concluded: "In clinical studies, while some positive results in parameters of nitrogen metabolism have been noted using BCAA-enriched solutions in the most severely ill patients, little or no major effect on outcome has yet been demonstrated."[121] Additional negative effects continue to be published.[122]

TAURINE

This amino acid, which has a sulfuric acid group replacing the carboxyl group of what would otherwise be alanine, is discussed in detail in Chapter 31, which notes abnormal vision in taurine-deficient cats. Considered a nonessential amino acid for humans, taurine is of nutritional interest with respect to parenteral nutrition because of depression of its plasma, platelet, and urine levels in children and adults who are maintained on long-term TPN. Other than these reduced taurine levels, substantial evidence for deficiency has not been forthcoming. In fact, despite the low levels in adult and pediatric patients receiving long-term TPN, there did not appear to be any correlation with any index of visual function.[122] Because LBW infants have a limited ability to synthesize taurine, and the low levels of precursor cysteine in TPN solutions and have a reduced capacity to reabsorb taurine (see Chap. 31), taurine has now been added to some pediatric formulas (see Chap. 66).

GLUTAMIC ACID AND GLUTAMINE

The central role of these compounds in metabolism is reviewed in Chapter 1. Although glutamic acid was present in the early parenteral protein hydrolysates, it was omitted from the succeeding free amino acid formulations. No evidence from early balance studies in healthy individuals indicated that it is an essential amino acid. The keto acid precursor of glutamic acid, α-ketoglutarate, is synthesized in the citric acid cycle and can be transaminated to glutamic acid, which in turn, can react with ammonia through the enzyme glutamine synthetase to form glutamine.

Certain observations over the past 20 years have increased interest in the clinical importance of glutamine. These observations include its abundance in plasma, its presence intracellularly in the free form, its importance as a transporter of nitrogen and carbon among tissues, and its role as a primary oxidative fuel in rapidly dividing cells (e.g., intestine and stimulated lymphocytes). The high intracellular free glutamine concentrations are labile, and under conditions that include hypercatabolic disease states, glutamine levels can decrease markedly. These conditions are discussed briefly in their various aspects in Chapters 65, 68, and 79 and in detail in an international glutamine symposium.[123]

The issues for parenteral nutrition relate to proof of stability in solutions, to safety, and to positive evidence of efficacy of glutamine added to standard formulas when given to hypercatabolic patients in terms of improved nitrogen balance, muscle protein kinetics, and other metabolic parameters.

Free glutamine has a limited solubility (35 g at 20° C). It is unstable in solution, hydrolyzing to yield ammonia and pyrolidone carboxylate (pyroglutamate) with increasing pH, temperature, and storage time. After infusion, it is initially metabolized enzymatically to ammonia and glutamic acid. Concern therefore arises as to the possible accumulation of ammonia and of elevated levels of potentially neurotoxic dicarboxylic acids. Lowe et al. observed healthy individuals in a metabolic unit who were given daily infusions of a TPN solution for over 5 days containing amounts of glutamine varying from 20 to 57 g (136 to 390 mmol).[124] Serum ammonia and glutamate concentrations did not change significantly from those during a control period without glutamine, and nitrogen balance, hormonal concentrations, mental status, and ophthalmologic examinations were normal and unchanged. In this study, the glutamine-amino acid solution was stored at −4° C after filtration for up to 8 days before being incorporated into the TPN formulation.

Sterile 2.5% glutamine solutions stored at 4° C lost this amino acid at a rate of less than 0.05% per day.[125] When added to a complete TPN solution including lipid and stored at 4° C for 30 days, the 18 g (124 mmol) glutamine decreased by 2.8±0.1% per day, and ammonia increased only 0.106 to 0.253 mmol/L; glutamate and pH were unchanged.

In an increasing but still limited number of clinical studies in stressed patients, L-glutamine has been given intravenously in TPN solutions as such,[126,127] in the form of the dipeptide L-alanyl-L-glutamine[127–130] or as its α-keto precursors, α-ketoglutarate or ornithine α-ketoglutarate.[128] In these studies, glutamine in its various forms was provided in daily amounts ranging from approximately 0.19 g (1.3 mmol)/kg body weight[128] to 0.2, 0.23, or 0.29 g/kg,[127] to 0.57 g/kg.[126] Given to postoperative patients in short 3- to 5-day studies, glutamine decreased the degree of negative nitrogen balance of the control subjects, increased intramuscular free glutamine concentration,[127,128,130] and maintained skeletal muscle ribosome concentrations.[127,130] After bone marrow transplantation, glutamine significantly decreased the negative nitrogen balance of the control subjects during the metabolic period of days 7 to 11; over 3 weeks, glutamine infusion raised plasma glutamine without increasing plasma glutamate or changing the ammonia concentration gradient between the groups. Fewer patients given glutamine developed clinical infection and microbial colonization, and their hospital stay was shortened.[126]

Issues remain to be resolved concerning the reported beneficial effects of glutamine in hypercatabolic patients. How much glutamine is necessary and safe to obtain optimum results? Fürst et al., on the basis of their work and that of others, suggest that in, routine postoperative patients, about 13 g (89 mmol) of glutamine per day meet the intestinal mucosal need for cell replication plus increased muscle needs, whereas severely injured or stressed patients may need glutamine in the range of 27 to 40 g (187 to 237 mmol) per day.[129]

How valid are the nitrogen balance data? Walser has pointed out that gains or losses of body free glutamine nitrogen should be included in overall nitrogen balance data, just as a net change in body urea nitrogen must be included in patients with renal disease.[131] Furthermore, changes in free glutamine nitrogen pools do not represent modification of protein nitrogen. This issue has raised some controversy.[132,133] Ziegler et al. acknowledge that about 25% of the improved nitrogen balance "may represent a relative increase in the free glutamine pool within skeletal muscle;" these investigators point out that direct measurement of intracellular glutamine concentrations in biopsy specimens is necessary to obtain confirmatory quantitative data.[126] Further data are needed on the effect of glutamine on quantitative changes in net protein synthesis in muscle.

CARNITINE

Derived either from the diet or formed de novo from lysine and methionine, carnitine plays a critical role in the intramitochondrial transport of fatty acids. Carnitine is reviewed in detail in Chapter 29. It is mentioned here because of the finding of its reduced levels in plasma and tissues of patients receiving TPN, compared to those of healthy individuals with usual oral intake; in addition are individual case reports of improved liver function and decreased muscle weakness with carnitine supplementation during TPN.[134] Subnormal levels do not per se indicate deficiency. In randomized studies of comparable groups receiving TPN with and without carnitine supplementation, contradictory results were obtained with LBW infants of 32 weeks' gestational age given high carnitine doses of 48 mg (300 μmol)/kg per day for 4 days[135] and those given 8.1 mg/kg per day for 1 week and 16.1 mg/kg per day for the second week.[136] In the first study, the RQ of the treated groups was slightly lower than that of the control group, both fat and protein oxidation were greater, nitrogen excretion was increased, and the time required to regain birth weight was delayed.[135] In the other study, increases in nitrogen accretion and growth in the carnitine group were modest as compared to control subjects; essentially no differences occurred over 6 hours in association with an initial 2-hour infusion of lipid with respect to triglycerides, FFA, or ketone bodies.[136] In adults randomized to carnitine (12 mg/kg per day) or no carnitine with TPN for 11 days starting the day after esophagectomy, no differences occurred between groups in their RQ or plasma levels of triglycerides, FFA, or ketone bodies before or after 11 days; all the infused carnitine was excreted by the end of the study.[137] In all these studies, total plasma carnitine levels rose with supplementation; this was primarily in the form of free carnitine.[136,137]

In a longitudinal study of the carnitine status of children given TPN without added carnitine, the low plasma carnitine values and relatively low fat intake common in the children appeared to be without clinical consequence even after 10 years of carnitine-free TPN. Although plasma total and free carnitine values were 50% lower in the TPN group than in an age-matched healthy group, values did not change over 3 years; no significant abnormalities were noted in FFA, triglycerides, or cholesterol.[138]

With the possible exception of the uncommon situation where the liver is so badly damaged that carnitine cannot be synthesized, there seems little reason for carnitine supplementation at any age with current amino acid formulas providing the precursors.

SHORT-CHAIN PEPTIDE UTILIZATION

Adibi has summarized the advantages of using short-chain peptides in place of free amino acids in TPN solutions as (1) increased utilizable nitrogen sources in more concentrated form minimizing fluid volume, (2) decreased osmolality with its advantage for PPN, and (3) perhaps most important, the increased solubility as dipeptides of poorly soluble amino acids or the increased stability of unstable free forms.[139]

How well are small peptides used when given intravenously? Adibi has summarized his studies in baboons, in which a series of free amino acids and their dipeptides were infused as the only nitrogen sources, and his studies of glutamine in peptide form.[139] In a 1-week crossover study and in 4-week studies, comparing free amino acids and dipeptides, no significant differences were noted with respect to nitrogen balance, plasma and muscle amino acid concentrations, urinary losses, plasma concentration of insulin, glucose, and lipids, and other parameters.[140]

Glycylglutamine has also been infused into human subjects in the postabsorptive period and after brief starvation; significant increases occurred in the arterial concentration of glycine and glutamine in both conditions, and less than 1% of the infused dipeptide was recovered in the urine.[141] Amino acid and dipeptide balances across muscle, splanchnic tissue, and kidney were calculated. As previously noted in rats, dogs, and baboons, human subjects can utilize glutamine peptides.

MINERALS

The minerals—sodium, potassium, calcium, magnesium, phosphate, and chloride—are essential nutrients. Because a significant proportion of patients receiving or needing parenteral nutrition have malabsorption with large fluid losses with their ionic constituents, a continuing concern in the care of such patients is the adequacy of fluid and electrolyte balance. These important issues are considered in some detail in many chapters of this book and earlier in this chapter.

The basic daily needs of patients with reasonable normal cardiovascular, intestinal, renal, hormonal, and hydration status are 50 to 60 mEq (mmol) of sodium, 40 mEq (mmol) of chloride and bicarbonate (including those associated with amino acids as acetate), and 40 to 60 mEq (mmol) of potassium. Excessive losses from the intestine or the kidney and abnormal retention require appropriate changes with suitable monitoring as specific situations indicate.

CALCIUM, PHOSPHORUS, AND MAGNESIUM

Calcium and phosphorus (as inorganic phosphate) present a special concern for infants who need relatively large amounts of each because of the problem of solubility with their presence together in the TPN solution. Investigators have recommended that glycerophosphate or glucose phosphate together with calcium gluconate[142] or calcium glycerophosphate[143] be utilized to provide more soluble forms of the needed calcium and phosphate. Reference curves have been developed to estimate calcium and phosphate compatibility in commonly used neonatal TPN solutions.[144] The electrolyte needs of infants and children per kilogram per day are given in Table 66–2. Recommended pediatric concentrations of calcium, phosphorus, and magnesium per liter of TPN solution are given in reference 145; daily amounts for children and adults are given in Table 80–7.[146] The direct relationships as calcium excretion of the amounts of infused calcium, amino acid, glucose, sodium, and aluminum and the inverse effect of potassium have been reviewed recently.

Negative calcium balance related to hypercalciuria may occur in adults receiving TPN, especially during the

TABLE 80–7. RECOMMENDED LEVELS FOR CALCIUM, PHOSPHORUS, AND MAGNESIUM

MINERALS*	PEDIATRIC†			ADULTS
	Preterm	Term	Children	(mEq/day)
	Infants (mg/L‡)	Infants (mg/L‡)	>1 Year (mg/L)	
Ca^{+}	500–600	500–600	200–400	10–25
P^{+}	400–450	400–450	150–300	300–450§
Mg^{+}	50–70	50–70	20–40	12–20§

*Equivalents: Ca: 100 mg = 2.5 mmol = 5 mEq; P: 100 mg = 3.3 mmol; Mg; 12 mg = 0.5 mmol = 1 mEq.
†Data from Greene, H.L., Hambidge, M., Schanler, R., et al.: Am. J. Clin. Nutr., *48*:1324–1342, 1988 (rev. reprint issued Dec. 1990).
‡To avoid Ca-P precipitation, recommended intakes are given per liter and assume an average fluid intake of approximately 120 to 150 ml/kg per day with 25 g amino acids/L of a pediatric formulation. Dosages for preterm infants are to be given in a central vein infusion.
§P and Mg needs vary from these ranges, depending on the extent of intestinal losses and of renal retention or losses.

infusion period of cyclic TPN;[147] supplementation with either sodium or potassium acetate (replacing equimolor amounts of NaCl or KCl) resulted in major decreases in urinary calcium in patients receiving 24-hour and cyclic TPN, attributable primarily to increased renal tubular reabsorption with reduced excretion to near-infusion levels.[147] Reports are contradictory concerning whether urine calcium excretion with 12-hour cyclic TPN is greater than that with continuous 24-hour infusion.[146] The need for these macrominerals varies among the basic ranges for all ages with excessive loss through a dysfunctional alimentary tract and/or kidneys or by abnormal renal retention. Hence, monitoring of these parameters is critical in estimating need in the formulation.

TRACE ELEMENTS

Currently, acceptable direct evidence indicates that iron, iodide, zinc, copper, chromium (Cr^{3+}), and selenium are essential human nutrients. Manganese (Mn^{2+}) has been found essential for all experimental species studied, but clear evidence for manganese deficiency in man is lacking. A single well-documented case of molybdenum deficiency has been noted in a patient receiving long-term TPN. The biochemical and physiologic roles of these trace elements and the effects of their depletion in humans and other species are reviewed in Chapters 9 to 15.

Several generalizations about essential trace elements are in order. The cationic trace elements (Fe, Cu, Cr, Mn) in their salt forms are variably and usually poorly absorbed by the normal intestine; when in excess in the body, all these elements are toxic. Giving them by the IV route imposes a risk of excessive retention. These elements tend to be poorly excreted. Copper and manganese, and to a much smaller extent molybdate, are excreted through the bile into the intestinal tract; hence administration of copper and manganese over long periods in the presence of obstructive jaundice imposes a risk. In contrast, all the anionic forms of trace elements (iodide, selenite, or molybdate) are well absorbed and excreted in the urine; again, excess imposes a risk of toxicity. Many of the trace elements are present as contaminants in TPN components and hence contribute variably to the imput. Finally, nonessential, potentially toxic trace elements, which may be contaminants, must be considered.

Iron. The IV requirement for the term infant is estimated to be about 100 μg per kg per day; the premature infant probably needs double that amount intravenously.[145] For older children, 1 to 2 mg per day are needed; for nonmenstruating females and for men whose condition is stable, about 1 mg; and double that for menstruating females. Estimates of iron loss through frequent venipuncture for various tests may be made on the basis that 1 mg of iron is lost for every 1 ml of packed red cells removed (see Chap. 6).

Contamination with iron of various TPN additives varies by item and by manufacturer; figures of complete formulations with free amino acids vary from 0.025 to 1.4 mg/L,[148] thus meeting on average the needs of those children and adults receiving their normal fluid and energy requirements who have no significant blood loss.

When evidence indicates iron depletion, this ion may be given by the IV route as dilute Imferon* (iron dextran) solution in varying amounts after one ensures that the patient has no hypersensitivity to a test dose; ferrous citrate may be used.[149] Because many adult patients

*Although Imferon had been temporarily withdrawn from the market, it is again available in a similar formulation by another pharmaceutical company.

receiving parenteral nutrition have had previous blood transfusions, it is essential to estimate body stores before instituting iron therapy in such patients, to avoid iron overload. This can be done by measuring serum iron or ferritin or staining for iron in a bone marrow biopsy.

Iodide. Serum iodides with no added iodide remain normal in infants[150] and adults.[151] In addition, over a period of 4 or more years of observation in patients receiving long-term TPN at home, the various parameters of thyroid function have remained within normal limits.[151] Contamination of various mineral salts with iodide occurs; to this is added the efficient absorption of iodides from any ingested diet in the upper gastrointestinal tract and any iodide-containing topical antimicrobial agent. For the occasional, previously depleted adult patient with malabsorption who may have a low serum iodide level, 1 μg/kg appears adequate during the repletion period. The same amount has been recommended for infants, to avoid any risk of deficiency or toxicity.[145]

Following the recommendation of an expert committee of the Nutrition Advisory Group (NAG) of the American Medical Association (AMA) to the FDA in 1979,[152] commercial intravenous solutions of zinc, copper, manganese, and chromium became available and ended a period in which such solutions were available only to physicians and pharmacists who personally prepared them. I have modified the committee's 1979 suggested intakes on the basis of available new information (Table 80–8); some data are reviewed briefly in the following paragraphs.

Zinc. Pediatric dosages have been more precisely defined by Greene et al.[145] (Table 80–8). The original recommendations of the AMA committee[152] for stable and for hypermetabolic patients remain reasonable.[148] As with adults, severe diarrhea secondary to infectious disease and the short bowel syndrome in children are associated with increased zinc losses and increased need.[153,154]

The zinc contamination of TPN additives is variable, depending on the specific sources. As a result, the total zinc in the formulation may be as high as 0.3 to 0.4 mg/L.[155] Data on specific components have been published.[152,156] When zinc losses are likely to be high, balance data based on the contents of the TPN solution used and stool (or fistula) fluid and urine outputs are advisable in addition to serum levels; special precautions to avoid extraneous contamination are essential.

Copper. The pediatric dose recommendations are the same as in the AMA recommendations.[152] It is clear from the work of Shike et al. that, unlike with zinc, increased stool volume losses are not associated with major increase in copper excretion, and urinary losses tend to be low; therefore, copper accumulation occurs in the body when infused in relatively low amounts.[157] On the basis of these and other findings,[155] it is suggested that the range for copper be lowered to 0.3 to 0.5 mg per day for stable patients; hence the upper limit of the revised recommendation is the lower limit of the AMA recommendation.[152] Caution in copper administration in obstructive jaundice is emphasized because the major

TABLE 80–8. RECOMMENDED LEVELS FOR TRACE ELEMENTS

	INFANTS (μg/kg/day)		CHILDREN* (μg/kg/day [‡])		ADULT (PER DAY)		
Trace Element†	Preterm*	Term*			Stable	Acute Hypermetabolic	With Intestinal Losses
Zinc	400	<3 mo–250 <3 mo–100	50§	[5000]‡	2.5–40‖ mg	2.0‖ mg	Add as per#
Copper**	20‖	20‖	20‖	[300]	0.3–0.5§††‡‡		Total 0.5††
Chromium§§	0.20‖	0.20‖	0.2‖ 0.05##	[50]	10–15‖	—	Add 20 μg‖
Manganese**	1.0	1.0	1.0§	[50]	60–100 μg§	—	—
Selenium§§	2.0	2.0	2.0	[30]	40–80‖‖		
Molybdenum§§	0.25	0.25	0.25	[5]	0 (see text		

*Data from Greene, H.L., Hambidge, M., Schanler, R., et al.: Am. J. Clin. Nutr., *48:*1324–1342, 1988 (rev. reprint issued Dec. 1990).
†Conversion factors: Zn: 1 μg = 0.0153 μmol; Cu: 1 μg = 0.0157 μmol; Cr: 1 μg = 0.0192 μmol; Mn: 1 μg = 0.0182 μmol; Se: 1 μg = 0.0127; Mo: 1 μg = 0.0104 μmol.
‡[ ] = maximum in micrograms per day.
§Lower range than in 1979 AMA recommendations; data from Shils, M.E., Burke, A.W., Greene, H.L., et al.: JAMA, *241:*2051–2054, 1979.
‖Unchanged from 1979 AMA recommendations; data from Shils, M.E., Burke, A.W., Greenne, H.L., et al.: JAMA, *241:*2051–2054, 1979.
#Add 12 mg/L of small bowel losses and 17 mg/kg of stool or ileostomy losses; data from Shils, M.E., Burke, A.W., Greene, H.L., et al.: JAMA, *241:*2051–2054, 1979.
**Decrease or omit with increasing severity of obstructive jaundice.
††Data from Phillip, G.D., Garnys, V.P.: JPEN J. Parenter. Enteral Nutr., *5:*11–18, 1981.
‡‡Data from Shike, M., Roulet, M., Kurian, R., et al.: Gastroenterology, *81:*291–297, 1981.
§§Decrease or omit with increasing severity of renal dysfunction.
‖‖Data from Berkelhammer, C.H., Wood, R.J., Sitrin, M.D.: Am. J. Clin. Nutr., *48:*1482–1489, 1988.
##Data from Moukarzel, A.A., Song, M.K., Buchman, A.L., et al.: Am. J. Clin. Nutr., *339:*385–388, 1992.

excretory route is through bile. The copper content of TPN additives is variable.

Manganese. Pediatric recommendations (1.0 μg/kg) are appreciably lower[145] than the 2 to 10 μg/kg of the AMA recommendation. For adults, more recent data on manganese content of various TPN additives have yielded a daily intake as contaminants of 8 to 22 μg.[158] Patients on long-term TPN receiving a total of 60 to 120 μg Mn^{2+} per day in TPN infusions have been found to have serum values within the normal range;[159] these data suggest the need for provision of this ion below AMA recommendations.[151]

Chromium. The literature has been reviewed through 1989 concerning the chromium (Cr^{3+}) content of TPN additives and the intakes, balances, and serum levels of TPN of this ion.[160] As noted in the 1979 AMA report,[152] as with manganese, quantitative data were lacking at that time, and the qualitative suggestions were based on estimates from balance data on healthy individuals. The situation to 1989 had not been clarified much,[160] except more analytic data on Cr^{3+} content of TPN additives were available, and since Cr^{3+} has been added widely to TPN solutions, reports of signs and symptoms attributable to Cr^{3+} deficiency have ceased.

In calculations from low and high values for a variety of TPN additives from different batches and sources, the total daily Cr^{3+} content of a high-glucose TPN formula ranged from 2.4 to 8.1 μg and that of a high-lipid formula from 2.6 to 10.5 μg.[160] Amino acids, especially those containing phosphate or with phosphate additives, accounted for 85 to 90% of the Cr^{3+}. Other investigators have found levels of 4 to 11 μg in 3 L of the TPN solution.[161] A pediatric formula containing 4.0 μg Cr^{3+} as contaminant that was given over 16 months did not produce signs or symptoms suggestive of chromium deficiency.[162] More recently, children aged 1.3 to 14 years who were receiving long-term TPN at 0.15±0.09 μg/kg per day had high serum chromium concentrations compared to control subjects (e.g., 2.1±1.2 versus 0.10±0.03 μg/L).[163] The Cr^{3+} intake of the drinking water was 4.3 to 5.7 μg/L. Cr^{3+} supplementation was discontinued for 1 year (during which time the Cr^{3+} intake was estimated to be 0.05±0.01 μg/kg per day), at which time the serum Cr^{3+} concentration was 0.5±0.3 μg/L. No signs of deficiency were present. It was suggested that the parenteral Cr^{3+} pediatric intake should be lowered to 0.05 μg/kg and that current values of Cr^{3+} as contaminants may be sufficient for adults.[163] Although this may indeed be correct, a period of 1 year of reduced Cr^{3+} intake following a period of high intake without signs or symptoms may not be an adequate test of need in long-term patients. I am of the opinion that, for children, the recommendations of Greene et al.[145] and, for long-term use in adults, the recommendations of the AMA in 1979 still appear valid pending further studies; however, for periods of 1 year or less, the recommendations of Moukarzel et al.[163] may be tried with adequate precautions.

Selenium. Recommendations for this trace element were not made in the 1979 AMA report. In that year appeared the first reports in English of the relation of selenium deficiency to Keshan disease in China (see Chap. 12) and the report of Van Rijn et al. of a case of selenium deficiency in a patient receiving TPN.[164] Considerable clinical and biochemical information has accrued since then, including selenium deficiency in patients receiving TPN, with some deaths associated with cardiomyopathy and reports of muscle tenderness and weakness (see Chap. 12). Selenium in TPN solutions as measured by fluorometric analysis is below its detection level (e.g., <10 μg/ml).[164,165] Although deaths may occur, low plasma levels of selenium (<10 μg/ml,< 0.13 μmol/L) may be present without symptoms.[165]

Selenious acid (as selenite salts) is available for IV use. The use of 40 μg per day in TPN will maintain normal plasma levels; 100 μg will raise low levels in previously depleted patients receiving TPN into a control range of 100 μg/ml (= 1.3 μmol/L mol).[164,165] The requirement for selenium is inversely related to the severity of jejunal malabsorption in patients ingesting a usual American diet. Americans have blood selenium levels much higher than those of healthy New Zealanders, who often have values lower than 0.63 μmol/L (see Chap. 12).

Molybdenum. This subject has been reviewed in Chapter 15. Some controversy exists as to whether a "true" molybdenum deficiency has been observed in several species of experimental laboratory animals because of the need to add tungsten to the diet as an antagonist to molybdenum uptake to induce depletion.[166] A well-documented case of molybdenum deficiency has been reported in a patient receiving long-term TPN; clinical and biochemical abnormalities were reversed by daily supplementation with 300 μg of ammonium molybdate.[167,168] Tissue levels of molybdenum and balance data were not obtained, nor were molybdenum-dependent enzyme activities measured. Balance data have been obtained on two patients with active Crohn's disease and malabsorption.[168] Ileostomy losses were large, 560 and 300 to 350 μg per day, respectively; intake data were not given. The molybdenum content of TPN solutions has been reported to be 244 μg per day, with half derived from amino acids and one quarter from dextrose.[169] In view of a time lapse of at least 6 months from the initiation of TPN to the development of symptoms in the single reported case, the availability of simple biochemical criteria as diagnostic clues, and molybdenum contamination reported, it is recommended that molybdenum not be added at present to TPN infusions in adults and that it be withheld in children, except those receiving long-term TPN.[145] If deficiency is suspected by the clinical picture, serum urate and urine sulfate measurements should be made periodically as guides to indicate a need for initiating this element; if deficiency is suspected in adults, a dose of 200 to 300 μg in the form of ammonium molybdate appears to be safe. More data on levels of molybdenum contamination are warranted.

Ultratrace elements. These elements are reviewed in detail in Chapter 15. Data have been presented on the contamination levels in TPN additives of boron, nickel, and vanadium.[169] At present, evidence is insufficient to warrant their addition to TPN solutions.

Potential Toxicity of Trace Elements. The issue of toxicity of parenteral lead, cadmium, and mercury merits consideration because of the large amounts of fluids administered that bypass the normal barriers of the gastrointestinal tract and lungs.[170] Twenty components of a TPN solution used by me were individually analyzed for mercury; all values were below the quantitative detection limit. The complete formulations had 0.001 μg/ml of mercury (the lower detection limit), whereas the cadmium content was 0.08 ng/ml, and that of lead was 2.0 ng/ml. Potassium chloride and phosphate solutions contained 135 and 77 ng/ml of lead, respectively. Another report notes cadmium levels at about 10 mg/ml.[169]

Aluminum is of special concern as a toxic element because of its adverse effects on neurologic, bone, and hematopoietic functions, as originally described in patients with renal disease who were treated with reduced dietary phosphate antacids and/or hemodialysis. Reports of serious metabolic bone disease in a group of patients receiving home TPN (HPN) for 6 to 72 months[170] was followed by the discovery that the casein hydrolysate used contained relatively large amounts of this element (e.g., 2313±149 μg L).[171] The aluminum concentrations in plasma, urine, and bone were markedly elevated in all patients studied, and the bone morphology was that of osteomalacia, ranging from mild to severe. Intense periarticular and lower extremity pain in long bones and weight-bearing joints developed within 5 months in 5 of the initial 11 patients despite improvement in their overall nutritional state. Patients with impaired renal clearance are at increased risk; Figure 52–25 is a photomicrograph of a bone biopsy showing aluminum staining and osteomalacia. Casein hydrolysate was replaced in July, 1981 by crystalline amino acid solutions. The effects of aluminum on various aspects of bone metabolism have been reviewed.[146]

Even though free amino acid solutions have much smaller amounts of aluminum (e.g., 26±20 μg/L of 10% solution), other TPN ingredients may have significant amounts and may contribute to the total burden. Premature infants are at increased risk because of their poor renal clearance.[145] Widely varying concentrations of aluminum have been found in the same component from different manufacturers or in different salts of the same mineral; careful selection can reduce aluminum contamination from 288 μ/L of TPN solution to 10.9 μg/L.[172] A joint working group on Standards for Aluminum Content of Parenteral Nutrition Solutions has supported the FDA proposal for setting an upper limit of 25 μg Al/L (0.93 μmol/L) in large volume parenteral infusions; it recommended that salts of calcium, phosphate, and magnesium, trace element solutions, multivitamin solutions, and heparin should require statements of the amount of aluminum on their label and that pharmacists and physicians be educated about the risk of aluminum.[173]

VITAMINS

The current parenteral multivitamin formulations in the United States are those proposed in 1975 by the Nutrition Advisory Group of the AMA for intravenous vitamin formulations.[174] The adult formulation was approved by the FDA in 1979 and is designated here as the AMA-FDA adult formula. In 1984, the recommended pediatric formula was approved. The vitamin content of the formulations per unit are the same regardless of manufacturer (Table 80–9). The pediatric formula provides all known essential vitamins, whereas the adult formula omits vitamin K; this must be added separately at a recommended dose of 5 mg once weekly in the TPN solution. The manufacturers add excess nutrients at production time (within limits set by the FDA), to meet label requirements at the expiration date.

Provision of lipid-soluble vitamins in aqueous suspension requires the presence of one or more synthetic solubizing agents. In addition, these parenteral multivitamins contain a variety of excipients serving as stabilizers, antioxidants, buffers, and preservatives. Their presence and concentrations in various commercial preparations of the AMA-FDA formulas are given in Table 80–10. The American Academy of Pediatrics has reviewed the issue of excipients as "inactive ingredients" in pharmaceutical products with particular reference to infants and children.[175]

In many other countries, particularly in Europe, an alternative formulation resulting from the work of Wretlind consists of two solutions. One (Vitalipid) contains fat-soluble vitamins dissolved in fractionated soybean oil emulsified with egg phospholipids similar to that used in Intralipid and can be infused with IV fat emulsions. The other is a solution of water-soluble vitamin C (Soluvit) (see Table 80–9).

The absorption and/or destruction of individual vitamins may occur in varying degree through contact with plastic containers and tubes and in passage through filters, exposure to light and heat, and interactions with other substances present in solutions. Factors affecting the solubility and stability of vitamins in various pharmaceutical preparations have been reviewed.[176]

Appreciable amounts of retinol appear to be lost from solution, particularly when flow through tubing is slow, by a combination of adsorption and photodegradation;

TABLE 80–9. PARENTERAL MULTIVITAMIN FORMULATIONS

	CHILDREN		ADULT (PER UNIT DOSE)		
Vitamin*	Very Low Birth Weight (per kg[†])	Term to 11 Yr: AMA-FDA (per day)	AMA-FDA[‡]	Soluvit	Vitalipid
A[§] (μg) (IU)	500.0 (167)	700.0 (2,300)	990.0 (3,300)	—	750.0 (2,500)
D_2 (μg) (IU)	4.0 (160)	10.0 (400)	5.0 (200)	—	3.0 (120)
E[#] (mg) (IU)	2.8 (2.8)	7.0 (5)	10.0 (10)	—	—
K_1 (μg)	80.0	200.0	0	—	150.0
Thiamin[‖] (mg)	0.35	1.2	3.0	1.24	—
Riboflavin** (mg)	0.15	1.4	3.6	2.47	—
Pyridoxine[‖]	0.18	1.0	4.0	2.43	—
Niacin[††] (mg)	6.8	17.0	40.0	10.0	—
Pantothenate (mg)	2.0[‡‡]	5.0[‡‡]	15.0[‡‡]	10.0	—
Biotin (μg)	6.0	20.0	60.0	300.0	—
Folate (μg)	56.0	140.0	400.0	200.0	—
Cobalamin (B_{12}) (μg)	0.3	1.0	5.0	2.0	—
Ascorbate (mg)	25.0	80.0	100.0	34.0	—

*For International System equivalent units, see Appendix Table A–1a.
[†]Proposed by Greene, H.L., Hambidge, M., Schanler, R., et al.: Am. J. Clin. Nutr., *48:*1324–1342, 1988 (rev. reprint issued Dec. 1990).
[‡]May be in divided form and different volumes (see Table 80–10).
[§]As retinol.
[#]As dl-α-tocopherol acetate.
[‖]As the hydrochloride.
**As the phosphate.
[††]As niacinamide.
[‡‡]As dexpanthenol.

TABLE 80–10. EXCIPIENTS AND DISTRIBUTION OF NUTRIENTS IN COMMERCIAL PARENTERAL MULTIVITAMIN SOLUTIONS (PER DAILY DOSE) IN THE UNITED STATES

INGREDIENT	FUNCTION	PEDIATRIC	ADULT	
		MVI-Pediatric* 5 ml[‡]	MVI-12* 10 ml[§]	MCV 9 + 3[†] 10 ml[‖]
Polysorbate 80 (mg)	Surfactant; emulsifier	50	80.0[#]	—
Polysorbate 20 (mg)	Surfactant; emulsifier	0.8	1.4[#]	240.0
Gentisic acid ethanolamide	Solubilizer; stabilizer; preservative	—	2.0[#]	1.0
Propylene glycol (%)	Stabilizer	—	30.0**	30.0
Butylated hydroxytoluene (mg)	Lipid antioxidant	0.058	0.1[#]	0.09
Butylated hydroxyanisole (mg)	Lipid antioxidant	0.014	0.025[†]	0.02
Citric Acid, sodium citrate, and/or sodium hydroxide	Buffer	Present	Present	Present
Mannitol (mg)	Lyophilization aid	375.0	—	—

*Manufactured by Armour, Kankakee, IL, for Astra Pharmaceutical Products, Westborough, MA.
[†]Lymphomed, Deerfield, IL.
[‡]On reconstitution of lyophilized product.
[§]In two vials of 5 ml: vial 2 contains biotin, folate, and B_{12}; vial 1 has the other vitamins (see Table 80–9).
[‖]In two-chambered vial mixed before using.
[#]In vial 1 only.
**In vials 1 and 2.

this situation is particularly true with procedures and increased light intensity in neonatal nurseries.[145] Use of polyolefin tubing rather than polyvinyl tubing reduces vitamin A loss.[145] Little loss of vitamin D occurs in plastic delivery systems.[145]

Addition of the multivitamin solution to TPN solutions presents the possibility of some losses of specific vitamins. Thiamin is split and so may lose biologic activity in the presence of sulfite compounds;[177] these remain, in one form or another, a component of amino acid solutions in the United States.[120] Hence multivitamin solutions should not be added directly to undiluted amino acid solutions, but rather to the ultimate solution shortly before infusing it into the patient. Ascorbic acid is progressively lost in the presence of Cu^{2+} and oxygen.[178] Folate is stable when the TPN solution has a pH between 5.0 and 6.0, as is the usual situation.[179] Riboflavin and pyridoxine are unstable when exposed to direct sunlight over a matter of hours.[180] Thiamin, folate, riboflavin, and pyridoxine are stable under fluorescent light.

ADULT NEEDS

The issue of vitamin needs for the sick and injured has long been of concern. Varying amounts of vitamins have been administered to postoperative and other patients who are receiving parenteral nutrition, with differing intervals between the times of vitamin infusion and those of blood sampling; blood levels have been the usual criteria, although some enzymatic methods have been used by some investigators. Few investigators have performed a complete survey of the 13 vitamins. Although many of the data obtained in seriously ill adult patients are based on short-term information of a few weeks to a few months, for most patients, this is the critical time range. These data indicate that the range of requirements for certain of these nutrients is relatively narrow and that adequate blood levels or related enzyme activities may be attained in hypercatabolic patients with daily infusion dosages for some that are appreciably less than those of the old MVI formula and, in some cases, below, at, or not far above the AMA-FDA adult dosages.[178,181–186]

The adequacy of the adult AMA-FDA formulation was tested in 16 adults with severe malabsorption or intestinal obstruction who had been receiving HPN for 1 to 9 years. These patients were studied serially over many months on this formulation (MVI-12).[178] Blood sampling was performed at least 36 hours after the preceding infusion of vitamins was terminated. Mean values for plasma vitamin A were near or above the upper limit of reference values, in part because of the presence of 5 subjects with renal insufficiency; the high values were associated with elevated retinol-binding protein levels. Thiamin, pyridoxine, niacin, biotin, riboflavin, vitamin B_{12}, and folate levels were within the reference ranges for all subjects; pantothenate levels tended to be within or above the reference ranges; thiamin tended to be toward the lower half of the reference range, as did vitamin E levels. In addition to the label amount of 10 mg/dl α-tocopherol acetate, a small amount of vitamin E was given as a part of the IV lipid, with an average of 1 mg of the α form and 3 mg of the γ form. The low plasma lipid levels of these patients tended to decrease circulating vitamin E levels. A few subjects had ascorbic acid values persistently below 0.3 mg/dl; this may have been caused by losses of this vitamin during storage for 30 hours of half of the solutions to be infused. Levels of 25-OH vitamin D and 1:25 $(OH)_2$ vitamin D in 8 individuals over 430 to 588 days on MVI-12 were within reference range, as were parathormone levels. Prothrombin times were normal, with 5 mg of vitamin K oxide added once every week.

In one study, the plasma (mean ± SD) vitamin E levels over 28 to 250 days on this formulation rose from 2.1±4.6 to 16.5±4.6 μmol/L.[180] In another study with some of the same patients receiving HPN,[178] the same multivitamins, and double the volume of Intralipid, the plasma α-tocopherol levels were 17.5 ± 6.6 μmol in 7 patients.[187]

In another report on vitamin E levels in patients receiving long-term HPN, the average plasma α-tocopherol level was 11.14 μmol/L, compared to normal values of 18.11 μmol/L; this finding was associated with significantly higher breath pentane levels in these patients.[188] Breath pentane was used as a measure of lipid peroxidation. A negative correlation was noted between pentane levels and those of plasma tocopherol.

A major function of vitamin D is to improve the efficiency of absorption of calcium and phosphate by the small intestine. Because parenteral nutrition annuls this route, why is this vitamin included in parenteral solutions? Calcitriol, as the active form of vitamin D, plays an intimate role with parathyroid hormone in the mobilization of calcium from bone, and the vitamin plays a role in cellular differentiation (see Chap. 17). Whether the current parenteral dosage recommendations are higher than necessary for these functions remains to be demonstrated.

THIAMIN DEFICIENCY

I am dismayed by the persistence of reports of severe thiamin deficiency in patients receiving TPN despite (1) the easy availability of its parenteral preparation in multivitamin or individual form, (2) the widespread knowledge of its increased need with use of high-glucose formulas, and (3) the fairly rapid onset (1 to 2 months) of life-threatening metabolic changes characteristic of its deficiency. Five reports have described 12 cases,[189–193] with 4 deaths;[189,193] 11 patients had severe lactic acidosis,[189–192] and 1 had peripheral neuropathy and ataxia.[193] A patient with Crohn's disease who was receiving long-term TPN was given a daily TPN formula containing 1.24 mg thiamin as Soluvit; this was added in the pharmacy and was sent to the outpatient, so a proportion of the solution was stored for several days before use.[193]

PEDIATRIC NEEDS

Greene et al. have summarized research on vitamin levels in term-gestation infants and children and problems related to the needs of preterm and underweight newborn infants.[145,194] These investigators have concluded that "the vitamin dosages suggested for children in the 1975 AMA report appear adequate for continued use in term infants and children up to 11 years of age." This formulation is commercially available as MVI-Pediatric (see Table 80–9). Use of this formulation for underweight infants was found to increase blood tocopherol to a high level; the manufacturer and the FDA then recommended that the daily dose be reduced successively to 65% and then to one third of a vial for infants <1000 g. The last level may prove to be too low. Further problems have surfaced in providing this formulation to very LBW infants; these include large losses of retinol through the delivery sets and elevated riboflavin and vitamin B_6 plasma levels.[194] Greene et al. have recommended a revised formulation for the very LBW infant (see Table 80–9); currently, this is not in production.

COMPLICATIONS IN HOSPITAL AND AT HOME

Relevant complications include (1) fluid and electrolyte abnormalities, (2) other nutrient deficiencies or excesses, (3) metabolic problems that increase or decrease normal nutrient needs, such as diabetes and various organ failures, and present problems in maintaining homeostasis, (4) sepsis, (5) difficulties associated with initiating or maintaining patent venous access,[195] and (6) certain disorders related directly to intravenous feeding, including liver dysfunction, gallstones, and decreased bone mass; these vary in degree and the causes are not completely known. Many of these complications can be prevented or minimized by having responsibility vested in experienced physicians, nurses, and pharmacists working as a team and by exercising close supervision of inpatients and outpatients.

HEPATIC DYSFUNCTION

Since the first description of TPN-associated cholestasis and early cirrhosis in 1971 in a premature infant,[196] a large and continuing literature has confirmed TPN as a contributing risk factor for hepatobiliary dysfunction of varying degree and incidence. Reviews of the biochemical, clinical, and histopathologic changes in adults and children have emphasized the multifactorial nature of the problem.[197,198,248] In children, the degree of prematurity, infection, the inability to consume food orally, the extent of intestinal dysfunction, the number of surgical procedures, the duration of TPN, and the long-term administration of excessive calories are associated risk factors.[197–200] Immaturity of the hepatic excretory function and of the enterohepatic circulation, particularly in the neonate, is one of the reasons for the development of cholestasis. Cholestasis has been reported in various series to occur from 7.4 to 42.1% of infants, with wide variations among differing populations, criteria, hospital practices, and clinical conditions.[201]

In adults, preexisting liver and other diseases, sepsis, preexisting malnutrition, extent of bowel resection and/or damage (such as from radiation), excess nonprotein calories, little or no oral intake, and duration on TPN are also associated risk factors. Increases may occur in serum transaminase, alkaline phosphatase, α-glutamyltransferase and, less frequently, bilirubin as indicators of hepatic dysfunction.

Fatty liver (steatosis), intrahepatic cholestasis, and portal inflammation can occur, particularly in children, but also in adults, it can progress to portal tract fibrosis and infiltration, liver failure, and death.

In adult patients receiving long-term TPN (median 18 months) who were given a relative excess of carbohydrate, abnormal fat, and amino acids, hepatic function tests and cholestatic changes were present; jaundice was reversed, liver function tests and histologic features improved when the amounts of these macronutrients were reduced.[202] Other investigators have noted increasing steatosis with administration of excess calories, either as carbohydrate or lipid, or both.[203,204]

What is the relationship between the extent of bowel resection and the development of serious hepatic dysfunction in patients receiving long-term TPN? Data from various studies suggest strongly that patients with little or no remaining small intestine are at increased risk of developing serious hepatic dysfunction with fibrotic changes;[205] the rapidity of development and the severity of the disease vary among series.

A variety of agents have been tested on patients receiving TPN who have developed evidence of associated significant hepatic dysfunction and who require continued TPN. Mention has been made previously that a mixture of MCT and LCT as the IV lipid source given to patients receiving TPN did not cause a change in liver size or gray-scale value (an indication of fat and connective tissue), whereas LCT infusion increased both.[113] On the grounds that metronidazole could depress the formation by intestinal bacteria of potentially damaging bile acids, this drug has been tested in patients receiving TPN and has been reported by some to reduce increases in liver enzymes as compared to untreated control subjects.[198,206] Ursodeoxycholic acid, (UDCA) an epimer of chenodeoxycholic acid, which is used for gallstone dissolution and has been found beneficial for patients with primary biliary cirrhosis, was given to a patient receiving TPN who had developed marked jaundice during previous treatment by reduction of TPN calories and in whom administration of metronidazole had been ineffective.[207] Jaundice and enzyme abnormalities regressed, and the patient's clinical condition improved; discontinuance of the UDCA resulted in a return of his jaundice, which again regressed when this drug was administered.

Choline in the form of lecithin was given orally in a double-blind, randomized study with a placebo control to patients receiving long-term TPN who had low plasma choline levels and hepatic steatosis, as determined by computed tomography (CT) scanning.[208] The lecithin supplement was associated with a significant and progressive decline in the CT evidence of steatosis. A more recent brief report notes regression of steatosis by CT scan with IV choline chloride at 1 to 4 weeks.[209] The number of patients given lecithin or choline was small. No liver biopsies were done in either report. Liver enzymes and other biochemical changes with lecithin were often within normal limits at baseline.[205] Although choline depletion may be a possible cause of steatosis in such patients, further studies are required to settle this issue. Choline is a constituent of the egg phosphatide in lipid emusions; 100 ml Intralipid, for example, supplies about 120 mg choline (in addition, choline is derived from methionine). If choline depletion occurs, some factors must increase choline needs.

GALLSTONES

Sludge in the gallbladder has been observed repeatedly as a TPN- and bowel rest-associated risk factor; this situation can progress to gallstone formation as the duration of TPN increases. Patients who receive long-term TPN maintenance usually malabsorb bile salt because of resection or disease of the terminal ileum. Thus, the body's bile salt pool decreases, and consequently, fewer bile salts accumulate in the gallbladder. This situation, in turn, increases the tendency of cholesterol to precipitate in the bile and thus form the nidus of gallstones. One also sees an increase in unconjugated bilirubin and calcium, and these substances are present in the stones that form from the sludge that accumulates in the gallbladder.[210,211] Stasis and resulting sludge were prevented in the prairie dog model given daily injections of cholecystokinin.[212]

Ultrasonography indicated development of biliary sludge within 12 days of starting TPN in 14 of 23 patients; by 6 weeks, all had sludge, with 6 developing stones and 3 requiring surgery. The sludge was noted to disappear 4 weeks after instituting oral feeding.[213] Nine of 29 children receiving TPN developed cholelithiasis; 64% of those with ileal disorders or resection developed stones.[214] Emergency cholecystectomy was performed in 35 patients with TPN-associated gallbladder disease (23 adults and 12 children; the operative morbidity was 54% and hospital mortality 11%).[215] The experience with infants is noted later. Because of such potential problems, the following suggestions have been made for management of such patients at risk: if food can be ingested safely, it should be taken orally or by tube routinely, in an effort to decrease biliary stasis; ultrasonic examination should be performed periodically to detect the development of biliary sludge and stones; when stones are first detected, elective cholecystectomy should be considered; if laparotomy is to be done for any reason, cholecystectomy should be performed at that time.

METABOLIC BONE DISEASE

Rickets has been described in infants who are receiving parenteral nutrition;[216] the need for more calcium and phosphate in the small fluid volume required by the neonate appeared to be the causative factor, rather than provision of more vitamin D.

Reference has been made to the role of aluminum contamination of casein hydrolysate and its effects on bone.[146,171] Patients on TPN were studied while receiving casein hydrolysate and again after conversion to TPN with crystalline amino acids.[217] The conversion was associated with increased bone formation and reduced osteoid area; reduced aluminum at the bone surface and plasma was noted, as was reduced calcium excretion.

Examination of the histomorphologic features of bone in relation to formula composition have been made in patients receiving long-term HPN (see Chap. 54 for a discussion of this technique). In a prospective study in Toronto, crystalline amino acids were used, although some of the patients had received casein hydrolysate some time previously. Bone biopsies initially showed a hyperkinetic pattern, possibly resulting from initial malnutrition;[218] at 6 to 73 months on HTPN, the histologic features changed; 12 of 16 patients had some degree of osteomalacia. Three had bone pain and 2 had lumbar vertebral compression. In this study, 500 IU (12.5 μg = 32.5 nmol) of vitamin D_2 were given every other day; all other vitamins were supplied with the exception of biotin. Because 7 of these patients were hypercalcemic and 6 had elevated 25(OH) vitamin D levels, further studies were performed on 11 patients before and after withdrawal of vitamin D_2 (and, by necessity, the accompanying vitamin A for 6 months).[219] Six of 10 patients had a lower osteoid elevation and increased tetracycline uptake with the vitamin modification, but there was continuing evidence of a high turnover rate. In the 3 symptomatic patients, bone pain subsided, fractures healed, and urinary loss of calcium and phosphate was decreased.[218,219] It was recommended that "vitamin D solutions not be added to total parenteral nutrition of home patients."[219] The mechanism of the postulated adverse role of this vitamin was not delineated.

Another study, in New York City, was of 12 patients who had been receiving HPN and had been taking crystalline amino acids (with the exception of 2 patients who had been transferred from casein hydrolysate 6 years earlier). Average vitamin D intake over the years had been 284 IU (7.1 μg) replaced 3 to 10 months earlier by 200 IU (5 μg) daily. Histomorphometry with tetracycline labeling revealed osteopenia, subnormal osteoid volume, and normal trabecular osteoid seam width; the calcification rate was normal. Of the 7 women, 4 were in the 66- to 77-year range, and at least 1 had been a heavy cigarette smoker for many years. Six patients had minor bone complaints associated with osteoarthritis or postmenopausal osteoporosis.[220] The reasons for the marked difference in the histologic features of bone between the Toronto and New York studies are not apparent. The TPN formulas in the New York study had appreciably fewer fat calories and proportionately more glucose calories and a different vitamin formulation including biotin; normal serum calcium, PTH, and calcitriol values were obtained.[220]

A group of 12 patients receiving long-term HPN who either had never been given casein hydrolysate or had received it for only a short while were compared to 16 healthy volunteers with respect to histomorphometry of iliac bone biopsies. Most subjects were women of postmenopausal age in both groups. A variety of abnormal histologic findings were noted in the patients receiving TPN indicating that neither increased tissue osteoid nor depressed bone formation was necessarily a concomitant of parenteral nutrition.[221]

Comparison of a group of patients receiving long-term HPN (mean 55, range 9.5 to 90 months) with a group of patients who had received TPN at home for appreciably shorter periods (mean 3.9, range 1 to 7.5 months) using dual-photon absorptiometry indicated that, in the first group, the vertebral bone mass was reduced but not that of the appendicular skeleton, presumably because most of the bone mass loss occurred in trabecular bone.[222] In a short-term study of seven patients on TPN for 7±2 months, a low-remodeling bone disease was noted with reduced bone formation, subnormal osteoclastic activity, low trabecular bone volume, decreased osteoid surface, and osteoid volume lower than normal. No aluminum stain was found, but aluminum ingestion was estimated at 253±84 μg/dl because of contamination of the phosphate.[223] Children receiving long-term TPN who had not been exposed to aluminum-contaminated casein hydrolysate and whose aluminum level was within normal limits were found to have more than a 35% loss of trabecular bone mineral but were asymptomatic.[224]

With the exception of the observation of the Toronto study,[218,219] osteomalacia was not present in bone biopsies of any of the other studies in which aluminum contamination was not a significant factor. The amounts of vitamin D given to adults in most studies were similar to the dosage given in the Toronto study. Serial histomorphometric examinations in prospective longitudinal studies of patients receiving long-term TPN in comparison with age-, sex-, and activity-matched healthy individuals are warranted to shed further light on this TPN-related and multifactorial bone disease.[146]

COMPATIBILITY OF DRUGS WITH TPN SOLUTIONS

The frequency of drug interventions for coexistent illnesses or complications of TPN requires assurances that administration of a drug as part of the TPN solution or in conjunction with that solution will not produce incompatibility or an adverse reaction. Significant information on this issue has been summarized.[225]

HOME PARENTERAL NUTRITION (HPN)

Since the first patients were discharged from hospital to home on parenteral nutrition in 1969 and the early 1970s,[226–228] this form of primary outpatient nutritional support has mushroomed. To collect and compile the data being obtained by an increasing number of medical centers who discharge patients on HPN, an HPN registry for the United States and Canada was activated at the New York Academy under my direction during the years 1978 to 1983. Some of this information was published.[229] In 1984, this registry became a joint effort of the Oley Foundation and the American Society for Enteral and Parenteral Nutrition and has been termed the OASIS Registry under the direction of Lyn Howard, M.B., in Albany, New York.

Issues related to suitability, training, formulations, and home support have been extensively studied,[230] and standards on organization, patient selection, and management have been developed.[231] Some current problems and complications are discussed in this and other chapters.

BENEFITS

A summary for the years 1984 to 1987 of 1594 patients receiving HPN in 7 disease categories has been published by the OASIS Registry.[232] Patients in disease categories of a stable nature for the most part, such as short bowel syndrome (resulting from resection for ischemic bowel disease, radiation enteritis, and Crohn's disease with resection) and congenital bowel dysfunction, have had fairly long-term clinical courses with a 3-year survival of 65 to 80%; 49% have had complete rehabilitation. These patients averaged 2.6 complications requiring hospitalization per year. On the other hand, those receiving HPN who had active cancer, AIDS, and certain bowel dysfunctions (other than massive bowel resection or radiation enteritis) had a mean survival of 6 months, 4.6 complications per year, and about 15% complete rehabilitation.

An analysis of 63 patients, aged 11 to 75 years, receiving HPN who had short bowel syndrome and chronic intestinal obstruction with or without intestinal resection indicated that body weight was well maintained on cyclic 8- to 12-hour overnight infusion; 78% returned to relatively normal life styles, with a 5% annual mortality.[233] Periodic abnormal biochemical test values occurred, and 73% needed readmission to hospitals, however, mainly for suspected catheter sepsis.

One of the more dramatic successes of HPN concerns its effectiveness in the management and outcome of the newborn with various abnormalities of the gastrointestinal tract requiring extensive intestinal resection. Parenteral nutrition has transformed the outcome of such infants and has allowed them to grow normally during the relatively long periods required for hyperplastic adaption of the remaining bowel; HPN has allowed them to be discharged home to continue their nutritional support in a supportive psychosocial environment.

In his major review of the literature prior to 1972, Wilmore noted that 11 infants with <15 cm of remaining jejunum and ileum (JI) died, as did all 5 with only 15 to 38 cm without an ileocolic valve (ICV); of 14 infants with

15 to 38 cm remaining, with and without a remaining ICV, 7 died.[234] Data from several experiences reveal major benefits ascribable in large part to parenteral nutrition in hospital and at home, but also to improvements in surgical procedures, intensive care, and supportive medications. In the management of such patients, the entry of food into the alimentary tract is necessary to achieve the earliest maximal bowel adaptation. Hence, when feasible, oral or tube feeding is a desirable accompaniment to the parenteral nutrition program.

In a Los Angeles HPN program for the years 1977 to 1984, 13 children were left with≦ 38 cm JI beginning in the first month of life: of these, 69% survived, as compared with 23% previously.[235] Five of these had HPN discontinued after 4 to 32 months and had normal growth and development, whereas 2 remained on partial HPN after 9 and 55 months, and 2 required TPN after 66 and 68 months; these 4 children have grown normally. Of those with 15 to 38 cm without an ICV and those with <15 cm with and without an ICV, 70% survived (compared to none in Wilmore's review); 3 of the 10 discontinued HPN. "Ultimate survival with normal growth and without HPN is now possible with as little as 11 cm residual JI and an intact ICV and as little as 25 cm JI without an ICV."[235]

The course of 87 children managed from 1970 to 1988 in a Paris hospital were analyzed. HPN was introduced in 1980. Fourteen of the 16 deaths occurred before 1980. Of those with less than 40 cm JI who were born before 1980, 42% survived. Of those born after 1980, 94% survived. The presence of an ICV did not significantly affect survival. The average time required for the acquisition of adequate bowel adaption was 27.3 months for those with <40 cm and 14 months for those with 40 to 80 cm.[236]

Gallstones were a significant problem. Of the 13 patients with ≦38cm in the Los Angeles study, 6 had to have a cholecystectomy.[235] In the Paris study, the frequent occurrence of gallstones led to the policy of routine cholecystectomy whenever total or subtotal resection of the terminal ileum was performed.[236]

COST EFFECTIVENESS

Estimates of the cost of HPN vary from $75,000 to $150,000 per patient year.[232] A patient who underwent HPN who compared costs from 10 providers in 1989 was reported to have found a cost range of $73,000 to $183,000.[233]

Many factors enter into the total cost of maintaining a patient on HPN; such charges vary considerably, depending in part on the method used in their estimations and on differences in the perspectives chosen for the analyses, particularly the matter of estimating benefits gained and/or the effectiveness gained. Goel has discussed these issues and has reviewed the pertinent literature relating to hospital TPN and to HPN.[237] Daily costs of HPN were lower than those of hospital TPN by an estimated 60 to 70%.

Goel has summarized factors involved in cost-effectiveness analysis, the variability in determining precise costs, and the inclusion of effectiveness as measured by quality-adjusted life-year (QALY);[237] the last is a composite measure of both life expectancy and morbidity. The only cost-effectiveness analysis of HPN that has been reported compared the cost of HPN in a cohort of 72 patients from 1970 to 1982 in Toronto, with the alternative cost basis being those that would have accrued from intermittent hospital care including TPN on each admission for the same patients not receiving HPN. It was concluded that HPN was cost effective.[238]

PSYCHOSOCIAL ISSUES

HPN presents certain stress factors to the patient and family members.[239] These begin with suddenly having to cope with the technical aspects and safety measures of HPN after hospital discharge. They include the issues of management of handicaps resulting from primary and secondary illness and their treatments and concerns about meeting costs and the patient's dependency, with the danger of excessive dependence on family members. Essential for a smooth transition to home care are (1) adequate predischarge assessment and training of the patient and family in HPN management and (2) assurance of and provision of close support by the health-care team by telephone contact and follow-up at home or in the physician's office to ensure that the patient's condition remains satisfactory. Dietary intake and other factors at home may require modification of the parenteral nutritional formulation from that deemed satisfactory in the hospital setting. Involvement both of the social worker, to ensure that all are coping satisfactorily, and of ancillary support personnel, such as the physical therapist, is often helpful in the postdischarge period. These issues are discussed in more detail elsewhere.[230–232,239]

Issues concerning nutrition support decision making for the competent and incompetent patient and for the terminally ill are reviewed in Chapters 73 and 81 and elsewhere.[230,231]

SMALL BOWEL TRANSPLANTATION

Successful small bowel transplantation was demonstrated to be technically feasible in the late 1950s.[240] Until the late 1980s, attempts were unsuccessful because the immunosuppressive drugs available in that period were unable to prevent rejection of the transplanted intestine.[240,241] With the availability of cyclosporine and other agents in 1989, single successful transplants (of several or more attempts) of isolated bowel were reported from Kiel and Paris,[241] and a successful combined liver-small bowel transplantation was performed in London, Ontario.[242]

Increasing numbers of successful combined transplants (e.g., liver and intestine) and transplants of small bowel only have been reported.[241,249] Because failure occurs as well as success and because the goal is a high rate of successful transplantation of small bowel alone, intestinal transplantation is still regarded as experimental for those primarily dependent on HPN.

EFFECT OF TROPHIC AGENTS

Standard TPN solutions do not appear to support a variable proportion of malnourished or hypercatabolic patients with trauma, surgery, sepsis, cancer, and AIDS (with a secondary infection) efficiently. The problem is epitomized by the failure to uniformly develop a net positive peripheral uptake of amino acids despite adequate provision of energy and known essential nutrients.[243–246] Strategies to improve this situation include (1) having the patient perform regular exercise,[243] (2) providing increased amounts of certain nutrients such as arginine,[244] BCAA,[244] and n-3 polyunsaturated fatty acids,[244] (3) providing certain nutrients not currently standard in most TPN formulations, such as glutamine,[123–130,244] (4) blocking the signals of interleukins, which initiate responses to inflammation,[244,246] and (5) providing hormones and related growth factors that appear to enhance protein retention such as recombinant human growth factor and insulin-like growth factor,[243,244] the β-adrenergic agonist clenbuterol (see Chap. 73), and low-dose bradykinin.[247] It remains to be conclusively demonstrated that exercise or any of these or related agents, singly or in combination, will have a persistent positive influence on amino acid flux in muscle without significant undesirable side effects in hypercatabolic patients receiving parenteral nutrition.

REFERENCES

1. Elman, R.: Parenteral Alimentation in Surgery. New York, Paul B. Hoeber, 1947.
2. Gamble, J.L.: Pediatrics, *11:*554–567, 1953.
3. Levenson, S.M., Hopkin, B.S., Waldron, M., et al.: Fed. Proc., *43:*1391–1406, 1984.
4. Seibert, F.B.: Am. J. Physiol., *67:*90–104, 1923.
5. DuBois, E.F.: Basal Metabolism in Health and Disease. Philadelphia, Lea & Febiger, 1924, pp. 237–288.
6. Cuthbertson, D.P.: Q. J. Med., *1:*233–246, 1932.
7. Spies, T.D. (Ed.): Med. Clin. North Am., *27:*273–600, 1943.
8. Levenson, S.M., Green, R.W., Lund, C.C.: Ann. Surg., *124:*840–856, 1946.
9. Ellison, E.H., McCleery, R.S., Zollinger, R.M., et al.: Surgery, *26:*374–383, 1949.
10. Schuberth, O., Wretlind, A.: Acta Chir. Scand., *278(Suppl.):*1–21, 1961.
11. Dudrick, S., Wilmore, D.W., Vars, H.M., et al.: Surgery, *64:*134–142, 1968.
12. Winters, R.W., Heird, W.C., Dell, R.B.: Fed. Proc., *43:*1407–1411, 1984.
13. Shils, M.E.: Fed. Proc., *43:*1412–1416, 1984.
14. Co Tui, Wright, A.M., Mulholland, J.H., et al.: Ann. Surg., *120:*99–122, 1944.
15. Co Tui, Wright, A.M., Mulholland, J.H., et al.: Gastroenterology, *5:*5–17, 1945.
16. Watkin, D.M., Steinfeld, J.L.: Am. J. Clin. Nutr., *16:*182–212, 1965.
17. Wolk, R.A., Rayburn, W.F.: Nutr. Clin. Pract., *5:*139–152, 1990.
18. Chin, D.E., Kearns, P.: Nutr. Clin. Pract., *6:*213–222, 1991.
19. Ott, L., Young, B.: Nutr. Clin. Pract., *6:*223–229, 1991.
20. Konvolinka, C.W., Morell, V.O.: Nutr. Clin. Pract., *6:*281–255, 1991.
21. Veterans Affairs Total Parenteral Nutrition Cooperative Study Group: N. Engl. J. Med., *325:*525–532, 1991.
22. Detsky, A.S.: N. Engl. J. Med., *325:*573–575, 1991 (Edit.).
23. Campos, A.C.L., Meguid, M.M.: Am. J. Clin. Nutr., *55:*117–130, 1992.
24. Freeman, J.B., Fairful-Smith, R.J.: Physiologic approach to peripheral parenteral nutrition. *In* Surgical Nutrition. Edited by J.E. Fischer. Boston, Little, Brown, 1983, pp. 703–717.
25. Hoshal, V.: Arch. Surg., *110:*644–646, 1975.
26. Dudrick, S.J., Wilmore, D.W., Vars, H.M., et al.: Ann. Surg., *169:*974–984, 1969.
27. Jeejeebhoy, K.N., Zohrab, W.J., Langer, B., et al.: Gastroenterology, *65:*811–820, 1973.
28. Broviac, J.W., Cole, J.J., Scribner, B.H.: Surg. Gynecol. Obstet., *136:*602–606, 1973.
29. Joyeux, J., Astruc, B., Martin, G., et al.: J. Chir. (Paris), *107:*335–366, 1974.
30. Zincke, H., Hirsche, B.L., Amamoo, D.G., et al.: Surg. Gynecol. Obstet., *139:*350–352, 1974.
31. Heizer, W.D., Orringer, E.P.: Gastroenterology, *72:*527–532, 1977.
32. Shils, M.E., Wright, W.L., Turnbull, A., et al.: N. Engl. J. Med., *283:*341–344, 1970.
33. Malt, R.A., Kempter, M.: JPEN J. Parenter. Enteral Nutr., *7:*580–581, 1983.
34. Krog, M., Gerdin, B.: JPEN J. Parenter. Enteral Nutr., *13:*666–667, 1989.
35. Fonkalsrud, E.W., Berquist, W., Burke, M., et al.: Am. J. Surg., *143:*209–211, 1982.
36. Oram-Smith, J.C., Muller, J.L., Harken, A.H., et al.: Surgery, *83:*274–276, 1979.
37. Lokich, J.J., Bothe, A., Jr., Benotti, P.: J. Clin. Oncol., *3:*710–717, 1985.
38. Belin, R.P., Koster, J.K., Bryant, L.J., et al.: Surg. Gynecol. Obstet., *134:*491–493, 1972.
39. Flowers, J.F., Ryan, J.A., Jr., Gough, J.A.: Catheter-related complications of total parenteral nutrition. *In* Total Parenteral Nutrition. 2nd Ed. Edited by J.E. Fischer. Boston, Little, Brown, 1991, pp. 25–45.

40. Clark-Christoff, N., Watters, V.A., Sparks, W., et al.: JPEN J. Parenter. Enteral Nutr., *16:*403–407, 1992.
41. Williams, W.W.: JPEN J. Parent. Enteral Nutr., *9:*735–746, 1985.
42. Shils, M.E.: Am. J. Clin. Nutr., *28:*1429–1435, 1975.
43. Newsome, H.H., Jr., Armstrong, C.W., Mayhall, G.C., et al.: JPEN J. Parenter. Enteral Nutr., *8:*560–562, 1984.
44. Keohane, P.P., Jones, B.J.M., Attrill, H., et al.: Lancet, *2:*1388–1390, 1983.
45. Press, O.W., Ramsey, P.G., Larson, E.B., et al.: Medicine, *63:*189–200, 1984.
46. Peterson, F.B., Clift R.A., Hickman, R.O., et al.: JPEN J. Parenter. Enteral Nutr., *10:*58–62, 1986.
47. Allwood, M.C.: Int. J. Pharm., *29:*233–236, 1986.
48. Seres, D.S.: Nutr. Clin. Pract., *5:*111–117, 1990.
49. McMahon, M., Manji, N., Driscoll, D.F., et al.: JPEN J. Parenter. Enteral Nutr., *13:*545–553, 1989.
50. Shaw, S.N., Elwyn, D.H., Askanazi, J., et al.: Am. J. Clin. Nutr., *37:*930–940, 1983.
51. Rudman, E., Millikan, W.J., Richardson, T.J., et al.: J. Clin. Invest., *55:*94–104, 1975.
52. Wolman, S.L., Anderson, G.H., Marliss, E.B., et al.: Gastroenterology, *76:*458–467, 1979.
53. Starker, P.M., LaSala, P.A., Askanazi, J., et al.: Ann. Surg., *198:*720–724, 1983.
54. Starker, P.M., LaSala, P.A., Forse, A., et al.: JPEN J. Parenter. Enteral Nutr., *9:*300–302, 1985.
55. Fryburg, D.A., Gelfand, R.A.: JPEN J. Parenter. Enteral Nutr., *14:* 535–537, 1990.
56. Woods, H.F., Alberti, K.G.M.M.: Lancet, *2:*1354–1357, 1972.
57. Georgieff, M., Moldawer, L.L., Bistrian, B.R., et al.: JPEN J. Parenter. Enteral Nutr., *9:*199–209, 1985.
58. Young, E.A., Drummond, A., Cool, D.A., et al.: J. Clin. Endocrinol. Metab., *50:*764–772, 1980.
59. Young, E.A., Fletcher, J.T., Cioletti, L.A., et al.: JPEN J. Parenter. Enteral Nutr., *5:*369–377, 1981.
60. Waxman, K., Day, A.T., Stellin, G.P., et al.: JPEN J. Parenter. Enteral Nutr., *16:*374–378, 1992.
61. Lev-Ram, A., Johnson, J., Hwang, D.L., et al.: JPEN J. Parenter. Enteral Nutr., *11:*271–274, 1987.
62. Byrne, W.J., Lippe, B.M., Strobel, C.T., et al.: Gastroenterology, *80:*947–956, 1981.
63. Wolfe, R.R., Allsop, J.R., Burke, J.F.: Metabolism, *28:*210–220, 1979.
64. Burke, J.F., Wolfe, R.R., Mullany, C.J., et al.: Ann. Surg., *190:*274–283, 1979.
65. Wolfe, R., O'Donnell, T.F., Jr., Stone, M.D., et al.: Metabolism, *29:*892–900, 1980.
66. Shaw, J.H.F., Wolfe, R.R.: Ann. Surg., *209:*63–72, 1989.
67. Flatt, J.P.: The biochemistry of energy expenditure. *In* Recent Advances in Obesity Research. Edited by G. Bray. London, Newman, 1978, pp. 211–228.
68. Elwyn, D.H., Grump, F.E., Munroe, H.N., et al.: Am. J. Clin. Nutr., *32:*1597–1611, 1979.
69. Askanazi, J., Carpentier, Y.A., Elwyn, D.H., et al.: Ann. Surg., *191:*40–46, 1980.
70. Nordenstrom, J., Carpentier, Y.A., Askanazi, J., et al.: Ann. Surg., *198:*725–735, 1983.
71. MacFie, J., Halmfield, J.H.M., King, R.F.G., et al.: JPEN J. Parenter. Enteral Nutr., *7:*1–5, 1983.
72. Askanazi, J., Rosenbaum, S.H., Hyman, A.I., et al.: JAMA, *243:*1444–1447, 1980.
73. Chait, A., Foster, D., Miller, D.G., et al.: Proc. Soc. Exp. Biol. Med., *168:*97–104, 1981.
74. Barr, L.H., Dunn, G.D., Brennan, M.F.: Surgery, *193:*304–311, 1981.
75. Carlsson, L.A.: Scand. Lab. Invest., *40:*139–144, 1980.
76. Carpentier, Y.A., Richelle, M., Haumart, D., et al.: Proc. Nutr. Soc., *49:*375–380, 1990.
77. Adamkin, D.H., Gelke, K.N., Andrews, B.F.: JPEN J. Parenteral. Enteral Nutr., *8:*563–567, 1984.
78. Jeejeebhoy, K.N., Marliss, E.B., Anderson, G.H., et al.: Lipid in parenteral nutrition: studies of clinical and metabolic features. *In* Fat Emulsions in Parenteral Nutrition. Edited by H.C. Meng and D.W. Wilmore. Chicago, American Medical Association, 1976, pp. 45–54.
79. Seidel, D., Alaupovic, P., Furman, R.: J. Clin. Invest., *48:*1211–1223, 1969.
80. Rigaud, D., Serog., P., Legrand, A., et al.: JPEN J. Parenter. Enteral Nutr., *8:*529–534, 1984.
81. Messing, B., Peynet, J., Poupon, J., et al.: Am. J. Clin. Nutr., *52:*1094–1100, 1990.
82. Tashiro, T., Mashima, Y., Yamamori, H., et al.: JPEN J. Parenter. Enteral Nutr., *15:*546–550, 1991.
83. Elwyn, D.H., Kinney, J.M., Gump, F.E., et al.: Metabolism, *29:*125–132, 1980.
84. Goodenough, R.D., Wolfe, R.R.: JPEN J. Parenter. Enteral Nutr., *8:*357–360, 1984.
85. Smith, R.D., Mackie, W., Kohlhardt, S.R., et al.: Surgery, *111:*12–20, 1992.
86. Elwyn, D.H.: Repletion of the malnourished patient. *In* Amino Acids: Metabolism and Medical Application. Edited by G.L. Blackburn, J.P. Grant, V.R. Young, et al. Boston, P.S.G., 1983, pp. 359–375.
87. Long, J.M., Wilmore, D.W., Mason, A.D., et al.: Ann. Surg., *185:*417–422, 1977.
88. Jeejeebhoy, K.N.: Lipid emulsions. *In* Total Parenteral Nutrition. 2nd Ed. Edited by J.E. Fischer. Boston, Little, Brown, 1991, pp. 410–413.
89. Davis, S.S.: The stability of fat emulsions for intravenous administration. *In* Advances in Clinical Nutrition. Edited by I.D.A. Johnson. Boston, MTP Press, 1983, pp. 214–239.
90. Rollins, C.J.: JPEN J. Parenter. Enteral Nutr., *16:*296–297, 1992 (lett.).
91. Bullock, L., Fitzgerald, J.F., Walter, W.V.: JPEN J. Parenter. Enteral Nutr., *16:*64–68, 1992.
92. Deitel, M., Friedman, K.L., Cunnane, S., et al.: J. Am. Coll. Nutr., *11:*5–10, 1992.
93. Simmons, B.P., Hooten, T.M., Wang, E.S., et al.: J. Natl. Intrav. Ther. Assoc., *5:*40–46, 1982.
94. Rubin, M., Bilik, R., Aserin, A., et al.: JPEN J. Parenter. Enteral Nutr., *13:*641–643, 1989.
95. Campbell, A.N., Freedman, M.H., Pencharz, P.B., et al.: JPEN J. Parenter. Enteral Nutr., *8:*447–449, 1984.
96. Greene, H.C., Hazlett, D., Demaree, R.: Am. J. Clin. Nutr., *29:*127–135, 1975.
97. Pereira, G.R., Fox, W.W., Stanley, C.A., et al.: Pediatrics, *66:*26–30, 1980.
98. Sundstrom, G., Zaunder, C.W., Arborelius, M., Jr.: J. Appl. Physiol., *34:*816–820, 1973.
99. Schmidt, B.F., Allen, R., Chandler, C., et al.: Surg. Forum, *37:*84–86, 1986.
100. Wolfe, B.M., Suda, S.A.: JPEN J. Parenter. Enteral Nutr., *12(Suppl. 6):*59S–61S, 1988.
101. Gutcher, G.R., Farrell, P.M.: Am. J. Clin. Nutr., *54:*1024–1028, 1991.
102. Kollef, M.H., McCormack, M.T., Caras, W.E., et al.: Ann. Intern. Med., *112:*545–546, 1990.

103. Fischer, G.W., Hunter, K.W., Wilson, S.R., et al.: Lancet, *1:*819–820, 1980.
104. Cleary, T.G., Pickering, L.K.: J. Clin. Lab. Immunol., *11:*21–26, 1983.
105. Sobrado, J., Moldawer, L., Pomposelli, J., et al.: Am. J. Clin. Nutr., *42:*855–863, 1985.
106. Ota, D.M., Jessup, J.M., Babcock, G.E., et al.: JPEN J. Parenter. Enteral Nutr., *9:*23–27, 1985.
107. Müller, J.M., Keller, H.W., Brenner, U., et al.: World J. Surg., *10:*53–63, 1986.
108. American College of Physicians Position Paper: Ann. Intern. Med., *110:*734–736, 1989.
109. Desai, T.K., Kinzie, J.: JPEN J. Parenter. Enteral Nutr., *14(Suppl.):*75, 1990 (abstr.).
110. Freeman, J., Goldmann, D.A., Smith, N.E., et al.: N. Engl. J. Med., *323:*301–308, 1990; *324:*268, 1991 (lett.).
111. Mascioli, E.A., Babayan, V.K., Bistrian, B.R., et al.: JPEN J. Parenter. Enteral, Nutr., *12(Suppl. 6):*127S–132S, 1988.
112. Babayam, V.K.: Lipids, *22:*417–420, 1987.
113. Baldermann, H., Wicklmayr, M., Rett, K., et al.: JPEN J. Parenter. Enteral Nutr., *15:*601–603, 1991.
114. Ball, M.J.: Am. J. Clin. Nutr., *53:*916–922, 1991.
115. Miles, J.M., Cattalini, M., Sharbrough, F.W., et al.: JPEN J. Parenter. Enteral Nutr., *15:*37–41, 1991.
116. Rossle, C., Carpentier, Y.A., Richelle, M., et al.: Am. J. Physiol., *258:*E944–E947, 1990.
117. Wan, J.M.-F., Teo, T.C., Babayan, V.K., et al.: JPEN J. Parenter. Enteral Nutr., *12(Suppl. 6):*43S–48S, 1988.
118. Wretlind, A.: The application of fat emulsions: history and future perspectives. *In* Nutrition in Clinical Practice. Proceedings of the 10th Congress of the European Society for Parenteral and Enteral Nutrition, Leipzig, 1988. Edited by Hartig, Dietze, Weiner, et al. Basel, Karger, 1989, pp. 71–76.
119. Spielmann, D., Bracco, V., Traitler, H., et al.: JPEN J. Parenter. Enteral Nutr., *12(Suppl. 6):*111S–123S, 1988.
120. Facts and Comparisons Loose Leaf Drug Information Service, St. Louis, 1992.
121. Brennan, M.F., Cerra, F., Daly, J.M., et al.: JPEN J. Parenter. Enteral Nutr., *10:*446–452, 1986.
122. Vinton, N.E., Heckenlively, J.R., Laidlaw, S.A., et al.: Am. J. Clin. Nutr., *52:*895–902, 1990.
123. Souba, W.W. (Ed.): JPEN J. Parenter. Enteral Nutr., *14(Suppl. 4):*39S–146S, 1990.
124. Lowe, D.K., Benfell, K., Smith, R.J., et al.: Am. J. Clin. Nutr., *52:*1101–1106, 1990.
125. Hardy, G., Grimble, G., McElroy, B.: JPEN J. Parenter. Enteral Nutr., *16(Suppl. 1):*30S, 1992 (abstr.).
126. Ziegler, T.R., Young, L.S., Benfell, K., et al.: Ann. Intern. Med., *116:*821–828, 1992.
127. Vinnars, E., Hammarqvist, F., von der Decken, A., et al.: JPEN J. Parenter. Enteral Nutr., *14(Suppl. 4):*125S–129S, 1990.
128. Stehle, P., Zander, J., Mertes, N., et al.: Lancet, *1:*231–233, 1989.
129. Fürst, P., Albers, S., Stehle, P.: JPEN J. Parenter. Enteral Nutr., *14(Suppl. 4):*118S–124S, 1990.
130. Hammarqvist, F., Wernerman, J., von der Decken, et al.: Ann. Surg., *212:*637–644, 1990.
131. Walser, M.: Am. J. Clin. Nutr., *53:*1337–1338, 1991 (edit.).
132. Fürst, P., Stehle, P., Rennie, M.J.: Am. J. Clin. Nutr., *56:*959–960, 1992. (lett.).
133. Walser, M.: Am. J. Clin. Nutr., *56:*960, 1992 (lett.).
134. Palombo, J.D., Schnure, F., Bistrian, B.R., et al.: JPEN J. Parenter. Enteral Nutr., *11:*88–91, 1987.
135. Sulkers, E.J., Lafeber, H.N., Degenhart, H.J., et al.: Am. J. Clin. Nutr., *52:*889–894, 1990.
136. Helms, R.A., Mauer, E.C., Hay, W.W., et al.: JPEN J. Parenter. Enteral Nutr., *14:*448–453, 1990.
137. Pichard, C., Roulet, M., Rössle, C., et al.: JPEN J. Parenter. Enteral Nutr., *12:*555–562, 1988.
138. Moukarzel, A.A.,Dahlstrom, K.A., Buchman, A.L., et al.: J. Pediatr., *120:*759–762, 1992.
139. Adibi, S.A.: Metab. Clin. Exp., *36:*1001–1011, 1987.
140. Vazquez, J.A. Paleos, G.A., Steinhardt, H.J., et al.: Am. J. Clin. Nutr., *44:*24–32, 1986.
141. Lochs, A., Hubl, W., Gasic, S., et al.: Am. J. Physiol., *25:*E155–E160, 1992.
142. Raupp, P., Dries, R., Pfahl, H.G., et al.: JPEN J. Parenter. Enteral Nutr., *15:*469–473, 1991.
143. Hanning, R.M., Atkinson, S.A., Whyte, R.K.: Am. J. Clin. Nutr., *54:*903–908, 1991.
144. Dunham, B., Marcuard, S., Khazanie, P.G., et al.: JPEN J. Parenter. Enteral Nutr., *15:*608–611, 1991.
145. Greene, H.L., Hambidge, M., Schanler, R., et al.: Am. J. Clin. Nutr., *48:*1324–1342, 1988 (rev. reprint issued Dec. 1990).
146. Klein, G.L., Coburn, J.W.: Annu. Rev. Nutr., *11:*93–119, 1991.
147. Berkelhammer, C.H., Wood, R.J., Sitrin, M.D.: Am. J. Clin. Nutr., *48:*1482–1489, 1988.
148. Fleming, C.R.: Am. J. Clin. Nutr., *49:*573–579, 1989.
149. Sayers, M.H., Johnson, K.D., Schumann, L.A., et al.: JPEN J. Parenter. Enteral Nutr., *7:*117–120, 1983.
150. Greene, H.L.: Personal communication.
151. Shils, M.E., Jacobs, D.H.: Personal communication.
152. Shils, M.E., Burke, A.W., Greene, H.L., et al.: JAMA, *241:*2051–2054, 1979.
153. Latimer, J.S., McClain, C.J., Sharp, H.L.: J. Pediatr., *97:*434–437, 1980.
154. Schwarz, K., Peden, V.H.: Nutr. Rev., *40:*81–83, 1982.
155. Solomons, N.W., Layden, T.J., Rosenberg, I.H., et al.: Gastroenterology, *70:*1022–1025, 1976.
156. Phillips, G.D., Garnys, V.P.: JPEN J. Parenter. Enteral Nutr., *5:*11–18, 1981.
157. Shike, M., Roulet, M., Kurian, R., et al.: Gastroenterology, *81:*290–297, 1981.
158. Kurkus, J., Alcock, N.W., Shils, M.E.: JPEN J. Parenter. Enteral Nutr., *8:*254–257, 1984.
159. Shike, M., Ritchie, M.E., Shils, M.E.: Clin. Res., *34:*804A, 1986 (abstr.).
160. Ito, Y., Alcock, N.W., Shils, M.E.: JPEN J. Parenter. Enteral Nutr., *14:*610–614, 1990.
161. Shenkin, A., Fell, G.S., Halls, D.G.: Selenium and chromium requirements during intravenous nutrition. *In* Essential and Toxic Trace Elements in Health and Disease. Edited by A.S. Prasad. New York, Alan R. Liss, 1988, pp. 479–488.
162. Kien, C.L., Veillon, C., Patterson, K.Y., et al.: JPEN J. Parenter. Enteral Nutr., *10:*662–664, 1986.
163. Moukarzel, A.A., Song, M.K., Buchman, A.L., et al.: Lancet, *339:*385–388, 1992.
164. Van Rijn, A.M., Thompson, C.D., McKenzie, J.M., et al.: Am. J. Clin. Nutr., *43:*2076–2085, 1979.
165. Shils, M.E., Levander, O.A., Alcock, N.W.: Am. J. Clin. Nutr., *35:*838, 1982 (abstr.).
166. Rajagopalan, K.V.: Annu. Rev. Nutr., *8:*401–427, 1988.

167. Abumrad, N.N., Schneider, A.J., Steel, D., et al.: Am. J. Clin. Nutr., *34:*2551–2559, 1981.
168. Abumrad, N.N.: Bull. N.Y. Acad. Med., *60:*163–171, 1984.
169. Berner, Y.N., Schuler, T.R., Nielsen, F.J., et al.: Am. J. Clin. Nutr., *50:*1079–1083, 1989.
170. Mahaffey, K.R.: Bull. N.Y. Acad. Med., *60:*196–209, 1984.
171. Klein, G.L., Alfrey, A.C., Miller, N.L., et al.: Am. J. Clin. Nutr., *35:*1425–1429, 1982.
172. Wu, W.W.K., Kaplan, L.A., Horn, J., et al.: JPEN J. Parenter. Enteral Nutr., *10:*591–595, 1986.
173. Klein, G.L., Alfrey, A.A., Shike, M., et al.: Am. J. Clin. Nutr., *53:*399–402, 1991.
174. Vanamee, P., Shils, M.E., Burke, A.W., et al.: JPEN J. Parenter. Enteral Nutr., *3:*258–262, 1979 (adapt. of the orig. AMA Guidelines for Multivitamin Preparations for Parenteral Use, 1977).
175. American Academy of Pediatrics Committee on Drugs: Pediatrics, *76:*635–643, 1985.
176. De Ritter, E.: J. Pharm. Sci., *71:*1073–1096, 1982.
177. Scheiner, J.M., Aranjo, M.M., DeRitter, E.: Am. J. Hosp. Pharm., *38:*1911–1913, 1982.
178. Shils, M.E., Baker, H., Frank, O.: JPEN J. Parenter. Enteral Nutr., *9:*179–188, 1985.
179. Barker, A., Hebron, B.S., Beck, P.R., et al.: JPEN J. Parenter. Enteral Nutr., *8:*3–7, 1984.
180. Chen, M.F., Boyce, H.W., Jr., Triplett, L.: JPEN J. Parenter. Enteral Nutr., *7:*462–464, 1983.
181. Nichoalds, G.E., Meng, H.C., Caldwell, M.D.: Arch. Surg., *112:*1061–1064, 1977.
182. Bradley, J.A., King, R.F.J.G., Schorah, C.J., et al.: Br. J. Surg., *65:*492–494, 1978.
183. Kishi, H., Nishii, S., Ono, T., et al.: Am. J. Clin. Nutr., *32:*332–338, 1979.
184. Stromberg, P., Shenkin, A., Campbell, R.A., et al.: JPEN J. Parenter. Enteral Nutr., *5:*295–299, 1981.
185. Kirkemo, A.K., Burt, M.E., Brennan, M.: Am. J. Clin. Nutr., *35:*1003–1009, 1982.
186. Jeppson, B., Gimmon, Z.: Vitamins. *In* Surgical Nutrition. Edited by J.E. Fischer. Boston, Little, Brown, 1983.
187. Steephen, A.C., Traber, M.G., Ito, Y., et al.: JPEN J. Parenter. Enteral Nutr., *15:*647–652, 1991.
188. Lemoyne, M., Gossum, A.V., Kurian, R., et al.: Am. J. Clin. Nutr., *48:*1310–1315, 1988.
189. Centers for Disease Control: MMWR, *38:*43–46, 1989.
190. Wilmanns, Witzigmann, H., Schlag, P., et al.: Chirurgie, *61:*183–186, 1990.
191. Klein, G., Behne, M., Probst, S., et al.: Dtsch. Med. Wochenschr., *115:*254–256, 1990.
192. Oriot, D., Wood, C. Gottesman, R., et al.: JPEN J. Parenter. Enteral Nutr., *15:*105–109, 1991.
193. Zak, J., III, Burns, D., Lingenfelser, T., et al.: JPEN J. Parenter. Enteral Nutr., *15:*200–201, 1991.
194. Greene, H.L., Smith, R., Pollack, P., et al.: J. Am. Coll. Nutr., *10:*281–288, 1991.
195. Flowers, J.F., Ryan, J.A., Jr., Gough, J.A.: Catheter-related complications of total parenteral nutrition. *In* Total Parenteral Nutrition. 2nd Ed. Edited by J.E. Fischer. Boston, Little, Brown, 1991.
196. Peden, Y., Witzleben, C., Shelton, M., et al.: J. Pediatrics, *78:*180, 1971 (lett.).
197. Bowyer, B.A., Fleming, C.R., Ludwig, J., et al.: JPEN J. Parenter. Enteral Nutr., *9:*11–17, 1985.
198. Payne-James, J.J., Silk, D.B.A.: Dig. Dis., *9:*106–124, 1991.
199. Kubota, A., Okada, A., Nezu, R., et al.: JPEN J. Parenter. Enteral Nutr., *12:*602–606, 1988.
200. Drongowski, R.A., Coran, A.G.: JPEN J. Parenter. Enteral Nutr., *13:*586–589, 1989.
201. Bell, R.L., Ferry, G.D., Smith, E.O., et al.: JPEN J. Parenter. Enteral Nutr., *10:*356–359, 1986.
202. Messing, B., Colombel, J.F., Heresbach, D., et al.: Nutrition, *8:*30–36, 1992.
203. Buzby, G.P., Mullen, J.L., Stein, P.T., et al.: J. Surg. Res., *31:*46–54, 1981.
204. Wagner, W.H., Lowry, A.C., Silberman, H.: Am. J. Gastroenterol., *78:*199–202, 1983.
205. Ito, Y., Shils, M.E.: JPEN J. Parenter. Enteral Nutr., *15:*271–276, 1989.
206. Lambert, J.P., Thomas, S.M.: JPEN J. Parenter. Enteral Nutr., *9:*501–503, 1985.
207. Lindor, K.D., Burnes, J.: Gastroenterology, *101:*250–253, 1991.
208. Buchman, A.L., Dubin, M., Venden, D., et al.: Gastroenterology, *102:*1363–1370, 1992.
209. Buchman, A.L., Dubin, M., Moukarzel, A.A., et al.: JPEN J. Parenter. Enteral Nutr., *17(Suppl. 1):*36S, 1993 (abstr.).
210. Allen, B., Berhorft, R., Blanckhaert, N., et al.: Am. J. Surg., *141:*51–56, 1981.
211. Muller, E.L., Grace, P.A., Pitt, H.A.: J. Surg. Res., *40:*55–62, 1986.
212. Doty, J.E., Pitt, H.A., Porter-Fink, V., et al.: Ann. Surg., *201:*76–80, 1985.
213. Messing, B., Bories, C., Kustlinger, F., et al.: Gastroenterology, *84:*1012–1019, 1983.
214. Roslyn, J.J., Berquist, W.E., Pitt, H.A., et al.: Pediatrics, *71:*784–789, 1983.
215. Roslyn, J.J., Pitt, H.A., Mann, L.L.: Am. J. Surg., *148:*58–63, 1984.
216. Kien, C.L., Brouring, C., Jona, J., et al.: JPEN J. Parenter. Enteral Nutr., *6:*152–156, 1982.
217. Vargas, J.H., Klein, G.L., Ament, M.E., et al.: Am. J. Clin. Nutr., *48:*1070–1078, 1988.
218. Shike, M., Harrison, J.E., Sturtridge, W.C., et al.: Ann. Intern. Med., *92:*343–350, 1980.
219. Shike, M., Sturtridge, W.C., Tam, C.S., et al.: Ann. Intern. Med., *95:*560–568, 1981.
220. Shike, M., Shils, M.E., Heller, A., et al.: Am. J. Clin. Nutr., *44:*89–98, 1986.
221. Lipkin, E.W., Ott, S.M., Klein, G.L.: Am. J. Clin. Nutr., *46:*673–680, 1987.
222. Lipkin, E.W., Ott, S.M., Chestnut, C.H., III, et al.: Am. J. Clin. Nutr., *47:*515–523, 1988.
223. de Vernejoul, M.C., Messing, B., Modrowski, D., et al.: J. Clin. Endocrinol. Metab., *60:*109–113, 1985.
224. Moukarzel, A., Ament, M.E., Vargas, J., et al.: Am. J. Clin. Nutr., *51:*520, 1990 (abstr.).
225. LaFrance, R.J., Miyagawa, C.I.: Pharmaceutical considerations in total parenteral nutrition. *In* Total Parenteral Nutrition. 2nd Ed. Edited by J.E. Fischer. Boston, Little, Brown, 1991.
226. Shils, M.E., Wright, W.L., Turnbull, A., et al.: N. Engl. J. Med., *283:*341–344, 1970.
227. Scribner, B.H., Cole, J.J., Christopher, T.G., et al.: JAMA, *212:*457–463, 1970.
228. Jeejeebhoy, K.N., Zohrab, W.J., Langer, B., et al.: Gastroenterology, *65:*811–820, 1973.
229. Howard, L., Michalek, A.V.: Annu. Rev. Nutr., *4:*69–99, 1984.

230. Grant, J.P. (Ed.): Home total parenteral nutrition. *In* Handbook of Total Parenteral Nutrition. 2nd Ed. Philadelphia, W.B. Saunders, 1992.
231. American Society of Parenteral and Enteral Support: Nutr., Clin. Pract., *7:*65–69, 1992.
232. Howard, L., Heaphey, L., Fleming, C.R., et al.: JPEN J. Parenter. Enteral Nutr., *15:*384–393, 1991.
233. Burnes, J.V., O'Keefe, S.J.D., Fleming, C.R., et al.: JPEN J. Parenter. Enteral Nutr., *16:*327–332, 1992.
234. Wilmore, D.W.: J. Pediatr., *80:*88–95, 1972.
235. Dorney, S.F.A., Ament, M.E., Berquist, W.E., et al.: J. Pediatr., *107:*521–525, 1985.
236. Goulet, O.J., Révillion, Y., Jan, D., et al.: J. Pediatr., *119:*18–23, 1991.
237. Goel, V.: The economics of total parenteral nutrition. *In* Evaluating Total Parenteral Nutrition. Background papers for Technology Assessment and Practice Guidelines Form. Program on Technology and Health Care. Washington, D.C., Georgetown University School of Medicine, 1989, pp. 41–51.
238. Detsky, A.S., McLaughlin, J.R., Abrams, H.B., et al.: JPEN J. Parenter. Enteral Nutr., *10:*49–57, 1986.
239. Gulledge, A.D., Srp, F., Sharp, J.W., et al.: Nutr., Clin. Pract., *2:*183–194, 1987.
240. Schraut, W.H.: Gastroenterology, *94:*525–538, 1988.
241. Wood, R.F.M., Ingraham-Clark, C.L.: Br. Med. J., *304:*1453–1454, 1992.
242. Grant, D., Wall, W., Mimeault, R., et al.: Lancet, *335:*181–184, 1990.
243. Ng, E.H., Lowry, S.F.: Hematol. Oncol. Clin. North Am., *5:*162–184, 1991.
244. Wilmore, D.W.: N. Engl. J. Med., *325:*695–702, 1991.
245. Möller-Loswick, A.C., Zachrisson, H., Bennegård, K., et al.: JPEN J. Parenter. Enteral Nutr., *15:*669–675, 1991.
246. Gruenfeld, C., Feingold, K.R.: N. Engl. J. Med., *327:*328–337, 1992.
247. Hartl, W.H., Jauch, K.W., Herndon, D.N., et al.: Lancet, *335:*69–71, 1990.
248. Quigley, E.A.A., Marsh, M.N., Shaffer, J.L., et al.: Gastroenterology, *104:*286–301, 1993.
249. Starzl, T.E., Todo, S., Tzakis, A., et al.: Gastroenterology, *104:*673–679, 1993.

CHAPTER **81**

Nutrition and Medical Ethics: The Interplay of Medical Decisions, Patients' Rights, and the Judicial System

Maurice E. Shils

Without clinical craftmanship, the physician-humanist is without authenticity. Incompetence is inhumane because it betrays the trust the patient places in the physician's capacity to help and not harm.—Edmund D. Pellegrino, M.D.[1]

Our current knowledge of human nutritional and dietary requirements and the widespread availability of essential nutrients in stable forms and the means to administer them orally, by tube or by vein have brought nutrition support into the arena of effective therapy in certain clinical situations. Much of this book is concerned with the causes and management of primary and secondary malnutrition.

Much attention has been devoted in recent years to the ethical, medical, and legal aspects of providing or withholding nutrition and fluids to patients with incurable disease, especially those who cannot make decisions for themselves. These issues are important and are considered in some detail in this chapter. Before doing so, however, one should note the important medical-ethical issues related to nutrition support for other types of patients.

THERAPEUTIC ROLE OF NUTRITION SUPPORT

Physicians have become significantly more sensitive in recent years to the need for remedial attention to the problem of hospital-based malnutrition. However, many physicians still either overlook the development of serious undernutrition in their patients or delay proper therapy on the basis of hope that the underlying disease will soon be controlled and the "patient will again eat well"—a hope often too long delayed.

At periodic intervals over many years, the prevalence of such hospital-based malnutrition with its increased morbidity, delayed convalescence, and increased mortality has been reported.[2] In addition to failing to recognize the need for instituting adequate nutrition support, some physicians have failed to exercise adequate oversight to ensure optimum nutrition support modalities, particularly total parenteral nutrition, with serious consequences.[3] There is obviously an ethical issue when serious undernutrition is either not anticipated in a patient who is at obvious risk of developing such a condition or else is ignored when it is present in a patient who is neither terminally ill nor incurable. For the nonterminal patient at home or in a nursing home who has a treatment-responsive disease, development of serious undernutrition also represents the physician's failure to recognize the problem and to take appropriate action.

The sequelae of serious undernutrition are many and are discussed in various chapters in this book (see especially Chaps. 55 to 59). The restoration of lean body mass, appropriate amounts of body fat, reasonable strength, and ability to return to gainful employment all may take considerable time. One way to do good for the patient deemed likely to respond appropriately is to prevent serious undernutrition.

NUTRITION IN THE PREVENTION OF CHRONIC ILLNESSES

Chronic diseases, particularly cardiovascular diseases, cancer, osteoporosis, hypertension, and diabetes, are major causes of morbidity and mortality in our population. In recent years, it has become increasingly apparent that certain diets instituted at appropriate times can play an important role as preventive or ameliorating factors. This is clearly the case for management of hyperlipidemias in controlling coronary artery disease (see Chaps. 72 and 87); for efforts to minimize or delay serious osteoporosis (see Chap. 89); for optimum management of insulin-independent diabetes mellitus, (see Chap. 70); and for assisting in controlling hypertension (see Chap. 71); in addition, because many of these diseases are exacerbated by overweight, weight management is important (see Chap. 59). The research data base on the role of diet for prevention of certain types of human cancer is less convincing because of difficulties in accruing accurate and consistent long-term data and in executing long-term intervention studies. However, recent advances in knowledge of genetic changes in various cancers give promise of a better understanding of the role of diet in prevention.

With such information, "doing good" for the individual must now include the physician's attention to the possible need for dietary and other interventions to delay, ameliorate, or prevent one or more diet-sensitive chronic illnesses. Neglect in obtaining the proper history (including dietary intakes in relation to need), in doing an adequate physical examination, and/or in ordering the indicated laboratory studies is as much a professional failure as is failure to diagnose an illness or prescribe the correct medication. The traditional responsibilities of the physician expand as the result of advances in biomedical knowledge.

NUTRITION SUPPORT OF THE COMPETENT PATIENT: ETHICAL AND PROFESSIONAL ISSUES

Prior to the practical application of artificial feeding techniques, the inability to maintain adequate nutrition by mouth meant progressive body wasting until death. Except for death occurring rapidly because of violence and trauma or acute and overwhelming infection with organ failure, dehydration and varying degrees of starvation were the usual direct causes of "natural" death. Under these circumstances, a physician could do little in maintaining a patient's good nutritional state.

With respect to overseeing medical care in general, the prevailing judicial position in the past was that of "compelling state interest," relevant examples including the preservation of life, the prevention of suicide, and the issuing of credentials to medical practitioners. The Fifth Amendment to the United States Constitution prohibits the federal government from enacting laws that infringe on an individual's fundamental rights. The Fourteenth Amendment prohibits state governments from enacting such laws. Whereas the right of privacy is a right not specifically enumerated in the Constitution, it has been deemed basic to ordered liberty. This is particularly the case when courts find that an individual's rights are superior in a situation when no compelling state interest is found.

AUTONOMY OF THE PATIENT

In recent years the term *autonomy* (originally referring to self-governance in Greek city-states) has been used frequently, signifying the right of the competent individual to freely make choices concerning medical care and the obligation of the health care provider to effectively communicate with the patient and solicit those decisions. As has been pointed out, this term has been used to refer to personal and political notions, so "it is doubtful that autonomy is a univocal concept in either ordinary English or contemporary philosophy."[4] As detailed by Beauchamp and Childress, autonomous actions require definitions, including criteria for someone to be able to give or refuse informed consent and to make other decisions; furthermore, the principle of respect for autonomy must be evaluated in given situations in competition with other principles, including those of nonmaleficence (the obligation not to inflict harm), beneficence (the obligation to promote the welfare of the patient while balancing benefits and harm), and justice (an area of diverse views often involving the other principles and elements of fairness and entitlement).[4]

The right to refuse medical treatment was established judicially in 1891 when the United States Supreme Court upheld the right of a personal injury plaintiff to refuse a medical examination.[5] This decision firmly endorsed the rights of individuals to make choices regarding bodily examination and treatment under the principle that common law guards the right of every individual to the possession and control of his own person on the basis of the doctrine of informed consent. However, state laws vary with respect to specific requirements defining informed consent. In general, there must be a basic understanding about the disease, purpose, nature, risks, and consequences of any proposed treatment, the probabilities of its success, the right to make choices about the type of medical care to be received, and finally, the ability to make a voluntary decision on the basis of such information, i.e., to give or withhold consent.

BIOMEDICAL ISSUES IN WITHHOLDING FOOD AND FLUID

With the development of effective life-support techniques with the potential for long-term effectiveness (such as mechanical ventilation, more effective antibiotics and other medications, hemodialysis, and enteral and parenteral nutrition), in conjunction with important changes in social and economic aspects of medical care, a new medical era was initiated and with it came new questions relating to ethics of practice, patient-physician relations, and patients' rights.

Before considering those patients with the capacity for long survival in the setting of irreversible, severe, and disabling neurologic and medical impairment, it is well to consider briefly the category of patients who are considered to be in a terminal condition or related designation. Cranford has summarized his position on this category as follows:

> Patients . . . include those whose disease processes are so overwhelming that death will occur within a relatively short period of time, regardless of the continued application of medical treatment. The problem with this category is that there is no widespread consensus on the definition of these terms, nor how to apply them in individual cases. Also, no one agrees on what a short period of time is—hours, days, a few weeks, 6 months, a year? To a large extent, limiting nutrition and hydration for patients in this category is more a medical, not a moral, decision. For example, in the terminally ill cancer patient, there is little conceivable benefit to starting artificial nutrition and hydration in someone who is going to die within a few hours, days, or weeks. These patients usually don't have any appetite during the final stages of their disease processes. In a hospice or other humane setting, these patients are usually given fluids and food by mouth as tolerated for comfort. . . .[6]

Dr. Cranford is considering here the issue of the medical benefit to the dying patient and I am in agreement. For the anorectic competent cancer or other patient who has failed therapy and whose expected demise from the underlying disease is probably a matter of months or a year with an acceptable quality of life and good family support, tube feeding is relatively safe and inexpensive and should be considered.

DEHYDRATION AS THE PRIMARY BIOLOGIC RESPONSE TO CESSATION OF FOOD AND FLUID

Mention has been made of the natural death of a patient unable to ingest food and fluid in the era before artificial feeding; dehydration with associated electrolyte changes was the usual immediate cause of death.

The conscious and competent patient with an advancing severe illness who is in little or no pain becomes progressively weaker—with or without food and fluid—with decreasing communication and desire for food and with progressive apathy. In the patient who is not receiving artificial nutrition, signs and symptoms of dehydration appear with dryness of skin and mouth, decreased urinary output, and occasional thirst.[6–9] Hospice workers report that they rarely encounter nausea, vomiting, or cramps in this situation, and the dehydrated patient rarely needs oral pharyngeal suction; this is in contrast to the hydrated patient.[9,10] Obtundation usually progresses to a peaceful death. Chemically, electrolytes and blood urea nitrogen become abnormal; however, Oliver noted that of 22 patients dying peacefully without intravenous or tube feedings within 48 hours of blood tests, 12 had essentially normal electrolytes, the only consistent abnormality being a slightly raised urea.[7]

Cranford pointed out that when food and fluid were discontinued in patients in the vegetative state, 1 died in 8 days, another in 10 days, and another in 2 weeks.[6] As noted later, Barber died in 6 days and Cruzan in 12 days. Such deaths differ markedly from the extended suffering of pure starvation when there is adequate fluid intake, such as occurred with the Irish Republican Army hunger strikers in 1981.[11]

AUTONOMY, LEGAL ISSUES, AND THE JUDICIARY

The issue of provision of nutrition and fluids has caused the most controversy and disagreements among adult patients, their surrogates, physicians, hospital administrations, and the courts. Notwithstanding the acceptance of the right of the competent individual to make a decision for or against receiving medical therapy, this right was not automatically granted upon request of an individual in the instance of withholding forced feeding.

THE BOUVIA CASE

In a celebrated relatively early case, the issue arose concerning the right of a competent individual to starve to death while hospitalized in California. Elizabeth Bouvia was a quadraplegic in her midtwenties with severe cerebral palsy and arthritic pain requiring morphine injection; while able to ingest food orally with assistance, she asked that such feeding be stopped. The hospital refused to accede to her wishes, and a lower court ruling in 1984 supported the hospital.[12] When her condition deteriorated to the point that she had to be fed by a nasogastric tube, the appellate court ruled in 1986 that her refusal of treatment was not a form of suicide, thus rejecting the arguments of hospital officials that removal of the tube would make them a party to suicide.[13] With the additional support given by the United States Supreme Court decision in the Cruzan case (discussed later), the right of an irreversibly ill but competent patient to refuse artificial feeding is not likely to be seriously challenged again.

Cranford classified Bouvia's condition—together with that of a group of clinically related patients in which life support was an issue—as being a state of severe and permanent paralysis.[6] This condition, which may acutely or progressively result in a "permanent locked-in state," was first described as a medical term in 1966. In his summary of this neurologic syndrome, Cranford listed irreversible loss of motor function, preservation of normal consciousness, possible long-term survival of years or even decades, and physical and psychologic suffering of a degree that may become extreme because of the patient's awareness of the condition.[6]

PATIENT-PHYSICIAN INTERACTION AND DECISION MAKING

In an incisive and compassionate essay, Pellegrino stated:

> that a more sensitive and compelling guide to the care of the sick is to be found in the fact of illness as a human experience than in the assigned role of the profession. Without supplanting traditional professional ethics, the intrinsic dehumanizing nature of illness imposes additional obligations of greater sensitivity.[14]

He reviewed the multiple changes in social attitudes, medical technology, fragmentation of the activities of physicians and other health professionals, and governmental and judicial involvement, all of which modify the patient-doctor relation. Furthermore, individuals with "illness as an acute event or as a chronic accompaniment of life are deprived in varying degrees of those things which distinguish humanity from other forms of existence." These include losses of freedom of action, of freedom to make choices, and of freedom from the power of others as well as threats to personal self-image. These disabilities "must be the infrangible base for the obligations of physicians and all others who profess to heal" and

> these obligations constitute the substance of professional medical ethics. . . . Its rooting in the existential situation is more authentic and more human . . . than the traditional one in the self-declared duties of the profession. . . . The professional can make a valid claim for technical authority but this no longer extends to moral authority. . . . The patient has the human right to his own moral agency if he or she wishes to exercise it. The physician has the moral obligation to ascertain the degree to which the patient wishes to exercise his moral prerogatives and to provide the fullest exposition which will enable the privilege to be exercised.[14]

Pellegrino had earlier emphasized the need for the physician to combine cognitive aspects of medical care with humanistic concern recognizing the specific conditions and needs of each patient.[1]

The principle of respect for autonomy of the competent patient may result in tension between patient and physician when the patient's decision appears inappropriate in the professional opinion of the physician. For example, disagreement may occur when the patient wishes parenteral feeding to be stopped and the physician believes that continuing feeding is in the patient's best interest, or conversely, when the patient wishes parenteral feeding continued although tube feeding would serve as well in the view of the physician. An example of an even more difficult situation requiring a decision by the patient, family, and others is that of stopping parenteral feeding in a patient with obstructive cancer who has failed all therapy but who is competent and not terminally ill (but with continuing fluid and electrolyte problems) and who has little or no health insurance (including Medicare or Medicaid).

What is legally a clear-cut situation, i.e., the rights of a competent patient, may be a complex and difficult situation for all concerned with the welfare of the individual. The old Spanish proverb quoted elsewhere in this general context is apt: *"The appearance of the bull changes as one leaves the grandstand and enters the ring."*[15] For example, the patient's viewpoint may or may not reflect some degree of an underlying psychologic and psychiatric problem, such as depression, other mental difficulty, or the side effect of medications,[16,17] or an unspoken social problem, or a strong family influence of one type or another, or the misunderstanding of the physician's intentions or the degree of the severity or irreversibility of the disease.

RECOMMENDATIONS OF THE PRESIDENT'S COMMISSION

In this connection, it is worth noting several conclusions published in 1983 by the President's Commission for the Study of Ethical Problems in Medicine and

Biomedical and Behavioral Research.[18] The Commission held that "health care professionals serve patients best by maintaining a presumption in favor of sustaining life while recognizing that competent patients are entitled to choose to forego any treatments, including those that sustain life" and that "the voluntary choice of a competent and informed patient should determine whether or not life-sustaining therapy will be undertaken," while "health care institutions and professionals should try to enhance patients' abilities to make decisions on their own behalf and to promote understanding of the available options."[18]

In such situations, members of the hospital clinical nutrition team, who are often and intimately involved in a major aspect of the patient's care, may be helpful in affording insight into the patient's status and expressed position. The physician's discussion of the medical situation with patient and family, the basis for the medical recommendations and the therapeutic alternatives with their probabilities of success, and the offer of a second opinion are all essential in the decision-making process.

The Commission laid great stress on the importance of shared decision making. It emphasized the need for improved communication between physician and terminally ill patient and noted that this aspect has improved in recent years. Despite advances in this relationship, evidence indicates that a physician's values may be a more decisive factor than a patient's values with respect to decisions about life-sustaining treatment. The general counsel of the American Medical Association reviewed recent surveys comparing advance directives with actual treatment decisions. He noted the frequent failure of physicians to discuss preferences on end-of-life decisions directly with hospitalized patients when they were competent and pointed out physicians' biases with respect to decision making in relation to the types of diseases and personal and other attributes of patients.[19]

> Some predominance of physician values may be explained by the fact that, in some cases, patients may desire treatment which is medically futile. Principles of patient autonomy do not include a right to receive futile treatment. However, unreasonable patient desires cannot provide a full explanation for the predominance of physician values. In many cases the patient will receive more treatment than is desired. In addition, physicians may view new treatment as undesirable even when it is not medically futile. . . . A reasonable argument can be made that professional resistance to patient autonomy has so far prevailed and that changes in the treatment of the dying reflect changes in physician attitudes more than changes in the way end-of-life decisions are made. Under this view, the real change has been a decreased willingness of physicians to offer life-sustaining treatment to hopelessly ill patients.[19]

Orentlicher's report concludes with a call (1) for physicians to examine their own practices in an effort to recognize how wittingly or unwittingly they may be imposing their own values, (2) for more vigorous and realistic educational efforts in this area for physicians in training, (3) for more legal protection of patients' autonomy, and (4) for better education of the public about the value of advance directives and the need for improved interactions with physicians including knowledge of their physicians' values concerning end-of-life decisions.[19]

The President's Commission re-examined the role of traditional moral distinctions as they relate to decisions about medical care and whether they are acceptable or unacceptable. The Commission noted that, from the viewpoint of most competent patients, decisions about alternative available courses of treatment are made on the basis of factors that include treatment benefits in terms of extension of their life, the nature and quality of that life, the degree of suffering involved, and the various costs to themselves and to others.

The Commission noted that, in addition to such key factors in decision making, other bases have been suggested for judging the acceptability or unacceptability of life-and-death decisions:

> These bases are traditionally presented in the form of opposing categories. Although the categories—causing death by acting versus by omitting to act; withholding versus withdrawing treatment; the intended versus the unintended but forseeable consequences of a choice; and ordinary versus extraordinary treatment—do reflect factors that can be important in assessing the moral and legal acceptability of decisions to forego life sustaining treatment, they are inherently unclear. Worse, their invocation is often so mechanical that it neither illuminates an actual case nor provides an ethically persuasive argument.[18]

The Commission presented its conclusions about such distinctions; several of these are relevant to the issue of nutrition and have, in fact, had a significant influence on the attitudes of various courts. Some of these conclusions are reproduced here:[18]

> The distinction between acting and omitting to act provides a useful rule-of-thumb by separating cases that probably deserve more scrutiny from those that are likely not to need it. . . . Nonetheless, the mere difference between acts and omissions—which is often hard to draw in any case—never by itself determines what is morally acceptable. Rather, the acceptability of particular actions or omissions turns on other morally significant considerations, such as the balance of harms and benefits likely to be achieved, the duties owed by others to a dying person, the risks imposed on others in acting or refraining, and the certainty of outcome. . . . A justification that is adequate for not commencing a treatment is also sufficient for ceasing it. Moreover, erecting a higher requirement for cessation might unjustifiably discourage vigorous initial attempts to treat seriously ill patients that sometimes succeed. . . . Whether care is "ordinary" or "extraordinary" should not determine whether a patient must accept or may decline it. To avoid misunderstanding, public discussion should focus on the underlying reasons for or against a therapy rather than on a simple categorization as "ordinary" or "extraordinary."[18]

The guidelines of the Hastings Center point out that the terms "extraordinary" and "ordinary" are often used as an ethical basis for distinguishing types of treatments that may be withheld or withdrawn. Its position is that "these terms obscure ethically important questions rather than helping to resolve them." Prevalence of a treatment or its degree of technological complexity is sometimes used to make the distinction between "ordinary" and "extraordinary."

> We reject the distinction. No treatment is intrinsically "ordinary" or "extraordinary." All treatments that impose undue burdens on the patient without overriding benefits or that simply provide no benefits may justifiably be withheld or withdrawn. While traditional definitions of "extraordinary" hinged on this comparison of benefits and burdens, the term has become so confusing that it is no longer useful.[20]

RECOMMENDATIONS OF THE LAW REFORM COMMISSION OF CANADA

This commission is an official agency charged with periodically evaluating and recommending reform of Canadian federal law; its proposed legal reforms were brief and concise with basic principles discussed in other documents in the Protection of Life series. The Law Reform Commission issued recommendations that included those on cessation of medical treatment.[21,22] In its final report these principles were summarized and were stated in part as follows:[21]

> The first is that in the medical context the presumption in favour of life should always be recognized. . . . The proposed system of rules should never depart from the principle that in the absence of reasons to the contrary the patient should always be presumed to want to live, and that the patient would prefer life to death even when unable to express that preference. In practical terms, this principle may be expressed by the rule that if a treatment is reasonable and useful for the purpose of preserving the health or life of a human being, it should be assumed that a patient unable to express a choice would choose to receive the treatment and not to refuse it. . . . This principle and presumption does not however oblige extraordinary measures. First of all, the presumption is not absolute and, secondly, it applies only if the proposed treatment is reasonable and useful. But according to this first principle the onus is on those who stop or do not initiate life-supporting treatment to provide justification for that decision.
>
> The second principle is that of the patient's autonomy and right to self-determination. . . . Within the bounds of public order, morality and the rights of others, human beings must remain masters of their fate. They should therefore have the right, based on the notion of free and informed consent, to make decisions concerning themselves.
>
> A third principle which any reform proposals should acknowledge is that human life should be considered not only from the "quantitative" perspective, but also from the "qualitative" perspective. . . . We believe that the law should now clearly recognize the right of patients, exercising their free and informed choice, not to undertake treatment if they feel it would deprive them of, or not provide, an adequate quality of life for the time remaining.[21]

RESOLVING DIFFERENCES BETWEEN PATIENT AND PHYSICIAN

When all the stated precautions and efforts have been honored in decision making and, nevertheless, the choice of the competent and informed patient is contrary to that of the physician, where does this leave the physician? "The physician too has a set of values to which he owes allegiance. He has a double obligation, to protect those of the patient and to be faithful to his own."[14] To deal in a humane way with those conflicts that must occasionally arise, "the physician must know enough about his own beliefs to decide when he can compromise, when he cannot, and when he must give the patient an opportunity to transfer his care to another physician whose values more closely coincide."[14] In a situation where a patient makes a decision that the physician cannot accept, the President's Commission took the position that "health care professionals or institutions may decline to provide a particular option because that choice would violate their conscience or professional judgment, though in doing so they may not abandon a patient."[18] This means that, in the case of the physician, responsibility for the care of the patient must be transferred to another physician who accepts the patient's decision and acts accordingly. In the case of opposition on the part of the institution's administration, possible solutions to this problem are to yield to staff pressure on behalf of the patient, to transfer the patient to another hospital willing to accept the patient, or finally, to yield to a court order supporting the patient.

Often, in the past, the reluctance of the hospital administration to discontinue tube feedings (because of fear of civil or criminal penalties or on religious grounds) has led to legal actions by patients or family members.

PATIENT SELF-DETERMINATION ACT

The President's Commission recommended that information about the existence and justification of constraints on patients' decisions be available to patients or their surrogates. As a result of this and other similar recommendations, federal legislation (the Patient Self-Determination Act) was enacted and became law on December 1, 1991.[23] This law applies to hospitals, nursing homes, hospices, health care maintenance organizations, and health care companies participating in Medicare and Medicaid. The institutions or organizations are required on admission, on enrollment, or on initiating home care to inform patients about their legal rights in that state to make decisions concerning their medical care and to formulate advance directives. Such a directive must be in the patient's medical record indicating whether life support has been rejected. This law, as well as most state laws and court decisions on this subject, also allows hospitals and nursing homes to express their beliefs to the patient before admission. One goal of the statute is to encourage but not require adults while competent to complete advanced directives in the form of treatment directives or a proxy appointment or both. Another goal is to influence both health care givers and institutions to honor advance directives.

Although agreement on the value of advance directives is widespread, significant problems arise in the implementation of this law because of the complexity and unpredictability of outcome of clinical situations and of issues with patient-proxy-physician-bureaucracy relations; these have been discussed.[19,24–26] The issue of proxy decision making is discussed further later.

As a result of the majority decision of the United States Supreme Court on the Cruzan case (see later) and of the 1990 Patient Self-Determination Act now in force, advance directives must be based on the legal requirements of individual states. Areen summarized relevant state laws as of October 1990 in relation to living will legislation, proxy appointments, durable power of attorney, and court decisions and legislation authorizing family members to withhold or withdraw treatment.[27]

NUTRITION AND THE INCOMPETENT PATIENT

The major medical, ethical, and legal issues concerning cessation of involuntary nutrition support have involved incompetent patients. Traditionally, the right of the state to preserve life in the incompetent patient has been manifest in the requirement for a court-appointed guardian or surrogate to act on behalf of the patient.

PATIENTS IN A PERSISTENT VEGETATIVE STATE

An important category of incompetent patients is that of the persistent vegetative state with permanent loss of cerebral function. About 40% of these patients have had severe head injury with disruption of white matter fibers to and from the cerebral cortex; another 40% have suffered massive loss of cortical cells because of hypoxia, usually after cardiorespiratory arrest due to disease, trauma, or medical accident. The others may have had various acute cerebral insults, including hypoglycemia, poisoning, or acute brain disease.[28–30] Patients with chronic dementing brain orders may eventually become vegetative, and some children with severe developmental abnormalities never surpass a vegetative state. Good recovery has never been documented beyond 1 to 3 months following a sustained period of lack of oxygen or of blood supply to the brain secondary to cardiac or respiratory arrest.[6] Two patients in the presumed persistent vegetative state recovered consciousness after periods of 15 and 20 months, respectively, but both were left severely and permanently paralyzed.[6]

Such patients may have long periods in which the eyes are open, with alternate periods of "sleep." For this reason, Jennett and Plum suggested using the term persistent vegetative state rather than the term coma.[28] Such patients when "awake" may, by reflex, follow a moving object with their eyes or look in the direction of a loud sound; despite limb spasticity, they can withdraw from painful stimuli and can have hand reflex groping or grasping. The face can grimace; groans and cries can occur but without words; if small amounts of food or fluid are put in the mouth, they may be swallowed. Inexperienced observers may interpret reflex movements as voluntary responses and vocal sound as words, but careful observation indicates no psychologically meaningful response to the environment. Breathing is spontaneous.

Criteria and prognosis of this condition have been periodically published.[28–30] The diagnosis depends on clinical observation over several weeks or longer, depending on the nature of the insult and age of the patient. Cranford noted a poor diagnostic correlation with the electroencephalogram, a good correlation with computed tomography or magnetic resonance imaging, and an excellent correlation with positron emission tomography.[6] The 50% of the patients surviving the first year may live for years, some up to 30 years. Progressive spasticity and bed rest lead to muscle atrophy and limb, hand, and foot contraction. Prolonged survival depends primarily upon continued feeding by a tube placed either through the nose or a gastrostomy and care either in a hospital, a nursing home, or at home, with periodic antibiotic treatment for infection.

THE QUINLAN CASE

The distress of the patient's relatives and friends is severe as they observe the loved one remaining unresponsive while weeks pass into months and into years. The economic, psychologic, and social consequences of this condition are enormous. Such issues attracted widespread attention in the case of Karen Ann Quinlan, a young woman in New Jersey who was in a persistent vegetative state and on a respirator. The state's Supreme Court, on a reversal of a lower court decision, made medical-legal history in 1976 when, despite the opposition of the patient's physician and hospital, it ruled, at the request of the parents, that the respirator could be discontinued.[31] When this was done, the patient was found to be able to breathe spontaneously and she survived for some years on tube feeding.

Withdrawal of tube feeding was not considered an option by the parents.[32] The position reflected a widely held view, namely, that food and hydration were not in the category of a special life support system but were rather a humanitarian action necessary for the comfort of the patient. Some physicians were and some still are of the opinion that the withholding of food and fluid is a violation of medical ethics,[32,33] and some judges have held that it is a form of assisted suicide.

Some cases have been related to the right of a surrogate to order cessation of tube feeding to an incompetent patient. Several of these are reviewed here, to delineate issues and the bases for rulings and also to illustrate the changes in attitudes of interested parties, especially the courts.

THE BARBER AND NEJDL CASE

Another troubling judicial issue is the question of legal liability of physicians when nutrition is withheld from an incompetent patient who is not terminally ill and who, while competent, had not clearly indicated in writing or verbally to a reliable witness a wish not to be force fed when terminally or incurably ill. This concern is well illustrated by legal developments resulting from the medical management of the patient, Clarence Herbert, who had suffered respiratory arrest in association with routine intestinal surgery;[34,35] following resuscitation, he remained comatose over the following several days. On the advice of physicians that prognosis for recovery was poor and with consent of family, the use of the respirator was stopped. The patient then breathed spontaneously but with no change in his comatose state. Two days later, again after consultation with the family, the attending physicians ordered removal of the nasogastric tube, intravenous nutrition, and air mist. The patient died 6 days later.

Herbert had not previously executed a formal directive under the California Natural Death Act, nor had written anything concerning his wishes in such circumstances; however, he had stated to his wife that he did not want to be kept alive by machine or "become another Karen Ann Quinlan." A nurse reported the actions of the physicians to local authorities, who then filed criminal charges for murder against the attending physicians Drs. Barber and Nejdl. Despite a municipal court magistrate ruling that the death had resulted from brain damage secondary to anoxia and that the conduct of the physicians was not "unlawful," the district attorney appealed the case to the Los Angeles Superior Court. The murder charge was reinstated by a judge who decided that there was no legal justification for the action of the physicians. The physicians then appealed to the California Court of Appeals, which then dismissed the criminal charges.

THE CONROY CASE

Another case, occurring in New Jersey at the same time, further delineated the complex relationships between the medical status of an incurably ill patient and legal and judicial issues arising in the minds of concerned jurists. Claire Conroy was an 84-year-old woman severely ill with advanced atherosclerosis, diabetes, and organic brain syndrome.[35,36] Although the case description stated that she was not in a persistent vegetative state, her described behavior approximated closely the clinical description of this state; the diagnosis is discussed further in the section dealing with incompetent patients in nonvegetative states. A nephew filed a petition to authorize removal of the nasogastric feeding tube from the patient, although there was no clear evidence of what the patient would have desired. A trial judge, after taking testimony and having visited the patient, authorized removal of the feeding tube, but not cessation of any voluntary or assisted oral feeding. The decision was appealed by the institution, and, pending the hearing, the tube feeding was continued to the patient's death.

Despite Conroy's death, the New Jersey Appellate Court heard the appeal. It reversed the earlier trial judges' decision and held that (1) she was neither comatose nor terminally ill, (2) the feeding tube was not a particularly invasive treatment such as the respirator in the Quinlan case, and (3) if the nasogastric tube had been removed in accordance with the trial judge's decision, Conroy would have died, not as a result of her condition, but from a "new and independent condition: dehydration and starvation and that this would constitute murder (euthanasia)." The case was appealed to the New Jersey Supreme Court, which sanctioned the withdrawal of artificial nutrition and hydration in this type of case but with a time constraint of expected survival of 1 year or less.

In discussing the final decision in the Conroy case in the context of criteria for guidelines on decisions in terminating care for incompetent patients, Emanuel noted:

> the court laid down three standards for terminating such care and stipulated that one of them be satisfied before treatment could be stopped. The court designated the first as a "subjective standard" which permits the termination of treatment when an incompetent patient had left clear indication, such as a living will, that he or she would have refused that treatment. It called the second a "pure objective standard" which permits the termination of life-sustaining treatment if the burden of the care outweighs the benefits, i.e., administering life-sustaining care would be inhumane because it would perpetuate severe pain. This standard is applied to patients who have not left indication of their preferences about life-sustaining care. Others label this the "best interests standard," in which the patient's surrogate objectively evaluates the benefits and risks of a treatment, opting for the care which most benefits the patient. The third standard, called by the court a "limited objective standard," is a combination of the first two and permits termination of care if there is some evidence (such as remarks made during a conversation) that the patient would not want the treatment and if the burden and pain of continued life outweigh the benefits.[37]

THE JOBES CASE AND SUBSTITUTED JUDGMENT

A subsequent ruling by the same court involved the case of a woman, Nancy Jobes, who was in a persistent vegetative state following hemorrhage.[38] Her husband and parents requested that a feeding tube be removed and that she be allowed to die. The nursing home refused to accede to this request. When the case was brought before the New Jersey Supreme Court, the court sanc tioned the removal of the feeding tube but rejected as "remote," "general," and "casual conversation" statements of the patient's friends and relatives that she had stated in conversation that she did not wish to be dependent on a respirator. In its decision making on the Jobes case the court eliminated its previous "Conroy" criteria and, instead, based its ruling on the Quinlan case; that is, it ruled that the "substituted judgment standard," exercised by the family, should apply to patients in a persistent vegetative state.

In reviewing this case, Emanuel noted that the substituted judgment standard means, in effect, that the surrogate for the incompetent patient is put into the position of attempting to make a decision for the patient as if that individual were competent; this standard thus differs from the best interest standard, which is based on an objective standard of benefits and burdens. He pointed out that the opinion of the President's Commission was that this standard not be used if there is no "reliable evidence" of the patient's views.

Some studies, mostly limited in scope and types of subjects, challenge the view that family members and physicians are able to make substituted judgment decisions in concordance with those of competent patients.[39,40] In a small series of medical journal letters to the editor commenting on the study of Seckler et al., the responding physicians for the most part were unhappy with the substituted judgment standard.[41] The judicial and legislative history and endorsement of decision making for incompetent patient by proxy or surrogate and the ethical justification for this were briefly reviewed by Emanuel and Emanuel.[40] Theoretic and empiric objections to proxy making are summarized as the basis for suggesting that "proxy decision makers cannot divine or implement the incompetent patient's wishes regarding the termination of life sustaining care."[40] Alternative solutions are suggested, with recognition that each has limitations. While agreeing with the array of concerns about proxy decision making, Lynn, in an accompanying editorial, takes the position that "a morally justifiable and pragmatic policy for decision making for incompetent adults, at this point, will have to rely heavily on appointed and family proxies, with a morally defensible and practical plan,"[42] which provides options similar to those suggested by the Coordinating Council on Life-Sustaining Medical Treatment Decision-Making by the Courts.[43]

AMA STATEMENT OF 1986

In the midst of these and other pertinent judicial decisions, the American Medical Association, through its Council on Ethical and Judicial Affairs, issued in 1984, and in revised form in 1986, statements on withholding or withdrawing life-prolonging medical treatment.[44] The 1986 statement consists of four short paragraphs, which includes the following key sentences that also relate to food and fluids:

> In the absence of the patient's choice or an authorized proxy, the physician must act in the best interest of the patient. . . . For humane reasons, with informed consent, a physician may do what is medically necessary to alleviate severe pain, or cease or omit treatment to permit a terminally ill patient whose death is imminent to die. Even if death is not imminent but a patient's coma is beyond doubt irreversible and there are adequate safeguards to confirm the accuracy of the diagnosis and with the concurrence of those with responsibility for the care of the patient, it is not unethical to discontinue all means of life-prolonging medical treatment. . . . Life-prolonging medical treatment includes medication and artificially or technologically supplied respiration, nutrition or hydration.[44]

The effect on attitudes of physicians of the widespread interest and discussion on these issues is evidenced by significant differences in the 1984 and 1986 statements; e.g., in the first version there was reference only to terminally ill patients, whereas the later one includes those in irreversible coma; the 1984 version did not define "life-prolonging medical treatment," whereas in 1986 these are specifically designated and include nutrition or hydration.

THE CRUZAN CASE

This case was the first to involve the United States Supreme Court on the issue of discontinuance of tube feeding of an incompetent patient. Like the Quinlan case, it aroused widespread public and professional interest and resulted in a decision with far-reaching implications. Cruzan was one of about 10,000 patients estimated to be in the permanent vegetative state.[45] The background is briefly as follows. In January 1983, at the age of 25 years, Nancy Cruzan suffered irreversible brain damage secondary to prolonged hypoxia following an automobile accident; she was then supported in hospital by food and fluid fed through a tube. In 1986 her parents requested discontinuance of the feedings but had to resort to legal action at the insistence of the Missouri state hospital administration. In July 1988 a trial court ruled that the tube feedings could be withheld;[46] however, on appeal, the Missouri Supreme Court, by a 4 to 3 decision, reversed the trial court decision on the grounds that no reliable evidence indicated that Cruzan would have refused artificial feedings.[47]

On June 25, 1990 the United States Supreme Court affirmed the latter Missouri ruling by a vote of 5 to 4.[48,49] The majority opinion centered on whether the United States Constitution prohibited Missouri from choosing to rule as it did. The five Justices answered in the negative with variations on this theme. Three of the four dissenting Justices stated that incompetent as well as competent patients had the constitutional right to be free of unwanted medical treatment; the fourth stated that the Constitution required that the best interest of the patient be followed and that a state may not override the patient's wishes or best interests. Six of the nine Justices explicitly found no distinction between fluids and nutrition, artificially delivered, and other medical treatments; none of the other three found a constitutionally relevant distinction.[49]

Nearly 8 years after Cruzan's accident, the judge in the Missouri Circuit Court, in a brief order, authorized the parents as co-guardians "to cause the removal of nutrition and hydration from our ward, Nancy Beth Cruzan."[50] This was done and Cruzan died 12 days later.

Differing reactions to the significance of the United States Supreme Court's decision are exemplified by the views of Bopp and Marzen[51] and of Annas.[49] There was widespread disappointment that the court had not recognized a constitutional right to refuse artificial means of prolonging life in the given circumstance; this was associated with the view that the court opinion would make such a right more difficult to achieve in the future.[52,53] Nevertheless, others believed that the decision had important positive aspects; these were summarized in a statement by physicians, nurses, lawyers, and bioethicists that concluded that (1) the decision affirmed the right of competent patients to refuse life-sustaining treatment, (2) it did not differentiate discontinuance of artificial nutrition and fluid from that of other forms of medical treatment, (3) the decision applied only to the Missouri requirement for explicit authorization to terminate treatment prior to the loss of capacity to make such a decision, (4) other states are not required to adopt Missouri's strict standard of proof, nor did the decision prevent Missouri from changing its standard, and (5) it did not alter the laws, ethical standards, or clinical practices permitting the foregoing of life-sustaining treatment that have evolved in the United States since the Quinlan case in 1976. The statement concluded by recommending that physicians continue to be guided by medical ethics and accepted clinical practices in this area, urged wider discussions on the use of life-sustaining treatment with patients' families and close friends, and encouraged preparation of advance directives.[54]

The best evidence of the impact of the Supreme Court's decision was the rapid collapse of the medical, institutional, surrogate, and legal opposition in Missouri to discontinuing Cruzan's feedings. The nature of Cruzan's condition and the widespread support of her parents' petition by many groups apparently was the tinder for further evaluation; the United States Supreme Court's decision was the spark for change, even though the court's decision upheld the state supreme court's position. Another effect of the Cruzan decision was the speed with which many states enacted health proxy legislation.[55] Unfortunately, the variability in important requirements among state laws creates potential problems for those moving from one state to another, commuting regularly between states, or living for different periods of the year in two or more states.

Cranford pointed out that as a result of publicity about the Cruzan case, families in similar situations are requesting physicians not to *start* artificial feedings because they and the patient may become prisoners of technology and state law. This type of situation presents a professional problem for physicians who are hesitant to start or to stop such treatment before the disease prognosis can be made with sufficient certainty. To help resolve this dilemma, Cranford proposed that assurance be given to the family

> that once a diagnosis and prognosis have been established with great certainty at some point in the future, physicians will then be willing to discontinue artificial nutrition and hydration, thus freeing the family of the fear that the patient and family will be held hostage by unthinking, unfeeling and dehumanizing medical technology.[6]

This position of Cranford's seems to me a satisfactory resolution to conflicting opinions on the issue of decision making for the incompetent patient. On the one hand, there is the opinion that, without a prior clear advance directive to the contrary, physicians and courts should automatically assume that the family has the authority to make decisions for that patient (with the burden of proof in court for those of the opinion that the family is not acting in the best interest of the patient).[56] On the other hand, there is the position that the legal definition of death should be extended to include the irreversible persistent vegetative state and that the withdrawal of life support from such patients does not require a family decision.[57]

The situation in the United Kingdom with respect to the withdrawal of life-sustaining treatment of patients in the vegetative state (without a prior assignment of power of attorney) had, up to 1991, not reached the British courts.[30,58] The British Medical Association accepts that patients may refuse treatment and that artificial feeding is such a treatment. In practice, physicians discontinue treatment in consultation with families without involving the courts and hence operate in a legal vacuum.

INCOMPETENT PATIENTS IN A NONVEGETATIVE STATE

Additional to the state of severe and permanent paralysis and the persistent vegetative state, which have been considered earlier, is a third syndrome in this category of disabling neurologic conditions with the potential for prolonged survival and the issue of life-sustaining medical treatment. This is *dementia*, which includes Alzheimer's disease, with its variable destruction of the neocortex, and multi-infarct dementia, with its variable destruction of subcortical white matter.[6,17] Both disorders are characterized by a gradual onset of progressive neurologic deterioration occurring over years to decades, with time to prognostic certainty of months to years and with suffering decreasing with increasing impairment of cortical function. The persistent vegetative state is the ultimate and most severe form of dementia as the result of complete loss of neocortical function.[6]

The estimate of 10,000 patients in the United States in the persistent vegetative state[45] pales in comparison with the estimate of 4 million patients in the United States at various stages of dementia,[6] of whom 1.3 to 1.9 million have Alzheimer's disease.[17]

The President's Commission,[59] the American College of Physicians,[60] the American Medical Association,[29] and other organizations draw a distinction between the incompetent patient in the permanent vegetative state and one in a "conscious" state but with severe, irreversible, and deteriorating mental impairment. The New Jersey Supreme Court also made a distinction of sorts in the case of Conroy, who, as noted previously, was not considered to be in a vegetative state but who had severe mental impairment. That decision permitted removal of the feeding tube from such patients, but only if the estimated maximum life expectancy was 1 year or less.

Emanuel discussed the relative lack of a significant medical distinction between patients in a permanent vegetative state and patients with severe mental impairment who are not terminally ill, such as patients with Alzheimer's disease or organic brain syndrome. He stated "as long as it seems legitimate to terminate treatments to a young vegetative patient, so it seems acceptable to withdraw nasogastric feeding from a non-terminal patient with advanced Alzheimer's disease."[38]

Cranford agreed that, in terms of consciousness and capacity for experiencing suffering, clinical distinction between no consciousness (the persistent vegetative state) and only minimal consciousness (profound dementia) is minor.[6] He then made the important point that

> from a legal and ethical standpoint, a major distinction should be drawn between these conditions, for the sake of future debates concerning the unique moral and legal status of the permanently unconscious (primarily the persistent vegetative state and infants with anencephaly) and whether these patients might be considered alive or dead, persons or non persons. . . . While it may be relatively easy in most cases for neurologic specialists to distinguish the persistent vegetative state from dementia, ascertaining various stages of dementia accurately may be difficult at times, even for the most experienced clinician.[6]

For the patient in the persistent vegetative state, it is more appropriate to withdraw treatment (food and fluid) when the family and physicians agree that the situation is hopeless; on the other hand, with respect to the slowly progressive neurologic deficits of Alzheimer's disease, Cranford was of the opinion that it may be more appropriate to consider withholding artificial nutrition and hydration at the stage where patients become so severely impaired that they cannot sustain themselves through voluntary intake of food and fluids.[6]

Undoubtedly, this issue will receive increasing medical-legal scrutiny as long as such conditions remain irreversible and as long as efforts are made by family members or surrogates to erase the distinction between the persistent vegetative state and severe dementia.

CAVEAT

> We are easily shocked by crimes that appear at once in their full magnitude, but the gradual growth of our wickedness, endeared by interest and palliated by the artifices of self-deceit gives us time to make distinctions in our own favour, and reason by degrees submits to absurdity, as the eye is in time accustomed to darkness. . . . —Dr. Samuel Johnson

This chapter briefly reviews the relatively rapid shift in attitudes about the provision of nutrition and hydration to competent patients who refuse it and similar rights accorded to incompetent patients in the permanent vegetative state. With this change in attitude the risks rise of unthinking, uncaring, or hasty decisions regarding cessation or continuance of life-support systems including nutrition. The President's Commission has properly devoted much space to the need for and the practice of careful decision making which involves the patient or surrogate, physician and associated health practitioners with others in reaching critical decisions.

Against the emerging consensus has stood a relatively small number of physicians and ethicists who, for one or another reason, oppose cessation of provision of food and fluid. Rosner, for example, takes the position that "the physician is given divine license to heal but not to hasten death" and that "when a physician has nothing further to offer medically or surgically, the physicians' license to heal ends and he becomes no different than a lay person."[61] In that capacity, the physician has a common obligation to provide various types of supportive care until the very end; i.e., nutrition and hydration by tube or vein is not medical treatment but a form of supportive care.

Siegler and Weisbard's stated concern, on the other hand, is neither the permanently unconscious patient nor the competent dying adult who directs his or her physician to stop various life-prolonging interventions; rather, it is concern about stopping nutrition and fluid for "patients possessing the capacity for consciousness who have not completely rejected such support. Patients must be protected against diagnostic errors. . . ., inadequate treatment, and unscrupulous care for financial or other reasons."[33] These authors admit that this particular concern is premature in the light of current safeguards. However, they foresee that economic trends, i.e., cost-containment strategies, may lead to unacceptable social consequences that result in a decline in standards of the medical profession and in social acceptance of classifications of "undesirable persons" that include a variety of groups including the terminally and incurably ill, various senile groups, the retarded, and the aged. These authors likely recall that before the Nazi government in Germany inflicted its lethal violence on Jews,

Poles, Russians, Gypsies, and others, its first victims put to death (besides the political opposition) were German "disabled" children and the elderly under the "euthanasia" projects established by Hitler,[62,63] following the earlier forced sterilization program.[63] Included in the killing program of "inferior" children was deliberate lethal starvation.

Moreover, prior to these events in Nazi Germany, there

> existed in much of the Western World, including the United States. . . . a history of coercive and sometimes illegal sterilization applied mostly to the underclass of our society. In the United States a relatively simple form of vasectomy was developed at a penal institution. . . . This, led, by 1920, to the enactment of laws in twenty-five states providing for compulsory sterilization of the criminally insane and other people considered genetically inferior.[63]

In addition to the increased support of the judiciary in upholding termination of life-support systems for the categories of competent and incompetent patients described previously, there has been an increasing acceptance by many individuals in the United States—on some issues a majority—for the withholding and withdrawal of life support for the terminally ill. The results of certain polls conducted by Louis Harris and Associates have been summarized in part as follows:

> (1) the majority of Americans who believe that "a patient with a terminal disease ought to be able to tell his doctor to let him die when no cure is in sight" increased from 62% to 85%. . . . (2) The minority of 37% of Americans who believed in 1973 that "a patient who is terminally ill with no cure in sight ought to have the right to tell his doctors to put him out of his misery" had increased to a majority of 61% by 1985.[64]

A more detailed analysis indicating the shift in American public opinion on these issues has been published recently.[65] Although the recent referendum in the state of Washington concerning assisted euthanasia was defeated, the relatively narrow margin of 54 to 46% indicates the strength of this viewpoint.[65]

These changes in attitude may be taken as evidence of an increased understanding of certain undesirable aspects of advanced medical technology together with an increased sophistication about dying and death. On the other hand, other factors may underlie these attitudinal changes. Without question, an increasingly large number of Americans are concerned about their inability to obtain and pay for adequate medical care for themselves and their loved ones. It is estimated that 35 million Americans have no health insurance coverage at work, nor do they qualify for Medicare, Medicaid, or any other health insurance coverage;[66] another 20 million are underinsured.[67] An important aspect of this is an increasing inability to care at home or in nursing homes for their infirm or incompetent elderly relatives. These serious personal concerns occur at the same time as the levels of payments by Medicare, Medicaid, and private health insurance are being reduced in association with an inability of most states to maintain their health services at previous levels.

The mounting budget items devoted to health care at the federal and state levels combined with serious overall budgetary problems are leading to various proposals for imposition of severe cost-control measures with rationing of health care services. Implicit in any rationing system is the likelihood of decreased availability of expensive life-support systems, particularly including parenteral nutrition support. Rationing health has been defined as the "societal toleration of inequitable access to health care services acknowledged to be necessary by reference to necessary care guidelines."[68] With rationing as a potential item on the national agenda for change, questions must be faced as to what will be rationed, by whom will it be rationed, who will be rationed, and who will supervise the rationing system.

Discussion about legal rationing of health care in the United States is no longer academic; a rationing system is part of the legislation approved by the Oregon legislature in 1989. In an effort to ensure all Oregonians third-party financing for needed health care, it expanded Medicaid coverage to include all poor in the state. That coverage includes only those services deemed to be of sufficiently high priority by a scale system and depending on legislative appropriation of funds;[69,70] it will begin in late 1992 if federal waivers are obtained. Ethical concerns about rationing in general and the Oregon proposal in particular have been expressed.[68–71]

Attention by all citizens to proposals for rationing health care and to those for modification of health insurance coverage is a prerequisite to ensure that any changes are more efficient, more widespread, fairer, and more ethical than those operating currently. As Sulmasy stated:

> cost-control efforts that place the physician either in the role of unilateral bedside rationer or restrictive gatekeeper threaten the integrity of medicine as a profession. . . . A morally sound system would attempt to control costs by honestly informing patients and assigning responsibility justly, would encourage physicians to act in the interests of patients, would foster truth and would recognize the great importance of equal treatment of patients. Such a system would depend on input from an informed public and would apply equally to all members of society.[72]

A continuing need exists for a combination of alert and concerned health care and legal professional, religious, and political leaders, a judiciary exercising proper safeguards, and an informed public cooperating to help ensure the strict ethical application of the two-edged sword of medical technology with its capability for the extension of life on one side and its extinction on the other.

REFERENCES*

1. Pellegrino, E.D.: JAMA, *227:*1288–1294, 1974.
2. Anon.: Nutr. Rev., *46:*315–317, 1988.
3. Centers for Disease Control: Morbid. Mortal. Weekly Rep., *38:*43–46, 1989.
4. Beauchamp, T.L., Childress, J.F.: Principles of Biomedical Ethics. 3rd Ed. New York, Oxford University Press, 1989, Chap. 3.
5. *Union Pacific Ry v. Botsford,* 141 US 250, 251 (1891).
6. Cranford, R.E.: Law Med. Health Care, *19:*13–22, 1991.
7. Oliver, D.J.: Lancet, *2:*631, 1984.
8. Printz, L.A.: Geriatrics, *43:*84–88, 1988.
9. Zerwekh, J.V.: Nursing, *83:*47–51, 1983.
10. Schmitz, P.: Law Med. Health Care, *19:*23–26, 1991.
11. O'Malley, P.: Biting at the Grave: The Irish Hunger Strikers and the Politics of Despair. Boston, Beacon Press, 1990, pp. 113–115 (cited by Cranford.[6]).
12. *Bouvia v. County of Riverside,* 159780 Riverside Co., CA Sup. Ct. (1984).
13. *Bouvia v. Superior Court (Glenchur),* 179 Cal. App. 3d 1127 225 Cal. Rpts. 297 (1986).
14. Pellegrino, E.D.: N.Y. State J. Med., *77:*1456–1462, 1977.
15. Nevins, M.: Am. Coll. Physicians Observer, *March:*13–16, 1986.
16. Appelbaum, P.S., Grisso, T.: N. Engl. J. Med., *319:*1635–1638, 1988.
17. Howe, E.G., Gordon, D.S., Valentin, M.: Law Med. Health Care, *19:*27–33, 1991.
18. President's Commission for the Study of Ethical Problems in Medicine and Biomedical and Behavioral Research: Deciding to Forego Life-Sustaining Treatment: A Report on the Ethical, Medical, and Legal Issues in Treatment Decisions. Washington, D.C., United States Government Printing Office, 1983, pp. 3, 61, and 62.
19. Orentlicher, D.: JAMA, *267:*2101–2104, 1992.
20. Hastings Center: Guidelines on the Termination of Life. Sustaining Treatment and the Care of the Dying. Briarcliff Manor, NY, Hastings Center, 1987, p. 5.
21. Law Reform Commission of Canada: Report on Euthanasia, Aiding Suicide and Cessation of Treatment. Report 20 to the Minister of Justice and Attorney General. Ottawa, Ministry of Supply and Services, 1983, pp. 11–12.
22. Curran, W.J.: N. Engl. J. Med., *310:*297–298, 1984.
23. The Patient Self-Determination Act, Sections 4206 and 4751 of the Omnibus Budget Reconciliation Act of 1990 P.L. 101–508, 11/5/90.

*The references to judicial decisions follow the form of citation generally used in legal writing. Following the case name, the initial numeric reference is to the volume of the reporter series for the decisional court. The reporter series then follows, represented by an abbreviation. The number following the abbreviation of the reporter series refers to the first page of the printed judicial decision cited. The year of the decision then follows. As an example, *Smith v. Jones,* 261 F.2d 448 (1990) can be found in Volume 261 of the second series of The Federal Reporter beginning on page 448.

Published court decisions are generally available to the public through state, county, or city bar association libraries or law school libraries. West Publishing Company and Mead Data Services also provide case text data bases on a fee-for-service basis to libraries and law firms.

24. Wolf, S.M., Boyle, P., Callahan, D., et al.: N. Engl. J. Med., *325:*1666–1671, 1991.
25. Letters to the Editor: N. Engl. J. Med., *326:*1501–1503, 1992.
26. Lynn, J.: Law Med. Health Care, *19:*101–104, 1991.
27. Areen, J.: Law Med. Health Care, *19:*91–100, 1991.
28. Jennett, B., Plum, F.: Lancet, *1:*734–737, 1972.
29. Council on Scientific Affairs, American Medical Association: JAMA, *263:*426–430, 1990.
30. Working Party on the Ethics of Prolonging Life and Assisting Death, Institute of Medical Ethics: Lancet, *337:*96–98, 1991.
31. *In re Quinlan* 70 NJ 10, 355 A2d 647 (1976).
32. Rosner, F.: N.Y. State Med J., *87:*591–593, 1987.
33. Siegler, M., Weisbard, A.J.: Arch. Intern. Med., *145:*129–131, 1985.
34. *People v. Barber* A025586 Los Angeles Sup. Ct. 1983; *Barber v. Superior Ct.* 147 CA 3d 1006 CA, 1983.
35. Myers, D.W.: Arch. Intern. Med., *145:*125–127, 1985.
36. *Matter of Claire Conroy,* 464 A 2d 303 (NJ App. 1983); cf also *in re Claire Conroy* 98 NJ 321 (1985).
37. Emanuel, E.J.: Lancet, *1:*170–171, 1988.
38. Emanuel, E.J.: Lancet, *1:*106–107, 1988.
39. Seckler, B.A., Meier, D.E., Mulvihill, M., et al.: Ann Intern. Med., *115:*92–98, 1991.
40. Emanuel, E.J., Emanuel, L.L.: JAMA, *267:*2067–2071, 1992.
41. Letters to the Editor: Ann. Intern. Med., *115:*743–745, 1981.
42. Lynn, J.: JAMA, *267:*2082–2084, 1992.
43. Coordinating Council on Life-Sustaining Medical Treatment Decision-Making by the Courts: Guidelines for State Court Decision-Making in Authorizing or Withholding Life Sustaining Medical Treatment. Williamsburg, VA, National Center for State Courts, 1991.
44. Council on Ethical and Judicial Affairs of the American Medical Association: Withholding or Withdrawing Life Prolonging Medical Treatment. Chicago, American Medical Association, 1986.
45. Angell, M.: N. Engl. J. Med., *322:*1226–1228, 1990.
46. Brief for petitioners, *Cruzan v. Missouri Department of Health* No. 89–1503 (July 1988).
47. *Cruzan v. Harmon* 760 SW 2d 408 (Nov. 1988).
48. *Cruzan v. Missouri Department of Health* 497–111 L. Ed. 2d 224, 110 St. Ct. 2841 (1990).
49. Annas, G.J.: Law Med. Health Care, *19:*52–59, 1991.
50. *Cruzan v. Mouton Estate* No. CV 384–9P Circ. Ct. Jasper Co. (filed Dec. 14, 1990) (Teel).
51. Bopp, J.J., Marzen, T.J.: Law Med. Health Care, *19:*37–51, 1991.
52. Lo, B., Steinbrook, R.: Ann. Intern. Med., *114:*895–901, 1991.
53. Annas, G.J.: N. Engl. J. Med., *323:*670–673, 1990.
54. Bioethicists' Statement on the U.S. Supreme Court's Cruzan Decision: N. Engl. J. Med., *323:*686, 1990.
55. Rouse, F.: Law Med. Health Care, *19:*83–90, 1991.
56. King, P.A.: Law Med. Health Care, *19:*76–79, 1991.
57. Baron, C.H.: Law Med. Health Care, *19:*73–76, 1991.
58. Jennett, B., Dyer, C.: Br. Med. J., *302:*1256–1258, 1991.
59. President's Commission for the Study of Ethical Problems in Medicine and Biomedical and Behavioral Research: Deciding to Forego Life-Sustaining Treatment: A Report on

the Ethical, Medical, and Legal Issues in Treatment Decisions. Washington, D.C., United States Government Printing Office, 1983, Chap. 2, p. 46.
60. American College of Physicians, Ethics Manual Pt. 2: Ann. Intern. Med., *111*:327–355, 1989.
61. Rosner, F.: Bull. N.Y. Acad. Med., *64*:363–375, 1988.
62. Gallagher, H.G.: By Trust Betrayed: Patients, Physicians and the License to Kill in the Third Reich. New York, Henry Holt, 1990.
63. Lifton, J.R.: The Nazi Doctors. New York, Basic Books, 1986.
64. Taylor, H.: N. Engl. J. Med., *322*:1891–1892, 1990.
65. Blendon, R.J., Szalay, U.S., Knox, R.A.: JAMA, *267*:2658–2662, 1992.
66. Dougherty, C.J.: Law Med. Health Care. *20*:82–91, 1992.
67. Bodenheimer, T.: N. Engl. J. Med., *327*:274–278, 1992.
68. Hadorn, D.C., Brook, R.H.: JAMA, *266*:3328–3331, 1991.
69. Hadorn, D.C.: JAMA, *265*:2218–2225, 1991.
70. Garland, M.J.: Law Med. Health Care, *20*:67–81, 1992.
71. Menzel, P.T.: Law Med. Health Care, *20*:57–66, 1992.
72. Sulmasy, D.P.: Ann. Intern. Med., *116*:920–926, 1992.

SELECTED READINGS

Beauchamp, T.L., Childress, J.F.: Principles of Biomedical Ethics. 3rd Ed. New York, Oxford University Press, 1989.
Faden, R.R., Beauchamp, T.L.: A History and Theory of Informed Consent. New York, Oxford University Press, 1986.
Lynn, J. (Ed): By No Extraordinary Means: The Choice to Forego Life-Sustaining Food and Water. Expanded Ed. Indianapolis, Indiana University Press, 1989.
Meisel, A.: Legal Myths About Terminating Life Support. Arch. Intern. Med., *151*:1497–1502, 1991.
Pellagrino, E.D., Thomasma, D.C.: For the Patient's Good: The Restoration of Beneficence in Health Care. New York, Oxford University Press, 1988.

PART V

Diet in the Health of Populations

CHAPTER **82**

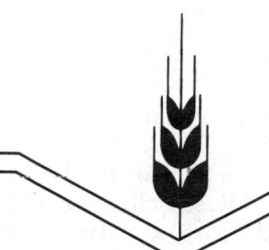

Recommended Dietary Intakes: Current and Future Approaches

Alfred E. Harper

To plan food supplies for large groups of people, make reliable public health recommendations for nutritionally adequate diets, formulate appropriate modifications of usual diets for therapeutic purposes, and assess the adequacy of diets consumed by individuals or populations, information about human needs for specific nutrients is essential. Recommended dietary intakes (RDI) are a set of reference standards—usually called dietary standards—developed to meet this need. RDI are defined as *amounts of essential nutrients considered sufficient to meet the physiologic needs of practically all healthy persons in a specified group and the average amount of food sources of energy needed by the members of the group.*[1–6] RDI for essential nutrients are not average requirements. They exceed the needs of most, if not all, individuals in the specified group, specified by age and sex.

The names used for such standards include Recommended Dietary Allowances (RDA) in the United States,[5] Recommended Intakes of Nutrients in the United Kingdom,[4] and Safe Intakes of Nutrients by the Food and Agriculture and World Health Organizations (FAO/WHO).[3] The definitions of dietary standards differ slightly from one organization to another, and values for some nutrients differ somewhat from one standard to another, but all are reference standards designed to accomplish the same objective: to provide physicians, health educators, and policy administrators with reliable scientific information about the amounts of essential nutrients and food sources of energy needed in diets. The terms and their abbreviations are used interchangeably in this chapter, but RDA is used when reference is made to U.S. standards.

EVOLUTION OF DIETARY STANDARDS

Knowledge of human nutritional needs and of relationships between diet and health was largely speculative until the nineteenth century. Only after Lavoisier had established that the body obtained energy through oxidation of foodstuffs and Magendie had recognized that protein was essential in the diet for survival, did science begin to impact on nutrition. The development by the mid-nineteenth century of respiration chambers for estimating energy expenditure and the nitrogen balance procedure for measuring nitrogen retention first made it possible to estimate energy and protein requirements accurately. As a result, during the economic recession of the 1860s, when the British Privy Council sought information about the amount of food that would be needed to relieve starvation and hunger among the unemployed, Dr. Edward Smith was able to respond, on the basis of experimental observations, that it would require food providing about 3000 kcal of energy and 80 g of protein per person per day. This was the first dietary standard proposed on scientific principles. During the next 50 years other recommendations were made for meeting energy and protein needs but, despite the experimental approach adopted by Edward Smith, most were based only on estimates of the amounts of energy and protein provided by the usual diets of healthy working men.[7–9]

Between 1910 and 1920, after several minor constituents of foods (vitamins and minerals) were discovered to be essential nutrients, new directions in dietary advice began to evolve and government agencies began to propose programs for preventing dietary deficiency diseases that were directed toward improving the health of the entire population. Toward the end of World War I, a Food Committee of the British Royal Society recommended that "protective foods" such as fruits and vegetables be included in all diets as sources of unidentified factors, and that milk be included in the diets of all children.[7] In the United States at that time, the Department of Agriculture (USDA) recommended that diets be selected from a wide variety of foods in order to encourage consumption of adequate quantities of the various essential nutrients. Dietary recommendations made through the 1920s and early 1930s were based on limited quantitative information, but both the League of Nations Health Organization and the USDA had recognized that scientific knowledge of human requirements for essential nutrients was needed to provide a reliable base for practical nutrition programs.[10,11] As knowledge of human requirements for essential nutrients began to accumulate, several health organizations realized that, in order to develop sound recommendations for a nutritionally adequate diet, it would be important to establish standards for the amounts of nutrients needed in diets. Standards for intakes of energy sources and protein had been proposed earlier, but had not been adopted formally. This is not surprising because prior to 1940, *no clear distinction had been made between dietary standards and health policy recommendations.*

ADOPTION OF RECOMMENDED DIETARY ALLOWANCES AND INTAKES

The first effort to distinguish clearly between dietary standards and health policy recommendations was made by Dr. Hazel Stiebling. She proposed a set of reference values for desirable nutrient intakes as a standard for ensuring that diets used in the food programs of the USDA during the great depression would be nutritionally adequate.[12] A few years later she and Dr. Esther Phipard[13] proposed a set of values for energy, protein, calcium, phosphorus, and iron based on current knowledge of human requirements.[10] Their standard included recommended intakes for different age groups and different degrees of physical activity. They adjusted the average requirement values for the various essential nutrients upward by 50% to allow for individual variations among the requirements of apparently healthy people.

Just after the beginning of World War II, the U.S. government asked the National Research Council/National Academy of Sciences (NRC/NAS) to form a Committee on Food and Nutrition to establish nutrition objectives for the nation. In 1941, this committee became the Food and Nutrition Board. One of the first tasks it undertook was to prepare a set of dietary standards for adequate intakes of known nutrients.[14] Standards for nine nutrients were adopted formally at a National Nutrition Conference in 1941; these were the first set of Recommended Dietary Allowances (RDA).[15] A similar Dietary Standard had been adopted by the Canadian Council on Nutrition the previous year.[16] These actions represented a shift in the basis for dietary advice from knowledge of patterns of food consumption of healthy people to scientific knowledge of human requirements for essential nutrients.

RDI have since been adopted by many countries, and most have revised their recommendations at intervals as new knowledge of human requirements has become available.[2] The tenth edition of the RDA bulletin of the NRC/NAS was published in 1989.[5] Over the years the number of nutrients for which RDA have been established has increased from 9 to 19, with tentative values for 7 others included in separate tables. The most recent table of RDA is included in Appendix Table A–2b.

RDI ARE NOT DIETARY GUIDELINES

RDI are not health policy recommendations or dietary guidelines for the public; they are, it is important to reiterate, reference values for intakes of essential nutrients and food sources of energy that will maintain health in practically all healthy individuals, for use by physicians, dietitians and other health professionals, educators, and administrators. To make this distinction clearer, the RDA for protein for adults in the United States is 0.8 g/kg of body weight per day, a standard for the amount judged adequate to maintain health; but the amount usually recommended in diets is about 12.5% (10 to 15%) of calories[4,6] or about 1.2 g/kg of body weight. The latter is a dietary guideline for the public, not just to meet protein needs, but to encourage consumption of high-protein foods, which are good sources of other nutrients and which contribute to the palatability of the diet.

Dietary guidelines, in contrast to RDI, are dietary recommendations for the public and a component of health policy; specific guidelines are described in Chapter 93. Dietary guidelines bear a distinct resemblance to rules of personal hygiene, which have been advocated since biblical times. Galen, about 1800 years ago, codified factors such as diet, exercise, rest, and sleep, which he considered important for health and over which the individual could exert some control. This concept of personal responsibility for health was a motivating force for many health movements during the nineteenth and early twentieth centuries[17] and underlies current dietary guidelines.

Dietary guidelines differ from RDI in several respects (Table 82–1). Guidelines deal primarily with the quantities of certain foods and nonessential dietary components, such as fiber and cholesterol, and the proportions and types of energy sources that are judged to be desirable in healthful diets. RDI deal mainly with meeting needs for essential nutrients. Also, the objective of most dietary guidelines is to reduce the risk of chronic and degenerative diseases in the population, rather than to ensure that intakes of essential nutrients will be adequate. Dietary guidelines designed to reduce the risk (commonly called "prevention") of chronic and degenerative diseases have been proposed by many organizations concerned with control of diseases such as heart disease and cancer. General dietary guidelines for the population as a whole that have less emphasis on disease prevention and more on promotion of health have been adopted by health departments in the United States[18] and in many countries as part of national health policy (see Chap. 93).

Associations observed among diet, health behaviors, and the occurrence of chronic and degenerative diseases, which have been the main impetus for proposing dietary guidelines, are highly complex; they are subject to various interpretations.[19,20] Unlike the situation with nutritional deficiency diseases, the causes of chronic and degenerative diseases are not clearly established; furthermore, susceptibility or resistance of individuals to these diseases is highly variable and cannot be predicted from knowledge of diet consumption alone. In contrast to the general agreement on the scientific validity of the basis for RDI, there is considerable controversy over the general applicability of the scientific evidence marshaled to support dietary guidelines for reducing risk of chronic and degenerative diseases. The limited effectiveness of dietary modifications and drug treatment to reduce serum cholesterol concentration in lowering mortality from heart disease in men judged to be at high risk for coronary heart disease has been one factor contributing to this controversy. In some 19 trials of this type involving about 30,000 men over a 5- to 10-year period, results have not been consistent and, overall, although the treatments produced a marginally significant reduction in heart attacks, no significant reduction in total mortality was observed.[20]

CURRENT APPROACHES TO RDI

The objective in establishing RDI is to identify intakes of essential nutrients that are high enough to maintain health in virtually all individuals in groups specified by age and sex. Responsibility for accomplishing this task is assigned to a committee of 8 to 15 scientists, each with special knowledge in one or more areas of nutrition. Committees that set the RDA in the United States and those that set RDI for other countries use essentially the same process. The initial step is to evaluate critically the international scientific literature on human requirements and, from this, to estimate for each essential nutrient average requirements of groups of different ages and in different physiologic states. Then, using information about individual variability of requirements, the value for each average requirement is increased to take into account, first, the range of requirements observed among individuals with similar characteristics and, second, the biologic availability and efficiency of utiliza-

TABLE 82–1. DIFFERENCES BETWEEN RDI AND DIETARY GUIDELINES

RDI	DIETARY GUIDELINES
Reference values for meeting needs for essential nutrients and energy	Advice on selecting foods to achieve a nutritionally adequate diet
Deal mainly with quantities of micronutrients and protein needed daily	Deal mainly with proportions of energy-yielding nutrients in diets
Do not deal with non-nutrients and nutrients that are not essential	Include advice on consumption of such non-nutrients as fiber and nonessential nutrients as cholesterol
Specific values are given for different age-sex groups	Recommendations are general, without specification for different segments of the population
Serve as standards for establishing health policy	Are health policy proposals
Designed to prevent impairment of health from nutritional inadequacy, which is directly related to diet and to which susceptiblity is universal	Directed toward prevention of chronic diseases for which diet is a potential modifying factor and to which susceptibility is highly variable
Firmly established on the basis of experimental evidence	Evidence mainly indirect from associations observed between diet and disease incidence

tion of the various essential nutrients from the foods usually consumed.[1] The basis for estimating RDI for energy is different from that for essential nutrients and is dealt with separately later in this chapter.

Although all committees use essentially the same process and the same basic information to establish RDI, values proposed for some nutrients differ from one RDI report to another (see Appendix Tables A–2 to A–6). The differences are usually attributable to (1) differences in judgement among the various committees as to the appropriate criteria for establishing when the requirement has been met, and (2) differences in the bioavailability of nutrients from the major food sources in the various national food supplies.

REQUIREMENTS FOR ESSENTIAL NUTRIENTS

The concept of a requirement for an essential nutrient is illustrated by the curve in Figure 82–1, which shows the relationship between level of intake and probability that intake is inadequate or excessive. The minimum intake at which the risk of inadequacy is judged to be essentially zero is taken as the requirement. FAO/WHO have proposed the term "safe range of intake" for intakes that fall between the safe level (RDI) and the level above which evidence of adverse effects can be detected.[3,21]

CHARACTERISTICS OF REQUIREMENTS

Requirements change with increasing age between birth and maturity. During periods of growth, when new tissue is being laid down, requirements are higher per unit of body weight than they are after growth has ceased. In the mature female, requirements increase during pregnancy as the fetus grows; they also increase during lactation in proportion to the amount of milk produced. With increasing age beyond 40, lean body mass and activity decline; hence, energy needs decline.[3,5] The available evidence, however, suggests that needs for essential nutrients do not decline as might be anticipated, despite the lowered rate of metabolism. Needs of the elderly for several essential nutrients, including thiamin, riboflavin, and protein, were found not to be appreciably different from those of younger age groups,[22] but the requirement for vitamin B_{12} appeared to be increased.[23] Reduced efficiency of gastrointestinal function may impair the utilization of some nutrients by a portion of the elderly population.[23]

Also, there are some differences in requirements, more apparent than real, between the sexes. Requirements of males appear to be higher than those of females when requirements are reported per person; but, when requirements are expressed per unit of body weight, except for iron, values for the two sexes are similar. For ages between menarche and menopause, loss of blood during menstruation increases iron requirements of females considerably above those for males (see Chap. 9),[21] (Appendix Table A–2b).

RDI established by these procedures are reported separately for different age-sex groups. The range of ages included in the specified groups for young children are narrowest because their rates of growth change rapidly. Values are expressed as the amount of each nutrient required per day by an individual of average weight and height in the specified group or, for adults, for a reference individual. The range of body weights included in the age-sex groups may be wide, so the average value for the

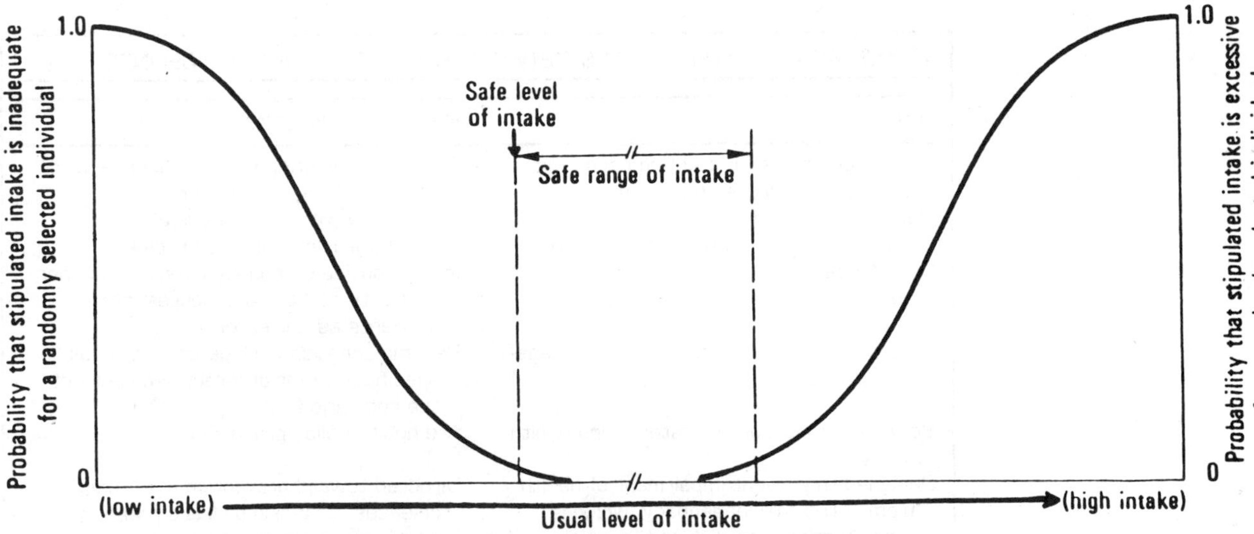

FIGURE 82–1. Relation between level of intake of an essential nutrient and probability that intake is inadequate or excessive. (From Food and Agriculture Organization (FAO)/World Health Organization (WHO)/United Nations University: Energy and Protein Requirements. WHO Technical Report Series 724. Geneva, World Health Organization, 1985.)

group will not apply directly to individuals at the extremes of the range. Requirements are considered to be a function of body size for individuals who are not overweight. In using requirement or RDI values as guides to the needs of persons whose body sizes deviate considerably from the average, the convention adopted is to adjust the values on the basis of body weight even though requirements for some nutrients may not be proportional to body weight.[21] For overweight individuals, adjustment on the basis of lean body mass is considered more appropriate.

INDIVIDUAL VARIABILITY OF REQUIREMENTS

Requirements, like other human characteristics, differ considerably among individuals owing to genetic differences. The distribution of requirements, illustrated in Figure 82–2 for protein requirements of adults,[3] is Gaussian, often called "normal." Values for 95% and 99.9% of the population fall within the range of the mean ±2 standard deviations (s.d.) and ±3 s.d, respectively.[3] Variability is often expressed as the coefficient of variation (CV), that is, the standard deviation expressed as a percentage of the mean. For most biologic variables, including nutrient requirements, the CV is about 15% (range = 10 to 20%); higher values are usually associated with inaccurate or unreliable methods for measuring the variable. With a CV of 15%, requirements of individuals in a single age-sex group will be expected to range from about 45% below to 45% above the average. Iron requirements of menstruating women are an exception. They are not normally distributed but are skewed toward the upper end of the range.[21]

Only for a few nutrients have sufficient data been obtained to formulate a reliable statistical estimate of variability. For many nutrients, it must be assumed that the CV of requirements does not differ greatly from that for nutrients for which satisfactory values have been obtained.

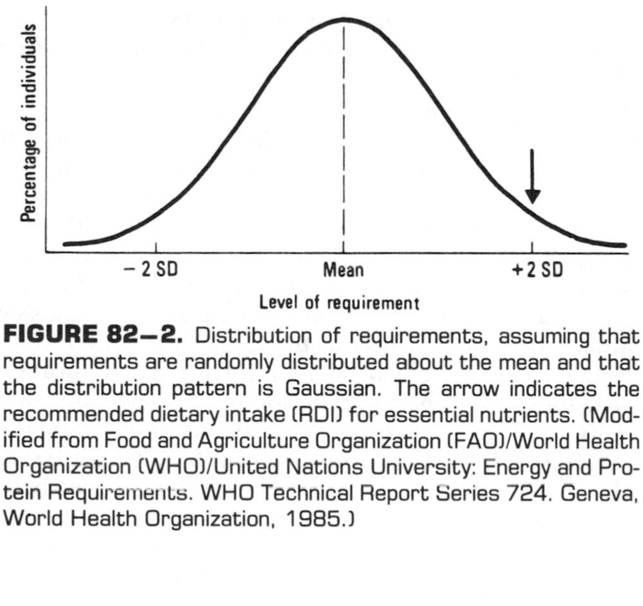

FIGURE 82–2. Distribution of requirements, assuming that requirements are randomly distributed about the mean and that the distribution pattern is Gaussian. The arrow indicates the recommended dietary intake (RDI) for essential nutrients. (Modified from Food and Agriculture Organization (FAO)/World Health Organization (WHO)/United Nations University: Energy and Protein Requirements. WHO Technical Report Series 724. Geneva, World Health Organization, 1985.)

ESTIMATION OF REQUIREMENTS

The number of methods for estimating requirements is limited, and methods that can be used differ from one nutrient to another. For age groups beyond infancy there is not always agreement on the criteria that should be used to establish either reliable requirements or how much weight should be given to different indicators of nutrient depletion. For infants and children, maintenance of satisfactory growth rates is accepted. For most nutrients, there is little information about the requirements of age groups between infancy and adulthood. It is therefore necessary to use information about rates of growth and the composition of the accumulating tissues to interpolate between infant and adult requirements in order to obtain estimates of requirements for intermediate age groups. Values for infants for the most part are estimated from the amount of each nutrient provided by the amount of human milk consumed by infants whose growth rates are satisfactory.

The objective of all methods for establishing requirements is to ensure that the quantity of the nutrient in tissues (body pool) will be high enough to protect against impairment of health even if intake is inadequate for a short period. For a few nutrients including ascorbic acid, vitamin B_{12}, and iron, it has been possible to estimate directly relationships among intake, body pool size, and occurrence of signs of deficiency. For several, especially those that have posed public health problems—thiamin, niacin, ascorbic acid, vitamin A, iron, and iodine—the quantities required to prevent or cure deficiencies have been established within narrow limits through both epidemiologic and experimental studies. For some—riboflavin, folic acid, and vitamins B_6 and E—similar but less extensive information has been obtained from depletion-repletion experiments on human subjects in which the amount of nutrient that will prevent or cure signs of deficiency has been established.

For several nutrients, indirect methods are used to estimate the state of the body pool and the requirement. The balance procedure (which consists of measuring intake and output of a nutrient, calculating the difference, and thus obtaining an estimate of the gain by, or loss from, the body) has been used to estimate requirements for protein, calcium, magnesium, zinc, copper, and other mineral elements. The accuracy of balance studies has been questioned because of an underlying assumption of this procedure that the state of the body pool, which is not measured directly, is appropriate and has not changed during the course of the experiment. Other methods used to obtain an indirect estimate of the state of body stores and requirements include measurements of changes, in response to changes in intake of the nutrient, in the blood concentration or urinary excretion of the nutrient or one of its metabolites, or changes in a metabolic function such as the activity of an enzyme for which the nutrient of interest is a cofactor or a component of the cofactor.

For many nutrients, neither the total amount of information nor the total number of subjects studied is as great as is desirable. The reliability of requirement values thus varies considerably from nutrient to nutrient, as is illustrated by the following examples.

For thiamin, requirements have been estimated by several methods, and the values obtained are in good agreement.[24,25] Thiamin is needed particularly for the metabolism of carbohydrates, and the need for it has been related to carbohydrate intake. However, because carbohydrate intake usually increases in proportion to energy intake, the requirement is expressed as a function of caloric intake. In early nutrition surveys, thiamin deficiency (beri-beri) was not encountered in populations with intakes of the vitamin in excess of 0.35 mg/1000 kcal per day, but the incidence increased steadily as intake fell progressively below this level. Thiamin excretion in urine was found to rise sharply as intake increased above 0.35 mg/1000 kcal (1.04 μmol/239kJ) per day, evidence that tissues were amply nourished by intakes at this level. Also, erythrocyte transketolase, an enzyme for which thiamin pyrophosphate is the coenzyme, was found to be adequately maintained by intakes of thiamin on the order of 0.4 mg/1000 kcal per day. Higher intakes of thiamin were required to achieve maximum enzyme activity, but this state, referred to as "saturation" of tissues, was not associated with any detectable health benefit. Because the requirement of adults for thiamin has been shown by three different approaches to be on the order of 0.35 mg/1000 kcal per day, there is considerable confidence that this is a reliable estimate.

Requirements of adults for calcium are estimated using the balance procedure. Inconsistencies among the results obtained in different studies have posed a continuing problem for committees assigned the task of setting requirements. Calcium intakes required to achieve zero balance (intake = output) in 10 separate studies on human adults have ranged from 200 to 975 mg (5 to 24.3 mmol) daily, with most values falling between 400 and 800 mg.[6,26] Individuals can adapt to a wide range of calcium intakes; however, after a change in intake, adaptation to the new level may occur only slowly. The fraction of ingested calcium absorbed declines as intake rises but the absolute amount absorbed increases. Calcium absorption is influenced by several dietary factors; it increases in the presence of lactose and decreases in the presence of phytic acid, a constituent of cereal grains. Also, urinary excretion of calcium is influenced by the amounts of sodium, phosphate, and protein in the diet. From a detailed analysis of the individual studies, taking these factors into account, Nordin has estimated the average requirement of young western adults to be 500 to 600 mg per day,[26] but the range of values observed indicates the need for a better method for determining calcium requirements.

The amount of vitamin E required by human subjects has not been established directly. In one human experiment, men consuming only 2 to 3 mg (4.6 to 7.0 μmol) of vitamin E per day for a year showed no ill effects except for an increase in the fragility of red blood cells. With increasing amounts of polyunsaturated fatty acids in the diet, blood concentration of vitamin E fell, suggesting that the requirement increased with increasing intakes of fats rich in these fatty acids. Observations on the amount of vitamin E required to maintain a blood concentration of 0.5 mg (1.2 μmol)/100 ml in subjects consuming usual diets suggest that the requirement for adults is 3 to 4 mg of α-tocopherol per day. Limited knowledge of the requirement has led to dependence on information about amounts of vitamin E consumed by groups of healthy individuals as a guide to recommendations for appropriate intakes of this vitamin.

This brings us to another important point. Requirements cannot be established directly from results of scientific experiments; an element of judgment is required. The patterns of response of biologic variables to changing inputs tend to be curvilinear; they rarely have sharp inflection points. Selection of the point on the curve for the response in pool size, urinary excretion, or nutrient retention in balance studies as nutrient intake increases that represents an adequate intake or body pool requires a measure of judgment. For ascorbic acid, for example, signs of scurvy begin to appear in adults if the body pool falls below 300 mg (1.7 mmol). This occurs if intake is less than 10 mg per day. If daily intake has been 60 mg (0.34 mmol) or more, the body pool will approach the maximum size (saturation) of about 1500 mg (8.5 mmol) and will not fall to the point at which signs of scurvy develop (300 mg) for at least 60 days, even if intake is negligible.[27,28] A daily intake of 10 mg is obviously insufficient to ensure an adequate reserve of the vitamin. An intake of 60 mg per day would be an appropriate recommendation for a sailor who is starting on an 80-day voyage with no expectation of obtaining fresh food throughout that time. But what, between these two values, is an appropriate intake for an adult who is consuming fresh food regularly? An intake of 30 mg per day, an amount that would maintain a body pool of about 1000 mg and provide a reserve lasting 20 to 30 days, should be ample. Differences in judgment on the size of the desirable reserve resulted in the FAO/WHO recommending 30 mg per day of ascorbic acid as a safe intake for men,[29] whereas the U.S. NRC/NAS recommends 60 mg per day or more, implying that saturation of tissues should be the criterion of adequacy and that individuals consuming between 30 and 60 mg daily are at risk from inadequate intakes, even though no evidence of a health benefit from the higher intake has been demonstrated.

PROCESS FOR ESTABLISHING RDI

FROM REQUIREMENTS TO RDI FOR ESSENTIAL NUTRIENTS

It is apparent that a recommendation for consumption of an amount of an essential nutrient equal to the average requirement of the population group under consideration is actually a recommendation for an intake that is below the requirements of half of that population. The pattern of distribution of individual requirements is, therefore, a major consideration in establishing RDI; namely, recommendations for meeting the needs of essentially all individuals. An intake two standard deviations above the mean, proposed by the FAO/WHO as an appropriate safe intake for public health recommendations (see Appendix Tables A–9 and A–10),[3,21] has been adopted widely as an acceptable first approximation for establishing RDI. An intake at this level would theoretically meet or exceed the needs of 97.5% of the population (Fig. 82–2) and includes the 95% whose requirements fall between the mean ±2 s.d. and the 2.5% whose requirements are more than 2 s.d. below the mean.[3] As noted earlier, for those nutrients for which there are too few individual requirement values to permit accurate adjustment for individual variability, the coefficient of variation of requirements is assumed either to resemble that for nutrients for which such information is available or variability is estimated from the range of requirements actually observed (despite their paucity). The latter procedure was used as a guide to the upper limit of requirements before the FAO/WHO approach was adopted.

For nutrients that are fully available from food, RDI based on the FAO/WHO approach are unlikely to be inadequate for anyone, for at least three reasons. First, committees estimating requirements or bioavailability of nutrients tend to select the higher of alternative values because consumption of a small excess of an essential nutrient is not known to be detrimental, whereas a small deficit over a long time will lead to depletion. Second, for some nutrients at least (protein, iron, calcium), individuals adapt to intakes below the estimated requirement by conserving the nutrient more efficiently or increasing efficiency of absorption. Thirdly, even if for some individuals the RDI is somewhat below their estimated requirement, the reserve of the nutrient in their body pools may be smaller than is considered desirable without depletion occurring to a point that impairs health.

The FAO/WHO concluded that if the distribution of requirements is skewed, as was noted for the iron requirements of menstruating females, setting the RDI at the 95th percentile of the distribution is an appropriate public health recommendation.[21] The alternative is to such as women with high menstrual losses, as clinical consider individuals with unusually high requirements, problems and propose the use of therapeutic supplements for them.

Finally, in setting RDI, the bioavailability of nutrients from the foods usually consumed, and efficiency of utilization of different forms or precursors of the nutrient in foods must be considered (see Chaps. 39, 90, and others on individual nutrients). The extent to which certain vitamins such as folic acid and vitamin B_6 and most minerals are released and absorbed from foods can vary greatly. The availability of iron from plant products may be only 3%, whereas from many animal products it may be as high as 20 to 25%. RDI for iron in India, where most diets are composed largely of foods of plant origin, are therefore much higher than in the United States where most diets contain a high percentage of meats. Several carotenoids are precursors of retinol (vitamin A), so RDI for vitamin A are expressed as "retinol equivalents" with factors for efficiency of conversion of carotenoids to retinol being provided to permit estimation of the retinol equivalents obtained from foods by using information about the relative proportions of carotenoids and retinol they contain (see Appendix Table A–1b).

RDI FOR INDIVIDUALS AND POPULATIONS

It is not always clear whether RDI are proposed as safe intakes for individuals or as appropriate average intakes for groups. RDI are derived from the observed average requirements of individuals grouped by similar characteristics, adjusted upward, as described above, to take into consideration the variability observed among the requirements of the individuals in the group. As stated earlier they are therefore considered to be high enough to cover the needs of almost all persons in such groups, and presumably the entire population of such persons. RDI are obviously appropriate safe intakes for individuals, because if the average intake of a nutrient by an individual equals or exceeds the RDI, that intake will exceed the requirement of almost every individual.

Are RDI appropriate average intakes for population groups? They are used as recommendations for groups on the assumption that, if each individual in the group consumes an amount of an essential nutrient equal to the RDI, all will be consuming an adequate or more than adequate amount. A problem with this assumption is that food, and hence nutrient, intakes of individuals vary even more widely than nutrient requirements. Thus, even when the average intake of a population equals or exceeds the RDI, intakes of a segment of the population are found to be below the RDI; this is illustrated in Figure 82–3 as the overlap between the requirement and intake curves, wherein the food intakes of some individuals in this segment are likely to be inadequate. Intakes of both food and individual nutrients may be low as the result of poverty, illness, alcoholism, inappropriate food selection, or bizarre food beliefs, as well as for many

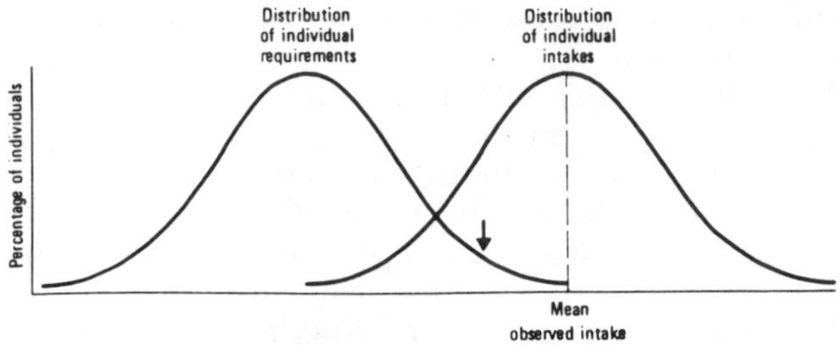

FIGURE 82–3. Comparison of distribution of individual requirements (left) with distribution of individual intakes (right). The arrow indicates the recommended dietary intake (RDI). The greater the overlap of the distribution curves, the greater will be the proportion of individuals with inadequate intakes. (From Food and Agriculture Organization (FAO)/World Health Organization (WHO)/United Nations University: Energy and Protein Requirements. WHO Technical Report Series 724. Geneva, World Health Organization, 1985.)

other reasons. In view of the probability that essential nutrient intakes of a portion of the population will be inadequate when average intake of the group equals or exceeds the RDI that is appropriate for individuals, questions have arisen as to whether RDI for populations should not exceed those for individuals in order to ensure that the incidence of inadequate intakes will be low (see Chap. 83).[21,30] When the average intake of a nutrient by a population exceeds the *average requirement* by twice or more the CV of the *average intake,* the probability of inadequate intakes should, on the basis of statistical considerations, be low. It should be recognized, however, that even if this approach were to be adopted, the causes of low intakes are unlikely to be influenced by increasing RDI for populations above those for individuals.

RDI values established by the procedures discussed are widely accepted as the best available reference values for dealing with nutrition problems of individuals whose intakes of nutrients are considered to be inadequate and for many aspects of nutrition and health policy. When the incidence of nutritional inadequacy is estimated from observations made in health and nutrition surveys, the incidence of intakes below the RDA for several nutrients greatly exceeds the incidence of clinical evidence of deficiency.[31] Such data suggest that RDI are more likely to be overestimates rather than underestimates of human needs for nutrients. RDI should not be considered as rigid daily requirements, but as average amounts to be consumed over a period of several days, because a small deficit on one day will be readily compensated for by a small surplus on another. Also, because of limited knowledge about possible beneficial or detrimental effects of many food constituents, RDI should be met from as wide a variety of foods as is possible. Nutritional problems are encountered mainly when diets are composed of a narrow selection of foods.

RDI FOR ENERGY

It is conventional to use the term energy as if energy were a nutrient. The body generates the energy it needs from carbohydrates, fats, and to a lesser extent, proteins; hence, the nutritional requirement is for these food components. The quantities required are often expressed as a percentage of total energy needs or intake—for example, 12% of energy as protein.

The situation in meeting requirements for essential nutrients is different from that of meeting energy needs; healthy individuals with ready access to palatable food will ordinarily meet their energy needs by adjusting their intake of food spontaneously and will maintain energy balance without conscious effort over considerable periods. Hence, the basis for establishing RDI for energy is different from that for essential nutrients. To establish the RDI for energy at the *upper end* of the requirement range is a prescription (if followed) for overweight or obesity for most people. *RDI for energy are not, therefore, recommended intakes for all individuals in the specified age-sex groups but are the estimated average requirement of each group.* Assuming that requirements for energy are distributed normally, RDI for energy will be represented by the mean in Figure 82–2. Total energy expenditure cannot fall below the resting requirement without inducing weight loss but it can rise very much above it for highly active individuals; therefore, the distribution for many populations will be skewed toward the upper end of the range.

Energy is needed to cover the cost of the resting (basal) energy expenditure, the thermic effect of food (TEF), and the energy expended for physical activity. Resting energy expenditure can be measured directly by calorimetry. It varies with body weight, age, and sex. Equations have been derived empirically from relationships among basal metabolic rate, body weight, age, sex, and height for predicting resting energy expenditure.[32] The FAO/WHO have proposed a set of equations for estimating resting energy metabolism for different age-sex groups based on analysis of several sets of measurements of weight, height, and energy expenditure.[3] The physical activity component is calculated by multiplying the amounts of time spent in different activities by an "activity factor" appropriate for the activity, expressed as a multiple of the resting expenditure[3–6] (see Appendix Table A–8d). For a more accurate estimate of requirements, an adjustment should be made for TEF (see Chap. 5).

RDI for energy, being average requirements of population groups, are not useful as standards for the energy needs of individuals. Energy requirements of individuals must be estimated separately for each person as outlined above. For individuals who are maintaining stable and appropriate body weight, the amount of food energy consumed provides a reasonably satisfactory estimate of energy requirements. Changes in patterns of energy intake over time can be detected reliably by monitoring body weight. Tables of appropriate body weight for age, included in most RDI publications serve as guides that can be used together with estimates of usual caloric intake for adjusting energy intake to correct undesirable weight changes (see Appendix Tables A–2 to A–6 and A–9b).

USES OF RDI

RDI have been used for many purposes since they became established as standards for planning food supplies. The uses have been categorized as *prescriptive* and *diagnostic*.[33] Uses related to planning diets, food supplies, dietary guidance about how to meet nutritional needs, and regulations to help ensure that they will be met are prescriptive. Uses related to evaluation of the adequacy of nutrient intakes or nutritional status are diagnostic. RDI are used frequently as standards for nutritional assessment, often without sufficient consideration being given to their limitations for this purpose, as is discussed later. Problems encountered in using dietary intake information to assess nutritional status have been re-examined by U.S.[30] and FAO/WHO[3] committees (see Chap. 83).

PRESCRIPTIVE USES

PLANNING FOOD SUPPLIES AND DIETS

The original purpose in establishing RDI was to provide a set of standards for nutrient intakes for planning nutritionally adequate food supplies for population groups such as the armed forces and the institutionalized.[14] They were and are also used by international agencies to estimate food needs of national populations.[3] For these purposes data about the composition of foods and the proportions of the population in the various age-sex groups are used in conjunction with RDI to estimate both the total amount of food energy sources needed and the amounts of various individual foods required to provide RDI levels of essential nutrients for the specified population.

Although RDI for energy, being average requirements, do not provide guidance about individual energy needs, they are appropriate standards for planning food supplies or diets for population groups. If food is available in an amount that will meet the RDI for energy, that amount should be adequate because approximately one-half of that population will be expected to eat more and one-half less than the RDI. The calculated amounts must cover estimated losses of essential nutrients that may occur during food preparation.

A nutritionally adequate diet should provide amounts of essential nutrients sufficient to meet or exceed the RDI in an amount of food that meets the RDI for energy. If the daily allotment of a diet provides less than the recommended amount of a nutrient when it is evaluated against the RDI, the diet planner will be alerted to the need to correct for the shortage by replacing poor food sources of the nutrient in question with better ones. Use of RDI in this way for evaluating the nutritional adequacy of diets should be distinguished clearly from the diagnostic uses of RDI (discussed later) for evaluating the adequacy of nutrient intakes of individuals or populations.

The objective in planning meals and food supplies is not to adjust the mix of foods so it provides just the amounts of essential nutrients needed to meet RDI but to ensure that, in selecting an acceptable mix of foods, the amounts do not fall below the RDI (see Chap. 52).[1] Some nutrients, protein for example, will usually considerably exceed the RDI because, where available, foods high in protein are used as important sources of other nutrients. The amount of vitamin A may greatly exceed the RDI on one day and be below it on another because relatively few foods are rich sources of vitamin A. Day-to-day variability of this type need not be avoided as long as the average amounts consumed over several days meet the RDI. In planning diets food should be selected for palatability and acceptability, not merely for its nutrient content.

DIETARY GUIDANCE AND NUTRITION EDUCATION

RDI, as was indicated earlier, are standards for nutrient intakes for use by health professionals, not recommendations for the public. To provide the population generally with meaningful information about nutritionally adequate diets, it is necessary to express RDI in terms of foods, not nutrients. An early application of RDA was their use as standards for developing a food guidance system that would enable people with little knowledge of nutrition to meet their nutritional needs by selecting diets from among a few groups of familiar foods. The USDA separated foods into four major groups based on nutrients of which the foods were rich sources. Then, using the RDA as a guide, the number of servings needed daily from each food group to meet essential nutrient needs of individuals of different ages was estimated.[34] The system was designed so that RDA for adults could be met by consuming quantities of foods that provided only about 1200 to 1600 kcal (5.0 to 6.7 MJ) of energy. They could then obtain any additional needed energy from among a wide selection of foods. The validity of this approach was established by determining that model diets provided the required amounts of nutrients.

This guidance system, based on scientific principles, has been used widely in nutrition education programs to illustrate the principles of a nutritionally adequate diet. Many modifications have been proposed to adapt it to meet the food preferences and needs of individuals and families with different cultural patterns and levels of income.[35] In use for several decades, it is the basis for the first two recommendations in most sets of dietary guidelines today—namely, to help assure (1) variety in food selection and (2) moderation in food consumption.[18]

The USDA has recently published a new food guide.[52] This guide differs from the previous one[34] in several respects. It provides little information about the essential nutrient contributions of foods. The food groups have been expanded from four to five by separating fruits and vegetables into two groups. It is now a guide for the total diet rather than for a basic diet that meets essential nutrient needs but only part of the energy (caloric) needs. The emphasis in the guide is on consuming a low-fat diet that conforms with the dietary guidelines for fat, fiber, sugar, starch, and cholesterol (see Table 82–1 and Chap. 93). Its purpose is not to educate the public about the essentials of a nutritionally adequate diet but to achieve conformity with a dietary policy purported to prevent chronic and degenerative diseases.

Nutrient Density. RDI also serve as the basis for using the "nutrient density" concept in providing guidance about food selection.[36] The nutrient density of a food is defined as the quantity of a given nutrient *contained* in the amount of a given food that provides 1000 kcal of energy. RDI, expressed as the amount of nutrient *required* per 1000 kcal of energy, are used as standards for assessing the nutritional adequacy of a diet or a food from knowledge of its nutrient density. To illustrate: if the ratio of nutrient density of thiamin in a diet to the RDI for thiamin per 1000 kcal is 1, then the thiamin requirement will be met when the amount of diet consumed meets the energy requirement. Nutrient density standards should be calculated separately for each age group if they are to correspond accurately with RDI. In practice, the value for the age group having the highest RDI per 1000 kcal is used to provide a single standard for diet planning because diets meeting this value will meet or exceed the nutrient needs of individuals of all ages. A serious shortcoming in using the nutrient density approach in comparing the nutrient contributions of foods is the failure to take into account the amounts of food usually consumed. If two foods have the same vitamin content per 1000 kcal but one contributes only 50 kcal and the other 250 kcal per day to the diet, their nutrient contributions to the total diet are not related to their nutritional value as assessed by this procedure.

The nutrient density concept can be useful for assessing the relative nutrient contributions of foods and diets if its shortcomings are clearly recognized. In addition to the problem just cited, an assumption underlying the concept is that nutrient needs are proportional to energy needs. This assumption is considered correct only for thiamin,[25] and possibly for niacin and riboflavin, whereas requirements for most other nutrients are a function of body size and growth rate. It should also be recalled that the RDI for essential nutrients are set high to cover almost all individuals, whereas the RDI for energy are average values. In addition, during aging, caloric requirements decline, and during weight reduction and illness, caloric intake is curtailed; hence, nutrient density of diets for these segments of the population must be higher than for healthy younger individuals who, because they consume large amounts of food, can meet their needs for essential nutrients with diets of lower nutrient density.

THERAPEUTIC DIETS—CLINICAL APPLICATIONS

Special nutritional needs that arise from clinical problems are not considered in establishing RDI. Acute and chronic infections of the gastrointestinal tract and other diseases that impair absorption increase nutritional needs but may affect the utilization of some nutrients such as iron, folate, and vitamin B_{12} more than others. In pancreatic insufficiency, treatment with a low-fat diet may lead to impaired absorption, specifically of the fat-soluble vitamins. Systemic infections, trauma, and burns increase metabolic losses of nitrogen and some vitamins and minerals. For the treatment of genetic diseases in which utilization of vitamins B_6, B_{12}, or biotin is impaired, doses of these vitamins greatly exceeding the RDI are required. Therapeutic nutritional needs differ greatly from one disease state to another and even from one individual to another; these diverse needs must therefore be dealt with individually as part of the clinical management of each patient.

For patients whose health problems do not alter nutrient requirements, RDI provide a guide to nutritional needs, just as they do for healthy persons. In the treatment of obesity by severe dietary restriction, for example, it is important that the recommended low-calorie diets provide amounts of essential nutrients that meet the RDI. Also, when protein intake must be restricted as a therapeutic measure for individuals with renal disease or certain inborn errors of amino acid metabolism, RDI can serve as a guide to the degree of restriction that can be imposed without creating the risk of protein deficiency.

Besides the impairment of absorption and metabolic waste of nutrients that occur in many disease states, the loss of appetite commonly associated with both chronic and acute illnesses can result in depletion of body stores of nutrients and wasting of tissues. Special dietary management is needed to ensure that these losses are replenished and to prevent complications from malnutrition. The period of repletion following illness or trauma during which body stores are being replenished should be considered comparable to a period of growth during which nutritional needs are increased.

Careful monitoring of nutritional status and clinical judgment are required in dealing with medical problems, many of which are discussed in other chapters. Drug-nutrient interactions that alter nutrient needs also are special clinical problems not covered by RDI (see Chap. 78).

STANDARDS FOR FOOD AND NUTRITION REGULATIONS AND HEALTH AND WELFARE POLICY

Reference values that can be related to nutrient requirements are needed for many food and nutrition regulations. The Food and Drug Administration (FDA) selected the highest values from among the 1968 RDA for 20 nutrients to serve as standards for food labeling and called these the U.S. RDA. They are not appropriate guides to nutrient needs of individuals other than adult males but serve as satisfactory regulatory standards. Expression of the nutrient contributions of foods as fractions of the U.S. RDA per serving simplifies comparisons of the nutrient contributions of different sources of a single food and of the quantities of nutrients contributed by different types of foods. U.S. RDA are also satisfactory standards for programs for fortifying foods with nutrients judged to be low in the food supply and for ensuring that foods designed for special dietary purposes, such as nutritional supplements or special diets for weight reduction, contain appropriate amounts of essential nutrients.

The FDA is currently proposing that a new standard be adopted for food and nutrition regulations: Reference Daily Intakes, which are defined as *population-weighted* averages of the 1989 RDA values for age-sex groups beyond 4 years of age. This proposal has created controversy because it is less directly related to RDA than the present U.S. RDA and will result in lower values for most nutrients. What the outcome of the debate over the proposal for a new standard will be is not clear, but pressure for action to modify the present standard makes it likely that a change can be anticipated.

RDI have also been used as standards for economic assistance programs by government agencies to ensure that foods or meals supplied through programs, such as school lunch, child feeding, and food programs for the elderly provide specified proportions of essential nutrient needs. RDI are appropriate standards for this. Also, meeting RDI has been an important consideration in developing the food plan that has served as the basis for allotment of coupons in the food stamp program and in establishing the poverty level of income.[37] This has created the impression that the economic implications of these uses of RDI should be considered in establishing RDI values. Were this to be done instead of creating independent standards, the scientific value of the RDI would be undermined.

DIAGNOSTIC USES: EVALUATING THE ADEQUACY OF NUTRIENT INTAKES

Dietary histories of individuals or surveys of dietary intakes of large numbers of individuals are used together with information about food composition to estimate intakes of essential nutrients by individuals or populations. These estimates are compared with reference standards such as RDI to determine, for individuals, how much intake deviates from the recommended intake and, for populations, the distribution of intakes and the proportion of individuals with intakes below the standard. The validity of conclusions drawn about the adequacy of essential nutrient intakes of either individuals or populations from this information depends on the reliability of estimates of food intake, accuracy of food composition tables, and appropriateness of the standard.[1,30] The discussion here is confined to the use of RDI as standards.

RDI were not originally intended to serve as standards for assessing the adequacy of individual nutrient intakes.[14] RDI exceed the requirements of most individuals; also, requirements of individuals are not known a priori and can be determined only by metabolic and biochemical studies of each individual. It is, therefore, not possible to evaluate the adequacy of nutrient intakes *below the RDI* by comparing dietary intake with RDI. The 1974 RDA committee concluded that "it is only within the framework of statistical probability that RDA can be used legitimately and meaningfully" for assessing the adequacy of nutrient intakes.[38]

What conclusions can be drawn from comparisons of nutrient intakes with RDI? If the intake of an individual exceeds the RDI, the probability of nutritional inadequacy is obviously remote. It is not appropriate, however, to conclude that an intake below the RDI is inadequate. All that can be said is that the greater the actual intake falls below the RDI, the more likely is the probability that intake is inadequate. Such information is useful in providing a basis for deciding the need for specific clinical and biochemical evaluations of individuals in such categories and for confirming and correcting nutritional problems that may be identified.

Figure 82–4 represents the cumulative distribution of requirements, assuming they are normally distributed, and illustrates the relationship between usual dietary intake of a nutrient below the maximum requirement and the probability that a particular intake is inadequate. If the usual intake of a nutrient by an individual (horizontal axis), is below the highest estimated requirement (mean +3 s.d.), the probability of that intake being inadequate is obtained from the vertical axis on the right.[3,21] For intakes falling between the average and the maximum requirement, the probability of inadequacy declines in curvilinear fashion from 50% to zero. This type of analysis makes it possible to express quantitatively the probability of the intake of an individual being inadequate; however, to maintain perspective, one should recall the caveats mentioned above and below that without specific biochemical data such quantification is comparable to the prediction of a meteorologist that the chance of rain in the future is, say, 30%.

In applying probability analysis to populations, it is important to recognize, as was mentioned earlier, that even if the average intake of an essential nutrient by a population exceeds the RDI this does not assure that all individuals in that population are meeting their require-

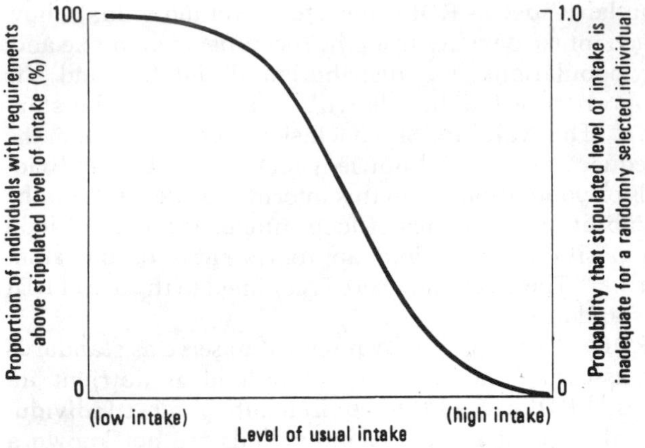

FIGURE 82–4. Cumulative distribution of requirements and relationship between usual intakes below the maximum requirement (zero on right-hand vertical axis) and the probability that intake is inadequate. (From Food and Agriculture Organization (FAO)/World Health Organization (WHO)/United Nations University: Energy and Protein Requirements. WHO Technical Report Series 724. Geneva, World Health Organization, 1985.)

ments. This conclusion is contrary to the following statement by the 1989 RDA committee: "If a population's habitual intake approximates or exceeds the RDA, the probability of deficiency is quite low."[5] The basis for the conclusion is illustrated in Figure 82–3, in which the distribution of individual requirements is shown on the left and the distribution of individual intakes on the right. The average intake of the nutrient by this particular population exceeds the RDI, so if this curve is representative of the curves for other essential nutrients, the total mixture of foods *available* for consumption provides more than adequate quantities of nutrients. However, the area of overlap of the two curves indicates that, despite the fact that average intake is well above the RDI, a portion of the population is consuming less than the RDI. Intakes of some in this portion may be inadequate. Because it is not possible to distinguish between individuals with high and those with low requirements, the problem of identifying individuals whose intakes are inadequate still remains.

With knowledge of the distribution of individual intakes, however, it is possible to estimate the *probable proportion of the population* with inadequate intakes, just as it is to estimate the likelihood of a particular intake being inadequate for an individual.[30] From an examination of Figure 82–4, for any given level of average intake below the maximum requirement, the proportion of individuals consuming less than their requirement can be estimated from the vertical axis on the left.[3] Probability analysis of the results of population dietary surveys that provide information about the distribution of nutrient intakes can alert public health officials to the likelihood of nutritional inadequacy being or becoming a problem. Use of RDI as standards for evaluating the adequacy of nutrient intakes has created misunderstanding of the RDI concept, but at the same time has created greater awareness of the problems involved in attempting to assess nutritional status from dietary survey information.[3,21,30,39] These issues of interpretation and application of requirement estimates are discussed in some detail in Chapter 83.

Although inability to quantify the degree of inadequacy of nutrient intakes below the RDI is disconcerting, it is not a shortcoming of the standard. It is a problem inherent in attempting to assess the adequacy of a variable (nutrient intake) using a reference standard (RDI) that exceeds the upper limit of the range of concern (intake less than requirement) when the specific standard needed (requirement of each individual) is not available. It is like trying to assess the appropriateness of body weight with a scale that registers only weights in excess of 100 kg.

FUTURE APPROACHES TO RDI

The persistence of a substantial proportion of people with inadequate incomes, the continuing increase in the proportion of people over 65 years of age, and the changes that have been occurring in the food supply are among the factors that have increased awareness of the importance of health and nutrition surveys and of the need for more accurate estimates of human requirements for nutrients and better methods and standards for assessing the adequacy of nutrient intakes.[3,21,31,39]

ALTERNATIVE STANDARDS FOR EVALUATING THE ADEQUACY OF NUTRIENT INTAKES

Despite discrepancies between different sets of RDI standards (which serve quite well as reference values for most prescriptive uses), their limitations for diagnostic uses are well documented.[30] Recognition of these limitations has provided the impetus for proposals for alternative standards.[21,40] Separate standards for prescriptive and diagnostic applications were proposed by a European nutrition group in 1976. Since then standards that represent lower limits of acceptable nutrient intake to be used only for evaluating the adequacy of nutrient intakes have been included in RDI reports of New Zealand, the Nordic countries, and Australia.[40] The FAO/WHO have published two sets of requirements for iron, one to prevent anemia, and a higher "basal" set to prevent impairment of function but that is associated with low tissue reserves.[21] For vitamin A, there is a "basal requirement" and a "Safe Level of Intake"; the latter is essentially the RDI.

The distribution of individual requirements around the mean is of prime importance in establishing RDI and provides the basis for methods of estimating the probability of individual intakes being inadequate (Fig. 82–2) and of the incidence of inadequacy in a population group (Fig. 82–4). The mean and the distribution curve may be shifted in either direction along the horizontal axis of Figure 82–2, depending on the criteria used for establishing the requirement, but any standard that may be selected for assessing the adequacy of nutrient intakes will be derived, either directly or indirectly, from an average requirement. Agreement is likely to be greater in setting lower limits of acceptable nutrient intake than in establishing RDI for which selection of criteria for appropriate reserves involves a substantial element of judgment. Furthermore, intakes below the lower standard are more likely to be associated with deficiency than is the case for intakes less than some arbitrary level below the RDI.[40] A table of average requirements with estimates of individual variability would be more useful than tables of RDI for diagnostic purposes.[33] The basic problem in assessing adequacy of nutrient intakes from dietary information, however, is not solved by establishing new standards. Conclusions about inadequacy of intake of an individual can be drawn only in terms of probability or risk using any standard derived from average requirements. What is actually needed is a specific, albeit unattainable, standard for each individual. Also, whatever standard may be proposed, the critical problem of establishing accurate and reliable average requirements remains.

IMPROVING ESTIMATES OF REQUIREMENTS

Current approaches to RDI are limited by the sparsity of information about many aspects of human requirements for nutrients, insufficiently sensitive criteria for establishing when a requirement has been met, and differences in the criteria used by committees in making decisions that cannot be made directly from the results of scientific studies.

These problems involve much more than merely collecting additional information about human requirements. If the standard used to evaluate the adequacy of nutrient intakes is too low, the incidence of inadequacy will be underestimated; if it is too high, the incidence will be overestimated. If the individual values are not established in a consistent manner, decisions about the relative importance of apparent problems will be unreliable. Differences in judgment about the criteria to be used for determining when a requirement has been met, and about the size of the adjustments needed to allow for unavailability of the nutrient from foods, are responsible for most differences between RDI set by different committees. These differences deserve careful examination.

Recognition of such problems has led to increased use of metabolic measurements as a way of improving the accuracy of estimates of requirements. Such studies have greatly increased knowledge of relationships between iron intake and the state of different iron reserves[21] and between ascorbic acid intake and body pool size.[27,28] Expanded use of metabolic approaches in the future will continue to enlarge knowledge of nutrient utilization and provide new criteria for establishing when requirements have been met. But, as with efforts to devise better standards for diagnostic uses of RDI, these advances will not solve the basic problem in estimating requirements: differences of opinion over the appropriate size of body reserves for healthy individuals who are consuming a mixed diet regularly. Recent committees have evaluated critically the available information on human requirements for vitamins A and C and have proposed RDI for these nutrients,[21,40,41] which are in close agreement but lower than those in the U.S. NRC/NAS report.[5] Their assessments place the amount of the tissue reserve at a level considered to be *adequate* for healthy people rather than on the assumption that higher tissue levels are more desirable (even if they cannot be shown to confer a health benefit). The former position points the way for selecting more realistic values for requirements in the future and may help in establishing more accurate and consistent standards for both prescriptive and diagnostic applications of RDI.

The proportion of the population found in U.S. health and nutrition surveys to have low blood ascorbic acid levels or impaired iron status was about one-fifteenth that with intakes below the RDA for these nutrients.[31] Beaton and Chery concluded from a model epidemiologic analysis that the incidence of protein deficiency in infants was much lower than would be predicted from current RDI values for protein requirements based on breast milk consumption.[42] The epidemiologic approach has potential for identifying questionable requirement estimates and should receive more attention in the future.

RDI FOR THE ELDERLY

Almost all recent committees on dietary standards have deplored their inability to establish RDI specifically for older age groups. Efficiency of physiologic processes such as digestion and renal reabsorption may decline with increasing age; hence, requirements for at least some essential nutrients may increase during aging. So far, there is little to indicate that nutrient needs of healthy elderly people differ greatly from those of younger adults,[22] but some evidence suggests that, for a portion of the elderly, requirements for vitamins B_{12} and some minerals may be elevated.[23]

The elderly are a highly heterogeneous population. They differ greatly in rates of deterioration of physiologic functions and susceptibility to chronic and degenerative diseases; also, their use of pharmaceutical preparations is extensive. In circumstances more likely to occur in the aged, an individual can move rapidly from a state of health to one of infirmity. In future approaches to RDI for the elderly, criteria will be required to distinguish between the effects of disease and senescence and to determine when nutrition for the elderly ceases to be a matter that can be dealt with through recommendations for healthy people and becomes a clinical problem.

PHARMACOLOGIC USES AND TOXIC EFFECTS OF NUTRIENTS

Commercial production of nutrients for fortification programs and as supplements has made vitamins and minerals readily available in pure form. Individuals can obtain and consume them in amounts greatly in excess of those that can be obtained from diets. Consumption of nutrients has been promoted by organizations that encourage belief in their use in very large doses with reported cases of overdosage (see Chaps. 74, 76, and 86).

Recently severe adverse effects have been reported from use of the amino acid tryptophan as a drug.[43] Whether these are attributable to the presence of an altered form as a contaminant or not, this tragedy points up the danger of self-medication with products that in the United States are classified as foods. As a result of Congressional action they are not subjected to the tests for efficacy and safety required for non-nutrient products used as drugs. Toxic effects observed with some trace elements led to inclusion of a table of "Safe but Adequate" intakes of several of these nutrients in the 1980 RDA report,[25] primarily to provide the FDA with reference values for safe upper limits of intake for regulatory purposes.

Potential toxic effects from excessive intakes of vitamins A and D and adverse effects observed from ingestion of high doses of many other nutrients are discussed in the text pertaining to each nutrient in most RDI publications. The International Union of Nutrition Sciences committee included values for upper levels of safe intake in its RDI report, and the Nordic Nutrition Regulations have a table of similar values.[40] The range between the RDI and the toxic dose ("Safe Range of Intake") varies greatly from nutrient to nutrient, from about 3 times the RDI for selenium to 25 to 50 times or more for folate and vitamins C and E. More emphasis on establishing safe ranges of intake is a likely future direction for RDI committees.

Investigation of nutrient toxicity has led to discoveries that, in high doses, several nutrients have pharmacologic actions. The use of niacin in doses 50 to 100 times the RDI as a serum triglyceride- and cholesterol-lowering agent is clearly an example of a nutrient used as a drug for a purpose unrelated to its nutrient function and to physiologic needs.[44] Observations suggest that vitamin E may be beneficial in large doses in preventing accumulation of oxidation products in tissues,[45] and that vitamin A or carotenoids may have some anticancer action[46]; however, such activities do not appear to be unique effects of these nutrients, because similar actions are observed with substances having no vitamin action.

The relation of such observations to RDI became a matter of controversy during review of the tenth edition of the RDA.[47] The committee preparing the revision, on the basis of a comprehensive evaluation of the scientific literature, proposed that values for vitamins A and C be lowered (see Appendix Table A–1d in the seventh edition of this book). This proposal was rejected by the NRC/NAS. It was considered to be inconsistent with the conclusion of another committee that consumption of sources of these vitamins should be encouraged as a health policy measure for prevention of cancer even though there were no supporting quantitative data.[47] As a result, publication of the tenth edition of the RDA report was withheld for 4 years while a new committee revised the revision to retain the previous higher 1980 values.[5]

The Australian, the FAO/WHO, and most other committees have not considered pharmacologic or prophylactic effects of nutrients in revising their RDI reports, and eventually such effects were not considered by the NRC/NAS as bases for adjusting RDI for vitamins A and C even though the values were not lowered. This approach is essential for maintaining the integrity of RDI as nutrient standards. Inclusion of information with an adequate scientific base concerning pharmacologic and prophylactic uses and toxic effects of nutrients as a separate section will be of value in future RDI reports.

Unless the scientific reports on which policies are based are prepared and published by organizations or committees that function independently of agencies involved in setting health policy, it is difficult to see how they can be objective evaluations of the scientific literature uninfluenced by the policy objectives of health administrators. To protect the scientific integrity of RDI and separate cleanly the process of establishing RDI from that of using them for health policy, a major future approach should be to restrict membership on RDI committees to scientists with no direct involvement with official health policy development and who have been selected by professional scientific societies solely on the basis of their expert knowledge. Furthermore, the review process should be limited strictly to evaluation of the adequacy of the scientific basis of the report.

CLARIFYING THE RELATION BETWEEN RDI AND DIETARY GUIDELINES

The question of the relationship between RDI and dietary guidelines will continue to be an important issue in future approaches to RDI. It has become an issue in large part because the word "recommended" in the term RDI is misunderstood or misconstrued to mean a recommendation for the public. Widespread adoption of the term "dietary standard," which was used in Canada for many years, might have avoided this problem. Substitution of the term "reference value" for RDI, as was proposed by Waterlow in 1979,[48] could help greatly to reduce misunderstanding of the purpose for which RDI are established. "Reference values for intakes of essential nutrients and food sources of energy" should be explicit enough to make misunderstanding of the concept of RDI unlikely. A step in this direction has been taken in the United Kingdom where the title of the most recent report on the subject is "Dietary Reference Values for Food Energy and Nutrients."[49]

The type of problem that arises when no clear distinction is made between dietary standards and dietary guidelines is illustrated by the new Canadian RDI report in which Recommended Nutrient Intakes are intermixed with dietary guidelines.[6] The nonessential dietary component cholesterol is included among the RDI for essential nutrients and is given more space than the five major water-soluble vitamins combined. This failure to distinguish between scientific dietary standards and health policy guidelines for the public makes it appear that both are part of health and nutrition policy. It also leads to confusion about the use of such documents by the public, politicians, and even professionals. The FAO/WHO, the Australian National Health and Medical Research Committee, and the NRC/NAS in the United States have published their RDI separately from reports relating to dietary guidelines. Continuation of this approach is necessary to maintain separation of the scientific basis for guidelines from their application in health policy.

This leads to a final issue, the one that created the conflict between the U.S. NRC, its Food and Nutrition Board, and the Ninth Committee on RDA, and which resulted in the rejection of the proposed ninth revision by the NRC/NAS. To what extent should evidence that a nutrient protects against specific chronic or other diseases be considered in establishing RDI? The bases for establishing RDI for nutrients have been (1) incontrovertible evidence of the essentiality of the nutrient, (2) the ability to establish a quantitative relationship between intake below a critical level and a specific physiologic or biochemical response, and (3) the determination that the quantity required to prevent the depletion is ordinarily met by diet (RDI are dietary standards) and does not depend on ingestion of amounts that must be obtained from pharmacologic doses.

Fluoride, which reduces the incidence of dental caries, is an example of a substance present in foods and water for which no RDI has been set because it has not been clearly established to be an essential nutrient; yet, because of its established beneficial effect on dental health, fluoride is discussed in RDI publications, and its inclusion in the water supply is recommended as a public health measure.[5] There is currently evidence suggestive of an essential role for ω-3-fatty acids for retinal development[50] and for effects on lipid metabolism that are increasingly being considered to be beneficial in reducing the risk of cardiovascular disease.[51] The state of knowledge of the biologic roles of these fatty acids is not sufficiently definitive at present to permit a decision as to how they should be dealt with in establishing RDI or dietary guidelines. If the criteria for essentiality can be clearly established, it will undoubtedly be appropriate to establish RDI for these fatty acids. If health benefits are firmly established independently of their essentiality and especially if the quantities required to produce the effects exceed the quantities ordinarily obtained from diets, they may be dealt with as fluoride is, especially if the range between health benefit and toxicity or undesirable side effects is narrow.

This problem is analogous to that discussed in relation to pharmacologic or prophylactic effects from ingestion of large quantities of nutrients. Such effects bear little relation to nutrition and are not appropriate for consideration in establishing RDI. They will undoubtedly continue to receive attention and should be discussed, just as the cholesterol-lowering effect of niacin is discussed, in RDI publications. Effects of this type should nonetheless be distinguished clearly from the physiologic effects of nutrients in diets.

REFERENCES

1. Harper, A.E.: Evolution of recommended dietary allowances—New directions. Annu. Rev. Nutr., 7:509–537, 1987.
2. Truswell, A.S.: Recommended dietary intakes around the world. Nutr. Abstr. Rev., *53*:939–1015, 1075–1119, 1983.
3. Food and Agriculture Organization (FAO)/World Health Organization (WHO)/United Nations University: Energy and Protein Requirements. WHO Technical Report Series 724. Geneva, World Health Organization, 1985.
4. Department of Health and Social Security (UK): Recommended Daily Amounts of Food Energy and Nutrients for Groups of People in the United Kingdom. London, Her Majesty's Stationery Office, 1985.
5. NRC/NAS: Recommended Dietary Allowances. 10th Ed. Washington, D.C., National Academy Press, 1989.
6. Health and Welfare Canada: Nutrition Recommendations, Report of the Sci. Review Committee. Ottawa, Canada, Canadian Govt. Publ. Centre, 1990.
7. Leitch, I.: Nutr. Abstr. Rev., *11*:509–521, 1942.
8. Harper, A.E.: Am. J. Clin. Nutr., *41*:140–148, 1985.
9. Truswell, A.S.: Am. J. Clin. Nutr., *45*:1060–1072, 1987.
10. U.S. Department of Agriculture: Food and Life Yearbook. Washington, D.C., USDA, 1939.
11. League of Nations: The Problem of Nutrition, Vol. II. Report on the Physiological Basis of Human Nutrition. Technical

Commission of the Health Committee. Official No. A 12(a) II B. Geneva, League of Nations, 1936.
12. Stiebling, H.K.: Food Budgets for Nutrition and Production Programs. USDA Misc. Publ. No. 183. Washington, D.C., USDA, 1933.
13. Stiebling, H.K., Phipard, E.F.: Diets of Families of Employed Wage Earners and Clerical Workers in Cities. USDA Circular 507. Washington, D.C., 1939.
14. Roberts, L.J.: N. Y. State J. Med., *44*:59–66, 1944.
15. American Dietetic Association: J. Am. Diet. Assoc., *17*:565–567, 1941.
16. Canadian Council on Nutrition: Natl. Health Rev., *8*:1–9, 1940.
17. Burnham, J.C.: How Superstition Won and Science Lost. New Brunswick, NJ, University Press, 1987.
18. USDA-USDHHS. Nutrition and your health: Dietary Guidelines for Americans. 3rd Ed. Home and Garden Bulletin No 232. Washington, D.C., U.S. Govt. Printing Office, 1990.
19. Harper, A.E.: Am. J. Clin. Nutr., *45*:1094–1107, 1987.
20. Smith, R.L., Pinckney, E.R.: Diet, Blood Cholesterol, and Coronary Heart Disease: A Relationship in Search of Evidence. Santa Monica, CA, Vector Enterprises, 1988.
21. FAO/WHO: Requirements of Vitamin A, Iron, Folate and Vitamin B_{12}. FAO Food and Nutrition Series No. 23. Rome, FAO, 1988.
22. Munro, H.N., Suter, P.M., Russell, R.M.: Annu. Rev. Nutr., 7:23–49, 1987.
23. Kassarjian, Z., Russell, R.M.: Annu. Rev. Nutr., *9*:271–285, 1989.
24. FAO/WHO: Requirements of Vitamin A, Thiamine, Riboflavine and Niacin. FAO Nutrition Meetings Report No. 41. Rome, FAO, 1967.
25. NRC/NAS: Recommended Dietary Allowances. 9th Ed. Washington, D.C., National Academy Press, 1980.
26. Nordin, B.E.C.: Calcium. *In* Recommended Nutrient Intakes Australian Papers. Edited by A.S. Truswell. Sydney, Australian Professional Publications, 1990.
27. Olson, J.A., Hodges, R.E.: Am. J. Clin. Nutr., *45*:693–703, 1987.
28. Read, R.S.D.: Vitamin C. *In* Recommended Nutrient Intakes Australian Papers. Edited by A.S. Truswell. Sydney, Australian Professional Publications, 1990.
29. FAO/WHO: Requirements of Ascorbic Acid, Vitamin D, Vitamin B_{12}, Folate and Iron. WHO Technical Report Series No. 452. Geneva, WHO, 1970.
30. NRC/NAS: Nutrient Adequacy: Assessment Using Food Consumption Surveys. Washington, D.C., National Academy Press, 1985.
31. USDA/USDHHS: Nutrition Monitoring in the United States—A Report from the Joint Nutrition Monitoring Evaluation Committee. DHHS Publ. No. (PHS) 86-1255. Washington, D.C., U.S. Govt. Printing Office, 1986.
32. Warwick, P.M.: Predicting food energy requirements from estimates of energy expenditure. *In* Recommended Nutrient Intakes Australian Papers. Edited by A.S. Truswell. Sydney, Australian Professional Publications, 1990.
33. Beaton, G.H.: Criteria of an adequate diet. *In* Modern Nutrition in Health and Disease. 7th Ed. Edited by M.E. Shils and V.R. Young. Philadelphia, Lea & Febiger, 1988.
34. U.S. Department of Agriculture. Essentials of an Adequate Diet. (Home Economics Research Report No. 3). Washington, D.C., USDA, 1957.
35. King, J.C., Cohenour, C.G., Correccini, C.G., et al.: J. Nutr. Educ., *10*:27–29, 1978.
36. Hansen, R.G., Wyse, B.W., Sorensen, A.W.: Nutritional Quality Index of Foods. Westport, CT, Avi Publ., 1979.
37. Smith, J., Turner, J.S.: Currents (Univ. N. Carolina), *2*:4–11, 1986.
38. NRC/NAS: Recommended Dietary Allowances. Washington, D.C., National Academy Press, 1974.
39. Beaton, G.H.: Nutr. Rev., *44*:349–358, 1986.
40. Truswell, A.S.: Recommended nutrient intakes: Some general principles and problems. *In* Recommended Nutrient Intakes Australian Papers. Edited by A.S. Truswell. Sydney, Australian Professional Publications, 1990.
41. Olson, J.A.: Am. J. Clin. Nutr., *45*:704–716, 1987.
42. Beaton, G.H., Chery, A.: Am. J. Clin. Nutr., *48*:1403–1412.
43. Centers for Disease Control: JAMA, *264*:1655–1660, 1990.
44. DiPalma, J.R., Thayer, W.S.: Annu. Rev. Nutr., *11*:169–187, 1991.
45. Burton, G.W., Taber, M.G.: Annu. Rev. Nutr., *10*:357–382, 1990.
46. NRC/NAS: Diet Nutrition and Cancer. Washington, D.C., National Academy Press, 1982.
47. Pellett, P.L.: Ecol. Food Nutr., *21*:315–320, 1988.
48. Waterlow, J.C.: Food Policy, *4*:107–114, 1979.
49. U.K. Dept. of Health: Dietary Reference Values for Food Energy and Nutrients for the UK. London, H.M. Stationery Office, 1992.
50. Neuringer, M., Anderson, G.J., Connor, W.E.: Annu. Rev. Nutr., *8*:517–541, 1988.
51. Nestel, P.: Annu. Rev. Nutr., *10*:149–167, 1990.
52. U.S. Department of Agriculture: Food Guide Pyramid. Home and Garden Bulletin No. 249. Washington, D.C., USDA, 1992.

CHAPTER 83

Criteria of an Adequate Diet

George H. Beaton

Since 1970 there has been a progressive evolution of understanding of nutrient requirements in relation to a number of areas of application. One such set of applications lies in the development of recommendations concerning suitable levels of nutrient intake. A second closely related area is the use of requirement estimates in the assessment of adequacy of observed intakes. The present chapter attempts to portray the current understanding of these applications and to provide illustrative examples. In addressing these concepts and approaches the chapter draws heavily upon a series of United Nations (UN) agency reports[1–7] and a National Research Council report.[8] As will be noted later, the information desired for implementation of the described approaches is not always available. Often this is more a function of failing to see the need for the particular parameter of requirements (e.g., the estimate of *average* requirement) than an inability to generate the needed estimates. As the framework for use of requirement estimates becomes more widely understood and more generally implemented, requirement reports can be expected to move toward inclusion of relevant parameters. The reader should see this chapter as describing an approach to interpretation and application of requirement estimates

REQUIREMENT TERMINOLOGY

This chapter places major emphasis on distinctions between "requirement" estimates derived for application to individuals and to populations. Terminology in current wide use does not make the necessary distinctions. For this chapter, designations developed by a recent FAO/WHO/IAEA committee have been applied.[7] These are explain thus:

E_R	average requirement of individuals for the nutrient element E
E_{SLmin}	Safe level of intake or recommended intake for an individual (often taken as $E_R + 2$ SD of individual requirements). Since there is actually a range of 'safe' intakes, it's counterpart, marking the beginning of risk associated with excess intake, would be E_{SLmax}
E_{PImin}	lower limit of safe range of group (or "population") mean intakes at which it would be expected that only 2 to 3% of individuals in the group would have intakes below their own true requirements. This estimate takes into account variation of intake as well as variation of requirement among individuals. The upper end of the range of group mean intakes, at which some individuals might be expected to show signs of effects of excess intake, has been designated E_{PImax}

Any of these terms may be associated with basal or normative requirements (see text for explanation) by addition of a superscript, such as E_R^{basal} and $E_R^{normative}$

that has been examined and defended but has not yet been widely implemented. It is an approach that, when implemented, should serve to diminish if not fully resolve some of the conflicts and contradictions now found in the nutrition literature.

Figure 83–1 provides a framework for this chapter. Whether one is developing recommendations for suitable levels of intake (the *prescriptive* mode) or assessing the probable adequacy of observed intakes (the *diagnostic* mode), there are major distinctions to be made between approaches to the *individual subject* and to the *population group.* These then constitute the four subdivisions of consideration in the chapter. Discussion of these is followed by some special applications including the derivation of nutrient energy ratios (nutrient densities) as sometimes applied in judging dietary quality.

Three important caveats must be stated as applying to all that follows. The first is that current requirement estimates as developed in FAO/WHO,[1–7] U.S.,[9,10] and Canadian[16] reports relate to the maintenance of health in already healthy individuals. Such estimates may or may not be applicable to patients with known diseases. They are certainly not intended to cover the needs of those recovering from nutritional deficiencies. The second caveat is that the approaches described relate to nutrients but *not* to energy. A basic assumption of the underlying statistical models is that the distributions of requirements and of intakes are essentially independent of one another (very low correlation). This is not a tenable assumption for energy intake.[2,4,8] Energy needs and the assessment of adequacy of energy intake are discussed in Chapter 5. A full discussion of the estimation of energy needs will be found in UN reports.[4,11] The final caveat is that "intake" as used in this chapter refers to the *usual intake* of an individual or group—the average intake persisting over moderate periods (i.e., weeks or months, not days). Application of the approaches to 1-day intakes could be seriously misleading except when the group mean intake is being used (see Chap. 52). When working with population group data it may be possible to estimate the between-subject (between person variation in usual intakes) and within-subject (day-to-day variation in intake within the same subject) variance components[12–14] and to apply appropriate statistical adjustments to estimate the distribution of usual intakes.[8,15]

PRESCRIPTIVE MODE—DEVELOPMENT OF INTAKE RECOMMENDATIONS

The most common use of requirement estimates, and that foreseen by most committees charged to describe human nutrient requirements, is in recommending appropriate dietary intakes. Confusion has arisen because the committees often were not explicit in specifying whether their recommendations were intended to apply to the diets of individuals or to the average diet of a

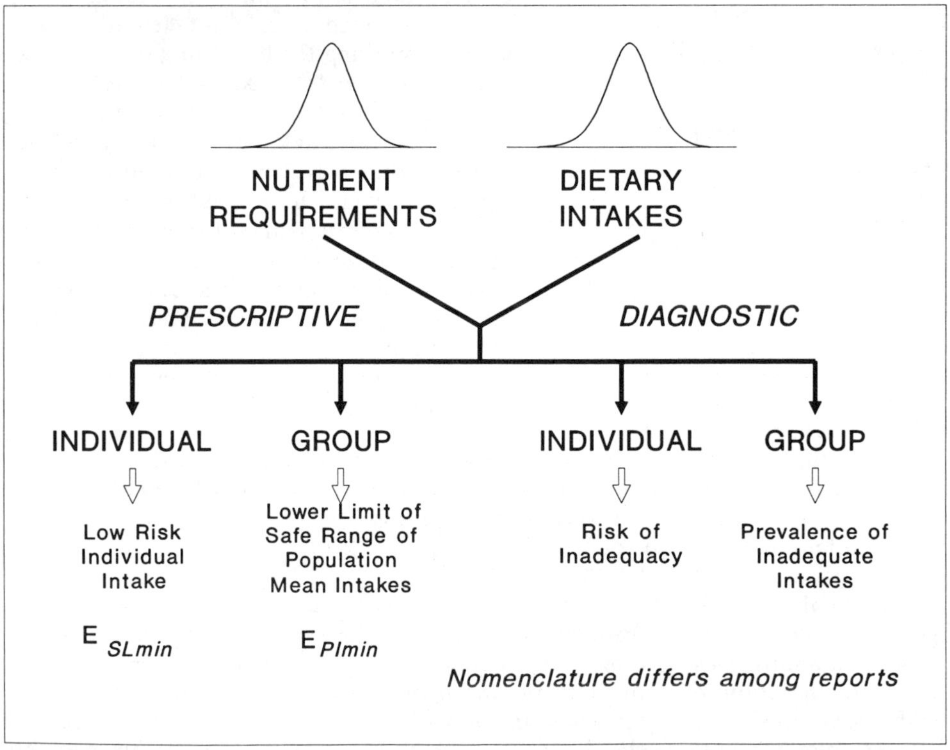

FIGURE 83–1. A construct of applications of nutrient requirement estimates.

group. Examination of many of the reports suggests that there may have been inconsistencies between nutrients in the intended application, regardless of what the introductory sections may have stated. That is, for some nutrients, the derivations suggest that the final numeric estimates represents the "recommended intake" for the individual (E_{SLmin}), whereas, for others the numeric estimate appears to represent what is deemed to be an adequate group mean intake (E_{PImin}). As indicated below there are major differences between individual and group applications. It is unfortunate that the distinctions have not always been explicitly recognized in national and international reports. The onus is on the user of such reports to examine the arguments and approaches applied in the derivation of each nutrient requirement estimate before he or she can have confidence in the actual meaning of the derived numeric estimate.

APPLICATION TO THE INDIVIDUAL

The principle underlying the prescriptive application of requirement estimates to the individual is that at the advocated level of intake, he or she should be at an acceptably *low risk of inadequate intake.* This is a probability statement relating to the randomly selected individual.[2,4] The acceptable level of risk is arbitrary, although existing conventions are consistent across reports. In simple terms, the advocated level will be in the upper tail of the distribution of individual requirements (Fig. 83–2*A*). Of necessity the advocated intake will exceed the actual requirements of all but a small proportion of individuals of the specified class.[2] The information needed to develop such an estimate is a knowledge or reasonable estimate of the *distribution of individual requirements* (average requirement and be-

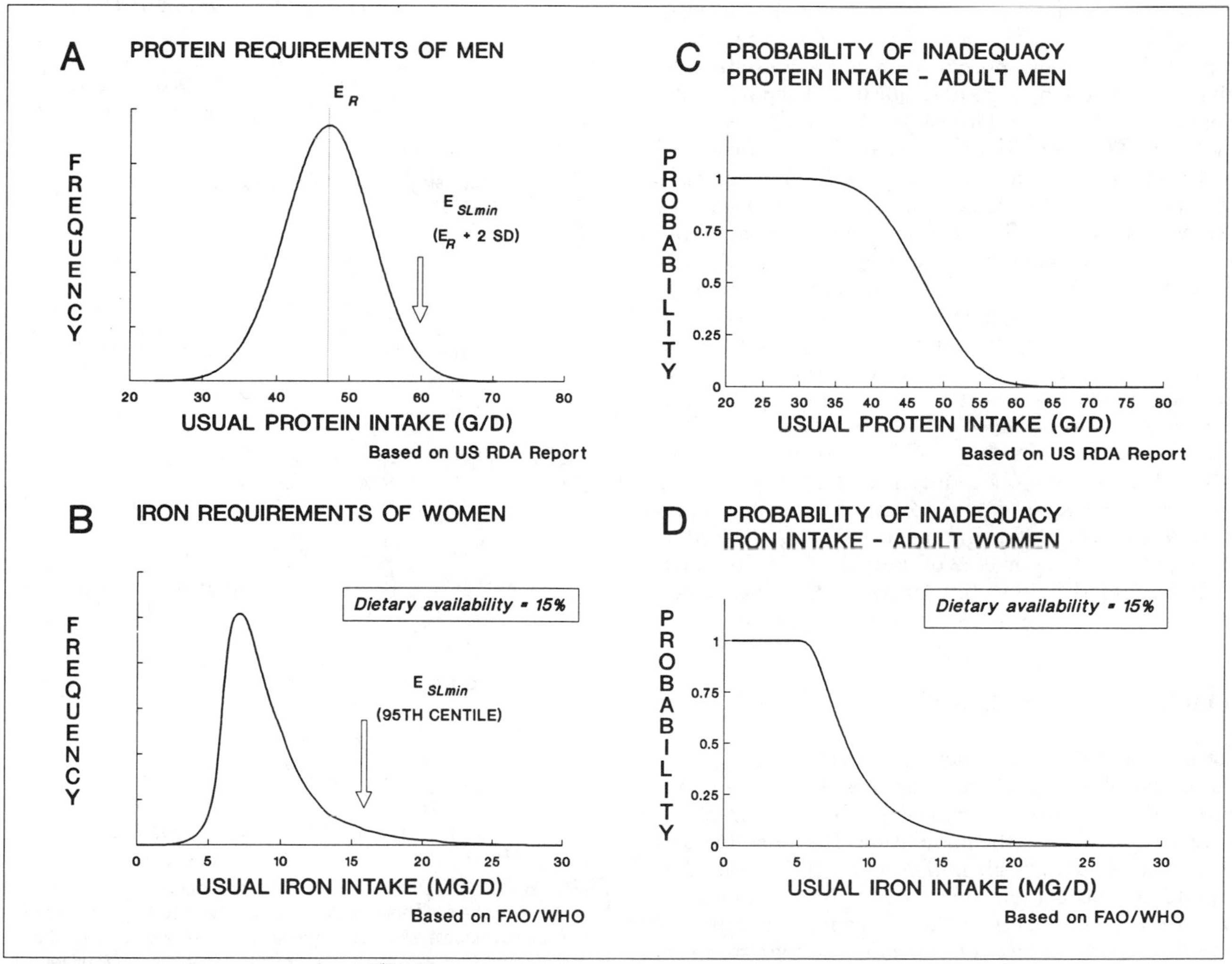

FIGURE 83–2. Application to the individual. *A* and *B* portray a normally distributed and a highly skewed distribution of requirements. The intake advocated to maintain an individual at low risk (E_{SLmin}) is indicated. *C* and *D* present the associated probability curves portraying the likelihood that a given level of usual intake is inadequate to meet the true needs of a randomly chosen individual.

tween-person variation in requirements). If the average requirement (E_R) and the variability of requirement can be estimated, and if the distribution is assumed to approximate normality, the "recommended dietary allowance,"[9] "recommended intake,"[1] or "safe level of intake"[3–5] now termed E_{SLmin}, usually is set at E_R + 2 SD (standard deviations) of requirement, theoretically covering all but 2 to 3% of individuals and, as noted, exceeding the actual need of 97 to 98% of individuals (illustrated for protein in Fig. 83–2*A*). When the requirement distribution is known to be skewed, as in the case of the strong positive skew in the distribution of iron requirements of menstruating women (Fig. 83–2*B*), the convention is to estimate the 95th percentile of the requirement distribution covering all but about 5% of normal women.[1,6] For the individual selected at random the risk that his or her own (unknown) requirement would not be met at the recommended level of intake would be about 2.5 and 5 chances in 100 for these 2 conventions described previously for protein and iron, respectively. These "risk" or probability levels have been accepted *de facto* as appropriate when counseling the individual, although there may not have been a specific rationale for the particular risk level selected.

In the absence of direct (experimental) information about requirements, the recommended intake may have been based on observations of population group intakes in situations where no signs of deficiency were seen, the lowest reported group mean intakes then being judged as adequate (an estimate of E_{PImin}). This approach requires special interpretation, which it has not always received (see the section on application of concepts to derivation of requirement estimates later for discussion of interpretation of such evidence). It has often been suggested that the recommended intakes "err on the side of safety" or include a "margin of safety." Whether or not this is an "error" depends on one's interpretation and desired application. If the intent is to counsel an individual toward a low risk dietary intake, the E_{SLmin}, derived as covering all but 97.5 or 95% of individuals, is appropriate. As indicated below, the serious error arises when such a numerical estimate is used in assessment.

APPLICATION TO THE GROUP

For some applications, such as the planning of group diets or the planning of food supplies for a population group, one needs to estimate the desirable mean intake of a group or subgroup of the population. The objective is to ensure that essentially all individuals will have intakes adequate to meet their own needs. In this mode of application, one must take into account the expected *variability of usual intakes of individuals* in that group, as well as the *variability of requirements.*

One could demand that each individual be at individual low risk of inadequacy, meeting the E_{SLmin} (see above). That would imply that the intake distribution should be positioned such that its lower tail would not overlap by very much the E_{SLmin}. Such an approach is illustrated in Figure 83–3*A*. Recall, however, that the E_{SLmin} actually exceeds the real requirement of almost all the individuals in the group. For the population planner that would seem to be an unwarranted approach. Given the implications for apparent food needs and the potential, with some nutrients, for undesirable effects of excessive intake, such an approach might be seen as imprudent, going well beyond "erring on the side of safety." Most planners would be satisfied if the population risk of inadequate intakes (the proportion of individuals expected to have intakes below their own requirements) was acceptably low. As discussed later under assessment mode and its application to the group, the relative positions of the requirement and intake

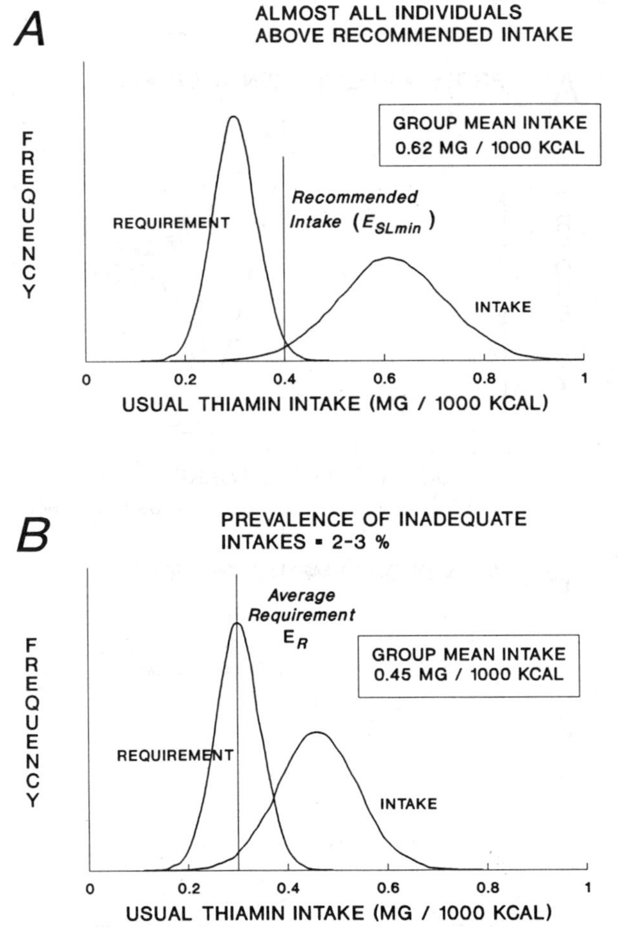

FIGURE 83–3. Derivation of safe or recommended population mean intake for thiamin. *A* portrays the situation that would hold if all individuals were to be maintained at low individual risk (almost all intakes above the "recommended intake"). *B* presents the situation in which the population risk (prevalence of inadequate intakes) is 2 to 3%. This would represent the lower limit of safe population group mean intakes. Note that the intake and requirement distributions can show considerable overlap.

distributions can overlap considerably before the expected prevalence of inadequate intakes rises to levels that should cause concern (Fig. 83–3*B*). A National Research Council committee demonstrated that, empirically, the proportion of individuals with usual intakes below the average requirement (E_R) provides a general approximation of the expected prevalence of inadequate intakes provided that the distribution of requirements is reasonably symmetrical.[8] The estimate is relatively insensitive to the variability of requirements, at least when the expected prevalence is low. If one has an estimate of the variability of usual *intakes* in the group, and can assume that the distribution approximates normality, it follows that if the population mean intake, E_{PImin}, is set 2 SD of *intake* above the E_R, the expected prevalence of inadequate intakes would be about 2 to 3%. This is an arbitrary risk level but may be acceptable for purposes of planning group intakes and requisite food supplies. This was the approach followed by a recent FAO/WHO/IAEA committee in arriving at the lower limit of the "safe range of population mean intakes," the E_{PImin}.[7] If intakes are skewed (most intake distributions show some positive skew) then the suggested margin will tend to err on the side of safety. That is, the expected prevalence of inadequate intakes will be lower than 2 to 3%. When intake distributions are highly skewed (e.g., those for vitamin A and vitamin C), the shape of the distribution must be taken into account (see footnotes to Table 83–1). More precise estimates of the desirable population mean intake can be obtained by statistical application of full probability approaches. For most users this would be an unnecessary level of refinement.

It is to be noted that derivation of recommendations for both individuals (E_{SLmin}) and population groups (E_{PImin}) start from an estimate of the *average requirement of individuals* (E_R). They differ in the estimate of variability that is applied. When dealing with recommendations for individuals, the *variability of individual* ***requirements*** is used. In addressing population groups, the *variability of individual* ***intakes*** is used. The last U.S. RDA committee may have been technically in error in suggesting that "if a population's habitual intake approximates or exceeds the RDA, the probability of deficiency is quite low," at least for those RDA that were developed in the manner described in the preceding section of this chapter (and set forth in the introduction of Recommended Dietary Allowances).[9] If the statement had read "if an individual's habitual intake. . . ," there would have been consistency with the introduction, although, as discussed later, perhaps not with all of the numeric estimates presented. This has been a continuing, and troubling, source of misinterpretation of published recommendations—how they apply to individuals and to groups or populations.

Table 83–1 presents some comparisons of derived recommendations directed toward the individual, E_{SLmin}, and the population group, E_{PImin}, for nutrients where explicit estimates of the average requirement and the variability of requirement have been offered. In the last edition of the U.S. *Recommended Dietary Allowances* explicit, or reasonably clear implicit, estimates of these parameters were offered for protein, iron (in males and children), zinc, and vitamin C.[9] The text describing the derivation of estimates for other nutrients does not make it clear whether the committee attempted to estimate the level of intake that conveyed low risk to the individual, E_{SLmin} (see Fig. 83–2), or the safe level of population mean intakes, E_{PImin} (see Fig. 83–3). The approach may have been inconsistent across nutrients, perhaps accounting for the apparent error in the assertion noted in the preceding paragraph.

Additional examples (Table 83–1) have been based on recent FAO/WHO reports. In some instances, those committees reached different conclusions about appropriate recommended or safe levels of intake than are found in the U.S. report. The table presents U.S. RDA figures for information. Intake distributions have been modeled on reported intakes in the United States, adjusted to remove the effect of day-to-day variation. The main import of this table is to illustrate the distinction between customary "recommended intakes" directed toward individuals, E_{SLmin}, and the population mean intake, E_{PImin}, that might be advocated in planning for control of apparent inadequacy of intake in the population. It is clear that the numeric values are different for most examples. (See later discussion of level of requirement.) An assumption of the population estimates in Table 83–1 was that the requirement distributions (but not necessarily the intake distributions) are reasonably symmetrical. If the requirement distribution is highly skewed (e.g., iron requirements of menstruating women) a more elaborate approach is needed; the simple approach underestimates the target group mean intake. In the particular case of iron for menstruating women, a group mean intake of about 20 mg (0.36 mmol) per day (with 25% CV) would be needed to achieve a 5% prevalence of inadequate intakes (applying the FAO/WHO definition of basal iron requirements[5]). In the FAO/WHO report, the intake required to meet the basal needs of all but 5% of women (i.e., the E_{SLmin}) was estimated to be 16 mg (0.29 mmol) per day.[5] This is numerically similar to U.S. RDA estimate 15 mg (0.27 mmol) per day).[10] However, the basis of derivation of the FAO/WHO and U.S. figures appear to be different, possibly implying different intended meanings of the numbers. Further, the U.S. report suggests that an intake of 15 mg (0.27 mmol) per day (E_{SLmin} or E_{PImin}?) would be sufficient to maintain reasonable stores of iron in most menstruating women; the FAO/WHO report refers its requirement estimate to the satiation of functional needs for iron but absence of significant iron stores. As noted earlier, a population group mean intake of about 20 mg (0.36 mmol) per day would be expected to meet the basal iron needs of all but about 5% of menstruating women. It would also serve to maintain iron stores in a much smaller proportion of women.

TABLE 83–1. A COMPARISON OF INTAKES RECOMMENDED FOR INDIVIDUALS AND FOR POPULATIONS—YOUNG ADULT MEN

	REQUIREMENT*			ADVOCATED INTAKE		
Nutrient	Average E_R	CV†	Intake CV‡	Individual E_{SLmin}	Group Mean E_{PImin}	CURRENT U.S. RDA
Protein						
g/kg	0.6[4,9]	12.5%		0.75		0.8
g per day (72 kg)	47	12.5%	25%	59	94	63
Iron	6.7[9]	15%	25%	8.7	13.5	10
mg per day§	6.1[5¶]	15%	25%	7.9	12	
Zinc						
mg per day	12.5[9]	10%	20%	15	21	15
Vitamin C						
mg per day	45[9]	15%	**	59	150††	60
Vitamin A						
RE per day	480[5]**	20%	**	675	1850††	1000
Thiamin						
mg/1000 kcal	0.3[16]	15%	17.5%	0.4	0.45	0.5
Folate						
μg per day	173[5]**	12.5%	20%	215	290	200

*Source of estimate referenced.
†Coefficient of variation = (Standard deviation/Mean) × 100.
‡The estimates are judgemental, based on examinations of intake distributions for males and females (examined separately) as seen in various USDA surveys. The effect of day- to-day variation within individuals has been removed. Note that this variability is applied to the mean intake, not to the average requirement.
§To convert metric and other units to SI units for Tables 83–1 and 83–2 (see also Appendix Tables A–1a and A–1b):

1. Iron. . . . . .mg/55.9 = mmol
2. Vitamin C. . . . . .mg/176 = mmol
3. Thiamin. . . . . mg/301 = mmol
4. Folate. . . . . μg/441 = μmol
5. Vitamin B_{12}. . . . . μg/1355 = μmol
6. Copper. . . . . mg/63.5 = mmol
7. Selenium. . . . . μg/79 = μmol
8. Zinc. . . . . mg/65.4 = mmol; μg/65.4 = μmol
9. Vitamin A:. . . . . . . 1 μg all-trans retinol = 3.49 nmol all-*trans* retinol

¶Basal requirement estimate; does not provide for maintenance of stores. Assumes high dietary availability (15%).
**Normative requirement estimate; body weight = 72 kg.
††The distributions of vitamin A and vitamin C intakes exhibit a strong positive skew. The variability estimate used is based on variability of a log transformation, and the population median, rather than mean, is estimated.

The message here is not only the importance of specification of whether low risk intakes for the individual, E_{SLmin}, or for the population group, E_{PImin}, are under discussion, but also the importance of specifying the target level of nutritional status. It is *not* enough to simply compare published numbers without asking what they are supposed to mean. In fact, on close scrutiny the U.S. and FAO/WHO reports appear to strongly disagree in the estimation of iron requirements of menstruating women. Similar discrepancies for female iron needs are found between the FAO/WHO report and the Canadian Recommended Nutrient Intake.[16] In the Canadian report, as in the U.S. report, it is difficult to be sure what was being estimated.

In this chapter, frequent reference is made to the U.S. RDA report. Because many of the references may be critical, this *might* be seen as an intended criticism of that report. That is *not* the intent. The U.S. RDA report is used only as a convenient familiar example. Similar issues, problems, and criticisms could be directed toward the recent Canadian report[16] and probably to most other national reports. The problems exemplified seem to be generic.

DIAGNOSTIC MODE

Many applications of nutritional requirement estimates are "diagnostic" in nature. Although one can never assess the state of health (nutritional status) from dietary data alone, the assessment of the likely adequacy of intakes is an important part of the more general assessment. This finds application in both individual assessment (literally as a part of diagnosis or as a background to counseling) and population assessment (as in nutrition monitoring and surveillance[18] or as a background to public health and food-related planning). Considerations pertaining to assessment of intake of the individual and of the population are different. In the material that follows, "group" and "population" are used almost interchangeably. This is not correct. The inference is that population groups should be seen as aggregates of physiologically and socioculturally similar individuals. Major dissimilarities would influence the distributions of requirements (e.g., across different age-sex classes) or distributions of self-selected intakes. It is assumed, there fore, that in applying requirement estimates to populations, the population will have been stratified into such groupings.

APPLICATION TO THE INDIVIDUAL

From the discussion of derivation of E_{SLmin}, directed toward individuals, it should be apparent that, in theory, an assessment of probable adequacy of any observed intake can be made. It is a matter of locating the usual intake of the target individual on the probability curves portrayed in Figure 83–2. With many existing statistical programs, this is accomplished very easily (see Addendum). It can also be accomplished by various categorization of the probabilities. Thus one could devise a system of high, moderate, and low risk intakes by simply defining probability intervals and reading the intake values from the risk or probability curve. An important point is that because the particular individual's requirement remains unknown except as a part of a distribution of requirements among similar individuals, there can never be an absolute classification of "adequate/inadequate" unless the observed intake is well above or well below the requirement distribution. No system of cutoffs can ever result in such categorization of individual dietaries falling within the range of variation of requirements.

In practice, individual assessment is fraught with other dangers. The real problem is not the definition of requirements or the probability curve. It is the difficulty of estimating the usual intake of the particular individual (see Chap. 52). It is relatively easy to understand the impact of day-to-day variation in intake on this estimation process. Suppose that one has estimated protein intake of an adult man using a 3-day record. The estimated mean intake is 50 g per day. The literature suggests that day-to-day variation in protein intake may have a CV (coefficient of variation = SD/average, expressed as a percentage) of about 25%. As one pools multiple days of observation, the CV for the pooled estimate decreases.[12–15] With a 3-day estimate it might be about 15%. This implies that the estimate of 50 g per day could be an erroneous estimate of the individual's real *usual intake*—the 95% confidence intervals might be about ± 30%, that is, 35 to 65 g per day. When these limits are transferred to the risk curve in Figure 83–2*C*, the true probability of inadequacy might be as high as 1 or as low as 0. One cannot place great confidence in such an assessment. To obtain a "reliable" estimate of the individual's *usual intake* (i.e., to narrow the confidence limits to useful levels) would require many days of intake data selected to represent the time frame of interest[17,18]—too many days for most practical applications. Conversely, if the observed intake were well above, or well below, the range spanned by the risk curve, one might be reasonably sure that intake is almost certainly adequate or inadequate, respectively. For nutrients such as iron or zinc, where the nature of the diet consumed at each eating event influences nutrient utilization and hence requirement, the problem of assessment of the individual is even greater. Another source of within-person variation has been added.

The implication is that in assessment of adequacy of intake of a particular individual, seldom is it possible to apply a probability assessment, or apply the RDA, in a literal sense. Only general conclusions about "likely to be adequate," "might be problematic," and "likely to pose a problem" can be offered. Unfortunately, this inference is not in accord with current practices in some areas.

Although one cannot assess nutrient adequacy of the diet of the individual with confidence, there are other valid reasons for estimating intake of individuals. It may be important to monitor a subject's intakes over time in the course of a therapeutic intervention. One might wish to use the information gained about dietary practices as a basis for counseling. In these situations, the requirement estimates may be useful as a reference point rather than being used in a true assessment mode. It need only be recognized that the information actually collected may not reflect the usual intake or pattern (and hence that one should expect substantial variations in repeated measurements over time).[17]

APPLICATION TO POPULATION GROUPS

Conceptually, assessment of adequacy of intakes in a population group involves application of the probability curves (see Fig. 83–2) to the intakes estimated for each of the individuals in the group. The population assessment, expressed as an expected prevalence of inadequate intakes (number of individuals with intakes below their own requirements, particular individuals not being identified) is simply a summation of individual probabilities. This is illustrated for iron in menstruating women in Figure 83–4*A*. Intakes have been grouped into small intervals, and a probability of inadequacy has been assigned to each interval. The expected number of individuals with inadequate intakes is then the summation of frequency × probability across all of the intervals; when divided by the total number of individuals examined, this becomes a prevalence estimate. Observed intakes are based on the USDA CSFII-85 data; requirements are based upon an FAO/WHO report.[5] With many currently available computer programs, this can be done for each observed intake without prior grouping into intervals (Fig. 83–4*B*) (see also Addendum). At first it would seem that population assessments face all the issues described previously for individual assessments. That is not true. There are extremely important differences that make population assessment more feasible than individual assessment.

In a population assessment one is concerned with the population or population group as a whole, not the particular individual. It follows that one is concerned with the distribution of usual intakes in the group, not with the usual intake of particular individuals. As discussed elsewhere,[8,15] statistical approaches can be

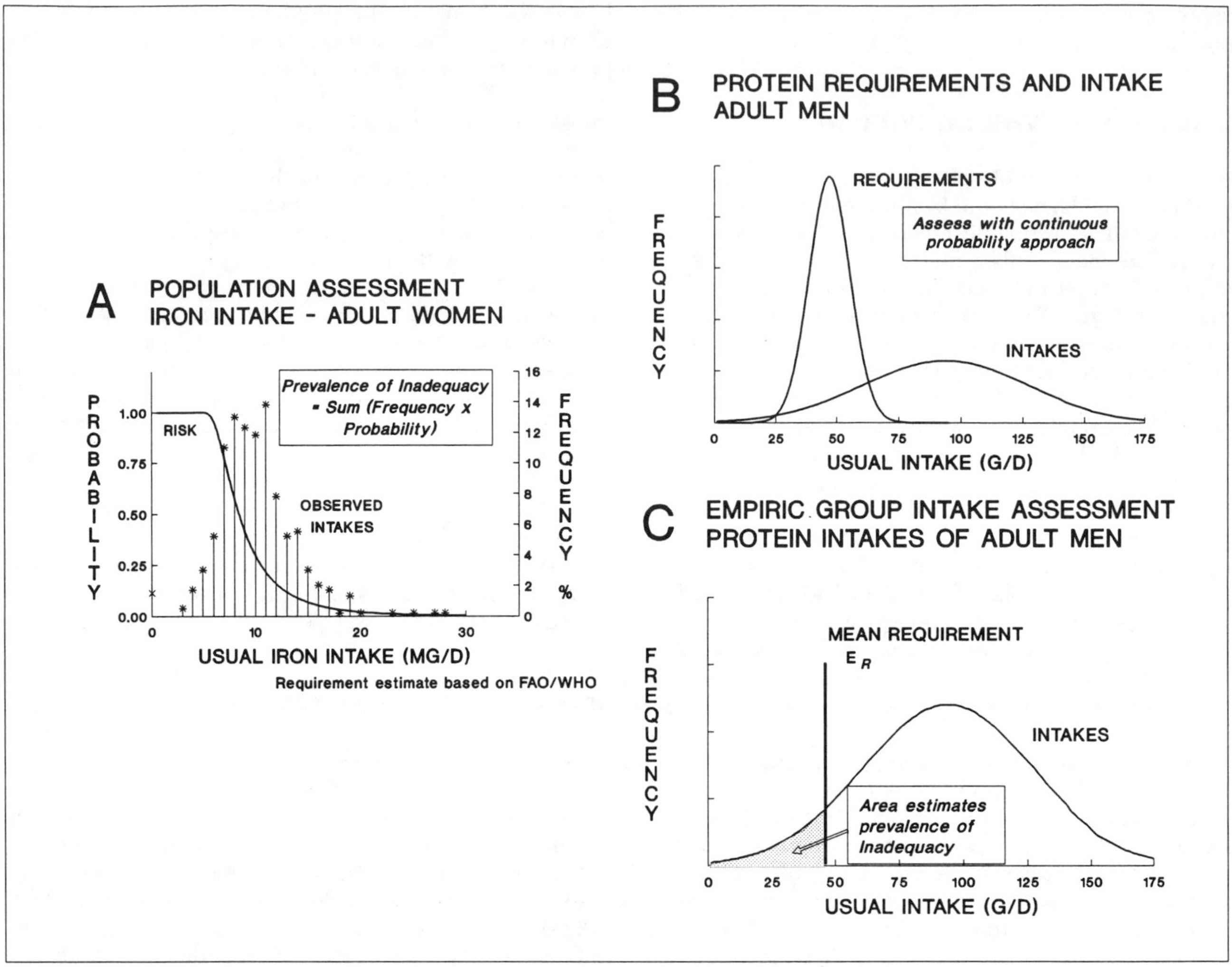

FIGURE 83–4. Assessment of population groups. *A* portrays application of the probability approach, using intervals of intake, to iron intakes of women. *B* represents application of the full probability approach, without grouping intakes, for protein in adult men. *C* presents a simple empiric approach to assessment of protein intakes in adult men. The proportion of intakes falling below the average requirement (shaded area) provides an estimate of the prevalence of inadequate intakes in the population. This does *not* identify the individuals with inadequate intakes.

applied to estimating the distribution of usual intakes as long as there is an adequate sample of replicated 1-day intake estimates. Further, if data are collected for multiple days (e.g., for 3 to 7 days) on all individuals, the distribution of subject means will be a reasonable approximation of the distribution of usual intakes unless within-person (day-to-day) variation is extreme. This is true even though the individual means are not good estimates of the intake of the particular individual—a difficult concept to grasp. A similar situation holds for variation in the nature of the diet consumed as it might affect utilization of a nutrient such as zinc or iron. As long as that variation is random across the group, it has but small impact on the estimate of prevalence of inadequate intakes. The estimate of utilizability of the "average diet" could be applied to all intake estimates. In a small series of Canadian subjects, it was shown that the dietary factors recognized as affecting iron utilizability did not associate with the absolute level of iron in the diet (unpublished analysis of data collected by Sabry et al.); this lends confidence that an assumption of independence (of random effect) was not being violated. Food composition variation similarly has minimal effect. Even random under- and over-reporting has less impact than might be thought. A full discussion of these issues has been presented elsewhere.[8]

Equally important is the realization that population assessments are *not* very sensitive to the variability of requirement within a class of individuals (e.g., adult men or adult women) as long as the requirement distribution is reasonably symmetrical. As pointed out by the National Research Council committee, simply estimating the proportion of usual intakes falling below the *average* requirement (E_R) provides a crude estimate of the prevalence of inadequate intakes in the population group.[8] This is illustrated for protein in Figure 83–4*C*. Such an estimate would be sufficient for most applications although it must be emphasized, as noted previously, that although this estimates the prevalence of inadequate intakes in the group, it does not identify the individuals with inadequate intakes. When the requirement distribution is known to be highly skewed, then the probability approach should be applied as illustrated for iron in Figure 83–4*A* or protein in Figure 83–4*B*. In this situation, simply estimating the proportion of intakes below the median requirement underestimates true prevalence when prevalence is low. As prevalence approaches 50%, the difference between approaches becomes small.

VOICED CRITICISMS OF THE PROBABILITY APPROACH APPLIED TO POPULATION GROUPS

Recently, application of the probability approach to assessment of intake was commended on a theoretical basis and condemned on a practical basis. The USHHS/USDA report on Nutrition Monitoring in the United States[19] suggested that limitations to application of the probability approach to population assessment as proposed by the NRC committee[8] included the following: (1) lack of information about the mean and shape of the requirement distributions, (2) constraint by the same systematic errors of intake estimation as affect any other approach to evaluation of nutrient adequacy, and (3) the necessary statistical assumption of low correlation between intake and requirement is violated for energy and for iron. It is worth considering these points in greater detail. That the probability approach is constrained by absence of *published* estimates of average requirements (E_R) is correct. However, this must be recognized as a circular argument. Up until very recently, committees charged with development of requirement estimates have seen little merit in estimating E_R; rather, attention has been focused on the much less useful "recommended intake" (E_{SLmin}). That the approach is constrained by absence of information about the magnitude and shape of the requirement distribution is an overstatement. Knowledge of the average requirement but not the variability of requirements is needed in empiric population assessment. It *is* required that there be knowledge or reasoned judgment concerning the general symmetry of the requirement distribution; it is not necessary that normality be assumed. That the approach is constrained by the same systematic biases in data collection as would be any other evaluative approach is correct (as long as biases are systematic for all individuals; if bias in estimation is random across individuals, the probability approach is not seriously constrained[8]).

That the approach is not applicable to energy because the assumption of low correlation between intake and requirement is violated is absolutely correct. The simple probability approach cannot be applied to energy without more information—information that is unlikely to be forthcoming and might only be addressed by important assumptions[4] (see statement in early paragraphs of this chapter).

The suggestion that the assumption of independence is violated for iron (because iron absorption increases as requirement increases) is an error on the part of the committee or a misconception about how iron requirements are or should be estimated. Iron requirement refers to the amount of dietary iron that would just balance iron needs driven by losses/utilization (retention in net tissue/blood formation) holding in that individual and that would maintain the individual's iron status at a defined level of nutriture. The FAO/WHO committee estimated dietary iron requirements from a distribution of physiologic needs (e.g., urinary, dermal, and endogenous fecal iron excretion plus menstrual iron losses in women or tissue iron deposition in children).[5] The assumption of the derivation was that individuals with different needs, but the same iron status, are absorbing at comparable efficiencies (i.e., that there is no systematic change in absorption with change in need). The FAO/WHO group then noted that there were major differences in the efficiency of iron absorption associated with changes in the level of iron nutriture (e.g., level of body iron stores). Thus, the FAO/WHO committee derived multiple dietary iron requirement distributions for predefined levels of iron nutriture—they addressed the key question "requirement for what?". The USHHS/USDA committee appears to have failed to make this conceptual distinction between variation in physiologic need and variation in iron nutriture.[19] Instead, that committee appears to have confused this conceptual approach to the definition of requirements with the well-documented fact that if intake is held constant, iron absorption varies with need (absorption is a major regulator of body iron flux) or that if need is held constant, proportional absorption varies with intake. The criticisms levied by the USHHS/USDA committee[19] and similar criticisms suggested by others (e.g., the minority report presented in the NRC report[8]) are sobering but seriously misleading. The real constraint in population assessment of dietary adequacy is the absence of published estimates of average requirements. As is argued throughout this chapter, it is now obvious that the estimate of average requirement is much more important for many applications than the estimate of a poorly understood and often misused "recommended intake." It is to be hoped that future requirement committees will address this problem seriously.

AN EXAMPLE OF CONFUSION IN INTERPRETATION—INDIVIDUAL VERSUS POPULATION

A current example of the confusion that can and does arise in considering recommendations for individuals and for population groups is illustrated by statements of goals concerning dietary fat intakes and chronic disease.

In 1989 and 1990, three reports were published by national and international bodies. All three proposed that the desirable level of total fat was below 30% of energy (and that the desirable level of saturated fatty acids was below 10% of energy). Two reports were explicit about their meaning but took opposite interpretations, although they had reviewed essentially the same evidence. A National Research Council report on diet and health specified that its recommendation pertained to individuals and that the desired population mean intake would be substantially lower than that.[10] A WHO report was equally explicit that its recommendation related to population mean intakes.[6] Both reports discussed the statistical issues to make their meanings absolutely clear. The third report, issued by Health and Welfare Canada, did not address the statistical questions and, unfortunately, the wording was left ambiguous, suggesting only that "the Canadian diet should contain no more than 30% of energy as fat. . . ."[16] Later clarification (J. Beare-Rogers, personal communication, 1991) suggested that the intended meaning was identical with the U.S. recommendation.[10] Figure 83–5 exemplifies the issue that arises from these discordant recommendations.

When the population goal described by the WHO committee[6] is achieved, one might expect that about half of the individuals would have intakes above this level. That would be an acceptable situation because that committee's judgment of the evidence reviewed related to the position of the population intake distribution without providing clear information about an upper limit of individual intakes. However, the U.S. committee stressed that in its judgment, intakes of individuals should fall below 30% of energy as fat.[10] As that committee noted, this implies that the population distribution would have to shift to a substantially lower level, as portrayed in Figure 83–5. The implications for both advocacy and assessment seem clear. There is a major difference between urging a modest reduction in fat intake in North America (from a current average of 36 to 38% of energy to 30%—a near 20% reduction) and advocacy of a major reduction (from an average of 36 to 38% to about 24%—a 35% reduction). An equally startling difference in the perception of the problem occurs in the assessment mode. If the goal of population mean intake = 30% of energy as fat were achieved (= "no problem"), one would still expect to see about half of the individuals with intakes above 30% (= "50% prevalence of excessive intakes"). Obviously, the difference has importance. Until recently, few of the source reports have been clear about the intended meaning of recommendations.

FURTHER REFINEMENTS AND APPLICATIONS

LEVELS OF REQUIREMENT

The National Research Council report pointed out that no dietary evaluation was interpretable unless there was an explicit statement of the basis of requirements (see

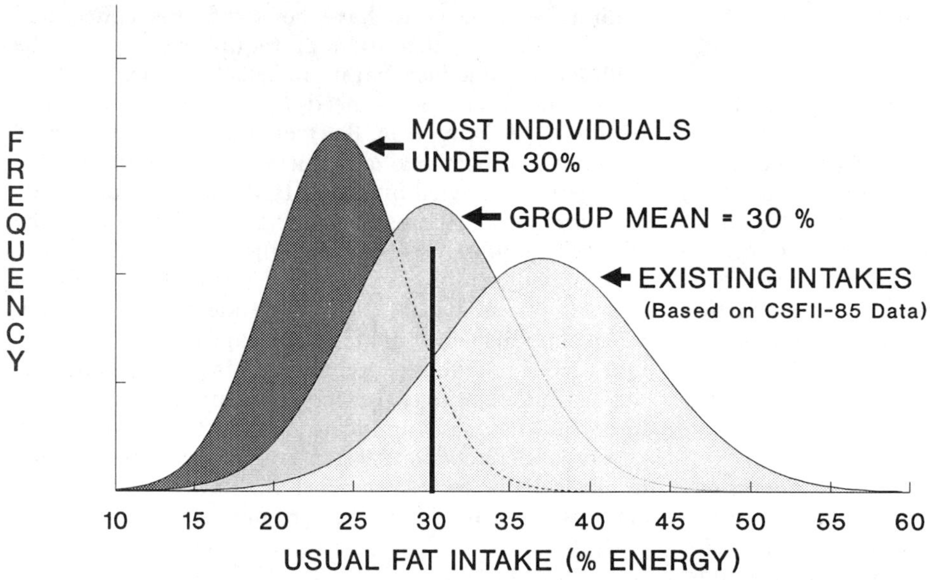

FIGURE 83–5. Goals for dietary fat intake: an example of confusion. The distribution of fat intakes that may exists in North America today is portrayed on the right (mean 37%; SD 4.6%). Although apparent consensus exists that "fat intake should be at or below 30% of energy", there are two interpretations. A United States report explicitly referred the 30% to individuals, implying the population distribution on the left (mean about 24%; assumes relative variability unchanged).[10] A World Health Organization (WHO) report explicitly referred the 30% to the group mean intake, implying the central distribution.[6] The shapes of the distributions are based on United States data reported in the USDA Continuing Survey of Food Intake of Individuals (CSFII), 1985.

previous discussion of iron).[8] That is, one could not offer meaningful statements about probable inadequacy of intake without also specifying "inadequacy for what?". The challenge offered by that committee has been taken up by recent FAO/WHO committees.[5–7] Unfortunately the challenge has not yet been taken up by U.S.[9] and Canadian[16] committees. In the FAO/WHO series, two (or three) levels of requirement have been defined, and requirements for each have been estimated. The traditional requirement estimate, providing for levels of storage or adaptive capacity (in the case of zinc) that are judged desirable but that are not seen as conveying identifiable functional advantage, has been designated *normative requirement,* the term "normative" implying judgmental. Conversely, the level of intake needed to satisfy all demonstrable functional needs has been termed *basal requirement.* In the case of iron, a third, lower level of requirement adequate to maintain hemoglobin at the level commonly recognized as marking the beginning of anemia but not adequate to fully maintain hematopoiesis was described as the *requirement to prevent anemia.*[5] These levels are listed in Table 83–2. With availability of such multiple estimates, each with clearly defined meaning, it is both feasible and desirable to carry out multi-tiered assessments of population groups and to set planning goals that address intermediate as well as long-term goals. Perhaps most important, with the specification of "requirement for what?" there is at least hope that dietary, biochemical, and clinical evaluations will come into closer agreement.[20]

Although not discussed in this chapter, parallel conceptual issues hold for the estimation of energy needs where one can consider energy intakes required to maintain a status quo condition, to establish a desirable (normative) body size, and to permit a defined level of physical activity (perhaps including normative levels of activity supportive of cardiovascular health).[4,11]

SAFE RANGES OF INTAKE—INDIVIDUAL AND POPULATION

For some nutrients there is documented reason for concern about excessive intakes. For many other nutrients, there is recognition that very high intakes confer no physiologic benefit and at least a potential for detrimental effects. Conceptually there is a risk curve associated with high intakes—a risk of detrimental effects—just as there is a risk of inadequacy associated with lower intakes. The concept of a safe range of intakes, minimizing risk of inadequacy and risk of excess for the individual, has been presented in several reports[4,8] even though information about the upper risk curve is often lacking. Recently, two committees addressed the estimation of lower (E_{PImin}) and upper (E_{PImax}) limits of population nutrient goals[6] and the safe range of population mean intakes.[7] The first group, addressing diet and noncommunicable disease, was particularly concerned with macronutrients such as fat. Because this group was addressing populations around the world, it was necessarily concerned not only with the association of excessive fat (and saturated fatty acid) intake with cardiovascular disease and cancer, but also with the undesirability of low fat intakes from the standpoint of energy density of diets (bulkiness of diet) and the effects of such intakes on utilization of other nutrients. It strove, therefore, to define a range of population mean intakes that would be consistent with both adequate and not-excessive intakes among individuals in those populations—a range for dietary goals. This approach was extended to several other macronutrients and to dietary fiber. The second group addressed trace element requirements.[7] The lower end of the safe range of intakes (E_{PImin}) was developed exactly as described in the present chapter and illustrated in Figure 83–3. In this report, the

TABLE 83–2. MULTIPLE LEVELS OF INDIVIDUAL REQUIREMENT OF ADULT MEN AS PRESENTED BY FAO/WHO COMMITTEES

	BASAL REQUIREMENT*		NORMATIVE REQUIREMENT*	
Nutrient (reference)	Average Requirement (E_R^{basal})	With Allowance for Variation in Requirements (E_{SLmin}^{basal})	Average Requirement ($R_R^{normative}$)	With Allowance for Variation in Requirements ($E_{SLmin}^{normative}$)
Vitamin A[5] (RE per day)	–	300	434	600
Folate[5] (μg total folate per day)*	60	(75)†	160	200
Vitamin B_{12}[5] (μg) per day	–	(0.9)†	–	1.0
Iron[5] (mg per day)	6.1‡	8‡	(9)‡**	(12)‡**
Copper[7] (mg per day)	0.7	***	0.8	***
Selenium[7] (μg per day)	(14)*	***	30	***

*See conversion chart in footnotes of Table 83–1.
†Not estimated directly; inferred from report.
‡Refers to a diet with high (15%) availability of iron. Estimates were offered for other diets.
**No estimate of normative requirements was offered. The figures shown are inferred from the report. The report did offer an estimate of the requirement to prevent anemia: average = 4.1 mg per day; variability = 5 mg per day.
***Variability of individual requirements was not presented. The report focused on estimation of safe ranges of population mean intakes.

upper end of the range (E_{PImax}) was concerned with potential detrimental physiologic effects.

In each of these examples, the explicit assumption is that there is no "optimal" intake. Rather, there is a range of intakes through which there is low risk of either inadequate or detrimentally high intake. The approaches differ in terms of whether the range is directed toward intakes of individuals (E_{SLmin} to E_{SLmax}) or of mean intakes of population groups (E_{PImin} to E_{PImax}), following the principles and constructs outlined in this chapter. Ranges applied to individuals are likely to be wider than ranges applied to population group mean intakes (see Table 83–2 for illustration of impact on the lower limit of these ranges; an analogous difference, but with opposite direction, would apply to the upper limit). The goal of counseling or of planning would be to position individual intakes (counseling) or population mean intakes (planning) within the appropriate range for specified age-sex groups.[6,7] An example of a practical application of this concept lies in the development of guidelines for water fluoridation where the objective is to achieve near-maximal benefit in terms of reduction of dental carries while avoiding detrimental effects as indexed by dental fluorosis. It is customary to specify a range of desirable fluoride concentrations in public water supplies.

The foregoing does not argue against the use of higher levels of nutrients for specific therapeutic purposes. Rather, as noted in the opening of this chapter, the discussion relates to the maintenance of health in already healthy individuals.

Most of the foregoing discussions relate to nutrient requirements defined in terms of established essential *nutrient* functions. There is growing evidence that some dietary components, for example ascorbic acid and carotenoids, may have *chemical* effects, distinct from their *nutrient* role, that are beneficial in the control of some forms of cancer. As a result, dietary guidelines and goals may suggest higher intakes than could be advocated on the basis of known nutrient functions (see Chaps. 82 and 93).

APPLICATION OF CONCEPTS IN DERIVATION OF REQUIREMENT ESTIMATES

Human nutrient requirement estimates usually have been estimated from the results of experimental depletion/repletion studies, balance studies, or similar investigations of individuals. Committees building from such data bases have had difficulty in attempting to relate these studies to population-based data. Conversely, in some instances experimental data may have served to establish linkages between the nutrient and human functions/diseases, but those studies may have been designed inappropriately for estimation of requirements. In this case, the available evidence for requirement estimation may relate to observed group intakes. A specific example, explored by Beaton and Chery, is the use of breast milk intake data in the estimation of infant requirements for protein or other nutrients.[21] Another recent example lies in the estimation of selenium requirements where the primary evidence comes from epidemiologic studies in China relating group mean intakes to the presence or absence of clinical evidence of functional abnormalities.[7]

The framework discussed in this chapter provides an approach to linking experimental and epidemiologic studies. It can be used in "testing" requirement estimates derived from experimental studies against epidemiologic data—do the requirement estimates make sense when tested against experience in populations?[22] The framework can also be used in inferring likely average requirements of individuals when only population information is available.[7,21] Here the first estimate is of the safe or appropriate population mean intake (E_{PImin}). The derived estimate, taking into account variability of intakes in the population and the observed prevalence of nutrient inadequacy (judged by biochemical or clinical criteria), is the likely position of the average nutrient requirement of individuals (E_R). This is merely a reversal of the derivations presented previously. Application of such approaches in the course of developing human nutrient requirement estimates would increase the scope of data available to support such activity. Perhaps much more important, it would mandate both a clarification of exactly what was being estimated (E_R, E_{SLmin}, E_{PImin}, or perhaps some other parameter) and the level of nutriture used to define requirement. By crossing the experimental and epidemiologic lines of evidence, it should enhance confidence in the derived estimates. Recent U.S.[9] and Canadian[16] requirement reports drew on population intake data in the estimation of suitable iron intakes for menstruating women. Unfortunately, in each case the committee failed to record either the process or logic of utilization of these data in a manner that was sufficiently clear for the reader to be sure what had actually been estimated. It would have been much better to merge factorial approaches to estimation (used for men and children) with population data in the derivation of clearly defined estimates of requirements. That is what one might hope to see emerging in future reports.

NUTRIENT DENSITY: ANOTHER TYPE OF DERIVATION

For certain areas of application it has been convenient to use estimates of the nutrient density of the diet. This description of diets is qualitative. The underlying concept is that individuals and groups consume food for satiation of energy needs rather than nutrient needs. It follows that an "adequate" diet would be one that meets nutrient needs when consumption by the individual or group stops because of satiation of energy needs. This is a function of the concentration of nutrients in the diet (expressed as nutrients per 1000 kcal or, for the energy sources, nutrient as percentage of energy). It will be recognized from the foregoing discussion that nutrient needs can be considered in terms of various levels of requirements (e.g., basal or normative needs). As noted previously, energy needs also can be considered in terms of maintenance of the status quo or achievement of a normative goal. Thus, one can envisage families of nutrient density distributions for each of the nutrients. An important recognition is that distributions of nutrient density requirements are involved for each nutrient, each level of requirement, and each age/sex group. This is illustrated in Figure 83–6 for protein for young adult males using protein and energy requirement estimates presented in the U.S. Recommended Dietary Allowances.[9] Figure 83–6*A* presents a bivariate distribution of protein needs and energy needs assuming independence of protein and energy requirements per kilogram of body weight. Each point represents an individual's own protein and energy requirement. Figure 83–6*B* then presents the distribution of the ratios of these individual requirements expressed as a percentage of energy from protein. This distribution is comparable in interpretation to those presented earlier for nutrient requirements. Direct estimation of the bivariate distribution shown in Figure 83–6*A* is not feasible because that would require the joint measurement of energy needs and protein needs in the same individuals. A key assumption in estimation of the theoretic joint distribution pertains to the correlation between nutrient and energy *requirements*. If it can be accepted that this correlation is low, it has minimal impact upon the derivations.[4] For protein and energy, a maximal estimate from the literature is a correlation of about 0.2.[23] The distribution shown in Figure 83–6*B* is a derivation from the estimated requirements for protein and for energy of moderately active people[9]; no further assumptions have been made; it is simply a frequency distribution of ratios. If we now wish to estimate the protein concentration that would suffice to meet the needs of almost all individuals (E_{SLmin}), it would be about 9 to 10% of energy (based on the distribution curve). An algorithm for estimation has been presented elsewhere.[4] Conversely, if we wish to estimate the population figure, E_{PImin}, then the variability of the protein/energy ratio in self-selected diets must be considered. Figure 83–6*C* presents a theoretic intake distribution for young adult males that modeled after the variability seen in the USDA CSFII-85 survey of adult women. If variation in the usual concentration of protein is of the order suggested (CV = 25%), then the E_{PImin} consistent with a low prevalence of inadequate protein intakes when energy needs are satiated would be on the order of 13% energy as protein. These estimates may be compared with the more often seen (but perhaps uninterpretable) ratio of the published requirement estimates (the recommended intake for protein and the average requirement for energy). Again using U.S. estimates,[9] that simple ratio would be 7.5% energy as protein. Note that this agrees with neither the E_{SLmin} nor the E_{PImin}.

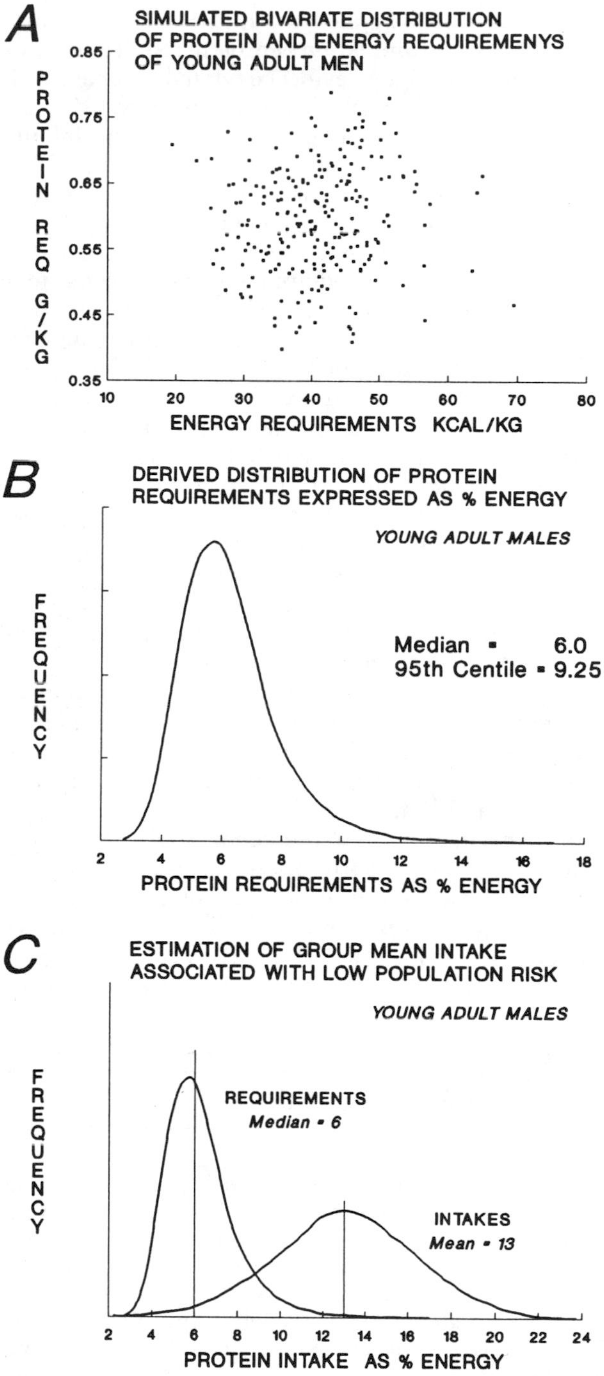

FIGURE 83–6. Derivation of nutrient density criteria for protein. *A* presents the joint distribution of protein requirements and energy requirements assuming 0 correlation. *B* presents the distribution of joint requirements expressed as a ratio (protein as percentage of energy). This is conceptually analogous to other requirement distributions. *C* presents the extension to estimation of the population mean intake consistent with a low prevalence of inadequate protein intakes given the condition that individuals eat to satiation of their own energy needs.

Beaton and Chery applied the illustrated conceptual framework in the examination of protein requirements of infants where the original evidence related to breast milk intake—that is, where the epidemiologic basis of requirement was the assumption that among infants nursed by well-nourished mothers, breast milk provided adequate intakes of energy (matched to individual needs by self demand) and at least adequate intakes of protein.[21] The question to be addressed was "what is the highest level of protein requirement that is consistent with that epidemiologic evidence?" The answer was "much lower than we currently estimate through an erroneous interpretation of the breast milk data." The concepts are important and useful. However, it must be determined whether a particular application (e.g., in food labeling or nutritional claims) best uses an average of the ratio for individuals (E_R), a ratio associated with low risk to the randomly selected individual (E_{SLmin}), or a group mean intake ratio associated with a low prevalence of inadequate intakes in the population (E_{PImin}). It must be recognized also that the ratios change from one age-sex group to the next because energy and nutrient requirements do not always move together.[24]

In conclusion, it has often been suggested that derivations of the type presented in this chapter are unjustified because of limitations of existing knowledge. It is true that our present knowledge of human nutrient needs is fragmentary and that any estimates we derive reflect a mix of experimental data, epidemiologic data, and informed judgment. It is true also that our estimates will change from time to time as our base of knowledge and understanding evolves. However, to suggest that we should not establish an underlying construct for estimation, and to suggest that we should not consider multiple estimates for different purposes, is a specious argument. Perhaps the greatest sin committed by the nutrition community has been to estimate single numbers—the recommended dietary allowance, safe level of intake, recommended intake, or whatever other term may have been applied—and to then use that unitary estimate for a range of purposes without first considering its conceptual suitability for the particular application. This failure has caused much confusion and may have led to a major loss of credibility in human nutrient requirement estimates. In many applications the recommended intake is patently inappropriate. The argument of this chapter is that estimates appropriate to specific applications *can* be derived with as much confidence as the conventional recommended intake has been derived. For many applications, such specific estimates would be greatly superior. There are strong initiatives in this direction in recent reports. Let us hope that those important initiatives will be followed through in the numerous applications of nutrient requirement estimates in the coming years. If this is done, perhaps we will reap the benefits of the major investment of time and effort that we have expended in the examination of human nutritional needs.

The concepts presented in this chapter are sometimes difficult to grasp and often difficult to apply in the first instance. It is not that the concepts are themselves challenging or their application mathematically obtuse. Rather, it is because they may challenge conventional wisdom and hence general experience. To aid in the evolution of thinking and practical implementation of the concepts, I am prepared to assist interested individuals or groups wishing to apply these approaches within the context of SAS programs.

REFERENCES

1. FAO/WHO: Requirements of Ascorbic Acid, Vitamin D, Vitamin B_{12}, Folate and Iron: Report of a Joint FAO/WHO Expert Group. FAO Nutrition Meetings Report Series No. 47, Rome. WHO Technical Report Series No. 452. Geneva, 1970.
2. FAO/WHO: Eighth Report of the Joint Expert Committee on Nutrition. WHO Technical Report Series No. 477. Geneva, 1971.
3. FAO/WHO: Energy and Protein Requirements: Report of a Joint FAO/WHO Ad Hoc Expert Committee. FAO Nutrition Meetings Report Series No. 52, Rome. WHO Technical Report Series No. 522. Geneva, 1973.
4. FAO/WHO/UNU: Energy and Protein Requirements: Report a Joint FAO/WHO/UNU Expert Consultation. WHO Technical Report Series No. 724. Geneva, 1985.
5. FAO/WHO: Requirements of Vitamin A, Iron, Folate and Vitamin B_{12}: Report of a Joint FAO/WHO Expert Consultation. FAO Food and Nutrition Series No. 23. Rome, 1988.
6. WHO: Diet, Nutrition and the Prevention of Chronic Diseases: Report of a WHO Study Group. WHO Technical Report Series No. 797. Geneva, 1990.
7. WHO/FAO/IAEA: Trace Elements in Human Nutrition: Report of a Joint WHO/FAO/IAEA Expert Consultation. FAO Nutrition Meetings Report Series. In press.
8. National Research Council Subcommittee on Criteria for Dietary Evaluation: Nutrient Adequacy: Assessment Using Food Consumption Surveys. Washington, D.C., National Academy Press, 1986.
9. Food and Nutrition Board, National Research Council: Recommended Dietary Allowances. 10th Ed. Washington, D.C., National Academy Press, 1989.
10. National Research Council: Diet and Health: Implications for Reducing Chronic Disease Risk. Washington, D.C., National Academy Press, 1989.
11. James, W.P.T., Schofield E.C.: Human Energy Requirements: A Manual for Planners and Nutritionists. Oxford, Oxford University Press, 1990.
12. Liu, K., Stamler, J., Dyer, A., et al.: J. Chronic Dis., *31*:399–418, 1978.
13. Beaton, G.H., Milner, J., McGuire, V., et al.: Am. J. Clin. Nutr., *32*:2546–2559, 1979.

14. Beaton, G.H., Milner, J., McGuire, V., et al.: Am. J. Clin. Nutr., *37:*986–995, 1983.
15. Life Sciences Research Office: Guidelines for Use of Dietary Data. Bethesda, MD, Federation of American Societies for Experimental Biology, 1986.
16. Health and Welfare Canada: Nutrition Recommendations: Report of the Scientific Review Committee. Ottawa, Minister of Supply and Services Canada, 1990.
17. Tarasuk, V., Beaton, G.H.: Am. J. Clin. Nutr., *54:*464–470, 1991.
18. Tarasuk, V., Beaton, G.H.: Am. J. Clin. Nutr., *55:* 22–27, 1992.
19. USDHHS/USDA: Nutrition Monitoring in the United States: An Update Report on Nutrition Monitoring. Department of Health and Human Services Publication No. (PHS) 89–1255. Hyattsville, MD, 1989.
20. Beaton, G.H.: Nutr. Rev., *44:*349–358, 1986.
21. Beaton, G.H., Chery, A.: Am. J. Clin. Nutr., *48:*1403–1412, 1988.
22. Beaton, G.H.: The epidemiology of iron deficiency. *In* Iron in Biochemistry and Medicine. Edited by A. Jacobs and M. Worwood. London, Academic Press, 1974.
23. Beaton, G.H., Swiss, L.: Am. J. Clin. Nutr., *27:*485–504, 1974.
24. Beaton, G.H.: Criteria of an adequate diet. *In* Modern Nutrition in Health and Disease. 7th Ed. Edited by M.E. Shils and V.R. Young. Philadelphia, Lea & Febiger, 1988.
25. SAS Institute: SAS/STAT Guide for Personal Computers, Version 6. Cary, NC, SAS Institute, 1987.

I take this opportunity to thank the many individuals who participated in working committees wherein these concepts were refined and developed over the past two decades. Without sound criticism and challenging questions, the approaches described in this chapter might well have suffered an early demise. The ideas are not new. In 1945 Pett et al. (Pett, L. B., Morrell, C.A., Hanley, F.W.: Can. J. Public Health, *36:* 232–239, 1945) outlined the elements of the probability approach to concurrent examination of intake and requirement distributions. A quarter of a century later Lorstad (Lorstad, M.H.: FAO Nutr. Newslett., 9: 18–31, 1971) described the bivariate distribution approach to this assessment and positioning of intake distributions to achieve a low population risk. The wheel has but turned again, but this time, I hope, on more fertile ground and before an audience more willing to consider the melding of biologic and statistical concepts.

ADDENDUM: IMPLEMENTATION OF PROBABILITY ASSESSMENT

Earlier reference was made to implementation of the probability approach in existing statistical programs. This is illustrated below for version 6 of Statistical Analysis System (SAS).[25] For application to the estimate habitual intake (INTK) of an individual, the likelihood of inadequacy (PROBINAD) would be estimated by the following SAS program lines:

```
PROBINAD = 1 − PROBNORM((INTK−MEANREQ)/
                    SDREQ)
```

where MEANREQ is the estimated average requirement of the class of individuals and SDREQ is the estimated standard deviation of requirements.

For a group, the predicted prevalence of intakes inadequate to meet the individual's requirement (PREVINAD) can be estimated by a process of summation:

(include in a data step):

```
PROBINAD = 1 − PROBNORM((INTK−MEANREQ)/
                    SDREQ)
PROC MEANS N MEAN; VAR PROBINAD;
```

The resultant mean of PROBINAD is an estimate of the prevalence of inadequate intakes among the individuals studied. If multiplied by 100 it yields the conventional form of prevalence estimate (percentage of individuals). Please see earlier sections for important caveats about this application and note in particular that the approach embodied in the SAS program example assumes normality of the requirement distribution but makes no assumption about the intake distribution other than that it indeed represents a distribution of usual or habitual intakes. If normality of the requirement distribution is not seen as a justifiable assumption, then other approaches can be applied.

CHAPTER 84

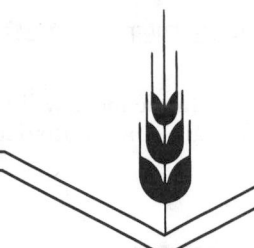

Nutrition Monitoring in the United States

Marie Fanelli Kuczmarski and Robert J. Kuczmarski

The efforts to monitor nutritional status in the United States are probably better than in any other nation. However, the present system is still developing and has known limitations. For example, it is unable to describe completely the current dietary and nutritional status of the United States population, particularly in subgroups of the population at high risk of malnutrition. This inability stems in part from insufficient coverage by current data collection systems of selected population groups, such as Native Americans residing on Indian reservations, persons who do not reside in households, and institutionalized persons, especially older adults. Although various national surveys have been conducted since the 1930s, not until 1990 did Congress and the executive branch of government mandate a comprehensive strategy for a coordinated program to strengthen existing national monitoring efforts. This strategy was designed to review and integrate the various federal surveys to provide timely, useful information that systematically addresses questions concerning the dietary and nutritional status of the American population. Thus, the National Nutrition Monitoring and Related Research Act of 1990, a public law (PL 101–445), was enacted to place the existing monitoring system, consisting of interacting federal groups, under an expanded program that includes related research. This program was designated to be guided by a specific 10-year plan under which action would be taken toward a goal of comprehensive national nutrition monitoring.

Although they are often used interchangeably, the terms dietary status and nutritional status have different connotations. Nutritional status encompasses anthropometric, biochemical, clinical, dietary, and sociodemographic factors. Dietary status is a more limited term that refers to intake of foods, beverages, both nonalcoholic and alcoholic, and nutrients, including supplements. Additionally, related health status, in the context of nutritional monitoring, refers to health conditions that may be associated with nutritional variables, such as diabetes and obesity, or osteoporosis and calcium.

The National Nutrition Monitoring and Related Research Act defines nutrition monitoring as "the set of activities necessary to provide timely information about the role and status of factors that bear on the contribution that nutrition makes to the health of the people in the United States."[1] Nutrition monitoring is characterized by regular data collection, analysis and interpretation to provide a description of nutrition conditions in the population, and linkages with policymaking and research. Monitoring provides a data base for public policy decisions related to such issues as public health intervention programs, fortification, safety and labeling of the food supply, food assistance programs, and federally supported food service programs.[2] It also assists in the identification of health and nutrition research priorities of public health significance such as food security/insecurity, thereby strengthening the research base for monitoring and policymaking. The five components of the United States National Nutrition Monitoring System (NNMS) were specified in the 1987 Operational Plan as follows: (1) nutritional and health status measurements; (2) food consumption measurements; (3) food composition measurements and nutrient data banks; (4) dietary knowledge and attitude measurements; and (5) food supply and demand determinations.[3] Although the titles of these components have been modified slightly in the 10-year plan for the National Nutrition Monitoring and Related Research Program (NNMRRP), the components remain the same (See Table 84–2 for revised names).

This chapter provides a brief account of the historical development of the NNMS and the current NNMRRP (Table 84–1), describes the cornerstone surveys of the NNMS, giving special attention to survey design, discusses some of the limitations of the current system, and recognizes provisions in PL 101–445 that may enhance the system.

HISTORICAL OVERVIEW

In the late 1960s, concerns about the nutritional status of the United States population emerged as reports about the existence of hunger and malnutrition were released.[4] Between 1969 and 1977, the Senate Select Committee on Nutrition and Human Needs investigated not only the extent to which hunger existed in the United States but also how effective the federal government was in measuring this problem. Recognizing serious deficiencies in the federal nutrition monitoring efforts and identifying the need for a coordinated comprehensive NNMS, Congress sought to remedy the situation by legislative action.

The Food and Agriculture Act of 1977 (PL 95–113) required the Secretary of Agriculture and the Secretary of Health, Education and Welfare (currently Health and Human Services) to:

> formulate and submit to Congress . . . a proposal for a comprehensive nutritional status monitoring system, to include: (1) an assessment of a system consisting of periodic surveys and continuous monitoring to determine: the extent of risk of nutrition-related health problems in the United States; which population groups or areas of the country face greatest risk; and the likely causes of risk and changes in the above risk factors over time; (2) a surveillance system to identify remediable nutrition-related health risks to individuals or for local areas, in such a manner as to tie detection to direct intervention and treatment . . . ; and (3) program evaluations to determine the adequacy, efficiency, effectiveness and side effects of nutrition-related programs in reducing health risks to individuals and populations.[5]

The proposal for a comprehensive NNMS was submitted by the Department of Health, Education and Welfare and the United States Department of Agriculture to Congress in 1978.[6] This proposal reviewed current federal, state, and local agency activities in the areas of nutritional and dietary status assessment, nutritional quality of foods, dietary practices and knowledge, and the impact of nutrition intervention programs. It acknowledged the deficiencies in existing nutritional and dietary assessment methods, recognized delays in data analysis and the publication of results, pointed out the inadequate coverage of certain target groups and geographic areas, and recognized the inadequate evaluation of nutrition intervention programs. Although the proposal contained a series of recommendations for improving and expanding the scope of federal nutrition monitoring activities, it lacked the following: a set of priorities; an assignment of tasks and a timetable for completion; a prospective plan; a reporting component to monitor progress of the NNMS; a timetable for publications; an assignment of responsibility for implementation; identification of costs; and identification of the relationship to the Joint Subcommittee on Human Nutrition Research.[7]

The proposal, at the request of the Committee on Science and Technology, was reviewed by the General Accounting Office, from which came the recommendation that the departments develop an implementation plan for a NNMS that would provide specific information on how and when the system could be implemented

TABLE 84–1. HISTORY OF NUTRITION MONITORING IN THE UNITED STATES

1977	Food and Agriculture Act (PL 95–113)
1978	Proposal to Congress for a comprehensive nutritional status monitoring system
1981	Joint Implementation Plan for a comprehensive national nutrition monitoring system
1986	First report to Congress: *Nutrition Monitoring in the United States: A Progress Report from the Joint Nutrition Monitoring Evaluation Committee*
1987	Operational plan for the National Nutrition Monitoring System
1988	Interagency Committee on Nutrition Monitoring formed
1989	Second report to Congress: *Nutrition Monitoring in the United States: An Update Report on Nutrition Monitoring*
1990	National Nutrition Monitoring and Related Research Act (PL 101–445)
1991	Interagency Board for Nutrition Monitoring and Related Research formed Draft comprehensive plan published in the Federal Register on October 29th
1992	National Nutrition Monitoring Advisory Council formed
1993	Comprehensive plan for the National Nutrition Monitoring and Related Research program signed by the president and transmitted to Congress

and on its cost. The Department of Health and Human Services and Department of Agriculture (DHHS–USDA) Joint Implementation Plan for a Comprehensive NNMS was submitted to Congress in 1981.[8] The plan assigned the Assistant Secretary for Food and Consumer Services, USDA, and the Assistant Secretary for Health, DHHS, as the parties responsible for implementing compatible survey plans. It also identified and described the current efforts in nutrition monitoring conducted by the USDA and DHHS and proposed major goals and objectives for the NNMS. The two major objectives were to (1) achieve the best possible coordination of the National Health and Nutrition Examination Survey (NHANES) and the Nationwide Food Consumption Survey (NFCS), and (2) develop a reporting system to translate the findings from these two national surveys and other monitoring activities into periodic reports to Congress on the nutritional status of the American population. The plan contained a description of activities to be accomplished to implement the first coordinated NHANES-NFCS survey in 1987. However, certain critical features were never completed, which inhibited the achievement of a comprehensive system.[7]

In 1982 and 1983, the Subcommittee on Science, Research, and Technology and the Subcommittee on Department Operations, Research, and Foreign Agriculture jointly held hearings to review the system. They noted that coordination had improved but was still inadequate. The NNMS lacked a central focus, a provision for continuous monitoring, and a mechanism for evaluating food assistance programs.

In 1983, the Joint Nutrition Monitoring Evaluation Committee (JNMEC) was appointed. This federal advisory committee, jointly sponsored by the USDA and DHHS, was responsible for the first progress report to the Congress, as stipulated in the Joint Implementation Plan. The report, published in 1986, contained information on the nutritional status of the United States population and made specific recommendations to improve the monitoring system.[9] The JNMEC reported that the principal nutrition-related health problems experienced by Americans arose from overconsumption of fat, saturated fat, cholesterol, and sodium. Intakes of iron and vitamin C were low in certain population groups. In addition to reviewing available data, the Committee made 14 recommendations on how to improve nutrition monitoring efforts.

In 1987, the DHHS and the USDA published an operational plan for the NNMS, a revision of the 1981 Joint Implementation Plan.[3] The operational plan described the goals of the operational phase, progress during the implementation phase (1981 to 1986) and proposed activities for the operational phase (1987 to 1996), including a calendar of events. The specific goals were to achieve a comprehensive system through coordination among NNMS components, improving information dissemination and exchange between data generators and users and Congress, and improving the research base for nutrition monitoring.

The operational plan did not provide a clear indication of dates for implementation of the comprehensive, coordinated system sought by the Congress. Given the lack of legislative mandate to establish such a system, it was unclear how this operational plan would be any more successful than the 1981 Joint Implementation Plan.

In 1988, the Interagency Committee on Nutrition Monitoring (ICNM) was formed.[10] The Committee was co-chaired by the Assistant Secretary for Health, DHHS, and the Assistant Secretary for Food and Consumer Services, USDA. The purpose of this committee was to increase the effectiveness and productivity of federal nutrition monitoring efforts by improving planning, coordination, and communication among the agencies engaged in nutrition monitoring. The membership included representatives from Public Health Service (DHHS) agencies, USDA agencies, the Agency for International Development, the Bureau of Labor Statistics, the Census Bureau, the Department of Defense, and the Veterans Administration.

In 1989, the second progress report on nutrition monitoring prepared by an ad hoc expert panel was transmitted to the Congress. This report provided (1) an update to the 1986 report on the dietary and nutritional status of the United States population, and (2) an indepth analysis of the contributions of the NNMS to the assessment of iron nutriture and dietary and nutritional factors related to cardiovascular disease.[11] The expert panel concluded that the principal nutrition-related health problems experienced by Americans were related to overconsumption of selected nutrients, particularly food energy, fat, saturated fatty acids, cholesterol, sodium, and alcohol. Iron deficiency was cited as the most common single nutrient deficiency. The expert panel also offered several recommendations for improvements in the NNMS.

Between 1984 and 1990, several attempts were made to pass a legislative bill to establish a coordinated national nutrition monitoring and related research program.[7,12] This proposed legislation included the development of a comprehensive plan for the assessment of the nutritional status and dietary intake of the United States population and the nutritional quality of the food supply with provisions for conducting scientific research. Finally, on October 22, 1990, the National Nutrition Monitoring and Related Research Act (PL 101–445) was signed into law.[1]

The key monitoring provisions of this bill (Titles I and II) were as follows:

1. Establish an Interagency Board for Nutrition Monitoring and Related Research, which is jointly chaired by an Assistant Secretary from the USDA and by an Assistant Secretary from the DHHS.

2. Establish a National Nutrition Monitoring Advisory Council of nine voting members who are not federal employees.

3. Develop and implement a 10-year comprehensive plan for a coordinated program that is designed to assess and report on a continuous basis the dietary and nutritional status of the United States population, particularly infants and children, the aged, disadvantaged persons, minorities, and women; to develop and update nutrient data banks; to sponsor/conduct research to develop uniform indicators and methods for conducting and reporting nutrition monitoring activities; and to assist state and local government agencies in developing procedures and networks for nutrition monitoring and surveillance.
4. Publish every 2 or 5 years a report to the Congress on the dietary, nutritional, and health-related status of the American population and the nutritional quality of food consumed in the United States.

NATIONAL NUTRITION MONITORING CORNERSTONE SURVEYS

Since 1896, when the first food composition tables were published, to 1991, there have been over 100 federal nutrition surveys and surveillance activities. A chronologic listing categorized by the measurement components has been published in the comprehensive plan for national nutrition monitoring and related research.[41,42] Although many surveys and surveillance activities have been sponsored by a variety of agencies in the federal government, three in particular, the Nationwide Food Consumption Survey (NFCS), the Continuing Survey of Food Intakes by Individuals (CSFII), and the National Health and Nutrition Examination Survey (NHANES), are regarded as the cornerstones of national nutrition monitoring. The NFCS and CSFII are sponsored by the Human Nutrition Information Service of the USDA and the NHANES, by the National Center for Health Statistics of the DHHS.

NATIONWIDE FOOD CONSUMPTION SURVEY

The involvement of the federal government in nutrition monitoring actually dates back to 1893, when the USDA received the first appropriation to conduct human nutrition research. The first national survey of household food consumption and dietary levels was conducted in 1936 to 1937 as part of the Consumer Purchases Study.[13] Between 1942 and 1955, three nationwide studies on household food consumption (NFCS) were conducted by the Human Nutrition Information Service.[14] These surveys included the collection of information on household food use over 7 days and reflected food use from an economic perspective; that is, it included food used whether it is eaten, discarded, or fed to pets. The person primarily responsible for food preparation in a given household provided this information. Food distribution among members of the household was not taken into account. In the 1965 and subsequent NFCS (1977 to 1978, 1987 to 1988), data were obtained on dietary intakes and patterns of individuals, as well as on household food use. Information on food consumed by individuals both at and away from home was collected for 1 day in the 1965 NFCS and for 3 consecutive days in the 1977 to 1978 and 1987 to 1988 NFCS. Nutrient content of food used by households and of food consumed by individuals was estimated from food composition data files developed from the National Nutrient Data Bank.[15]

The objectives of the NFCS are to describe current food consumption behavior to identify changes in diet that have occurred since the previous NFCS and to assess the nutritional content of diets for their implications on policies relating to food production and marketing, food safety, food assistance, and nutrition education. More specifically, data from the NFCS have been used to develop the Dietary Guidelines for Americans[16] and the Thrifty Food Plan,[17] which is used as the statutory basis for the Food Stamp Program; to evaluate the achievement of the 1990 Health Objectives for the Nation;[18] and to help develop the nutrition objectives included in Healthy People 2000.[19]

The NFCS is designed to provide a multistage stratified area probability sample representative of the 48 conterminous states.[15] The stratification plan takes into account geographic location and degree of urbanization. In the 1987 to 1988 NFCS, households were drawn from 9 geographic divisions and 3 urbanization classes as defined by the Bureau of the Census.[20] This NFCS included 2 probability samples—one for the general population, the basic survey (households and individuals with all incomes), and one for the low-income survey (households and individuals with incomes consistent with eligibility for the Food Stamp Program).

The 1987 to 1988 NFCS involved three visits with participants.[21] The initial visit identified respondents and provided them with materials needed to keep notes on household food used during the survey period. The next visit, scheduled 7 days later, consisted of a 2- to 3-hour personal interview to conduct the household phase of the survey, to obtain a 1-day dietary recall from individual members, and to leave these individuals a 2-day dietary record to complete. The final contact with respondents was 2 days later to collect the 2-day dietary record. In addition to obtaining information on food use/intake, questions were posed concerning household characteristics, individual characteristics, such as self-reported height, weight, and health status; participation in food assistance programs; and diet-related topics such as supplement use, alcohol consumption, use of salt at the table, and dieting.[20] To reduce data processing time and to make NFCS results more readily available, interviews in the 1987 to 1988 NFCS household component were conducted with the use of a laptop computer.

The basic survey provided information from about 5000 households and their approximately 10,000 individual members; the low-income survey, from 2500 households and about 6000 individual members.[15] The household response rate was 38% for the basic sample and 42% for the low-income sample. The individual response rate for the basic sample was 31%.[22]

CONTINUING SURVEY OF FOOD INTAKES BY INDIVIDUALS

The first Continuing Survey of Food Intakes by Individuals was conducted in 1985, the second in 1986. These two surveys constitute Series I. Series II began in 1989 and includes the 1990 and the 1991 CSFII. Series III is scheduled to begin in 1994 and will continue through 1996. The purpose of these surveys is to provide information on the dietary status of the United States population and to monitor changes in dietary intakes. In addition, individuals identified as the main meal planner/preparer in the 1989 to 1991 CSFII were contacted to participate in the Diet and Health Knowledge Survey, another NNMS activity sponsored by the USDA. The dietary data collected in the CSFII was then linked to an individual's nutrition knowledge and attitudes.

"Usual" intakes were assessed in the 1985 and 1986 CSFII by multiple 24-hour dietary recalls over a 1-year period. A 1-day dietary recall in an in-person interview and a self-administered 2-day dietary record were the methods selected for use in the second CSFII series.[23] Similar to NFCS, nutrient intakes were calculated from the National Nutrient Data Bank. The dietary data collection method for the 1994–1996 CSFII is scheduled to consist of 2 nonconsecutive 1-day recalls of food intake through in-person interviews.

The target population for Series I and II CSFII consisted of individuals selected by sex and age residing in the 48 conterminous States in households with incomes at all levels (basic sample) and with incomes at or below 130% of poverty guidelines (low-income sample). The 1985 CSFII included men and women aged 19 to 50 years and children 1 to 5 years of age,[24–26] whereas the 1986 CSFII included women 19 to 50 years of age and children 1 to 5 years of age.[27,28] For the Series I CSFII, the basic sample included approximately 1300 households and their 2000 individual members. The 1985 low-income sample included about 1900 households and their 3400 individual members, whereas the 1986 low-income sample had about 1200 households and 2100 individual members. Individual response rates for women and children completing 1-day recalls were 71% for the basic sample and 65% for the low-income sample in 1985 and 66% for the basic sample and 75% for the low-income sample in 1986.[29]

The 1989 to 1991 CSFII were designed to obtain information on food intakes from all household members (men, women, and children of all ages). Approximately 1500 households and their 3500 individual members were included in the basic sample, and approximately 750 households and their 1600 individual members were included in the low-income sample.[22] The household response rates were 63% for the basic sample in both the 1989 and 1990 CSFII, whereas they were 73% and 69% for the low-income households in 1989 and 1990 CSFII, respectively. Individual response rates were 56% for the basic sample and 66% for the low-income sample in the 1989 CSFII. In the 1990 CSFII, individual response rates were 54% for the basic sample and 60% for the low-income sample.[22]

The sample size for the 1994–1996 CSFII is projected to include approximately 15,000 to 16,000 respondents. Notable design changes from the first two series include a target population of noninstitutionalized persons in all 50 states, an oversampling of the low-income population, and subsampling within households.

NATIONAL HEALTH AND NUTRITION EXAMINATION SURVEY

In 1967, the Senate Subcommittee on Employment, Manpower, and Poverty of the Committee on Labor and Public Welfare noted in a letter to President Lyndon Johnson that the conditions of malnutrition and widespread hunger had reached emergency proportions. In response to the concerns regarding the existence of hunger and malnutrition and the lack of a monitoring system to determine the magnitude of the problem, Congress mandated, in Section 14 of the Partnership for Health Amendments of 1967, that the Secretary of Health, Education, and Welfare, in collaboration with other federal government and state officials, was to conduct a comprehensive survey to assess the incidence and location of serious hunger, malnutrition, and health problems. This action authorized the National Nutrition Survey, better known as the Ten State Nutrition Survey.

The Ten State Nutrition Survey, 1968 to 1970, was designed to select families randomly from the 1960 Bureau of Census enumeration districts, where the highest percentage of families had incomes below the Orshansky Poverty Index in the states of California, Kentucky, Louisiana, Massachusetts, Michigan, New York, South Carolina, Texas, Washington, and West Virginia. The sample population included middle- and upper-income persons who, because of changes in residential patterns subsequent to 1960, were living in selected enumeration districts. Nutritional status was assessed on the basis of dietary intakes and food patterns, dental examinations, and anthropometric and biochemical measurements. Information on non-nutritional factors that affect food intake, such as socioeconomic characteristics, health status, and income, was also gathered. The findings of the Ten State Survey indicated nutritional problems in selected age and sex groups.[30]

While the Ten State Survey was still underway, in 1969, President Richard Nixon asked the Secretary of the Department of Health, Education, and Welfare to expand this survey to provide a description of the extent of hunger and malnutrition in the entire United States. In response, a Task Force on Nutritional Surveillance at the National Center for Health Statistics (NCHS) was formed and asked to plan and implement a survey that would provide an effective nutrition surveillance system. To minimize duplication with other surveys conducted by the NCHS and to permit relating nutritional variables to other health status measurements already being collected in the National Health Examination Survey (NHES), a nutritional assessment component was added to the NHES to create the first National Health and Nutrition Examination Survey (NHANES I). Conducted between 1971 and 1974, this health survey was the first to assess dietary intake and other measures of nutritional status in a representative sample of the civilian, noninstitutionalized population in the United States.[31,32]

A major objective of the NHANES is the periodic assessment of the health and nutritional status of the United States population and the monitoring of changes in status over time. The second NHANES was conducted in 1976 to 1980,[33] and the third NHANES was fielded in 1988 and will be completed in 1994. The Hispanic HANES (HHANES) was conducted in the period 1982 to 1984.[34] This special survey included three Hispanic groups consisting of Mexican Americans residing in five southwestern states, Cubans in Dade County, Florida, and Puerto Ricans in the New York City metropolitan area.

Each of the NHANES surveys has used complex, multistage, probability, cluster sampling to select a representative sample of the civilian, noninstitutionalized population residing in households in the United States. Special oversampling techniques were used to ensure adequate representation of subgroups considered to be at high risk of malnutrition. NHANES II statistically selected for a sample of 27,805 individuals to represent the entire United States population and selected subgroups. About 91% of those selected agreed to be interviewed and 73% agreed to be interviewed and examined.[29] In the first 3 years of data collection for the NHANES III, about 20,000 individuals were selected, among whom 86% were interviewed and 77% were examined. The age range for the third NHANES has been expanded, beginning at 2 months, with no upper age limit.

The NHANES is unique in that it collects data on the health and nutritional status of Americans through interviews and direct physical examinations. The household interview is administered in four parts:

1. Household screener questionnaire to determine household eligibility and select sample persons.
2. Family questionnaire to determine relationships of persons in the household, obtain basic demographic data, and assess participation in income assistance programs, including the Food Stamp Program.
3. Adult household questionnaire to assess health status including dental conditions and care, use of health services, meal program participation, and use of vitamin/mineral supplements and medications.
4. Child household questionnaire, with items similar to those asked of adults, and the addition of questions on infant feeding practices, weight status, breast-feeding, time of introduction of solid foods, and other nutrition-related questions.

After completing the household interview, sample persons are invited to Mobile Examination Centers where the NHANES staff administer standardized examination and laboratory tests.

Nutritional status is evaluated from data generated through interviews and direct physical examinations. Listings of the major parameters measured by sex and age have been published.[35] Briefly, the interviews include a single 24-hour dietary recall, a food frequency questionnaire, questions related to eating habits, life style, and other nutrition-related practices, and a medical history. The third NHANES includes a quantitative measure of intake of vitamins and minerals from supplements and a series of food sufficiency questions. Physical examinations include components such as anthropometric measurements, hematologic and biochemical assessments, and physical and dental examinations. The survey design and implementation strategies have been described in various reports,[35,36] and a compendium of all data collection instruments for the NHANES III has been published.[37]

The NHANES is designed as a multipurpose survey. Some examples of the major uses of the data include the assessment of selected conditions such as growth retardation, prevalence of overweight,[38] hypertension,[39] high blood cholesterol level,[40] evaluation and development of nutrition policy such as Healthy People 2000[19] and the Dietary Guidelines for Americans,[16] and assessment of food fortification policies.

OTHER NUTRITION MONITORING ACTIVITIES

In addition to the core components, i.e., NFCS, CSFII and NHANES, several other survey and surveillance activities constitute the NNMRRP. Approximately 50 monitoring activities that will provide information on the 5 measurement components are planned between 1992 and 2002.[41] The activities conducted on a regular basis and sponsoring federal agency are shown in Table 84–2. The periodicity of the activities does vary. For example, the Total Diet Study is conducted annually, whereas the Food Label and Package Survey is done biennially. Many special surveys, such as the Vitamin and Mineral Intake Survey, the Navajo Health and Nutrition Survey, and the National Maternal and Infant Health Survey, are also conducted. A comprehensive

TABLE 84–2. PRINCIPAL NNMRRP ACTIVITIES, SPONSORING FEDERAL AGENCIES AND SURVEY DESIGNS

ACTIVITY	AGENCY	SURVEY DESIGN
Nutrition and related Health Measurements		
National Ambulatory Medical Care Survey	National Center for Health Statistics	Multistage, stratified, probability sample of licensed physicians in office-based patient care
National Health and Nutrition Examination Survey	National Center for Health Statistics	Complex, multistage, stratified, probability cluster sample of households
NHANES I Epidemiologic Follow-up Study	National Center for Health Statistics	Follow-up on NHANES I participants, aged 25 to 74 years in 1971–1975
Pediatric Nutrition Surveillance System	Centers for Disease Control	Convenience population of low-income children, 0–17 years of age, who participate in publicly funded health, nutrition, and food assistance programs
Pregnancy Nutrition Surveillance System	Centers for Disease Control	Convenience population of low-income, high-risk pregnant women who participate in publicly funded prenatal nutrition and food assistance programs
Vital Statistics Program	National Center for Health Statistics	Vital registration system
Food and nutrient consumption measurements		
Continuing Survey of Food Intakes by Individuals	Human Nutrition Information Service	Multistage, stratified area probability sample of defined populations
Military Feeding Systems and Military Populations	United States Army Research Institute of Environmental Medicine	Varies with specific study
Nationwide Food Consumption Survey	Human Nutrition Information Service	Multistage, stratified area probability sample of defined populations
Knowledge, attitudes, and behavior assessments		
Behavioral Risk Factor Surveillance System	Centers for Disease Control	Multistage, cluster telephone survey based on Waksberg method
Diet-Health Knowledge Survey	Human Nutrition Information Service*	Follow-up of CSFII meal planners using telephone interview
Health and Diet Survey	Food and Drug Administration	Telephone interviews with a national probability Waksberg sample selected by random digit dialing method
National Health Interview Survey	National Center for Health Statistics	Complex, multistage, stratified, probability cluster sample of households
Food composition and nutrient data bases		
Food Label and Package Survey	Food and Drug Administration	Biennial probability survey of retail packaged foods using commercial market research data bases (A.C. Nielsen Scantrack)
National Nutrient Data Bank	Human Nutrition Information Service	NA
Nutrient Composition Laboratory	Agricultural Research Service	NA
Survey Nutrient Data Base	Human Nutrition Information Service	NA
Food supply determinations		
A.C. Nielsen Scantrack	Economic Research Service*	NA
Total Diet Study	Food and Drug Administration	NA
United States Food and Nutrition Supply Series	Economic Research Service*	NA

*Primary sponsor.

compilation of all NNMRRP activities with descriptions about survey design and objectives, sample sizes, and response rates is provided in the Directory of Federal and State Nutrition Monitoring Activities[22] and the comprehensive plan for national nutrition monitoring and related research.[41]

LIMITATIONS OF THE NATIONAL NUTRITION MONITORING SYSTEM

The five components of the NNMRRP provide a considerable amount of valuable information. However, there is a need for improvement, especially with regard to components that have not been functionally integrated into a coordinated and comprehensive system. Both the USDA and the DHHS have made serious efforts to improve and coordinate their individual nutrition monitoring activities. The National Nutritional Monitoring and Related Research Act (PL 101–445) will result in a re-evaluation of departmental efforts and the development of a plan designed to correct past limitations. The proposed 10-year Comprehensive Plan for the National Nutrition Monitoring and Related Research Program was designed to cover national nutrition monitoring activities for the period 1992 to 2002. This plan was compiled by members of a DHHS/USDA working group and was published on October 29, 1991.[42] After subsequent public comment and departmental revision periods, the finalized plan was signed by the President and forwarded to Congress in January, 1993, and submitted for publication in the Federal Register.[41] This plan is intended to be the guidance mechanism that will provide direction to the federal and state agencies participating in the national nutritional monitoring program. It discusses a tentative course of action designed to address some of the recognized deficiencies in the NNMS. For a detailed presentation of the proposed national nutritional monitoring activities and the agencies responsible, the reader is encouraged to refer to the 10-year comprehensive plan.[41] Some of the shortcomings of the NNMS are discussed subsequently.

POPULATION SUBGROUP COVERAGE

The core components (NFCS, CSFII, and NHANES) provide data representative of the civilian, noninstitutionalized population in the United States. Groups excluded from these surveys include active-duty military personnel and persons in institutions, such as long-term care hospitals, homes for the aged, convents, monasteries, and penal and mental institutions. Homeless people who do not have an address are excluded from all household surveys because lists of addresses within census tracts are used as the basic unit for sampling.

As shown in Table 84–2, a complex, multistaged, stratified probability method of sampling is used in the core surveys. This method either limits or eliminates the size of some subgroups that may be at higher risk for nutritional problems. For example, selected subgroups, such as pregnant or lactating women and ethnic minority groups such as Asians and selected Hispanic subgroups, do not occur in the population in sufficient numbers to appear in the survey sample with adequate representation to make reliable estimates of their nutritional and health status. Both the NFCS and NHANES exclude nursing homes, so the estimates of food and nutrient intake of older adults may not be sufficiently representative of that age group. To capture all population subgroups, other approaches need to be implemented.[43] Special surveys, such as the Hispanic HANES or the CSFII low-income sample, can be conducted. Oversampling, a technique used to increase sample size, can help to improve the precision of estimates for nutritional and health variables. For example, the third NHANES is designed to oversample black and Mexican American persons, young children less than 6 years of age, and adults aged 74 years or older.

The nutrition objectives in Healthy People 2000, the Year 2000 Health Promotion and Disease Prevention Objectives for the Nation, identify as a high priority the need for data on the nutritional status of seven selected groups. These groups are people in hospitals, nursing homes, convalescent centers, and institutions such as those for the developmentally disabled; physically, mentally, and developmentally disabled individuals in community settings; children in child care facilities; Native Americans on reservations; old and very old individuals living independently; people in correctional facilities; and the homeless.[19] PL 101–445 also cites the need to gather data on these groups.[1] More specifically, this current legislation mandates that the comprehensive plan include components to incorporate, in survey design, military and (where appropriate) institutionalized populations; to sample representative subsets of identifiable low-income populations such as Native Americans and the homeless; and to collect dietary and nutritional status measurements on preschool and school-age children, pregnant and lactating women, elderly individuals, low-income populations, blacks, and Hispanics.

Even though a survey is designed to be representative of the United States population, if response rates are extremely low, it is questionable whether or not the data will provide an unbiased estimate of the dietary and nutritional status of the nation. Reports have documented such problems in a national survey and point out potential limitations to the intended utility of the collected data.[44,45]

GEOGRAPHIC COVERAGE

Many users of NNMS data request that federal agencies provide information on defined geographic areas, such as cities, counties, and individual states. The design of federal surveys uses primary sampling units, consisting of a county or a contiguous group of small counties that are stratified by characteristics such as urbanization and income. However, confidentiality restrictions generally prohibit release of data with identification of limited geographic areas. Areas are selected randomly within regions to provide the most representative sample while minimizing operational costs. Both NHANES and NFCS are designed to provide a picture of the nation. The USDA also reports the findings from NFCS and CSFII by the four major geographic regions of the country (Northeast, North Central, South, and West), as defined by the Bureau of the Census. It is anticipated that data from the third NHANES will be reported by these four regions. Data from the first and second NHANES were available by region; however, the regions were not identical to those defined by the Census Bureau. Although regional data are available, representative state and local (city) data are not obtainable from the core surveys.

The surveillance activities at the Centers for Disease Control (CDC) effectively target high-risk populations in narrow geographic areas. These activities include the Pediatric Nutrition Surveillance System (PedNSS) and the Pregnancy Nutrition Surveillance System (PregNSS). The target populations for PedNSS and PregNSS consist of a convenience sample of low-income children and pregnant women, respectively, who participate in publically funded health, nutrition, and food assistance programs. Participation in the CDC system is voluntary. In 1990, 40 states, 2 Indian tribes, Washington, D.C., and Puerto Rico participated in the PedNSS, and 18 states, Washington, D.C., and American Somoa participated in the PregNSS.[22] The states involved in these two surveillance activities receive the data analysis results on a monthly, quarterly, or annual basis for use in program planning, management, and evaluation.

The comprehensive plan for the NNMRRP in Public Law 101–445 requires the federal government to provide scientific and technical assistance, training, and consultation to state and local governments for the purpose of obtaining dietary and nutritional status data; developing related data bases; and promoting the development of regional, state, and local data collection services to become an integral component of a national nutritional status network. A grants program to encourage and assist state and local governments in developing the capacity to conduct monitoring and surveillance of nutritional status, food consumption, and nutrition knowledge and to enhance nutrition services is also a provision of PL 101–445.[1] As part of the related research provision of this law, innovative ways need to be developed to help smaller areas meet their needs for information about the nutritional status and health of their residents.

TIMELINESS OF DATA

Timely data are essential to both policymakers and researchers. National surveys involve large sample sizes and oftentimes relatively long periods for data collection. In the past, one of the major limitations of the NNMS has been inordinate delays in the processing and release of data from both the core and ancillary surveys.[46] With improvements in technology and the use of automated data collection systems, such as an automated system for assigning food codes that is used in the NHANES III, the time required to disseminate data of future NNMRRP activities should be shorter. For faster data release and publication, the results from the third NHANES, a 6-year survey, will be analyzed and published in two phases. Preliminary analysis can be accomplished after the first 3 years of data collection. Approximately 2 years after the completion of the entire survey, data should be available for analysis on public release data tapes.

In conclusion, the future direction of the NNMRRP will be determined in large part by the interpretation of the National Nutrition Monitoring and Related Research Act of 1990 (PL 101–445), by the various federal agencies that sponsor monitoring activities and contribute to the 10-year comprehensive plan. The law does provide many windows of opportunity to enhance the current NNMRRP by increasing the involvement at the state and local levels. The law provides authorization to carry nutrition monitoring activities into nonfederal areas, with the potential to expand monitoring beyond the core components of DHHS and USDA. The plan is ambitious and includes new activities. The extent to which these proposed initiatives are carried out and realized will largely depend upon the adequate allocation of resources. Although the legislation did not carry with it additional appropriations to support new monitoring initiatives, included in the coordinated program and the comprehensive plan is a provision for a competitive grants program to be implemented to the extent funds are available. This grants program may have an impact on the direction and extent of research accomplished in the monitoring arena between 1992 and 2002, the 10-year period covered by the comprehensive nutrition monitoring plan.

REFERENCES

1. National Nutrition Monitoring and Related Research Act of 1990 (PL 101–445), Congressional Record, 136, October 22, 1990.

2. Forbes, A.L., Stephenson, M.G.: J. Am. Diet. Assoc., *84:*1189–1193, 1984.

3. U.S. Department of Health and Human Services and U.S. Department of Agriculture: Operational Plan for the National Nutrition Monitoring System. Unpublished government report, 1987.

4. Ostenso, G.L.: J. Am. Diet. Assoc., *84:*1181–1185, 1984.

5. Food and Agriculture Act of 1977 (PL 95–113), Sec. 1428. Congressional Record, 123, September 29, 1977.

6. Department of Health, Education and Welfare and U.S. Department of Agriculture: Proposal—A Comprehensive Nutritional Status Monitoring System. Unpublished government report, 1978.

7. Porter, D.: A National Nutrition Monitoring System: Brief Background and Bill Review. CRS Report for Congress no. 88–199 SPR. Washington, D.C., Congressional Research Service, 1988.

8. U.S. Department of Health and Human Services and U.S. Department of Agriculture: Joint Implementation Plan for a Comprehensive National Nutrition Monitoring System. Unpublished government report, 1981.

9. U.S. Department of Health and Human Services and U.S. Department of Agriculture: Nutrition Monitoring in the United States: A Progress Report from the Joint Nutrition Monitoring Evaluation Committee. DHHS Publ. no. (PHS) 86–1255. Washington, D.C., U.S. Government Printing Office, 1986.

10. U.S. Department of Health and Human Services, Interagency Committee on Nutrition Monitoring: Announcement of Committee Formation. 53 FR 26505 no. 134. Washington, D.C., U.S. Government Printing Office, 1988.

11. Life Sciences Research Office, Federation of American Societies for Experimental Biology: Nutrition Monitoring in the United States: An Update Report on Nutrition Monitoring. DHHS Publ. no. (PHS) 89–1255. Washington, D.C., U.S. Government Printing Office, 1989.

12. Nestle, M.: J. Nutr. Ed., *22:*141–144, 1990.

13. Stiebeling, H.K., Monroe, D., Coons, C.M., et al.: Family Food Consumption and Dietary Levels Five Regions. Consumer Purchases Study. USDA Misc. Publ. no. 405. Washington, D.C., U.S. Government Printing Office, 1941.

14. Woteki, C.E., Fanelli-Kuczmarski, M.T.: The National Nutrition Monitoring System. *In* Present Knowledge in Nutrition. 6th Ed. Edited by M.L. Brown. Washington, D.C., International Life Sciences Institute, 1990.

15. Peterkin, B.B., Rizek, R.L., Tippett, K.S.: Nutr. Today, *23:*18–24, 1988.

16. U.S. Department of Agriculture and Department of Health and Human Services: Nutrition and Your Health: Dietary Guidelines for Americans. 3rd Ed. Washington, D.C., U.S. Government Printing Office, 1990.

17. Human Nutrition Information Service: USDA Family Food Plans, 1983: Low-cost, Moderate-cost, and Liberal. Hyattsville, MD, United States Department of Agriculture, 1983.

18. U.S. Department of Health and Human Services: The 1990 Health Objectives for the Nation: A Midcourse Review. Washington, D.C., U.S. Government Printing Office, 1986.

19. Department of Health and Human Services: Healthy People 2000: National Health Promotion and Disease Prevention Objectives. DHHS Publ. No. (PHS) 91–50212. Washington, D.C., U.S. Government Printing Office, 1991.

20. Hamma, M.Y., Riddick, H.A.: Family Economic Review, *2:*24–27, 1988.

21. National Analysts: Nationwide Food Consumption Survey 1987/88, Survey Operations Report. Philadelphia, National Analysts, 1991.

22. Interagency Board for Nutrition Monitoring and Related Research: Nutrition Monitoring in the United States: The Directory of Federal and State Nutrition Monitoring Activities. DHHS Publ. No. (PHS) 92-1255-1. Washington, D.C., U.S. Government Office, 1992.

23. National Analysts: The Continuing Survey of Food Intakes by Individuals and the Diet and Health Knowledge Survey: 1989, Survey Operations Reports. Philadelphia, National Analysts, 1991.

24. U.S. Department of Agriculture: Nationwide Food Consumption Survey: Continuing Survey of Food Intakes By Individuals, Women 19–50 Years and Their Children 1–5 Years, 1 Day, 1985. NFCS, CSFII Report no. 85–1. Washington, D.C., U.S. Government Printing Office, 1985.

25. U.S. Department of Agriculture: Nationwide Food Consumption Survey: Continuing Survey of Food Intakes By Individuals, Low-Income Women 19–50 and Their Children 1–5 Years, 1 Day, 1985. NFCS, CSFII Report no. 85–2. Washington, D.C., U.S. Government Printing Office, 1986.

26. U.S. Department of Agriculture: Nationwide Food Consumption Survey: Continuing Survey of Food Intakes By Individuals, Men 19–50 Years, 1 Day, 1985. NFCS, CSFII Report no. 85–3. Washington, D.C., U.S. Government Printing Office, 1986.

27. U.S. Department of Agriculture: Nationwide Food Consumption Survey: Continuing Survey of Food Intakes By Individuals, Women 19–50 Years and Their Children 1–5 Years, 1 Day, 1986. NFCS, CSFII Report no. 86–1. Washington, D.C., U.S. Government Printing Office, 1987.

28. U.S. Department of Agriculture: Nationwide Food Consumption Survey: Continuing Survey of Food Intakes By Individuals, Low-Income Women 19–50 and Their Children 1–5 Years, 1 Day, 1986. NFCS, CSFII Report no. 86–2. Washington, D.C., U.S. Government Printing Office, 1987.

29. Interagency Committee on Nutrition Monitoring: Nutrition Monitoring in the United States: The Directory of Federal Nutrition Monitoring Activities. DHHS Publ. no. (PHS) 89-1255-1. Washington, D.C., U.S. Government Printing Office, 1989.

30. U.S. Department of Health, Education and Welfare: Ten-State Nutrition Survey 1968–1970. DHEW Publ. no. (HSM) 72-8130–72-8133. Washington, D.C., U.S. Government Printing Office, 1972.

31. National Center for Health Statistics: Plan and Operation of the Health and Nutrition Examination Survey, United States, 1971–1973 (Part A —Development, plan, and operation) Vital and Health Statistics. Series 1, No. 10a. DHEW Publ. No. (PHS) 79–1310. Washington, D.C., U.S. Government Printing Office, 1973.

32. National Center for Health Statistics: Plan and Operation of the Health and Nutrition Examination Survey, United States, 1971–1973 (Part B-Data Collection Forms of the Survey) Vital and Health Statistics. Series 1, No. 10b. DHEW Publ. No. (PHS) 79–1310. Washington, D.C., U.S. Government Printing Office, 1977.

33. National Center for Health Statistics: Plan and Operation of the Second National Health and Nutrition Examination Survey, 1976–80. Vital and Health Statistics. Series 1, No. 15. DHHS Publ. No. (PHS) 81–1317. Washington, D.C., U.S. Government Printing Office, 1981.

34. National Center for Health Statistics: Plan and Operation of the Hispanic Health and Nutrition Examination Survey, 1982–1984. Vital and Health Statistics. Series 1, No. 19.

DHHS Publ. No. (PHS) 85–1321. Washington, D.C., U.S. Government Printing Office, 1985.

35. Woteki, C.E., Briefel, R.B., Kuczmarski, R.: Am. J. Clin. Nutr., *47*:320–328, 1988.

36. Woteki, C.E., Briefel, R.B. Hitchcock, D., et al.: J. Nutr., *120*:1440–1445, 1990.

37. National Center for Health Statistics: National Health and Nutrition Examination Survey III Data Collection Forms. Hyattsville, MD, 1990.

38. Najjar, M.F., Rowland, M.: Anthropometric Reference Data and Prevalence of Overweight, United States, 1976–1980. Vital and Health Statistics. Series 11, No. 238. DHHS Publ. No. (PHS) 87–1688. Washington, D.C., U.S. Government Printing Office, 1987.

39. Drizd, T., Dannenberg, A.L., Engel, A.: Blood Pressure Levels in Persons 18–74 Years of Age in 1976–80, and Trends in Blood Pressure from 1960 to 1980 in the United States. Vital and Health Statistics. Series 11, No. 234. DHHS Publ. No. (PHS) 86–1684. Washington, D.C., U.S. Government Printing Office, 1986.

40. Fulwood, R., Kalsbeek, W., Rifkind, B., et al.: Total Serum Cholesterol Levels of Adults 20–74 Years of Age: United States, 1976–1980. Vital and Health Statistics. Series 11, No. 236. DHHS Publ. No. (PHS) 86–1686. Washington, D.C., U.S. Government Printing Office, 1986.

41. Department of Health and Human Services and United States Department of Agriculture: Fed. Register. In press.

42. Department of Health and Human Services and United States Department of Agriculture: Fed. Register, *56*:55,716–55,767, 1991.

43. Lepkowski, J.M.: J. Nutr., *121*:416–423, 1991.

44. Life Sciences Research Office, Federation of American Societies for Experimental Biology: Impact of Nonresponse on Dietary Data from the 1987–88 Nationwide Food Consumption Survey. Bethesda, MD, LSRO/FASEB, 1991.

45. United States General Accounting Office: Nutrition Monitoring: Mismanagement of Nutrition Survey has Resulted in Questionable Data. GAO/RCED 91–117. Gaithersburg, MD, U.S. General Accounting Office, 1991.

46. Callaway, C.W.: J. Am. Diet. Assoc., *84*:1179–1180, 1984.

SELECTED READINGS

Department of Health and Human Services and United States Department of Agriculture: Ten-Year Comprehensive Plan for the National Nutrition Monitoring and Related Research Program. Fed. Register. In press.

Interagency Board for Nutrition Monitoring and Related Research: Nutrition Monitoring in the United States: The Directory of Federal and State Nutrition Monitoring Activities. DHHS Publ. No. (PHS) 92-1255-1. Washington, D.C., U.S. Government Printing Office, 1992.

Life Sciences Research Office, Federation of American Societies for Experimental Biology: Nutrition Monitoring in the United States: An Update Report on Nutrition Monitoring. Prepared for the U.S. Department of Agriculture and U.S. Department of Health and Human Services. DHHS Publ. no. (PHS) 89–1255. Washington, D.C., U.S. Government Printing Office, 1989.

National Nutrition Monitoring and Related Research Act of 1990 (PL 101–445). Congressional Record, October 20, 1990.

United States Department of Health and Human Services and United States Department of Agriculture: Nutrition Monitoring in the United States: A Progress Report from the Joint Nutrition Monitoring Evaluation Committee. DHHS Publ. no. (PHS) 86–1255. Washington, D.C., U.S. Government Printing Office, 1986.

Woteki, C.E., Fanelli-Kuczmarski, M.T.: The National Nutrition Monitoring System. *In* Present Knowledge in Nutrition. 6th Ed. Edited by M.L. Brown. Washington, D.C., International Life Sciences Institute, 1990.

CHAPTER **85**

Nutritional Anthropology: An Integrated Approach to Pregnancy and Delivery

Louis E. Grivetti

Nutritional anthropology is an ill-defined, eclectic, diverse field. If considered in a narrow sense, it comprises research on food and diet-related topics conducted by anthropologists, or studies on cultural food-related themes by nutritionists. If these limits are accepted, the field begins as a distinct specialization from anthropology during the middle of the twentieth century with the pioneering research on African diet by Richards.[1,2]

In this chapter, however, nutritional anthropology is extended to encompass a range of academic disciplines in the humanities, social sciences, biologic and medical sciences, engineering and applied sciences, law, and politics that link topics of culture, diet, food, and nutrition. The discussion includes a brief examination of selected publications represented by this expanded definition of nutritional anthropology, approaches and methods used in the field, and examination of pregnancy and delivery, drawing on a broad range of cultural, historical, ethical, legal, and technologic viewpoints and integrated by nutritional anthropology.

CONTRIBUTIONS TO NUTRITIONAL ANTHROPOLOGY

Within the humanities, art historians have described the geographic distribution and stylistic representations of goiter and cretinism in ancient and Medieval paintings.[3] Folklorists have traced the introduction of various food-related myths from Europe into the Americas.[4] Religious scholars have compiled lists of chemical compounds and food additives and then considered ethical and practical difficulties of maintaining Jewish or Islamic codes in the twentieth century.[5] Philosophers have examined moral issues of inconsistent economic and political behavior in food assistance programs and debated essential human rights to food.[6,7]

Social scientists, other than anthropologists, regularly contribute to nutritional anthropology. Economists have analyzed food price support systems and entitlements and their impacts on food access and nutritional status.[8] Geographers have mapped the cultural boundaries of human lactase deficiency,[9] described historical and political implications of repeated famine,[10] evaluated hypotheses for the origins of religious dietary practices,[11] and documented cultural response to drought in Africa.[12] Historians interested in food and culture have contributed thousands of diverse works that range from analysis of hospital diets prescribed in sixteenth century Spain,[13] to water supply and food distribution methods implemented after the 1906 San Francisco earthquake,[14] to nutritional evaluation of rations served in World War II concentration camps.[15] Psychologists working in tandem with physiologists have reported on cultural-physiologic responses to chili pepper consumption,[16] and associations between appetite, brain serotonin level, and meal selection.[17] Sociologists have conducted research on alcohol abuse and impact on felony drunk driving legislation,[18] factors that attract people to religious cults and associated dietary practices,[19] and feeding the homeless in American cities.[20]

Biologic and medical scientists, other than nutritionists, have produced elegant accounts that fit well within a broad definition of nutritional anthropology. Clinical physicians and radiologists have described contamination of human food and resulting consumption of toxic foods after the destruction of Hiroshima[21] and the Chernobyl reactor accident.[22] Herpetologists have reported dietary and nutritional roles of snake as human food,[23] and ichthyologists and toxicologists have considered human behavior and cultural practices that contribute to outbreaks of ciguatera[24] and puffer-fish intoxication.[25] Pediatricians have described cultural and economic factors leading to kwashiorkor in Native American Navajo children,[26] and social-environmental determinants of infantile diarrhea in tropical nations.[27] Physiologists have integrated themes of culture and mythology as both relate to human athletic performance, especially use of beverages, drugs, and foods believed by consumers to provide a competitive edge.[28,29] Zoologists interested in entomology have documented human use of edible insects and cultural factors that either promote or hinder consumption.[30,31]

Engineers interested in food processing and quality control have examined cultural factors when creating new ethnic foods.[32] Other engineering research has assured food quality and adherence to aesthetic standards,[33] improved the safety of the food supply and reduced microbial contamination,[34] and addressed packaging technology, potential criminal behavior, and the reality of food tampering.[35]

Lawyers and food technologists have written reports on cultural-social and economic-political factors that influence food labeling,[36] and have identified and differentiated categories of legislation for food, food additives, drugs, and so-called medical foods.[37] More telling, however, is the emerging body of legal opinion on the ethics of international food relief.[38] Lawyers regularly debate food, diet, and nutrition problems associated with pregnancy and fetal outcome,[39] exposure of pregnant and lactating women to toxic environments,[40] and patient rights versus medical ethics and requests to withhold food and hydration to terminal and nonterminal patients.[41] Other topics have included human rights issues and policies that derive from forced-feeding of hunger strikers,[42] and relationships between alcoholism and food intake, homicide, the legal argument of diminished capacity, and appropriate length of jail sentences.[43]

THEORETIC APPROACHES

Nutritional anthropology, broadly defined, encompasses a vast sweep from the present to the dawn of writing. The field is traceable to descriptive, classical texts produced in ancient Egypt, Greece, Rome, Mesopotamia, India, China, and elsewhere.[44] Despite this diversity in topic and historical depth, three theoretic approaches are used to describe and analyze food practices and the nutritional consequences of human behavior.[45]

CULTURAL-HISTORICAL

The approach of culture-history draws on a wide array of data available from archeology and ethnography, archive, and library texts, especially diaries and travel accounts, film and photography, observations, and interviews. Such studies usually document origins and dispersals of food and associated food-related traits, identify human food behavior, how behavior is related to nutrition and health conditions, and historical changes that have occurred.

CULTURAL-ECOLOGICAL

Cultural ecology holds that both culture and the environment exert influence on human food-related behavior. One objective of cultural ecologists is to determine the relative role of each component by focusing on food-related activities during a single time period, usually the present. Food-related practices are documented by observation, interview, and questionnaire, sometimes by film, and two paradigms are used to differentiate cultural from environmental determinants.

Cultural contributions are isolated by conducting the investigation in geographic areas that exhibit cultural homogeneity, but ecologic diversity. Both requirements are met, for example, in mountainous regions occupied by a single ethnic group. Conversely, environmental contributions are identified by setting the research in geographic areas represented by ethnic diversity, but ecologic homogeneity. Such locations would include midlatitude prairies and flat desert lands occupied by diverse cultures.

FUNCTIONALISM

Functional studies identify how food supply systems work and document the multiplicity of food uses within society. Incorporating a wide range of methods, data are collected on food availability, food procurement, and how consumable goods ultimately reach and are shared by individuals, families, and different social groups. Functionalists direct their attention to nonnutritional uses of food that provide food security and practices that either stabilize or fragment society, and ultimately document how foods are used to promote ethnic identity by defining age, gender, and social relationships.

METHODS: A-G SYSTEM

Nutritional anthropologists use a wide range of methods drawn from many disciplines. Several important works describe the most common method categories, easily remembered by the letter sequence A to G.[46–51]

Anthropometric: including height-weight relationships, skinfold measurements, and waist-hip and upper arm circumferences.

Biochemical: including hemoglobin, hematocrit, serum albumin, alkaline phosphatase, various mineral and vitamin determinations from blood and excretory products.

Clinical: including signs of malnutrition associated with skull-skeleton, hair, face, eyes, gums-lips, tongue, neck, skin, and extremities.

Dietary: including food intake protocols such as food histories, food-frequency, household inventory, menu evaluation, recall, record keeping, and weighed intake.

Ecologic: including measurement and analysis of climate, weather, soil and vegetation patterns; measurement of geologic structure and relief; and description, measurement, and analysis of human-animal associations.

Food Habit: including description and analysis of everyday and special dietary components by observation, interview, and questionnaire; determination of primary, secondary, tertiary, and peripheral elements of diet, foods associated with feasts and the seasonal timing of fasts, dietary prohibitions and taboos and associations with age, gender, religious practices, and life events (birth, coming-of-age, engagement-marriage, death); and description and analysis of food procurement systems (hunting, gathering, agriculture, horticulture, animal husbandry, barter, gift, cash exchanges), energy flow in food transportation systems, storage and preservation techniques, cooking and waste disposal, and relationships to human health and nutritional status.

Geographic: including production, use, and interpretation of maps, aerial photographs, satellite data (remote sensing), quantitative methods and computer-generated graphics to determine spatial patterns of food-related behavior and nutritional status; description and analysis of human land use patterns, especially as they relate to food production; and identification of appropriate historical documents (archive and library research) to determine changes in agricultural and food intake patterns and the nutritional consequences of human food-related behavior.

Methods and topics in nutritional anthropology have been considered in a wide range of textbooks[52–57] and review articles.[58–60] Readers are introduced to an enormous volume of creative, descriptive, and analytic work on hundreds of culture-nutrition topics conducted among thousands of human groups in numerous geographic areas. Managing this vast resource is an enormous task facilitated by four important annotated bibliographies, indexed by author and topic, that provide ready access to more than 10,000 nutritional anthropology citations.[61–64]

PREGNANCY AND DELIVERY

The reproductive cycle of conception, gestation, and birth generates wide ranges of emotion and behavior from anxiety, frustration, and sorrow to elation, joy, and thanksgiving. Pregnancy and delivery, as a theme within nutritional anthropology, illustrates the diversity of research viewpoints taken by contributors in the humanities, social sciences, biologic medical, and technologic sciences.

CONCEPTION

The wonder of conception has captured human imagination since remote antiquity. Few life events express such a range of cultural and technologic perspectives than conception, ranging from mythologic views that pregnancies were caused by "fire from heaven," or "insects," to twentieth century technology exhibited by sperm banks, fertility drugs, in vitro fertilization, surrogate conception, and associated ethical, legal, and moral implications.[65,66]

Numerous American beliefs hold that should men or women consume certain foods, such as onions, conception will occur; other myths to improve fertility have husbands premasticate bread, then pass the bolus to his wife to remove sterility and create, in essence, a "magic bullet."[67] Misinformed American teenagers frequently state that conception cannot occur with first intercourse, if both partners remain vertical, or if one partner is "too young."[68]

In many traditional societies, it is considered especially auspicious if a new wife becomes pregnant during the first marriage year. Early conception bonds relatives and in-laws closely, the reproductive role of wife as conceiver and bearer of the next generation is validated, and the specter of sterility-based divorce is banished.[69] In such societies, food may play important roles in marriage customs.

Among rural Nubians in southern Egypt, grooms must provide demonstrations of marital strength, vitality, and vigor to assembled guests on their wedding nights by crushing toasted bread in one hand. Inability to do so is considered a sign of marital weakness and portends problems in siring children. Such toasted breads are provided to grooms by their close male friends; knowing what is expected, grooms request the breads be baked lightly. Not unexpectedly, however, mischief reigns at this time as the bread usually is toasted to the consistency of granite. But recognizing this possibility, in turn, grooms and their brides usually prepare softening solutions in advance, hide them, turn the joke, then retire to their bridal chambers.[70]

In sharp juxtaposition to conception lies sterility and the poignant search of couples to have children. Here, too, folklore and mythology are deeply ingrained and numerous food-related prescriptions and behaviors are implemented to remove barrenness. The literature abounds with descriptions of concoctions prepared in the belief that consumption of these foods will lead to conception. In contemporary Egypt, for example, chick pea (Cicer arietinum), plaster from ancient Egyptian tombs and beverages prepared from the palm pollen are used to counter sterility.[71]

GENDER PREDICTION

While modern medical procedures of amniocentesis, tissue typing, and ultrasonography allow accurate gender determination, an ancient Egyptian papyrus dated more than 3000 years ago shows that the wish to know fetus gender is as ancient as humanity. Egyptian women provided a urine sample to their physician; he then poured it into separate bowls containing either seeds of barley or wheat planted in Nile mud. The physician then recorded emergence of cereal sprouts in each receptacle: if neither cereal grew, the woman was not pregnant; if barley grew first, the fetus would be male; if wheat grew, then the child would be female.[72]

This ancient Egyptian gender prediction technique was tested and evaluated empirically under controlled laboratory conditions; urine from nonpregnant women always inhibited cereal growth, and that from pregnant women stimulated growth in 40% of test cases. No association was found, however, between first emergence of barley or wheat and fetal gender.[73]

CRAVINGS-AVERSIONS

Human folklore is rich with examples of food cravings of women expressed during pregnancy.[67] Dietary cravings commonly are viewed by the lay public as expressions of natural physiologic demands placed on the mother by the growing fetus that reflect unfulfilled physiologic needs for specific nutrient requirements.[67] Psychologists and sociologists, however, suggest that dietary cravings for specific items of unusual food combinations are not physiologically based but are cultural devices designed to evoke attention and involve partners or friends in the pregnancy process.[67]

The cultural phenomenon of pica, or eating nonfood items, sometimes is associated with pregnancy.[74] Pica frequently is subdivided into specific categories of items, whether geophagia (earth eating),[75] amylophagia (starch eating),[76] pagophagia (ice eating),[77] or miscellaneous.[78] Researchers debate whether or not humans have "felt" physiologic needs for items consumed, and if consumption is related to specific nutrient deficiencies.

Careful review of the vast pica literature, however, leads to three conclusions. First, pica is not specifically associated with pregnancy. It is practiced widely by males and females on all inhabited continents, some women practice pica during their first pregnancy but not during subsequent ones, and religious pica is described extensively in the literature. Second, pica is not nutritionally based. When dietary assessments are made, and serologic data are correlated, minerals contained in edible clays do not provide "missing" nutrients to consumers. The practice of amylophagia, furthermore, provides extensive carbohydrate calories but essentially no minerals to the diet and the phenomenon of pagophagia adds neither energy or nutrients. Third, pica is not a response to anemia. Review of nutritional and physiologic data suggest the reverse, that consumption of inordinate quantities of clay, for example, produces anemia.[79,80]

Because human behavior ultimately is neurologic and biochemical, dietary cravings are linked with brain function. But separating physiologic and psychologic components of behavior, especially dietary cravings, is a challenging task. Classic experiments conducted by physiologists provided paradigms to differentiate between experience, memory, and taste in regulating food intake,[81,82] whereas more recent work has demonstrated inter-relationships between hormonal balance and alteration in ability to smell and taste foods.[83] The question of how taste signals influence human behavior and are translated as cravings or, conversely, food aversions during pregnancy, remains unanswered.

What foods attract or repel one consumer or another during pregnancy is not universal. Common dietary aversions exhibited during pregnancy in American and European women reveal rejection of alcohol, coffee or tea, the avoidance of some meat and vegetable items, sometimes onions and strong-smelling foods such as broccoli and cabbage, as well as spicy dishes and "greasy-fried" foods. Foods high or low in protein, vitamins, or minerals are not specifically sought or rejected.[84,85]

DIETARY MANAGEMENT

Once pregnancy is confirmed, many Western-trained physicians advise women to maintain regular activities, exercise, eat a balanced diet, take a vitamin-mineral supplement, and enjoy their condition. Such advice, however, is not universally accepted. Mineral supplements frequently are rejected by some women who believe that difficult pregnancies and hard labors would follow. Indeed, millions of Americans practice age-old traditions of humoral balance during pregnancy and postpartum periods, practices that originated between two and three thousand years ago in three regions of the ancient world: the Mediterranean basin, India, and China.[86]

HUMORAL MEDICAL PRACTICES

Within the classical non-Western humoral systems, good health and physiologic conditions such as pregnancy and lactation are perceived as balances between physical elements and body humors. Whether in the ancient Mediterranean, Indian, or Chinese systems, available foods and disease conditions are assigned temperature and moisture qualities or attributes.[87] Usually, foods and diseases are categorized as hot or cold, wet or dry; hot illness is treated by consuming cold foods and a wet disease is treated by dry foods. Ambient temperature is not the basis for temperature designations. In simplest form, Mediterranean medicine takes two dimensions, usually temperature and moisture, although the Chinese system, expresses other dimensions of gender, light, and time.[88]

Within the Chinese hot-cold system, pregnancy is considered a "hot" condition, and diet management is based on intake of "cold" foods, items commonly high in water content and low in caloric density and protein.[89] Chinese dietary management of pregnancy, not unexpectedly, results in smaller babies compared to Western weight values. Tradition holds that babies born of mothers following the system are delivered more easily.[90,91]

In the Chinese system, the postpartum period is one of intense "cold," one to be balanced by foods designated "hot." A review of "hot" foods appropriate during lactation show many are calorically dense and high in energy and protein. Dietary management at this time permits the mother to restore her strength and increase breast milk production.[92]

Within contemporary America, numerous ethnic groups practice hot-cold, humoral medicine. Representatives from Mediterranean lands influenced more than two thousand years ago by ancient Greek and Roman medicine and by Medieval Moslem and Jewish medicine include Arabs, Cypriots, Greeks, Israelis (Ashkhanazi and Sephardic Jews), Italians, Maltese, Portuguese, Spanish, and Turks. But any American ethnic group with historical roots to countries colonized by Spain and Portugal, whether in the Caribbean, Central and South America, Africa (Angola and Mozambique), mainland Asia (Goa and Macao), or the Philippines, may also practice the Mediterranean system of humoral medicine. Other American ethnic groups from the Indian subcontinent, those practitioners of humoral Ayurvedic medicine that evolved in ancient India perhaps 3500 years ago, also practice the hot-cold method. Other Asiatic ethnic groups in addition to Chinese-Americans influenced by the humoral hot-cold (Yang-Yin) systems of ancient China include Burmese, Cambodians, Laotians, Malay, Thai, and Vietnamese.[93]

Such ethnic Americans who seek medical or nutritional advice during pregnancy exhibit three categories of behavior. Some reject, categorically, the Western medical model based on germ theory and accept only hot-cold dietary management. Others reject hot-cold concepts and accept most Western-based medical and nutritional advice. The largest group of women, however, are syncritic and blend both medical systems. This group, perhaps more than the other two, present the most exciting, educational challenge to physician and nutrition educator. With care and understanding, Western physicians can offer sound medical and nutritional advice during pregnancy to their ethnic clients. This advice will be taken and followed, if the information is set within basic, easily understood principles of hot-cold.[94]

INCONSISTENT BEHAVIORS

Radio and television advertising, public announcements, and popular and scientific literature regularly provide nutrition education to pregnant women to avoid alcohol,[95] tobacco products,[96] and street-drugs.[97] Such warnings, while accepted and followed by most women, are ignored or rejected by others because of physiologic addiction, ignorance, or lack of confidence in "establishment" medicine and nutrition.

Use of toxic or teratogenic substances or foods during pregnancy occurs widely. What moral and legal issues, therefore, follow when drug addicts use heroin during pregnancy? Are such prospective mothers responsible for their addictions? If women understand relationships between substance abuse and fetal outcome, and the inconsistent behavior is maintained, is fetal abuse ultimately child abuse?[98,99]

What arguments logically follow when a woman refuses the medical-nutritional advice of her physicians to eat a balanced diet during pregnancy, chooses not to take vitamin-mineral supplements, eats poorly, drinks alcohol, and the delivered child does not exhibit fetal alcohol syndrome? Can the state represent such behavior during pregnancy as child abuse, without adverse fetal outcome?[100] Who, ultimately, should enforce legal precedents delineating maternal and fetal rights? Should a cadre of pregnancy police be formed?[101] Should the same moral, ethical condemnation of pregnant drug addicts be extended to other women accidentally exposed to toxic substances, or who unknowingly ingest teratogenic foods?[102]

The literature regarding inconsistent behavior during pregnancy differentiates deliberate from nonpurposeful actions. Numerous papers document food habit and cultural behavior during pregnancy beyond control of the pregnant woman, for example, consumption of mercury-labeled wheat sent to Iraq[103] and polybrominated biphenyls (PBB) and polychlorinated biphenyls (PCB) contamination of the human food supply in Wisconsin[104] and northern Canada.[105] In recent years, there has been radioactive contamination of meat, milk, and vegetables and increased risk to pregnant women by nuclear reactor accidents at Three Mile Island in Pennsylvania[106] and at Chernobyl in the Soviet Union.[107]

Beyond accidental exposure to teratogenic substances, what implications follow if educated women evaluate evidence, then carefully practice a regimen during pregnancy that in fact produces nutritional or teratogenic effects? Are fetal and child rights violated in instances of religious cult practices, where the faith promotes dietary practices accepted by practitioners, but the practices are deemed medically and nutritionally unsound by scientists?[108] Because California law allows the arrest of parents for failure to provide food to their children, could these statutes be interpreted to include failure to provide food of the right type during fetal development?[109]

All humans take risks and practice inconsistent behavior. When risks are known, prospective outcome may be evaluated and weighed, and decisions are taken. But if nutrition risks are not anticipated, considered, or recognized, and cultural behavior leads to spontaneous abortion or delivery of malformed neonates, who is to blame? In one widely publicized California case, several women delivered children with severe deformities. Distraught families feared that environmental exposure to the herbicide 2,4-D was the cause. Investigative work by epidemiologists and toxicologists, however, revealed that several cultural factors linked these women: they raised goats, kept them unpenned to range and browse freely, and all the women had consumed fresh goat milk during the first trimester of pregnancy. Fresh goat milk was believed to be a "natural product," good for the developing fetus. Tragically, the unpenned goats had foraged on lupine (Lupinus latifolius), which contains anagyrine, a powerful teratogen.[110]

Uninformed or misguided consumers regularly practice "dietary roulette." Incautious consumption of "natural" food, items from "nature's bounty," sometimes pose risks during pregnancy. Herbal teas prepared from catnip (Nepta cataria) or mandrake (Mandragora officinarum) contain psychoactive agents,[111] and other teas brewed from devil's claw root (Harpagophytum procumbens) contain compounds that find regular use as abortifacients and should be avoided during pregnancy.[112] Teas prepared from comfrey (Symphytum officinale) have been contaminated with atropine,[113] whereas tea from sassafras (Sassafras spp.) consumed in inordinate quantity poses risk as a potential hepatocarcinogen.[114]

Patterns of behavior inconsistent with medical and nutritional principles are common in "new age" communities of highly educated, pregnant and/or lactating American women. In one study conducted in northern California, pregnant women abandoned use of commercial coffee and tea during pregnancy believing that caffeine compounds led to low-birth-weight babies. These same women then substituted herbal teas of unknown composition because they were "natural." One women in the same study stopped smoking tobacco cigarettes during pregnancy, but continued to smoke marijuana and explained her behavior as a "reasoned response" to alleviate nausea.[115]

DELIVERY AND CELEBRATION

Delivery of a baby in some societies is immediately accompanied by cultural traditions that favorably influence both mother and neonate. In many African societies, for example, a laying-in period may last 3 to 6 months. Recently delivered BaTlokwa mothers in the Republic of Botswana, for example, are tended by elderly female relatives beyond childbearing years whose duties are to prepare and serve all food and restrict visitors. The mothers are "fattened" at this time and family members willingly donate portions of their food to assist in this process. During the laying-in period, mothers are not permitted to eat with bare hands and are served by a female attendant. Restriction of visitors allows the mothers to rest and regain strength quickly, and reduces exposure to communicable diseases.[116]

In the United States today, the number of in-home births attended by midwives is increasing. Also present may be the father, other members of the immediate family, and close friends and neighbors. Also associated with this increase in home births are "birthing ceremonies" infrequently witnessed by practicing physicians. One such custom is placentophagia and eating the "meat of life." After the neonate has been delivered, shown, and displayed to all in attendance, the expelled placenta is carefully washed, cooked, and shared as a dietary treat among those attending. Placentophagia is explained by practitioners as a natural process, one with biologic, cultural, and religious functions. Biologically, the practice is widespread in mammals, so it is "natural" to do so. Eating is explained as a means to provide the new mother with her own lost nutrients so to gain strength more quickly. Culturally, the practice is seen as wonderfully human, a blend of folklore, mythology, and religion that stresses ethical behavior and the sanctity of life. The placenta is viewed as a tissue produced and ultimately eaten in love; it is a meat produced by life, not by animal slaughter. Culturally, the practice is bonding and links consumers to one another, thus forging a strong support network among those who have shared in the miracle of life. Religiously, sharing the "meat of life" is viewed as a eucharistic "first supper," a functional means of defining ethical-social identity. But stepping back from functional interpretations and taking a detached view, is not placentophagia a form of ritual cannibalism practiced today in twentieth century America?[117]

In conclusion, nutritional anthropology defined in this chapter and explored using the theme of pregnancy and delivery is a broad continuum linking the humanities with the physical sciences. Elsewhere, it has been described as a tapestry created by the threads of cultural nutrition.[118] Thus conceived, the field extends beyond anthropology and nutrition to encompass diverse researchers interested in a wide range of cultural, environmental, historical, and geographic connections between food, diet, and nutrition. Within this broad definition is place for all, whether one is interested in depiction of food on ancient and contemporary coins, or attracted to food terms used by Homer, Shakespeare, or modern writers. Welcomed, too, are those interested in human response to drought, how foods are shared within and between members of different societies, or how food selection may or may not affect athletic performance. Invited to participate are chemists, physicians, and physiologists interested in the biology of human starvation, and problems of re-feeding civilian populations during famine. Described in this chapter are important contributions by lawyers and politicians. The field has room too for technical engineers, astrophysicists, and physicians interested in the management of sound nutrition under conditions of extended human space flight. It is fitting to conclude this essay, still building on the theme of pregnancy and delivery, by considering what basic nutritional problems might be faced by women who conceive elsewhere, beyond earth:

Recall the biologic and engineering evidence for human fragility, recognizing that during weightlessness of spaceflight, calcium does not easily remain within bone matrix; recall the pioneering efforts of Klaus Schwarz and others who determined the essentiality of nutrients such as chromium, fluorine, selenium, silicon, and tin, using closed environmental chambers, akin to spaceships, and how laboratory animals fed purified diets, distilled water, and triple-filtered air languished in those chambers while their experimental counterparts flourished on purified diets, distilled water, and standard California urban smog;[119] recall the compound pyrroloquinoline quinone (PQQ) was determined essential to mammalian life only in 1989,[120] raising questions about the viability of prolonged spaceflight in closed environmental chambers. Because PQQ and related compounds appear widely on earth under normal conditions, and spaceflight is not a normal condition, can astronauts survive extended journeys to Mars or beyond? How will human diet be managed?

Are all essential nutrients known? In the centuries to come, will women be able to conceive and manage safe pregnancies with limited adverse fetal outcome? Nutritional anthropology, explored broadly in this chapter, may contribute solutions to these still-imagined medical-nutritional problems.

REFERENCES

1. Richards, A.I.: Hunger and Work in a Savage Tribe. A Functional Study of Nutrition among the Southern Bantu. London, Routledge, 1932.
2. Richards, A.I.: Land, Labor and Diet in Northern Rhodesia. An Economic Study of the Bemba Tribe. Oxford, Oxford University Press, 1939.
3. Matovinovic, J.: Annu. Rev. Nutr., *3*:341–412, 1983.
4. Dorson, R.M.: Peasant Customs and Savage Myths. Vol. 1., pp. 223–224. Chicago, University of Chicago Press, 1968.
5. Regenstein, J.M., Regenstein C.E.: Food Tech., *33*:89–99, 1979.
6. Singer, P.: Philosophy and Public Affairs, *1*:229–243, 1972.
7. Stumpf, S.E.: Annu. Rev. Nutr., *1*:1–15, 1981.
8. Sen, A.K.: Food Entitlements and Economic Chains. *In* Science, Ethics, and Food. Papers and Proceedings of a Colloquium Organized by the Smithsonian Institution. Edited by B.W.J. LeMay. Washington, D.C., Smithsonian Institution Press, 1988., pp. 58–70.
9. Simoons, F.J.: Mod. Probl. Pediatr., *15*:125–141, 1974.
10. Dando, W.A.: The Geography of Famine. New York, Wiley, 1980.
11. Grivetti, L.E., Pangborn, R.M.: J. Am. Diet. Assoc., *65*:634–638, 1974.
12. Grivetti, L.E.: Ecol. Food Nutr., *7*:235–256, 1979.
13. Vincent, B.: Ann. Econ. Soc. Civ., *30*:445–453, 1975.
14. Voorsanger, J.: Western States Jewish Hist. Quart., *8*:243–250, 1976.
15. Pilichowski, C.: Studia Historiae Oeconomicae, *17*:205–215, 1982.
16. Rozin, P., Vollmecke, T.A.: Annu. Rev. Nutr., *6*:433–456, 1986.
17. Blundell, J.E., Hill, A.J.: Int. J. Obes., *3*:141–155, 1987.
18. Kingsnorth, R., Jungsten, M.: Crime and Delinquency, *34*:3–27, 1988.
19. Roth, J.A.: Health Purifiers and Their Enemies. New York, Prodist, 1977.
20. Bungton, T., Breton, M.: Women Health, *16*:43–62, 1990.
21. The Committee For the Compilation of Materials on Damage Caused by the Atomic Bombs in Hiroshima and Nagasaki. *In* Hiroshima and Nagasaki. The Physical, Medical, and Social Effects of the Atomic Bombings. Translated by E. Ishikawa, D.L. Swain. New York, Basic Books, 1981, pp. 270–271.
22. Gale, R.P.: JAMA, *258*:625–628, 1987.
23. Irvine, F.R.: Br. J. Herpt., *1*:183–189, 1954.
24. Ruff, T.A.: Lancet, *1*:201–205, 1989.
25. Sims, J.K., Ostman, D.C.: Ann. Emerg. Med., *15*:1094–1098, 1986.
26. Van Duzen, J., Carter, J.P., Secondi, J., et al.: Am. J. Clin. Nutr., *22*:1362–1370, 1969.
27. Black, R.E., Lopez de Romana, G., Brown, K.H., et al.: Am. J. Epidemiol., *129*:785–799, 1989.
28. Hickson Jr., J.F., Johnson, T.E., Lee, W., et al.: J. Am. Diet. Assoc., *90*:264–267, 1990.
29. Weight, L.M., Myburgh, K.H., Noakes, T.D.: Am. J. Clin. Nutr., *47*:192–195, 1988.
30. Bodenheimer, F.S.: Insects as Human Food. The Hague, W. Junk, 1951.
31. Taylor, R.L.: Butterflies in My Stomach. Or: Insects in Human Nutrition. Santa Barbara, California, Woodbridge Press, 1975.
32. Twaigery, S., Spillman, D.: Food Tech., *43*:88–90, 1989.
33. Elias, P.S.: Food Tech., *43*:81–83, 1989.
34. Linnan, M.J., Masoda, L., Lou, X.D., et al.: N. Engl. J. Med., *319*:823–828, 1988.

35. Penhanich, M.: Dairy Foods, *88:*64–68, 1987.
36. Mermelstein, N.H.: Food Tech., *44:*86–91, 1990.
37. Hutt, P.B.: Food Tech., *43:*288–295, 1989.
38. Weber, J.A.: Brooklyn J. Int. Law, *15:*369–397, 1989.
39. Thompson, E.L.: Indiana Law J., *64:*357–374, 1989.
40. Duncan, A.D.: North Carolina Law Rev., *18:*67–86, 1989.
41. Derr, P.G.: Issues in Law and Med., *2:*25—38, 1986.
42. O'Conner, A., Johnson-Sabine, E.: Med. Sci. Law, *28:*62–64, 1988.
43. Hardyman, D.: Glendale Law Rev., *3:*311–321, 1978.
44. Grivetti, L.E.: Annu. Rev. Nutr., *1:*47–68, 1981.
45. Grivetti, L.E.: pangborn, R.M.: J.Nutr. Ed., *5:*204-207, 1973.
46. Jelliffe, D.B.: The Assessment of the Nutritional Status of the Community. Geneva, World Health Association, 1966.
47. Jelliffe, D., Jelliffe, P., Naylor, A., et al.: J. Hum. Lact., *5:*68–73, 1989.
48. Krantzler, N.J., Mullen, B.J., Comstock, E.M., et al.: J. Nutr. Ed., *14:*108–119, 1982.
49. Naroll, R., Cohyen, R.: A Handbook of Method in Cultural Anthropology. new York, Columbia University Press, 1970.
50. Quandt, S.A., Ritenbaugh, C.: Training Manual in Nutritional Anthropology. Washington, D.C., American Anthropological Association, 1986.
51. Pelto, G.H., Pelto, P.J., Messer, E.: Research Methods in Nutritional Anthropology. Food and Nutrition Bulletin Supplement, Number 11. Tokyo, United Nations University, 1989.
52. Fitzgerald, T.K.: Nutrition and Anthropology in Action. Amsterdam, Van Gorcum, 1977.
53. Jerome, N.W., Kandel, R.F., Pelto, G.H.: Nutritional Anthropology. Contemporary Approaches to Diet and Culture. Pleasantville, NY, Redgrave, 1980.
54. Farb, P., Armelagos, G.: Consuming Passions. The Anthropology of Eating, Boston, Houghton-Mifflin, 1980.
55. Fieldhouse, P.: Food and Nutrition, Customs and Culture. London, Croom Helm, 1986.
56. Johnston, F.E.: Nutritional Anthropology. New York, Alan R. Liss, 1987.
57. Harris, M., Ross, E.B.: Food and Evolution. Toward a Theory of Human Food Habits. Philadelkphia, Temple University Press, 1987.
58. Haas, J.D., Harrison, G.G.: Annu. Rev. Anthropol., *6:*69–101, 1977.
59. Grivetti, L.E.: Biosci. Rep., *28:*171–177, 1978.
60. Messer, E.: Annu. Rev. Anthropol., *13:*205–249, 1984.
61. Wilson, C.S.: J. Nutr. Ed., *5(Suppl.):*39–72, 1973.
62. Wilson, C.S.: J. Nutr. Ed. *11(Suppl.):*210–264, 1979.
63. Freedman, R.L.: Human Food Uses. A Cross-Cultural, Comprehensive Annotated Bibliography. London, Greenwood, 1981.
64. Freedman, R.L.: Human Food Uses. A Cross-Cultural, Comprehensive Annotated Bibliography. Supplement. London, Green, 1983.
65. Annas, G.J., Elias, S.: Clin. Obstet. Gynecol., *32:*614–621, 1989.
66. Robertson, J.A.: Case Western Reserve Law Rev., *39:*1–38, 1988.
67. Hand, W.D., Casseta, A., Thiederman, S.B.: Popular Beliefs and Superstitions. A Compendium of American Folklore. Vol. 1. Boston, G.K. Hall, 1981.
68. Zelnik, M., Kantner, J.F.: Fam. Plann. Perspect., *11:*289–296, 1979.
69. Lane, E.W.: Manners and Customs of the Modern Egyptians. London, Alexander Gardner, 1895, pp. 69–70.
70. Darby, W.J., Ghalioungui, P., Grivetti, L.: Food. The Gift of Osiris. Vol. 1. London, Academic Press, 1977, p. 333.
71. Blackman, W.S.: The Fellahin of Upper Egypt. London, George G. Harrap, 1927.
72. Wrezinski, W.: *In* Der grosse medizinische Papyrus des Berliner Museums (pap. Berlin 3038) mit Uebersetzung, Kommentar and Glossar. Leipzig, Hinrichs, 1909, folio page 199.
73. Ghalioungui, P., Khalil, S., Ammar, A.R.: Med. Hist., *7:*241–246, 1963.
74. Cooper, M.: Pica. Springfield, IL, Charles C Thomas, 1957.
75. Loveland, C.J., Furst, T.H., Lauritzen, G.C.: Food Foodways, *3:*333–356, 1989.
76. Keith, L., Evenhouse, H., Webster, A.: Obstet. Gynecol., *32:*415–418, 1968.
77. Coltman, C.A.: JAMA, *207:*513–516, 1969.
78. Danford, D.E.: Annu. Rev. Nutr., *2:*303–322, 1982.
79. Halsted, J.A.: Am. J. Clin. Nutr., *21:*1384–1393, 1968.
80. Vermeer, D.E., Frate, D.A.: Am. J. Clin. Nutr., *32:*2129–2135, 1979.
81. Richter, C.P.: J. Compar. Physiol. Psychol., *40:*129–141, 1947.
82. Harris, L.J., Clay, J., Hargreaves, J., et al.: Proc. R. Soc., SEries B., *113:*161–190, 1933.
83. Dickens, G., Trethowan, W.H.: J. Psychiatr. Res., *15:*259–268, 1971.
84. Hook, E.B.: Am. J. Clin. Nutr., *31:*1355–1362, 1978.
85. Finley, D.A., Dewey, K.G., Lonnerdal, B., et al.: J. Am. Diet. Assoc., *85:*678–685, 1985.
86. Logan, M.: med. Anthropol. newsletter, *6:*8–14, 1975.
87. Wilson, C.S.: Nutrition in Two Cultures. Mexican-American and Malay Ways with Food. *In* Gastronomy. The Anthropology of Food and Food Habits. Edited by M. Arnott. The Hague, Mouton, 1975, pp. 131–144.
88. Manderson, L.: Soc. Sci. Med., *25:*329–330, 1987.
89. Andersen Jr., E.N.: Soc. Sci. Med., *25:*331–337, 1987.
90. Veith, I.: Huang Ti Nei Ching Su Wen. The Yellow Emperor's Classic of Internal Medicine. Baltimore, Williams & Wilkins, 1949.
91. Anderson, Jr., E.N., Anderson, M.L.: Modern China: South. *In* Food in Chinese Culture. Anthropological and Historical Perspectives. Edited by K.C. Chang. London, Yale University Press, 1977, pp. 317–382.
92. Pillsbury, B.L.K.: Soc. Sci. Med., *12:*11–22, 1978.
93. Grivetti, L.E.: Nutrition and Health. Historical Perspectives on Non-Scientific Nutrition. *In* Proceedings, Fourth Ethel Austin Martin Visiting Professorship in Human Nutrition at South Dakota State University. Edited by J.W. Howard. Brookings, South Dakota, Human Nutrition Fund Committee, South Dakota University, 1985, pp. 111–129.
94. Grivetti, L.E.: Nutrition Today. January/February, pp. 13–24, 1991.
95. Waterson, E.J., Murray-Lyon, I.M.: Soc. Sci. Med., *30:*349–364, 1990.
96. Aaronson, L.S., Macnee, C.L.: J. Obstet. Gynecol. Neonatal Nurs., *18:*279–287, 1989.
97. Briggs, G.G., Freeman, R.K., Yaffee, S.J.: Drugs in Pregnancy and Lactation. A Reference Guide to Fetal and Neonatal Risk. 2nd Ed. Baltimore, Williams & Wilkins, 1986.
98. Roberts, I.F., West, R.J., Ogilvie, D., et al.: BMJ, *1:*296–298, 1979.
99. Shain, R.N.: Clin. Obstet. Gynecol., *13:*1–17, 1986.
100. Burton IV, C.R.: Willamette Law Rev., *25:*223–242, 1989.

101. McNutty, M.: N. Y. Univ. Rev. Law Soc. Change, *16:*277–319, 1988.
102. Pettinger, G., Duggan, M.B., Forrest, A.R.: Med. Sci. Law, *28:*310–311, 1988.
103. Marsh, D.O., Myers, G.J., Clarkson, T.W., et al.: Ann. Neurol., *7:*348–353, 1980.
104. Senn, C.L.: The Firemaster Incident. *In* Adverse Effects of Foods. Edited by E.F.P. Jelliffe and D.B. Jelliffe. New York, Plenum, 1982, pp. 129–134.
105. Kinloch, D., Kuhnlein, H.: Arctic Med. Res., *47:*159–162, 1988.
106. Upton, A.C.: Impact of the Three Mile Island Accident. *In* The Three Mile Island Nuclear Accident. Lessons and Implications. Edited by T.H. Moss, D.L. Sills. Vol. 365. New York, New York Academy of Sciences, 1981, pp. 63–75.
107. Guskova, A.K., Barabanova, A.V., Baranov, A.Y., et al.: Acute Radiation Effects in Victims of the Chernobyl Nuclear Power Plant Accident. *In* Sources, Effects and Risks of Ionizing Radiation. United Nations Scientific Committee on the Effects of Atomic Radiation. Report to the General Assembly with Annexes. New York, United Nations, 1988, pp. 613–647.
108. Robson, J.R.K., Konlande, J.E., Larkin, F.A., et al.: Pediatrics, *53:*326–329, 1974.
109. Food. *In* West's California [Law] Digest 2D. Volume 46. Descriptive-Word Index F-O. St. Paul, West Publishing, 1982, pp. 62–63.
110. Kilgore, W.W., Crosby, D.G., Craigmill, A.L., et al.: Calif. Ag., *35*(Nov.-Dec.):6, 1981.
111. Siegel, R.K.: JAMA, *236:*473–476, 1976.
112. Abramowicz, M.: Med. Lett. Drugs Ther., *21:*29–31, 1979.
113. Routledge, P.A., Spriggs, T.L.B.: Lancet, *1:*963–964, 1989.
114. Tyler, V.E.: The Honest Herbal. A Sensible Guide to the Use of Herbs and Related Remedies. Philadelphia, George F. Stickley, 1981.
115. Finley, D-A.C.: Breast Milk and Diet Composition of Vegetarian and Non-Vegetarian Lactating Women. Ph.D. Dissertation, Department of Nutrition, University of California, Davis, 1985.
116. Grivetti, L.E.: Am. J. Clin. Nutr., *31:*1204–1220, 1978.
117. Janszen, K.: Sci. Digest, Nov-Dec., pp. 78–81, 122, 1980.
118. Grivetti, L.E., Lamprecht, S.J., Rocke, H.J., et al.: Prog. Food Nutr. Sci., *11:*249–306, 1987.
119. Schwarz, L.: New Essential Trace Elements (Sn, V,F,Si): Progress Report and Outlook. *In* Trace Element Metabolism in Animals–2. Edited by W.G. Hoekstra, J.W. Suttie, H.E. Ganther, et al. Baltimore, University Park Press, 1974, pp. 355–380.
120. Killgore, J., Smidt, C., Duich, L., et al.: Science, *245:*850–852, 1989.

SELECTED READINGS:

Freedman, R.L.: Human Food Uses. A Cross-Cultural, Comprehensive Annotated Bibliography. London, Greenwood, 1981.
Freedman, R.L.: Human Food Uses. A Cross-Cultural, Comprehensive Annotated Bibliography. Supplement. London, Greenwood 1983.
Grivetti, L.E.: Cultural Nutrition. Anthropological and Geographical Themes. Annu. Rev. Nutr., *1:*47–68, 1981.
Grivetti, L.E., Lamprecht, S.J., Rocke, H.J., et al.: Threads of Cultural Nutrition. Arts and Humanities. Prog. Food Nutr. Sci., *11:*249–306, 1987.
Johnston, F.E.: Nutritional Anthropology. New York, Alan R. Liss, 1987.
Wilson, C.S.: Food — Custom and Nurture. An Annotated Bibliography on Sociocultural and Biocultural Aspects of Nutrition. J. Nutr. Ed., *11(Suppl.):*210–264, 1979.

CHAPTER **86**

Fads, Frauds, and Quackery

Stephen Barrett and Victor Herbert

Food faddism can be defined as an unusual pattern of food behavior enthusiastically adopted by its adherents.[1] It is commonly expressed by: (1) beliefs that particular foods or food substances can cure diseases; (2) elimination of certain foods from the diet; and/or (3) emphasis on "natural" foods.

Quackery can be defined as the promotion for profit of a medical scheme or remedy that is unproven or known to be false. This definition seeks to distinguish folk practices and neighborly advice from practices done for financial gain. "Health fraud" has been defined in a similar way. However, because most people regard "fraud" as a deliberate attempt to deceive, "health fraud" is most appropriate when deliberate deception is involved.

Quack methods are sometimes referred to as "alternatives." Because ineffective methods are not true alternatives to effective ones, the terms "unscientific" or "dubious" are preferable.

Faddists and quacks urge everyone to distrust large food companies, government regulators, and scientific health professionals. This negative philosophy is essential because without it, consumers would have no reason to buy health food industry products or to consult "alternative" practitioners.

VULNERABILITY TO QUACKERY

Victims of quackery usually have one or more of the following characteristics.

1. They are not suspicious enough. Many people believe that if something appears in print or in a broadcast, it must be true, or somehow it would not be allowed. People also tend to believe what others tell them about personal experience.
2. They believe in magic. Some people are easily taken in by the promise of an easy solution to their problem. Those who buy one fad diet book after another fall into this category.
3. They are desperate. Many people faced with a serious health problem that doctors cannot solve become desperate enough to try almost anything that arouses hope. Many victims of cancer, arthritis, multiple sclerosis, and acquired immunodeficiency syndrome (AIDS) are vulnerable in this regard.
4. They are alienated. Some people feel deeply antagonistic toward scientific medicine but are attracted to methods that are "natural" or otherwise unorthodox. They may also harbor extreme distrust of the medical profession, the food industry, drug companies, and government agencies.

MISLEADING CLAIMS

Nutrition faddism and quackery are promoted with the following four basic fallacies. (1) *Our food supply is nutritionally inadequate because our soils are depleted and important nutrients are removed by food processing.* These claims encourage the purchase of "organic," "natural," and "health" foods. (2) *Most health problems result from faulty diet and can be treated with "nutritional" methods.* These types of claims are used to market hundreds of "food supplements," "health foods," and quack dietary methods. (3) *Americans are in danger of being poisoned by food additives and pesticide residues.* This claim is used to promote the sale of "organic" and "natural" foods. (4)

Personal experience is the best way to tell whether something is effective. This claim encourages people to disregard scientific studies and rely on testimonial evidence.

CLAIMS FOR FOODS

Many foods are promoted with slogans suggesting that they are safer, are more nutritious, or have special therapeutic value. "Organically grown" foods are said to be foods grown without the use of "artificial" fertilizers or pesticides. The foods themselves usually are indistinguishable from "ordinary" foods but they cost more. Studies comparing "organically grown" and conventionally grown foods have found that their pesticide content is similar.[2] Food and Drug Administration (FDA) market basket studies indicate that pesticide residues are insignificant in the overall diet.[3] Nutrients are absorbed by the plant in their inorganic chemical state regardless of whether the soil has been prepared with manure, compost, or manufactured fertilizer. Plants grow only if they receive enough nutrients, and their vitamin content is determined by their genes. Fertilizers can influence the mineral composition of plants, but these variations are rarely significant in the overall diet. Despite these facts, several states have established standards for organic food "certification," and a federal law calling for national standards has been passed. The industry has gained considerable political support by affiliating with "alternative agriculture," and loosely defined movement focused on protecting soil quality and the environment.[4]

The word "natural" is said by its proponents to represent foods that are minimally processed and contain no artificial additives or preservatives. This definition implies that these substances pose a health risk. Actually, they help make our food supply safe, abundant, and palatable. Although an additive is occasionally found to pose a health hazard (sulfites, for example), the vast majority appear safe, and the overall level in our food supply should not be a cause for concern or a reason to buy "natural" foods.

Although the term "health food" cannot actually be defined, it is used to suggest that certain foods have special health-giving properties not found in "ordinary" foods. Some "health" foods are rich in various nutrients and can be a valuable part of a balanced diet. But no food has any special health-promoting property beyond those of the nutrients it contains.

Recent scientific developments and lax FDA enforcement have inspired many food companies to make false or exaggerated claims that their products have special value in preventing various diseases. In 1991, the FDA proposed to permit messages on product labels regarding: (1) calcium and osteoporosis; (2) sodium and high blood pressure; (3) dietary fats and heart disease; and (4) dietary fats and cancer. The proposal would permit claims that are truthful and not misleading. The claims must be limited to the relationship between these conditions and a particular food component, rather than the specific product. The recommendation must also be consistent with sound total diet.[5] It remains to be seen how effectively this program will be developed and enforced. (See also Chapter 94.)

PROMOTION OF SUPPLEMENTS

Americans waste several billion dollars a year on worthless or unnecessary "dietary supplements." These products are promoted with scare tactics and false promises. The most common sales pitch is "nutrition insurance," the idea that everyone needs vitamin and mineral supplements to be sure of getting enough. Some promoters suggest that it is difficult to achieve a balanced diet; others insist that our food supply is inadequate.

Another common ploy is the suggestion that supplementation is advisable to help deal with "stress." This idea was commercialized by distorting a 1952 National Academy of Sciences Report. The report noted that people who lose their appetite because of serious illness might benefit from supplementation to prevent depletion of water-soluble vitamins, which have limited storage. However, in 1976, a major vitamin manufacturer began falsely advertising that "stress robs the body of vitamins" and that water-soluble vitamins must be replaced daily because the body cannot store them. Other manufacturers embellished further by suggesting that extra vitamins are needed to cope with emotional stress, the stress of a busy lifestyle, or life's other stressful events. Some manufacturers made no claims for their "stress" products but assumed that consumers would know what they are for.

In the mid-1980s, the New York State Attorney General secured consent agreements with two major "stress supplement" manufacturers to stop misrepresenting the need for their products. Since that time, there has been much less direct advertising of "stress supplements." However, the Council for Responsible Nutrition (CRN), a trade organization that represents major supplement manufacturers and suppliers, has advertised that a busy lifestyle places Americans at nutritional risk. The advertisement included a narrowly worded "Vitamin Gap Test," which suggested that virtually everyone may have one or more "gaps." At a hearing held by the National Advertising Review Board, CRN representatives maintained that everyone needs supplements. In 1990, the Federal Trade Commission secured a consent agreement barring another large manufacturer from making unsubstantiated claims that any vitamin product is needed to replace nutrients lost as a result of athletic activities or "the stress of daily living."

Some manufacturers advertise that β-carotene or other antioxidants are being studied as cancer preventives, implying that supplements may be beneficial. This claim is misleading, because it has never been demonstrated that Americans fail to get adequate amounts of these nutrients from foods. Several manufacturers falsely suggest that being active and elderly creates special needs for which their products are supposedly designed.

During the past few years, many health food industry manufacturers have developed "ergogenic aids"—amino acid supplements falsely claimed to increase stamina, endurance, and muscle development. Some of these products are claimed to be "natural steroids" that release growth hormone. No scientific evidence exists that these products actually release growth hormone, which is fortunate, because acromegaly might result if they did.

ADVICE FROM RETAILERS

Health Foods Business estimates that in 1991, there were about 7300 health food stores in the United States with total sales of 3.9 billion dollars.[6] Several large studies have found that the proprietors of these stores often give advice that is irrational, unsafe, and illegal:

- In 1983, investigators from the American Council on Science and Health made 105 inquiries at stores in New York, New Jersey, and Connecticut. Asked about eye symptoms characteristic of glaucoma, 17 of 24 suggested a wide variety of products for a person not seen; none recognized that urgent medical care was needed. Asked over the telephone about sudden, unexplained 15-pound weight loss over 1 month, 9 of 17 recommended products sold in their store; only 7 suggested medical evaluation. Seven of 10 stores carried "starch blockers" despite an FDA ban. Nine stores contacted made false claims of effectiveness for bee pollen, and 10 stores did so for RNA.[7]
- In 1987, a registered dietitian posed five similar questions to 10 health food store proprietors in eastern Pennsylvania and concluded that only 23 of 50 (46%) were correct.[8]
- In 1989, volunteers of the Consumer Health Education Council telephoned 41 Houston-area health food stores and asked to speak with the person who provided nutritional advice. The callers explained that they had a brother with AIDS who was seeking an effective alternative against human immunodeficiency virus (HIV). The caller also explained that the brother's wife was still having sex with her husband and wanted to reduce her risk of being infected, or make it impossible. All 41 retailers offered products they said could benefit the brother's immune system, improve the woman's immunity, and protect her against harm from the HIV virus. Thirty said they sold products that would cure AIDS. None recommended abstinence or use of a condom.[9]

Several dozen companies market supplements through person-to-person (multilevel) sales. Virtually anyone can become a distributor by filling out a one-page application and buying a distributor kit for less than $50. Most multilevel companies claim their products can prevent or cure a wide range of diseases. A few companies merely suggest that people will feel better, look better, or have more energy if they use supplements.

Although pharmacists receive scientific training in nutrition, a study by *Consumer Reports* magazine has cast considerable doubt on the ability of community pharmacists to give appropriate advice about supplements. When 30 pharmacists were asked by undercover reporters whether vitamins could relieve their nervousness or fatigue, 17 recommended vitamins, one recommended L-tryptophan, and only 9 mentioned the possibility of seeing a doctor.[10]

Actually, few supplement products have any usefulness against disease, and most that do, such as niacin for cholesterol control, should never be taken without competent medical supervision.

UNSCIENTIFIC PRACTICES

Many practitioners use nutritional methods inconsistent with current scientific knowledge. Their approaches include dubious tests, fad diagnoses, unproven nutritional remedies, and fad diets. Many of these practitioners make inappropriate diagnoses of food allergies, hypoglycemia, hypothyroidism, and chronic fatigue syndrome. Some label their approach holistic, complementary, or nutritional medicine.

Many companies market supplement concoctions to chiropractors with claims that they are suitable for treating almost anything. The claims, which would not be legal on product labels, do not appear on the labels. Rather, they are made in literature distributed by mail or provided at seminars in which use of the products is described. Although this marketing strategy is illegal, government agencies have done little to counter it.

DUBIOUS TESTS

Unscientific practitioners use a variety of tests as a basis for prescribing supplements and/or making dietary recommendations. The most common of these tests is hair analysis, which is purported to detect mineral imbalances or the presence of toxic minerals. The test usually is obtained by sending a small amount of hair from the nape of the neck to a commercial laboratory for analysis. The laboratory then issues a computerized report suggesting what supplements might be prescribed.

When 52 hair samples from two healthy teenagers were sent under assumed names to 13 commercial hair analysis laboratories, the reported levels of minerals varied considerably between identical samples sent to the same laboratory and from one laboratory to another. The laboratories also disagreed about what was normal or usual for many of the minerals. Literature from most of the laboratories suggested falsely that their reports were useful against a wide variety of diseases and supposed nutrient imbalances.[11] Properly performed, hair analysis has limited value as a research tool, but little if any clinical application.[12]

Nutrient deficiency tests are sometimes used by nutrition quacks to help them decide what their customers need. One type involves completion of a dietary history; another involves completion of a questionnaire about common symptoms that supposedly are signs of deficiency. The answers are then fed into a computer programmed to recommend supplements for everyone.

Some practitioners use data from legitimate laboratory tests but misrepresent their meaning. The SMAC-24, which measures 24 different chemical characteristics of the blood, is a valuable screening test in scientific medical practice. But dubious practitioners misuse the test by narrowing the normal ranges so that healthy individuals appear to have abnormalities, which are then used to recommend expensive supplements or special diets.

Iridology is based on the idea that each area of the body is represented by a corresponding area in the iris (pupil) of the eye. Practitioners claim to diagnose nutritional imbalances that can be treated with vitamins, minerals, herbs, and similar products. In a scientific test, three iridologists showed no statistically significant ability to detect which patients had kidney disease and which did not.[13]

Live-cell analysis is performed by examining a drop of blood under a dark-field microscope to which a television monitor has been attached. Both practitioner and patient can then see blood cells and debris, which appear as dark bodies outlined in white. Proponents claim that the procedure is useful in diagnosing vitamin and mineral deficiencies, tendencies toward allergic reactions, liver weakness, and many other health problems that are treatable with food supplements. Although videomicroscopy is a legitimate technique, live-cell analysis is useless in diagnosing most of the conditions its practitioners claim to treat.[14]

"Provocation" and "neutralization" are performed by having the patient report symptoms that occur within 10 minutes after suspected substances are administered under the tongue or injected into the skin. If any symptoms occur, the test is considered positive and lower concentrations are given until a dose is found that "neutralizes" the symptoms.

Researchers at the University of California have demonstrated that these procedures are not valid.[15] In a double-blind study, 18 patients each received three injections of suspected food extracts and nine of normal saline over 3 hours. The tests were carried out in the offices of proponents who had been treating them. In unblinded tests, these patients had consistently reported symptoms when exposed to food extracts and no symptoms when given saline injections. But during the experiment, they reported as many symptoms after saline injections as they did after food extract injections, indicating that their symptoms were nothing more than placebo reactions. "Neutralizing" doses were equally effective whether they were food extracts or saline. The symptoms included nasal stuffiness, dry mouth, nausea, fatigue, headaches and/or feelings of disorientation or depression.

PSEUDOSCIENTIFIC APPROACHES

Clinical ecology, also called "environmental medicine," is practiced by several hundred physicians. It is based on the notion that hypersensitivity to tiny amounts of common foods and chemicals can trigger a wide range of symptoms—a condition they call "environmental illness." Their principal diagnostic procedure is provocation-neutralization, but elimination diets and isolation in special "environmentally safe" facilities are also used. Their usual treatment involves elimination of exposure to foods and environmental substances to which they consider the patient hypersensitive.

Similar numbers of physicians practice "orthomolecular therapy" (sometimes referred to as megavitamin therapy), which is based on the idea that most ailments respond to correct doses of nutrients. This approach began in the 1950s when a few psychiatrists began using large doses of niacin to treat severe mental problems. Later, the treatment regimen was expanded to include other vitamins, minerals, hormones, and diets, any of which may be combined with standard drug therapy and/or electroshock treatments. In 1973, an American Psychiatric Association task force report noted that megavitamin proponents used unconventional methods not only in treatment, but also in diagnosis. The report concluded that, "the credibility of the megavitamin proponents is low," and "is further diminished by a consistent refusal over the past decade to perform controlled experiments and to report their new results in a scientifically acceptable fashion."[16]

Applied kinesiology is based on the notion that every organ dysfunction is accompanied by a specific muscle weakness, which enables diseases to be diagnosed through muscle-testing procedures. Its practitioners, most of whom are chiropractors, also claim that nutritional deficiencies, allergies, and other adverse reactions to food substances can be detected by placing substances in the mouth so that the patient salivates. "Good" substances make specific muscles stronger, whereas "bad" substances cause specific weaknesses. "Treatment" then consists of expensive vitamin supplements or a special diet. Double-blind studies have found no difference between the results with test substances and with placebos.[17]

Macrobiotics is a quasi-religious philosophic system that advocates a vegetarian diet in which animal foods are used as condiments rather than full-fledged menu items. The optimal diet is said to be achieved by balancing "yin" and "yang" foods. The yin/yang classification does not correspond to nutrient composition but to activity characteristics of the universe as defined by

Oriental philosophy. Macrobiotic theory claims that improper diet and inadequate elimination of waste result in constitutional or metabolic contamination and cause cancer, and that cure results from righting the balance and cleansing the body with special vegetarian diets, appropriate spiritual attitudes, and other measures. These notions often lead to radical dietary changes that can compromise nutrient adequacy in patients whose nutritional status is already precarious.[18]

Naturopathy is a system of healing that is said to rely on "nature." Naturopaths purport to "identify and relieve the underlying cause of illness rather than to eliminate or merely suppress symptoms." Naturopaths believe that virtually all diseases are within the scope of their practice. Their methods include fasting, "natural food" diets, vitamins, herbs, homeopathic remedies, tissue minerals, spinal manipulation, massage, remedial exercise, colonic enemas, and the use of natural forces such as rest, heat, cold, air, and sunlight.

Natural Hygiene is a philosophy of health and natural living that denounces most medical treatment and advocates eating a raw food diet of vegetables, fruits, and nuts. It also advocates periodic fasting and food combining (avoiding food combinations it considers detrimental).[19]

"FAD" DIAGNOSES

Years ago, many nervous or tired people were said to have adrenal insufficiency, a serious glandular disorder that is rare. The vast majority of these people were not only misdiagnosed but also were treated with adrenal gland extract, a substance they did not need and that is potentially harmful. Today, a diagnosis of hypoglycemia (low blood sugar) is sometimes used to explain certain symptoms of neurotic nervousness or fatigue. True believers in hypoglycemia are apt to diagnose it in many of their patients. The diagnosis should be reserved for patients who develop symptoms 2 to 4 hours after eating, have blood glucose levels below 45 mg per 100 ml whenever symptoms occur, and are immediately relieved of symptoms when blood sugar levels are increased.

The glucose tolerance test is not reliable for evaluating most cases of suspected hypoglycemia.[20] Low blood sugar levels without symptoms occur commonly in normal individuals fed large amounts of sugar and are of no diagnostic significance. The only way to diagnose hypoglycemia reliably is to prove that blood sugar is low whenever symptoms occur during the patient's usual living pattern. The most practical way to do this assessment is with a home testing device.

"Candidiasis hypersensitivity," another fad diagnosis, is based on the notion that multiple common symptoms are caused by allergy to the common yeast Candida albicans and can be treated with vitamins, antifungal drugs, and special diets that "starve" the yeast. The American Academy of Allergy and Immunology regards the concept of "candidiasis hypersensitivity" as "speculative and unproven." In a double-blind trial, the antifungal drug nystatin did no better than a placebo in relieving systemic or psychologic symptoms of "candidiasis hypersensitivity syndrome."[21]

"Mercury-amalgam toxicity" is diagnosed by a small number of dentists who claim that the mercury in silver-mercury fillings is toxic and causes a wide range of illnesses. These dentists recommend replacement of these fillings with other materials, which can cost thousands of dollars. Some recommend an elaborate program of supplements to minimize negative effects claimed to occur when the mercury-containing fillings are removed. The American Dental Association considers it unethical to remove amalgam fillings "for the alleged purpose of removing toxic substances."

DUBIOUS CREDENTIALS

During the past decade, several individuals and groups have developed credentials intended to resemble those of established medical and nutritional organizations. During this period, unaccredited correspondence schools and other organizations have issued a steady stream of degrees and other certificates intended to suggest that the recipient is a qualified expert in nutrition. The schools typically issue bachelor of science, master of science, and/or doctor of philosophy "degrees" based on study of unscientific writings plus open-book tests that are scored liberally. The professional organizations typically grant immediate professional memberships and a fancy certificate for a modest fee. Household pets and nonexistent individuals have achieved membership in several of these groups.

Bogus nutritionists typically use hair analysis to diagnose "imbalances" and computerized questionnaires to diagnose "deficiencies." The American Dietetic Association is striving for government regulation of nutritionists and has gained passage of laws in about one half of the states.

OBESITY QUACKERY

Many weight-reduction schemes are promoted to the public as a solution to obesity. Fad diet books typically have several things in common. They claim to offer a revolutionary new idea based on the author's personal experience. They suggest that certain nutrients, foods, or food combinations are either the key to weight reduction or villains that prevent it. And they contain inaccurate information about biochemistry. Many fad diets are unbalanced and lack important nutrients. During the past two decades, many best-selling diet plans have emphasized proteins, some recommending unlimited amounts and others using small amounts. Food-combining schemes also have been popular. *Fit for Life,* which sold over 3 million copies, claims that obesity caused the accumulation of "toxic waste" from incomplete assimilation of foods eaten in the wrong combinations.

Many people who use fad diets achieve rapid weight loss. However, most regain the lost weight, and sometimes more, when they resume normal eating.

Mail-order diet pills typically are "guaranteed" to produce effortless, rapid, and permanent weight loss. Dozens of such pills are offered each year through direct mail solicitations and newspaper advertising. Some of these, as well as others sold over-the-counter, contain phenylpropanolamine (PPA), a nasal decongestant that can have a temporary effect on appetite. However, no evidence proves that PPA offers any long-term benefit for weight control, and several young adults have suffered a stroke after using it.

Other mail-order pills supposedly block the absorption of starch, fat, or calories; flush fat out of the body; or step up the body's "fat-burning system." Some contain a fiber, such as glucomannan or guar gum, that is claimed to curb appetite by absorbing water and swelling to fill the stomach. However, the amount of fiber is too small to actually fill the stomach, and even if it could, that would not necessarily curb a person's appetite. In 1990, guar gum was banned as a diet aid after the FDA received 17 reports of individuals whose esophagus became blocked as a result of using tablets of "Cal-Ban 3000," a widely promoted guar gum product.[22]

Spirulina, a dark-green powder or pill derived from algae, is said by its promoters to suppress appetite. However, no scientific evidence supports this claim.

Products containing Gymnema sylvestre are being touted as weight-control aids with claims that they block the absorption of sugar. The leaves of this plant, when chewed, can prevent the taste sensation of sweetness, but no evidence exists that Gymnema sylvestre blocks absorption of sugar into the body.

DANGERS OF QUACKERY

The harm of quackery can be classified as economic, indirect, direct, psychologic, and societal.[23] Economic damage can range from a few dollars a year for "nutrition insurance" to many thousands of dollars wasted on quack cures for serious disease. Because everyone must eat, the potential market for nutrition quackery is immense. Indirect harm occurs when the use of an ineffective approach diverts someone from effective care. Direct harm occurs when a dubious method causes death, serious injury, and unnecessary suffering. Psychologic harm arises when individuals blame themselves for the failure of an ineffective remedy or when they reach the mistaken conclusion that they have been helped and become more vulnerable to future deception. Quackery can also harm our democratic society when large numbers of people hold erroneous beliefs about the nature of disease and the best way to deal with it. Limited resources can be wasted if funds are used to follow leads based on data that are inadequate or faked.

From 1986 to 1989, the American Dietetic Association collected case reports of people harmed by inappropriate nutrition advice from bogus nutritionists, health food store operators, and others. More than 500 such cases were documented.

The recent tryptophan tragedy illustrates how inappropriate use of supplements can lead to disaster. In 1989, an L-tryptophan product was implicated in an outbreak of eosinophilia-myalgia syndrome, a previously rare disorder characterized by severe muscle and joint pain, weakness, swelling of the arms and legs, fever, and skin rash. This amino acid had been promoted by the health food industry to treat insomnia, depression, premenstrual syndrome, and overweight, although it had not been proven safe and effective for these purposes. More than 1500 cases were reported, with 27 deaths and more than 100 hospitalizations.[24]

CONSUMER PROTECTION

Three federal agencies have responsibility for fighting quackery. The Postal Service has jurisdiction over products sold through the mail with false claims. When a scheme is detected, the Postal Service can use an administrative procedure to block transfer of money and orders through the mail. The Postal Service has a vigorous enforcement program but is hampered by loopholes in its law.

The Federal Trade Commission (FTC) has jurisdiction over the advertising of nonprescription products and services. It files complaints and negotiates settlements, going to court when necessary. It has a powerful law but insufficient manpower to act against the majority of violations it encounters.

The United States FDA has jurisdiction over the labeling of foods and drugs. Under federal law, any product "intended for use in the cure, mitigation, treatment or prevention of disease" is a drug. If a product is marketed with drug claims that lack FDA approval, the agency can issue a warning letter, initiate a seizure, obtain an injunction, and/or seek criminal penalties. The claim does not have to be on the product label itself. Any claim traceable to the manufacturer is considered part of the label. The FDA has a powerful law but has not always used it effectively.

Several state attorneys general have been active in combating quackery, but their actions may not stop promoters from continuing their schemes out of state. State and federal laws pertaining to quackery need strengthening.[25]

The primary antiquackery force in the United States is the National Council Against Health Fraud, Inc., a nonprofit organization of health and nutrition professionals, educators, researchers, attorneys, and other concerned citizens wishing to actively oppose misinformation, fraud, and quackery in the health marketplace. Information about the Council and its publications can be obtained by writing to P.O. Box 1276, Loma Linda, CA 92354.

REFERENCES

1. Schafer, R., Yetley, E.A.: J. Am. Diet. Assoc., *66:*129–133, 1975.
2. Institute of Food Technologists Expert Panel on Food Safety and Nutrition. Food Tech., *44:*123–130, 1990.
3. Food and Drug Administration Pesticide Program. Residues in foods—1989. Rockville, MD, Food and Drug Administration, 1990.
4. Pesek, J. et al.: Alternative Agriculture. Washington D.C., National Academy Press, 1989.
5. Federal Register, *56:*60366–60878, 1991.
6. Anon.: Health Foods Business, *38:*25–40, 1992.
7. Stookey, H.E., Miller, B., Meister, K. ACSH News & Views, *4:*1, 8–9, 13–14, 1983.
8. Aigner, C.: Nutr. Forum, *5:*1–3, 1988.
9. Martin, N.: Nutr. Forum, *7:*16, 1990.
10. Consumer Reports, *51:*170–175, 1986.
11. Barrett, S.: JAMA, *254:*1041–1045, 1985.
12. Hambidge, K.M.: Am. J. Clin. Nutr., *36:*943–949, 1982.
13. Simon, A., Worthen, D.M., Mitas, J.A.: JAMA, *242:*1385–1389, 1979.
14. Lowell, J.: Nutr. Forum, *3:*81–85, 1987.
15. Jewett, D.L., Fein, G., Greenberg, M.H.: N. Engl. J. Med., *323:*429–433, 1990.
16. Lipton, M., et al.: Task Force Report on Megavitamin and Orthomolecular Therapy in Psychiatry. Washington, D.C., American Psychiatric Association, 1973.
17. Kenny, J.J., Clemens, R., Forsythe, K.D.: J. Am. Dietetic Assoc., *88:*698–704, 1988.
18. Dwyer, J.: Nutr. Forum, *7:*9–11, 1990.
19. Raso, J.: Nutr. Forum, *7:*33–36, 1990.
20. Benion, L.J.: Hypoglycemia, Fact or Fad? New York, Crown Publishers, 1983.
21. Dismukes, W.E., Wade, S., Lee, J.Y., et al.: N. Engl. J. Med., *323:*1717–1723, 1990.
22. Barrett, S.: Nutrition Today, *25:*24–28, 1990.
23. Jarvis, W.: How quackery harms. *In* Dubious Cancer Treatment. Edited by S. Barrett, B.R. Cassileth. Tampa, American Cancer Society, Florida Division, 1991.
24. Swyert, L.A., Maes, E.F., Sewell, L.E., et al.: JAMA, *264:*1698–1703, 1990.
25. Barrett, S.: Priorities, Fall 1990, pp. 35–36.

SELECTED READINGS

Barrett, S., and the editors of Consumer Reports: Health Schemes, Scams, and Frauds. New York, Consumer Reports Books, 1990.

Barrett, S., Cassileth, B.R. (eds.): Dubious Cancer Treatment. Tampa, American Cancer Society, Florida Division, 1991.

Fried, J.J.: Vitamin Politics. Buffalo, Prometheus Books, 1984.

Herbert, V., Barrett, S.: Vitamins and "Health" Foods: The Great American Hustle. Philadelphia, George F. Stickley, 1981.

Herbert, V., Suback-Sharpe, G.J., Hammock, D.A. (eds.): The Mount Sinai School of Medicine Complete Book of Nutrition. New York, St. Martin's Press, 1990.

Yetiv, J.: Popular Nutritional Practices: Sense and Nonsense. New York, Dell Publishing, 1988.

CHAPTER **87**

Cardiovascular Disease

Donald J. McNamara

CARDIOVASCULAR DISEASE

It is estimated that 67 million Americans, one out of every four, have some form of cardiovascular disease (CVD). In 1987, CVD accounted for nearly 1 million deaths in the United States, almost one half of the total deaths, with 18% of these deaths occurring in patients under 65 years of age. The estimated cost of CVD in the United States is $94.5 billion for 1990. Although the numbers are of epidemic proportions, the age-adjusted death rates between 1977 and 1987 from all forms of CVD declined 23.3% (coronary heart disease [CHD] down 28.7%, stroke down 36.6%). The extent of CVD morbidity and mortality in the population clearly makes it a major public health concern, and extensive epidemiologic and clinical research efforts have resulted in the identification of a number of life-style and genetic risk factors for CVD. Major risk factors such as genetic predisposition, gender, and advanced age are not modifiable by intervention, whereas the life-style risk factors that include cigarette smoking, hypertension, elevated plasma cholesterol levels, excessive body weight, diabetes mellitus, and long-term physical inactivity can be modified by intervention.

Federal and private public health agencies have recommended that Americans have their plasma cholesterol levels and blood pressure measured and institute dietary modifications to reduce their risk for CVD.[1–4] The recommended approaches to reduce CVD mortality and morbidity involve a combined strategy of interventions directed at high-risk patients coupled with a general-population community approach to reduce the overall population risk of CVD. This two-phase approach attempts to address a basic paradox in the public health approach to disease prevention. Whereas concentrating on high-risk individuals may confer large benefit to them, the overall benefit to the population may be small, whereas the community-based approach provides a relatively small risk reduction for the individual while the population as a whole achieves a large theoretic benefit. A patient at high risk for CVD certainly should receive aggressive intervention to reduce their overall risk profile. If a patient does have hypercholesterolemia, then a fat-modified diet should be prescribed in an attempt to reduce the high plasma cholesterol level, and the primary emphasis should be on lowering the atherogenic low-density lipoprotein (LDL) cholesterol concentration. The rationale and approaches to dietary intervention in the hyperlipidemic patient are addressed in a separate chapter in this volume. The focus of this chapter is on the role of population-based dietary interventions directed at CVD prevention as related to blood cholesterol levels, with particular attention to aspects of efficacy in lowering plasma cholesterol levels and CVD risk and applicability to special populations.

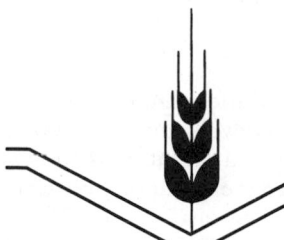

Numerous reviews of the role of dietary factors in the etiology and prevention of hypercholesterolemia and CVD risk have been published,[1–6] and these reviews provide extensive listings of primary references for the interested reader. The primary goal of this chapter is to evaluate the evidence regarding the efficacy of recommended dietary changes in lowering plasma cholesterol levels; the benefits of such changes in terms of lowering CVD morbidity and mortality; and the potential consequences of institution of the recommended dietary changes with respect to the population as a whole.

PLASMA CHOLESTEROL LEVELS AND CORONARY HEART DISEASE RISK

The National Cholesterol Education Program (NCEP) defined categories of coronary heart disease (CHD) risk according to three levels of plasma total cholesterol and, if available, levels of plasma LDL cholesterol (Table 87–1). On the basis of currently available data, approximately one half the population has cholesterol levels within the desirable range, one fourth in the borderline-high range, and one fourth can be classified at high CHD risk. The NCEP Adult Treatment Panel recommended that dietary interventions were appropriate for the high-risk group and for the borderline-high patient if an individual had two or more additional risk factors.[3] The recommendations include two stages of dietary intervention (Table 87–2), with implementation of the step 2 diet for high-risk individuals who do not lower their cholesterol levels below 6.2 mmol/L (240 mg/dl) on the step 1 diet. After publication of the recommendations of the Adult Treatment Panel, the NCEP Population-Based Panel put forth the recommendation that everyone, irrespective of plasma cholesterol levels, initiate dietary changes to reduce dietary fat, saturated fat, and cholesterol and follow the recommended step 1 dietary pattern.

The bases of these recommendations[1–4] come from epidemiologic and metabolic studies that demonstrated that certain dietary factors have significant influences on plasma cholesterol levels and, potentially, on CVD risk. Studies carried out under controlled metabolic ward conditions indicate that the major dietary determinants of plasma cholesterol levels are percent of calories from saturated and polyunsaturated fatty acids and the amount of dietary cholesterol. The quantitative impact of these dietary factors on plasma cholesterol levels can be estimated from the equations developed by Keys and Hegsted (Table 87–3). By using these equations as guidelines, it is possible to estimate the effects of the proposed dietary modifications on plasma cholesterol levels, which can be used to calculate potential changes in CHD risk and mortality. More recent data show that many other dietary factors also affect plasma lipid levels to varying degrees, and these other dietary variables also should be considered in evaluating the efficacy of dietary modifications for reducing CHD morbidity and mortality.

TABLE 87–1. NCEP ADULT TREATMENT PANEL CLASSIFICATION OF CHD RISK

CLASSIFICATION	TOTAL CHOLESTEROL mmol/L	TOTAL CHOLESTEROL mg/dl	LDL CHOLESTEROL mmol/L	LDL CHOLESTEROL mg/dl
Desirable	<5.17	<200	<3.36	<130
Borderline high	5.17–6.18	200–239	3.36–4.11	130–159
High	≥6.19	≥240	≥4.12	≥160

(Adapted from Report of the National Cholesterol Education Program Expert Panel on Detection, Evaluation, and Treatment of High Blood Cholesterol in Adults. Arch. Intern. Med., *148:*36–69, 1988.)

TABLE 87–2. NCEP DIETARY RECOMMENDATIONS

NUTRIENT	CURRENT INTAKE*	RECOMMENDED INTAKE Step 1		RECOMMENDED INTAKE Step 2
Total fat (%)	37%	<30%		<30%
Saturated	13%	<10%		< 7%
Monounsaturated	14%		10–15%	
Polyunsaturated	7%		≤10%	
Carbohydrate	46%		50–60%	
Protein	16%		10–20%	
Cholesterol (mg/day)	370	<300		<200
Calories		To achieve/maintain desirable weight		

*As percentage of total ingested calories.

(Adapted from Report of the National Cholesterol Education Program Expert Panel on Detection, Evaluation, and Treatment of High Blood Cholesterol in Adults. Arch. Intern. Med., *148:*36–69, 1988.)

TABLE 87–3. EQUATIONS TO ESTIMATE CHANGES IN PLASMA CHOLESTEROL LEVELS RESULTING FROM MODIFICATIONS IN DIETARY FAT AND CHOLESTEROL

Keys equation: $\Delta Chol = 1.35\ (2\Delta S - \Delta P) + 1.5\Delta Z$
Hegsted equation:
$\Delta Chol = 2.16\Delta S - 1.65\Delta P + 0.097\Delta C$
in which ΔS and ΔP are the changes in percentage of calories from saturated (S) and polyunsaturated (P) fat, ΔZ is the difference between the square root of the initial and subsequent intake of cholesterol (mg/1000 kcal), and ΔC is the difference in cholesterol intake (mg/1000 kcal).

(Adapted from National Research Council Committee on Diet and Health: Diet and Health; Implications for Reducing Chronic Disease Risk. Washington, D.C., National Academcy Press, 1989.)

IMPACT OF DIETARY FACTORS ON PLASMA LIPIDS

DIETARY FAT

SATURATED FAT

A consistent finding of epidemiologic and clinical studies is that plasma cholesterol levels are positively correlated with the percentage of saturated fat calories in the diet. As shown in Figure 87–1, epidemiologic studies demonstrate a significant interpopulation relationship between the percentage of saturated fat calories and CHD mortality. What is of interest in evaluating these data is that 13 of the 18 countries average between 13 and 15% of total calories from saturated fat yet exhibit over a fourfold range of CHD mortality. It is also important to recognize that the correlation coefficient between CHD mortality and percentage of calories from saturated fat decreases from 0.713 to 0.559 if Italy and Japan, the countries with the lowest saturated fat intake, are deleted from consideration. Thus, although a statistically significant international correlation exists between saturated fat calories and CHD mortality, most countries exhibit a relatively narrow range of saturated fat intake while exhibiting a wide range of CHD death rates.

Metabolic ward studies indicate that the average change in plasma cholesterol levels is 0.06 mmol/L (2 mg/dl) for every 1% change in saturated fat calories (see Table 87–3). On the basis of this estimate, decreasing saturated fat intake from 13 to 10% of calories would result in an average decrease of 0.19 mmol/L (7 mg/dl) in plasma total cholesterol levels. Saturated fat calories represent the single most prominent dietary determinant of plasma cholesterol levels for most individuals, and most individuals experience some degree of plasma cholesterol lowering by decreasing saturated fat intake. Recent studies have shown, however, that the plasma cholesterol response to changes in saturated fat intake are highly variable and that some individuals do not experience such a decrease.[8]

Although the effects of saturated fat intake on plasma cholesterol levels have been studied extensively, recent investigations have demonstrated that not all saturated fat in the diet raises blood cholesterol levels. In metabolic ward studies, using well-defined diets, intake of stearic acid (18:0), as compared to palmitic acid (16:0), did not increase plasma cholesterol levels, and actually resulted in a decrease.[9] Considering the dietary saturated fats consumed in a typical diet, the evidence from clinical studies indicates only three saturated fatty acids appear to elevate plasma cholesterol levels; lauric acid (12:0), myristic acid (14:0), and palmitic acid (16:0), which together constitute approximately 26% of the total dietary fat consumed. The finding that intake of stearic acid does not increase plasma cholesterol levels suggests that recommending that patients reduce intake of hydrogenated vegetable oils derived from oils rich in oleic and linoleic acids is not justified because the major saturated fat generated is stearic acid.

POLYUNSATURATED FAT

In contrast to the effects of dietary saturated fat on plasma cholesterol levels, studies have shown that plasma total cholesterol levels fall as the percentage of calories from polyunsaturated fat increase. Results of epidemiologic studies suggest that as the percentage of calories from polyunsaturated fats increase, CHD mortality decreases,[7] but this relationship is not statistically significant ($r=-0.342$, $P>0.05$). On the basis of findings from metabolic ward studies, it has been estimated that for every 1% increase in polyunsaturated fat calories, plasma cholesterol levels are lowered an average of 0.04 mmol/L (1.5 mg/dl) for most individuals (see Table 87–3). A population-based change in polyunsaturated fat intake from 7 to 10% of calories would therefore be predicted to result in a 0.12 mmol/L (5 mg/dl) decrease in the mean plasma cholesterol level.

A great deal of research has been directed toward the effects of ω-3 fatty acids on plasma lipids and the potential role these long-chain highly unsaturated fats might have on modifying CVD risk.[10,11] Intake of ω-3 fatty acids can reduce platelet aggregation and monocyte adherence, increase erythrocyte deformability, alter prostaglandin synthesis, lower blood pressure, and modify plasma lipids.[11] Intake of these fatty acids can lower elevated plasma triglyceride levels, but under most conditions, moderate intake has little effect on plasma LDL cholesterol concentrations. Some evidence suggests that intake of fish, as part of a normal diet, may reduce CHD mortality,[12] whether this effect is related to changes in thrombosis and platelet aggregation; the plasma lipoprotein profile, either directly or the result of replacement of high saturated fat foods in the diet; or by some combination of these multiple effects on the process of atherogenesis remains uncertain. What is clear is that both the beneficial effects and the potential

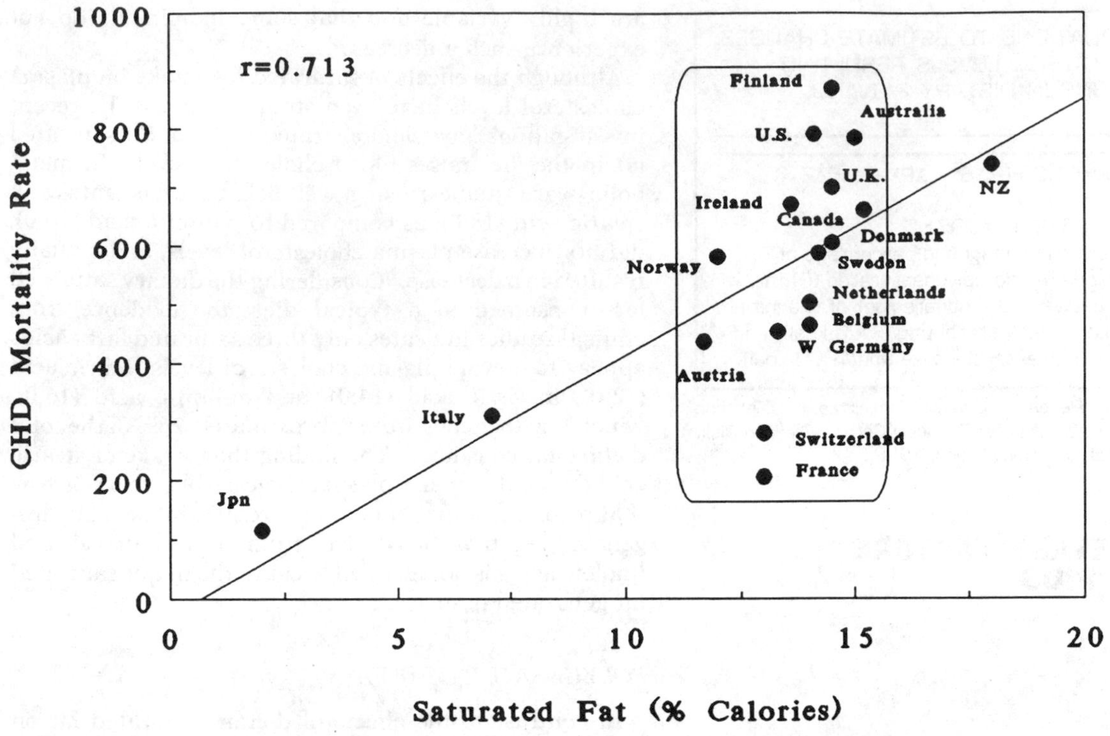

FIGURE 87–1. Relationship between the percentage of calories from saturated fatty acids and coronary heart disease (CHD) mortality. Epidemiologic studies have demonstrated a significant positive correlation between the percentage of calories from saturated fatty acids and the rate of CHD mortality ($P<0.001$). (Redrawn from Hegsted, D.M., Ausman, L.M.: J. Nutr., *118*:1184–1189, 1988.)

harmful effects of ω-3 fatty acid intake need to be determined and, until such time as these are clearly defined, it seems reasonable to encourage people to consume fish in the diet, but not to consume concentrated ω-3 fatty acids in an attempt to modify CHD risk.

MONOUNSATURATED FAT

Results of early metabolic ward studies suggested that intake of monounsaturated fat had no effect on plasma cholesterol levels; however, more recent findings demonstrated that substitution of saturated fat in the diet with monounsaturated fat does have a plasma cholesterol-lowering effect.[13] These observations are consistent with epidemiologic data that indicate that intake of monounsaturated fatty acids is negatively correlated with CHD mortality and with total mortality.[14] The interest in monounsaturated fatty acids as a substitute for saturated fat in the diet results in part from its common usage in Mediterranean countries, which have a low rate of CHD, and the fact that intake of monounsaturated fatty acids does have certain advantages, in terms of the plasma lipoprotein profile, over polyunsaturated fat and may in fact be a better substitute. As discussed in detail subsequently, the observed hypocholesterolemic effect of monounsaturated fatty acids raises questions regarding the need for dietary interventions to require significant reduction in total fat intake versus substitution of saturated fat with monounsaturated fat.[13]

TOTAL FAT

A common misperception is that any reduction in total fat intake has beneficial effects by lowering plasma cholesterol levels. The available data indicate that the key to reducing total and LDL cholesterol levels is to lower saturated fat intake, primarily myristic and palmitic acids; little LDL cholesterol-lowering benefit is achieved by reducing unsaturated fatty acid intake as a means to reduce total fat intake to very low levels. Too often, the advice to reduce total fat intake results in significant reductions in visible fat intake, often the major source of unsaturated dietary fat, and saturated fat remains as the predominant fat in the low-fat diet. Reductions of total fat from 37% to less than 30% of total calories, while keeping the ratio of polyunsaturated to saturated fat constant, or often even lower than found in the current diet, have little if any effect on plasma LDL cholesterol levels and may in fact result in a reduction in levels of the antiatherogenic high-density lipoprotein (HDL).

DIETARY CHOLESTEROL

Despite much media concern regarding dietary cholesterol intake and its role in high blood cholesterol levels, dietary cholesterol has a minimal effect on plasma cholesterol levels for most individuals.[15] The average change in plasma cholesterol levels is 0.06 mmol/L (2.2 mg/dl) for every 100-mg change in the daily dietary cholesterol intake. It would thus be predicted that a decrease in dietary cholesterol intake from 385 to 300 mg per day would result in a 0.05 mmol/L (2 mg/dl) decrease in the average plasma cholesterol level, a 1% decrease in the population average. Analysis of the available data reveals no interactive effect between the amount of dietary cholesterol and the type or amount of fat in the diet.[15]

Although the average change in plasma cholesterol levels in response to changes in dietary cholesterol are small, evidence is substantial for a large degree of heterogeneity of responses to dietary cholesterol within the population.[15] The results from numerous studies indicate that the response of most individuals to an increase in dietary cholesterol intake is to reduce endogenous cholesterol synthesis, which under physiologic conditions, can maintain constant plasma cholesterol levels (dietary cholesterol compensators); however, some individuals lack this feedback response and, when challenged with a high-cholesterol diet, experience a significant increase in plasma cholesterol concentrations (noncompensators). Results from various studies indicate that approximately two thirds of the population have sufficiently precise regulatory responses to compensate effectively for changes in dietary cholesterol intake whereas one third lack this feedback response.[15] As discussed subsequently, the apoprotein E phenotypic pattern exhibited by an individual is associated with noncompensation in response to dietary cholesterol.

DIETARY CARBOHYDRATES

Replacement of fat calories with complex carbohydrates has a number of effects on plasma lipids, including (1) an increase of plasma triglyceride concentrations; (2) a fall in HDL cholesterol levels, and (3) minimal change in LDL cholesterol.[13,16] Findings of metabolic studies indicate that a shift from fat to carbohydrate calories results in an increased plasma very low-density lipoprotein (VLDL) concentration, because of an increase in VLDL synthesis and reduced turnover, and lower plasma HDL levels resulting from an increased turnover of HDL apoprotein A-1.[5] The reported changes in the plasma lipoprotein profile resulting from decreasing fat and increasing carbohydrates have prompted some investigators to question the rationale of recommending that everyone adhere to a low-fat, high-carbohydrate diet as a means to reduce CHD risk.[13,17,18] A moderate-fat diet, rich in monounsaturated fat, may be a more suitable diet for lowering the atherogenic LDL while maintaining levels of the protective HDL cholesterol.[13] Whether a low-fat diet, or possibly a moderate-fat diet, represents the most acceptable and effective dietary intervention to reduce plasma LDL cholesterol levels and CHD risk needs further study and evaluation. Ample evidence is available that the low-fat, low-cholesterol diet now recommended to the public is not the only effective plasma cholesterol-lowering diet, and some studies suggest that a moderate-fat diet may be more effective in altering the overall plasma lipoprotein profile toward a less atherogenic pattern. Clearly, the population benefits from having more than one plasma cholesterol-lowering diet available to address problems of compliance failure and lack of a blood cholesterol-lowering response.

DIETARY FIBER

One benefit of decreasing dietary saturated fat and increasing complex carbohydrates is that this change results in an increased intake of dietary fiber, which can contribute to plasma cholesterol lowering. The water-soluble fiber fractions lower plasma cholesterol levels in humans and the associated increased intake of fiber in a low-saturated fat diet augments the cholesterol-lowering benefits of a low-fat diet. It should be noted, however, that significant lowering of plasma cholesterol levels in response to fiber intake requires intakes of 15 to 30 g per day; such levels of intake are not obtained easily by intake of the popular high-fiber cereals or fiber supplements in the market place. Although dietary fiber can lower plasma cholesterol levels, the amount of fiber intake required is significant. The most reasonable approach is to recommend intake of fiber-rich foods but not fiber supplementation.[2]

ALCOHOL

A considerable amount of interest has focused on the relationship between alcohol consumption and CHD risk based on the observations that intra- and interpopulation epidemiologic data indicate that CHD incidence and mortality are decreased by moderate alcohol intake.[7] Analysis of epidemiologic data indicate that the three most significant dietary determinants of CHD mortality are percentage of calories from saturated and polyunsaturated fats and alcohol intake. The mechanism by which moderate alcohol intake lowers CHD incidence is unclear and, whereas it may relate to alcohol-mediated increases in plasma HDL levels, the available data do not delineate the mechanisms involved. Two important points to consider regarding alcohol intake and CHD risk are that alcohol intake can raise plasma triglyceride levels in patients who exhibit carbohydrate-induced hypertriglyceridemia, and that alcohol consumption has been linked to hypertension in some patients. Considering the many health-related problems attributed to overconsumption of alcohol, it is not advisable to make any recommendations at this time regarding alcohol intake and CHD risk. However, if a patient consumes alcohol in moderation and is not hypertensive or hypertriglyceridemic, little reason exists to recommend abstinence for this individual.

CALORIC INTAKE AND BODY WEIGHT

The question of whether obesity is an independent risk factor for CHD is more theoretic than practical, because obesity is related to a number of well-documented CHD risk factors: hypertension, hypercholesterolemia, hypertriglyceridemia, glucose intolerance, low plasma HDL levels, and a sedentary life style. In addition, data from various epidemiologic studies indicate that obesity itself is a risk factor independent of its associated metabolic effects.[19] Every 1 kg/m^2 increase in the body mass index is associated with a corresponding increase in the total plasma cholesterol of 0.20 mmol/L (7.7 mg/dl) and a 0.02 mmol/L (0.8 mg/dl) decrease in the level of HDL cholesterol.[20] Metabolic studies have documented that obesity results in an increased rate of endogenous cholesterol synthesis, 20 mg per day for every kilogram of excess body weight, and increased VLDL apoprotein B and triacylglycerol production rates.[5] From a quantitative perspective, it can be estimated that an individual 10 kg overweight will produce an additional 200 mg of cholesterol every day, and this cholesterol directly enters the body's pool of cholesterol; in comparison, reducing dietary cholesterol intake from 385 to 300 mg per day reduces the amount of absorbed cholesterol (assuming an average 60% absorption) by only 45 mg per day. For the overweight patient, reducing excess body weight has a more significant quantitative impact on the mass of cholesterol the body must transport, metabolize, and excrete daily than can be achieved by reducing dietary cholesterol intake.

Evidence is growing that the distribution of body fat is itself a significant determinant of CHD risk. Central fat mass distribution characteristic of upper trunk android obesity contributes to a more atherogenic plasma lipoprotein profile and increased risk for CHD.[21] On the basis of accumulated data, it is clear that obesity increases plasma lipid levels, alters endogenous cholesterol and lipoprotein metabolism, and contributes to CHD risk.

Obesity may well be one of the most prevalent diet-related health problems in the United States, affecting 26% of adult males and 29% of adult females, about 34 million adults ages 20 to 74 years.[1] It is essential that any population-based approach to CHD prevention must address the importance of maintaining an ideal body weight as a major risk reduction tool. Although one argument is that a low-fat diet results in weight loss for many individuals, maximal efficacy of any dietary intervention to reduce CHD risk cannot depend solely on changes in caloric distribution of the diet to facilitate weight maintenance; it also must involve a decrease in total calories not only from fat but also from all sources when treating the overweight patient.

EFFICACY OF DIETARY INTERVENTIONS

Using the Keys and Hegsted equations, it is possible to predict the extent of plasma cholesterol lowering that could be achieved when the current dietary pattern is changed to the recommended NCEP step 1 diet. The proposed changes in the type and amount of dietary fat and in dietary cholesterol intake would be predicted to result in an average 0.36 mmol/L (14 mg/dl) decrease in plasma total cholesterol levels, equivalent to a reduction in the mean plasma cholesterol of 6.7%. The plasma cholesterol reduction is attributable primarily to the decrease in saturated fat calories (52% of change) coupled with the increased intake of polyunsaturated fat (33%) and a small decrease resulting from the reduction in dietary cholesterol (17%). Various predictions have been made as to the potential reduction in CHD mortality that might be achieved from such a reduction in plasma cholesterol levels. The most widely quoted estimate is that every 1% reduction in plasma cholesterol levels is associated with a predicted 2% reduction in CHD mortality.[22] Because this approximation was derived from intervention studies primarily in hypercholesterolemic high-risk male populations, the question of whether similar benefits will be gained by individuals with average plasma cholesterol levels must be addressed.

The current population distribution of plasma cholesterol levels in 40- to 49-year-old American men,[23] and the theoretic distribution after dietary intervention and a 0.36 mmol/L (14 mg/dl) reduction in plasma cholesterol levels, are shown in Figure 87–2. Also presented in Figure 87–2 is the age-adjusted risk of CHD mortality (6-year mortality rate per 1000).[24] When the data are analyzed to determine the relative reduction in CHD mortality from initiation of the dietary recommendations, the 6-year mortality rate decreases from 59.3 to 50.8 per 10,000 treated subjects; this finding equates to a saving of 8.5 lives over 6 years per 10,000 individuals treated. The composite data indicate that the average 6.7% reduction in plasma cholesterol levels (0.36 mmol/L, 14 mg/dl) should result in a 14.3% reduction in CHD mortality. The theoretic data are consistent with findings of intervention studies that indicate that a 2% reduction in CHD mortality is achieved for every 1% reduction in plasma cholesterol.[22] If the mortality data are evaluated within specific risk groups as defined by the NCEP guidelines,[3] the result of treatment of the 52% of the population with cholesterol levels in borderline-high and high-risk groups accounts for 92.9% (decrease of 6-year mortality rate by 7.9 deaths per 10,000) of the reduction in total CHD mortality for the entire group; 3.2 deaths in the high-risk group and 4.7 deaths in the borderline-high group (Fig. 87–3). The effects of the dietary intervention in 48% of the population classified as having an average risk are relatively modest (7.1%), because this group has a relatively small risk to begin with and intervention results in a decrease in the 6-year mortality rate of 0.6 lives.

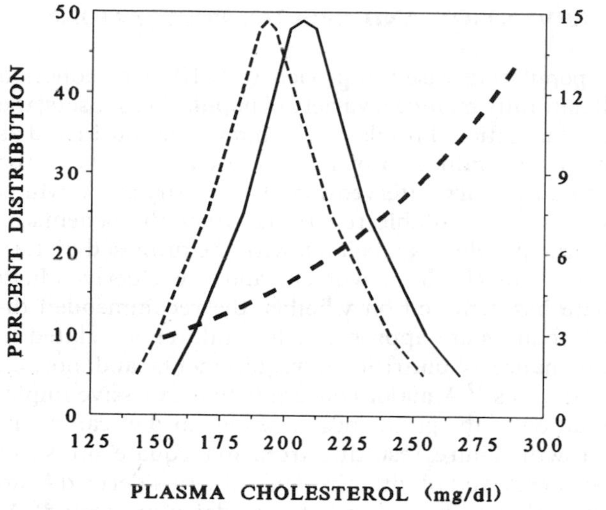

FIGURE 87–2. Population distribution of plasma cholesterol levels in men aged 40 to 49 years. This figure illustrates the present distribution of plasma total cholesterol levels in a middle-aged male population (solid line) and the theoretic distribution following a 14-mg/dl (0.36 mmol/L) reduction in plasma cholesterol after institution of the recommended diet (short dashed line). (Current distribution derived from data provided in the Lipid Research Clinics Population Studies Data Book. Vol. 1: The Prevalence Study. NIH Publication No. 80–1527. Washington, D.C., U.S. Department of Health and Human Services, 1980; also shown in this figure is the 6-year coronary heart disease (CHD) mortality data per 1000 (long dashed line) as reported from the Multiple Risk Factor Intervention Trial (MRFIT) in Stamler, J., Wentworth, D., Neaton, J.D.: JAMA, *256*:2823–2828, 1986.)

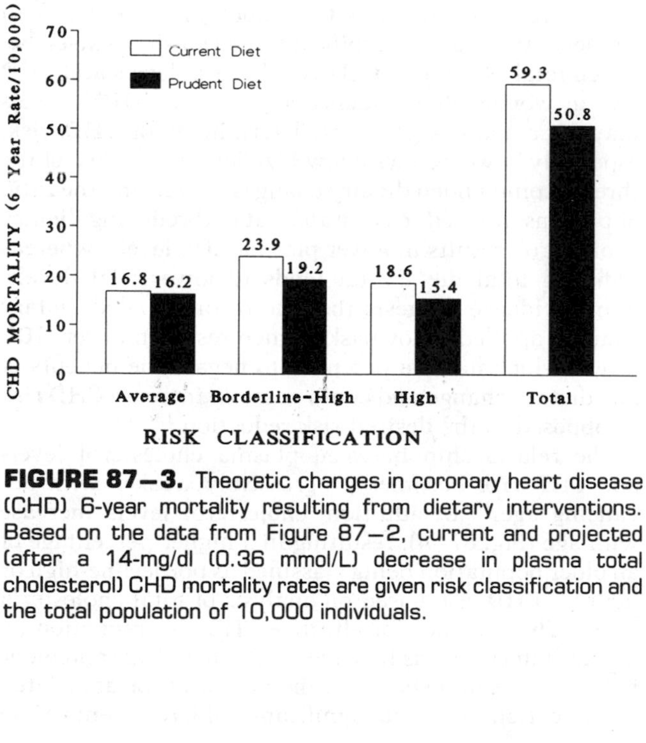

FIGURE 87–3. Theoretic changes in coronary heart disease (CHD) 6-year mortality resulting from dietary interventions. Based on the data from Figure 87–2, current and projected (after a 14-mg/dl (0.36 mmol/L) decrease in plasma total cholesterol) CHD mortality rates are given risk classification and the total population of 10,000 individuals.

This analysis reveals that the major impact of dietary intervention to lower plasma cholesterol levels and CHD mortality occurs in the borderline-high and high-risk groups. Does this finding then indicate that only the high-risk approach to interventions should be used, to the exclusion of a population-based approach? Two points to note before coming to such a conclusion are that the data only consider mortality and not potential changes in morbidity resulting from intervention, and that the data only consider changes in plasma total cholesterol levels without associated changes in body weight, plasma LDL and HDL profiles, or any other reductions in CHD risk factors. What the data do indicate is that identification of those individuals in the borderline-high and high CHD risk groups and initiation of effective dietary intervention have the greatest theoretic potential for reducing overall CHD mortality in the population. It is disturbing, however, that the actual numbers of lives saved is relatively modest, 8.5 lives per 6 years for every 10,000 interventions.

CONCERNS AND CONSIDERATIONS

HETEROGENEITY OF RESPONSES AND GENETICS

Interindividual variations in plasma lipid levels are the result of two interactive factors: genetics and environment. About 50 to 60% of the interindividual variability of plasma total, LDL, and HDL cholesterol levels can be attributed to genetic factors;[25] recent studies of genetic profiles by analysis of restriction fragment length polymorphisms (RFLP) have identified genetic patterns associated with elevated plasma lipids and in some individuals with increased CHD risk even in the absence of hyperlipidemia.[26–28] The results of analysis of RFLP as related to CHD risk, along with the well-characterized rare genetic variations that affect lipid transport and increase CHD risk,[25] demonstrate the strong impact of genetics in determining CHD risk and raise the question of whether dietary interventions in "normolipidemic" individuals who have a high-risk genetic profile will have any effect on CHD incidence.

Many clinical studies of the effects of dietary interventions on plasma lipid levels have revealed a high degree of patient-to-patient heterogeneity of responses to the intervention,[8,29,30] which no doubt arises from variations in genetic factors. A recent study revealed that subjects with an apoprotein E4 allele exhibit increased serum cholesterol levels, enhanced cholesterol absorption, and failure to exhibit metabolic compensation when challenged with dietary cholesterol.[31] In the United States, the apoprotein E4 allele has a frequency of 14%, and population studies indicate that it is more prevalent in Caucasians than in Asians.[32] The need to confirm and expand these observations is clear in order to define the efficacy of dietary interventions in the population as a whole and in subsets of the population to determine whether specific genetic profiles make some individuals more or less responsive to dietary interventions and the extent to which diet can reduce CHD risk in these population subsets.

GOOD CHOLESTEROL–BAD CHOLESTEROL

Dietary changes not only affect plasma levels of atherogenic LDL cholesterol but also can result in changes in the protective HDL cholesterol concentrations. Data from the Framingham Study indicate that the protective effect of HDL cholesterol is almost twice as strong as the atherogenic effect of LDL cholesterol relative to CHD risk.[33] Other studies have obtained similar results,[34] and indicate that the ratio of plasma total to HDL cholesterol is a better determinant of CHD risk, especially at low total cholesterol levels, than the total plasma cholesterol value alone. One consistent observation of decreasing total fat calories is a decrease in plasma HDL cholesterol levels, often associated with an increase in plasma triacylglycerol concentrations because of a carbohydrate-induced increase in triglycerides.[13,18] Because some individuals have total cholesterol levels within the average range and low levels of HDL cholesterol, it is uncertain what effect additional HDL lowering, by compliance with a low-fat diet, will have on their relative CHD risk.

The emphasis of a plasma cholesterol-lowering diet is to reduce the concentration of atherogenic particles in the plasma, primarily LDL cholesterol. As noted previously, genetic factors play a significant role in determining CHD risk, and studies have shown that abnormalities in lipoprotein composition and in generation of abnormal lipoproteins particles also play a significant role in CHD incidence. One example is lipoprotein (a) [Lp(a)], a lipoprotein consisting of an apoprotein(a) molecule covalently bonded to the apoprotein B of LDL. The atherogenicity of Lp(a) appears to relate to its ability to increase fibrinolysis time because of an interference with the interaction of plasmin with fibrin and effects on plasminogen activation. Increased Lp(a) levels are associated with a two- to three-fold increased risk for CHD and stroke,[28] and plasma concentrations do not appear to be altered by dietary intervention. CHD risk is also increased in some patients who exhibit increased rates of LDL synthesis and catabolism even though plasma LDL levels are not elevated.[35] This finding appears to be characteristic of hyperapobetalipoproteinemia, defined as increased plasma LDL apolipoprotein B levels with normal plasma LDL cholesterol concentrations.[36] The effects of dietary interventions, in terms of reducing the underlying metabolic abnormality associated with increased CHD risk, have not been defined in patients with hyperapobetalipoproteinemia.

INTERVENTION AND SPECIAL POPULATIONS

A population-based approach to CHD risk reduction will naturally include a variety of population subsets, the special nutritional needs of which must be considered as part of the evaluation of the efficacy and safety of the proposed dietary intervention. Three groups for which few data are available regarding either the benefits or potential problems associated with the proposed dietary changes are children, women, and the elderly. Much debate has centered on whether the recommended dietary changes are appropriate for children as related to maintenance of nutritional requirements and normal growth rates.[37] A major concern is that excessive implementation of the guidelines for a low-fat diet can result in growth failure resulting from inadequate intake of total energy and of vitamins and minerals derived from such foods as eggs, red meat, and dairy products.[37] At present, uncertainty remains regarding the CHD risk reduction benefits relative to questions of overall nutritional balance associated with initiating a low-fat, low-cholesterol diet during the first two decades of life. The soon to be released report of the NCEP Expert Panel on Blood Cholesterol Levels in Children and Adolescents should provide additional insight and direction regarding the suitability of dietary modifications in this age group. However, the basic principles of good nutrition must be emphasized when advising dietary restrictions to parents to ensure maintenance of the overall nutritional balance necessary for normal growth and development in this age group.

Most clinical studies have been directed at determining the efficacy of CHD risk reduction interventions in male populations and data are limited on which to base dietary recommendations for reduction of CHD risk in women. Although a significant relationship exists between total plasma and LDL cholesterol levels and CHD risk in women, the evidence suggests that HDL levels may be a more significant determinant of CHD risk, especially in women with low LDL levels.[18,33] Two of the three recommended dietary changes, increasing the ratio of polyunsaturated to saturated fat and reducing dietary cholesterol, results in lower plasma LDL levels, whereas reducing total dietary fat tends to lower HDL levels. Some evidence suggests that the recommended dietary changes applied to low-risk women result in lower HDL levels, which has the potential to negate the benefits of any dietary change and could possibly increase CHD risk as opposed to the desired risk reduction.[13,16,18]

The relationship between plasma cholesterol levels and CHD risk becomes progressively weaker with advancing age.[38] In addition, cholesterol levels increase with age (Fig. 87–4), resulting in a higher percentage of an older population being classified as borderline-high or high for CHD risk based on analysis of total cholesterol levels. The evidence for effective CHD risk reduction by dietary interventions in persons 65 years of age and older is far from established and the potential for associated complications may be significant. Older patients have

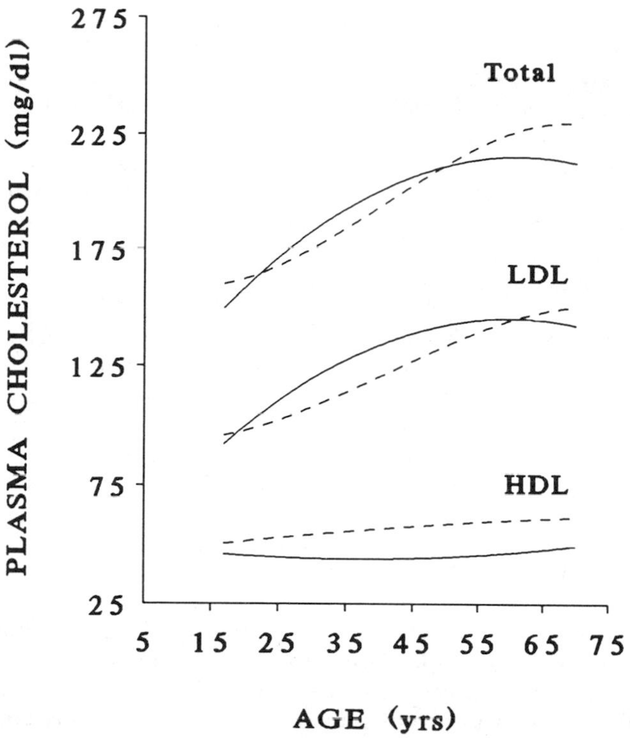

FIGURE 87–4. Age-related changes in plasma total, LDL, and HDL cholesterol levels in males (solid lines) and females (dashed lines). (Data represent the fiftieth percentile values for males and females as reported by the Lipid Research Clinics Population Studies Data Book. Vol. 1: The Prevalence Study. NIH Publication No. 80–1527. Washington, D.C., U.S. Department of Health and Human Services, 1980.)

special dietary needs that may not be met by a low-fat, low-cholesterol diet and the increased carbohydrate intake could exacerbate existing mild glucose intolerance resulting in postprandial hyperglycemia and hyperinsulinemia, which are in themselves CHD risk factors.[17]

CORONARY HEART DISEASE AND TOTAL MORTALITY

Sufficient data are available to support the thesis that reduction of elevated plasma LDL cholesterol levels by drugs can reduce CHD incidence and mortality,[22,39] and analysis of all the intervention trials carried out to date support intervention in high-risk subjects (Table 87–4). The argument that a 1% reduction in plasma cholesterol levels results in a 2% reduction in CHD deaths appears justified on the basis of both theoretic and direct applications.[22] Even with this evidence in hand, it is worth asking whether intervention will have a minor or major effect on CHD mortality and whether changes will occur in total mortality rates.

Table 87–4 is a summary of the results of the major dietary and drug trials designed to investigate the effect of plasma cholesterol lowering on CVD mortality (adapted from reference 40). Included are the sample sizes for the intervention (I) and control (C) groups, designations as to diet or drug trials, primary or secondary intervention trials, years duration, percentage change in plasma total cholesterol levels, and the number and percentage of CVD deaths in the intervention

TABLE 87–4. CARDIOVASCULAR DISEASE (CVD) AND TOTAL MORTALITY IN CLINICAL TRIALS

	SIZE						NUMBER (%) OF DEATHS			
							CVD		Total	
TRIAL	I	C	Diet/Rx	1°/2°	Yrs	ΔTC	I	C	I	C
LA Veterans	424	422	Diet	1°	8	−14%	57 (13.4)	81 (19.2)	174 (41.0)	177 (41.9)
Oslo Heart Study	206	206	Diet*	2°	5	−15%	38 (18.4)	52 (25.2)	41 (19.9)	55 (26.7)
LRC-CPPT	1906	1900	Rx	1°	7	− 9%	37 (1.9)	47 (2.5)	68 (3.6)	71 (3.7)
Helsinki Heart	2051	2031	Rx	1°	5	−10%	22 (1.1)	23 (1.1)	45 (2.2)	42 (2.1)
WHO-clofibrate	5331	5296	Rx	1°	5	− 8%	68 (1.3)	62 (1.2)	162 (3.0)	127 (2.3)
CDP-clofibrate	1103	2789	Rx	2°	6	− 6%	241 (21.8)	633 (22.7)	281 (25.5)	709 (25.4)
Stockholm	279	276	Rx	2°	5	−13%	54 (19.4)	75 (27.2)	61 (21.9)	82 (29.7)
CDP-niacin	1119	2789	Rx	2°	6	−10%	238 (21.3)	633 (22.7)	273 (24.4)	709 (25.4)

I, Intervention group; C, control group; Diet/Rx, diet or drug trial; 1°/2°, primary or secondary intervention trial; yrs, years duration; ΔTC, percent change in plasma total cholesterol; LA, Los Angeles; LRC-CPPT, Lipid Research Clinics–Coronary Primary Prevention Trial; WHO, World Health Organization, CDP, Coronary Drug Project.

*Oslo Heart Study included both dietary intervention and cigarette smoking cessation.

and control populations. Also presented in Table 87–4 are the number and percentage of total deaths. The data are for CVD and total mortality and do not indicate nonfatal events. As can be seen, CVD deaths are reduced in most of the studies; however, total mortality rates are similar for both the intervention and control groups in most studies. Analysis of the data from both lipid-lowering and multiple risk factor intervention trials indicate similar findings and leaves unresolved the question of whether interventions to lower plasma cholesterol levels have any significant effect on overall mortality.[41]

In an attempt to determine the magnitude of benefit attained from adherence to a dietary program to lower serum cholesterol levels, Taylor et al. developed a model based on multiple risk factors to determine probable gains in life expectancy from risk factor interventions.[42] The data from the model indicate that a person at low risk (10th percentile for smoking habit and systolic blood pressure and 90th percentile for HDL cholesterol) would gain 3 days to 3 months in life expectancy from a lifelong program of diet-mediated cholesterol reduction.[42] For persons at high risk (90th percentile for smoking and blood pressure and 10th percentile for HDL cholesterol), the calculated gain in life expectancy from achieving a 6.7% reduction in plasma cholesterol ranges from 18 days to 12 months. In another model analysis of clinical data determining CVD attributable risk reduction by dietary intervention, the results suggest that treatment of hypercholesterolemia is effective in absolute terms, but the benefit is relatively modest and the trend is for treatment to be less effective at older ages.[43] Similar estimates of benefit have been reported by Browner et al., in that a reduction in dietary fat intake from 37 to 30% of calories would in theory result in a 2% benefit and would thereby defer 42,000 of the 2.3 million deaths in adults each year and increase average life expectancy by 3 to 4 months.[44]

Although these reports suggest that the effects of intervention on CVD and total mortality are relatively modest, a reduction in total mortality is not necessarily the best indicator of the value of plasma cholesterol lowering in that preventing the incidence of nonfatal heart attacks results in a reduction in chronic CHD. Even if life expectancy cannot be extended, decreasing the likelihood of a morbid event or preventing its early onset constitutes a worthwhile goal. Unfortunately, insufficient data exist to allow estimation of the efficacy of dietary interventions in reducing nonfatal CHD events.

RISKS OF RISK REDUCTION

Any recommended population-wide dietary change must be both effective in lowering plasma cholesterol levels and free from negative side effects. To date, no evidence shows that the proposed dietary changes have any deleterious side effects; however, areas of concern need to be monitored if a population-wide change to a lowfat, high-carbohydrate diet is accomplished. As noted previously, dietary changes to lower saturated fat, increase polyunsaturated fat, and increase carbohydrate intake have significant effects on plasma HDL cholesterol levels. Increasing carbohydrate intake can result in higher levels of plasma triglyceride and lower HDL cholesterol. In a similar manner, it has been estimated that HDL cholesterol is reduced 1% for every 2% of calories in which polyunsaturated fatty acids are substituted for saturated or monounsaturated fat.[13,45] Considering the significant protective role of HDL in CHD incidence, such changes could result in an unacceptable shift in the LDL to HDL ratio resulting in minimal change in the CHD risk profile.

Other concerns include the observation that populations with a high-carbohydrate intake often have a high prevalence of hypertension, which is thought to result from the tendency of high-carbohydrate diets to cause salt retention.[13,45] Also of concern is that a low-fat, high-carbohydrate diet could increase the risk for osteoporosis, either directly or indirectly, by decreasing calcium intake, interference with calcium absorption, and/or promotion of renal excretion of calcium.[13,45] And finally, high intake of polyunsaturated fatty acids has been shown to decrease immune functions, which could be of special concern in the elderly population in whom the immune system may already be compromised.[13,45] The long-term consequences of institution of the population-based dietary guidelines remain unclear; only by appropriate follow-up studies addressing these potential problem areas will we be able to define the consequences of these changes relative to these other health questions. As with any intervention, the risk-to-benefit ratio of the proposed dietary change must be investigated thoroughly and established scientifically.

Any population-based approach to dietary change and plasma cholesterol lowering will shift the overall plasma cholesterol distribution of the population toward a lower level, as shown in Figure 87–2. Data from the Multiple Risk Factor Intervention Trial (MRFIT) demonstrate that, at low levels of plasma cholesterol, total mortality rates increase,[46] as shown in Figure 87–5. The increased total mortality at the low end of the plasma cholesterol distribution appear to result from a variety of causes, including intracranial hemorrhage[46] and cancer, primarily colon cancer.[47] Although debate continues over the significance of these data, whether because of existing hypertension or subclinical malignancy, the inverse relationship between low cholesterol and cancer and the observed increased mortality rates in those with very low cholesterol levels raises the troubling question of what the long-range consequences of having those with already low cholesterol levels achieve additional lowering through dietary change. The potential relationship between low plasma cholesterol levels and increased cancer risk, especially in men, needs to be evaluated thoroughly and its significance given serious consider-

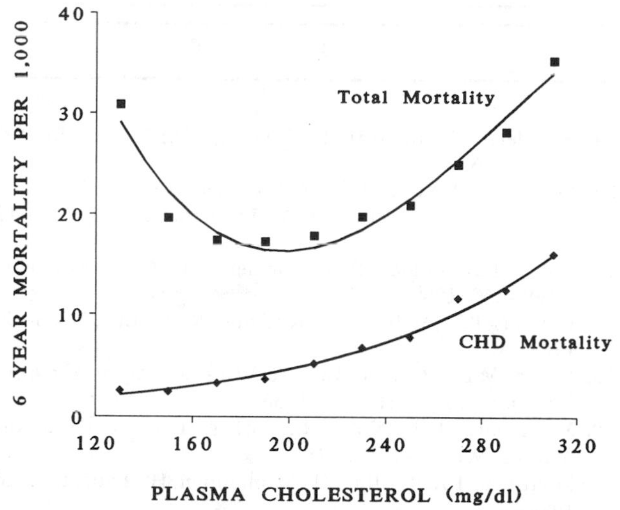

FIGURE 87–5. Relationship among plasma cholesterol levels, coronary heart disease (CHD) mortality, and total mortality. (Data for CHD and total mortality derived from the Multiple Risk Factor Intervention Trial reports in Iso, H., Jacobs, D.R., Jr., Wentworth, D., et al.: N. Engl. J. Med., *320*:904–910, 1989.)

ation in the evaluation of a population-based approach to dietary interventions for CHD risk reduction.

In summary, any attempt to modify the dietary pattern of an entire population must be based on evidence that the proposed intervention will have a significant impact on overall CHD morbidity and mortality and be free of any potentially harmful side effects. The basic question is whether the proposed community-based, population approach to reducing plasma cholesterol levels will significantly lower CHD incidence while maintaining overall nutritional health and well being. The answer is that it probably will have a lowering affect on CHD incidence and mortality, although quantitatively it will be a relatively small effect overall. The question of safety of the proposed changes will continue to be investigated and debated for some time.

A large body of evidence supports the hypothesis that obesity contributes significantly to the "mass hypercholesterolemia" typical of the United States and other affluent societies. The most significant dietary intervention the population could initiate to reduce CHD risk would be to attain and maintain ideal body weight. This approach has the potential to decrease CHD risk substantially not only by reducing android obesity but also to reduce plasma lipids, both cholesterol and triglyceride; increase HDL cholesterol levels; reduce blood pressure; reduce blood insulin levels and correct glucose intolerance; and often increases the exercise potential. Weight loss for the overweight patient represents a significant multiple risk factor intervention approach to CVD risk reduction.

The relative importance of blood cholesterol as a CHD risk factor also must be kept in perspective with regard to the other major CHD risk factors such as cigarette smoking and hypertension. An analysis of the potential increase in life expectancy resulting from changes in risk factors among persons at high risk for CHD[42] indicates that a 40-year-old man who lowers his cholesterol level 6.7% by diet will gain 7 months in life expectancy, whereas if that patient reduces an elevated blood pressure, he gains 34 months, and if he stops smoking, he gains 63 months. Whether these estimates accurately reflect the degree of benefit achieved by risk reduction can be debated; however, the relative importance of interventions aimed at specific CHD risk factors is apparent and obvious.

In making dietary recommendations to the public, the programs must minimize the national obsession to have as low a cholesterol level as possible. Also, the public must recognize that the cholesterolphobia promoted in advertising is not necessarily the best or most effective approach to dietary changes, because the type and amount of fat in the diet plays the major role in determining blood cholesterol levels. More emphasis on achieving and maintaining normal body weight and the benefits of regular exercise need to be communicated to the public as part of an overall nutritional approach to CHD risk reduction. The mixed messages that the public receives from the media, health reports, and various proponents of wellness leave many individuals confused and frustrated, whereas others often make dietary modifications that are of little benefit in CHD risk reduction and may actually be harmful. Extremely low-fat diets, with associated reductions in HDL levels, represent just one example of how an individual can make potentially harmful changes in their dietary pattern in the hope of reducing CHD risk. The public needs to know the most effective dietary changes and to what extent both the individual and the population can expect to benefit from such changes in terms of CVD risk reduction. Indeed, the projected reductions in CHD mortality are relatively small on a percentage basis; however, considering that almost 1 million Americans died of CVD in 1987, a 14% reduction in the 6-year mortality rate does result in a significant number of lives saved. What remains uncertain are the consequences of changing the dietary pattern of 125 million Americans to achieve this rather modest reduction in CVD deaths.

REFERENCES

1. Surgeon General's Report on Nutrition and Health. Washington, D.C., U.S. Government Printing Office, 1988.
2. National Research Council Committee on Diet and Health: Diet and Health: Implications for Reducing Chronic Disease Risk. Washington, D.C., National Academy Press, 1989.
3. Report of the National Cholesterol Education Program Expert Panel on Detection, Evaluation, and Treatment of High Blood Cholesterol in Adults. Arch. Intern. Med., *148:*36–69, 1988.
4. Report of the Expert Panel on Population Strategies for Blood Cholesterol Reduction: Circulation, *83:*2154–2232, 1991.
5. McNamara, D.J.: Annu. Rev. Nutr., *7:*273–290, 1987.
6. Goldberg, A.C., Schoenfeld, G.: Annu. Rev. Nutr., *5:*195–212, 1985.
7. Hegsted, D.M., Ausman, L.M.: J. Nutr., *118:*1184–1189, 1988.
8. Grundy, S.M., Vega, G.L.: Am. J. Clin. Nutr., *47:*822–824, 1988.
9. Bonanome, A., Grundy, S.M.: N. Engl. J. Med., *318:*1244–1248, 1988.
10. Nestel, P.J.: Annu. Rev. Nutr., *10:*149–167, 1990.
11. Connor, W.E., Connor, S.L.: Adv. Intern. Med., *35:*139–172, 1990.
12. Kromhout, D., Bosschieter, E.B., de Lezenne Coulander, C.: N. Engl. J. Med., *312:*1205–1209, 1985.
13. Grundy, S.M.: J. Nutr., *119:*529–533, 1989.
14. Keys, A., Menotti, A., Karvonen, M.J., et al.: Am. J. Epidemiol., *124:*903–915, 1986.
15. McNamara, D.J.: Adv. Meat Sci., *6:*63–87, 1990.
16. Wolf, R.N., Grundy, S.M.: J. Nutr., *113:*1521–1528, 1983.
17. Reaven, G.M.: J. Nutr., *116:*1143–1147, 1986.
18. Crouse, J.R.: Lancet, *1:*318–320, 1989.
19. Gotto, A.M., Jr., LaRosa, J.C., Hunninghake, D., et al.: Circulation, *81:*1721–1733, 1990.
20. Berns, M.A.M., de Vries, J.H.M., Katan, M.B.: Am. J. Epidemiol., *130:*1109–1122, 1989.
21. Larsson, B., Svardsudd, K., Welin, L., et al.: Br. Med. J., *288:*1401–1404, 1984.
22. Lipid Research Clinics Program: JAMA, *251:*351–364, 365–374, 1984.
23. Lipid Research Clinics Population Studies Data Book. Volume I: The Prevalence Study. NIH Publication No. 80–1527. Washington, D.C., U.S. Department of Health and Human Services, 1980.
24. Stamler, J., Wentworth, D., Neaton, J.D.: JAMA, *256:*2823–2828, 1986.
25. Lusis, A.J.: J. Lipid Res., *29:*397–429, 1988.
26. Wallace, R.B., Anderson, R.A.: Epidemiol. Rev., *9:*95–119, 1987.
27. Fisher, E.A., Coates, P.M., Cortner, J.A.: Annu. Rev. Nutr., *9:*139–160, 1989.
28. Hopkins, P.N., Williams, R.R.: Annu. Rev. Nutr., *9:*303–345, 1989.
29. Katan, M.B., Beynen, A.C., de Vries, J.H.M. et al.: Am. J. Epidemiol., *123:*221–234, 1986.
30. McNamara, D.J., Kolb, R., Parker, T.S., et al.: J. Clin. Invest., *79:*1729–1739, 1987.
31. Miettinen, T.A., Gylling, H., Vanhannen, H.: Lancet, *ii:*1261, 1988.
32. Davignon, J., Gregg, R.E., Sing, C.F.: Arteriosclerosis, *8:*1–21, 1988.
33. Kannel, W.B.: Am. Heart J., *114:*413–419, 1987.
34. Goldbourt, U., Holtzman, E., Neufeld, H.N.: Br. Med. J., *290:*1239–1243, 1985.
35. Kesaniemi, Y.A., Grundy, S.M.: Arteriosclerosis, *3:*40–46, 1983.
36. Sniderman, A., Shapiro, S., Marpole, D., et al.: Proc. Natl. Acad. Sci. USA, *77:*604–608, 1980.
37. Lifshitz, F., Moses, N.: Am. J. Dis. Child., *143:*537–542, 1989.
38. Anderson, K.M., Castelli, W.P., Lvy, D.: JAMA, *257:*2176–2180, 1987.
39. Frick, M.H., Elo, O., Haapa, K., et al.: N. Engl. J. Med., *317:*1237–1245, 1987.
40. Rossouw, J.E., Rifkind, B.M.: Endocrinol. Metab. Clin. North Am., *19:*279–297, 1990.
41. McCormick, J., Skrabanek, P.: Lancet, *ii:*839–841, 1988.
42. Taylor, W.C., Pass, T.M., Shepard, D.S. et al.: Ann. Intern. Med., *106:*605–614, 1987.
43. Malenka, D.J., Baron, J.A.: Arch. Intern. Med., *149:*1981–1985, 1989.
44. Browner, W.S., Westenhouse, J., Tice, J.A.: JAMA, *265:*3285–3291, 1991.
45. Grundy, S.M., Denke, M.A.: J. Lipid Res., *31:*1149–1172, 1990.
46. Iso, H., Jacobs, D.R., Jr., Wentworth, D., et al.: N. Engl. J. Med., *320:*904–910, 1989.
47. Cowan, L.D., O'Connell, D.L., Criqui, M.H., et al.: Am. J. Epidemiol., *131:*468–482, 1990.

SELECTED READINGS

Garber, A.M., Sox, H.C., Jr., Littenberg, B.: Screening asymptomatic adults for cardiac risk factors: The serum cholesterol level. Ann. Intern. Med., *110:*622–639, 1989.

Grundy, S.M., Denke, M.A.: Dietary influences on serum lipids and lipoproteins. J. Lipid Res., *31:*1149–1172, 1990.

Kwiterovich, P.: Beyond Cholesterol. Baltimore, Johns Hopkins University Press, 1989.

McNamara, D.J.: Effects of fat-modified diets on cholesterol and lipoprotein metabolism. Annu. Rev. Nutr., *7:*273–290, 1987.

Moore, T.J.: Heart Failure. New York, Random House, 1989.

CHAPTER 88

Diet, Cancer, and Food Safety

Michael W. Pariza

HISTORICAL BACKGROUND

The discovery of effects of nutritional status on cancer development in experimental animals accompanied the emergence of nutritional science as an independent academic discipline. The earliest experiments established that an effective means of reducing cancer incidence was "underfeeding," that is, giving the test animals less food than controls ate ad libitum. Although underfeeding reduced the intake of all nutrients, it is now accepted that its anticancer effect is largely if not completely due to the restriction of calories. Indeed, calorie restriction remains the most generally effective anticarcinogen in rodents that we know of.[1]

As information was accumulating on the relationship between nutrient status and cancer in experimental animals (with an eye toward eventual human application), a separate body of knowledge was emerging on food safety. The latter effort was led by microbiologists pursuing the causes of food poisoning.[2] The two research areas—the nutritional aspects of cancer and the microbiologic aspects of food safety—found a common course in the early 1960s with the discovery of aflatoxin B_1, a metabolite of certain molds (e.g., Aspergillus flavus). Aflatoxin B_1, which can contaminate nuts and cereal grains, is an extremely potent carcinogen for the rat.[3] Hence, the discovery of aflatoxin B_1 underscored the complex interdisciplinary nature of diet/cancer relationships.

Meanwhile, on a separate front, politicians had become increasingly concerned about reports of carcinogens in the food supply. Because of this the United States Congress included in the Food Additives Amendment of 1958 the well-known Delaney Clause, which stipulated that a substance shown to induce cancer in man or animals cannot be intentionally added to food.

In 1969 the federal government banned cyclamates, which were used as synthetic sweeteners. What had actually been tested was a mixture of cyclamates and saccharin. It now seems probable that the tumors in the test rats were produced by the saccharin, not the cyclamates, in the mixture.[4] Saccharin remains a legal food additive in the United States because of a special congressional exemption. (Interestingly, Canadian authorities elected to ban saccharin but to retain cyclamates.) The decision in 1969 to ban cyclamates in the United States is seen as giving impetus to the "consumer movement," which aims to free the food supply of all synthetic chemicals.[5]

The outcome of these separate developments is the concept of food safety as it exists today, encompassing as it does much more than bacterial food poisoning. Dietary aspects of cancer embody a large segment of what the public perceives as a growing food safety problem. There is a considerable gulf between what the public believes about food safety and what has been established scientifically.[5,6]

DEFINITIONS AND MECHANISMS

CARCINOGENS

Carcinogens are substances that induce cancer in man or animals. They include chemical agents, biologic agents (e.g., certain oncogenic viruses), and ionizing radiation.

Today, experiments in animals are used to screen for potential carcinogens. However, the earliest reports of environmental carcinogens were based on human observations. Tobacco was first implicated as a human carcinogen in 1761.[7] Forty years later Percival Pott established that young boys forced to serve as chimney sweeps were at risk of developing scrotal cancer. Today we recognize that this was the result of exposure to carcinogenic hydrocarbons in the smoke residue.[8]

METABOLIC ACTIVATION

Figure 88–1 depicts the structures of five chemical carcinogens, substances that will produce cancer when fed to rodents. The structures include a polynuclear arene (benzo[a]pyrene), an aromatic amine (2-acetylaminofluorene, referred to by the acronym AAF), a mycotoxin (aflatoxin B_1), a substituted benzene (safrole), and a relatively simple compound (urethan) that resembles urea, an important byproduct of nitrogen metabolism. Four of these carcinogens (benzo[a]pyrene, aflatoxin B_1, safrole, and urethan) are produced by natural processes and undoubtedly predate by eons the appearance of humans on this planet. Only AAF is solely a product of human synthesis.

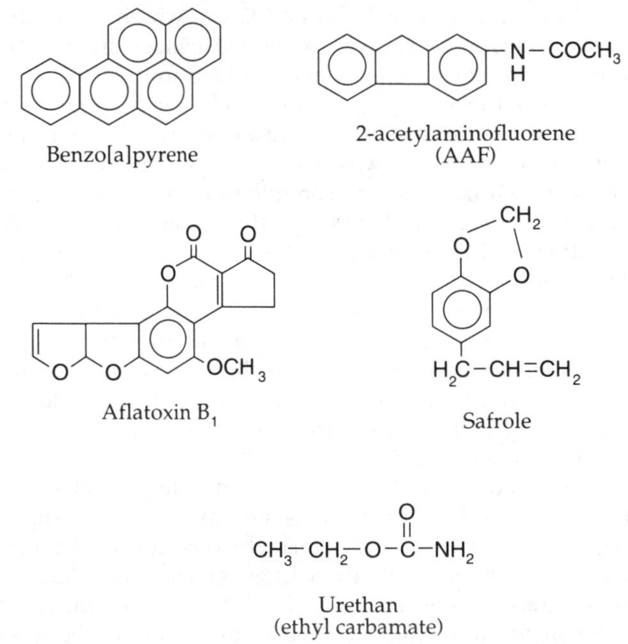

FIGURE 88–1. Chemical structures of representative carcinogens.

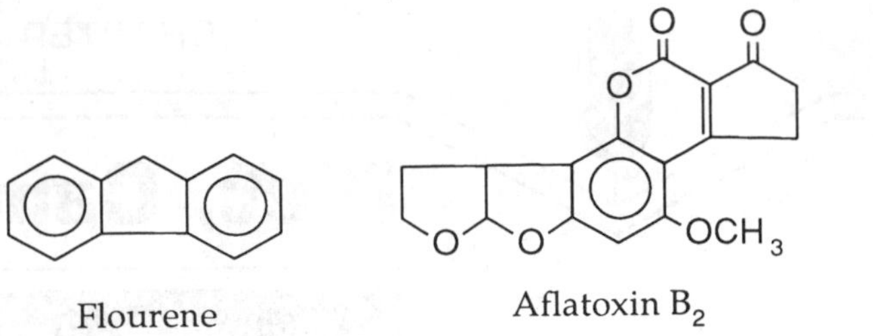

FIGURE 88–2. Compounds with little or no carcinogenic activity.

On first approaching the matter, one might expect carcinogens to be chemically similar to one another. However, perusal of structures such as those depicted in Figure 88–1 reveals no such similarity. Moreover, for any one compound, slight changes in structure may have marked effects on carcinogenic potential. For example, removing the acetylamino function from AAF yields fluorene (Fig. 88–2), which is not carcinogenic. Likewise, moving the functional group to another position may also reduce or eliminate carcinogenic activity. For aflatoxin B_1, reducing the double bond between carbon atoms 2 and 3 produces aflatoxin B_2 (Fig. 88–2), which is only weakly carcinogenic. Hence, even though there are no key structural similarities among chemical carcinogens, there is something unique about each structure that imparts carcinogenic activity.

Another seemingly puzzling observation is that most carcinogens are chemically stable. They do not react when mixed with cellular constituents, such as DNA. How, then, are carcinogens able to induce cancer?

The key to the puzzle was discovered by James A. and Elizabeth C. Miller.[8] They showed that it was not the inert chemical structures per se that cause cancer, but rather metabolites of the carcinogens produced by cell enzymes, most notably the class of enzymes known collectively as cytochrome P-450.

Actually the cytochrome P-450 enzymes (also known as mixed function oxidases) represent one of the body's principal means of protection against xenobiotics (foreign chemicals that do not serve as nutrients, many of which are toxic to animals). Xenobiotics occur naturally in the environment. For example, virtually all food plants contain xenobiotics produced to ward off insects and other predators. Cytochrome P-450 enzymes are designed to detoxify xenobiotics, usually metabolizing them to water-soluble metabolites that can be excreted.

However, the diverse nature of xenobiotics makes it imperative that cytochrome P-450 enzymes be inherently adaptable. This feature, in turn, leads to a diverse array of potential xenobiotic metabolites. The enzymes must be able to cope with the vast number of xenobiotics potentially present in food, water, and air. It is not surprising, then, that the enzymes sometimes make what amount to biologic mistakes.

With some xenobiotics the cytochromes P-450 produce one or more highly reactive metabolites as well as a variety of less toxic products. Such highly reactive metabolites may be capable of carcinogenic initiation, particularly if they are electrophilic (electron-poor, capable of covalent bonding with nucleophilic regions in DNA.) In this way cytochrome P-450 enzymes produce carcinogenic intermediates in the course of metabolizing certain xenobiotics. We call such xenobiotics carcinogens, but more precisely they are procarcinogens, whereas the carcinogenic metabolites produced from them are the true ultimate carcinogens. The process whereby procarcinogens are converted to ultimate carcinogens is referred to as metabolic activation.

Pathways for the metabolic activation by rat liver of AAF[8] and aflatoxin B_1[9] to ultimate carcinogens are shown in Figure 88–3. In both cases the activated products are highly reactive, chemically unstable electrophiles capable of covalent bonding to DNA, RNA, and protein. Reaction of these ultimate carcinogens with DNA leads to mutations and other types of genetic damage.

It should be noted that the pathways for activation are species-specific. Hence, the guinea pig is resistant to carcinogenesis by AAF because it lacks the hepatic hydroxylase enzyme required for catalyzing the first step in the AAF activation pathway. Likewise the mouse is

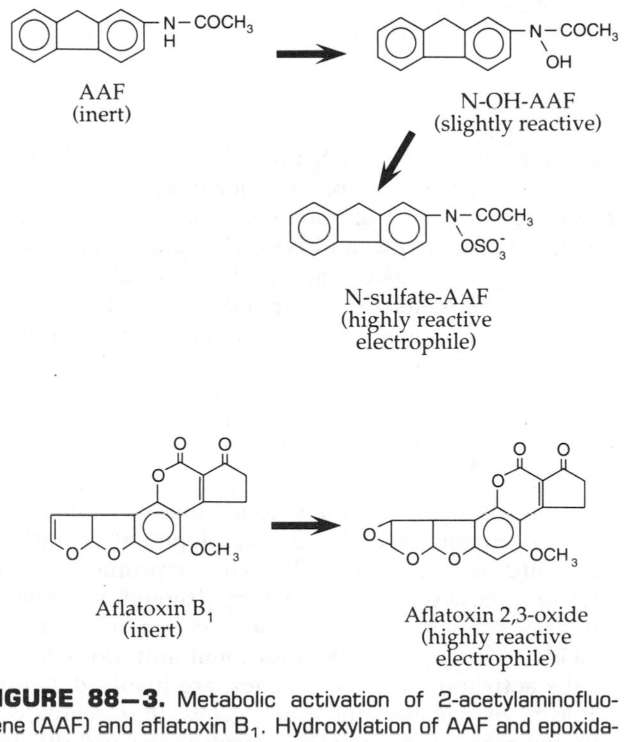

FIGURE 88–3. Metabolic activation of 2-acetylaminofluorene (AAF) and aflatoxin B_1. Hydroxylation of AAF and epoxidation of aflatoxin B_1 are effected by cytochrome P-450 enzymes. The sulfation of N-OH-AAF is produced by a soluble enzyme.

highly resistant to aflatoxin B_1 carcinogenesis, probably because it rapidly saturates the key double bond rather than forming an epoxide at that position. Enzyme diversity among tissues is the major reason for carcinogen tissue specificity. Hence, AAF and aflatoxin B_1 do not induce epidermal carcinogenesis because epidermal cells lack the enzymes needed for activation.

PROTECTIVE FACTORS

Given the potentially catastrophic consequences of uncontrolled metabolic activation of carcinogens, it is not surprising that the body has developed many layers of defense. For example, detoxification by cytochrome P-450 enzymes is a major method for removing carcinogens from the body. Moreover, continued exposure to a xenobiotic, be it a carcinogen or not, leads to the induction of cytochrome P-450. Characteristically the detoxification pathways predominate in such induced states. The biochemical effect of increased detoxification is to reduce substrate for activation.

Ultimate carcinogens (potent electrophiles) initiate carcinogenesis by damaging nucleophilic centers in DNA. Fortunately the critical DNA targets represent only a small fraction of the nucleophilic sites in a cell. Proteins, RNA, and even noncritical segments of DNA may serve as nucleophilic sinks with which ultimate carcinogens may react without producing genetic damage leading to cancer. There are also numerous small molecules, such as glutathione, ascorbic acid, and other antioxidants, which may serve to trap or otherwise inactivate ultimate carcinogens.

Another important protective mechanism is found in the DNA repair system. Humans deficient in DNA repair enzymes are prone to developing certain kinds of cancer. Epithelial surfaces that are exposed to the outside environment readily turn over and are shed on a continual basis. Evolution has provided higher organisms with layer upon layer of biologic defense against xenobiotics, including carcinogens.

CARCINOGENESIS

Carcinogenesis, the biologic process whereby normal cells are transformed into cancerous tumor cells, is exceedingly complicated. As depicted in Figure 88–4, carcinogenesis is characterized by several experimentally distinct phases through which cells go following exposure to a carcinogen: initiation, tumor promotion, and tumor progression. (The terms "initiation" and "promotion" as defined here are distinct from their context of use in molecular biology parlance.)

INITIATION

Initiation is the first step in carcinogenesis. It is caused by a specific interaction between a carcinogen and a living cell. The nature of the interaction leading to

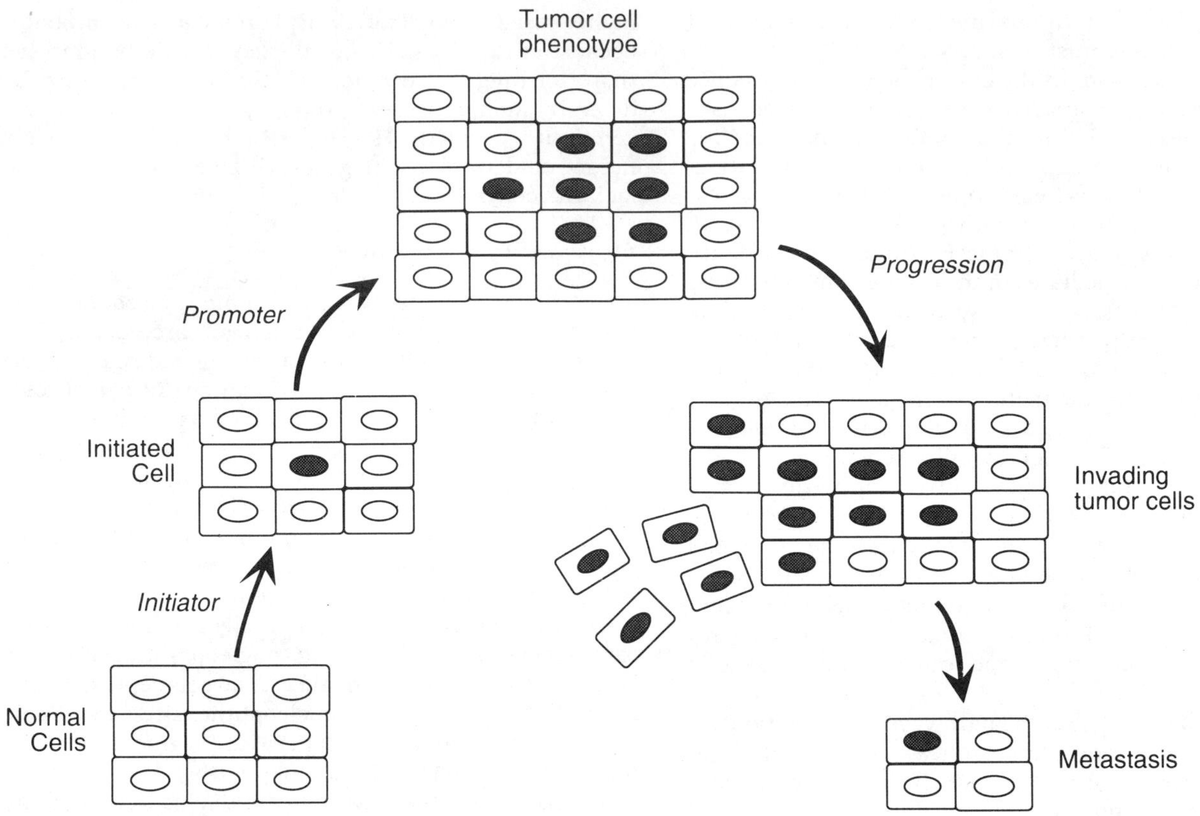

FIGURE 88–4. The process of carcinogenesis. A normal cell is initiated by exposure to low levels of a carcinogen (initiator); exposure to a promoter causes the initiated cell to proliferate and form a benign tumor, which can then progress by undergo further mutations to become invading tumor cells that ultimately metastasize. (Redrawn from Boutwell, R.K.: Tumor promoters in human carcinogenesis. *In* Important Advances in Oncology. Edited by V.T. DeVita, S. Hellman, and S.A. Rosenberg. Philadelphia, J.B. Lippincott, 1985.)

initiation is not yet completely understood, but it is evident that the result is a heritable change that imparts the potential for further development and ultimate progression to malignancy. For example, initiation may result from mutations in oncogenes, the genetic regulatory sequences that govern their expression, or both. Because initiation involves genetic damage it would be difficult if not impossible to reverse in an absolute sense, a conclusion supported by experimental data.

Experimentally, initiation is accomplished by treating an animal with a subcarcinogenic dose of a carcinogen (a dose too small to produce cancer by itself). Two well-studied models are epidermal carcinogenesis in mice and hepatocarcinogenesis in rats. The mouse skin model is particularly sensitive to polycyclic hydrocarbon carcinogens such as benzo[a]pyrene, whereas in the rat liver model aromatic amines such as AAF are often used.

In both models, a sufficiently high dose of carcinogen will produce neoplasms. However, smaller doses of carcinogen produce more subtle changes that can be detected only by careful examination at the cellular level. Such altered cells lack the capacity to become foci for tumor masses (either benign or malignant), but they have been affected by the carcinogen and consequently exhibit a spectrum of modified phenotypes, each reflecting its respective (and possibly unique) carcinogen-modified genotype. A certain, probably small, number of the carcinogen-altered cells are initiated and possess the capacity to become tumor foci, depending on other conditions.

PROMOTION

Tumor promotion is the second stage of carcinogenesis. It is characterized by the development of initiated cells into benign tumor cells. Tumor promotion is an area of intense scientific research; although the molecular events essential for the process are not yet fully elucidated, it appears that additional mutations, as well as the activation of altered genes, are involved. Central subjects of current study are genes that regulate or otherwise influence growth control and/or cell differentiation.

Evidence indicates that tumor promotion is much more easily reversed than initiation or progression is. Hence, promotion appears to be a particularly important candidate for chemopreventive intervention.

PROGRESSION

The stage of tumor promotion culminates in the appearance of cells capable of growing autonomously and forming benign tumors. From there progression proceeds, driven by additional mutation-like changes, leading eventually to the expression of a fully malignant phenotype that includes the capacity for tissue invasion and metastasis.

MODULATION OF CARCINOGENESIS

The multistage nature of carcinogenesis, and the complexity of the biologic events that characterize each stage, leads to multiple opportunities for modulation—that is, altering the process so that the endpoint (number of neoplasms) is affected.

ENHANCEMENT

Carcinogenesis can be enhanced in several ways. For example, a substance that increases the uptake of a carcinogen would be seen as an enhancer of initiation. However, most examples of enhancers of carcinogenesis act on the tumor promotion stage.

Tumor promoters are chemical substances that enhance carcinogenesis by effecting tumor promotion. They stimulate promotion principally through gene activation. The most thoroughly studied tumor promoter is 12-0-tetradecanoylphorbol-13-acetate (TPA). TPA is a potent mouse skin tumor promoter that was originally isolated from a plant used in southeast Asia as a medicinal herb. TPA effects tumor promotion by binding to a specific membrane receptor, thereby activating protein kinase C, an important cellular regulatory enzyme. Other genes are then activated, leading to cell growth. Both normal and initiated skin cells are stimulated by TPA, but the initiated cells serve as foci for the development of benign tumor masses called papillomas. Papillomas begin appearing about 10 weeks after TPA administration is begun. By 20 weeks or so some of the papillomas will have progressed to frank carcinomas. It is worth noting, though, that most papillomas do not progress to carcinomas. It is likely that additional mutation-like events are required to transform a papilloma cell into a fully competent cancer cell capable of invasive growth.

Endogenously generated substances may also serve as tumor promoters. For example the polypeptide hormone prolactin, anabolic steroids, and bile salts all exhibit tumor promoting activity in model systems. Butylated hydroxytoluene (BHT), a synthetic antioxidant used as a food additive, also exhibits tumor promoting activity for rat liver when fed continuously at high levels that far exceed human dietary exposure.

An important feature of tumor promoters is that they exhibit "thresholds." Any given promoter is effective only when used at concentrations above its respective threshold dose. Moreover, repeated dosing is required. Treating animals once with a tumor promoter is not sufficient to enhance or accelerate tumor appearance.

Timing is also important. The promoter must come after the carcinogen. If the promoter is given prior to the initiating dose of the carcinogen it is not effective.

INHIBITION

Many substances will inhibit carcinogenesis, acting either as anti-initiators or antipromoters. For example, most xenobiotics induce cytochrome P-450 enzymes, which in turn degrade the very substances that induced them as well as related xenobiotics, including carcinogens. Feeding such xenobiotics before a carcinogen is administered will result in fewer tumors. In this way edible plants that contain relatively high levels of xenobiotics, such as cruciferous vegetables, inhibit carcinogenesis in rodents.[10]

There are also a variety of diet-derived antipromoters. Particularly prominent examples include substances in onion and garlic extracts, vitamin A (especially some synthetic derivatives), D-limonine (a bitter substance in citrus fruits), protease inhibitors, and calcium. Whereas anti-initiators serve to prevent initiation from occurring, antipromoters may actually reverse the process of promotion after it has begun.[7]

Some inhibitors act at more than one stage of carcinogenesis. D-Limonine is an example.[11] We have obtained evidence that an anticarcinogenic derivative of linoleic acid (referred to by the acronym CLA) is effective as an anti-initiator and probably as an antipromoter in some model carcinogenesis systems.[12,13] CLA is a potent antioxidant, which may explain at least in part its anticarcinogenic activity. The discovery of CLA as an anticarcinogen is of interest because the parent compound, linoleic acid, is the only fatty acid that has been unequivocally shown to enhance carcinogenesis under some experimental conditions.

Some modulators inhibit carcinogenesis under one set of conditions but enhance the process under different conditions (compare the findings in references 14 and 15). Dose is a central factor in determining whether inhibition or enhancement will predominate. For xenobiotics that are not enzymatically activated to carcinogenic metabolites, inhibition of carcinogenesis is the likely outcome from exposure to levels usually found in the diet.[10,15]

CARCINOGEN DETECTION

The discovery that some chemicals cause cancer led to proposals for reducing human cancer risk through carcinogen detection and subsequent reduction in exposure. This has had considerable beneficial impact in the area of occupation-associated cancer where exposure can be high. However, extending the approach to reducing or eliminating minute quantities of suspect carcinogens that may occur in food (e.g., pesticide residues) is of doubtful relevance to public health.

ANIMAL FEEDING STUDIES

Long-term feeding studies using normal animals are the mainstay of carcinogen screening programs. Such feeding tests are conducted routinely by the United States federal government's National Toxicology Program (NTP).[16,17]

A typical NTP test begins with the establishment of the maximum tolerated dose, or MTD, for a test substance. The MTD is defined operationally as the highest dose level that produces no obvious signs of toxicity and no more than a 10% drop in body weight. For relatively toxic substances the MTD is low, but most substances tested by the NTP are relatively nontoxic. Therefore, the MTD is often large, 1% or more of the diet. For example, the highest dose of saccharine tested in long-term feeding studies was 5% of the diet. A feeding regimen is developed using the MTD and a lower dose equivalent to one-half the MTD. Ideally an additional exposure level, one-fourth the MTD, is also employed. Ames and Gold have commented that one-half the MTD is still a high dose,[17] an observation that would in many instances also hold for one-fourth the MTD.

Rodent strains are selected for study, usually one strain of mice and one strain of rats. Test groups consist of 100 animals each, 50 females and 50 males. Hence, testing a single chemical requires 400 animals at minimum (2 dose levels times 2 strains times 100 animals per group), not counting controls. Animals are fed the test substance for 2 years and then sacrificed, after which each is subjected to a complete autopsy, including histologic analysis as needed.

Experience shows that about half the time a tested chemical is positive—that is, one or more of the test groups exhibits an increased incidence of neoplasia at some site. This conclusion may seem particularly startling. Does it mean that every other chemical substance is a carcinogen? The answer depends on how one defines the term carcinogen.

Chemical carcinogens that induce cancer following exposure of susceptible animals to relatively low levels for limited periods are substances that either are highly reactive electrophiles or are capable of being metabolized to intermediates that are highly reactive electrophiles (i.e., activated to ultimate carcinogens). Virtually all of these substances are mutagens in one or more test systems.

However, available knowledge about most substances determined to be "carcinogens" in high-dose long-term rodent feeding studies indicates that they are neither chemically reactive substances nor substances capable of being metabolized to such species. Moreover, few if any are mutagens under any test condition. These "carcinogens" seem to induce neoplasia through secondary mechanisms related to the nature of the feeding regimen itself. For example, adrenal, thyroid, and pituitary tumors are common. Biologic stress related to housing and ad libitum feeding may be an important factor in the cause of such tumors. Moreover, feeding substances at or near the MTD can induce abnormally high cell proliferation, a manifestation of toxicity that leads to increased chances for mutation and DNA replication errors.[18,19]

SHORT-TERM TESTS

Given the cost and time required for 2-year animal feeding studies, various short-term test systems have been developed. Such tests offer savings, but they suffer from drawbacks too, usually in the sense of yielding less complete data.

For example, there are various short-term animal models that can be used for carcinogen screening. The initiation of epidermal carcinogenesis in mice is one such model, offering the advantages of relative speed (6 months or less) and the appearance of external tumors (papillomas) that can be easily seen and quantified. The disadvantage is that the skin is insensitive to many potent carcinogens, such as aflatoxin B_1 and AAF, because it lacks the cytochrome P-450 enzymes needed for activation of the carcinogens to their ultimate forms. Hence a bioassay system based on the induction of mouse epidermal tumors would generate many falsely negative results.

Systems involving cultured animal cells have also been developed. Some are based on morphologic transformation that in some ways mimics tumorigenesis in animals; others are based on mutagenesis as a marker for genetic damage (genotoxicity). In general these systems work well only for carcinogens belonging to certain chemical classes, in part because cultured animal cells exhibit only a limited repertoire of enzymes capable of activating procarcinogens.

Various systems involving lower organisms such as fruit flies, molds, yeasts, and bacteria have also been developed. Because these organisms do not develop cancer the assays are based on the detection of genotoxicity, usually induced mutations. Such organisms are not able to activate most procarcinogens either, so their use is limited. Ames and colleagues approached this problem by incorporating a rat liver–derived extract ($9000 \times g$ supernatant fraction) into their bacterial mutagenesis test system.[20] Required cofactors are also included so that the rat liver enzymes can activate procarcinogens for mutagenesis in vitro. The activated metabolites then diffuse into the test bacteria and produce mutations in the *his* locus (the pathway producing histidine).

The test developed by Ames and colleagues became widely available in the mid-1970s. It was soon discovered that bacterial mutagens were ubiquitous in the environment, and further that most of the mutagens were of natural, not man-made, origin. These observations led Ames to publish a landmark paper in which he argued that synthetic chemicals are only a very small part of the "carcinogen/mutagen burden" to which all life on Earth is continuously exposed.[21]

At one time it was thought that a battery of short-term tests might replace the 2-year feeding study, but this has not proved to be the case. Virtually all of the "carcinogens" detected in high-dose feeding studies as conducted today yield negative results in short-term assays.

RISK ASSESSMENT

Once data have been obtained from carcinogen screening tests, the process of risk assessment may commence. In the simplest case, data from a high-dose rodent feeding study are plotted and extrapolated downward, to conditions of human exposure. It is then assumed that the humans are just as sensitive as the test animals, and a risk calculation is made.

For example, suppose that feeing substance Z at its MTD, 5 g per kg body weight, induced neoplasia in five mice from a group of 50. The cancer "risk" at the MTD would be 10%. But Z is a food additive that is used sparingly, and typical daily ingestion by a person is 3.5 mg per day. Hence, an "average" person weighing 70 kg is exposed to 50 μg of Z per kg body weight per day. By linear extrapolation, the cancer risk to the public is 1×10^{-6}, one extra cancer per million individuals.

The two principal assumptions implicit in this risk assessment should be noted. It is assumed that mice and humans metabolize Z in exactly the same fashion, and that this is true whether the exposure level to Z is 5 g per kg body weight per day or 0.00005 g per kg body weight per day. We know the first assumption is rarely correct, and the second probably never. Moreover, the calculation takes no account of the mechanism whereby cancer is induced or of modulating factors that may also be in the diet. Nonetheless, this method, with a few refinements,[22] is commonly used.

HERP INDEX

The problem with such simplistic cancer risk assessments is that the numbers often take on lives of their own, divorced from the reasoning and assumptions that went into their creation. This becomes particularly difficult when the estimates are communicated to the public. Using the example cited previously, it may be inferred that because Z increases cancer risk by one in a million, and because there are 250 million people in the United States, then the continued use of Z will produce 250 additional cancer deaths. This kind of "personalization" of cancer risk assessment data leads to distorted perceptions and policy decisions.

In an attempt to address this issue, Ames and colleagues developed the HERP (*h*uman *e*xposure / *r*odent *p*otency) index.[23] A HERP is calculated by dividing human exposure to a substance by the rodent TD_{50} for that substance (defined as the amount of the substance required to produce neoplasia in half of a group of test rats or mice). The result is then multiplied by 100. To correct for differences in body size between rodents and humans, both human exposure and rodent potency are based on *mg per kg body weight per day*.

The HERP is a ratio. As such it avoids the perceptual difficulties associated with the usual approach to risk assessment (i.e., so much cancer per so much exposure). In this respect it discourages the temptation to personalize the data. Moreover, the HERP permits comparison among various putative food-associated cancer risks.

Table 88–1 presents HERP ratios for some substances to which consumers are commonly exposed. It is readily apparent that some risks often taken for granted (e.g., alcohol consumption) far exceed many that receive a lot of media attention (e.g., trace contamination of drinking

TABLE 88–1. HERP VALUES FOR COMMONLY ENCOUNTERED CARCINOGEN EXPOSURES

DAILY HUMAN EXPOSURE	HERP (%)
PCBs, daily dietary intake	0.0002
EDB*, daily dietary intake	0.0004
Tap water, 1 L (chloroform)	0.001
6 ounces of apple juice (Alar*)	0.0017
Cooked bacon, 100 g (nitrosamines)	0.003
Worst well water in Silicon Valley (trichloroethylene)	0.004
Peanut butter (one sandwich) (aflatoxin)	0.03
One glass of wine (ethanol)	4.7

*Banned because of health concerns; HERP value based on exposure prior to ban.
(Data from Ames, B.N., Magaw, M., Gold, L.S.: Science, *236*:271–280, 1987.)

water or fruit juice with industrial byproducts or pesticides). Such comparisons may provide the basis for a more rational approach to setting public health priorities.

DIETARY ASPECTS OF CANCER

It is clear that lifestyle influences cancer risk. Diet is an important component of lifestyle, and because of this it would seem logical to expect that there might be important dietary effects on cancer risk. A major problem with separating and defining such effects lies in the complexity of the diet itself as well as in the process of carcinogenesis, influenced as it is by genetic and physiologic factors as well as by life style.

CARCINOGENS IN FOOD

METABOLITES OF EDIBLE PLANTS

Carcinogens enter the food supply in numerous ways, mostly the result of natural processes. In fact it would be virtually impossible to eat a diet totally devoid of traces of naturally occurring carcinogens.

Carcinogens occur among the normal metabolites of edible plants. One such substance is safrole (Figure 88–1). Safrole is representative of a class of alkenylbenzene derivatives, the natural flavor components of many spices and herbs.[24] For example, safrole itself is found in sassafras, sweet basil, and cinnamon. Estragole, a related carcinogenic alkenylbenzene, is found in tarragon, sweet basil, and anise. Methyleugenol, yet another carcinogenic alkenylbenzene, is found in sweet bay, cloves, and lemongrass.

There are also a number of alkenylbenzene derivatives that appear to be noncarcinogens in rodents: anethole, eugenol, elemicin, myristicin, dill apiol, and parsley apiol. In general the overall dietary levels are low, in the parts-per-million range or less.

The carcinogenic alkenylbenzenes are examples of carcinogens found among the natural products of edible plants. Many such non-nutritive minor components are produced to ward off pests. For example, carcinogens are known to exist among the natural metabolites of parsley, celery, figs, mustard, parsnips, pepper, and citrus oil.[25–27] Some known carcinogenic pesticidal plant products are shown in Table 88–2.

It should be emphasized that all the compounds shown in Table 88–2 are natural. The doses required to produce cancer in rodents greatly exceed dietary exposure. Moreover, many of these xenobiotic rodent carcinogens are known or hypothesized to be anticarcinogens.[10]

MUTAGEN-CARCINOGENS FORMED BY COOKING

Carcinogens also enter the food chain as a result of cooking practices. In particular, cooking meats can generate an array of carcinogenic substances present in the final food at parts-per-billion levels. If, during charcoal grilling, fat from the meat drips onto hot coals and is incinerated, benzo[a]pyrene forms (Fig. 88–1). Smoke containing this carcinogen may then be absorbed to the surface of the meat.

Cooking may also result in the formation of carcinogenic heterocyclic amines that are chemically related to AAF. These carcinogens are particularly potent bacterial mutagens. They readily form in cooked meat, depending on temperature. In general, lower cooking temperatures generate fewer such mutagen-carcinogens.

This discussion is not meant to be exhaustive but rather to illustrate the importance of naturally occurring carcinogens when considering the background "carcinogen burden" that we all are exposed to. Even though ingestion of natural carcinogens is very low, it exceeds the intake of synthetic carcinogens by a factor of at least 10,000.[22,26–28]

MODULATORS OF CARCINOGENESIS IN FOOD

ENHANCEMENT

Non-nutritive Factors. Some non-nutritive dietary substances exhibit tumor-promoting properties in high-dose rodent feeding studies. Examples include certain terpenes found in citrus fruits.[27] However, it is unlikely that such factors exert much influence on human cancer risk. The reasons for this conclusion are that tumor promoters exhibit a threshold below which they are not effective, and exposure to a dose above the threshold must be continual for a prolonged period. There are no known examples of non-nutritive tumor promoters in the United States diet that fulfill these criteria.

Nutrients. Some nutrients exhibit tumor-enhancing properties in model carcinogenesis systems. Usually it is necessary to feed the nutrient at greatly excessive levels. An example is ascorbic acid which, when fed at 5% of the diet, enhances bladder carcinogenesis in rats.[29] But there are exceptions to the high-dose requirement, the most important being the essential fatty acid, linoleic acid. Linoleic acid enhances the development of neoplasia at least at three sites in rodents: mammary gland, pancreas, and colon.[1] Of these, the most thoroughly studied is the enhancement of mammary neoplasia in rats.[30]

The rat mammary neoplasia model system involves giving young female rats a single intragastric dose of 7,12-dimethylbenz[a]anthracene (DMBA), a synthetic polynuclear arene carcinogen that is structurally related to benzo[a]pyrene. DMBA administered in this manner initiates mammary carcinogenesis. The animals are then put on various dietary regimens that may accelerate or slow tumor appearance. Neoplasia is not affected in an absolute sense because virtually all of the DMBA-treated rats will eventually develop carcinomas, irrespective of postcarcinogen treatment. Rather, the model is used to reveal enhancers or inhibitors of tumor appearance.

TABLE 88–2. SOME NATURAL PESTICIDAL CARCINOGENS IN FOOD

RODENT CARCINOGEN	PLANT FOOD	CONCENTRATION (PPM)
5-/8-Methoxypsoralen	Parsley	14
	Parsnip, cooked	32
	Celery	0.8
	Celery, new cultivar	6.2
	Celery, stressed	25
p-hydrazinobenzoate	Mushrooms	11
Glutamyl *p*-hydrazinobenzoate	Mushrooms	42
Sinigrin (allyl isothiocyanate)	Cabbage	35–590
	Collard greens	250–788
	Cauliflower	12–66
	Brussels sprouts	110–1560
	Mustard (brown)	16,000–72,000
	Horseradish	4,500
Estragole	Basil	3,800
	Fennel	3,000
Safrole	Nutmeg	3,000
	Mace	10,000
	Pepper, black	100
Ethyl acrylate	Pineapple	0.07
Sesamol	Sesame seeds (heated oil)	75
α-Methylbenzyl alcohol	Cocoa	1.3
Benzyl acetate	Basil	82
	Jasmine tea	230
	Honey	15
Catechol	Coffee (roasted beans)	100
Caffeic acid	Apple, carrot, celery, cherry, eggplant, endive, grapes, lettuce, pear, plum, potato	50–200
	Absinthe, anise, basil, caraway, dill, marjoram, rosemary, sage, savory, tarragon, thyme	>1,000
	Coffee (roasted beans)	1,800
Chlorogenic acid (caffeic acid)	Apricot, cherry, peach, plum	50–500
	Coffee (roasted beans)	21,600
Neochlorogenic acid (caffeic acid)	Apple, apricot, broccoli, brussels sprouts, cabbage, cherry, kale, peach, pear, plum	50–500
	Coffee (roasted beans)	11,600

(From Ames, B.N., Gold, L.S.: Proc. Natl. Acad. Sci. U.S.A., *87*:7777–7781, 1990.)

In this model linoleic acid is required for mammary tumor development. Moreover, the amount of linoleic acid required for optimal tumor development is about five times the amount required for optimal body growth. The mechanism of linoleic acid enhancement is a subject of much debate and research.

Linoleic acid is the only fatty acid that has been unequivocally shown to enhance mammary carcinogenesis in rats. Although much has been said and written about the effects of "fat type" on carcinogenesis in rodents, these effects seem invariably to come down to linoleic acid content. Those fats with higher levels of linoleic acid (e.g., corn oil) enhance carcinogenesis more than fats with less linoleic acid (e.g., coconut oil, beef tallow, fish oils).[31]

INHIBITION

Both nutrients and non-nutritive factors in foods may exhibit cancer-inhibiting activity in animal experiments. Food-derived xenobiotics may induce cytochrome P-450 enzymes and inhibit carcinogenesis by increasing carcinogen detoxification. Nutrients such as vitamins C and E may act to prevent the formation of carcinogenic nitrosamines in the gastrointestinal tract.[10]

Other nutrients and non-nutritive factors act as antipromoters. Many antipromoters also exhibit anti-initiation activity. That substances that inhibit carcinogenesis under one set of conditions may induce cancer under other conditions greatly complicates the development of an effective strategy for using food-derived anticarcinogens as drugs. Clearly, it is imperative that biochemical mechanisms be thoroughly understood before public health programs based on dietary anticarcinogens are undertaken.

CALORIE EFFECT

Of all the reported effects of diet on experimental carcinogenesis the most effective, generally consistent anticarcinogen that we know of is the calorie effect. Simply put, restricting caloric intake retards the onset of senescence, prolongs life, and lowers the incidence of neoplasia in rodents.

The calorie effect was first demonstrated in the 1930s, and was subsequently reproduced and expanded upon by numerous investigators during the 1940s. It was shown that calorie restriction was effective in inhibiting, at virtually every organ site, neoplasia that developed "spontaneously" or was induced by chemicals, radiation, or viruses. The anticarcinogenic nature of the calorie effect is supported by literally hundreds of independent studies, most of which were conducted prior to 1950. Some selected results are shown in Table 88–3.

More recent investigations with rats by Ross and co-workers established that the risk of developing a spontaneous neoplasm is directly proportional to calorie intake and growth rate *early in life.*[38–40] Protein consumption also appears to be important but in a more complex way. Given that calorie restriction increases life span in rodents it is important to consider cancer risk in terms of longevity. In other words, does calorie restriction decrease cancer risk in an absolute sense, or does it just prolong the period of life prior to cancer development? The data of Ross and co-workers indicate that for rats it is the former—that is, restricted rats developed fewer tumors, developed tumors later in life, lived longer, and died of causes other than cancer.

TABLE 88–3. INHIBITION OF NEOPLASIA BY THE CALORIE EFFECT

INCIDENCE OF NEOPLASIA		
Ad Libitum Feeding	Restricted Feeding	Reference
67%	0%	32
100%	20%	33
50%	30%	34
65%	10%	35
87%	7%	36
82%	18%	37

In investigating the calorie effect, calories are restricted relative to ad libitum feeding (allowing animals free access to food). Historically the restrictions were considerable, up to 60% of the ad libitum consumption level, which was interpreted by some to mean that calorie restriction was unnatural, that calorie-restricted animals were deprived of sufficient food. But calorie-restricted animals, even those restricted to 60% of the ad libitum level of food, are observed to be more active and generally healthier than their counterparts fed ad libitum.

Moreover, one should consider that rodents in the wild do not encounter ad libitum feeding conditions. In fact the survival instinct dictates that when food is freely available rodents will eat to excess. This, in turn, leads to obesity as well as to profound physiologic changes. In their landmark review Doll and Peto commented that "more interest might have been aroused [in the calorie effect] if the freely fed mice had been described as obese instead of the mice on the restricted diet being described as small."[41]

In animals fed ad libitum the adrenal glands atrophy. There is no need to convert amino acids to glucose because eating at will substitutes for the redistribution of body caloric stores, controlled in part by glucocorticoids. Calorie restriction reverses such undesirable effects. A consequence of calorie restriction is increased production of adrenocorticotropic hormone (ACTH) as well as decreased production of gonadotropins, changes viewed as beneficial in terms of cancer protection. For example, Boutwell established that carcinogen-induced skin neoplasia was inhibited by topically applied or systemically administered cortisone,[42] thereby establishing a link between optimal adrenal gland function and the inhibition of tumor formation. On the other hand, prolactin has been shown to promote the development of tumors in the DMBA rat mammary cancer model.[43] It is known that under ad libitum feeding conditions corticosteroid levels are decreased whereas prolactin is increased. Both of these observations would be expected to increase cancer risk, and both are reversed by restricted feeding. Undoubtedly there are other favorable hormonal changes induced as well by calorie restriction. Additionally, in postmenopausal women excessive body fat serves as a source of estrogen, which, when unopposed by progesterone, increases endometrial cancer risk.[1]

A particularly important question concerns the relationship between the calorie effect and the putative enhancement of carcinogenesis in some model systems by dietary fat. The data in Table 88–4 are from an experiment designed to address this issue.[44] The system used is the DMBA rat mammary cancer model.

In this experiment rats were fed one of two isonutrient diets: a low-fat diet containing 5% corn oil by weight, or a high-fat diet containing 30% corn oil by weight. Two

TABLE 88–4. THE EFFECT OF DIETARY FAT LEVEL AND RESTRICTED FEEDING ON CARCINOGEN-INDUCED RAT MAMMARY CARCINOGENESIS

	DIETARY REGIMEN		
	High-Fat Ad Libitum	Low-Fat Ad Libitum	High-Fat Restricted
Kilocalories consumed per day	41	42	34
Fat consumed per day	2.7	0.6	2.2
Carcass weight (g)	217	190	182
Percentage of body fat	24%	16%	25%
Linoleic acid consumed per day (g)	1.5	0.3	1.2
Tumor incidence	73%	43%	7%

(Data from Boissonneault, G.A., Elson, C.E., Pariza, M.W.: J. Natl. Cancer Res., *76*:335–338, 1986.)

feeding conditions were used: ad libitum and modestly restricted (calorie intake was more than 80% of control levels).

Let us first compare the groups fed ad libitum. Calorie consumption was similar, but corn oil supplied most of the calories in the high-fat group whereas most of the calories in the low-fat group were from carbohydrate (because the diets were isonutrient, protein intake was identical). Animals on the high-fat diet weighed more than those on the low-fat diet because of differences in body fat stores. More mammary tumors developed in the high-fat group (73% versus 43%), probably a reflection of differences in linoleic acid intake.

The high-fat restricted group adds a new dimension to the experiment. This group ate about 20% fewer calories (roughly the human equivalent of giving up a midnight snack) yet substantially more fat and linoleic acid than the low-fat group fed ad libitum. This group matured at a smaller body size, but was proportionately just as "fat" as the high-fat rats fed ad libitum. The tumor incidence for this group was just 7%.

The data given in Table 88–4, which have been verified in other studies,[45] clearly show that the calorie effect is far more important in determining mammary cancer risk in this model than are the intakes of dietary fat or linoleic acid.

EPIDEMIOLOGY

To this point we have considered experimental data derived principally from rodent models. Animal experiments can be conducted with great precision using defined diets and rigorously controlled conditions. However, one must use caution in extrapolating the data to man. By contrast the great strength of epidemiologic studies is that they are conducted with human subjects. This strength, however, is also a weakness in that confounding variables are difficult to control.

There are many types of epidemiologic investigations. In the simplest case the incidence of cancer in various countries is compared with differences in the per capita consumption of selected foods or food components. These are called international correlational studies. Using this technique a relationship between fat consumption and the incidence of breast cancer is observed. However, epidemiologists consider the international correlational study to be the weakest kind of epidemiologic investigation because of the numerous uncontrolled, confounding variables that are inherently present in the data. Hence, the correlations observed in such studies should not be taken as causal. The correlation between fat consumption and breast cancer seen in international correlational studies does not necessarily mean that eating fat increases a woman's risk of developing that disease. (In fact, the great preponderance of epidemiologic evidence now indicates that dietary fat intake does not correlate with breast cancer risk,[41,46–49] as discussed later.)

Another type of epidemiologic investigation is the case-control study. In this design, the eating habits of individuals with cancer are compared with the eating habits of cancer-free controls matched for age, sex, and ethnic background. This type of epidemiologic investigation is considered stronger than the international correlational studies because more variables can be identified and accounted for. Interestingly the relationships between dietary factors (including fat) and cancer risk (including breast cancer) are much weaker in case-control investigations than in international correlational studies. For example, of 13 case control studies conducted between 1975 and 1986, an association between fat intake and breast cancer was observed in only one.[48]

The strongest type of epidemiologic investigation is the prospective (or cohort) study, where dietary habits of subjects are determined prior to cancer development. The prospective studies to date have provided virtually no support for a causal link between fat consumption and breast cancer risk.[47,49]

By contrast evidence is emerging that body size and stature, as well as energy expenditure, may play a role in determining risk. Specifically, smaller body size and mass, and regular exercise, may be protective. These findings fit well with the experimental data discussed previously.

Epidemiologic observations indicate that alcohol consumption may also be positively associated with breast cancer risk. In developed populations alcohol accounts for extra caloric intake.[49]

Although support has steadily waned over the past decade for the hypothesis that dietary fat increases breast cancer risk, the question of colon cancer risk versus fat intake is still open. A review of 24 epidemiologic studies revealed no consistent trend.[50] The uncertainty within the data was underscored by Kolonel and LeMarchand, who wrote ". . . one cannot firmly conclude that dietary fat either promotes or has no effect on colon carcinogenesis in humans."[51]

Willett et al. completed a prospective epidemiologic study among women.[52] They reported a positive association between colon cancer and the consumption of red meat (beef, pork, and lamb). No association was found between red meat or fat consumption and breast cancer, or between dairy fat intake and cancer risk of either the colon or the breast.

At almost the same time a smaller case-control study of colorectal cancer and adenoma in Japan was published. This report concluded that ". . . intakes of animal and vegetable fat-rich foods, especially meats, were associated with decreases in risks of both adenoma and cancer, though the association with cancer was not statistically significant."[53]

In the Japanese study "meat" apparently included chicken as well as pork and beef. In the study of Willett and co-workers chicken was correlated with decreased colon cancer risk. Moreover, moderate meat consumption for an American is no doubt high for a Japanese national. However, the findings of these two reports that appeared in the literature at about the same time point up the difficulties of reaching specific conclusions concerning fat and colon cancer risk, particularly for populations consuming very different diets. Dietary calcium and fiber, total caloric intake, physical activity, and genetics are among the additional factors that should be considered. For example, if excessive dietary fat is involved in the cause of colon cancer then perhaps this effect is offset by adequate dietary levels of calcium and fiber. Obviously, it is difficult to observe the entire range of such interactions in any single epidemiologic study.

TABLE 88–5. DIETARY RECOMMENDATIONS TO MINIMIZE CANCER RISK

1. Reduce intake of both saturated and unsaturated fats, from 40 to 30% of total calories.
2. Include fruits, vegetables, and whole-grain cereal products in daily diet, especially citrus and carotene-rich and cabbage family vegetables; avoid high-dose supplements of individual nutrients.
3. Minimize consumption of cured, pickled, and smoked foods.
4. Drink alcohol only in moderation.

(From Committee on Diet, Nutrition and Cancer, Assembly of Life Sciences, National Research Council: Diet, Nutrition and Cancer. Washington, D.C., National Academy Press, 1982.)

PERSPECTIVE

In 1982 the Diet, Nutrition and Cancer committee of the National Research Council developed a set of specific dietary guidelines for the purpose of reducing cancer risk (Table 88–5).[54] These recommendations were incorporated with few changes in the 1989 NRC "Diet and Health" reports which presented a set of dietary guidelines for reducing the risk of chronic diseases.[54,55] In light of the many new research findings of the past 10 years it may be instructive to review these recommendations.

The first, to reduce dietary fat intake as a means of reducing cancer risk, was considered by the committee to be the strongest. The underlying evidence, however, was far from clear-cut.[46] Since then, support has declined substantially for the hypothesis that fat ingestion increases the risk of developing breast cancer.[41,46–49] A possible role for dietary fat in the cause of colon cancer remains open but unproved. For example, in the study of Willett et al. red meat was correlated with increased colon cancer risk.[52] However, animal fat was less strongly correlated, in part because there was no relation between cancer risk and the intake of dairy fat. Fat from plant sources was not linked to increased risk either. There are many good reasons to moderate fat intake in accordance with life style, but one might wonder if a continued emphasis on dietary fat, implying that it is proved to be a principal etiologic factor for cancer in humans, is in fact warranted.

Although the dietary fat/cancer link remains open, scientific support for the second recommendation (Table 88–5), to eat adequate amounts of fruit, vegetables, and cereal grains as a means of reducing risk, has grown.[45,56] Substantial epidemiologic evidence now indicates that fruit and vegetable consumption is protective. The reasons may be many, including the presence of numerous anticarcinogens in plant-based foods and the fact that plant-based foods are generally lower in calories.

The third recommendation of the Diet, Nutrition and Cancer committee (Table 88–5), to minimize consumption of cured, pickled, and smoked foods, was the most controversial of the set.[46] The confusion it engendered persists to this day. The recommendation was based on the observation that in some parts of the world where large amounts of heavily smoked, pickled, and/or salt-cured foods are consumed daily, the death rate from certain cancers, especially stomach cancer, is high.

Traditional methods of food preservation used in those areas are also known to contaminate food with carcinogenic heterocyclic amines, polynuclear arenes, and nitrosamines.[57]

In the United States, however, stomach cancer is much less common. Additionally there are few if any foods routinely available in American supermarkets that are preserved by the methods of smoking, pickling, or salt-curing used in those parts of the world where stomach cancer risk is high. Commercial food preservation methods used in the United States are carefully controlled so as to preclude carcinogen contamination.[46] Hence the advice in recommendation 3 might make sense for some parts of the world, but the United States is not among them.

The final recommendation, to minimize alcohol consumption (Table 88–5), makes sense for a lot of reasons. As discussed previously there is good reason to conclude that excessive alcohol consumption is linked to increased cancer risk.

A year before the National Research Council's Diet, Nutrition and Cancer committee report was issued, Doll and Peto summarized their exhaustive review on the causes of human cancer by saying that "by far the largest reliably known percentage is the 30% of current U.S. cancer deaths that are due to tobacco, although it is possible that some nutritional factor(s) may eventually be found to be of comparable importance."[41]

Although much experimental and epidemiologic research has been conducted since, we still have not identified a nutritional factor that is central in determining cancer risk. It may be that the key to the diet/cancer puzzle lies in nutrient interactions coupled with individual response to dietary factors, determined in turn by genetic, physiologic, and life-style factors. Given the recent rapid strides in the areas of cancer biochemistry and molecular biology, we may look forward to the day when optimal dietary and lifestyle guidelines can be tailored on an individual basis.

What might be done in the interim? Doll suggests a strategy of encouraging increased consumption of fruits, vegetables, and fiber.[56] He cautions that this approach may be justified so long as care is taken to distinguish between advice based on established knowledge and that based on best guesses. Henderson et al. recommend moderating animal fat intake as a possible means of reducing colon cancer risk while pointing out that this approach is unlikely to affect the risk of developing breast or prostate cancer.[58] This advice is advocated by others as well.[45] It fits with major dietary goals and guidelines (see Chap. 93). One might add only that in light of the public confusion that surrounds this issue a certain amount of reassurance also seems in order, particularly in areas where concern is misplaced, such as pesticides and smoked, pickled, or salted foods.

REFERENCES

1. Pariza, M.W., Simopoulos, A.P. (eds.): Am. J. Clin. Nutr., *45(Suppl.)*:149–372, 1987.
2. Cliver, D.O. (ed.): Foodborne Diseases. New York, Academic Press, 1990.
3. Hsieh, D.P.H.: Carcinogenic potential of mycotoxins in food. *In* Food Toxicology. Edited by S.L. Taylor and R.A. Scanlan. New York, Marcel Dekker, 1989.
4. Munro, I.C.: A case study: The safety of artificial sweeteners. *In* Food Toxicology. Edited by S.L. Taylor and R.A. Scanlan. New York, Marcel Dekker, 1989.
5. Foster, E.M.: Food Tech., *6*:82–93, 1982.
6. Sato, S.: Regulatory perspective: Japan. *In* Mutagens and Carcinogens in the Diet. Edited by M.W. Pariza, H.-U. Aeschbacher, J.S. Felton, and S. Sato. New York, Wiley-Liss, 1990.
7. Boutwell, R.K.: Tumor promoters in human carcinogenesis. *In* Important Advances in Oncology. Edited by V.T. DeVita Jr., S. Hellman, and S.A. Rosenberg. Philadelphia, J.B. Lippincott, 1985.
8. Miller, J.A.: Cancer Res., *30*:559–576, 1970.
9. Swenson, D.H., Lin, J.K., Miller, E.C., et al.: Cancer Res., *37*:172–181, 1976.
10. Wattenberg, L.W.: Cancer Res., *43*:2448s–2453s, 1983.
11. Gould, M.N., Wacker, W.D., Maltzman, T.H.: Chemoprevention and chemotherapy of mammary tumors by monoterpenoids. *In* Mutagens and Carcinogens in the Diet. Edited by M.W. Pariza, H.-U. Aeschbacher, J.S. Felton, and S. Sato. New York, Wiley-Liss, 1990.
12. Ha, Y.L., Storkson, J., Pariza, M.W.: Cancer Res., *50*:1097–1101, 1990.
13. Ip, C., Chin, S.F., Scimeca, J.A., et al.: Cancer Res., *51*:6118–6124, 1991.
14. Peraino, C., Fry, R.J.M., Staffeldt, E., et al.: Cancer Res., *35*:2884–2890, 1975.
15. Wattenberg, L.W., Loub, W.D., Lam, L.K., et al.: Fed. Proc., *35*:1327–1331, 1976.
16. Chhabra, R.S., Huff, J.E., Schwetz, B.S., et al.: Environ. Health Perspect., *86*:313–321, 1990.
17. Ames, B.N., Gold, L.S.: Science, *251*:12–13, 1991.
18. Ames, B.N., Gold, L.S.: Science, *249*:970–971, 1990.
19. Cohen, S.M., Ellwein, L.B.: Science, *249*:1007–1011, 1990.
20. Ames, B.N., McCann, J., Yamasaki, E.: Mutation Res., *331*:347–364, 1975.
21. Ames, B.N.: Science, *221*:1256–1264, 1983.
22. Hall, R.L., Dull, B.J., Henry, S.H., et al.: Comparison of the carcinogenic risks of naturally occurring and adventitious substances in food. *In* Food Toxicology. Edited by S.L. Taylor and R.A. Scanlan. New York, Marcel Dekker, 1989.
23. Ames, B.N., Magaw, M., Gold, L.S.: Science, *236*:271–280, 1987.

24. Miller, E.C., Swanson, A.B., Phillips, D.H., et al.: Cancer Res., *43:*1124–1134, 1983.
25. Ames, B.N., Gold, L.S.: Proc. Natl. Acad. Sci. U.S.A., *87:*7772–7776, 1990.
26. Ames, B.N., Gold, L.S.: Proc. Natl. Acad. Sci. U.S.A., *87:*7777–7781, 1990.
27. Ames, B.N., Gold, L.S.: Proc. Natl. Acad. Sci. U.S.A., *87:*7781–7786, 1990.
28. Roe, F.J.C., Pierce, W.E.H.: J. Natl. Cancer Inst., *24:*1389–1403, 1960.
29. Fukushima, S., Imaida, K., Sakata, T., et al.: Cancer Res., *43:*4454–4457, 1983.
30. Ip, C., Carter, C.A., Ip, M.M.: Cancer Res., *45:*1997–2001, 1985.
31. Pariza, M.W.: Annu. Rev. Nutr., *8:*167–183, 1988.
32. Visscher, M.B., Ball, Z.B., Barnes, R.H., et al.: Surgery, *11:*48–55, 1942.
33. White, F.R., White, J.: J. Natl. Cancer Inst., *5:*41–42, 1944.
34. Larsen, C.D., Heston, W.E.: J. Natl. Cancer Inst., *6:*31–40, 1945.
35. Saxton, J.A., Boon, M.C., Furth, J.: Cancer Res., 401–409, 1944.
36. Rusch, H.P., Kline, B.E., Baumann, C.A.: Cancer Res., *5:*431–435, 1945.
37. Boutwell, R.K., Brush, M.K., Rusch, H.P.: Cancer Res., *9:*741–746, 1949.
38. Ross, M.H., Bras, G.: J. Nutr., *87:*245–260, 1965.
39. Ross, M.H., Bras, G.: J. Nutr., *103:*944–963, 1973.
40. Ross, M.H., Lustbader, E.D., Bras, G.: J. Natl. Cancer Inst., *71:*947–954, 1983.
41. Doll, R., Peto, R.: J. Natl. Cancer Inst., *66:*1191–1308, 1981.
42. Boutwell, R.K.: Prog. Exp. Tumor Res., *4:*207–250, 1964.
43. Clifton, K.H., Crowley, J.J.: Cancer Res., *38:*1507–1513, 1978.
44. Boissonneault, G.A., Elson, C.E., Pariza, M.W.: J. Natl. Cancer Res., *76:*335–338, 1986.
45. Boutwell, R.K.: Opportunities for nutritional scientists in cancer prevention. *In* Mutagens and Carcinogens in the Diet. Edited by M.W. Pariza, H.-U. Aeschbacher, J.S. Felton, and S. Sato. New York, Wiley-Liss, 1990.
46. Pariza, M.W.: JAMA, *251:*1455–1458, 1984.
47. Willett, W.: Nutritional Epidemiology. New York, Oxford University Press, 1990.
48. Goodwin, P.J., Boyd, N.F.: J. Natl. Cancer. Inst., *79:*473–485, 1987.
49. Kritchevsky, D.: Cancer, *66:*1321–1325, 1990.
50. Rogers, A.E., Longnecker, M.P.: Lab. Invest., *59:*729–759, 1988.
51. Kolonel, L.N., LeMarchand, L.: Prog. Clin. Biol. Res., *222:*69–91, 1986.
52. Willett, W.W., Stampfer, M.J., Colditz, G.A., et al.: N. Engl. J. Med., *323:*1664–1670, 1990.
53. Kato, I., Tominaga, S., Matsuura, A., et al.: Jpn. J. Cancer Res., *81:*1101–1108, 1990.
54. Committee on Diet, Nutrition and Cancer, Assembly of Life Sciences, National Research Council: Diet, Nutrition and Cancer. Washington, D.C., National Academy Press, 1982.
55. Committee on Diet and Health, Food and Nutrition Board, Commission on Life Sciences National Research Council: Diet and Health: Implications for Reducing Elsonic Disease Risk. Washington, D.C., National Academy Press, 1989.
56. Doll, R.: J. Cancer Res. Clin. Oncol., *114:*447–458, 1988.
57. Knudsen, I. (ed.): Genetic Toxicology of the Diet. New York, Alan R. Liss, 1986.
58. Henderson, B.E., Ross, R.K., Pike, M.C.: Science, *254:*1131–1138, 1991.

SELECTED READINGS

CARCINOGENS IN FOOD AND CARCINOGEN RISK ASSESSMENTS

Ames, B.N., Gold, L.S.: Chemical carcinogenesis: too many rodent carcinogens. Proc. Natl. Acad. Sci. U.S.A., *87:*7772–7776, 1990.
Ames, B.N., Profet, M., Gold, L.S.: Nature's chemicals and synthetic chemicals: comparative toxicology. Proc. Natl. Acad. Sci. U.S.A., *87:*7782–7786, 1990.
Ames, B.N., Profet, M., Gold, L.S.: Dietary pesticides (99.99% all natural). Proc. Natl. Acad. Sci. U.S.A., *87:*7777–7781, 1990.
Pariza, M.W.: A new approach to evaluating carcinogenic risk. Proc. Natl. Acad. Sci. U.S.A., *89:*860–861, 1992.

NUTRITION AND CANCER

Doll, R.: Epidemiology and the prevention of cancer: some recent developments. J. Cancer Res. Clin. Oncol., *114:*447–458, 1988.
Henderson, B.E., Ross, R.K., Pike, M.C.: Toward the primary prevention of cancer. Science, *254:*1131–1138, 1991.
Willett, W.: Nutritional Epidemiology. New York, Oxford University Press, 1990.
Willett, W.C., Stampfer, M.J.: Dietary fat and cancer: another view. Cancer Causes Control, *1:*103–109, 1990.

CHAPTER 89

Osteoporosis

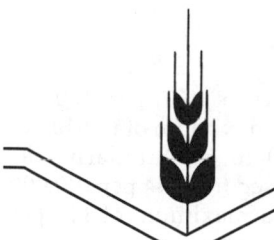

Elizabeth A. Krall and Bess Dawson-Hughes

Osteoporosis is a reduction in bone mass that renders an individual susceptible to fracture with a moderate degree of trauma. Osteoporosis and its link to the menopause were described by Albright 50 years ago.[1] At the time, immobilization, metabolic disease, and diet were recognized causes. Bone mass throughout the life span is determined by a number of environmental and genetic factors including age of menopause, body height and weight, physical activity, smoking, and alcohol use in addition to dietary intake of calcium, vitamin D, and other nutrients. The mechanisms by which these factors influence bone mass are diverse and not completely understood. However, it is apparent that the influences of the individual risk factors vary with age, sex, and ethnicity. Furthermore, a number of risk factors are interactive. For example, smoking has been associated with decreased absorption of calcium. Osteoporosis can also develop secondary to conditions such as hyperparathyroidism, hyperthyroidism, or hypogonadism. Thyroid hormone, glucocorticoids, and anticonvulsants are some of the medications known to accelerate bone loss. Nutrition, however, remains of critical interest in this multifactorial disease because diet can be safely modified.

BONE COMPOSITION

Bone tissue is a matrix of collagen fibers and other proteins onto which minerals are deposited. Calcium and phosphorus, which together with water constitute the hydroxyapatite crystals of bone, are the two most abundant minerals in bone. Two types of bone structure exist, cortical and trabecular. Outer surfaces of the appendicular and much of the axial skeleton are composed of cortical bone. This compact bone forms a thin covering at certain skeletal sites and composes the majority of bone tissue at others. Trabecular bone derives its name from the network of plates and rods (trabeculae) that interconnect the interior surfaces of cortical layers and surround the spaces in which marrow is found.

Bone undergoes continuous remodeling in cycles of resorption, formation, and quiescence. Osteoclasts resorb bone, forming localized cavities on a bone surface. During the formation phase, osteoblasts refill the cavities by laying down bone matrix proteins, which then become mineralized. Net bone loss occurs when, throughout the skeleton, the amount of bone resorbed exceeds the amount formed.

Bone remodeling is influenced by several hormones. Parathyroid hormone (PTH) stimulates and calcitonin inhibits bone resorption. Both of these hormones are regulated by the serum calcium level. PTH is secreted in response to low, and calcitonin to high, calcium concentrations. In addition to its bone resorbing action, PTH stimulates the formation of 1,25-dihydroxyvitamin D ($1,25(OH)_2D$), which in turn enhances intestinal calcium absorption. PTH also reduces calcium loss via the urine. The functions of these hormones are described in more detail in the chapters on calcium and vitamin D.

EPIDEMIOLOGY OF BONE LOSS AND FRACTURES

For several years after longitudinal growth has ceased, bones continue to increase in mass, reaching a peak during the third or fourth decade of life. The age of onset of bone loss varies by skeletal site. Bone loss occurs in both sexes and in different ethnic groups, although studies of white women provide the most extensive data on the pattern of bone loss.

PATTERNS OF BONE LOSS

Longitudinal studies confirm that some loss from the spine occurs before menopause.[2,3] Accelerated rates of loss at the spine, approximately 3 to 6% annually, have been reported during the first 5 years after cessation of menses, with a reduction in the rate thereafter.[2,4] Cross-sectional studies suggest that women also lose bone from the hip before menopause (approximately 10% between ages 20 and 40 years), and that the rate of bone loss increases around the time of menopause.[5] Longitudinal studies are not yet available to confirm this. Bone loss at the radius among women appears to be negligible before menopause and to occur at the rate of about 1% per year after menopause.[6]

Men between the ages of 20 and 90 years lose bone at a fairly constant rate. Cross-sectional data indicate that bone loss from the femoral neck and Ward's triangle are 0.5 and 0.7% per year, respectively.[7] Age-related loss from the trochanter region is less. Longitudinal data reveal that men lose bone at annual rates of 2% from the spine and 1% from the radius.[8] Thus, the rates of bone loss in men are fairly similar to those of women who are 6 or more years beyond menopause.

FRACTURES

The majority of fractures among children and adults under age 30 result from severe trauma so that the probability of fracture at these ages is not highly dependent on bone mass. After age 30, incidence rates rise sharply and an increasing proportion of fractures occur with moderate trauma. At most skeletal sites, rates of fracture are higher in white women than in white men or black women, reflecting gender and ethnic variations in average bone density. Rates at specific sites are discussed in more detail.

Radius. The white female-to-male incidence ratios of forearm fracture range from 2:1 at age 35 to more than 8:1 after age 80.[9] The incidence of fractures of the distal radius (Colles' fracture) among women in Rochester, Minnesota increased from a rate of 107 per 100,000 person-years at ages 35 to 39 to a maximum of to 640 per 100,000 person-years at ages 60 to 64. Similarly, the radial fracture rate in men increased from 44 per 100,000 person-years at ages 35 to 39 to a maximum of 118 per 100,000 person-years at ages 50 to 54.

Femur. Beginning at age 40, the rate of hip fracture doubles about every 6 or 7 years in men and women in the United States.[10] At ages 80 to 84, the annual incidence rate of femoral fracture in white women is 1731 per 100,000 compared to 735 per 100,000 in white men. This excess risk associated with gender is observed in whites, but among blacks in the United States, the difference in hip fracture rates between women and men is small (940 and 610 per 100,000 per year, respectively).[10] International comparisons indicate variability in the rates of femoral fractures among ethnic groups. For example, the prevalence of hip fracture among Chinese women in Hong Kong was intermediate between those of blacks and whites in other countries.[11] Of all osteoporotic fractures, those at the hip are associated with the highest risk of death and disability.

Spine. Spine fractures associated with osteoporosis often take the form of compression fractures or loss of vertebral height. Among white women living in Rochester, Minnesota, the fracture rate increased from 500 per 100,000 person-years at ages 50 to 54 to 3800 per 100,000 person-years above age 80.[12] The true incidence of spinal osteoporosis may be underestimated because, unlike fractures at other sites, vertebral compression fractures do not necessarily cause severe symptoms and thus may remain undiagnosed.

The prevalence of spine fractures in women in the United States increases from 5% at ages 50 to 54 to over 50% in women over age 80.[12] In a randomly chosen population in Israel, the prevalence of vertebral fractures among women was 3% in the 65 to 74 age group and 6% in the 75 to 84 age group.[13] In comparison, the prevalence of vertebral fractures in men aged 65 to 84 was consistently less than 1%.

Other Sites. Rates of pelvic fractures occurring with moderate trauma in women in Rochester, Minnesota rose from 27 per 100,000 at ages 35 to 54 to 250 per 100,000 over age 75.[14] In men, the rates rose from 0 to 64 per 100,000 in comparable age strata. Fractures of the humerus displayed a similar gender-specific pattern, rising from 120 at ages 50 to 69 to 317 per 100,000 after age 70 in women, and from 27 to 51 per 100,000 men of the same ages.[15] Exceptions to this pattern of excess risk in women have been noted for ankle fracture among persons over age 65,[16] and for femoral fractures in two districts in Yugoslavia.[17]

BONE MINERAL DENSITY AND FRACTURE RISK

A reduction in bone mass or bone density is associated with diminished bone strength and with an increase in fracture risk. Low bone mass is not the only characteristic that influences fracture risk. Others include thinning and discontinuity of trabeculae and accumulation of microfracture damage. The propensity to fall and the protective effect of muscle and fat tissue also influence probability of fracture.

Fracture is the most important event that defines osteoporosis. Although the ranges of bone mineral density (BMD) values of osteoporotic patients overlap those of healthy age-matched controls, the ability of bone mass measurements to predict fracture risk at the same site or other sites has been demonstrated.[18–21] Fractures at nonspine sites are predicted by distal radius mass[18–21] and heel density,[18,20] often more effectively than knowledge of many other known risk factors except age.[21] Because of this, bone mass measurements are widely used in the investigation of causes and treatment of osteoporosis.

NUTRITIONAL DETERMINANTS OF BONE MASS AND FRACTURE RISK

A number of nutritional factors have been investigated in relation to osteoporosis risk because of their presence in bone or their influence on calcium metabolism. Calcium, phosphorus, and trace minerals are mineral components of bone; thus, at different times in the lifespan, intakes of these nutrients might be expected to affect bone mass. Protein and trace minerals can also influence calcium and phosphorus balance. It is helpful to examine associations between diet and bone mass in terms of developmental stage, menopausal status, and habitual intakes of the subjects studied. Because longitudinal studies measure bone loss directly and randomly selected control groups reflect influences of extraneous factors, studies of this design (randomized, controlled) provide the most valid means of assessing the effects of nutrient or other interventions on change in bone density.

CALCIUM

Calcium Intake and Peak Bone Mass. Although a positive effect is expected, it has not been demonstrated in a prospective study that increasing calcium intake of children and adolescents will increase their peak bone mass. Evidence suggesting that calcium is important comes from cross-sectional studies. In two districts of Yugoslavia, men and women in the district with average calcium intakes of 20.3 to 27.1 mmol (812 to 1087 mg) per day had higher metacarpal bone density than those in the district where average intakes were 8.6 to 12.9 mmol (343 to 517 mg) calcium daily.[17] Differences in bone density in the two communities became less pronounced with age. One interpretation of these findings was that calcium intake had more influence on development of peak bone mass than on subsequent rates of loss.

Estimated calcium intake in early adulthood was positively correlated with bone density of the radius and vertebrae of premenopausal women.[22,23] Errors associated with retrospective diet assessment and presence of other influences on bone that occur in intervening years do not allow firm conclusions to be made from these studies, however. Because of increasing evidence that bone mass continues to build for several years after full height is achieved, and the likelihood that higher calcium intake results in higher peak bone mass, the recommended dietary allowance (RDAs) of calcium for adults between the ages of 18 and 24 years was recently raised from 20 mmol (800 mg) to 29.9 mmol (1200 mg) per day.[24]

Calcium Intake and Bone Loss in Premenopausal and Postmenopausal Women.

Premenopausal. Prospective studies have now demonstrated that increasing calcium intake from food sources from 22.5 to 37.4 mmol (900 to 1500 mg) daily prevents bone loss from the spine in premenopausal adult women (Fig. 89–1).[25] A similar level of calcium supplementation retarded bone loss at the humerus but not at the radius or ulna.[26] The effect of added calcium on hip density in this age group is unknown.

Cross-sectional[27–29] and observational[30] studies of

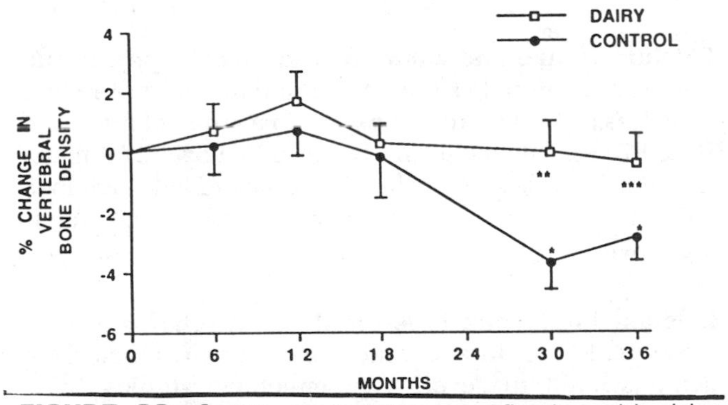

FIGURE 89–1. Effect of dietary modification with dairy products on vertebral bone density in premenopausal women. Values represent the mean ± s.e. of the bone density as a percentage of initial density. * Significantly different from baseline, $p<0.001$; ** significantly different from control, $p<0.02$; *** significantly different from control, $p = 0.05$. (From Baran, D., Sorensen, A., Grimes, J., et al.: Dietary modification with dairy products for preventing vertebral bone loss in premenopausal women: a three-year prospective study. J. Clin. Endocrinol. Metab., *70*:264–270, 1989, by permission of the Endocrine Society.)

bone mass and calcium intake in premenopausal women offer conflicting results that may have resulted in part from different diet assessment methods and the presence of other environmental factors that impact on bone density.

Early Menopausal. Not only do rates of bone loss in early menopause differ from those in later years,[4] but the responsiveness of bone to calcium and other interventions appears to be affected by menopausal age as well. In women within the first few years of menopause, the addition of 49.9 mmol (2000 mg) of calcium to a mean habitual intake of about 25.0 mmol (1000 mg) per day slowed the rate of bone loss from the proximal radius slightly, but had no effect on loss from the spine or distal radius.[31] Similarly, a limited responsiveness to added calcium has been observed in women with low, i.e., under 16.2 mmol (650 mg),[32] and moderate (16.2 to 21.2 mmol; (650 to 850 mg)[33] usual intakes.

Later Menopausal. As women pass beyond the perimenopausal period of rapid bone loss, they become more responsive to supplementation with calcium, at least in those with low usual intakes. In healthy women 12 years beyond menopause with low usual calcium intakes, daily supplementation for 2 years with 12.5 mmol (500 mg) of elemental calcium as citrate malate prevented bone loss from the spine, femoral neck, and radius.[32] A similar dose of calcium carbonate was effective at the femoral neck and radius. A less striking effect of supplementation is seen in women with higher usual dietary intakes of calcium.[32,34] In older women with a previous history of Colles' fracture, those taking placebo lost more from the femoral neck than a group supplemented with 25 mmol (1 g) of calcium daily.[35]

Calcium Intake and Bone Loss in Men. Supplementation with 25 mmol (1 g) of calcium daily did not reduce bone loss from the radius or spine in a group of men aged 30 to 87 years who habitually consumed over 27.4 mmol (1100 mg) per day.[8] The effectiveness of added calcium in men with lower usual dietary intakes of calcium is unknown.

Calcium Intake and Fracture Rates. A relationship between calcium intake and bone fractures has been demonstrated in several epidemiologic studies.[17,36,37] During a follow-up period of 14 years, individuals over age 50 who fractured a hip were found to have consumed less calcium at entry into the study than those who remained fracture-free.[36] Men and women who consumed less than 11.7 mmol (470 mg) daily had fracture rates two and one half times greater than those who consumed 19.1 mmol (765 mg) or more. Among women in Yugoslavia over 75 years of age, hip fractures occurred at a rate of 15 per 10,000 persons per year in the high-calcium district compared to 54 per 10,000 in the low-calcium district.[17] Rates of hip fracture among men of the same age were 11 and 30 per 10,000 per year in the high- and low-calcium districts, respectively. Forearm fracture rates were not different in the two districts. Among men aged 50 and older in Britain, calcium intakes less than 26.0 mmol (1041 mg) per day were associated with about a sixfold elevation in relative risk of hip fracture compared to intakes over 26.0 mmol when other risk factors were taken into account.[37] However, no association between calcium intake and fracture risk was seen in the women.

Summary of Calcium Intake and Bone Mass. It is unknown whether increasing calcium intake of children and adolescents will have an impact on peak bone density or future risk of fracture. In premenopausal adult women, increased dairy food intake appears to slow the rate of vertebral bone loss. Increasing calcium intake of women within the first 5 years after menopause is effective in slowing but not eliminating bone loss from the radius. Vertebral bone loss in these women is unresponsive to calcium, and the effect of calcium on loss at the hip is unknown. These variations in the responsiveness may be related to differing proportions of trabecular and cortical tissue or to differences in weight-bearing or hormonal sensitivity at different skeletal sites. In older postmenopausal women with low usual calcium intakes, added calcium reduced bone loss from the spine, femoral neck, and radius. In older women with higher usual intakes, the effect of different doses of added calcium on rate of bone loss from the spine and hip is unknown.

VITAMIN D

Vitamin D is obtained from the diet and is also synthesized in the skin after exposure to sunlight. It is hydroxylated to 25-hydroxyvitamin D (25(OH)D) in the liver and then to $1,25(OH)_2D$ in the kidney. The active metabolite, $1,25(OH)_2D$, stimulates calcium absorption from the intestine and is also necessary for the maintenance of normal bone. The most widely used clinical indicator of vitamin D status is the plasma level of 25(OH)D. Although plasma 25(OH)D reflects both dietary and endogenous contributions, sunlight exposure appears to have a stronger influence on 25(OH)D level than diet at vitamin D intakes typical in the United States and Europe. However, diet takes on increased importance in wintertime at high latitudes in healthy adults, and throughout the year in individuals who have limited sun exposure or a diminished ability to synthesize the vitamin cutaneously. In the United States and Europe, older persons ingest an average of around 2.5 μg (100 IU) per day, a value far below the recommended dietary allowance in the United States of 5 μg (200 IU) per day.[24]

With age, serum PTH concentration rises and plasma levels of both 25(OH)D and $1,25(OH)_2D$ decline. These hormonal changes coincide with age-related bone loss, but a causal relationship has not been established.

The concentrations of 25(OH)D, $1,25(OH)_2D$, and PTH also vary with the season. In winter, at least at higher latitudes, PTH rises and 25(OH)D, and probably also $1,25(OH)_2D$, decline. The wintertime changes in 25(OH)D and PTH are most striking in those with vitamin D intakes below 5 μg (200 IU).[38] The significance to bone remodeling rate of seasonal variation in calcium-regulating hormones has not been established. Although it has been reported by some,[39,40] not all investigators have observed seasonal variation in bone mass or rates of bone loss.[41] Such variation in rates of bone loss may occur only if calcium intake is low or may be related to other environmental factors such as level of physical activity.

A role for vitamin D insufficiency in the evolution of osteoporosis has been postulated. Blood levels of 25(OH)D and $1,25(OH)_2D$, as well as intestinal calcium absorption, are frequently lower in osteoporotic patients than in age-matched controls.[42,43] Both the $1,25(OH)_2D$ level and calcium absorption can be increased by administration of $1,25(OH)_2D$. If vitamin D insufficiency is a cause of osteoporosis, then supplementation with vitamin D would be expected to retard bone loss and prevent fractures. The results of several controlled $1,25(OH)_2D$ intervention trials in postmenopausal women are summarized in Table 89–1. Because $1,25(OH)_2D$ supplementation is sometimes associated with hypercalciuria and hypercalcemia, doses of $1,25(OH)_2D$ and calcium intake differ among subjects within some studies. Although the number of years since menopause was reported in only two studies,[44,45] the mean ages in others were over age 64, so it may be assumed most subjects were in the later menopausal period.

In osteoporotic women, positive effects of $1,25(OH)_2D$ treatment on incidence of vertebral fractures and on rate of bone loss have been observed by some investigators[44,46] but not by others.[47]

Rates of bone loss in healthy women in early menopause did not appear responsive to $1,25(OH)_2D$ treatment,[45] and in older, mostly healthy women, treatment resulted in a slight reduction in vertebral height.[18] Failure to find consistent effects of $1,25(OH)_2D$ treatment on bone mass and fracture incidence may reflect differences in dietary vitamin D and calcium status of the study subjects or differences in their capacity to produce $1,25(OH)_2D$. Providing more $1,25(OH)_2D$ to individuals who are vitamin D replete may offer no additional benefit. Similarly, administration of $1,25(OH)_2D$ without adequate calcium may not retard bone resorption.

PHOSPHORUS

Unlike calcium, phosphorus intake is rarely deficient because this mineral is available in a large variety of foods. Although a small proportion of the population may be at risk of phosphate depletion, excessive phosphorus intake rather than deficiency has been a greater concern with regard to osteoporosis. This concern stems from observations that a high phosphorus intake raises the serum phosphorus level, which in turn suppresses production of $1,25(OH)_2D$. This causes a decrease in intestinal calcium absorption. The resulting calcium deficiency and increase in PTH secretion are expected to affect bone adversely. However, no effect of high phosphorus intake on bone loss has been demonstrated in humans. In addition, a high phosphorus intake reduces the amount of calcium lost in the urine; thus, significant alterations in calcium balance in humans do not occur.[49,50]

OTHER NUTRIENTS

Other nutrients have been implicated in osteoporosis because of their effects on calcium metabolism. With the exception of fluoride, no human studies have been conducted that manipulate intakes of these nutrients and directly observe the effect on rates of bone loss or fracture.

Protein. Because an increase in nitrogen intake is known to increase urinary calcium excretion,[51,52] a high protein diet is often regarded as a risk factor for osteoporosis. The source of this calcium is presumed to be skeletal because protein has no demonstrable effect on calcium absorption.[52,53]

In the typical American diet, major sources of protein are also rich in phosphorus. When a diet using meat to boost protein content from 857 mmol of nitrogen (12 g) to 1499 mmol (21 g) was evaluated in a study, no significant increase in urinary calcium excretion was observed, nor did an overall negative calcium balance ensue.[53] The lack of significant calciuria on this high-meat-protein diet was attributed to the simultaneous increase in phosphorus intake. Furthermore, despite an increase in urinary calcium excretion on a high-meat diet supplying 1571 mmol (22 g) of nitrogen daily, a positive calcium balance was maintained because of a decline in fecal calcium excretion.[51] Thus, although large increases in protein intake at calcium and phosphorus intake levels commonly consumed in this country enhance urinary calcium loss, the significance to bone loss is uncertain because of interactive effects of nutrients in a mixed diet. Small increases in calcium excretion could be important. Increasing the protein content of the diet from 785 mmol (11 g) to 1178 mmol (16.5 g) of nitrogen daily is estimated to raise daily calcium excretion by 0.80 mmol (0.032 g), an amount that would account for a large proportion of the bone lost annually in normal men and women.[50]

Fluoride. Fluoride stimulates the activity of osteoblasts and increases bone mass at some skeletal sites.[54] Fluoride can also replace hydroxyl ions in the hydroxyapatite structure. This substitution results in bone with increased crystalline size but decreased elasticity. Thus, although the compression strength of fluorotic bone may increase, the quality of tension is lessened so that it is not necessarily more resistant to fracture than normal bone. An association between a naturally occurring high fluo-

TABLE 89–1. SUMMARY OF RANDOMIZED, PLACEBO-CONTROLLED STUDIES OF 1,25(OH$_2$D IN POSTMENOPAUSAL WOMEN

REFERENCE	SUBJECTS	1,25(OH)$_2$D (μG/DAY)	DURATION	CALCIUM (MG/DAY)*	METHOD†	SITE	RESULT IN 1,25(OH)$_2$D GROUP COMPARED TO PLACEBO
Gallagher[46]	N = 62 Mean age 62 1 or more vertebral fractures	0.5–1.0	1 year‡	Not reported	NF	Vertebrae	↓ incidence, $p<0.05$
Alola[44]	N = 27 Mean age 64, range 50–80. Postmenopausal osteoporosis	0.5–1.0 (mean 0.8)	2 years	P: 1000 mg D: 500 mg	NA DPA SPA RA NF	Total body Spine L2-L4 Distal radius Phalanges Vertebrae	↓ loss, $p<0.05$ ↓ loss, $p<0.05$ ↓ loss, $p<0.01$ ↓ loss, $p<0.03$ No difference
Ott[47]	N = 56 Mean age 67, range 50–80 2 or more vertebral fractures	0.5–2.0 (mean 0.43)	2 years	823 mg at entry D ~ 200 mg less, P ~ 200 mg more during study	NA DPA SPA NF	Total body Spine L1-L2 Distal radius Vertebrae T4-L4	No difference No difference No difference No difference
Christiansen[45]	N = 84 Mean age 50 Healthy	0.25	1 year	Diet unknown 500 mg given as supplement	SPA	Radius	No difference
Jensen[48]	N = 70 Age 70 Mix of healthy and spine fractures	0.12–0.5 (mean 0.4)	1 year	Diet unknown 500 mg given as supplement	Loss in vertebral height	Vertebrae T6-L5	↑ loss, $p<0.05$

*P refers to placebo group, D to group treated with 1,25(OH)$_2$D.
†NA = neutron activation; DPA = dual photon absorptiometry; SPA = single photon absorptiometry; RA =radiographic absorptiometry; NF = new fracture defined as a decrease in anterior vertebral height of at least 15%.
‡Placebo controlled during first year only.

ride level in drinking water and increased bone density on radiographs was observed in 1966 by Bernstein.[55]

Although fluoride initially appeared to be effective in treating osteoporosis,[56] a recent 4-year controlled trial in osteoporotic women indicates that it is not.[54] Fluoride at a relatively high dose increased lumbar spine BMD by approximately 10% per year but had no effect on the vertebral fracture rate. At the radius, where fluoride did not increase BMD, the fracture rate was higher than the rate in a group treated with calcium alone. An increase in hip fracture rate among women treated with fluoride has also been reported.[57] It has been suggested that lower doses of fluoride may have antifracture efficacy, but this remains to be demonstrated.

Boron. Calcium and phosphorus excretion respond to alterations in boron intake. Increasing boron intake from a level of 23 μmol (0.25 mg) to 301 μmol (3.25 mg) per day resulted in a drop in urinary excretion of calcium, phosphorus, and magnesium, and in a simultaneous increase in serum estradiol concentration.[58] These responses appeared more marked when dietary magnesium was low. Such findings suggest that boron may play a role in maintaining calcium balance. Although the mechanism is unknown, it is postulated that boron is necessary for the formation of certain steroid hormones or in the hydroxylation of 25(OH)D. More information is needed on usual dietary intakes and boron requirements before its importance in the development of osteoporosis can be assessed.

Magnesium. Bone tissue contains approximately half of the body stores of magnesium. About one-third of this magnesium is on the bone surface in a freely exchangeable form, which can equilibrate with serum during acute hypomagnesemia. The remainder of bone magnesium is incorporated into hydroxyapatite. In animals, dietary magnesium restriction is associated with increased bone resorption and decreased formation. When magnesium depletion has been induced in human volunteers, decreased parathyroid hormone (PTH) secretion, hypocalcemia, hypocalciuria, and a positive calcium balance result.

Studies of bone magnesium content in postmenopausal women with osteoporosis report conflicting findings. Hip biopsy studies revealed higher magnesium as well as sodium content among osteoporotics compared to age-matched controls,[59] suggesting that during hypocalcemia, other metal ions such as magnesium and sodium may displace calcium in the bone. Other studies have not confirmed this finding. As with boron, any association of magnesium with osteoporosis requires further definition.

DRUG THERAPIES

Dietary factors have not proven to be effective in treating individuals in whom osteoporosis has already developed. The commonly prescribed medications for osteoporosis are described briefly.

ESTROGEN

The accelerated bone loss seen in women in the first several years of menopause can be prevented by estrogen replacement therapy.[60] Recently, estrogen receptors have been identified in normal human osteoblast-like bone cells.[61] This discovery provides a means by which estrogen can directly affect bone turnover. Estrogen also enhances calcium absorption through its trophic effect on $1,25(OH)_2D$.

Estrogen in a replacement dosage (0.625 mg of conjugated estrogens or 92 nmol (25 μg) of ethinyl estradiol) prevents bone loss from the spine,[31] radius,[31,62] metacarpals,[60] ulna,[62] and total body,[31] and reduces the rate of vertebral compression fracture.[63] Supplementation with calcium appears to reduce the amount of estrogen needed to maintain bone mineral.[33] A combination of 0.3 mg of conjugated estrogens and 37.4 mmol (1500 mg) of calcium per day was effective at preventing bone loss at the spine, radius, and metacarpals in a group of women within 3 years of the onset of menopause (Fig. 89–2). When estrogen treatment is discontinued, rapid bone loss, similar to that observed in perimenopausal women, occurs.[64] Although the value of estrogen for women beyond the period of rapid bone loss is less well established, estrogen does appear to be an effective treatment in older women.

CALCITONIN

Calcitonin, a small peptide hormone produced by the C cells of the thyroid gland, is secreted in response to an increase in serum calcium level. The main function of calcitonin is to inhibit bone resorption. Women with osteoporosis have an attenuated calcitonin response to a calcium challenge.

Because salmon calcitonin is a more potent inhibitor of bone resorption than human calcitonin, it is more effective therapeutically. Treatment with this hormone prevented bone loss from the proximal radius and reduced bone loss at the distal radius by 65% in osteoporotic patients.[65] A similar trend was seen at the spine. In another 2-year study, bone resorption surfaces decreased and total body calcium increased during calcitonin treatment.[66] Calcitonin can now be administered as a nasal spray rather than by injection. Evaluation of the effectiveness of the nasal preparation in the treatment of osteoporosis is in progress.

DIPHOSPHONATES

Because of their effects on calcium and bone metabolism, diphosphonates have been evaluated as therapeutic agents in a number of disorders of calcification, including Paget's disease, ectopic calcification, heterotopic calcification, metastatic disease of the skeleton and,

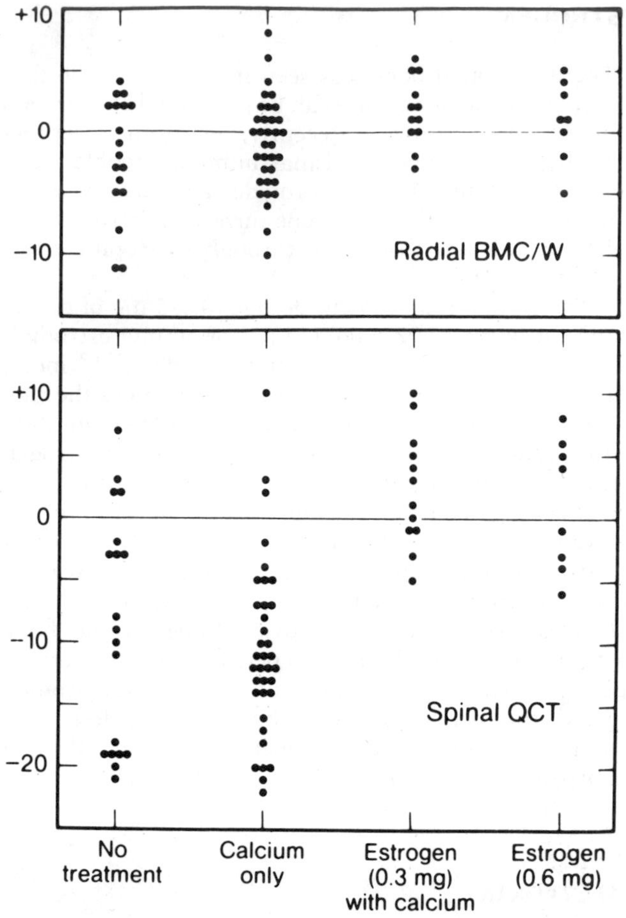

FIGURE 89–2. Distributions of percentage of change in radial bone mineral content (BMC)/width and in vertebral BMC after 2 years in early postmenopausal women (within 3 years of cessation of menses). Women taking estrogen + calcium or estrogen alone showed no changes in mineral content at the radius or spine. Women taking calcium or placebo lost mineral content at these sites. (From Ettinger, B., Genant, H.K., Cann, C.E.: Postmenopausal bone loss is prevented by treatment with low-dosage estrogen with calcium. Ann. Intern. Med., *106*:40–45, 1987.)

more recently, osteoporosis. Diphosphonates are structural analogues of pyrophosphate. Their metabolic effects include inhibition of hydroxyapatite formation and dissolution, inhibition of bone resorption through a direct effect on osteoclasts, dose-related inhibition of bone mineralization, and alteration in serum phosphate levels. Only one diphosphonate, etidronate, is commercially available in the United States, whereas the newer generation analogues, dichloromethylene diphosphonate and 3-amino-1-hydroxy-propane-1,1,diphosphate (APD), are available in Europe. At a dose of 20 nmol (5 μg) per kg body weight per day, etidronate blocks bone resorption but not bone formation.

In recently published controlled studies, osteoporotic women on intermittent cyclic etidronate therapy along with continuous calcium supplementation showed increases in vertebral mass of 4 to 5% over 2 to 3 years, and a greater than 50% reduction in new spinal deformities[67] and vertebral fractures.[68] Etidronate therapy did not alter density of the forearm[67,68] or Ward's triangle[68] in these studies. Given its demonstrated effectiveness at the spine, even among women with advanced osteoporosis, and the minimal side effects, etidronate is a promising treatment for spinal osteoporosis.

In summary, the development of low bone mass that characterizes osteoporosis is influenced by a host of genetic and environmental factors. Inadequate calcium intake has been implicated as a contributor to osteoporosis, both at the stage of peak bone formation and in later years when bone loss occurs. There are many in the population who would benefit by increasing their calcium intake. The importance of vitamin D intake in preventing and treating osteoporosis is uncertain and needs to be established. Excess phosphorus intake is not thought to play a significant role. Protein, boron, and other nutrients, through influences on calcium balance, may play roles in bone loss, but the magnitude of their roles is unknown.

Diet modification alone is not sufficient treatment for established osteoporosis. For patients with osteoporosis, the most promising treatments are estrogen replacement, diphosphonates, calcitonin, and perhaps other drugs. The effectiveness of these therapeutic agents may depend on nutritional status, however. Progress in answering many of the remaining questions about nutrition and bone health will be aided by recent improvements in techniques to precisely measure bone density and to track changes in bone mass over time.

REFERENCES

1. Albright, F., Smith, P.H., Richardson, A.M.: JAMA, *116*:2465–2474, 1941.
2. Krolner, B., Pors Nielsen, S.: Clin. Sci., *62*:329–336, 1982.
3. Riggs, B.L., Wahner, H.W., Melton, L.J., et al.: J. Clin. Invest., *77*:1487–1491, 1986.
4. Gallagher, J.C., Goldgar, P., Moy, A.: J. Bone Min. Res., *2*:491–496, 1987.
5. Mazess, R.B., Barden, H.S., Ettinger, M., et al.: Bone Min., *2*:211–219, 1987.

6. Ambrey, B.J., Jacobsen, P.C., Grubb, S.A., et al.: J. Orthop. Res., *2:*314–321, 1984.
7. Mazess, R.B., Barden, H.S., Drinka, P.J., et al.: J. Bone Min. Res., *5:*645–652, 1990.
8. Orwoll, E.S., Oviatt, S.K., McClung, M.R., et al.: Ann. Intern. Med., *112:*29–34, 1990.
9. Owen, R.A., Melton, L.J., Johnson, K.A., et al.: Am. J. Public Health, *72:*605–607, 1982.
10. Farmer, M.E., White, L.R., Brody, J.A., et al.: Am. J. Public Health, *74:*1374–1380, 1984.
11. Chalmers, J., Ho, K.C.: J. Bone Joint Surg., *52:*667–674, 1970.
12. Melton, L.J., Kan, S.H., Frye, M.A., et al.: Am. J. Epidemiol., *129:*1000–1011, 1989.
13. Pogrund, H., Makin, M., Rubin, G., et al.: Clin. Orthop., *124:*165–172, 1977.
14. Melton, L.J., Sampson, J.M., Morrey, B.F., et al.: Clin. Orthop., *155:*43–47, 1981.
15. Rose, S.H., Melton, L.J., Morrey, B.F., et al.: Clin. Orthop., *168:*24–30, 1982.
16. Daly, P.J., Fitzgerald, R.H., Melton, L.J., et al.: Acta Orthop. Scand., *58:*539–544, 1987.
17. Matkovic, V., Kostial, K., Simonovic, J., et al.: Am. J. Clin. Nutr., *32:*540–549, 1979.
18. Wasnich, R.D., Ross, P.D., Heilbrun, L.K., et al.: Am. J. Obstet. Gynecol., *153:*745–751, 1985.
19. Hui, S.L., Slemenda, C.W., Johnston, C.C.: Ann. Intern. Med., *111:*355–361, 1989.
20. Cummings, S.R., Black, D.M., Nevitt, M.C., et al.: JAMA, *263:*665–668, 1990.
21. Gardsell, P., Johnell, O., Nilsson, B.E.: Calcif. Tissue Int., *44:*235–242, 1989.
22. Halioua, L., Anderson, J.J.B.: Am. J. Clin. Nutr., *49:*534–541, 1989.
23. Picard, D., Ste-Marie, G., Coutu, D., et al.: Bone Min., *4:*299–309, 1988.
24. Food and Nutrition Board, National Research Council: Recommended Dietary Allowances. 10th Ed. Washington, D.C., National Academy Press, 1989.
25. Baran, D., Sorensen, A., Grimes, J., et al.: J. Clin. Endocrinol. Metab., *70:*264–270, 1989.
26. Smith, E.L., Gilligan, C., Smith, P.E., et al.: Am. J. Clin. Nutr., *50:*833–842, 1989.
27. Kanders, B., Dempster, D.W., Lindsay, R.: J. Bone Min. Res., *3:*145–149, 1988.
28. Stevenson, J.C., Lees, B., Devenport, M., et al.: Br. Med. J., *298:*924–928, 1989.
29. Johnell, O., Nilsson, B.E.: Calcif. Tissue Int., *36:*354–356, 1984.
30. Riggs, B.L., Wahner, H.W., Melton, L.J., et al.: J. Clin. Invest., *80:*979–982, 1987.
31. Riis, B., Thomsen, K., Christiansen, C.: N. Engl. J. Med., *316:*173–177, 1987.
32. Dawson-Hughes, B., Dallal, G.E., Krall, E.A., et al.: N. Engl. J. Med., *323:*878–883, 1990.
33. Ettinger, B., Genant, H.K., Cann, C.E.: Ann. Intern. Med., *106:*40–45, 1987.
34. Recker, R.R., Saville, P.D., Heaney, R.P.: Ann. Intern. Med., *87:*649–655, 1977.
35. Lamke, B., Sjoberg, H.-E., Sylven, M.: Acta Orthop. Scand., *49:*143–146, 1978.
36. Holbrook, T.L., Barrett-Conner, E., Wingard, D.L.: Lancet, *2:*1046–1049, 1988.
37. Cooper, C., Barker, D.J.P., Wickham, C.: Br. Med. J., *297:*1443–1446, 1988.
38. Krall, E.A., Sahyoun, N., Tannenbaum, S., et al.: N. Engl. J. Med., *321:*1777–1783, 1989.
39. Krolner, B.: Calcif. Tissue Int., *35:*145–147, 1983.
40. Aitken, J.M., Anderson, J.B.: Nature, *241:*59–60, 1973.
41. Overgaard, K., Nilas, L., Sidenius Johansen, J., et al.: Bone, *9:*285–288, 1988.
42. Gallagher, J.C., Riggs, B.L., Eisman, J., et al.: J. Clin. Invest., *64:*729–736, 1979.
43. Lips, P., van Ginkel, F.C., Jongen, M.J.M., et al.: Am. J. Clin. Nutr., *46:*1005–1010, 1987.
44. Aloia, J.F.: Am. J. Med., *84:*401–408, 1988.
45. Christiansen, C., Christensen, M.S., Rodbro, P., et al.: Eur. J. Clin. Invest., *11:*305–309, 1981.
46. Gallagher, J.C., Riggs, B.L., Recker, R.R., et al.: Proc. Soc. Exp. Biol. Med., *191:*287–292, 1989.
47. Ott, S.M., Chesnut, C.H.: Ann. Intern. Med., *110:*267–274, 1989.
48. Jensen, G.F., Meinecke, B., Boesen, J., et al.: Clin. Orthop., *192:*215–221, 1985.
49. Spencer, H., Kramer, L., Osis, D., et al.: J. Nutr., *108:*447–457, 1978.
50. Heaney, R.P., Recker, R.R.: J. Lab. Clin. Med., *99:*46–55, 1982.
51. Cummings, J.H., Hill, M.J., Jivraj, T., et al.: Am. J. Clin. Nutr., *32:*2086–2093, 1979.
52. Allen, L.H., Oddoye, E.A., Margen, S.: Am. J. Clin. Nutr., *32:*741–749, 1979.
53. Spencer, H., Kramer, L., Osis, D., et al.: Am. J. Clin. Nutr., *31:*2167–2180, 1978.
54. Riggs, B.L., Hodgson, S.F., O'Fallon, W.M., et al.: N. Engl. J. Med., *322:*802–809, 1990.
55. Bernstein, D.S., Sadowsky, N., Hegsted, D.M., et al.: JAMA, *198:*499–504, 1966.
56. Riggs, B.L., Seeman, E., Hodgson, S.F., et al.: N. Engl. J. Med., *306:*446–450, 1982.
57. Hedlund, L.R., Gallagher, J.C.: J. Bone Min. Res., *4:*223–225, 1989.
58. Nielsen, F.H., Hunt, C.D., Mullen, L.M., et al.: FASEB J., *1:*394–397, 1987.
59. Burnell, J.M., Baylink, D.J., Chesnut, C.H., et al.: Metabolism, *31:*1113–1120, 1982.
60. Lindsay, R., Hart, D.M., Aitken, J.M., et al.: Lancet, *1:*1038–1041, 1976.
61. Eriksen, E.F., Colvard, D.S., Berg, N.J., et al.: Science, *241:*84–86, 1988.
62. Horsman, A., Gallagher, J.C., Simpson, et al.: Br. Med. J., *2:*789–792, 1977.
63. Lindsay, R., Hart, D.M., Forrest, C., et al.: Lancet, *2:*1151–1154, 1980.
64. Lindsay, R., Hart, D.M., MacLean, A., et al.: Lancet, *1:*1325–1327, 1978.
65. Overgaard, K., Riis, B.J., Christiansen, C., et al.: Clin. Endocrinol., *30:*435–442, 1989.
66. Gruber, H.E., Ivey, J.L., Baylink, D.J., et al.: Metabolism, *33:*295–303, 1984.
67. Storm, T., Thamsborg, G., Steiniche, T., et al.: N. Engl. J. Med., *322:*1265–1271, 1990.
68. Watts, N.B., Harris, S.T., Genant, H.K., et al.: N. Engl. J. Med., *323:*73–79, 1990.

SELECTED READING

Parfitt, A.M.: Bone remodeling: Relationship to the amount and structure of bone, and the pathogenesis and prevention of fractures. *In* Osteoporosis. Etiology, Diagnosis, and Management. Edited by B.L. Riggs and L.J. Melton III. New York, Raven Press, 1988.

CHAPTER **90**

Factors Affecting Nutritive Value in Processed Foods

John W. Erdman, Jr., and Angela G. Poneros-Schneier

Mankind's attempts to preserve food go back for centuries. One of the earliest examples of food preservation is the curing of meat, which involves drying, salting, and smoking. This practice dates from 1500 B.C. Sun drying is another early method of preserving food. A more recent advancement in food preservation came in the late eighteenth century in France. Napoleon's armies were hindered by inadequate supplies of food, and prizes were offered as an incentive for developing useful methods of preserving food for soldiers. In this competition, Nicholas Appert showed that a food, if sufficiently heated in a sealed container and then stored unopened, could be preserved. He was awarded 12,000 francs and honored in 1809. Thus, canning was born. The work of Louis Pasteur some 50 years later helped to explain the effectiveness of Appert's canning by showing that the growth of microorganisms was the major cause of food spoilage.[1]

Since the late 1800s, society has changed from a largely rural way of life to modern urban living. Improvements in farm production and yields, and the development of a food processing industry, have both had a marked impact on societal change. Today relatively few people live on farms. Thus, processing, storage and transportation systems are all critical for providing food for urban populations. Additionally, more and more women are joining the working force, leaving less time for home food preparation. This has created an increasing demand for convenience foods.

Many consumers are health conscious and are increasingly insistent that these foods also be highly nutritious. Although most food processing is done in such a way as to minimize nutrient loss while assuring maximum product safety, there is still a need to evaluate processing techniques continually and to look for ways to improve nutrient retention. As food processing technology continues to advance, it will be possible to produce processed foods with improved nutritive value.

OVERVIEW OF FOOD PROCESSING

Foods are processed for several reasons: to preserve the food and to extend its shelf-life, to increase the digestibility of the food, to improve the palatability and texture, to prepare foods for serving, to eliminate microorganisms, to destroy toxins, to remove inedible parts, to destroy antinutritional factors, and to create new types of foods. Of these reasons, perhaps the most important is safety. Although processing may decrease the overall nutrient content of a food, this is a necessary price to pay for safety. Additionally, processing can increase the bioavailability of some nutrients. Other advantages of food processing to the consumer include increased convenience and availability of a variety of foods year-round.

There are three major causes of food spoilage: microbial growth, chemical changes, and enzymatic changes. Because raw foods are living biologic systems that often contain enzymes that may contribute to rapid spoilage, inactivation of these enzymes can often greatly extend the shelf-life of a food. This is especially important for foods with a high moisture content, because they deteriorate more rapidly than those with a low moisture content.

Environmental conditions such as pH, temperature, light, and oxygen all can affect the shelf-life and nutrient retention in a stored food. Manipulation of these environmental conditions can minimize spoilage and nutrient damage. Riboflavin is an example of a nutrient that is greatly affected by environmental conditions. It is very sensitive to light, and its rate of destruction increases as the temperature and pH increase.

Food processing can have both positive and negative effects on nutrient retention. An example of a positive effect is the lime-[$Ca(OH)_2$] treatment of corn during tortilla making. The added calcium has been shown to be highly bioavailable.[2] Also, this process increases the bioavailability of niacin. Niacin is tightly bound to the corn proteins, but can be liberated from this bound form under alkaline conditions.[3] Alkaline treatment of corn greatly helps in eliminating pellagra in populations in which corn is the mainstay of the diet.[4] Unfortunately, the alkaline conditions associated with lime treatment are damaging to another B vitamin, thiamin.

An example of a negative effect of food processing is nutrient destruction during extrusion of food materials. Extrusion can be destructive to heat-labile nutrients such as thiamin and ascorbic acid. Significant losses of the amino acids lysine and methionine can occur as well.

Appropriate processing of foods is always a question of balance. Some nutrient loss is inevitable, especially with certain vitamins. For example, in a breakfast cereal one would want sufficient heat treatment to maximize the digestibility of the cereal and destruction of heat-labile antinutrients, while minimizing the loss of heat-labile vitamins and amino acids.

Several factors should be considered when determining if a nutrient loss is significant. The degree of concern depends on whether the nutrient in question is abundant or scarce in the total average diet and on whether that food is generally relied on as a major source of that nutrient. Vitamin C is destroyed in the pasteurization of milk, but milk is not an important source of this vitamin when compared with other foods such as citrus fruits and juices. Conversely, milk is an important source of riboflavin; thus, its destruction due to light or heat would be important to populations consuming low levels of riboflavin.

A common misconception is that commercially processed foods are always nutritionally inferior to freshly prepared foods. In fact, nutrient losses in commercially processed products are often in place of, rather than in addition to, those that would inevitably accompany preparation of "fresh produce" in the home.[5] Unprotected raw food material can rapidly deteriorate in nutritional value after harvest if not preserved. For example, the procedures used during harvesting and the ensuing handling and storage period can dramatically affect both nutritional value and sensory properties of fruits and vegetables. Ascorbic acid, thiamin, and folic acid are especially susceptible to both enzymatic and nonenzymatic oxidation during this period. Enzymatic destruction of ascorbic acid can begin as soon as a crop is harvested. Storage under both cool and humid conditions reduces wilting and improves retention of ascorbic acid during storage. Other preprocessing conditions that influence nutrient content of the final prepared food are genetic variation, soil composition, fertilizer use, type of feed, and degree of maturity when picked or killed.[6]

Vitamin C and thiamin are readily lost in the processing of foods because they are thermally labile and water-soluble (susceptible to leaching during processing). It is generally assumed that if these two vitamins are well retained during processing and storage, other nutrients also are well retained.[7] Vitamin stability during processing is largely related to heat, pH, oxygen, and light. The presence of trace elements can accelerate the loss of some vitamins. Factors that affect vitamin loss are presented in Table 90–1.

Minerals are relatively heat-stable, but are easily leached from food when exposed to excess water. Also, during processing their bioavailability may be altered as a result of interactions with other components of the food.

Of the amino acids, lysine is the most labile. All amino acids are sensitive to dry heat. Thus, in the roasting and

TABLE 90–1. FACTORS AFFECTING VITAMIN LOSS

NUTRIENT	LOSSES MAINLY DUE TO:
Ascorbic acid*	Water leaching, oxidation: accelerated by heat, light, copper, and iron
Biotin	Alkaline conditions
Carotene (pro-A)	Oxidation and isomerization: accelerated by heat and light
Cobalamin (B_{12})	Alkaline and acid conditions, oxidation
Folic acid	Light and heat
Niacin	Water leaching
Pantothenic acid	Alkaline and acidic conditions: accelerated by heat
Pyridoxine (B_6)	Light: accelerated by alkaline conditions
Riboflavin (B_2)	Light and heat: accelerated by alkaline conditions, heat-stable in acid solution
Thiamin (B_1)*	Alkaline conditions, water leaching, oxidation: accelerated by heat and light
Tocopherol (E)	Oxidation
Vitamin A	Oxidation and isomerization: accelerated by heat and light
Vitamin D	Alkaline conditions: accelerated by light and oxygen
Vitamin K	Light and alkaline conditions

*Considered to be one of the more heat-labile vitamins.

toasting of legumes, cereals, and prepared dry mixtures of foodstuffs, a significant reduction in the biologic value of the respective proteins may occur.[8]

Essential fatty acids can isomerize when heated in alkali and are sensitive to oxygen and light, especially at high temperatures. When oxidized they become biologically inactive and can produce off-flavors and free radicals.

THERMAL PROCESSING

Heat processing is one of the most important processes for food preservation. Generally, for any thermal process, exposure of foods to high temperature for a short time is less damaging to nutrients than a moderate temperature for a longer time. For many foods, heat will increase digestibility of protein, carbohydrates, and other nutrients, thereby enhancing the nutritive value of the food. Heat treatment can also inactivate some of the naturally occurring enzymes, such as pectinase and lipoxygenase, in fruits and vegetables, thereby protecting against off flavors, loss of color, and poor texture in the food product. Thermal processing can also enhance the bioavailability of vitamins B_6, niacin, folacin, and certain carotenoids, because heat can release these vitamins from poorly digested complexes. Another advantage of thermal processing is inactivation of antinutritional factors in certain foods. In these foods, nutritional value is greatly enhanced by processing[9] (Table 90–2). On the other hand, thermal processing does have several adverse effects. During thermal processing and subsequent storage, thiamin and ascorbic acid are especially susceptible to depletion due to leaching and thermal degradation. Carotene and folacin are also heat-labile. Lipids, minerals, vitamin K, biotin, and niacin are normally stable during heating.

Maillard browning (nonenzymatic browning) is commonly induced during thermal processing conditions. It can occur in foods containing reducing sugars (glucose, fructose, lactose) and protein. Foods that undergo Maillard browning include bread and other baked items, dried fruits, gravy mixes, maple syrup, dried milk, cocoa, and extruded products (e.g., cereals). During heat processing, the free aldehyde or ketone groups of sugars can react with amino groups of certain amino acids to create poorly digested complexes. Maillard browning can destroy many of the amino acids, in particular the basic amino acids. Because of the presence of an ϵ-amino group, lysine is one of the most labile of the amino acids. Because lysine is typically in low concentration in plant foods, any loss is of concern. Loss of arginine and methionine also occur. Thus, Maillard browning will reduce the protein quality of plant foods.[10] The results of the Maillard reaction include decreased caloric content, increased color and flavor, and reduction in essential amino acids and total nitrogen digestibility. For foods such as breads, cocoa, and maple syrup, a certain amount of Maillard browning is desirable to improve appearance and flavor. On the other hand, for a food such as milk, Maillard browning is undesirable because it produces a "cooked" flavor and undesirable color. The Maillard reaction can be minimized by decreasing the concentration of reducing sugars, increasing the moisture content, reducing heat, and lowering pH.

In addition to the Maillard reaction, thermal processing at high temperatures can also cause other undesirable reactions to protein. Such reactions include the oxidation of amino acids (particularly sulfur amino acids), altered peptide linkages between amino acids, which delay or impair amino acid release during digestion, and formation of new amino acid structures or dipeptides that are not subject to normal digestion and absorption processes.

BLANCHING

Blanching is frequently used before freezing, drying, or canning of foods. Blanching prior to canning is used to wilt the food tissue to facilitate packing, to increase the temperature of the tissue prior to can closing, to remove tissue gases, and to inactivate many enzymes. Blanching before freezing is used to inactivate enzymes that cause undesirable changes during storage such as browning, rancidity, off-flavor development, and vitamin destruc-

TABLE 90–2. HEAT-LABILE ANTINUTRITIONAL FACTORS

ANTINUTRITIONAL FACTOR	COMMON FOOD SOURCES	EFFECTS OF ANTINUTRITIONAL FACTOR
Avidin	Egg whites	Binds biotin making it biologically unavailable
Hemagglutinins	Red kidney beans, yellow wax beans	Induces clumping of red blood cells
Lathyrogens	Chick peas	Disrupts collagen structure
Goitrogens	Sweet potatoes, beans, cabbage, turnips	Causes goiters by interfering with iodine absorption
α-Amylase inhibitors	Cereal grains, peas, beans	Slows starch digestion
Trypsin inhibitor	Legumes, egg whites, potatoes	Inhibits the activity of digestive enzyme trypsin
Thiaminases	Fish, shellfish, brussel sprouts, red cabbage	Destroys thiamin

tion in food. Microbial destruction is not a primary objective of blanching. Even though some loss of vitamins is inevitable during blanching, it is a necessary price to pay to ensure a stored product of higher quality.

The loss of vitamin C during water blanching and cooling of vegetables ranges from about 10 to 50%, and losses of thiamin are about 9 to 60%. Actual losses depend on the product and processing conditions, such as how much water is used and whether the water is discarded.[7] Water blanching causes an average loss of 30% of niacin from lima beans and a 14% loss of riboflavin from green beans. This loss is primarily due to the leaching of water-soluble vitamins rather than to their chemical degradation. In contrast, no significant loss of fat-soluble carotene from broccoli, corn, squash, carrots, and collards occurs because of leaching.[7]

The growing use of steam blanching results in substantial improvement in the retention of water-soluble nutrients as compared to the more traditional method of water blanching.[11] This is especially true for products with a large surface/volume ratio (e.g., spinach).[12] Additionally, microwave blanching results in even smaller losses of nutrients than steam blanching does;[7] however, this method is relatively expensive.[13]

PASTEURIZATION

The main objectives of pasteurization are to reduce the population of spoilage microorganisms and to inactivate pathogenic microorganisms and deteriorative enzymes. Because the food is not rendered sterile, pasteurization must be used in conjunction with other preservation methods such as refrigeration (e.g., milk) or fermentation (e.g., pickles). It may be used alone if the food is highly acidic (e.g., wine and some fruit juices) and the packaging is adequate. Because most heat-labile nutrients are relatively stable in acidic conditions, nutrient losses during pasteurization of acidic products are minor.[13]

Milk is pasteurized by one of three methods: (1) Low-temperature-long-time (LTLT), 63° C (145° F) for 30 minutes, (2) High-temperature-short-time (HTST), 72° C (161° F) for 15 seconds, and (3) Ultra-high temperature (UHT, sterilization), ≥135° C (≥275° F) for less than 10 seconds, an aseptic process. As can be seen above, increased processing temperature dramatically reduces processing time. This results in a product with greater nutrient retention because, as Lund said, "an increase in process temperature (with an appropriate decrease in process time) will have a greater effect in increasing the rate of microbial destruction than it will on the rate of nutrient destruction."[13] As an example, the Institute of Food Technologist's Expert Panel said, "an 18° F rise in processing temperature usually produces a tenfold increase in bacterial destruction, while only doubling the chemical reactions which lead to the destruction of certain nutrients and flavors."[11] So, theoretically, the higher the process temperature, the better the product quality and nutrient retention. In the United States, HTST is most frequently used and results in better nutrient retention than LTLT processing.[11]

Pasteurization of milk is geared towards the elimination of the most heat-resistant pathogen, Coxiella burnetti, the rickettsial organism responsible for Q fever in milk. Both HTST and UHT processes destroy harmful microorganisms without adversely affecting most nutrients to any great extent. All the fat-soluble vitamins and certain water-soluble vitamins such as riboflavin, pantothenic acid, biotin, and nicotinic acid are stable during pasteurization. On the other hand, folic acid, thiamin, and vitamins B_6, B_{12}, and C are more susceptible to heat and oxidative degradation. Methods to exclude oxygen during processing and storage will serve to protect folic acid and vitamins C and B_{12}.[14]

CANNING

Canning ("commercial sterilization") produces food products with a much longer shelf-life than pasteurization does. Canning is a widely used process that destroys all pathogenic and toxin-forming organisms. Because some nonpathogenic microorganisms and spores are extremely heat-resistant, it is not usually practical to render food completely sterile without unacceptably altering sensory qualities and the nutritive value of food. Therefore, commercial sterilization is used in conjunction with other preservation techniques such as packaging and control of storage temperature. These further preservation techniques ensure that the remaining dormant microorganisms or their spores will not grow under the conditions of storage.[13]

Canning is widely used for many fruits, vegetables, and juices. Unpeeled fruit shows high nutrient retention during canning. In canned vegetables, water-soluble vitamins and minerals are distributed between the solids and liquids. The liquid, usually discarded by the consumer, contains significant quantities of nutrients. For example, approximately 30% of the available thiamin is found in the liquid portion.[15] Also, more than 50% of the manganese, cobalt, and zinc may end up in the liquid portion of canned spinach, beans, and tomatoes.[11] Consumption of this liquid by incorporating it into soups, sauces, and gravies is a way for the consumer to overcome these losses.

RETORT POUCHES

This relatively new processing technique results in improved nutrient retention compared to traditional thermal processing techniques. A retort pouch is a flexible, heat-sealable, relatively flat container made of polymeric laminates capable of withstanding the high temperatures required during thermal processing. Polymeric laminates are thinly layered materials such as plastics, paper, or aluminum that are tightly joined together.[10] The thinner slab-like geometry of a retort pouch increases the surface-to-volume ratio of the packaged food product compared to glass or metal cans. Because of the geometry of the pouch, the product temperature increases much more rapidly than it does in a traditional container. Improved heat transfer due to an increased surface area generally decreases process time by one third to one half the time required for metal cans. As in HTST processing, retention of heat-labile vitamins is significantly enhanced because of the shorter process time. For example, a study showed that retorted sweet potato puree had a thiamin retention of 77% whereas heated cans with equal volume retained only 60% of the thiamin.[10]

ASEPTIC PROCESSING

Aseptic processing (UHT processing, approximately 149° C (300° F) for a few seconds) is a process whereby sterile products are filled and sealed into sterile containers under aseptic conditions. It is used extensively for packaging of puddings and of fruit juices and drinks. Aseptic processing provides food products that are superior to retorted versions in flavor, texture, and nutrition. In particular, the retention of pyridoxine and thiamin is significantly improved.[11]

BAKING

Baking is a major heat-processing technique used by the food industry. It causes some destruction of nutrients, especially basic amino acids (because of Maillard browning) and water-soluble vitamins (particularly thiamin). Baking may improve the absorption and utilization of other nutrients through inactivation or destruction of antinutrients and mineral complexes. Thermal destruction of nutrients is most pronounced in the crust portion of baked foods, where the temperature is the highest. Other factors that influence nutrient retention and stability are time, pH, oxygen, light, metals, enzymes, and moisture content.

During the fermentation of dough for yeast products, chemical changes in the food occurs through the action of enzymes derived from microorganisms. Ideally, fermentation is the controlled growth of desirable microorganisms. The loss of nutrients due to fermentation is small; indeed, the nutrient level may even increase through vitamin and protein synthesis by the yeast and through liberation of nutrients locked into plant structures and cells by indigestible materials.[16]

The heat of baking denatures protein, thus enhancing digestibility, but also fostering Maillard browning. Milk solids, milk replacers, or sugars added to bread dough mix will intensify the Maillard reaction. Loss of lysine is most significant in the crust portion of the bread.

Thiamin is highly susceptible to baking losses. Thiamin is relatively stable during the fermentation process in bread making because the pH is mildly acidic. Thiamin losses during bread making generally do not exceed 25%. However, in chemically leavened goods (such as cookies and crackers), where the pH generally rises above 6, nearly all the thiamin is destroyed.[17,18] One study on high-protein cookies revealed thiamin losses of more than 90%, whereas losses of riboflavin and niacin were only modest. Lower baking temperatures may improve thiamin retention in baked goods. Thiamin loss is highly variable depending on the particular baked product; thus no universal loss factor can be used.[18]

Much of the niacin in grain products, especially from unrefined flours, is present as bound niacin. Bound niacin is essentially unutilizable by humans. Baking appears to have a beneficial effect by releasing bound niacin. It has been shown that the proportion of free niacin was higher in bread, cakes, and crackers than from the flours from which they were made.[17,18] Alkali treatment of corn in the making of tortillas improves niacin availability, probably through hydrolysis of bound niacin during the baking stage of tortilla making. In the United States, much of the white bread and many of the variety breads are made with enriched flour; thiamin, riboflavin, niacin, iron, and possibly calcium are added. No significant losses of these added vitamins occur during bread making.[17]

Baking is unlikely to affect adversely the mineral content of foods.[18] However, enzymes present during fermentation of bread dough and the heat of baking may have a beneficial effect on mineral bioavailability by breaking up the organic complexes of minerals, such as phytate.[17] Phytic acid, a much studied organic chemical, is a chief storage form of phosphate and inositol in whole-grain cereals such as corn and wheat. It is a strong chelating agent that can bind to monovalent and divalent metal ions to form the complex phytate. Numerous studies have shown poor mineral bioavailability from foods high in phytate.[19] When chemical leavening instead of yeast leavening is used, phytate hydrolysis may not be of significance. In this case, phytic acid will probably continue to adversely affect mineral bioavailability.[17]

EXTRUSION

Extrusion is the process of forcing a dough-like material (usually at high temperature and pressure) through a small opening called a die. Extrusion-processed foods include breakfast cereals, snack foods, textured vegetable proteins, infant food formulas, soup bases, and precooked starches. Time-temperature conditions are comparable to other HTST processes. However, the product is also subjected to high pressure and severe shear. Extrusion has both beneficial and undesirable effects on the nutritional value of food. The benefits include the destruction of antinutritional factors and undesirable microorganisms, gelatinization of starch, and improved digestibility. Some undesirable effects are reduced protein quality due to Maillard browning and loss of heat-labile vitamins.

Extruders consist of either a single or two rotating flighted screws tightly fitted into a barrel.[10] A granular mix is fed into the hopper and conveyed forward in the channels between the flights of the rotating screw(s). Water is usually introduced after the dry mixture. While moving forward, the mixture is heated by friction, mechanical energy, steam injection, and heat transfer from the barrel. The mixture is transformed into a continuous dough. During this process, the starch granules are disrupted and protein is denatured. At the barrel exit, the heated and pressurized dough is forced through a die to produce the desired product shape. A spinning blade can be used to cut the product to appropriate lengths. If a puffed product is desired, high temperature and pressure inside the barrel is required so that when the dough passes through the die into a cooler environment at atmospheric pressure, the water changes to steam causing rapid expansion of the product.[10]

In studies of model systems for extrusion processing, it has been shown that extensive loss of lysine occurs before much visual brown color is noticed.[20] Loss of lysine was found to be comparable or worse to that during baking. As either the temperature of extrusion increases or the moisture content decreases, lysine losses usually increase.[20] For example, retention of available lysine was shown to be 93% at a processing temperature of 170° C, but only 63% at a processing temperature of 210° C.[10] Also, a decrease in the amino acids arginine and tryptophan occurs with increasing severity of process conditions.

High shear rates in the extruder also are detrimental to vitamin retention.[20] Vitamins that are negatively affected include ascorbic acid, vitamin A, and carotene;[10] however, in processed foods, vitamins are often added to the surface of the product after extrusion. For vitamin E, one study showed minimal tocopherol destruction in extruded full-fat soy flour. Vitamin E is sometimes added before extrusion to protect sensitive materials from undergoing oxidation during extrusion.[21] Niacin, pyridoxine, and folic acid appear to be relatively stable during extrusion cooking.[22]

MICROWAVE COOKING

In conventional cooking, heat is applied to the exterior of the food and is conducted inward toward the interior. During microwave processing, heat is generated within the food product by microwave-induced molecular vibrations. Microwave cooking can be used for pasteurization, sterilization, precooking, dehydration, baking, blanching, and tempering (used to raise temperature in frozen foods to just below the freezing point of water). Combining traditional heating methods with microwave exposure can offer both sensory and nutritional benefits. In conventional ovens, microwaves are used to achieve internal heating, and conventional heating methods are used to produce the desired surface browning and crispness. The most highly developed commercial applications include the tempering of frozen foods (frozen meat and fish blocks), precooking of meat products (bacon, poultry, and beef patties), and dehydration of low-moisture solids (pasta).[23]

Generally, microwave cooking can be as good as the best conventional processes for a food product. However, the amount of cook "drip" loss while microwave cooking of meats can result in higher losses of minerals, protein, water-soluble vitamins, and some fats as compared to conventional methods.[10] Loss of ascorbic acid is generally less with microwave cooking as compared to conventional methods.[24] In 1987, the Institute of Food Technologist's Expert Panel on Food Safety and Nutrition reported that vitamin retention in microwave foods is improved because of a shorter cooking time than with conventional methods.[23] However, retention varies depending on cooking time, internal temperature, product type, and oven size, type, and power. Also, because of a shorter length of heating time, foods blanched or cooked at higher wattage levels retain greater amounts of heat-labile nutrients than foods heated by other methods.[23]

FREEZING

Freezing is generally considered the best method of food preservation with regard to sensory qualities and retention of nutrients. Nutrient losses from fruits and vegetables can be minimal if blanching procedures are adequate, proper packaging is provided, and storage temperatures are low and constant. Any nutrient loss that occurs usually takes place during blanching or frozen storage, not during the actual freezing process. In general, the lower the storage temperature and the greater the temperature stability, the greater the nutrient retention and product quality. The loss of vitamins during frozen storage varies greatly depending on the product and packaging. Loss of ascorbic acid is greatly influenced by the oxygen permeability of the packaging material. The lower the oxygen permeability, the greater the retention of vitamin C. Additionally, the shorter the frozen storage period, the greater the nutrient retention.

The storage temperature has a significant effect on nutrient retention. For example, in one study vegetables stored at −7° C almost invariably had greater losses of vitamin C, β-carotene, folic acid, and pantothenic acid compared to those stored at −18° C. No significant effect on niacin, riboflavin, thiamin, vitamin B_6, and minerals was observed.[7] For maximum nutrient retention, storage temperatures should remain below −18° C.

During the entire freezing process, blanching is responsible for a major share of the loss of water-soluble nutrients in vegetables that occurs.[7] This loss could be minimized significantly if vegetables were blanched and cooled by means that do not involve liquid water, such as microwaving or steaming. For fruits and meats, the biggest losses of vitamins occur during prolonged storage and thawing (significant amounts of water-soluble vitamins and minerals end up in the syrup or thaw-exudate).

MOISTURE REMOVAL

Methods of moisture removal include both dehydration and concentration processes. Multiple factors prior to the drying or concentration will influence ultimate nutrient retention. For example, the presence of sulfur dioxide will adversely affect thiamin, but will protect ascorbic acid. However, the presence of copper, iron, light, or dissolved oxygen can decrease ascorbic acid concentration. Also, heavy metals can catalyze the oxidation of carotenes.[25] The temperature during drying or concentration varies greatly depending on the process and the product. Temperatures can range from −30° C to above 100° C. Generally, low-temperature processing such as freeze-drying should produce products with the least amount of chemical deterioration. However, low-temperature processing is usually more expensive because of the longer processing time.[25]

DEHYDRATION

Methods for dehydration include sun drying, tunnel drying, spray drying, drum drying, and freeze drying. Metabolism of microorganisms requires a sufficient concentration of free (not bound) water. Removing the biologically active water by drying or dehydration will prevent the growth of microorganisms and reduce the rate of enzymatic activity and chemical reactions, if the product is stored under proper conditions.

For most types of drying, heat is supplied to the food and moisture in the vapor state is removed. Dehydrated foods are susceptible to loss of vitamin A and provitamin A activity during storage if oxygen is present (they will undergo oxidation). Vitamin C, as well as other vitamins, is also susceptible to losses during drying.

Sun Drying. One of the least expensive methods of drying is sun drying. It is used to dry grapes, prunes, apricots, dates, figs, spices, grain, and other foods. This is a time-consuming method of drying that usually takes 3 to 4 days. Sun drying is often accompanied by a large vitamin loss. Additional problems such as mold growth can occur (if rain or high humidity is present), resulting in an increase in mold toxins such as aflatoxin. For best results, a warm, dry climate is necessary.

Tunnel Drying. Tunnel driers are an important class of driers. Fruits and vegetables can be dried by this method. The food is placed onto trays or a conveyor and passed into a stream of high-velocity air. This method is often used to dry pasta. It is an LTLT process.

Spray Drying. Spray drying is an HTST process used for nonfat dry milk, eggs, tea, and coffee. It is more expensive than tunnel drying, but product quality is generally better. Little or no loss of vitamin A or D occurs during the spray drying of milk. Additionally, spray-dried milk powder has negligible loss of available lysine. Most dried milk available to the consumer is further processed by rewetting and drying to produce an instant powder that dissolves well in water. During this rewetting and drying process, losses of amino acids are minimal.[25]

Drum Drying. A fairly inexpensive process, drum drying is generally used for foods that are relatively heat-insensitive, such as potatoes. Mashed potatoes are processed by drum drying to produce "instant" potatoes. Most of the vitamin C in potatoes is lost during drum drying and subsequent storage of the product.[5] Milk can also be processed by drum drying. Little or no loss of vitamin A or D occurs during the drum drying of milk.[25] Deterioration of heat-sensitive nutrients is greater than that from spray or tunnel drying because the heat treatment is harsher owing to the high temperature and direct contact between the food and the hot drum. Drum drying of milk results in lysine losses of 3 to 16%.[25]

Freeze Drying. Although freeze drying is the most expensive drying process, it produces foods of very high quality. The food is frozen in sheets and placed in a chamber with very low atmospheric pressure. Water leaves directly from the ice phase (sublimation). The process takes about 6 to 8 hours. The effect of temperature on product quality and nutrient retention is minimal. Because freeze drying is carried out in the absence of oxygen, even vitamin C is not adversely affected.[25]

CONCENTRATION

Evaporation, freeze concentration, and membrane processes are commonly used by the food industry to concentrate foods and juices.

Evaporation. Evaporation is both the most common method of concentrating food products and the least expensive. Basically, this process consists simply of boiling off water at temperatures that depend on the product and process. Foods processed by this method include condensed milk, fruit juices, candy, jam, and jelly. Even though the temperature is high, processing time can be very short so that nutrient destruction can be minimal. The loss of lysine due to nonenzymatic browning is probably the only deterioration of any consequence. One study showed a 20% reduction in lysine when evaporated milk was retorted at 113° C for 15 minutes. However, when sweetened condensed milk was evaporated at 50 to 55° C, only 3% of the lysine was destroyed.[25] When performed under a partial vacuum, nutrient retention is improved because of lower boiling temperatures and a lower concentration of atmospheric oxygen.

Freeze Concentration. Freeze concentration is a low-temperature moisture removal method that is used commercially for the manufacture of orange juice concentrate. This process involves the freezing of water to produce large ice crystals, which are then separated from the concentrate. Excellent nutrient retention is expected because it is a low-temperature process. Only adhering solutes that are removed with the ice are lost.[25]

Membrane Processes. Both ultrafiltration and reverse osmosis are food processing methods that use membranes. They are nonthermal processes. Reverse osmosis is a concentration process designed to remove only water. Ultrafiltration is a less specific concentration and purification process. With both processes, the liquid solution to be concentrated is passed through equipment holding a membrane. The membrane allows the selective passage of water with or without other compounds of low molecular weight.[25] Ultrafiltration results in a substantial loss of the water-soluble vitamins and minerals. Reverse osmosis has a much smaller pore size so that nutrients are not lost.

Of the concentration methods discussed, ultrafiltration shows the highest nutrient losses (particularly water-soluble vitamins and minerals). Drying processes generally offer good nutrient retentions, with the exception of β-carotene and ascorbic acid. The losses of water-soluble vitamins, other than ascorbic acid, during drying average approximately 5%. For dried carrots, loss of β-carotene is significant. The loss of β-carotene is small in freeze-dried orange juice. Other fat-soluble vitamins are not lost to any significant degree during spray drying, drum drying, or evaporation of milk. Loss of ascorbic acid during concentration is minimal. Freeze concentration should offer excellent nutrient retention.[25]

OTHER PROCESSES

IONIZING RADIATION

Other names for ionizing radiation are irradiation, cold-pasteurization, radurization, and cold-sterilization. Ionizing radiations include electrons, x rays, or γ rays produced by radioactive isotopes of either cesium or cobalt (^{137}Cs or ^{60}Co). Irradiation causes only a slight increase in food temperature; however, free radicals and peroxides can be formed. No increase in radioactivity of food has ever been observed in samples irradiated with ^{60}Co or ^{137}Cs. Irradiation is effective in destroying microorganisms, and the extent of vitamin destruction is similar to that caused by thermal processes.[5] Enzymes are not inactivated and therefore need to be heat-inactivated.[26] The applications of irradiation can be divided into five general categories: Sprout inhibition, delayed ripening, control of insect infestation, shelf-life extension, and sterilization.

The effects of ionizing irradiation on the nutrient content of food is comparable to that of conventional heat-processed foods.[11] Also, holding the food at low temperature and excluding free oxygen during irradiation can aid in protecting the nutritional quality of the food. Even though irradiation of food has been shown to be safe, approval for its use in foods has been limited in the United States. Consumer mistrust of the process and time-consuming procedures and the cost required to obtain Food and Drug Administration (FDA) clearances have prevented substantial commercial use in the United States thus far.[27] The use of ionizing radiation has recently been approved for use with eggs but it is not expected to be used commercially. In Florida, irradiated strawberries have reached the marketplace.

MILLING

Milling is a process by which bran and germ are removed from cereal grains. It is commonly used to refine wheat to make white flour. In the United States, milling of wheat to produce white flour results in a 40 to 60% loss of vitamins and minerals. Most wheat flour and breads are enriched with thiamin, niacin, riboflavin, and iron (addition of calcium and other nutrients is optional) in accordance with a standard identity as defined by the FDA.[11,28] Degermination of grains results in a loss of vitamin E.

Milling is also used to remove bran and germ from rice. For thousands of years, rice has been traditionally extracted from the husk by pounding it in a stone or wooden mortar. The outerhusk is broken and separated from the grain by winnowing, although some of the germ and pericarp are removed at the same time. Machine milling can produce an even more refined product with an even greater loss of bran. Brown rice may contain about 15.0 nM/g (4 μg) thiamin/g rice, whereas highly polished rice may contain as little as 2.63 nM/g (0.7 μg/g) rice. Other B vitamins are also lost. Additionally, the Asian practice of washing the rice before cooking results in additional losses of water-soluble thiamin. Thiamin losses are of most concern in areas of the world where polished rice is the staple food. Thiamin deficiency can result in beriberi, at one time a major cause of death in many countries.[5] Now, white rice is usually enriched with niacin, thiamin, and iron.

EFFECT OF HOME AND INSTITUTIONAL PREPARATION

A discussion of nutrient loss during processing would not be complete without mentioning the losses that commonly occur in the home or food service establishment. Because the greatest nutrient losses are due to excess heat and leaching into cooking water and cook-drip, improper home or institutional cooking practices cause large nutrient losses. Often, the primary factors responsible for vitamin and mineral losses in foods are the final preparation steps.

Because of the large vitamin losses that occur during home cooking, the final vitamin content among table-ready foods may be similar, regardless of whether the food was commercially processed or was freshly purchased. Losses in the home can be minimized by using less cooking water, by reducing trimming of fruits and vegetables, by chopping food less finely, by cooking in covered pans (to lessen cooking time and water use), by cooking vegetables only until tender, and by using cooking water for soups. Steaming or stir-frying will result in greater nutrient retention than boiling or typical pan frying.[11,29]

In conclusion, the most common food processing methods generally do not cause major losses of nutrients. Some loss of nutrients is necessary to assure product safety. Major nutrient losses are incurred with excessive use of heat and water during cooking. As more sophisticated food processing methods are developed, even greater nutrient retention during commercial processing becomes possible. Extrusion tends to have a negative effect on nutrient retention whereas retort pouches and the use of HTST thermal processes have a positive effect. Other factors that influence nutrient retention are the adequacy of food storage and distribution, institutional food preparation, and the handling of food by the home consumer. Thiamin and vitamin C are the most labile nutrients in foods. Monitoring the retention of these nutrients and of lysine in high-protein foods will provide an index of the overall nutrient retention in the food after processing.

REFERENCES

1. Potter, N.N.: Food Science. 3rd Ed. Westport, CT, AVI Publishing, 1978.
2. Poneros, A.G., Erdman, J.W. Jr.: J. Food Sci., *53:*208–210, 1988.
3. Darby, W.J., McNutt, K.W., Todhunter, E.N.: Nutr. Rev., *33:*289–297, 1975.
4. Wall, J.S., Carpenter, K.J.: Food Technol. *42(10):*198–204, 1988.
5. Bender, A.E.: Food Processing and Nutrition. New York, NY, Academic Press, 1978.
6. Committee on Nutritional Misinformation: Nutr. Rev., *34:*316–317, 1976.
7. Fennema, O.: Effects of freeze preservation on nutrients. *In* Nutritional Evaluation of Food Processing. 3rd Ed. Edited by E. Karmas and R.S. Harris. New York, AVI Publishing, 1988, pp. 269–317.
8. Harris, R.S.: General discussion on the stability of nutrients. *In* Nutritional Evaluation of Food Processing. 3rd Ed. Edited by E. Karmas and R.S. Harris. New York, AVI Publishing, 1988, pp. 3–5.
9. Nelson, P.E.: Hortscience, *7(2):*13–15, 1972.
10. Dietz, J.M., Erdman, J.W. Jr.: Nutr. Today, *24(4):*6–15, 1989.
11. IFT: Food Technol., *40(12):*109–116, 1986.
12. Lamb, F.C., Farrow, R.P., Elkins, E.R.: Effect of processing on nutritive value of food: Canning. *In* Handbook of Nutritive Value of Processed Food. Vol. 1. Edited by M. Rechcigl Jr. Boca Raton, FL, CRC Press, 1982, pp. 11–30.
13. Lund, D.: Effects of heat processing on nutrients. *In* Nutritional Evaluation of Food Processing. 3rd Ed. Edited by E. Karmas and R.S. Harris. New York, AVI Publishing, 1988, pp. 319–354.
14. Swaisgood, H.E.: Characteristics of edible fluids of animal origin: Milk. *In* Food Chemistry. New York, Marcel Dekker, 1985, pp. 791–827.
15. Borenstein, B., LaChance, P.A.: Effects of processing and preparation on the nutritive value of foods. *In* Modern Nutrition in Health and Disease. 7th Ed. Edited by M.E. Shils and V.R. Young. Philadelphia, Lea & Febiger, 1988, pp. 672–684.
16. Adams, C.E., Erdman, J.W. Jr.: Effects of home food preparation practices on nutrient content of foods. *In* Nutritional Evaluation of Food Processing. 3rd Ed. Edited by E. Karmas and R.S. Harris. New York, AVI Publishing, 1988.
17. Ranhotra, G.S., Bock, M.A.: Effects of Baking on Nutrients. *In* Nutritional Evaluation of Food Processing. 3rd Ed. Edited by E. Karmas and R.S. Harris. New York, AVI Publishing, 1988, pp. 355–364.
18. Ranhotra, G.S., Gelroth, J.A.: Cereal Chem., *63:*401–403, 1986.
19. Erdman, J.W. Jr.: J. Am. Oil Chem. Soc., *56:*736–741, 1979.
20. Harper, J.M.: Effects of extrusion processing on nutrients. *In* Nutritional Evaluation of Food Processing. 3rd Ed. Edited by E. Karmas and R.S. Harris. New York, AVI Publishing, 1988, pp. 365–391.
21. Camire, M.E., Camire, A., Krumhar, K.: Crit. Rev. Food Sci. Nutr., *29:*35–57, 1990.
22. Björck, I., Asp, N.-G.: J. Food Engin., *2:*281–308, 1983.
23. IFT: Food Technol., *43(1):*117–126, 1989.
24. Klein, B.P.: Contemp. Nutr., *14(2)*, 1989.
25. Bluestein, P.M., Labuza, T.P.: Effects of moisture removal on nutrients. *In* Nutritional Evaluation of Food Processing. 3rd Ed. Edited by E. Karmas and R.S. Harris. New York, AVI Publishing, 1988, pp. 393–422.
26. Karmas, E.: The major food Groups, their nutrient content, and principles of food processing. *In* Nutritional Evaluation of Food Processing. 3rd Ed. Edited by E. Karmas and R.S. Harris. New York, AVI Publishing, 1988, pp. 7–19.

27. Thomas, M.H.: Use of ionizing radiation to preserve food. *In* Nutritional Evaluation of Food Processing. 3rd Ed. Edited by E. Karmas and R.S. Harris. New York, AVI Publishing, 1988, pp. 457–490.

28. Tannenbaum, S.R., Young, V.R.: Vitamins and minerals. *In* Food Chemistry. New York, Marcel Dekker, 1985, pp. 477–544.

29. Erdman, J.W. Jr.: Food Technol., *33(2)*:38–48, 1979.

SELECTED READINGS

Bender, A.E.: Food Processing and Nutrition. London, Academic Press, 1978.

Karmas, E., Harris, R.S. (eds.): Nutritional Evaluation of Food Processing. 3rd Ed. New York, AVI Publishing, 1988.

Labuza, T.P., Erdman, J.W. Jr.: Food Science and Nutritional Health: An Introduction. St. Paul, West Publishing, 1984.

Rechcigl, M. Jr. (ed.): Handbook of Nutritive Value of Processed Food. Vol. 1. Boca Raton, FL, CRC Press, 1982.

CHAPTER **91**

Nutrification of Foods

J. Christopher Bauernfeind

For some time, humans have been nourished by consuming a variety of foods selected from available plant, animal, marine, and inorganic sources in the environment. Early humans probably ate an average share of the digestible portion of whole living matter as influenced by variation in food availability with seasons of the year and other prevailing factors. As humans began to control and modify animal and plant life to better accommodate human needs, food development became more integral to the economic and social life of the community. In the historic struggle for food humans ate primarily whole foods or so-called natural foods, which underwent little processing except prior to consumption. To preserve food for longer periods and to provide variety, food preservation and food processing programs were introduced. Today the emphasis of food is on its nutritive values and its role in the maintenance of optimal health and resistance to disease.

According to the 1976 Nutrition Bill of Rights framed by the American Dietetic Association,[1] every person has (1) the right to optimum nutritional health, (2) the right to safe foods that will promote good nutrition and improve resistance to disease, and (3) the right to make informed choices from available foods and to be protected against nutritional misinformation.

Authoritative food guides have been issued that deal with preventive health and nutritional approaches, whereby foods can combat or prevent some disease problems.[2–4] Another U.S. approach to food guides for better health and nutrition was the voluntary adoption of food nutritional labeling laws for some foods almost two decades ago. Although this was a progressive step for providing quantitative information on nutrients in a given food serving, there have been mixed reviews on the ability of the consumer to use the information in preparing nutritionally balanced meals. As a result of the U.S. Nutrition Labeling and Education Act of 1990, food labeling may be moving from a voluntary toward a mandatory basis and would then apply to more food products.[5] Consumer nutrient labeling issues including current consumer nutritional knowledge were reviewed in 1991.[6]

NUTRITION, FOOD SCIENCE, AND DIETARY PRACTICES

Food science and technology predate the concept of modern nutrition.[7] While an awareness of the importance of nutrition was evolving, marked changes had been taking place in the food supply system. Food technological advances in the developed countries have imposed on the consumer the burden of selecting a balanced diet not only from the traditional, natural, processed, and refined food, but also from the new convenience, fabricated, and novel foods, some of which simulate known foods and others that have no past traditional counterpart.

The nutrient content of food usually decreases when it is processed (see Chap. 90) because (1) some nutrients are sensitive to heat, oxygen, light, or a combination thereof, (2) some nutrients are extracted by liquids (solvents) or gases (water vapor), (3) some nutrients are altered by enzyme action, and (4) nutrients are lost by physically removing part of the food or fractionating it into two or more parts.[8,9] Nutrient content may change then through harvesting, storing, washing, trimming or peeling, blanching, extracting, straining, pasteurizing, boiling, sterilizing or canning, baking, dehydrating, irradiating, fermenting, brining, milling, bleaching, curing, frying, roasting, and steam table holding practices. The nutrient content of a food at the time of consumption, not that of the raw food product, is important.

Over the past two decades in the United States dynamic changes have been made in living and market place patterns influencing calorie intakes, eating habits, food purchasing practices, and meal preparation, which have in turn influenced diet nutrient adequacy.[3,10] Eating-out habits influence dietary intake. Skipped meals, high-fat snacks, high-sugar sweets and soft drinks, and high alcohol consumption may lower micronutrient consumption. Unsound food faddism programs may also contribute to dietary insufficiencies (see Chap. 86).

About 50 nutrients are now known to be needed for life. Nutrient daily allowances for humans exist for approximately half of them[11] (see Appendix Tables A–2b and A–2c). The nutrients have been identified by chemical structure and by chemical reactions. Assay methods have been developed to determine the content of the nutrients in foods,[12] thereby establishing the potential contribution that an individual serving of any food product makes in meeting the daily allowance for that nutrient. No single food, even whole or natural, supplies all the nutrients required for human nutrition or in the correct proportions to meet the daily nutrient needs. Hence, the earlier admonition to eat a variety of different foods is valid. If all the people in the world had a sufficient array and quantity of plant, animal, marine, and inorganic foods and chose to eat a correctly selected diet, there probably would be little or no insufficiency of required nutrient consumption. In reality, however, an insufficient volume of food and/or poor dietary practices bring about certain nutrient deficiencies of varying degrees of severity in the developing countries, including vitamin A,[13] iron,[14] energy, and protein. In developed countries, furthermore, there are also marginal insufficiencies of vitamins and minerals.[15] Until consumers become more knowledgeable about nutrition, it is wise to concentrate on the limiting nutrients consumed within population groups, whether in developed or developing countries, and to adopt a nutrient delivery system that requires minimal nutritional education.[3]

Advances in chemical and microbial engineering have produced relatively pure inorganic and organic nutrients (the vitamins and amino acids) cheaply enough and in adequate volume to permit their consideration as components of the human diet. It has been apparent for some time that part of the solution of the world's need for a nourishing food supply will depend on maximizing the combined benefits from food technologic and nutritional knowledge[3,7] and adapting these towards human needs as influenced by social and political pressures within individual countries.

NUTRIFICATION: DEFINITION AND OBJECTIVES

Nutrification is defined as the addition of one or more nutrients to one or more commonly consumed foods or food mixtures that can, if properly introduced and controlled, improve the dietary intake of a given population.[16,17] To "nutrify" is merely to make a food more nutritious. Nutrification is used here as a replacement term for fortification, enrichment, restoration, supplementation, etc., terms that originally were borrowed from other disciplines or applications than food use.

In 1989 nutrification of food was listed among the top 10 food science innovations of the past 50 years by the Institute of Food Technologists. Nevertheless, the great potential offered by wise use of industrially produced nutrients, vitamins, minerals, amino acids, and protein isolates rarely has been fully realized.[18] Richardson has noted that many nutrition surveys in developed and developing countries continue to indicate that an appreciable fraction of the population, particularly young children, adolescents, the elderly, and women of childbearing age, can suffer from nutrient deficiencies at a borderline or pathologic level. In the developed nations, nutrient needs and food choices of these specific population groups, the increasing use of dietetic and low-energy products, the overall trend towards consuming fewer calories, and the greater reliance on commercially prepared foods are just some of the reasons why it is essential to re-examine policies and guidelines for the addition of nutrients to foods.[19]

When considering a program of food nutrification other alternatives for improved nutritional status need be examined simultaneously. Each may have inherent advantages and disadvantages with respect to certain criteria. These include costs, delivery system infrastructure, personnel, degree of skill required, role of the beneficiary including acceptability, time necessary to make an impact or achieve the goal, the assurance of continuation of the intervention, and appropriateness of the intervention for the target population. From time to time, attempts have been made to evaluate and rank different interventions; one such reported attempt[20] is illustrated in Table 91–1.

Nutrification has a long history of civilian use in both developed and developing countries since Boussingault first proclaimed the virtues of this concept by suggesting, in 1831, that iodine be added to table salt to prevent the development of goiter.[21] USDA food assistance programs include nutrified foods used in the WIC (Women, Infant, and Children) distribution plan.[22] Under U.S. Public Law 480, donated low-cost nutrified foods are exported to combat malnutrition and hunger in developing countries and to encourage their economic development. Nutrification is practiced by the U.S. Armed Forces.[3]

Nutrification of food could not be undertaken until the necessary active ingredients[23,24] could be produced in sufficient quantities at commercially feasible prices. A technology has been developed over the years to make feasible the addition of nutrients to many foods or food ingredients.[10,25–32] In 1939 the Council on Foods and Nutrition of the American Medical Association (AMA) first published a policy on the addition of specific nutrients to foods, followed in 1941 by one from the Food and Nutrition Board of the National Research Council (NRC). The latest policy revision, issued in 1982, calls for evidence that the nutrified food would be nutritionally and economically beneficial for the population, that the food selected would be a proper carrier for effective distribution of the added nutrient, and that the added

TABLE 91–1. TABLE COMPARISON OF ALTERNATIVE INTERVENTIONS

CRITERIA	FORTIFICATION	TABLETS	INJECTIONS	NUTRITION EDUCATION	HOME GARDENS	PLANT BREEDING
Costs						
Initial capital investments	Moderate	Low	Low	Low	Low	High
Continuing personnel	Low	High	High	High	Low	High
Continuing materials	Low*	Low	Moderate	Low	Moderate	High
Personnel Requirements						
Skill level	Moderate	Moderate	High	Low	Moderate	High
Numbers	Low	High	High	Moderate	High	Low
Administrative Requirements						
Supervision	Moderate	High	High	Moderate	Moderate	High
Health system organization	Low	High	High	Moderate	Low	Low
Technical Feasibility						
Technology dependability	High†	High	Moderate	Moderate	High	Moderate
Side effects risk	Low	Moderate	High	Low	Low	Moderate
Beneficiary Rule						
Acceptability	High	Moderate	Moderate	Moderate	Moderate	Moderate
Community involvement	Low‡	Moderate	Moderate	High	High	Low
Impact						
Population coverage	High	Moderate§	Moderate§	Moderate	Moderate	Moderate
Time needed to show benefit	Moderate	Low	Low	Moderate	Low	High
Permanency of benefit	High	Low	Low	Moderate	High	High

*An exception is protein fortification, which is expensive compared to micronutrient fortification.
†Iron fortification has encountered technical difficulties, but recent improvements appear to have resolved these.
‡In contrast to a central processing plan, village-level fortification could have high community participation.
§Direct-dosage coverage is a function of the outreach capacity of the delivery system, but coverage is constrained by the one-to-one system.
(Adapted from World Food Council 1977 in Austin, J.E., Hitt, C.: Nutrition Intervention in the United States. Cambridge, MA, Ballinger, 1977).

nutrient would be physiologically available, chemically stable, capable of being monitored, and nontoxic under usual conditions of dietary use.[33] Improved food processing techniques were recommended. Snack foods were recognized as contributors to the total food intake and thereby as potential carriers of nutrients in some circumstances. Guideline regulations for food nutrification are available by the U.S. Food and Drug Administration[34] and by appropriate regulatory divisions in other countries.

Bioavailability of added vitamins to food is usually very good, and is good or acceptable for mineral sources that have been tested for the intended application.[23,24,35] There are no toxicity problems from the consumption of nutrified foods. Because food nutrification continues at daily nutrient levels in the recommended dietary allowance (RDA) tables and in the FDA USRDA tables or slightly above those values, nutrient toxicity should not be a deterrent because minimum toxic dose levels[4] are not approached (Table 91–2).

Nutrification is the most rapidly applied, the most flexible, and a socially acceptable intervention method of changing the nutrient intake without a vast educational effort and without a change in the current food intake pattern of a given population. It usually has a favorable cost/benefit ratio compared to other methods. Once a nutrification program involving the addition of a single nutrient has been initiated, adding a second one or subsequent ones becomes easier, and unit costs are lower. An educational effort along with any nutrification plan may be helpful to explain the goal of the program and to introduce, if warranted, other long-range interventions such as improved agricultural and public health practices.

PROGRAM CONSIDERATIONS

Any contemplated program to be undertaken will depend on (1) local circumstances and (2) a consideration of alternative approaches. Once a nutrification policy is adopted it should remain dynamic, open to revision and to periodic updating of nutritional knowledge and standards. The foods to nutrify and other aspects to be considered prior to initiating a nutrification program are discussed in the following paragraphs.

Food Vehicle(s) or Food Carrier(s) for Added Nutrient(s). The carrier should be a food or food ingredient universally consumed by the targeted population, preferably with relatively little variation in consumption pattern. More than one food carrier may be chosen. In early nutrification practices the food carrier was usually a staple food product, one that passed through central,

TABLE 91–2. VITAMIN AND MINERAL SAFETY INDEXES

NUTRIENT	HIGHEST RECOMMENDED ADULT INTAKE*	SOURCE OF RECOMMENDED INTAKE	ESTIMATED DAILY ADULT ORAL MINIMUM TOXIC DOSE
Vitamin A	5,000 IU	USRDA	25,000 to 50,000 IU
Vitamin D	400 IU	USRDA	50,000 IU
Vitamin E	30 IU	USRDA	1,200 IU
Vitamin C	60 mg	RDA	1,000 to 5,000 mg
Thiamin	1.5 mg	USRDA	300 mg
Riboflavin	1.7 mg	USRDA	1,000 mg†
Niacin (nicotinamide)	20 mg	USRDA	1,000 mg
Pyridoxine	2.0 mg	RDA	2,000 mg‡
Folacin	0.4 mg	USRDA	400 mg
Biotin	0.3 mg	USRDA	50 mg
Pantothenic acid	10 mg	USRDA	1,000 mg
Calcium	1,200 mg	RDA	12,000 mg
Phosphorus	1,200 mg	RDA	12,000 mg
Magnesium	400 mg	USRDA	6,000 mg
Iron	18 mg	USRDA	100 mg
Zinc	15 mg	USRDA	500 mg
Copper	3 mg	ESAADDI	100 mg
Fluoride	4 mg	ESAADDI	4 to 20 mg
Iodine	0.15 mg	USRDA	2 mg
Selenium	0.2 mg	ESAADDI	1 mg

*Figures represent the highest published value for each nutrient, either the Recommended Dietary Allowances (RDA) (except those for pregnancy and lactation) or Estimated Safe and Adequate Daily Dietary Intakes (ESAADDI) (NRC, 1980), or the U.S. Recommended Daily Allowances (USRDA).

†However, only ~25 mg of riboflavin can be absorbed in a single oral dose given to an adult.

‡More recent data suggest that the toxic dose of pyridoxine for some individuals is much lower.

(From Food and Nutrition Board, National Research Council: Diet and Health: Implications for Reducing Chronic Disease Risk. Washington, D.C., National Academy Press, 1989.)

communal, or regional processing centers where the nutrification technique could be introduced. When a staple food product is not available, an alternative may be a sweetening, seasoning agent, or beverage. In other instances village nutrification may have merit over a state or country program. Special foods or ingredients imported into a country for uniform distribution to the populace may open another opportunity for nutrification at the site of export.[3]

Sources of the Added Nutrient(s). Added nutrients should possess acceptable chemical, physical, and organoleptic properties. More than one nutrient may be considered. The physical form of the nutrient, its ease of incorporation into the end product, its stability characteristics, and its acceptability under the specific conditions of intended use can be critical to the success of the project. A pilot trial under the expected field conditions to be encountered is a safe-guard to possible future disaster without such a preliminary measure. The amount of added nutrient must be adequate to fulfill the need, yet protect against nutrient imbalance and unsafe use.

Voluntary or Mandated Program. If the program is to be undertaken by government decree, it must be determined that there is popular support for such action. Acceptance of the program is of utmost importance.

Assurance of Adequacy of the Nutrification Program.

The addition of the nutrient(s) to the food carrier(s) in a uniform fashion and production of adequate volume is necessary to serve the intended purpose. Adequate equipment operated with required expertise is necessary whether operations are carried out by the batch system or on a continuous basis.[36]

Production Controls for the Nutrified Food(s). Qualitative control procedures at the site of the nutrification process and quantitative laboratory procedures, periodically applied, are necessary to provide assurance of proper operations.

Distribution of Nutrified Product. Marketplace and home use checkpoints are desirable to observe intended and continued patterns of use.

Overall Program Monitoring. If the program is to remedy an existing health problem, monitoring of the targeted population at suitable intervals will confirm whether the program is correcting the problem. A baseline study prior to the nutrification program is highly desirable.

Cost of Program. Costs need to be weighted with a comparison of expected benefits of the program against not instituting the program in regard to the well-being of the population. Prior decisions are necessary to determine whether the consumer, the food industry or government pays for the program. If the food industry is to absorb the cost initially, an early understanding is advisable with government on prevailing policy.

POTENTIAL BENEFITS

Nutrification of food can be considered one possible intervention measure in which a substantial segment of a population would benefit from the incorporation of a nutrient or nutrients in the diet, but preferably in which the total caloric needs for food are reasonably adequate. Nutrification with micronutrients adds to the nutritional quality of the diet, with little or no change in the quantity of the diet. The following are situations that might call for nutrification with industrially produced nutrients.

Changing Economic Conditions. Industrially produced nutrients, appropriately used in combination with agricultural products, offer protective safeguards or alternative products in changing economic conditions. Amino acids and more vegetable protein extenders are now used in fabricated foods in Japan and the United States, although the initial impetus for the increased use of vegetable protein concentrates in human foods came from the earlier concern of meeting the protein crises in the developing countries by supplementing local calorie food products[25] rather than importing more expensive food sources.

Inadequate Intake of Protective Foods. Some populations in the world do not have access to a sufficient quantity of protective foods or do not consume such foods because of beliefs and taboos. Both conditions can lead to dietary deficiencies. Although long-range approaches need to be considered under these circumstances, in many instances a nutrification program can quickly introduce the missing nutrient or nutrients. Examples are the insufficient consumption of foods containing vitamin A, iron, and iodine in some of the developing countries. These nutrients can even be added to condiments.[26] Vitamin A and iron may also be added to a sweetening agent such as sucrose.[27]

Overconsumption of High-Calorie Foods. With the passage of time a greater percentage of the populations in developed countries has become involved in more-sedentary occupations, the result of which is lowered caloric needs. On the other hand, advances in food technology have generated more kinds of high-energy food products, many of which are of a refined or highly processed character or have been fabricated from refined food components. Hence, they do not contain an appropriate level of essential micronutrients relative to their energy contribution. Examples of these high-energy items are high-calorie beverages and sweets made from sucrose, fructose, glucose, corn sugar syrups, and table syrups; high-calorie items made with fats, shortenings, and vegetable oils, some of which also have added sugar and/or starch; and alcoholic (ethanol) drinks. Substantial consumption of these high-calorie items can lead to underconsumption of important micronutrients.[3,10]

Making Food Metabolically Self-Sufficient. If all foods contained the required micronutrients at levels comparable to their caloric contribution to the diet, there would be less difficulty with nutritional insufficiencies. Certain high-calorie foods fit less well into a meal pattern and fall more into a category of "snack, fun, or pleasure foods"—that is, they are more frequently consumed between meals.[10] Soft drinks can make up 30 to 35% of the caloric intake of children 10 to 15 years old.[37] How should they be considered in nutrification programs?[38] Where there is no recognized serving size or weight for the food, the program could add nutrients relative to caloric content.[39] Nutrified confectionary products have been developed.[10,40]

Food Class Standardization. If a natural food in a given class of foods serves as a substantial source of a micronutrient and another food that contains little or none of that nutrient is promoted or recommended for the same purpose, some justification exists for adding the missing nutrient(s) to the latter. One case in point is use of cranberry juice (naturally low in vitamin C) in place of citrus juice as a breakfast beverage. Because a goodly portion of the daily vitamin C needs is consumed at breakfast, there is merit to standardizing the vitamin C level in cranberry and other juices low in natural vitamin C (e.g., apple, apricot, grape, pineapple, and prune juice).[28] The consumer can then have variety without forfeiting nutritional value.

Another case is the protein food analogues adapted to serve as replacements for animal protein products wherein the vegetable product can be nutrified to simulate the composition of the product imitated.[25]

A third example are the meal replacers. When either a dietetic, instant, frozen, or dried meal product is developed and promoted to replace a regular meal, a suitable approach to micronutrient nutrification would be to have the new product provide about one-third of the daily allowance of micronutrients. Similarly, when food products are developed to replace an existing food, the new products could contain a reasonably complete array of micronutrients found in the natural product to avoid nutritional inferiority.[3,33]

Restoration of Lost Nutrients. Under the restoration concept, some micronutrients originally present in a whole natural food but lost in processing are returned to a processed food. For example, when peanuts are roasted in the usual manufacture of peanut butter, the process destroys the thiamin naturally present. It is technically feasible to add pure thiamin back to the butter during the grinding operation.

Large amounts of natural tocopherols are lost in the bleaching, deodorization, and further refining treatment of vegetable oils preliminary to margarine production. As a restoration step vitamin E can be added back to margarine in the manner practiced in some countries during the past decade.[29]

Because of the volume consumed, freshly cooked white potatoes have made a substantial contribution of vitamin C and other nutrients to some populations. Currently more potatoes are consumed in manufactured forms such as fries, powders, buds, flakes, chips, or crisps. In many instances, processing and storage on supermarket shelves degrade much of the natural vitamin C. Restoring vitamin C, for example, to these processed potato products is nutritionally justifiable under this concept.[30]

As has been known for nearly half a century, when butterfat is removed from whole fluid milk for the production of fluid skim milk or dry nonfat milk (dry skim milk), the natural carotenes, vitamin A, and tocopherols are also removed. A technology exists for the addition of β-carotene and vitamins A, D, and E to these low-fat dairy products.[31]

From the early days of the addition of synthetic nutrients to processed foods, two positions were advanced: (1) to restore nutrient levels only to the level of the unprocessed food and (2) to add nutrients at levels to prevent disease and produce optimal health based on the use of the food product in the daily diet.[41] In the past decade it has become apparent that the trend is shifting from the former to the latter view as human needs and goals are more realistically recognized.

Deficiencies in Geochemical Environments. Soils in many areas of the world are deficient in certain minerals; this can result in low concentrations of major or trace minerals in drinking water, plant crops, and even tissues of farm animals, thus contributing to marginal or deficient dietary intakes of humans.[42] Minerals in this category are fluoride, iodide, molybdenum, and selenium; in some countries, the first two are added back to the diet in the form of fluoride-treated water and iodized salt.[24,43] Certain areas of the United States, Finland, New Zealand, and China are known to have soils low in selenium. Because estimated safe intakes of selenium have been determined, nutrification with selenium in selected areas may be a consideration in the future. Copper, chromium, magnesium, and zinc likewise may become future additives under certain prevailing conditions.[42,44]

Improvement in Bioavailability. When one is dealing with an insufficiency of a mineral element in the diet, two approaches are possible: (1) increase the mineral content by the addition of a proper mineral source, and (2) attempt to improve the bioavailability of the mineral already in the diet. For example, one can improve the biologic availability of existing dietary iron supplies or added iron by incorporating some facilitating substance in the diet such as L-ascorbic acid or its sodium salt.[24,25] Enhancement by ascorbic acid is dose-dependent; an intake as little as 25 mg (143 μM) at a meal may be significant, but intakes of 100 mg or more daily may be the goal in severely iron-deficient populations.[24,82]

Improvement of Cereal Grain Products. Cereal grains account for 52% of the global average per capita intake for calories and 47% of the average protein intake.[46] About 26% of the daily caloric intake in the United States comes from products based on cereal grains.[47] This intake does not vary greatly relative to income and geographic region. In some developing countries cereal grain products provide up to 70% of the caloric intake. As a class of foods, cereal grains have considerable merit because (1) they are universally consumed, (2) they are prime suppliers of calories and protein, (3) they provide variety in the diet through industrial and home processing for consumption, (4) they contain complex carbohydrates (indigestible fiber) that are believed to function as a health maintenance aid, and (5) they are a form of food easily stored if moisture content and insect infestation are controlled.[32] Because cereal grains enjoy wide acceptability as a food and contain some vitamins, minerals, and amino acids, they can be further improved by nutrification to make them into superior food products; in short they are logical food products to serve as carriers of added nutrients to populations of both developed and developing countries. The number and amount of additives, vitamins, minerals, amino acids, and/or vegetable protein concentrates to be added to specific cereal grain meal or fractional grain products depends on geographic location and local problems.

A major contribution to an increased food supply can be made through developing nutritionally designed processed products based on cereal, tuber, and other primarily carbohydrate crops and using nutrients that are produced by chemical and microbial processes.[18,30,32] In the United States, the Food and Nutrition Board of the National Research Council, on reviewing nutrition and dietary survey data, found evidence of potential risk of deficiencies of vitamin A, thiamin, riboflavin, niacin, vitamin B_6, folacin, iron, calcium, magnesium, and zinc among some segments of the population. Believing cereal grain products to be suitable nutrient carriers, the Board proposed in 1974 that these 10 nutrients be added to all products based on the major cereal grains (wheat, corn, and rice) where technically feasible[47] (Table 91–3).

Between 1974 and 1985 studies were conducted to determine the technical feasibility of the proposed 10-nutrient addition to wheat flour, farina, pasta, refrigerated and frozen dough, prepared mixes, corn flour, grits, corn meal, and white rice. The data generated so far indicate that with small modifications on specific carriers the proposed program is feasible.[32,48,49] Riboflavin, because of its yellow color and high calcium and magnesium additions, may have to remain in an optional classification for white rice until further technologic advances work out feasible procedures. Even so, in 1992 the 10-nutrient addition proposal has yet to be implemented.

Over the past decades it has been the expectation that the lower-quality proteins of the cereal grains would be supplemented with amino acids, with protein isolates, or with legume or oilseed meals to provide improved protein quality more in line with human needs. At present the trend is toward the preparation of blended food mixtures of a cereal grain product with a plant protein concentrate, such as a soybean product; this has merit where there is insufficiency of food, thus meeting both protein and calorie needs.[25]

Limitation of the Gastrointestinal Tract. In young children consideration is not always given to the physical limitation of the size of the stomach or entire gastrointestinal (GI) tract. If rice is the only dietary source of certain essential amino acids for the very young child, it is not possible for the stomach to hold the amount of rice needed to meet the daily allowance.[50]

Retardation of Chronic Degenerative Diseases. The last few decades have produced increasing evidence of an interrelationship between nutrition and chronic degenerative diseases. There is also the realization that certain subgroups—namely, alcohol abusers, oral contraceptive users, pregnant and lactating women, smokers, strict vegetarians, the elderly, those with digestive tract disorders, and weight-loss dieters—may be consuming less than recommended daily allowances of micronutrients. It may now be more possible to manipulate the diet over the life cycle toward the goal of better health.[4,51–57]

Nutrients possessing dual roles (an essential physiologic role and a role as an antioxidant or inhibitor of free radical damage)—namely, β-carotene, vitamin C, vitamin E, and selenium—appear to have greater significance in the nutrient-health equation, although other nutrients may be involved also. A higher intake of β-carotene may reduce the risk of certain cancers, vitamin A having a somewhat more limited role. Vitamin C intake has been associated with improvement of immune response, lower serum cholesterol levels, and retardation of cataract formation. Calcium and vitamin D appear to have a role in preventing colon cancer.[58] Vitamin E intake has been reviewed as to its health benefits in the case of cancer, cardiovascular disease, cataracts, certain anemias, immunity development, and infections.[57]

Malnutrition predisposes to infection as immunity is lowered.[59] The fifth world food survey (60) has indicated that one-third to half a billion humans suffer from malnutrition.[60] Vitamin A is one nutrient in short supply in developing world countries. Not only is it needed for maintenance of eyesight but when consumed in insufficient amounts it is associated with more respiratory

TABLE 91–3. COMPARISON OF NUTRIFICATION OF FLOUR WITH FOUR NUTRIENTS VS. TEN NUTRIENTS

	USED AT PRESENT[b]		PROPOSED[c]	
Nutrients[a]	In Flour	In Bread[d]	In Flour	In Bread
Thiamin	2.9	1.8	2.9	1.8
Riboflavin	1.8	1.1	1.8	1.1
Niacin	24.0	15.0	24.0	15.0
Iron	13.0–16.5	8.0–12.5	40.0[e]	—
Calcium	—	—	900	562
Vitamin A[f]	None	None	1.3 (4,300 IU)[g]	0.8 (2,700 IU)
Pyridoxine	None	None	2.0	1.2
Folic acid	None	None	0.3	0.18
Magnesium	None	None	200.0	125.0
Zinc	None	None	10.0	6.2

[a]Expressed as milligrams per pound of flour.
[b]Minimums and maximums in Code of Federal Regulations. Title 21, Parts 136–137.
[c]NAS, NRC (1974). As of 1992 values are still in proposed status for flour & bread.
[d]Bread is considered to contain 62.5% wheat flour based on the conversion of 100 lb of flour to 160 lb of bread.
[e]November 18, 1977, the FDA restored the provision for 13.0–16.5 mg lb.
[f]Retinol equivalent.
[g]The originally proposed level of 2.2 mg/lb (7,300 IU) was lowered to 1.3 mg/lb (4,300 IU).
(From Emodi, A.S., Scialpi, L., Cereal Chem., *57*:1–3, 1980, by permission of Cereal Chemistry.)

diseases, measles, parasitic diseases, and diarrhea.[61,62] In refugee camps, these health problems multiply and nutrification of food or use of nutrient supplements should have a high priority.[63] Food fortification and/or nutrient supplements are offered as one approach of four major categories offered to address malnutrition in developing countries.[60]

Foods with health messages have been on the market in the United States for several years now, but new federal regulations are pending on such products[34] (see Chap. 94). Food modified in macronutrient and/or micronutrient content with appropriate messages in developed countries is another approach toward improvement of health.

Special Purpose Alimentation. A number of unique dietary foods have been designed to meet specific physiologic states or life cycle stages. They may be sole sources of nutrient supplies for the period in question or may be supplemental to the diet. Examples are diets for pregnancy and lactation, for diabetics, for allergy control, for control of hypertension, for weight control, for preoperative or postoperative periods, and for infants.[64] The diets that influence the most adult individuals are those for weight control. Diets containing 900 to 1200 calories need close scrutiny regarding adequacy in essential amino acids, vitamins, and minerals.

Technological Applications. Several nutrients have multiple properties; in addition to serving as dietary essentials they contribute technological advantages to the food product to which they are added. L-Ascorbic acid (vitamin C) may act as (1) an oxygen-scavenging agent in bottled and canned food products, (2) an inhibitor of oxidative rancidity in frozen fish, (3) a stabilizer of color and flavor and an inhibitor of nitrosamine formation in cured meats, (4) a flour-maturing agent and dough conditioner, (5) an oxygen acceptor in beer production, and (6) a reducing agent in wine.[65,66] α-Tocopherol (vitamin E) serves as a fat-soluble antioxidant in fats and oils[65,67] and a retardant to nitrosamine formation. β-carotene and β-apo-8′-carotenal, carotenoid vitamin A precursors, also serve as food colors.[68] Under certain conditions β-carotene can quench singlet oxygen and act as an unusual antioxidant when added to vegetable oils.[29]

SUCCESSFUL NUTRIFICATION PROGRAMS

Over the past decades a large number of publications have appeared on the nutrification of foods, including those cited in references 3, 41, and 69 through 72. Iodine addition in the form of potassium iodide or iodate to salt (NaCl) as a goiter preventive is a practice still carried on in the United States and certain other countries.[26] Instances of the effectiveness of iodine nutrification are the 1980 Thailand study in which potassium iodate nutrification of salt reduced iodine deficiency in school children from 84% to practically zero within 6 years,[73] and the effect of mandatory iodization based on health and nutrition survey observations in Central America[72] (Fig. 91–1). Another mineral, fluoride, has been added to drinking water to reduce dental caries. Although this practice has successfully lowered tooth decay for several decades,[74] it remains a moot subject in some parts of the world.

Now vitamin D is added directly to fluid milk, a more economical and better controlled practice than direct irradiation with ultraviolet light or feeding irradiated ergosterol to cows. The nutrification of cows' milk with vitamin D has been credited as the major factor in the disappearance of infantile rickets as a public health problem.[41] Nonfat milk (skim milk) in many instances has added vitamins A and D, whether in dry or fluid form. Today the major portion of the world's margarine production is nutrified with vitamin A[75] (Table 91–4). Vitamin A nutrification of margarine and wheat flour enrichment have been credited with significant health improvement in the people of Newfoundland.[76]

The addition of three vitamins and one mineral to processed white flour and other processed cereal-grain

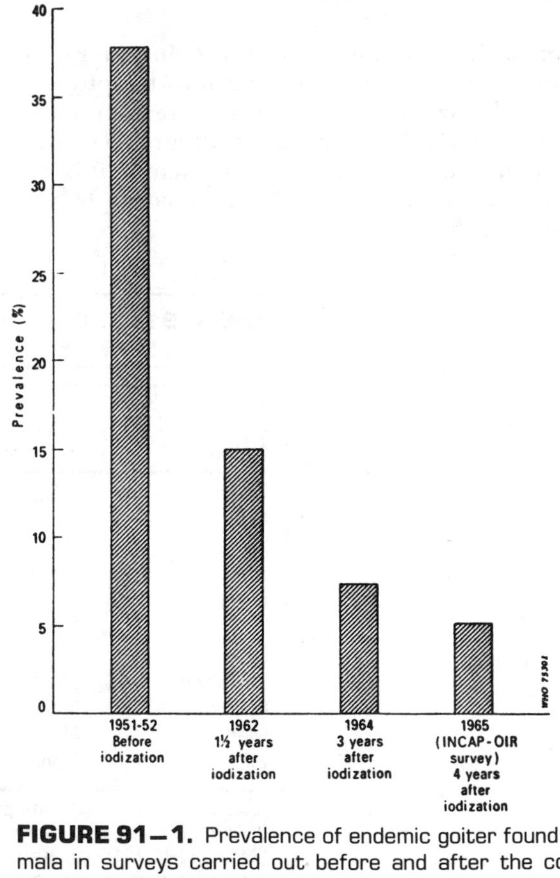

FIGURE 91–1. Prevalence of endemic goiter found in Guatemala in surveys carried out before and after the compulsory iodization of salt. Data provided by the Institute of Nutrition of Central America and Panama (INCAP), Guatemala. (From Beaton, G.H.: Food fortification. *In* Nutrition in Preventive Medicine. Edited by G.H. Beaton and J.M. Bengoa. Geneva, World Health Organization, 1976.)

TABLE 91–4. VITAMIN POTENCY OF NUTRIFIED MARGARINE

VITAMINS A AND D COMMONLY ADDED TO MARGARINE

Country	Vitamin A (IU/kg)	Vitamin D IU/kg
Australia	30,000	4,000
Austria	20,000	1,000
Belgium	20,000	1,000
Brazil	15,000–50,000	500–2,000
Canada	33,000	
Chile	14,000–18,000	1,000
Columbia	20,000–30,000	2,000–4,000
Denmark	20,000	625
Finland	20,000	2,500–3,500
Germany	20,000–30,000	1,000
Greece	25,000	1,500
Israel	30,000	3,000
Japan	30,000–40,000	
Mexico	20,000	2,000
Netherlands	20,000	2,000
Norway	20,000	2,500
Philippines*	22,000	1,100
Portugal	20,000–35,000	875–1,000
South Africa	20,000	1,000
Sweden	30,000	1,500
Switzerland	30,000	1,000
Turkey	20,000	1,000
United Kingdom	30,000–33,000	2,900–3,500
United States	33,000	4,400

*100 mg vitamin B_1 also added.

(From Morton, R.A., R. Soc. Health J., *90:*21–28, 1970, by permission.)

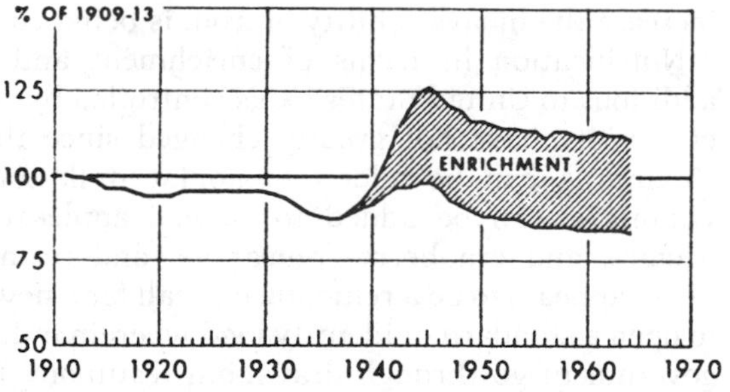

FIGURE 91–2. Value of nutrification of cereal grain products in improving thiamin (vitamin B_1) intake. These figures are based on per capita civilian consumption. (Reprinted with permission from LeBovit, C.J.: Agric. Food Chem., *16:*153–157, 1968. Copyright 1968 by the American Chemical Society.)

products in the United States has been credited with substantial dietary increases of these nutrients, such as thiamin[77] (Fig. 91–2), as well as with the virtual disappearance of pellagra in the South[78] and beriberi and pellagra in urban centers (Fig. 91–3), in association with the influence of enrichment and other factors. In 1972 it was estimated that nutrification provided 40% of thiamin, 25% of iron, 20% of niacin, and 15% of riboflavin in the 1970 U.S. nutrient supplies.[79] A number of countries currently add these nutrients to cereal-grain products[32] (Table 91–5).

Flour enriched in Israel with riboflavin is credited with improved status in that vitamin. Enrichment of rice with thiamin was shown to solve the beriberi problem in Bataan. Enrichment of maize meal with riboflavin and niacin during milling was shown to be highly effective in improving vitamin nutritional states in Africa and was recommended for national initiation.[3]

Retention of nutrients added to cereal grains is good during storage. The loaf volume, crumb color, grain, and proof time of nutrified bread compare favorably with those of non-nutrified bread. For years, micronutrients have been added to U.S. breakfast cereals. A developed technology allows the addition of micronutrients in a stable and biologically available form without influencing flavor or color of the cereal product.[32,48]

Successful nutrification projects have been underway in other parts of the world. The commercial production of amino acids, largely centered in Japan, has enabled nutrification of cereal grain products with them.[3,23,32] During the past decades, oilseed protein mixtures have been prepared with wheat, corn, sorghum, oats, and bulgur and have been incorporated in various cooked or baked foods.[25] In these products, the oilseed or vegetable proteins supplement the proteins from cereal grains, which are inferior. For some years a nutrified bun (Nutribun) made from soy-wheat flour and added micronutrients has been successfully used in the school nutrition program in the Philippines. In India and Ecuador a soy-wheat flour has been used with success in the production of bread.

Other cereal-grain products that are improved through the addition of oilseed protein are CSM (corn-soymilk blend), WSB (wheat-soy blend), SFSG (soy-fortified sorghum grits), SFCM (soy-fortified cornmeal), and WSDM (whey soy drink mix)[25]; these are designed to be used for infants, children, and pregnant and lactating women. Processing cereal grain–vegetable protein mixtures in low-cost extrusion cookers has introduced an appropriate technology in the production of nutritious food supplements. High-protein pasta and high-protein cookies have elicited some interest. Blends of cereal products that have achieved some success in retail sales are Incaparina in Guatemala and Pronutro in South Africa.[25]

One form of blindness, xerophthalmia, occurs in infants and young children in areas of the world such as Asia, the Middle East, Africa, and Latin and South America where the intakes of vitamin A are inadequate.[13] As many as 500,000 or more children around the

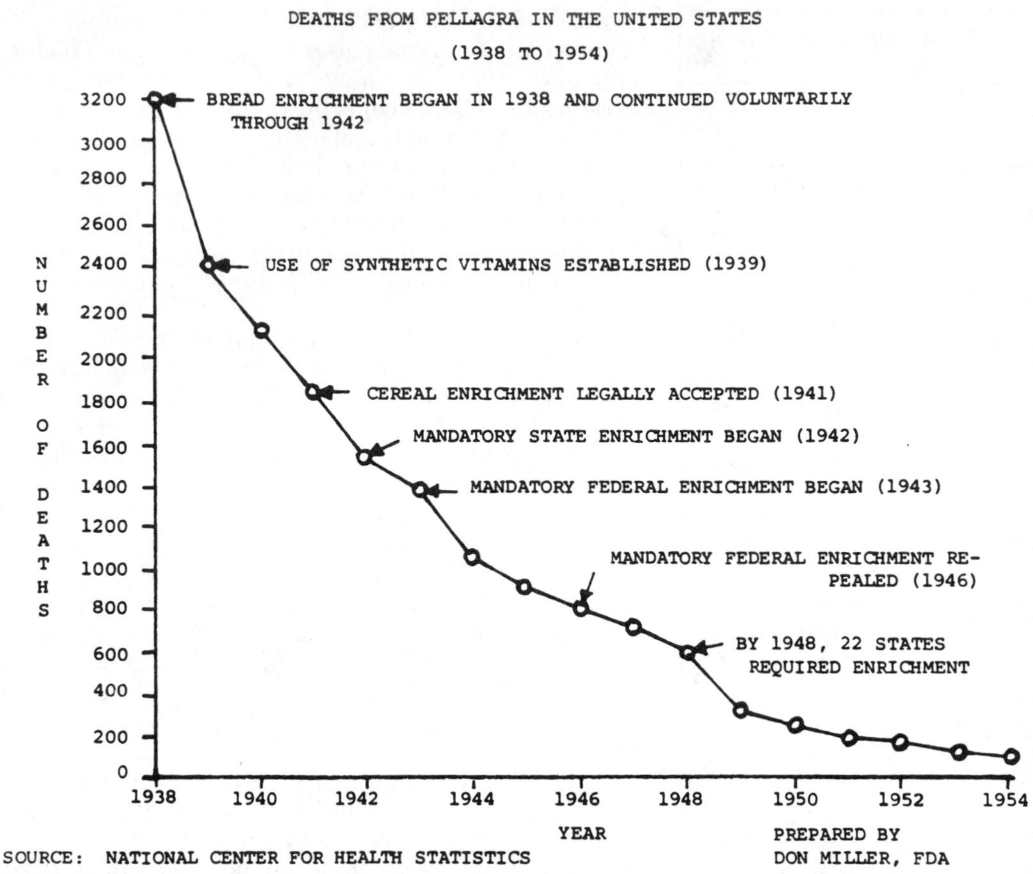

FIGURE 91–3. Deaths from pellagra in the United States from 1938 to 1954. (From Miller, D.F.: Food Product Dev., *12(4)*:30, 1978, by permission of the American Association of Cereal Chemists.)

world may go blind annually as a result of this nutritional deficiency. In addition to eye symptoms, other signs of vitamin A deficiency are growth impairment, greater susceptibility to disease and, in many instances, eventual death. Through the cooperative efforts of the Agency for International Development, the World Health Organization, UNICEF, the International Vitamin A Consultative Group, the international blindness societies, and national groups, a concerted effort has been made to eradicate vitamin A deficiency. As many as 70 countries have the problem to some degree, and programs of various types are underway in India, Africa, Indonesia, Bangladesh, Pakistan, Sri Lanka, Haiti, Guatemala, Panama, Costa Rica, El Salvador, Brazil, the Philippines, and elsewhere. Part of these programs deals with distribution of foods nutrified with vitamin A. Among the foods are dried milk, cereal grain products, sugar (sucrose), and seasonings such as monosodium glutamate and salt.[80] The nutrification of sugar with vitamin A, developed by INCAP[27,81] and practiced in Guatemala (Fig. 91–4), is an outstanding example of the nutrification concept converted to successful practice.

Similar programs are underway for nutrifying foods with available forms of iron to combat another worldwide problem, iron deficiency anemia.[82] Some plans call for putting both vitamin A and iron in the same food carrier. Elsewhere the addition of vitamin C, known to increase the bioavailability of iron, is being considered.

Nutrification in terms of enrichment and nutrient additions to United States foods controlled by standards of identity have not greatly changed since the 1940s. Vitamin A can be added to nonfat milk solids, and vitamin C can be added to canned applesauce, fruit nectars, and cranberry, pineapple, and prune juices. There appears to be a reluctance to call for a new hearing to open a standard of identity food wherein industry and government go through drawn-out testimony that may focus simultaneously on other changes in the standard not favored by one group of participants. Additional nutrients to cereal-grain products (foods under standards of identity) were proposed in 1974 that as of 1992 have yet to be implemented. Years ago, however, another country, Canada, permitted nine nutrients to be added to flour and bread.[32] At the 1969 White House Conference on Nutrition, the panel on new foods, the food quality panel, and the panel on food manufacturing and processing all favored accelerated efforts to expand the nutrification of food.[83]

TABLE 91–5. NUTRIFICATION OF WHEAT FLOUR* (MG/KG)

Country	VITAMIN B_1 Min.	VITAMIN B_1 Max.	VITAMIN B_2 Min.	VITAMIN B_2 Max.	NIACIN Min.	NIACIN Max.	IRON Min.	IRON Max.	CALCIUM Min.	CALCIUM Max.
Australia	1.5	—	2.2	—	15	—	14	—	1,000	
Canada†	4.4	7.7	2.7	4.8	35	64	29	43	1,100	1,400
Chile	6.3	—	1.3	—	13	—	30	—	—	—
Congo	4	6	2.5	3.5	32	45	26	35	1,000	1,500
Costa Rica‡	4.4	5.5	2.6	3.3	35	44	28	36	1,100	1,400
Denmark	5	—	5	—	—	—	30	—	2,000	—
Dominican Republic	4.4	5.5	2.6	3.3	35	44	29	38	1,100	1,400
Guatemala‡	4.4	—	2.6	—	35	—	29	—	1,700	—
Guyana	4.4	5.5	2.7	3.3	35	44	29	36	1,100	1,400
Israel	—	—	2.5	—	—	—	—	—	—	—
Japan	5	8	3	5	—	—	—	—	1,500	3,000
Kenya	4.5	5.5	2.7	3.3	35	44	29	36	—	—
Mexico	4.4	8.8	2.6	5.2	35	70	29	57	—	—
Nigeria	5	—	3.5	—	50	—	35	—	—	—
Panama‡	4.4	—	2.6	—	35	—	29	—	1,100	—
Peru	4	—	4	—	30	—	20	—	1,000	—
Philippines	4.4	5.5	2.6	3.3	35	44	29	36	1,100	1,400
Portugal	4.4	5.5	2.6	3.3	35	44	28	36	—	—
Puerto Rico	4.4	5.5	2.6	3.3	35	44	28	36	1,100	—
Sweden	4	8	1.5	3	40	80	65	90	—	—
Switzerland	4.4	—	2	—	50	—	29	—	—	—
United Kingdom	2.4	—	—	—	16	—	16.5	—	940	1,560
USA§	6.4	—	4	—	55	—	44	—	2,120	—
USSR	2	4	4	—	10	30	—	—	—	—
West Indies	4.4	5.5	2.6	3.3	35	44	28	36	1,100	1,400

*Specifications exist in some countries for other cereal grain products such as white rice, maize meal, corn grits, pasta products, and breakfast cereals.

†Other nutrients permitted are vitamin B_6, 2.5–3.1; folic acid, 0.40–0.50; D-pantothenic acid, 11–13; and magnesium 1,500–1,900 mg/kg.

‡Guatemala and Costa Rica started to add vitamin A palmitate (50 IU of 15 μg or retinol equivalent per gram) to refined sugar (sucrose) in 1975. Panama initiated the practice in 1976. El Salvador, Honduras, and Nicaragua are planning to introduce this nutrification practice.

§FDA regulations do not allow marketing U.S. enriched bread (see Table 91–3) containing added vitamin A, vitamin B_6, folic acid, magnesium, and zinc in addition to the above-listed nutrients. Nutrified food sent abroad from the USA under the USA-AID or Food for Peace (PL 480) have the following specifications: nonfat dried milk, 2,200 IU vitamin A and 440 IU vitamin D per 100 g: soy-fortified corn meal, 2–3 mg thiamin, 1.2–1.3 mg riboflavin, 16–24 mg niacin, 4,000–6,000 IU vitamin A, 13–26 mg iron, and 500–700 mg calcium per lb; soy-wheat flour blend, 2–2.5 mg thiamin, 1.2–1.5 mg riboflavin, 16–20 mg niacin, 4,000–6,000 IU vitamin A, and 500–1,107 mg (for 6% soy) or 750–1,364 mg (for 12% soy) calcium per lb: other foods have other specifications.

Note: This table of values taken from the literature serves as a guide. Up-to-date values need to be confirmed with the regulatory agency of the specific country.

FUTURE TRENDS

Foods without a standard of identity, such as ready-to-eat breakfast cereals and meal replacers, have evolved substantial profiles of added nutrients. Yet too many new foods today do not deliver a sufficient array of micronutrients relative to their caloric contribution in low-total-calorie diets consumed daily by sedentary and/or weight-watching subjects, thereby bringing about potential marginal nutrient insufficiencies.[84] Beverages substituted for milk at a meal constitute one such food group.[28] The current trend is for more nutrification of new fabricated foods formulated from partitioned components of natural foods and components obtained from industrial processes.

Following the lead of the United States in the years 1940 through 1945, many countries now add four or five nutrients to flour (Table 91–5). Various scientifically crafted cereal grain–plant protein concentrate blends have been formulated with added minerals and vitamins, at times with amino acids for feeding children, pregnant women, and other undernourished persons in developing countries, either manufactured in the particular country or imported from the United States and other developed countries.[25] In developing countries, three specific nutrient deficiency problems stand out (iodine, iron, and vitamin A); for this reason international organizations have been formed to coordinate and to expand food nutrification programs to correct these deficiencies. The International Council for Control of

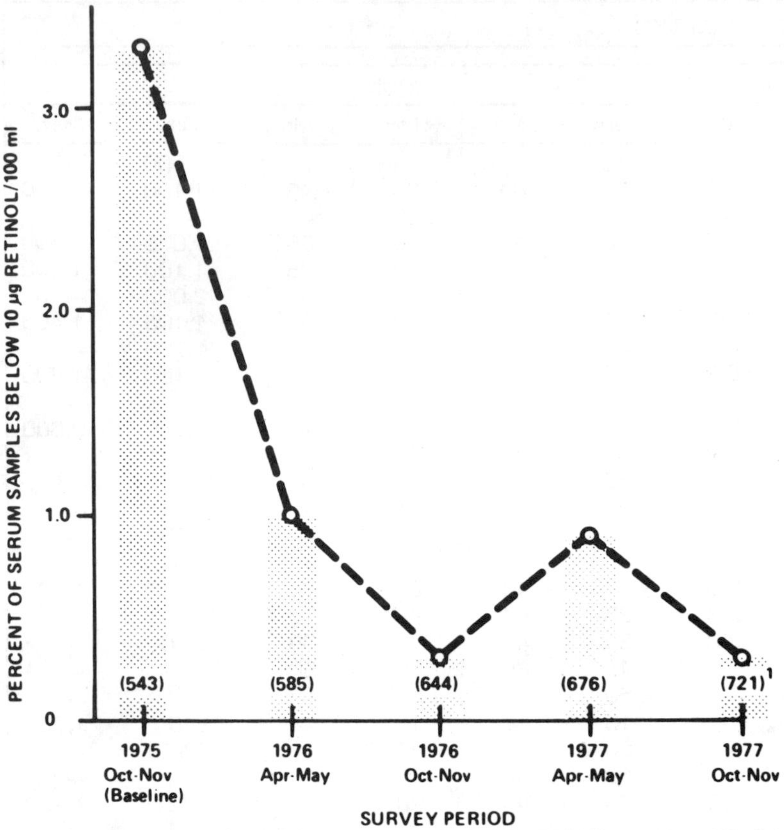

FIGURE 91–4. Decrease in the percentage of children with "deficient" serum retinol levels as a result of nutrification of sugar with vitamin A initiated after the baseline period. (From Arroyave, G., Aguilar, J.R., Flores, M., et al.: Evaluation of sugar fortification with vitamin A at the National Level. Scientific Publication No. 384. Washington, D.C., Pan American Health Organization, 1979.)

Iodine Deficiency Disorders, the International Nutritional Anemia Consultative Group, and the International Vitamin A Consultative Group pursue iodine, iron, and vitamin A projects, respectively; the World Health Organization is pursuing all three problems plus other nutritional concerns. Efforts are being made internationally to eliminate iodine and vitamin A deficiency by the year 2000.[13,85]

Although food purveyors in the past have accepted the obligation to ensure the attractiveness, cleanliness, and safety of their products, greater responsibility in the future must be shown for the nutritive and health value of products marketed to consumers in all countries.[84]

Knowledge of the requirements for and function of the essential nutrients is incomplete. The larger gaps in our knowledge of the major minerals are being filled, and in the future more trace minerals may be included in the nutrification programs. Greater use of the pure amino acids as additives as well as new sugars and fats may be involved in future programs. New micronutrients can be incorporated only after detailed assessment of their past intake, the human requirement, the nutritional status of the population, their safe use, and benefits to be derived. The possibility that more micronutrients will be incorporated into nutrification programs in the future brings with it the following concerns:

Continued pressures on the ingenuity of the chemist and food technologist to develop application forms that allow the nutrient to be uniformly incorporated and stable in food during market distribution without altering flavor biologic availability and safety.

Continued biologic evaluation by the nutritionist of potential interactions among nutrients and among food components that might alter metabolic performance in the body.

Continued search for nutrifying food carriers that minimize changes in the consumer's food habits and hence reach an increasing percentage of the population.

Overcoming past barriers, real and created, to nutrification.

REFERENCES

1. Nutrition bill of rights: J. Am. Diet. Assoc., *69:*cover page, 1976.
2. Haughton, B., et al.: J. Nutr. Educ., *19:*169–174, 1987.
3. Lachance, P.A., Bauernfeind, J.C.: Concepts and practices of nutrifying foods. *In* Nutrient Additions to Food: Nutritional, Technological and Regulatory Aspects. Edited by J.C. Bauernfeind and P.A. Lachance. Trumbull, CT, Food and Nutrition Press, 1991.
4. Food and Nutrition Board, National Research Council: Diet and Health: Implications for Reducing Chronic Disease Risk. Washington, D.C., National Academy Press, 1989.
5. Dept. of Health and Human Services, Food and Drug Administration: Food Labeling; Reference Daily Intakes, etc. Fed. Reg., *55:*29476, 1990.
6. Gregory, J.: Consumer nutrient labeling issues. *In* Nutrient Additions to Food: Nutritional, Technological and Regulatory Aspects. Edited by J.C. Bauernfeind and P.A. Lachance. Trumbull, CT, Food Nutrition Press, 1991.
7. Chichester, C.O., Darby, W.J.: Food Technol., *29(1):*38–42, 1975.
8. Borenstein, B., Lachance, P.A.: Effects of processing preparation on the nutritive value of food. *In* Modern Nutrition in Health and Disease. 7th Ed. Edited by M. Shils and V. Young. Philadelphia, Lea & Febiger, 1988.
9. Pederson, B., et al.: Nutritive value of cereal products with emphasis on the effect of milling. *In* Nutritional Value of Cereal Products, Beans and Starches. Edited by G.H. Bourne. Basel, Karger, 1989.
10. Ranhotra, G., Vetter, J.: Food considered for nutrient addition: Snacks and confectioneries. *In* Nutrient Additions to Food: Nutritional, Technological and Regulatory Aspects. Edited by J.C. Bauernfeind and P.A. Lachance. Trumbull, CT, Food Nutrition Press, 1991.
11. Anonymous: Recommended Dietary Allowances. 10th Ed. Nutr. Today, *24:*32–33, 1989.
12. Agricultural Handbooks: Composition of Food Nos. 8-4 to 8-21. Washington, D.C., U.S. Dept. Agric., 1979–1989.
13. Bauernfeind, J.C.: Vitamin A Deficiency and Its Control. Orlando, FL, Academic Press, 1986.
14. WHO: Control of Nutritional Anemia with Special Reference to Iron Deficiency. Tech. Report 580. Geneva, World Health Organization, 1975.
15. Brin, M.: Marginal micronutrient deficiency. *In* Nutrient Additions to Food: Nutritional, Technological and Regulatory Aspects. Edited by J.C. Bauernfeind and P.A. Lachance. Trumbull, CT, Food and Nutrition Press, 1991.
16. Bauernfeind, J.C.: Proceedings of the 3rd International Congress Food Science and Technology. Washington, D.C., August 9–14, 1970, pp. 217–232.
17. Lachance, P.A.: Food Technol., *24(6):*100, 1970.
18. Darby, W.J., Hambraeus, L.: Nutr. Rev., *36:*65–71, 1978.
19. Richardson, D.P.: Proc. Nutr. Soc., *49:*39–50, 1990.
20. Austin, J.E., Hitt, C.: Nutrition Intervention in the United States. Cambridge, MA, Ballinger, 1979.
21. Boussingault, M.: Ann. Chem. Phys., *54:*163–177, 1833.
22. Jarrett, M.C.: Food Eng., *54(3):*123–124, 1982.
23. Bailey, L.: Vitamin and amino acid additives. *In* Nutrient Additions to Food: Nutritional, Technological and Regulatory Aspects. Edited by J.C. Bauernfeind and P.A. Lachance. Trumbull, CT, Food Nutrition Press, 1991.
24. Clydesdale, F.: Mineral additives. *In* Nutrient Additions to Food: Nutritional, Technological and Regulatory Aspects. Edited by J.C. Bauernfeind and P.A. Lachance. Trumbull, CT, Food Nutrition Press, 1991.
25. Phillips, R., Eitenmiller, R.: Foods considered for nutrient addition: Food analogs and extruded or blended food mixtures. *In* Nutrient Additions to Food: Nutritional, Technological and Regulatory Aspects. Edited by J.C. Bauernfeind and P.A. Lachance. Trumbull, CT, Food Nutrition Press, 1991.
26. Bauernfeind, J.C.: Food considered for nutrient addition: Condiments. *In* Nutrient Additions to Food: Nutritional, Technological and Regulatory Aspects. Edited by J.C. Bauernfeind and P.A. Lachance. Trumbull, CT, Food Nutrition Press, 1991.
27. Molina, M.: Food considered for nutrient addition: Sugars. *In* Nutrient Additions to Food: Nutritional, Technological and Regulatory Aspects. Edited by J.C. Bauernfeind and P.A. Lachance. Trumbull, CT, Food Nutrition Press, 1991.
28. De Ritter, E., Bauernfeind, J.C.: Food considered for nutrient addition: Juices and beverages. *In* Nutrient Additions to Food: Nutritional, Technological and Regulatory Aspects. Edited by J.C. Bauernfeind and P.A. Lachance. Trumbull, CT, Food Nutrition Press, 1991.
29. Bauernfeind, J.C.: Foods considered for nutrient addition: Fats and oils. *In* Nutrient Additions to Food: Nutritional, Technological and Regulatory Aspects. Edited by J.C. Bauernfeind and P.A. Lachance. Trumbull, CT, Food Nutrition Press, 1991.
30. Bauernfeind, J.C.: Foods considered for nutrient addition: Roots and tubers. *In* Nutrient Additions to Food: Nutritional, Technological and Regulatory Aspects. Edited by J.C. Bauernfeind and P.A. Lachance. Trumbull, CT, Food Nutrition Press, 1991.
31. De Ritter, E.: Food considered for nutrient addition: Dairy products. *In* Nutrient Additions to Food: Nutritional, Technological and Regulatory Aspects. Edited by J.C. Bauernfeind and P.A. Lachance. Trumbull, CT, Food Nutrition Press, 1991.
32. Bauernfeind, J.C., De Ritter, E.: Food considered for nutrient addition: Cereal grain products. *In* Nutrient Additions to Food: Nutritional, Technological and Regulatory Aspects. Edited by J.C. Bauernfeind and P.A. Lachance. Trumbull, CT, Food Nutrition Press, 1991.
33. Anonymous: Nutr. Rev., *40:*93–96, 1982.
34. Iannarone, A.: Regulation of food fortification: United States. *In* Nutrient Additions to Food: Nutritional, Technological and Regulatory Aspects. Edited by J.C. Bauernfeind and P.A. Lachance. Trumbull, CT, Food Nutrition Press, 1991.
35. Roe, D.A.: Bioavailability of nutrients added to human foods. *In* Nutrient Additions to Food: Nutritional, Technological and Regulatory Aspects. Edited by J.C. Bauernfeind and P.A. Lachance. Trumbull, CT, Food Nutrition Press, 1991.
36. Lund, D.: Engineering aspects of nutrifying foods. *In* Nutrient Additions to Food: Nutritional, Technological and Regulatory Aspects. Edited by J.C. Bauernfeind and P.A. Lachance. Trumbull, CT, Food Nutrition Press, 1991.
37. MacDonald, I.: Food Chem., *2:*193–197, 1977.

38. Morgan, K.J.: Cereal Food World, *28:*305–306, 1983.
39. Borenstein, B.: CRC Crit. Rev. Food Technol., *2:*171–186, 1971.
40. Richardson, T.: Manufact. Confect., *60(10):*47–48, 50, 53–54, 1980.
41. Sebrell, W.H. Jr.: The concept of the fortification of foods with synthetic vitamins. *In* Amino Acid Fortification of Protein Foods. Edited by N.W. Scrimshaw and A.A. Altschul. Cambridge, MA, MIT Press, 1971.
42. Mertz, W.: Ann. N. Y. Acad. Sci., *300:*151–160, 1977; J. Am. Diet Assoc., *77:*258–263, 1980.
43. Dunn, J.T., Van Der Harr, F.A.: Practical Guide to the Correction of Iodine Deficiency. International Council for Control of Iodine Deficiency Disorders. Charlottesville, VA, University of Virginia Health Sciences Center, 1990.
44. Gibson, R.S.: Prog. Food Nutr. Sci., *13:*67–111, 1989.
45. Hallberg, L.: The role of vitamin C in improving the critical iron balance situation in women. *In* Vitamins: Nutrients and Therapeutic Agents. Edited by A. Hanck and F. Hornig. Int. J. Vitamin Nutr. Res. Suppl., *27:*177–187, 1985.
46. Austin, J.E.: Cereal Food World, *23:*229–233, 265, 1978.
47. NRC: Proposed fortification policy for cereal-grain products. Publ. ISBN 0-309-02232-0. Washington, D.C., National Academy of Sciences, 1974.
48. Emodi, A.S., Scialpi, L.: Cereal Chem., *57:*1–3, 1980.
49. Vetter, J.L.: Adding Nutrients to Foods. St. Paul, American Association of Cereal Chemists, 1982.
50. Huang, P.C., Tung, T.C.: J. Formosan Med. Assoc., *70:*135, 1971.
51. Somogyi, J.C., Hejda, S.: Nutrition in the prevention of disease. Bibl. Nutr. Dieta, *44:*54–84, 1989.
52. Christakis, G.: Nutrient influence on health. *In* Nutrient Additions to Food: Nutritional, Technological and Regulatory Aspects. Edited by J.C. Bauernfeind and P.A. Lachance. Trumbull, CT, Food and Nutrition Press, 1991.
53. Conference Reports; Antioxidant Vitamins and β-Carotene in Disease Prevention: Am. J. Clin. Nutr., *53*(Suppl.):189S–395S, 1991.
54. Bendich, A., Butterworth, C.E. Jr.: Micronutrients in Health and in Disease Prevention. New York, Marcel Dekker, 1991.
55. Moon, T.E., Micozzi, M.S.: Nutrition and Cancer Preventions: Investigating the Role of Micronutrients. New York, Marcel Dekker, 1989.
56. Bendich, A., et al.: Micronutrients and Immune Functions Ann. N.Y. Acad. Sci. 587:1–375, 1990.
57. Gaby, S.K., et al.: Vitamin Intake and Health: A Scientific Review. New York, Marcel Dekker, 1990.
58. Lipkin, M., et al.: Cancer Res., *51:*3069–3070, 1991.
59. Tomkins, A., Watson, F.: ACC/SCK News, *4:*7–11, 1989; *4:*20–21, 1990.
60. Dichter, C.R.: J. Am. Diet. Assoc., *87:*668–672, 1987.
61. Wittpen, J., Sommer, A.: Clinical aspects of vitamin A deficiency. *In* Vitamin A Deficiency and its Control. Edited by J.C. Bauernfeind. Orlando, FL, Academic Press, 1986.
62. Rahmathullah, M.B., et al.: N. Engl. J. Med., *323:*929–987, 1990.
63. Harrell-Bond, B.E., et al.: Lancet, *1:*1392, 1989; ACC/SCN News, *4:*29–30, 1989.
64. Hagen, R., et al.: Formulated special purpose foods. *In* Nutrient Additions to Food: Nutritional, Technological and Regulatory Aspects. Edited by J.C. Bauernfeind and P.A. Lachance. Trumbull, CT, Food Nutrition Press, 1991.
65. Johnson, L., Mergens, W.: Added ascorbates and tocopherols as antioxidants and food improvers. *In* Nutrient Additions to Food: Nutritional, Technological and Regulatory Aspects. Edited by J.C. Bauernfeind and P.A. Lachance. Trumbull, CT, Food Nutrition Press, 1991.
66. Bauernfeind, J.C.: Ascorbic acid technology in agricultural, pharmaceutical, food and industrial applications. *In* Ascorbic Acid: Chemistry, Metabolism and Uses. Edited by P.A. Seib and B. Tolbert. Washington, D.C., American Chemical Society, 1982.
67. Bauernfeind, J.C.: Tocopherols in food. *In* Vitamin E: A Comprehensive Treatise. Edited by L.J. Machlin. New York, Marcel Dekker, 1980.
68. Bauernfeind, J.C.: Carotenoids as Colorants and Vitamin A Precursors: Technology and Applications. Orlando, FL, Academic Press, 1981.
69. Miller, S.A., Stephenson, M.G.: Bibl. Nutr. Dieta, *40:*82–95, 1987.
70. Quick, J.A., Murphy, E.W.: The Fortification of Foods: A Review. USDA Agricultural Handbook No. 598. Washington, D.C., United States Department of Agriculture, 1982.
71. Austin, J.E., et al.: Nutrition Intervention in Developing Countries: Fortification and Formulated Foods. Cambridge, MA, Oelgsschlager, Gunn and Hain Publishers, 1981.
72. Beaton, G.H.: Food fortification. *In* Nutrition in Preventive Medicine. Edited by G.H. Beaton and J.M. Bengoa. Geneva, World Health Organization, 1976.
73. Suwanik, R.J.: Natl. Res. Counc. (Thailand), *12(2):*1–45, 1980.
74. Present Knowledge in Nutrition. 6th Ed. Washington, D.C., Nutrition Foundation, 1990.
75. Morton, R.A.: R. Soc. Health J., *90:*21–28, 1970.
76. Miller, L.A.: Bakers Weekly, July 14, 1952; What's New in Home Economics, *16:*60–61, 144, 1952.
77. LeBovit, C.: J. Agric. Food Chem., *16:*153–157, 1968.
78. Miller, D.F.: Food Product Dev., *12(4):*30, 1978.
79. Friend, B.: Enrichment and fortification of foods, 1966–1970. National Food Situation USDA-ARS, Form CFE (Adm.)-282, Jan., 1973. Hyattsville, MD, U.S. Department of Agriculture, 1973.
80. Bauernfeind, J.C.: World Rev. Nutr. Diet., *41:*110–199, 1983.
81. Arroyave, G., Aguilar, J.R., Flores, M., et al.: Evaluation of Sugar Fortification with Vitamin A at the National Level. Scientific Publication No. 384. Washington, D.C., Pan American Health Organization, 1979.
82. Clydesdale, F.M., Weimer, K.L.: Iron Fortification of Foods. Boca Raton, FL, Academic Press, 1985.
83. Kline, O.L.: What foods should be fortified? *In* Nutrients in Processed Foods: Vitamins, Minerals. Chicago, American Medical Association Publishing Sciences Group, 1974.
84. Lachance, P.A.: Food Technol., *43(4):*144–150, 1989.
85. Anonymous: IDD Newsletter, *6(4):*1–2, 1990.

CHAPTER **92**

Food Additives, Contaminants, and Natural Toxins

John N. Hathcock and Jeanne I. Rader

Human foods contain a wide variety of chemicals with the potential for adverse effects if consumed in excess. These substances may occur naturally in foods, may be added directly or indirectly during food processing, or may contaminate foods as a result of their use in agricultural or livestock production activities.[1] Direct food additives are intentionally added to foods to perform a variety of technical functions. Other chemicals (indirect food additives) are present in foods as a result of their use in some phase of food production, processing, storage, etc. Contaminants such as mercury, arsenic, selenium, and cadmium enter foods or forages via the soil or the marine environment in which they occur naturally or to which they have been added as a result of human agricultural or industrial activities. Proteinase inhibitors, goitrogens, alkaloids, allergens, oxalates, phytates, and other such substances are natural, innate components of particular foods, whereas other compounds (e.g., aflatoxins, paralytic shellfish toxins) are products of the metabolism of fungi, molds, or marine dinoflagellates. Some of these toxicants or contaminants are found in foods that are common in the human diet, whereas others are found only in unusual food sources. As might be expected, the potential hazard to human health posed by such varied compounds ranges from virtually nil to substantial.

FOOD ADDITIVES: FOOD CHEMICALS AND FOOD ADDITIVES

The broadest use of the term *food additive* would include all natural or synthetic, nutritive or non-nutritive, physiologically active or inert chemicals added directly to indirectly to foods. Such a definition is far more inclusive than, for example, the legal definition of food additive as used in the Food Additive Amendment to the Federal Food, Drug, and Cosmetic Act. For regulatory purposes, distinctions are made between *direct* and *indirect* food additives, and between food additives and *Generally Recognized as Safe (GRAS) substances.*[1] Direct food additives include chemicals added to foods during processing to perform a specific function. From a functional viewpoint, examples of direct additives include antioxidants, antispoilage agents, vitamins, minerals, flavoring agents, coloring agents, emulsifiers, stabilizers, bleaching agents, acidulants, nutritive and non-nutritive sweeteners, leavening agents, and others; some of these food additives are GRAS substances and others are not. Indirect additives include chemicals that become components of foods indirectly or unintentionally via, for example, contact of food with processing equipment or packaging containers. Food contaminants include substances such as products of molds (e.g., aflatoxins), agricultural chemicals (e.g., pesticide residues), and environmental chemicals (e.g., dioxin and lead).

Safety considerations for food chemicals begin with the axiom that any substance can be toxic if consumed in a sufficiently high quantity. The intake necessary to generate a toxic response, however, varies greatly from one substance to another. Some substances, such as sucrose, have such low toxic potential and such a long history of widespread use as direct food additives that they are known as GRAS substances for defined uses, with the amount limited only by good manufacturing practice. Contaminants such as aflatoxins and dioxin have such high toxicity that they are stringently regulated in foods.

Certain categories of food chemicals have generated much interest and debate because of their widespread use, their relatively common occurrence in foods, or the uncertain degree of health risk associated with them. Selected categories that meet these criteria will be discussed in detail.

NUTRIENTS

There is growing interest in the value of treating specific diseases with vitamins and minerals in larger than nutritionally required quantities. Clinical uses of iron, iodine, and fluoride have long been recognized and are well described.[2] The safety of vitamins and minerals, whether used as food ingredients, dietary supplements or, in some cases, drugs depends on (1) the inherent toxicodynamic potency of the specific compound, (2) its chemical form, (3) total daily intake, (4) the duration and regularity of consumption, and (5) the biologic characteristics of the person consuming the compound.[2,3]

Generally, fat-soluble vitamins are much more toxic than water-soluble vitamins because of their extensive tissue storage and slow rate of metabolism. It does not follow, however, that all fat-soluble vitamins present an equal and high toxic hazard or that all water-soluble vitamins are innocuous. There are large differences in inherent toxic potency within each category.

Vitamin A. Among the vitamins, vitamin A is one of few for which substantial numbers of human cases of intoxication have been reported.[4-6] To assess toxic potential, the total intake of preformed vitamin A from all sources must be considered; these include foods with naturally high levels (e.g., eggs and liver), foods fortified with vitamin A (milk and many ready-to-eat cereals), and nutrient supplements. Almost all reported toxic intakes have resulted from consumption of single-nutrient supplements of vitamin A rather than from consumption of conventional or fortified foods. The toxicity of vitamin A is discussed in Chapter 16.

Vitamin E. Two uses of vitamin E in food are as a nutrient and as an antioxidant. Vitamin E is considered relatively innocuous with no side effects at intakes up to 300 IU (201 mg α-TE) per day (tenfold the U.S. Recommended Dietary Allowance, or RDA)[7] and with few side effects at intakes of 3200 IU (2148 mg α-TE) per day.[8] Food additive uses of vitamin E are not known to generate intakes near the possibly adverse range, although there may be reason for concern if all synthetic antioxidants in foods were replaced by vitamin E. The toxicity of vitamin E is discussed in Chapter 18.

Pyridoxine. Water-soluble vitamins usually have been considered virtually nontoxic because of their solubility and rapid excretion. Reports of toxic effects of pyridoxine have proven such assumptions to be unjustified.[6] No toxicity has been reported from food-ingredient uses of pyridoxine. The toxicity of pyridoxine is discussed in Chapter 23.

Vitamin C. Two uses of vitamin C in foods are as a nutrient and as an antioxidant. Intakes resulting from such uses of vitamin C are modest in comparison to intakes which can cause adverse effects.[2,7,10-18] Most high intakes result from supplement use.[10] Apparently, vitamin C has a low order of toxicity, or intoxications would be common because of the widespread use of supplements. Although large intakes may cause adverse effects in some individuals, some of the widely reported and often-cited adverse effects have little apparent basis.[2] The toxicity of vitamin C is discussed in Chapter 27.

Niacin. Niacin is nutritionally required. At high dosages it is an effective drug for lowering blood cholesterol levels.[19,20] This latter use of niacin has led to nearly all cases of niacin toxicity. An error in preparation of niacin-containing bagel dough has resulted in accidental overfortification, with adverse reactions (skin flushing) in consumers.[21] Niacin toxicity is discussed in Chapter 22.

Copper. Copper is among the most inherently toxic of the essential trace elements. At the low levels found naturally in foods or added by food-additive (GRAS substance) uses, dietary copper causes no known toxicity, except in persons with Wilson's disease.[17] In general, humans are less sensitive to copper intoxication than are some animals, such as sheep. The toxicity of specific levels of copper are affected by dietary iron and zinc as well as protein. Copper toxicity is discussed in Chapter 11.

Iron. Iron oxides are used as food coloring agents. Ferric phosphate and pyrophosphate, ferrous gluconate, lactate, sulfate, and reduced iron are classified as GRAS substances for use as food ingredients in the United States. Absorption of nonheme iron is closely regulated by the intestinal mucosa. Diets high in heme iron or high in promoters of nonheme iron absorption may occasionally lead to iron overload and resulting disease.[22-24] The degree to which added dietary iron may contribute to iron overload in some individuals is uncertain. The toxicity of iron is discussed in Chapter 9.

Zinc. Several zinc compounds are used as food additives. Prophylactic supplementation of poultry and livestock feeds with zinc is common. Individual tolerances for zinc sulfate vary widely.[3] Chronic ingestion of large doses of supplements may have adverse effects, but no toxicity seems to have occurred as a result of ingestion of the moderate levels from food-additive uses.[3,27,28] Zinc toxicity is discussed in Chapter 10.

Selenium. Selenium is one of the most toxic of the essential elements. Consequently, there are currently no approved uses for selenium in human foods in the United States. Intoxications have been caused by extremely high-potency supplements and may be caused by high dietary intakes in some geographic areas.[17,24-26] Selenium toxicity is discussed in Chapter 12.

ARTIFICIAL SWEETENERS

Much of the use of non-nutritive sweeteners is prompted by the accompanying reductions in calorie intake. Also, a motivating interest for some consumers may be the absence of a procariogenic effect. Safety concerns center around possible carcinogenicity of some artificial sweeteners and about neurologic effects of others.

Saccharin. Saccharin is 300 to 500 times sweeter than sucrose. There is no apparent tissue accumulation or metabolism, the ingested material being excreted unchanged in the feces or urine. Mutagenicity studies have been all negative. Carcinogenicity studies in animals have produced positive results in certain experimental designs.[29,30] The ability of saccharin to produce bladder cancer has been seen in two-generation studies in which exposure began in utero by dietary treatment of the pregnant rat and continued through the diet for 2 years following birth. The doses used ranged up to 7.5% of the diet. No adverse effects have been observed with less than 1% dietary saccharin. Epidemiologic studies have given relative risk ratios close to unity (no significant risk).

Cyclamate. The metabolism of cyclamate depends on the intestinal microflora. It is excreted largely unaltered in test animals treated for the first time. Pretreatment with cyclamate, however, may alter the microflora by selection of microbes capable of converting cyclamate to cyclohexylamine, dicyclohexylamine, and cyclohexanone. These metabolites have been found in rats, dogs, guinea pigs, monkeys, and humans. The results of toxicity studies with cyclamate have been largely negative.[29,30] In the rat, bladder tumors have occurred when cyclamate and saccharin were fed in a 10:1 ratio in conjunction with cyclohexylamine. Also, dietary cyclamate appears to promote bladder cancer initiated by intravenous doses of methylnitrosourea (MNU) in the rat. The results of carcinogenicity studies in mice, dogs, hamsters, and primates have been negative. The United States Food and Drug Administration (FDA) banned food use of cyclamate in 1969.

Aspartame. Considering its structure and constituent parts, there are many hypothetical possibilities for adverse effects by aspartame. Thus far, however, extensive investigation has not shown side effects from aspartame.[29,30] Aspartame is metabolized to several products, including phenylalanine and aspartic acid. Thus, aspartame is a very low calorie sweetener, not a zero calorie sweetener. Diketopiperazine occurs as a contaminant in aspartame, at about 1%. Aspartame is metabolized to phenylalanine, and consequently carries a risk for persons with phenylketonuria (PKU) proportional to consumption of equivalent amounts of phenylalanine. Claims of risk for other consumers, however, have not been substantiated. Such claims relate mainly to purported adverse neurologic effects of phenylalanine or aspartame. Phenylalanine is a precursor of the neuroactive substances norepinephrine and epinephrine. Adverse neurologic effects might logically be related to overproduction of either or both of these compounds. Concrete evidence for such effects, however, has not been found.

FOOD COLOR ADDITIVES

Food colorants include both natural substances and synthetic compounds.[31] Natural substances that have been used as food colorants include carmine, paprika, saffron, and turmeric. Certain nutrients when used to impart color (for example, β-carotene and riboflavin) are regarded as color additives, as are fruit or vegetable juices, carrot oil, and beet extract. Synthetic compounds that are permitted for food use under good manufacturing practices and subject to certification by the FDA include FD&C (Food, Drug & Cosmetic Act) Yellow No. 5 (tartrazine), Red No. 3 (erythrosine), Red No. 40, Blue No. 1, and Citrus Red No. 2. Provisionally listed colors include FD&C Blue No. 2, Yellow No. 6, and Green No. 3.

The safety evaluation and history of use and regulation for food colors are complex.[31] For several of the food colors, such as FD&C Red No. 2 (amaranth) and FD&C Red No. 3, the crucial safety issue is that of possible carcinogenicity. Use of FD&C Red No. 2 was banned because of concerns about carcinogenicity that were not addressed by available data. For FD&C Red No. 3 (a synthetic compound with a high content of iodine), the possibility of indirect carcinogenicity has provoked much controversy about whether this should be sufficient reason for banning it from food uses. Erythrosine causes hypertrophy, hyperplasia, adenomas, and carcinomas of the thyroid glands. These changes may be associated with secondary (indirect) oncogenesis. Whether hypertrophy and hyperplasia from any cause in any organ would carry risk for increased tumors remains an unanswered question. The FDA concluded that the data were insufficient to determine that erythrosine-induced carcinogenicity was caused by an indirect mechanism.

Synthetic food colors and some flavoring agents such as methyl salicylate (oil of wintergreen) have been alleged to cause hyperactivity in some children.[32] This concept was promoted by Feingold in 1975 and stimulated research in hyperactivity in both humans and animals. Various chemical insults to the central nervous system can result in hyperactivity in brain-damaged animals. Some dyes, such as FD&C No. 3, inhibit uptake of neurotransmitters in rat striatal synaptosomes, but this effect may be nonspecific and may not account for any selective behavioral effects. The ease with which hyperactivity can be induced in brain-damaged rats suggests that this model should not be used for evaluation of the hyperactive child. Clinical trials of salicylates and other food additives in children have yielded little or no information in elucidating the cause of or in identifying therapy for hyperactivity in children.

The viewpoint that the only functions of food colors are to provide aesthetic appeal to foods overlooks the psychologic value of food color in diet therapy. Alteration of the average American diet to meet the dietary goals in the Surgeon General's Report on Diet and Health is a difficult objective. Food colors may have a positive role in dietary management,[31] but few argue that this role is essential.

PRESERVATIVES

Chemical preservatives include both antioxidants and antimicrobial agents. Antioxidants are used to inhibit changes in flavor, nutritive value, and appearance that result from the oxidation of fatty acids, amino acids, and vitamins. Antimicrobial agents are used to prevent the growth of bacteria, yeasts, and molds that may generate food-borne intoxications or infections or that may cause undesirable alterations in flavor, appearance, or nutritive value. Although refrigeration obviates the need for some preservatives, it is comparatively expensive and is not available under many circumstances. Food irradiation as an alternative to chemical preservatives has received relatively little acceptance because of the technical requirements and public controversy.

Antioxidants. Common antioxidant food additives include ascorbic acid, ascorbyl palmitate, tocopherols, butylated hydroxyanisole (BHA), butylated hydroxytoluene (BHT), ethoxyquin, propyl gallate, and t-butylhydroquinone (TBHQ). The common antimicrobial agents nitrite and sulfite also have antioxidant activity, as well as other properties.

BHA and BHT. BHA and BHT have been the subject of considerable controversy about their safety. Both are lipid-soluble antioxidants and are capable of inducing increased blood concentrations and activities of several liver enzymes that are involved in the detoxification of foreign compounds. Each of these properties, antioxidant and inducing agent, can provide protection against chemically induced carcinogenesis under certain experimental conditions.

Antioxidants can provide protection against the reactivity of electrophilic chemicals that may, following binding to DNA, cause mutations and initiate carcinogenesis. Many carcinogens are actually procarcinogens that are metabolized to electrophilic ultimate carcinogens. Some carcinogens are electrophilic and do not require metabolic activation. Inducers of liver enzymes that metabolize foreign compounds may have either anticarcinogenic or procarcinogenic activities, depending on the dose and timing in relation to exposure to the initiating carcinogen. If treatment with the inducer occurs before treatment with the carcinogen, the resulting induction usually results in more-rapid metabolism of the carcinogen to inactive forms and decreased net carcinogenicity. If exposure to the carcinogen occurs first, followed by treatment with high doses of the inducing agent, the resulting hyperplasia and hypertrophy can result in promotion of the carcinogenesis caused by the carcinogen. With certain carcinogens, there may be inhibition of carcinogenesis by late treatment with high doses of inducing antioxidants.

BHA treatment alone in high doses (2% of the diet) has produced hyperplasia, papilloma, and squamous cell carcinoma in the forestomachs of rats and hamsters.[33] No evidence of carcinogenicity was found when BHT was included in diets of male and female mice at a level of 0.5% in one study.[33] Both BHA and BHT provide protection against the early neoplastic changes in the liver caused by diethylnitrosourea.

The relationships between antioxidants and carcinogenesis are complex, and no generalization can be accurate. The effect of antioxidants on cancer depend on the carcinogen, organ and tumor type, and timing and dose of the antioxidant.

Nitrite. Sodium nitrite is used as an antimicrobial preservative, a flavoring agent, and a color fixing agent (via its reactivity with myoglobin). Nitrite is effective in preventing the growth of Clostridium botulinum, and thereby decreases the risk of botulism.

Nitrite reacts with primary amines and amides to form the corresponding N-nitroso derivatives.[34,35] Many but not all N-nitroso compounds are carcinogenic. Ascorbic acid and other reducing agents inhibit the nitrosation reactions of nitrite; ascorbic acid is an especially effective inhibitor in the acid environment of the stomach where much nitrosation takes place. Some nitrosamines are formed in foods during processing, but the largest part of nitrosamine exposure occurs via the nitrosation reactions in the stomach. Food additive sources of nitrite are significant but a substantial portion of total nitrite exposure comes from bacterial reduction of nitrate to nitrite in the mouth. Food nitrate, principally from vegetables, is absorbed and then slowly released into saliva. This slow reconsumption of nitrate allows ample time for reduction to nitrite in the mouth and subsequent nitrosation reactions in the stomach. Safety evaluation of nitrite as a food additive must take into account this major additional endogenous source.

The question of possible direct carcinogenicity by nitrite has been addressed through studies of nitrite "alone." Biologic systems, however, always contain a variety of amines, and thus any studies to compare the carcinogenicity of nitrite with that of nitrosamines must take this into account.

Nitrite is capable of causing some toxicities not related to carcinogenesis, but the dose required to cause these effects is relatively large. Persons chronically exposed to large amounts of nitrite may develop methemoglobinemia, but this problem is not common.

Sulfite and Sulfur Dioxide. Sulfur dioxide and its salts are commonly used as inhibitors of enzymatic and nonenzymatic browning, broad-spectrum antimicrobial agents, dough conditioners, bleaching agents for certain products, and antioxidants. Sulfites are very reactive, and consequently little free sulfite remains in foods. Sulfites have been used for centuries with little evidence of adverse reactions in consumers.

Asthma is the most common and severe adverse reaction attributed to sulfite ingestion.[36,37] An association has been recognized between sulfite ingestion and the onset of asthma in sensitive individuals. To date, more than 20 deaths have been attributed to this idiosyncratic reaction. Sensitive individuals are more likely to respond to acidified, sulfited beverages than to sulfited foods, perhaps because of the volatilization of sulfur dioxide in the beverages. Challenge tests indicate that only 1 to 2% of asthmatics are sensitive to sulfite. In one large test, none of the mild asthmatics were sensitive to sulfite.

The pathogenesis of sulfite-induced asthma is not understood. The mechanism(s) may involve IgE-mediated reactions, hyper-reactivity to inhaled sulfur dioxide, or sulfite oxidase deficiency. Sulfite-sensitive individuals are especially sensitive to sulfite-containing acidified beverages and to sulfite-treated lettuce. Lettuce contains a preponderance of free sulfite. Regulations to limit sulfite concentrations and for labeling requirements have been strengthened in recent years.

Toxicity studies in animals indicate rapid metabolism to sulfate by sulfite oxidase and excretion. At high concentrations in vitro, sulfite causes some mutations and sister chromatid exchanges in Chinese hamster ovary cells. At high doses (more than 600 mg/kg), there is no evidence of sulfite genotoxicity in Chinese hamsters.

GRAS SUBSTANCES

The Food, Drug and Cosmetic Act has been much amended since its passage in 1938.[38] One of these amendments, the Food Additives Amendment of 1958, used the phrase "generally recognized as safe," from which the term GRAS arose. The amendment required prior approval from the FDA for all substances intended to be added to foods. At the time of passage of this amendment, several hundred substances that were previously sanctioned or that were already in common use as food additives were exempted from the requirements of the amendment. A listing of "Substances Generally Recognized as Safe" for their intended use was first published in the early 1960s. Among the several hundred substances on the diverse GRAS list were a variety of nutrients, general purpose food chemicals, emulsifying agents, anticaking agents, stabilizers, spices, and flavorings.

The Food Additives Amendment of 1958 exempted GRAS substances from the premarketing clearance required for food additives; thus GRAS substances are not officially food additives. In presuming GRAS substances to be safe when used in the amounts and manner intended and in accordance with good manufacturing practice, the Food Additives Amendment effectively negated the need for the FDA to require a demonstration of safety before these ingredients could be used in food. Consequently, the 1958 amendment required the FDA to demonstrate that a GRAS substance was no longer generally recognized as safe before its use in food could be prohibited. In 1972, reevaluation of the safety data available on GRAS substances was undertaken by a Select Committee on GRAS Substances, in coordination with the FDA and the Federation of American Societies for Experimental Biology (FASEB). The conclusions reached by the committee supported continued GRAS status for many substances, suggested further studies for some, and rescinded the GRAS status for others. Because the safety and toxic potential for any substance depends on intake, the GRAS reviews have prompted considerable study of the consumption levels for many substances in food.

CONTAMINANTS

Food contaminants may include minerals and heavy metals, mycotoxins, shellfish toxins, pesticide residues, and environmental organic chemicals.

MINERALS AND HEAVY METALS

A number of minerals present in foods are of concern because of their potential toxicity. Because plant materials are the primary source of minerals for both animals and humans, the complex factors influencing the mineral content of plants are also important as major determinants of dietary intakes of certain elements. The literature relating to the metabolism of essential and nonessential minerals, the interrelationships among environmental factors and plant and seafood content of minerals, and the toxic and carcinogenic effects of excessive mineral intake is extensive.[39-41] Only a few examples of toxicities related to high levels of specific minerals in foods will be described here.

Arsenic. Arsenic (As) is ubiquitous in the environment and occurs in inorganic and organic compounds in the trivalent or pentavalent form.[42,43] Levels of arsenic in most foods are low (normally below 0.25 mg/kg).[44] Meats, poultry, and fish contribute most of the arsenic consumed by human populations. Analysis of a special diet excluding seafood gave a calculated average intake of 0.04 mg As per day whereas a more typical diet contributed 0.19 mg As per day.[45] The degree of arsenic uptake by plants is related to the type of plant, chemical composition of the soil, and concentration of soluble arsenic in the soil. Arsenic concentrations in marine organisms and seaweed, in which arsenic occurs in a variety of organic methylated forms, are generally much higher than are those in other foods. These methylated compounds are considerably less toxic than are inorganic arsenic compounds. Symptoms of acute and chronic arsenic toxicity from various arsenic compounds have been reviewed by Anke[42] and Nielsen.[43] Carcinogenic effects of arsenic were recognized more than 100 years ago through examination of workers in the smelting industry. It has been suggested that arsenic alone is not able to produce malignant changes and should therefore be considered a co-carcinogen.[46,47]

Selenium. Selenium (Se) is among the most toxic of the essential trace elements. Like arsenic, it is ubiquitous in the environment but is unevenly distributed over the earth's surface. Areas of both selenium deficiency, such as New Zealand and parts of China, and selenium-excess, such as North Dakota and parts of China, are now recognized. "Accumulator" (or "converter") plants play major roles in determining the effects of soil conditions on selenium availability to livestock in selenium-rich areas. These plants absorb selenium from soils that contain selenium in forms that are relatively unavailable to other plants. The absorbed selenium is converted to organic forms that are returned to the soil and then become available to other plants. Cereal grains may accumulate high levels of selenium in selenium-rich areas. Interest in selenium in the food chain is related in part to its known toxicity to grazing animals. Well-defined symptoms and lesions following acute or chronic ingestion of high-selenium forages are now recognized.[48] The discovery of selenium as the cause of the "blind stagger" syndrome and "alkali disease" in livestock led to concerns about possible deleterious effects of human dietary overexposure to selenium. Liver dysfunction resulting from excessive selenium intake was proposed as a possible cause of a high incidence of gastrointestinal disturbances and skin discolorations reported in a group of people living in a high-selenium area of North Dakota.[49,50] Endemic human selenium intoxication has been reported in China.[51] During the peak prevalence years of 1961 to 1964, morbidity approached 50% in the most severely affected villages. The main symptoms were brittle hair, lack of pigment in new hair, and brittle nails with spots and longitudinal streaks. Skin lesions also occurred frequently and symptoms of neurological disturbances were reported in about half of the afflicted persons. Similar symptoms have been reported among persons living in a seleniferous area of Venezuela.[52]

Mercury. With the exception of fish, food products generally contain inorganic mercury (Hg) at levels below 50 ng/g. Fish can contain 10 to 1500 ng/g in the form of methyl mercury.[53] Even higher levels can be found in fish following ingestion of methylmercury formed from mercury released into lakes from chloroalkali plants.[54] The hazardous nature of residues of mercury in fish is well recognized. Recent episodes of serious poisonings include those of Minamata Bay (1953 to 1960)[55] and the Niigata area (1965) in Japan. In 1971 to 1972, ingestion of bread prepared from alkyl mercury–treated wheat seed caused widespread mercury intoxication in Iraq. These acute poisonings were widely publicized. However, chronic effects of low level exposure are harder to identify and evaluate. "Late onset" symptoms have been recognized in individuals not thought to have been affected in the original poisonings in the Niigata area in Japan, for example, and these findings raise concerns about injuries that are not detectable using current procedures and about determination of "lowest effect" levels. Marketing limits of 0.4 to 1.0 mg/kg for mercury in fish have been established in several countries including the United States, Canada, Finland, Sweden, and Japan.

Cadmium. Cadmium (Cd) is a highly toxic element that accumulates in biologic systems and has a long half-life. There is increasing concern regarding the potential for renal damage from long-term, low-level exposures to cadmium. The kidney is a critical target organ for cadmium accumulation, and the half-life of the element in this tissue is about 30 years.[56] Food is one of the principal environmental sources of cadmium. Cadmium in soil can be increased by application of sewage sludge and phosphatidic fertilizers, all of which contain some cadmium. Wheat and the edible portions of fruits and vegetables grown on soil heavily fertilized with superphosphate have higher levels of cadmium than those grown on less heavily treated soil. Atmospheric cadmium contamination may also play a role in increasing the cadmium in foods. Daily intakes of 25 to 60 μg cadmium for a 70-kg individual have been estimated for typical diets in Europe and the United States.[57] Cadmium accumulates primarily in the kidney, liver, lungs, and pancreas; the kidney is the organ most sensitive to long-term, low-level exposures. Cadmium toxicity is manifested by a variety of syndromes. Effects include kidney dysfunction, hypertension, hepatic injury, reproductive toxicity, lung damage after inhalation exposure, and bone effects.[56,58] Itai-itai ("ouch-ouch") disease was first reported in Japan in 1955 and resulted from industrial contamination of the food and water supply.[59] The poisoning occurred primarily in postmenopausal, multiparous women who consumed diets poor in calcium and protein. Symptoms included bone pain, lumbago, and a duck-like gait. Pathologic changes associated with the progressive disease included osteomalacia and osteoporosis, and renal atrophy and degeneration. The disease appeared to be caused by a combination of low dietary calcium, mobilization of bone calcium during pregnancy, and a cadmium-induced calciuria. Cadmium-induced calciuria and radiologic signs of osteomalacia have been reported in occupationally exposed workers.[60] The bone changes caused by ingestion of cadmium in rats are more severe when the animals are fed calcium-deficient diets low in protein.[61]

PESTICIDES

The most common types of pesticides are fungicides, herbicides, insecticides, and rodenticides. Pesticides may also be classified by chemical type, such as organochlorine, organophosphorus, pyrethrins, and carbamates.

Pesticides are, by definition, toxic to living organisms, and this property leads to the possibility that other organisms, including humans, will also be harmed.[62-64] Pesticides are deliberately introduced into the environment, in contrast to other types of environmental and food contaminants. Humans may be exposed through air, water, or direct contact, as well as through residues in foods.

Selective Exposure. Because it is not usually feasible to administer a pesticide directly to organisms of the pest species, the pesticide is applied to the particular part of the environment that a pest is likely to occupy. Most pesticides are unstable to a considerable degree in the environment, thereby allowing the substance to be applied at higher concentrations during the times the pest species is likely to be present and at much lower concentrations when the food is harvested.[64,65] This strategy is highly effective for most pesticides in current use. In contrast, the organochlorine insecticides, such as dichlorodiphenyltrichloroethane (DDT) and lindane, are environmentally persistent pesticides for which this strategy is not very successful. For these substances, selective exposure is helpful but not sufficient to prevent harm to nontarget species.

Selective Toxicity. Selective toxicity may be based on species differences in either toxicokinetic or toxicodynamic characteristics, or both. These changes influence the distribution of the substance into tissues, rate of elimination, type of toxic reactivity, and toxicodynamic potency of the molecule.[62,63]

When humans or other inadvertently exposed species have responsive systems or receptors essentially identical to those for the pesticide in the target species, the relationships of toxicity and potency to the effective exposure (tissue concentration) may be similar even though responsiveness to the total exposure may be different. Toxicity in humans may also involve effects on structures and systems that are not found in the target species.

Most pesticides are active as the parent compound; metabolic changes generally result in detoxification. Phase I metabolism usually introduces functional groups into the pesticide molecule or exposes existing functional groups. Toxicity and potency may or may not be decreased, but responsiveness to phase II metabolism is dramatically increased. Phase II, which is conjugation with another substance, ordinarily causes marked decreases in reactivity and usually large increases in water solubility and rate of excretion.

The difference between pest species and humans or other nontarget species in rate of metabolism of the pesticide chemical is a common basis of selective toxicity. More-rapid metabolism in most instances decreases toxic potency. If the rate of metabolism is high enough, the compound may never reach the threshold toxic concentration in the exposed organism. In general, organophosphorus insecticides are hydrolyzed much faster by mammals than by insects, causing mammals to be relatively resistant to these toxicants. Some compounds such as aldicarb are exceptions to this generalization.

Because of resistance to metabolic degradation, some substances bioaccumulate. These substances may also be resistant to environmental breakdown—that is, resistant to light, heat, water, oxygen, and other factors. Also, highly bioaccumulative substances usually are lipid-soluble and readily absorbed by organisms ingesting them. Bioaccumulation involves gradual increases in the concentration of a substance in an organism with continuing exposure. This is reflected in magnification of the concentration at succeeding steps in the food chain. The environmental behavior of DDT is an excellent example of bioaccumulation and food chain magnification with resulting toxicity in the species at the top of the exposed food chain.

Acute Effects. The organophosphate and carbamate insecticides produce their lethal effects in insects by inhibiting acetylcholine esterase, an enzyme essential to the function of nerves that utilize the neurotransmitter acetylcholine.[62,63] Humans and other mammals also have essential nerve functions based on acetylcholine, and thus organophosphorus and carbamate pesticides are potent toxicants in these nontarget species. Toxicity in humans is limited by selective (lower) exposure and by the toxicokinetic difference of more-rapid metabolism, and not by any inherent resistance to the toxic action of these pesticides. Both types of cholinesterase-inhibiting pesticides can be powerful acute toxicants in vertebrate species. The most important difference between organophosphorus and carbamate pesticides is the rate at which the phosphoryl and carbamoyl groups are released from the active site of acetylcholine esterase. The release step, which occurs very quickly (in milliseconds) with the natural substrate acetylcholine, proceeds at a moderate rate (seconds or minutes) for carbamates, but proceeds at very slow rates (hours or days) for organophosphorus compounds. Thus, carbamate poisoning is a reversible inhibition, whereas organophosphorus poisoning is essentially irreversible, even though both result from competitive inhibition of the active center of the enzyme. Although a crisis phase in poisoning may be reached rapidly following exposure to a high level of either type of insecticide, the more-rapid recovery of acetylcholine esterase from carbamate inhibition makes this type of poisoning more survivable.

Pyrethroid compounds, notably the natural pyrethrum extracted from certain chrysanthemums, have multiple toxic actions.[62] The effect on neuron Na^+ channels is similar to that of DDT, and ATPases and Cl^- uptake are inhibited in much the same way they are by the other organochlorine insecticides.

A wide variety of other compounds have been used as pesticides, and the types of toxicity they may produce are numerous. In general, the herbicides, being designed for toxicity to plants, are relatively nontoxic to humans. Notable exceptions are paraquat and diquat, which have high toxic potency in mammals (LD_{50} values of 100 to 250 mg/kg).

The practical importance of food-borne pesticides as a cause of acute toxicity seems to be limited to the occasional heavy contamination related to a spill, and not to the usual residue levels in foods.

Neurotoxicity. Chronic neurotoxicity of gradually increasing severity may be caused by continued exposure to pesticides. Also, many pesticides causing chronic toxicity are bioaccumulative and can be accumulated in nerve and adipose tissues. If dietary energy intake is suddenly reduced to a level substantially below expenditures, mobilization of energy stores from body fat may increase blood levels of stored fat-soluble pesticides sufficiently to cause toxicity.[66]

Gradual accumulation of alkylmercury compounds in nerve tissue may cause gradual-onset central nervous system toxicity with symptoms of tremors, incoordination, paralysis, and behavioral/emotional changes. For example, ingestion of wheat treated with a methylmercury fungicide resulted in an outbreak of methylmercury poisoning among Iraqi farmers.[62]

Certain organophosphorus compounds cause a delayed toxic response.[63] In experimental animals, the toxic symptoms are irreversible and may start 10 days or more after a single dose of certain phenylphosphonothioates. The mechanism of this delayed neurotoxicity is uncertain but may involve inhibition of the synthesis of microtubules in neurons. Thus, neurotoxicity is delayed until deficits in microtubule replacement impair function.

The significance of pesticide residues in foods as a cause of neurotoxicity is intensely debated, but the preponderance of available scientific evidence indicates that they are not a problem for most individuals. Some individuals are claimed to be extremely sensitive to such effects, but evidence of such susceptibility is lacking.

Mutagenicity. Many pesticides are mutagenic in various tests.[62] Mechanisms of these changes in genetic information include DNA alkylation, base substitution, intercalation of the mutagen molecule into the DNA helix, chromosome breakage, and chromosome cross-linking. Some pesticides are directly mutagenic, whereas others require activation through formation of a derivative that reacts with nucleic acids. Although mutagenesis itself may be considered a toxic effect, a major concern is the possibility that carcinogenesis may result from exposure to a mutagen. The significance, if any, of mutagenesis caused by pesticide residues in food and the clinical importance of such mutagenicity are not known.

Carcinogenicity. Some organochlorine pesticides cause malignant tumors in mammals.[62,63,67] Carcinogenic nitrosamine contaminants occur in nitroaniline herbicides. The potent carcinogen ethylene thiourea is a degradation product of the ethylene bisdithiocarbamate fungicides. The pesticides mirex, aminotriazole, and daminozide (Alar) produce positive results in multiple carcinogenesis test systems. The degree of threat to the public health generated by exposure to carcinogenic pesticides in foods is the subject of continuing debate over both exposure estimates and risk assessment methods.

Teratogenicity. Adverse effects on embryonic and fetal development caused by maternal exposure have been experimentally demonstrated for a wide variety of pesticides.[62,63] The chlorinated hydrocarbons mirex, Kepone, and DDT have teratogenic activity. Some organophosphorus pesticides, notably dimethoate and monocrotophos, have some teratogenic potency. The teratogenic effects of pesticides include impaired growth, neurologic defects, biochemical abnormalities, and deformed structures of the skeleton, skull, and viscera. Pesticide residues in foods are not known to cause such effects.

Reproductive Toxicity. Adverse reproductive effects, other than teratogenesis, can result from high exposures to some pesticides. The effects include fetotoxicity, decreased female fertility, lowered sperm count, and decreased male libido.[62,63] Some chlorinated hydrocarbons or related compounds, such as methoxychlor and *o,p'*-DDT, have estrogenic activity, thereby altering reproduction. The fumigant dibromochloropropane (DBCP) has caused spermatogenesis to fail in factory workers and in experimental animals. A variety of other toxic reproductive effects may be caused by a few pesticides. Reproductive problems associated with pesticides relate to pesticide workers, and are not known to be associated with the pesticide residues in foods.

Behavioral Toxicity. As might be expected for substances that are neurotoxic or concentrated in nerve tissue, many pesticides can cause behavioral alterations.[62] Very low levels of exposure can cause decreased learning and memory functions, hyperactivity, altered aggressive and defensive behaviors, and other behavioral changes. Two main issues are of importance: (1) alterations in higher-order functions such as memory and learning, and (2) the extremely low dose threshold for behavioral effects.

Impairments in physical behavioral tests such as swimming, walking, and balance seem directly attributable to neurotoxic effects. The importance of behavioral effects in evaluating the safety of pesticide residues at levels commonly found in foods is not established.

Enzyme Induction. Pesticides can induce increased enzyme activity in many species. Different types of enzymes are involved but the most commonly affected are those involved in detoxification processes, namely, the cytochrome P-450–dependent mixed-function oxidases (mono-oxygenases) and the transferases (conjugating enzymes).[62,63] The effects include increased cellular concentrations of the endoplasmic reticulum membrane, the most common location for cytochrome P-450 and some of the transferases, and increased expression of the genes for these enzymes. Enzyme induction not only causes increased rates of pesticide metabolism and hence usually increased rates of pesticide detoxification, but also causes increased metabolism of essential substances such as hormones.

Enzyme induction cannot be categorically considered harmful because it is often protective, but it does indicate that exposure is sufficient to elicit a response. Whether any enzyme induction whatever should be considered evidence of excessive exposure is an unsettled issue, but the usual conclusion is that it should not.

Sources of Exposure. The total exposure to pesticides may occur through air, water, food, or direct contact. Determination of the risk associated with a specific level of exposure through food must take account of the additional contributions of the other routes of exposure. In some instances the contribution of food to the total may be relatively small compared with exposure through the other routes, especially for pesticide workers.[68]

There are few basic sources of pesticide residues in foods; these include approved applications in registered uses, unapproved applications (use of an approved pesticide in excessive amounts or at times too near harvest), and environmental contamination (accidental spillage, contamination from a source such as nearby application or manufacturing facility in the vicinity, and persistence from previous use). In general, accidents cause massive and possibly highly toxic contamination in localized areas, inappropriate applications cause higher-than-normal and perhaps higher-than-permitted residue levels, and environmental persistence can result in low levels of residues of substances no longer in use.

Risk Assessment. The term "risk assessment," although seemingly general, is most often used to mean quantative assessment of cancer risk. The science of assessment of carcinogenic risk is well developed, compared with that of risk assessment for other types of toxicity such as reproductive effects and neurotoxicity. A recent National Research Council report titled "Regulating Pesticides in Food" focuses specifically on carcinogenic risk from herbicides, insecticides, and fungicides that the Environmental Protection Agency (EPA) has found to be oncogenic.

The basic steps in risk assessment are (1) determination of carcinogenicity and the dose-response relationship in animal studies, (2) estimation of human exposure, and (3) calculation of the human risk from human exposure data and animal dose-response data.[67,69] After these steps are completed, a decision must be made as to whether the calculated risk is at an acceptable level. Although the basics of risk assessment may be conceptualized in simple terms, the actual process is complex.

Carcinogenicity and Dose-Response Studies. The validity of extrapolation from animal data to humans is uncertain because of possible species differences in reactivity and the potency of the carcinogen. Calculation of equivalent dosages for different body sizes may be performed on several bases, including dose per weight and dose per surface area. Animal studies of practical size (tens to no more than hundreds of animals per treatment group) must use dosage levels that will give statistically significant results with the numbers of animals used. In practice, a treatment group of about 50 is needed to detect a tumor rate of about 10%; the specific number depends on the background tumor rate and the uniformity of response. Induced tumor rates far lower than 10% would, of course, be important in assessing the impact of the pesticide on human health. This is the reason that high doses far in excess of anticipated human exposure levels are necessary in animal studies.

Estimation of Risk to Humans. Many procedures have been proposed for extrapolation from the high-dose, high-response range in test animals to the low-dose, low-response range of interest in human health and pesticide regulation. Although the mathematical models and procedures used to estimate carcinogenic potency in humans make the assumption that effects seen at higher doses in animals extend to lower doses in humans, the data do not exclude the possibility that a threshold exists. The assumption is usually made in risk assessment that there is no threshold or, if it is concluded that one logically must exist, that it cannot be identified with present data and methods.[67,70] This is among several conservative assumptions used to preclude underestimation of risk. Thus, a risk assessment usually does not attempt to assess actual risk, but maximum risk. Risk assessment may be used to estimate the risk that may be associated with a specific residue intake. Conversely, risk assessment may be used to calculate the dose associated with an agreed-to upper limit of acceptable risk, for example, 1×10^{-6} in a lifetime.

SYNTHETIC ENVIRONMENTAL ORGANIC CHEMICALS

Several types of synthetic organic chemicals in addition to pesticides are present in the environment at detectable concentrations and may become incorporated into food. Dioxin is a contaminant in certain chlorinated pesticides, combustion products, and bleached paper. Polyaromatic hydrocarbons occur in soot, diesel smoke, and many coal tar–derived chemicals. Polychlorinated biphenyls (PCB) and polybrominated biphenyls (PBB) are used in a wide variety of industrial applications, and spillage may result in their entry into the food chain.[71]

Polychlorinated Biphenyls (PCB). PCBs caused food contamination problems after their use became widespread as heat-transfer liquids in applications such as electrical transformers. Because PCB are environmentally stable, resistant to metabolism, lipid-soluble, and readily absorbed, they strongly bioaccumulate. The environmental contamination and migration patterns of these substances caused the greatest exposure to persons who consumed fresh water fish. Few adverse health effects have been clearly related to PCB exposure. In the late 1960s in Japan, a heat exchanger leaked PCB into rice oil, resulting in massive contamination and heavy exposure of consumers.[71] Many exposed persons, including newborn babies exposed in utero, developed a variety of symptoms, including chloracne, increased skin pigmentation, eye discharges, transient visual disturbances, lethargy, tactile sensory loss in extremities, and decreased liver function. The affected adults showed protracted effects and slow regression of the symptoms.

Polybrominated Biphenyls (PBBs). A major contamination of food occurred in Michigan in 1972 when a PBB-containing flame retardant sold under the trade name FireMaster was mistakenly used in place of a dairy feed supplement sold under the trade name NutriMaster.[71] Both products contained the same level of magnesium, which may have contributed to the mix-up. The contamination was first noticed when cattle in several dairy herds refused to eat, decreased milk production, lost body weight, and developed abnormal hoof growth and lameness; affected cattle and swine aborted. No acute human intoxications occurred but contamination of humans was confirmed by blood analysis. Long-term effects of exposure include some alterations in liver functions and decrease in immune competence.

TOXICANTS PRODUCED DURING COOKING OF FOODS

Many cooking methods involve intense heat and limited availability of oxygen at the site of highest heat, conditions that cause pyrolytic decomposition of some food components. Major types of pyrolytic products are the poly(cyclic)aromatic hydrocarbons (PAH)[72] and the heterocyclic amines (HCA).[73] The PAH are produced during cooking mainly by pyrolysis of fats, and HCA are pyrolysis products of amino acids, especially tryptophan. PAH also originate from environmental sources such as wood-burning stoves, diesel exhaust, oil-burning heaters, and boilers.

A high rate of food component pyrolysis occurs during char-broiling of meats. In addition to direct pyrolysis of the fats or amino acids in the meat, melted fat and water drip into the flame or onto the hot charcoal where oxygen supplies probably are low, and the searing heat pyrolyses the fat and any amino acids in the water. Steam from the water steam-distills the pyrolysis products, which may then come in contact with the meat.

A large number of PAH have been identified as pyrolysis products in foods; those most likely to pose problems are benzo[a]pyrene (BP) and 7,12-dimethylbenzanthrene (DMBA). These PAHs and many others are potent carcinogens that are active after metabolic conversion to electrophilic epoxide derivatives.

HCA produced by food pyrolysis include several carbolines, quinolines, and quinoxalines. The carbolines Trp-P-2 and Trp-P-1 are tryptophan pyrolysis products, and they are considerably more potent in mutagenesis test systems than are BP and DMBA. The quinolines IQ and MeIQ and the quinoxalines MeIQx and two dimethyl MeIQx derivatives have mutagenic potencies similar to those of the Trp-P compounds.

These HCA occur in very small quantities but their mutagenic potencies raise concerns about their possible carcinogenicity.[74] For several years after their discovery, the HCA were not available in sufficient amounts to permit carcinogenesis bioassays. Carcinogenicity of several of the HCA has been confirmed in animal test systems. An epidemiologic survey indicated a higher risk of stomach cancer in people who frequently ate broiled fish. Thus, HCA may be related to some types of cancer in humans.

CONTAMINANTS FROM NATURAL SOURCES

MYCOTOXINS

A wide variety of fungal toxins are now recognized as contaminants of humans foods and animal forages. These include aflatoxins, patulin, ochratoxin, penicillic acid, trichothecene toxins, zearalenone, slaframine, and swainsonine.[75-79]

The first reports of aflatoxin contamination of plant products followed large-scale poisonings of turkeys in the early 1960s.[80] The birds had consumed Brazilian ground nut meal contaminated with the mold Aspergillus flavus. The responsible fungal metabolites were identified and collectively termed "aflatoxins." These highly substituted coumarins were further classified as "B" or "G" depending on their fluorescence (blue or green, respectively) in ultraviolet light. Aflatoxin B_1 is the most potent hepatocarcinogen known,[81] and the Fischer 344 rat is the most sensitive to aflatoxin-induced carcinogenesis among the wide variety of species tested.

Acute poisonings in man by foodstuffs contaminated with aflatoxin-producing A. flavus and A. parasiticum have been described, with primary effects relating to hepatotoxicity. One study showed that feeding of contaminated ground nut meal to rats resulted in formation of liver tumors.[82] A role for aflatoxin as a human liver carcinogen is based on epidemiologic data. Epidemiologic associations between the level of staple food contamination by aflatoxin-producing molds and the incidence of primary liver cancer have been found in parts of Africa and Asia but not in the United States.[81,83] Because epidemiologic studies have also indicated a high correlation between primary hepatocellular carcinoma and exposure to hepatitis B virus, a combined role for aflatoxin and hepatitis B virus in hepatic carcinogenesis has also been suggested.

Some 400 different metabolites have been shown to be produced by Penicillium species.[84] These include the nephrotoxins citrinin and ochratoxin A (produced by various species of Aspergillus and Penicillium) and patulin and penicillic acid (produced by P. expansum and P. aurantiogriseum, respectively).

Patulin, an aflatoxin produced by species of Penicillium, Aspergillus, and Byssochlamys, is found in apples and other fruits subject to soft rot.[85] Penicillium species are the predominant sources of patulin, whose structure (4-hydroxy-4H-furo[3,2-c] pyran-2(6H)-one) is that of a highly reactive unsaturated lactone. Patulin was initially intended for use as an antibiotic because it was found to be bacteriostatic to Staphylococcus, Streptococcus, Corynebacterium, Neisseria, and Haemophilis. Its antibiotic activity was eliminated when patulin was treated with cysteine. Subsequent toxicologic studies concluded that the compound was too toxic for therapeutic use.[86] Patulin was found to be carcinogenic in 100-g rats,[87] but a later study apparently did not confirm this result.[88]

Ochratoxins are produced by several Penicillium and Aspergillus fungi and may be found in grains and related foodstuffs. Ochratoxin A has been identified as the major causative factor in outbreaks of porcine nephropathy in Denmark, which occur in association with unusually wet climatic conditions. Histologic similarity between the nephropathy described in pigs and "Balkan nephropathy" in humans suggests a role for ochratoxin in the latter.[89] Balkan nephropathy occurs endemically in Bulgaria, Romania, and Yugoslavia. Levels of ochratoxins in foodstuffs, like those of other mycotoxins, are affected by heavy rainfalls, especially during harvest. A significant association between the number of individuals dying of nephropathy over a 2-year period and excess rainfall during two previous harvest periods has been reported.[90] Ochratoxin levels of 3 to 5 ng/g serum were measured in 6.5% of blood samples obtained from individuals living in an endemic area.[91] These data together with epidemiologic data linking rainfall and death rates from the nephropathy support a possible link between ochratoxin contamination and the disease. Ochratoxin produces a similar renal disease in animals.[92] The nephrotoxicity of other metabolites of some Penicillium strains was recognized in the course of studies of endemic Balkan nephropathy.[92,93] The role of other mycotoxins such as penicillic acid in the disease remains to be determined.

Many Fusarium species produce trichothecene toxins, all of which have a tetracyclic 12,13-epoxytrichothec-9-ene skeleton. Mouldy barley may contain the trichothecene "vomitoxin" (deoxynivalenol), which causes vomiting in pigs, deaths with hemorrhagic lesions in the gut in cattle, and necrosis of the mucosa of the esophagus and gizzard in ducks and geese.

Zearalenone is a fungal metabolite found in feed grains, maize, and soybeans and is related to periodic infection of the plants by F. roseum. Estrogenic syndromes in pigs fed mouldy grains have been described for many years. Enlargement of the mammary glands and vulva are the primary signs of the disorder. Feeding studies in animals have confirmed these findings. There are at present no confirmed reports of effects in man.

"Slobbers" in ruminants is caused by consumption of forage that has been infected with Rhizoctonia leguminocola. Various clovers, soybean, Kudzu, cow pea, blue lupine, and alfalfa may be infected. Conditions favoring the growth of R. leguminicola include wet weather and high humidity. Outbreaks of the disease have been reported in the northwestern, midwestern, and southeastern United States. Pathologic effects of ingestion of the fungus include excessive salivation, lacrimation, diarrhea, and frequent urination. The structure of the toxin is L-acetoxy-6-aminooctahydroindolizine, and total synthesis of the compound has been achieved.[94] Slaframine is activated in the liver following ingestion; a ketoimmine derivative is thought to be the active metabolite.[95]

Consumption of legumes of the genus Swainsonia by cattle, horses, and sheep produces a chronic disease characterized by neurologic disturbances, weight loss, and addiction to the plant.[96] Mortality is high among young animals, whereas older animals may survive for months in poor condition. Swainsonine, the active toxicant of the plant, is a strong inhibitor of mannosidase. Swainsonine has been identified in hays that are known to cause slobbers. Its role, if any, in sporadic outbreaks of the slobber syndrome is unknown.

A number of potent neurotoxins, termed "tremorgenic" mycotoxins, have been identified as metabolites of Aspergillus flavus, Penicillium crustosum, and Paspalum dilatatum.[75] These metabolites at low doses cause sustained, incapacitating whole-body trembling in susceptible animals. Higher doses can lead to convulsive seizures that may be fatal.

CIGUATERA TOXINS

Ciguatera poisoning is a serious human intoxication that may be caused by ingestion of over 400 species of marine fishes, many of which are highly valued as food.[97] The poisoning results from eating certain tropical and subtropical fish associated with coral reefs and nearby coastal waters. Symptoms observed in humans following ingestion of contaminated fish are varied but generally include moderate to severe gastrointestinal disorders, moderate to severe neurologic problems and, in extreme cases, death due to respiratory failure. Gastrointestinal symptoms are of relatively short duration, whereas the neurologic problems may persist for weeks or months. The poisoning involves multiple toxins acquired by fish in regions where ciguatera is endemic. The toxins are subsequently transferred to humans who consume the fish.

Numerous species of marine bacteria and dinoflagellates are accessible to herbivorous fish. In recent studies, various species of dinoflagellates from the Caribbean were grown in large-scale culture and assayed for toxicity.[98] Five of nine species examined produced one or more toxin fractions that killed mice within 48 hours. Specific toxigenic dinoflagellates may produce up to seven separate toxins that may enter the fish food chain. Studies are continuing on the toxins and how they are ultimately transmitted to humans via fish.

The isolation and characterization of okadaic acid from the Caribbean dinoflagellate P. concavum was reported recently.[99] The discovery of okadaic acid from another dinoflagellate, P. lima, represented the first toxin to be isolated from a dinoflagellate implicated as a source of ciguatera-related toxins. Further studies of the nature and extent of toxin production by dinoflagellates and the relationships between these toxins and those occurring in fish should aid in understanding the complexities of ciguatera poisonings.

PARALYTIC SHELLFISH TOXINS

Poisonings of shellfish have been recorded in Atlantic and Pacific coastal waters and in waters around South Africa, New Zealand, and a number of Western European countries for many years. The poisonings, which primarily affect mussels and clams, are associated with the growth of dinoflagellates in the waters. The dinoflagellates produce a toxin that is retained in the hepatopancreas of the shellfish. The toxic principle, "saxitoxin," has been isolated from Alaskan butter clams and from cultured dinoflagellates and appears to block nerve transmission in the motor axon. Hazardous levels of toxin accumulate in shellfish feeding in waters in which the dinoflagellates are undergoing rapid growth ("blooms"). The associated conditions are referred to as "red tides." Symptoms of toxicity, which develop within several hours of eating infected shellfish, include numbness of the lips and fingertips and an ascending paralysis. Death from respiratory paralysis may occur in as many as 8.5% of cases.[100,101]

NATURAL TOXINS INNATE IN CERTAIN FOODS

The literature on naturally occurring toxicants of the types mentioned above is extensive, and it was necessary to select specific topics to be covered. The toxicities of specific foods arise from lipids, antivitamins, plant phenolics, estrogens, hallucinogens, and a variety of other components.[102-109] Two National Research Council volumes review the available information on the carcinogenicity of a variety of naturally occurring toxicants.[81,109]

PROTEINASE INHIBITORS

Legumes are the source of compounds that inhibit the proteolytic activity of enzymes such as trypsin and chymotrypsin. Proteinase inhibitors have been found in many varieties of beans, peas, and peanuts. Potatoes and sweet potatoes also contain proteinase inhibitors. The trypsin inhibitor found in soybeans is perhaps the best studied of this type of compound.[110] Soybeans contain two major types of trypsin inhibitors, the Kunitz inhibitor (molecular weight approximately 20,000 daltons) and the smaller extensively disulfide cross-linked Bowman-Birk inhibitor (molecular weight approximately 8000 daltons). Enzyme activity assays for trypsin inhibitors do not distinguish between the two types of inhibitors. Progress is being made in the development and application of an enzyme-linked immunosorbent assay that should permit rapid determination of the amounts of the two types of inhibitors in raw and processed soy products.[111]

Chicks, rats, and mice fed raw soy meal experience reduced growth, decreased fat absorption, increased size of pancreas, and hypersecretion of pancreatic enzymes. Metabolizable energy from the diet is also reduced. It has long been recognized that the nutritive value of soy protein is enhanced by heat treatment, with the increased nutritive value paralleling the loss of trypsin inhibitor activity.[110] The observation that feeding raw soybeans or trypsin inhibitor concentrates led to hypertrophy and hyperplasia of the pancreas and increased output of proteolytic enzymes explained the effects of trypsin inhibitors on protein nutrition: fecal losses of nitrogen as digestive enzymes would serve as a substantial drain on protein supply. Although heat treatment improves the nutritional quality of soybean products through destruction of trypsin inhibitor activity, standard heat processing methods often leave 5 to 20% of the original trypsin inhibitor content.[112]

The rat responds to treatment with trypsin inhibitor with increased secretion of trypsin and chymotrypsin. Continued treatment with trypsin inhibitor leads to hypertrophy and hyperplasia of the pancreas.[113,114] No overtly neoplastic changes are observed unless the animals are also treated with a pancreatic carcinogen such as azaserine.[113,115] Both adenomas and adenocarcinomas have been observed in the pancreas after about a year of trypsin inhibitor treatment following azaserine initiation. In these studies, trypsin inhibitor appears to act as a promoter of azaserine-initiated pancreatic cancer. Long-term feeding of trypsin inhibitor (1 to 2 years) without treatment with azaserine or other initiators may result in progression of hypertrophy and atypical acinar cell foci to adenoma and carcinoma.[113]

The relationship between trypsin inhibitors and pancreatic carcinogenesis and the species differences in response to such inhibitors are not fully understood. Species that respond to trypsin inhibitor with increased pancreatic enzyme secretion, hypertrophy, and hyperplasia include rats, mice, and chickens; species that are reported to be unresponsive include the calf, pig, dog, Rhesus monkey, Cebus monkey, and marmoset.[115] A recent study with humans indicated that a single dose of the soybean Bowman-Birk inhibitor elicited increased pancreatic secretion of trypsin and chymotrypsin.[116] Present knowledge is insufficient for risk assessment of residual trypsin inhibitors in foods.[117]

HEMAGGLUTININS

The terms "phytohemagglutinins," "phytagglutinins," and "lectins" are used interchangeably to refer to plant proteins that can agglutinate red blood cells. Plant sources of hemagglutinins include castor beans (ricin), soybeans, peanuts, red kidney beans (phytohemagglutinin A), black beans (phaseolatoxin, phaseotoxin A), yellow wax beans (hemagglutinin), and jack beans (concanavalin A).[104,118] Rats fed purified kidney bean agglutinin at 0.5% of the diet died within 2 weeks in one study.[119] Differences in oral toxicity among various hemagglutinins may be related to susceptibility of some (but not of others) to inactivation by pepsin or other proteolytic enzymes. Most purified plant hemagglutinins are carbohydrate-containing proteins. Concanavalin A from jack beans is free of sugars.[120] The phytohemagglutinins have marked effects on cell division: lymphocytes respond with the induction of mitosis. Some phytohemagglutinins have become useful tools in studies related to immunocompetence in which exposure to specific lectins causes increased DNA synthesis.

AMINONITRILES AND RELATED COMPOUNDS

Seeds of various vetches (Lathyrus sativus, L. cicera, and L. clymenum) contain potent compounds that cause neurologic diseases in humans, cattle, and horses. Neurolathyrism is characterized by progressive muscle weakness and irreversible paralysis of the legs, and may be fatal. Outbreaks of neurolathyrism are generally associated with periods of famine during which large quantities of Lathyrus meal are eaten for lack of other food.[121] Toxic compounds isolated from Lathyrus species include various diaminobutyric acids, diaminopropionic acid, oxalylaminoalanine, and B-cyanoalanine.[105]

The condition of osteolathyrism, as distinct from neurolathyrism, is observed in domestic fowl (chickens, turkeys) and experimental animals (rats) following ingestion of L. odoratus, and is characterized by significant disturbances in the development of bones and connective tissue. The toxic component responsible for this disease has been isolated from seeds of L. odoratus and L. pusillus and identified as B-N-(-L-glutamyl)-aminopropionitrile. The β-aminopropionitrile moiety is thought to be the active component of this toxicant.[122]

PYRROLIZIDINE ALKALOIDS FROM SENECIO SPECIES

A large number of inedible plants may contaminate animal forages and human food grains. For example, a variety of Senecio species produce toxic alkaloids, and "Senecio disease" has been reported in human populations eating breads containing seeds from the poisonous plants.[123] The genera Senecio (ragworts), Crotalaria (rattleboxes), and Heliotropium (heliotropes) contain specific alkaloids in amounts ranging from trace to as much as 5% of the dry weight of the plant. A major feature of intoxications by the pyrrolizidine alkaloids in man and animals is delayed liver damage.[124] Veno-occlusive disease and cirrhosis have been reported in humans, and induction of liver cancer has been reported in animals.[125,126]

Consumption of teas prepared from plants of the Senecio genus has been associated with several forms of cancer, but data are not conclusive. In one study the mutagenic activities of seneciphylline and senkirkine, two pyrrolizidine alkaloids that occur in animal forages and medicinal teas, respectively, appeared to act as indirect mutagens.[127] Transfer of mutagenic activity via milk following treatment of lactating rats with seneciphylline was also reported.[127] The hepatocarcinogenicity of the pyrrolizidine alkaloids may be due to promoting effects on initiated hepatocytes rather than to their weak initiating activity.[128]

GOITROGENS

A number of food-borne compounds interfere with utilization of iodine or with the functioning of the thyroid gland.[129] The type of goiter induced by goitrogens is due to inhibition of organic binding of iodine and is not alleviated by increased iodine intake. Goitrogens are widely distributed in many food species, particularly cruciferous vegetables. Rutabaga, turnip, cabbage, peach, pear, strawberry, spinach, and carrot were shown to be active in reducing the rate of uptake of radioactive iodine by human thyroid glands.[130] Goitrogens such as sinigrin (allylthioglucoside), glucobrassicin (3-indoylmethylthioglucoside), progoitrin (2-hydroxy-3-butenylthioglucoside), and gluconapin (3-butenylthioglucoside) are among the compounds isolated and characterized from various Brassica species (cabbage, kale, Brussels sprouts, cauliflower, broccoli, kohlrabi).

ALLERGENS

In some individuals, complex interactions among ingested food antigens, the digestive tract, tissue mast cells, circulating basophils, and food antigen-specific IgE lead to food hypersensitivity.[131-133] Foods such as peanuts, nuts, eggs, milk, soy, fish and other seafood, bananas, and chicken have been implicated in immediate hypersensitivity reactions in children. Symptoms may include atopic eczema, asthma, and rhinitis.[134-136] The number of foods that have been studied in attempts to characterize specific food allergens includes codfish,[137] peanuts,[138] shrimp,[139] and eggs.[140] Food allergies are discussed in more detail in Chapter 77.

Gluten, a protein found in wheat, rye, barley, and oats, elicits a severe enteropathy ("gluten-sensitive enteropathy" or "nontropical sprue") in sensitive individuals. The complex and heterogeneous nature of wheat proteins has hindered attempts to identify the component of gluten responsible for the intestinal damage that occurs in sensitive individuals. Gliadin, an alcohol-soluble component of gluten, appears to be the primary toxic component. A more detailed discussion of gluten enteropathy is found in Chapter 62.

OXALATES

High levels of oxalates are found in a number of vegetables. The oxalates generally occur as soluble sodium or potassium salts or as insoluble calcium salts.[142] Leafy portions of plants usually contain higher concentrations of oxalates than do stalks. Insoluble calcium oxalate crystals are readily visible on microscopic examination of leaves of high-oxalate plants.[143] The percentage of oxalate content of some plant foods is as follows (fresh-weight basis): beet tops and cocoa leaves, 0.3 to 0.9%; spinach and rhubarb, 0.2 to 1.3%; tea leaves 0.3 to 2.0%. Ingestion of oxalate-containing plants can cause acute poisoning; plants of the rhubarb and sorrel grass species are particularly harmful. Symptoms of mild oxalate poisoning (for example, following ingestion of rhubarb) include abdominal pain and gastroenteritis. Symptoms of severe poisoning include diarrhea, vomiting, convulsions, noncoagulability of the blood, and coma.[143] Calcium oxalate kidney stones have been found in Thai children consuming native plants of high oxalate content.[144]

PHYTATES

Phytate (myoinositol 1,2,3,4,5,(6-hexakis) (dihydrogen phosphate) is widely distributed in plants. Its location in specific plants varies: for example, the phytate of seed plants such as corn is contained primarily in the bran and germ. The primary adverse effects of dietary phytate are due to its activity in decreasing the bioavailability of essential minerals such as zinc, calcium, iron, and manganese.[145] The bioavailability of zinc appears to be the most severely affected. Extensive studies in the Middle East resulted in recognition of the seriousness of this effect in humans. Zinc deficiency with delayed sexual development and growth retardation observed in certain populations was attributable to the high amounts of phytate ingested in whole-grain bread that served as the main dietary staple.

Much of the phytate of plants goes into the byproducts of flour milling and may become concentrated in high-protein flours.[146] The concentration of protein from seeds, particularly soybeans, and the use of plant protein to supplement or replace meat products is an important activity of the food industry. The processes used to obtain plant protein from seeds include adjustments in pH, aqueous washes, drying, and hot pressure extrusion to yield a wide range of products varying in protein, fiber, phytic acid, and essential mineral content. Other food processes result in the hydrolysis of phytate to yield lower inositol phosphates or inorganic phosphate and myo-inositol. Processing of seeds to prepare protein concentrates and isolates results in some mineral loss and sometimes in decreased bioavailability of the remaining minerals. The decreased bioavailability of minerals resulting from food processing can be counterbalanced to some extent by the large amount of minerals occurring in most whole seeds. Areas of current interest in relation to phytates in foods include (1) methods of removing phytate, (2) beneficial and adverse effects of smaller inositol phosphates, (3) differences in sensitivity among varying age groups, and (4) adaptation to dietary phytates.

CYCAD

High-incidence foci of amyotrophic lateral sclerosis (ALS) and Parkinsonism-dementia (PD) occur on Guam, the Kii peninsula of Japan, and southern West New Guinea in the Western Pacific. The original incidence rates of ALS in the foci on Guam and in West New Guinea were 50 and 1300 per 100,000 population, respectively, versus a rate of 1 per 100,000 population in the United States.[147] These foci have provided unique opportunities to study the cause and mechanisms of pathogenesis of fatal neurodegenerative disorders. Attempts to identify an infectious agent in ALS and PD have been unsuccessful. Several studies have attempted to identify a relationship between the high incidence of ALS and ingestion of cycad plant material. In tropical and subtropical regions, including the foci mentioned previously, nuts of the palm-like cycad trees provide food for humans and livestock. Because ingestion of cycad fruits was known to produce motor neuron toxicity in foraging domestic animals, the cycad became a major candidate for a causative role in the human disorders. Rats fed diets containing 2% of a crude flour prepared from unwashed nuts of the cycad developed liver and kidney tumors.[148,149] A neurologic disease was not observed.[150] Extensive efforts to implicate cycad in the neurologic disease have not been successful.[147]

A toxic substance was extracted from cycad nuts and identified as methylazoxymethanol-B-glucoside (cycasin). Cycasin is one of the most potent carcinogens found in plants. Macrozamin, a related glucoside, is also found in cycad nuts. Because liver cancer also occurs at high rates in Guam and Okinawa, ingestion of cycasin in cycad nuts has been proposed an etiologic factor in this disease. The available information does not allow a definitive conclusion to be drawn.[151]

Studies with experimental animals support the hypothesis that a basic metabolic defect, provoked by a chronic nutritional deficiency of calcium, leads to increased absorption of toxic minerals and to the deposition of calcium, aluminum, and silicon in neurons of patients with ALS.[147] Although the deposition of toxic minerals in neurons in patients with ALS is now recognized, the process by which neuronal degeneration occurs is not understood.

BRACKEN FERN TOXINS

Bracken fern is consumed by both humans and animals in several parts of the world. Damage to the bone marrow and intestinal mucosa of cattle has been associated with ingestion of this plant. In one study a high risk of esophageal cancer was associated with daily intake of bracken fern.[109] Rats fed fresh or powdered milk from cows that had consumed bracken fern daily (1 g/kg body weight) for about 2 years developed carcinomas of the intestine, urinary bladder, and kidney.[152] In another study, however, dietary administration of quercetin, which occurs as a conjugate in the fern, did not lead to increased incidence of tumors in ACI rats.[126] A highly mutagenic substance has been isolated from bracken fern and identified as aquilide-A.[153]

PHYTOALEXINS

Several plants, including the sweet potato, are capable of producing "stress metabolites" (phytoalexins) in response to fungal infections, mechanical damage, and insect invasion. These compounds accumulate at levels that are fungitoxic at sites of infection and are thought to be part of the mechanisms by which potatoes resist disease. Some of these metabolites are toxic to animals consuming infected roots. Because sweet potatoes serve as a food staple for large numbers of people, the toxicities of these metabolites are of considerable importance.[75,104] One of the most abundant of these metabolites, ipomeamarone, produces liver necrosis in mice when fed or injected intraperitoneally. In large-scale outbreaks of mouldy sweet potato poisoning, however, the predominant manifestation is lung edema leading to death from asphyxiation rather than liver damage. The fatal pulmonary disease has been described as acute interstitial pneumonia, acute bovine pulmonary emphysema (ABPE), or pulmonary edema.[154] Components of mouldy sweet potatoes other than ipomeamarone, when fed to mice, reproduce certain features of the bovine disease and cause death of the animals from asphyxiation within 24 hours.

ABPE can be caused by other toxic plant components.[155] Outbreaks of ABPE occur in animals grazing pastures that contain a variety of plant species, but no single plant type or combination of plants has been consistently associated with the disease.[156] The most common observation associated with outbreaks of the disease is a sudden change from relatively dry to lush forage. Ruminal microorganisms can convert L-tryptophan via indoleacetic acid to 3-methylindole, which can cause pulmonary lesions in cattle, goats, and sheep. Presumably, tryptophan contained in lush pasture plants can be converted to enough 3-methylindole to induce ABPE. Observations that ABPE is associated with changes from dry to wetter pastures may also support a role for mycotoxins or stress metabolites.

VASOACTIVE AMINES

Certain foods, notably aged cheeses, contain vasoactive amines such as tyramine, dopamine, norepinephrine, serotonin, and histamine. These compounds can cause large increases in blood pressure when administered intravenously to humans. Levels of tyramine may be as high as 2000 μg/g in Camembert cheese; somewhat lower levels have been reported in cheddar (120 to 1500 μg/g) and Emmenthaler (225 to 1000 μg/g) cheeses. Pickled herring may contain as much as 3000 μg tyramine/g.[157] The foregoing amines are normally metabolized rapidly in the human body by monamine oxidase (MAO). Tyramine has been found to produce serious effects in persons taking drugs that inhibit MAO. Such inhibitors are often prescribed for depressive illnesses. Episodes of hypertension, intense headaches, and intracerebral hemorrhage have been reported following ingestion of high-tyramine food by individuals taking MAO inhibitors. Hypertensive reactions are not limited to cheese or to ingestion of tyramine only and have been reported in persons taking MAO inhibitors following ingestion of pickled herring, chicken liver, stewed bananas, and beef liver. Other chemically effective antidepressants without the "cheese effect" have been described.[158,159]

REFERENCES

1. Gilchrist, A.: Foodborne Disease & Food Safety. Chicago, American Medical Association, 1981.
2. Hathcock, J.N., Rader, J.I.: Ann. N.Y. Acad. Sci., *587:*257–266, 1990.
3. Hathcock, J.N.: J. Nutr., *119:*1779–1784, 1989.
4. Hathcock, J.N., Hattan, D.G., Jenkins, M.Y., et al.: Am. J. Clin. Nutr., *52:*183–202, 1990.
5. Krasinski, S.D., R.M. Russell, C.L. Otradovec, et al.: Am. J. Clin. Nutr., *49:*112–120, 1989.
6. Bendich, A., Langseth, L.: Am. J. Clin. Nutr., *49:*358–371, 1989.
7. Miller, D.R., Hayes, K.C.: Vitamin excess and toxicity. *In* Nutritional Toxicology. Edited by J. Hathcock. Vol. I. New York, Academic Press, 1982, pp. 81–133.
8. Bendich, A., Machlin. L.J.: Am. J. Clin. Nutr., *48:*612–619, 1988.
9. Cohen, M., Bendich, A. Toxicol. Lett., *34:*129–139, 1986.
10. Stewart, M.L., McDonald, J.T., Levy, A.S., et al.: J. Am. Diet. Assoc., *85:*1585–1590, 1985.
11. Cochrane, W.A.: Can. Med. Assoc. J., *93:*893–899, 1965.
12. Seigel, C., Barker, B., Kunstadrt, M.: J. Peridontol., *53:*453–455, 1982.
13. Hoffer, A.: Can. Med. Assoc. J., *132:*320, 1985.
14. Ringsdorf, W.M., Cheraskin, E.: South. Med. J., *74:*41–46, 1981.
15. Schrauzer, G.N., Ishmael, D., Kiefer, G.W.: Ann. N.Y. Acad. Sci., *258:*377–381, 1975.
16. Guinta, J.L.: J. Am. Diet. Assoc., *107:*253–256, 1983.
17. National Nutrition Consortium.: Vitamin-Mineral Safety, Toxicity, and Misuse. Chicago, American Dietetic Association, 1978.
18. Metz, J., Hundertmark, U., Pevny, I.: Contact Dermat., *6:*172–174, 1980.
19. Henkin, Y., Johnson, K.C., Segrest, J.P.: JAMA, *264:*241–243, 1990.
20. Hodis, H.N.: JAMA, *264:*181, 1990.
21. Patterson, D.J., Dew, E.W., Gorkey, F., et al.: South. Med. J., *76:*239–241, 1983.
22. Cantinieaux, B., Boelaert, J., Hariga, C., et al.: J. Lab. Clin. Med., *111:*524–528, 1988.
23. Akbar, A.N., Fitzgerald-Bocarsly, P.A., DeSousa, M., et al.: J. Immunol., *136:*1635–1640, 1986.
24. McEnery, J.T.: Clin. Toxicol., *4:*603–616, 1971.
25. Fox, M.R.S., Jacobs, R.M.: Human nutrition and metal ion toxicity. *In* Metal Ions in Biological Systems. Concepts on Metal Ion Toxicity. Edited by H. Sigel. New York, Marcel Dekker, 1986.
26. Food and Nutrition Board, National Research Council: Recommended Dietary Allowances. 10th Ed. Washington, D.C., National Academy Press, 1989.
27. Chandra, R.K.: JAMA, *252:*1443–1446, 1984.
28. Beisel, W.R.: Am. J. Clin. Nutr., *35:*417–468, 1982.
29. Conning, D.M.: Artificial sweeteners—a long running saga. *In* Food Toxicology—Real or Imaginary Problems? Edited by G.G. Gibson and R. Walker. London, Taylor and Francis, 1985.
30. Munro, I.C.: A case study: The safety evaluation of artificial sweeteners. *In* Food Toxicology: A Perspective on the Relative Risks. Edited by S.L. Taylor and R.A. Scanlan. New York, Marcel Dekker, 1989.
31. Berdick, M.: Safety of food colors. *In* Nutritional Toxicology. Vol. 1. Edited by J.N. Hathcock. New York, Academic Press, 1982.
32. Norton, S.: Effects of food chemicals on behavior of experimental animals. *In* Nutritional Toxicology. Vol. 1. Edited by J.N. Hathcock. New York, Academic Press, 1982.
33. Ito, N., Fukushima S, Tsuda H., et al.: Antioxidants: Carcinogenicity and modifying activity in tumorigenesis. *In* Food Toxicology—Real or Imaginary Problems? Edited by G.G. Gibson and R. Walker. London, Taylor and Francis, 1985.
34. Archer, M.C.: Hazards of nitrate, nitrite and N-nitroso compounds in human nutrition. *In* Nutritional Toxicology. Vol. 1. Edited by J.N. Hathcock. New York, Academic Press, 1982.
35. Hotchkiss, J.H.: Relative exposure to nitrite, nitrate, and n-nitroso compounds from ednogenous and exogenous sources. *In* Food Toxicology: A Perspective on the Relaltive Risks. Edited by S.L. Taylor and R.A. Scanlan. New York, Marcel Dekker, 1989.
36. Taylor, S.L.: Allergic and sensitivity reactions to food components. *In* Nutritional Toxicology. Vol. 2. Edited by J.N. Hathcock. New York, Academic Press, 1987.
37. Taylor, S.L., J.A. Nordlee, J.H. Rupnow. *In* Food Toxicology: A Perspective on the Relative Risks. Edited by S.L. Taylor and R.A. Scanlan. New York, Marcel Dekker, 1989.
38. Irving, G.W. Jr.: Determination of the GRAS status of food ingredients. *In:* Nutritional Toxicology. Vol. 1. Edited by J.N. Hathcock. New York, Academic Press, 1982.
39. Oehme, F.W.: Toxicity of Heavy Metals in the Environment. Part 1 and Part 2. New York, Marcel Dekker, 1978 and 1979.
40. Mertz, W.: Trace Elements in Human and Animal Nutrition. 5th Ed. Vols. 1 and 2. New York, Academic Press, 1986 and 1987.
41. Smith, K.T.: Trace Minerals in Foods. New York, Marcel Dekker, 1988.
42. Anke, M.: Arsenic *In* Trace Elements in Human and Animal Nutrition. 5th Ed. Edited by W. Mertz. New York, Academic Press, 1986.
43. Nielsen, F.H.: The ultratrace elements. *In* Trace Minerals in Foods, Edited by K.T. Smith. New York, Marcel Dekker, 1988.
44. Jelinek, C.F., Corneliussen, P.E.: Environ. Health Perspect., *19:*83–87, 1977.
45. Schroeder, H.A., Balassa, J.J.: J. Chronic Dis., *19:*85–106, 1966.
46. Axelson, O., Dahlgren, E., Jansson, C.-D., et al.: Br. J. Ind. Med., *35:*8–15, 1978.
47. Mabuchi, K., Lilienfeld, A.M., and Snell, L.M.: Arch. Environ. Health, *34:*312–319, 1979.
48. Levander, O.A.: Selenium. *In* Trace Elements in Human and Animal Nutrition. 5th Ed. Edited by W. Mertz. New York, Academic Press, 1986.
49. Smith, M.J., Franke, K.W., and Westfall, B.B.: Public Health Rep., *51:*1496, 1936.
50. Smith, M.J., Westfall, B.B.: Public Health Rep., *52:*1375, 1937.
51. Yang, G., Wang, S., Zhou, R., Sun, S.: Am. J. Clin. Nutr., *37:*872–881, 1983.

52. Jaffee, W.G.: Effect of selenium intake in humans and rats. *In* Proceedings of the Symposium on Selenium-Tellurium in the Environment. Notre Dame, IN, University of Notre Dame, 1976, pp. 188–193. Industrial Health Foundation, 1976.

53. Bennett, B.G.: Exposure Commitment Assessments of Environmental Pollutants. Vol. 1, No. 2. London, Monitoring and Assessment Research Center, 1981.

54. Environmental Protection Agency: Mercury Health Effects Update. U.S. Research Triangle Park, NC, Environmental Protection Agency, 1984.

55. Tsubaki, T., Irukuyama, K.: Minamata Disease. Tokyo, Kodansha, 1977.

56. Friberg, L., Kjellstrom, T. Nordberg, G.: Cadmium. *In* Handbook of the Toxicology of Metals. 2nd Ed. Vol. 2. Edited by L. Friberg, G.F. Nordberg, and V.B. Vouk. New York, Elsevier, 1986, pp. 130–183.

57. Dunnick, J.K., Fowler, B.A.: Cadmium. *In* Handbook on Toxicity of Inorganic Compounds. Edited by H.G. Seiler, H. Sigal, and A. Sigal. New York, Marcel Dekker, 1988.

58. Kostial, K.: Cadmium. *In* Trace Elements in Human and Animal Nutrition. Edited by W. Mertz. New York, Academic Press, 1986.

59. Kobayashi, J., Morii, F., Muramoto, S., et al.: Jpn. J. Hyg., *25:*364–367, 1970.

60. Kazantzis, G.: Environ. Health Perspect., *28:*155–160, 1979.

61. Itokawa, Y., Tomoko, A., Tanaka, S.: Arch. Environ. Health, *26:*241–247, 1973.

62. Coats, J.R.: Toxicology of pesticide residues in foods. *In* Nutritional Toxicology. Vol. II. Edited by J.N. Hathcock. Orlando, FL, Academic Press, 1987.

63. Murphy, S.D.: Toxic effects of pesticides. *In* Casarett's and Doull's Toxicology. Edited by C.D. Klaassen, M.O. Amdur, and J. Doull. New York, Macmillan, 1986.

64. Büchel, K.H.: Regul. Toxicol. Pharmacol., *4:*174–191, 1984.

65. Turnbull, G.J.: J. R. Soc. Med., *77:*932–935, 1984.

66. Ariens, E.J., Simonis, A.M.: General principles of nutritional toxicology. *In:* Nutritional Toxicology. Vol. 1. Edited by J.N. Hathcock. New York, Academic Press, 1982.

67. Roberts, L.: Science, *243:*1430, 1989.

68. Hathcock, J.N., Zarba-Vary, A: Standards for pesticide residues in foods: A workshop report. *In* Proceedings of the XIII International Congress of Nutrition. Edited by T.G. Taylor and N.K. Jenkins. London, John Libby, 1986.

69. National Research Council: Regulating Pesticides in Foods. Washington, D.C., National Academy Press, 1987.

70. Fan, A.M., Jackson, R.J.: Regul. Toxicol. Pharmacol., *9:*158–174, 1989.

71. Cordle, F., Kolbye, A.C.: Environmental contaminants in food. *In* Nutritional Toxicology. Vol. 1. Edited by J.N. Hathcock. New York, Academic Press, 1982.

72. Santodonato, J., Howard, P., Basu, D.: J. Environ. Pathol. Toxicol., *5:*1–364, 1981.

73. Hargraves, W.A.: Mutagens in cooked foods. *In* Nutritional Toxicology. Vol. 2. Edited by J.N. Hathcock. Orlando, FL, Academic Press, 1987.

74. Sugimura, T., Wakabayashi, K., Nagao, M., et al.: Heterocyclic amines in food. *In* Food Toxicology: A Perspective on the Relative Risks. Edited by S.L. Taylor and R.A. Scanlan. New York, Marcel Dekker, 1989.

75. Wilson, B.J.: Mycotocins and toxic stress metabolites of fungus-infected sweet potatoes. *In* Nutritional Toxicology. Vol. 1. Edited by J.N. Hathcock. New York, Academic Press, 1982.

76. Berry, C.L.: J. Pathol., *154:*301–311, 1988.

77. Schlatter, C.: Bibl. Nutr. Dieta., *41:*55–65, 1988.

78. Krogh, P.: J. Appl. Bacteriol., *Symposium Supplement:* 99s–104s, 1989.

79. Mantle, P.G.: J. Appl. Bacteriol., *Symposium Supplement:* 83s–88s, 1989.

80. Blount, W.T.: Turkeys, *9:*53, 1961.

81. National Research Council: Diet, Nutrition and Cancer. Washington, D.C., Academy Press, 1982.

82. Goldblatt, L.A.: Aflatoxin. New York, Academic Press, 1969.

83. Stoloff, L.: Nutr. Cancer, *5:*165–186, 1983.

84. Mantle, P.G.: Secondary metabolites of *Penicillium* and *Acremonium. In* Penicillium and Acremonium, Biotechnology Handbooks. Vol. 1. New York, Plenum, 1987.

85. Doores, S.: CRC Crit. Rev. Food Sci. Nutr., *19:*133–149, 1983.

86. Broom, W.A., Bulbring, E., Chapman, C.J., et al.: Br. J. Exp. Pathol., *25:*95–100, 1944.

87. Dickens, F., Jones, H.E.H.: Br. J. Cancer, *15:*85–92, 1961.

88. Anonymous: Food Chem. News, *22:*9, 1980.

89. Krogh, P.: Mycotoxic porcine nephropathy: A possible model for Balkan endemic nephropathry. *In* Endemic Nephropathy. Edited by A. Puchlev. Proceedings of the Second International Symposium on Endemic Nephropathy, Sofia, November 9–11, 1972. Sofia, Bulagarian Academy of Sciences, 1974.

90. Austwick, P.K.C., Carter, R.L., Greig, J.M., et al.: Contrib. Nephrol., *16:*154–160, 1979.

91. Hult, K., Plestina, R., Hzbazin-Novak, et al.: Arch. Toxicol., *51:*313–321, 1982.

92. Barnes, J.M., Austwick, P.K.C., Carter, R.L., et al.: Lancet, *1:*671–675, 1977.

93. Yeulet S.F., Mantle, P.G., Rudge, M.S., Greig, J.B.: Mycopathologia, *102:*21–30, 1988.

94. Broquist, H.: Annu. Rev. Nutr., *5:*391–409, 1985.

95. Aust, S.D., Broquist, H.P., Rinehart, K.L. Jr.: Biotechnol. Bioengin., *10:*408–412, 1968.

96. Hartley, W.J.: A comparative study of Darling pea *(Swainsona spp.)* poisoning in Australia with locoweed (*Astragalus* and *Oxytropis spp.*) poisoning in North America. *In* Effects of Poisonous Plants on Livestock. Edited by R.E. Keeler, K.R. VanKampen, and L.F. James. New York, Academic Press, 1978.

97. Halstead, B.: Poisonous and Venomous Marine Animals of the World. Vol. 2. Washington, D.C., U.S., Government Printing Office, 1967.

98. Tindall, D.R., Dickey, R.W., Carlson, R.D., et al.: Ciguatoxigenic dinoflagellates from the Caribbean Sea. *In* Seafood Toxins. Edited by E.P. Ragelis. Washington, D.C., American Chemical Society, 1984.

99. Dickey, R.W., Bobzin, S.C., Faulkner, D.J., et al.: Toxicon, *28:*371–377, 1990.

100. Halstead, B.W.: Fish as Food. Vol. 2. Edited by G. Borgstrom. New York, Academic Press, 1962.

101. Baden, D.G.: Int. Rev. Cytol., *82:*99–150, 1983.

102. National Research Council: Toxicants Occurring Naturally in Foods. Washington, D.C., National Academy of Sciences, 1973.

103. Morton, I.D.: J. Hum. Nutr., *31:*53–60, 1977.

104. Salunkhe, D.K., Wu, M.R.: Toxicants in plants and plant products. CRC Crit. Rev. Food Sci. Nutr., *12:*265–324, 1977.

105. Somogyi, J.C.: Bibl. Nutr. Dieta, *29:*110–127, 1980.

105. Furihata, C., MatsushiMa, T.: Annu. Rev. Nutr., *6:*67–94, 1986.

106. Ory, R.L.: Antinutrients and Natural Toxicants in Foods. Westport, CT, Food and Nutrition Press, 1981.
107. deWolff, F.A.: Hum. Toxicol., *7*:443–447, 1988.
108. Newberne, P.M.: Naturally occurring food-borne toxicants. *In* Modern Nutrition in Health and Disease. Edited by M.E. Shils and V.R. Young. Philadelphia, Lea & Febiger, 1988.
109. National Research Council: Diet and Health: Implications for Reducing Chronic Disease Risk. Washington, D.C., National Academy Press, 1989.
110. Rackis, J.J.: Biologically active components. *In* Soybeans: Chemistry and Technology. Vol. 1. Edited by A.K. Smith and S.J. Circle. Westport, CT, Avi Publishing, 1978.
111. Brandon, D.L., Bates, A.H., Friedman, M.: J. Food. Sci., *53*:102–106, 1988.
112. Rackis, J.J., Gumbmann, M.R.: Protease inhibitors: physiological properties and nutritional significance. *In* Antinutrients and Natural Toxicants in Foods. Edited by R.L. Ory. Westport, CT, Food and Nutrition Press, 1981.
113. Roebuck, B.: J. Nutr., *117*:398–404, 1987.
114. Smith, J.C., Wilson, F.U., Allen, P.V., et al.: J. Appl. Toxicol., *9*:175–179, 1989.
115. Liener, I.E.: J. Nutr., *116*:920–923, 1986.
116. Liener, I.E., Goodale, R.L., Desmukh, A., et al.: Gastroenterology, *94*:419–427, 1988.
117. Hathcock, J.N.: Residual trypsin inhibitor. *In* Nutritional and Toxicological Consequences of Food Processing. Edited by M. Friedman. New York, Plenum Press, 1991, pp. 273–279.
118. Jaffe, Y.: Hemagglutins and Toxic Constituents of Plant Foodstuffs. Edited by I. Liener. New York, Academic Press, 1969.
119. Honavar, P.M., Shih, C.V., Liener, L.E.: J. Nutr., *77*:109–114, 1962.
120. Olsen, M.O.J., Liener, L.E.: Biochemistry, *6*:105–111, 1967.
121. Bell, E.A.: Aminonitriles and aminoacids not derived from proteins. *In* Toxicants Occurring Naturally in Foods. Washington, D.C., National Academy of Sciences, 1973.
122. Dasler, W.: Science, *120*:307–308, 1954.
123. Selzer, G., Parker, G.F.: Am. J. Pathol., *27*:S85, 1951.
124. Bull, L., Culvenor, I., Dick, A.T.: The Pyrrolizidine Alkaloids. New York, John Wiley and Sons, 1968.
125. Schoental, R.: Cancer Res., *28*:2237–2246, 1968.
126. Hirono, I., Ueno, I., Hosaka, S., et al.: Cancer Lett., *13*:15–21, 1981.
127. Canadrian, U., Luthy, J., Graf, U., et al.: Food Chem. Toxicol., *22*:223–225, 1984.
128. Hayes, M.A., Roberts, E., Farber, E.: Cancer Res., *45*:3726–3734, 1985.
129. Van Etten, C.H.: Goitrogens. *In* Toxic Constituents of Plant Foodstuffs. 2nd Ed. Edited by I.E. Liener. New York, Academic Press, 1980.
130. Greer, M.A., Astwood, E.B.: Endocrinology, *43*:105–109, 1948.
131. Berrens, L.: Monogr. Allergy, *13*:164–193, 1971.
132. Spies, J.R.L.: J. Agri. Food Chem., *22*:30–36, 1974.
133. Metcalfe, D.D.: Clin. Rev. Allergy, *3*:331–349, 1985.
134. Van Metre, T.E., Anderson, S.A., Barnard, J.H., et al.: J. Allergy, *41*:195–208, 1968.
135. Bock, S.A., May, C.D.: Adverse reactions to food caused by sensitivity. *In* Allergy: Principles and Practice. Edited by E. Middleton, C.E. Reed, and E.F. Ellis. St. Louis, C.V. Mosby, 1983.
136. Sampson, H.: J. Allergy Clin. Immunol., *71*:473–480, 1983.
137. Aas, K.: Int. Arch. Allergy Appl. Immunol., *31*:239–260, 1967.
138. Sachs, M.I., Jones, R.T., Yunginger, J.W.: J. Allergy Clin. Immunol., *67*:27–34, 1981.
139. Hoffman, D.R., Day, E.D., Miller, J.S.: Ann. Allergy, *47*:17–22, 1981.
140. Langeland, T., Harbitz, O.: Allergy, *38*:131–139, 1983.
141. Jos, J., Charbonnier, L., Mosse, J., Olives, J.P., et al.: Clin. Chim. Acta, *119*:263–274, 1982.
142. Gleason, M.N., Gosselin, R.E., Hodge, H.C.: Clinical Toxicology of Commercial Products. Baltimore, Williams & Wilkins, 1963.
143. Jeghers, H., Murphy, R.: N. Engl. J. Med., *233*:208–215, 1945.
144. Valyesevi, A., Dhanamitta, S.: Am. J. Clin. Nutr., *27*:877–882, 1974.
145. Fox, M.R.S., Tao, S.-H.: Antinutritive effects of phytate and other phosphorylated derivatives. *In* Nutritional Toxicology. Vol. 3. Edited by J.N. Hathcock. New York, Academic Press, 1989.
146. Ferrell, R.E., Wheeler, E.L., Pence, J.W.: Cereal Sci. Today, *14*:110, 1969.
147. Garruto, R.M., Yanagihara, R., Gajdusek, D.C.: Environ. Geochem. Health, *12*:137–151, 1990.
148. Hirono, I.: CRC Crit. Rev. Toxicol., *8*:235–277, 1981.
149. Zedeck, M.S.: Hydrazine derivatives, azo and azoxy compounds and methylazoxymethanol and cycasin. *In* Chemical Carcinogenesis. 2nd Ed. ACS Monograph 182. Edited by C.E. Searle. Washington, D.C., American Chemical Society, 1984.
150. Laqueur, G.L., Spatz, M.: Cancer Res., *28*:2262–2267, 1968.
151. Hirono, I., Kachi, H., Kato, C.: Acta Pathol. Jpn., *20*:327–337, 1970.
152. Pamukcu, A.M., Yalciner, S., Hatcher, J.F., et al.: Cancer Res., *40*:3468–3472, 1980.
153. Van der Hoeven, J.C.M., Lagerweg, W.J., Posthumus, M.A., et al.: Carcinogenesis, *4*:1587–1590, 1983.
154. Peckham, J.C., Mitchell, F.E., Jones, O.H., et al.: J. Am. Vet. Med. Assoc., *160*:169–172, 1972.
155. Linnabary, R.D., Tarrier, M.P.: Vet. Hum. Toxicol., *30*:255–256, 1988.
156. Hammond, A.C., Bradley, B.J., Yokoyama, M.T., et al.: Am. J. Vet. Res., *40*:1398–1401, 1978.
157. Kuhn, D.M., Lovenberg, W.: Psychoactive and vasoactive substances in food. *In* Nutritional Toxicology. Vol. 1. Edited by J.N. Hathcock. New York, Academic Press, 1982.
158. Larochelle, P., Hamet, P., Enjalberg, M.: Clin. Pharmacol. Ther., *26*:24–30, 1979.
159. Marley, E.: Monamine-oxidase inhibitors and drug interactions. *In* Drug Interactions. Edited by D.G. Grahame-Smith. Baltimore, University Park Press, 1977.

This chapter was written by John Hathcock and Jeanne Rader in their private capacities. No official support or endorsement by the Food and Drug Administration is intended or should be inferred.

SELECTED READINGS

Archer, M.C.: Hazards of nitrate, nitrite and N-nitroso compounds in human nutrition. *In* Nutritional Toxicology. Vol. 1. Edited by J.N. Hathcock. New York, Academic Press, 1982.

Ariens, E.J., Simonis, A.M.: General principles of nutritional toxicology. *In* Nutritional Toxicology. Vol. 1. Edited by J.N. Hathcock. New York, Academic Press, 1982.

Hathcock, J.N. Nutritional toxicology: basic principles and actual problems. Food Addit. Contam., *7:*S12–S18, 1990.

Hathcock, J.N. Toxicology of pesticide residues in foods. *In* Encyclopedia of Human Biology. Vol. 7. San Diego, Academic Press, 1991.

Hathcock, J.N., Rader, J.I. Micronutrient safety. Ann. N.Y. Acad. Sci., *587:*257–266, 1990.

Mertz, W. Trace Elements in Human and Animal Nutrition. 5th Ed. New York, Academic Press, 1986.

National Research Council: Toxicants Occurring Naturally in Foods. Washington, D.C., National Academy Press, 1973.

Rackis, J.J., Gumbmann, M.R. *Antinutrients and Natural Toxicants in Foods.* Edited by R.L. Ory. Westport, CT, Food and Nutrition Press, 1981.

Ragelis, E.P.: Seafood Toxins. Washington, D.C., American Chemical Society, 1984.

Salunke, D.K., Wu, M.R.: Toxicants in plant and plant products. CRC Crit. Rev. Food Sci. Nutr., *12:*265–324, 1977.

Sugimura, T., Wakabayashi, K., Nagao, M., et al.: Heterocyclic amines in food. *In* Food Toxicology: A Perspective on the Relative Risks. Edited by S.L. Taylor and R.A. Scanlan. New York, Marcel Dekker, 1989.

CHAPTER **93**

Dietary Goals and Guidelines: National and International Perspectives

A. Stewart Truswell

NEED FOR DIETARY GUIDELINES

In public health nutrition there are two major sets of messages from the consensus of nutritional scientists to the rest of the population—that is, to politicians, economists, government departments, food industry, farmers, health professionals, journalists, school teachers, supermarkets, caterers, shoppers, and consumers. Recommended dietary intakes (RDI; see Chaps. 82 and 83) are the first and older set. They advise quantities of the essential nutrients that people ought to consume. These technical numbers have to be replaced for ordinary people by educational devices such as food groups, meal plans, or exchange lists, or by food enrichment, subsidies etc. In underdeveloped countries and communities food and nutritional policy must concentrate on striving to reach the RDIs for as many people and as many nutrients as possible.

But in affluent countries achievement of intakes near the RDIs can be taken for granted for most people. Other sets of authoritative statements, called *dietary guidelines,* have emerged since the late 1960s; these guidelines advise consumers how to select from the many combinations of foods in adequate diets to give the best chances of long-term health. The variety of food products is bewildering and there is, as it were, a Tower of Babel of nutritional breakthroughs and threats. The whole food system needs signposts—guidelines to healthier diets that can be used in nutrition education, in planning by food companies, and in national nutrition policy.

In the early 1970s opinions on human nutrition seemed adrift. There were open disputes between leading nutrition scientists about basic concepts. The first era of vitamin research was over. Some experts thought there were no more nutritional problems to solve.[1] Efforts to meet the protein gap in developing countries were criticized as a fiasco.[2] Public advice on dietary prevention of coronary heart disease was in conflict between the fat and sucrose theories.[3–5] The new dietary fiber hypothesis was attracting popular enthusiasm ahead of a scientific basis for it.[6] Carbohydrates had gotten a bad press,[7] and low-carbohydrate diets were fashionable for obesity.[8]

The rational response to this threat of nutritional information anarchy was for an authoritative body to convene a committee of experts to try to formulate a statement on the role of nutrition in diseases of affluence and what these mean in terms of food choice. A parallel response was to collect the votes of experts on key questions by postal questionnaire[9] or at a meeting[10] or by statistical analysis of ballots by a panel.[11]

FEATURES OF DIETARY GUIDELINES OR GOALS

These guidelines aim not to provide enough of the essential nutrients (that is the purpose of RDI) but to reduce the chances of developing chronic degenerative diseases. While there is never more than one RDI (or Recommended Dietary Allowance—RDA) committee and report in a country, there can be and have been several sets of dietary guidelines at a time.

Dietary goals or guidelines start not from zero intake (as RDI do) but from the present estimated national average diet. They deal not with energy requirements but with the optimal proportions of the energy-yielding macronutrients: how much carbohydrate? fat? protein? alcohol? and which type? They are not usually expressed as nutrients, but as food components, or as food groups or even as food behavior. They are often a hybrid collection of recommendations.

Dietary goals or guidelines are not expressed as weight of nutrient per day, but as change from the present consumption of a food component or from people's eating behavior. If expressed quantitatively this is mostly as percentage of total energy, that is, nutrient density (e.g., total fat intake should be 30 to 35% of total energy).

Dietary guidelines are targets for the population to aim for some time in the future; in some sets the year is given (such as the year 2000[12]) or goals are progressive (e.g., for total fat the intermediate goal is 35% energy, and the ultimate goal is 20 to 30%[13]). RDI by contrast are needed now and every day (although there are reserves in the body, large for some nutrients, small for others, all of which vary among individuals).

In a few sets of dietary guidelines a distinction is made between general advice for the whole population and (usually more radical) advice for groups at risk. For example, the U.S. Surgeon General's Report has five recommendations for most people and another four for some people.[14] The recommendations of the World Health Organization (WHO) Europe give intermediate goals separately for the general population and for the cardiovascular high-risk group.[13]

Although most RDI are relatively well established scientifically, guidelines are more provisional, being based on indirect evidence about the complex role of food components in the cause of multifactorial diseases with long incubation periods. As the U.S. Senate Select Committee on Nutrition and Human Needs put it, "Nutritionists have greater confidence in their conclusions concerning micronutrients than in their observations about macronutrients."[15] Dietary goals and guidelines, which primarily examine macronutrients, rely more on epidemiologic data than RDI do. In addition, they depend on using food consumption patterns. In the concluding chapter of their review the National Research Council (NRC) Committee on Diet and Health observed that

> the term *insufficient data* could perhaps be applied to most issues concerning nutrition and health. In particular it characterizes many of the relationships between diet and certain chronic diseases. The lack of certainty about causal associations and mechanisms of action is common and stems in part from attempts to relate a complex mixture such as diet to complex, multifactorial chronic diseases for which the pathophysiological, environmental, and genetic predisposing factors are imprecisely understood. . . . Despite such limitations, a large body of evidence has emerged in the past four decades concerning chronic diseases and their relationship to general dietary patterns or specific dietary components.[16]

Unlike RDI, which give separate numbers for males and females and for different age groups and physiologic states, dietary guidelines usually appear to be the same for every man, woman, and child. Of course at the implementation stage adjustments have to be made. Although they are newer than RDI, dietary guidelines are already better known by the general public. Their summary recommendations, written in deliberately simple language about major food components or food habits, appeal to journalists, consumer organizations, and cook book writers.

GOALS OR GUIDELINES?

The classic "Dietary Goals for the United States" formulated by a select committee of the United States Senate was addressed to the nation,[15] and the recommendations were expressed in such technical terms as "increase the consumption of complex carbohydrates and naturally occurring sugars from about 28% of energy intake to about 48% of energy intake"[15]—this is not a calculation the shopper can manage in the aisle of a supermarket! These recommendations were followed by "Dietary Guidelines for Americans" published by the Department of Agriculture in which the corresponding recommendation is headed "Eat foods with adequate starch and fiber."[17] Similarly in Australia the first recommendations of this type were in a paper on food and nutrition policy called "Dietary Goals for Australia."[18] One of them was "Increase consumption of complex carbohydrates and dietary fibre. . . ."[18] Three years later the Department of Health published the same eight recommendations in a mass-produced booklet entitled "Dietary Guidelines for Australians" written in less technical language—for example, "Eat more bread and cereals (preferably wholegrain), vegetables and fruit."[19] In both these examples dietary goals were part of food and nutrition policy and were expressed in technical language, whereas dietary guidelines were written for consumers in simpler language about, for example, selection of food groups. Helsing suggests that recommendations are needed at three levels: nutrient level goals for scientists and professionals, food level goals for politicians and producers, and dietary guidelines that are expressed as advice to the public.[20] In usage around the world, especially when committees prepare English translations from recommendations first written in another language, these nice distinctions sometimes may be blurred. They have not been authoritatively defined.

HISTORY OF DIETARY GOALS AND GUIDELINES

NORDIC *SYNPUNKTER* (1968)

The first set of dietary goals were *Mediciniska synpunkter på folkkosten i de Nordiska länderna* (medical viewpoints on people's food in the Nordic countries*) published in Sweden in 1968.[21,22] Ancel Keys arranged for an English translation to be printed in *Nutrition Reviews* 4 months later.[23] These goals were further disseminated in the major British textbook[24] (Table 93–1).[1]

The goals were developed by A. Wretlind, G. Blix, S. Bergstrom and, I. Westin (Sweden),[25] who were subsequently joined by P. Roine (Finland), E. Uhl (Denmark), R. Nicolaysen, N. Eeg-Larsen (Norway), M. Malmros, and B. Isaakson (Sweden).[22] Wretlind described the ideas behind these recommendations. In modern Sweden mechanization had reduced physical work and with it calorie consumption. Consumers with low calorie intakes need to increase the density of iron, calcium, and other nutrients per 1000 kcal if they are to obtain their RDI. Meanwhile the proportion of fat in the diet had risen in Sweden from 29% of energy at the end of the nineteenth century to 42% in the mid-1960s.[26] "Simple calculations showed that a diet ensuring the micronutrient requirements of the low-calorie groups is practically impossible to achieve without reduction of the fat consumption . . . to, at most, 35% of calories."[27]

After a review of different diets, additional reasons were put forward for the proposed changes. "The fat reduction might help to counteract a too high supply of calories. In view of the correlation between consumption of saturated fats and the frequency of atherosclerotic heart disease it might also help to prevent this disease, especially if part of the saturated fat were at the same time replaced by polyunsaturated fat. The reduction of sugar consumption, particularly in the form of confectionery, should further be a valuable measure in the fight against dental caries."[27] The Nordic viewpoints were the foundation for the Swedish Diet and Exercise campaign and the Norwegian Nutrition policy. There was, however, some professional opposition in Scandinavia to these proposals, which prompted the professor of nutrition at the University of Oslo to send out questionnaires about coronary disease and diet to over 200 experts in 22 different countries.[9,28] The 192 replies that Kaare Norum received were reassuring: 92% of respondents said that knowledge *was* sufficient to recommend moderate change in the diet of affluent communities, and they voted for reduced saturated fat.

*"Nordic" and "Scandinavian" are used often interchangeably, but the original meaning of "Scandinavia" was the peninsula comprising Norway and Sweden. Nordic also includes Denmark, Finland, and Iceland.

TABLE 93–1. MEDICAL VIEWPOINTS ON PEOPLE'S FOOD IN THE NORDIC COUNTRIES

The calorie supply in the diet should in many cases be reduced to prevent overweight.
Total fat consumption should be reduced from the present around 40% to between 25 and 35% of total calories.
The use of saturated fat should be reduced, and consumption of polyunsaturated fat should be increased simultaneously.
Consumption of sugar and sugar-containing products should be reduced.
One should increase consumption of vegetables, fruit, potatoes, skimmed milk, fish, lean meat, and cereal products.
From the medical and nutritional standpoint it is essential to emphasize the importance of regular exercise habits from childhood for all individuals with mainly sedentary work.

(Data translated from Mediciniska synpunkter på folkkosten i de Nordiska länderna. Vår. Föda., *20:*3–5, 1968; and Mediciniska synpunkter på folkkosten i de Nordiska länderna. Lakartidningen, *65:*2012–2013, 1968.)

ACCUMULATING DIETARY RECOMMENDATIONS FOR PREVENTION OF CORONARY HEART DISEASE

Meanwhile, evidence was accumulating for the dietary fat hypothesis of coronary heart disease (CHD) that Ancel Keys started to develop around 1952.[29,30] The American Heart Association has been publishing diet-heart statements every few years since 1961, and they have become progressively less tentative, with a larger scientific infrastructure.[31,32] Other bodies in the United States made their own statements with dietary advice on prevention of CHD since 1970: the Inter-Society Commission for Heart Disease Resources (1970),[33] the American Medical Association/National Research Council (1972),[34] and the American Health Foundation (1972).[35] In other countries authoritative statements were made between 1971 and 1976 by committees of the National Heart Foundation of Australia,[36] the Royal Society of New Zealand,[37] the New Zealand Heart Foundation,[38] the Netherlands Nutrition Council,[39] the International Society of Cardiology,[40] the U.K. Department of Health and Social Security,[3] the Royal College of Physicians (London),[41] the Federal Health Office in West Germany,[42] and Health & Welfare Canada.[43]

All these committees had a different starting point from that of the Nordic group, concentrating on dietary modifications to reduce the risk of CHD. Some took the clinical viewpoint: find individuals with a high plasma cholesterol level and prescribe a modified diet for them.[34,36] Others gave advice to the whole community.[35,39] They agreed that total fat intake should be reduced, and most recommended an increased proportion of polyunsaturated fatty acid intake and some restriction of dietary cholesterol.

So, by the mid-1970s, there were two lines of reasoning for dietary advice to the public in affluent countries. The Nordic nutrition professors aimed primarily to replace empty-calorie foods (fats and sugar) with a variety of more nutritious foods because people in these countries were expending less energy and so eating less food than their grandparents. The followers of Ancel Keys aimed primarily to bring down the plasma (total) cholesterol concentration. Their advice concentrated on eating less saturated fat and cholesterol.

DIETARY GOALS FOR THE UNITED STATES (1977)

A third group of miscellaneous ideas, less well established, also went into *Dietary Goals for the United States,* which is a central document in the history of dietary guidelines. Most important were the dietary fiber hypothesis (for which there was one reference in the report[44]), the possible relation of high fat intake to breast and large bowel cancer (without a cited reference), and the possible role of salt in causing high blood pressure (quoting Meneely and Battarbee[45]). These three concepts were poorly documented in the report, but each has turned out to be a powerful hypothesis for which the evidence continued to grow.[2]

The first edition of *Dietary Goals for the United States*[46] (Table 93–2) was a revolutionary Senate committee report. Its appearance and content took nutritionists by surprise. It was written by a group of political activists with a nonprofessional interest and knowledge of nutrition, but just before its publication Mark Hegsted, Professor of Nutrition at Harvard University, was consulted. The final report contains no major follies, although the references are few and sometimes unconventional.

Dietary Goals met strong and polarized reactions from nutrition scientists and various other groups and individuals in the United States (Table 93–3). A revised edition was published before the end of the same year with some important additions and corrections[15] (Table 93–2). A new goal was added about overweight persons and the salt goal was increased up to 5 g per day. Alcohol was discussed in the introduction. These changes went a considerable way to answer the objections in group 8 of Table 93–3. The other objections are of a more philosophic nature and have tended to recur after the publication of subsequent sets of dietary guidelines in the United States and in other countries. Committees that draft dietary guidelines have to keep in mind these possible objections and try to minimize them. There have never again been so many published commentaries and criticisms as those following the first edition of *Dietary Goals for the United States*. One collection of commentaries runs to 889 pages.[47]

TABLE 93–2. DIETARY GOALS FOR THE UNITED STATES AND DIETARY GUIDELINES FOR AMERICANS (IN ABBREVIATED FORM AND IN ORIGINAL ORDER)

DIETARY GOALS FOR THE UNITED STATES, FEB. 1977*	DIETARY GOALS FOR THE UNITED STATES, DEC. 1977†	DIETARY GUIDELINES FOR AMERICANS, 1980‡
↑Carbohydrate	Avoid overweight	Eat variety
↓Total fat	↑Complex carbohydrates	Desirable weight
↓Saturated fatty acids, ↑PUF	↓Sugars	Not too much fat, saturated fatty acids, and cholesterol
↓Cholesterol	↓Total fat	Eat starch and fiber
↓Sugar	↓Saturated fatty acids ↑PUF	Not too much sugar
↓Salt to 3 g/d	↓Cholesterol	Not too much sodium
	↓Salt to 5 g/d	Moderate alcohol

PUF, Polyunsaturated fatty acids.

*Data from Select Committee on Nutrition and Human Needs, United States Senate: Dietary Goals for the United States. Washington, D.C., United States Government Printing Office, 1977.

†Data from Select Committee on Nutrition and Human Needs, United States Senate: Dietary Goals for the United States. 2nd Ed. Washington, D.C., United States Government Printing Office, 1977.

‡Data from United States Department of Agriculture: Dietary Guidelines for Americans. Home and Garden Bulletin No. 232. Hyattsville, MD, Human Nutrition Information Service, United States Department of Agriculture, 1980.

TABLE 93–3. OBJECTIONS TO DIETARY GOALS FOR THE UNITED STATES*

1. *Reasoning not scientific enough.* Based more on intuition than on scientific reasoning. Not a scientifically sound review. Should be re-examined by expert bodies, such as the NIH, FDA, USDA, and NAS.
2. *Not needed.* America's health is improving. The Committee has perpetrated a hoax by claiming that Americans are suffering from an epidemic of killer diseases.
3. *We need more research.* Too soon. The lipid hypothesis of coronary heart disease not yet proven; the relation between salt and hypertension not yet proven. We are only on the threshold of discovery in nutrition. It is unwise to base recommendations on food disappearance data. Promises too much. The politicians are overselling nutrition.
4. *Political.* Politically motivated. A puritanical, big brother approach. Its unwise to tamper with the diets of the great majority of people. For high-risk groups diets should be individually prescribed by medical practitioners or dietitians.
5. *Problem of recommending for all age-sex groups.* These look like guidelines for food intake by overweight, middle-aged men. Neglects children.
6. *Vested interests.* My advice was not asked, or that of our professional association. Our industry may be affected (salt, dairy, sugar, egg, cattlemen).
7. *There could be adverse effects.* We are concerned that increased intake of polyunsaturated fat could have side effects. If less meat is eaten, iron deficiency may increase.
8. *Major issues were omitted and corrections are required.* Should add a goal about obesity. Should add encouragement of water fluoridation. The goal of 3 g NaCl per day is far too low.

*Many of the commentaries were a mixture of positive and (some of the above) negative comments. Individual commentators often made criticisms in several of the above groups.

(Data from Select Committee on Nutrition and Human Needs, United States Senate: Dietary Goals for the United States: Supplemental Views. Washington, D.C., United States Government Printing Office, 1977; Twenty Commentaries on the McGovern Dietary Goals: Nutr. *Today,* November/December:10–13, 20–27, 1977; and Harper, A.E.: Am. J. Clin. Nutr., *31:*310–321, 1978.)

Notwithstanding the criticisms, many of the principal U.S. researchers on diet and atherosclerosis and on dentistry approved of *Dietary Goals* on balance. Overseas, the first comment came in an editorial in *The Lancet,* which thought that "The Committee shows its professionalism by starting with what should be increased (carbohydrates) to compensate for the reductions entailed by the other five goals. . . . The first goal will surprise those (one hopes few of them are medical people) who still imagine that starchy foods are unhealthy or that bread and potatoes are especially fattening."[50] The goal of 30% energy intake from fat, continued the editorial, "is rather less than was available in Britain during the 1939–1945 war but more than the content in traditional Mediterranean cooking. . . . The American goals will be welcomed by people who have thought seriously about the diet of modern Western man. Their major blind spot is to ignore alcohol consumption. . . ."[50]

Dietary Goals for the United States was never withdrawn, nor was it ever an official U.S. government statement, although most nutritionists outside the country probably did not realize this. The ideas in the *Dietary Goals* have been modified and re-used—or rediscovered—in official or authoritative sets of recommendations in the United States and in many national sets of guidelines around the world.

APPEARANCE OF TWO NEW SETS OF RECOMMENDATIONS IN 1980

One comment on *Dietary Goals* was that the task of developing dietary recommendations for the population should be reallocated to a more authoritative scientific body.[46] The Food and Nutrition Board of the National Research Council (the body responsible for Recommended Dietary Allowances) produced a report called "Toward Healthful Diets" (Table 93–4).[51] The Board's recommendations were conservative, except for the one on salt, which was widely criticized because the evidence about fats and health is stronger than that about salt.[52]

At about the same time, the U.S. Department of Agriculture (USDA) and the Department of Health and Human Services (DHHS) combined to publish "Dietary Guidelines for Americans,"[17] a pamphlet of 24 half-pages written in simplified language for the general public (Table 93–4). The recommendations were similar to Dietary Goals (Table 93–2), with an extra recommendation to eat a variety of foods and another urging moderate alcohol consumption.[4]

The contrast between these two sets of recommendations appearing the same year in the same country led to confusion in the media, and scientists took sides. Congress held separate hearings on each.[53,54] The two hearings reports make interesting reading. There was no official judgment at the time but the criticisms seemed to be stronger against "Toward Healthful Diets." The USDA-DHHS guidelines were revised by a fresh committee, which made only small changes for the second edition (1985).[55] The third edition of the guidelines was published in 1990 (Table 93–4). A later NRC Food and Nutrition Board appointed a new Committee on Diet and Health. It spent 5 years writing a 750-page report that reaches recommendations similar to but more comprehensive than *Dietary Goals* and "Dietary Guidelines for Americans."[16]

TABLE 93–4. COMPARISON OF DIFFERENT DIETARY RECOMMENDATIONS IN THE UNITED STATES

TOWARD HEALTHFUL DIETS*	DIETARY GUIDELINES FOR AMERICANS (1ST ED.) (1980)†	DIETARY GUIDELINES FOR AMERICANS (3RD ED.) (1990)‡
1. Select a nutritionally adequate diet from the four food groups	1. Eat a variety of foods	1. Eat a variety of foods
2. Vary diet as widely as practicable in each of the major groups	2. Maintain desirable weight	2. Maintain healthy weight
3. Maintain or achieve appropriate weight for height	3. Avoid too much fat, saturated fat, and cholesterol	3. Choose a diet low in fat, saturated fat, and cholesterol
4. If energy requirement is low (e.g., reducing diet), reduce consumption of alcohol, sugars, fats, and oils, which provide calories but few other essential nutrients	4. Eat foods with adequate starch and fiber	4. Choose a diet with plenty of vegetables, fruits, and grain products
5. Use salt in moderation—3 to 8 g NaCl per day	5. Avoid too much sugar	5. Use sugars only in moderation
	6. Avoid too much sodium	6. Use salt and sodium only in moderation
	7. Drink alcohol in moderation (if you drink)	7. If you drink alcholic beverages, do so in moderation

*Data from Food and Nutrition Board, National Research Council: Toward Healthful Diets. Washington, D.C., National Academy of Sciences, 1980.
†Data from United States Department of Agriculture: Dietary Guidelines for Americans. Home and Garden Bulletin No. 232. Hyattsville, MD, Human Nutrition Information Service, United States Department of Agriculture, 1980.
‡Data from United States Department of Agriculture: Nutrition and Your Health; Dietary Guidelines for Americans. 3rd Ed. Home and Garden Bulletin No. 232. Hyattsville, MD, Human Nutrition Information Service, United States Department of Agriculture, 1980.

DEVELOPMENT OF DIETARY GUIDELINES ELSEWHERE

In Canada, the Committee on Diet and Cardiovascular Disease of Health and Welfare Canada published in 1976 a report on nutrition and health that looked beyond the committee's title.[43,56] The dietary guidelines for the general public were as follows: (1) consume a nutritionally adequate diet (i.e., four food groups); (2) avoid overweight; (3) limit amount of total fat (to 30 to 35% of calories), cholesterol (to <400 mg per day), sugar, alcohol, and salt in the diet; and (4) reduce the total amount of saturated fat in the diet and replace some of this with polyunsaturated fats. These were published 3 months before *Dietary Goals for the United States*, but do not appear to have influenced the latter.

In Quebec a different set of objectives was included in a book on that Canadian province's nutrition policy.[57] They are as follows: (1) three well-balanced meals each day should cover 80% of calorie requirements (only 20% from snacks); (2) reduce sugar (sucrose) intake by 50%; (3) reduce fat consumption by 25%; (4) increase breastfeeding; (5) increase cellulose intake (i.e., fruits, vegetables, and cereals); (6) preserve the nutritive value of foods (by good food preparation); and (7) vary the diet.

After this came a succession of sets of national dietary guidelines (Table 93–5).[5] Most of the earlier committees knew of *Dietary Goals for the United States,* even if they chose to develop their own guidelines by independent reasoning. In Britain, *Dietary Goals for the United States* was quoted in publications in 1977,[50,58] and in Australia it was discussed in nutrition circles in 1978. In the later 1980s, *Dietary Goals* had been superseded in the United States; by then national nutrition authorities knew that other countries had their own dietary guidelines and realized that a set in their own country would be useful for nutrition education and policy.

TABLE 93–5. FIRST APPEARANCE OF NATIONAL DIETARY GUIDELINES OUTSIDE THE UNITED STATES

Canada, 1976[43*]
Quebec, 1977[57]
Australia, 1979[18*]
France, 1981[59]
Sweden, 1981[60*]
Norway, 1981[61*]
New Zealand, 1982[62*]
Denmark, 1983[63]
UK—NACNE, 1983[64*]
UK—COMA, 1984[65]
Eire, 1984[66]
Netherlands, 1984–1985[67]
Federal Republic of Germany, 1985[68]
Japan, 1984[69]
Korea, 1987[70]
Finland, 1987[71]
Hungary, 1988[72]
India, 1988–1989[73]
Singapore, 1989[74]

*Now replaced by more recent guidelines.

A SELECTION OF NATIONAL DIETARY GUIDELINES IN INDUSTRIAL COUNTRIES

There is only space to record the headings and add a few brief notes.

AUSTRALIA (1979, REVISED 1992)

The first set of dietary guidelines was published in 1979.[19] They were well accepted by nutritionists, health authorities, and the food industry. In the (following) revised set of guidelines (1992), the elements have been reordered and reworded with more emphasis on a low-fat diet, and two guidelines on specific nutrients have been added:[91] (1) Enjoy a wide variety of nutritious foods. (2) eat plenty of breads and cereals (preferably whole-grain), vegetables (including legumes), and fruits; (3) eat a diet low in fat and, in particular, low in saturated fat; (4) maintain a healthy body weight by balancing food intake and regular physical activity; (5) if you drink alcohol, limit your intake; (6) eat only a moderate amount of sugars and foods containing added sugars; (7) use salt sparingly and choose foods with little added salt; (8) encourage and support breast-feeding; (9) eat foods containing calcium; this is particularly important for girls and women; and (10) Eat foods containing iron; this is particularly important for girls, women, vegetarians, and athletes.

FRANCE (1981)[59]

Recommendations are to: (1) adapt alimentary consumption to needs; (2) eat three good meals each day; (3) consume a varied and diversified diet; (4) with regard to drinks, soft drinks contain sugar, that is, energy; alcohol abuse can cause diseases; (5) with regard to lipids, everyone should reduce intake, especially of foods rich in saturated fatty acids; (6) with regard to proteins, vegetable proteins should be used more; (7) sugar consumption has not increased since 1973; we must avoid a new increase; (8) for sufficient fiber take wholemeal breads, vegetables, cereals, (dry) legumes, and dried fruits; and (9) it is sensible to add less salt in food preparation or while eating.

These guidelines come towards the back of the French book on recommended nutrient intakes.[59]

NEW ZEALAND (1982 AND 1991)

The first (1982) set of dietary guidelines[62] was revised by the Nutrition Taskforce for the New Zealand Department of Health and was published in 1991.[92] They are: (1) eat a variety of foods from each of the four major food groups each day; (2) prepare meals with minimal added fat (especially saturated fat), salt, and sugar; (3) choose preprepared foods, drinks, and snacks that are low in fat (especially saturated fat), salt, and sugar; (4) maintain a healthy body weight by regular physical activity and by healthy eating; (5) drink plenty of liquids each day; and (6) if drinking alcohol, do so in moderation.

In the major report, for professionals, quantitative targets are suggested.[92] For example, by the year 2000, total fat should be 30 to 33% of energy, saturated fatty acids (including *trans*) should be not more than 12%, polyunsaturated fatty acids should be in the range of 6 to 10% of energy, with monounsaturated fatty acids making up the rest of the fat. For carbohydrates the targets are: total carbohydrate, 50 to 55% of energy; dietary fiber, 25 to 30 g per day (of which one quarter should be soluble fibre); and sucrose and other free sugars, no more than 15% of energy. Targets are set for obesity, alcohol, and all the major nutrients. Fluoridation of water supplies is generally recommended.

DENMARK (1983)[63]

Recommendations are to: (1) *eat lean;* save on sugar; eat coarse food; eat a variety of foods; do not eat too much; (2) *eat more* bread and corn products, potatoes, vegetables, and fruit; (3) *eat less* butter, margarine, fat, sugar, meat fat and fewer fatty meat products and full-cream dairy products.

UNITED KINGDOM

Official recommendations for the United Kingdom for prevention of coronary heart disease are in the 1984 report of the Committee on Medical Aspects of Food Policy (COMA).[65] These have been generally accepted,[76] and they are as follows: (1) eat less total fat; 35% food energy recommended; (2) eat less saturated fatty acids; 15% of food energy recommended, including *trans*-fatty acids (which provide about 1.5% of energy); (3) polyunsaturated fatty acids may be increased from 5 to 7% of energy (P/S ratio up to 0.45); (4) "there are no specific recommendations about the dietary intake of cholesterol;" (5) "intake of simple sugars (sucrose, glucose, and fructose) should not be increased further;" (6) "an excessive intake of alcohol is to be avoided;" (7) consider ways and means of decreasing salt intake; (8) increase fiber-rich carbohydrate foods; and (9) avoid or treat obesity.

The other British recommendations by NACNE (1983)[64] are not official and have been controversial.[77–79] They are difficult to summarize because the moderate early changes were for the 1980s. The long-term proposals include targets of 30% energy from total fat, 10% from saturated fat, and 4% from alcohol. Sucrose intake should be halved; the target for salt is not clear. Fiber intakes should rise to 30 g per day.

In 1991, the revised recommended intakes of essential nutrients for the United Kingdom were published in a completely rewritten report in which new terms were introduced and recommendations for fat and carbohydrate intake included.[93] For essential nutrients, the new term corresponding to RDA in the United States is Reference Nutrient Intake. For fats and carbohydrates, the "dietary reference values" (average contribution to energy intake for groups of people) are as follows: total fat, 33% energy; saturated fatty acids, 10%; monounsaturated fatty acids, 12%; polyunsaturated fatty acids, 6% (not more than 10% for individuals); *trans* fatty acids, 2%. Available carbohydrates are presented in two groups: (1) starches plus intrinsic sugars and lactose in milk and milk products—dietary reference value, 37%; and (2) "non-milk extrinsic sugars" (mainly sucrose)—dietary reference value, 10%. The dietary reference value for nonstarch polysaccharides (i.e., dietary fiber except lignin) is 18 g/day for adults. All these figures assume an average alcohol intake of 5% and protein intake of 15%. If these are substantially less, the average intakes of fats and carbohydrate should be a little higher.

FEDERAL REPUBLIC OF GERMANY

In Ten Guidelines for Sensible Nutrition (1985),[68] recommendations are to: (1) use variety in the choice of foods; (2) eat not too much and not too little; (3) eat small meals more often; (4) eat sufficient protein; (5) avoid too much fat; (6) eat sweets seldom; (7) eat fresh food (fruits, juices, vegetables, milk) and whole-grain products daily; (8) prepare foods properly; (9) use salt sparingly; and (10) use restraint with alcohol.

JAPAN (1985)[69]

Recommendations are as follows: (1) obtain well-balanced nutrition with a variety of foods; eat 30 foodstuffs a day; take staple food, main dish, and side dish together; (2) take energy corresponding to daily activity; (3) consider the amount and the quality of the fats and oils you eat: avoid too much; eat more vegetable oils than animal fat; (4) avoid too much salt, not more than 10 g a day; and (5) happy eating makes for happy family life; sit down and eat together and talk; treasure family taste and home cooking.

NETHERLANDS 1985[67]

Recommendations are: (1) achieve or maintain a normal bodyweight; (2) balance the diet; supply adequate amounts of all essential nutrients; (3) ensure an average total fat intake of 30 to 35% of dietary energy; (4) make sure that saturated fat consumption is around 10% of total energy and polyunsaturated fat is 50 to 100% of saturated fat; (5) do not let dietary cholesterol exceed 33 mg/MJ; (6) maintain carbohydrate (total) consumption at 50 to 60% of energy; (total) sugars, 15 to 25 en%; (7) maintain protein consumption at 10 to 15% of energy (as at present); (8) eat dietary fiber, target 3 g/MJ; (9) realize that current alcohol consumption is far too high in many cases; and (10) eat no more than 8 g salt (NaCl) per day.

There is also advice for special groups (e.g., about vitamin D and fluoride for children).

KOREA (1986)[70]

These recommendations are: (1) eat a variety of foods; (2) keep ideal body weight; (3) consume enough protein; (4) keep fat consumption at 20% of energy intake; (5) drink milk every day; (6) reduce salt intake; (7) keep in good dental health; (8) moderate alcohol and caffeine consumption; (9) keep harmony between diet and daily life; and (10) enjoy meals. (Those in Western countries who think a target of 30% energy from total fat too stringent should ponder the fourth Korean recommendation.)

HUNGARY (1988)[72]

Recommendations are to: (1) eat a variety of foods; (2) avoid too much fat; use vegetable oil and margarine; (3) avoid too much salt; (4) reduce sugary snacks; (5) drink half a liter of low-fat milk per day; (6) eat fresh fruits, vegetables, and salads more often; (7) always have whole-grain bread on the table; choose potatoes over rice; (8) eat four or five meals daily, none too rich or too light; (9) quench thirst with water; it's best to avoid alcohol, and alcohol is forbidden for children and pregnant women; and (10) good nutrition means a balanced diet—in other words, no food is prohibited, but some are to be preferred and others to be eaten less frequently.

SINGAPORE (1989)[74]

Recommendations are to: (1) eat a variety of foods; (2) maintain desirable body weight; (3) restrict total fat intake to 20 to 30% of total energy intake; (4) modify composition of fat in the diet to one third polyunsaturated, one third monounsaturated, and one third saturated; (5) reduce cholesterol intake to less than 300 mg per day; (6) maintain intakes of complex carbohydrates at about 50% of total energy intake; (7) reduce salt intake to less than 4.5 g a day (1800 mg Na); (8) reduce intake of salt-cured, preserved, and smoked foods; (9) reduce intake of refined and processed sugar to less than 10% of energy; (10) increase intake of fruit and vegetables and whole-grain cereal products, thereby increasing vitamins A and C and fiber; (11) for those who drink, have not more than 2 to 3 standard drinks (about 40 g alcohol) per day; and (12) encourage breast-feeding in infants until at least 6 months of age.

NORDIC NUTRITION RECOMMENDATIONS (1989)[80]

These are the first set of guidelines agreed on for the countries of a region (Denmark, Finland, Norway, and Sweden). The report contains RDI as well as guidelines. For adults and children over 3 years of age: (1) protein ought to provide 10 to 15% of the total energy intake; (2) fat should not provide more than 30% of the total energy intake; the decrease from most people's present intake should be primarily by reducing saturated fat, which will generally be accompanied by a desirable decrease in dietary cholesterol; total fat should not, however, be below 20 to 25% energy; essential fatty acids should contribute 3 to 10% (at least 4.5% for pregnancy and 6% for lactation); both linoleic (ω-6) and linolenic (ω-3) acids are essential, but the requirement of the former is greater; Linolenic and long-chain ω-3 acids should provide at least 0.5% energy; (3) carbohydrates should provide 55 to 60% of energy; sugar should not provide more than 10% of energy (i.e., refined, not naturally occurring); the intake of dietary fiber should be at least 3 g/MJ (12.5 g/1000 kcal), which for adults comes to 25 to 30 g per day; (4) it is desirable that the sodium intake should gradually decrease to a level corresponding to 5 g NaCl per day; and (5) the consumption of alcohol should be avoided or be moderate; during pregnancy, alcohol should be avoided entirely.

CANADA (1990)[81]

The Canadian diet should: (1) provide energy consistent with maintenance of body weight within the recommended range; (2) include essential nutrients in amounts recommended; (3) include no more than 30% of energy as fat and no more than 10% as saturated fat; (4) provide 55% of energy as carbohydrate from a variety of sources; (5) contain reduced sodium; (6) include no more than 5% of total energy as alcohol, or two drinks daily, whichever is less; (7) contain no more caffeine than the equivalent of four regular cups of coffee per day; and (8) ensure fluoridation of community water supplies containing less than 1 mg/L fluorine to that level.

GUIDELINES FOR LOW-INCOME COUNTRIES

Dietary guidelines were originally introduced to meet the nutritional problems of affluent communities. Until the end of the 1980s, there were no (published) proposals to apply them in developing countries, where the biggest nutritional problem is that many people cannot afford or cannot grow the food they need. However, in these developing countries, the following facts must be kept in mind: (1) coronary heart disease and cancers are increasing their share of mortality as infections come under control;[82] now is a good time to try and prevent the consequences of further increase of fat intake; (2) the affluent middle class in a country such as India may only be 5% of the population, but it comprises 40 million individuals who play a major part in the development of the country;[83] (3) developing countries had a bad experience when they followed industrial countries, as in the case of abandoning breast-feeding; (4) low-income countries cannot afford to add the burden of medical care of degenerative diseases to their health budgets. Dietary guidelines are a low-cost measure. If they have official status, such guidelines can be written into nutrition material adopted by multinational companies for their staff and by voluntary and international agencies, as well as by national health workers. Two conditions that make formulation of dietary guidelines especially challenging in low-income countries are the scarcity of food composition data—food analysis is expensive—and the wide range of nutritional status, from undernutrition among the poor to overnutrition in the affluent.

For India, Gopalan proposed two sets of guidelines.[83] For the relatively poor, diets should be least expensive and conform to tradition and cultural practices as far as possible. Some pulses (legumes) should be eaten along with the high-cereal diet, and at least 150 ml of milk per day and 150 g of leafy vegetables per day. Energy from fat and oil need not exceed 15%, and that from sugar need not exceed 5% of total calories.

For affluent Indians,[73,83] he proposed restriction of energy intake to levels commensurate with sedentary occupations; giving preference to undermilled cereals; inclusion of green leafy vegetables in the diet; restriction of edible fat to 20% of total energy and of ghee (clarified butter) to special occasions; restriction of intake of sugar and sweets; and avoidance of high salt intake, especially by those prone to hypertension.

For Latin America, Scrimshaw and Bengoa proposed an alternative model, dietary goals that can apply to all, rich and poor, "metas nutricionales."[84] These general goals then have to be converted into focused guidelines for different segments of the population. Energy and protein requirements are derived from the FAO/WHO/UNU report.[85] Fat should be 20 to 25% of dietary energy; the ratio of fatty acids should be as follows: saturated to monounsaturated to polyunsaturated = 1:1:1. ω-3 fatty acids should be 10% of total polyunsaturated fat. Carbohydrates should provide 60 to 70% of total energy, with the emphasis on less-refined cereals and products. Sugar contributes to dental caries, but it has a role in increasing the caloric density of diets, particularly for young children. Most adults in Latin America can only take moderate amounts of milk because of lactase insufficiency. Fiber only needs to be encouraged for the more affluent (the recommendation is 8 to 10 g per 1000 kcal). Attention to biologic interactions among nutrients can enhance availability of limited micronutrients. Salt intake should be less than 10 g per day. There are separate recommendations for different age groups, including of course breast-feeding for infants and adequate calcium for adolescents and pregnant women.

With goals like these, some people need to be helped to eat, for example, more fat, whereas other sections of society need to bring their fat intake down to 20 to 25% energy, which Scrimshaw and Bengoa think is the optimal range for health. Such dietary goals might eventually be developed, after wide consultation, into International Dietary Goals. Such a set was put forward at the Toronto conference.[86] A WHO study group has also proposed population nutrient goals for the whole world,[86a] expressed as ranges, including total fat between 15% of energy (lower limit) and 30% of energy (interim goal); saturated fatty acids between 0% (lower limit) and 10% (upper limit); polyunsaturated fatty acids 3 to 7% of energy; total protein 10 to 15% of energy; total carbohydrate 55 to 75% of energy; "complex" carbohydrates 50 to 70% of energy; dietary fiber (expressed as nonstarch polysaccharides) 16 to 24 g per day; fruits and vegetables (lower limit) 400 g per day; salt 0 to 6 g per day.

CURRENT GUIDELINES FOR THE UNITED STATES

Dietary Guidelines for Americans of the USDA and USDHHS is now in its third revised edition (Table 93–4).[87] Work continues to distribute and help implement these guidelines, which will be updated every 5 to 10 years.[55]

Guidelines to Prevent Cancer were developed by an NRC committee to reduce dietary factors that appear to contribute to development of cancers; these recommendations were published initially in a large review in 1982[88] and updated in 1989. Summarized briefly, they are as follows:

1. Reduce fat (unsaturated as well as saturated) to 30% total energy or less.
2. Frequently consume fruits (e.g., citrus) and vegetables (especially carotene-rich and cruciferous).
3. Reduce consumption of salt-cured and smoked foods.
4. Continue efforts to minimize contamination of foods with carcinogens from any source.
5. Further efforts to identify mutagens in foods, test them for carcinogenicity, and minimize their concentration.
6. Consume alcohol in moderation, if at all.

The Surgeon General's Report on Nutrition and Health is a large review of 727 pages that has 90 contributors and 171 reviewers.[14] There are five recommendations *for most people:*

1. Reduce consumption of fat (especially saturated) and cholesterol.
2. Adjust energy for weight control.
3. Increase consumption of whole-grain cereal foods, vegetables, and fruits.
4. Reduce intake of sodium.
5. Take alcohol in moderation (no more than two drinks per day), if at all.

There are another four recommendations *for some people:*

1. Community water systems should be fluoridated.
2. Children should limit consumption and frequency of use of foods high in sugars.
3. Adolescent girls and adult women should increase consumption of foods high in calcium.
4. Children, adolescents, and women of childbearing age should be sure to eat foods that are good sources of iron.

The National Research Council's *Diet and Health* review is a substantial, large-format book of 749 pages written by a committee of 33.[16] Contributions or advice from 93 persons are acknowledged. Its recommendations are as follows:

1. Reduce total fat intakes to 30% of calories or less. Reduce saturated fatty acid intake to less than 10% of calories and dietary cholesterol to less than 300 mg daily. Polyunsaturated fatty acid intake should stay about the present 7% of calories (and not be above 10% of calories in individuals). Concentrated fish oils are not recommended (for the general public.)
2. Eat five or more servings of vegetables and fruits each day (especially green and yellow vegetables and citrus fruits). Also increase intake of starches and complex carbohydrates as breads, cereals, and legumes. Increase of added sugars is not recommended.
3. Maintain protein intake at moderate levels, that is, at less than twice the RDA.
4. Balance food intake and physical activity to maintain appropriate body weight. All healthy people should maintain physical activity at a moderate level.
5. The Committee does not recommend alcohol consumption. For those who do drink, limit consumption to two standard drinks a day. Pregnant women and women attempting to conceive should avoid alcoholic beverages.
6. Limit total daily salt intake to 6 g NaCl or less.
7. Maintain adequate calcium intake, but the potential benefits of calcium above the RDA are not well documented.
8. Avoid taking dietary supplements in excess of the RDA.
9. Maintain an optium intake of fluoride, particularly during the years of primary and secondary tooth formation and growth—that is, consume fluoridated water or (if not available) fluoride tablets.

The United States is a large and democratic country and has by far the largest investment in nutrition research in the world. It is not surprising that there have been more than one set of authoritative dietary guidelines in the country since 1980. Other important sets are not reviewed here, such as those of the American Heart Association and the American Dietitians Association for women. There is close agreement now among the different sets of recommendations, and no serious conflict between them.

WHERE DIFFERENT SETS OF GUIDELINES (AMERICAN AND WORLDWIDE) AGREE AND WHERE THEY DISAGREE

There is almost complete agreement on the following six recommendations:

1. Eat a nutritionally adequate diet composed of a variety of foods.
2. Eat less fat, particularly saturated fat.
3. Adjust energy intake for weight control; exercise.

4. Eat more foods containing complex carbohydrates and fiber.
5. Reduce salt intake.
6. Drink alcohol in moderation, if at all.

The Japanese recommendations suggest 30 different foods a day to give a numeric expression to the concept of variety.[69] A more usual way to explain variety is to advise consumers to eat foods from each of four (or more) nutritional groups each day and to make regular changes of foods within each group. The target for total fat is sometimes not quantitative.[19,62,68,69] If it is stated it ranges between 35[65] and 20%[70] of total energy. The recommendation to increase complex carbohydrates and fiber is stated in different ways and is less likely to be expressed quantitatively.

The recommendation to reduce salt is often not expressed quantitatively, but when it is the target ranges between 4.5[74] and 10 g NaCl[69] (75 to 166 mmol Na) per day. The NRC limit is 6 g salt per day,[16] and in Australia the upper limit of RDI of 2.3 g (100 mmol) sodium corresponds to this.

Where the quantity of alcohol is stated (for those who are not pregnant), it is two drinks per day.

A *second group* of recommendations is more controversial; these give advice about polyunsaturated fats, dietary cholesterol, and sugar. Where polyunsaturated fats are mentioned, the usual upper limit is 10% of energy,[16,67,74,80] but guidelines more often concentrate only on reduction of saturated fat.

Some guidelines in the United States, the Netherlands, and Singapore recommend reduction of dietary cholesterol (to less than 300 mg per day[74,87] or a similar amount expressed per MJ[67]), but most committees do not mention dietary cholesterol in their headings, and U.K. guidelines spell out that they are not making specific recommendations about cholesterol intake.[65]

On sugar(s) (other than naturally occurring sugars), there appears to be the largest difference of opinion. Canada recommends 55% of energy from a variety of sources and does not mention sugar.[81] Japan[69] and Korea[70] do not mention sugar. At the other extreme the recommendations of the Nordic countries[80] and of Singapore[74] advise the restriction of refined sugar to less than 10% of energy. In between are several different opinions: "Do not increase sugar consumption,"[16,59,65] "Decrease" (not quantified),[62,63] "Eat only a moderate amount of sugars and sugary foods,"[87,91] "Intake less than 15% of energy,"[92] and "Cut down sugary snacks and sweets between meals."[68,72]

A *third group* of recommendations appears only in a small number of guideline sets: Do not eat too much protein,[16,62] preserve (by good preparation) the nutritive value of foods,[57,68] eat three good meals a day,[57,59] drink fluoridated water (or fluoride tablets),[14,16,62,81] make sure you get enough calcium (or milk),[14,16,70,72] reduce intake of salt-cured and smoked foods,[74] limit caffeine intake,[81] and eat happily for happy family life.[69]

BRIEF CRITIQUE

The original hypotheses underlying dietary guidelines were mentioned in describing their history. After 15 years of evolution, how well are current guidelines justified by scientific knowledge? The 6 guidelines on which there is general agreement have clearly been reasoned by large numbers of experienced scientists independently in about 20 different countries, and examined at greater length than is possible in this chapter. The evidence they used is, of course, also discussed in different places in this textbook. The following brief notes are intended to help link the 6 major guidelines with these scientific bases.

1. *Eat a Nutritionally Adequate Diet from a Variety of Foods.* A nutritionally adequate diet means eating all (or nearly all) the recommended nutrient intakes (RDA) of those nutrients for which there is an RDA. A varied diet, if built around the food groups of nutrition education, is a fundamental principle of nutrition, older than dietary guidelines. It maximizes the probability of eating all the RDA as well as minor nutrients that do not have an RDA. At the same time variety minimizes the risk of toxins and pathogens from food and drink.

2. *Eat Less Fat, Particularly Saturated Fat.* Fats in food provide more calories than any other food component, and much of it is hidden in tempting dishes and products. To reduce fat is the most important way of reducing excess energy intake. Many fatty ingredients in foods contain few other nutrients. If they are replaced by lean meat, low-fat milk, and vegetables, the intake of essential nutrients will be improved. Saturated fat raises plasma total and LDL (low-density lipoprotein) cholesterol. The importance of limiting these is explained in Chapters 72 and 87.

3. *Adjust Energy (Calorie) Intake to Expenditure and Avoid Overweight and Underweight.* "Don't eat too much or too little" is the fundamental quantitative principle of nutrition; it long antedates dietary guidelines. Mortality and morbidity are increased in people who are too thin (see Chaps. 56 and 57) or too fat (see Chap. 59).

4. *Eat More Foods Containing Complex Carbohydrates and Fiber.* Both terms are imprecise. "Complex carbohydrates" is used here to mean starchy foods and naturally occurring sugars, and some sets head this recommendation: eat more cereals, vegetables (including legumes), and fruits, that is, the foods containing these carbohydrates and fiber. From the preceding guidelines these should be eaten in variety and without added fat. They should also be eaten as whole foods because they are intended not only to replace fat-rich foods but also to provide generous intakes of such nutrients as carotenes, vitamin C, and fiber. These last three components are all under investigation as possible protective factors against certain types of cancer (see Chap. 88). In the meantime it can do no harm to eat more of them.

5. *Reduce Salt Intake.* The idea behind this is to try and reduce the prevalence of essential hypertension and (a harder epidemiologic index) mortality from cerebral hemorrhage. The evidence is not as strong (see Chap. 71) as that for saturated fat and plasma cholesterol. But a taste for salty food is an acquired one. Most societies consume several times more sodium than is needed. No harm, and possibly some benefit, could result from intakes of 50 to 100 mmol sodium per day (3 to 6 g NaCl).

6. *Drink Alcohol in Moderation, if at All.* Alcoholic drinks in excess cause road accidents, raised blood pressure, cirrhosis of the liver, and other complications (see Chap. 64), depending on the pattern of excess drinking.

GUIDELINES FOR GUIDELINES

1. *Dietary guidelines must be seen to be based on an objective review of the best available evidence.* Any individual organization or company can concoct their own dietary guidelines, but confusion and conflict can only be avoided if the process is fair, objective, and authoritative. Production of the Nordic guidelines included an open session for interested scientists.[80] Development of the Canadian guidelines was preceded by an international conference.[75,82–84,86] The Surgeon General's report[14] and the NRC recommendations[16] in the United States are both excellent models of guideline development. There was input by many scientists into both, and the evidence is well presented in thorough, well-referenced reviews.

2. *It may be helpful to differentiate dietary goals, explained at some length in scientific and quantitative language, from dietary guidelines written in a pamphlet in simple language for consumers.*

3. *More care is needed with the meaning and understanding of words* like "limit," "avoid too much," "restrict," "use in moderation," "reduce," "eat less." "Eat less fat," advice for the whole population, assumes that the experts know that everyone in the country is eating more than is good for them. Although this may be so for a great majority, it cannot apply to all. Some committees have recently expressed the primary scientific recommendation directly, without reference to the present diet; for example, "Include no more than 30% of energy as fat"[81] or "Choose a diet low in fat, saturated fat, and cholesterol."[87]

4. *It may be helpful to differentiate guidelines for the majority,* (e.g., reduce saturated fat) *from those for special or at risk groups,* (e.g., for infants and for those at increased risk of heart disease).

5. *A structure is needed in which dietary guidelines can be regularly reconsidered and updated.* Guidelines are provisional and should not be treated as if engraved on tablets of stone. The United States, Canada, the Nordic countries, Australia and New Zealand have each revised their original sets.

6. *Dietary guidelines can't apply equally to everyone in the population.* Even within the same sex, age, and occupational subgroup there are genetic variations in susceptibility to different dietary components.[90]

7. *Difficulties and quarrels come when people translate dietary guidelines into judgments about individual foods.* Items within a food category, group, or subgroup can vary greatly in composition. "No food is prohibited but some are to be preferred and others less frequent."[72]

8. *Finally, we ought to find out how many consumers know about a country's guidelines,* what they think they mean, and to what extent they are changing their food habits.

REFERENCES

1. Dubois, R.: The intellectual basis of nutritional science and practice. *In* Critical Food Issues of the Eighties. Edited by M. Chou and D.P. Harman. New York, Pergamon, 1979, pp. 95–102.
2. McLaren, D.S.: Lancet, *2:*93–95, 1974.
3. Department of Health and Social Security: Diet and Coronary Heart Disease. Report of the Advisory Panel of the Committee on Medical Aspects of Food Policy (Nutrition). Report on Health and Social Subjects 7. London, H.M. Stationery Office, 1974.
4. Yudkin, J.: Lancet, *2:*4–8, 1964.
5. Keys, A.: Atherosclerosis, *14:*193–202, 1971.
6. Burkitt, D.P., Walker, A.R., Painter, N.S.: Lancet, *2:*1408–1412, 1972.
7. Brody, J.: Carbohydrates have gotten a bad press. *In* Jane Brody's Nutrition Book. Edited by J. Brody. New York, Bantam Books, 1981, pp. 94–118.
8. Atkins, R.C.: Dr. Atkins Diet Revolution. Toronto, New York, London, Bantam Books, 1973.
9. Norum, K.R.: Nutrition and Metabolism, *22:*1–7, 1978.
10. Truswell, A.S.: [Appendix to article.] Proc. Nutrition Soc., *36:*314–315, 1977.
11. Symposium. The evidence relating six dietary factors to the nation's health: Consensus statements. Am. J. Clin. Nutrition, *32:*2627–2748, 1979.
12. Commonwealth Department of Health: Towards Better Nutrition for Australians. Report of Nutrition Taskforce of the Better Health Commission. Canberra, Australian Government Publishing Service, 1987.
13. James, W.P.T., Ferro-Luzzi, A., Isaksson, B. et al.: Healthy Nutrition. Preventing nutrition-related diseases in Europe. Copenhagen, WHO Regional Office for Europe, 1988.
14. The Surgeon General's Report on Nutrition and Health. United States Department of Health and Human Services

Publication PHS 88-50210. Washington, D.C., United States Government Printing Office, 1988.
15. Select Committee on Nutrition and Human Needs, United States Senate: Dietary Goals for the United States. 2nd Ed. Washington, D.C., United States Government Printing Office, December, 1977.
16. Committee on Diet and Health, Food and Nutrition Board, National Research Council: Diet and Health: Implications for Reducing Chronic Disease Risk. Washington, D.C., National Academy Press, 1989.
17. United States Department of Agriculture and United States Department of Health & Human Services: Dietary Guidelines for Americans. Home and Garden Bulletin No. 232. Hyattsville, MD, Human Nutrition Information Service, United States Department of Agriculture, 1980.
18. Langsford, W.A.: Food and Nutrition Notes and Reviews (Australian Commonwealth Department of Health), *36:*100–103, 1979.
19. Commonwealth Department of Health: Dietary Guidelines for Australians. Canberra, Australian Government Publishing Service, 1982.
20. Helsing, E.: Nutrition targets in the EEC. *In* Important Components for a Food and Nutrition Policy in the EEC (Corfu, Greece, 6–8 October, 1988). Report of a Workshop. Athens, Department of Nutrition & Biochemistry, 1989, p. 15.
21. Mediciniska synpunkter på folkkosten i de Nordiska länderna. Vår föda, *20:*3–5, 1968.
22. Mediciniska synpunkter på folkkosten i de Nordiska länderna. Lakartidningen, *65:*2012–2013, 1968.
23. Keys, A.: Nutr. Rev., *26:*259–263, 1968.
24. Davidson, S., Passmore, J.F., Brock, J.F.: Human Nutrition & Dietetics. 5th Ed. Edinburgh & London, Churchill Livingstone, 1972, p. 329.
25. Blix, G., Wretlind, A., Bergström, S., et al.: Vår Föda, *17:*7, 1965.
26. Wretlind, A.: Nutrition problems in healthy adults with low activity and low caloric consumption. *In* Nutrition and Physical Activity. Edited by G. Blix. Symposia of the Swedish Nutrition Foundation No. 5. 1967, pp. 114–130.
27. Blix, G., Isaksson, B., Wretlind, A.: Bibl. Nutr. Diet., *19:*154–165, 1973.
28. Norum, K.R.: Tidsskift for den Norske laegerforening, *7:*363–364, 1977 and (in English) Nutr. Metab., *22:*1–7, 1978.
29. Keys, A.: Voeding, *13:*535–556, 1952.
30. Keys, A.: JAMA, *164:*1912–1919, 1957.
31. Central Committee for Medical and Community Program of the American Heart Association: Circulation, *23:*133, 1961.
32. Grundy, S.M., Bilheimer, C., Blackburn, H., et al.: Circulation, *65:*839A–854A, 1982.
33. Inter-Society Commission for Heart Disease Resources: Circulation, *42:*55A–95A, 1970.
34. Joint Statement of the AMA Council on Foods & Nutrition and the Food & Nutrition Board of the National Academy of Sciences-National Research Council: JAMA, *222:*1647, 1972.
35. American Health Foundation: Prevent. Med., *1:*255–286, 1972.
36. National Heart Foundation of Australia: Med. J. Aust., *1:*1155–1160, 1971.
37. Royal Society of New Zealand: Coronary Heart Disease. Wellington, New Zealand, Royal Society, 1971.
38. Report to the National Heart Foundation of New Zealand: Coronary Heart Disease. A New Zealand report. Dunedin, John McIndoe, 1971.
39. Voedingsraad: Advies over hoeveelheid en/of aard der vetten in de voeding. Volksgesondheid 25, Ministerie van Volksgezondheid en Milieuhygiene. s'Gravenhage, Staatsuitgeverij, 1973.
40. Council on Rehabilitation, International Society of Cardiology: Myocardial Infarction: How to Prevent, How to Rehabilitate. Mannheim, Boehringer, 1973.
41. Joint Working Party of the Royal College of Physicians of London and the British Cardiac Society. J. R. Coll. Physicians Lond., *10:*213–275, 1976.
42. Editorial: Nutr. Metab., *18:*113–115, 1975.
43. Health and Welfare Canada: Report of the Committee on Diet and Cardiovascular Disease. Ottawa, Department of National Health and Welfare, 1976.
44. Burkitt, D.P.: Nutr. Today, January/February, 1976.
45. Meneely, G.R., Batterbee, H.D.: Sodium and potassium. *In* Present Knowledge in Nutrition. 4th Ed. Washington, D.C., Nutrition Foundation, 1976, pp. 259–279.
46. Select Committee on Nutrition and Human Needs, United States Senate: Dietary Goals for the United States. Washington, D.C., United States Government Printing Office, February, 1977.
47. Select Committee on Nutrition and Human Needs, United States Senate: Dietary Goals for the United States: Supplemental Views. Washington, D.C., United States Government Printing Office, 1977.
48. Twenty Commentaries on the McGovern Dietary Goals: Nutr. Today, *November/December:* 10–13, 20–27, 1977.
49. Harper, A.E.: Am. J. Clin. Nutr., *31:*310–321, 1978.
50. Editorial: Lancet, *1:*887–888, 1977.
51. Food and Nutrition Board, National Research Council: Toward Healthful Diets. Washington, D.C., National Academy Press, 1980.
52. Connor, T.P., Campbell, T.C.: Dietary guidelines. *In* Dietary Fat and Cancer. Edited by C. Ip, D.F. Birt, A.E. Rogers, et al. New York, A.R. Liss, 1986, pp. 731–771.
53. Hearings before the Subcommittee on Domestic Marketing, Consumer Relations, and Nutrition of the Committee on Agriculture, House of Representatives, 90th Congress. National Academy of Sciences Report on Healthful Diets. Washington, D.C., United States Government Printing Office, 1980.
54. Senate Hearings before the Committee on Appropriations, 96th Congress: Dietary Guidelines for Americans. Washington D.C., United States Government Printing Office, 1980.
55. Welsh, S., Davis, C., Cronin, F.: Background paper on the Dietary Guidelines for Americans. *In* Dietary Guidelines: Proceedings of an International Conference, Toronto, June 26–27, 1988. Edited by M.C. Latham and M.S. van Veen. Cornell International Nutrition Monograph Series, No. 21, 1989, pp. 158–184.
56. Murray, T.K., Rae, J.: Can. Med. Assoc. J., *120:*1241, 1979.
57. Ministère des Affaires sociales: Quebec's Policy on Nutrition. Quebec City, Ministère des Affaires sociales, May, 1977.
58. Truswell, A.S.: Proc. Nutr. Soc., *36:*307–316, 1977.
59. Dupin, H., et al.: Apports Nutritionnels Conseillés pour la population francaise. Paris, Technique et Documentation, 1981.
60. Swedish Food Regulations: Swedish Nutrition Recommendations. Uppsala, Swedish National Food Administration, 1981.
61. Royal Ministry of Health and Social Affairs: Report No. 11 to the Storting (1981–1982). On the Follow-Up of the Norwegian Nutrition Policy, Oslo.

62. Nutrition Advisory Committee: Nutrition goals for New Zealanders. Health (quarterly magazine of the New Zealand Department of Health), *34:*11–12, 1982.

63. Oplaeg om Ernaeringspolitik. Søborg, Miljøministeriet, 1983.

64. A discussion paper on proposals for nutritional guidelines for health education in Britain prepared by the National Advisory Committee on Nutrition Education (NACNE), Health Education Council, London, 1983.

65. Committee on Medical Aspects of Food Policy, Department of Health and Social Security: Diet and Cardiovascular Disease. Report of the Panel on Diet in Relation to Cardiovascular Disease. Report of Health and Social Subjects 28. London, Her Majesty's Stationery Office, 1984.

66. Department of Health (Ireland): Nutritional Guidelines. Dublin, Department of Health, 1984.

67. Guidelines for a Healthy Diet [In English]. Den Haag (The Hague), Netherlands Nutrition Council, 1985.

68. Deutsche Gesellschaft für Ernährung: Die IO Es der DGE. English translation of "Ten Guidelines for Sensible Nutrition." Frankfurt am Main, Deutsche Gesellschaft für Ernährung, 1985.

69. Ministry of Health and Welfare, Dietary guidelines for health promotion in Japan [English translation]. Tokyo, Ministry of Health & Welfare, 1985.

70. Korean Dietary Guideline: Seoul, Korean Nutrition Society, 1986.

71. Resumé of the Committee Report of the State Advisory Board on Nutrition (1987). Dietary Guidelines and Their Scientific Principles [English translation]. Helsinki, Government Printing Centre, 1989.

72. Complex Committee on Food Science of the Hungarian Academy of Sciences and of the Ministry of Food and Agriculture; National Institute of Food Hygiene: Dietary Guidelines for Hungarians. Budapest, Hungarian Society of Nutrition, 1988.

73. Gopalan, C.: Bull. Nutr. Found. India, *9* (3), 1988.

74. Guidelines for a Healthy Diet. Recommendations of the National Advisory Committee on Food Nutrition. Singapore, Training and Health Education Department, Ministry of Health, 1989.

75. Truswell, A.S.: Objectives and uses of dietary guidelines with emphasis on the Australian experience. *In* Dietary Guidelines: Proceedings of an International Conference, Toronto, June 26–27, 1988. Edited by M.C. Latham and M.S. van Veen. Cornell International Nutrition Monograph Series No. 21, 1989, pp. 69–87.

76. Truswell, A.S.: Br. Med. J., *289:*509–510, 1984.

77. Walker, C., Cannon, G.: The Food Scandal. London, Century Publishing, 1984.

78. Passmore, R.: J. R. Coll. Gen. Pract., *35:*387–389, 1985.

79. Anderson, D. (ed.): A Diet of Reason. London, The Social Affairs Unit, 1986.

80. Nordisk Ministerråd, Standing Nordic Committee on Food: Nordic Nutrition Recommendations, 2nd Ed. [English version]. Uppsala, National Food Administration, 1989.

81. Health and Welfare Canada: Nutrition Recommendations . . . A Call for Action. Summary report of the Scientific Review Committee and the Communications/Implementation Committee. Ottawa, Department of National Health and Welfare, 1990.

82. Solon, M.A.: Dietary guidelines for non-industrialized countries. *In* Dietary Guidelines: Proceedings of an International Conference, Toronto, June 26–27, 1988. Edited by M.C. Latham and M.S. van Veen. Cornell International Nutrition Monograph Series No. 21, 1989, pp. 45–68.

83. Gopalan, C.: Dietary guidelines from the perspective of developing countries. *In* Dietary Guidelines: Proceedings of an International Conference Toronto, Canada, June 26–27, 1988. Edited by M.C. Latham and M.S. van Veen. Cornell International Nutrition Monograph Series No. 21, 1989, pp. 88–111.

84. Scrimshaw, N.S., Bengoa, J.M.: Dietary goals and guidelines for health in Latin America. *In* Dietary Guidelines: Proceedings of an International Conference, Toronto, June 26–27, 1988. Edited by M.C. Latham and M.S. van Veen. Cornell International Nutrition Monograph Series No. 21, 1989, pp. 133–150.

85. Report of a Joint FAO/WHO/UNU Expert Consultation: Energy and Protein Requirements. WHO Technical Report Series 724. Geneva, World Health Organization, 1985.

86. Latham, M.C.: Afterword. *In* Dietary Guidelines: Proceedings of an International Conference, Toronto, June 26–27, 1988. Edited by M.C. Latham and M.S. van Veen. Cornell International Monograph Series No. 21, 1989, pp. 202–207.

86a. Report of a WHO Study Group: Diet, Nutrition and the Prevention of Chronic Diseases. Technical Report Series 797. Geneva, World Health Organization, 1990.

87. United States Department of Agriculture and United States Department of Health & Human Services: Nutrition and Your Health: Dietary Guidelines for Americans. 3rd Ed. Home and Garden Bulletin No. 232. Hyattsville, MD, Human Nutrition Information Service, United States Department of Agriculture, 1990.

88. Committee on Diet, Nutrition and Cancer, National Research Council: Diet, Nutrition and Cancer. Washington, D.C., National Academy Press, 1982.

89. Truswell, A.S.: Am. J. Clin. Nutr., *45:*1060–1072, 1987.

90. Velázquez, A., Bourges, H. (Eds.): Genetic Factors in Nutrition. Orlando, FL, Academic Press, 1984.

91. Commonwealth Department of Health: Dietary Guidelines for Australians. Revised Ed. Canberra, Australian Government Publishing Service, 1992.

92. Report of the Nutrition Taskforce: Food for Health. Wellington, New Zealand Department of Health, 1991.

93. Panel on Dietary Reference Values of the Committee on Medical Aspects of Food Policy, Department of Health: Dietary Reference Values for Food Energy and Nutrients for the United Kingdom. Report on Health and Social Subjects 41. London, Her Majesty's Stationery Office, 1991.

CHAPTER **94**

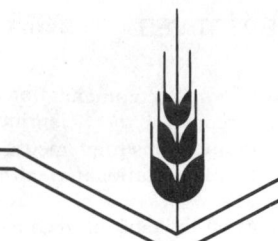

National Nutrition Policy, Food Labeling, and Health Claims

Allan L. Forbes

This textbook illustrates the complexity of nutrition science in today's world. Public policy aspects are equally complex. The truism "we are what we eat" still holds. The largest single industry in the world is the American food production system. We spend 16% of our expendable income on food. The Department of Defense (DOD) is the largest single purchaser of food in the world. No other segment of medical science is as diversified and far reaching as nutrition, because every soul practices it every day; because it is the union of a biomedical science with our national food supply and distribution system; because it is particularly dependent on industry; and because, understandably, a great many "players" are involved. This chapter focuses on two specific topics that are direct examples of public health nutrition policies, i.e., nutritional aspects of food labeling and health claims in food labeling. However, to put these topics into perspective, it is essential to understand who the key players are in establishing overall policies (Table 94–1), how the system works, and where the major benefits and deficits lie. This information should serve as a reference point as new issues, problems, and solutions arise in the future, which is inevitable as the science base continues to improve and our society evolves.

NATIONAL NUTRITION POLICY

The inception of nutrition policy occurred in World War I, with the need to sustain the Army in Europe and to assist in feeding large population segments in the devastated, post-war areas. During the years between World War I and the onset of World War II, nutrition policy per se languished, but enormous advances in nutrition science were made by the discovery of vitamins, essential minerals, and essential amino acids. World War II reawakened the concept of nutrition policy

TABLE 94–1. GLOSSARY OF ACRONYMS APPEARING IN THIS CHAPTER (ACRONYMS FOLLOWING THOSE UNDERLINED SHOW AFFILIATIONS)

AAP	American Academy of Pediatrics
ABMS	American Board of Medical Specialties
ABN	American Board of Nutrition
ACS	American Cancer Society
ACSH	American Council on Science and Health
ADA	American Dietetic Association
ADAMHA/DHHS	Alcohol, Drug Abuse, and Mental Health Administration
AHA	American Heart Association
AIN/FASEB	American Institute of Nutrition
AMA	American Medical Association
AMS/USDA	Agricultural Marketing Service
ANL/DA	Army Nutrition Laboratory
ARS/USDA	Agricultural Research Service
ASCN/AIN/FASEB	American Society for Clinical Nutrition
ASPEN	American Society for Parenteral and Enteral Nutrition
ASTPHO	Association of State and Territorial Public Health Officials
BRFSS/DON/CCDPHP/CDC	Behavioral Risk Factor Surveillance System
CCDPHP/CDC	Center for Chronic Disease Prevention and Health Promotion
CCFL/CODEX	Committee on Food Labeling
CCNFSDU/CODEX	Committee on Nutrition and Foods for Special Dietary Uses
CDC/USPHS/DHHS	Centers for Disease Control
CEHIC/CDC	Center for Environmental Health and Injury Control
CFN/AMA	Council on Foods and Nutrition
CFR	Code of Federal Regulations
CFSAN/FDA	Center for Food Safety and Applied Nutrition
CNI	Community Nutrition Institute
CNRU/NIH	Clinical Nutrition Research Units
CODEX/WHO and FAO	Joint FAO/WHO Codex Alimentarius Commission
CRIS/USDA	Current Research Information Service
CRN	Council for Responsible Nutrition
CSFII/USDA	Continuing Surveys of Food Intake by Individuals
CSPI	Center for Science in the Public Interest
CSRS/USDA	Cooperative State Research Service
DA/DOD	Department of the Army
DEHLS/CEHIC/CDC	Division of Environmental Health Laboratory Sciences
DHHS	Department of Health and Human Services
DNRC/NIH	Division of Nutrition Research Coordination
DOC	Department of Commerce
DOD	Department of Defense
DOE	Department of Education
DON/CDC	Division of Nutrition
DON/FDA	Division of Nutrition
DRR/NIH	Division of Research Resources
DRV/FDA	Daily Reference Values
EPA	Environmental Protection Agency
ERS/USDA	Economics Research Service
ES/USDA	Extension Service
ESADDI/FNB/IOM	Estimated Safe and Adequate Daily Dietary Intakes
FAO/UN	United Nations Food and Agricultural Organization
FASEB	Federation of American Societies for Experimental Biology
FDA/USPHS/DHHS	Food and Drug Administration
FDCA	Food, Drug, and Cosmetic Act
FDLI	Food and Drug Law Institute
FLAPS/FDA	Food Label and Package Survey

TABLE 94–1. GLOSSARY OF ACRONYMS APPEARING IN THIS CHAPTER (ACRONYMS FOLLOWING THOSE UNDERLINED SHOW AFFILIATIONS) *(continued)*

FMI	Food Marketing Institute
FNB/IOM/NAS	Food and Nutrition Board
FNIC/NAL/USDA	Food and Nutrition Information Center
FNS/USDA	Food and Nutrition Service
FR	Federal Register
FSIS/USDA	Food Safety and Inspection Service
FTC	Federal Trade Commission
GAO	Government Accounting Office, the Congress
GMA	Grocery Manufacturers of America
GRAS	"generally recognized as safe"
HHANES/NCHS/CDC	Hispanic Health and Nutrition Examination Survey
HNIS/USDA	Human Nutrition Information Service
HNRIMS/NIH	Human Nutrition Research Information Management System
HPB/Canada	Health Protection Branch, Health and Welfare Canada
HR	House of Representatives, Congress of the United States
HRSA/DHHS	Health Resources and Services Administration
HUD	Department of Housing and Urban Development
IBNMR	Interagency Board for Nutrition Monitoring and Research
ICHNR	Interagency Committee on Human Nutrition Research
ICNM	Interagency Committee on Nutrition Monitoring
ICNND/NIAMD/NIH	Interdepartmental Committee on Nutrition for National Defense
IFT	Institute of Food Technologists
ILSI/NF	International Life Sciences Institute/Nutrition Foundation
INACG/USAID	International Nutritional Anemia Consultative Group
IOM/NAS	Institute of Medicine
IUNS	International Union of Nutritional Sciences
JECFA/CODEX	Joint Expert Committee on Food Additives
LSRO/FASEB	Life Sciences Research Office
NAL/USDA	National Agricultural Library
NAMCS/NCHS/CDC	National Ambulatory Medical Care Survey
NAS	National Academy of Sciences
NASA	National Aeronautics and Space Administration
NBB/DEHLS/CEHIC/CDC	Nutritional Biochemistry Branch
NCC/NIH	Nutrition Coordinating Committee
NCHS/CDC	National Center for Health Statistics
NCI/NIH	National Cancer Institute
NETSS/DON/CCDPHP/CDC	Nutrition Education Training Surveillance System
NFCS/USDA	Nationwide Food Consumption Surveys
NFPA	National Food Processors Association
NHANES/NCHS/CDC	National Health and Nutrition Examination Surveys
NHDS/NCHS/CDC	National Hospital Discharge Survey
NHEFS/NCHS/CDC	NHANES I Epidemiological Followup Study
NHIS/NCHS/CDC	National Health Interview Survey
NHLBI/NIH	National Heart, Lung, and Blood Institute
NIAMD/NIH	National Institute of Arthritis and Metabolic Diseases
NICHD/NIH	National Institute of Child Health and Human Development
NIDDK/NIH	National Institute of Diabetes and Digestive and Kidney Diseases
NIH/USPHS/DHHS	National Institutes of Health
NLEA	Nutrition Labeling and Education Act of 1990
NLM/USPHS/DHHS	National Library of Medicine
NMFS/DOC	National Marine Fisheries Service
NMIHS/NCHS/CDC	National Maternal and Infant Health Survey
NMNFS/NCHS/CDC	National Mortality and Natality Followback Survey

TABLE 94–1. GLOSSARY OF ACRONYMS APPEARING IN THIS CHAPTER (ACRONYMS FOLLOWING THOSE UNDERLINED SHOW AFFILIATIONS) *(continued)*

NNHS/NCHS/CDC	National Nursing Home Survey
NNMRRA	National Nutrition Monitoring and Related Research Act of 1990
NNMS	National Nutrition Monitoring System
NRICGP/CSRS/USDA	National Research Initiative Competitive Grants Program
NSDA	National Soft Drink Association
NSF	National Science Foundation
NSFG/NCHS/CDC	National Survey of Family Growth
NTIS/DOC	National Technical Information Service
ODPHP/DHHS	Office of Disease Prevention and Health Promotion
OMB	Office of Management and Budget, The White House
ONFS/CFSAN/FDA	Office of Nutrition and Food Sciences
OSTP	Office of Science and Technology Policy, The White House
OTA	Office of Technology Assessment, The Congress
PedNSS/DON/CCDPHP	Pediatric Nutrition Surveillance System
PNSS/DON/CCDPHP/CDC	Enhanced Pregnancy Nutrition Surveillance System
QMF and CI/DA-DOD	Quartermaster Food and Container Institute
R and D	research and development
RDA/FNB/NAS	Recommended Dietary Allowances
RDI/FDA	Reference Daily Intakes
S	Senate, Congress of the United States
TDS/FDA	Total Diet Survey
UN	United Nations
USAID	U.S. Agency for International Development
USAMRNL/DA	U.S. Army Medical Research and Nutrition Laboratory
USARIEM/DA	U.S. Army Research Institute of Environmental Medicine
USDA	U.S. Department of Agriculture
USPHS/DHHS	U.S. Public Health Service
USRDA/FDA	U.S. Recommended Daily Allowances
VA	Veterans Administration
WHO/UN	World Health Organization
WIC/FNS/USDA	Supplemental Food Program/Women, Infants and Children
YRBSS	Youth Risk Behavior Surveillance System

and was associated with or followed by the founding of a number of important agencies.*

These agencies, together with the academic and industrial communities, accomplished a great deal in a remarkably short period, including the following: institution of enrichment of basic staples, particularly bread, flour, and milk; initiation of the concept of recommended physical performance, energy expenditure, and nutrient requirements; establishment of federal support for nutrition research; and establishment of official methods for analysis of nutrients in foods. Collectively, these efforts established the birth of our current multifactorial approach to nutrition policy. The history of nutrition for almost 3000 years is replete with examples of major advances in nutrition and food processing brought about by the exigencies of war. World War II was no exception.

The momentum was lost in the postwar period. The arrival of victory and the discovery of the essential nutrients resulted in a general sense of complacency, with a few exceptions from the middle 1940s through the middle 1960s. The academic community and a few foundations kept nutrition science alive, even if at a modest level. Internationally, the Marshall Plan put us in the forefront of providing for the nutritional needs of continental Europe for a decade (the British looked after themselves with little help from us). This effort then led

*(NIH); Food and Nutrition Board/NAS; (QMF and CI) (later the Army Natick Laboratories); (ANL) (later the Army Medical Research and Nutrition Laboratory); (CFN/AMA); DN/FDA.

to the Food for Peace Program focused on the developing world, vestiges of which still persist. Then came the Korean conflict. At an early stage, it became evident that Korean youth conscripted into the Army were seriously malnourished to the point of being militarily ineffective. Corrective measures were instituted, and at the end of the conflict, the Interdepartmental Committee on Nutrition for National Defense (ICNND) was founded, supported largely by the Department of Defense with its secretariat in the National Institute of Arthritis and Metabolic Disease (NIAMD) at NIH. In collaboration with the academic community and the Army Nutrition Laboratory (ANL), the ICNND conducted extensive nutrition surveys in over 30 developing countries during the next decade, becoming the cornerstone of nutrition activities at the federal level. Practically every Institute of Nutrition developed in these 30 plus countries owes its birthright to the ICNND.

The White House Conference on Food, Nutrition, and Health in December 1969, called by President Nixon, was the birthing of our current approach to nutrition policy.[1] It came about mainly for two reasons: (1) it was recognized that complacency was inappropriate because malnutrition persisted in vulnerable population segments right in the United States, and (2) the relationships between diet and degenerative diseases were beginning to take on real substance.

Turning to current affairs, it sounds perfectly rational to say that a monolithic national nutrition policy is a good idea and should exist. If I have learned anything in over 30 years in the federal nutrition bureaucracy, I cannot think of anything worse than a "nutrition czar" with the power to govern nutrition affairs for our nation. Bureaucratic centralization of things that do not fit together is also a bad idea. Such a system would be like having a national transportation policy covering everything from nuts and bolts to speeding tickets. Things simply do not work that way in our complex multifactorial society. What we do have is a long series of separate policies in many areas of nutrition that are loosely coordinated, at least at the federal level. Putting them all together yields a semblance of order, with a few glaring exceptions.

We now turn to the "key players," with the thought that one cannot understand how the organ systems work without first examining the body as a whole. This chapter does not include discussion of dietary guidelines, except in passing, because this topic is covered in Chapters 82, 83, and 93. It is impossible to include all the groups involved as key players, so the following is limited to those that play major roles in overall nutrition policies.

KEY PLAYERS

THE CONGRESS

The Congress has an enormously important role in establishing nutrition policy. In 1990, for example, two fundamental acts were passed, both of which are reviewed in detail elsewhere in this chapter. They are the Nutrition Labeling and Education Act of 1990 (NLEA)[2] and the Nutrition Monitoring and Related Research Act of 1990 (NMRRA).[3] It is important to keep in mind that the Congress in essence does three things: (1) it authorizes, i.e., it requires that specific parts of the executive branch do certain things; (2) it appropriates, i.e., it provides the funds for operation of the government; and (3) it oversees, i.e., it reviews problems and progress. Most of these functions are pursued through the use of congressional hearings, which go on continuously and are labor intensive from the point of view of the executive branch. In the field of human nutrition, many committees and subcommittees are involved one way or the other, specifically 11 committees with 14 subcommittees in the House of Representatives (HR) and 9 committees with 11 subcommittees in the Senate (S).*

*House of Representatives: (1) Committee on Agriculture. Subcommittee on Department Operations, Research and Foreign Agriculture: authorizes research components in food and agriculture; Subcommittee on Domestic Marketing, Consumer Relations and Nutrition: authorizes food stamps and related food distribution programs. (2) Committee on Appropriations. Subcommittee on Labor, Health and Human Services, Education: appropriations for all of the DHHS (e.g., NIH) except for FDA; Subcommittee on Rural Development, Agriculture and Related Agencies: appropriations for USDA and FDA; Subcommittee on VA, HUD, and Independent Agencies: appropriations for the VA, NASA, and NSF; Subcommittee on Commerce, Justice, State and Judiciary: appropriations for the AID). (3) Committee on Armed Services. Subcommittee on Appropriations: provides nutrition research funds; Subcommittee on Research and Development: authorizes research and development in the DOD including food and nutrition research and development. (4) Committee on Energy-Commerce. Subcommittee on Health and the Environment: authorizes all programs within DHHS, e.g., the Nutrition Labeling and Education Act of 1990 arose from this subcommittee. (5) Committee on Government Operations. Subcommittee on Human Resources and Intergovernmental Relations: oversight functions, e.g., FDA food safety and labeling activities. (6) Committee on Science, Space and Technology. Subcommittee on Science, Research and Technology: authorizes major science agencies except those in DHHS and USDA; oversight for all federal research and development except in DOD. The NNMRA arose from this subcommittee. (7) Committee on Veterans' Affairs. Subcommittee on Hospitals and Health Care: authorizes VA medical care, including nutrition support. (8) Committee on Ways and Means. Subcommittee on Health: oversight for programs such as Medicare and Medicaid, including nutrition components. (9) Select Committee on Aging. Subcommittee on Health and Long-term Care: oversight for such issues as health fraud through the mails (including nutrition-related issues), and nursing home care. (10) Select Committee on Children, Youth and Families: oversight for such areas as Head Start. (11) Select Committee on Hunger: oversight for such areas as temporary food assistance programs in USDA, and measurement of hunger prevalence, both domestically and internationally.

(continued . . .)

The only way to describe the role of the Congress in the field of nutrition is to say it is a maze. There is no central focal point for nutrition. The subject is literally scattered all over the Congress. At any given time, a half-dozen activities may be underway within the Congress relative to nutrition, through the hearing process, other forms of consultation (including much lobbying), the drafting of proposed legislation, and the management of such proposals through the intricacies of the two houses, and ultimately joint final revisions of legislation. To the best of the author's knowledge, only one individual currently on the congressional staffs is recognized as an authority in human nutrition.

THE WHITE HOUSE

Three components of the Office of the President can and do become directly involved in nutrition policy. The Office of Management and Budget (OMB) reviews and often requires significant changes in major regulatory proposals and final orders before publication in the Federal Register (FR). For example, OMB required major changes in FDA "Advance Notice of Proposed Rulemaking" concerning health messages in food labeling, published in the FR in 1987[4] (see the section on health claims in food labeling). The OMB also reviewed the massive proposals by the FDA to revise food labeling, published in the FR in 1991[5] (see the section on nutritional aspects of food labeling). This time, OMB did not make major changes in the original document as proposed by The Food and Drug Administration (FDA) of the Department of Health and Human Services (DHHS). A second arm of the White House is the Office of Science and Technology Policy (OSTP), which is the office of the Science Advisor to the President. During the 1970s and early 1980s, OSTP maintained the Joint Subcommittee on Human Nutrition Research until the Interagency Committee on Human Nutrition Research (ICHNR) was founded in 1983 (see the sections on NIH and on coordination). In recent years, OSTP has not been particularly active in nutrition-related matters. The third component is the White House Council on Competitiveness, chaired by the Vice-President. In March 1991, the Council initiated a massive review of all major regulatory proposals, final orders, and related policy documents throughout the government, primarily for purposes of analysis of costs and benefits. The Council is also requiring preparation of detailed Regulatory Impact Analyses by the operating agencies of the government, specifically including the FDA and the United States Department of Agriculture (USDA). Review of FDA proposals to implement the provisions of the NLEA[2] is part of the Council's work at this writing, the ultimate outcome of which is not clear.

Senate. (1) Committee on Agriculture, Nutrition and Forestry. Subcommittee on Agricultural Research and General Legislation: authorizes all research and development in USDA; Subcommittee on Nutrition and Investigations: authorizes the food stamp program, and related food distribution programs. (2) Committee on Appropriations subcommittees and functions exactly the same as in the House. Subcommittee on Labor, Health and Human Services, Education; Subcommittee on Rural Development, Agriculture and Related Agencies; Subcommittee on VA, HUD and Independent Agencies. (3) Committee on Armed Services. Subcommittee on Manpower and Personnel: authorizes food and nutrition programs. (4) Committee on Commerce, Science and Transportation. Subcommittee on the Consumer: authorizes FTC functions, including food and nutrition advertising. (5) Committee on Government Affairs. Subcommittee on Oversight for Government Management: oversight throughout government; the Senate role in the National Nutrition Monitoring and Related Research Act of 1990 stemmed from this Subcommittee. (6) Committee on Labor and Human Resources: authorizes all functions in DHHS, including FDA; the Senate role in the NLEA of 1990 stemmed from this Committee. Subcommittee on Aging: authorizes related programs including for nutrition; Subcommittee on Children, Family, Drugs and Alcoholism: authorizes nutrition activities in these areas. (7) Committee on Veterans' Affairs: authorizes health support, including nutrition. (8) Special Committee on Aging: oversight of all related programs. (9) Joint Economic Committee (with the House). Subcommittee on Education and Health: involved with nutrition education.

DEPARTMENT OF HEALTH AND HUMAN SERVICES

The DHHS with its multiple agencies provides the national leadership in nutrition in research and development, epidemiology and monitoring, and regulation. The Office of Disease Prevention and Health Promotion (ODPHP) in the Office of the Assistant Secretary for Health provides department-wide coordination of all nutrition activities. The coordination system used in DHHS for nutrition is comprehensive and is discussed in the section on coordination.

The National Institutes of Health. From a purely medical point of view, the NIH collectively is the most important single entity at the federal level in the field of nutrition. The reason is simple: NIH provides about three quarters of all federal dollars to support nutrition research and training. In fiscal year (FY) 1988, this support amounted to $276,195,000. This amount sounds impressive, which it is, but it accounts for slightly more than 4% of NIHs total support for biomedical research. These figures represent the combined individual contributions of the 12 NIH institutes, 2 centers, and 1 division. Three institutes account for about two thirds of the total in approximately equal proportions: the National Heart, Lung, and Blood Institute (NHLBI); the National Institute of Diabetes and Digestive and Kidney Diseases (NIDDK); and the National Cancer Institute (NCI), each providing about $60 million. The other two biggest supporters are the National Institute of Child Health and Human Development (NICHD) at about $34 million, and the Division of Research Resources (DRR) at about $22 million. Only about $3 million of the total is for individual training per se, or about 1%. Part of this total expenditure provides support for 8 clinical nutrition research units (CNRU). These units at university clinical centers are supported by 2 institutes: NIDDK and NCI. In FY 88, this support amounted to about $13 million.

The NIH plays a key role in coordination of nutrition research and action programs throughout the federal government in a number of different ways. At a policy level, the most important structure is the Interagency Committee on Human Nutrition Research (ICHNR), which is chaired jointly by the Assistant Secretary for Health, DHHS, and the Assistant Secretary for Science and Education, USDA. This Committee regularly brings together everybody at the federal level involved in human nutrition research.* All members are at policy levels in their respective agencies, and the Committee really does make fundamental decisions concerning nutrition policies. The ICHNR fosters communication among federal research agencies through four subcommittees: 1. Subcommittee on Research and the RDA; 2. Subcommittee on Technology, Nutrition, and Food Production; 3. Subcommittee on Nutrition Monitoring Research; and 4. Subcommittee on the HNRIM System (discussed subsequently).

A sister committee to the ICHNR is the Interagency Committee on Nutrition Monitoring (ICNM), established in 1988 to improve the planning, coordination, and communication among agencies engaged in nutrition monitoring. This committee is chaired jointly by the Assistant Secretary for Health, DHHS, and the Assistant Secretary for Food and Consumer Services, USDA.† The Committee monitors the overall effectiveness and productivity of nutrition monitoring efforts of the National Nutrition Monitoring System (NNMS), which includes all federally supported or conducted surveys on human nutritional status, and food consumption and surveillance of the food supply. The Committee has three working groups: the Survey Complementarity Group, the Federal-State Relations and Information Dissemination and Exchange Group, and the Food Composition Data Group.

The NIH has maintained an active Nutrition Coordinating Committee (NCC) since 1975. The NCC operates as an NIH-wide forum and locus to review, stimulate, and encourage the support of nutrition research and training in order to better define the role of nutrition in the promotion and maintenance of health and in prevention and treatment of disease. Other DHHS agencies, such as FDA and USDA, have liaison representatives to the NCC, and are also in regular attendance. The NCC plays a key role in the development of nutrition research policy at the NIH. Currently, the NIH nutrition research policy consists of eight areas. Research is emphasized in four of these areas: clinical nutrition throughout the life cycle, and nutritional factors in the development of disease, prevention of disease, and treatment of disease. The other four areas are related to education and technology transfer: the transfer of modern nutrition technology, nutrition education for professionals and the public, nutrition research training and research manpower development in nutrition, and trans-NIH and interagency coordination. Each year, the Division of Nutrition Research Coordination (DNRC) publishes a detailed report entitled "Program in Biomedical and Behavioral Nutrition Research and Training,"[7] which provides a detailed review of nutrition activities in each segment of NIH plus overall fiscal resources.

In addition, the NIH operates the Human Nutrition Research Information Management System (HNRIMS), a unique computerized data base system that contains information on all nutrition research and research training supported by the federal government. Developed in 1982, the system is maintained and updated by the DNRC, under the auspices of the ICHNR. The HNRIMS data base resides on-line in the NIH mainframe computer and is available for purchase by the general public through the National Technical Information Service (NTIS/DOC). The data base is also accessible to the public through Dialog Information Retrieval Service, as a subfile of the USDA Current Research Information Service (CRIS) data base. In addition, each fiscal year, the DNRC prepares a progress report to the Congress on the HNRIMS.

The NIH not only is the biomedical research center of the nation, but also conducts large-scale risk reduction programs that involve nutrition to a major degree. Two such programs are particularly outstanding—both operated by the NHLBI. The National High Blood Pressure Education Program has been in place since 1972. Since 1988, greater emphasis has been placed on the role of nonpharmacologic therapy, particularly weight reduction, sodium restriction, and moderation of alcohol consumption. The National Cholesterol Education Program has been in existence since 1985, and has developed specific guidelines for the detection, evaluation, and treatment of high blood cholesterol levels. Lastly, the NHLBI has collaborated with the NCI to develop a text entitled "Eating for Life," which addresses food choices and eating patterns that help reduce the risk of developing both cardiovascular disease and some types of cancer.

To put federal nutrition research policy into perspective, a few comments are in order relative to other parts of the federal establishment. The only other large nutrition research capability resides within the USDA (amounting to $68 million in FY 1988). All other agencies combined expended a total of $28 million (FY 88). Most NIH nutrition research is extramural. Most USDA research is intramural. All of that by the FDA is intramural, and practically all by the CDC is also intramural, except for state contracts for cooperative data collection.

*Members include: DHHS (NIH; FDA); USDA (ARS, HNIS); NSF; USAID; VA; NASA; OSTP, at the White House level; DOD; and the Department of Commerce (the NMFS). The NIH, through the DNRC in the Office of the Director of NIH, currently serves as the Executive Secretariat for the ICHNR. The secretariat rotates periodically between DHHS and USDA.

†Members include: DHHS (NIH; FDA; Centers for Chronic Diseases and Health Promotion [CDC]; and USDA (HNIS; ARS; FNS; ERS; AID; Bureau of the Census (Bureau of Statistics); DOD; and the VA.

Three other major contributions to the nutrition science base are in the epidemiologic area, and not accounted for under the "research" rubric, but all of which cost many millions of dollars: (1) The National Health and Nutrition Examination Surveys, conducted by the National Center for Health Statistics (NCHS), an arm of the CDC; (2) The Nationwide Food Consumption Surveys (NFCS), conducted by the USDA; and (3) The Continuing Surveys of Food Intake by Individuals (CSFII), also conducted by the USDA.

In summary, the NIH is indeed the major supporter of human clinically related nutrition research in the nation. However, this agency also performs an invaluable service by providing coordinating services to the entire government. In addition, NIH operates several major intervention-type action programs. As a result, NIH provides a vast proportion of the science base underlying all nutrition policies at the federal level.

The Food and Drug Administration. The FDA has been in the nutrition business since 1938 when the first federal laboratory for development of nutrient analytic methods was established within the predecessor to the FDA (which at that time was a part of USDA). The stimulus behind this effort was the need for good methods as enrichment of basic staples such as wheat flour with vitamins and iron was beginning.

The principal statute under which the FDA operates is the Food, Drug, and Cosmetic Act (FDCA). The food portions of the act are fundamentally directed to labeling. For example, if the FDA takes legal action against a food product, it usually does so because the food is adulterated, i.e., it contains an unapproved ingredient listed in the ingredient statement on the label, or because the food is misbranded, i.e., the label bears information deemed to be false or misleading. The FDA does not depend on the act alone. The act is implemented by hundreds of FDA regulations issued over the years, mostly through public rule making. All of these regulations are encoded in the Code of Federal Regulations, Volume 21 (21 CFR), updated annually. Most of the pertinent regulations can be found in parts 1 through 199.

The nutrition activities of the FDA are in the FDA Center for Food Safety and Applied Nutrition (CFSAN), except for fewer than 10 inspectors in the FDA field forces. Total staffing is of the order of 100 within CFSAN, divided into 5 groups within the Office of Nutrition and Food Sciences: (ONFS):

1. Research. This group allows the Center to keep abreast of current nutrition science by actual hands-on research. Much of the work focuses on mineral metabolism.
2. Clinical Nutrition. Most of this effort is devoted to nutrition epidemiology and analysis of consumption of specific food ingredients, such as sugars, aspartame, sulfites, and tropical oils.
3. Methods Development. This group supports the need for the best methodology for nutrient and ingredient analysis of foods, primarily to steadily improve capabilities to ensure compliance with the law and regulations.
4. Consumer and Marketing Research. This group permits the Center to track food labeling in the retail marketplace, and changing public attitudes and knowledge relative to nutrition over time. It is the only such consumer research capability in the entire federal government.
5. Regulatory Affairs. This group provides the focal point for development of new regulations, and for coordination between the nutrition components and the other parts of the Center, particularly those concerned with compliance and enforcement.

One of the most fundamental nutrition policy activities at the federal level during the past two decades is now under way at FDA. The Nutrition Labeling and Education Act of 1990 (NLEA)[2] requires a massive restructuring of the food label as related to health issues. Regulatory proposals to implement the act have now been developed as of 1991,[5] requiring practically all of the resources in nutrition of the agency. All such regulations are proposed in the FR for public comment (which will result in thousands of comments), and then finalized. The comment period closed on February 25, 1992. This slow and arduous process may well take up to 5 years to complete. The key matters that must be covered by these regulatory proposals are as follows: revision of ingredient labeling requirements; nutrition labeling of raw fruit, vegetables, and fish; revision of nutrition labeling (including revision of the USRDA, derived from the RDA of the National Academy of Sciences); adjectival descriptors (e.g., "low," "reduced," etc.); nutrition labeling format; standardized serving sizes; health claims (i.e., disease-specific claims for conventional foods); and adjectival descriptors for cholesterol and fat. Every segment of our society will comment, because these issues affect everybody, and the comments will be diverse, argumentative, and contradictory. All must be responded to in developing final regulations, an awesome task because of the differences between state and local governments, the food industry, the scientific community, the consumer advocate community, and the general citizenry. The NLEA requires that FDA finalize its regulatory proposals by November 8, 1992 (or the proposals themselves will become the final regulations). In spite of these problems, it is reasonable to anticipate that, by the middle 1990s, we will see profound changes in the health and nutrition aspects of the food label, which will benefit all consumers.

A particularly troublesome issue involved in labeling is created by the fact that the USDA regulates meat and poultry products (including, for example, pizzas containing sausages), whereas the FDA regulates all the rest of the food supply. This situation is analogous to the dichotomy between food labeling invested in FDA and food advertising invested in the Federal Trade Commission (FTC). The key problem has to do with the definition of "low fat" or "reduced fat." The basic premise should be that the two agencies end up with the same definitions. Given the enormous power of the meat and poultry lobbies on the one hand (USDA) and the dairy lobbies on the other hand (FDA), reaching a consensus is not going to be easy. Yet the public needs consistent definitions to minimize confusion derived from the label itself.

Some most positive events unfolded in 1991 in addition to the labeling revisions, stemming from the strengthened leadership of the FDA. After years of hesitation, the agency took strong action against "no cholesterol" claims on vegetable-derived fats and oils as being misleading, implying to the public that these foods are of value in reducing risk of heart disease, whereas reduction of total fat in the diet is perhaps the most prominent component of current nutrition thinking. FDA Commissioner David A. Kessler also publically announced that he intends to pursue appropriate regulation of two major segments of the food supply: (1) dietary supplements of vitamins, minerals, and amino acids; and (2) medical foods, i.e., those specially formulated products used in the dietary management of critically ill or severely incapacitated patients. The L-tryptophan episode of 1990 associated with eosinophilia-myalgia syndrome is an example of problems with dietary supplements. Medical foods need major attention as well. These issues are discussed in more detail in the section on food labeling.

Centers for Disease Control (CDC). The three components of CDC that are major players in helping establish the scientific base for nutrition policy are: (1) the National Center for Health Statistics (NCHS); (2) the Division of Nutrition (DON) in the National Center for Chronic Disease Prevention and Health Promotion (CCDPHP); and (3) the Division of Environmental Health Laboratory Sciences (DEHLS) in the Center for Environmental Health and Injury Control (CEHIC). With other components of the federal government, they are involved in implementation of the NMRRA of 1990,[3] which is discussed elsewhere in this chapter, as is the ICNM. The NCHS headquarters is in Hyattsville, MD; the remainder of the CDC is in Atlanta, GA.

The NCHS provides the fundamental data base for nutritional status in the United States. It conducts huge surveys contributing to this knowledge base, and is the repository of data tapes on all of its surveys, which are readily available at minimal cost. Currently, there are 17 such data bases.*

Although almost 50 individual surveys collectively make up the NNMS, the huge surveys just described form the core. As discussed elsewhere in this chapter, other agencies involved in the NNMS include multiple components of the USDA, FDA, several institutes at NIH, other components of the CDC, the Bureau of the Census, and the Bureau of Labor Statistics. Without question, the survey efforts of NCHS provide the most extensive and comprehensive evaluation of nutritional status over time of any population in the world.

The mission of the Division of Nutrition (DON), National Center for Chronic Disease Prevention and Health Promotion (CCDPHP), is "to improve the quality of life by preventing nutrition-related disease, disability, and premature death and by promoting health through good nutrition." The DON accomplishes its mission by activities that include applied research in nutrition epidemiology and nutrition intervention, demonstration, and evaluation; training and professional development, consultation, and technical and financial support; setting and evaluating standards and guidelines for nutri tion assessment, nutrition intervention, and nutrition surveillance; surveillance and data management by

*(1) National Health and Nutrition Examination Survey I (NHANES I), conducted from 1971 to 1974, involving complete clinical, biochemical, dietary, and anthropometric examinations of over 20,000 individuals representing a national probability sample. (2) NHANES II, conducted from 1976 to 1980, patterned after NHANES I, again involving over 20,000 individuals. (3) Hispanic Health and Nutrition Examination Survey (HHANES), conducted from 1982 to 1984, patterned after the NHANES surveys, involving over 11,000 individuals representing the Mexican American, Cuban, and Puerto Rican segments of the population. (4) NHANES III, being conducted 1988 to 1994, with a sample size of approximately 40,000, from which the first phase data will be available in 1992. (5) National Health Interview Survey (NHIS), Core Survey, conducted annually, involving about 135,000 individuals. (6) NHIS Supplement on Aging, conducted in 1984, on over 16,000 individuals. (7) NHIS Supplement on Health Promotion and Disease Prevention, conducted in 1985 on over 33,000 individuals. (8) NHIS Supplement on Vitamin and Mineral Supplements, conducted in 1986 in collaboration with FDA on over 13,000 individuals. (9) NHIS Supplement on Cancer Epidemiology and Cancer Control, conducted in 1987 on about 45,000 individuals. (10) NHANES I Epidemiological Followup Study (NHEFS), conducted from 1982 to 1984, 1986, and 1987, involving over 12,000 individuals with the purpose of examining the relationship of baseline clinical, nutritional, and behavioral factors assessed in NHANES I to subsequent morbidity and mortality. (11) National Survey of Family Growth (NSFG), conducted from 1973 to 1974, 1976, 1982, and 1988, involving about 8,000 women of reproductive age. (12) National Maternal and Infant Health Survey (NMIHS), conducted from 1988 to 1990, involving a total of 60,000 mothers, focusing on live births, fetal deaths of 28 weeks or more of gestation, and infant deaths. (13) National Mortality and Natality Followback Survey (NMNFS), conducted in 1987, involving over 18,000 decedents, focusing on cause of death, height, weight, medical history, dietary patterns, lifestyle behaviors, and demographic characteristics. (14) Vital Statistics System, conducted annually, involving all births and deaths, and focusing on age, race, sex, occupation, marital status, birth weight, weight gain during pregnancy, educational status, and cause of death. (15) National Hospital Discharge Survey (NHDS), conducted annually on all in-patients, providing among other things information on hospitalizations resulting from nutrition-related diseases. (16) National Ambulatory Medical Care Survey (NAMCS), performed annually since 1989, involving 40,000 patient visits to office-based physicians, with data on reasons for visits and diagnosis. (17) National Nursing Home Survey (NNHS), conducted from 1973 to 1974, 1977, and 1985, involving over 1,000 nursing homes and over 11,000 patients, with emphasis on diagnoses, functional status, charges for care, and discharge status, including nutritional parameters.

developing methods and software, managing and enhancing nutrition surveillance systems, and analyzing and interpreting surveillance data; and development of a long-term cooperative plan for industry and public health nutrition action. The CDC can do these sorts of things, whereas the FDA can only do so to a limited degree, because the latter must retain a certain distance from the regulated industry.

Several specific activities of the DON include obesity epidemiology research, chronic disease nutrition intervention guidelines, and enhanced pregnancy nutrition surveillance (PNSS). In addition to PNSS, the DON operates other surveillance activities, including the Behavioral Risk Factor Surveillance System (BRFSS), the Pediatric Nutrition Surveillance System (PedNSS), the Nutrition Education Training Surveillance System (NETSS) and the nutrition component of the Youth Risk Behavior Surveillance System (YRBSS). The DON/CDC chairs the steering committee for the Criteria Coalition, an effort originally founded by the American Heart Association (AHA), the purpose being to work with voluntary organizations, professional groups, the FDA, and the USDA to develop criteria for foods and food products that meet the dietary guidelines for Americans, and to disseminate the results widely in the private and public sectors. The Division is finalizing *Nutrition Education Guidelines in Comprehensive School Health.* This effort constitutes one of the few at the federal level to improve nutrition education in our schools per se. Guidelines will also involve development of criteria for evaluating existing nutrition education curricula for use by classroom teachers. These criteria will be used as the basis for a CDC Teacher Training Institute to acquaint teachers with outstanding nutrition education curricula.

The Nutritional Biochemistry Branch Division of Environmental Health Laboratory Sciences, Center for Environmental Health and Injury Control (NBB/DEHLS/CEHIC), has been in existence since 1971, and was originally patterned after the approaches established by the ICNND, starting in the middle 1950s. It provides all of the nutritional biochemical support for the NHANES surveys. It is also involved in support of other programs in nutrition, such as osteoporosis risk factors; the Eye Disorder Case Control Study; and the Age-Related Eye Disease Study sponsored by the National Eye Institute of NIH. They provide quality control support for the NCI in its studies of the role of micronutrients in the etiology of cancer, and laboratory support to NHLBI for children with hyperlipidemias participating in the Dietary Intervention Study in Children.

DEPARTMENT OF AGRICULTURE

The USDA plays an enormous role in nutrition policy and human nutrition research, and has an impact on maintenance of nutritional well-being that touches practically every citizen and resident of our country every day. Its budget for 1990 for research, education, and information on nutrition was $233.3 million; of this amount, only $65.5 million was allocated to human nutrition research, mostly managed and conducted by the Agricultural Research Service (ARS). All of the USDA nutrition-related activities are coordinated by the Department's Subcommittee for Human Nutrition of the Research and Education Committee of the Secretary's Policy and Coordination Council. All such activities also fall under the ultimate authority of five individuals: the Assistant Secretary for Food and Consumer Services; the Assistant Secretary for Science and Education; the Assistant Secretary for Marketing and Inspection Services; the Assistant Secretary for Economics; and the Undersecretary for International Affairs and Commodity Programs. The most fundamental component of all nutrition policy, i.e., the *Dietary Guidelines for Americans,* is approved at the secretarial level in the USDA, as well as in the DHHS.

Agricultural Research Service. The ARS is the principal intramural research agency of the USDA. *Promoting Optimal Health and Well-Being Through Improved Nutrition* is one of six major objectives of the ARS, and the nutrition objective is pursued through four basic approaches: (1) Define nutrient requirements at all stages of life; (2) Determine the nutrient content of agricultural commodities and processed foods as eaten, and establish the bioavailability of nutrients in these foods; (3) Improve human nutrition status by making available techniques to assess the effectiveness of nutrition programs; and (4) Integrate knowledge of human nutritional needs into the agricultural/food system. The ARS specifically does not pursue disease-specific research. This effort is the responsibility at the federal level of the USPHS, the NIH in particular. The ARS nutrition research program is conducted principally at five separate Human Nutrition Research Centers, and to a lesser extent in their Regional Research Centers.*

*The five centers are as follows. (1) Beltsville Human Nutrition Research Center, Beltsville, MD. Research is conducted on nutrient composition and nutritional qualities of food. Dietary strategies are developed to delay the onset of nutritionally related chronic diseases. (2) Grand Forks Human Nutrition Research Center, Grand Forks, ND. Their focus is on defining human requirements for trace elements and the physiologic and biochemical factors that influence those requirements. (3) Western Human Nutrition Research Center, Presidio of San Francisco, CA. Improved methods are developed for monitoring and evaluating nutritional status and factors that lead to malnutrition are investigated, as well as studies on human nutritional requirements. (4) Human Nutrition Research Center on Aging, Tufts University, Boston, MA. Research is conducted on the special nutritional needs of persons as they age with a view toward enhancing the quality of later life through improved nutrition and health. (5) Children's Nutrition Research Center, Houston, TX. The focus is on determining the unique nutrient needs of pregnant and lactating women, and of children from conception through early years of development.

Another ARS laboratory directly involved in nutrition research is the Plant, Soil, and Nutrition Laboratory, Ithaca, NY, in which investigators study the cause and effect relationships between plants, soil, and nutrition. An additional five ARS regional laboratories are generally commodity oriented, and focus on specific areas of research directed at food production, food processing, food storage, distribution and marketing, and food safety.

Food Safety and Inspection Service (FSIS). The primary role of FSIS in nutrition is the approval of all labels of packaged meat and poultry products before such products enter the marketplace. Such labeling approval includes nutrition labeling. As pointed out elsewhere in this chapter, the USDA has had a voluntary and simplified type of nutrition labeling in the marketplace for many years (as compared with the FDA nutrition labeling requirements), and, on November 8, 1991, joined with the FDA in proposing mandatory nutrition labeling for most packaged products under their jurisdiction. This joint effort occurred even though the USDA is not subject to the provisions of the NLEA,[2] and because the USDA determined that they had the statutory authority in previously existing legislation to do so.

Food and Nutrition Service (FNS). The FNS was established in 1969 to administer the food assistance programs of the USDA. The goals of the agency are to provide needy people with access to a more nutritious diet, to improve the eating habits of the nation's children, and to stabilize farm prices through the distribution of surplus foods. Some members of the nutrition science community may argue that these are not nutrition programs, but rather are part of our welfare system. Be that as it may, they warrant mention in a chapter concerned with nutrition policy. In addition, the enormity of these efforts needs to be understood by anyone interested in nutrition. Congress appropriated $27.5 billion in FY 1991 for the 13 programs administered by the FNS (about 47% of the total USDA budget), and the budget continues to grow in spite of the current efforts to curtail government spending.*

Human Nutrition Information Service (HNIS). HNIS conducts applied research in the following four general areas.

1. Nutrient composition. The HNIS collects and evaluates information on the nutrient composition of all foods important in American diets. Data are processed through the computerized National Nutrient Data Bank and published in *Agriculture Handbook No. 8* and its supplements.
2. Food consumption. The HNIS monitors the diets of the United States population and of subpopulations at nutritional risk, providing information on household food use, food costs, dietary practices of individual household members, nutritional quality of diets, and socioeconomic variables. It conducts the Nationwide Food Consumption Survey (NFCS) about every 10 years, and the annual Continuing Survey of Food Intakes by Individuals (CSFII), as well as the Diet-Health Knowledge Survey in collaboration with the FDA.
3. Dietary appraisal. The HNIS conducts and interprets food and nutrition research to solve practical problems faced by government policy makers, educators, health professionals, and consumers; e.g., annual studies are made of the nutrient content of the national food supply to show trends over time in nutrient availability and food sources of nutrients.
4. Nutrition education. The HNIS publishes many consumer-oriented information pieces each year with DHHS. It also coordinates the review and publication of the *Dietary Guidelines for Americans,*[8] jointly published by the USDA and DHHS every 5 years, and

*These 13 programs are: (1) Food Stamp Program. Served over 20 million people in 1990, for a total cost of $18 billion in FY 1991. The program received additional state-derived contributions as well. (2) Nutrition Assistance Program (Puerto Rico and the Northern Marianas). FY 1991 budget: $974 million. (3) National School Lunch Program. Participation is over 24 million children in more than 91,000 schools and residential institutions. FY 1991 budget: $3.4 billion. (4) School Breakfast Program. School breakfast participation approximates 3.8 million in over 40,000 schools and institutions. FY 1991 budget: $656 million. (5) Child and Adult Food Program. Provides cash and commodity assistance to child and adult care centers and family day care homes. FY 1991 budget: $1.04 billion. (6) Special Supplemental Food Program for Women, Infants and Children (WIC). The goal of the program is to improve the health of pregnant, breast-feeding, and postpartum women, and infants and children up to 5 years old, by providing supplemental foods, nutrition education, and access to health services. Much of the program is actually administered through public health clinic facilities, supported by USPHS and state programs. WIC reaches 90 to 95% of eligible infants, plus 90% of eligible pregnant women. This is one of the few assistance programs of which the nutritional impact has actually been clinically measured by the CDC and other epidemiologic efforts, the results being measurably positive. FY 1991 budget: $2.4 billion. (7) Commodity Supplemental Food Program. A direct food distribution program with a target population similar to WIC, this agency operates primarily in areas without a WIC program. FY 1991 budget: $81.9 million. (8) Food Distribution Program on Indian Reservations and the Trust Territories. Provides commodity foods to Native American Families who live on or near Indian reservations, and to Pacific islanders. Also known as the Needy Family Program, this is the oldest FNS program, going back to the Great Depression of the 1930s. It was the main form of food assistance until the Food Stamp Program was expanded in the early 1970s. FY 1991 budget: $78.2 million. (9) Nutrition Program for the Elderly. Provides cash and commodity foods for meals for senior citizens. Food is served in senior citizen centers or delivered by meals-on-wheels programs. The program served an average of over 929,000 meals daily in FY 1990. FY 1991 budget: $149.9 million. (10) Commodity Distribution to Charitable Institutions. Commodities are provided to nonprofit, charitable institutions that serve meals to needy persons regularly. Almost $60 million worth of USDA commodities went to charitable institutions in FY 1990, plus another $32 million specifically for soup kitchens and food banks. (11) The Emergency Food Assistance Program. The program was initiated in 1981 to reduce inventories and storage costs of surplus commodities through distribution to needy households. About 12 million people participated in 1990. FY 1990 budget: $169.4 million. (12) FNS participates in the National Advisory Council on Women, Infants and Children, established by Congress in 1975. (13) FNS participates in the National Advisory Council on Food Distribution, established by the Congress in 1987.

conducts a corollary program entitled *Eating Right . . . The Dietary Guidelines Way* to help the consuming public to become aware of the guidelines and put them into practice.

Cooperative State Research Service (CSRS). This agency is responsible for administering and coordinating funds appropriated under the Hatch Act and the 1977 Food and Agriculture Act to 54 state agricultural experiment stations, to 16 "1890 land-grant colleges," and to Tuskegee Institute to carry out research on food and agricultural issues, including human nutrition research. Matching funds, often in excess of the amount of federal funds, are provided by the states. This total activity is complementary to the in-house research efforts of the USDA through the ARS.

The CSRS also administers the National Research Initiative Competitive Grants Program (NRICGP). For practical purposes, this is the only actual research grant program at the federal level other than the huge programs of NIH. The amount devoted to nutrition research in FY 1991 approximated $4 million. In the broad national perspective, federal dollars for support of nutrition research derive from the NIH or from the various USDA programs. All other agencies are small in comparison. Other than state matching funds, the only other major source of funds in support of nutrition research is industry.

Economic Research Service (ERS). Since 1909, the ERS has provided a fundamental piece of information for the nutrition scientific community annually by developing annual estimates of the per capita quantity of foods available for domestic consumption in the United States. These food availability or disappearance data are used widely to examine trends over time. Although through no fault of the ERS, these data are often misused by the scientific community, by referring to them as consumption or intake data, which they are not. We now have extensive data of actual consumption through the NHANES and NFCS, eliminating the need to use disappearance data for intake estimates.

The ERS also conducts research on factors that influence consumer demand for major food products and individual food items. Socioeconomic factors that are analyzed include regional population shifts, increasing life expectancy, rising incomes, declining birth rates, and health and nutrition concerns. In addition, the agency analyzes the effects of alternative government food policies on both producers and consumers.

Extension Service (ES). The ES disseminates research-based nutrition, food science, and food safety principles and concepts through the Cooperative Extension Service (CES). More than 25% of all resources allocated to home economics is directed to human food and nutrition education programs.

Agricultural Marketing Service (AMS). This agency provides a service of particular relevance to nutrition, i.e., they develop quality grade standards and provide grading and certification services to industry. These quality standards appear on labels of many foods, particularly meat, eggs and dairy products, e.g., grade A milk and grade A large eggs. Meat grades frequently reflect fat content, and the USDA is now developing new standards of leanness, which clearly will benefit the consumer in terms of moderating fat intakes.

National Agricultural Library (NAL). The NAL in Beltsville, MD has a unit within the library called the Food and Nutrition Information Center (FNIC) to serve persons seeking information or educational materials in the area of food and nutrition. The items in the FNIC collection are listed in AGRICOLA, the computerized bibliographic data base and are readily available through numerous channels.

THE FOOD INDUSTRY

Next to the Congress, the food industry probably has more to do with nutrition policy than any other segment of our society, and, in fact, much of what the Congress does is influenced heavily by the food industry. The nutrition scientific community plays a decidedly tertiary role in establishing such policy. The only thing that "salvages" the nutrition scientific community is the impact of the nutrition scientists and administrators within the federal establishment itself, and those serving in advisory capacities through various committees within and without the government. Generally, the food industry is reasonably responsible in its actions, but never underestimate its power. Such influence is to be expected, because the food industry molds the nature of our food supply, particularly at the retail level in the supermarkets of the land. This is what we eat, and the industry makes it. Industry performs its role in a number of ways:

1. Billions of dollars are expended per year in food advertising.
2. Billions of dollars are expended per year in research and development of new products.
3. Hundreds of millions of dollars are expended per year in support of trade associations, the primary function of which is to influence the Congress and the regulatory agencies.
4. Similar expenditures are made on lobbyists for individual firms and commodity groups, most frequently derived from law firms specializing in food law.
5. Moderately strong support is provided to the scientific community through sponsorship of professional organizations and their major meetings, symposia, and texts in the food and nutrition field.
6. It supports consumer information programs.
7. It employs more people than any other segment of our society.

Most of these activities are self-evident. A few words about the at least 100 trade associations in the food and nutrition business in Washington might be helpful.* No day goes by at the FDA, for example, where representatives of these and similar groups fail to appear to discuss some issue. The same situation occurs at the USDA. They play a fundamental role in drafting legislation, in commenting on regulatory proposals, in building cases in courts against specific government actions, and the like. They are staffed by highly trained and motivated personnel whose views are not to be taken lightly.

The influence of the food industry on our daily lives is obvious. Perhaps the most prominent elements of public nutrition policy currently are achievement and maintenance of normal body weight, and reduction of fat intake. The *Dietary Guidelines for Americans* say so,[8] but it is the food industry that makes the changes in our food supply to facilitate achieving such objectives. Way and by far the largest single endeavor today in the food industry is development and marketing of calorie-reduced foods and lower fat foods. Supermarkets are loaded with such items, whereas such was not the case a decade ago. Huge expenditures are going into research and development at industry level to come up with more and better products. In parallel, research is ongoing in an effort to develop new artificial sweeteners for purposes of reducing caloric content of specific foods.

The author is a devotee of the American food industry. We are way ahead of everyone else in the world in the diversity and nutritional quality of our food supply, despite the break from time to time with common sense in promotional activities in labeling and advertising.

OTHER ORGANIZATIONS

The Federal Trade Commission (FTC). The FTC has one major role in nutrition policy: it regulates food advertising, as distinct from the FDA, which regulates food labeling. Herein lies an odd dicotomy. By its nature, the FDA is a health protection agency, and its policies evolve from a science base. As a result, the concept of scientific consensus governs policy. On the other hand, the FTC is a legal agency staffed primarily by lawyers. FTC policies have evolved on a basis of "substantiation," i.e., if advertising claims are made and they can be reasonably "substantiated," such claims are likely to be deemed satisfactory, whether or not there is scientific consensus. In addition, the congressional statutes under which these two agencies operate are entirely different, and neither sets of laws directly address this matter of consensus versus substantiation. Hence, the dicotomy that exists has come about more as a matter of internal policy making in the two agencies, rather than being forced by specific stipulations of law. This results in major differences between health-related food label claims as contrasted with advertising claims on the same subject. Generally, label claims are more restricted than advertising claims. To the best of my knowledge, no other country has this split between agencies for regulation of food labeling and food advertising.

Other Federal Agencies. Although this chapter puts emphasis on the USPHS and USDA as the focal points for nutrition within the executive branch, other federal agencies with active research and/or action programs are concerned with nutrition.

The VA has been actively involved in clinical nutrition research for many years. Examples include research in hematology, obesity, and iron metabolism.

The Department of Defense (DOD), primarily through the Department of the Army (DA), played a major role in keeping human nutrition research alive during the post-World War II era for several decades, and continues to have a small research effort. Since 1982, the Army has supported the Committee on Military Nutrition Research, a function of the FNB/IOM/NAS. The Committee has prepared numerous reports to the Surgeon General of the Army on topics such as water, electrolyte, and carbohydrate requirements in environmental extremes; the design and testing of new combat rations; and reviews of the total Army nutrition research effort.

The National Aeronautics and Space Administration (NASA) maintained a substantial nutrition research effort during the 1960s and 1970s to develop feeding systems for the astronaut programs (see Chap. 43). Some results of the NASA effort have "filtered" into the domestic food supply, e.g., fortified fabricated foods and products for use by sports enthusiasts.

The National Marine Fisheries Services (NMFS) of the Department of Commerce (DOC) works collaboratively with the FDA on many aspects of fish and shellfish quality and safety. Recently, NMFS compiled new tables of nutrient composition of many of the common seafood items in the American diet.

The National Science Foundation (NSF) does not have a specific program in nutrition, but periodically supports some basic research in the area of nutrition.

Occasionally, the Department of Education (DOE) becomes involved in nutrition education development efforts, e.g., in collaboration with the CDC.

The United States Agency for International Development (USAID) supports substantial efforts in the nutrition field in developing countries. Most of this involvement has little to do with domestic nutrition issues, but the expertise is derived from our domestic scientific community. In addition, development efforts by USAID

*Examples include: (1) The Grocery Manufacturers of America (GMA), representing primarily the food processors. (2) The National Food Processors Association (NFPA), representing primarily the canned and frozen food segments of industry. (3) The Council for Responsible Nutrition (CRN), representing the dietary supplement industry. (4) The Salt Institute, representing the salt industry. (5) The Sugar Association, representing the natural sweetener industry. (6) The National Soft Drink Association (NSDA), representing the soft drink industry. (7) The National Dairy Council, representing the dairy industry. (8) The Food Marketing Institute (FMI), representing primarily the food retailers. (9) The Infant Formula Council (IFC), representing the infant formula industry.

do have domestic relevance, e.g., their support over the years of the International Nutritional Anemia Consultative Group (INACG) in cooperation with WHO. This group, managed by the International Life Sciences Institute/Nutrition Foundation (ILSI/NF), has produced a long series of reports focused primarily on iron deficiency, both domestic and international, and they have acted as a stimulus for research in both government laboratories, e.g., FDA, and at the medical school and food science levels in our academic institutions.

Advisory Institutions. The government, both the Congress and the Administration, rely on many authoritative institutions in the nation for advice relative to nutrition. However, two are most prominent.

The Food and Nutrition Board (FNB) of the Institute of Medicine (IOM), National Academy of Sciences (NAS), in Washington, D.C. has played a lead advisory role since before World War II. To quote from the 1989 Annual Report of the IOM, "The Food and Nutrition Board was established to address issues of national importance that pertain to the safety and adequacy of the nation's food supply, to establish principles and guidelines of adequate dietary intake, and to render authoritative judgments on the relationships among food intake, nutrition, and health. FNB is a multidisciplinary group of biomedical scientists with expertise in various aspects of nutrition, food science, biochemistry, medicine, public health, epidemiology, food toxicology, policy, and food safety." Three recent publications make the value of their efforts in shaping nutrition policy clear.*

The Life Sciences Research Office (LSRO) of the Federation of American Societies for Experimental Biology (FASEB) in Bethesda, MD was established in the 1960s under federal government contracts to provide reviews of topics in the life sciences with particular emphasis on nutrition issues. This arrangement permitted the federal government to tap the resources of the over 30,000 biomedical scientists that constitute the membership of the various societies belonging to FASEB, including the American Institute of Nutrition (AIN) and the American Society for Clinical Nutrition (ASCN). Their biggest undertaking was the review for the FDA of the hundreds of substances previously determined to be generally recognized as safe (GRAS), accomplished through the Select Committee on GRAS Substances, which functioned for over a decade. The most recent effort of the LSRO was a complete review in 1991[12] of the 12 topics identified in the NLEA as potentially suitable for "health messages" or, more correctly, disease-specific health claims in food labeling. This review was also performed under contract with the FDA. Although the LSRO performs studies primarily for the federal government, it also undertakes reviews through a peer review system for other clients, including private industry. Their analyses have provided solid scientific evaluation and recommendations for future research without management advice, a helpful approach when working from a government perspective.

*(1) *Recommended Dietary Allowances*, 10th Ed., 1989.[9] (2) *Diet and Health: Implications for Reducing Chronic Disease Risk*, 1989.[10] This publication, along with *The Surgeon General's Report on Nutrition and Health* (1988),[6] provides the foundation for all current nutrition policies concerned with the relationships between diet and risk reduction from degenerative diseases. Both reports are well reflected in the provisions of the NLEA of 1990. (3) *Nutrition Labeling: Issues and Directions for the 1990s*,[11] 1990. This report will play a major role in shaping the implementing regulations for the 1990 Act.

Scientific Societies and Organizations. Many scientific and professional societies and organizations significantly influence national nutrition policy. Space does not permit an exhaustive review of all of them, so the focus of the following discussion is on a limited number of key groups.

The three major scientific societies devoted entirely to nutrition are the American Institute of Nutrition (AIN) and its clinical division, the American Society for Clinical Nutrition (ASCN), headquartered in Bethesda, MD; and the American Society for Parenteral and Enteral Nutrition (ASPEN), headquartered in Silver Spring, MD. The first two are part of FASEB. These societies play a huge role by providing a large part of the total scientific foundation for nutrition science through their various journals and annual and regional meetings. The AIN encompasses the entire science of nutrition, with emphasis on basic science, and applied animal and human nutrition; its membership is predominantly composed of doctors of philosophy (PhD), and its annual meeting is attended by many thousands. The ASCN focuses on clinical nutrition research, with the majority of members being physicians. ASPEN is clinically oriented, and its membership is primarily composed of physicians, Ph.Ds, dietitians, nurses, and pharmacists.

Starting before World War II and until about 15 years ago, the American Medical Association (AMA) was a major player in national nutrition policy through its Council on Foods and Nutrition. This council was most influential in establishing and maintaining our fortification policy for basic staples, e.g., enriched flours and breads. Regrettably, the AMA has withdrawn almost entirely from nutrition science in recent years. The American Academy of Pediatrics (AAP), headquartered in Elk Grove, IL, on the other hand, has been and remains active in the field through its Committee on Nutrition. For example, their reviews of dietary management of inborn errors of metabolism, sponsored primarily by the FDA for many years, have provided the fundamental guidance to the federal establishment for such disorders, in terms not only of clinical management but also relative to inclusion in food assistance programs and to insurance coverage.

The American Dietetic Association (ADA), headquartered in Chicago, is another key player, obviously focusing on the dietetics side of the application of nutrition science. Their approach is highly applied, and they rarely fail to testify authoritatively before Congress when hearings are held and nutrition-related bills are under consideration. Their huge membership of over 60,000 and their concomitant fiscal resources give them a substantial voice in public forums. Other organizations with major commitments to nutrition are the American Heart Association (AHA), particularly for its efforts to develop and publicize diet plans to reduce risk of atherosclerotic disease, and the American Cancer Society (ACS), which in like manner publicizes dietary approaches to reduction of risk of various forms of cancer, focusing particularly on reduction of fat intakes and augmentation of fiber intakes.

A unique organization is the International Life Sciences Institute-Nutrition Foundation (ILSI/NF), headquartered in Washington, D.C. The ILSI/NF is basically industry supported but independent, and performs a number of efforts that strongly influence national nutrition policy. They support nutrition research in terms of millions of dollars per year, hold many nutrition-related conferences each year, and publish numerous monographs on nutrition topics, e.g., on carbohydrates (sucrose, starches, and fructose) and on minerals (e.g., zinc and calcium). They have expanded worldwide in recent years as well, as a result of which they have an outstanding international network in the nutrition field. In addition, they publish the journal *Nutrition Reviews.*

Several professional organizations focus primarily on foods. The Institute of Food Technologists (IFT), headquartered in Chicago, is a huge organization of food scientists and technologists, primarily from academia and industry. They play a major role in nutrition policy, because they provide the forum for dissemination of knowledge in food science and technology, assisting in the beneficial revolution in our processed food supply directed toward facilitating dietary reduction of risk of various degenerative diseases. Another institution is the Food and Drug Law Institute (FDLI), headquartered in Washington, D.C. It is primarily supported by industry, and is a highly professional organization focused, as its name implies, on law and regulations. Undoubtedly, they will be intimately involved in the evolution of national policy stemming from the NLEA. They also have been involved in governmental consideration of medical foods.

Two other organizations having to do with medical "politics" warrant mention. The American Board of Nutrition (ABN) has existed since 1948 for purposes of certifying physicians and Ph.Ds as specialists in clinical nutrition and human nutrition, respectively. The examinations have now become rigorous, similar to those of other certifying bodies in medical specialties. It has been active in cooperation with the ASCN in negotiating with the American Board of Medical Specialties (ABMS) to achieve specialty status by certificates of competence in nutrition with certain recognized medical specialties. To date, this has not been effected with adverse consequences on the entire science of clinical nutrition at the policy level. It is hoped that the situation will be corrected in the foreseeable future.

International Organizations. Some international organizations have major impacts on domestic nutrition policy. At the United Nations (UN) level, the World Health Organization (WHO) in Geneva, Switzerland has two small groups concerned with nutrition: a food safety group and a nutrition group. The United Nations Food and Agriculture Organization (FAO) in Rome, Italy has a large unit, the Food Policy and Nutrition Division. Within this Division is the Secretariat for the Joint FAO/WHO Codex Alimentarius Commission (the Codex). The United States belongs to all three by formal international agreements. Over 130 nations specifically belong to the Codex, which has been in existence for about 30 years for the primary purpose of facilitating world trade in food. The Codex develops and disseminates standards and guidelines for quality and safety of foods. As these standards and guidelines are finalized and approved by the commission, treaty obligations require each nation to respond to them, by adopting them as laws or regulations; modifying them to meet national needs with appropriate explanations for any departures; or publicly announcing that any food that meets the standard or guideline may be imported.

Three committees of the Codex have major impacts on United States nutrition policy. The Committee on Nutrition and Foods for Special Dietary Uses (CCNFSDU) has developed many standards and guidelines that affect the United States, e.g., standards for infant formulas and baby foods, low sodium foods, medical foods, and formula foods for use in weight control diets, as well as guidelines, e.g., for weaning foods, and for addition of essential nutrients to foods. The Committee on Food Labeling (CFL) has finalized provisions for nutrition labeling. The new United States law on nutrition labeling and education, and the proposed implementing regulations, are in conflict with the Codex labeling standard. At this writing, it is not clear how this conflict is going to be resolved. The third committee is the Joint Expert Committee on Food Additives (JECFA), operated from FAO headquarters. Among other things, this committee establishes acceptable daily intakes (ADI) for many substances of nutritional significance, e.g., artificial sweeteners and preservatives. In promulgating food additive regulations, the FDA uses JECFA positions as a fundamental base for such regulations.

An informal group, known only as the Tripartite, is used to bring together regulators of food safety and quality, including nutritional quality, among the United States, Canada, and the United Kingdom, specifically involving the FDA's Center for Food Safety and Applied Nutrition (CFSAN), Canada's Health Protection Branch (HPB), and Britain's Department of Health and the Ministry of Agriculture, Fisheries, and Food. Their forums permit free exchange of policies with the purpose of harmonizing such policies wherever possible. The recent free trade agreement between the United States and Canada also has provisions that affect nutritional quality and labeling. Working groups currently are busy developing appropriate implementing approaches in accord with the agreement.

The International Union of Nutritional Sciences (IUNS) has the United States as an official member, through the Department of State. The IUNS is the union of nutrition scientists on a worldwide basis, and holds the International Congresses of Nutrition every 4 years. It also has many committees, e.g., the Committee on Nutritional Aspects of Food Standards (chaired by the author). The IUNS is officially advisory to WHO, FAO, and the Codex, and position statements developed by the IUNS do in fact influence outcomes from the Codex, e.g., relative to medical foods and nutrient additions to foods. These in turn influence United States policies.

State and Local Organizations. Thousands of committees on nutrition in the country at state, county, and local levels focus on all aspects of applied nutrition in their jurisdictions. Many individual school boards also have committees on nutrition, focusing particularly on the adequacy of school lunch and breakfast programs in the school systems for which they are responsible. At these same levels, the ES of the USDA operates agricultural extension programs in cooperation with state and county authorities. This USDA effort has long been influential at the local level, particularly through the county extension workers, with oversight provided by the land grant universities. Historically, their impact on nutritional well-being has been enormous, e.g., providing the foundation for teaching of home economics in schools and programs to teach youth the best farming practices. These USDA efforts continue today in much the same manner they have for many decades.

At the state level, one organization deserves special mention, i.e., the Association of State and Territorial Public Health Officials (ASTPHO). They have a functional nutrition committee that frequently consults at the federal level in matters concerning dietary guidelines, other public educational efforts in nutrition, and food safety issues related to nutrition.

The enormity of the nutrition activities at state and local levels through the abovementioned organizations, coupled with their individual independence, makes effective coordination difficult. Nevertheless, the totality of these organizations provides for networking, which does in fact occur, particularly through ASTPHO and the land grant universities.

Consumer Organizations. A great many consumer organizations in the United States are concerned with nutrition. Collectively, they are referred to as the "consumer advocacy community." Four such organizations are The Center for Science in the Public Interest (CSPI), headquartered in Washington, D.C.; the Community Nutrition Institute (CNI), in Washington; Public Voice for Food and Health Policy in Washington; and the American Council on Science and Health (ACSH), in New York, NY. All four take strong positions on various nutrition issues, and their voices are heard in the Congress, the federal courts, and the Administration, as well as before the public through the electronic and printed media. They all publish newsletter types of periodicals that receive wide circulation. The CSPI and CNI often take positions that are against recent governmental proposals or policies, and often question the adequacy of regulations on food safety and quality. The ACSH often takes the opposite tack, supporting the position that our food supply is of high quality and safety. In general, the positions of Public Voice are in between the extremes. A great deal of effort is devoted by the FDA and other regulatory agencies to responding to their petitions concerning regulatory proposals involving nutrition. They will likely have a lot to say about the regulatory proposals stemming from the new nutrition labeling and education law.

The Media. The media plays a huge role in shaping nutrition policies. In fact, in the author's opinion, the greatest power bases for such policies are the food industry, the Congress, and the media. Such influence by the media comes in multiple forms in both printed and electronic approaches.

Food advertising is a multibillion dollar industry, and advertising tends to be somewhat overstated as contrasted with labeling, which is more tightly constrained. No day goes by without publicity in the media for new food products claimed to have special nutritional attributes, particularly for reduction of risk of degenerative diseases. Hopefully, as the regulations stemming from the NLEA are implemented, the FTC will take a more constrained approach in this arena. A major positive phenomenon is also happening in the media; i.e., improvement in the quality of articles published by the nation's food editors in newspapers and major magazines. Creation of public fear is being replaced by more positive approaches to the public. Much of their detailed articles are also being reflected in condensed form in the electronic media.

One publication that deserves special mention is *Food Chemical News*, privately published in Washington, D.C., which, as stated on the masthead, is "a weekly publication providing indepth information regarding regulation of food, including additives, labeling, standards, contaminants, and feed." Each issue provides exactly what the authors say it does—up-to-date information on what is happening in Washington relative to food; it is remarkably authoritative.

THE SYSTEM

From the foregoing, it is clear no system for nutrition policy exists per se, nor is there likely to be one in the foreseeable future. What one has to learn, often the hard way, is that, if you want to play the game, you have to touch a lot of bases. Yet, as already noted, the bits and pieces when collected together do reveal a semblance of order. One can also separate the key components in a functional sense as distinct from an organizational sense. Such an overview follows.

LEGISLATION AND LOBBYING

One could reasonably expect that the Congress would be a major source of fundamental nutrition-related policies. Such leadership is sorely lacking and has been lacking for many years. The only really substantive congressional efforts go back to the Johnson and Nixon eras, with legislation for entitlement programs such as food stamps and the WIC Program. The value of these programs remains controversial, with three different points of view being expressed: (1) they are basic nutrition programs to reach the disadvantaged segments of society; (2) they are welfare programs with little or nothing to do with improvement of nutritional health; and (3) they are economic programs to assist in disposing of surplus food commodities such as butter, cheese, and dried milk accumulated by the USDA (Commodity Credit Corporation) from subsidized programs for the agricultural sector. I think they are all of these things concurrently, for better or worse. In defense of the WIC Program, the CDC developed data that demonstrate improved nutritional status of mothers and infants participating in the program as compared with controls, i.e., families eligible for participation but not participating. These programs are superimposed on the congressionally mandated School Lunch Program, which, in one form or another, has been in existence for over 40 years, and is now an ingrained part of our societal fabric.

No substantive efforts have been made to provide more resources for nutrition research, e.g., by requiring NIH to reprioritize to place more emphasis on nutrition, or to improve nutrition education in our public schools or in our health professional schools.

Four amendments to the FDCA have been passed during this period, all of which border on the bizarre for different reasons. In 1976, the Congress passed an amendment, commonly known as "the Proxmire Amendment," which in essence took away FDA authority to regulate the potency and composition of most vitamin, mineral, and other nutrient supplements. This action came about largely because of a massive lobbying campaign by the supplement industry, based on the incorrect argument that the FDA was trying by regulation to ban supplements from the marketplace. Actually, the FDA was trying to control potency and composition to minimize risk of nutrient intoxication and imbalances. Subsequent history has vindicated the FDA's position, e.g., recall the serious neurologic consequences of vitamin B_6 intoxication. The Proxmire Amendment is now section 411 (Vitamins and Minerals) of the FDCA.

Two other actions were the passage of the Infant Formula Act of 1980 and its amendment in 1986. It is now section 412 (Requirements for Infant Formulas) of the FDCA. It came about because, in 1978, one manufacturer made an error in formulation relative to sodium and chloride content, resulting in a number of cases of failure-to-thrive syndrome. Inherently, at first glance, nothing is wrong with the provisions of law. On closer examination, the amendments are not laws, they are detailed regulations right down to the amount of riboflavin that must be present per 100 kilocalories. The first result is that the FDA has had to promulgate 23 regulations to implement the law, and the regulatory process is not over yet. The second result is that the American infant formula industry is over-regulated. Everybody involved, from the industry, to the pediatric community, to the FDA, learned about human chloride deficiency the hard way, but 23 regulations and the huge expenditure of FDA and industry people resources are not needed to fix the problem. It was fixed the day the cause of this new syndrome was recognized and understood.

Finally, the NLEA of 1990,[2] commonly known as the "Metzenbaum/Hatch Amendment" to the FDCA, was passed on the last day of the 101st Congress, second session, while the Congress was trying to reconcile differences between the Congress and the administration over the national budget for FY 1991. It too is not a law in the conventional sense, i.e., authorizing legislation to proceed with mandatory nutrition labeling for most foods, but rather is a detailed regulation right down to the specific nutrients that must be declared as well as a long list of specific diseases that must be considered as to appropriateness for disease-specific claims on food labels, many of which were still clearly in the research phase, e.g., the role of folic acid in reduction of risk of neural tube defects. All of this is superimposed on actions by the FDA to accomplish the same objectives within the regulatory procedures of public rulemaking as is already required by law. The key FDA action was the proposed rule published July 19, 1990 in the FR and entitled, "Food Labeling; Mandatory Status of Nutrition Labeling and Nutrient Content Revision."[13] The details of the FDA proposal and the new law as they pertain to nutrition labeling and health messages are discussed subsequently. Two final points are worthy of note: (1) not one word is about education in the new law, so its name is a misnomer; and (2) at the last minute, without debate, additions to the draft amendment were made, e.g., by lobbyists representing the supplement industry, so the Proxmire Amendment surfaces again in different clothing.

On the other hand, another act, the National Nutrition Monitoring and Related Research Act (NNMRRA) of 1990,[3] is a constructive piece of legislation, as discussed in several other sections of this chapter.

RESEARCH

The specific activities of the many federal agencies conducting and/or supporting nutrition research are described elsewhere in this chapter. This discussion focuses on the nature of the overall system relative to nutrition research.

As described previously, the NIH and ARS are the cornerstones of federal nutrition research, accounting for a total of approximately $350 million annually in financial support. The level of support by the NIH is about three times that of the ARS. Comparatively speaking, all other parts of the federal establishment are small in this regard. The majority of NIH support is extramural, i.e., through their grant mechanisms, with grant approval occurring through the traditional NIH study section review process. Hence, in academia, most nutrition research supported federally is derived from the NIH. The ARS is the other way around; most USDA nutrition research is intramural in their various research centers located all over the country. The ARS and other USDA research focuses on the normal population and is generally of an applied nature. The NIH focuses primarily on basic mechanisms and on specific disease states. All of the other federal agencies, e.g., FDA, CDC, DOD, etc., conduct research in narrower areas related to their specific missions and to retain scientific competence within their walls. To this effort one must add the unmeasured but large investments by industry in nutrition research, both within their own establishments and in academia and much smaller amounts from private foundations.

Members of the nutrition science community frequently complain that the NIH expends only approximately 4% of its budget in support of nutrition research. Nevertheless, it is a fact that over the past decade or more, both the NIH and ARS support of nutrition research has increased gradually in addition to keeping up with inflation. There are, however, three "missing links." One is training. Little purpose is served in arbitrarily increasing funding levels unless people are available who can put it to use wisely. In FY 1988 for example, the NIH budget for training grants and fellowships in nutrition research amounted to just above $2.5 million. No specific nutrition research training program exists elsewhere at the federal level, although the USDA plays a significant role through its support of the land grant colleges and universities that have many of the nation's best departments of nutrition, food science, and food technology. This problem deserves serious attention, both within the executive branch and by the Congress.

A second "missing link" is the continuing decrease in fiscal and personnel support for nutrition research and epidemiology conducted by in-government agencies, particularly to components of the USPHS such as the FDA, CDC (including NCHS), and NIH. Recall for the latter that the level of intramural nutrition research is small. Even though the budgets themselves have remained fairly stable over the past decade, the actual "purchasing power," i.e., what you can get done with the resources available, has gone down badly, and little effort has been made to keep up with inflation. Intramural research and epidemiology are absolutely essential to maintaining scientific competence to achieve the specific missions of these agencies in pursuit of improvement of the public's health. In this regard, ARS has done a better job of keeping up their level of effort.

A third "missing link" is the absence of appropriations, i.e., money and people, as the Congress assumes the role as the basic instrument for establishment of nutrition policies for the nation. It is fundamentally important to reiterate that the Congress passes two kinds of laws, i.e., those that authorize and those that appropriate. One says "thou shalt," and the other provides resources. The flurry of activity in the Congress over the past few years has focused on authorizing, i.e., requiring, the executive branch to do many things, including nutrition research. Keep in mind the Nutrition Labeling and Education Act of 1990 (NLEA)[2] and the National Nutrition Monitoring and Related Research Act of 1990 (NNMRRA).[3] But appropriations to facilitate implementation are lacking. The end result is that the involved agencies "take it out of their hides" to free up the personnel to implement the requirements of the acts. The bureaucratic side of these agencies increases and research decreases—nothing unusual in the course of human events. For example, in a recession, industry cuts way back on research and development, including in the areas of food and nutrition. But it is a penny wise and pound foolish approach by both government and industry, particularly when the level of resources required is modest indeed, as is the case relative to nutrition research and epidemiology.

EPIDEMIOLOGY AND MONITORING

The reader is referred to discussions of specific agencies for details of epidemiologic and monitoring activities elsewhere in this chapter, with particular reference to the CDC, USDA, and FDA. Note also the section on nutrition policy, wherein the specific nutrition objectives for the nation for the year 2000 are outlined, most of which are based on epidemiologic and monitoring data. In fact, developing these objectives would have been impossible were it not for our extensive epidemiologic data bases.

Relative to food consumption, the only data on a national scale we had for many years were related to food disappearance, so there was no choice but to try to interpret these data in terms of human consumption. This situation remained until the middle 1970s, when we began to have multiple surveys of food intake combined with measurements of nutritional status, which allows review over time with multiple data points. Six surveys have been completed over a 25-year period, and in the next several years, a seventh set of data will become available. These have been mentioned in the sections on the CDC, FDA, and USDA, and in the following section. So at last, in the field of nutrition, we can virtually abandon disappearance data (except for trends concerning food commodities), and focus on interpretation of actual intake data combined with data on clinical nutritional status with physical, anthropometric, biochemical, radiologic, electrocardiographic, and similar data. This interpretation is precisely what led to developing the nutrition objectives for the year 2000.

In this regard, the United States is unique. Canada has had only one national nutrition survey, done in the early 1970s. The British are just beginning to develop data. It is extraordinary that most European nations still use commodity disappearance data to estimate human food consumption, because it is all they have with which to work. In so doing, huge errors can be made. To illustrate with a domestic problem in the United States, opponents of the use of sugars as a significant caloric source in our diet frequently use disappearance data and conclude that consumption is of the order of 155 g per person daily on a per capita basis, equivalent to about 125 pounds per year. To correct this absurd conclusion, from 1984 to 1986, the FDA undertook an exhaustive review of actual consumption data and published a report in 1986 providing the correct conclusion that consumption of sugars in the United States approximates 53 g per person daily, equivalent to about 43 pounds per year, i.e., a threefold difference compared with the use of disappearance data.[14] The same type of gross misuse of disappearance data applies to calories, and many nutrients. As another example, caloric availability is approximately 3400 calories per person daily, whereas average daily consumption for the total population is about 1800 calories per person.[14]

The passage of the NNMRRA in 1990 makes it crystal clear that nutrition epidemiology and monitoring are fundamental components of nutrition policy by both the Congress and the executive branch. The law itself requires many things.* It is self-evident that the requirements of this Act, coupled with those of the NLEA, are resource-intensive activities for the agencies involved. Let us hope that the resources required are forthcoming before the system collapses under its own weight.

*Requirements are as follows: (1) Development of a 10-year coordinated program and plan jointly by DHHS and USDA, including: continuation of the existing coordinating functions in each department; update of the 1981 implementation plan; establishment of a competitive grants program (from existing resources); establishment of a grants program to assist state and local governments to enhance their capacities (from existing resources); submission by the President of an annual interagency report on budgetary matters to the Congress; and submission to the Congress of a biennial report from the secretaries of DHHS and USDA on progress, policies, and priorities. (2) Establishment of a nine-member advisory council consisting of five members appointed by the President with recommendations from the secretaries, and four members appointed by the Congress. This Council has been established and the law requires that it submit annual reports to the secretaries. (3) The *Dietary Guidelines for Americans*[8] shall be updated by DHHS and USDA every 5 years. The dietary guidance portion of the law also requires secretary-level review of all guidance materials for the general public, and a report on the federal role in assuring that nutrition is a significant component of medical education for medical students and physicians.

The National Nutrition Monitoring System. Many nutrition-related efforts are made throughout the federal government to implement nutrition policies, and many of these are shared among various agencies. Only one such program is truly comprehensive and coordinated, i.e., the NNMS, a large activity that involves expenditures of many tens of millions of dollars per year.

Historically, our national capability to monitor the nutritional status of the American population actually started internationally as the result of war and was fostered in large measure by the defense establishment. By 1953, during the Korean conflict, a severe malnutrition problem among recruits into the Korean Army became patently obvious. Shortly thereafter, a similar problem was recognized in the Nationalist Chinese Army in Taiwan. The Army Nutrition Laboratory (ANL) in Denver assembled a team of nutrition experts to measure nutritional status of both military population groups. Problems such as calorie, thiamin, riboflavin, and vitamin A deficiencies were quickly documented, and corrective measures were instituted. Under the leadership of the late Frank B. Berry, then Assistant Secretary for Health of DOD, the ICNND was established in 1955, with the basic purpose of measuring the nutritional status of civilian and military populations in friendly developing countries.* The underlying premise of the ICNND was that malnutrition breeds insurrection and international instability, but corrective actions must be based on understanding nutritional status. During its 12-year life, the ICNND did nutrition surveys in over 30 developing countries all over the world. When it "died," the same cadre of leaders and experts had already undertaken surveys domestically, particularly among the Indian and Eskimo populations, and these same individuals set up and performed the Ten-State Nutrition Survey in the late 1960s, the first attempt to get a national picture of nutritional status in the United States. The results, coupled with the media-driven program called "Hunger USA," were fundamental factors in President Nixon's call for the White House Conference on Food, Nutrition and Health, which completed its report in late 1969. The Army and the ICNND deserve enormous credit for helping keep nutrition science and epidemiology alive during those years.

By 1970, the National Center for Health Statistics (NCHS) had absorbed the ICNND and Ten-State Nutrition Survey concepts, and organized the first truly national survey, i.e., The First National Health and Nutrition Examination Survey (NHANES I).[15] The NHANES program is based on national probability samples derived from the census, and has the basic purpose of collection and dissemination of data that can be obtained best or only by direct physical examination, clinical and laboratory tests, and related measurement

*The first director of the ICNND was Colonel Harold Sandstead, USAMC. After his untimely death, he was succeeded by Arnold Schaefer who recently also passed away.

procedures. Prevalence data are collected for specifically defined diseases or conditions of ill health, and normative health-related measurement data are collected to describe the health characteristics within the total population.

Subsequent to NHANES I, the concept of a NNMS gradually developed. In 1988, the administration-wide Interagency Committee on Nutrition Monitoring (ICNM) was established to enhance the effectiveness and productivity of federal nutrition monitoring activities. Cochairs are the Assistant Secretary for Health, DHHS, and the Assistant Secretary for Food and Consumer Services, USDA. Thirteen agencies are represented (NIH; FDA; two parts of CDC; four parts of USDA; AID; Bureau of the Census; Bureau of Labor Statistics; DOD; and the VA). In 1989, the ICNM published *Nutrition Monitoring in the United States: The Directory of Federal Nutrition Monitoring Activities,*[15] which provides a detailed description of the 50 individual programs that form the NNMS. The comprehensive nature of the NNMS is best illustrated by a list of its activities.*

The end result is an enormous data base concerning nutrition monitoring in the United States that is far more extensive than anywhere else in the world. Most of the individual data bases are readily available in data tape form as well as in the published literature.

The national policy to maintain this comprehensive monitoring system took on even greater significance by passage of the NNMRRA, enacted on October 22, 1990 (see previous description). The Interagency Board for Nutrition Monitoring and Related Research (IBNMRR) has now been put in place (and replaces the former Interagency Committee on Nutrition Monitoring). The chairmanships and memberships remain much the same, with some additions. It is splendid to have such strong congressional recognition of the importance of nutrition monitoring and related research. It is equally important to emphasize that this legislation is authorizing, not appropriating. Hence, no additional dollars are provided by the Act.

REGULATION

As pointed out previously, five agencies are involved in food and nutrition regulation. To summarize:

1. The FDA regulates food safety, quality, and labeling of all foods except meat and poultry, except as noted below.
2. The USDA regulates the safety, quality, and labeling of meat, poultry, and of eggs, until the egg is minimally processed. Thereafter, as the egg enters the food supply, the FDA takes over. The USDA also regulates the actual production of fresh produce. The FDA takes over when it reaches the consumer level.
3. The FTC regulates all food advertising.
4. The Environmental Protection Agency (EPA) regulates water, until such time as it enters interstate com-

*(1) Health and Nutrition Status Measurements. National Health and Nutrition Examination Survey: NHANES I (1971–1974) (by NCHS), NHANES II (1976–1980) (by NCHS), Hispanic HANES (1982–1984) (by NCHS), NHANES III (1988–1994) (by NCHS); National Health Interview Survey-Core Survey (annual) (by NCHS): Supplement on Aging (1984) (by NCHS), Supplement on Health Promotion and Disease Prevention (1985) (by NCHS), Supplement on Vitamin and Mineral Supplements (1986) (by NCHS), Supplement on Cancer Epidemiology and Cancer Control (1987) (by NCHS); NHANES I Epidemiologic Followup Study (1982–1984; 1986; 1987) (by NCHS); National Survey of Family Growth (1973–1974; 1976; 1982; 1988) (by NCHS); National Maternal and Infant Health Survey (1988–1990) (by NCHS); National Mortality and Natality Followback Survey (1987) (by NCHS); Vital Statistics System (annual) (by NCHS); National Hospital Discharge Survey (annual) (by NCHS); National Ambulatory Medical Care Survey (annual) (by NCHS); National Nursing Home Survey (1973–1974; 1977; 1985) (by NCHS); Pregnancy Nutrition Surveillance System (continuous) (by CDC); Pediatric Nutrition Surveillance System (continuous) (by CDC); Surveillance of Severe Pediatric Undernutrition (continuous) (by CDC); Behavioral Risk Factor Surveillance System (annual) (by CDC); Nutritional Evaluation of Military Feeding Systems and Military Populations (continuous) (by the Army Research Institute of Environmental Medicine [USARIEM]); Nutritional Status Surveys and Surveillance Systems (periodic) (by AID). (2) Food and Nutrient Consumption Measurements. Nationwide Food Consumption Survey (NFCS) (every 10 years, most recently 1987–1988) (by HNIS/USDA); Continuing Survey of Food Intakes by Individuals (CFSII) (1985–1986; 1986–1987) (by HNIS/USDA); Continuing Survey of Food Intakes by Individuals (CFSII) (1989–1996) (by HNIS/USDA); Total Diet Study (annual) (by FDA); Vitamin and Mineral Intake Survey (1980) (by FDA); Survey of Infant Feeding Practices (1989) (by FDA); NHANES Surveys (see Health and Nutritional Status Measurements); Nutritional Evaluation of Military Feeding Systems and Military Populations (see Health and Nutritional Status Measurements). (3) Food Composition Measurements. Food Label and Package Survey (FLAPS) (biennially) (by FDA); National Nutrient Data Bank (continuous) (by HNIS/USDA); Nutrient Composition Laboratory (continuous) (ARS/USDA); Total Diet Study (see Food and Nutrient Consumption Measurements). (4) Dietary Knowledge and Attitude Assessment. Health and Diet Survey (1982; 1984; 1986; 1988) (by FDA); Survey of Weight Loss Practices (1989) (by FDA); Diet-Health Knowledge Survey; Follow-on Survey to the Continuing Survey of Food Intakes by Individuals (annual) (by HNIS/USDA); Cholesterol Awareness Survey-Public Survey (1983; 1986; 1989) (by NHLBI/NIH); Cholesterol Awareness Survey-Physicians' Survey (1983; 1986; 1989) (by NHLBI/NIH); Nationwide Survey of Nurses' and Dietitians' Knowledge, Attitudes, and Behavior Regarding Cardiovascular Disease Risk Factors (1989) (by NHLBI/NIH); Basic Office of Cancer Communications National Knowledge, Attitude, and Behavior Survey (1988–1991) (by NCI/NIH); Cancer Prevention Awareness Survey: Wave I (1984) (by NCI/NIH); Cancer Prevention Awareness Survey: Wave II (1986) (by NCI/NIH); Prospective Survey of Infant Feeding Practices Among Primipara (1984–1986) (by NICHD/NIH). (5) Food Supply Determinations. U.S. Food and Nutrition Supply Series (annual since 1909) (by ERS/USDA); A.C. Nielsen Scantrack (monthly since 1985) (by USDA and FDA); Food Needs Assessment Project (1987–1990) (by AID). (6) Sociodemographic Measurements and Economic Indicators. Consumer Expenditure Survey (continuous) (by Bureau of Labor Statistics); Survey of Income and Program Participation (continuous) (by Bureau of the Census.

merce, e.g., on trains, airplanes, ships, etc. Then, the FDA takes over.

5. The NMFS regulates fish and shellfish production to a limited extent, but in practice, the FDA does most such regulation.

The actual statutes under which these agencies operate are often not explicit as to who has what responsibility. Some of these arbitrary dividing lines have come about through the passage of many years, plus informal agreements between agencies. Hence, the regulatory arrangements among agencies are not neat and tidy. In addition, at the level of the Congress, both oversight and appropriations are handled entirely differently for each of the agencies, further compounding the uncertainty. Nevertheless, the statutes and the regulations issued by these multiple agencies have a uniform theme, i.e., they are aimed at safety, quality, and the provision of information to the public that is truthful and neither false nor misleading. The most important element of these themes from a nutritional point of view is the provision of information to the public through labeling and advertising. Keep in mind, however, that nutrition does become involved in matters concerning safety and quality.

Safety surfaces in many different ways. One example is the decision-making process relative to approval or disapproval of artificial sweeteners and nonabsorbable or partially absorbable fat substitutes. Another is the banning or seizure of unsafe food substances, e.g., the elimination of a specific form of L-tryptophan from the marketplace because it proved to be the cause of numerous cases of eosinophilia-myalgia syndrome in 1990. A third type of approach is the FDA effort to reduce the iodine content of the American food supply, because the total amount in our diets far exceeds the RDA for iodine, and if it should increase further, we could reach potentially toxic levels. The FDA also has the authority to seize or ban dietary supplements if the potency of one or more nutrients exceeds safe levels.

Quality also has nutritional implications. The fat content of many meat products is regulated by the USDA according to a series of quality standards. Many food products regulated by the FDA must meet specific nutritional quality standards, e.g., infant formulas, enriched bread, milk and margarine, and iodized salt. All foods must be produced under the provisions of the Good Manufacturing Practices regulations of both the FDA and the USDA. In essence, these regulations require strict adherence to the use of "safe and suitable" ingredients, avoidance of microbiologic and environmental contamination, and the use of specific additives only at levels either prescribed by regulation as to upper permissible limits or at levels "not to exceed that required for its intended purpose." Such ingredients include many with nutritional attributes, e.g., everything from protein to salt. In the final analysis, however, the American public decide most quality issues, without regard to regulations. For the most part, they assume that, if the product is on the shelf, it is safe, suitable for human consumption, and nutritious. Remarkably, the food supply at the supermarket level is so diversified and tasty that it is difficult to procure and consume a diet that will not sustain life in the short term. Reduction of risk of contributing by dietary means to degenerative diseases is another matter.

EDUCATION

As noted several times in this chapter, all the components of a comprehensive national nutrition program with a relatively clear policy base exist, and function remarkably well in spite of the complexity of the overall system with one major exception—nutrition education. It is clear from recent legislation and the development of nutrition objectives for the year 2000 that nutrition education is a major part of our nutrition policy. The USDA has had this mission for many decades, the DHHS only recently.

Americans as a whole remain nutritionally illiterate. Whatever we have been doing is either wrong or grossly insufficient. We as a people seem to be incredibly susceptible to the massive amount of nutrition misinformation available through the media and from innumerable pressure groups. Every piece of nutrition quackery seems to get headlines, at the expense of solid scientific fact.

It seems strange that nutrition appears to be viewed as boring in educational settings, whereas, when asked, the citizenry in attitudinal surveys stress how important nutrition is to them in terms of maintaining good health. Americans have a fundamental understanding that nutrition is important and part of life every day, but no specific knowledge as to why this is so. The public already has difficulty understanding the nutrition information provided through nutrition and ingredient labeling, compounded by the overstatements found in advertising. I fear for the citizenry when confronted with the increased information that will appear on practically all foods in the marketplace over the next several years. How will they understand the significance of polyunsaturated and saturated fatty acid content labeling to their health, given their weak educational background? How will they understand that labeling of sugars content is aimed at reduction of dental caries, but not to reduction of risk of diabetes?

Approximately 30% of medical schools now have mandatory nutrition components in their curricula, and an additional 70% have nutrition incorporated in other courses often without student recognition of the importance of nutrition.

Nutrition education in public schools is generally nonexistent or poor, with some exceptions in individual communities. Where it does exist, it is rarely a part of overall health education, as called for in the nutrition objectives for the year 2000.

Why has the Department of Education not taken a leadership role in improving nutrition education in our country? Nutrition is part of science. Cannot it become part of national efforts to improve science education? The nutrition science community should bear a major responsibility for improving nutrition education at all educational levels, but particularly in our public schools. It certainly has not been involved in this area to any significant extent. Nutrition scientists, the teaching profession, and the Department of Education should join forces in a constructive manner to accomplish this objective.

PUBLIC ACTION PROGRAMS

The reader is referred to the various sections of this chapter addressing specific agencies for details of their action programs directed toward the public at large. It is virtually impossible to list them all, and it would be redundant. As in so many other areas of nutrition, the United States surely has the largest and most diversified levels of efforts of anywhere else in the world. The most important such efforts are: (1) The huge food assistance programs managed by the USDA, coupled with the food bank and other meal service programs derived from the private sector, including industry contributions. (2) The current efforts by the FDA and FSIS to improve food labeling. (3) Efforts by DHHS and USDA to publicize the *Dietary Guidelines for Americans.* (4) The National Cholesterol Education Program by NHLBI. (5) The National High Blood Pressure Education Program by NHLBI. (6) The efforts of the DOD to incorporate national nutritional concepts into military feeding systems and commissary systems worldwide for military personnel and their families. (7) Primary sustenance of the nutrition science base in support of all public health nutrition efforts.

COORDINATION

The Interagency Committee on Human Nutrition Research (ICHNR) was established in 1983 to coordinate and increase overall effectiveness and productivity of federally supported and federally conducted research in human nutrition. It was described in the section on the NIH. The ICHNR meets three times per year and manages the Human Nutrition Research Information Management System (HNRIMS) (a computerized system containing abstracts of every federally supported nutrition research effort). The ICHNR also sponsors biennial conferences on federally supported human nutrition research centers and units (e.g., the Clinical Nutrition Research Units or [CNRU] supported by the NIH), and prepares reports, including the Federal Five-Year Plan for Human Nutrition Research. The Division of Nutrition Research Coordination, NIH, has served as the Executive Secretariat since 1986. As the former FDA representative, I attest to the fact that it is truly effective.

The NNMRRA, enacted in 1990,[3] requires the Secretaries of DHHS and USDA to implement a 10-year coordinated nutrition monitoring and related research program, including a comprehensive plan, an interagency board, an advisory council, an annual budget report, and related reports to Congress, as well as other interagency collaboration. All of these requirements are being implemented. The new Interagency Board for Nutrition Monitoring and Related Research (IBNMRR) has replaced the former ICNM, originally established in 1988 to enhance the effectiveness and productivity of federal nutrition monitoring activities. The IBNMRR was described in the preceding section concerning epidemiology and monitoring.

As noted in the section concerning the USDA, coordination of nutrition activities is achieved in that department through their Subcommittee for Human Nutrition, a function of the Research and Education Committee of the Secretary's Policy and Coordination Council. All of the agencies involved with human nutrition participate in the work of the subcommittee.

In like manner, the DHHS has a Nutrition Policy Board, chaired by the Deputy Assistant Secretary for Health (Disease Prevention and Health Promotion), which meets regularly. Membership includes NIH, CDC, FDA, ADAMHA, HRSA, the Indian Health Service, the Administration on Aging, the Administration for Children and Families, and the Office of Consumer Affairs for the Department. Again, this Board is highly effective. For many years, the NIH has had its own Nutrition Coordinating Committee (NCC), which operates directly out of the Office of the Director, NIH.

Although DHHS and USDA are the central focal points for nutrition at the federal level, great efforts have been made in recent years to bring other agencies of government into the arena. Nutrition activities today at the federal level are about as well coordinated as one could reasonably expect. Certainly, no other country in the world has such a sophisticated and workable coordination effort.

THE POLICY

In spite of the enormous complexity of nutrition science and its application stemming from the federal establishment, all the pieces are there and do in fact come together in a recognizable way as national nutrition policy. I will not further comment on the role of the Congress, except to remind the reader that they are always there. As stated previously, the basic tenets of the policy must be, and usually are, the health and safety of our citizens.

For many decades, the United States has made a clear-cut commitment to nutrition research and epidemiology, as well as to regulation, action programs, and coordination. The weakest part of the overall commitment is in education. This latter component is beginning to get attention, but it has a long way to go.

The science base for our current policy rests on two basic documents: *The Surgeon General's Report on Nutrition and Health,* 1988[6] and *Diet and Health: Implications for Reducing Chronic Disease Risk,* 1989.[10] The policy itself is articulated in *Dietary Guidelines for Americans, 1990*[8] and the nutrition chapter of *Healthy People 2000, National Health Promotion and Disease Prevention Objectives*, 1990.[17]

The *Dietary Guidelines for Americans*, 1990 (3rd. Ed.)[8] is available in a 27-page brochure in lay language. Recommendations are as follows: (1) Eat a variety of foods. (2) Maintain healthy weight. (3) Choose a diet low in fat, saturated fat, and cholesterol. (4) Choose a diet with plenty of vegetables, fruits, and grain products. (5) Use sugars only in moderation. (6) Use salt and sodium only in moderation. (7) If you drink alcoholic beverages, do so in moderation. Canada has recently issued a similar set of dietary guidelines.[16]

Healthy People 2000 is a unique attempt to pull together all of the nation's health objectives for the year 2000, and is 692 pages in length.[17] The total document encompasses everything from oral health to tobacco to sexually transmitted diseases to clinical preventive services. No other nation has ever undertaken such a comprehensive review of preventive medical needs. The nutrition chapter is 24 pages in length; its key nutrition-related components are listed in Appendix Table A–16d.

Healthy People 2000 is concerned with keeping people well, not treating the sick. It is a statement of national opportunities. Although the USPHS facilitated its development, it is not intended as a statement of federal standards or requirements. That is why it is labeled "national," not just a federal, initiative to focus existing knowledge, resources, and commitment to capitalize on our opportunities to prevent premature death and needless disease and disability. It is a remarkable compilation of all the various aspects of nutrition from basic research to teaching in schools and providing services in the workplace, within the limits of what we know now. Presumably, it will be updated for the year 2010.

Nutrition generally is an arm of preventive medicine. Nevertheless, in many areas, nutrition is a component of therapeutic medicine. The NIH program has many activities concerned with patient treatment, undertaken also as part of federal nutrition policy. Lastly, in the latter category, industry supports and performs much of the research and development involved in nutritional management of critically ill patients, e.g., parenteral and enteral feeding, and the dietary management of low birth-weight infants and patients with inborn metabolic errors.

NUTRITIONAL ASPECTS OF FOOD LABELING

Many people think only of the nutrition label when the subject comes up. In reality, the food label has at least six separate, readily identifiable, nutrition-related components. These are: (1) the nutrition label itself (which in turn has three major components: the nutrients declared; the quantitative units used to declare the content; and serving sizes); (2) ingredient labeling; (3) adjectival descriptors, e.g., "low sodium;" (4) health claims; (5) labeling of foods for special dietary use, which frequently is substantially different from labeling of conventional foods; and (6) warning labeling. All are discussed subsequently. Health claims, or more correctly, disease-specific claims, are discussed in detail elsewhere in this chapter. Under law, "labeling" includes the food label itself along with associated materials, e.g., in-store placards and restaurant menus providing nutrition information; shelf labeling, e.g., using adjectival descriptors; and even pamphlets or books if made available to the public in close proximity to the point of sale of a specific food mentioned in the text. Many law suits initiated by the FDA have been won (or lost) on this legal definition of "labeling." This discussion of food labeling is limited to labeling of foods under the jurisdiction of the FDA that, for practical purposes, includes all food items except meat and poultry. The latter are under the jurisdiction of the USDA by law. The labeling approach by the USDA is similar to that of the FDA, but it differs in two major respects: (1) the current USDA system is more flexible, because of law and regulations; and (2) the USDA preapproves every label for meat and poultry products before marketing; the FDA does not have this authority under law (nor does it want such authority).

HISTORY

Consumer and professional interest in nutrition labeling came into focus in late 1969 at the White House Conference on Food, Nutrition, and Health. Different ways to present nutrition information on food labels were studied during 1970 and 1971. In 1972, the FDA proposed a system for nutrition labeling. Many comments from consumers, scientists, industry, and other government agencies were received, and the proposal was modified accordingly and issued as a final regulation in 1973.[18] Nutrition labeling began to appear in a substantive way in grocery stores in 1973, and its use has expanded greatly since then.[19] Hence, we have now had virtually 20 years of experience with nutrition labeling, and it has stood the test of time. Today, about 60% of the packaged food supply bears nutrition labeling, two thirds of which is voluntary by industry and one third is mandatory because the food is fortified with nutrients or a nutrition claim is made. As will be discussed, much is happening to alter this situation.

Ingredient labeling, i.e., the declaration of all ingredients in descending order of predominance, has been required on most foods for over 40 years. The only exceptions are certain standardized foods, i.e., foods with standards of identity for which the ingredients are fixed by regulation, but most such foods (e.g., enriched bread, mayonnaise) bear full ingredient labeling, either voluntarily by industry or because the FDA has modified the standards of identity to require such labeling.

The concept of defining the specific meaning of adjectival descriptors by regulation started in 1977 by a proposal to define "low" and "reduced" relative to calories for products promoted for reducing or maintaining body weight. The proposal was revised as a result of comments received and issued as a final order in 1978.[20] Next came a proposal in 1982 to define "low" and similar terms relative to sodium content. The proposal was revised and finalized in 1984,[21] providing definitions of "sodium-free," "very low sodium," "low sodium," and "reduced sodium." Finally, in 1986, the FDA proposed definitions of "cholesterol-free," "low cholesterol," and "cholesterol reduced."[22] The agency is trying to finalize the proposal currently (which must also be pursued under the provisions of the new NLEA.[2])

NUTRITION LABELING

The required contents and format for nutrition labeling are straightforward, as delineated in the Code of Federal Regulations.[23] Minor variations are permitted by the regulation. Currently, information must be declared in the order indicated in the footnote on this page.* The USRDA were developed specifically for food labeling purposes and are a simplified version of the recommended dietary allowances published by the Food and Nutrition Board of the National Academy of Sciences.[9] If a nutrient required to be declared is present in an amount of less than 2% of the USRDA, the percentage declaration can be replaced with an asterisk and a footnote added at the end of the list stating: "contains less than 2% of the USRDA of this (these) nutrient (nutrients)." There are many minor specifications in the regulation, but the core items are as noted here.

In July 1990, on its own initiative, the FDA issued proposals for major revisions in nutrition labeling.[13] Although the proposals contain innumerable details, the core items are listed in the footnote on this page.† These proposed changes were designed to provide consumers with information more in keeping with the current *Dietary Guidelines for Americans*[8] and similar recommendations. The macronutrient requirements were increased, and the required micronutrient requirements decreased. Also, in July 1990,[13] the FDA proposed related regulations. The RDA would be replaced with two new sets of reference values: (1) reference daily intakes (RDI) to replace the former USRDA, but still based on the Food and Nutrition Board RDA; and (2) daily reference values (DRV) to replace the Food and Nutrition Board's Estimated Safe and Adequate Daily Dietary Intakes (ESADDI). The new proposed DRV are for vitamins and trace minerals for which no RDA have been established, e.g., biotin and molybdenum. The ESADDI were difficult to deal with in labeling because they are ranges of values; the proposed DRV are single reference values. The FDA also proposed standardized serving sizes for a huge list of conventional foods, and proposed procedures for setting fixed serving sizes for other foods.

The Congress passed the NLEA late in 1990.[2] In fact, the new law is similar to the earlier 1990 FDA proposals. The only really fundamental differences between the act and the FDA proposals is the mandatory declaration under the law of complex carbohydrates and sugars. In addition, the act requires the secretary to issue voluntary nutrition labeling guidelines for raw agricultural commodities and raw fish, which was done in the FR of November 27, 1991.[5] These guidelines apply to 20 varieties of vegetables, 20 varieties of fruits, and 20 varieties of fish that are most frequently consumed. The act also sets up a procedure whereby, if compliance in due time is deemed inadequate, the secretary must by regulation make the guidelines mandatory. The act does not cover labeling of foods regulated by the USDA, but does exempt restaurant foods and foods prepared directly in retail establishments, e.g., salad bars in supermarkets. The basic problem with the existence of the law is that it is detailed, almost like a regulation itself. Regulations are difficult enough to change over time, but it can be done. Laws have a habit of staying unchanged unless some major event causes the Congress to reopen the matter.

The FDA issued a massive set of proposals in compliance with the requirements of the NLEA on November 27, 1991[5]; these collectively are the most voluminous proposals ever issued by FDA. The most fundamental point is that nutrition labeling will become mandatory for practically all packaged foods. The actual proposals emphasize: (1) the addition of sugars and complex carbohydrates to the list of required nutrients; (2) the prescription of a simplified form of nutrition labeling and the circumstances in which such simplified nutrition

*NUTRITION INFORMATION (CFR[23]):
Content: serving size in ordinary household measures, or per unit such as a slice; number of servings per container; macronutrients per serving (calories; protein [in grams and as percentage of the USRDA]; carbohydrate [in grams]; fat [in grams]; fatty acids [optional] [in grams as saturated and polyunsaturated]; cholesterol [optional] [in milligrams]; sodium [in milligrams]; potassium [optional] [in milligrams]; micronutrients per serving (all as percentage of the USRDA) (vitamin A; vitamin C; thiamin; riboflavin; niacin, calcium; iron; other vitamins and minerals [optional]).

†NUTRITION INFORMATION (July 1990 proposal[13]):
Content: serving size in ordinary household measures or per unit such as a slice; number of servings per container; macronutrients per serving (calories; calories from fat [not required if less than 1 g]; calories from saturated and unsaturated fatty acids [voluntary] [monounsaturated fatty acids can be separated from polyunsaturated fatty acids]; fat [in grams]; cholesterol [in milligrams]; carbohydrates [in grams]; calories from carbohydrate [voluntary]; complex carbohydrate [voluntary] [in grams]; sugar content [voluntary] [in grams]; fiber [in grams]; soluble and insoluble fiber [voluntary] [in grams]; protein [in grams]; calories from protein [voluntary]; sodium [in milligrams]; potassium [voluntary] [in milligrams]; micronutrients per serving (all as percentage of the RDI) (vitamin A; vitamin C; calcium; iron; other vitamins and minerals [optional]).

labeling must be used (i.e., when the food makes only trivial contributions to nutrient intakes); (3) allowing specified products to be exempt from nutrition labeling as indicated previously; and (4) the establishment of regulations for the nutrition labeling of vitamin and mineral supplements.

The FDA published the final orders concerning food labeling on January 6, 1993 effective at the retail level by 1994. The key provisions of the regulations are: (1) nutrition labeling becomes mandatory for practically all packaged foods (except meat and poultry); (2) nutrients will be declared in terms of RDI and DRV instead of USRDA; (3) the format of the nutrition label has been modified; (4) serving sizes for most foods have been standardized; and (5) label statements concerning macronutrients such as saturated fat and perjorative statements concerning competitive sources of fat will be tightly controlled.[47]

INGREDIENT LABELING

For about 50 years, the FDA has required that ingredients be listed on the label of all packaged foods regulated by the agency in descending order of predominance. Hence, for most products, consumers could figure out what was actually in the foods they purchased. A major medical reason for such ingredient listings is the ability to avoid ingredients to which an individual may be allergic, e.g., peanut-derived ingredients. However, a loophole in the actual FDCA allowed for ingredients of standardized foods to omit mandatory ingredients specified in food standard regulations, e.g., mayonnaise, ice cream, and bread. This issue is now almost moot for two reasons: (1) in the 1980s, the FDA by regulation modified the standards of identity for many foods, making all but the absolute basic ingredients optional; and (2) the 1990 NLEA closed this loophole except for spices and flavorings; colors must now be listed. Hence, virtually no packaged foods in the marketplace are without full ingredient disclosure. The USDA regulations for meat and poultry products are similar to those of the FDA in this regard.

Another facet of ingredient labeling relates to the presence of specific fats and oils. Since the middle 1980s, the FDA permitted so-called "and/or" labeling, i.e., a manufacturer could list that a product may contain one or more fats or oils, e.g., "may contain corn oil, cottonseed oil, soybean oil, and/or canola oil," following the statement that it does contain vegetable oil. This is a purely economic matter, because many manufacturers of processed food change the specific sources of oils in their products based on market price, and they may change many times per year. However, many complaints have been raised, particularly from the consumer advocacy communities, opposing this practice. Industry says rescinding this practice creates a labeling nightmare. The consumer advocacy community says that the consumer has no way of knowing if the product contains "tropical oils," for example, because sometimes it may, and other times it may not. The FDA has taken the position that the new requirement for declaration of total saturated fatty acid content renders the issue moot, and "and/or" labeling should be retained to minimize labeling costs that ultimately are borne by the consumer. The FDA plans to issue its proposal in this regard at a later date, but it will inevitably be controversial.

In 1989, the FDA also issued a policy that in essence said that for those ingredients present in a food at a level of less than 2% by weight, such ingredients could be listed at the end of the ingredient list without specifically being in descending order of predominance, because such ingredients are present in very small amounts.

A final matter concerning ingredient listing is the format. Currently, labels simply say "ingredients," followed by the list. Consumer studies have revealed that many individuals do not know that the list is in descending order of predominance, and that the phraseology could also be confusing. The FDA probably will propose that the ingredient list include something like, "from most to least." An ingredient deemed harmful to health if consumed in large amounts, e.g., highly saturated fats, can still sensibly be present in the food if the amount is small. Understanding this "from most to least" idea will help reduce the level of unnecessary concerns in the mind of the consumer.

ADJECTIVAL DESCRIPTORS

For many years, "low-fat" milks and similar dairy products have been available in the marketplace. The definitions of "low fat" for such products was established by standards of identity promulgated at both state and federal levels. For practical purposes, these were the only adjectival descriptors in existence until 1970. After the FDA developed the nutrition labeling regulation, it proceeded to consider regulations to define the meaning of additional adjectival descriptors. Two sets of such definitions have now been established by public rulemaking—one for calories and one for sodium.

CALORIES[24]

1. Foods may be labeled as "low calorie" only if a serving of the food supplies no more than 40 calories and not more than 0.4 calories per gram. The latter provision exists to prevent foods with small serving sizes such as candies from being labeled as "low calorie."
2. Foods may be labeled as "reduced calorie" only if a comparison of the calorie content of a specified serving of the food with the calorie content of an equivalent serving of the same food without the fabrication or alteration of special dietary significance reveals a calorie reduction of at least one third. In addition, the "reduced calorie" food must be nutri-

tionally equivalent to the food with which it is being compared.

SODIUM[25]

1. The term "sodium free" may be used on the label and in labeling of foods that contain less than 5 mg of sodium per serving.
2. The term "very low sodium" may be used for foods that contain 35 mg or less of sodium per serving.
3. The term "low sodium" may be used for foods that contain 140 mg or less of sodium per serving.
4. The term "reduced sodium" may be used for foods that have been formulated to serve and are represented as direct replacements for foods containing at least four times the sodium content (i.e., a 75% reduction).

CHOLESTEROL

The FDA has been struggling with definitions concerning cholesterol for at least a decade. In July 1990, the FDA proposed certain definitions.[26]

1. The terms "free of cholesterol," "cholesterol-free," or "no cholesterol" may be used for foods that contain less than 2 mg of cholesterol per serving, and 5 g or less total fat per serving, 20% or less total fat on a dry weight basis, 2 g or less saturated fatty acids per serving, and 6% or less saturated fatty acids on a dry weight basis. This proposal is a bit complicated, but two basic principles are involved: "cholesterol-free" labeling is linked to fat content so that such labeling would be prohibited on foods relatively high in fat content, and such labeling is also similarly linked to the saturated fatty acid content. The term "cholesterol-free" may also be used on foods that inherently contain no cholesterol, provided a label statement clearly refers to all foods of that type, e.g., "applesauce, a cholesterol-free food."
2. The terms "low in cholesterol" or "low cholesterol" may be used for foods that contain 20 mg or less of cholesterol per serving, 0.2 mg or less cholesterol per gram of food, and 5 g or less total fat per serving, 20% or less total fat on a dry weight basis, 2 g or less saturated fatty acids per serving, and 6% or less saturated fatty acids on a dry weight basis. The rationale for this complex definition is the same as for "low calorie" and "cholesterol-free." As for "cholesterol-free," the term "low cholesterol" may be used for foods that are inherently low in cholesterol provided a label statement clearly refers to all foods of that type, e.g., "low-fat cottage cheese, a low cholesterol food."
3. The terms "cholesterol reduced" or "reduced cholesterol" may be used for a food that has been specifically formulated or processed to reduce its cholesterol content by 75% or more from the food it resembles in organoleptic properties and for which it substitutes, provided that the label of such a food also bears clear and concise quantitative information comparing the product's per serving cholesterol content with that of the food it replaces, e.g., "cholesterol content has been reduced from 100 to 25 mg per serving." However, this complex history of cholesterol labeling became intertwined with the NLEA, and the whole concept was reproposed again in 1991.[27]

The biggest problem for the future in the area of so-called "avoidance characteristics" of foods is definition of terms pertaining to fat and saturated fat. The FDA has an informal definition of "low-fat," i.e., 2 g or less fat per serving and less than 10% fat on a dry weight basis, but it has not proposed this definition by rulemaking. The problem is compounded by two particular factors: (1) the old definitions of "low fat" for dairy products, which may no longer be valid for dietary control of fat intakes; and (2) differences of positions between the FDA and the USDA. The FDA has to deal with the dairy-derived foods, and the USDA has to deal with meat and poultry. From the USDA's perspective, it is difficult to visualize a low-fat chicken that would meet the FDA's informal definition. The controversy is in full swing at this writing. Not just the regulatory agencies are involved. The dairy, meat, and poultry industries are big and powerful, and the Congress is deeply involved. It may turn out that the term "low fat" may simply be unsuitable for meat and poultry products, and some form of standards of "leanness" may be needed, because it is unrealistic for meat and poultry products to be truly low in fat. This whole issue, including cholesterol labeling, is compounded by the uncertain state of the science base as it pertains to saturated fatty acids. Current research suggests that each individual fatty acid has its own metabolic role distinct from other fatty acids, and yet currently, they are all lumped together. We are in for a stormy decade on this issue.

As mentioned previously, the Congress is involved. The NLEA of 1990 specifically requires the secretary of DHHS to define by regulation the following terms, "used to characterize the level of any nutrient in food": (1) free; (2) low; (3) light or lite; (4) reduced; (5) less; and (6) high. The FDA has now issued extremely detailed proposals to define these terms.[28]

Until these regulations are finalized, no regulations are available for adjectival descriptors for the positive attributes of foods such as vitamins, minerals, protein, and fiber, as contrasted with avoidance characteristics of foods. The FDA does have informal positions (but keep in mind that the Congress now requires definition of "high"): (1) Vitamins and minerals (per serving): "source of" means 10% or more of the USRDA; "good source of" means 25% or more of the USRDA; "excellent source of" means 40% or more of the USRDA. (2) Protein (per serving): same as for vitamins and minerals. (3) Fiber (per serving): "fair source of" means 2 g or more; "good source of" means 5 g or more; "excellent source of" means 8 g or more.

This discussion of adjectival descriptors would be incomplete without mentioning the international scene. In the political era of free trade, the largest single item of commerce internationally is food for man and animals. At the UN level, the matter of adjectival descriptors is under debate currently, primarily in two committees of the Joint FAO/WHO Codex Alimentarius Commission (the Codex): the Committee on Nutrition and Foods for Special Dietary Uses (CCNFSDU) chaired by Germany, and the Committee on Food Labeling (CCFL) chaired by Canada. Only one set of definitions has been approved to date by the Codex, specifically for sodium, as follows: (1) "low sodium" means 120 mg/100 g of the food or less; "very low sodium" means 40 mg/100 g of the food or less. The dilemma is apparent because the sodium levels are different from the United States definitions, and the food quantity is different. We use servings; most of the rest of the world uses a 100-g basis. The United States has argued against the 100-g basis as a unique method of expression for years, but with little success. Sooner or later, these differences must be resolved to facilitate world trade.

FOODS FOR SPECIAL DIETARY USE

This category of foods has existed in regulations since World War II, and means exactly what it implies. The regulations governing such foods are codified in three parts of the Code of Federal Regulations in 21 CFR 105, 106, and 107 (the latter two covering infant formulas).[29–31] The term "special dietary use" means particular uses of food as follows:

1. Uses for supplying particular dietary needs that exist by reason of a physical, physiologic, pathologic, or other condition, including but not limited to the conditions of disease, convalescence, pregnancy, lactation, allergic hypersensitivity to food, underweight, and overweight.
2. Uses for supplying particular dietary needs that exist by reason of age.
3. Uses for supplementing or fortifying the ordinary or usual diet with any vitamin, mineral, or other dietary property.

Hence, the regulations govern labeling of foods such as dietary supplements, infant formulas and infant foods, hypoallergenic foods, and foods for reducing or maintaining caloric intake or body weight. Medical foods also fall under this category, but no governing regulations have been applied to date. Generally, if the food is in the form of a conventional food, e.g., diet soft drinks, the label bears conventional nutrition labeling. If they are in another form, such as tablets or liquid formulas, the label bears detailed information on actual nutrient composition. All such foods also disclose ingredients on the label.

INFANT FORMULAS

These deserve special mention. As noted previously, a manufacturer of infant formulas marketed two formulas in 1979 that had been formulated to reduce the sodium content as low as possible, at the height of professional and public concern relative to sodium and hypertension. The result was that the formulas were grossly deficient in chloride, and the first clinically recognized cases of failure-to-thrive syndrome associated with hypochloremic metabolic alkalosis in babies because of chloride deficiency were documented.[32] Some of the affected infants are still being followed by the NIH, and some appear not to have fully recovered. This event became a national incident and quickly resulted in Congressional action. The Infant Formula Act of 1980 became law as an amendment to the FDCA, and was expanded further by the Infant Formula Act of 1986. This action in turn resulted in the necessity for the FDA to propose and finalize eight separate regulations pertaining to quality control procedures,[30] and 15 separate regulations pertaining to labeling, exempt infant formulas, nutrient requirements, and infant formulas recalls.[31] Establishment of these regulations took the entire decade of the 1980s, and at this writing in 1992, more regulations remain to be finalized. The labeling requirements are detailed, both in terms of nutrient information and directions for use. The latter includes required pictograms for preparation and prominent statements such as, "The health of your infant depends on carefully following the directions for preparation and use," and "Use as directed by a physician."

The term *exempt infant formulas* is a bit of a misnomer, because these formulas are represented and labeled for use by an infant who has an inborn error of metabolism or low birth weight or who otherwise has an unusual medical or dietary problem. These formulas, however, are not exempt from any of the regulations, except for the nutrient requirements established for normal healthy infants, because the actual nutrient requirements for these special babies may differ from those of the normal infant. As noted previously, the end result is that the American infant formula industry is the most severely regulated component of the food processing industry. In fact, no segment of this industry anywhere in the world is so strictly regulated by any government. It is a perfect illustration of the enormous role of the Congress in establishing nutrition policy in the United States.

MEDICAL FOODS

Medical foods, which are almost identical in principle to infant formulas, are unregulated except for the general good manufacturing practices regulations that govern all processed foods. Medical foods are now defined in law, specifically by the Orphan Drug Amendments of 1988, which amended the FDCA and defined these foods as, "The term 'medical food' means a food which is formulated to be consumed or administered enterally under the supervision of a physician and which is intended for the specific dietary management of a disease or condition for which distinctive nutritional requirements, based on recognized scientific principles, are established by medical evaluation." In other words, these are the formulas used in every hospital usually for seriously ill patients, and are most frequently administered by the nasogastric, gastrostomy, or jejeunostomy route. Hence, they may be viewed as life-support systems, and are based on the medical concept that if the gastrointestinal tract is functional, use it, in preference to parenteral feeding.

Current thinking suggests five different types of products are involved: (1) nutritionally complete formulas; (2) modular formulas (i.e., formulas put together at the diet kitchen or pharmacy level from several or more components, but ultimately nutritionally complete); (3) inborn error products (as covered by regulation of exempt infant formulas, but for infants only); (4) oral rehydration solutions (mostly for severe diarrhea); and (5) very low calorie diets (fewer than 400 calories daily), because they too should be administered only under medical supervision. These products make explicit disease-related claims in labeling, and generally are marketed only through professional medical channels. They are therefore completely different from the matter of conventional foods bearing "health claims" in their labeling. The whole idea of medical foods is an American phenomenon, first conceived in 1971 by the author in the context of getting inborn error products out from under drug law and regulation and into regulation as foods for special dietary use. This in turn was based on the concepts that: (1) the nutritional principles on which such foods are based are well established, unlike the situation that exists for new drugs; and (2) the cost of approval through the drug route is enormous compared with the food route. So, today they are recognized as a type of food for special dietary use, even though, after 20 years, governing regulations are still lacking. In 1991, the Codex Committee on Nutrition and Foods for Special Dietary Uses (CCNFSDU) approved an international standard for these foods. Sooner or later, appropriate regulation of these products in the United States will result, because of the new CCNFSDU standard, because of unjustifiable manufacturer health claims for one or more commercial formulas, or because we have a medical catastrophe similar to the spark for the infant formula legislation and implementing regulations. That does not mean that regulation need be as detailed and severe as in the case of infant formulas, but some kind of assurance of safety and suitability for their intended uses is needed. The FDA is now taking steps to develop a regulatory policy for medical foods that most likely will come about through public rulemaking sometime in 1992 or 1993.

WARNING LABELING

The FDA and USDA have been conservative in the use of warning labeling on conventional foods, and wisely so. The primary motive in such conservatism is avoidance of creation of unnecessary fear in the minds of consumers. Therefore, strikingly few examples of use of such labeling can be cited. The presence of a food ingredient not deemed safe in a public health sense is illegal in the first place. Only three warnings are of any significance (plus two consumer alerts).

1. Saccharin warning labeling. By act of Congress, all food products that contain saccharin must bear a prominent label statement as follows: "Use of this product may be hazardous to your health. This product contains saccharin, which has been determined to cause cancer in laboratory animals." This statement is specifically required by section 403(o)(2) of the FDCA, and in turn stems from the infamous Delaney Clause, codified as section 409(c)(3)(A), which states, "no additive shall be deemed to be safe if it is found to induce cancer when ingested by man or animal." The labeling requirement by Congress is in fact contrary to the Delaney Clause. When the FDA tried to ban saccharin because of the extreme nature of the Delaney Clause, Congress promptly pre-empted the agency by permitting saccharin to be used as a food additive with the accompanying warning statement. The Delaney Clause issue has received a great deal of attention over the past decade, and sooner or later, it may be rescinded or modified because the science base no longer supports it.

2. Protein product warning. In the late 1970s, a series of sudden deaths of obese individuals, mostly young women, consuming high protein, very low calorie diets (VLCD) occurred. Use of such diets resulted from popularization in the lay press of the idea of achieving rapid weight loss with such a regimen. For those cases in which cause of death could be determined, it proved to be from acute ventricular tachycardia. The actual mechanism of death remains unclear, although perhaps the best working hypothesis is that the basic cause is probably acute cardiomyofibrillar protein depletion. To date, proceedings against promoters of these diets continue in the courts. As a result of these deaths, the FDA promulgated warning labeling requirements for such products. Specifically, "The label and labeling of any food product in liquid, powered, tablet, capsule, or similar forms that derives more than 50% of its total caloric value from either whole protein, protein hydrolysates, amino acid mixtures, or a combination of these, and that is represented for use in reducing weight shall bear the following warning: *Warning: Very low calorie protein diets (below 400 calories per day) may cause serious illness or death. Do not use for weight reduction in such diets without medical supervision. Not for use by infants, children, or pregnant or nursing women.*"[33] The regulation goes on to point out that such protein products represented as part of a nutritionally balanced diet plan providing 400 or more calories per day and the label or labeling provides *information about the total diet are exempt from this strong warning statement, but the label or labeling must bear the following statement: "For weight reduction, use only as directed in the accompanying diet plan. Do not use in diets supplying less than 400 calories per day without medical supervision."* The FDA originally proposed that the caloric limit should be 800 calories rather than 400, because, although no documented deaths occurred in association with diets over 400 calories, a margin of safety would be desirable, as is the case with most other medical issues. Nevertheless, when the issue was before the federal courts, the FDA lost and the court decided on the 400 calorie value. Fortunately, few of these VLCD are now marketed in the United States.

3. Phenylalanine warning. When the sweetener aspartame was approved as a food additive in 1983, the FDA required that all products containing the additive bear a conspicuous label statement, "Phenylketonurics: Contains Phenylalanine."[34] The reason is straightforward, i.e., aspartame is a dipeptide consisting of aspartic acid and phenylalanine with a methyl group in between, and, phenylketonuric individuals must avoid unnecessary intakes of phenylalanine. Fortunately, such persons and/or their families are thoroughly familiar with this dietary requirement.

4. Sulfite alert. In the middle 1980s, sudden deaths, usually of an anaphylactic type, occurred in otherwise healthy people that ultimately proved to be associated with exposure to sulfites used in a variety of foods for preservation of freshness and color or for prevention of browning or melanosis. The FDA established a tracking system to document all suspected cases, which continues. Once the cause was known and widely publicized, the number of new cases declined precipitously. Few reports of injury have occurred since 1986; the latest death was noted in 1988. Of a total of 27 deaths, 17 were clearly attributable to sulfite exposure. In 1985, the FDA decided to regulate the use of sulfites on a commodity-by-commodity basis, and proposed a ban on the use of sulfites to preserve color and freshness of fresh fruits and vegetables. The ban was finalized in 1986, resulting in the cessation of spraying in supermarkets and salad bars. Concurrently, the FDA required that the ingredient list for canned and dehydrated fruits and vegetables include the presence of sulfites if used. The FDA also retained the maximum level of sulfites in shrimp at 100 ppm, used to prevent melanosis (black spotting), and tightened its compliance activities in this regard. However, in these proceedings, the FDA excluded potatoes at that time because of the lack of viable alternatives to the use of sulfites. In 1987, the FDA proposed to revoke the GRAS (generally recognized as safe) status of sulfites used on fresh, unpackaged, and unlabeled potatoes. This action would have had the effect of banning its use until such time as a food additive petition for its safe use was approved. This rule was finalized in 1990, but the FDA was sued in court and lost. In 1991, after appeal, the FDA lost again, largely on the basis that the legal record was deemed inadequate. The FDA now plans to repropose, with the thought that the legal record is now solid. One other facet of the sulfite matter is that in 1989, the Bureau of Alcohol, Tobacco and Firearms (BATF) of the Department of the Treasury required that all wine in which sulfites are used bear a label that declares "contains sulfites." With this phrase, the latter becomes a type of warning labeling, whereas where permitted in foods regulated by FDA, sulfites must simply be declared in the ingredient list. In spite of the complexity of the issue, the sulfite alert is a good example of a lethal health hazard being brought under control by regulation and publicity in a relatively short time.

5. Radiation alert. When a food has been treated with ionizing radiation, the label must bear the international logo indicating that such treatment has been applied, plus the statement "treated with radiation" or "treated with irradiation." Technically, this is not a warning statement because of the lack of health implications, but rather is simply a consumer alert because many consumers are still apprehensive about the idea of consuming irradiated food. The FDA began to approve specific uses of food irradiation in 1983. As of 1986, the following uses had been approved[35]: (1) for control of *Trichinella spiralis* in pork at a maximum dose of 0.3 kGy; (2) for growth and maturation inhibition of fresh foods at a maximum dose of 1 kGy; (3) for disinfestation of arthropod pests in food at a maximum dose of 0.3 kGy; (4) for microbial disinfection of dry or dehydrated enzyme preparations at a maximum dose of 10 kGy; and (5) for microbial disinfection of dry or dehydrated aromatic vegetable substances (herbs and spices) at a maximum dose of 30 kGy. These values represent relatively low-dose applications of irradiation and are not for purposes of sterilization. More recently, low-dose irradiation of fresh chicken has also been approved, primarily for salmonella control. In fact, little irradiated food is present in the American marketplace, largely because of the widespread false belief that irradiation renders the food radioactive. Nevertheless, it is reasonable to predict the eventual widespread use of irradiation, particularly for disinfestation of flours, prolongation of shelf life of fresh produce, and salmonella control in poultry. It is already applied in many parts of Europe and elsewhere in the world. As of January 25, 1992, irradiation-preserved strawberries appeared on supermarket shelves in the Miami Beach, Florida area. Many hospital and home use medical products, such as gauzes, band-aids, etc., are treated with high-dose irradiation to achieve sterility, and whole diets treated with sterilizing doses are now permitted in hospital settings for patients with compromised immunity who are in a germ-free environment.

HEALTH CLAIMS IN FOOD LABELING

BASIC FACTS

Health claims in food labeling is a bureaucratic description of disease-specific claims in labeling of conventional foods, e.g., claims that consumption of certain high-fiber cereals will reduce the risk of some forms of cancer. The term *health claims* has now superseded but is synonymous with "health messages."

The FDCA governs food labeling, except for meat and poultry, and the enforcement agency is the FDA. The FDA also acts in labeling under the authority of the Federal Fair Packaging and Labeling Act, but it does not have premarketing label approval authority. The FDA regulates about three quarters of the packaged food supply, the remaining quarter being meat and poultry, which is regulated by the USDA. This agency regulates its labeling under the authority of the Federal Meat Inspection Act, the Poultry Products Inspection Act, and the Federal Fair Packaging and Labeling Act. The USDA does have premarket label approval authority, and, in fact, reviews every label before it enters the marketplace. The philosophies behind the two sets of laws for the two agencies are different in many respects. Neither of these agencies has authority over food advertising. This arena is regulated by the FTC, and again, the basic legal foundation for this agency is different indeed from the other two, because each of the three agencies exist for different purposes. However, all three agencies operate under laws that prohibit false and misleading labeling or advertising.

Another basic factor, often poorly understood, is that laws require that implementing regulations be promulgated by public rulemaking in the case of labeling. In other words, the details of what is expected of industry must be spelled out along with compliance criteria, i.e., what FDA and USDA will do in the case of infractions of the regulations. Regulations have the force of law unless overturned by federal courts. A fact of life stemming from our enormously complicated system of checks and balances is that public rulemaking is difficult and time consuming. At a minimum, such rulemaking requires that the agencies publish proposals in the FR for public comment, the comments are reviewed in infinite detail, and a final rule is published that must also respond to the comments received. If the concept behind the proposal is complex, it frequently is necessary to publish a series of proposals, before a final rule can be fully designed. Even then, final rules are subject to suits in federal courts. Final rules are rarely adopted in less than 2 years, and the process can take 5 to 10 years. Ultimately, all final rules are incorporated into the Code of Federal Regulations (CFR).

HISTORY OF "HEALTH MESSAGES"

Relative to labeling, the FDCA remained unchanged since 1938, until recently. Before 1970, the FDA prohibited any form of nutrition-related claim in food labeling (except for foods for special dietary use, e.g., infant formulas and dietary supplements to prevent deficiency diseases). Up to the moment, the issue of "health messages" in labeling is limited to the FDA, i.e., it has not spilled over into the meat and poultry areas regulated by the USDA. Labeling was limited to providing the common or usual name of the food, plus its fanciful name, the ingredients, the name of the manufacturer, directions for preparation, and the like. The White House Conference on Food, Nutrition and Health in 1969 substantially changed this status quo, and we entered the era of "implicit health claims" consisting primarily of nutrition labeling and the use of adjectival descriptors such as "reduced calorie." Still, specific diseases were not mentioned, because it was generally understood that disease-specific claims would render the product a drug.

Food labeling changed precipitously in October 1984 when the Kellogg Company, in cooperation with the National Cancer Institute (NCI) of the NIH made, on its own initiative, specific claims on several high-fiber cereals inferring a link between high-fiber intakes and reduction of risk of certain cancers. This action caught the FDA off guard. The basic question arose as to whether we should practice medicine on the back of the cereal box or elsewhere in labeling. Shortly thereafter, numerous other firms entered the disease-specific labeling arena and the subjects expanded to include calcium and osteoporosis, fat and heart disease, sodium and hypertension, etc. This author publicly raised the dimension of the issue in 1985.[19] A perception arose that the FDA was not going to do much about it. Much public debate surfaced, and in 1987, the FDA issued an "Advance Notice of Proposed Rulemaking" concerning health messages.[4] This publication laid out a number of options for public comment. Finally, in February 1990, the FDA issued a Reproposed Rule on health messages,[36] which proposed criteria that must be met to avoid false or misleading claims, e.g., "The label statement is consistent with generally recognized medical and nutritional principles for a sound total dietary pattern." This proposal also laid out a multicomponent scheme on how to reach a satisfactory consensus on what would be appropriate for labeling claims. This scheme included: (1) development of authoritative scientific summaries for specific diet-nutrient-disease relationships; (2) consumer health message summaries, which would be a consumer-oriented summary of the scientific summaries; (3) development of model label statements to guide industry; (4) development of a comprehensive consumer guide to the health-related aspects of food labeling; and (5) establishment of a PHS Committee on Health Messages to provide general oversight to the whole process. The proposal specifically identified six topics deemed appropriate for possible labeling claims. Concurrently, the FDA issued proposed rules and tentative final rules designed to strengthen parts of the earlier era of "implicit health claims" relating to cholesterol labeling, new USRDA for labeling purposes, mandatory nutrition labeling, and standardized serving sizes.

THE PRESENT

In November of 1990, Congress passed and President Bush signed into law the NLEA,[2] the first major labeling amendment to the FDCA in many years. Five major components of the act impact on "health claims": (1) It significantly modifies most of the FDA proposals issued earlier in 1990, requiring reconsideration of many specific topics by the FDA; (2) It retains the original six disease-specific topics, and adds four more for consideration; (3) It requires the secretary of the DHHS to consider separate rules for "health claims" for dietary supplements of vitamins, minerals, herbs, or other similar substances. (4) It requires the establishment of a public petition process for issuing regulations for new "health claims"; (5) It establishes rigid time requirements for the FDA to propose and finalize implementing regulations.

On January 6, 1993, the FDA also finalized its positions on disease-specific health claims, which are briefly summarized; (1) fiber and cancer[39]: *not authorized* (but claims are authorized for cereal grains, fruits, and vegetables); (2) fiber and cardiovascular disease[40]: *not authorized* (but claims are authorized for cereal grains, fruits, and vegetables); (3) folic acid and neural tube defects[42]: *not authorized;* (4) antioxidant vitamins and cancer[37]: *not authorized* (but claims are authorized for fruits and vegetables; (5) Zinc and immune function[46]: *not authorized;* (6) calcium and osteoporosis[38]: *authorized;* (7) omega-3 fatty acids and coronary heart disease[44]: *not authorized;* (8) saturated fat, cholesterol, and coronary heart disease[43]: *authorized;* (9) fat and cancer[41]: *authorized;* (10) Sodium and hypertension[45]: *authorized.*

On the one hand, the NLEA implies strict control by the FDA and DHHS over any disease-specific claims. On the other hand, it adds four topics for review that most authorities consider to be in the area of continuing biomedical research with varying degrees of consensus. In addition, it implies a looser control over dietary supplements, a troublesome area for the FDA for many years. The tight time constraints for proposals and final orders is most difficult to attain given the complexity of public rulemaking.

The FDA contracted with the LSRO of FASEB to prepare reviews of the total of 12 disease-specific areas[12] that will contribute to the development of the scientific summaries just specified. The LSRO reviews were issued in February 1992; their conclusions are similar but not the same as the FDA proposals. No doubt, these differences will be brought out as the debate toward final rules unfolds. The FDA issued in the FR its proposals for "health claims," including review of all 10 issues required by the NLEA;[37–46] its key decision on each issue.

The passage of the Dietary Supplement Act of 1992 provides for a moratorium on FDA actions against disease-specific claims on dietary supplements until December 31, 1993. The FDA is required by the Act to publish a proposal on such claims for supplements by June 15, 1993 and to finalize such regulations by December 31, 1993. It is also likely that the Congress will introduce permanent legislation in 1993 to reduce the FDA's authority to control disease-specific claims and nutrient potencies for dietary supplements (including herbal products). If the legislation passes, the nutrition science community will have a big problem.

Both the earlier FDA proposals and the new NLEA have made the food industry more cautious about making disease-specific claims in labeling for the moment, but it remains to be seen how long this trend will last. It is also reasonable to anticipate that efforts by the FDA and DHHS to finalize rules governing health claims will be contested in federal court. Hence, the decade of the 1990s will be controversial relative to the label of conventional foods as a means of giving advice to the public on dietary means of reducing risk of degenerative and other diet-related diseases.

REFERENCES

1. White House Conference on Food, Nutrition and Health—Final Report (1970). Superintendent of Documents, (1970; 0-378-473). Washington, D.C., Government Printing Office, 1970.
2. Nutrition Labeling and Education Act of 1990. Public Law 101-535, November 8, 1990, 104 Stat. 2353, 21 USC,301 note, 321, 337, 343, 343 notes, 343-1, 343-1 note, 345, 371.
3. National Nutrition Monitoring and Related Research Act of 1990. Public Law 101-445, October 22, 1990, 104 Stat. 1034, 7 USC, 5301. 5301 note, 5302, 5311-5316, 5331, 5332, 5341, 5342.
4. Food labeling; public health messages on food labels and labeling; notice of proposed rulemaking. 52 Federal Register 28843, August 4, 1987.
5. Food labeling; general provisions; nutrition labeling; nutrient content claims; health claims; ingredient labeling; state and local requirements; and exemptions; proposed rules. 56 Federal Register 60366, November 27, 1991.
6. The Surgeon General's Report on Nutrition and Health (1988). U.S. Department of Health and Human Services, Public Health Service, DHHS (PHS) Publ. No. 88-50210. Superintendent of Documents, Stock No. 017-001-00465-1. Washington, D.C., Government Printing Office, 1988.
7. 12th Annual Report of the National Institutes of Health Program in Biomedical and Behavioral Nutrition Research and Training, Fiscal Year 1988. National Institutes of Health, NIH Nutrition Coordinating Committee, Division of Nutrition Research Coordination, NIH Publ. No. 89-2092, September 1989.
8. Dietary Guidelines for Americans. USDA Home and Garden Bulletin No. 232. 3rd Ed. Washington, D.C., Government Printing Office (1990-272-930), 1990.
9. Recommended Dietary Allowances. 10th Ed. Washington, D.C., National Academy Press, 1989.
10. Diet and Health: Implications for Reducing Chronic Disease Risk, 1989. Washington, D.C., National Academy Press, 1989.
11. Nutrition Labeling—Issues and Directions for the 1990s, 1990. Washington, D.C., National Academy Press, 1990.
12. Life Sciences Research Office, Federation of American Societies for Experimental Biology: Evaluation of Publicly Available Scientific Evidence Regarding Certain Nutrient-

Disease Relationships. Prepared under FDA Contract No. 223-88-2124. Bethesda, MD, 1991. (a) Roe, D.A.: Folic acid and neural tube defects; (b) Beisel, W.R.: Zinc and immune function in the elderly; (c) Heaney, R.P.: Calcium and osteoporosis; (d) Kotchen, T.: Sodium and hypertension; (e) Kritchevsky, D.: Dietary fiber and cancer; (f) Kritchevsky, D.: Dietary fiber and cardiovascular disease; (g) Connor, W.E.: Omega-3 fatty acids and heart disease; (h) Ross, A.C.: Vitamin A and cancer; (i) Sauberlich, H.E.: Vitamin C and cancer; (j) Chow, C.K.: Vitamin E and cancer; (k) Grundy, S.M.: Lipids and cardiovascular disease; (l) Carroll, K.K.: Lipids and cancer.

13. Food labeling; mandatory status of nutrition labeling and nutrient content revision; proposed rule. 55 Federal Register 29487, July 19, 1990.
14. Glinsmann, W. H., Irausquin, H., Park, Y.K.: J. Nutr., *116:*S1, 1986.
15. Nutrition Monitoring in the United States: The Directory of Federal Nutrition Monitoring Activities. National Center for Health Statistics. DHHS Publ. No. (PHS) 89-1255-1.
16. Nutrition Recommendations—The Report of the Scientific Review Committee, Health and Welfare Canada (1990). Ottawa, Canadian Government Publishing Centre, Cat. No. H49-42/1990 E; ISBN: 0-660-13417-9, 1990.
17. Nutrition. *In* Healthy People 2000—National Health Promotion and Disease Prevention Objectives. Washington, D.C., Government Printing Office (287-302/21332, S/N 017-001-00474-0), 1991.
18. Part I. Regulations for the enforcement of the Federal Food, Drug and Cosmetic Act and the Fair Packaging and Labeling Act; nutrition labeling. 38 Federal Register 2125, January 19, 1973.
19. Forbes, A.L.: Am. J. Clin. Nutr., *43:*629, 1986.
20. Part 105—Foods for special dietary use; label statements; final order. 43 Federal Register 43248, September 22, 1978.
21. Food labeling; declaration of sodium content of foods and label claims for foods on the basis of sodium content; final rule. 49 Federal Register 15510, April 18, 1984.
22. Food labeling; definitions of cholesterol free, low cholesterol and reduced cholesterol; proposed rule. 51 Federal Register 42584, November 25, 1986.
23. Nutrition labeling of food. Title 21, Code of Federal Regulations, Section 101.9.
24. Label statements relating to usefulness in reducing or maintaining caloric intake or body weight. Title 21, Code of Federal Regulations, Section 105.66.
25. Sodium labeling. Title 21, Code of Federal Regulations, Section 101.13.
26. Food labeling; definitions of the terms cholesterol free, low cholesterol, and reduced cholesterol; tentative final rule. 55 Federal Register 29456, July 19, 1990.
27. Food labeling; "cholesterol free", "low cholesterol", and "________ percent fat free" claims; proposed rule. 56 Federal Register 60507, November 27, 1991.
28. Food labeling; nutrient content claims, general principles, petitions, definition of terms; proposed rule. 56 Federal Register 60421, November 27, 1991.
29. Part 105. Foods for special dietary use. Title 21, Code of Federal Regulations, Sections 105.3 through 105.69.
30. Part 106. Infant formula quality control procedures. Title 21, Code of Federal Regulations, Sections 106.1 through 106.120.
31. Part 107. Infant formula. Title 21, Code of Federal Regulations, Sections 107.3 through 107.280.
32. Willoughby, A., Moss, H.A., Hubbard, V.S., et al.: Pediatrics, *79:*851, 1987.
33. Food labeling warning and notice statements. Title 21, Code of Federal Regulations, Section 101.17(d).
34. Aspartame. Title 21, Code of Federal Regulations, Section 172.804.
35. Ionizing radiation for the treatment of food. Title 21, Code of Federal Regulations, Section 179.26.
36. Food labeling; health messages and label statements; reproposed rule. 55 Federal Register 5176, February 13, 1990.
37. Food labeling; health claims and label statements; antioxidant vitamins and cancer; proposed rule. 56 Federal Register 60624, November 27, 1991.
38. Food labeling; health claims; calcium and osteoporosis; proposed rule. 56 Federal Register 60689, November 27, 1991.
39. Food labeling; health claims; dietary fiber and cancer; proposed rule. 56 Federal Register 60566, November 27, 1991.
40. Food labeling; health claims; dietary fiber and cardiovascular disease; proposed rule. 56 Federal Register 60582, November 27, 1991.
41. Food labeling; health messages; dietary lipids and cancer; proposed rule. 56 Federal Register 60764, November 27, 1991.
42. Food labeling; health claims and label statements; folic acid and neural tube defects; proposed rule. 56 Federal Register 60610, November 27, 1991.
43. Food labeling; health claims and label statements; lipids and cardiovascular disease; proposed rule. 56 Federal Register 60727, November 27, 1991.
44. Food labeling; health claims and label statements; omega-3 fatty acids and coronary artery disease. 56 Federal Register 60663, November 27, 1991.
45. Food labeling; health claims and label statements; sodium/hypertension. 56 Federal Register 60825, November 27, 1991.
46. Food labeling; health claims; zinc and immune function in the elderly. 56 Federal Register 60652, November 27, 1991.
47. Fed. Reg., *58:*2066–2941, 1993.

Appendix

Abby Stolper Bloch and Maurice E. Shils

The Appendix for this edition has been appreciably revised and updated since the seventh edition. It has been divided into two segments. The first part provides basic reference data, various national and international recommendations, energy and nutrient requirements, and height and weight as well as body composition data. The second part is composed of tabular information on nutrient contents of various foods and diets for various disease entities. As always, such dietary prescriptions may require modification in accordance with the clinical status and reactions of the individual patient. An expanded section on supplemental exchange lists has been included in this edition. In addition, a listing of current commercially available nutrition formulations with manufacturer information is provided.

Past editions have included detailed formulations of commercially available dietary products for oral and tube-feeding purposes. Because such listings have been widely adopted and widely circulated by various companies and because revisions of such formulations are frequent, we have decided to eliminate such detailed data. Instead, Table A–37 simply lists the types and names of current formulas and provides the addresses and phone numbers where the latest information may be obtained.

In the following Appendix table of contents, section and subsection titles are given with designating numbers. The specific tables under these headings are designated by letter and/or number. In the text, each table has a designation specifying the section, subsection, and table.

APPENDIX CONTENTS

TABLE A—1A. CONVERSION FACTORS BETWEEN TRADITIONAL AND SI UNITS

Factors for converting nutrients expressed in metric or millequivalent units into International System (SI) units.

1. Definitions

- **a.** Equivalent weight (EW) = atomic weight of element/valence of ionic form. Example with magnesium: atomic wt = 24, valence = 2+; therefore EW = 12
- **b.** Quantity of an electrolyte in milliequivalents per liter (mEq/1) = mg of electrolyte/L/EW. Example: 48 mg of magnesium/L/12 = 4 mEq/L
- **c.** Quantity of an electrolyte in mg/dl = (mEq/L × EW)/10
- **d.** To convert mg/dl (= mg%) of an electrolyte to mEq/L mg/dl × 10/EW = mEq/L
- **e.** 1 mol = 1 molecular or atomic weight of element or compound in grams (GMWt). In solutions this is usually expressed as moles per liter; i.e., 1 mol/L = 1 M; 1 mM (mmol) = 1 mol × 10^{-3}; 1 μM (μmol) = 1 mol × 10^{-6}; 1 nM (nmol) = 1 mol × 10^{-9}
- **f.**
  - **(1)** To convert mEq/L of an electrolyte or other ions in solution to mmol/L: mEq/L divided by valence = mmol/L; e.g., (a) 2 mEq/L of magnesium (Mg^{2+}) = 2/2 = 1 mmol/L; e.g., (b) 140 mEq Na^+/L = 140/L = 140 mmol/L
  - **(2)** To convert mg/dl to mmol/L: (mg/dl × 10/EW) divided by valence = mmol/L; e.g., 2 mg/dl of magnesium = (2 × 10/12) divided by 2 = 0.83 mmol/L
  - **(3)** For organic substances: mmol/L = wt in mg/L/MW (in mg)

2. SI units for expressing clinical laboratory data

These units are now widely used and are increasingly required for publication of scientific data in physical, biologic, and biomedical publications. Extensive SI conversion tables have been published together with an explanation of the rationale for their use and technical aspects of usage.[1–3]

a. The base units of interest in physical quantities used in clinical chemistry are:

Quantity	Base Unit
mass	kilogram
time	second
amount	mole
length	meter

A derived unit for energy is the kjoule(kJ) 4.18 kJ = 1 kcal

1 MJ = 239 kcal

b. Prefixes and symbols for decimal multiples and submultiples include:

Factor	Prefix	Symbol	Factor	Prefix	Symbol
10^9	giga	G	10^{-3}	milli	m
10^6	mega	M	10^{-6}	micro	u
10^3	kilo	k	10^{-9}	nano	n
10^2	hecto	h	10^{-12}	pico	p
10^1	deka	da	10^{-15}	femto	f
10^{-1}	deci	d	10^{-18}	atto	a
10^{-2}	centi	c			

3. Conversion factors for selected compounds of nutrition interest*				
	(1)	(2)	(3)	(4)
Component	Present Unit	Conversion Factor	SI Unit Symbol	Mass Conversion Factor
Albumin (s)	g/dl	10	g/L	—
Aluminum (s)	µg/L	37.04	nmol/L	µg/27 = mol
Amino acids	(see ref. 3, p. 119 for individual amino acids)			
Amino acid nitrogen (p)	mg/dl	0.714	mmol/L	mg/14 = mmol
Ascorbic acid (p)	mg/dl	56.78	µmol/L	mg/176 = mmol
Calcium (s)	mg/dl	0.250	mmol/L	mg/40 = mmol
Calcium (s)	mEq/dl	0.500	mmol/L	mEq/2 = mmol
β-Carotene† (s)	µ/dl	0.0186	µmol/L	ug/536.85 umol
Chloride (s)	mEq/L	1.00	mmol/L	mEq = mmol
Cholesterol (p)	mg/dl	0.0259	mmol/L	mg/386.6 = mmol
Copper (s)	µg/dl	0.157	µmol/L	µg/63.5 = umol
Cyanocobalamin (B_{12})	pg/ml	0.738	pmol/L	pg/1355 = pmol
Ethanol (p)	mg/dl	0.217	mmol/L	mg/46 = mmol
Folic acid	ng/ml	2.265	nmol/L	ng/441.4 = nmol
Glucose (p)	mg/dl	0.0555	mmol/L	mg/180.2 = mmol
Iron (s)	µg/dl	0.179	µmol/L	µg/55.9 = umol
Phosphate (p) (as phosphorus)	mg/dl	0.323	mmol/L	mg/31 = mmol
Potassium (s)	mEq/L	1.000	mmol/L	mEq = mmol
Potassium	mg/dl	0.256	mmol/L	mg/39.1 = mmol
Magnesium (s)	mg/dl	0.411	mmol/L	mg/24.3 = mmol
Pyridoxal (B)	ng/ml	5.981	nmol/L	ng/167 = nmol
Retinol† (p,s)	µg/dl	0.0349	µmol/L	µg/286 = umol
Riboflavin (s)	µg/dl	26.57	nmol/L	µg/376 = nmol
Sodium (s)	mEq/L	1.00	mmol/L	mEq = mmol
Thiamin HCl (U)	µg/24 hr	0.00298	µmol/d	µg/337 = umol
α-Tocopherol (p)	mg/dl	23.22	µmol/L	µg/431 = umol
Vitamin D_3	µg/dl	26.01	nmol/L	µg/384 = umol
Calcidiol	ng/ml	2.498	nmol/L	ng/400 = nmol
Zinc (s)	µg/dl	0.153	µmol/L	µg/65.4 = umol

*To convert metric or equivalent unit per unit volume (column 1) to S.I. units per liter (column 3), multiply by the conversion factor in column 2. p = plasma; s = serum; B = blood; U = urine.

†See Appendix table A—1b for detailed conversion figures for retinol and carotene

REFERENCES

1. Young, D.S.: Ann. Intern. Med., *106*:114, 1987.
2. Lundberg, G.D., Iberson, C., Radulescu, G.: JAMA, *255*: 2329, 1986.
3. Monsen, E.R.: J. Am. Diet. Assoc., *87*:356, 1987.

TABLE A–1B. FACTORS AND FORMULAS USED IN INTERCONVERTING UNITS OF VITAMIN A AND CAROTENOIDS

Factors

1 nmol retinol = 286.42 ng
1 nmol retinoic acid = 300.42 ng
1 nmol β-carotene = 536.85 ng

1 μg retinol equivalent (μg RE)
= 1 μg all-*trans* retinol
= 3.49 nmol all-*trans* retinol
= 6 μg all-*trans* β-carotene
= 11.18 nmol all-*trans* β-carotene
= 12 μg other all-*trans* provitamin A carotenoids
= 3.33 IU_a (the international unit of all-*trans* retinol)
= 10 IU_c (the international unit of all-*trans* β-carotene)

1 IU_a
= 0.3 μg all-*trans* retinol
= 0.3 μg RE
= 1.05 nmol all-*trans* retinol
= 1.8 μg all-*trans* β-carotene
= 3.35 nmol all-*trans* β-carotene
= 3 IU_c
= 3.6 μg other all-*trans* provitamin A carotenoids

1 IU_c
= 0.6 μg all-*trans* β-carotene
= 1.12 nmol all-*trans* β-carotene
= 0.1 μg RE
= 0.33 IU_a
= 1.2 μg other all-*trans* provitamin A carotenoids

Formulas and Examples: All-*trans* configurations of retinol and carotenoids are assumed

1. μg RE = μg retinol + μg β-carotene/6
A diet contains 500 μg retinol and 1800 μg β-carotene. Then,

$$\mu g\ RE = 500 + 1800/6 = 800\ \mu g\ RE$$

2. μg RE = $IU_a/3.33 + IU_c/10$
A diet contains 1667 IU_a of retinol and 3000 IU_c of β-carotene. Then,

$$\mu g\ RE = 1667/3.33 + 3000/10 = 800\ \mu g\ RE$$

3. μg RE = μg β-carotene/6 + μg other provitamin A carotenoids/12
A serving of sweet potato contains 2400 μg of β-carotene and 480 μg of other provitamin A carotenoids. Then,

$$\mu g\ RE = 2400/6 + 480/12 = 440\ \mu g\ RE$$

(continued)

TABLE A–1B. (continued)

4.

$$\% \ \mu g \text{ RE as retinol} = \left[1.5 - \frac{0.15 \text{ total IU}}{\text{total RE}} \right] \times 100$$

$$\% \ \mu g \text{ RE as carotenoids} = \left[\frac{0.15 \text{ total IU}}{\text{total RE}} - 0.5 \right] \times 100$$

A 100-g portion of cheese contains a total of 300 μg RE and a total of 1200 IU, in which 1 IU_a has been *assumed* to equal 1 IU_c. Then,

$$\% \text{ RE as retinol} = \left[1.5 - \frac{0.15 \times 1200}{300} \right] \times 100 = 90\%$$

$$\% \text{ RE as carotenoids} = \left[\frac{0.15 \times 1200}{300} - 0.5 \right] \times 100 = 10\%$$

In this sample of cheese, therefore, 270 μg (270 μg RE) is present as retinol and 180 μg, or 30 μg RE, is present as β-carotene or its equivalent of other provitamin A carotenoids.

5.

$$IU_a = \frac{10 \ \mu g \text{ RE} - \text{total IU}}{2}$$

$$IU_c = \frac{3 \text{ total IU} - 10 \ \mu g \text{ RE}}{2}$$

In a cheese sample containing a total of 300 μg RE and a total of 1200 IU, in which 1 IU_a is *assumed* to equal 1 IU_c,

$$IU_a = \frac{10 \times 300 - 1200}{2} = 900$$

$$IU_c = \frac{3 \times 1200 - 10 \times 300}{2} = 300$$

Note: Assumptions used from revised sections of the United States Department of Agriculture's *Handbook 8* (i.e., 8.1–8.10) are *(a)* that 1 IU_a = 1 IU_c and *(b)* that 1 RE = 1 μg of retinol = 6 μg of β-carotene = 12 μg of other provitamin A carotenoids.

In some cases, small negative values for IU_c are obtained when the values for total IU and total RE are given for foods containing only preformed vitamin A_1 particularly in fortified foods like margarine. This aberrant calculation results from the rounding of analytic values. Similarly, small negative values for IU_a may result for foods containing only carotenoids. In both cases, the negative values should be taken as zero.

Prepared by J.A. Olson. For further discussion of these interconversions, see Chapter 16.

TABLE A–1C. ATOMIC WEIGHTS (ALPHABETIC ORDER)

ELEMENT	SYMBOL	ATOMIC NUMBER	ATOMIC WEIGHT	ELEMENT	SYMBOL	ATOMIC NUMBER	ATOMIC WEIGHT
Actinium	Ac	89	227.0278*	Neodymium	Nd	60	144.24
Aluminum	Al	13	26.981539	Neon	Ne	10	20.1797
Americium	Am	95	243.0614*	Neptunium	Np	93	237.0482*
Antimony	Sb	51	121.75	Nickel	Ni	28	58.69
Argon	Ar	18	39.948	Niobium	Nb	41	92.90638
Arsenic	As	33	74.92159	Nitrogen	N	7	14.00674
Astatine	At	85	209.9871*	Nobelium	No	102	259.1009*
Barium	Ba	56	137.327	Osmium	Os	76	190.2
Berkelium	Bk	97	247.0703*	Oxygen	O	8	15.9994
Beryllium	Be	4	9.012182	Palladium	Pd	46	106.42
Bismuth	Bi	83	208.98037	Phosphorus	P	15	30.973762
Boron	B	5	10.811	Platinum	Pt	78	195.08
Bromine	Br	35	79.904	Plutonium	Pu	94	244.0642*
Cadmium	Cd	48	112.411	Polonium	Po	84	208.9824*
Calcium	Ca	20	40.078	Potassium	K	19	39.0983
Californium	Cf	98	251.0796*	Praseodymium	Pr	59	140.90765
Carbon	C	6	12.011	Promethium	Pm	61	144.9127*
Cerium	Ce	58	140.115	Protactinium	Pa	91	231.0359*
Cesium	Cs	55	132.90543	Radium	Ra	88	226.0254*
Chlorine	Cl	17	35.4527	Radon	Rn	86	222.0176*
Chromium	Cr	24	51.9961	Rhenium	Re	75	186.207
Cobalt	Co	27	58.93320	Rhodium	Rh	45	102.90550
Copper	Cu	29	63.546	Rubidium	Rb	37	85.4678
Curium	Cm	96	247.0703*	Ruthenium	Ru	44	101.07
Dysprosium	Dy	66	162.50	Samarium	Sm	62	150.36
Einsteinium	Es	99	252.083*	Scandium	Sc	21	44.955910
Erbium	Er	68	167.26	Selenium	Se	34	78.96
Europium	Eu	63	151.965	Silicon	Si	14	28.0855
Fermium	Fm	100	257.0951*	Silver	Ag	47	107.8682
Fluorine	F	9	18.9984032	Sodium	Na	11	22.989768
Francium	Fr	87	223.0197*	Strontium	Sr	38	87.62
Gadolinium	Gd	64	157.25	Sulfur	S	16	32.066
Gallium	Ga	31	69.723	Tantalum	Ta	73	180.9479
Germanium	Ge	32	72.61	Technetium	Tc	43	97.9072*
Gold	Au	79	196.96654	Tellurium	Te	52	127.60
Hafnium	Hf	72	178.49	Terbium	Tb	65	158.92534
Helium	He	2	4.002602	Thallium	Tl	81	204.3833
Holmium	Ho	67	164.93032	Thorium	Th	90	232.0381
Hydrogen	H	1	1.00794	Thulium	Tm	69	168.93421
Indium	In	49	114.82	Tin	Sn	50	118.710
Iodine	I	53	126.90447	Titanium	Ti	22	47.88
Iridium	Ir	77	192.22	Tungsten	W	74	183.85
Iron	Fe	26	55.847	Unnilquadium	Unq	104	261.11*
Krypton	Kr	36	83.80	Unnilpentium	Unp	105	262.114*
Lanthanum	La	57	138.9055	Unnilhexium	Unh	106	263.118*
Lawrencium	Lr	103	262.11*	Unnilseptium	Uns	107	262.12*
Lead	Pb	82	207.2	Uranium	U	92	238.0289
Lithium	Li	3	6.941	Vanadium	V	23	50.9415
Lutetium	Lu	71	174.967	Xenon	Xe	54	131.29
Magnesium	Mg	12	24.3050	Ytterbium	Yb	70	173.04
Manganese	Mn	25	54.93805	Yttrium	Y	39	88.90585
Mendelevium	Md	101	258.10*	Zinc	Zn	30	65.39
Mercury	Hg	80	200.59	Zirconium	Zr	40	91.224
Molybdenum	Mo	42	95.94				

*Relative atomic mass of the isotope of that element with the longest known half-life.

(Based on 1987 IUPAC Table of Standard Atomic Weights of the Elements. *In* The Merck Index. 11th Ed. Rahway, NJ, Merck & Co., 1989.)

TABLE A–1D. WEIGHTS AND MEASURES

VOLUMES:

Apothecaries' Measure	Metric	Household
1 fluid dram (fl dr)	4 milliliter (ml)	1 teaspoon (tsp)
2 fl dr	8 ml	1 dessert spoonful
½ fluid ounce (fl oz)	15 ml	1 tablespoon (Tbsp) (3 tsp)
1 fl oz.	30 ml	2 Tbsp (⅛ cup)
1-½ fl oz	45 ml	1 jigger
2 fl oz	59 ml	4 Tbsp (¼ cup)
2-⅔ fl oz	80 ml	5-⅓ Tbsp (⅓ cup)
4 fl oz	118 ml	8 Tbsp (½ cup)
8 fl oz	237 ml	1 cup
16 fl oz	473 ml	1 pint (pt)
32 fl oz	947 ml	1 quart (qt)
128 fl oz	3,785 ml	1 gallon (gal)
3.38 fl oz	1 deciliter (dl) (100 ml)	
2.11 pt	1 liter (L) (1,000 ml)	

WEIGHTS:

Avoirdupois	Metric
	1 femtogram (fg) (10^{-15} g)
	1 picogram (pg) (10^{-12} g)
	1 nanogram (ng) (10^{-9} g)
	1 microgram (μg) (10^{-6} g)
1 grain (gr)	0.065 g (65 mg)
1 gram (0.035 oz)	15.432 gr
1 scruple (20 gr)	1.296 g
1 dram (dr) (= drachm) (27.3 gr)	1.77 g
1 oz (16 dr)	28.35 g
1 lb (16 oz)	453.59 g
1 ton (2,000 lb)	0.91 metric tons
1.015 gr	1 milligram (mg) (10^{-3} g)
	1 centigram (cg) (10^{-2} g)
	1 decigram (dg) (10^{-1} g)
15.4 gr (0.035 oz)	1 gram (g)
2.2 lb	1 kilogram (kg) (10^{3} g)

LENGTH/AREA:

	Metric
1 angstrom (A)	10 millimeter (mm)
1/2500 inch (in)	1 micron (μ) (10^{-3} mm) = micrometer (μm)
0.039 in	1 mm
0.39 in	1 centimeter (cm)
1 in	2.54 cm
1 foot (ft) (12 in)	30.5 cm
39.4 in	1 meter (m)
1 yard (yd) (3 ft)	0.9 m
1 rod (5.5 yd)	4.95 m
1093.6 yd (0.62 mile)	1 kilometer (km)
1 mile (mi) (5280 ft)	1.61 km
1 acre (160 square rods)	0.4 hectare

TEMPERATURE CONVERSIONS:

F to C: $5/9\,(F - 32)$
C to F: $(9/5 \times C) + 32$

TABLE A—1D. WEIGHTS AND MEASURES

ELECTROLYTE DATA:

Ion		Atomic Wt (1)	Valence (2)	Equivalent Wt* 1 ÷ 2
Bicarbonate	HCO_3^-	61.0	1	61.0
Calcium	Ca^{2+}	40.1	2	20.0
Chloride	Cl^-	35.5	1	35.5
Magnesium	Mg^{2+}	24.3	2	12.2
Phosphate†	HPO_4^{2-}	96.0	2	48.0†
Potassium	K^+	39.1	1	39.1
Sodium	Na^+	23.0	1	23.0
Sulfate	SO_4^{2-}	96.1	2	48.0

*Milliequivalent (mEq) = equivalent weight in milligrams (mg). To convert mg quantities of all electrolytes to mEq:

$$\frac{\text{mg of electrolyte}}{\text{equivalent weight in mg}} = \text{mEq}$$

To convert mEq quantities of all electrolytes to mg:

$$\text{mEq} \times \text{equivalent wt} = \text{mg}$$

To convert mg/dl to mEq/L:

$$\frac{\text{mg/dl} \times 10}{\text{equivalent wt in mg}} = \text{mEq/L}$$

To convert mEq/L to mg/dl: mEq/L × equivalent wt in mg × 0.1

†At the normal pH of plasma, 20% of the total inorganic phosphate radical is combined with one equivalent of base as BH_2PO_4, and 80% with two equivalents of base as B_2HPO_4. Under these conditions, base equivalence is therefore 0.2 + (0.8 × 2) = 1.8, and the equivalent weight of 53.3 is obtained by dividing the ionic weight by 1.8 instead of by 2. For phosphorus content of phosphate solutions, 1 mEq provides approximately 15 mg, and 1 mmol provides approximately 31 mg.

TABLE A–2A. MEDIAN HEIGHTS AND WEIGHTS AND RECOMMENDED ENERGY INTAKE IN THE UNITED STATES[a]

CATEGORY	AGE (YEARS) OR CONDITION	WEIGHT (kg)	WEIGHT (lb)	HEIGHT (cm)	HEIGHT (in)	REE[b] (kcal/day)	AVERAGE ENERGY ALLOWANCE (kcal)[c] Multiples of REE	Per kg	Per day[d]
Infants	0.0–0.5	6	13	60	24	320		108	650
	0.5–1.0	9	20	71	28	500		98	850
Children	1–3	13	29	90	35	740		102	1,300
	4–6	20	44	112	44	950		90	1,800
	7–10	28	62	132	52	1,130		70	2,000
Males	11–14	45	99	157	62	1,440	1.70	55	2,500
	15–18	66	145	176	69	1,760	1.67	45	3,000
	19–24	72	160	177	70	1,780	1.67	40	2,900
	25–50	79	174	176	70	1,800	1.60	37	2,900
	51+	77	170	173	68	1,530	1.50	30	2,300
Females	11–14	46	101	157	62	1,310	1.67	47	2,200
	15–18	55	120	163	64	1,370	1.60	40	2,200
	19–24	58	128	164	65	1,350	1.60	38	2,200
	25–50	63	138	163	64	1,380	1.55	36	2,200
	51+	65	143	160	63	1,280	1.50	30	1,900
Pregnant	1st trimester					—			+0
	2nd trimester								+300
	3rd trimester								+300
Lactating	1st 6 months								+500
	2nd 6 months								+500

[a]Median Height/Weight used by the RDA are those which are the medians for the U.S. population of designated age as reported in NHANES II.
[b]Calculations based on WHO equation derived from BMR data (Table A–7a), then rounded.
[c]In the range of light to moderate activity, the coefficient of variation is ±20%.
[d]Figure is rounded.
(From Food and Nutrition Board, National Research Council: Recommended Dietary Allowances. 10th Ed. Washington, D.C., National Academy Press, 1989, p. 33.)

TABLE A–2B. RECOMMENDED DIETARY ALLOWANCES[a], REVISED 1989 (DESIGNED FOR THE MAINTENANCE OF GOOD NUTRITION OF PRACTICALLY ALL HEALTHY PEOPLE IN THE UNITED STATES)

		WEIGHT[b]		HEIGHT[b]			FAT-SOLUBLE VITAMINS			
CATEGORY	AGE (YEARS) OR CONDITION	(kg)	(lb)	(cm)	(in)	PROTEIN (G)	Vitamin A (μg RE)[c]	Vitamin D (μg)[d]	Vitamin E (mg α-TE)[e]	Vitamin K (μg)
Infants	0.0–0.5	6	13	60	24	13	375	7.5	3	5
	0.5–1.0	9	20	71	28	14	375	10	4	10
Children	1–3	13	29	90	35	16	400	10	6	15
	4–6	20	44	112	44	24	500	10	7	20
	7–10	28	62	132	52	28	700	10	7	30
Males	11–14	45	99	157	62	45	1,000	10	10	45
	15–18	66	145	176	69	59	1,000	10	10	65
	19–24	72	160	177	70	58	1,000	10	10	70
	25–50	79	174	176	70	63	1,000	5	10	80
	51+	77	170	173	68	63	1,000	5	10	80
Females	11–14	46	101	157	62	46	800	10	8	45
	15–18	55	120	163	64	44	800	10	8	55
	19–24	58	128	164	65	46	800	10	8	60
	25–50	63	138	163	64	50	800	5	8	65
	51+	65	143	160	63	50	800	5	8	65
Pregnant						60	800	10	10	65
Lactating	1st 6 months					65	1,300	10	12	65
	2nd 6 months					62	1,200	10	11	65

[a]The allowances, expressed as average daily intakes over time, are intended to provide for individual variations among most normal persons as they live in the United States under usual environmental stresses. Diets should be based on a variety of common foods in order to provide other nutrients for which human requirements have been less well defined. See text for detailed discussion of allowances and of nutrients not tabulated.

[b]Weights and heights of reference adults are actual medians for the U.S. population of the designated age, as reported by NHANES II. The median weights and heights of those under 19 years of age were taken from Hamill et al. (1979). The use of these figures does not imply that the height-to-weight ratios are ideal.

[c]Retinol equivalents. 1 retinol equivalent = 1 μg retinol or 6 μg β-carotene. See text for calculation of vitamin A activity of diets as retinol equivalents.

[d]As cholecalciferol. 10 μg cholecalciferol = 400 IU of vitamin D.

[e]α-Tocopherol equivalents. 1 mg d-α tocopherol = 1 α-TE. See text for variation in allowances and calculation of vitamin E activity of the diet as α-tocopherol equivalents.

[f]1 NE (niacin equivalent) is equal to 1 mg of niacin or 60 mg of dietary tryptophan.

(From Food and Nutrition Board, National Research Council: Recommended Dietary Allowances. 10th Ed. Washington, D.C., National Academy Press, 1989.)

TABLE A–2B. (CONTINUED)

WATER-SOLUBLE VITAMINS							MINERALS						
Vitamin C (mg)	Thiamin (mg)	Riboflavin (mg)	Niacin (mg NE)[f]	Vitamin B_6 (mg)	Folate (μg)	Vitamin B_{12} (μg)	Calcium (mg)	Phosphorus (mg)	Magnesium (mg)	Iron (mg)	Zinc (mg)	Iodine (μg)	Selenium (μg)
30	0.3	0.4	5	0.3	25	0.3	400	300	40	6	5	40	10
35	0.4	0.5	6	0.6	35	0.5	600	500	60	10	5	50	15
40	0.7	0.8	9	1.0	50	0.7	800	800	80	10	10	70	20
45	0.9	1.1	12	1.1	75	1.0	800	800	120	10	10	90	20
45	1.0	1.2	13	1.4	100	1.4	800	800	170	10	10	120	30
50	1.3	1.5	17	1.7	150	2.0	1,200	1,200	270	12	15	150	40
60	1.5	1.8	20	2.0	200	2.0	1,200	1,200	400	12	15	150	50
60	1.5	1.7	19	2.0	200	2.0	1,200	1,200	350	10	15	150	70
60	1.5	1.7	19	2.0	200	2.0	800	800	350	10	15	150	70
60	1.2	1.4	15	2.0	200	2.0	800	800	350	10	15	150	70
50	1.1	1.3	15	1.4	150	2.0	1,200	1,200	280	15	12	150	45
60	1.1	1.3	15	1.5	180	2.0	1,200	1,200	300	15	12	150	50
60	1.1	1.3	15	1.6	180	2.0	1,200	1,200	280	15	12	150	55
60	1.1	1.3	15	1.6	180	2.0	800	800	280	15	12	150	55
60	1.0	1.2	13	1.6	180	2.0	800	800	280	10	12	150	55
70	1.5	1.6	17	2.2	400	2.2	1,200	1,200	320	30	15	175	65
95	1.6	1.8	20	2.1	280	2.6	1,200	1,200	355	15	19	200	75
90	1.6	1.7	20	2.1	260	2.6	1,200	1,200	340	15	16	200	75

TABLE A–2C. ESTIMATED SAFE AND ADEQUATE DAILY DIETARY INTAKES OF SELECTED VITAMINS AND MINERALS*

CATEGORY	AGE (years)	VITAMINS: BIOTIN (μg)	VITAMINS: PANTOTHENIC ACID (mg)
Infants	0–0.5	10	2
	0.5–1	15	3
Children and adolescents	1–3	20	3
	4–6	25	3–4
	7–10	30	4–5
	11+	30–100	4–7
Adults		30–100	4–7

CATEGORY	AGE (years)	TRACE ELEMENTS†: COPPER (mg)	MANGANESE (mg)	FLUORIDE (mg)	CHROMIUM (μg)	MOLYBDENUM (μg)
Infants	0–0.5	0.4–0.6	0.3–0.6	0.1–0.5	10–40	15–30
	0.5–1	0.6–0.7	0.6–1.0	0.2–1.0	20–60	20–40
Children and adolescents	1–3	0.7–1.0	1.0–1.5	0.5–1.5	20–80	25–50
	4–6	1.0–1.5	1.5–2.0	1.0–2.5	30–120	30–75
	7–10	1.0–2.0	2.0–3.0	1.5–2.5	50–200	50–150
	11+	1.5–2.5	2.0–5.0	1.5–2.5	50–200	75–250
Adults		1.5–3.0	2.0–5.0	1.5–4.0	50–200	75–250

*Because there is less information on which to base allowances, these figures are not given in the main table of RDA and are provided here in the form of ranges of recommended intakes.

†Because the toxic levels for many trace elements may be only several times usual intakes, the upper levels for the trace elements given in this table should not be habitually exceeded.

(From Food and Nutrition Board, National Research Council: Recommended Dietary Allowances. 10th Ed. Washington, D.C., National Academy Press, 1989, p. 284.)

TABLE A–3A. SUMMARY OF EXAMPLES OF RECOMMENDED NUTRIENTS BASED ON ENERGY EXPRESSED AS DAILY RATES, CANADA

AGE	SEX	ENERGY (kcal)	THIAMIN (mg)	RIBOFLAVIN (mg)	NIACIN (ne[b])	n-3 PUFA[a] (g)	n-6 PUFA (g)
Months							
0–4	Both	600	0.3	0.3	4	0.5	3
5–12	Both	900	0.4	0.5	7	0.5	3
Years							
1	Both	1100	0.5	0.6	8	0.6	4
2–3	Both	1300	0.6	0.7	9	0.7	4
4–6	Both	1800	0.7	0.9	13	1.0	6
7–9	M	2200	0.9	1.1	16	1.2	7
	F	1900	0.8	1.0	14	1.0	6
10–12	M	2500	1.0	1.3	18	1.4	8
	F	2200	0.9	1.1	16	1.2	7
13–15	M	2800	1.1	1.4	20	1.5	9
	F	2200	0.9	1.1	16	1.2	7
16–18	M	3200	1.3	1.6	23	1.8	11
	F	2100	0.8	1.1	15	1.2	7
19–24	M	3000	1.2	1.5	22	1.6	10
	F	2100	0.8	1.1	15	1.2	7
25–49	M	2700	1.1	1.4	19	1.5	9
	F	1900	0.8[c]	1.0[c]	14[c]	1.1[c]	7[c]
50–74	M	2300	0.9	1.2	16	1.3	8
	F	1800	0.8[c]	1.0[c]	14[c]	1.1[c]	7[c]
75+	M	2000	0.8	1.0	14	1.1	7
	F[d]	1700	0.8[c]	1.0[c]	14[c]	1.1[c]	7[c]
Pregnancy (additional)							
1st trimester		100	0.1	0.1	1	0.05	0.3
2nd trimester		300	0.1	0.3	2	0.16	0.9
3rd trimester		300	0.1	0.3	2	0.16	0.9
Lactation (additional)		450	0.2	0.4	3	0.25	1.5

[a]PUFA, Polyunsaturated fatty acids.
[b]NE, Niacin equivalents.
[c]Level below which intake should not fall.
[d]Assumes moderate (more than average) physical activity.
(From Health and Welfare Canada: Nutrition Recommendations. The Report of the Scientific Review Committee. Ottawa; Supply and Services Canada, 1990. Reproduced with permission of the Minister of Supply and Services Canada 1992.)

TABLE A–3B. SUMMARY OF EXAMPLES OF RECOMMENDED NUTRIENT INTAKE BASED ON AGE AND BODY WEIGHT EXPRESSED AS DAILY RATES, CANADA

AGE	SEX	WEIGHT (kg)	PROTEIN (g)	VIT. A (RE)[a]	VIT. D (μg)	VIT. E (mg)	VIT. C (mg)	FOLATE (μg)	VIT. B_{12} (μg)	CALCIUM (mg)	PHOSPHORUS (mg)	MAGNESIUM (mg)	IRON (mg)	IODINE (μg)	ZINC (mg)
Months															
0–4	Both	6.0	12[b]	400	10	3	20	25	0.3	250[c]	150	20	0.3[d]	30	2[d]
5–12	Both	9.0	12	400	10	3	20	40	0.4	400	200	32	7	40	3
Years															
1	Both	11	13	400	10	3	20	40	0.5	500	300	40	6	55	4
2–3	Both	14	16	400	5	4	20	50	0.6	550	350	50	6	65	4
4–6	Both	18	19	500	5	5	25	70	0.8	600	400	65	8	85	5
7–9	M	25	26	700	2.5	7	25	90	1.0	700	500	100	8	110	7
	F	25	26	700	2.5	6	25	90	1.0	700	500	100	8	95	7
10–12	M	34	34	800	2.5	8	25	120	1.0	900	700	130	8	125	9
	F	36	36	800	2.5	7	25	130	1.0	1100	800	135	8	110	9
13–15	M	50	49	900	2.5	9	30[e]	175	1.0	1100	900	185	10	160	12
	F	48	46	800	2.5	7	30[e]	170	1.0	1000	850	180	13	160	9
16–18	M	62	58	1000	2.5	10	40[e]	220	1.0	900	1000	230	10	160	12
	F	53	47	800	2.5	7	30[e]	190	1.0	700	850	200	12	160	9
19–24	M	71	61	1000	2.5	10	40[e]	220	1.0	800	1000	240	9	160	12
	F	58	50	800	2.5	7	30[e]	180	1.0	700	850	200	13	160	9
25–49	M	74	64	1000	2.5	9	40[e]	230	1.0	800	1000	250	9	160	12
	F	59	51	800	2.5	6	30[e]	185	1.0	700	850	200	13	160	9
50–74	M	73	63	1000	5	7	40[e]	230	1.0	800	1000	250	9	160	12
	F	63	54	800	5	6	30[e]	195	1.0	800	850	210	8	160	9
75+	M	69	59	1000	5	6	40[e]	215	1.0	800	1000	230	9	160	12
	F	64	55	800	5	5	30[e]	200	1.0	800	850	210	8	160	9
Pregnancy (additional)															
1st trimester			5	0	2.5	2	0	200	0.2	500	200	15	0	25	6
2nd trimester			20	0	2.5	2	10	200	0.2	500	200	45	5	25	6
3rd trimester			24	0	2.5	2	10	200	0.2	500	200	45	10	25	6
Lactation (additional)			20	400	2.5	3	25	100	0.2	500	200	65	0	50	6

[a]Retinol Equivalents.

[b]Protein is assumed to be from breast milk and must be adjusted for infant formula.

[c]Infant formula with high phosphorus should contain 375 mg calcium.

[d]Breast milk is assumed to be the source of the mineral.

[e]Smokers should increase vitamin C by 50%.

(From Health and Welfare Canada: Nutrition Recommendations. The Report of the Scientific Review Committee. Ottawa, Supply and Services Canada, 1990. Reproduced with permission of the Minister of Supply and Services Canada 1992.)

TABLE A–4A. ESTIMATED AVERAGE REQUIREMENTS (EAR) FOR ENERGY, UNITED KINGDOM

AGE	EAR MJ/D (KCAL/D) Males	Females
0–3 months	2.28 (545)	2.16 (515)
4–6 months	2.89 (690)	2.69 (645)
7–9 months	3.44 (825)	3.20 (765)
10–12 months	3.85 (920)	3.61 (865)
1–3 years	5.15 (1,230)	4.86 (1,165)
4–6 years	7.16 (1,715)	6.46 (1,545)
7–10 years	8.24 (1,970)	7.28 (1,740)
11–14 years	9.27 (2,220)	7.92 (1,845)
15–18 years	11.51 (2,755)	8.83 (2,110)
19–50 years	10.60 (2,550)	8.10 (1,940)
51–59 years	10.60 (2,550)	8.00 (1,900)
60–64 years	9.93 (2,380)	7.99 (1,900)
65–74 years	9.71 (2,330)	7.96 (1,900)
75+ years	8.77 (2,100)	7.61 (1,810)
Pregnancy		+0.80*(200)
Lactation:		
1 month		+1.90 (450)
2 months		+2.20 (530)
3 months		+2.40 (570)
4–6 months (Group 1)		+2.00 (480)
4–6 months (Group 2)		+2.40 (570)
>6 months (Group 1)		+1.00 (240)
>6 months (Group 2)		+2.30 (550)

*last trimester only

(From Report on Health and Social Subjects: Dietary Reference Values for Food and Energy and Nutrients for the United Kingdom. London, Her Majesty's Stationery Office, 1991.)

TABLE A–4B. REFERENCE NUTRIENT INTAKES FOR PROTEIN, UNITED KINGDOM

AGE	REFERENCE NUTRIENT INTAKE[a] (g/d)	
0–3 months	12.5[b]	
4–6 months	12.7	
7–9 months	13.7	
10–12 months	14.9	
1–3 years	14.5	
4–6 years	19.7	
7–10 years	28.3	
Males		
11–14 years	42.1	
15–18 years	55.2	
19–50 years	55.5	
50+ years	53.3	
Females		
11–14 years	41.2	
15–18 years	45.0	
19–50 years	45.0	
50+ years	46.5	
Pregnancy[c]		+ 6
Lactation[c]		
0–4 months		+11
4+ months		+ 8

[a]These figures, based on egg and milk protein, assume complete digestibility.

[b]No values for infants 0 to 3 months are given by WHO. The reference nutrient intake is calculated from the recommendations of Committee on Medical Aspects of Food Policy (COMA).

[c]To be added to adult requirement through all stages of pregnancy and lactation.

(From Report on Health and Social Subjects: No. 41, Dietary Reference Values for Food Energy and Nutrients for the United Kingdom, Report of the Panel on Dietary Reference Values of the Committee on Medical Aspects of Food Policy. London, Her Majesty's Stationery Office, 1991.)

TABLE A–4C. REFERENCE NUTRIENT INTAKES FOR VITAMINS, UNITED KINGDOM

AGE	THIAMIN (mg/d)	RIBOFLAVIN (mg/d)	NIACIN (NICOTINIC ACID EQUIVALENT) (mg/d)	VITAMIN B_6 (mg/d[a])	VITAMIN B_{12} (μg/d)	FOLATE (μg/d)	VITAMIN C (mg/d)	VITAMIN A (μg/d)	VITAMIN D (μg/d)
0–3 months	0.2	0.4	3	0.2	0.3	50	25	350	8.5
4–6 months	0.2	0.4	3	0.2	0.3	50	25	350	8.5
7–9 months	0.2	0.4	4	0.3	0.4	50	25	350	7
10–12 months	0.3	0.4	5	0.4	0.4	50	25	350	7
1–3 years	0.5	0.6	8	0.7	0.5	70	30	400	7
4–6 years	0.7	0.8	11	0.9	0.8	100	30	500	—
7–10 years	0.7	1.0	12	1.0	1.0	150	30	500	—
Males									
11–14 years	0.9	1.2	15	1.2	1.2	200	35	600	—
15–18 years	1.1	1.3	18	1.5	1.5	200	40	700	—
19–50 years	1.0	1.3	17	1.4	1.5	200	40	700	—
50+ years	0.9	1.3	16	1.4	1.5	200	40	700	**
Females									
11–14 years	0.7	1.1	12	1.0	1.2	200	35	600	—
15–18 years	0.8	1.1	14	1.2	1.5	200	40	600	—
19–50 years	0.8	1.1	13	1.2	1.5	200	40	600	—
50+ years	0.8	1.1	12	1.2	1.5	200	40	600	**
Pregnancy	+0.1[b]	+0.3	*	*	*	+100	+10	+100	10
Lactation									
0–4 months	+0.2	+0.5	+2	*	+0.5	+ 60	+30	+350	10
4+ months	+0.2	+0.5	+2	*	+0.5	+ 60	+30	+350	10

*No increment
**After age 65 the RNI is 10 μg/d for men and women
[a]Based on protein providing 14.7% of EAR for energy
[b]For last trimester only
(From Report on Health and Social Subjects: No. 41, Dietary Reference Values for Food Energy and Nutrients for the United Kingdom, Report of the Panel on Dietary Reference Values of the Committee on Medical Aspects of Food Policy. London, Her Majesty's Stationery Office, 1991.)

TABLE A–4D. REFERENCE NUTRIENT INTAKES FOR MINERALS, UNITED KINGDOM

AGE	CALCIUM (mmol/d)	PHOSPHORUS[1] (mmol/d)	MAGNESIUM (mmol/d)	SODIUM (mmol/d[2])	POTASSIUM (mmol/d[3])	CHLORIDE[4] (mmol/d)	IRON (μmol/d)	ZINC (μmol/d)	COPPER (μmol/d)	SELENIUM (μmol/d)	IODINE (μmol/d)
0–3 months	13.1	13.1	2.2	9	20	9	30	60	5	0.1	0.4
4–6 months	13.1	13.1	2.5	12	22	12	80	60	5	0.2	0.5
7–9 months	13.1	13.1	3.2	14	18	14	140	75	5	0.1	0.5
10–12 months	13.1	13.1	3.3	15	18	15	140	75	5	0.1	0.5
1–3 years	8.8	8.8	3.5	22	20	22	120	75	6	0.2	0.6
4–6 years	11.3	11.3	4.8	30	28	30	110	100	9	0.3	0.8
7–10 years	13.8	13.8	8.0	50	50	50	160	110	11	0.4	0.9
Males											
11–14 years	25.0	25.0	11.5	70	80	70	200	140	13	0.6	1.0
15–18 years	25.0	25.0	12.3	70	90	70	200	145	16	0.9	1.0
19–50 years	17.5	17.5	12.3	70	90	70	160	145	19	0.9	1.0
50+ years	17.5	17.5	12.3	70	90	70	160	145	19	0.9	1.0
Females											
11–14 years	20.0	10.0	11.5	70	80	70	260[5]	140	13	0.6	1.0
15–18 years	20.0	20.0	12.3	70	90	70	260[5]	110	16	0.8	1.1
19–50 years	17.5	17.5	10.9	70	90	70	260[5]	110	19	0.8	1.1
50+ years	17.5	17.5	10.9	70	90	70	160	110	19	0.8	1.1
Pregnancy	*	*	*	*	*	*	*	*	*	*	*
Lactation											
0–4 months	+14.3	+14.3	+2.1	*	*	*	*	+90	+5	+0.2	*
4+ months	+14.3	+14.3	+2.1	*	*	*	*	+40	+5	+0.2	*
0–3 months	525	400	55	210	800	320	1.7	4.0	0.2	10	50
4–6 months	525	400	60	280	850	400	4.3	4.0	0.3	13	60
7–9 months	525	400	75	320	700	500	7.8	5.0	0.3	10	60
10–12 months	525	400	80	350	700	500	7.8	5.0	0.3	10	60
1–3 years	350	270	85	500	800	800	6.9	5.0	0.4	15	70
4–6 years	450	350	120	700	1,100	1,100	6.1	6.5	0.6	20	100
7–10 years	550	450	200	1,200	2,000	1,800	8.7	7.0	0.7	30	110
Males											
11–14 years	1,000	775	280	1,600	3,100	2,500	11.3	9.0	0.8	45	130
15–18 years	1,000	775	300	1,600	3,500	2,500	11.3	9.5	1.0	70	140
19–50 years	700	550	300	1,600	3,500	2,500	8.7	9.5	1.2	75	140
50+ years	700	550	300	1,600	3,500	2,500	8.7	9.5	1.2	75	140
Females											
11–14 years	800	625	280	1,600	3,100	2,500	14.8[5]	9.0	0.8	45	130
15–18 years	800	625	300	1,600	3,500	2,500	14.8[5]	7.0	1.0	60	140
19–50 years	700	550	270	1,600	3,500	2,500	14.8[5]	7.0	1.2	60	140
50+ years	700	550	270	1,600	3,500	2,500	8.7	7.0	1.2	60	140
Pregnancy	*	*	*	*	*	*	*	*	*	*	*
Lactation											
0–4 months	+550	+440	+ 50	*	*	*	*	+6.0	+0.3	+15	*
4+ months	+550	+440	+ 50	*	*	*	*	+2.5	+0.3	+15	*

*No increment

[1]Phosphorus RNI is set equal to calcium in molar terms

[2]1 mmol sodium = 23 mg

[3]1 mmol potassium = 39 mg

[4]Corresponds to sodium 1 mmol = 35.5 mg

[5]Insufficient for women with high menstrual losses where the most practical way of meeting iron requirements is to take iron supplements

(From Report on Health and Social Subjects: No. 41, Dietary Reference Values for Food Energy and Nutrients for the United Kingdom, Report of the Panel on Dietary Reference Values of the Committee on Medical Aspects of Food Policy. London, Her Majesty's Stationery Office, 1991.)

TABLE A—4E. SAFE INTAKES, UNITED KINGDOM

NUTRIENT	SAFE INTAKE
Vitamins	
Pantothenic acid	
adults	3–7 mg/d
infants	1.7 mg/d
Biotin	10–200 μg/d
Vitamin E	
men	above 4 mg/d
women	above 3 mg/d
infants	0.4 mg/g polyunsaturated fatty acids
Vitamin K	
adults	1 μg/kg/d
infants	10 μg/d
Minerals	
Manganese	
adults	1.4 mg (26 μmol)/d
infants and children	16 μg (0.3 μmol)/d
Molybdenum	
adults	50–400 μg/d
infants, children, and adolescents	0.5–1.5 μg/kg/d
Chromium	
adults	25 μg (0.5 μmol)/d
children and adolescents	0.1–1.0 μg (2–20 μmol)/kg/d
Fluoride (for infants only)	0.05 mg (3 μmol)/kg/d

For some nutrients, which are known to have important functions in humans, the Panel found insufficient reliable data on human requirements and were unable to set any dietary reference values for these. However, they decided on grounds of prudence to set a safe intake, particularly for infants and children. The safe intake was judged to be a level or range of intake at which there is no risk of deficiency and below a level where there is risk of undesirable effects. They are not therefore intended as a "toxic level," and although exceeding these safe intakes would not necessaily result in undesirable effects, equally there is no evidence for any benefits. The Panel agreed that the safe range of intakes set for the nutrients need not be exceeded.

(From Report on Health and Social Subjects: No. 41, Dietary Reference Values for Food Energy and Nutrients for the United Kingdom, Report of the Panel on Dietary Reference Values of the Committee on Medical Aspects of Food Policy. London, Her Majesty's Stationery Office, 1991.)

TABLE A–5A. RECOMMENDED DIETARY ALLOWANCES FOR PERSONS WITH LOW ACTIVITY, JAPAN

AGE	ENERGY (kcal) M	ENERGY (kcal) F	PROTEIN (g) M	PROTEIN (g) F	FAT (%)	CALCIUM (g) M	CALCIUM (g) F	IRON (mg) M	IRON (mg) F	VITAMIN A (IU) M	VITAMIN A (IU) F	VITAMIN B_1 (mg) M	VITAMIN B_1 (mg) F	VITAMIN B_2 (mg) M	VITAMIN B_2 (mg) F	NIACIN (mg) M	NIACIN (mg) F	ASCORBIC ACID (mg)	VITAMIN D (IU)
15~	2,350	2,000	85	70		0.8						0.9	0.8	1.3	1.1	16	13		
16~	2,400	1,950	80	70								1.0	0.8	1.3	1.1	16	13		
17~	2,400	1,900	80	70	25~30			12	12			1.0	0.8	1.3	1.0	16	13		
18~	2,350	1,850	75	65		0.7						0.9	0.7	1.3	1.0	16	12		
19~	2,300	1,850	75	60								0.9	0.7	1.3	1.0	15	12		
20~29	2,250	1,800	70	60								0.9	0.7	1.2	1.0	15	12		
30~39	2,200	1,750	70	60			0.6		12	2,000	1,800	0.9	0.7	1.2	1.0	15	12	50	100
40~49	2,150	1,700	70	60								0.9	0.7	1.2	0.9	14	11		
50~59	2,000	1,650	70	60								0.8	0.7	1.1	0.9	13	11		
60~64	1,850	1,550	70	60	20~25	0.6		10				0.7	0.6	1.0	0.9	12	10		
65~69	1,800	1,500	70	60								0.7	0.6	1.0	0.9	12	10		
70~74	1,650	1,450	65	55					10[†]			0.7	0.6	1.0	0.9	12	10		
75~79	1,600	1,400	65	55								0.7	0.6	1.0	0.9	12	10		
80~	1,500	1,250	65	55								0.7	0.6	1.0	0.9	12	10		
1st Half Pregnancy*		+150		+10			+0.4		+3		+0		+0.1		+0.1		+1	+10	+300
Last Half Pregnancy		+350		+20	25~30		+0.4		+8		+200		+0.2		+0.2		+2	+10	+300
Lactation		+700		+20			+0.5		+8		+1,400		+0.3		+0.4		+5	+40	+300

*Pregnancy increases are shown for convenience; however, values apply to each activity level.

†Decrease to 10 mg after menopause.

(From the Health Promotion and Nutrition Division, Health Policy Bureau, Ministry of Health and Welfare, Tokyo, Japan, 1991.)

TABLE A–5B. RECOMMENDED DIETARY ALLOWANCES FOR PERSONS WITH MEDIUM ACTIVITY OR GROWTH STAGES, JAPAN

AGE	AVERAGE HEIGHT (CM) M	AVERAGE HEIGHT (CM) F	AVERAGE WEIGHT (kg) M	AVERAGE WEIGHT (kg) F	ENERGY (kcal) M	ENERGY (kcal) F	PROTEIN (g) M	PROTEIN (g) F	FAT (%)	CALCIUM (g) M	CALCIUM (g) F	IRON (mg) M	IRON (mg) F	VITAMIN A (IU) M	VITAMIN A (IU) F	VITAMIN B₁ (mg) M	VITAMIN B₁ (mg) F	VITAMIN B₂ (mg) M	VITAMIN B₂ (mg) F	NIACIN (mg) M	NIACIN (mg) F	ASCORBIC ACID (mg)	VITAMIN D (IU)
0~mo					120/kg		3.3/kg		45	0.4		6		1,300		0.2		0.3		4			
2~mo					110/kg		2.5/kg		45	0.4		6		1,300		0.3		0.4		6			
6~mo					100/kg		3.0/kg		30~40	0.4		6		1,000		0.4		0.5		6			
1~yr	80.7	79.6	10.95	10.35	960	910	30	30				7	7			0.4	0.4	0.5	0.5	6	6		400
2~	90.0	89.1	13.24	12.74	1,200	1,150	35	35								0.5	0.5	0.7	0.6	8	8		
3~	97.3	96.6	15.04	14.70	1,400	1,350	40	40						1,000	1,000			0.8	0.7	9	9		
4~	104.3	103.7	16.97	16.69	1,550	1,450	45	45		0.4	0.4	8	8			0.6			0.8	10			
5~	110.8	110.3	19.04	18.78	1,600	1,500	50	50									0.6	0.9			10	40	
6~	117.0	116.5	21.35	21.04	1,700	1,600	55	50								0.7				11			
7~	122.7	122.2	23.85	23.44	1,800	1,650	60	55			0.5	9	9	1,200	1,200			1.0	0.9	12	11		
8~	128.3	127.9	26.70	26.24	1,900	1,750	65	60		0.5							0.7		1.0	13	12		
9~	133.5	133.6	29.76	29.50	1,950	1,850	65	65			0.6					0.8							
10~	138.8	139.8	33.21	33.54	2,050	1,950	70	70		0.6		10	10					1.1	1.1		13		
11~	144.6	146.5	37.26	38.46	2,150	2,100	75	75	25~30	0.7	0.7			1,500	1,500	0.9	0.8	1.2	1.2	14	14		
12~	151.4	151.9	42.29	43.31	2,350	2,250	80	80		0.8								1.3		15			
13~	159.0	155.4	48.34	47.43	2,500	2,300	85	80		0.9						1.0			1.3	16			
14~	164.9	157.1	53.87	50.32	2,600	2,300	85	75										1.4		17	15		
15~	168.5	157.6	57.98	51.99	2,700	2,250	85	70									0.9						
16~	169.9	158.0	60.21	52.87	2,700	2,200	80	70		0.8		12	12			1.1		1.5	1.2	18			
17~	170.8	158.1	61.55	52.92	2,700	2,150	80	70															100
18~	171.3	158.1	62.18	52.52	2,650	2,100	75	65		0.7													
19~	171.5	158.1	62.41	52.02	2,600	2,050	75	60													14		
20~29	171.1	157.7	64.00	51.83	2,550	2,000	70	60								1.0	0.8	1.4	1.1	17		50	
30~39	169.8	156.7	65.48	54.09	2,500	2,000	70	60			0.6		12	2,000	1,800								
40~49	167.8	154.6	65.10	55.14	2,400	1,950	70	60												16	13		
50~59	164.2	151.9	61.93	54.13	2,250	1,850	70	60					*			0.9		1.3		15			
60~64	162.1	149.8	59.41	52.49	2,100	1,750	70	60	20~25	0.6		10											
65~69	160.8	148.3	57.61	51.02	2,000	1,700	70	60											1.0				
70~74	159.7	145.7	55.83	49.26	1,850	1,600	65	55					10			0.8	0.7	1.2		14	12		
75~79	158.7	145.0	54.07	47.22	1,750	1,550	65	55															
80~	157.6	142.4	52.38	44.53	1,650	1,400	65	55															

*Decrease to 10 mg after menopause.

(From the Health Promotion and Nutrition Division, Health Policy Bureau, Ministry of Health and Welfare, Tokyo, Japan, 1991.)

TABLE A–5C. RECOMMENDED DIETARY ALLOWANCES FOR PERSONS WITH MEDIUM-HIGH ACTIVITY, JAPAN

AGE	ENERGY (kcal) M	ENERGY (kcal) F	PROTEIN (g) M	PROTEIN (g) F	FAT (%)	CALCIUM (g) M	CALCIUM (g) F	IRON (mg) M	IRON (mg) F	VITAMIN A (IU) M	VITAMIN A (IU) F	VITAMIN B_1 (mg) M	VITAMIN B_1 (mg) F	VITAMIN B_2 (mg) M	VITAMIN B_2 (mg) F	NIACIN (mg) M	NIACIN (mg) F	ASCORBIC ACID (mg)	VITAMIN D (IU)
15~	3,200	2,650	100	85		0.8						1.3	1.1	1.8	1.5	21	17		
16~	3,200	2,600	95	80								1.3	1.0	1.8	1.4	21	17		
17~	3,200	2,550	95	80				12	12			1.3	1.0	1.8	1.4	21	17		
18~	3,150	2,500	90	75		0.7						1.3	1.0	1.7	1.4	21	17		
19~	3,100	2,450	90	70								1.2	1.0	1.7	1.3	20	16		
20~29	3,050	2,400	85	70	25~30		0.6			2,000	1,800	1.2	1.0	1.7	1.3	20	16	50	100
30~39	2,950	2,350	85	70					12			1.2	0.9	1.6	1.3	19	16		
40~49	2,850	2,300	85	70								1.1	0.9	1.6	1.3	19	15		
50~59	2,700	2,200	85	70		0.6		10	*			1.1	0.9	1.5	1.2	18	15		
60~64	2,450	2,050	80	70								1.0	0.8	1.3	1.1	16	14		
65~69	2,350	2,000	80	70					10			1.0	0.8	1.3	1.1	16	14		

*Decrease to 10 mg after menopause.
(From the Health Promotion and Nutrition Division, Health Policy Bureau, Ministry of Health and Welfare, Tokyo, Japan, 1991.)

TABLE A–5D. RECOMMENDED DIETARY ALLOWANCES FOR PERSONS WITH HIGH ACTIVITY, JAPAN

AGE	ENERGY (kcal) M	ENERGY (kcal) F	PROTEIN (g) M	PROTEIN (g) F	FAT (%)	CALCIUM (g) M	CALCIUM (g) F	IRON (mg) M	IRON (mg) F	VITAMIN A (IU) M	VITAMIN A (IU) F	VITAMIN B_1 (mg) M	VITAMIN B_1 (mg) F	VITAMIN B_2 (mg) M	VITAMIN B_2 (mg) F	NIACIN (mg) M	NIACIN (mg) F	ASCORBIC ACID (mg)	VITAMIN D (IU)
15~	3,750	3,100	115	95		0.8						1.5	1.2	2.1	1.7	25	20		
16~	3,750	3,050	110	95								1.5	1.2	2.1	1.7	25	20		
17~	3,750	2,950	110	95				12	12			1.5	1.2	2.1	1.6	25	19		
18~	3,700	2,900	105	90		0.7						1.5	1.2	2.0	1.6	24	19		
19~	3,700	2,850	105	85								1.5	1.1	2.0	1.6	24	19		
20~29	3,550	2,800	100	85	25~30		0.6			2,000	1,800	1.4	1.1	2.0	1.5	23	18	50	100
30~39	3,450	2,750	100	85					12			1.4	1.1	1.9	1.5	23	18		
40~49	3,350	2,700	100	85		0.6		10	*			1.3	1.1	1.8	1.5	22	18		
50~59	3,150	2,600	100	85								1.3	1.0	1.7	1.4	21	17		
60~64	2,850	2,400	95	80								1.1	1.0	1.6	1.3	19	16		
65~69	2,750	2,300	95	80					10			1.1	1.0	1.6	1.3	19	16		

*Decrease to 10 mg after menopause.
(From the Health Promotion and Nutrition Division, Health Policy Bureau, Ministry of Health and Welfare, Tokyo, Japan, 1991.)

Comments

1. These general guidelines are not for individual daily values. For individual nutrient requirements, other tables must be used.
2. An individual should take no more than 10 mg sodium daily.
3. Vitamin E: Males should have at least 8 mg, females should have at least 7 mg.
4. For those in the low activity category, more exercise is recommended. The values in Table A–5c represent the ideal intake for adults. These values are reflective of individuals who exercise accordingly.

TABLE A–6. RECOMMENDED DAILY DIETARY ALLOWANCES, KOREA*

CATEGORY	AGE (years)	WEIGHT (kg)	HEIGHT (cm)	ENERGY (kcal)	PROTEIN (g)	VITAMIN A (re)†	Vitamin B_1 (mg)	VITAMIN B_2 (mg)	NIACIN (mg)	VITAMIN C (mg)	VITAMIN D (μg)‡	CALCIUM (mg)	IRON (mg)§
Infants													
	0–3 mo	5.5	58.5	800	25	350	0.40	0.48	6.4	35	10	400	10
	4–6 mo	8.4	67.5	900	25	350	0.45	0.54	7.2	35	10	400	10
	7–9 mo	9.5	76.0	1,000	30	350	0.50	0.60	8.0	35	10	400	15
	10–12 mo	10.4	79.0	1,100	30	350	0.55	0.66	8.0	35	10	400	15
Children													
	1–3	12.6	87.0	1,200	35	350	0.60	0.72	8.0	40	10	500	15
	4–6	19.0	110.0	1,300	40	400	0.75	0.90	10.0	40	10	600	10
	7–9	26.0	130.0	1,800	50	500	0.90	1.08	12.0	40	10	700	10
Males													
	10–12	36.0	144.0	2,100	60	600	1.05	1.26	14.0	50	10	800	15
	13–15	51.0	161.0	2,600	80	700	1.30	1.36	17.0	50	10	800	18
	16–19	59.0	169.0	2,500	75	700	1.25	1.50	16.5	55	10	800	18
	20–29	64.0	170.5	2,500	70	700	1.25	1.50	16.5	55	5	600	10
	30–49	65.0	168.5	2,500	70	700	1.25	1.50	16.5	55	5	600	10
	50–64	63.0	168.0	2,200	70	700	1.10	1.32	14.5	55	5	600	10
	65 or older	61.0	167.0	1,900	70	700	1.00	1.20	13.0	55	5	600	10
Females													
	10–12	37.0	145.0	2,000	60	600	1.00	1.20	13.0	50	10	800	18
	13–15	48.0	155.0	2,300	65	700	1.15	1.38	15.0	50	10	800	18
	16–19	52.0	158.0	2,200	60	700	1.10	1.32	14.5	55	10	700	18
	20–29	52.5	159.5	2,000	60	700	1.00	1.20	13.0	55	5	600	18
	30–49	55.0	158.0	2,000	60	700	1.00	1.20	13.0	55	5	600	18
	50–64	54.0	156.0	1,900	60	700	1.00	1.20	13.0	55	5	600	10
	65 or older	53.0	156.0	1,600	60	700	1.00	1.20	13.0	55	5	600	10
Pregnancy													
		First half		+150	+30	+ 0	+0.40	+0.30	+2.0	+15	+5	+400	+2
		Second half		+350	+30	+100	+0.40	+0.30	+2.0	+15	+5	+400	+2
Lactation													
				+700	+30	+300	+0.60	+0.50	+6.0	+35	+5	+500	+2

*The allowances for energy are based on individuals of moderate activity. Data in this table are intended to provide only a standard figure under usual environment and given conditions.

†Retinol equivalent: 1 RE = 1 μg retinol = 6 μg β-carotene

‡Vitamin D : 10 μg = 400 IU.

§Supplemental iron should be taken to meet the increased requirement during pregnancy and lactation.

(From the Ministry of Health and Social Affairs, Kyonggi, Korea, 1989.)

TABLE A–7A. EQUATIONS FOR PREDICTING BASAL METABOLIC RATE FROM BODY WEIGHT (W)*

AGE RANGE (years)	$KCAL_{th}$/DAY	CORRELATION COEFFICIENT	SD†	MJ/DAY	CORRELATION COEFFICIENT	SD
Males						
0–3	60.9 W − 54	0.97	53	0.255 W − 0.226	0.97	0.222
3–10	22.7 W + 495	0.86	62	0.0949 W + 2.07	0.86	0.259
10–18	17.5 W + 651	0.90	100	0.0732 W + 2.72	0.90	0.418
18–30	15.3 W + 679	0.65	151	0.0640 W + 2.84	0.65	0.632
30–60	11.6 W + 879	0.60	164	0.0485 W + 3.67	0.60	0.686
> 60	13.5 W + 487	0.79	148	0.0565 W + 2.04	0.79	0.619
Females						
0–3	61.0 W − 51	0.97	61	0.255 W − 0.214	0.97	0.255
3–10	22.5 W + 499	0.85	63	0.0941 W + 2.09	0.85	0.264
10–18	12.2 W + 746	0.75	117	0.0510 W + 3.12	0.75	0.489
18–30	14.7 W + 496	0.72	121	0.0615 W + 2.08	0.72	0.506
30–60	8.7 W + 829	0.70	108	0.0364 W + 3.47	0.70	0.452
> 60	10.5 W + 596	0.74	108	0.0439 W + 2.49	0.74	0.452

*Since the present report was compiled, the data base for the equations contained in Schofield, W. N., et al.: Hum. Nutr. Clin. Nutr. *39(Suppl.),* 1985 has been slightly expanded. They therefore differ from the equations shown in this table, but the differences are negligible.

†Standard deviation of differences between actual BMR and predicted estimates.

(From Energy and Protein Requirements: Report of a Joint FAO/WHO/UNU Expert Consultation. Technical Report Series No. 724. Geneva, World Health Organization, 1985, p. 71.)

TABLE A–7B. EXAMPLES OF PREDICTED BASAL METABOLIC RATE (BMR) IN SUBJECTS OF THE SAME HEIGHT BUT DIFFERENT WEIGHTS, PREDICTED FROM ACTUAL WEIGHT AND FROM MEDIAN ACCEPTABLE WEIGHT FOR HEIGHT

	MAN, AGE 40, HEIGHT 1.8 M			WOMAN, AGE 25, HEIGHT 1.5 M		
	Position in range*			Position in range*		
	Upper	Median	Lower	Upper	Median	Lower
BMI†	25	22	20	24	21	19
Wt(kg)	81.0	71.3	64.8	54.0	47.2	42.7
BMR‡ from actual wt						
$kcal_{th}$/day	1,820	1,710	1,630	1,290	1,190	1,120
MJ/day	7.61	7.15	6.82	5.39	4.98	4.68
BMR from median wt						
$kcal_{th}$/day	1,710	1,710	1,710	1,190	1,190	1,190
MJ/day	7.15	7.15	7.15	4.97	4.97	4.97

*Acceptable range of BMI (see Annex 2A in original reference).

†Body mass index = $wt(kg)/ht^2(m)$.

‡Predicted from equations in Table A–7a.

(From Energy and Protein Requirements: Report of a Joint FAO/WHO/UNU Expert Consultation. Technical Report Series No. 724, Geneva, World Health Organization, 1985, p. 72.)

TABLE A—7C. BASAL METABOLIC RATES OF ADOLESCENT BOYS AND GIRLS

			BMR‡			
			Total		per kg	
AGE (years)	HEIGHT* (cm)	WEIGHT† (kg)	($kcal_{th}$/day)	(MJ/day)	($kcal_{th}$/day)	(MJ/day)
Boys						
10–11	140	32.2	1215	5.08	37.7	0.16
11–12	147	37.0	1300	5.43	35.1	0.15
12–13	153	40.9	1370	5.73	33.4	0.14
13–14	160	47.0	1465	6.12	31.4	0.13
14–15	166	52.6	1570	6.57	29.9	0.12
15–16	171	58.0	1665	6.96	28.7	0.12
16–17	175	62.7	1750	7.32	27.9	0.12
17–18	177	65.0	1790	7.48	27.5	0.12
Girls						
10–11	142	33.7	1160	4.85	34.3	0.14
11–12	148	38.7	1220	5.10	31.5	0.13
12–13	155	44.0	1280	5.38	29.1	0.12
13–14	159	48.8	1340	5.60	27.5	0.12
14–15	161	51.4	1375	5.75	26.7	0.11
15–16	162	53.0	1395	5.83	26.3	0.11
16–17	163	54.0	1405	5.87	26.0	0.11
17–18	164	54.4	1410	5.89	25.9	0.11

*Median height for age from NCHS standards.

†Median weight for height and age from Baldwin's standards (Annex 2(B) of original reference.

‡Boys: BMR = 17.5 W + 651 $kcal_{th}$/day (2.72 MJ/day). Girls: 12.2 W + 746 $kcal_{th}$/day (3.12 MJ/day).

(From Energy and Protein Requirements: Report of a joint FAO/WHO/UNU Expert Consultation. Technical Report Series No. 724. Geneva, World Health Organization, 1985, p. 72.)

TABLE A—7D. BASAL METABOLIC RATE IN ADULT MEN AND WOMEN IN RELATION TO HEIGHT AND MEDIAN ACCEPTABLE WEIGHT FOR HEIGHT* (VALUES GIVEN IN $KCAL_{TH}$ WITH MJ IN PARENTHESES)

		18–30 YEARS		30–60 YEARS		>60 YEARS	
HEIGHT (m)	WEIGHT† (kg)	Per kg per day	Per day	Per kg per day	Per day	Per kg per day	Per day
Men							
1.5	49.5	29.0 (121)	1440 (6.03)	29.4 (123)	1450 (6.07)	23.3 (98)	1150 (4.81)
1.6	56.5	27.4 (115)	1540 (6.44)	27.2 (114)	1530 (6.40)	22.2 (93)	1250 (5.23)
1.7	63.5	26.0 (109)	1650 (6.90)	25.4 (106)	1620 (6.78)	21.2 (89)	1350 (5.65)
1.8	71.5	24.8 (104)	1770 (7.41)	23.9 (99)	1710 (7.15)	20.3 (85)	1450 (6.07)
1.9	79.5	23.9 (100)	1890 (7.91)	22.7 (95)	1800 (7.53)	19.6 (82)	1560 (6.53)
2.0	88	23.0 (96)	2030 (8.49)	21.6 (90)	1900 (7.95)	19.0 (80)	1670 (6.99)
Women							
1.4	41	26.7 (112)	1100 (4.60)	28.8 (120)	1190 (4.98)	25.0 (105)	1030 (4.31)
1.5	47	25.2 (105)	1190 (4.98)	26.3 (110)	1240 (5.19)	23.1 (97)	1090 (4.56)
1.6	54	23.9 (100)	1290 (5.40)	24.1 (101)	1300 (5.44)	21.6 (90)	1160 (4.85)
1.7	61	22.9 (96)	1390 (5.82)	22.4 (94)	1360 (5.69)	20.3 (85)	1230 (5.15)
1.8	68	22.0 (92)	1500 (6.28)	20.9 (87)	1420 (5.94)	19.3 (81)	1310 (5.48)

*BMR from eqquations in Table A—7a rounded to 10 $kcal_{th}$.

†Weight taken as median acceptable weight for height: body mass index (wt/ht^2) = 22 in men, 21 in women.

(From Energy and Protein Requirements: Report of a joint FAO/WHO/UNU Expert Consultation. Technical Report Series No. 724. Geneva, World Health Organization, 1985, p. 72.)

TABLE A–8A. CALCULATED ENERGY REQUIREMENTS OF INFANTS FROM BIRTH TO 1 YEAR

	INTAKE*		CALCULATED ENERGY REQUIREMENT†		MEDIAN BODY WEIGHT‡		TOTAL REQUIREMENT			
							Boys		Girls	
AGE (months)	($kcal_{th}$/kg per day)	(kJ/kg per day)	($kcal_{th}$/kg per day)	(kJ/kg per day)	Boys (kg)	Girls (kg)	($kcal_{th}$/day)	(kJ/day)	($kcal_{th}$/day)	(kJ/day)
0.5	118	494	124	519	3.8	3.6	470	1,965	445	1,860
1–2	114	477	116	485	4.75	4.35	550	2,300	505	2,115
2–3	107	448	109	456	5.6	5.05	610	2,550	545	2,280
3–4	101	423	103	431	6.35	5.7	655	2,740	590	2,470
4–5	96	402	99	414	7.0	6.35	695	2,910	630	2,635
5–6	93	389	96.5	404	7.55	6.95	730	3,055	670	2,800
6–7	91	381	95	397	8.05	7.55	765	3,220	720	3,010
7–8	90	377	94.5	395	8.55	7.95	810	3,390	750	3,140
8–9	90	377	95	397	9.0	8.4	855	3,580	800	3,350
9–10	91	381	99	414	9.35	8.75	925	3,870	865	3,620
10–11	93	389	100	418	9.7	9.05	970	4,060	905	3,790
11–12	97	406	104.5	437	10.05	9.35	1,050	4,395	975	4,080
12	102	427								

*Observed intakes at ages indicated, from data of sources given in original publication. Average intake predicted from equation (age in months): 1 ($kcal_{th}$/kg) = 123 − 8.9 age + 0.59 age. See original reference.

†Requirement over interval indicated, calculated as predicted intake + 5%. See original reference.

‡NCHS median weights at midpoint of month.

(From Energy and Protein Requirements: Report of a Joint FAO/WHO/UNU Expert Consultation. Technical Report Series No. 724. Geneva, World Health Organization, 1985, p. 91.)

TABLE A—8B. ESTIMATED AVERAGE DAILY ENERGY INTAKES AND REQUIREMENTS, AGES 1 TO 10 YEARS

Age (years)	BOYS Intake* (kcal$_{th}$/day)	Intake* (MJ/day)	Requirement† (kcal$_{th}$/day)	Requirement† (MJ/day)
1–2	1,140	4.76	1,200	5.02
2–3	1,340	5.60	1,410	5.89
3–4	1,490	6.23	1,560	6.52
4–5	1,610	6.73	1,690	7.07
5–6	1,720	7.19	1,810	7.57
6–7	1,810	7.57	1,900	7.94
7–8	1,895	7.92	1,990	8.32
8–9	1,970	8.24	2,070	8.66
9–10	2,045	8.55	2,150	8.99

Age (years)	GIRLS Intake* (kcal$_{th}$/day)	Intake* (MJ/day)	Requirement† (kcal$_{th}$/day)	Requirement† (MJ/day)	REQUIREMENT BY WEIGHT‡ Boys (kcal$_{th}$/kg per day)	Boys (kJ/kg per day)	Girls (kcal$_{th}$/kg per day)	Girls (kJ/kg per day)
1–2	1,090	4.56	1,140	4.76	104	435	108	452
2–3	1,250	5.23	1,310	5.48	104	410	102	427
3–4	1,370	5.73	1,440	6.02	99	414	95	397
4–5	1,465	6.12	1,540	6.44	95	397	92	385
5–6	1,550	6.48	1,630	6.81	92	385	88	368
6–7	1,620	6.77	1,700	7.11	88	368	83	347
7–8	1,685	7.05	1,770	7.40	83	347	76	318
8–9	1,740	7.28	1,830	7.65	77	322	69	268
9–10	1,795	7.51	1,880	7.86	72	301	62	259

*From data of Ferro-Luzzi and Durnin, Rome, FAO, 1981 (Document ESN: FAO/WHO/UNU/EPR/81/9).

†Intakes +5%. See original reference.

‡From NCHS median weights at midyear.

(From Energy and Protein Requirements: Report of a Joint FAO/WHO/UNU Expert consultation. Technical Report Series No. 724. Geneva, World Health Organization, 1985, pp. 94 and 95.)

TABLE A–8C. CALCULATED AVERAGE ENERGY EXPENDITURE AND OBSERVED INTAKES AND COMPARISON WITH RECOMMENDATIONS OF 1971 COMMITTEE FOR ADOLESCENTS AGED 10 TO 18 YEARS

AGE	EXPENDITURE	EXPENDITURE		INTAKE†		1971 COMMITTEE‡ RECOMMENDED REQUIREMENT	
(years)	(× BMR)*	($kcal_{th}$/day)	(MJ/day)	($kcal_{th}$/day)	(MJ/day)	($kcal_{th}$/day)	(MJ/day)
Boys							
10–11	1.76	2,140	8.95	2,110	8.82	2,500	10.46
11–12	1.73	2,240	9.37	2,170	9.07	2,600	10.87
12–13	1.69	2,310	9.66	2,200	9.20	2,700	11.29
13–14	1.67	2,440	10.20	2,280	9.53	2,800	11.71
14–15	1.65	2,590	10.83	2,340	9.79	2,900	12.13
15–16	1.62	2,700	11.29	2,390	9.99	3,000	12.55
16–17	1.60	2,800	11.71	2,440	10.20	3,050	12.76
17–18	1.60	2,870	12.0	2,490	10.41	3,100	12.97
Girls							
10–11	1.65	1,910	7.99	1,850	7.74	2,300	9.62
11–12	1.63	1,980	8.28	1,890	7.90	2,350	9.83
12–13	1.60	2,050	8.57	1,930	8.07	2,400	10.04
13–14	1.58	2,120	8.87	1,970	8.24	2,450	10.25
14–15	1.57	2,160	9.03	2,010	8.40	2,500	10.46
15–16	1.54	2,140	8.95	2,050	8.57	2,500	10.46
16–17	1.53	2,130	8.91	2,080	8.70	2,420	10.12
17–18	1.52	2,140	8.95	2,120	8.87	2,340	9.79

*Expenditure calculated as in original publication.

†Intakes from reference in original publication.

‡Reference in original 1971 publication. (cf ref. d)

(From Energy and Protein Requirements: Report of a Joint FAO/WHO/UNU Expert consultation. Technical Report Series No. 724. Geneva, World Health Organization, 1985, p. 98.)

TABLE A–8D. DERIVATION OF AVERAGE VALUES OF THE ENERGY COST OF THREE GRADES OF PHYSICAL ACTIVITY AT WORK FOR WOMEN AND MEN*

	WOMEN†				MEN‡			
	Cost/min ($kcal_{th}$)	(kJ)	Average cost × BMR (gross)	(net)	Cost/min ($kcal_{th}$)	(kJ)	Average cost × BMR (gross)	(net)
Light work								
75% of time sitting or standing	1.51	6.3			1.79	7.5		
25% of time standing and moving	1.70	7.1			2.51	10.5		
Average	1.56	6.5	1.7	0.7	1.99	8.3	1.7	0.7
Moderate work								
25% of time sitting or standing	1.51	6.3			1.79	7.5		
75% of time spent on specific occupational activity	2.20	9.2			3.61	15.1		
Average	2.03	8.5	2.2	1.2	3.16	13.2	2.7	1.7
Heavy work								
40% of time sitting or standing	1.51	6.3			1.79	7.5		
60% of time spent on specific occupational activity	3.21	13.4			6.22	26.0		
Average	2.54	10.6	2.8	1.8	4.45	18.6	3.8	2.8

*Times and energy costs of sitting, standing, moving around, and work tasks are composite values derived from published and unpublished data (Annex 5) in original reference.

†Based on young adult females (18–30 years). Wt 55 kg, BMR 0.90 $kcal_{th}$(3.8) kJ)/min (Table A–7a.)

‡Based on young adult males (18–30 years). Wt 65 kg, BMR 1.16 $kcal_{th}$(4.9 kJ)/min (Table A–7a.)

(From Energy and Protein Requirements: Report of a Joint FAO/WHO/UNU Expert Consultation. Technical Report Series No. 724. Geneva, World Health Organization, 1985, p. 76.)

TABLE A–8E. AVERAGE DAILY ENERGY REQUIREMENT OF ADULTS WHOSE OCCUPATIONAL WORK IS CLASSIFIED AS LIGHT, MODERATE, OR HEAVY, EXPRESSED AS A MULTIPLE OF BASAL METABOLIC RATE

	LIGHT	MODERATE	HEAVY
Men	1.55	1.78	2.10
Women	1.56	1.64	1.82

(From Energy and Protein Requirements: Report of a Joint FAO/WHO/UNU Expert Consultation. Technical Report Series No. 724. Geneva, World Health Organization, 1985, p. 78.)

TABLE A–8F. NOMOGRAM FOR ESTIMATION OF CALORIC REQUIREMENTS

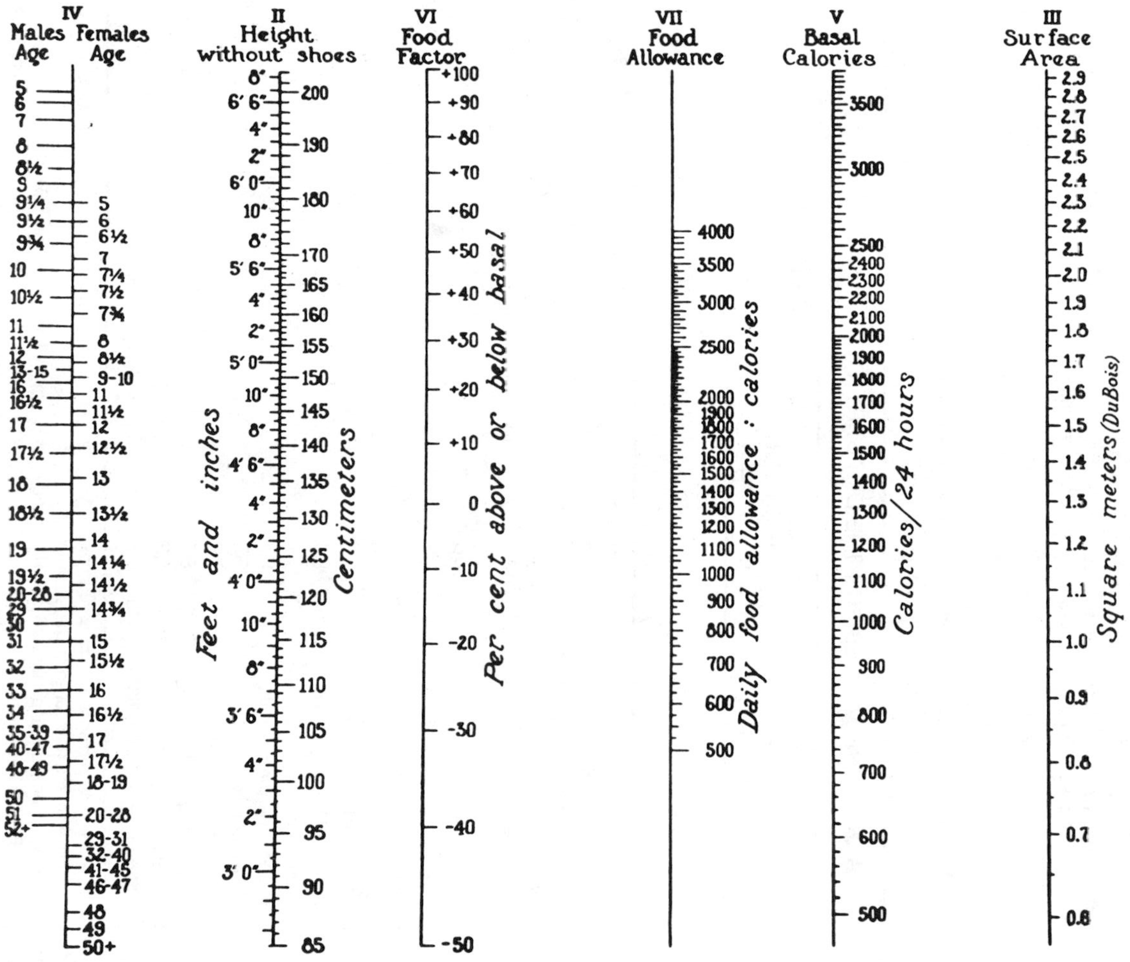

FOOD

NOMOGRAM

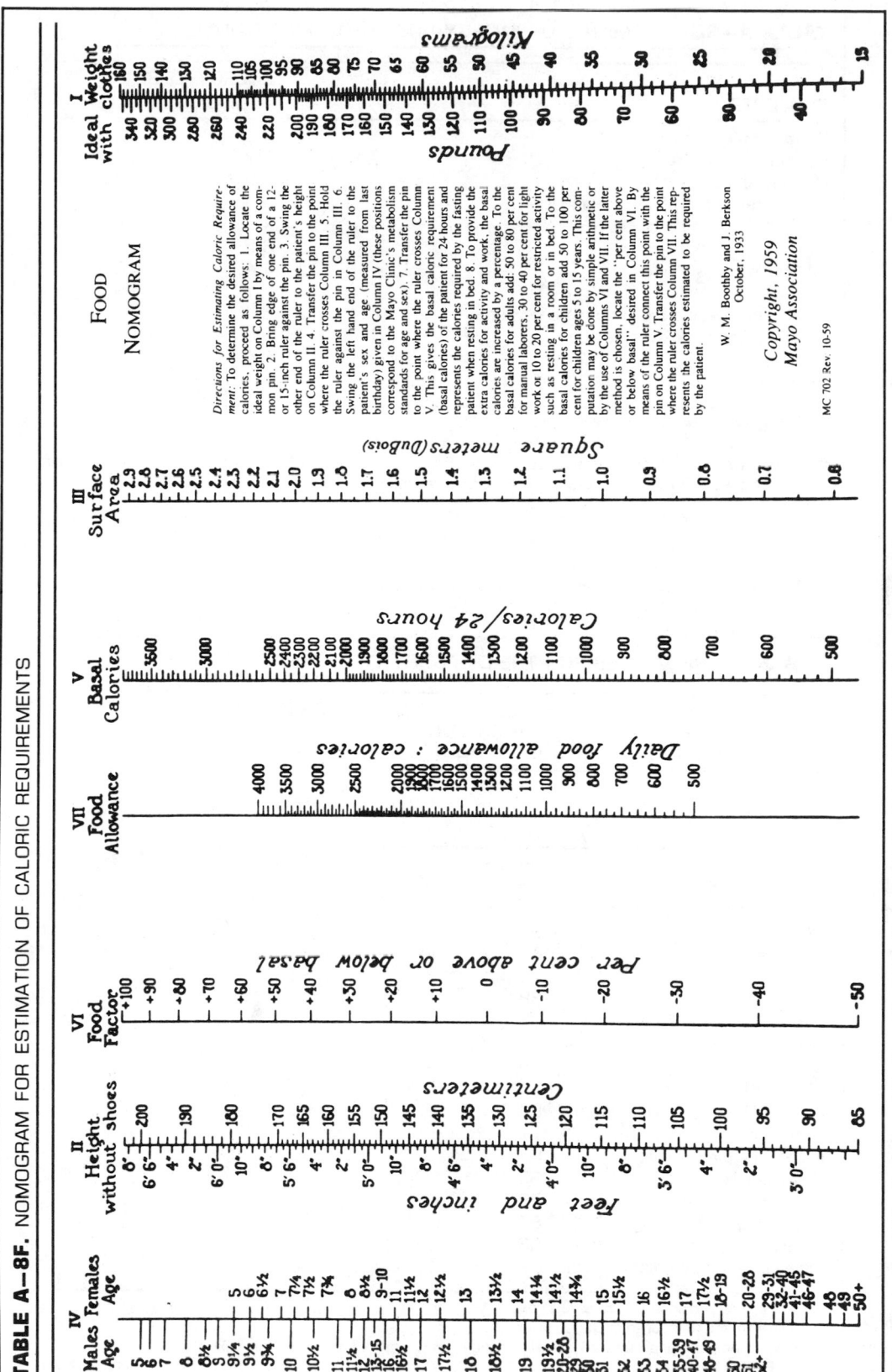

Directions for Estimating Caloric Requirement: To determine the desired allowance of calories, proceed as follows: 1. Locate the ideal weight on Column I by means of a common pin. 2. Bring edge of one end of a 12- or 15-inch ruler against the pin. 3. Swing the other end of the ruler to the patient's height on Column II. 4. Transfer the pin to the point where the ruler crosses Column III. 5. Hold the ruler against the pin in Column III. 6. Swing the left hand end of the ruler to the patient's sex and age (measured from last birthday) given in Column IV (these positions correspond to the Mayo Clinic's metabolism standards for age and sex). 7. Transfer the pin to the point where the ruler crosses Column V. This gives the basal caloric requirement (basal calories) of the patient for 24 hours and represents the calories required by the fasting patient when resting in bed. 8. To provide the extra calories for activity and work, the basal calories are increased by a percentage. To the basal calories for adults add: 50 to 80 per cent for manual laborers, 30 to 40 per cent for light work or 10 to 20 per cent for restricted activity such as resting in a room or in bed. To the basal calories for children add 50 to 100 per cent for children ages 5 to 15 years. This computation may be done by simple arithmetic or by the use of Columns VI and VII. If the latter method is chosen, locate the "per cent above or below basal" desired in Column VI. By means of the ruler connect this point with the pin on Column V. Transfer the pin to the point where the ruler crosses Column VII. This represents the calories estimated to be required by the patient.

W. M. Boothby and J. Berkson
October, 1933

MC 702 Rev. 10-59

(From Pemberton, C.M., Gastineau, C.F.: Mayo Clinic Diet Manual. 5th Ed. Philadelphia, W.B. Saunders, 1981.)

TABLE A–8G. ESTIMATES OF ENERGY COST OF WEIGHT GAIN*

SUBJECTS		ENERGY COST ($kcal_{th}$/g)	(kJ/g)
Premature infants		4.9	20.5
Premature infants		5.7	23.8
Normal infants		5.6	23.4
Infants recovering from malnutrition		5.55	23.2
		4.6	19.2
		3.5	14.6
		4.4	18.4
		7.1	29.7
Adults, recovering from anorexia nervosa		6.4	26.7
Adults, intentional overfeeding		8.2	34.3
Pregnancy	Theoretic estimate†	6.4	26.7

*See original references for data sources.

†Calculated as 80,000 $kcal_{th}$ (335 mJ) stored for 12.5 kg of weight gain.

(From Energy and Protein Requirements: Report of a Joint FAO/WHO/UNU Expert Consultation. Technical Report Series No. 724. Geneva, World Health Organization, 1985, p. 185.)

TABLE A–9A. VALUES FOR THE DIGESTIBILITY OF PROTEIN IN MAN*

PROTEIN SOURCE	TRUE DIGESTIBILITY (mean ±SD)		DIGESTIBILITY RELATIVE TO REFERENCE PROTEINS
Egg	97 ± 3		
Milk, cheese	95 ± 3	95	100
Meat, fish	94 ± 3		
Maize	85 ± 6		89
Rice, polished	88 ± 4		93
Wheat, whole	86 ± 5		90
Wheat, refined	96 ± 4		101
Oatmeal	86 ± 7		90
Millet	79		83
Peas, mature	88		93
Peanut butter	95		100
Soyflour	86 ± 7		90
Beans	78		82
Maize + beans	78		82
Maize + beans + milk	84		88
Indian rice diet	77		81
Indian rice diet + milk	87		92
Chinese mixed diet	96		98†
Brazilian mixed diet	78		82
Filipino mixed diet	88‡		93
American mixed diet	96‡		101
Indian rice + bean diet	78‡		82

*See original reference for data sources.

†Relative to egg measured in the same study.

‡Recalculated from apparent digestibility, using F_K = 12 mg N/kg (see original text).

(From Energy and Protein Requirements: Report of a Joint FAO/WHO/UNU Expert Consultation. Technical Report Series No. 724. Geneva, World Health Organization, 1985, p. 119.)

TABLE A–9B-1. DAILY AVERAGE (PER KG) ENERGY REQUIREMENTS AND SAFE LEVEL OF PROTEIN INTAKE FOR INFANTS AND CHILDREN AGED 3 MONTHS TO 10 YEARS (SEXES COMBINED UP TO 5 YEARS)

AGE	MEDIAN WEIGHT (kg)	ENERGY REQUIREMENT ($kcal_{th}$/kg)		ENERGY REQUIREMENT (kJ/kg)		SAFE LEVEL OF PROTEIN INTAKE (g/kg)*
Months						
3–6	7.0	100		418		1.85
6–9	8.5	95		397		1.65
9–12	9.5	100		418		1.50
Years						
1–2	11.0	105		439		1.20
2–3	13.5	100		418		1.15
3–5	16.5	95		397		1.10
		Boys	Girls	Boys	Girls	
5–7	20.5	90	85	377	356	1.00
7–10	27.0	78	67	326	280	1.00

*Minimum level considered safe.

(From Diet, Nutrition and the Prevention of Chronic Diseases: Report of a WHO Study Group. Technical Report Series No. 797. Geneva, World Health Organization, 1990, pp. 167–168.

TABLE A–9B-2. DAILY AVERAGE ENERGY REQUIREMENTS AND SAFE LEVEL OF PROTEIN INTAKE FOR ADOLESCENTS AGED 10 TO 18 YEARS

AGE (years)	MEDIAN WEIGHT (kg)	ENERGY REQUIREMENT ($kcal_{th}$)	ENERGY REQUIREMENT (kJ)	SAFE LEVEL OF PROTEIN INTAKE (g/kg)*
Boys				
10–12	34.5	2,200	9,200	1.00
12–14	44.0	2,400	10,000	1.00
14–16	55.5	2,650	11,100	0.95
16–18	64.0	2,850	11,900	0.90
Girls				
10–12	36.0	1,950	8,200	1.00
12–14	46.5	2,100	8,800	0.95
14–16	52.0	2,150	9,000	0.90
16–18	54.0	2,150	9,000	0.80

*Minimum level considered safe.

(From Diet, Nutrition and the Prevention of Chronic Diseases: Report of a WHO Study Group. Technical Report Series No. 797. Geneva, World Health Organization, 1990, pp. 167–168.)

TABLE A–9B-3. DAILY AVERAGE ENERGY REQUIREMENTS AND SAFE LEVEL OF PROTEIN INTAKE FOR ADULTS*

	ENERGY REQUIREMENT						SAFE LEVEL OF PROTEIN INTAKE
WEIGHT	18–30 years		30–60 years		Over 60 years		
(kg)	(kcal$_{th}$)	(kJ)	(kcal$_{th}$)	(kJ)	(kcal$_{th}$)	(kJ)	(g/day)†
Men							
50	2,300	9,700	2,350	9,700	1,850	7,700	37.5
55	2,400	10,100	2,450	10,100	1,950	8,300	41.0
60	2,550	10,600	2,500	10,400	2,100	8,600	45.0
65	2,700	11,300	2,600	10,900	2,200	9,100	49.0
70	2,800	11,700	2,700	11,200	2,300	9,600	52.5
75	2,900	12,300	2,800	11,800	2,400	10,000	56.0
80	3,050	12,900	2,900	12,000	2,500	10,400	60.0
Women							
40	1,700	7,200	1,900	7,900	1,650	6,800	30.0
45	1,850	7,700	1,950	8,300	1,700	7,100	34.0
50	1,950	8,200	2,050	8,500	1,800	7,500	37.5
55	2,100	8,600	2,100	8,800	1,900	7,900	41.0
60	2,200	9,200	2,200	9,000	1,950	8,200	45.0
65	2,300	9,800	2,250	9,400	2,050	8,500	49.0
70	2,450	10,300	2,300	9,600	2,150	8,900	52.5
75	2,550	10,800	2,400	10,000	2,200	9,300	56.0

*For a basal metabolic rate factor of 1.6.

†Minimum level considered safe.

(From Diet, Nutrition and the Prevention of Chronic Diseases: Report of a WHO Study Group. Technical Report Series No. 797. Geneva, World Health Organization, 1990, pp. 167–168.)

TABLE A–10. RECOMMENDED DIETARY ALLOWANCES OF VITAMINS AND MINERALS

AGE	VITAMIN A[a,b] SAFE LEVEL (μg retinol/day)		FOLATE[a] (μg/day)		VITAMIN B_{12}[a] (μg/day)		VITAMIN C[c] (mg/day)		VITAMIN D[c] (μg/day)		IRON[a,d] ABSORBED (μg/kg per day)		ZINC[e] (mg/day)	
	M	F	M	F	M	F	M	F	M	F	M	F	M	F
Infants (months)														
0–3	350		16		0.1		20		10		120		3.1	
4–6	350		24		0.1		20		10		120		3.1	
7–9	350		32		0.1		20		10		120		2.8	
10–12	350		32		0.1		20		10		120		2.8	
Children and adults (years)														
1–2	400		50		1.0		20		10		56		4.0	3.9
3–4	400		50		1.0		20		10		44		4.0	3.9
5–6	400		102		1.0		20		10		40		4.0	3.9
7–10	400		102		1.0		20		2.5		40		4.0	3.9
11–12	500		102		1.0		20		2.5		40		7.0	6.6
13–14	600		170		1.0		30		2.5		34	40	7.0	6.6
15–16	600	500	170		1.0		30		2.5		34	40	7.0	5.5
17–18	600	500	200	170	1.0		30		2.5		34	40	7.0	5.5
19+	600	500	200	170	1.0		30		2.5		18	43	5.5	5.5
Pregnant women		600		370 to 470		1.4		50		10		[f]		6.4 to 7.5
Lactating women		850		270		1.3		50		10		24		13.7
Postmenopausal women		500		170		1.0		30		2.5		18		5.5

[a]Adapted from reference 1.
[b]Minimum level considered safe.
[c]Adapted from reference 2; 2.5 μg of cholecalciferol are equivalent to 100 IU of vitamin D.
[d]The amount of absorbed iron is a variable proportion of the intake, depending on the type of diet.
[e]Adapted from reference 3.
[f]Requirements during pregnancy depend on the woman's iron status before pregnancy.

REFERENCES

1. FAO Food and Nutrition Series No. 23. Rome, Food and Agriculture Organization, 1988.
2. WHO Technical Report Series No. 452. Geneva, World Health Organization, 1970.
3. WHO Technical Report Series No. 532. Geneva, World Health Organization, 1973.

(From Diet, Nutrition and the Prevention of Chronic Diseases; Report of a WHO Study Group. Technical Report Series No. 797. Geneva, World Health Organization, 1990, p. 169.)

The Metropolitan Life Insurance Company presented their height and weight tables derived from data of the Build Study, 1979.[1] Metropolitan Life had previously utilized data from life insurance mortality studies compiled in the early 1900s and late 1950s to develop desirable weight tables in 1942,[2] 1943,[3] and 1959.[4] These studies reported the prevalence of mortality among insured persons according to variations in body build (height and weight) and also presented the average weight for height of persons by age. Such studies were designed to determine which groups (those underweight or overweight) showed a proportionately higher prevalence of mortality to yield information for underwriting purposes and for warranting changes in insurance policy premiums.

AVERAGE WEIGHT BY HEIGHT TABLES AND AGE-GROUP

Mortality Studies. In the American life insurance industry, interest in build (height and weight) as factors that influence mortality dates back to 1885. In that year, the Union Mutual Life Insurance Company published a pamphlet containing the results of a study of the company's records on mortality in relation to build.[5] The first indepth study on the subject was presented in 1901 by a representative of the New York Life Insurance Company at the twelfth annual meeting of the Association of Life Insurance Medical Directors of America.[6] In this presentation it was pointed out that a certain amount of overweight had previously been looked on favorably. Nonetheless, the summary of this report noted that: "First among life insurance risks [is that] the [health] hazard increases in proportion to the degree of over- or underweight, second, whereas among overweights the mortality to be expected increases with [the] increased age of [the] applicant, among underweights the mortality decreases with advancing years."

Height-Weight Tables. The first height-weight table based on a considerable volume of statistics and taking age into account was the "Shepherd Table." This table was prepared in 1897 and was based on 74,162 male applicants accepted for life insurance in the United States and Canada.[7]

The basic study of height and weight based on life insurance statistics, however, was made as part of the Medico-Actuarial Mortality Investigation of 1912.[8] This study and the tables derived therefrom were the basis of the height-weight tables prepared for the general population. In addition to the study of the prevalence of mortality of certain groups of the insured population, the 1912 investigation included a study of the height and weight of a sample of persons insured from 1885 to 1900. The height and weight were recorded with the subjects wearing shoes and street clothes. A total of 221,819 men residing in the United States and Canada were included in this sample. At least 40% of the weights were estimated by the medical examiners. The data as tabulated were then smoothed to provide the figures for the height-weight age tables, and the adjusted tables became the basis for height-weight tables for males in the United States at this time.

Substantially the same procedure was employed to develop height-weight tables for women, but to secure enough cases for the preparation of tables it was necessary to add 126,504 policies issued after 1900 to the 10,000 included in the 1885 to 1900 sample.

In the Medical Impairment Study of 1929,[9] height-weight data were again collected on 667,000 men and 85,000 women. The average weights of both men and women in the 1929 study were not significantly different from those observed in the Medico-Actuarial Mortality Investigation. In fact, differences were so small that it was decided not to revise the standard height-weight tables except for those individuals younger than age 15.

TABLES OF "IDEAL" OR "DESIRABLE" WEIGHTS

An article presented in 1920, "Is the 'Average' the Same as the 'Normal' for Weight and Blood Pressure?"[10] illustrates an important development in the preparation of height-weight tables. In this paper the "normal" weight group is defined as that having the lowest mortality rate. The article presented a table of "normal" weights, so defined, for medium-sized men averaging 68 inches in height, and several discussants added their tables of similarly defined normal weights for men of small, medium, and tall height. In 1922, complete height-weight tables were presented that showed this normal weight for each inch of height and for each age group.[11] In general, all such tables of normal weight indicated that the ideal weight in terms of mortality was the average weight for height at age 30.

METROPOLITAN LIFE DEVELOPS "IDEAL" HEIGHT-WEIGHT TABLES

Desirable Weight Tables, 1942 and 1943. The concept of a "normal" weight, represented by the average weight of men at age 30, plus an awareness of the shortcomings of height and weight alone as complete indications of obesity, led to the development of "ideal" weight tables by the Metropolitan Life Insurance company.[2,3] Al-

(From Clinical Consultations in Nutrition Support, *3*:5–8, 1983. Reprinted with permission of Sidney Abraham and Clinical Consultants in Nutrition Support.)

though employed for many purposes, these tables were originally intended for use in health education. The basic data were derived from the standard height-weight tables of the Medico-Actuarial Study of 1912, using the average weight for each inch of height at age 30 for men and at age 25 for women. Arbitrary ranges were then developed, using the base figures as reference points. These ranges are approximately the standard deviation of average weights for a given height and include the lightest weight for persons with small frames to the heaviest weight for persons with large frames. The total was then arbitrarily divided into three overlapping ranges, and the resulting figures represented ideal weights for individuals of small, medium, and large frames. However, no definition of frame size was presented.

These tables were intended to aid people in achieving a weight below the average for their height. Before these tables were developed, only average weights for each inch of height by age and sex were available. The new approach represented a change in concept between average weight (assuming that the average value is optimal for health) and desirable weight (weight based on the criterion of longevity). The concept underlying these tables deemphasized the use of a single average at each height and refuted the popular notion that weight increments attendant with advancing age were normal and therefore not harmful.

Desirable Weight Tables, 1959. The next study of build in relation to mortality was made in conjunction with the Build and Blood Pressure Study of 1959.[4] This investigation was based on the combined experience of 26 life insurance companies in the United States and Canada from 1935 to 1954 and involved observation of nearly 5 million insured persons for periods up to 20 years. Only those insured persons ages 15 through 69 were included. The height and weight data were recorded with the subjects wearing street shoes and indoor clothing. More than 90% of the insured persons were reported to have been actually weighed and measured at the time of examination for life insurance. The study presented average weights for men and women for each inch of height, ranging from 62 to 76 inches for men and from 58 to 72 inches for women. To provide some indication of the sole effect of weight on mortality, persons with heart disease, cancer, or diabetes were excluded.

When the Build and Blood Pressure Study was completed, the "ideal weight" table, originally developed by the Metropolitan Life Insurance company in 1942 and 1943, was revised to conform to the latest data. The new table, called the "desirable weight" table (Table A–11b) was derived directly from weights associated with lowest mortality. Ranges of "desirable weight" for individuals 25 years and older with small, medium, and large frames were given, but again, no definition of frame size was included.

1983 Metropolitan Height-Weight Tables. Data published by the Society of Actuaries and the Association of Life Insurance Medical Directors of America in the Build Study, 1979,[1] are the source for the 1983 Metropolitan Life Insurance Height-Weight Tables (Table A–11c). The data are from 25 life insurance companies in the United States and Canada and show the prevalence of mortality from 1954 to 1972 of approximately 4.2 million insured men and women. Almost 90% of the recorded weights submitted for the study was obtained by actually weighing the applicants. As in the 1959 Build and Blood Pressure Study, applicants with major disease conditions at the time of policy issuance were excluded from the study. The terms "ideal body weight" and "desirable body weight," used in the earlier tables were not applied to the new height and weight tables because of the various misinterpretations of their meaning.

The findings from the Build Study, 1979, showed that the gap between the weights based on lowest mortality and average weights has narrowed considerably since the 1959 Build and Blood Pressure Study. Metropolitan Life considered this factor in developing the 1983 height-weight tables. Weight for height has increased in contrast to the 1959 tables, but the increased weights are still less than the average weights (see Table A–11f). Additionally, the increases in weight are not uniformly distributed throughout the 1983 height-weight tables. For each frame size, the weight increases for tall men or women were not as large as those for short men or women or for those of medium height.

In conjunction with investigations based on the life insurance data previously enumerated, long-term studies such as the Framingham Heart Study[12] and the Manitoba Study[13] all indicate that the weight associated with the greatest longevity tends to be below the average weight of the population under consideration and that "slimmer is better," provided that the underweight is not associated with a medical history of significant impairment.

FRAME SIZE

The 1983 Metropolitan height-weight tables relate weight to body frame size. A distinction is made among persons with small, medium, and large frames. The previous Metropolitan height-weight tables also related weight to body frame size, but although the body frame sizes were statistically defined, no generally accepted method of measuring frame size was provided. Body frame size is an integral factor in considering variation in weight, assuming that persons with larger frames have larger lean body mass and therefore weigh more. In the 1983 tables, elbow breadth is now used to determine frame size in men and women (Table A–11d). The frame sizes were developed from elbow breadth measurements taken from the first National Health and Nutrition Examination Survey, 1971 to 1975,[14] and were distributed so that 50% of the population falls within the medium frame and 25% each falls within the small and large frames.

SUMMARY

Major insurance mortality studies on insured populations in the United States and Canada conducted in 1912 by the Actuarial Society of America[8] and in 1959 and 1979 by the Society of Actuaries and the Association of Life Insurance Medical Directors of America[1,4] analyzed the mortality experience among insured persons according to variations of weight by height. The studies also presented data on the distribution of weight and height. The earliest study showed that the lowest mortality by build (weight for height) was found for those somewhat overweight at younger ages and among those underweight at older ages. In later mortality studies, it was generally found that insured persons whose weight was below the average lived longer than those whose weights were above average.

Since 1942, the Metropolitan Life Insurance Company has developed weight tables from data derived from each of the three major studies. The weights in each of the tables at given heights for men and women are classified according to frame size and refer to the weights associated with lowest mortality of policyholders. The weights were those obtained when the individual was originally insured. Because it is recognized that height and weight alone are incomplete indicators of excess weight, the weight tables also considered measurements of body build. In the tables issued in the 1940s,[2,3] 1959,[4] and 1983, three groups of frame size were identified. In each frame size, weight was given as a range rather than as a single value. However, no objective method was presented to estimate frame size in the earlier two tables. In the 1983 Metropolitan Height-Weight Tables, elbow breadth, unaffcted by degree of adiposity and closely representative of bony dimension, was suggested to estimate frame size in the three categories of body build.

The views herein are solely those of the author and do not necessarily represent those of the National Center for Health Statistics.

REFERENCES

1. Build Study, 1979: Society of Actuaries and Association of Life Insurance Medical Directors of America. Philadelphia, Recording and Statistical Corporation, 1980.
2. Ideal Weight for Men: Stat. Bull. Metropol. Life Insur. Co., *23*:6, 1942.
3. Ideal weights for Woman: Stat. Bull. Metropol. Life Insur. Co., *24*:6, 1943.
4. New Weight Standards for Men and Women: Stat. Bull. Metropol. Life Insur. Co., *40*:1, 1959.
5. Grant, F. S.: Proc. Assoc. Life Insur. Med. Dir. Am., *2*:323–327, 1902.
6. Rogers, O. H.: Proc. Assoc. Life Insur. Med. Dir. Am., *1*:280–288, 1901.
7. Shepherd, G. R.: Proc. Assoc. Life Insur. Med. Dir. Am., *6*:46–58, 1912.
8. Medico-Actuarial Mortality Investigation. New York, Actuarial Society of America, 1912.
9. Medical Impairment Study, 1929. New York, The Association of Life Insurance Medical Directors of America and the Actuarial Society of America, 1931.
10. Hunter, A.: Trans. Actuar. Soc. Am., *21*:365–370, 1920.
11. Knight, A. S.: Proc. Assoc. Life Insur. Med. Dir. Am., *9*:193–199, 1922.
12. Hubert, H. B., Feinleib, M., McNamara, P. M., et al.: Circulation, *5*:968–977, 1983.
13. Rabkin, S. W., Mathewson, F. A. L., Hsu, P. H.: Am. J. Cardiol., *39*:452–458, 1977.
14. Public Use Data Tape, NHANES I—Anthropometry, goniometry, skeletal age, bone density, and cortical thickness, ages 1–74. Tape No. 4111, National Health and Nutrition Examination Survey, 1971–1975. Hyattsville, MD, National Center for Health Statistics.

TABLE A–11B. DESIRABLE WEIGHTS FOR MEN AND WOMEN AGED 25 AND OVER (IN POUNDS BY HEIGHT AND FRAME, IN INDOOR CLOTHING), 1959

MEN (IN SHOES, ONE-INCH HEELS)					WOMEN (IN SHOES, TWO-INCH HEELS)				
HEIGHT					HEIGHT				
FEET	INCHES	SMALL FRAME	MEDIUM FRAME	LARGE FRAME	FEET	INCHES	SMALL FRAME	MEDIUM FRAME	LARGE FRAME
5	2	112–120	118–129	126–141	4	10	92–98	96–107	104–119
5	3	115–123	121–133	129–144	4	11	94–101	98–110	106–122
5	4	118–126	124–136	132–148	5	0	96–104	101–113	109–125
5	5	121–129	127–139	135–152	5	1	99–107	104–116	112–128
5	6	124–133	130–143	138–156	5	2	102–110	107–119	115–131
5	7	128–137	134–147	142–161	5	3	105–113	110–122	118–134
5	8	132–141	138–152	147–166	5	4	108–116	113–126	121–138
5	9	136–145	142–156	151–170	5	5	111–119	116–130	125–142
5	10	140–150	146–160	155–174	5	6	114–123	120–135	129–146
5	11	144–154	150–165	159–179	5	7	118–127	124–139	133–150
6	0	148–158	154–170	164–184	5	8	122–131	128–143	137–154
6	1	152–162	158–175	168–189	5	9	126–135	132–147	141–158
6	2	156–167	162–180	173–194	5	10	130–140	136–151	145–163
6	3	160–171	167–185	178–199	5	11	134–144	140–155	149–168
6	4	164–175	172–190	182–204	6	0	138–148	144–159	153–173

(Data adapted from new weight standards for men and women. Stat. Bull. Metropol. Life Insur. Co., *40*:1, 1959.)

TABLE A–11C. HEIGHT-WEIGHT TABLES, 1983

MEN					WOMEN				
HEIGHT					HEIGHT				
FEET	INCHES	SMALL FRAME	MEDIUM FRAME	LARGE FRAME	FEET	INCHES	SMALL FRAME	MEDIUM FRAME	LARGE FRAME
5	2	128–134	131–141	138–150	4	10	102–111	109–121	118–131
5	3	130–136	133–143	140–153	4	11	103–113	111–123	120–134
5	4	132–138	135–145	142–156	5	0	104–115	113–126	122–137
5	5	134–140	137–148	144–160	5	1	106–118	115–129	125–140
5	6	136–142	139–151	146–164	5	2	108–121	118–132	128–143
5	7	138–145	142–154	149–168	5	3	111–124	121–135	131–147
5	8	140–148	145–157	152–172	5	4	114–127	124–138	134–151
5	9	142–151	148–160	155–176	5	5	117–130	127–141	137–155
5	10	144–154	151–163	158–180	5	6	120–133	130–144	140–159
5	11	146–157	154–166	161–184	5	7	123–136	133–147	143–163
6	0	149–160	157–170	164–188	5	8	126–139	136–150	146–167
6	1	152–164	160–174	168–192	5	9	129–142	139–153	149–170
6	2	155–168	164–178	172–197	5	10	132–145	142–156	152–173
6	3	158–172	167–182	176–202	5	11	135–148	145–159	155–176
6	4	162–176	171–187	181–207	6	0	138–151	148–162	158–179

Weight according to frame (ages 25 to 59) for men wearing indoor clothing weighing 5 lb, shoes with one-inch heels; for women, indoor clothing weighing 3 lb, shoes with one-inch heels.

Reprinted with permission from the Metropolitan Life Insurance Company, New York.)

TABLE A–11D. HEIGHT AND ELBOW BREADTH FOR MEN AND WOMEN*

HEIGHT IN ONE-INCH HEELS	ELBOW BREADTH
Men	
5′2″–5′3″	2½″–2⅞″
5′4″–5′7″	2⅝″–2⅞″
5′8″–5′11″	2¾″–3″
6′0″–6′3″	2¾″–3⅛″
6′4″	2⅞″–3¼″
Women	
4′10″–4′11″	2¼″–2½″
5′0″–5′3″	2¼″–2½″
5′4″–5′7″	2⅜″–2⅝″
5′8″–5′11″	2⅜″–2⅝″
6′0″	2½″–2¾″

*See Table A–11f; see Table A–11g for data on frame size by elbow breadth from NHANES I and II.

Extend your arm and bend the forearm upward at a 90° angle. Keep fingers straight and turn the inside of your wrist toward your body. If you have a caliper, use it to measure the space between the two prominent bones on either side of your elbow. Without a caliper, place thumb and index finger of your other hand on these two bones. Measure the space between your fingers against a ruler or tape measure. Compare it with these tables that list elbow measurements for medium-frame men and women. Measurements lower than those listed indicate you have a small frame. Higher measurements indicate a larger frame.

TABLE A–11E. HEIGHT-WEIGHT TABLES (METRIC UNITS), 1983*

	MEN				WOMEN		
HEIGHT (cm)	SMALL FRAME (kg)	MEDIUM FRAME (kg)	LARGE FRAME (kg)	HEIGHT (cm)	SMALL FRAME (kg)	MEDIUM FRAME (kg)	LARGE FRAME (kg)
157.5	58.2–60.9	59.4–64.1	62.7–68.2	147.5	46.4–50.5	49.5–55.0	53.6–59.5
160	59.1–61.8	60.5–65.0	63.6–69.5	150	46.8–51.4	50.5–55.9	54.5–60.9
162.5	60.0–62.7	61.4–65.9	64.5–70.9	152.5	47.3–52.3	51.4–57.3	55.5–62.3
165	60.9–63.7	62.3–67.3	65.5–72.7	155	48.2–53.6	52.3–58.6	56.8–63.6
167.5	61.8–64.5	63.2–68.6	66.4–74.5	157.5	49.1–55.0	53.6–60.0	58.2–65.0
170	62.7–65.9	64.5–70.0	67.7–76.4	160	50.5–56.4	55.0–61.4	59.5–66.8
173	63.6–67.3	65.9–71.4	69.1–78.2	162.5	51.8–57.7	56.4–62.7	60.9–68.6
175	64.5–68.6	67.3–72.7	70.5–80.0	165	53.2–59.1	57.7–64.1	62.3–70.5
178	65.4–70.0	68.6–74.1	71.8–81.8	167.5	54.5–60.5	59.1–65.5	63.6–72.3
180	66.4–71.4	70.0–75.5	73.2–83.6	170	55.9–61.8	60.5–66.8	65.0–74.1
183	67.7–72.7	71.4–77.3	74.5–85.6	173	57.3–63.2	61.8–68.2	66.4–75.9
185.5	69.1–74.5	72.7–79.1	76.4–87.3	175	58.6–64.5	63.2–69.5	67.7–77.3
188	70.5–76.4	74.5–80.9	78.2–89.5	178	60.0–65.9	64.5–70.9	69.1–78.6
190.5	71.8–78.2	75.9–82.7	80.0–91.8	180	61.4–67.3	65.9–72.3	70.5–80.0
193	73.6–80.0	77.7–85.0	82.3–94.1	183	62.3–68.6	67.3–73.6	71.8–81.4

*The 1983 Metropolitan Height-Weight Tables are based on the 1979 Build Study.

The values are statistical computations from individuals ranging from 25 to 59 years of weights by height and body frame at which mortality has been found to be lowest or longevity the highest. Metropolitan Life does not advocate the use of the term "ideal," which has different meanings to various individuals, because the term was used originally in their 1942 to 1943 tables. If one wishes to use these tables in the sense that they are "ideal" in terms of lowest mortality, they are "appropriate" in that context. These tables do not provide weights related to minimizing illness, optimizing job performance, or creating the best appearance.

TABLE A–11F. AVERAGE WEIGHTS BY HEIGHT AND AGE GROUP: 1959 AND 1979 BUILD AND BLOOD PRESSURE STUDIES

	HEIGHT														
MEN	5′2″	5′3″	5′4″	5′5″	5′6″	5′7″	5′8″	5′9″	5′10″	5′11″	6′0″	6′1″	6′2″	6′3″	6′4″
15–16 Years*															
1959 Study	107	112	117	122	127	132	137	142	146	150	154	159	164	169	†
1979 Study	112	116	121	127	133	137	143	148	153	159	162	168	173	178	184
Weight Change	+5	+4	+4	+5	+6	+5	+6	+6	+7	+9	+8	+9	+9	+9	—
17–19 Years															
1959 Study	119	123	127	131	135	139	143	147	151	155	160	164	168	172	176
1979 Study	124	129	132	137	141	145	150	155	159	164	168	174	179	185	190
Weight Change	+5	+6	+5	+6	+6	+6	+7	+8	+8	+9	+8	+10	+11	+13	+14
20–24 Years															
1959 Study	128	132	136	139	142	145	149	153	157	161	166	170	174	178	181
1979 Study	130	136	139	143	148	153	157	163	167	171	176	182	187	193	198
Weight Change	+2	+4	+3	+4	+6	+8	+8	+10	+10	+10	+10	+12	+13	+15	+17
25–29 Years															
1959 Study	134	138	141	144	148	151	155	159	163	167	172	177	182	186	190
1979 Study	134	140	143	147	152	156	161	166	171	175	181	186	191	197	202
Weight Change	+0	+2	+2	+3	+4	+5	+6	+7	+8	+8	+9	+9	+9	+11	+12
30–39 Years															
1959 Study	137	141	145	149	153	157	161	165	170	174	179	183	188	193	199
1979 Study	138	143	147	151	156	160	165	170	174	179	184	190	195	201	206
Weight Change	+1	+2	+2	+2	+3	+3	+4	+5	+4	+5	+5	+7	+7	+8	+7
40–49 Years															
1959 Study	140	144	148	152	156	161	165	169	174	178	183	187	192	197	203
1979 Study	140	144	149	154	158	163	167	172	176	181	186	192	197	203	208
Weight Change	+0	+0	+1	+2	+2	+2	+2	+3	+2	+3	+3	+5	+5	+6	+5
50–59 Years															
1959 Study	142	145	149	153	157	162	166	170	175	180	185	189	194	199	205
1979 Study	141	145	150	155	159	164	168	173	177	182	187	193	198	204	209
Weight Change	−1	+0	+1	+2	+2	+2	+2	+3	+2	+2	+2	+4	+4	+5	+4
60–69 Years															
1959 Study	139	142	146	150	154	159	163	168	173	178	183	188	193	198	204
1979 Study	140	144	149	153	158	163	167	172	176	181	186	191	196	200	207
Weight Change	+1	+2	+3	+3	+4	+4	+4	+4	+3	+3	+3	+3	+3	+2	+3

(Continued)

TABLE A—11F. (continued)

WOMEN	HEIGHT 4′10″	4′11″	5′0″	5′1″	5′2″	5′3″	5′4″	5′5″	5′6″	5′7″	5′8″	5′9″	5′10″	5′11″	6′0″
15–16 Years*															
1959 Study	97	100	103	107	111	114	117	121	125	128	132	136	†	†	†
1979 Study	101	105	109	112	117	121	123	128	131	135	138	142	146	149	152
Weight Change	+4	+5	+6	+5	+6	+7	+6	+7	+6	+7	+6	+6	—	—	—
17–19 Years															
1959 Study	99	102	105	109	113	116	120	124	127	130	134	138	142	147	152
1979 Study	103	108	111	115	119	123	126	129	132	136	140	145	148	150	154
Weight Change	+4	+6	+6	+6	+6	+7	+6	+5	+5	+6	+6	+7	+6	+3	+2
20–24 Years															
1959 Study	102	105	108	112	115	118	121	125	129	132	136	140	144	149	154
1979 Study	105	110	112	116	120	124	127	130	133	137	141	146	149	155	157
Weight Change	+3	+5	+4	+4	+5	+6	+6	+5	+4	+5	+5	+6	+5	+6	+3
25–29 Years															
1959 Study	107	110	113	116	119	122	125	129	133	136	140	144	148	153	158
1979 Study	110	112	114	119	121	125	128	132	134	138	142	148	150	156	159
Weight Change	+3	+2	+1	+3	+2	+3	+3	+3	+1	+2	+2	+4	+2	+3	+1
30–39 Years															
1959 Study	115	117	120	123	126	129	132	135	139	142	146	150	154	159	164
1979 Study	113	115	118	121	124	128	131	134	137	141	145	150	153	159	164
Weight Change	−2	−2	−2	−2	−2	−1	−1	−1	−2	−1	−1	0	−1	0	0
40–49 Years															
1959 Study	122	124	127	130	133	136	140	143	147	151	155	159	164	169	174
1979 Study	118	121	123	127	129	133	136	139	143	147	150	155	158	162	168
Weight Change	−4	−3	−4	−3	−4	−3	−4	−4	−4	−4	−5	−4	−6	−7	−6
50–59 Years															
1959 Study	125	127	130	133	136	140	144	148	152	156	160	164	169	174	180
1979 Study	121	125	127	131	133	137	141	144	147	152	156	159	162	166	171
Weight Change	−4	−2	−3	−2	−3	−3	−3	−4	−5	−4	−4	−5	−7	−8	−9
60–69 Years															
1959 Study	127	129	131	134	137	141	145	149	153	157	161	165	†	†	†
1979 Study	123	127	130	133	136	140	143	147	150	155	158	161	163	167	172
Weight Change	−4	−2	−1	−1	−1	−1	−2	−2	−3	−2	−3	−4	—	—	—

*Height in shoes (feet and inches) and weight in indoor clothing (pounds).

†Average weights omitted in classes with too few cases for analysis.

(Data from Association of Life Insurance Medical Directors of America and Society of Actuaries. Compiled by Seltzer, F.: Dietetic Currents, *10*:17–22, 1983. Reprinted with permission of Ross Laboratories, Columbus, Ohio.)

TABLE A–11G. FRAME SIZE BY ELBOW BREADTH (cm) OF UNITED STATES MALE AND FEMALE ADULTS DERIVED FROM THE COMBINED NHANES I AND II DATA SETS*

AGE (YEARS)	FRAME SIZE SMALL	MEDIUM	LARGE
MEN			
18–24	≤6.6	>6.6 AND <7.7	≥7.7
25–34	≤6.7	>6.7 AND <7.9	≥7.9
35–44	≤6.7	>6.7 AND <8.0	≥8.0
45–54	≤6.7	>6.7 AND <8.1	≥8.1
55–64	≤6.7	>6.7 AND <8.1	≥8.1
65–74	≤6.7	>6.7 AND <8.1	≥8.1
WOMEN			
18–24	≤5.6	>5.6 AND <6.5	≥6.5
25–34	≤5.7	>5.7 AND <6.8	≥6.8
35–44	≤5.7	>5.7 AND <7.1	≥7.1
45–54	≤5.7	>5.7 AND <7.2	≥7.2
55–64	≤5.8	>5.8 AND <7.2	≥7.2
65–74	≤5.8	>5.8 AND <7.2	≥7.2

*The tenth and ninetieth percentiles, respectively, represent the predicted mean ±1.282 times the SE. Similarly, the fifteenth and eighty-fifth percentiles are the predicted mean minus and plus, respectively, 1.036 times the SE of the regression equation. There were significant black-white population differences in weight and body composition when age and height were considered. However, when the comparisons were made with reference to age, height, and frame size, there were only minor interpopulation differences. For this reason, all races (white, black, and other) included in the NHANES I and II surveys were merged together for the purpose of calculating percentiles of anthropometric measurements.

(Combined NHANES I and II data sets from Frisancho, A.R.: Am, J. Clin. Nutr., *40*:808–819, 1984, with permission.)

TABLE A–11H. COMPARISON OF THE WEIGHT-FOR-HEIGHT TABLES FROM ACTUARIAL DATA (BUILD STUDY): NON-AGE-CORRECTED METROPOLITAN LIFE INSURANCE COMPANY AND AGE-SPECIFIC GERONTOLOGY RESEARCH CENTER RECOMMENDATIONS*

	METROPOLITAN 1983 WEIGHTS FOR AGES 25–59†		GERONTOLOGY RESEARCH CENTER WEIGHT RANGE FOR MEN AND WOMEN BY AGE (YEARS)				
HEIGHT	MEN	WOMEN	25	35	45	55	65
ft-in	lb						
4–10	—	100–131	84–111	92–119	99–127	107–135	115–142
4–11	—	101–134	87–115	95–123	103–131	111–139	119–147
5–0	—	103–137	90–119	98–127	106–135	114–143	123–152
5–1	123–145	105–140	93–123	101–131	110–140	118–148	127–157
5–2	125–148	108–144	96–127	105–136	113–144	122–153	131–163
5–3	127–151	111–148	99–131	108–140	117–149	126–158	135–168
5–4	129–155	114–152	102–135	112–145	121–154	130–163	140–173
5–5	131–159	117–156	106–140	115–149	125–159	134–168	144–179
5–6	133–163	120–160	109–144	119–154	129–164	138–174	148–184
5–7	135–167	123–164	112–148	122–159	133–169	143–179	153–190
5–8	137–171	126–167	116–153	126–163	137–174	147–184	158–196
5–9	139–175	129–170	119–157	130–168	141–179	151–190	162–201
5–10	141–179	132–173	122–162	134–173	145–184	156–195	167–207
5–11	144–183	135–176	126–167	137–178	149–190	160–201	172–213
6–0	147–187	—	129–171	141–183	153–195	165–207	177–219
6–1	150–192	—	133–176	145–188	157–200	169–213	182–225
6–2	153–197	—	137–181	149–194	162–206	174–219	187–232
6–3	157–202	—	141–186	153–199	166–212	179–225	192–238
6–4	—	—	144–191	157–205	171–218	184–231	197–244

*Values in this table are for height without shoes and weight without clothes. To convert inches to centimeters, multiply by 2.54; to convert pounds to kilograms, multiply by 0.455.

†The weight range is the lower weight for small frame and the upper weight for large frame.

(Gerontology Research Center data from Andres, R.: Mortality and obesity: the rationale for age-specific height-weight tables. *In* Principles of Geriatric Medicine. Edited by R. Andres, E. Bierman, and W. R. Hazzard. New York, McGraw-Hill, 1985, pp. 311–318.)

TABLE A–11I. NOMOGRAPH FOR ESTIMATING BODY MASS INDEX (kg/m²)*

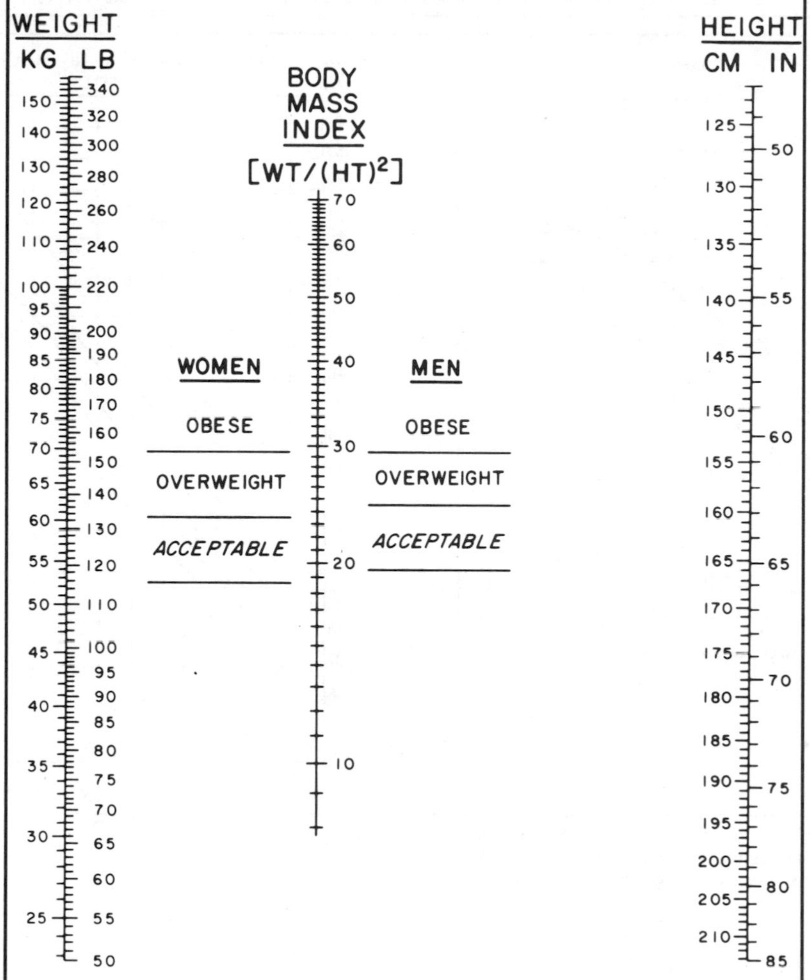

*The ratio of weight/height² emerges from varied epidemiologic studies as the most generally useful index of relative body mass in adults. This nomograph facilitates use of this relationship in clinical situations. While showing the range of weight given as desirable in life insurance studies, the scale expresses relative weight as a continuous variable. This method encourages use of clinical judgment in interpreting "overweight" and "underweight" and in accounting for muscular and skeletal contributions to measured mass.

(From G. A. Bray, 1978.)

TABLE A–11J. DESIRABLE BODY MASS INDEX (BMI) IN RELATION TO AGE

Age (years)	BMI (kg/m²)
19–24	19–24
25–34	20–25
35–44	21–26
45–54	22–27
55–65	23–28
>65	24–29

(From Committee on Diet and Health, Food and Nutrition Board, National Research Council. Diet and Health: Implications for Reducing Chronic Disease Risk. Washington, D.C., National Academy Press, 1989, p. 564.)

TABLE A–12A. FETAL GROWTH STANDARDS: INTRAUTERINE WEIGHT* AND LENGTH† CHARTS

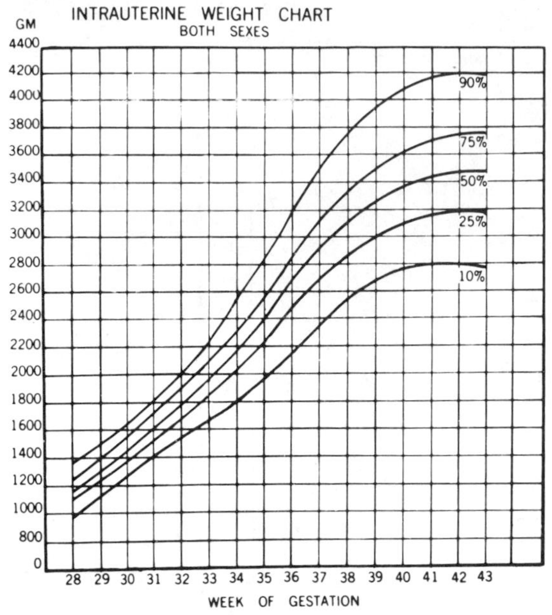

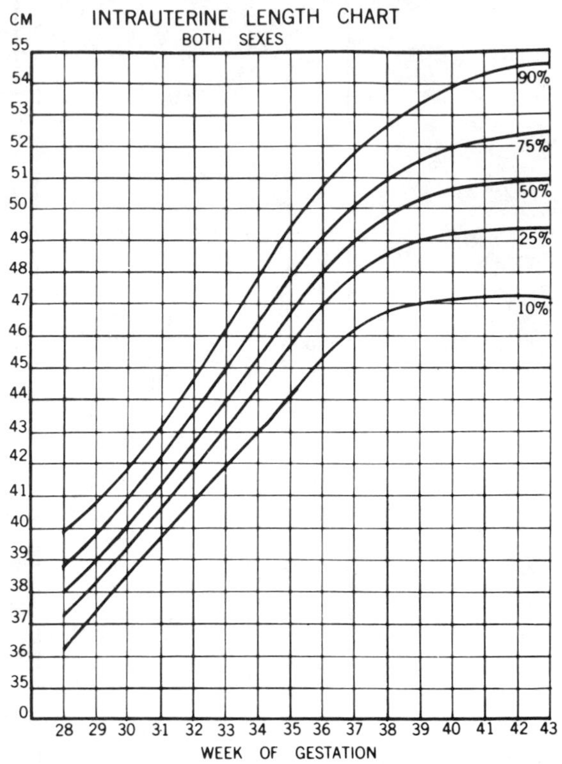

*Fetal body weight percentiles from 28 to 43 weeks of gestation.
†Fetal body length percentiles from 28 to 43 weeks of gestation.
(From Naeye, R.L., Dixon J.B.: Pediatr. Res., *12*:989, 1978.)

TABLE A–12B-1. PHYSICAL GROWTH NCHS PERCENTILES: GIRLS FROM BIRTH TO 36 MONTHS

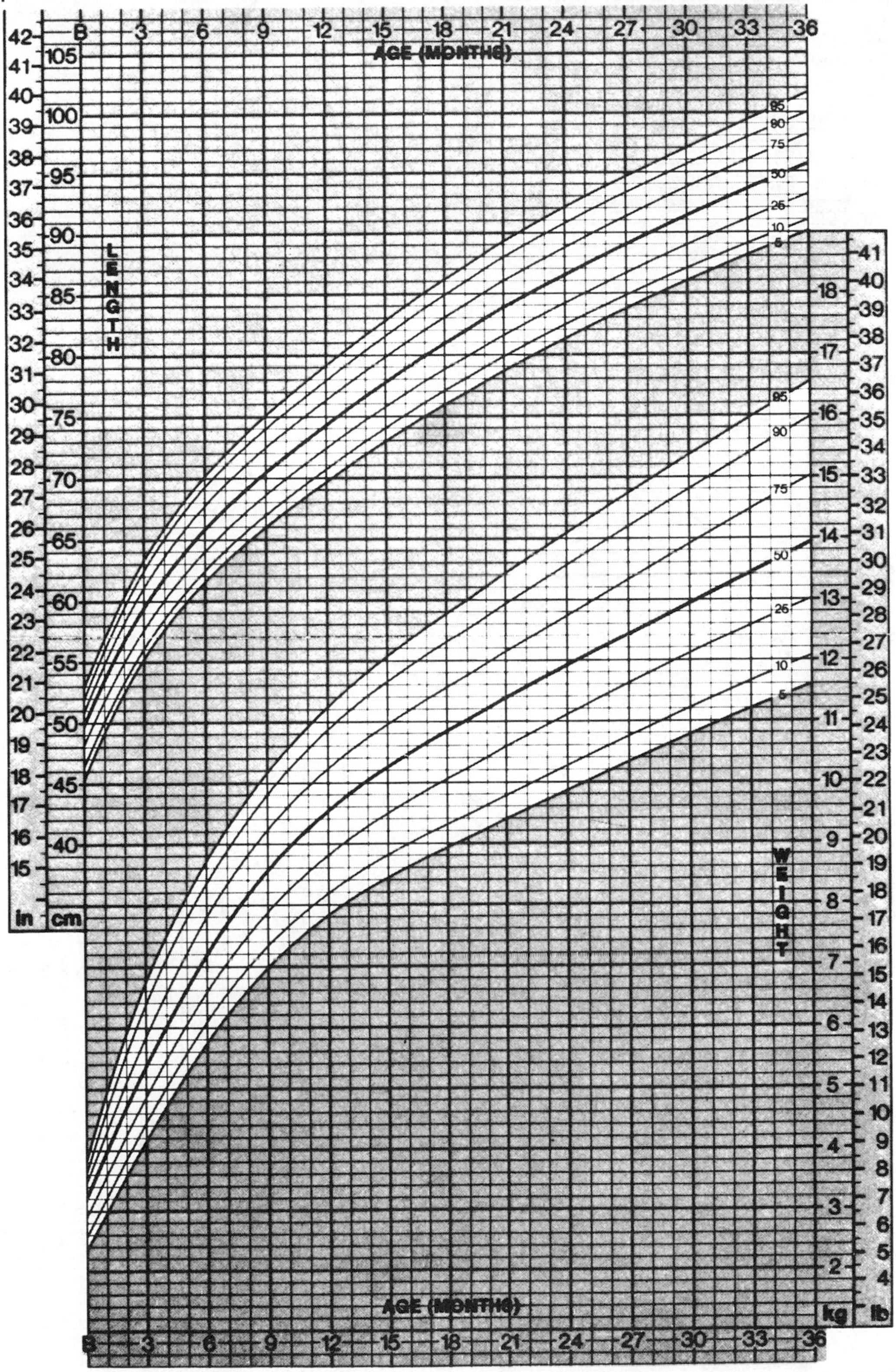

(Courtesy of Ross Laboratories, who adapted the growth curves from the original data: National Center for Health Statistics, NCHS Growth Charts, 1976. Monthly Vital Statistics Report, Vol. 25, No. 3, Suppl. (HRA) 76–1120. Rockville, MD, Health Resources Administration, June, 1976. Data from The Fels Research Institute, Yellow Springs, Ohio.)

TABLE A–12B-2. PHYSICAL GROWTH NCHS PERCENTILES: BOYS FROM BIRTH TO 36 MONTHS

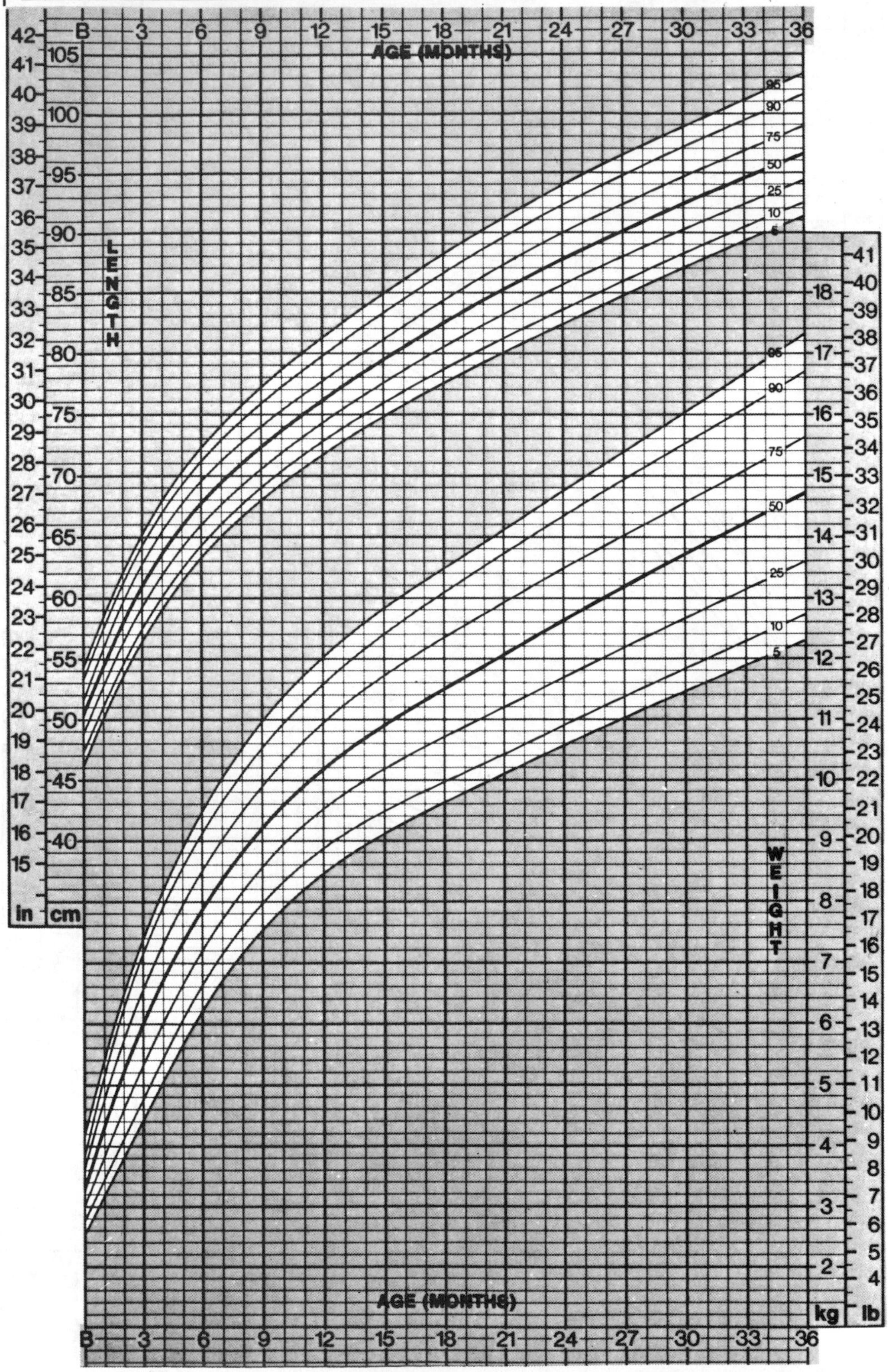

(Courtesy of Ross Laboratories, who adapted the growth curves from the original data: National Center for Health Statistics, NCHS Growth Charts, 1976. Monthly Vital Statistics Report, Vol. 25, No. 3, Suppl. (HRA) 76–1120. Rockville, MD, Health Resources Administration, June, 1976. Data from The Fels Research Institute, Yellow Springs, Ohio.)

TABLE A–12C-1. PHYSICAL GROWTH NCHS PERCENTILES: GIRLS FROM 2 TO 18 YEARS

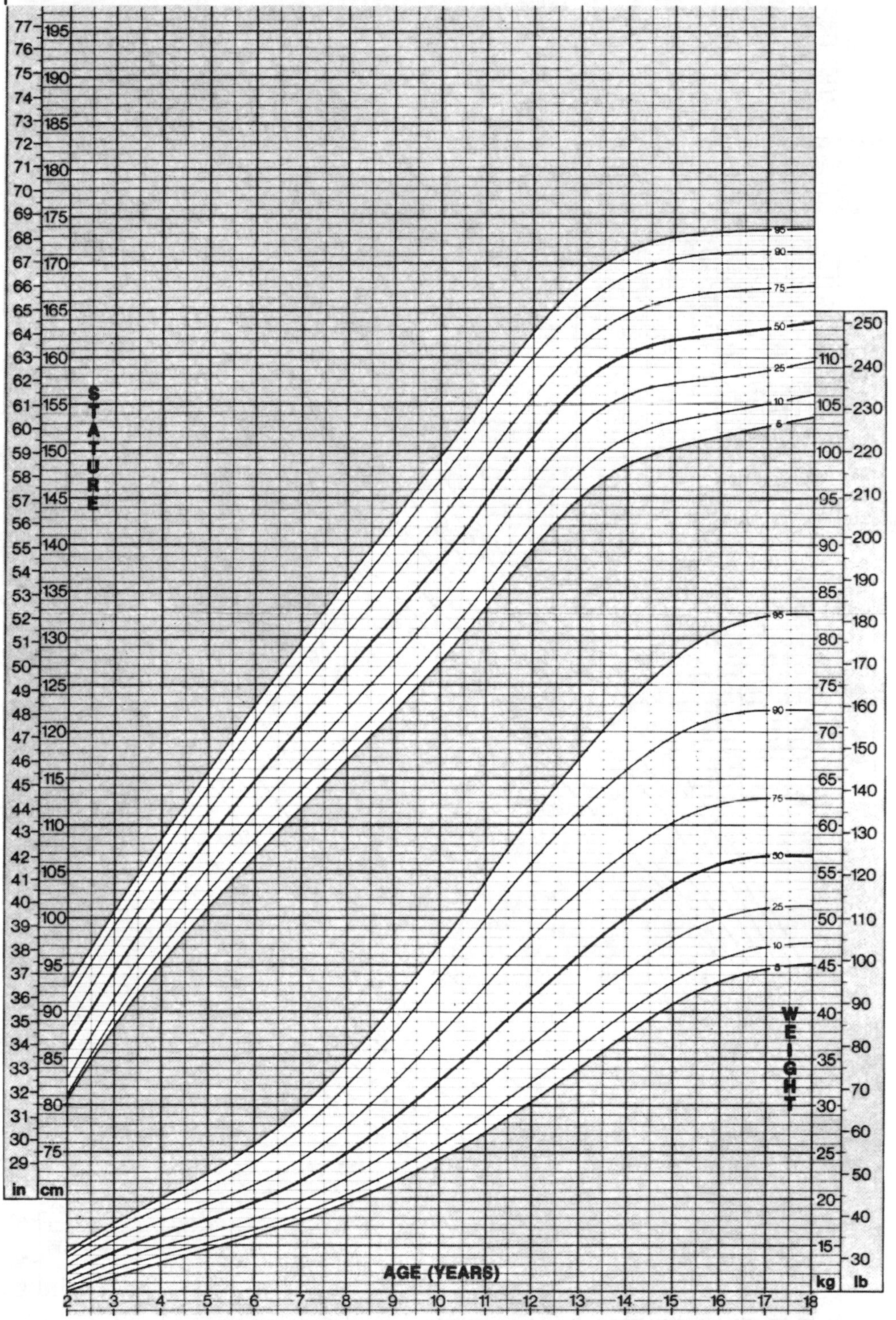

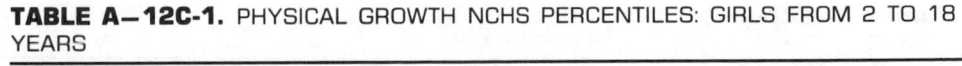

(Courtesy of Ross Laboratories, who adapted the growth curves from the original data: National Center for Health Statistics, NCHS Growth Charts, 1976. Monthly Vital Statistics Report, Vol. 25, No. 3, Suppl. (HRA) 76–1120. Rockville, MD, Health Resources Administration, June, 1976. Data from The Fels Research Institute, Yellow Springs, Ohio.)

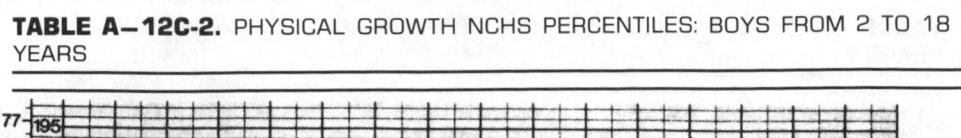

TABLE A–12C-2. PHYSICAL GROWTH NCHS PERCENTILES: BOYS FROM 2 TO 18 YEARS

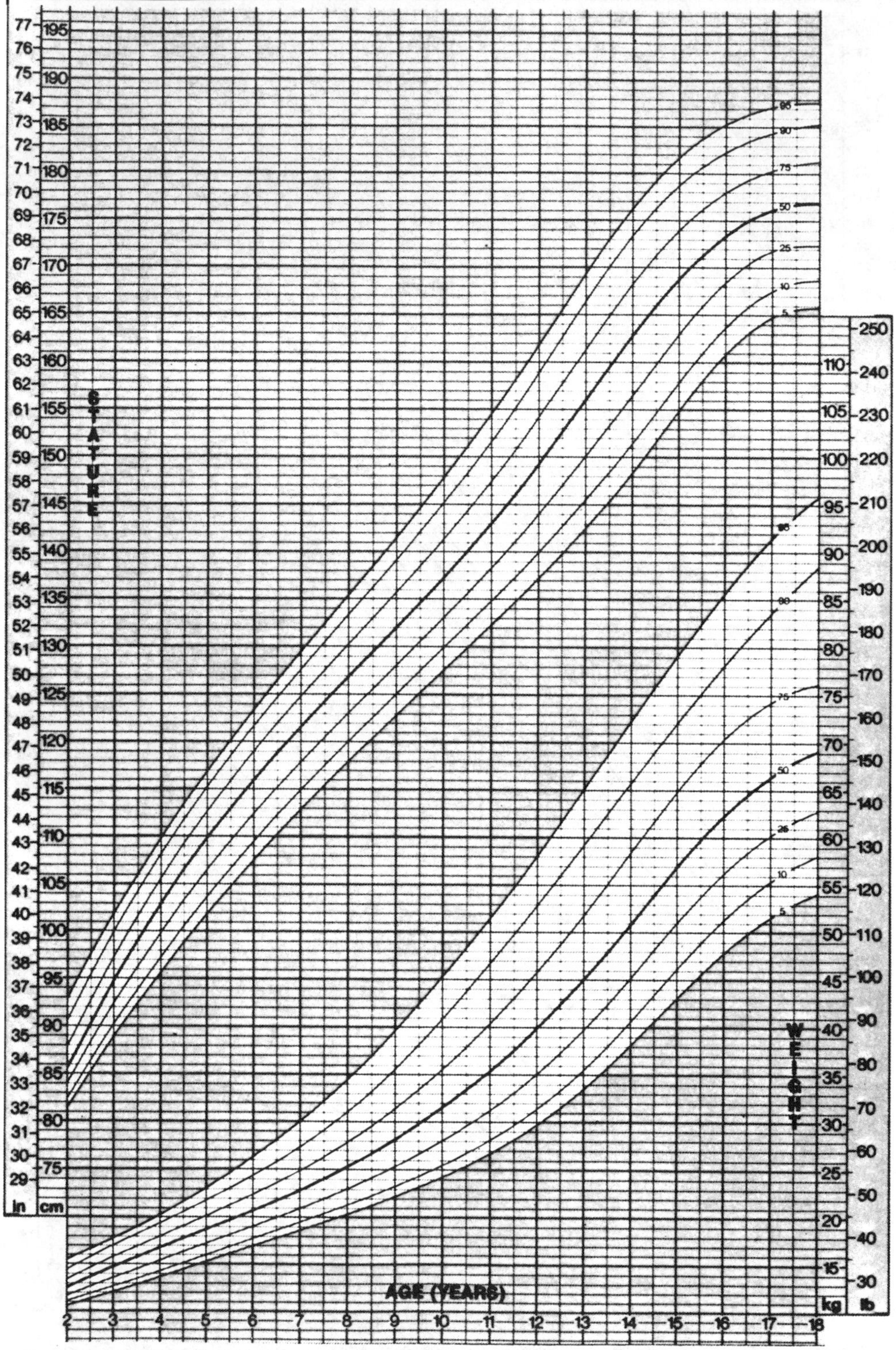

(Courtesy of Ross Laboratories, who adapted the growth curves from the original data: National Center for Health Statistics, NCHS Growth Charts, 1976. Monthly Vital Statistics Report, Vol. 25, No. 3, Suppl. (HRA) 76–1120. Rockville, MD, Health Resources Administration, June, 1976. Data from The Fels Research Institute, Yellow Springs, Ohio.)

TABLE A–12D. HEIGHT IN CENTIMETERS FOR PERSONS 2 TO 19 YEARS OF AGE: NUMBER EXAMINED, MEAN, STANDARD DEVIATION, AND SELECTED PERCENTILES BY SEX AND AGE, UNITED STATES, 1976 TO 1980*

SEX AND AGE (years)	NUMBER OF EXAMINED PERSONS	MEAN	STANDARD DEVIATION	PERCENTILE 5th	10th	15th	25th	50th	75th	85th	90th	95th
Male												
2	375	91.2	4.3	84.5	85.8	85.5	88.2	91.3	94.2	95.8	96.6	97.6
3	418	99.2	4.5	92.0	94.3	94.9	96.5	98.8	102.0	103.9	105.0	107.0
4	404	106.0	5.2	97.8	99.5	100.5	102.5	106.4	109.2	111.0	112.4	115.0
5	397	112.6	5.4	104.0	105.8	107.2	109.4	112.6	115.6	118.1	119.6	121.2
6	133	119.5	5.1	111.2	112.6	114.5	115.9	120.1	122.6	124.7	125.5	126.8
7	148	125.1	5.9	115.4	117.6	119.1	121.8	125.9	128.1	130.2	131.5	133.6
8	147	129.9	7.0	118.6	122.0	123.5	125.3	130.6	134.1	136.5	138.0	142.0
9	145	135.5	5.8	125.9	126.4	129.4	131.2	136.1	139.6	141.2	143.1	144.7
10	157	141.6	7.3	130.3	132.8	134.0	137.0	141.5	146.4	149.6	150.6	153.0
11	155	146.0	7.8	133.1	135.9	138.0	141.1	145.6	151.2	153.9	155.2	160.2
12	145	152.5	7.9	139.0	142.6	144.9	147.5	152.0	158.0	160.5	162.0	164.4
13	173	158.9	8.3	144.4	147.6	149.7	152.6	159.7	165.0	168.7	169.5	171.6
14	186	167.5	8.3	153.9	156.5	159.1	162.5	167.5	173.1	176.5	178.7	180.6
15	184	170.8	6.7	160.1	162.0	162.6	165.7	171.1	175.5	177.5	178.2	181.9
16	178	173.8	6.4	163.0	164.7	167.4	169.8	173.7	178.1	180.3	182.6	186.1
17	173	175.1	7.1	164.1	167.3	168.4	170.6	174.9	179.7	182.8	184.3	187.5
18	164	176.9	6.7	166.5	168.8	169.9	172.3	176.9	180.9	183.9	185.1	189.6
19	148	176.5	6.7	164.5	168.2	169.4	171.8	176.9	181.1	183.5	184.8	187.2
Female												
2	336	89.7	4.2	83.1	84.4	85.5	86.7	89.8	92.2	93.6	94.9	97.2
3	366	97.5	4.8	89.6	91.1	92.5	94.5	97.6	100.8	102.5	103.4	104.5
4	396	104.6	5.0	96.1	98.2	99.5	101.5	104.5	108.2	109.8	110.7	112.4
5	364	111.6	5.3	103.0	105.1	106.4	108.1	111.6	115.2	116.5	118.8	120.3
6	135	118.4	6.1	109.9	111.1	111.5	113.3	118.5	122.2	124.5	126.5	128.7
7	157	123.7	6.7	113.3	116.6	117.4	119.6	124.1	128.1	130.1	132.2	134.7
8	123	130.2	5.7	120.8	123.4	124.4	125.8	130.6	133.2	135.4	137.5	140.5
9	149	134.4	7.6	124.0	126.4	127.8	129.0	134.8	139.0	140.7	142.6	147.1
10	136	141.9	6.5	131.6	133.6	135.1	137.6	141.6	146.3	148.1	150.4	153.8
11	140	147.9	7.8	134.7	139.3	140.6	142.2	147.9	152.2	154.7	156.9	162.7
12	147	154.4	7.2	143.9	145.7	146.7	149.2	154.8	158.6	161.9	164.7	165.9
13	162	158.9	6.6	149.0	150.3	152.7	155.3	159.0	163.0	164.5	166.9	170.3
14	178	160.8	6.4	151.0	152.7	154.5	156.7	160.9	165.1	166.9	168.2	172.3
15	145	163.2	6.2	153.0	155.2	157.1	159.1	163.1	167.1	170.2	172.4	173.5
16	170	162.9	6.1	152.0	154.5	157.2	159.1	163.2	166.4	169.4	171.4	173.3
17	134	163.5	5.7	153.8	156.8	158.5	160.4	163.1	166.7	169.7	170.7	172.2
18	170	162.4	6.8	150.7	154.2	155.6	158.0	162.7	166.2	169.1	171.5	174.0
19	158	163.5	5.6	153.8	156.8	157.7	159.7	163.7	167.2	169.5	170.4	172.1

*Height without shoes.

(From National Center for Health Statistics: Anthropometric Reference Data and Prevalence of Overweight, United States 1976–1980. DHHS Publication No. 87–1688. Hyattsville, MD, U.S. Department of Health and Human Services, Public Health Service, 1987.)

TABLE A–12E. WEIGHT IN KILOGRAMS FOR PERSONS 6 MONTHS TO 19 YEARS OF AGE: NUMBER EXAMINED, MEAN, STANDARD DEVIATION, AND SELECTED PERCENTILES BY SEX AND AGE, UNITED STATES, 1976 TO 1980*

SEX AND AGE	NUMBER OF EXAMINED PERSONS	MEAN	STANDARD DEVIATION	PERCENTILE 5th	10th	15th	25th	50th	75th	85th	90th	95th
Male												
6–11 months	179	9.4	1.3	7.5	7.6	8.2	8.6	9.4	10.1	10.7	10.9	11.4
1 year	370	11.8	1.9	9.6	10.0	10.3	10.8	11.7	12.6	13.1	13.6	14.4
2 years	375	13.6	1.7	11.1	11.6	11.8	12.6	13.5	14.5	15.2	15.8	16.5
3 years	418	15.7	2.0	12.9	13.5	13.9	14.4	15.4	16.8	17.4	17.9	19.1
4 years	404	17.8	2.5	14.1	15.0	15.3	16.0	17.6	19.0	19.9	20.9	22.2
5 years	397	19.8	3.0	16.0	16.8	17.1	17.7	19.4	21.3	22.9	23.7	25.4
6 years	133	23.0	4.0	18.6	19.2	19.8	20.3	22.0	24.1	26.4	28.3	30.1
7 years	148	25.1	3.9	19.7	20.8	21.2	22.2	24.8	26.9	28.2	29.6	33.9
8 years	147	28.2	6.2	20.4	22.7	23.6	24.6	27.5	29.9	33.0	35.5	39.1
9 years	145	31.1	6.3	24.0	25.6	26.0	27.1	30.2	33.0	35.4	38.6	43.1
10 yars	157	36.4	7.7	27.2	28.2	29.6	31.4	34.8	39.2	43.5	46.3	53.4
11 years	155	40.3	10.1	26.8	28.8	31.8	33.5	37.3	46.4	52.0	57.0	61.0
12 years	145	44.2	10.1	30.7	32.5	35.4	37.8	42.5	48.8	52.6	58.9	67.5
13 years	173	49.9	12.3	35.4	37.0	38.3	40.1	48.4	56.3	59.8	64.2	69.9
14 years	186	57.1	11.0	41.0	44.5	46.4	49.8	56.4	63.3	66.1	68.9	77.0
15 years	184	61.0	11.0	46.2	49.1	50.6	54.2	60.1	64.9	68.7	72.8	81.3
16 years	178	67.1	12.4	51.4	54.3	56.1	58.7	64.4	73.6	78.1	82.2	91.2
17 years	173	66.7	11.5	50.7	53.4	54.8	58.7	65.8	72.0	76.8	82.3	88.9
18 years	164	71.1	12.7	54.1	56.6	60.3	61.9	70.4	76.6	80.0	83.5	95.3
19 years	148	71.7	11.6	55.9	57.9	60.5	63.8	69.5	77.9	84.3	86.8	92.1
Female												
6–11 months	177	8.8	1.2	6.6	7.3	7.5	7.9	8.9	9.4	10.1	10.4	10.9
1 year	336	10.8	1.4	8.8	9.1	9.4	9.9	10.7	11.7	12.4	12.7	13.4
2 years	336	13.0	1.5	10.8	11.2	11.6	12.0	12.7	13.8	14.5	14.9	15.9
3 years	366	14.9	2.1	11.7	12.3	12.9	13.4	14.7	16.1	17.0	17.4	18.4
4 years	396	17.0	2.4	13.7	14.3	14.5	15.2	16.7	18.4	19.3	20.2	21.1
5 years	364	19.6	3.3	15.3	16.1	16.7	17.2	19.0	21.2	22.8	24.7	26.6
6 years	135	22.1	4.0	17.0	17.8	18.6	19.3	21.3	23.8	26.6	28.9	29.6
7 years	157	24.7	5.0	19.2	19.5	19.8	21.4	23.8	27.1	28.7	30.3	34.0
8 years	123	27.9	5.7	21.4	22.3	23.3	24.4	27.5	30.2	31.3	33.2	36.5
9 years	149	31.9	8.4	22.9	25.0	25.8	27.0	29.7	33.6	39.3	43.3	48.4
10 years	136	36.1	8.0	25.7	27.5	29.0	31.0	34.5	39.5	44.2	45.8	49.6
11 years	140	41.8	10.9	29.8	30.3	31.3	33.9	40.3	45.8	51.0	56.6	60.0
12 years	147	46.4	10.1	32.3	35.0	36.7	39.1	45.4	52.6	58.0	60.5	64.3
13 years	162	50.9	11.8	35.4	39.0	40.3	44.1	49.0	55.2	60.9	66.4	76.3
14 years	175	54.8	11.1	40.3	42.8	43.7	47.4	53.1	60.3	65.7	67.6	75.2
15 years	145	55.1	9.8	44.0	45.1	46.5	48.2	53.3	59.6	62.2	65.5	76.6
16 years	170	58.1	10.1	44.1	47.3	48.9	51.3	55.6	62.5	68.9	73.3	76.8
17 years	134	59.6	11.4	44.5	48.9	50.5	52.2	58.4	63.4	68.4	71.6	81.8
18 years	170	59.0	11.1	45.3	49.5	50.8	52.8	56.4	63.0	66.0	70.1	78.0
19 years	158	60.2	11.0	48.5	49.7	51.7	53.9	57.1	64.4	70.7	74.8	78.1

*Includes clothing weight, estimated as ranging from 0.09 to 0.28 kilogram.

(From National Center for Health Statistics: Anthropometric Reference Data and Prevalence of Overweight, United States 1976–1980. DHHS Publication No. 87–1688. Hyattsville, MD, U.S. Department of Health and Human Services, Public Health Service, 1987.)

TABLE A—12F-1. WEIGHT IN KILOGRAMS OF YOUTHS AGED 12 YEARS AT LAST BIRTHDAY BY SEX AND HEIGHT GROUP IN CENTIMETERS: SAMPLE SIZE, ESTIMATED POPULATION SIZE, MEAN, STANDARD DEVIATION, STANDARD ERROR OF THE MEAN, AND SELECTED PERCENTILES, UNITED STATES, 1966 TO 1970

SEX AND HEIGHT	n	N	$\bar{X}$	s	$s_{\bar{x}}$	PERCENTILE 5th	10th	25th	50th	75th	90th	95th
Male						in kilograms						
Under 130	5	15	*	*	*	*	*	*	*	*	*	*
130.0–134.9	4	8	*	*	*	*	*	*	*	*	*	*
135.0–139.9	34	111	32.50	3.741	0.727	26.6	27.6	30.2	31.6	34.7	37.7	39.4
140.0–144.9	80	241	34.28	3.635	0.601	28.1	30.0	31.8	34.1	36.5	38.6	40.7
145.0–149.9	123	386	39.27	6.243	0.615	32.1	33.2	35.7	38.2	40.9	46.1	52.5
150.0–154.9	156	513	42.90	6.314	0.480	34.9	36.1	38.2	42.1	46.0	51.6	56.3
155.0–159.9	135	432	47.35	7.551	0.769	38.3	39.4	41.9	46.2	50.5	57.4	61.9
160.0–164.9	65	201	50.82	8.735	1.388	42.1	42.7	44.9	48.4	56.0	61.1	67.1
165.0–169.9	29	88	55.75	8.811	2.031	43.3	46.4	49.0	54.4	59.9	68.3	76.6
170.0–174.9	8	21	62.37	4.503	1.993	54.0	58.1	60.1	61.0	66.0	69.1	69.5
175.0–179.9	3	10	*	*	*	*	*	*	*	*	*	*
180.0–184.9	1	2	*	*	*	*	*	*	*	*	*	*
185.0–189.9	—	—	—	—	—	—	—	—	—	—	—	—
190.0–194.9	—	—	—	—	—	—	—	—	—	—	—	—
195.0 and over	—	—	—	—	—	—	—	—	—	—	—	—

TABLE A—12F-1. (continued)

Sex and Height	n	N	$\bar{X}$	s	$s_{\bar{x}}$	PERCENTILE 5th	10th	25th	50th	75th	90th	95th
Female						in kilograms						
Under 130	—	—	—	—	—	—	—	—	—	—	—	—
130.0–134.9	3	10	*	*	*	*	*	*	*	*	*	*
135.0–139.9	12	44	29.41	3.372	0.914	25.0	25.0	26.4	28.9	32.1	34.1	34.2
140.0–144.9	32	116	38.30	7.314	1.194	28.8	30.6	33.3	36.8	41.4	49.2	55.1
145.0–149.9	72	258	39.78	6.205	0.975	31.8	32.8	35.5	38.5	42.8	48.3	50.6
150.0–154.9	147	517	44.00	7.421	0.677	34.4	35.8	38.9	42.8	47.4	52.9	57.4
155.0–159.9	144	525	48.74	8.369	0.714	37.9	39.2	43.0	46.8	53.8	60.7	63.5
160.0–164.9	95	336	53.06	8.010	0.658	42.5	43.9	47.2	51.1	57.2	65.6	69.6
165.0–169.9	31	117	54.89	7.022	1.384	43.9	47.1	50.4	53.1	59.7	64.5	71.3
170.0–174.9	11	42	63.66	14.501	6.214	48.7	50.1	50.8	56.7	82.2	86.0	86.1
175.0–179.9	—	—	—	—	—	—	—	—	—	—	—	—
180.0–184.9	—	—	—	—	—	—	—	—	—	—	—	—
185.0–189.9	—	—	—	—	—	—	—	—	—	—	—	—
190.0–194.9	—	—	—	—	—	—	—	—	—	—	—	—
195.0 and over	—	—	—	—	—	—	—	—	—	—	—	—

n, Sample size; *N*, estimated number of youths in population in thousands; $\bar{X}$, mean; *s*, standard deviation; $s_{\bar{x}}$, standard error of the mean.
(From National Center for Health Statistics: Height and weight of youths 12–17 years, United States. *In* Vital and Health Statistics, Series 11, No. 124, Health Services and Mental Health Administration. Washington, D.C., U.S. Government Printing Office, 1973, pp. 282–288.)

TABLE A—12F-2. WEIGHT IN KILOGRAMS OF YOUTHS AGED 13 YEARS AT LAST BIRTHDAY BY SEX AND HEIGHT GROUP IN CENTIMETERS: SAMPLE SIZE, ESTIMATED POPULATION SIZE, MEAN, STANDARD DEVIATION, STANDARD ERROR OF THE MEAN, AND SELECTED PERCENTILES, UNITED STATES, 1966 TO 1970

SEX AND HEIGHT	n	N	$\overline{X}$	s	$s_{\overline{x}}$	PERCENTILE						
						5th	10th	25th	50th	75th	90th	95th
Male						in kilograms						
Under 130	—	—	—	—	—	—	—	—	—	—	—	—
130.0–134.9	2	5	*	*	*	*	*	*	*	*	*	*
135.0–139.9	6	25	32.62	5.624	7.716	27.2	27.6	28.9	31.0	34.9	43.1	43.2
140.0–144.9	18	56	36.54	5.852	1.607	30.0	30.5	32.1	36.1	39.2	41.7	53.2
145.0–149.9	65	204	39.03	5.270	0.662	32.4	33.9	36.1	37.9	41.2	44.5	46.4
150.0–154.9	99	312	42.58	6.724	0.865	34.8	36.2	37.9	41.0	45.5	49.4	61.0
155.0–159.9	131	421	47.27	7.482	0.717	37.8	39.2	41.7	45.8	51.1	58.7	61.7
160.0–164.9	125	393	53.01	9.324	0.916	41.5	43.7	46.9	50.4	58.2	64.4	72.5
165.0–169.9	91	285	55.92	8.560	0.833	46.3	47.5	49.3	53.6	59.4	69.0	75.0
170.0–174.9	63	215	62.01	10.362	1.033	51.2	51.6	53.7	60.1	67.0	76.0	85.0
175.0–179.9	19	68	67.92	12.085	3.428	56.3	57.9	60.1	63.3	70.3	88.3	89.0
180.0–184.9	5	15	*	*	*	*	*	*	*	*	*	*
185.0–189.9	—	—	—	—	—	—	—	—	—	—	—	—
190.0–194.9	—	—	—	—	—	—	—	—	—	—	—	—
195.0 and over	—	—	—	—	—	—	—	—	—	—	—	—
Female												
Under 130	—	—	—	—	—	—	—	—	—	—	—	—
130.0–134.9	1	3	*	*	*	*	*	*	*	*	*	*
135.0–139.9	—	—	—	—	—	—	—	—	—	—	—	—
140.0–144.9	15	51	37.13	7.317	2.259	26.6	27.5	30.5	36.7	40.1	44.5	56.1
145.0–149.9	47	165	42.23	6.880	0.888	34.7	35.6	38.2	40.5	44.2	53.6	57.6
150.0–154.9	98	329	44.32	7.029	0.787	35.6	36.5	39.2	42.9	47.3	53.7	57.9
155.0–159.9	152	499	49.75	8.757	0.699	39.1	39.9	43.8	48.4	53.8	61.0	65.9
160.0–164.9	156	515	53.16	8.399	0.522	41.2	43.9	47.7	52.2	57.0	63.8	68.5
165.0–169.9	86	284	58.17	9.125	0.921	46.2	47.4	52.2	58.1	61.5	69.3	76.2
170.0–174.9	24	87	58.11	13.209	2.343	46.2	47.1	48.4	52.9	65.3	68.6	96.8
175.0–179.9	3	10	*	*	*	*	*	*	*	*	*	*
180.0–184.9	—	—	—	—	—	—	—	—	—	—	—	—
185.0–189.9	—	—	—	—	—	—	—	—	—	—	—	—
190.0–194.9	—	—	—	—	—	—	—	—	—	—	—	—
195.0 and over	—	—	—	—	—	—	—	—	—	—	—	—

n, Sample size; *N*, estimated number of youths in population in thousands; $\overline{X}$, mean; *s*, standard deviation; $s_{\overline{x}}$, standard error of the mean.

(From National Center for Health Statistics: Height and weight of youths 12–17 years, United States. *In* Vital and Health Statistics, Series 11, No. 124, Health Services and Mental Health Administration. Washington, D.C., U.S. Government Printing Office, 1973, pp. 282–288.)

TABLE A—12F-3. WEIGHT IN KILOGRAMS OF YOUTHS AGED 14 YEARS AT LAST BIRTHDAY BY SEX AND HEIGHT GROUP IN CENTIMETERS: SAMPLE SIZE, ESTIMATED POPULATION SIZE, MEAN, STANDARD DEVIATION, STANDARD ERROR OF THE MEAN, AND SELECTED PERCENTILES, UNITED STATES, 1966 TO 1970

SEX AND HEIGHT	n	N	$\overline{X}$	s	$s_{\overline{x}}$	PERCENTILE 5th	10th	25th	50th	75th	90th	95th
Male						in kilograms						
Under 130	—	—	—	—	—	—	—	—	—	—	—	—
130.0–134.9	—	—	—	—	—	—	—	—	—	—	—	—
135.0–139.9	2	7	*	*	*	*	*	*	*	*	*	*
140.0–144.9	3	13	*	*	*	*	*	*	*	*	*	*
145.0–149.9	11	42	40.51	1.829	0.644	36.9	38.6	39.6	40.6	42.0	42.5	42.7
150.0–154.9	45	135	43.63	6.277	1.182	36.2	37.0	39.0	41.4	48.0	51.7	55.3
155.0–159.9	83	261	47.42	7.822	0.872	37.7	38.7	41.8	46.1	51.2	58.0	62.7
160.0–164.9	96	299	52.28	6.785	0.584	42.5	44.0	47.5	52.1	56.3	61.5	65.1
165.0–169.9	134	432	58.07	9.416	1.054	47.7	49.3	51.6	55.4	62.3	70.6	75.7
170.0–174.9	144	435	62.37	11.516	1.095	49.7	51.0	55.0	59.4	65.6	79.2	86.3
175.0–179.9	71	228	65.54	9.704	1.306	50.9	55.1	58.5	64.7	69.9	74.5	84.0
180.0–184.9	25	81	72.44	13.014	2.298	59.6	60.0	65.1	69.4	77.0	83.0	94.3
185.0–189.9	3	9	*	*	*	*	*	*	*	*	*	*
190.0–194.9	1	3	*	*	*	*	*	*	*	*	*	*
195.0 and over	—	—	—	—	—	—	—	—	—	—	—	—
Female												
Under 130	—	—	—	—	—	—	—	—	—	—	—	—
130.0–134.9	—	—	—	—	—	—	—	—	—	—	—	—
135.0–139.9	1	2	*	*	*	*	*	*	*	*	*	*
140.0–144.9	2	6	*	*	*	*	*	*	*	*	*	*
145.0–149.9	17	52	42.00	5.879	1.683	32.0	35.3	36.3	42.3	47.5	49.5	51.1
150.0–154.9	64	196	48.26	6.797	0.926	37.7	39.2	42.5	47.9	53.3	55.9	58.8
155.0–159.9	157	508	51.35	7.705	0.520	41.2	43.4	46.3	49.6	55.6	62.2	64.3
160.0–164.9	186	603	54.59	8.810	0.707	43.0	45.0	48.4	53.0	59.7	66.7	70.7
165.0–169.9	114	372	58.46	10.185	0.955	45.9	47.5	52.1	56.8	61.8	70.5	76.4
170.0–174.9	36	121	64.37	15.821	2.814	49.2	52.1	56.2	59.8	70.5	72.9	99.4
175.0–179.9	7	28	61.33	5.496	2.620	51.7	52.0	57.7	59.8	64.6	70.2	70.6
180.0–184.9	2	7	*	*	*	*	*	*	*	*	*	*
185.0–189.9	—	—	—	—	—	—	—	—	—	—	—	—
190.0–194.9	—	—	—	—	—	—	—	—	—	—	—	—
195.0 and over	—	—	—	—	—	—	—	—	—	—	—	—

n, Sample size; N, estimated number of youths in population in thousands; $\overline{X}$, mean; s, standard deviation; $s_{\overline{x}}$, standard error of the mean.
(From National Center for Health Statistics: Height and weight of youths 12–17 years, United States. *In* Vital and Health Statistics, Series 11, No. 124, Health Services and Mental Health Administration. Washington, D.C., U.S. Government Printing Office, 1973, pp. 282–288.)

TABLE A—12F-4. WEIGHT IN KILOGRAMS OF YOUTHS AGED 15 YEARS AT LAST BIRTHDAY BY SEX AND HEIGHT GROUP IN CENTIMETERS: SAMPLE SIZE, ESTIMATED POPULATION SIZE, MEAN, STANDARD DEVIATION, STANDARD ERROR OF THE MEAN, AND SELECTED PERCENTILES, UNITED STATES, 1966 TO 1970

SEX AND HEIGHT	n	N	$\overline{X}$	s	$s_{\overline{x}}$	PERCENTILE 5th	10th	25th	50th	75th	90th	95th
Male						in kilograms						
Under 130	—	—	—	—	—	—	—	—	—	—	—	—
130.0–134.9	—	—	—	—	—	—	—	—	—	—	—	—
135.0–139.9	—	—	—	—	—	—	—	—	—	—	—	—
140.0–144.9	—	—	—	—	—	—	—	—	—	—	—	—
145.0–149.9	1	2	*	*	*	*	*	*	*	*	*	*
150.0–154.9	10	30	45.72	8.582	3.550	35.7	39.2	42.6	44.7	46.0	48.7	76.1
155.0–159.9	34	99	52.81	10.552	1.695	40.3	43.1	46.7	49.2	56.7	69.6	76.3
160.0–164.9	71	206	53.01	8.417	0.986	42.7	44.1	46.9	51.5	56.3	65.3	68.8
165.0–169.9	132	404	57.72	8.503	0.819	48.0	48.8	53.1	56.4	61.3	67.1	73.3
170.0–174.9	176	574	62.88	8.464	0.633	51.6	53.4	56.7	61.9	67.2	72.9	78.1
175.0–179.9	118	374	65.80	9.457	1.045	53.1	55.6	59.7	64.3	69.5	80.2	89.2
180.0–184.9	51	144	72.00	11.928	1.724	54.6	60.3	64.4	70.2	78.4	84.4	96.6
185.0–189.9	14	48	74.21	15.035	5.200	58.3	58.5	62.9	70.7	84.6	92.4	110.8
190.0–194.9	6	15	83.39	16.431	10.332	66.4	66.7	69.6	73.8	103.0	105.7	106.2
195.0 and over	—	—	—	—	—	—	—	—	—	—	—	—
Female												
Under 130	—	—	—	—	—	—	—	—	—	—	—	—
130.0–134.9	—	—	—	—	—	—	—	—	—	—	—	—
135.0–139.9	—	—	—	—	—	—	—	—	—	—	—	—
140.0–144.9	2	5	*	*	*	*	*	*	*	*	*	*
145.0–149.9	15	51	47.91	7.875	3.623	36.0	39.4	42.1	45.4	52.7	55.7	66.3
150.0–154.9	69	242	49.69	8.895	1.190	39.1	40.6	44.3	48.1	52.8	60.5	68.3
155.0–159.9	111	400	51.52	8.473	0.934	41.4	43.5	46.3	50.8	55.1	59.8	65.2
160.0–164.9	137	509	57.03	10.828	0.875	45.1	47.3	50.2	55.0	60.2	71.7	77.7
165.0–169.9	109	398	60.71	10.357	1.053	47.5	49.3	55.1	58.4	65.7	74.1	81.0
170.0–174.9	49	188	65.27	10.730	1.880	49.7	53.6	57.2	61.2	71.6	85.3	86.4
175.0–179.9	7	23	63.30	8.872	4.807	49.7	49.9	53.8	62.4	71.1	71.9	79.2
180.0–184.9	3	26	*	*	*	*	*	*	*	*	*	*
185.0–189.9	1	3	*	*	*	*	*	*	*	*	*	*
190.0–194.9	—	—	—	—	—	—	—	—	—	—	—	—
195.0 and over	—	—	—	—	—	—	—	—	—	—	—	—

n, Sample size; N, estimated number of youths in population in thousands; $\overline{X}$, mean; s, standard deviation; $s_{\overline{x}}$, standard error of the mean.
(From National Center for Health Statistics: Height and weight of youths 12–17 years, United States. *In* Vital and Health Statistics, Series 11, No. 124, Health Services and Mental Health Administration. Washington, D.C., U.S. Government Printing Office, 1973, pp. 282–288.)

TABLE A—12F-5. WEIGHT IN KILOGRAMS OF YOUTHS AGED 16 YEARS AT LAST BIRTHDAY BY SEX AND HEIGHT GROUP IN CENTIMETERS: SAMPLE SIZE, ESTIMATED POPULATION SIZE, MEAN, STANDARD DEVIATION, STANDARD ERROR OF THE MEAN, AND SELECTED PERCENTILES, UNITED STATES, 1966 TO 1970

SEX AND HEIGHT	n	N	$\overline{X}$	s	$s_{\overline{x}}$	PERCENTILE 5th	10th	25th	50th	75th	90th	95th
Male						in kilograms						
Under 130	—	—	—	—	—	—	—	—	—	—	—	—
130.0–134.9	—	—	—	—	—	—	—	—	—	—	—	—
135.0–139.9	—	—	—	—	—	—	—	—	—	—	—	—
140.0–144.9	—	—	—	—	—	—	—	—	—	—	—	—
145.0–149.9	1	1	*	*	*	*	*	*	*	*	*	*
150.0–154.9	4	12	*	*	*	*	*	*	*	*	*	*
155.0–159.9	11	33	49.89	7.323	3.572	42.0	42.2	44.7	46.8	54.4	59.8	67.2
160.0–164.9	32	108	53.09	6.459	1.273	44.2	44.9	48.2	51.4	58.0	60.9	66.1
165.0–169.9	87	275	59.39	9.178	0.981	48.5	49.8	52.7	58.0	63.9	69.3	75.9
170.0–174.9	166	552	62.66	7.556	0.629	51.6	53.8	57.5	61.6	67.1	73.1	78.0
175.0–179.9	149	511	67.33	9.018	0.856	56.3	58.2	61.0	65.4	72.5	80.1	83.8
180.0–184.9	72	227	72.38	12.485	1.993	58.3	59.3	64.4	68.9	76.5	90.2	96.9
185.0–189.9	29	95	81.06	14.268	3.265	63.7	66.6	69.7	78.4	90.3	97.0	111.4
190.0–194.9	3	10	*	*	*	*	*	*	*	*	*	*
195.0 and over	2	7	*	*	*	*	*	*	*	*	*	*
Female												
Under 130	—	—	—	—	—	—	—	—	—	—	—	—
130.0–134.9	—	—	—	—	—	—	—	—	—	—	—	—
135.0–139.9	—	—	—	—	—	—	—	—	—	—	—	—
140.0–144.9	2	5	*	*	*	*	*	*	*	*	*	*
145.0–149.9	10	33	52.58	8.198	3.191	43.9	44.1	44.9	51.0	54.5	72.0	72.1
150.0–154.9	57	178	51.79	10.457	1.053	41.4	42.0	45.8	48.9	54.1	61.5	83.3
155.0–159.9	117	354	53.20	7.766	0.734	44.0	45.6	48.4	51.6	56.4	61.9	69.0
160.0–164.9	160	547	57.71	11.129	1.246	46.1	47.3	51.5	55.5	61.2	69.5	75.1
165.0–169.9	122	450	61.72	11.998	0.802	47.1	48.8	53.3	59.1	67.3	78.7	86.7
170.0–174.9	53	170	63.61	8.734	1.126	52.9	53.8	58.1	62.1	66.8	73.8	84.2
175.0–179.9	14	45	72.55	15.012	5.224	58.6	58.8	61.7	65.9	80.6	99.1	105.5
180.0–184.9	1	2	*	*	*	*	*	*	*	*	*	*
185.0–189.9	—	—	—	—	—	—	—	—	—	—	—	—
190.0–194.9	—	—	—	—	—	—	—	—	—	—	—	—
195.0 and over	—	—	—	—	—	—	—	—	—	—	—	—

n, Sample size; *N*, estimated number of youths in population in thousands; $\overline{X}$, mean; *s*, standard deviation; $s_{\overline{x}}$, standard error of the mean.
(From National Center for Health Statistics: Height and weight of youths 12–17 years, United States. *In* Vital and Health Statistics, Series 11, No. 124, Health Services and Mental Health Administration. Washington, D.C., U.S. Government Printing Office, 1973, pp. 282–288.)

TABLE A—12F-6. WEIGHT IN KILOGRAMS OF YOUTHS AGED 17 YEARS AT LAST BIRTHDAY BY SEX AND HEIGHT GROUP IN CENTIMETERS: SAMPLE SIZE, ESTIMATED POPULATION SIZE, MEAN, STANDARD DEVIATION, STANDARD ERROR OF THE MEAN, AND SELECTED PERCENTILES, UNITED STATES, 1966 TO 1970

SEX AND HEIGHT	*n*	*N*	$\overline{X}$	*s*	$s_{\overline{x}}$	PERCENTILE 5th	10th	25th	50th	75th	90th	95th
Male						in kilograms						
Under 130	—	—	—	—	—	—	—	—	—	—	—	—
130.0–134.9	—	—	—	—	—	—	—	—	—	—	—	—
135.0–139.9	—	—	—	—	—	—	—	—	—	—	—	—
140.0–144.9	—	—	—	—	—	—	—	—	—	—	—	—
145.0–149.9	—	—	—	—	—	—	—	—	—	—	—	—
150.0–154.9	1	3	*	*	*	*	*	*	*	*	*	*
155.0–159.9	11	39	54.63	9.397	3.414	43.8	46.4	48.2	49.7	57.8	69.9	73.2
160.0–164.9	25	81	57.75	6.503	1.355	49.7	51.1	52.5	56.9	61.6	70.1	70.8
165.0–169.9	63	248	62.57	8.344	1.224	50.2	53.2	56.4	61.5	66.9	72.7	77.3
170.0–174.9	115	396	67.06	11.163	0.704	53.3	55.5	59.5	64.6	71.9	80.9	91.6
175.0–179.9	151	537	68.37	9.907	0.831	56.9	58.9	61.5	66.5	73.6	79.4	88.4
180.0–184.9	80	297	73.31	12.454	1.335	59.6	61.0	65.1	71.2	78.4	91.8	102.7
185.0–189.9	36	133	76.03	9.171	1.301	62.4	66.3	70.5	75.3	80.8	90.3	92.9
190.0–194.9	7	25	81.40	10.985	7.588	62.9	62.9	67.8	87.3	90.3	90.6	90.6
195.0 and over	—	—	—	—	—	—	—	—	—	—	—	—
Female												
Under 130	—	—	—	—	—	—	—	—	—	—	—	—
130.0–134.9	—	—	—	—	—	—	—	—	—	—	—	—
135.0–139.9	—	—	—	—	—	—	—	—	—	—	—	—
140.0–144.9	2	5	*	*	*	*	*	*	*	*	*	*
145.0–149.9	8	26	43.49	3.939	1.604	38.6	38.8	40.1	45.1	45.7	51.1	51.2
150.0–154.9	43	151	49.96	6.508	0.827	41.6	42.3	44.6	48.9	53.5	59.2	64.1
155.0–159.9	103	385	54.71	9.903	0.775	44.4	45.5	48.7	53.2	57.7	61.6	76.2
160.0–164.9	133	506	57.79	10.620	1.028	46.8	48.0	50.2	55.4	61.5	72.3	82.3
165.0–169.9	116	433	60.63	10.117	1.182	47.9	50.3	55.1	59.3	65.1	69.4	71.6
170.0–174.9	51	186	62.18	9.132	1.407	50.6	52.9	55.5	60.2	65.7	76.1	82.7
175.0–179.9	12	47	65.76	8.405	2.229	54.9	56.7	60.1	61.7	75.2	75.9	83.0
180.0–184.9	1	2	*	*	*	*	*	*	*	*	*	*
185.0–189.9	—	—	—	—	—	—	—	—	—	—	—	—
190.0–194.9	—	—	—	—	—	—	—	—	—	—	—	—
195.0 and over	—	—	—	—	—	—	—	—	—	—	—	—

n, Sample size; *N*, estimated number of youths in population in thousands; $\overline{X}$, mean; *s*, standard deviation; $s_{\overline{x}}$, standard error of the mean.

(From National Center for Health Statistics: Height and weight of youths 12–17 years, United States. *In* Vital and Health Statistics, Series 11, No. 124, Health Services and Mental Health Administration. Washington, D.C., U.S. Government Printing Office, 1973, pp. 282–288.)

TABLE A–13A. WEIGHT IN KILOGRAMS FOR WOMEN 18 TO 74 YEARS OF AGE: NUMBER EXAMINED, MEAN, STANDARD DEVIATION, AND SELECTED PERCENTILES BY RACE AND AGE, UNITED STATES, 1976 TO 1980*

RACE AND AGE (years)	NUMBER OF EXAMINED PERSONS	MEAN	STANDARD DEVIATION	PERCENTILE								
				5th	10th	15th	25th	50th	75th	85th	90th	95th
All races†												
18–74	6,588	65.4	14.6	47.7	50.3	52.2	55.4	62.4	72.1	79.2	84.4	93.1
18–24	1,066	60.6	11.9	46.6	49.1	50.6	53.2	58.0	65.0	70.4	75.3	82.9
25–34	1,170	64.2	15.0	47.4	49.6	51.4	54.3	60.9	69.6	78.4	84.1	93.5
35–44	844	67.1	15.2	49.2	52.0	53.3	56.9	63.4	73.9	81.7	87.5	98.9
45–54	763	68.0	15.3	48.5	51.3	53.3	57.3	65.5	75.7	82.1	87.6	96.0
55–64	1,329	67.9	14.7	48.6	51.3	54.1	57.3	65.2	75.3	82.3	87.5	95.1
65–74	1,416	66.6	13.8	47.1	50.8	53.2	57.4	64.8	73.8	79.8	84.4	91.3
White												
18–74	5,686	64.8	14.1	47.7	50.3	52.2	55.2	62.1	71.1	77.9	83.3	91.5
18–24	892	60.4	11.6	47.3	49.5	50.8	53.3	57.9	64.8	69.7	74.3	82.4
25–34	1,000	63.6	14.5	47.3	49.5	51.3	54.0	60.6	68.9	76.3	81.5	89.7
35–44	726	66.1	14.5	49.3	51.8	52.9	56.3	62.4	71.9	79.7	85.8	94.9
45–54	647	67.3	14.4	48.6	51.3	53.4	57.0	65.0	74.8	81.1	85.6	94.5
55–64	1,176	67.2	14.4	48.5	50.7	53.7	57.1	64.7	74.5	81.8	86.2	92.8
65–74	1,245	66.2	13.7	47.2	50.7	52.9	57.2	64.3	72.9	79.2	84.3	91.2
Black												
18–74	782	71.2	17.3	48.8	51.6	55.1	59.1	67.8	80.6	87.4	94.9	105.1
18–24	147	63.1	13.9	46.2	49.0	50.6	53.8	60.4	70.0	75.8	79.1	89.3
25–34	145	69.3	16.7	48.3	50.8	53.1	57.8	65.3	80.2	87.1	91.5	102.7
35–44	103	75.3	18.4	50.7	55.2	57.2	63.0	70.2	85.2	95.3	103.5	113.1
45–54	100	77.7	18.8	55.1	60.3	60.8	64.5	74.3	83.6	94.5	98.2	117.5
55–64	135	75.8	16.4	54.2	55.2	57.6	65.4	74.6	83.4	91.9	95.5	108.5
65–74	152	72.4	13.6	52.9	56.4	60.3	64.0	70.0	82.2	84.4	86.5	98.1

*Includes clothing weight, estimated as ranging from 0.09 to 0.28 kilogram.

†Includes all other races not shown as separate categories.

(From National Center for Health Statistics: Anthropometric Reference Data and Prevalence of Overweight, United States 1976–1980. DHHS Publication No. 87–1688. Hyattsville, MD, U.S. Department of Health and Human Services, Public Health Service, 1987.)

TABLE A–13B. WEIGHT IN KILOGRAMS FOR MEN 18 TO 74 YEARS OF AGE: NUMBER EXAMINED, MEAN, STANDARD DEVIATION, AND SELECTED PERCENTILES BY RACE AND AGE, UNITED STATES, 1976 TO 1980*

RACE AND AGE (years)	NUMBER OF EXAMINED PERSONS	MEAN	STANDARD DEVIATION	PERCENTILE								
				5th	10th	15th	25th	50th	75th	85th	90th	95th
All races†												
18–74	5,916	78.1	13.5	58.6	62.3	64.9	68.7	76.9	85.6	91.3	95.7	102.7
18–24	988	73.8	12.7	56.8	60.4	61.9	64.8	72.0	80.3	85.1	90.4	99.5
25–34	1,067	78.7	13.7	59.5	62.9	65.4	69.3	77.5	85.6	91.1	95.1	102.7
35–44	745	80.9	13.4	59.7	65.1	67.7	72.1	79.9	88.1	94.8	98.8	104.3
45–54	690	80.9	13.6	60.8	65.2	67.2	71.7	79.0	89.4	94.5	99.5	105.3
55–64	1,227	78.8	12.8	59.9	63.8	66.4	70.2	77.7	85.6	90.5	94.7	102.3
65–74	1,199	74.8	12.8	54.4	58.5	61.2	66.1	74.2	82.7	87.9	91.2	96.6
White												
18–74	5,148	78.5	13.1	59.3	62.8	65.5	69.4	77.3	85.6	91.4	95.5	102.3
18–24	846	74.2	12.8	56.8	60.5	62.0	65.0	72.4	80.6	85.5	91.0	100.0
25–34	901	79.0	13.1	59.9	63.7	65.9	69.8	78.0	85.6	91.3	95.3	102.7
35–44	653	81.4	12.8	62.3	66.6	68.8	72.9	80.1	88.2	94.6	98.7	104.1
45–54	617	81.0	13.4	62.0	66.1	67.3	71.9	79.0	89.4	94.2	99.0	104.5
55–64	1,086	78.9	12.4	60.5	64.5	66.6	70.6	78.2	85.6	90.4	94.5	101.7
65–74	1,045	75.4	12.4	55.5	59.5	62.5	67.0	74.7	83.0	87.9	91.2	96.0
Black												
18–74	649	77.9	15.2	58.0	61.1	63.6	67.2	75.3	85.4	92.9	98.3	105.4
18–24	121	72.2	12.0	58.3	60.9	62.3	64.9	70.8	77.1	81.8	83.7	93.6
25–34	139	78.2	16.3	58.7	63.4	64.9	68.4	75.3	84.4	90.6	92.2	106.3
35–44	70	82.5	15.4	*	61.7	65.2	69.7	83.1	94.8	100.4	104.2	*
45–54	62	82.4	14.5	*	64.7	67.0	73.2	81.8	93.0	100.0	102.5	*
55–64	129	78.6	14.7	56.8	61.4	64.3	68.0	77.0	86.5	93.8	98.6	104.7
65–74	128	73.3	15.3	52.5	56.7	58.0	61.0	71.2	81.1	90.8	97.3	105.1

*Includes clothing weight, estimated as ranging from 0.09 to 0.28 kilogram.

†Includes all other races not shown as separate categories.

(From National Center for Health Statistics: Anthropometric Reference Data and Prevalence of Overweight, United States 1976–1980. DHHS Publication No. 87–1688. Hyattsville, MD, U.S. Department of Health and Human Services, Public Health Service, 1987.)

TABLE A–13C. HEIGHT IN CENTIMETERS FOR WOMEN 18 TO 74 YEARS OF AGE: NUMBER EXAMINED, MEAN, STANDARD DEVIATION, AND SELECTED PERCENTILES BY RACE AND AGE, UNITED STATES, 1976 TO 1980*

RACE AND AGE (years)	NUMBER OF EXAMINED PERSONS	MEAN	STANDARD DEVIATION	PERCENTILE								
				5th	10th	15th	25th	50th	75th	85th	90th	95th
All races[†]												
18–74	6,588	161.8	6.6	150.9	153.6	155.2	157.4	161.7	166.3	168.6	170.3	172.6
18–24	1,066	163.4	6.6	152.9	155.2	156.7	159.0	163.7	167.6	170.0	171.6	174.0
25–34	1,170	163.1	6.3	153.2	155.2	156.6	158.7	163.1	167.6	169.9	171.3	173.7
35–44	844	162.8	6.3	152.6	155.5	156.7	158.5	162.5	167.0	169.3	171.0	173.5
45–54	763	161.3	6.4	150.5	152.9	154.5	156.8	161.3	165.6	167.7	169.4	171.8
55–64	1,329	160.1	6.4	149.2	151.8	153.7	155.9	160.3	164.5	166.7	168.0	170.3
65–74	1,416	158.1	6.2	147.9	150.0	151.7	154.1	158.4	162.2	164.5	166.0	167.7
White												
18–74	5,686	161.9	6.5	151.3	153.8	155.4	157.6	161.9	165.4	168.7	170.3	172.7
18–24	892	163.7	6.4	153.1	155.7	157.1	159.4	163.9	167.7	170.1	171.8	174.0
25–34	1,000	163.3	6.2	153.5	155.4	156.6	158.9	163.3	167.8	170.1	171.5	173.7
35–44	726	162.9	6.3	152.6	155.6	156.7	158.4	162.6	167.0	169.4	171.2	173.5
45–54	647	161.5	6.2	151.5	153.6	155.2	157.2	161.3	165.7	167.6	169.4	171.7
55–64	1,176	160.1	6.3	149.6	151.9	153.9	156.1	160.3	164.4	166.5	167.7	170.1
65–74	1,245	158.1	6.2	147.8	150.1	151.7	154.1	158.5	162.2	164.5	166.0	167.7
Black												
18–74	782	162.1	6.7	150.6	154.2	155.2	157.6	162.2	166.6	168.9	170.4	173.0
18–24	147	163.2	6.9	152.8	155.1	156.4	158.6	163.0	168.1	170.2	171.1	174.8
25–34	145	162.3	6.3	151.3	154.8	156.3	158.1	162.5	166.2	168.6	170.4	174.1
35–44	103	163.3	5.5	155.2	156.9	157.3	159.7	162.5	167.0	168.7	170.1	171.7
45–54	100	161.7	6.9	150.4	152.6	154.4	155.2	162.1	167.5	169.3	170.5	171.9
55–64	135	161.0	7.4	148.7	149.2	153.4	155.8	161.8	166.5	169.1	171.0	174.5
65–74	152	158.8	6.2	148.2	150.4	152.6	155.6	159.1	163.0	164.7	166.4	169.4

*Height without shoes.

[†]Includes all other races not shown as separate categories.

(From National Center for Health Statistics: Anthropometric Reference Data and Prevalence of Overweight, United States 1976–1980. DHHS Publication No. 87–1688. Hyattsville, MD, U.S. Department of Health and Human Services, Public Health Service, 1987.)

TABLE A—13D. HEIGHT IN CENTIMETERS FOR MEN 18 TO 74 YEARS OF AGE: NUMBER EXAMINED, MEAN, STANDARD DEVIATION, AND SELECTED PERCENTILES BY RACE AND AGE, UNITED STATES, 1976 TO 1980*

RACE AND AGE (years)	NUMBER OF EXAMINED PERSONS	MEAN	STANDARD DEVIATION	PERCENTILE 5th	10th	15th	25th	50th	75th	85th	90th	95th
All races†												
18—74	5,916	175.5	7.2	163.9	166.4	168.2	171.1	175.7	180.4	182.9	184.5	187.0
18—24	988	177.0	7.1	165.8	168.3	169.8	172.2	177.0	181.6	183.9	186.0	189.6
25—34	1,067	176.7	6.7	165.5	167.9	170.0	172.2	176.8	181.2	183.6	185.3	187.4
35—44	745	176.3	7.3	164.1	166.4	168.8	172.2	176.5	181.2	183.6	185.2	188.0
45—54	690	175.2	6.6	164.5	167.2	168.3	170.7	175.1	179.8	182.5	184.3	185.7
55—64	1,227	173.7	6.9	162.1	165.4	166.8	169.2	173.7	178.5	180.6	182.2	184.6
65—74	1,199	171.3	7.1	159.3	162.3	164.1	166.3	171.5	176.1	178.6	180.4	183.1
White												
18—74	5,148	175.7	7.1	164.2	166.7	168.6	171.2	175.9	180.5	183.0	184.6	187.2
18—24	846	177.2	7.0	166.3	168.6	170.1	172.4	177.1	181.9	184.1	186.4	189.7
25—34	901	177.0	6.6	165.8	168.2	170.6	172.5	177.0	181.4	183.8	185.4	187.7
35—44	653	176.7	7.3	164.5	166.7	169.6	172.6	176.8	181.7	183.7	185.8	188.0
45—54	617	175.4	6.8	164.6	167.3	168.9	171.2	175.3	179.8	182.5	184.3	185.7
55—64	1,086	173.8	6.8	163.1	165.6	167.2	169.5	173.6	178.5	180.7	182.2	184.5
65—74	1,045	171.6	6.9	159.6	162.9	164.6	166.9	171.6	176.4	178.7	180.5	183.3
Black												
18—74	649	175.5	7.0	164.3	166.5	168.1	171.1	175.7	180.3	183.0	184.5	186.5
18—24	121	176.7	7.0	165.1	167.6	169.9	172.5	177.9	181.0	183.8	185.0	186.4
25—34	139	176.7	6.9	165.5	168.5	169.6	172.4	177.1	181.8	183.2	184.7	187.1
35—44	70	176.5	6.4	*	167.6	170.7	172.8	175.2	179.9	181.9	185.1	*
45—54	62	174.2	6.7	*	167.6	167.7	169.1	172.8	178.4	183.2	184.5	*
55—64	129	174.2	6.9	162.7	165.3	166.8	168.6	174.6	178.8	180.7	182.8	186.8
65—74	128	171.2	6.5	161.2	162.6	163.8	165.9	171.6	175.3	177.7	180.8	182.2

*Height without shoes.

†Includes all other races not shown as separate categories.

(From National Center for Health Statistics: Anthropometric Reference Data and Prevalence of Overweight, United States 1976—1980. DHHS Publication No. 87—1688. Hyattsville, MD, U.S. Department of Health and Human Services, Public Health Service, 1987.)

TABLE A—13E. PROVISIONAL AGE- AND SEX-SPECIFIC REFERENCE VALUES FOR WEIGHT IN KILOGRAMS (POUNDS) IN ELDERLY SUBJECTS*,†

AGE GROUP (YEARS)	5%	50%	95%
Men			
65	62.6 (138.0)	79.5 (175.0)	102.0 (224.9)
70	59.7 (131.6)	76.5 (168.7)	99.1 (218.5)
75	56.8 (125.2)	73.6 (162.3)	96.3 (212.3)
80	53.9 (118.8)	70.7 (155.9)	93.4 (205.9)
85	51.0 (112.4)	67.8 (149.5)	90.5 (199.5)
90	48.1 (106.0)	64.9 (143.1)	87.6 (193.1)
Women			
65	51.2 (112.9)	66.8 (147.3)	87.1 (192.0)
70	49.0 (108.0)	64.6 (142.4)	84.9 (187.2)
75	46.8 (103.2)	62.4 (137.6)	82.8 (182.5)
80	44.7 (98.5)	60.2 (132.7)	80.6 (177.7)
85	42.5 (93.7)	58.0 (127.9)	78.4 (172.8)
90	40.3 (88.8)	55.9 (123.2)	76.2 (168.0)

*Data from 119 men and 150 women. The subjects were all ambulatory.

†See Tables A—14b-1 through A—14b-6 for data compiled by Frisancho (Am. J. Clin. Nutr., *40*:808—819, 1984) from NHANES I and II.

(From Chumlea, W.C., Roche, A.F., Mukherjee, D.: Nutritional Assessment of the Elderly through Anthropometry. Ohio, Wright State University School of Medicine, 1984.)

TABLE A–14A-1. TRICEPS SKINFOLD THICKNESS: GIRLS, 1 TO 17 YEARS, UNITED STATES, 1971 TO 1974

RACE AND AGE IN YEARS	NUMBER IN SAMPLE	ESTIMATED POPULATION IN THOUSANDS	MEAN†	STANDARD DEVIATION	PERCENTILE 5th	10th	15th	25th	50th	75th	85th	90th	95th
All Races*					Triceps Skinfold in Millimeters								
1	267	1,620	10.1	2.8	6.0	6.5	7.0	8.0	10.0	12.0	13.0	14.0	15.0
2	272	1,708	10.5	2.5	7.0	7.5	8.0	9.0	10.0	12.0	13.5	14.0	15.0
3	292	1,701	10.9	2.7	6.0	7.0	8.0	9.0	11.0	12.5	13.5	14.0	15.0
4	281	1,599	10.5	2.7	7.0	7.5	8.0	8.0	10.0	12.0	13.0	14.0	15.0
5	314	1,695	10.5	3.8	6.0	7.0	7.0	8.0	10.0	12.0	13.0	15.0	17.5
6	176	1,787	10.3	3.3	6.0	6.5	7.0	8.0	10.0	12.0	13.0	13.5	15.0
7	169	1,754	10.8	4.2	4.0	6.0	7.0	8.0	10.5	12.0	15.0	16.0	18.0
8	152	1,800	12.3	4.8	6.5	8.0	8.0	9.0	11.0	15.0	17.0	18.0	22.5
9	171	2,017	13.2	4.8	7.0	7.5	8.0	10.0	12.5	16.0	18.0	20.0	22.0
10	197	2,173	13.1	5.0	7.0	8.0	8.0	9.5	12.0	15.5	19.0	20.0	23.0
11	166	1,911	14.5	6.2	7.0	8.0	8.5	10.0	13.0	18.0	20.5	23.5	28.5
12	177	1,812	15.0	5.9	7.5	8.0	9.0	10.5	14.0	18.5	20.0	23.0	27.0
13	198	2,175	16.2	6.8	7.0	8.0	10.0	11.5	15.0	20.0	24.0	25.0	30.0
14	184	2,036	17.5	7.3	8.5	9.5	10.0	13.0	16.0	21.0	24.0	27.0	33.0
15	171	2,163	17.0	7.0	8.0	10.0	11.0	12.0	16.0	20.5	23.0	25.0	28.5
16	175	2,145	18.2	6.7	10.0	10.5	12.0	13.5	17.0	21.0	24.0	26.0	32.5
17	157	1,804	19.6	8.1	10.0	11.5	12.0	13.0	19.0	24.0	26.5	29.5	35.0
White													
1	189	1,328	10.2	2.8	6.0	7.0	7.0	8.0	10.0	12.0	13.0	13.5	15.5
2	203	1,434	10.6	2.6	7.0	7.5	8.0	9.0	10.0	12.0	13.5	14.0	15.0
3	211	1,438	11.1	2.6	7.0	8.0	8.5	9.0	11.0	13.0	13.5	14.0	15.0
4	204	1,339	10.8	2.6	7.5	8.0	8.0	9.0	10.5	12.0	13.0	14.5	16.0
5	224	1,416	10.7	3.7	6.0	7.0	8.0	8.5	10.0	12.0	13.0	15.0	17.5
6	125	1,445	10.6	3.3	6.5	7.0	7.5	8.0	10.5	12.0	13.0	14.0	16.0
7	122	1,507	10.9	4.2	4.0	6.0	7.0	8.0	11.0	12.0	15.0	15.5	17.5
8	117	1,507	12.4	4.7	7.0	8.0	8.0	9.0	11.5	15.0	16.5	18.0	22.0
9	129	1,751	13.6	4.6	7.5	8.0	9.0	10.0	13.0	16.0	18.0	20.0	22.0
10	148	1,855	13.4	4.8	7.5	8.0	8.5	10.0	12.5	15.5	19.0	20.0	23.0
11	122	1,569	14.9	6.1	8.0	8.5	9.0	10.0	13.0	17.5	20.5	24.5	28.5
12	128	1,506	15.2	5.6	8.0	9.0	10.0	11.0	14.0	18.5	20.0	23.0	26.0
13	153	1,886	16.2	6.8	7.0	8.0	10.0	11.5	15.0	20.0	24.0	25.0	28.5
14	132	1,731	17.8	7.3	9.0	9.5	10.5	13.0	16.7	21.0	24.0	28.5	33.0
15	125	1,752	17.7	6.7	9.0	10.5	11.0	13.0	17.0	21.0	24.0	25.0	28.5
16	141	1,933	18.2	6.6	10.0	10.5	12.5	14.0	17.0	21.0	24.0	26.0	32.1
17	117	1,549	19.8	8.0	10.0	12.0	12.5	13.5	19.0	24.0	26.5	29.5	35.0
Black													
1	73	257	10.0	3.0	5.5	5.5	7.0	8.0	10.0	12.0	13.0	14.0	15.0
2	66	261	10.0	2.3	7.0	8.0	8.0	8.0	10.0	11.0	12.0	14.0	15.5
3	78	245	9.7	2.9	6.0	7.0	7.0	8.0	10.0	11.0	12.0	13.0	14.0
4	73	246	8.8	2.7	5.0	6.0	7.0	7.0	8.0	10.5	12.0	13.0	14.0
5	88	265	9.4	3.9	5.0	5.0	6.5	7.0	8.0	10.0	12.0	13.5	17.0
6	50	336	9.0	3.1	5.5	6.0	6.0	8.0	8.0	10.0	11.5	12.0	13.0
7	46	241	10.1	4.0	5.0	6.0	7.0	7.5	9.0	11.0	17.5	18.0	18.0
8	35	293	11.5	5.1	5.0	6.5	7.0	8.0	10.0	13.5	18.0	18.0	23.0
9	41	247	10.2	5.1	5.5	6.0	6.0	6.5	8.0	12.0	18.0	18.0	20.0
10	48	303	11.7	5.6	6.5	6.5	7.0	7.5	10.0	16.0	18.0	19.0	24.0
11	42	315	12.7	6.4	4.0	5.0	6.5	7.5	10.0	18.0	22.0	23.0	23.0
12	47	284	13.6	7.6	5.5	6.0	6.0	7.5	12.0	17.0	22.0	25.0	30.0
13	44	287	16.1	7.0	7.0	8.5	10.0	11.0	14.0	18.0	24.0	24.0	33.5
14	50	265	15.9	6.7	8.0	8.0	9.0	10.5	14.0	20.5	24.0	24.5	24.5
15	46	411	14.0	7.6	6.5	6.5	8.0	10.0	12.5	16.0	16.5	20.0	32.8
16	33	203	18.9	8.0	8.0	8.0	10.0	12.0	19.0	24.0	24.5	33.0	33.1
17	39	239	16.9	6.6	7.5	9.0	11.0	12.0	14.5	20.0	24.0	28.0	31.0

*Includes data for races that are not shown separately.

†Measurements made in the right arm.

(From the National Center for Health Statistics, Department of Health and Human Services. See also Bishop, C.W., Bowen, P.E., Ritchey, S.J.: Am. J. Clin. Nutr., *34*:2530–2539, 1981.)

TABLE A–14A-2. SUBSCAPULAR SKINFOLD THICKNESS: GIRLS, 1 TO 17 YEARS, UNITED STATES, 1971 TO 1974

RACE AND AGE IN YEARS	NUMBER IN SAMPLE	ESTIMATED POPULATION IN THOUSANDS	MEAN†	STANDARD DEVIATION	PERCENTILE 5th	10th	15th	25th	50th	75th	85th	90th	95th
All Races*					Subscapular Skinfold in Millimeters								
1	267	1,620	6.2	1.9	4.0	4.0	4.0	5.0	6.0	8.0	8.0	9.0	9.0
2	272	1,708	6.2	2.4	4.0	4.0	4.0	5.0	6.0	7.0	8.0	9.0	10.0
3	292	1,701	5.8	2.0	4.0	4.0	4.0	4.5	5.5	6.5	7.0	8.0	9.0
4	281	1,599	5.6	1.9	3.5	4.0	4.0	4.5	5.0	6.0	7.0	8.0	9.0
5	314	1,695	6.2	3.3	3.5	4.0	4.0	4.0	5.0	6.5	8.0	9.0	15.0
6	176	1,787	6.0	2.8	3.0	4.0	4.0	4.5	5.5	6.5	7.0	8.0	10.0
7	169	1,754	6.2	3.3	3.0	4.0	4.0	4.5	5.0	7.0	9.0	10.5	11.5
8	152	1,800	7.7	5.5	3.5	4.0	4.0	4.5	5.5	8.0	12.5	14.5	19.5
9	171	2,017	8.5	5.0	4.0	4.0	4.5	5.0	7.0	10.0	13.0	17.0	19.0
10	197	2,173	8.6	5.1	4.0	4.5	5.0	5.5	6.5	10.0	13.0	18.0	20.0
11	166	1,911	10.1	6.4	4.0	5.0	5.0	6.0	8.0	13.0	16.0	19.0	25.5
12	177	1,812	11.1	6.8	5.0	5.0	5.5	6.0	9.5	13.0	16.0	20.0	25.0
13	198	2,175	11.9	7.1	5.0	6.0	6.0	7.0	9.5	15.0	19.0	23.4	26.0
14	184	2,036	13.0	8.0	5.0	6.0	6.5	8.0	10.0	16.0	19.0	24.0	28.0
15	171	2,163	12.2	7.2	6.0	6.5	7.0	7.5	10.0	14.0	18.0	20.0	27.0
16	175	2,145	13.4	7.8	6.0	7.0	7.5	8.0	10.5	15.0	21.0	25.5	29.0
17	157	1,804	15.6	9.4	6.5	7.0	7.5	9.0	12.5	20.0	25.5	27.0	34.1
White													
1	189	1,328	6.3	1.9	3.5	4.0	4.0	5.0	6.0	8.0	8.0	9.0	9.5
2	203	1,434	6.0	2.1	4.0	4.0	4.0	5.0	6.0	7.0	8.0	8.5	10.0
3	211	1,438	5.8	1.9	4.0	4.0	4.0	5.0	5.5	6.5	7.0	8.0	9.0
4	204	1,339	5.7	1.9	3.5	4.0	4.0	4.5	5.0	6.0	7.0	8.0	9.0
5	224	1,416	6.2	3.2	3.5	4.0	4.0	4.5	5.5	6.5	8.0	10.0	15.0
6	125	1,445	6.0	2.7	3.0	3.5	4.0	4.5	6.0	6.5	7.0	8.0	10.0
7	122	1,507	6.2	3.4	3.0	3.5	4.0	4.5	5.0	7.0	8.5	10.0	12.5
8	117	1,507	7.6	5.6	3.5	4.0	4.0	4.5	6.0	8.0	10.0	13.0	21.0
9	129	1,751	8.5	4.7	4.0	4.5	5.0	5.0	7.0	10.0	13.0	16.0	18.0
10	148	1,855	8.8	5.1	4.0	4.5	5.0	5.5	7.0	10.0	13.0	18.0	20.0
11	122	1,569	10.3	6.7	4.0	5.0	5.0	6.0	8.0	13.0	16.5	20.5	25.5
12	128	1,506	11.1	6.4	5.0	5.0	6.0	6.5	9.5	13.5	17.0	20.0	22.0
13	153	1,886	11.6	6.9	5.0	5.5	6.0	7.0	9.0	15.0	19.0	21.0	25.0
14	132	1,731	13.2	8.2	5.0	6.0	6.5	8.0	10.5	16.0	20.0	24.0	30.0
15	125	1,752	12.4	6.9	6.0	7.0	7.0	8.0	10.0	14.5	18.0	20.0	27.0
16	141	1,933	12.9	7.3	6.0	7.0	7.5	8.0	10.0	15.0	20.5	25.0	28.5
17	117	1,549	15.2	9.3	6.0	7.0	7.5	8.0	12.5	18.0	25.0	26.5	34.0
Black													
1	73	257	6.1	2.0	4.0	4.0	4.0	5.0	5.5	8.0	8.5	9.0	9.0
2	66	261	6.8	3.3	4.0	4.0	4.5	5.0	6.0	7.5	9.5	12.0	15.5
3	78	245	5.5	2.0	4.0	4.0	4.0	4.5	5.0	6.0	7.0	7.0	8.0
4	73	246	5.2	1.7	3.0	3.5	4.0	4.0	5.0	6.0	6.0	8.0	8.5
5	88	265	5.8	3.5	4.0	4.0	4.0	4.0	5.0	6.0	6.5	7.0	13.0
6	50	336	6.0	3.3	3.0	4.0	4.0	4.5	5.0	7.0	7.5	7.5	10.0
7	46	241	6.4	2.6	3.0	4.0	4.0	5.0	5.5	8.0	11.0	11.0	11.0
8	35	293	8.2	5.2	4.0	4.0	4.0	4.5	5.0	14.0	15.0	16.0	17.5
9	41	247	8.3	6.4	4.0	4.0	4.0	4.5	5.5	7.5	14.5	24.0	24.0
10	48	303	8.1	5.5	4.0	4.0	4.5	5.0	6.0	8.0	12.5	14.3	22.0
11	42	315	9.2	4.5	4.0	5.0	5.0	5.5	8.0	11.0	14.5	14.5	15.5
12	47	284	10.7	8.6	4.5	5.0	5.0	5.5	7.0	11.5	16.0	28.0	31.0
13	44	287	13.9	8.1	6.0	6.0	6.5	8.0	12.0	15.0	26.0	26.0	28.4
14	50	265	12.5	7.3	6.0	6.0	6.5	7.0	10.0	16.5	23.0	23.0	25.0
15	46	411	11.2	8.4	5.5	5.5	6.0	6.5	7.5	10.5	19.0	20.0	33.4
16	33	203	17.8	10.7	6.0	7.0	8.0	10.5	15.0	24.5	31.0	38.0	38.0
17	39	239	16.4	8.4	7.0	7.5	8.0	9.0	12.5	23.5	27.0	28.0	30.0

*Includes data for races that are not shown separately.

†Measurements made in the right arm.

(From the National Center for Health Statistics, Department of Health and Human Services. See also Bishop, C.W., Bowen, P.E., Ritchey, S.J.: Am. J. Clin. Nutr., *34*:2530–2539, 1981.)

TABLE A–14A-3. TRICEPS SKINFOLD THICKNESS: BOYS, 1 TO 17 YEARS, UNITED STATES, 1971 TO 1974

RACE AND AGE IN YEARS	NUMBER IN SAMPLE	ESTIMATED POPULATION IN THOUSANDS	MEAN†	STANDARD DEVIATION	PERCENTILE								
					5th	10th	15th	25th	50th	75th	85th	90th	95th
All Races*					Triceps Skinfold in Millimeters								
1	286	1,693	10.4	3.1	6.0	7.0	7.5	8.0	10.0	12.0	14.0	15.0	16.0
2	298	1,747	10.0	2.7	6.0	6.5	7.0	8.0	10.0	12.0	12.5	13.5	15.0
3	308	1,807	9.9	2.7	6.5	7.0	7.0	8.0	10.0	11.0	12.5	13.1	14.5
4	304	1,815	9.4	2.5	5.0	6.5	7.0	8.0	9.0	11.0	12.0	12.5	14.0
5	273	1,563	9.5	3.3	5.0	6.0	7.0	7.0	9.0	11.0	12.5	13.5	15.0
6	179	1,673	8.6	3.0	5.0	5.5	6.0	6.5	8.0	10.0	12.0	12.0	14.0
7	164	1,979	8.9	3.5	4.0	5.0	6.0	6.5	8.0	10.0	12.0	13.0	15.5
8	152	1,861	9.0	3.3	5.0	5.5	6.0	6.5	8.0	10.0	12.0	13.0	16.0
9	169	2,019	10.6	4.8	5.0	6.0	6.5	7.0	9.0	14.0	17.0	17.0	19.0
10	184	2,205	10.9	4.4	5.5	6.0	6.0	8.0	10.0	13.5	15.0	17.0	19.5
11	178	2,177	11.9	6.4	5.0	6.0	6.0	7.5	10.0	14.5	18.0	20.0	24.0
12	200	2,304	11.9	6.3	4.5	6.0	6.5	8.0	10.5	13.5	16.5	20.0	27.0
13	174	1,978	11.2	6.6	5.0	5.0	5.5	7.0	10.0	13.0	19.0	22.0	25.0
14	174	2,030	10.3	6.2	4.0	5.0	5.5	6.5	8.0	12.0	16.5	19.0	22.5
15	171	2,093	10.0	6.1	4.0	5.0	5.0	6.0	8.0	11.5	15.0	19.0	23.5
16	169	2,019	9.7	5.2	4.0	5.0	5.0	6.0	8.0	12.0	14.0	17.0	22.0
17	176	2,095	9.2	5.4	4.0	5.0	5.0	6.0	7.5	11.0	12.5	15.0	19.0
White													
1	211	1,402	10.7	3.0	7.0	7.0	7.5	8.0	10.0	12.0	14.0	15.0	16.5
2	217	1,461	9.9	2.6	6.0	6.5	7.0	8.0	10.0	12.0	12.5	13.0	14.7
3	226	1,536	9.9	2.6	6.5	7.0	7.0	8.0	10.0	11.0	12.5	13.5	14.5
4	229	1,547	9.6	2.4	6.0	7.0	7.0	8.0	10.0	11.0	12.0	12.5	14.0
5	207	1,319	9.8	3.2	6.0	6.5	7.0	7.5	9.0	11.0	12.5	13.5	15.0
6	126	1,343	8.9	3.1	5.5	5.6	6.0	7.0	9.0	10.0	12.0	12.5	14.0
7	125	1,718	9.1	3.5	5.0	6.0	6.0	7.0	8.0	10.5	12.0	13.5	17.0
8	116	1,644	9.1	3.3	5.0	5.5	6.0	7.0	8.5	10.5	12.0	13.0	16.0
9	117	1,636	11.1	4.8	5.5	6.5	6.5	7.5	10.0	14.0	17.0	17.0	19.0
10	148	1,909	11.1	4.2	5.5	6.0	7.0	8.0	10.0	14.0	15.5	17.0	19.5
11	132	1,823	12.5	6.5	6.0	6.0	7.0	8.0	10.0	15.0	19.0	20.5	24.5
12	152	1,970	12.4	6.1	6.0	6.0	7.0	8.5	11.0	14.0	18.0	21.0	27.0
13	129	1,697	11.7	6.7	5.0	5.0	6.0	7.0	10.0	14.0	19.0	22.0	25.5
14	134	1,730	10.9	6.4	4.0	5.0	6.0	7.0	9.0	13.0	18.0	20.0	24.0
15	124	1,728	10.2	6.1	4.0	5.0	6.0	6.0	8.0	12.0	15.0	19.0	24.0
16	128	1,752	10.1	5.2	4.0	5.0	5.0	6.5	9.0	12.5	15.0	17.0	22.0
17	139	1,831	9.3	5.4	4.5	5.0	5.5	6.0	7.5	11.0	13.0	15.0	19.0
Black													
1	72	280	9.4	3.4	4.5	6.0	7.0	8.0	8.0	11.0	12.0	13.0	15.0
2	77	267	10.1	3.2	4.5	6.0	6.5	8.0	10.0	12.0	14.0	15.0	15.0
3	72	212	9.1	2.6	6.0	6.5	6.5	7.0	9.0	10.5	12.0	12.0	13.0
4	74	260	8.0	2.6	5.0	5.0	5.0	6.5	7.0	9.0	10.0	10.5	15.0
5	64	226	7.7	3.4	4.5	5.0	5.0	5.0	7.0	9.0	10.0	12.0	15.5
6	52	321	7.1	1.8	4.0	4.0	5.0	6.0	7.0	8.0	9.0	9.0	9.0
7	38	253	7.5	3.2	4.0	4.0	4.0	5.0	6.5	9.0	11.5	13.0	15.0
8	33	203	7.8	3.4	4.0	5.0	5.0	6.0	6.5	10.0	11.0	11.0	12.5
9	52	383	8.2	3.9	3.5	4.0	4.5	6.0	7.0	8.0	12.0	13.0	18.0
10	33	251	9.1	5.3	5.0	5.0	6.0	6.0	7.5	10.0	13.0	15.0	20.0
11	43	313	8.0	5.0	4.0	4.0	5.0	5.0	6.0	8.5	11.0	12.0	15.0
12	47	316	9.4	7.0	4.0	4.0	4.5	6.0	7.5	10.7	11.0	15.0	24.0
13	45	281	8.2	4.4	4.0	5.0	5.0	5.0	7.0	8.5	11.0	19.0	19.0
14	39	282	6.6	2.6	3.5	3.5	3.5	5.0	6.5	7.0	8.0	9.0	12.0
15	43	310	8.9	6.1	4.0	4.5	5.0	5.0	6.5	9.0	10.0	21.0	21.0
16	41	267	7.2	4.8	4.0	4.0	4.0	5.0	6.0	7.5	8.0	11.0	15.0
17	35	235	8.7	5.8	3.5	3.5	5.0	5.0	7.0	10.5	12.0	12.0	23.2

*Includes data for races that are not shown separately.

†Measurements made in the right arm.

(From the National Center for Health Statistics, Department of Health and Human Services. See also Bishop, C.W., Bowen, P.E., Ritchey, S.J.: Am. J. Clin. Nutr., *34*:2530–2539, 1981.)

TABLE A–14A-4. SUBSCAPULAR SKINFOLD THICKNESS: BOYS, 1 TO 17 YEARS, UNITED STATES, 1971 TO 1974

RACE AND AGE IN YEARS	NUMBER IN SAMPLE	ESTIMATED POPULATION IN THOUSANDS	MEAN†	STANDARD DEVIATION	PERCENTILE 5th	10th	15th	25th	50th	75th	85th	90th	95th
All Races*					Subscapular Skinfold in Millimeters								
1	286	1,693	6.2	1.9	4.0	4.0	4.0	5.0	6.0	7.0	8.0	8.5	10.0
2	298	1,747	5.7	2.0	3.0	4.0	4.0	4.5	5.0	6.5	7.0	8.0	10.0
3	308	1,807	5.4	2.0	3.5	4.0	4.0	4.0	5.0	6.0	6.8	7.0	9.5
4	304	1,815	5.1	1.7	3.0	3.5	4.0	4.0	5.0	6.0	6.0	7.0	7.0
5	273	1,563	5.3	2.7	3.0	3.5	4.0	4.0	5.0	6.0	7.0	7.0	8.0
6	179	1,673	5.1	2.4	3.0	3.0	3.5	4.0	4.5	5.0	6.0	7.0	9.0
7	164	1,979	5.5	3.0	3.0	3.0	3.5	4.0	4.5	6.0	7.0	9.0	11.0
8	152	1,861	5.1	2.3	3.0	3.0	3.5	4.0	4.5	6.0	6.0	7.5	9.0
9	169	2,019	7.1	5.1	3.5	3.5	4.0	4.0	5.0	8.0	11.0	14.0	14.0
10	184	2,205	6.8	4.5	3.5	4.0	4.0	4.0	5.5	7.0	10.0	12.0	18.0
11	178	2,177	8.0	6.2	4.0	4.0	4.0	4.5	6.0	8.5	13.0	15.0	19.0
12	200	2,304	8.0	6.0	3.5	4.0	4.5	5.0	6.0	9.0	11.0	14.0	20.5
13	174	1,978	8.8	6.9	3.5	4.0	4.5	5.0	6.5	9.0	13.5	17.0	26.0
14	174	2,030	8.5	6.1	4.0	4.5	5.0	5.0	6.5	9.0	13.0	16.0	20.0
15	171	2,093	9.1	6.5	4.0	5.0	5.0	5.5	7.0	10.0	13.0	15.5	23.0
16	169	2,019	9.8	6.2	5.0	5.5	6.0	6.5	8.0	10.5	13.5	16.5	23.5
17	176	2,095	9.7	5.9	5.0	5.5	6.0	7.0	8.0	10.0	13.0	16.0	23.0
White													
1	211	1,402	6.3	2.0	4.0	4.0	4.0	5.0	6.0	7.0	8.0	8.5	10.0
2	217	1,461	5.6	1.9	3.0	3.5	4.0	4.0	5.0	6.0	7.0	7.5	10.0
3	226	1,536	5.4	2.0	3.5	4.0	4.0	4.0	5.0	6.0	6.5	7.0	10.0
4	229	1,547	5.2	1.8	3.0	4.0	4.0	4.0	5.0	6.0	6.0	7.0	7.0
5	207	1,319	5.3	2.7	3.0	3.5	4.0	4.0	5.0	6.0	7.0	7.0	8.0
6	126	1,343	5.1	2.4	3.0	3.5	3.5	4.0	4.5	5.5	6.0	7.0	10.0
7	125	1,718	5.6	3.1	3.0	3.0	3.5	4.0	5.0	6.0	7.0	8.0	11.5
8	116	1,644	5.1	2.3	3.0	3.0	3.0	4.0	4.5	6.0	6.0	7.5	11.0
9	117	1,636	7.2	4.7	3.5	4.0	4.0	4.0	5.0	8.5	11.5	14.0	14.0
10	148	1,909	6.8	4.5	3.0	4.0	4.0	4.0	5.5	7.0	9.5	12.0	18.0
11	132	1,823	8.2	6.4	3.5	4.0	4.0	4.5	6.0	9.0	14.0	15.0	20.0
12	152	1,970	8.1	5.8	3.5	4.0	4.0	5.0	6.0	9.0	11.5	14.0	21.0
13	129	1,697	9.0	7.1	3.5	4.0	4.0	5.0	6.5	9.0	14.0	17.0	27.0
14	134	1,730	9.0	6.5	4.0	5.0	5.0	5.5	6.5	9.0	14.0	16.0	20.0
15	124	1,728	8.8	6.4	4.0	5.0	5.0	5.5	7.0	9.0	13.0	15.0	22.0
16	128	1,752	9.9	6.4	5.0	5.0	6.0	6.5	8.0	11.0	13.5	17.0	23.5
17	139	1,831	9.7	6.1	5.0	5.5	6.0	6.5	8.0	10.0	13.0	16.0	23.0
Black													
1	72	280	6.0	1.6	4.0	4.0	4.0	5.0	6.0	7.0	7.5	8.0	9.0
2	77	267	6.5	2.4	4.0	4.0	4.0	5.0	5.5	7.0	10.0	11.5	11.5
3	72	212	5.3	1.6	3.5	4.0	4.0	4.0	5.0	6.0	6.5	6.5	9.0
4	74	260	4.8	1.2	3.0	3.0	3.5	4.0	5.0	5.1	6.0	6.0	8.0
5	64	226	5.1	2.5	2.5	3.0	3.0	4.0	4.5	5.0	7.0	7.0	8.5
6	52	321	4.9	2.1	3.0	3.0	3.5	4.0	5.0	5.0	5.5	7.0	7.0
7	38	253	5.2	2.4	3.0	3.0	3.0	3.5	4.0	6.0	8.0	10.0	11.0
8	33	203	5.5	2.1	3.5	3.5	4.0	4.0	5.0	6.0	7.5	9.0	9.0
9	52	383	6.6	6.3	3.0	3.0	3.0	4.0	5.0	6.0	8.0	8.0	30.0
10	33	251	6.7	3.8	4.0	4.0	4.0	4.5	5.0	7.0	9.0	12.0	18.5
11	43	313	6.7	4.9	4.0	4.0	4.0	5.0	5.5	6.5	8.0	8.0	12.5
12	47	316	7.4	6.9	4.0	4.0	4.5	4.5	5.0	7.0	7.0	17.0	19.0
13	45	281	7.6	5.9	4.0	4.5	4.5	5.0	6.0	7.0	8.0	18.5	26.0
14	39	282	6.1	2.1	4.0	4.0	5.0	5.0	6.0	7.0	7.0	7.5	12.0
15	43	310	10.6	6.7	4.0	5.0	5.5	7.0	9.0	12.0	12.0	24.0	24.0
16	41	267	8.5	4.2	5.5	5.5	6.5	6.5	7.0	9.0	9.5	10.0	16.0
17	35	235	9.6	5.2	6.0	6.0	6.0	7.0	8.0	10.0	12.0	16.0	16.0

*Includes data for races that are not shown separately.

†Measurements made in the right arm.

(From the National Center for Health Statistics, Department of Health and Human Services. See also Bishop, C.W., Bowen, P.E., Ritchey, S.J.: Am. J. Clin. Nutr., *34*:2530–2539, 1981.)

TABLE A–14B-1. SELECTED PERCENTILES OF WEIGHT, TRICEPS AND SUBSCAPULAR SKINFOLDS, AND BONE-FREE UPPER ARM MUSCLE AREA (AMA) FOR UNITED STATES MEN AND WOMEN WITH SMALL FRAMES (25 TO 54 YEARS OLD)

HT			WT (kg)							TRICEPS (mm)							SUBSCAPULAR (mm)							BONE-FREE AMA (cm²)						
in	cm	n	5	10	15	50	85	90	95	5	10	15	50	85	90	95	5	10	15	50	85	90	95	5	10	15	50	85	90	95
Men																														
62	157	23	46*	50*	52*	64	71*	74*	77*				11							16							52			
63	160	43	48*	51*	53	61	70	75*	79*			6	10	17					8	12	20					32	48	54		
64	163	73	49*	53	55	66	76	76	80*		5	5	10	16	18			7	7	15	25	29			37	38	49	58	63	
65	165	112	52	53	58	66	77	81	84	4	5	6	11	17	19	21	7	8	9	14	25	28	35	31	35	37	47	60	63	71
66	168	129	56	57	59	67	78	83	84	5	6	6	11	18	18	20	7	8	8	14	26	26	32	31	36	38	49	60	62	71
67	170	132	56	60	62	71	82	83	88	5	6	6	11	18	20	22	6	7	9	15	23	25	30	35	39	41	49	58	60	62
68	173	107	56	59	62	71	79	82	85	5	6	6	10	15	16	20	7	8	9	13	24	30	40	33	37	40	49	59	62	69
69	175	97	57*	62	65	74	84	87	88*		6	6	11	17	20			7	7	13	24	26			36	40	58	61	63	
70	178	46	59*	62*	67	75	87	86*	90*			7	10	17					9	14	23					35	48	57		
71	180	49	60*	64*	70	76	79	88*	91*			7	10	16					8	13	22					39	47	52		
72	183	21	62*	65*	67*	74	87*	89*	93*				10							14							45			
73	185	9	63*	67*	69*	79*	89*	91*	94*																					
74	188	6	65*	68*	71*	80*	90*	92*	96*																					
Women																														
58	147	53	37*	43	43	52	58	62	66*		12	13	24	30	33			10	12	23	34	38			22	24	29	36	44	
59	150	108	42	43	44	53	63	69	72	8	11	14	21	29	36	37	6	9	10	17	29	32	34	17	20	22	28	38	39	43
60	152	142	42	44	45	53	63	65	70	8	11	12	21	28	29	33	6	7	8	18	27	32	39	19	21	22	28	36	40	44
61	155	218	44	46	47	54	64	66	72	11	12	14	21	28	31	34	7	8	9	16	28	32	36	20	21	23	28	38	39	42
62	157	255	44	47	48	55	63	64	70	10	12	14	20	28	31	34	6	7	8	14	22	27	32	20	21	21	27	33	35	37
63	160	239	46	48	49	55	65	68	79	10	11	13	20	27	30	36	6	7	7	14	27	29	31	20	21	22	27	33	35	38
64	163	146	49	50	51	57	67	68	74	10	13	13	20	28	30	34	6	7	8	13	24	27	34	22	23	23	28	34	38	42
65	165	113	50	52	53	60	70	72	80	12	13	14	22	29	31	34	7	8	8	15	26	30	33	21	22	23	28	37	39	47
66	168	47	46*	49*	54	58	65	71*	74*			12	19	30					9	12	25					23	27	35		
67	170	18	47*	50*	52*	59	70*	72*	76*				18							13							26			
68	173	18	48*	51*	53*	62	71*	73*	77*				20							15							25			
69	175	5	49*	52*	54*	63*	72*	74*	78*																					
70	178	1	50*	53*	55*	64*	73*	75*	79*																					

*Value estimated through linear regression equation.

(From Frisancho, A. R.: Am. J. Clin. Nutr., *40*:808–819, 1984, with permission.)

TABLE A–14B-2. SELECTED PERCENTILES OF WEIGHT, TRICEPS AND SUBSCAPULAR SKINFOLDS, AND BONE-FREE UPPER ARM MUSCLE AREA (AMA) FOR UNITED STATES MEN AND WOMEN WITH MEDIUM FRAMES (25 TO 54 YEARS OLD)

HT			WT (kg)							TRICEPS (mm)							SUBSCAPULAR (mm)							BONE-FREE AMA (cm²)						
in	cm	n	5	10	15	50	85	90	95	5	10	15	50	85	90	95	5	10	15	50	85	90	95	5	10	15	50	85	90	95
Men																														
62	157	10	51*	55*	58*	68	81*	83*	87*				15							13							58			
63	160	30	52*	56*	59*	71	82*	85*	89*				11							18							55			
64	163	71	54*	60	61	71	83	84	90*		6	6	12	18	20			7	9	17	30	32			43	47	56	67	71	
65	165	154	59	62	65	74	87	90	94	5	7	8	12	20	22	25	8	9	10	16	26	29	32	40	43	45	56	67	69	70
66	168	212	58	61	65	75	85	87	93	5	6	7	11	16	18	22	7	7	9	16	25	27	33	38	42	44	55	69	72	78
67	170	409	62	66	68	77	89	93	100	5	7	7	13	21	23	28	8	9	10	18	26	30	33	39	42	44	53	66	69	73
68	173	478	60	64	66	78	89	92	97	4	5	7	11	18	20	24	7	8	9	16	25	28	31	41	44	45	55	67	71	76
69	175	464	63	66	68	78	90	93	97	5	6	7	12	18	20	24	7	8	9	16	25	27	31	38	41	44	54	66	69	73
70	178	419	64	66	70	81	90	93	97	5	6	7	12	18	20	23	7	8	9	15	24	27	30	39	42	43	55	65	68	72
71	180	282	62	68	70	81	92	96	100	4	5	7	12	19	21	25	7	8	9	14	24	27	30	37	41	44	54	67	68	73
72	183	231	68	71	74	84	97	100	104	5	7	7	12	20	22	26	7	8	9	15	26	30	32	40	42	44	56	65	67	74
73	185	106	70	72	75	85	100	101	104	6	7	8	12	20	24	27	8	9	9	15	25	29	32	39	42	43	55	67	69	73
74	188	50	68*	76	77	88	100	100	104*		6	9	13	21	23			7	9	14	25	30			43	43	55	62	63	
Women																														
58	147	40	41*	46*	50	63	77	75*	79*			20	25	40					15	23	38					24	35	42		
59	150	104	47	50	52	66	76	79	85	15	19	21	30	37	40	40	10	12	13	29	38	39	43	23	24	26	33	43	45	49
60	152	208	47	50	52	60	77	79	85	14	15	17	26	35	37	41	8	10	11	22	35	37	41	22	25	25	32	42	45	49
61	155	465	47	49	51	61	73	78	86	11	14	15	25	34	36	42	7	9	10	19	32	36	42	21	24	25	31	42	45	51
62	157	644	49	50	52	61	73	77	83	12	14	16	24	34	36	40	7	9	10	18	33	37	40	21	23	25	31	40	43	48
63	160	685	49	51	53	62	77	80	88	12	13	15	24	33	35	38	7	8	10	18	31	34	38	22	23	25	32	41	43	50
64	163	722	50	52	54	62	76	82	87	11	14	15	23	33	36	40	7	7	8	16	31	35	38	21	23	24	31	40	43	48
65	165	628	52	54	55	63	75	80	89	12	14	15	22	31	34	38	7	8	8	15	29	33	38	21	23	24	31	40	43	49
66	168	428	52	54	55	63	75	78	83	11	13	14	22	31	33	37	7	8	9	14	28	30	35	21	23	24	30	39	41	44
67	170	257	54	56	57	65	79	82	88	12	13	15	21	29	30	35	7	8	8	15	28	32	37	22	24	25	30	40	43	48
68	173	119	58	59	60	67	77	85	87	10	14	15	22	31	32	36	8	8	9	15	29	33	35	22	24	25	30	37	38	39
69	175	59	49*	58	60	68	79	82	87*		11	12	19	29	31			8	8	12	25	29			23	24	30	36	39	
70	178	15	50*	54*	57*	70	80*	83*	87*				19							20							32			

*Value estimated through linear regression equation.

(From Frisancho, A. R.: Am. J. Clin. Nutr., *40*:808–819, 1984, with permission.)

TABLE A–14B-3. SELECTED PERCENTILES OF WEIGHT, TRICEPS AND SUBSCAPULAR SKINFOLDS, AND BONE-FREE UPPER ARM MUSCLE AREA (AMA) FOR UNITED STATES MEN AND WOMEN WITH LARGE FRAMES (25 TO 54 YEARS OLD)

HT			WT (kg)							TRICEPS (mm)							SUBSCAPULAR (mm)							BONE-FREE AMA (cm^2)						
in	cm	n	5	10	15	50	85	90	95	5	10	15	50	85	90	95	5	10	15	50	85	90	95	5	10	15	50	85	90	95
Men																														
62	157	1	57*	62*	66*	82*	99*	103*	108*																					
63	160	1	58*	63*	67*	83*	100*	104*	109*																					
64	163	5	59*	64*	68*	84*	101*	105*	110*																					
65	165	15	60*	65*	69*	79	102*	106*	111*				14							21							62			
66	168	37	60*	65*	75	84	103	106*	112*			9	14	30					13	22	36					48	58	76		
67	170	54	62*	70	71	84	102	111	113*		7	7	11	23	27			8	11	20	36	40			50	52	61	73	78	
68	173	84	63*	74	76	86	101	104	114*		9	10	14	22	23			12	14	20	31	35			51	53	65	78	86	
69	175	126	68	71	74	89	103	105	114	6	7	8	15	25	29	31	9	10	11	18	31	32	38	46	48	49	61	73	78	83
70	178	150	68	72	74	87	106	112	114	7	7	7	14	23	25	30	7	10	11	17	31	35	38	43	47	50	61	75	77	86
71	180	123	73	78	82	91	113	116	123	6	8	10	15	25	27	31	9	11	11	20	35	40	46	47	48	50	62	75	81	83
72	183	114	73	76	78	91	109	112	121	5	6	7	12	20	22	25	8	9	9	19	28	30	36	45	48	50	61	77	80	86
73	185	109	72	77	79	93	106	107	116	5	6	7	13	19	22	31	7	9	9	18	27	28	30	47	49	51	66	79	83	86
74	188	37	69*	74*	82	92	105	115*	120*			8	12	19					9	18	32					53	66	78		
Women																														
58	147	6	56*	63*	67*	86*	105*	110*	117*																					
59	150	19	56*	62*	67*	78	105*	109*	116*				36							35							45			
60	152	32	55*	62*	66*	87	104*	109*	116*				38							42							44			
61	155	92	54*	64	66	81	105	117	115*		25	26	36	48	50			17	17	35	48	53			29	33	41	62	74	
62	157	135	59	61	65	81	103	107	113	16	19	22	34	48	48	50	13	16	18	32	48	51	55	26	28	31	44	56	63	72
63	160	162	58	63	67	83	105	109	119	18	20	22	34	46	48	51	11	14	16	32	44	48	50	27	30	32	43	60	65	77
64	163	196	59	62	63	79	102	104	112	16	20	21	32	43	45	49	10	12	15	28	42	46	50	26	28	29	39	50	55	63
65	165	242	59	61	63	81	103	109	114	17	20	21	31	43	46	48	10	12	14	29	42	48	52	27	28	29	39	56	59	67
66	168	166	55	58	62	75	95	100	107	13	17	18	27	40	43	45	8	9	11	25	36	40	45	23	24	27	35	49	53	69
67	170	144	58	60	65	80	100	108	114	13	16	17	30	41	43	49	7	10	11	25	41	46	55	25	28	30	37	50	53	55
68	173	81	51*	66	66	76	104	105	111*		16	20	29	37	40			10	12	21	45	48			28	30	38	51	54	
69	175	39	50*	57*	68	79	105	104*	111*			21	30	42					11	20	43					27	35	49		
70	178	17	50*	56*	61*	76	99*	104*	110*				20							16							37			

*Value estimated through linear regression equation.

(From Frisancho, A. R.: Am. J. Clin. Nutr., *40*:808–819, 1984, with permission.)

TABLE A–14B-4. SELECTED PERCENTILES OF WEIGHT, TRICEPS AND SUBSCAPULAR SKINFOLDS, AND BONE-FREE UPPER ARM MUSCLE AREA (AMA) FOR UNITED STATES MEN AND WOMEN WITH SMALL FRAMES (55 TO 74 YEARS OLD)

HT			WT (kg)							TRICEPS (mm)							SUBSCAPULAR (mm)							BONE-FREE AMA (cm²)						
in	cm	n	5	10	15	50	85	90	95	5	10	15	50	85	90	95	5	10	15	50	85	90	95	5	10	15	50	85	90	95
Men																														
62	157	47	45*	49*	56	61	68	73*	77*			6	9	12					11	16	23					38	46	52		
63	160	78	47*	49	51	62	71	71	79*		5	5	10	16	17			6	6	12	21	22			34	35	43	54	55	
64	163	107	47	50	54	63	72	74	80	4	4	4	9	20	21	22	6	7	7	14	24	25	29	26	30	31	44	53	54	56
65	165	132	48	54	59	70	80	90	90	5	6	7	11	18	19	24	6	8	8	16	28	28	29	26	30	34	48	57	60	62
66	168	112	51	55	59	68	77	80	84	5	6	7	11	16	20	20	7	7	8	15	25	26	30	25	31	35	45	54	58	64
67	170	128	55	60	61	69	79	81	88	5	6	6	10	15	17	25	7	8	9	13	22	25	31	30	36	37	45	53	55	59
68	173	95	54*	54	58	70	79	81	86*		5	5	10	15	17			7	7	13	21	22			35	35	43	55	60	
69	175	47	56*	59*	63	75	81	84*	88*			8	10	15					10	16	27					38	47	62		
70	178	29	57*	61*	63*	76	83*	86*	89*				11							13							48			
71	180	14	59*	62*	65*	69	85*	87*	91*				9							10							43			
72	183	6	60*	64*	66*	76*	86*	89*	92*																					
73	185	1	62*	65*	68*	78*	88*	90*	94*																					
74	188	1	63*	67*	69*	77*	89*	92*	95*																					
Women																														
58	147	85	39*	46	48	54	63	65	71*		14	16	21	31	34			8	9	18	32	33			22	23	29	40	42	
59	150	122	41	45	48	55	66	68	74	11	13	15	21	30	31	33	6	7	9	19	29	30	33	22	23	24	30	39	40	44
60	152	157	43	45	47	54	67	70	73	10	11	13	20	29	31	35	5	7	8	15	27	32	36	20	22	23	30	37	41	44
61	155	145	43	43	45	56	65	70	71	10	12	14	22	29	29	32	6	7	8	17	29	31	34	18	21	23	28	36	40	42
62	157	158	47	49	52	58	67	69	73	11	11	12	21	29	30	32	7	8	9	17	25	26	30	20	23	24	30	37	40	43
63	160	89	42*	45	49	58	67	68	74*		12	13	20	29	30			6	7	14	25	27			19	20	27	35	36	
64	163	50	43*	47	49	60	68	70	75*		12	13	21	27	29			6	7	18	24	25			21	21	28	37	42	
65	165	26	43*	47*	49*	60	69*	72*	75*				18							13							28			
66	168	12	44*	48*	50*	68	70*	72*	76*				23							13							33			
67	170	1	45*	48*	51*	61*	71*	73*	77*																					
68	173	1	45*	49*	51*	61*	71*	74*	77*																					
69	175	0	46*	49*	52*	62*	72*	74*	78*																					
70	178	0	47*	50*	52*	63*	73*	75*	79*																					

*Value estimated through linear regression equation.

(From Frisancho, A. R.: Am. J. Clin. Nutr., *40*:808–819, 1984, with permission.)

TABLE A–14B-5. SELECTED PERCENTILES OF WEIGHT, TRICEPS AND SUBSCAPULAR SKINFOLDS, AND BONE-FREE UPPER ARM MUSCLE AREA (AMA) FOR UNITED STATES MEN AND WOMEN WITH MEDIUM FRAMES (55 TO 74 YEARS OLD)

HT			WT (kg)							TRICEPS (mm)							SUBSCAPULAR (mm)							BONE-FREE AMA (cm²)						
in	cm	n	5	10	15	50	85	90	95	5	10	15	50	85	90	95	5	10	15	50	85	90	95	5	10	15	50	85	90	95
Men																														
62	157	49	50*	54*	59	68	77	81*	85*			5	12	25					11	19	27					39	48	61		
63	160	89	51*	57	60	70	80	82	87*		7	7	11	20	23			8	10	15	26	28			36	38	50	60	63	
64	163	210	55	59	62	71	82	83	91	5	6	6	10	17	20	26	6	7	9	15	25	27	35	35	39	40	51	64	66	71
65	165	335	56	60	64	72	83	86	89	5	6	7	11	17	19	24	7	8	9	17	25	29	31	35	38	41	52	63	65	72
66	168	405	57	62	66	74	83	84	89	6	6	7	12	18	19	22	7	9	10	16	25	28	31	34	39	42	51	60	62	67
67	170	509	59	64	66	78	87	89	94	5	6	7	12	18	20	23	7	9	10	17	26	29	34	35	39	42	52	65	67	70
68	173	413	62	66	68	78	89	95	101	6	7	8	12	18	21	23	7	9	10	17	26	29	32	37	40	42	52	65	67	70
69	175	366	62	66	68	77	90	93	99	5	6	7	12	19	22	25	6	8	9	16	25	28	30	31	36	40	51	62	65	72
70	178	248	62	68	71	80	90	95	101	6	7	7	11	18	19	21	7	9	10	16	25	27	30	36	41	44	53	63	65	68
71	180	146	68	70	72	84	94	97	101	5	6	6	11	16	17	20	7	9	10	15	25	26	31	36	42	44	56	65	67	71
72	183	81	66*	65	69	81	96	97	101*		6	8	11	19	20			8	10	16	28	30			27	39	50	58	59	
73	185	35	68*	72*	79	88	93	99*	103*			8	13	16					10	15	26					43	56	67		
74	188	11	69*	73*	76*	95	98*	101*	104*				11							18							56			
Women																														
58	147	105	40	44	49	57	72	82	85	5	13	17	28	40	40	41	3	7	10	25	37	43	48	21	23	25	32	46	47	51
59	150	198	47	49	52	62	74	78	86	12	15	18	26	34	38	41	8	9	11	23	32	36	43	24	26	27	35	44	48	48
60	152	358	47	50	52	65	76	79	86	13	17	18	25	33	34	38	8	10	12	22	34	36	40	21	24	26	35	45	49	57
61	155	543	49	51	54	64	78	81	86	13	16	18	25	35	37	42	8	10	10	20	33	36	42	22	24	26	34	44	49	52
62	157	576	49	53	54	64	78	82	88	13	15	17	24	33	36	39	7	8	10	20	33	36	38	24	25	26	35	45	47	54
63	160	551	52	54	55	65	79	83	89	12	14	16	24	32	35	38	8	8	10	18	32	37	41	24	26	27	35	44	45	51
64	163	406	51	54	57	66	78	81	87	12	14	16	25	33	34	37	7	9	10	17	30	33	38	21	24	26	33	44	46	49
65	165	307	54	56	59	67	78	84	88	14	16	17	24	33	35	39	7	8	9	17	30	35	37	24	25	27	34	44	45	50
66	168	119	54	57	57	66	79	85	88	12	13	16	24	33	33	36	6	7	8	16	30	31	34	24	26	27	33	41	43	49
67	170	63	51*	59	61	72	82	85	89*		17	17	27	35	35			9	10	19	35	35			27	28	32	41	43	
68	173	28	52*	56*	59*	70	83*	86*	90*				25							16							36			
69	175	5	53*	57*	60*	72*	84*	87*	91*																					
70	178	1	54*	58*	61*	73*	85*	88*	92*																					

*Value estimated through linear regression equation.

(From Frisancho, A. R.: Am. J. Clin. Nutr., *40*:808–819, 1984, with permission.)

TABLE A–14B-6. SELECTED PERCENTILES OF WEIGHT, TRICEPS AND SUBSCAPULAR SKINFOLDS, AND BONE-FREE UPPER ARM MUSCLE AREA (AMA) FOR UNITED STATES MEN AND WOMEN WITH LARGE FRAMES (55 TO 74 YEARS OLD)

HT			WT (kg)							TRICEPS (mm)							SUBSCAPULAR (mm)							BONE-FREE AMA (cm²)						
in	cm	n	5	10	15	50	85	90	95	5	10	15	50	85	90	95	5	10	15	50	85	90	95	5	10	15	50	85	90	95
Men																														
62	157	7	54*	59*	63*	77*	91*	95*	100*																					
63	160	12	55*	60*	64*	80	92*	96*	101*				15							20							57			
64	163	20	57*	62*	65*	77	94*	97*	102*				21							31							44			
65	165	36	58*	63*	73	79	89	98*	103*			11	14	22					14	19	27					44	59	66		
66	168	58	59*	67	73	80	101	102	105*		7	8	13	21	25			9	11	20	31	35			43	47	56	67	72	
67	170	114	65	71	73	85	103	108	112	6	8	9	16	21	25	27	8	11	12	20	35	35	38	41	43	44	56	71	73	79
68	173	128	67	71	73	83	95	98	111	6	7	8	13	20	21	23	8	10	11	18	27	30	32	41	43	46	57	69	70	74
69	175	131	65	70	74	84	96	98	105	6	7	8	12	18	20	23	7	11	11	19	27	30	33	40	45	45	58	70	72	79
70	178	144	68	73	77	87	102	104	117	5	6	8	14	22	25	31	9	11	13	20	30	33	37	43	48	50	59	70	71	87
71	180	95	65*	70	70	84	102	109	111*		6	6	13	18	22			8	9	15	30	30			46	47	54	70	75	
72	183	72	67*	76	81	90	108	112	112*		8	8	13	23	26			8	9	20	28	31			47	48	59	73	78	
73	185	23	68*	73*	76*	88	105*	108*	113*				11							19							59			
74	188	15	69*	74*	78*	89	106*	109*	114*				12							15							54			
Women																														
58	147	14	53*	59*	63*	92	95*	99*	104*				45							44							50			
59	150	26	54*	59*	63*	78	95*	99*	105*				36							31							49			
60	152	72	54*	65	69	78	87	88	105*		25	26	35	44	45			19	21	31	42	45			28	33	41	58	60	
61	155	117	64	68	69	79	94	95	106	18	22	24	33	40	44	46	13	16	19	29	40	43	48	31	32	34	44	59	61	71
62	157	126	59	61	63	82	93	101	111	19	24	24	32	40	43	50	13	19	22	30	39	48	53	28	29	34	43	59	63	76
63	160	154	61	65	67	80	100	102	118	20	24	25	33	41	43	45	13	15	16	29	40	45	51	27	32	33	41	56	62	67
64	163	147	60	65	67	77	97	102	119	18	22	23	29	42	46	50	10	12	16	24	41	46	55	28	29	32	41	54	60	78
65	165	117	60	66	69	80	98	102	111	15	17	20	30	43	44	46	8	9	12	26	42	46	48	29	32	32	42	53	57	65
66	168	64	57*	60	63	82	98	105	109*		18	18	27	35	40			9	12	26	34	36			31	31	40	57	58	
67	170	40	58*	64*	68	80	105	104*	109*			22	32	44					14	25	46					30	40	58		
68	173	17	58*	64*	68*	79	100*	104*	110*				26							21							48			
69	175	7	59*	65*	69*	85*	101*	105*	110*																					
70	178	2	60*	65*	69*	85*	101*	105*	111*																					

*Value estimated through linear regression equation.
(From Frisancho, A. R.: Am. J. Clin. Nutr., *40*:808–819, 1984, with permission.)

TABLE A–14C-1. MIDARM MUSCLE CIRCUMFERENCE IN ADULTS (18 TO 74 YEARS), UNITED STATES*†

AGE GROUP (years)	SAMPLE SIZE	ESTIMATED POPULATION (millions)	MEAN (cm)	PERCENTILE 5th	10th	25th	50th	75th	90th	95th
Men										
18–74	5,261	61.18	28.0	23.8	24.8	26.3	27.9	29.6	31.4	32.5
18–24	773	11.78	27.4	23.5	24.4	25.8	27.2	28.9	30.8	32.3
25–34	804	13.00	28.3	24.2	25.3	26.5	28.0	30.0	31.7	32.9
35–44	664	10.68	28.8	25.0	25.6	27.1	28.7	30.3	32.1	33.0
45–54	765	11.15	28.2	24.0	24.9	26.5	28.1	29.8	31.5	32.6
55–64	598	9.07	27.8	22.8	24.4	26.2	27.9	29.6	31.0	31.8
65–74	1,657	5.50	26.8	22.5	23.7	25.3	26.9	28.5	29.9	30.7
Women										
18–74	8,410	67.84	22.2	18.4	19.0	20.2	21.8	23.6	25.8	27.4
18–24	1,523	12.89	20.9	17.7	18.5	19.4	20.6	22.1	23.6	24.9
25–34	1,896	13.93	21.7	18.3	18.9	20.0	21.4	22.9	24.9	26.6
35–44	1,664	11.59	22.5	18.5	19.2	20.6	22.0	24.0	26.1	27.4
45–54	836	12.16	22.7	18.8	19.5	20.7	22.2	24.3	26.6	27.8
55–64	669	9.98	22.8	18.6	19.5	20.8	22.6	24.4	26.3	28.1
65–74	1,822	7.28	22.8	18.6	19.5	20.8	22.5	24.4	26.5	28.1

*Measurements made in the right arm.
†See Tables A–14b-1 through A–14b-6 for data compiled by Frisancho (Am. J. Clin. Nutri., *40*:808–819, 1984) from NHANES I and II.
(From Bishop. C. W., Bowen, P.E., Ritchey, S.J.: Am. J. Clin. Nutr., *34*:2530–2539, 1981 [NHANES 1].)

TABLE A–14C-2. MIDARM MUSCLE AREA IN ADULTS (18 TO 74 YEARS), UNITED STATES*†

AGE GROUP (years)	SAMPLE SIZE	ESTIMATED POPULATION (millions)	MEAN (cm)	PERCENTILE 5th	10th	25th	50th	75th	90th	95th
Men										
18–74	5,261	61.18	62.4	45.1	49.0	55.1	62.0	69.8	78.5	84.1
18–24	773	11.78	59.8	44.0	47.4	53.0	58.9	66.5	75.5	83.1
25–34	804	13.00	63.8	46.6	51.0	55.9	62.4	71.7	80.0	86.2
35–44	664	10.68	66.0	49.8	52.2	58.5	65.6	73.1	82.0	86.7
45–54	765	11.15	63.3	45.9	49.4	55.9	62.9	70.7	79.0	84.6
55–64	598	9.07	61.5	41.4	47.4	54.7	62.0	69.8	76.5	80.5
65–74	1,657	5.50	57.2	40.3	44.7	51.0	57.6	64.7	71.2	75.0
Women										
18–74	8,410	67.84	39.2	27.0	28.7	32.5	37.8	44.3	53.0	59.8
18–24	1,523	12.89	34.8	24.9	27.2	30.0	33.8	38.9	44.3	49.4
25–34	1,896	13.93	37.5	26.7	28.4	31.8	36.5	41.8	49.4	56.3
35–44	1,664	11.59	40.3	27.2	29.4	33.8	38.5	45.9	54.2	59.8
45–54	836	12.16	41.0	28.1	30.3	34.1	39.2	47.0	56.3	61.5
55–64	669	9.98	41.4	27.5	30.3	34.4	40.7	47.4	55.1	62.9
65–74	1,822	7.28	41.4	27.5	30.3	34.4	40.3	47.4	55.9	62.9

*Measurements made in the right arm.
†See Tables A–14b-1 through A–14b-6 for data compiled by Frisancho (Am. J. Clin. Nutri., *40*:808–819, 1984) from NHANES I and II.
(From Bishop. C. W., Bowen, P.E., Ritchey, S.J.: Am. J. Clin. Nutr., *34*:2530–2539, 1981 [NHANES 1].)

TABLE A–14C-3. AGE CORRECTION FOR ESTIMATES OF WEIGHT, TRICEPS AND SUBSCAPULAR SKINFOLD THICKNESSES, AND BONE-FREE UPPER ARM MUSCLE AREA (AMA)

AGE GROUP: FRAME SIZE	MEDIAN AGE	WEIGHT	TRICEPS SKINFOLD	SUBSCAPULAR SKINFOLD	ARM MUSCLE AREA
Men					
25–54					
Small	39	0.074	0.016	0.080	0.030
Medium	39	0.080	0.005	0.083	0.055
Large	40	0.000	−0.024	0.049	0.026
55–74					
Small	66	−0.329	−0.036	−0.115	−0.407
Medium	67	−0.435	−0.040	−0.125	−0.521
Large	67	−0.562	−0.054	−0.185	−0.644
Women					
25–54					
Small	37	0.165	0.166	0.142	0.087
Medium	37	0.234	0.189	0.214	0.191
Large	37	0.284	0.191	0.233	0.270
55–74					
Small	67	−0.027	−0.072	−0.013	0.036
Medium	66	−0.196	−0.210	−0.221	−0.033
Large	67	−0.466	−0.370	−0.515	−0.378

(From Frisancho, A.R.: Am. J. Clin. Nutr., *40*:808–819, 1984, with permission.)

TABLE A–14D-1. PROVISIONAL PERCENTILES FOR TRICEPS SKINFOLD THICKNESS IN THE ELDERLY*†

AGE GROUP (Years)	PERCENTILE 5th	50th	95th
Men			
65	8.6	13.8	27.0
70	7.7	12.9	26.1
75	6.8	12.0	25.2
80	6.0	11.2	24.3
85	5.1	10.3	23.4
90	4.2	9.4	22.6
Women			
65	13.5	21.6	33.0
70	12.5	20.6	32.0
75	11.5	19.6	31.0
80	10.5	18.6	30.0
85	9.5	17.6	29.0
90	8.5	16.6	28.0

*Data are from 119 men and 150 women. All subjects were ambulatory, and measurements were made in the recumbent position on the left side.

†See Tables A–14b-1 and A–14b-2 for data compiled by Frisancho (Am. J. Clin. Nutr., *40*:808–819, 1984) from NHANES I and II.

(From Chumlea, W.C., Roche, A.F., Mukherjee, D.: Nutritional Assessment of the Elderly Through Anthropometry. Ohio, Wright State University School of Medicine, 1984.)

TABLE A–14D-2. PROVISIONAL PERCENTILES FOR MIDARM MUSCLE AREA (cm^2) IN THE ELDERLY*†

AGE GROUP (Years)	PERCENTILE 5th	50th	95th
Men			
65	43.2	59.4	77.1
70	41.4	57.7	75.3
75	39.6	55.9	73.5
80	37.8	54.1	71.7
85	36.0	52.3	69.9
90	34.3	50.5	68.2
Women			
65	33.5	44.5	66.4
70	33.0	44.1	65.9
75	32.6	43.6	65.5
80	32.2	43.2	65.1
85	31.8	42.8	64.7
90	31.3	42.4	64.2

*Data are from 119 men and 150 women. All subjects were ambulatory, and measurements were made in the recumbent position on the left side.

†See Tables A–14b-1 and A–14b-2 for data compiled by Frisancho (Am. J. Clin. Nutr., *40*:808–819, 1984) from NHANES I and II.

(From Chumlea, W.C., Roche, A.F., Mukherjee, D.: Nutritional Assessment of the Elderly Through Anthropometry. Ohio, Wright State University School of Medicine, 1984.)

TABLES A–15A TO C. BODY FAT ESTIMATIONS FROM SKINFOLD DATA

Various investigators have developed equations for predicting the proportions of body fat by anthropometric measures of specific regions. Durnin and Womersley used four different skinfolds (Table A–15-b). Pollock, Schmidt, and Jackson have prepared tables based on three sites, including thigh skinfolds (Tables A–13-b and A–15-c). Because some technicians have difficulty in obtaining consistent results with thigh skinfold measurements, data also are available based on other equations that do not use this skinfold. These data are included in the following sources:

Golding, L.A., Meyers, C.R., Sinning, W.E.: Y's Way to Physical Fitness: The Complete Guide to Fitness Testing and Instruction. 3rd Ed. Champaign, IL, Human Kinetics Publishers, 1989.

Pollock, M.L., Schmidt, D.H., Jackson, A.S.: Compr. Ther., *6*:12–27, 1980.

Jackson, A.S. and Pollock, M.L.: Phys. Sportsmed., *13*:76–90, 1985.

TABLE A–15A. EQUIVALENT FAT CONTENT, AS PERCENTAGE OF BODY WEIGHT, FOR A RANGE OF VALUES FOR THE SUM OF FOUR SKINFOLDS*

SKINFOLDS (mm)	MEN (AGE IN YEARS) 17–29	30–39	40–49	50+	WOMEN (AGE IN YEARS) 16–29	30–39	40–49	50+
15	4.8				10.5			
20	8.1	12.2	12.2	12.6	14.1	17.0	19.8	21.4
25	10.5	14.2	15.0	15.6	16.8	19.4	22.2	24.0
30	12.9	16.2	17.7	18.6	19.5	21.8	24.5	26.6
35	14.7	17.7	19.6	20.8	21.5	23.7	26.4	28.5
40	16.4	19.2	21.4	22.9	23.4	25.5	28.2	30.3
45	17.7	20.4	23.0	24.7	25.0	26.9	29.6	31.9
50	19.0	21.5	24.6	26.5	26.5	28.2	31.0	33.4
55	20.1	22.5	25.9	27.9	27.8	29.4	32.1	34.6
60	21.2	23.5	27.1	29.2	29.1	30.6	33.2	35.7
65	22.2	24.3	28.2	30.4	30.2	31.6	34.1	36.7
70	23.1	25.1	29.3	31.6	31.2	32.5	35.0	37.7
75	24.0	25.9	30.3	32.7	32.2	33.4	35.9	38.7
80	24.8	26.6	31.2	33.8	33.1	34.3	36.7	39.6
85	25.5	27.2	32.1	34.8	34.0	35.1	37.5	40.4
90	26.2	27.8	33.0	35.8	34.8	35.8	38.3	41.2
95	26.9	28.4	33.7	36.6	35.6	36.5	39.0	41.9
100	27.6	29.0	34.4	37.4	36.4	37.2	39.7	42.6
105	28.2	29.6	35.1	38.2	37.1	37.9	40.4	43.3
110	28.8	30.1	35.8	39.0	37.8	38.6	41.0	43.9
115	29.4	30.6	36.4	39.7	38.4	39.1	41.5	44.5
120	30.0	31.1	37.0	40.4	39.0	39.6	42.0	45.1
125	31.0	31.5	37.6	41.1	39.6	40.1	42.5	45.7
130	31.5	31.9	38.2	41.8	40.2	40.6	43.0	46.2
135	32.0	32.3	38.7	42.4	40.8	41.1	43.5	46.7
140	32.5	32.7	39.2	43.0	41.3	41.6	44.0	47.2
145	32.9	33.1	39.7	43.6	41.8	42.1	44.5	47.7
150	33.3	33.5	40.2	44.1	42.3	42.6	45.0	48.2
155	33.7	33.9	40.7	44.6	42.8	43.1	45.4	48.7
160	34.1	34.3	41.2	45.1	43.3	43.6	45.8	49.2
165	34.5	34.6	41.6	45.6	43.7	44.0	46.2	49.6
170	34.9	34.8	42.0	46.1	44.1	44.4	46.6	50.0
175	35.3					44.8	47.0	50.4
180	35.6					45.2	47.4	50.8
185	35.9					45.6	47.8	51.2
190						45.9	48.2	51.6
195						46.2	48.5	52.0
200						46.5	48.8	52.4
205							49.1	52.7
210							49.4	53.0

*Biceps, triceps, subscapular, and suprailiac of men and women of different ages.
(From Durnin, J.V.G.A., Womersley, J.: Br. J. Nutr., *32*:77–97, 1974, with permission.)

TABLE A–15B. PERCENTAGE OF BODY FAT ESTIMATION FOR WOMEN FROM AGE AND TRICEPS, SUPRAILIUM, AND THIGH SKINFOLDS*

SUM OF SKINFOLDS (mm)	AGE TO THE LAST YEAR								
	Under 22	23 to 27	28 to 32	33 to 37	38 to 42	43 to 47	48 to 52	53 to 57	Over 58
23–25	9.7	9.9	10.2	10.4	10.7	10.9	11.2	11.4	11.7
26–28	11.0	11.2	11.5	11.7	12.0	12.3	12.5	12.7	13.0
29–31	12.3	12.5	12.8	13.0	13.3	13.5	13.8	14.0	14.3
32–34	13.6	13.8	14.0	14.3	14.5	14.8	15.0	15.3	15.5
35–37	14.8	15.0	15.3	15.5	15.8	16.0	16.3	16.5	16.8
38–40	16.0	16.3	16.5	16.7	17.0	17.2	17.5	17.7	18.0
41–43	17.2	17.4	17.7	17.9	18.2	18.4	18.7	18.9	19.2
44–46	18.3	18.6	18.8	19.1	19.3	19.6	19.8	20.1	20.3
47–49	19.5	19.7	20.0	20.2	20.5	20.7	21.0	21.2	21.5
50–52	20.6	20.8	21.1	21.3	21.6	21.8	22.1	22.3	22.6
53–55	21.7	21.9	22.1	22.4	22.6	22.9	23.1	23.4	23.6
56–58	22.7	23.0	23.2	23.4	23.7	23.9	24.2	24.4	24.7
59–61	23.7	24.0	24.2	24.5	24.7	25.0	25.2	25.5	25.7
62–64	24.7	25.0	25.2	25.5	25.7	26.0	26.7	26.4	26.7
65–67	25.7	25.9	26.2	26.4	26.7	26.9	27.2	27.4	27.7
68–70	26.6	26.9	27.1	27.4	27.6	27.9	28.1	28.4	28.6
71–73	27.5	27.8	28.0	28.3	28.5	28.8	28.0	29.3	29.5
74–76	28.4	28.7	28.9	29.2	29.4	29.7	29.9	30.2	30.4
77–79	29.3	29.5	29.8	30.0	30.3	30.5	30.8	31.0	31.3
80–82	30.1	30.4	30.6	30.9	31.1	31.4	31.6	31.9	32.1
83–85	30.9	31.2	31.4	31.7	31.9	32.2	32.4	32.7	32.9
86–88	31.7	32.0	32.2	32.5	32.7	32.9	33.2	33.4	33.7
89–91	32.5	32.7	33.0	33.2	33.5	33.7	33.9	34.2	34.4
92–94	33.2	33.4	33.7	33.9	34.2	34.4	34.7	34.9	35.2
95–97	33.9	34.1	34.4	34.6	34.9	35.1	35.4	35.6	35.9
98–100	34.6	34.8	35.1	35.3	35.5	35.8	36.0	36.3	36.5
101–103	35.3	35.4	35.7	35.9	36.2	36.4	36.7	36.9	37.2
104–106	35.8	36.1	36.3	36.6	36.8	37.1	37.3	37.5	37.8
107–109	36.4	36.7	36.9	37.1	37.4	37.6	37.9	38.1	38.4
110–112	37.0	37.2	37.5	37.7	38.0	38.2	38.5	38.7	38.9
113–115	37.5	37.8	38.0	38.2	38.5	38.7	39.0	39.2	39.5
116–118	38.0	38.3	38.5	38.8	39.0	39.3	39.5	39.7	40.0
119–121	38.5	38.7	39.0	39.2	39.5	39.7	40.0	40.2	40.5
122–124	39.0	39.2	39.4	39.7	39.9	40.2	40.4	40.7	40.9
125–127	39.4	39.6	39.9	40.1	40.4	40.6	40.9	41.1	41.4
128–130	39.8	40.0	40.3	40.5	40.8	41.0	41.3	41.5	41.8

*Percentage of fat calculated by the formula of Siri: percentage of fat = $(4.95/D_b - 4.5) \times 100$, where D_b = body density.

(Reprinted with permission from Pollock, M.L., Schmidt, D.H., and Jackson, A.S.: Measurement of cardiorespiratory fitness and body composition in the clinical setting. Compr. Ther., *6*:12–27, 1980.)

TABLE A–15C. PERCENTAGE OF BODY FAT ESTIMATION FOR MEN FROM AGE AND THE SUM OF CHEST, ABDOMINAL, AND THIGH SKINFOLDS*

SUM OF SKINFOLDS (mm)	AGE TO THE LAST YEAR								
	Under 22	23 to 27	28 to 32	33 to 37	38 to 42	43 to 47	48 to 52	53 to 57	Over 58
23–25	9.7	9.9	10.2	10.4	10.7	10.9	11.2	11.4	11.7
26–28	11.0	11.2	11.5	11.7	12.0	12.3	12.5	12.7	13.0
29–31	12.3	12.5	12.8	13.0	13.3	13.5	13.8	14.0	14.3
32–34	13.6	13.8	14.0	14.3	14.5	14.8	15.0	15.3	15.5
35–37	14.8	15.0	15.3	15.5	15.8	16.0	16.3	16.5	16.8
38–40	16.0	16.3	16.5	16.7	17.0	17.2	17.5	17.7	18.0
41–43	17.2	17.4	17.7	17.9	18.2	18.4	18.7	18.9	19.2
44–46	18.3	18.6	18.8	19.1	19.3	19.6	19.8	20.1	20.3
47–49	19.5	19.7	20.0	20.2	20.5	20.7	21.0	21.2	21.5
50–52	20.6	20.8	21.1	21.3	21.6	21.8	22.1	22.3	22.6
53–55	21.7	21.9	22.1	22.4	22.6	22.9	23.1	23.4	23.6
56–58	22.7	23.0	23.2	23.4	23.7	23.9	24.2	24.4	24.7
59–61	23.7	24.0	24.2	24.5	24.7	25.0	25.2	25.5	25.7
62–64	24.7	25.0	25.2	25.5	25.7	26.0	26.7	26.4	26.7
65–67	25.7	25.9	26.2	26.4	26.7	26.9	27.2	27.4	27.7
68–70	26.6	26.9	27.1	27.4	27.6	27.9	28.1	28.4	28.6
71–73	27.5	27.8	28.0	28.3	28.5	28.8	29.0	29.3	29.5
74–76	28.4	28.7	28.9	29.2	29.4	29.7	29.9	30.2	30.4
77–79	29.3	29.5	29.8	30.0	30.3	30.5	30.8	31.0	31.3
80–82	30.1	30.4	30.6	30.9	31.1	31.4	31.6	31.9	32.1
83–85	30.9	31.2	31.4	31.7	31.9	32.2	32.4	32.7	32.9
86–88	31.7	32.0	32.2	32.5	32.7	32.9	33.2	33.4	33.7
89–91	32.5	32.7	33.0	33.2	33.5	33.7	33.9	34.2	34.4
92–94	33.2	33.4	33.7	33.9	34.2	34.4	34.7	34.9	35.2
95–97	33.9	34.1	34.4	34.6	34.9	35.1	35.4	35.6	35.9
98–100	34.6	34.8	35.1	35.3	35.5	35.8	36.0	36.3	36.5
101–103	35.3	35.4	35.7	35.9	36.2	36.4	36.7	36.9	37.2
104–106	35.8	36.1	36.3	36.6	36.8	37.1	37.3	37.5	37.8
107–109	36.4	36.7	36.9	37.1	37.4	37.6	37.9	38.1	38.4
110–112	37.0	37.2	37.5	37.7	38.0	38.2	38.5	38.7	38.9
113–115	37.5	37.8	38.0	38.2	38.5	38.7	39.0	39.2	39.5
116–118	38.0	38.3	38.5	38.8	39.0	39.3	39.5	39.7	40.0
119–121	38.5	38.7	39.0	39.2	39.5	39.7	40.0	40.2	40.5
122–124	39.0	39.2	39.4	39.7	39.9	40.2	40.4	40.7	40.9
125–127	39.4	39.6	39.9	40.1	40.4	40.6	40.9	41.1	41.4
128–130	39.8	40.0	40.3	40.5	40.8	41.0	41.3	41.5	41.8

*Percentage of fat calculated by the formula of Siri: percentage of fat = $(4.95/D_b - 4.5) \times 100$, where D_b = body density.

(Reprinted with permission from Pollock, M.L., Schmidt, D.H., and Jackson, A.S.: Measurement of cardiorespiratory fitness and body composition in the clinical setting. Compr. Ther., *6*:12–27, 1980.)

TABLE A–16A. DIETARY RECOMMENDATIONS IN INDUSTRIALIZED AND DEVELOPING COUNTRIES, 1977 TO 1989*

Country/region or Source of Recommendation	Target Group(s)	Maintain Appropriate Body Weight, Exercise	Limit or Reduce Total Fat (% Energy)	Reduce Saturated Fatty Acids (% Energy)
Australia 1983	GP	Yes	Yes	NC
1987, targets for 1995	GP	Reduce obesity prevalence to 30%	35%	NS
1987, targets for 2000	GP	To 25%	33%	NS
Canada 1982	GP	Yes	35%	Yes
Czechoslovakia 1988	GP	Yes, reduce by 10–15%	Yes, reduce by 15 g/day	Yes
France 1981	GP	Yes	30–35%	Yes
Germany, Federal Republic of, 1985	GP	Yes	Yes	NS
Hungary 1988	GP	Yes	Avoid too much	Use vegetable oil
India 1988	HR (affluent people)	Yes	15–20%	NC
Ireland 1984	GP	Yes	≤35%	Yes
Japan 1985	GP	Yes	20–25%	Yes
Latin America 1988	GP	Yes	20–25%	≤8
Netherlands 1983–1984	GP	Yes	30–35%	Yes
1986	GP	Yes	30–35%	Yes
New Zealand 1982	GP HR	Yes	Yes	Yes
Norway 1981–1982	GP	NC	<35%	Yes
Poland 1988	GP	Yes	≈30%	Yes
Sweden 1981	GP	Yes	25–35%	Yes
1985	GP	Yes	Reduce by 5% energy by 1990; to ≈30% by 2000	NS
United Kingdom 1983	GP	Yes	30%	10
United States of America 1977	GP	Yes	27–33%	Yes
1979	GP	Yes	Yes	Yes
1985	GP	Yes	Yes	Yes
1988	GP HR	Yes	Yes	Yes
1989	GP	Balance energy intake and expenditure	≤30%	<10% for individuals, 7–8% population mean
WHO 1988				
Intermediate goals	GP	BMI	35%	15%
Ultimate goals		20–25	20–30%	10–15%

*BMI = Body-mass index; GP = General population; HR = High-risk groups; NC = No comment; NS = Not specified; P/S = Ratio of polyunsaturated to saturated fatty acids; RDA = Recommended dietary allowance.

(From Diet, Nutrition and the Prevention of Chronic Diseases. Report of a WHO Study Group. Technical Report Series No. 797. Geneva, WHO, 1990, pp. 180–181.)

TABLE A–16A. CONTINUED.

Increase Polyunsaturated Fatty Acids (% Energy)	Limit Cholesterol (mg/day)	Limit Free Sugars (% Energy)	Increase Complex Carbohydrates (% Energy for Total Carbohydrates)
NC	NC	Yes	Yes
NS	NS	<14%	Indirectly
NS	NS	<12%	Indirectly
Yes	No	Yes	Yes
No	NS	Yes	Yes, more plant foods, vegetables, cereals, legumes
NS	NS	Yes	50–55%
NS	NS	Avoid excess	Yes; fresh fruits and vegetables, whole-grain cereals
NS	NS	Yes	Yes, fresh vegetables, salads, whole-grains
Balance (*n*-3)/(*n*-6) ratio	NC	Yes	Yes; avoid refined and polished grains
NC	NC	Moderation; ≤7 g/day for weight reduction	Yes
Use vegetables and fish oils	NC	NC	NC
P/S ≈1.0	<100 mg/1000 $kcal_{th}$ in children, up to 300 mg/day	Yes	Yes
Maximum 10%	Yes	Yes	NS
P/S = 1.0	<30 mg/MJ	Mono- and disaccharides 15–25%	45–55%
NS	NS	Yes	Yes
P/S = 0.5	NS	<10%	Yes; 50–60%
NS	Yes, <300 mg	≤10%	Yes
P/S = 0.5	Yes	<10%	Yes; 50–60%
P/S = >0.5	NS	Decrease by 3% energy by 1990	Yes; increase starch to 45–50% energy by 2000
NS	No	To 20 kg/year	Through whole grains, vegetables, cereals, fruits
Yes	250–350	Yes	Yes
NS	Yes	Yes	Yes
No	Yes	Yes	Adequate starch and fiber
No	Yes	Yes	Yes
Up to 10 for individuals and ≈7 population mean	<300	Yes	≥55%; ≥5 servings/day vegetables and fruits; ≥6 daily servings cereals, breads, and legumes
P/S ≥0.5	<100 mg/1000 $kcal_{th}$	10%	>40%
P/S = 1.0			45–55%

TABLE A–16A. CONTINUED.

Increase Dietary Fiber (g/day)	Restrict Sodium Chloride (g/day)	Moderate Alcohol Intake (% energy)	Other Recommendations
Yes	Yes	Yes	Promote breast-feeding; variety
25	130 mmol/day	<5%	Promote water fluoridation, increase prevalence of breast-feeding
30	100 mmol/day	<5%	
Yes	Yes	Yes	Exercise
Yes	Yes	Yes	Increase vitamin C intake; more plant foods; nutrition education; variety
Yes	Yes	<10%	Water fluoridation
Yes	Yes	Yes	Variety; small, frequent meals, proper cooking; sufficient protein
Yes	Yes	Yes	Variety; focus on cooking methods; consume milk and cheese as skimmed-milk products; 4 or 5 even meals daily; food labelling
Include grains, leafy vegetables, and whole grains	Yes	NC	Breast-feeding; water fluoridation upper limit 1 mg/L; different recommendation for general, poorer population
To 20–35	<9	<5%	Reduce protein to 1 g/kg of body weight daily; more vegetable protein
NC	<10	NC	Varied diet (at least 30 different foods daily); home cooking; pleasant eating environment
>8 g/1000 $kcal_{th}$	≤5; in profuse sweating, up to 10	NC	Protein 10–12% energy; variety; dietary interactions; vitamin C with iron-containing foods; calcium intake
NC	NC	Yes	Variety
3 g/MJ	Yes	<9 g/day	Variety
Yes	Yes	Yes	Variety; less animal protein; water fluoridation
Yes	NC	NC	Maintain adequate nutrient intake
Yes	?	?	?
>30	≈7–8	Yes	Varied diet, exercise, regular meals
Increase by 7–8 g/day by 1990 and to 30–35 g by 2000	Reduce by 1–2 g/day by 1990 to 7–8 g by 2000	Yes	Year 1990 and year 2000 goals
To 30	Decrease by 3 g/day	<4%	Long-term proposals: food labeling; nutrition education; greater proportion of vegetable protein
Yes	<8	Yes	Limit additives and processed foods
NS	Yes	Yes	More fish, poultry, legumes; less red meat
Yes	Yes	Yes	Variety in diet; consider high-risk groups
Yes	Yes	Yes	Fluoridation of water; adolescent girls and women increase intake of calcium-rich foods; children, adolescents, and women of child-bearing age increase intake of iron-rich foods
Indirectly through vegetables, fruits, and cereals	≤6 with a goal of 4.5	<30 g of ethanol or <2 drinks/day	Population and individual goals; avoid dietary supplements in excess of RDAs; drink fluoridated water; limit protein intake to less than twice the RDA; comments on future goals
>30	7–8	Yes	Increase nutrient density of food; water fluoridation; iodine prophylaxis
	5		

TABLE A–16B. DIETARY RECOMMENDATIONS TO REDUCE CORONARY HEART DISEASE RISK IN INDUSTRIALIZED COUNTRIES*

COUNTRY/REGION OR SOURCE OF RECOMMENDATION	TARGET GROUP(S)	BODY WEIGHT/EXERCISE	TOTAL FAT (% ENERGY)
Australia			
1979	HR	Avoid obesity	Reduce to 30–35
Canada			
1977	GP	Maintain appropriate body weight	Reduce to 35
1988	GP HR	Adjust energy intake and expenditure	<30
Europe			
1987	GP HR	Control obesity; increase exercise	≤30
Finland			
1987	GP HR	Avoid excess weight; exercise	<30
Finland, Norway, Sweden			
1968	GP	Reduce energy intake to avoid obesity; exercise	Reduce to 25–35
Germany, Federal Republic of			
1975	GP	NC	Reduce
Japan			
1983	GP	NC	20–25
Netherlands			
1973	GP	Maintain appropriate body weight	33
New Zealand			
1976	GP HR	Maintain appropriate body weight	35
United Kingdom			
1982	GP	Avoid obesity; increase exercise	30
1984	GP	Avoid obesity; exercise	Reduce to 35
United States of America			
1984	GP	Control obesity	<30
1985	GP HR	Maintain appropriate body weight	<30
1988	GP	Maintain appropriate body weight	<30
WHO			
1982	GP	Avoid obesity	Reduce to 20–30
1988	HR	BMI 20–25, regular exercise	20–30

*BMI = Body-mass index; GP = General population; HR = High-risk groups; NC = No comment; NS = Not specified; P:S = Ratio of polyunsaturated to saturated fatty acids.

(From Diet, Nutrition and the Prevention of Chronic Diseases. Report of a WHO Study Group. Technical Report Series No. 797. Geneva, WHO, 1990, pp. 182–183. With permission.)

TABLE A–16B. CONTINUED.

SATURATED FAT (% ENERGY)	POLYUNSATURATED FAT (% ENERGY)	CHOLESTEROL (MG/DAY)	COMPLEX CARBOHYDRATES AND FIBER
P:S = 1.0	P:S = 1.0	Restrict	Eat enough
10	10	NC	Increase
<10	<10	Restrict through less meats and egg yolks; for HR <300	Increase
<10	Increase oleic and linoleic acids	<300	Increase, especially vegetables, fruits, cereals, legumes
<10	P:S >0.5	Reduce	NC
Reduce	Increase	NC	Increase vegetables, fruits, potatoes
Reduce	Increase	Reduce	NC
NC	Cook with vegetable oil	NC	Increase
Restrict	10–13	250–300	Increase to make up energy need
Reduce especially for HR	HR should substitute for saturated fatty acids	Reduce	NC
<10	NC	NC	Increase
Reduce to 15	P/S≈0.45	NS	Increase breads, cereals, vegetables, fruits
8	<10	<250	Increase to make up energy loss
10	Up to 10	250–300	Endorsed earlier recommendations
<10	Up to 10	<300	Increase, ≥50% energy from total carbohydrates
<10	Up to 10	<300	Increase
10	Up to 10 P/S >1.0	<100 mg/1000 $kcal_{th}$	45–55% energy >30 g fiber/day

TABLE A–16B. CONTINUED.

FREE SUGARS	SODIUM CHLORIDE (G/DAY)	ALCOHOL INTAKE	OTHER RECOMMENDATIONS
Use less	Restrict	Moderation	Focus on HR groups; food labelling; recommendations safe for GP
NC	Restrict	NC	Variety of foods
NC	Limit	Limit	Focus on HR groups; limit protein to 10–15 % energy
Reduce	Moderation	Moderation, <25–30 g/day	Nutrition education; collaboration among government and other groups; food labelling
NC	Reduce; for HR <5	Moderation	Avoid trace element deficiencies; food labelling; focus on HR groups
Decrease	NC	NC	10–12% of energy from protein; 30–50% of animal origin
NC	NC	NC	NC
Reduce	Limit to <10	Avoid too much	Variety; eat enough protein, half from vegetables and half from animal sources; eat enough potassium, especially from green vegetables; eat lean meat and fish and fewer sweets
Use little	NC	NC	NC
Restrict to reduce weight	NC	Restrict to reduce weight	NC
NC	NC	NC	Special attention to children
Do not increase	Decrease	Avoid excess; <90 ml/day men; <65 ml/day women	Special recommendations for governments, professionals, industry
NC	5	NC	NC
	NC	NC	Guidelines for health professionals, industry, and public
NS	<3 (as sodium)	30–50 g ethanol/day	Protein to make up remainder of energy; wide variety of foods
NC	<5	Drink less	Emphasis on plant foods, fish, poultry, lean meats, low-fat dairy products, and fewer whole eggs
10% energy	<5	Limit	Increase nutrient density; water fluoridation 0.7–1.2 mg/L; iodine prophylaxis; intermediate and ultimate goals

TABLE A–16C. DIETARY RECOMMENDATIONS TO REDUCE CANCER RISK IN INDUSTRIALIZED COUNTRIES*

COUNTRY/ REGION	MAINTAIN APPROPRIATE BODY WEIGHT, EXERCISE	LIMIT OR REDUCE TOTAL FAT (% ENERGY)	MODIFY RATIO OF DIETARY FATS	PROMOTE FRUIT AND VEGETABLE INTAKE	INCREASE COMPLEX CARBOHYDRATE/ FIBER INTAKE
Canada					
1985	Yes	Reduce	Decrease saturated fatty acids and cholesterol	Yes	More fiber-containing foods
Europe					
1986	Yes	To ≈30	NC	Yes	Yes
Japan					
1983	NC	Avoid excess	NC	Especially green/ yellow vegetables, oranges, carotene, and fungi	Unrefined cereal, seafood, fiber-rich legumes
United States of America					
1982	NC	To ≈30	NC	Especially citrus fruits, green and yellow and cruciferous vegetables	Whole-grain products, vegetables, and fruits
1984	Yes	To ≈30	NC	Especially vitamin A- and C-rich foods and cruciferous vegetables	High-fiber foods, whole-grain cereals
1987	Yes	To ≈30	NC	Vitamin A-rich, green and yellow vegetables, citrus fruits	Whole-grain products, 20–30 g fiber/day

*NC = No comment; NS = Not specified.

(From Diet, Nutrition and the Prevention of Chronic Diseases. Report of a WHO Study Group. Technical Report Series No. 797. Geneva, World Health Organization, 1990, pp. 184–185.)

TABLE A–16C. CONTINUED

RESTRICT SODIUM CHLORIDE	FOOD PREPARATION METHODS	ALCOHOL INTAKE	OTHER RECOMMENDATIONS
NS	Minimize cured, pickled, and smoked foods	Two or fewer drinks per day, if any	NC
To <5 g/day	As above; avoid frying and high-temperature cooking	Drink less, if at all	Varied diet; no food supplements; recommendations to government, scientists, and industry
Yes	Avoid hot drinks and burned foods	Drink less, if at all	Varied diet; chew food well
Minimize cured and pickled foods	Minimize cured, pickled, and smoked foods	Drink less, if at all	Avoid food supplements; monitor and test mutagens and carcinogens; recommendations to government, scientists, and industry
NS	As above	As above	NC
NS	As above, avoid frying and high-temperature cooking	As above	Balanced diet; read labels

TABLE A–16D. NATIONAL NUTRITION OBJECTIVES FOR THE YEAR 2000

A. *Health Status Objectives*

1. Reduce deaths from coronary heart disease to no more than 100 per 100,000 persons (age-adjusted baseline: 135 per 100,000 in 1987).

2. Reverse the rise in deaths from cancer to achieve a rate of no more than 130 per 100,000 persons (age-adjusted baseline: 133 per 100,000 in 1987).

3. Reduce the overweight population to no more than 20% among adults aged 20 years and older and no more than 15% among adolescents aged 12 through 19 years (baseline: 26% for adults aged 20 through 74 years in 1976 to 1980, 24% for men and 27% for women; 15% for adolescents aged 12 through 19 years in 1976 to 1980).

4. Reduce growth retardation among low-income children aged 5 years and younger to less than 10% (baseline: up to 16% among low-income children in 1988, depending on age and race/ethnicity).

B. *Risk Reduction Objectives*

5. Reduce dietary fat intake to an average of 30% of calories or less and reduce average saturated fat intake to less than 10% of calories among persons aged 2 years and older (baseline: 36% of calories from total fat and 13% from saturated fat for persons aged 20 through 74 years in 1976 to 1980; 36% and 13% for women aged 19 through 50 years in 1985).

6. Increase complex carbohydrates and fiber-containing foods in the diets of adults to 5 or more daily servings for vegetables (including legumes) and fruits, and to 6 or more daily servings for grain products (baseline: 2.5 servings of vegetables and fruits and 3 servings of grain products for women aged 19 through 50 years in 1985).

7. Increase to at least 50% the proportion of overweight persons aged 12 years and older who have adopted sound dietary practices combined with regular physical activity to attain an appropriate body weight (baseline: 30% of overweight women and 25% of overweight men for people aged 18 years and older in 1985).

8. Increase calcium intake so that at least 50% of youth aged 12 through 24 years and at least 50% of pregnant and lactating women are consuming 3 or more servings daily of foods rich in calcium, and at least 50% of adults aged 25 years and older are consuming 2 or more servings daily (baseline: 7% of women and 14% of men aged 19 through 24 years and 24% of pregnant and lactating women consumed 3 or more servings daily, and 15% of women and 23% of men aged 25 through 50 years consumed 2 or more servings daily in 1985 to 1986).

9. Decrease salt and sodium intake so that at least 65% of those who prepare home-cooked meals do so without adding salt, at least 80% of persons avoid using salt at the table, and at least 40% of adults regularly purchase foods modified or lower in sodium (baseline: 54% of women aged 19 through 50 years who prepared most of the meals did not use salt in food preparation, and 68% of women aged 19 through 50 years did not use salt at the table in 1985; 20% of all persons aged 18 years and older regularly purchased foods with reduced salt and sodium content in 1988).

10. Reduce iron deficiency to less than 3% among children aged 1 through 4 years and among women of childbearing age (baseline: 9% for children aged 1 through 2 years, 4% for children aged 3 through 4 years, and 5% for women aged 20 through 44 years in 1976 to 1980).

11. Increase to at least 75% the proportion of mothers who breast-feed their babies in the early postpartum period and to at least 50% the proportion who continue to breast-feed until their babies are 5 to 6 months old (baseline: 54% at discharge from birth site and 21% at 5 to 6 months in 1988).

12. Increase to at least 75% the proportion of parents and caregivers who use feeding practices that prevent baby-bottle tooth decay.

13. Increase to at least 85% the proportion of persons aged 18 years and older who use food labels to make nutritious food selections (baseline: 74% used labels to make food selections in 1988).

C. *Service and Protection Objectives*

14. Achieve useful and informative nutrition labeling for virtually all processed foods and for at least 40% of fresh meats, poultry, fish, fruits, vegetables, baked foods, and ready-to-eat carry-out foods (baseline: 60% of processed foods regulated by the Food and Drug Administration had nutrition labeling in 1988; baseline data on fresh and carry-out foods are unavailable).

15. Increase the available processed food products that are reduced in fat and saturated fat to at least 5000 brand items (baseline: 2500 brand items reduced in fat in 1986).

16. Increase to at least 90% the proportion of restaurants and institutional service operations than offer identifiable low-fat, low-calorie food choices, consistent with the nutrition principles in the *Dietary Guidelines for Americans.*

17. Increase to at least 90% the proportion of school lunch and breakfast services and child-care food services that offer menus consistent with the nutrition principles in the *Dietary Guidelines for Americans.*

18. Increase to at least 80% the receipt of home food services by people aged 65 years and older who cannot prepare their own meals or are otherwise in need of home-delivered meals.

19. Increase to at least 75% the proportion of schools in the United States that provide nutrition education from preschool through 12th grade, preferably as part of quality school health education.

20. Increase to at least 50% the proportion of worksites with 50 or more employees that offer nutrition education and/or weight management programs for employees (baseline: 17% offered nutrition education activities and 15% offered weight-control activities in 1985).

21. Increase to at least 75% the proportion of primary care providers who provide nutrition assessment and counseling and/or referral to qualified nutritionists or dietitians (baseline: physicians provided diet counseling for an estimated 40 to 50% of patients in 1988).

(From Nutrition in Healthy People 2000. *In* National Health Promotion and Disease Prevention Objectives. Washington, D.C., U.S. Government Printing Office, 1991.)

TABLE A–16E. RECOMMENDED DIET MODIFICATIONS TO LOWER BLOOD CHOLESTEROL

For Table A–16e, National Cholesterol Education Program (NCEP) Recommendations and Diets in the United States, see Table A–28, Recommendations for Phased Dietary Modification in the Prevention and Therapy of Hyperlipidemia (NCEP Step-One and Step-Two Diets).

TABLE A–17. BEVERAGES AND ALCOHOLIC DRINKS: CALORIES AND SELECTED ELECTROLYTES (PER 100 ML)*

BEVERAGE	CALORIES	SODIUM (mg)	SODIUM (mEq)	POTASSIUM (mg)	POTASSIUM (mEq)	PHOSPHORUS (mg)
Cola (avg.)	48.1–55.0†	0.8–4.7 (mg)†		0–4.4 (mg)†		18.1–25†
Diet cola (avg.)	0.1–0.5†	0.8–13.0 (mg)†		0–33.2 (mg)†		8.5–17.6†
Patio grape/orange	52	11.2	0.5	4.1	0.1	—
Mountain Dew	49	8.7	0.4	2.7	0.1	—
Teem	41	8.6	0.4	—	—	—
Root beer	45	1	0.1	3.9	0.1	—
Club soda	0	21.9	1.0	—	—	0
Sprite	48	15.4	0.7	0.4	—	—
Fanta (avg.)	53	6.4	0.3	0.6	—	—
Fresca	1	12.1	0.5	—	—	—
Fanta ginger ale	42	9.4	0.4	—	—	—
Slice	45	3	0.1	27.6	0.7	—
Apricot nectar	56	3	0.1	114	2.9	9
Apple juice	47	3	0.1	119	3	7
Cranberry juice	58	4	0.2	24	0.6	1
Grape juice, canned	61	3	0.1	132	3.4	11
Grapefruit juice, unsweetened	38	trace	—	153	3.9	11
Orange juice, unsweetened or fresh	45	1	0.1	200	5.1	17
Pear nectar	60	4	0.2	13	0.3	3
Peach nectar	54	7	0.3	40	1	6
Pineapple juice, unsweetened	56	trace	—	134	3.4	0
Tomato juice	20	200.7	8.7	227	5.8	16.5
Fruit-flavored beverage	45	—	—	—	—	—
Beer, regular	41	5.3	0.2	25	0.6	12.4
Beer, light	28	2.8	0.1	18.1	0.5	12.1
Gin, rum, vodka, whiskey (86 proof)	250	trace	—	3.6	0.1	—
Table wine, 12.2% alcohol/vol.	86	3.5	0.1	93.1	2.4	10.3
Dessert wine, 18.5% alcohol/vol.	137	3.3	0.1	76.7	2	—

Alcoholic beverages are customarily served in special glassware, the size of which tends to standardize the alcoholic content:

1 cordial glass	= 20 ml	1 burgundy glass	= 120 ml
1 brandy glass	= 30 ml	1 champagne glass	= 150 ml
1 jigger	= 45 ml	1 tumbler	= 240–360 ml
1 sherry glass	= 60 ml	1 mixing glass	= 360 ml
1 cocktail glass	= 90 ml		

*Brand name data supplied by the commercial producer of the product. Other data obtained from Composition of Foods, Fruits, and Fruit Juices: Raw, Processed, Prepared. Agriculture Handbook No. 8–9. Consumer Nutrition Center, Washington, U.S. Department of Agriculture, 1982.

†Range.

TABLE A–18A. DIETARY FIBER CONTENT OF SELECTED FOODS*,† (g/100 g EDIBLE PORTION)

FOOD ITEM	MOISTURE	TOTAL DIETARY FIBER (AOAC)‡
Breads, Crackers, and Cakes		
Bagels, plain	31.6	2.1
Biscuits, made from refrigerated dough, baked	28.7	1.5
Bread		
Bran	37.7	8.5
Cornbread mix, baked	34.4	2.4
Cracked-wheat	35.9	5.3
French	33.9	2.7
Hollywood-type, light	37.8	4.8
Italian	34.1	3.1
Mixed-grain	38.2	7.1
Oatmeal	36.7	3.9
Pita		
White	32.1	1.6
Whole-wheat	30.6	7.5
Pumpernickel	38.3	5.9
Reduced-calorie, high-fiber		
Wheat	43.7	11.3
White	41.8	9.3
Rye	37.0	6.2
Wheat	37.0	4.3
White	37.1	2.3
Whole-wheat	38.3	6.9
Bread crumbs, plain or seasoned	5.7	4.2
Bread stuffing, flavored, from dry mix	65.1	2.9
Cake mix		
Chocolate, prepared	33.3	2.2
Yellow, prepared	40.0	0.8
Cakes		
Boston cream pie	47.6	1.3
Coffeecake		
Crumb topping	22.3	3.3
Fruit	31.7	2.5
Fruitcake, commercial	22.0	3.5
Gingerbread, from dry mix	38.5	3.2
Cheesecake		
Commercial	44.6	2.1
From no-bake mix	44.4	1.9
Cookies		
Brownies	12.6	2.4
Brownies with nuts	12.6	2.6
Butter	4.7	2.4
Chocolate chip	4.0	2.7
Chocolate sandwich	2.2	3.0
Fig bar	16.7	4.6
Fortune	8.0	1.6
Oatmeal	5.7	3.1
Oatmeal, soft-type	—	2.7
Peanut butter	6.7	1.8
Shortbread with pecans	3.3	1.8
Vanilla sandwich	2.1	1.5
Crackers		
Cheese, sandwich with peanut butter filling	4.0	1.1
Crisp bread, rye	6.1	16.2
Graham		
Regular	4.1	2.7
Honey	4.1	2.7

TABLE A–18A. CONTINUED

FOOD ITEM	MOISTURE	TOTAL DIETARY FIBER (AOAC)‡
Matzoh		
Plain	6.1	3.0
Egg/onion	8.0	5.0
Whole-wheat	3.0	11.6
Melba toast		
Plain	5.6	6.5
Rye	6.7	8.0
Wheat	6.1	7.4
Rye	7.2	15.8
Saltines	—	2.7
Snack-type	4.2	2.0
Wheat	3.2	5.5
Whole-wheat	2.7	10.4
Croutons, plain or seasoned	5.6	5.0
Doughnuts		
Cake	19.7	1.7
Yeast-leavened, glazed	26.7	2.1
English muffin, whole-wheat	45.7	6.3
French toast, commercial, ready-to-eat	48.1	2.8
Ice cream cones		
Sugar, rolled-type	3.0	4.6
Wafer-type	5.3	4.1
Muffins, commercial		
Blueberry	37.3	3.6
Oat bran	35.0	7.5
Pancake, waffle mix, prepared	50.4	1.3
Pastry, Danish		
Fruit	27.6	1.9
Plain	19.3	1.2
Pies, commercial		
Apple	51.7	1.7
Cherry	46.2	0.8
Chocolate, cream	43.5	2.0
Egg custard	46.5	1.2
Fruit and coconut	—	0.9
Lemon meringue	41.7	1.2
Pecan	19.8	3.5
Pumpkin	58.1	2.7
Rolls, dinner, egg	30.4	3.8
Taco shells	6.0	8.1
Toaster pastries	8.9	1.0
Tortillas		
Corn	43.6	5.2
Flour, wheat	26.2	3.1
Waffles, commercial, frozen, ready-to-eat	45.0	2.4
Breakfast Cereals, Ready-to-Eat		
Bran		
High-fiber	2.9	35.3
Extra fiber	—	45.9
Bran flakes	2.9	18.8
Bran flakes with raisins	8.3	13.4
Corn flakes		
Frosted or sugar-sparkled	1.9	2.2
Plain	2.8	2.0
Fiber cereal with fruit	—	14.8
Granola	3.3	10.5
Oat cereal	5.0	10.6
Oat flakes, fortified	3.1	3.0
Puffed wheat, sugar-coated	1.5	1.5
Rice, crispy	2.4	1.2

TABLE A–18A. CONTINUED

FOOD ITEM	MOISTURE	TOTAL DIETARY FIBER (AOAC)‡
Wheat and malted barley		
Flakes	3.4	6.8
Nuggets	3.2	6.5
with raisins	—	6.0
Wheat flakes	4.3	9.0
Cereal Grains		
Barley	9.4	17.3
Bulgur, dry	8.0	18.3
Corn flour, whole-grain	10.9	13.4
Cornmeal		
Degermed	11.6	5.2
Whole-grain	10.3	11.0
Cornstarch	8.3	0.9
Farina, regular or instant, cooked	85.8	1.4
Hominy, canned	79.8	2.5
Millet, hulled, raw	—	8.5
Oat bran, raw	6.6	15.9
Oat flour	7.8	9.6
Oats, rolled or oatmeal, dry	8.8	10.3
Rice, brown, long-grain, cooked	73.1	1.7
Rice, white		
glutinous, raw	10.0	2.8
Long-grain		
Parboiled, cooked	—	0.5
Precooked or instant, cooked	76.4	0.8
Rye flour, medium or light	9.4	14.6
Semolina	12.7	3.9
Tapioca, pearl, dry	12.0	1.1
Wheat bran, crude	9.9	42.4
Wheat flour		
White, all-purpose	11.8	2.7
Whole-grain	10.9	12.6
Wheat germ, toasted	2.9	12.9
Wild rice, raw	7.8	5.2
Fruits and Fruit Products		
Apples, raw:		
With skin	83.9	2.2
Without skin	84.5	1.9
Apple juice, unsweetened	87.9	0.1
Applesauce, unsweetened	88.4	1.5
Apricots, dried	31.1	7.8
Apricot nectar	84.9	0.6
Bananas, raw	74.3	1.6
Blueberries, raw	84.6	2.3
Cantaloupe, raw	89.8	0.8
Figs, dried	28.4	9.3
Fruit cocktail, canned in heavy syrup, drained	—	1.5
Grapefruit, raw	90.9	0.6
Grapes, Thompson, seedless, raw	81.3	0.7
Kiwifruit, raw	83.0	3.4
Nectarines, raw	86.3	1.6
Olives		
Green	—	2.6
ripe	—	3.0
Orange, raw	86.8	2.4
Orange juice, frozen concentrate, prepared	88.1	0.2

TABLE A—18A. CONTINUED

FOOD ITEM	MOISTURE	TOTAL DIETARY FIBER (AOAC)‡
Peach		
Canned in juice, drained	—	1.0
Dried	31.8	8.2
Raw	87.7	1.6
Pears, raw	83.8	2.6
Pineapple		
Canned in heavy syrup, chunks, drained	79.0	1.1
Raw	86.5	1.2
Prune		
Dried	32.4	7.2
Stewed	—	6.6
Prune juice	81.2	1.0
Raisins	15.4	5.3
Strawberries	91.6	2.6
Watermelon	91.5	0.4
Legumes, Nuts, and Seeds		
Almonds, oil-roasted	3.3	11.2
Baked beans, canned		
Barbecue-style	—	5.8
Sweet or tomato sauce, plain	72.6	7.7
Beans, Great Northern, canned, drained	69.9	5.4
Cashews, oil-roasted	5.4	6.0
Chickpeas, canned, drained	68.2	5.8
Coconut, raw	47.0	9.0
Cowpeas (black-eyed peas), cooked, drained	70.0	9.6
Hazelnuts, oil-roasted	1.2	6.4
Lima beans, cooked, drained	69.8	7.2
Miso	47.4	5.4
Mixed nuts, oil-roasted, with peanuts	—	9.0
Peanut		
Dry-roasted	1.6	8.0
Oil-roasted	2.0	8.8
Peanut butter		
Chunky	1.1	6.6
Smooth	1.4	6.0
Pecans, dried	4.8	6.5
Pistachio nuts	3.9	10.8
Sunflower seeds, oil-roasted	2.6	6.8
Tahini	3.0	9.3
Tofu	84.6	1.2
Walnuts, dried		
Black	4.4	5.0
English	3.6	4.8
Pasta		
Noodles, Chinese, chow mein	0.7	3.9
Noodles, egg, regular, cooked	68.7	2.2
Noodles, Japanese, dry		
Somen	9.2	4.3
Udon	8.7	5.4
Spaghetti and macaroni, cooked	64.7	1.6
Spaghetti, dry		
Spinach	8.7	10.6
Whole-wheat	7.1	11.8
Snacks		
Banana chips	4.3	7.7
Corn cakes	4.6	1.9

TABLE A–18A. CONTINUED

FOOD ITEM	MOISTURE	TOTAL DIETARY FIBER (AOAC)‡
Corn-based, extruded		
Chips		
Barbecue-flavor	1.2	5.2
Plain	1.0	4.4
Puffs or twists, cheese-flavor	1.5	1.0
CORNNUTS		
Barbecue-flavor	1.6	8.4
Nacho-flavor	2.1	8.0
Plain	1.3	6.9
Crisped rice bar		
Almond	6.7	3.6
Chocolate chip	7.0	2.2
Granola bars		
Hard		
Chocolate chip	2.4	4.4
Plain	3.9	5.3
Soft		
Milk-chocolate–coated, chocolate chip	3.6	3.4
Uncoated		
Chocolate chip	5.4	4.8
Chocolate chip, graham, and marshmallow	6.0	4.0
Nut and raisin	6.1	5.6
Peanut butter	7.3	4.3
Peanut butter and chocolate chip	5.9	4.2
Plain	6.4	4.6
Raisin	6.4	4.3
Popcorn		
Air-popped	4.1	15.1
Caramel-coated		
With peanuts	3.3	3.8
Without peanuts	2.8	5.2
Cheese-flavor	2.5	9.9
Oil-popped	2.8	10.0
Potato chips		
Barbecue-flavor	1.9	4.4
Plain	1.9	4.8
Sour-cream-and-onion–flavor	1.8	5.2
Potato chips, made from dried potatoes, plain	1.4	3.6
Potato sticks	2.2	3.4
Pretzels, hard, plain	3.3	2.8
Rice cakes, brown rice		
Buckwheat	5.9	3.8
Corn	5.9	2.9
Multigrain	6.3	3.0
Plain	5.8	4.2
Rye	6.8	4.0
Tortilla chips		
Nacho-flavor	1.7	5.3
Plain	1.8	6.5
Sweets		
Baking chocolate, unsweetened, squares	1.3	15.4
Candies		
ALPINE WHITE Bar With Almonds	1.1	5.4

TABLE A–18A. CONTINUED

FOOD ITEM	MOISTURE	TOTAL DIETARY FIBER (AOAC)‡
BABY RUTH Bar	5.0	2.9
BUTTERFINGER Bar	5.6	2.7
Caramels	8.5	1.2
CHUNKY Bar	2.9	4.8
Milk chocolate	1.3	2.8
Milk chocolate, with almonds	1.5	6.2
M&M's Plain Chocolate Candies	1.4	3.1
NESTLE CRUNCH Milk Chocolate With Crisp Rice	1.7	2.6
O'HENRY	5.9	3.5
Cocoa, dry powder, unsweetened	3.0	29.8
Jams and preserves	34.5	1.2
Jellies	28.4	0.6
Pie fillings, canned		
Apple	73.4	1.0
Cherry	69.7	0.6
Vegetables and Vegetable Products		
Artichokes, raw	84.4	5.2
Beans, snap		
Canned, drained, solids	93.3	1.3
Raw	90.3	1.8
Beets, canned, drained, solids	91.0	1.7
Broccoli		
Cooked	90.2	2.6
Raw	90.7	2.8
Brussel sprouts, boiled	87.3	4.3
Cabbage, Chinese		
Cooked	95.4	1.6
Raw	94.9	1.0
Cabbage, red		
Cooked	93.6	2.0
Raw	91.6	2.0
Cabbage, white, raw	91.5	2.4
Carrots		
Canned, drained, solids	93.0	1.5
Raw	87.8	3.2
Cauliflower		
Cooked	92.5	2.2
Raw	92.3	2.4
Celery, raw	94.7	1.6
Chives	92.0	3.2
Corn, sweet		
Canned		
Brine pack, drained, solids	76.9	1.4
Cream-style	78.7	1.2
Cooked	69.6	3.7
Cucumbers		
Raw	96.0	1.0
Pared	—	0.5
Lettuce		
Butterhead or iceberg	95.7	1.0
Romaine	94.9	1.7
Mushrooms		
Boiled	91.1	2.2
Raw	91.8	1.3
Onions, raw	90.1	1.6
Parsley, raw	88.3	4.4

TABLE A–18A. CONTINUED

FOOD ITEM	MOISTURE	TOTAL DIETARY FIBER (AOAC)‡
Peas, edible, podded		
Cooked	88.9	2.8
Raw	88.9	2.6
Peas, sweet, canned, drained, solids	81.7	3.4
Peppers, sweet, raw	92.8	1.6
Pickles		
Dill	93.8	1.2
Sweet	68.9	1.1
Potatoes		
Baked		
Flesh	75.4	1.5
Skin	47.3	4.0
Boiled	77.0	1.5
French-fried, home-prepared from frozen	52.9	4.2
Hashed brown	56.1	2.0
Spinach		
Boiled	91.2	2.2
Raw	91.6	2.6
Squash		
Summer, cooked	93.7	1.4
Winter, cooked	89.0	2.8
Sweet potatoes		
Canned, drained, solids	72.5	1.8
Cooked	72.8	3.0
Tomato, raw	94.0	1.3
Tomato products		
Catsup	—	1.6
Paste	74.1	4.3
Puree	87.3	2.3
Sauce	89.1	1.5
Turnip greens		
Boiled	93.2	3.1
Raw	91.1	2.4
Turnips, boiled	93.6	2.0
Vegetables, mixed, frozen, cooked	83.2	3.8
Water chestnuts, canned, drained, solids	87.9	2.2
Watercress	95.1	2.3

*Modified from the Provisional Table on the Dietary Fiber Content of Selected Foods, HNIS/PT-106, 1988 and from updated Appendix Tables 8–19, Aug. 1991, and 8–20, Oct. 1989.

†Appreciation is expressed to the U.S. Department of Agriculture, Human Nutrition Information Service, Nutrition Monitoring Division for assistance in obtaining these data.

‡The total dietary fiber in foods is measured by the enzymatic-gravimetric method (the Association of Official Analytical Chemists (AOAC) official method of analysis). Duplicate samples of dried foods, with fat extracted if containing >10% fat, are gelatinized with Termamyl (heat-stable α-amylase) and then enzymatically digested with protease and amyloglucosidase to remove protein and starch. (When analyzing mixed diets, fat is always extracted prior to determining total dietary fiber.) Four volumes of ethyl alcohol (EtOH) are added to precipitated soluble dietary fiber. Total residue is filtered and then washed with 78% EtOH, 95% EtOH, and acetone. After drying, residue is weighed. One duplicate is analyzed for protein; the other is incinerated at 525° and ash is determined.

Total dietary fiber = weight residue − weight (protein + ash)

TABLE A–18B. NONSTARCH POLYSACCHARIDE CONTENT OF SELECTED FOODS

FOOD ITEM	TOTAL g/100g FRESH WEIGHT
Vegetables and Legumes	
Beans, baked, canned	3.5
Beans, French, cooked	3.1
Beans, red kidney, cooked	6.7
Cabbage, red, cooked	3.3
Carrots, raw	2.4
Lentils, red, cooked	1.9
Onion, cooked	1.8
Peas, garden, canned	4.0
Potato, boiled, fresh	1.1
Potato Crisps	4.9
Sprouts, Brussel, boiled	4.8
Fruits and Nuts	
Apple, Golden Delicious with skin	1.7
Apricots, fresh	2.3
Avocado, fresh	4.4
Canteloupe	0.6
Coconut, fresh	7.3
Figs, dried	7.5
Kiwi fruit, no skin	1.7
Peanuts, roasted	6.2
Raisins, dried	2.1
Cereal Products	
Bran flakes	11.3
Corn flakes	0.9
Oatmeal, coarse	7.0
Popcorn	9.8
Pumpernickel bread	7.5
Shredded wheat	9.8
Spaghetti, white, cooked	1.7
Spaghetti, whole-wheat, cooked	3.5
White bread	1.6
Wholemeal bread (average)	5.0

(From references 23 and 24 in Chapter 4. Courtesy of Dr. Barbara Schneeman.)

TABLE A–19A. AVERAGE VALUES FOR TRIGLYCERIDES, FATTY ACIDS (FA), AND CHOLESTEROL IN SELECTED FOODS AND OILS (INCLUDING OMEGA-3 FA) (PER 100 g EDIBLE PORTION)

	FAT (g)	SFA (g)	MFA (g)	PFA (g)	M18:1 (g)	P18:2 (g)	P18:3 (g)	P:S	CHOL (mg)	S14:0 (g)	S16:0 (g)	S18:0 (g)	P20:5 (g)	P22:5 (g)	P22:6 (g)
Meats															
Liver calf	6.90	2.56	1.49	1.09	1.28	.61	0.08	0.43	561.00	0.00	1.40	1.16	0.00	0.00	0.00
Liver pork	4.40	1.41	0.63	1.05	0.56	0.42	0.04	0.74	355.00	0.02	0.53	0.84	0.00	0.04	0.03
Kidney, beef	3.44	1.09	0.74	0.74	0.61	0.40	0.01	0.68	387.00	0.06	0.47	0.51	0.00	0.00	0.00
Kidney pork	4.70	1.51	1.55	0.38	1.40	0.25	0.01	0.25	480.00	0.05	0.85	0.60	0.00	0.00	0.00
Brains, beef	12.53	2.92	2.50	1.44	2.00	0.03	0.00	0.49	2054.00	0.06	1.51	1.27	0.00	0.30	0.67
Brains, pork	9.51	2.15	1.72	1.47	1.10	0.09	0.12	0.68	2552.00	0.04	1.06	1.03	0.00	0.22	0.46
Beef, 5% fat, cooked	4.90	1.68	1.90	0.22	1.75	0.17	0.02	0.13	84.00	0.11	1.02	0.54	0.00	0.00	0.00
Beef, 26% fat, cooked	25.98	10.52	11.16	0.90	10.04	0.61	0.27	0.09	84.00	0.85	6.45	3.07	0.00	0.00	0.00
Lamb, 9% fat, cooked	9.17	3.28	4.02	0.60	3.72	0.49	0.05	0.18	92.00	0.29	1.76	1.13	0.00	0.00	0.00
Lamb, 36% fat, cooked	36.00	16.80	14.68	2.10	13.80	1.36	0.68	0.13	98.00	1.45	8.28	6.18	0.00	0.00	0.00
Veal, 6% fat, cooked	5.81	2.31	2.16	0.43	1.87	0.32	0.04	0.19	109.00	0.21	1.23	0.77	0.00	0.00	0.00
Veal, 25% fat, cooked	21.20	9.21	9.24	1.30	7.82	0.87	0.33	0.14	101.00	0.94	4.84	3.19	0.00	0.00	0.00
Chicken, light meat, unknown part, skin removed before cooking	3.87	1.15	1.05	0.92	0.88	0.66	0.02	0.80	77.00	0.03	0.67	0.32	0.00	0.03	0.03
Duck, domestic, skin removed before cooking	11.94	4.37	4.02	1.49	3.56	1.34	0.15	0.34	92.50	0.05	2.53	1.34	0.00	0.00	0.00
Ground beef, unknown % fat	22.56	8.86	9.88	0.84	8.63	0.62	0.09	0.09	89.00	0.64	5.10	2.66	0.00	0.00	0.00
Bologna, beef, regular	28.49	12.07	13.80	1.09	12.16	0.85	0.24	0.09	58.00	0.87	6.64	4.05	0.00	0.00	0.00
Pork, fresh, 25% fat, cooked	25.13	9.08	11.52	2.84	10.59	2.29	0.45	0.31	82.00	0.32	5.60	2.94	0.00	0.00	0.00
Frankfurter, all beef (Kosher), regular	28.54	12.05	13.62	1.38	11.99	1.11	0.27	0.11	61.00	0.94	6.52	3.96	0.00	0.00	0.00
Frankfurter, chicken	17.70	5.89	5.58	5.00	5.30	6.46	0.36	0.85	107.00	0.30	3.62	1.83	0.00	0.00	0.00
Frankfurter, regular, beef and pork	29.15	10.76	13.67	2.73	12.36	2.34	0.39	0.25	50.00	0.53	6.45	3.65	0.00	0.00	0.00
Pork, cured, 23% fat, cooked	23.48	8.38	11.03	2.51	10.15	2.15	0.36	0.30	67.00	0.25	5.12	2.93	0.00	0.00	0.00
Salami, pork	33.72	11.89	16.00	3.74	14.67	3.27	0.28	0.31	79.00	0.52	7.64	3.56	0.00	0.00	0.00
Bacon, regular cut	49.24	17.42	23.69	5.81	21.96	4.89	0.79	0.33	85.00	0.62	10.98	5.67	0.00	0.00	0.00
Fish															
Mussel, cooked from fresh or frozen	1.95	0.19	0.17	0.55	0.07	0.03	0.01	2.89	67.00	0.03	0.12	0.04	0.14	0.10	0.15
Fish, 0 to 2.9% fat	1.53	0.36	0.31	0.63	0.15	0.01	0.02	1.75	68.00	0.06	0.23	0.05	0.24	0.05	0.26
Fish, 3.0 to 6.9% fat	4.31	0.83	1.33	1.54	0.79	0.32	0.15	1.86	73.00	0.09	0.49	0.17	0.18	0.13	0.55
Fish, 7.0 to 10.9% fat	7.54	1.39	2.61	2.20	1.52	0.32	0.24	1.58	49.00	0.35	0.79	0.24	0.41	0.27	0.62
Fish, 11.0 to 14.9% fat	12.14	4.50	3.31	1.46	0.75	0.05	0.00	0.32	64.00	0.21	0.95	0.35	0.13	0.11	0.03
Herring, smoked/ kippered, canned and drained	12.37	2.79	5.11	2.92	2.07	0.18	0.14	1.05	82.00	0.76	1.85	0.15	0.97	0.07	1.18

Salmon, canned, drained, with salt	6.05	1.53	1.81	2.05	1.07	0.06	0.06	1.34	55.00	0.05	1.35	0.13	0.84	0.05	0.81
Sardines, canned in oil, drained	11.45	1.53	3.87	5.15	2.14	3.54	0.50	3.37	142.00	0.19	0.99	0.34	0.47	0.00	0.51
Tuna, canned, oil pack, regular, drained	8.21	1.53	2.95	2.88	2.84	2.68	0.07	1.88	18.00	0.03	1.41	0.09	0.03	0.00	0.10
Tuna, canned, water pack, regular, drained, not rinsed	0.50	0.16	0.14	0.13	0.07	0.00	0.00	0.81	18.00	0.03	0.11	0.02	0.04	0.01	0.07
Clams, cooked from fresh or frozen	1.95	0.19	0.17	0.55	0.07	0.03	0.01	2.89	67.00	0.03	0.12	0.04	0.14	0.10	0.15
Crab, hardshell, Alaskan King	1.77	0.23	0.28	0.68	0.15	0.03	0.02	2.96	100.00	0.02	0.14	0.06	0.24	0.05	0.23
Lobster, cooked from fresh or frozen	0.59	0.11	0.16	0.09	0.09	0.00	0.00	0.82	72.00	0.01	0.08	0.02	0.05	0.00	0.03
Oyster, cooked from fresh or frozen, Pacific	4.95	1.26	0.50	1.48	0.19	0.10	0.07	1.17	109.00	0.22	0.87	0.12	0.42	0.10	0.46
Scallops	1.40	0.15	0.07	0.48	0.03	0.01	0.00	3.20	31.81	0.02	0.10	0.02	0.17	0.03	0.20
Shrimp, cooked from fresh or frozen	1.08	0.29	0.20	0.44	0.11	0.02	0.01	1.52	195.00	0.02	0.14	0.10	0.17	0.02	0.14
Caviar	17.90	4.21	5.86	5.66	2.94	0.99	0.55	1.34	588.00	0.90	1.87	0.72	1.03	0.81	1.35
<u>Eggs Dairy</u>															
Eggs, whole, cooked	10.02	3.10	3.81	1.36	3.47	1.15	0.03	0.44	425.00	0.03	2.23	0.78	0.00	0.00	0.04
Eggs, yolk only, cooked	30.87	9.55	11.74	4.20	10.70	3.54	0.10	0.44	1281.00	0.10	6.86	2.42	0.01	0.00	0.11
Eggs, white only, cooked	0.00	0.00	0.00	0.00	0.00	0.00	0.00	0.00	0.00	0.00	0.00	0.00	0.00	0.00	0.00
Cream, coffee creamer, liquid/frozen	9.97	9.30	0.11	0.00	0.11	0.00	0.00	0.00	0.00	1.00	0.43	0.60	0.00	0.00	0.00
Cream, coffee creamer, powder, regular	35.48	32.52	0.97	0.01	0.97	0.00	0.01	0.00	0.00	5.99	3.75	6.34	0.00	0.00	0.00
Cream, coffee creamer, liquid/frozen	11.28	1.68	4.85	4.25	4.79	3.94	0.29	2.53	0.00	0.01	1.10	0.56	0.00	0.00	0.00
Cream, half and half, 10 to 12% fat	11.50	7.16	3.32	0.43	2.89	0.26	0.17	0.06	36.90	1.16	3.02	1.39	0.00	0.00	0.00
Cream, light/coffee cream, 20% fat	19.31	12.02	5.58	0.72	4.86	0.44	0.28	0.06	66.10	1.94	5.08	2.34	0.00	0.00	0.00
Milk, buttermilk, 1% fat	0.88	0.55	0.25	0.03	0.22	0.02	0.01	0.05	3.50	0.09	0.23	0.11	0.00	0.00	0.00
Milk, skim	0.18	0.12	0.05	0.01	0.04	0.00	0.00	0.08	1.80	0.02	0.05	0.02	0.00	0.00	0.00
Milk, 1% fat	1.06	0.66	0.31	0.04	0.27	0.02	0.01	0.06	4.00	0.11	0.28	0.13	0.00	0.00	0.00
Milk, 2% fat	1.92	1.19	0.55	0.07	0.48	0.04	0.03	0.06	7.50	0.19	0.50	0.23	0.00	0.00	0.00
Milk, whole, 3.5 to 4% fat	3.34	2.08	0.96	0.12	0.84	0.07	0.05	0.06	13.60	0.34	0.88	0.40	0.00	0.00	0.00
Parmesan cheese, dry	30.02	19.07	8.73	0.66	7.74	0.32	0.34	0.03	78.70	3.38	8.10	2.67	0.00	0.00	0.00
American cheese, processed	31.25	19.69	8.95	0.99	7.51	0.61	0.38	0.05	94.40	3.21	9.10	3.80	0.00	0.00	0.00
Cottage cheese, lowfat, 2% fat	1.93	1.22	0.55	0.06	0.45	0.04	0.02	0.05	8.40	0.20	0.58	0.22	0.00	0.00	0.00
Cottage cheese, regular or creamed, 4% fat	4.51	2.85	1.28	0.14	1.06	0.10	0.04	0.05	14.90	0.47	1.36	0.51	0.00	0.00	0.00
Cream cheese, Neufchatel	23.43	14.80	6.77	0.65	5.66	0.45	0.20	0.04	76.10	2.35	6.88	2.98	0.00	0.00	0.00
Cheddar cheese, natural	33.14	21.09	9.39	0.94	7.90	0.58	0.36	0.04	104.90	3.33	9.80	4.01	0.00	0.00	0.00
Swiss cheese, natural	27.45	17.78	7.27	0.97	6.02	0.62	0.35	0.05	91.70	3.06	7.79	3.25	0.00	0.00	0.00

TABLE A–19A. AVERAGE VALUES FOR TRIGLYCERIDES, FATTY ACIDS (FA), AND CHOLESTEROL IN SELECTED FOODS AND OILS (INCLUDING OMEGA-3 FA) (PER 100 g EDIBLE PORTION) (CONTINUED)

Monterey Jack cheese, natural	30.04	19.11	8.71	0.66	7.34	0.43	0.23	0.03	95.60	3.07	9.22	3.57	0.00	0.00	0.00
Mozzarella cheese, part skim milk	17.12	10.88	4.85	0.51	4.17	0.36	0.15	0.05	54.00	1.72	5.22	2.08	0.00	0.00	0.00
Brie cheese	24.26	15.26	7.02	0.72	5.75	0.45	0.27	0.05	72.00	2.69	7.23	2.52	0.00	0.00	0.00
Cheese, Kraft Light N' Lively Singles, American flavor	15.50	9.77	4.44	0.49	3.73	0.30	0.19	0.05	52.91	1.59	4.51	1.88	0.00	0.00	0.00
Cheese, Borden Lite-Line Singles, American flavor	8.20	4.99	2.34	0.26	1.94	0.19	0.07	0.05	45.00	0.82	2.47	0.88	0.00	0.00	0.00
Yogurt, frozen, fruit or vanilla, whole milk, 3 to 4% fat	3.24	2.10	0.90	0.09	0.75	0.06	0.03	0.04	9.74	0.33	0.87	0.30	0.00	0.00	0.00
Yogurt, frozen, fruit or vanilla, low fat, 1 to 2% fat	1.08	0.70	0.30	0.03	0.25	0.02	0.01	0.04	4.20	0.11	0.29	0.10	0.00	0.00	0.00
Yogurt, plain, lowfat, 1 to 2% fat	1.55	1.00	0.43	0.04	0.35	0.03	0.01	0.04	6.10	0.16	0.42	0.15	0.00	0.00	0.00
Yogurt, fruit, nonfat, <1% fat	0.20	0.12	0.05	0.01	0.00	0.00	0.00	0.08	2.00	0.00	0.00	0.00	0.00	0.00	0.00
Yogurt, fruit, whole milk, 3 to 4% fat	3.24	2.10	0.90	0.09	0.75	0.06	0.03	0.04	9.74	0.33	0.87	0.30	0.00	0.00	0.00
Ice cream and frozen desserts, regular, 10% fat, other flavors include chocolate chip	10.77	6.70	3.11	0.40	2.71	0.24	0.16	0.06	44.70	1.08	2.83	1.30	0.00	0.00	0.00
Sherbet, plain	1.98	1.23	0.57	0.07	0.50	0.04	0.03	0.06	7.30	0.20	0.52	0.24	0.00	0.00	0.00
Ice cream and frozen desserts, regular 5% fat, other flavors include chocolate chip	4.30	2.68	1.24	0.16	1.08	0.10	0.06	0.06	13.90	0.43	1.13	0.52	0.00	0.00	0.00
Fats/Oils															
Oils, canola	100.00	7.10	58.90	29.60	56.10	20.30	9.30	4.17	0.00	0.00	4.00	1.80	0.00	0.00	0.00
Oils, corn	100.00	12.70	24.20	58.70	24.20	58.00	0.00	4.62	0.00	0.00	10.90	1.80	0.00	0.00	0.00
Oils, sunflower	100.00	10.30	19.50	65.70	19.50	65.70	0.00	6.38	0.00	0.00	5.90	4.50	0.00	0.00	0.00
Oils, cottonseed	100.00	25.90	17.80	51.90	17.00	51.50	0.20	2.00	0.00	0.80	22.70	2.30	0.00	0.00	0.00
Oils, safflower	100.00	9.10	12.10	74.50	11.70	74.10	0.40	8.19	0.00	0.10	6.20	2.20	0.00	0.00	0.00
Oils, sesame	100.00	14.20	39.70	41.70	39.30	41.30	0.30	2.94	0.00	0.00	8.90	4.80	0.00	0.00	0.00
Oils, soybean (partially hydrogenated)	100.00	14.90	43.00	37.60	42.50	34.90	2.60	2.52	0.00	0.10	9.80	5.00	0.00	0.00	0.00
Oils, olive	100.00	13.50	73.70	8.40	72.50	7.90	0.60	0.62	0.00	0.00	11.00	2.20	0.00	0.00	0.00
Oils, peanut	100.00	16.90	46.20	32.00	44.80	32.00	0.00	1.89	0.00	0.10	9.50	2.20	0.00	0.00	0.00
Oils, coconut	100.00	86.50	5.80	1.80	5.80	1.80	0.00	0.02	0.00	16.80	8.20	2.80	0.00	0.00	0.00
Oils, palm	100.00	49.30	37.00	9.30	36.60	9.10	0.20	0.19	0.00	1.00	43.50	4.30	0.00	0.00	0.00

Oils, palm kernel	100.00	81.40	11.40	1.60	11.40	1.60	0.00	0.02	0.00	16.40	8.10	2.80	0.00	0.00	0.00
Shortening, vegetable	100.00	25.00	44.50	26.10	44.50	24.50	1.60	1.04	0.00	0.40	14.10	10.60	0.00	0.00	0.00
Margarine, regular, stick, salted, corn oil	80.50	19.85	36.48	18.62	36.48	18.62	0.00	0.94	0.00	1.08	11.54	7.23	0.00	0.00	0.00
Lard	100.00	39.20	45.10	11.20	41.20	10.20	1.00	0.29	95.00	1.30	23.80	13.50	0.00	0.00	0.00
Butter, regular, salted	81.11	50.49	23.43	3.01	20.40	1.83	1.18	0.06	218.90	8.16	21.33	9.83	0.00	0.00	0.00
Oils, medium chain triglyceride	100.00	94.50	0.00	0.00	0.00	0.00	0.00	0.00	0.00	0.00	0.00	0.00	0.00	0.00	0.00
Mayonnaise/mayo-type dressing, real, regular, commercial	79.40	11.80	22.70	41.30	22.50	37.10	4.20	3.50	59.00	0.10	8.50	3.10	0.00	0.00	0.00
Oils, rapeseed	100.00	6.80	55.50	33.30	53.80	22.10	11.10	4.90	0.00	0.00	4.80	1.60	0.00	0.00	0.00
Miscellaneous															
Peanuts, peanut butter, with salt	49.98	9.59	23.58	14.36	22.96	14.10	0.08	1.50	0.00	0.05	5.50	2.14	0.00	0.00	0.00
Almonds, roasted, dry roasted, salted	56.53	5.27	36.71	11.86	36.03	11.36	0.40	2.25	0.00	0.32	3.74	1.11	0.00	0.00	0.00
Cashews, roasted, dry roasted, salted	48.21	9.70	28.41	8.15	27.89	7.97	0.17	0.84	0.00	0.36	4.53	3.09	0.00	0.00	0.00
Peanuts, roasted, dry roasted, salted	49.30	6.84	24.46	15.58	23.79	15.58	0.00	2.28	0.00	0.02	5.16	1.10	0.00	0.00	0.00
Walnuts	61.87	5.59	14.17	39.13	13.30	31.76	6.81	7.00	0.00	0.19	4.24	1.08	0.00	0.00	0.00
Olives, black	10.68	1.41	7.89	0.91	7.77	0.85	0.06	0.65	0.00	0.00	1.18	0.24	0.00	0.00	0.00
Candy, chocolate pieces, fudge, plain	10.78	4.93	4.53	0.93	4.48	0.86	0.06	0.19	3.92	0.10	2.29	2.35	0.00	0.00	0.00
Avocado, unknown type	15.32	2.44	9.61	1.95	8.96	1.84	0.11	0.80	0.00	0.00	2.40	0.03	0.00	0.00	0.00
Coconut, fresh	33.49	29.70	1.42	0.37	1.42	0.37	0.00	0.01	0.00	5.87	2.84	1.73	0.00	0.00	0.00
Soybeans, cooked from dried	8.97	1.30	1.98	5.06	1.96	4.46	0.60	3.89	0.00	0.02	0.95	0.32	0.00	0.00	0.00
Peas, black-eyed, cooked from dried	0.53	0.14	0.04	0.22	0.04	0.14	0.08	1.57	0.00	0.00	0.11	0.02	0.00	0.00	0.00
Split peas, yellow or green, cooked from dried	0.39	0.05	0.08	0.16	0.08	0.14	0.03	3.20	0.00	0.00	0.04	0.01	0.00	0.00	0.00

SFA = saturated fatty acid, MFA = monounsaturated fatty acid, PFA = polyunsaturated fatty acid, M18:1 = oleic acid, P18:2 = linoleic acid, P18:3 = linolenic acid, S14:0 = myristic acid, S16:0 = palmitic acid, S18:0 = stearic acid, P20:5 = omega-3 (eicosapentaenoic acid), P22:5 = omega-3 (docosapentaenoic acid), P22:6 = omega-3 (docosahexaenoic acid).

(With appreciation to the Nutrition Coding Center, University of Minneapolis, Minneapolis, MN for the compilation and preparation of these tables. Data are based on Version 19 of the NCC Nutrient Data Base.)

TABLE A–19B. AVERAGE VALUES FOR TRIGLYCERIDES, FATTY ACIDS (FA), AND CHOLESTEROL OF MARINE FOODS AND OILS (INCLUDING OMEGA-3 FA)

FISH (100 g)	FAT (g)	CHOL (mg)	SFA (g)	MFA (g)	PFA (g)	M18:1 (g)	P18:2 (g)	P18:3 (g)	P20:5 (g)	P22:5 (g)	P22:6 (g)
Anchovy, European, raw	4.84	—	1.28	1.19	1.64	0.62	0.10	—	0.50	—	0.90
Bass, striped, raw	2.33	80.00	0.51	0.66	0.78	0.45	0.02	0.02	0.17	—	0.59
Bluefish, raw	4.24	58.82	0.92	1.79	1.06	0.68	0.06	trace	0.25	0.06	0.52
Burbot, raw	0.81	60.00	0.16	0.13	0.30	0.10	0.01	—	0.07	0.03	0.10
Carp, raw	5.60	65.88	1.08	2.33	1.44	1.15	0.52	0.27	0.24	0.08	0.11
Catfish, wild, raw	2.82	58.00	0.72	0.84	0.87	0.59	0.10	0.07	0.13	0.10	0.23
Catfish, farmed, raw	7.59	47.00	1.77	3.59	1.57	3.17	0.88	0.10	0.07	0.09	0.21
Cod, Atlantic, raw	0.67	43.53	0.13	0.09	0.23	0.06	0.01	trace	0.10	—	0.20
Eel, all varieties, raw	11.66	126.00	2.35	7.19	0.95	2.78	0.20	0.70	0.10	—	0.10
Flounder, unspecified, raw	1.00	46.00	0.20	0.30	0.30	—	—	trace	0.10	—	0.10
Haddock, raw	0.72	57.65	0.13	0.12	0.24	0.07	0.01	trace	0.10	—	0.10
Halibut, raw	2.29	31.77	0.33	0.65	0.84	0.36	0.03	0.07	0.07	0.09	0.29
Herring, Atlantic, raw	9.04	60.00	2.03	3.74	2.13	1.52	0.13	0.10	0.70	—	0.90
Mackerel, Atlantic, raw	13.87	70.07	3.26	4.06	4.76	2.28	0.22	0.16	0.90	0.21	1.40
Mussel, blue, raw	2.20	38.00	0.40	0.50	0.60	trace	—	—	0.20	1.03	0.37
Octopus, raw	1.01	—	0.30	0.10	0.30	—	—	—	0.10	—	0.10
Oyster, Eastern, wild, raw	2.46	53.00	0.77	0.31	0.97	0.12	0.06	0.05	0.27	0.06	0.29
Oyster, Eastern, farmed, raw	1.55	25.00	0.44	0.15	0.59	0.07	0.03	0.04	0.19	—	0.20
Perch, all varieties, raw	0.92	89.41	0.19	0.15	0.37	0.07	0.01	0.10	0.90	—	1.60
Pike, walleye, raw	1.21	85.88	0.25	0.29	0.45	0.20	0.03	0.01	0.09	0.04	0.23
Pollock, Atlantic, raw	0.98	71.06	0.14	0.11	0.48	0.07	0.01	—	0.07	0.02	0.35
Sablefish, raw	15.30	49.00	3.20	8.06	2.04	4.07	0.17	0.10	0.68	0.17	0.72
Salmon, Chinook, raw	10.45	65.88	2.51	4.48	2.08	2.80	0.11	0.09	0.79	0.23	0.57
Salmon, coho, wild, raw	5.93	45.00	1.26	2.13	1.99	1.20	0.21	0.16	0.43	0.23	0.66
Salmon, coho, farmed, raw	7.67	51.00	1.82	3.33	1.86	1.72	0.35	0.08	0.39	—	0.82
Sea bass, all, raw	2.00	41.18	0.51	0.42	0.74	0.29	0.02	trace	0.10	—	0.30
Smelt, rainbow, raw	2.58	75.00	0.48	0.68	0.94	0.43	0.05	0.10	0.30	—	0.40
Squid, short, finned, raw	1.50	0.40	0.42	0.09	0.52	—	—	trace	0.16	0.52	0.36
Red snapper, raw	1.34	37.06	0.29	0.25	0.46	0.17	0.02	trace	trace	—	0.20
Sole, European, raw	1.20	50.00	0.30	0.40	0.20	—	0.00	trace	trace	—	0.10
Sturgeon, all, raw	4.04	—	0.92	1.94	0.69	1.44	0.07	0.10	0.19	0.05	0.09
Swordfish, raw	4.01	38.82	1.10	1.54	0.92	1.09	0.03	—	0.10	0.00	0.10
Trout, rainbow, wild, raw	3.46	59.00	0.72	1.13	1.24	0.61	0.24	0.12	0.17	0.11	0.42
Trout, rainbow, farmed, raw	5.40	59.00	1.55	1.54	1.81	1.06	0.71	0.06	0.26	—	0.67
Tuna, bluefin, fresh, raw	4.91	37.65	1.26	1.37	1.67	0.92	0.05	—	0.40	—	1.20
Whitefish, all, raw	5.85	60.00	0.91	2.00	2.15	1.35	0.27	0.18	0.32	0.16	0.94
Cod liver oil	100.00	570.00	22.61	46.71	22.54	20.65	0.94	0.94	6.90	0.94	10.97
Herring oil	100.00	766.00	21.29	56.56	15.60	11.96	1.15	0.76	6.27	0.62	4.21
Menhaden oil	100.00	521.00	30.43	26.69	34.20	14.53	2.15	1.49	13.17	4.92	8.56
Max EPA conc fish body oil	100.00	600.00	25.40	28.30	41.10	—	—	0.00	17.80	—	11.60
Salmon oil	100.00	485.00	19.87	29.04	40.32	16.98	1.54	1.06	13.02	2.99	18.23

SFA = saturated fatty acid, MFA = monounsaturated fatty acid, PFA = polyunsaturated fatty acid, M18:1 = oleic acid, P18:2 = linoleic acid, P18:3 = linolenic acid, P20:5 = omega-3 (eicosapentaenoic acid), P22:5 = omega-3 (docosapentaenoic acid), P22:6 = omega-3 (docosahexaenoic acid).

(From Provisional Table on the Content of Omega-3 Fatty Acids and Other Fat Components in Selected Foods, U.S. Department of Agriculture, Human Nutrition Information Service, HNIS/PT-103, 1988. Other data obtained from Composition of Finfish and Shellfish Products, Agriculture Handbook No. 8-15, 1991 Supplement. Consumer Nutrition Center, Washington, U.S. Department of Agriculture, 1991.)

Trace is less than 0.05 g/100 g food.

— denotes Lack of reliable data for nutrient known to be present.

TABLE A–20. PROTEIN, SODIUM, POTASSIUM, CALCIUM, PHOSPHORUS, AND MAGNESIUM CONTENT OF SELECTED COMMON FOODS PER SERVING PORTION

FOOD NAME	SERVING PORTION	Pro (g)	Na (mg)	K (mg)	Ca (mg)	PO_4 (mg)	Mg (mg)
Dairy Products							
Egg, whole, raw, large	1.0 Item	6.250	63.000	60.000	25.000	89.000	5.000
Cheese, cottage, uncreamed	1.0 Oz	4.888	3.715	9.189	8.994	29.523	1.173
Cream, coffee, table, light	1.0 Tbsp	0.405	5.937	18.250	14.437	12.000	1.312
Cream, sour, cultured	1.0 Tbsp	0.454	7.687	20.687	16.750	12.187	1.625
Milk, buttermilk, fluid	1.0 Cup	8.110	257.000	371.000	285.000	219.000	27.000
Milk, whole, 3.3% fat, fluid	1.0 Cup	8.030	120.000	370.000	291.000	228.000	33.000
Milk, nonfat/skim, fluid	1.0 Cup	8.350	126.000	406.000	302.000	247.000	28.000
Milk, whole, low sodium	1.0 Cup	7.560	6.000	617.000	246.000	209.000	12.000
Fats							
Butter, regular	1.0 Tbsp	0.119	116.000	3.640	3.360	3.220	0.280
Vegetable oil, corn	1.0 Tsp	0.000	0.000	0.000	0.000	0.000	0.000
Vegetable oil, olive	1.0 Tsp	0.000	0.002	0.000	0.008	0.055	0.000
Shortening, veg, soybn/cottnsd	1.0 Tsp	0.000	0.000	0.000	0.000	0.000	0.000
Margarine, reg, hard, unsalted	1.0 Tsp	0.000	0.100	1.160	0.820	0.630	0.070
Mayonnaise, soy, commercial	1.0 Tsp	0.067	26.133	1.667	0.667	1.333	0.047
Cereals							
Bran flakes, Kellogg's	0.5 Cup	2.455	152.000	124.000	9.550	96.000	35.500
Corn flakes, Kellogg's	0.5 Cup	0.920	116.000	10.450	0.341	7.150	1.360
Cream of rice, cooked	1.0 Cup	2.200	2.440	48.800	7.320	41.500	7.320
Cream of wheat, instant	1.0 Cup	4.400	6.000	48.000	59.000	43.000	14.000
Farina, cooked, enriched	1.0 Cup	3.260	0.000	30.300	4.660	28.000	4.660
Oatmeal, cooked	1.0 Cup	6.080	2.340	131.000	18.700	178.000	56.200
Wheat, puffed, plain	0.5 Cup	0.880	0.240	20.900	1.680	21.300	8.700
Wheat, shredded, biscuit	1.0 Item	2.600	0.472	77.000	9.680	86.000	40.100
Rice Krispies	0.5 Cup	0.965	170.000	14.750	1.990	17.200	5.100
Breads, Cookies, Crackers							
Bread, white, soft	1.0 Slice	2.070	129.000	28.000	31.500	27.000	5.250
Bread, whole-wheat, soft	1.0 Slice	2.690	178.000	49.300	20.200	72.800	26.000
Crackers, graham, plain	1.0 Item	0.500	33.000	27.500	3.000	10.500	3.570
Crackers, sodium free/whole wheat	1.0 Serving	1.000	1.000	35.000	—	—	—
Crackers, saltines	1.0 Item	0.250	36.800	3.250	0.500	2.500	0.770
Muffin, English, plain	0.5 Item	2.215	179.000	157.000	45.350	31.350	5.300
Bread, Italian, enriched	1.0 Slice	3.000	152.000	22.000	5.000	23.000	—
Roll, hard, enriched	0.5 Item	2.500	156.000	24.500	12.000	23.000	5.750
Roll, hamburger/hotdog	1.0 Item	3.430	241.000	36.800	53.600	32.800	7.600
Cookies, vanilla wafer	5.0 Items	1.000	50.000	14.500	8.000	12.500	3.400
Meat, Fish							
Pot roast, arm, beef, cooked	1.0 Oz	9.355	18.711	81.931	2.551	75.978	6.804
Hamburger patty, beef/lean	1.0 Oz	7.004	21.679	85.384	3.002	44.693	6.004
Steak, sirloin, lean, broiled	1.0 Oz	8.606	18.731	114.000	3.119	69.356	9.062
Chicken, leg, no skin, roasted	1.0 Oz	7.669	25.963	68.637	3.402	51.925	6.864
Chicken, breast, roasted	1.0 Oz	8.447	19.961	69.429	4.050	60.750	7.811
Lamb, all cuts, lean/fat, cooked	1.0 Oz	6.971	20.345	87.718	4.669	53.365	6.671
Turkey, dark meat, no skin	1.0 Oz	8.100	22.275	82.215	9.113	57.915	6.885
Turkey, light, no skin, roasted	1.0 Oz	8.485	18.023	86.265	5.468	62.168	7.898
Veal, all cuts, lean, cooked	1.0 Oz	9.039	25.348	96.056	6.671	71.042	8.005
Bluefish	1.0 Oz	5.689	17.010	105.000	1.890	64.449	9.450
Flatfish, raw	1.0 Oz	5.336	23.014	102.000	5.003	52.031	9.005
Cod, cooked, dry heat	1.0 Oz	6.473	22.050	69.143	3.969	39.060	11.970
Halibut, broiled, dry	1.0 Oz	7.571	19.578	163.000	17.010	80.714	30.351
Shrimp, raw, mixed species	1.0 Oz	5.751	42.525	52.650	15.188	58.725	10.125
Tuna, can/oil, drained	1.0 Oz	8.272	100.000	58.701	3.702	88.052	8.805
Tuna, diet, low sodium	1.0 Oz	7.656	11.380	73.670	1.418	62.390	9.074
Sweets							
Honey, strained/extracted	1.0 Tbsp	0.000	1.000	11.000	1.000	1.000	0.630
Ice milk, van, hard, 4.3% fat	0.5 Cup	2.580	52.500	133.000	88.000	64.500	9.500
Ice cream, van, hard, 10% fat	0.5 Cup	2.400	58.000	129.000	88.000	67.000	9.000

TABLE A–20. CONTINUED

FOOD NAME	SERVING PORTION	Pro (g)	Na (mg)	K (mg)	Ca (mg)	PO_4 (mg)	Mg (mg)
Sweets							
Ice cream, van, hard, 16% fat	0.5 Cup	2.065	54.000	111.000	75.500	57.500	8.000
Jams/preserves, regular	1.0 Tbsp	0.000	2.000	18.000	4.000	2.000	—
Sherbet, orange, 2% fat	0.5 Cup	1.080	44.000	99.000	51.500	37.000	7.500
Sugar, brown, pressed down	0.5 Cup	0.000	33.000	379.000	93.500	21.000	—
Sugar, white, granulated	1.0 Tbsp	0.000	0.120	0.000	0.000	0.000	—
Juices							
Apple juice, can and bottle	3.5 Fl ozs	0.066	3.062	129.000	7.612	7.875	3.500
Apricot nectar, can	3.5 Fl ozs	0.402	3.937	125.000	7.700	9.887	5.687
Cranberry juice, bottle	3.5 Fl ozs	0.000	4.375	19.906	3.321	2.214	2.214
Grape juice, can	3.5 Fl ozs	0.000	0.000	38.500	3.500	3.500	—
Grapefruit juice, can, unsweetened	3.5 Fl ozs	0.560	1.081	165.000	7.569	11.900	10.806
Lemon juice, can and bottle	3.5 Fl ozs	0.427	22.400	109.000	11.725	9.625	8.531
Orange juice, can	3.5 Fl ozs	0.643	2.179	191.000	8.706	15.268	11.987
Pear nectar, can	3.5 Fl ozs	0.120	4.375	14.219	5.469	3.281	3.281
Pineapple juice, can	3.5 Fl ozs	0.350	1.094	147.000	18.593	8.750	14.219
Prune juice, can and bottle	3.5 Fl ozs	0.682	4.462	309.000	13.431	28.000	15.662
Tomato juice, can	3.5 Fl ozs	0.809	385.000	235.000	9.625	20.300	11.725
Tomato juice, low sodium	3.5 Fl ozs	0.809	10.675	235.000	9.625	20.300	11.725
Vegetables							
Asparagus, can, spears	0.5 Cup	2.590	472.000	208.000	19.350	52.000	12.100
Asparagus, can, low sodium	0.5 Cup	2.195	425.000	187.000	17.100	46.350	11.000
Beans, snap, green, can, cuts	0.5 Cup	0.775	170.000	73.500	17.550	12.850	8.800
Beans, green, can, low sodium	0.5 Cup	0.780	1.360	74.000	16.000	13.000	9.000
Beans, snap, wax, raw, boiled	0.5 Cup	1.180	1.875	187.000	28.750	24.000	15.650
Beets, can, whole	0.5 Cup	1.025	324.000	175.000	17.200	19.700	19.700
Beets, can, diet, low sodium	0.5 Cup	1.025	324.000	175.000	17.200	19.700	19.700
Broccoli, raw, boiled, drained	0.5 Cup	2.310	20.150	227.000	35.650	45.750	18.600
Cabbage, common, boiled, drained	0.5 Cup	0.695	13.800	149.000	23.950	18.150	10.900
Carrots, can, sliced, drained	0.5 Cup	0.467	176.000	131.000	18.250	17.500	5.850
Carrots, can, low sodium	0.5 Cup	0.750	47.950	213.000	30.750	24.600	11.050
Carrot, raw, whole, scraped	1.0 Item	0.740	25.200	233.000	19.400	31.700	10.800
Cauliflower, raw, boiled, drained	0.5 Cup	1.160	4.000	200.000	17.000	22.000	7.000
Celery, Pascal, raw, stalk	1.0 Item	0.300	34.800	115.000	16.000	10.000	4.400
Corn, sweet, can, drained	0.5 Cup	2.160	267.000	161.000	4.125	53.500	16.500
Corn, sweet, can, low sodium	0.5 Cup	2.480	3.840	196.000	5.100	65.500	20.500
Cucumber, raw, sliced	0.5 Cup	0.281	1.040	77.500	7.300	8.850	5.700
Peas, green, can, drained	0.5 Cup	3.755	186.000	147.000	17.000	57.000	14.450
Peas, green, can, low sodium	0.5 Cup	3.755	1.700	147.000	17.000	57.000	14.450
Tomato, raw, red, ripe	1.0 Item	1.050	11.100	273.000	6.150	29.500	13.500
Tomato, red, can, stewed	0.5 Cup	1.185	324.000	305.000	42.100	25.500	15.300
Tomato, can, low sodium, diet	0.5 Cup	1.115	15.600	265.000	31.200	22.800	14.400
Potato, boiled, peeled before cooked	1.0 Item	2.310	6.750	443.000	10.800	54.000	27.000
Noodles, egg, enriched, cooked	0.5 Cup	3.500	1.500	35.000	8.000	47.000	21.600
Rice, white, parboiled, cooked	0.5 Cup	2.005	2.625	32.400	16.650	36.750	10.500
Fruits							
Apples, raw, unpeeled	1.0 Item	0.262	1.000	159.000	10.000	10.000	6.000
Apples, raw, peeled	1.0 Item	0.190	0.000	144.000	5.000	9.000	4.000
Applesauce, can, unsweetened	0.5 Cup	0.208	2.440	91.500	3.660	8.550	3.660
Apricots, can, light syrup	0.5 Cup	0.675	5.000	175.000	13.900	17.000	10.500
Bananas, raw, peeled	1.0 Item	1.170	1.140	451.000	6.840	22.000	33.000
Blueberries, raw	0.5 Cup	0.486	4.350	64.500	4.350	7.250	3.625
Cherries, sweet, can/juice	0.5 Cup	1.140	3.750	164.000	17.500	27.500	15.000
Grapefruit, red/pnk/wht, raw	0.5 Cup	0.725	0.500	161.000	13.500	10.000	9.500
Oranges, raw, all varieties	1.0 Item	1.230	0.000	237.000	52.400	18.300	13.100
Peaches, raw, whole	1.0 Item	0.609	0.000	171.000	4.350	10.400	6.090
Peaches, can, light syrup	0.5 Cup	0.565	6.500	122.000	4.500	13.500	6.000
Pears, raw, bartlet, unpeeled	1.0 Item	0.647	0.000	208.000	18.300	18.300	9.960
Pineapple, can/juice	0.5 Cup	0.525	2.000	153.000	17.500	7.500	17.500
Strawberries, raw, whole	0.5 Cup	0.455	0.745	124.000	10.450	14.150	7.450

Pro = protein, Na = sodium, K = potassium, Ca = calcium, PO_4 = phosphorus, Mg = magnesium.

(Created on Nutritionist III, Version 7, N-Squared Computing, 1991. Data compiled from U.S. Department of Agriculture Handbook 8- Series, manufacturers' data, published journals, and industry sources. Appreciation expressed to Ms. Lori Cohen, M.S., R.D., for her assistance in preparing this table.)

TABLE A–21A. VITAMIN A, VITAMIN E, α-TOCOPHEROL (TOC), VITAMIN C, THIAMIN, RIBOFLAVIN, NIACIN, VITAMIN B_6, VITAMIN B_{12}, AND FOLATE CONTENT OF SELECTED COMMON FOODS PER SERVING PORTION

FOOD NAME	SERVING PORTION	A* (RE)	E† (mg)	α-TOC (mg)	C (mg)	THIAMIN (mg)	RIBO (mg)	NIACIN (mg)	B_6 (mg)	B_{12} (µg)	FOLATE (µg)
Dairy Products											
Egg, whole, raw, large	1.0 Item	95.200	0.700	0.350	0.000	0.031	0.254	0.037	0.070	0.500	23.000
Cheese, cottage, uncreamed	1.0 Oz	2.581	—	0.181	0.000	0.007	0.040	0.044	0.023	0.235	4.106
Cream, coffee, table, light	1.0 Tbsp	32.437	0.094	—	0.114	0.005	0.022	0.009	0.005	0.033	0.375
Cream, sour, cultured	1.0 Tbsp	34.124	—	—	0.124	0.005	0.021	0.010	0.002	0.043	1.562
Milk, buttermilk, fluid	1.0 Cup	24.300	0.980	—	2.400	0.083	0.377	0.142	0.083	0.537	12.300
Milk, whole, 3.3% fat, fluid	1.0 Cup	92.200	0.220	0.146	2.290	0.093	0.395	0.205	0.102	0.871	12.000
Milk, nonfat/skim, fluid	1.0 Cup	150.000	0.221	0.147	2.400	0.088	0.343	0.216	0.098	0.926	13.000
Milk, whole, low sodium	1.0 Cup	95.200	0.220	0.146	2.290	0.049	0.256	0.105	0.083	0.876	12.200
Fats											
Butter, regular	1.0 Tbsp	105.000	0.221	0.221	0.000	0.001	0.005	0.006	0.000	0.018	0.420
Vegetable oil, corn	1.0 Tsp	0.000	3.771	0.650	0.000	0.000	0.000	0.000	0.000	0.000	0.000
Vegetable oil, olive	1.0 Tsp	0.000	0.569	0.535	0.000	0.000	0.000	0.000	0.000	0.000	0.000
Shortening, veg, soybn/cottnsd	1.0 Tsp	0.000	2.771	0.342	0.000	0.000	0.000	0.000	0.000	0.000	0.000
Margarine, reg, hard, unsalted	1.0 Tsp	47.000	2.710	0.423	0.004	0.000	0.001	0.001	0.000	0.003	0.030
Mayonnaise, soy, commercial	1.0 Tsp	3.900	2.667	0.967	0.000	0.000	0.000	0.000	0.027	0.012	0.360
Cereals											
Bran flakes, Kellogg's	0.5 Cup	258.000	0.412	0.082	0.000	0.254	0.293	3.430	0.351	1.050	69.000
Corn flakes, Kellogg's	0.5 Cup	150.000	—	0.012	6.000	0.148	0.171	2.000	0.205	0.000	40.050
Cream of rice, cooked	1.0 Cup	0.000	—	—	0.000	0.000	0.000	0.976	0.066	0.000	7.320
Cream of wheat, instant	1.0 Cup	0.000	—	—	0.000	0.200	0.100	1.800	0.029	0.000	11.000
Farina, cooked, enriched	1.0 Cup	—	2.190	—	—	0.186	0.117	1.280	0.023	0.000	4.660
Oatmeal, cooked	1.0 Cup	4.680	5.400	3.530	—	0.257	0.047	0.304	0.047	0.000	9.360
Wheat, puffed, plain	0.5 Cup	0.000	—	0.040	0.000	0.012	0.014	0.650	0.010	0.000	1.920
Wheat, shredded, biscuit	1.0 Item	0.000	0.508	0.085	0.000	0.070	0.060	1.080	0.060	0.000	12.000
Rice Krispies	0.5 Cup	188.000	0.040	0.006	7.550	0.185	0.213	2.500	0.256	0.000	50.000
Breads, Cookies, Crackers											
Bread, white, soft	1.0 Slice	0.000	0.298	0.030	0.000	0.118	0.078	0.938	0.009	0.000	8.750
Bread, whole-wheat, soft	1.0 Slice	0.000	0.252	0.028	0.000	0.098	0.059	1.070	0.052	0.000	15.400
Crackers, graham, plain	1.0 Item	0.000	0.128	0.026	0.000	0.010	0.040	0.250	0.006	0.000	0.910
Crackers, sodium free/ whole-wheat	1.0 Serving	—	—	—	—	—	—	—	—	—	—
Crackers, saltines	1.0 Item	0.000	0.050	0.010	0.000	0.125	0.013	0.100	0.001	0.000	0.495
Muffin, English, plain	0.5 Item	0.000	—	—	0.000	0.129	0.090	1.050	0.011	0.000	8.950
Bread, Italian, enriched	1.0 Slice	0.000	0.357	0.036	0.000	0.120	0.070	1.000	0.016	0.000	10.500
Roll, hard, enriched	0.5 Item	0.000	0.133	0.010	0.000	0.100	0.060	0.850	0.009	0.000	14.750
Roll, hamburger/hotdog	1.0 Item	0.000	0.212	0.016	0.000	0.196	0.132	1.580	0.014	—	14.800
Cookies, vanilla wafer	5.0 Items	5.000	1.090	0.515	0.000	0.050	0.045	0.400	—	—	—
Meat, Fish											
Pot roast, arm, beef, cooked	1.0 Oz	0.000	—	0.040	0.000	0.023	0.082	1.055	0.094	0.964	3.118
Hamburger patty, beef, lean	1.0 Oz	3.005	0.172	0.101	0.000	0.014	0.060	1.464	0.073	0.667	2.668
Steak, sirloin, lean, broiled	1.0 Oz	1.519	0.156	0.037	0.000	0.036	0.084	1.215	0.128	0.810	2.835
Chicken, leg, no skin, roasted	1.0 Oz	5.372	0.156	0.099	0.000	0.021	0.066	1.791	0.104	0.093	2.387

TABLE A–21A. CONTINUED

FOOD NAME	SERVING PORTION	A* (RE)	E† (mg)	α-TOC (mg)	C (mg)	THIAMIN (mg)	RIBO (mg)	NIACIN (mg)	B_6 (mg)	B_{12} (μg)	FOLATE (μg)
Meat, Fish											
Chicken, breast, roasted	1.0 Oz	7.912	0.156	0.099	0.000	0.019	0.034	3.602	0.156	0.093	0.868
Lamb, all cuts, lean/ fat, cooked	1.0 Oz	—	—	—	—	0.027	0.073	1.888	0.037	0.724	5.003
Turkey, dark meat, no skin	1.0 Oz	0.000	—	0.181	0.000	0.018	0.070	1.035	0.101	0.105	2.552
Turkey, light, no skin, roasted	1.0 Oz	0.000	—	0.026	0.000	0.017	0.037	1.938	0.152	0.105	1.620
Veal, all cuts, lean, cooked	1.0 Oz	—	—	—	—	0.017	0.097	2.388	0.093	0.470	4.336
Bluefish	1.0 Oz	33.831	—	—	0.016	0.016	0.023	1.688	0.114	1.529	0.454
Flatfish, raw	1.0 Oz	2.668	—	—	—	0.025	0.022	0.820	0.059	0.430	—
Cod, cooked, dry heat	1.0 Oz	3.969	—	—	0.283	0.025	0.022	0.712	0.080	0.298	2.300
Halibut, broiled, dry	1.0 Oz	15.309	—	—	0.000	0.020	0.026	2.021	0.112	0.387	3.902
Shrimp, raw, mixed species	1.0 Oz	—	—	—	—	0.008	0.012	0.725	0.028	0.328	0.810
Tuna, can/oil, drained	1.0 Oz	6.537	—	0.474	0.000	0.011	0.034	3.502	0.031	0.624	1.504
Tuna, diet, low sodium	1.0 Oz	6.898	0.799	—	—	0.009	0.014	3.514	0.105	0.397	0.000
Sweets											
Honey, strained/ extracted	1.0 Tbsp	0.000	—	—	0.000	0.000	0.010	0.100	0.004	0.000	—
Ice milk, van, hard, 4.3% fat	0.5 Cup	26.000	0.230	0.040	0.380	0.038	0.174	0.059	0.043	0.438	1.500
Ice cream, van, hard, 10% fat	0.5 Cup	66.500	0.233	0.040	0.350	0.026	0.165	0.067	0.031	0.313	1.500
Ice cream, van, hard, 16% fat	0.5 Cup	104.000	0.259	0.045	0.305	0.022	0.142	0.058	0.027	0.269	1.000
Jams/preserves, regular	1.0 Tbsp	0.000	—	0.018	0.000	0.000	0.010	0.000	0.004	0.000	1.600
Sherbet, orange, 2% fat	0.5 Cup	19.500	—	—	1.930	0.016	0.045	0.066	0.013	0.079	7.000
Sugar, brown, pressed down	0.5 Cup	0.000	—	—	0.000	0.010	0.035	0.200	—	—	—
Sugar, white, granulated	1.0 Tbsp	0.000	—	—	0.000	0.000	0.000	0.000	—	—	—
Juices											
Apple juice, can and bottle	3.5 Fl ozs	0.087	—	0.011	1.006	0.023	0.018	0.108	0.032	0.000	0.108
Apricot nectar, can	3.5 Fl ozs	144.000	—	—	0.661	0.010	0.015	0.286	—	0.000	1.426
Cranberry juice, bottle	3.5 Fl ozs	0.000	—	—	39.199	0.010	0.010	0.039	0.021	0.000	0.221
Grape juice, can	3.5 Fl ozs	0.000	—	—	17.500	0.010	0.010	0.109	0.021	0.000	1.050
Grapefruit juice, can, unsweetened	3.5 Fl ozs	0.787	0.195	0.043	31.543	0.045	0.021	0.250	0.021	0.000	11.244
Lemon juice, can and bottle	3.5 Fl ozs	1.619	—	—	26.468	0.044	0.010	0.210	0.046	0.000	10.762
Orange juice, can	3.5 Fl ozs	19.118	0.218	0.044	37.493	0.065	0.031	0.342	0.096	0.000	19.731
Pear nectar, can	3.5 Fl ozs	0.044	—	—	1.203	0.002	0.014	0.140	0.015	0.000	1.312
Pineapple juice, can	3.5 Fl ozs	0.525	—	—	11.725	0.060	0.024	0.281	0.105	0.000	25.287
Prune juice, can and bottle	3.5 Fl ozs	0.394	—	—	4.594	0.018	0.078	0.879	0.244	0.000	0.446
Tomato juice, can	3.5 Fl ozs	59.936	0.757	0.234	19.556	0.050	0.033	0.717	0.119	0.000	21.262
Tomato juice, low sodium	3.5 Fl ozs	59.936	0.757	0.235	19.556	0.050	0.033	0.717	0.119	0.000	21.262
Vegetables											
Asparagus, can, spears	0.5 Cup	64.000	—	0.460	22.250	0.074	0.121	1.155	0.133	0.000	116.000
Asparagus, can, low sodium	0.5 Cup	57.500	—	0.464	20.000	0.066	0.109	1.040	0.120	0.000	104.000

TABLE A–21A. CONTINUED

FOOD NAME	SERVING PORTION	A* (RE)	E† (mg)	α-TOC (mg)	C (mg)	THIAMIN (mg)	RIBO (mg)	NIACIN (mg)	B_6 (mg)	B_{12} (μg)	FOLATE (μg)
Vegetables											
Beans, snap, green, can, cuts	0.5 Cup	23.650	0.034	0.021	3.240	0.010	0.038	0.135	0.025	0.000	21.450
Beans, green, can, low sodium	0.5 Cup	—	0.034	0.021	3.200	0.010	0.038	0.137	—	0.000	21.600
Beans, snap, wax, raw, boiled	0.5 Cup	41.900	—	0.182	6.050	0.047	0.061	0.384	0.035	0.000	20.800
Beets, can, whole	0.5 Cup	1.238	—	0.037	4.795	0.013	0.047	0.186	0.068	0.000	35.650
Beets, can, diet, low sodium	0.5 Cup	1.238	—	0.037	4.795	0.013	0.047	0.186	0.068	0.000	35.650
Broccoli, raw, boiled, drained	0.5 Cup	108.000	0.496	0.357	58.000	0.043	0.088	0.445	0.111	0.000	38.750
Cabbage, common, boiled drained	0.5 Cup	6.550	1.210	1.210	17.600	0.042	0.040	0.165	0.047	0.000	14.700
Carrots, can, sliced, drained	0.5 Cup	1005.000	0.336	0.307	1.970	0.013	0.022	0.403	0.082	0.000	6.700
Carrots, can, low sodium	0.5 Cup	1620.000	0.565	0.515	3.445	0.024	0.033	0.520	0.138	0.000	9.950
Carrot, raw, whole, scraped	1.0 Item	2025.000	0.367	0.317	6.700	0.070	0.042	0.668	0.106	0.000	10.100
Cauliflower, raw, boiled, drained	0.5 Cup	0.900	0.057	0.019	34.300	0.039	0.032	0.342	0.125	0.000	31.700
Celery, Pascal, raw, stalk	1.0 Item	5.200	0.292	0.144	2.800	0.018	0.018	0.129	0.035	0.000	11.200
Corn, sweet, can, drained	0.5 Cup	13.200	0.510	0.033	7.000	0.027	0.065	0.990	0.039	0.000	40.100
Corn, sweet, can, low sodium	0.5 Cup	15.350	0.795	0.051	8.600	0.033	0.078	1.200	0.048	0.000	48.750
Cucumber, raw, sliced	0.5 Cup	2.600	0.161	0.078	2.445	0.016	0.010	0.156	0.027	0.000	7.250
Peas, green, can, drained	0.5 Cup	65.500	2.235	0.017	8.150	0.103	0.066	0.620	0.055	0.000	37.650
Peas, green, can, low sodium	0.5 Cup	65.500	2.235	0.017	8.150	0.103	0.066	0.620	0.055	0.000	37.650
Tomato, raw, red, ripe	1.0 Item	76.300	0.603	0.418	23.500	0.073	0.059	0.772	0.098	0.000	18.500
Tomato, red, can, stewed	0.5 Cup	70.000	0.905	0.281	16.950	0.059	0.045	0.910	0.022	0.000	6.900
Tomato, can, low sodium, diet	0.5 Cup	72.000	—	0.264	18.150	0.054	0.037	0.880	0.108	0.000	9.350

TABLE A–21A. CONTINUED

FOOD NAME	SERVING PORTION	A* (RE)	E† (mg)	α-TOC (mg)	C (mg)	THIAMIN (mg)	RIBO (mg)	NIACIN (mg)	B_6 (mg)	B_{12} (μg)	FOLATE (μg)
Vegetables											
Potato, boiled, peeled before cooked	1.0 Item	0.000	0.081	0.041	9.990	0.132	0.026	1.770	0.363	0.000	12.000
Noodles, egg, enriched cooked	0.5 Cup	5.500	—	—	0.000	0.110	0.065	0.950	0.071	0.000	9.600
Rice, white, parboiled, cooked	0.5 Cup	0.000	0.342	0.097	0.000	0.219	0.016	1.225	0.016	0.000	3.000
Fruit											
Apple, raw, unpeeled	1.0 Item	7.400	0.911	0.814	7.800	0.023	0.019	0.106	0.066	0.000	3.900
Apple, raw, peeled	1.0 Item	5.600	0.845	0.346	5.120	0.022	0.013	0.116	0.059	0.000	0.500
Applesauce, can, unsweetened	0.5 Cup	3.500	—	0.110	1.465	0.016	0.031	0.230	0.032	0.000	0.730
Apricots, can, light syrup	0.5 Cup	167.000	—	1.125	3.415	0.020	0.026	0.385	0.069	0.000	2.150
Bananas, raw, peeled	1.0 Item	9.200	0.365	0.308	10.400	0.051	0.114	0.616	0.659	0.000	21.800
Blueberries, raw	0.5 Cup	7.250	—	—	9.450	0.035	0.037	0.261	0.026	0.000	4.640
Cherries, sweet, can/juice	0.5 Cup	15.650	—	—	3.125	0.023	0.030	0.510	0.038	0.000	5.250
Grapefruit, red/pnk/wht, raw	0.5 Cup	14.500	—	—	39.550	0.042	0.023	0.288	0.049	0.000	11.700
Oranges, raw, all varieties	1.0 Item	26.900	0.314	0.314	69.700	0.114	0.052	0.369	0.079	0.000	39.700
Peaches, raw, whole	1.0 Item	46.500	—	0.087	5.740	0.015	0.036	0.861	0.016	0.000	2.960
Peaches, can, light syrup	0.5 Cup	44.500	—	—	2.950	0.012	0.032	0.745	0.024	0.000	4.100
Pears, raw, bartlet, unpeeled	1.0 Item	3.300	—	0.820	6.640	0.033	0.066	0.166	0.030	0.000	12.100
Pineapple, can/juice	0.5 Cup	4.750	0.125	0.125	11.900	0.119	0.024	0.355	0.093	0.000	6.000
Strawberries, raw, whole	0.5 Cup	2.050	0.194	0.090	42.250	0.015	0.049	0.172	0.044	0.000	13.200

*RE = μg retinol + μg β-carotene (0.167) + μg other carotenes (0.083)

1 RE = 3.33 IU from vitamin A (retinol)
10 IU from β-carotene

†mg of vitamin E represents mg of total tocopherol including α-tocopherol.
— denotes Lack of reliable data for nutrient to be present.
(Created on Nutritionist III, Version 7, N-Squared Computing, 1991. Data compiled from U.S. Department of Agriculture Handbook 8- Series, manufacturers' data, published journals, and industry sources. Appreciation expressed to Ms. Lori Cohen, M.S., R.D., for her assistance in preparing this table.)

TABLE A–21B. RETENTION OF NUTRIENTS IN COOKED VEGETABLES[1]

	ASCORBIC ACID (%)	THIAMIN (%)	RIBOFLAVIN (%)	NIACIN (%)	PANTOTHENIC ACID[6] (%)	VITAMIN B_6 (%)	FOLACIN[7] (%)	VITAMIN A (%)
Potatoes								
Prepared from raw								
Baked in skin	80	85	95	95	90	95	90	—[8]
Boiled in skin	75	80	95	95	90	95	90	—
Boiled without skin	75	80	95	95	90	95	75	—
Fried	80	80	95	95	90	95	75	—
Hashed-brown[2]	25	40	85	80	—	—	65	—
Mashed	75	80	95	95	90	95	75	—
Scalloped and au gratin	80	80	95	95	90	95	75	—
Prepared from frozen								
French fried, heated	50	75	95	95	90	95	75	—
Baked, stuffed, heated	80	85	95	95	90	95	80	—
Hashed-brown	80	80	95	95	90	95	80	—
Sweet Potatoes								
Prepared from raw								
Baked in skin	80	85	95	95	90	95	90	90
Boiled in skin	75	80	95	95	90	95	90	85
Prepared from frozen								
Baked	80	80	95	95	90	95	80	90
Boiled	75	80	95	95	90	95	80	85
Tomatoes								
(prepared from raw, baked, boiled, or stewed)	95	95	95	95	95	95	70	95
Other Vegetables								
(cooked in small or moderate amount of water until tender)								
Prepared from raw, drained								
Greens, dark and leafy[3]	60	85	95	90	95	90	65	95
Roots, bulbs, other vegetables of high starch and/or sugar content[4]	70	85	95	95	90	95	70	90
Other[5]	80	85	95	90	90	90	70	90
Prepared from frozen, drained								
Greens, dark and leafy[3]	60	90	95	90	95	90	55	95
Roots, bulbs, other vegetables of high starch and/or sugar content[4]	70	90	95	95	90	95	70	90
Other[5]	80	90	95	90	90	90	70	90

[1] $\% \text{ True Retention} = \frac{\text{Nutrient content per g of cooked food} \times \text{g of food after cooking}}{\text{Nutrient content per g of raw food} \times \text{g of food before cooking}} \times 100$

[2] Potatoes were pared, boiled, and held overnight before hashed-browning.

[3] Vegetables such as beet greens, Chinese cabbage, collards, mustard greens, spinach, Swiss chard, turnip greens, and other wild greens.

[4] Vegetables such as beets, carrots, green peas, lima beans, onions, parsnips, rutabagas, salsify, turnips, summer and winter squash, and other immature seeds of the legume group.

[5] Vegetables such as asparagus, bean sprouts, broccoli, brussels sprouts, cabbage, cauliflower, eggplant, kohlrabi, okra, and sweet peppers.

[6] Because of limited data, values are based on nutrient retention data from other cooked plant products.

[7] Values are based on limited data.

[8] Dashes denote lack of reliable data.

(From Composition of Foods, Raw, Processed, Prepared. 1990 Supplement. Washington, D.C., U.S. Department of Agriculture, Human Nutrition Information Service, Agriculture Handbook No. 8.)

TABLE A–22. IRON, ZINC, COPPER, SELENIUM, AND MANGANESE CONTENT OF SELECTED FOODS, IN MG (100 g = 3½ oz)*

FOOD NAME	Fe	Zn	Cu	Se	Mn
Dairy Products					
Egg, whole, raw, large	1.440	1.100	0.014	0.044	0.024
Cheese, cottage, uncreamed	0.228	0.469	0.028	0.023	0.003
Cream, coffee, table, light	0.042	0.271	0.008	0.000	0.001
Cream, sour, cultured	0.061	0.270	0.019	—	0.003
Milk, buttermilk, fluid	0.049	0.420	0.011	0.001	0.002
Milk, whole, 3.3% fat, fluid	0.049	0.381	0.010	0.001	0.004
Milk, nonfat/skim, fluid	0.041	0.400	0.011	0.003	0.002
Milk, whole, low sodium	0.050	0.380	0.010	0.001	0.004
Fats					
Butter, regular, tablespoon	0.157	0.050	0.014	0.000	0.007
Vegetable oil, corn	0.000	0.000	0.000	—	0.000
Vegetable oil, olive	0.384	0.060	0.074	—	—
Shortening, veg, soybn/cottnsd	0.000	0.000	0.000	—	0.000
Margarine, reg, hard, unsalted	0.000	0.000	—	0.000	—
Mayonnaise, soy, commercial	0.714	0.143	0.243	—	—
Cereals					
Bran flakes, Kellogg's	63.590	13.205	0.741	0.010	4.333
Corn flakes, Kellogg's	6.300	0.282	0.066	0.004	0.084
Cream of rice, cooked	0.200	0.160	0.034	—	0.144
Cream of wheat, instant	4.979	0.170	0.038	—	—
Farina, cooked, enriched	0.502	0.070	0.011	—	—
Oatmeal, cooked	0.679	0.491	0.055	0.009	0.585
Wheat, puffed, plain	4.733	2.358	0.408	—	1.758
Wheat, shredded, biscuit	3.136	2.500	0.500	—	3.072
Rice Krispies	6.303	1.690	0.250	0.014	0.989
Breads, Cookies, Crackers					
Bread, white, soft	2.840	0.620	0.140	0.028	0.280
Bread, whole-wheat, soft	3.373	1.655	0.338	0.046	—
Crackers, graham, plain	3.571	0.757	0.857	0.014	—
Crackers, sodium free/ whole-wheat	—	—	—	—	—
Crackers, saltines	4.545	0.618	0.182	0.145	—
Muffin, English, plain	2.821	0.720	0.311	0.027	—
Bread, Italian, enriched	2.333	—	—	0.027	—
Roll, hamburger/hotdog	2.975	0.620	0.165	0.030	—
Cookies, vanilla wafer	1.500	—	—	0.000	—
Meat, Fish					
Pot roast, arm, beef, cooked	3.790	8.660	0.164	0.006	0.019
Hamburger patty, beef/lean	2.106	5.365	0.066	0.024	0.014
Steak, sirloin, lean, broiled	3.357	6.518	0.146	0.034	0.018
Chicken, leg, no skin, roasted	1.305	2.853	0.080	0.014	0.021
Chicken, breast, roasted	1.061	1.020	0.050	0.027	0.018
Lamb, all cuts, lean/fat, cooked	1.871	4.459	0.119	—	0.022
Turkey, dark meat, no skin	2.336	4.464	0.160	0.025	0.023
Turkey, light, no skin, roasted	1.343	2.036	0.042	—	0.020
Veal, all cuts, lean, cooked	1.165	5.094	0.120	—	0.038
Bluefish	0.480	0.807	0.053	—	0.021
Flatfish, raw	0.353	0.459	0.032	—	0.016
Cod, cooked, dry heat	0.490	0.578	0.036	0.045	0.020
Halibut, broiled, dry	1.071	0.529	0.035	0.060	0.020
Shrimp, raw, mixed species	2.400	1.114	0.271	—	0.057
Tuna, can/oil, drained	1.388	0.900	0.071	0.072	0.015
Tuna, diet, low sodium	1.201	0.500	0.060	0.116	0.039
Sweets					
Honey, strained/extracted	0.476	0.095	0.038	0.005	0.029
Ice milk, van, hard, 4.3% fat	0.137	0.420	0.023	0.002	0.009
Ice cream, van, hard, 10% fat	0.090	1.060	0.019	0.002	0.006
Ice cream, van, hard, 16% fat	0.068	0.818	0.019	0.002	0.006
Jams/preserves, regular	1.000	—	0.310	0.000	—
Sherbet, orange, 2% fat	0.161	0.689	0.030	—	0.011
Sugar, brown, pressed down	3.409	—	0.350	0.001	—
Sugar, white, granulated	0.000	0.050	0.017	0.000	—

TABLE A–22. CONTINUED

FOOD NAME	Fe	Zn	Cu	Se	Mn
Juices					
Apple juice, can and bottle	0.371	0.028	0.022	0.001	0.113
Apricot nectar, can	0.382	0.092	0.073	—	0.032
Cranberry juice, bottle	0.150	0.070	0.018	0.000	0.193
Grape juice, can	0.096	—	—	—	—
Grapefruit juice, can, unsweetened	0.200	0.090	0.038	0.000	0.020
Lemon juice, can and bottle	0.130	0.060	0.037	0.000	0.020
Orange juice, can	0.442	0.070	0.057	0.000	0.014
Pear nectar, can	0.260	0.070	0.067	0.000	0.030
Pineapple juice, can	0.260	0.110	0.090	0.001	0.992
Prune juice, can and bottle	1.180	0.210	0.068	0.000	0.151
Tomato juice, can	0.582	0.140	0.101	0.000	0.077
Tomato juice, low sodium	0.582	0.140	0.101	0.000	0.077
Vegetables					
Asparagus, can, spears	1.831	0.400	0.096	0.004	0.170
Asparagus, can, low sodium	0.582	0.471	0.107	0.001	0.152
Beans, snap, green, can, cuts	0.904	0.290	0.038	0.001	0.200
Beans, green, can, low sodium	0.897	0.294	0.038	0.001	0.200
Beans, snap, wax, raw, boiled	1.280	0.360	0.103	0.001	0.294
Beets, can, whole	0.671	0.230	0.097	0.000	0.241
Beets, can, diet, low sodium	0.671	0.230	0.097	0.001	0.241
Broccoli, raw, boiled, drained	0.839	0.380	0.043	0.002	0.218
Cabbage, common, boiled, drained	0.390	0.160	0.028	0.002	0.129
Carrots, can, sliced, drained	0.640	0.260	0.104	0.001	0.450
Carrots, can, low sodium	0.610	0.290	0.103	0.001	0.451
Carrot, raw, whole, scrapd	0.500	0.200	0.047	0.003	0.142
Cauliflower, raw, boiled, drained	0.419	0.242	0.090	0.001	0.177
Celery, pascal, raw, stalk	0.400	0.130	0.035	0.000	0.035
Corn, sweet, can, drained	0.861	0.390	0.058	0.001	0.173
Corn, sweet, can, low sodium	0.350	0.359	0.056	0.000	0.033
Cucumber, raw, sliced	0.280	0.230	0.040	0.001	0.061
Peas, green, can, drained	0.953	0.712	0.082	0.001	0.303
Peas, green, can, low sodium	0.953	0.712	0.082	0.001	0.303
Tomato, raw, red, ripe	0.450	0.089	0.074	0.001	0.105
Tomato, red, can, stewed	0.729	0.170	0.112	0.001	0.059
Tomato, can, low sodium, diet	0.608	0.160	0.110	0.001	—
Potato, boiled, peeled before cooked	0.310	0.270	0.167	0.001	0.140
Noodles, egg, enriched, cooked	0.875	—	0.169	0.059	—
Rice, white, parboiled, cooked	1.126	0.310	0.094	0.020	0.260
Fruits					
Apples, raw, unpeeled	0.181	0.036	0.041	0.001	0.045
Apple, raw, peeled	0.070	0.039	0.031	0.001	0.023
Applesauce, can, unsweetened	0.119	0.030	0.026	0.000	0.075
Apricots, can, light syrup	0.391	0.107	0.079	0.000	0.052
Bananas, raw, peeled	0.307	0.160	0.104	0.001	0.152
Blueberries, raw	0.170	0.110	0.061	0.001	0.282
Cherries, sweet, can/juice	0.580	0.100	0.073	0.000	0.061
Grapefruit, red/pnk/wht, raw	0.087	0.070	0.047	—	0.012
Oranges, raw, all varieties	0.100	0.069	0.045	0.002	0.025
Peaches, raw, whole	0.110	0.140	0.068	0.001	0.047
Peaches, can, light syrup	0.359	0.088	0.052	—	0.046
Pears, raw, Bartlet, unpeeled	0.250	0.120	0.113	0.001	0.076
Pineapple, can/juice	0.280	0.100	0.086	0.001	1.120
Strawberries, raw, whole	0.380	0.130	0.049	0.001	0.290

*Values for five trace elements have been provided in this table. Other trace elements have been analyzed and can be found in the following article by Hunt and Mullen: Concentration of boron and other elements in human foods and personal-care products, J. Am. Diet Assoc., *91*:558–568, 1991. These authors report the analyzed concentrations of boron and molybdenum, as well as of calcium, copper, iron, magnesium, and manganese in selected foods and personal-care products (analgesics, antibiotics, decongestants, antihistamines, dental hygiene products, gastric antacids, and laxatives). For those interested in obtaining data on these nutrients, this article may serve as a helpful reference.

Fe = iron, Zn = zinc, Cu = copper, Se = selenium, Mn = manganese.

— denotes Lack of reliable data for nutrient known to be present.

(Created on Nutritionist III, Version 7, N-Squared Computing, 1991. Data compiled from U.S. Department of Agriculture Handbook 8- Series, manufacturers' data, published journals, and industry sources. Appreciation expressed to Ms. Lori Cohen, M.S., R.D., for her assistance in preparing this table.)

TABLE A–23A. STANDARD EXCHANGE LISTS*,†

The reason for dividing food into six different groups is that foods vary in their carbohydrate, protein, fat, and calorie content. Each exchange list contains foods that are alike; each choice contains about the same amount of carbohydrate, protein, fat, and calories.

The following chart shows the amount of these nutrients in one serving from each exchange list.

Exchange List	*Carbohydrate (g)*	*Protein (g)*	*Fat (g)*	*Calories*
Starch/bread	15	3	trace	80
Meat (lean)	—	7	3	55
(medium-fat)	—	7	5	75
(high-fat)	—	7	8	100
Vegetable	5	2	—	25
Fruit	15	—	—	60
Milk (skim)	12	8	trace	90
(low-fat)	12	8	5	120
(whole)	12	8	8	150
Fat	—	—	5	45

As you read the exchange lists, you will notice that one choice often is a larger amount of food than another choice from the same list. Because foods are so different, each food is measured or weighed so the amount of carbohydrate, protein, fat, and calories is the same in each choice.

*The exchange lists are based on material in the *Exchange Lists for Meal Planning* prepared by Committees of the American Diabetes Association, Inc., and the American Dietetic Association in cooperation with the National Institute of Arthritis, Metabolism, and Digestive Diseases and the National Heart and Lung Institutes of Health, Public Health Service, U.S. Department of Health and Human Services.

†From the American Diabetes Assoc., 1986, with permission.

TABLE A—23A. CONTINUED

STARCH/BREAD LIST

Each item in this list contains about 15 g of carbohydrate, 3 g of protein, a trace of fat, and 80 calories.

Whole-grain products average about 2 g of fiber per serving. Some foods are higher in fiber. Those foods that contain 3 or more g of fiber per serving are identified with the fiber symbol.†

You can choose your starch servings from any of the items on this list. If you want to eat a starch food that is not on this list, the general rule is that:

- ½ cup of cereal, grain, or pasta is one serving
- 1 ounce of a bread product is one serving

Cereals/Grains/Pasta	
Bran cereals†, flaked	½ cup
Bran cereals†, concentrated (such as Bran Buds, All Bran	⅓ cup
Puffed cereal	1½ cup
Grapenuts	3 Tbsp
Shredded wheat	½ cup
Other ready-to-eat unsweetened cereals	¾ cup
Cooked cereals	½ cup
Bulgur (cooked)	½ cup
Grits (cooked)	½ cup
Pasta (cooked)	½ cup
Rice, white or brown (cooked)	⅓ cup
Cornmeal (dry)	2½ Tbsp
Wheat germ†	3 Tbsp
Dried Beans, Peas/Lentils	
Beans† and peas† (cooked), e.g., kidney, white, split, blackeye	⅓ cup
Lentils† (cooked)	⅓ cup
Baked beans†	¼ cup
Starchy Vegetables	
Corn†	½ cup
Corn on cob†, 6″ long	1
Lima beans†	½ cup
Peas, green† (canned or frozen)	½ cup
Plantain†	½ cup
Potato, baked	1 small (3 oz)
Potato, mashed	½ cup
Squash, winter† (acorn, butternut)	¾ cup
Yam, sweet potato, plain	⅓ cup
Bread	
Whole wheat	1 slice (1 oz)
Pita, 6″ across	½
Raisin, unfrosted	1 slice (1 oz)
Rye†, pumpernickel†	1 slice (1 oz)
White (including French, Italian)	1 slice (1 oz)
Bagel	½ (1 oz)
Bread sticks, crisp, 4″ long × ½″	2 (⅔ oz)
Croutons, low-fat	1 cup
English muffin	½
Plain roll, small	1 (1 oz)
Frankfurter or hamburger bun	½ (1 oz)
Tortilla, 6″ across	1
Crackers/ Snacks	
Animal crackers	8
Graham crackers, 2½″ square	3
Matzoth	¾ oz
Melba toast	5 slices
Oyster crackers	24
Popcorn (popped, no fat added)	3 cups
Pretzels	¾ oz
Rye crisp, 2″ × 3½″	4
Saltine-type crackers	6
Whole-wheat crackers, no fat added (crispbreads, such as Finn, Kavli, Wasa)	2–4 slices (¾ oz)
Starch Foods Prepared With Fat (Count as 1 starch/bread serving plus 1 fat serving)	
Biscuit, 2½″ across	1
Chow mein noodles	½ cup
Cornbread, 2″ cube	1 (2 oz)
Cracker, round butter type	6
French fried potatoes, 2″ to 3½″ long	10 (1½ oz)
Muffin, plain, small	1
Pancake, 4″ across	2
Waffle, 4½″ square	1
Stuffing, bread (prepared)	¼ cup
Taco shell, 6″ across	2
Whole-wheat crackers, fat added (such as Triscuits)	4–6 (1 oz)

†3 g or more of fiber per serving.

TABLE A—23A. CONTINUED

MEAT LIST

Each serving of meat and substitutes on this list contains varying amounts of fat and calories. The list is divided into three parts based on the amount of fat and calories: lean meat, medium-fat meat, and high-fat meat. One ounce (one meat exchange) of each of these includes:

	Carbohydrate (g)	*Protein (g)*	*Fat (g)*	*Calories*
Lean	0	7	3	55
Medium-fat	0	7	5	75
High-fat	0	7	8	100

You are encouraged to use more lean and medium-fat meat, poultry, and fish in your meal plan. This will help decrease your fat intake, which may help decrease your risk for heart disease. The items from the high-fat group are high in saturated fat, cholesterol, and calories. You should limit your choices from the high-fat group to three (3) times per week. Meat and substitutes do not contribute any fiber to your meal plan. Meat and meat substitutes that have 400 mg or more of sodium are identified with a § symbol.

Tips:

1. Bake, roast, broil, grill, or boil these foods rather than frying them with added fat.
2. Use a nonstick pan spray or a nonstick pan to brown or fry these foods.
3. Trim off visible fat before and after cooking.
4. Do not add flour, bread crumbs, coating mixes, or fat to these foods when preparing them.
5. Weigh meat after removing bones and fat, and after cooking. Three ounces of cooked meat is about equal to 4 ounces of raw meat. Some examples of meat portions are:

   2 oz meat (2 meat exchanges) = 1 small chicken leg or thigh
   ½ cup cottage cheese or tuna

   3 oz meat (3 meat exchanges) = 1 medium pork chop
   1 small hamburger
   ½ chicken breast (1 side)
   1 unbreaded fish fillet
   cooked meat, about the size of a deck of cards
6. Restaurants usually serve prime cuts of meat, which are high in fat and calories.

Lean Meat and Substitutes

(One exchange is equal to any one of the following items)

Beef:	USDA Good or Choice grades of lean beef, such as round, sirloin, and flank steak, tenderloin, and chipped beef§	1 oz
Pork:	Lean pork, such as fresh ham; canned, cured, or boiled ham; Canadian bacon§, tenderloin	1 oz
Veal:	All cuts are lean except for veal cutlets (ground or cubed). Examples of lean veal are chops and roasts.	1 oz
Poultry:	Chicken, turkey, Cornish hen (without skin)	1 oz
Fish:	All fresh and frozen fish	1 oz
	Crab, lobster, scallops, shrimp, clams (fresh, or canned in water§)	2 oz
	Oysters	6 medium
	Tuna§ (canned in water)	¼ cup
	Herring (uncreamed or smoked)	1 oz
	Sardines (canned)	2 medium
Wild Game:	Venison, rabbit, squirrel	1 oz
	Pheasant, duck, goose (without skin)	1 oz
Cheese:	Any cottage cheese	¼ cup
	Grated Parmesan	2 Tbsp
	Diet cheese§ with less than 55 calories per oz	1 oz
Other:	95% fat-free luncheon meat§	1 oz
	Egg whites	3 whites
	Egg substitutes with less than 55 calories per ¼ cup	¼ cup

TABLE A–23A. CONTINUED

Medium-Fat Meat and Substitutes		
(One exchange is equal to any one of the following items)		
Beef:	Most beef products fall into this category. Examples are all ground beef, roast (rib, chuck, rump), steak (cubed, Porterhouse, T-bone), and meatloaf	1 oz
Pork:	Most pork products fall into this category. Examples are chops, loin roast. Boston butt, cutlets	1 oz
Lamb:	Most lamb products fall into this category. Examples are chops, leg, and roast	1 oz
Veal:	Cutlet (ground or cubed, unbreaded)	1 oz
Poultry:	Chicken (with skin), domestic duck or goose (well-drained of fat), ground turkey	1 oz
Fish:	Tuna§ (canned in oil and drained), salmon§ (canned)	¼ cup
Cheese:	Skim or part-skim milk cheeses, such as	
	Ricotta	¼ cup
	Mozzarella	1 oz
	Diet cheeses§ with 56–80 calories per oz	1 oz
Other:	86% fat-free luncheon meat§	1 oz
	Egg (high in cholesterol, limit to 3 per week)	1
	Egg substitutes with 56–80 calories per ¼ cup	¼ cup
	Tofu (2½″ × 2¾″ × 1″)	4 oz
	Liver, heart, kidney, sweetbreads (high in cholesterol)	1 oz
High-Fat Meat and Substitutes		
Remember, these items are high in saturated fat, cholesterol, and calories, and should be used only three (3) times per week.		
(One exchange is equal to any one of the following items)		
Beef:	Most USDA Prime cuts of beef, such as ribs, corned beef§	1 oz
Pork:	Spareribs, ground pork, pork sausage§ (patty or link)	1 oz
Lamb:	Patties (ground lamb)	1 oz
Fish:	Any fried fish product	1 oz
Cheese:	All regular cheese,§ such as American, Blue, Cheddar, Monterey, Swiss	1 oz
Other:	Luncheon meat,§ such as bologna, salami, pimento loaf	1 oz
	Sausage,§ such as Polish, Italian, knockwurst, smoked	1 oz
	Bratwurst§	1 oz
	Frankfurter§ (turkey or chicken)††	1 frank (10/lb)
	Peanut butter (contains unsaturated fat)	1 Tbsp

§400 mg or more of sodium per exchange.
††Frankfurter (beef, pork or combination). Count as one high-fat meat plus one fat exchange: 1 frank (10/lb).

TABLE A–23A. CONTINUED

VEGETABLE LIST

Each vegetable serving on this list contains about 5 g of carbohydrate, 2 g of protein, and 25 calories. Vegetables contain 2–3 g of dietary fiber. Vegetables that contain 400 mg or more of sodium per serving are identified with a § symbol.

Vegetables are a good source of vitamins and minerals. Fresh and frozen vegetables have more vitamins and less added salt. Rinsing canned vegetables will remove much of the salt.

Unless otherwise noted, the serving size for vegetables is:

- ½ cup of cooked vegetables or vegetable juice
- 1 cup of raw vegetables

Artichoke (½ medium)	Eggplant	Rutabaga
Asparagus	Greens (collard, mustard, turnip)	Sauerkraut§
Beans (green, wax, Italian)	Kohlrabi	Spinach, cooked
Bean sprouts	Leeks	Summer squash (crookneck)
Beets	Mushrooms, cooked	Tomato (1 large)
Broccoli	Okra	Tomato/vegetable juice§
Brussels sprouts	Onions	Turnips
Cabbage, cooked	Pea pods	Water chestnuts
Carrots	Peppers (green)	Zucchini, cooked
Cauliflower		

Starchy vegetables, such as corn, peas, and potatoes, are found on the Starch/Bread list.

For free vegetables, see Free Food list.

FRUIT LIST

Each item on this list contains about 15 g of carbohydrate and 60 calories. Fresh, frozen, and dry fruits have about 2 g of fiber per serving. Fruits that have 3 g or more of fiber per serving have a † symbol. Fruit juices contain very little dietary fiber.

The carbohydrate and calorie contents for a fruit serving are based on the usual serving of the most commonly eaten fruits. Use fresh fruits, or fruits frozen or canned without sugar added. Whole fruit is more filling than fruit juice, and may be a better choice for those who are trying to lose weight. Unless otherwise noted, the serving size for fruit is:

- ½ cup of fresh fruit or fruit juice
- ¼ cup of dried fruit

Fresh, frozen, and unsweetened canned fruit

Apple (raw, 2″ across)	1 apple
Applesauce (unsweetened)	½ cup
Apricots (medium, raw)	4 apricots
Apricots (canned)	½ cup, or 4 halves
Banana (9″ long)	½ banana
†Blackberries (raw)	¾ cup
†Blueberries (raw)	¾ cup
Cantaloupe (5″ across)	⅓ melon
(cubes)	1 cup
Cherries (large, sweet, raw)	12 cherries
Cherries (canned)	½ cup
Figs (raw, 2″ across)	2 figs
Fruit cocktail (canned)	½ cup
Grapefruit (medium)	½ grapefruit
Grapefruit (segments)	¾ cup
Grapes (small)	15 grapes
Honeydew melon (medium)	⅛ melon
(cubes)	1 cup
Kiwi (large)	1 kiwi
Mandarin oranges	¾ cup
Mango (small)	½ mango
†Nectarine (1½″ across)	1 nectarine
Orange (2½″ across)	1 orange
Papaya	1 cup
Peach (2¾″ across)	1 peach, or ¾ cup
Peaches (canned)	½ cup, or 2 halves
Pear	½ large, 1 small
Pears (canned)	½ cup, or 2 halves
Persimmon (medium, native)	2 persimmons
Pineapple (raw)	¾ cup
Pineapple (canned)	⅓ cup
Plum (raw, 2″ across)	2 plums
†Pomegranate	½ pomegranate
†Raspberries (raw)	1 cup
†Strawberries (raw, whole)	1¼ cup
†Tangerine (2½″ across)	2 tangerines
Watermelon (cubes)	1¼ cup

Dried Fruit

†Apples	4 rings
†Apricots	7 halves
Dates	2½ medium
†Figs	1½
†Prunes	3 medium
Raisins	2 Tbsp

Fruit Juice

Apple juice/cider	½ cup
Cranberry juice cocktail	⅓ cup
Grapefruit juice	½ cup
Grape juice	⅓ cup
Orange juice	½ cup
Pineapple juice	½ cup
Prune juice	⅓ cup

§400 mg or more of sodium per serving.
†3 g or more of fiber per serving.

TABLE A–23A. CONTINUED

MILK LIST

Each serving of milk or milk products on this list contains about 12 g of carbohydrate and 8 g of protein. The amount of fat in milk is measured in percent (%) of butterfat. The calories vary, depending on what kind of milk you choose. The list is divided into three parts based on the amount of fat and calories: skim/very low-fat milk, low-fat milk, and whole milk. One serving (one milk exchange) of each of these includes:

	Carbohydrate (g)	*Protein (g)*	*Fat (g)*	*Calories*
Skim/Very low-fat	12	8	trace	90
Low-fat	12	8	5	120
Whole	12	8	8	150

Milk is the body's main source of calcium, the mineral needed for growth and repair of bones. Yogurt is also a good source of calcium. Yogurt and many dry or powdered milk products have different amounts of fat. If you have questions about a particular item, read the label to find out the fat and calorie content.

Milk is good to drink, but it can also be added to cereal and to other foods. Many tasty dishes, such as sugar-free pudding, are made with milk (see the Combination Foods list). Plain yogurt is delicious with one of your fruit servings mixed with it.

Skim and Very Low-fat Milk

- 1 cup skim milk
- 1 cup ½% milk
- 1 cup 1% milk
- 1 cup low-fat buttermilk
- ½ cup evaporated skim milk
- ⅓ cup dry nonfat milk
- 8-oz carton plain nonfat yogurt

Low-Fat Milk

- 1 cup fluid 2% milk
- 8-oz carton plain low-fat yogurt (with added nonfat milk solids)

Whole Milk

The whole milk group has much more fat per serving than the skim and low-fat groups. Whole milk has more than 3¼% butterfat. Try to limit your choices from the whole milk group as much as possible.

- 1 cup whole milk
- ½ cup evaporated whole milk
- 8-oz carton whole plain yogurt

FAT LIST

Each serving on the fat list contains about 5 g of fat and 45 calories.

The foods on the fat list contain mostly fat, although some items may also contain a small amount of protein. All fats are high in calories and should be carefully measured. Everyone should modify their fat intake by eating unsaturated fats instead of saturated fats. The sodium content of these foods varies widely. Check the label for sodium information.

Unsaturated Fats

Avocado	⅛ medium
Margarine	1 tsp
Margarine, diet#	1 Tbsp
Mayonnaise	1 tsp
Mayonnaise, reduced-calorie#	1 Tbsp
Nuts and seeds:	
Almonds, dry roasted	6 whole
Cashews, dry roasted	1 Tbsp
Pecans	2 whole
Peanuts	20 small, 10 large
Walnuts	2 whole
Other nuts	1 Tbsp
Seeds, pine nuts, sunflower (without shells)	1 Tbsp
Pumpkin seeds	2 tsp
Oil (corn, cottonseed, safflower, soybean, sunflower, olive, peanut)	1 tsp
Olives#	10 small, 5 large
Salad dressing, mayonnaise-type	2 tsp
Salad dressing, mayonnaise-type, reduced-calorie	1 Tbsp
Salad dressing (all varieties)#	1 Tbsp
Salad dressing, reduced-calorie (2 Tbsp of low-calorie is a free food)§	2 Tbsp

Saturated Fats

Butter	1 tsp
Bacon	1 slice
Chitterlings	½ oz
Coconut, shredded	2 Tbsp
Coffee whitener, liquid	2 Tbsp
Coffee whitener, powder	4 tsp
Cream (light, coffee, table)	2 Tbsp
Cream, sour	2 Tbsp
Cream (heavy, whipping)	1 Tbsp
Cream cheese	1 Tbsp
Salt pork	¼ oz

#If more than one or two servings are eaten, foods have 400 mg or more of sodium.
§400 mg or more of sodium per serving.

TABLE A—23A. CONTINUED

FREE FOODS

A free food is any food or drink that contains 20 calories or less per serving. You can eat as much as you want of those items that have no serving size specified. You may eat 2 or 3 servings per day of those items that have a specific serving size. Be sure to spread them out through the day.

Drinks	*Vegetables (raw, 1 cup)*	*Sweet Substitutes*
Bouillon§ or broth without fat†	Cabbage	Candy, hard, sugar-free
Bouillon, low-sodium	Celery	Gelatin, sugar-free
Carbonated drinks, sugar-free	Chinese cabbage†	Gum, sugar-free
Carbonated water	Cucumber	Jam/jelly, sugar-free (2 tsp)
Club soda	Green onion	Pancake syrup, sugar-free (¼ cup)
Cocoa powder, unsweetened (1 Tbsp)	Hot peppers	Sugar substitutes (saccharin, Equal)
Coffee/Tea	Mushrooms	Whipped topping, low calorie
Drink mixes, sugar-free	Radishes	*Condiments*
Mineral water	Zucchini†	Catsup (1 Tbsp)
Tonic water, sugar-free	Salad greens	Horseradish
	Endive	Mustard
Nonstick pan spray	Escarole	Pickles§, dill, unsweetened
Fruit	Lettuce	Salad dressing, low-calorie (2 Tbsp)
Cranberries, unsweetened (½ cup)	Romaine	Taco sauce (1 Tbsp)
Rhubarb, unsweetened (½ cup)	Spinach	Vinegar

Seasonings can be very helpful in making food taste better. Be careful of how much sodium you use. Read the label and choose those seasonings that do not contain sodium or salt.

Basil (fresh)	Garlic	Onion powder
Celery seeds	Garlic powder	Oregano
Cinnamon	Herbs	Paprika
Chili powder	Hot pepper sauce	Pepper
Chives	Lemon	Pimento
Curry	lemon juice	Spices
Dill	Lemon pepper	Soy sauce§
Flavoring extracts (e.g., vanilla, lemon, almond, walnut, peppermint, butter)	Lime	Soy sauce, low-sodium
	Lime juice	Wine, used in cooking (¼ cup)
	Mint	Worcestershire sauce

COMBINATION FOODS

Much of the food we eat is mixed together in various combinations. These combination foods do not fit into only one exchange list. It can be difficult to tell what is in a certain casserole dish or baked food item. This is a list of average values for some typical combination foods. This list will help you fit these foods into your meal plan. Ask your dietitian for information about any other foods you would like to eat. The *American Diabetes Association/American Dietetic Association Family Cookbooks* and the *American Diabetes Association Holiday Cookbook* have many recipes and further information about many foods, including combination foods. Check your library or local bookstore.

Food	*Amount*	*Exchanges*
Casseroles, homemade	1 cup (8 oz)	2 starch, 2 medium-fat meat, 1 fat
Cheese pizza§ thin crust	¼ of 15 oz or ¼ of 10″	2 starch, 1 medium-fat meat, 1 fat
Chili with beans†§ (commercial)	1 cup (8 oz)	2 starch, 2 medium-fat meat, 2 fat
Chow mein† (without noodles or rice)	2 cups (16 oz)	1 starch, 2 vegetable, 2 lean meat
Macaroni and cheese§	1 cup (8 oz)	2 starch, 1 medium-fat meat, 2 fat
Soup		
Bean†	1 cup (8 oz)	1 starch, 1 vegetable, 1 lean meat
Chunky, all varieties	10¾ oz can	1 starch, 1 vegetable, 1 medium-fat meat
Cream§ (made with water)	1 cup (8 oz)	1 starch, 1 fat
Vegetable§ or broth§	1 cup (8 oz)	1 starch
Spaghetti and meatballs§ (canned)	1 cup (8 oz)	2 starch, 1 medium-fat meat, 1 fat
Sugar-free pudding (made with skim milk)	½ cup	1 starch
If beans are used as a meat substitute:		
Dried beans,† peas,† lentils†	1 cup (cooked)	2 starch, 1 lean meat

†3 g or more of fiber per serving.
§400 mg or more of sodium per serving.

TABLE A–23A. CONTINUED

FOODS FOR OCCASIONAL USE

Moderate amounts of some foods can be used in your meal plan, in spite of their sugar or fat content, as long as you can maintain blood glucose control. The following list includes average exchange values for some of these foods. Because they are concentrated sources of carbohydrate, you will notice that the portion sizes are very small. Check with your dietitian for advice on how often and when you can eat them.

Food	*Amount*	*Exchanges*
Angel food cake	1/12 cake	2 starch
Cake, no icing	1/12 cake, or a 3″ square	2 starch, 2 fat
Cookies	2 small (1 3/4″ across)	1 starch, 1 fat
Frozen fruit yogurt	1/3 cup	1 starch
Gingersnaps	3	1 starch
Granola	1/4 cup	1 starch, 1 fat
Granola bars	1 small	1 starch, 1 fat
Ice cream, any flavor	1/2 cup	1 starch, 2 fat
Ice milk, any flavor	1/2 cup	1 starch, 1 fat
Sherbet, any flavor	1/4 cup	1 starch
Snack chips,§ all varieties	1 oz	1 starch, 2 fat
Vanilla wafers	6 small	1 starch, 1 fat

MANAGEMENT TIPS

Some food you buy uncooked will weigh less after you cook it. This is true of most meats. Starches often swell in cooking, so a small amount of uncooked starch will become a much larger amount of cooked food. The following table shows some of the changes:

Food (Starch Group)	*Uncooked*	*Cooked*
Oatmeal	3 level Tbsp	1/2 cup
Cream of wheat	2 level Tbsp	1/2 cup
Grits	3 level Tbsp	1/2 cup
Rice	2 level Tbsp	1/3 cup
Spaghetti	1/4 cup	1/2 cup
Noodles	1/3 cup	1/2 cup
Macaroni	1/4 cup	1/2 cup
Dried beans	3 Tbsp	1/3 cup
Dried peas	3 Tbsp	1/3 cup
Lentils	2 Tbsp	1/3 cup
Food (Meat Group)		
Hamburger	4 oz	3 oz
Chicken	1 small drumstick	1 oz
	1/2 breast (1 side)	3 oz

- Read food labels. Remember—*dietetic* does not mean *diabetic!* When you see the word "dietetic" on a food label, it means that something has been changed or replaced. It may have less salt, less fat, or less sugar. It does not mean that the food is sugar-free or calorie-free. Some dietetic foods may be useful. Those that contain 20 calories or less per serving may be eaten as many as 3 times a day as free foods.
- Know your sweeteners. Two types of sweeteners are on the market: those with calories and those without calories. Sweeteners with calories, such as fructose, sorbitol, and mannitol, when used in large amounts, may cause cramping and diarrhea. Remember, these sweeteners do have calories that add up. Sweeteners without calories include saccharin and aspartame (Equal, Nutrasweet) and may be used in moderation.

§If more than one serving is eaten, these foods have 400 mg or more of sodium.

TABLE A–23B. DIABETIC EXCHANGES FOR AFRICAN-AMERICAN (SOUTHERN) COOKERY

FOOD EXCHANGE GROUP	FOOD	PORTION	SODIUM CONTENT
Starch/Bread			
(80 calories per exchange)	Biscuit, 2″ diameter	1 (add 2 fat)	262 mg
	Cornbread, 2″ × 2″ × 1″	1 (add 1 fat)	220 mg
	Corn muffin, 2″ diameter	1 (add 1 fat)	250 mg
	Crackling bread, 2″ × 2″ × 1″	1 (add 2 fat)	High
	CooCoo (cornmeal, okra, butter, salt, and water)	(equals 1 veg/1 fat)	High
	Cornmeal	2 Tbsp	Low
	Black-eyed peas	½ cup (add ½ lean meat)	6 mg
	Pinto beans	¼ cup (add ½ lean meat)	2 mg
	Baked beans (no pork)	¼ cup	239 mg
	Grits (instant/cooked)	½ cup	385 mg
	Hoe cake, 2″ × 2″ × 1″	1 (add 2 fat)	Medium
	Hominy (canned)	½ cup	720 mg
	Hoppin john (frozen)	½ cup (add 1 fat, ½ bread)	High
	Hush puppies	2 small pieces (add 2 fats)	High
	Spoon bread	½ cup (add 1 lean meat, 1 fat)	High
	Pound cake, 3½″ × 3″ × ½″	1 (add 2 fat)	Low
	Custard (baked)	½ cup (add 1 lean meat, ½ fat)	Medium
Meat			
Lean Meat (55 calories per ounce)	Chicken gizzard	1 oz	19 mg
	Pork		
	Hog maw, stomach	⅓ cup	30 mg
	Sousemeat	3″ × 2″ × ¼″	High
	Pig ear	1 medium	Low
	Fish		
	Catfish, 4″ × 2″ × ¼″	1	Low
	Mullet, 4″ × 2″ × ¼″	1	Low
	Perch, 4″ × 2″ × ¼″	1	Low
	Snapper, 4″ × 2″ × ¼″	1	Low
	Sardines	3 drained	High
Medium-Fat Meat (75 calories per ounce)	Pork		
	Chipped ham	1 oz	High
	Fresh butt	1 oz	High
	Neck bones	½ cup	High
	Pork cubes (lean)	1 oz	High
	Tongue	1 oz	High
	Organ meats		
	Heart (beef)	1 oz	35 mg
	Kidney	1 oz	71 mg
	Liver (pork)	1 oz	14 mg
	Sweetbreads	1 oz	32 mg
	Fish		
	Eel, American (fresh)	1 oz	25 mg
	Mackerel (fresh)	1 oz	17 mg
High-Fat Meat (100 calories per ounce)	Barbecued ribs	1 oz	High
	Country ham	1 oz	High
	Devild ham (canned)	1 oz	High
	Pork belly (fresh)	1 oz	
	Hock (smoked)	1 oz	
	Pig's feet	1 (equals 2 exchanges)	
	Pork shank	1 oz	
	Pork tail	1 oz	
	Sausage (bulk, patties, link)	1 oz	High
	Pig snout	1 (equals 2 exchanges)	

TABLE A—23B. CONTINUED

FOOD EXCHANGE GROUP	FOOD	PORTION	SODIUM CONTENT
Luncheon Meats (100 calories per ounce)	Bologna	1 oz	High
	Frankfurter (hot dogs)	1 oz	High
	Sausage link (canned or frozen)	1 oz (add 1 fat)	215 mg
	Sausage links (brown and serve)	1 oz (add 1 fat)	High
	Small Vienna sausage	3 (add 1 fat)	High
	Spam	1 oz	High
	Treat	1 oz	High
	Scrapple	1 oz	High
Organ Meats	Brains	¼ cup	70 mg
Combination Meats	Chicken and dumplings	3 oz (equals 2 lean meat, 1 veg, 1 bread, 1 fat)	High
	Chili, 1 cup	(equals 2 medium-fat meat, 2 bread, 2 fat)	High
	Smothered chicken (no skin)	¼ broiler (equals 4 lean meat, ½ bread)	High
	Steamed fish with butter	3 oz (equals 4 lean meat, ½ fat)	Low
Vegetable (25 calories per exchange)	Collard (cooked without fat)	½ cup	25 mg
	Kale (cooked without fat)	½ cup	29 mg
	Mustard (cooked without fat)	½ cup	18 mg
	Turnip (cooked withou fat)	cup	8.5 mg
	Poke salad (cooked without fat)	1 cup	High
	Rape	½ cup (add 2 fat)	High
	Greens (cooked with fat)	½ cup	High
	Okra	8-9 pods	High
	Chickory (raw)	1 cup	6 mg
	Cressie greens (raw)	1 cup	5 mg per 10 sprigs
Fruit (60 calories per exchange)	No additions		
Milk (90 calories per exchange)	Buttermilk (skim milk)	1 cup	257 mg
	Buttermilk (whole milk)	1 cup (omit 2 fat)	250 mg
Fats (Saturated) (45 calories per teaspoon)	Bacon (thick sliced, crisp)	1 strip	High
	Bacon (thin/medium sliced, crisp)	1 strip	High
	Bacon grease	1 tsp	High
	Chitterlings, fried	2 Tbsp	High
	Crackling, pork	1½ tsp	High
	Fat back	¾″ cube	High
	Salt pork	¾″ cube	High
	Slab of bacon, 1″ × 1″ × ¼″	1 slice	High
	Streak o'lean, 1″ × 1″ × ¼″	1 slice	High

(Adapted with permission from The American Diabetes Association, Washington, D.C. Area Affiliate, Inc.: Exchange Lists for Meal Planning: Black American Cookery. 1987.)

TABLE A–23C. SUPPLEMENTARY EXCHANGE LISTS FOR CHINESE-AMERICAN FOODS

FOOD EXCHANGE GROUP	FOOD	PORTION
Starch/Bread	Cellophane or mung bean noodles (cooked)	¾ cup
	Ginkgo seeds	½ cup
	Lotus root, ¼″-thick slice, 2½″ diameter	10 slices
	Mung beans or green gram beans (cooked)	⅓ cup
	Red beans (cooked)	⅓ cup
	Rice congee or soup	¾ cup
	Rice vermicelli or noodles (cooked)	½ cup
	Taro (cooked)	⅓ cup
Meat and Meat Substitutes		
Lean Meat	Beef jerky, 3½″ × 1″*	½ oz
	Dried scallop	1 large
	Dried shrimp	1 Tbsp or 10 medium shrimp
	Soybeans (cooked)	3 Tbsp
	Squid	2 oz
	Tripe (beef)	2 oz
Medium-fat Meat and Substitutes	Beef tongue	1 oz
	Tofu or soybean curd, 2½″ × 2¾″ × 1″†	4 oz or ½ cup
High-fat Meat	Salted duck egg‡§	1
	Thousand-year-old or preserved limed duck egg‡§	1
High-fat Meat + 1 Fat	Chinese sausage (pork and spices and/or liver)*§	1 (2 oz)
Vegetables (½ cup cooked or 1 cup raw unless indicated otherwise)	Amaranth or Chinese spinach (cooked)	
	Arrowheads, or fresh corms (raw), 3½″ diameter	
	Baby corn (canned)*	
	Bamboo shoots	
	Bitter melon or bitter gourd	
	Chayote	
	Chinese celery	
	Chinese eggplant (white or purple)	
	Chinese or black mushroom (dried)	2 medium
	Hairy melon or hairy cucumber	
	Leeks†	
	Luffa (angled or smooth)	
	Mung bean sprouts	
	Mustard greens†	
	Peapods or sugar peas†	
	Soybean sprouts (cooked or raw)	½ cup
	Straw mushrooms	
	Turnip†	
	Water chestnuts (canned)†	½ cup
	Winter melon or wax gourd	
	Yard-long beans	
Fruits	Carambola or star fruit (raw)	2 medium
	Chinese banana (raw)	1 dwarf
	Guava (raw)	1 medium
	Kumquats (raw)	5 medium
	Litchi or lychee (raw)	10
	Litchi or lychee (canned, drained)	½ cup
	Longan (raw)	30
	Longan (canned, drained)	¾ cup
	Mango (raw)†	½ small
	Papaya (raw), 3½″ diameter, 5⅛″ hight†	½
	Persimmon, Japanese (soft type) (raw)	½
	Pummelo (raw)	¾ cup
Milk	Soybean milk (unsweetened)	1 cup
Fats	Coconut milk	1 Tbsp
	Sesame paste	1½ tsp
	Sesame seeds (whole, dried)	1 Tbsp

TABLE A–23C. CONTINUED

FOOD EXCHANGE GROUP	FOOD	PORTION
Free Foods	Amaranth or Chinese spinach	
	Bok choy	
	Chili pepper (raw)†	1
	Chinese or Peking cabbage†	
	Choy sum or Chinese flowering cabbage	
	Coriander	
	Garland chrysanthemum	
	Ginger	¼ cup
	Mustard greens (salted and soured)	2 Tbsp
	Oriental radish or daikon	
	Watercress	
Combination	Mock duck or wheat gluten (canned)	½ cup (equals ½ starch/bread, 1 lean meat)

*400 mg or more of sodium per serving.
†Foods are included in *Exchange Lists for Meal Planning,* 1986. © American Diabetes Association and The American Dietetic Association.
‡Probably 400 mg or more of sodium per serving, based on author's estimate.
§Limit high-fat meat choices to 3 times per week.
(From The American Dietetic Association and The American Diabetes Association, Inc.: Ethnic and Regional Food Practices: A Series. Chinese Food Practices, Customs and Holidays. 1990. With permission.)

TABLE A–23D. SUPPLEMENTARY EXCHANGE LISTS FOR HMONG-AMERICAN FOODS

FOOD EXCHANGE GROUP	FOOD	PORTION
Starch/Bread	Cellophane or mung bean noodles (cooked)	¾ cup
	Rice vermicelli or noodles (cooked)	½ cup
	Rice soup	¾ cup
Meat and Meat Substitutes		
Lean Meat	Pheasant†	1 oz
	Squirrel†	1 oz
	Venison†	1 oz
Medium-fat Meat and Substitutes	Pig's feet	2½ oz (equals 2 exchanges)
	Tofu or soybean curd, 2½″ × 2¾″ × 1″	4 oz or ½ cup
High-fat Meat	Ground pork†‡	1 oz
Vegetables (½ cup cooked or 1 cup raw unless indicated otherwise)	Bamboo shoots	
	Bitter melon or bitter gourd	
	Chinese onion (leeks†)	
	Cucuzzi squash (spaghetti squash)	
	Luffa gourd/squash	
	Mustard greens†	
	Mung bean sprouts	
	Pumpkin	
	Sugar peas, snow peas, sweet peas, peapods†	
	Yard-long beans, pod and seeds	½ cup
Fruits	Apple pear, Asian pear (raw), 2¼″ high, 2½″ diameter	1
	Guava (raw)	1½ medium
	Jackfruit (raw)	½ cup
	Mango (raw)†	½ small
	Papaya (raw), 5⅛″ high, 3½″ diameter†	½ or 1 cup
Fats	Beef fat	1 tsp
	Chicken fat	1 tsp
	Coconut cream or milk	1 Tbsp
	Coconut (raw)†	2 Tbsp
	Pork lard	1 tsp
	Pork intestine, chitterlings†	½ oz
Free Foods	Fish sauce*	
	Pumpkin or squash blossom	
	Soy sauce*†	
	Tender vines and leaves of pumpkin, squash, luffa gourd, and pea plants	
Occasional Foods	Condensed milk, sweetened	1 oz (equals 1½ starch/bread)

*400 mg or more of sodium per serving.

†Foods are included in *Exchange Lists for Meal Planning,* 1986. © American Diabetes Association and The American Dietetic Association.

‡Limit high-fat meat choice to 3 times per week.

(From The American Dietetic Association and The American Diabetes Association, Inc.: Ethnic and Regional Food Practices, a Series. Hmong Food Practices, Customs and Holidays. 1992. With permission.)

TABLE A–23E. DIABETIC EXCHANGES FOR AN INDIAN DIET

FOOD EXCHANGE GROUP	FOOD	PORTION
Starch/Bread	Arrowroot flour (uncooked)	2 Tbsp
	Barley (uncooked)	1½ Tbsp
	Colacassia (cooked)	¼ cup
	Indian breads*	
	Chapati, 5″–6″ diameter	1 medium
	Dosa, 5″–6″ diameter	1 medium
	Idli, 2½″–3″ diameter	1 medium
	Puri, 5″ diameter	1 large (omit 2½ fat)
	Phulka, 5″ to 6″ diameter	1 medium
	Phoa (rice flakes, Indian style) (uncooked)	3 Tbsp
	Plantain (raw)	½ medium
	Rice flour (uncooked)	2 Tbsp
	Sago (uncooked)	1¼ Tbsp
	Suji (cream of wheat) (uncooked)	2 Tbsp
	Upma (plain without vegetable) (cooked)	½ cup
	Vermicelli (thinner than very thin spaghetti) (uncooked)	½ cup
	Whole-wheat flour	2½ Tbsp
Meat and Meat Substitutes		
Lean Meat and Substitutes (omit 1 starch/bread for each)	Bengal gram dhal (Chana, whole, split) (uncooked)	2 Tbsp
	Bengal gram dhal (roasted) (uncooked)	3 Tbsp
	Black gram dhal (Urad dhal) (uncooked)	2 Tbsp
	Green gram dhal (Mung dhal) (uncooked)	2 Tbsp
	Masur dhal (uncooked)	2 Tbsp
	Toordhal (uncooked)	2 Tbsp
	Besan (chick pea flour) (uncooked)	3 Tbsp
High-Fat Meat and Substitute	Pannir (cheese) made with whole milk	¼ cup
Vegetables (½ cup cooked or 1 cup raw unless indicated otherwise)	Ashgourd (cooked)	
	Bitter gourd (cooked)	
	Bottle gourd (cooked)	1⅓ cup
	Chow-chow (cooked)	
	Cluster beans (cooked)	
	Drumstick (cooked)	
	Fenugreek leaves (cooked)	
	Ladies fingers (cooked) (okra)	
	Ridge gourd (cooked)	
	White radish (cooked)	
Fruits	Guava (fresh)	½ cup
Milk	Curds (yogurt) made from skim milk (plain)	1 cup
Fats	Coconut (grated) (unsweetened)	2 Tbsp
	Coconut chutney	2 Tbsp
	Coconut oil	1 tsp
	Ghee (clarified butter)	1 tsp
	Mustard oil	1 tsp
	Sesame oil	1 tsp

*Exchange values for Indian breads from *Diabetic Diet,* Dietetic Department, Christian Medical College and Hospital, Vellore, India.

(Adapted with permission from The American Diabetes Association, Washington, D.C. Area Affiliate, Inc.: Supplement to Exchange Lists for Meal Planning: Indian Cookery.)

TABLE A–23F. SUPPLEMENTARY EXCHANGE LISTS FOR EASTERN EUROPEAN (JEWISH) FOODS*

FOOD EXCHANGE GROUP	FOOD	PORTION
Starch/Bread	Bagel† or bialy	½ small, 1 oz
	Bulgur (cooked)†	½ cup
	Bulke	½ medium
	Farfel (dry)	½ cup
	Hallah	1 slice, 1 oz
	Kasha (cooked)	½ cup
	Kasha (raw)	2 Tbsp
	Lentils†	⅓ cup
	Matzoh†	¾ oz
	Matzoh meal	2½ Tbsp
	Potato starch (flour)	2 Tbsp
	Pumpernickel bread†	1 slice, 1 oz
	Rye bread†	1 slice, 1 oz
	Split peas†	⅓ cup
Starch/Bread Prepared with Fat	Matzoh ball‡	3 balls, 1½ oz (equals 1 starch/bread + 1 fat)
	Potato pancake	½ pancake (equals 1 starch/bread + 1 fat)
Meat		
Lean meat	Flanken†	1 oz
	Gefilte fish	2 oz
	Herring† (smoked, uncreamed)	1 oz
	Lox†	1 oz
	Sardines† (canned, drained)	2 medium
	Smelts	1 oz
Medium-fat meat	Beef tongue	1 oz
	Brisket	1 oz
	Chopped liver§	¼ cup
	Corned beef†	1 oz
	Sablefish (smoked)	1 oz
	Salmon† (canned)	¼ cup
High-fat meat	Pastrami	1 oz
Vegetables	Borscht (no sugar or sour cream)	½ cup
	Sorrel	½ cup
Fats	Cream cheese†	1 Tbsp
	Nondairy creamer† (liquid)	2 Tbsp
	Nondairy creamer† (powder)	4 tsp
	Schmaltz	1 tsp
	Sour cream†	2 Tbsp
Free Foods (in reasonable amounts)	Horseradish†	
	Pickles, dill†	
Occasional Foods	Sweet kosher wine	½ cup (equals 2 fat)

*Unless otherwise specified, all foods are 1 exchange.

†Foods are included on the American Diabetes Association and American Dietetic Association *Exchange Lists for Meal Planning.* 1986. © American Diabetes Association and The American Dietetic Association.

‡High in sodium.

§No additional salt in recipe.

(From The American Dietetic Association and The American Diabetes Association, Inc. Ethnic and Regional Food Practices, a Series. Jewish Food Practices, Customs and Holidays, 1989. With permission.)

TABLE A—23G. SUPPLEMENTARY EXCHANGE LISTS FOR MEXICAN-AMERICAN FOODS*

FOOD EXCHANGE GROUP	FOOD	PORTION
Starch/Bread	Bolillo (French roll), 4½" to 5" long	¼
	Frijoles cocidos† (cooked beans)	⅓ cup
	Frijoles cocidos	1 cup (equals 2 starch/bread + 1 lean meat)
	Frijoles refritos (refried beans) (no fat added)	⅓ cup
	Tortilla, corn, 7½" across (ready to bake)‡	1
	Tortilla, flour, 7" across (ready to bake)‡	1 (equals 1½ starch/bread)
	Tortilla, flour, 9" across (ready to bake)‡	⅓
Starch/Bread Prepared with Fat	Frijoles refritos (fat added)	⅓ cup (equals 1 starch/bread + 1 fat)
	Taco shell, 5" across (ready to use)	2 (equals 1 starch/bread + 1 fat)
	Tortilla, flour, 7" across (fried with added fat)	1 (equals 1½ starch/bread + 1 fat)
	Tortilla, corn, 7½" across (fried with added fat)	1 (equals 1 starch/bread + 1 fat)
	Tortilla, flour, 9" across (fried with added fat)	1 (equals 3 starch/bread + 2 fat)
Meat		
Lean meat	Menudo (tripe soup)	½ cup
Medium-fat meat	Queso fresco (cheese made with skim milk)	¼ cup (2 oz)
High-fat meat	Chorizo (Mexican sausage)	1 oz (equals 1 high-fat meat + 1 fat)
Vegetables	Chayote (squash) (cooked)	½ cup
	Jícama (yambean root) (raw)	½ cup
	Nopales (cactus) (raw)	½ cup
Fruits	Mango†	½ small
	Papaya†	1 cup
Fats	Avocado†	⅛ medium
Free Foods	Jalapeño chilis	
	Salsa de chile (chili/taco sauce)	
	Verdolagas (purslane)	
Occasional Foods	Pan dulce (sweet bread), 4½" across	1 (equals 4 starch/bread + 1 fat)

*Unless otherwise specified, all foods are 1 exchange.

†Food and amount are same as in 1986 *Exchange Lists for Meal Planning.* © American Diabetes Association, Inc., The American Dietetic Association.

‡Food, amount, or both differ from 1986 *Exchange Lists for Meal Planning* because of new information.

(From The American Dietetic Association and The American Diabetes Association, Inc. Ethnic and Regional Food Practices, a Series. Mexican Food Practices, Customs and Holidays, 1989. With permission.)

TABLE A—23H. SUPPLEMENTARY EXCHANGE LISTS FOR TRADITIONAL NAVAJO FOODS*

FOOD EXCHANGE GROUP	FOOD	PORTION
Starch/Bread	Blue corn mush	¾ cup
	Flour tortilla, 8" diameter	¼
	Steamed corn hominy (cooked)	½ cup
Meat		
Lean meat	Mutton, flesh (lean only) (cooked without added fat)	1 oz
High-fat meat	Mutton, flesh (lean and fat) (cooked without added fat)	1 oz
Fats	Piñon nuts	1 Tbsp (about 25 nuts)

*Nutrition practitioners who work with Navajo clients with noninsulin-dependent diabetes mellitus do not often use the Exchange system in client education sessions. This listing is presented for the few occasions when supplementary Exchange values may be needed.

(From The American Dietetic Association and The American Diabetes Association, Inc. Ethnic and Regional Food Practices, a Series. Navajo Food Practices, Customs and Holidays, 1991. With permission.)

TABLE A—231. DIABETIC EXCHANGES FOR A GENERAL ASIAN-AMERICAN DIET

FOOD EXCHANGE GROUP	FOOD	PORTION
Starch/Bread	Arrowroot	3 small
	Arrowroot starch	2 Tbsp
	Cellophane noodles (cooked)	½ cup
	Chestnuts (shelled)	¼ cup
	Chowmein noodles	½ cup (omit 1 fat)
	Congee (rice soup)*	1 cup
	Cornstarch*	2 Tbsp
	Fungi (woodears) (dried)	1 oz (omit 1 Fruit)
	Gingko seeds (dried)	1½ oz
	Glutinous rice, (cooked)*	¼ cup
	Glutinous rice flour*	1 Tbsp
	Lanka (jackfruit)	⅓ cup
	Lotus root	⅔ segment
	Lotus seeds (dried)	1 oz
	Millet	1 oz (omit ½ Bread)
	Mung bean noodles	½ cup
	Rice noodles (sticks)	
	Cooked	½ cup
	Dry	1 oz
	Tamarind	1 oz
	Tapioca pearles (dry)	1 Tbsp
	Taro (dasheen)	¼ cup
Meat and Meat Substitutes		
Lean Meat and Substitutes	Dried beans and peas (cooked)	½ cup (omit 1 Bread)
	Black-eyed peas	
	Broad beans (horse beans)	
	Garbanzo	
	Kidney	
	Lentils	
	Lima	
	Mung	
	Navy	
	Pinto	
	Abalone	1 oz
	Chicken wings	1 wing
	Dried duck feet	½ oz
	Gefilte fish	1 oz
	Octopus	1¾ oz
	Shrimp (dried)	½ oz
	Squid (calamares)	1¾ oz
Medium-Fat Meat and Substitutes	Bean curd cheese	2 oz
	Fishmaw (fish stomach)	2 oz
	Oxtail	1 oz
	Soybeans (cooked)	⅓ cup
	Tofu (soybean curd) 2½″ × 2¾″ × 1″	1 portion
High-Fat Meat and Substitutes	Anchovies	10
	Chinese sausage	1 oz
	Eel	1 oz
	Pork feet (fresh)	2 oz (omit 1 Fat)
	Preserved duck egg	⅔ egg

TABLE A–23I. CONTINUED

FOOD EXCHANGE GROUP	FOOD	PORTION
Vegetables	Bok choy (cooked)	1 cup
	Bamboo shoots (canned, drained)	¾ cup
	Banana flower	½ cup
	Bitter melon (balsam pear)	½ cup
	Chinese radish (daikon)	1 cup
	Dried Chinese mushrooms (soaked)	½ cup
	Green beans (Chinese)	½ cup
	Hairy cucumber	½ cup
	Kohlrabi	¾ cup
	Leek (Chinese onion)	½ cup
	Lotus seeds	1 oz
	Mung bean sprouts	1 cup
	Mustard green root	½ cup
	Pear squash (chayote)	½ medium
	Salted celery cabbage	Free
	Salted Chinese cabbage	½ cup
	Scallions, 5″ × ½″	3
	Seaweed (dried, soaked, drained)	½ cup
	Snow peas	½ cup
	Straw mushrooms	½ cup
	Water chestnuts	4
	White eggplant (Chinese)	½ cup
	Winter melon (Wax gourd)	1 cup
Fruit	Carambola (star fruit)	1
	Dried red dates	4
	Guava (fresh)	½ cup
	Kumquats (fresh)	3
	Litchis (dried or fresh)	6
	Longans (dried)	5
	Pomegranate	½
Milk	Coconut milk*	1 cup (omit 12 fats)
	Soymilk	1 cup (add ½ starch/bread)
Fats	Chicken fat or pork fat	1 tsp
	Nuts	
	Cashew	7 large (omit 1 Vegetable)
	Macadamia	6
	Pine	⅓ oz
	Pistachio (shelled)	⅓ oz
	Oils	1 tsp
	Peanut	
	Safflower	
	Sesame	
	Soy (tou yo)	
	Seeds (dried)	
	Pumpkin	1 Tbsp
	Sesame	1 Tbsp
	Watermelon	½ oz
	Sesame seed paste	1 tsp
Miscellaneous Foods		
YES! YES! YES!	Anise, curry powder, flower spice, ground ginger, mustard sauce, oyster sauce, parsley, soy sauce, tangerine peel, tea, vinegar, 5-spices powder.	
NO! NO! NO!	Brown sugar, hoisin sauce, molasses, moon cake, plum sauce, red preserved ginger, rock sugar, sweet buns, sweet coconut tarts, sweet mung bean soup.	

*See Professional Guidelines, *In* American Diabetes Association, Washington, D.C. Area Affiliate, Inc.: Supplement to Exchange Lists for Meal Planning Oriental Cookery, 1979, p. 18.

(Adapted with permission from The American Diabetes Association, Washington, D.C. Area Affiliate, Inc.: Supplement to Exchange Lists for Meal Planning Oriental Cookery. 1979.)

TABLE A–23J. DIET EXCHANGES FOR A VEGETARIAN DIET*

FOOD EXCHANGE GROUP	FOOD	PORTION
Starch/Bread	Brown rice (cooked)	1/3 cup
	Buckwheat flour (dark)	3 Tbsp
	Bulgur wheat	2 Tbsp
	Millet (cooked)	1/2 cup
	Miso	3 Tbsp
	Oats (dry)	1/4 cup
	Pita (Syrian) bread	1/2 of a 2 1/2-oz loaf
	Rye flour	3 Tbsp
	Wheat berries (cooked)	1/3 cup
	Wild rice (cooked)	1/2 cup
Meat and Meat Substitutes		
Lean Meat and Substitutes	Dried beans and peas (cooked) (omit 1 bread for each listing)	1/2 cup
	Black-eyed peas	
	Broad beans	
	Garbanzo	
	Kidney	
	Lentils	
	Lima	
	Mung	
	Navy	
	Pinto	
	Soy flour	1/4 cup (omit 1/2 bread)
Medium-fat Meat and Substitutes†	Cheeses	
	Camembert	1 oz
	Edam	1 oz
	Liederkranz	1 oz
	Soybeans	1/3 cup
	Tofu, 2 1/2″ × 2 3/4″ × 1″	1 portion
High-fat Meat and Substitutes	Cheeses	
	Blue, Roquefort	1 oz
	Brick	1 oz
	Gorgonzola	1 oz
	Gouda	1 oz
	Gruyère	1 oz
	Limburger	1 oz
	Muenster	1 oz
	Parmesan	1 oz
	Swiss	1 oz
	Hummus	4 Tbsp (omit 1 bread)
	Peanuts‡	4 Tbsp (omit 1/2 bread and 2 fat)
	Pignolia nuts‡	6 Tbsp (omit 1/2 vegetable and 1 fat)
	Pumpkin seeds‡	4 Tbsp (omit 1/2 bread and 1 1/2 fat)
	Sesame seeds‡	4 Tbsp (omit 1/2 bread and 2 fat)
	Sunflower seeds‡	4 Tbsp (omit 1/2 bread and 2 fat)
Vegetables	Bamboo shoots	3/4 cup
	Bean sprouts (raw or cooked)	
	Alfalfa	1 cup
	Mung	1 cup
	Soy	1 cup
	Water chestnuts	4
Fruit	Carrot juice	1/2 cup
Milk	Kefir	1 cup (omit 2 fats)
	Soy milk (fortified)	1 cup (add 1/2 bread)
Fats	Tahini	1 tsp

TABLE A—23J CONTINUED

Food containing complementary proteins may be eaten together, thereby increasing protein quality. Examples of foods that may be complemented to yield high-quality protein are listed below.

FOOD	COMPLEMENTARY PROTEIN
Grains	Combine rice with: cheese, legumes, sesame
	Combine wheat with: legumes, peanuts and milk, sesame, and soybean
	Combine corn with: legumes
Legumes	Combine beans with: wheat, corn
	Combine soybeans with: rice and wheat, corn and milk, wheat and sesame, peanuts and sesame, peanuts and wheat and rice
Nuts and seeds	Combined sesame with: beans, peanuts and soybeans, soybeans and wheat
	Combine peanuts with: sunflower seeds

DIET PATTERNS

Lacto-Ovovegetarian	Strict Vegetarian
Calories: 1,500	Calories: 1,500
CH_2O—190 g 50%	CH_2O—190 g 50%
Protein—75 g 20%	Protein—75 g 20%
Fat—47 g 30%	Fat—47 g 30%
Daily Food Allowance	Daily Food Allowance
3 Skim Milk Exchanges	3 Soybean Milk Exchanges (Note: Add ½ bread for each cup)
2 Vegetable Exchanges	2 Vegetable Exchanges
4 Fruit Exchanges	4 Fruit Exchanges
7 Bread Exchanges	7 Bread Exchanges
4 Lean Meat Exchanges	4 Lean Meat Exchanges
1 Medium-fat Meat Exchange	1 Medium-fat Meat Exchange
6 Fat Exchanges	6 Fat Exchanges
Meal Pattern	Meal Pattern
Breakfast	*Breakfast*
1 Fruit Exchange	1 Fruit Exchange
2 Bread Exchanges	2 Bread Exchanges
1 Medium-fat Meat Exchange	1 Medium-fat Meat Exchange
2 Fat Exchanges	2 Fat Exchanges
1 Skim Milk Exchange	1 Milk Exchange
Lunch	*Lunch*
2 Lean Meat Exchanges	2 Lean Meat Exchanges
2 Bread Exchanges	2 Bread Exchanges
1 Vegetable Exchange	1 Vegetable Exchange
2 Fruit Exchanges	2 Fruit Exchanges
2 Fat Exchanges	2 Fat Exchanges
Dinner	*Dinner*
2 Lean Meat Exchanges	2 Lean Meat Exchanges
2 Bread Exchanges	2 Bread Exchanges
1 Vegetable Exchange	1 Vegetable Exchange
1 Fruit Exchange	1 Fruit Exchange
2 Fat Exchanges	2 Fat Exchanges
1 Skim Milk Exchange	1 Milk Exchange
Bedtime Snack	*Bedtime Snack*
1 Skim Milk Exchange	1 Milk Exchange
1 Bread Exchange	1 Bread Exchange

TABLE A–23J. CONTINUED

GUIDELINES FOR THE PROFESSIONAL

You may revise the patient's meal plan to allow more calories from carbohydrate (50 to 60%) because of the high consumption of complex carbohydrates by vegetarians.

Many vegetarians use butter instead of margarine because it is considered a natural food.

The commercial meat analogues are very high in sodium, ranging in values from 300 mg to 3,000 mg/100 g edible portion. Nutritional analyses of these products are available upon request from Loma Linda Foods, Riverside, California 92505, and Worthington Foods, Miles Laboratories, Worthington, Ohio 43085.

Some vegetarians use diet supplements, such as wheat germ and brewer's yeast. Include these in the diet as follows:

Brewer's yeast, powder: 1 level Tbsp = ½ Lean Meat Exchange
Wheat germ: ¼ cup = 1 Bread Exchange

Vegetarian diets, unless fortified, could be deficient in iron. Iron absorption is enhanced by the inclusion of a vitamin C–rich food at each meal.

Vegetarian diets excluding dairy products may be inadequate in riboflavin and calcium. Two cups daily of fortified soybean milk or appropriate supplements should prevent deficiency.

For the strict vegetarian, vitamin B_{12} is also required as a vitamin supplement if 2 cups of fortified soybean milk are not consumed daily.

SUGGESTED READING FOR VEGETARIANS

1. Position of the American Dietetic Association: Vegetarian Diets, J. Am. Diet. Assoc., *88*:3, 351–355, 1988.
2. Lappe, F.M.: Diet for a Small Planet. New York, Ballantine Books, 1991.
3. Robertson, L., Flinders, C., Ruppenthal, B.: The New Laurel's Kitchen. Berkeley, CA, Ten Speed Press, 1986.
4. Hodgkin, G., Maloney, S.: Diet Manual Utilizing a Vegetarian Diet Plan. 7th Ed. Loma Linda, CA, The Seventh Day Adventist Dietetic Association, 1990.
5. Hinman, B., Snyder, N.: Lean and Luscious and Meatless. Prima Publications, Rocklin, CA, 1992.
6. Mangum, K.: Life's Simple Pleasures: Fine Vegetarian Cooking for Sharing and Celebration. Pacific Press Publications, Boise, ID, 1990.
7. Baird, P.: Quick Harvest: A Vegetarian's Guide to Microwave Cooking. New York, Prentice-Hall, 1991.

*Supplement to Exchange Lists for Meal Planning Vegetarian Cookery. American Diabetes Association, Washington, D.C. Area Affiliate, Inc., Food and Nutrition Committee, 1978. See Table A–23a for Standard Exchange lists.

†Meat analogs: Vegetable protein foods that closely duplicate the flavor, texture, and appearance of meat—"meatless" meats. See company information in the Guidelines for the Professional given above.

‡Seeds and nuts can be considered a "High-fat Meat" exchange and a complete protein only when they are complemented.

TABLE A–24A. GLYCEMIC INDEX VALUES OF SOME FOODS ADJUSTED SO THE GLYCEMIC INDEX OF WHITE BREAD IS 100*

FOOD	MEAN
Breads	
Rye (crispbread)	95
Rye (wholemeal)	89
Rye (whole grain, i.e., pumpernickel)	68
Wheat (white)	100
Wheat (wholemeal)	100
Pasta	
Macaroni (white, boiled 5 min)	64
Spaghetti (brown, boiled 15 min)	61
Spaghetti (white, boiled 15 min)	67
Star pasta (white, boiled 5 min)	54
Cereal Grains	
Barley (pearled)	36
Buckwheat	78
Bulgur	65
Millet	103
Rice (brown)	81
Rice (instant, boiled 1 min)	65
Rice (polished, boiled 5 min)	58
Rice (polished, boiled 10-25 min)	81
Rice (parboiled, boiled 5 min)	54
Rice (parboiled, boiled 15 min)	68
Rye kernels	47
Sweet corn	80
Wheat kernels	63
Breakfast Cereals	
"All Bran"	74
Cornflakes	121
Muesli	96
Porridge oats	89
Puffed rice	132
Puffed wheat	110
Shredded wheat	97
"Weetabix"	109
Cookies	
Digestive	82
Oatmeal	78
"Rich tea"	80
Plain crackers (water biscuits)	100
Shortbread cookies	88
Root Vegetables	
Potato (instant)	120
Potato (mashed)	98
Potato (new/white boiled)	80
Potato (Russett, baked)	116
Potato (sweet)	70
Yam	74
Legumes	
Baked beans (canned)	70
Bengal gram dal	12
Butter beans	46
Chick peas (dried)	47
Chick peas (canned)	60
Green peas (canned)	50
Green peas (dried)	65
Garden peas (frozen)	65
Haricot beans (white, dried)	54
Kidney beans (dried)	43
Kidney beans (canned)	74
Lentils (green, dried)	36
Lentils (green, canned)	74
Lentils (red, dried)	38
Pinto beans (dried)	60
Pinto beans (canned)	64
Peanuts	15
Soya beans (dried)	20
Soya beans (canned)	22
Fruit	
Apple	52
Apple juice	45
Banana	84
Orange	59
Orange juice	71
Raisins	93
Sugars	
Fructose	26
Glucose	138
Honey	126
Lactose	57
Maltose	152
Sucrose	83
Dairy Products	
Custard	59
Ice cream	69
Skim milk	46
Whole milk	44
Yogurt	52
Snack Foods	
Corn chips	99
Potato chips	77

*Glycemic index is defined as the blood glucose repsonse to a 50-g available carbohydrate portion of a food expressed as a percentage of the response to the same amount of carbohydrate from a standard food, in this case white bread (see Chap. 39). (From Wolever, T. M. S.: World Rev. Nutr. Diet., *62*:120–185, 1990.)

TABLE A–24B. DIETS FOR WEIGHT REDUCTION AND FOR DIABETIC PERSONS*

	TOTAL DAILY INTAKE (kcal)			
NUTRIENT CLASS	800	1,200	1,800	2,250
Carbohydrate (g)	109 (54%)	154 (51%)	249 (55%)	309 (55%)
Protein	54 (27%)	60 (20%)	84 (19%)	107 (19%)
Fat (g)	17 (19%)	40 (29%)	54 (27%)	65 (26%)
FOOD GROUP	TOTAL EXCHANGES FOR ONE DAY (see Table A–23)			
Skim milk	2	2	2	2
Vegetable	2	2	3	6
Fruit	3	4	5	7
Bread†	2	4	9	10
Meat	4‡	4	5	7
Unsaturated Fat	1	4	4	4
MEAL	SAMPLE MEAL PATTERN (servings based on exchanges)			
Breakfast				
Skim milk	½	1	1	1
Fruit	1	1	1	1 + 1 midmeal
Bread	1	1	2	2 + 1 midmeal
Meat	0	0	0	1
Unsaturated fat	1	1	1	1
Lunch				
Skim milk	1	½	0	0
Vegetable	0	1	1	2 + 2 midmeal
Fruit	1	1	2	1 + 1 midmeal
Bread	½	1	3	2
Meat	1	1	2	2
Unsaturated fat	0	1	1	1
Dinner				
Skim milk	½	0	0	0
Vegetable	2	1	2	2
Fruit	1	1	1	2
Bread	½	1	2	3
Meat	3	3	3	4
Unsaturated fat	0	1	1	1
Evening				
Skim milk	0	½	1	1
Vegetable	0	0	0	0
Fruit	0	1	1	1
Bread	0	1	2	2
Meat	0	0	0	0
Unsaturated fat	0	1	1	1

*This table, prepared by us with assistance from Ms. Lori Cohen, R.D., is based on the dietary recommendations in Nutrition Guide for Professionals: Diabetes Education and Meal Planning, Powers, M. (Ed.), American Diabetes Association, Inc., and The American Dietetic Association, 1988. See Table A–25 for nutrition guidelines.

†In Exchange lists, trace fat is listed for breads. For calculation purposes, 1 g fat can be used when amount of breads contribute significantly to diet (i.e., > 6 servings per day).

‡Lean meat exchanges are used to calculate the 800-kcal meal pattern. All other meal patterns are based on medium-fat meat exchange.

TABLE A—25. NUTRITION GUIDELINES FOR PERSONS WITH NONINSULIN-DEPENDENT DIABETES MELLITUS

	LEAN PERSONS	OBESE PERSONS
Energy	Enough to maintain desirable body weight	Enough to achieve reasonable body weight*
	Men and physically active women require 30 kcal/kg desirable body weight	20 kcal/kg desirable body weight
	Sedentary persons and persons older than 55 years require 28 kcal/kg desirable body weight	
Carbohydrate	Up to 55 to 60% of total energy	Same
Sucrose	Can be included with an individualized diet plan†	Low nutrient density; limit on low-calorie diets
Fiber	Up to 40 g/day, with emphasis on water-soluble fiber	25 g/1,000 kcal
Protein	Recommended dietary allowance is 0.8 g/kg body weight	Minimum of 60 g when restricted to ≤1,200-kcal diet‡
Fat	Ideally <30% of energy	Same
Polyunsaturated fats	Up to 10% of energy	
Saturated fats	<10% of energy	
Monounsaturated fats	10 to 15% of energy	
Cholesterol	<300 mg/day	
Alternative Sweeteners	Use is acceptable	Same
Sodum	Not to exceed 3,000 mg/day	Same
Alcohol	Occasional or no use; limit to 1 to 2 alcohol equivalents 1 to 2 times per week	Same
Vitamins/Minerals	No evidence that diabetes causes increased need	
Snacks	Individualized on the basis of preferences and glucose patterns; snack should be coordinated with insulin schedule if on insulin	Not necessary; if desired, should be included in total day's meal plan. If on insulin, coordinate with insulin schedule or adjust insulin as needed.

*Reasonable body weight is that which is achievable and maintainable for the patient, although it may not be in the range considered desirable. For example, a reasonable weight goal for a patient weighing 105 kg may be 95 kg, although desirable body weight may actually be closer to 84 kg. Losing 4.5 to 9 kg may dramatically improve a person's glucose intolerance and may be a maintainable weight loss. Individual weight goals should be discussed and set.

†Individualization should be based on nutritional adequacy, promotion of diet adherence, and glucose and lipid control. Postprandial glucose response to a high-sucrose snack or meal should be evaluated; use of food and glucose records is helpful.

‡For example, 12% of a 1,200-kcal diet is only 36 g protein, which is less than the Recommended Dietary Allowance (9) for a 163-cm-tall woman; 20% of a 1,200-kcal diet will provide the recommended 60 g protein.

(From Beebe, C. A., Pastors, J. G., Powers, M. A., et al.: Nutrition management for individuals with noninsulin-dependent diabetes mellitus in the 1990's: A review by the Diabetes Care and Education dietetic practice group. J. Am. Diet. Assoc., *91*:199, 1991. With permission.)

TABLE 1–26A. RENAL DIETS

Purpose: The diet for chronic renal insufficiency (CRI) is designed to slow the progression of kidney disease and possibly delay the need for maintenance dialysis. The diet for chronic renal failure (CRF) is designed to meet nutritional requirements, minimize uremic complications, and maintain acceptable blood chemistries, blood pressure, and fluid status in patients with impaired renal function.

Use: The CRI diet (often called the predialysis diet) is indicated for patients with chronic renal insufficiency who do not yet require dialysis. The CRF diet is used for patients requiring hemodialysis or peritoneal dialysis treatments.

Modifications: The CRI diet is restricted in two major areas—protein and phosphorus. Restrictions of sodium, potassium, fluid, and calories are based on individual needs.[1-5] Generally, the CRF diet reflects controlled intake of protein, potassium, sodium, phosphorus, and fluids. Additional modifications of fat, cholesterol, triglycerides, and fiber may be necessary based on individual requirements.[6,7] Certain underlying conditions may require the adjustment of kilocalories.

SUMMARY OF NUTRIENT RECOMMENDATIONS FOR ADULT PATIENTS WITH CRI, HEMODIALYSIS, AND PERITONEAL DIALYSIS[4-12]

Nutrient	CRI	Hemodialysis	Peritoneal Dialysis
Protein	0.6-0.8 g/kg ideal body weight	1.1-1.4 g/kg ideal body weight; at least 60% high biologic value	1.2-1.5 g/kg ideal body weight 1.2-1.3 maintenance 1.5 repletion 1.2 reduction or with diabetes
Energy	Normal weight: 35 kcal/kg ideal body weight Obese: 20-30 kcal/kg ideal body weight Underweight or catabolic: 45 kcal/kg ideal body weight	30-35 kcal/kg ideal body weight	20-50 kcal/kg ideal body weight 25-35 maintenance 35-50 repletion 20-25 reduction 35 with diabetes (for CAPD and CCPD, include dialysate calories)*
Phosphorus	5-10 mg/kg ideal body weight (IBW)	< 17 mg/kg IBW or approximately 800-1,200 mg/day	< 17 mg/kg IBW or approximately 1,200 mg/day
Sodium	1,000-3,000 mg/day if necessary; additional sodium may be required with salt-losing nephropathic conditions	1,000-3,000 mg/day	Individualized based on blood pressure and weight; CAPD and CCPD, 3,000-4,000 mg/day; IPD, 2,000-3,000 mg/day*
Potassium	Generally not restricted unless potassium is elevated and urine output is < 1 L/d	40 mg/kg ideal body weight or approximately 50-80 mEq/day	Generally unrestricted with CAPD and CCPD; IPD, 2,000-3,000 mg/day*
Fluid	Generally unrestricted; balance fluid intake with urine output in patients with edema or congestive heart failure	500-750 ml/day plus urine output or approximately 750-1,500 ml/day	CAPD and CCPD, approximately 2,000-3,000 ml/day based on daily weight fluctuations and blood pressure; IPD, same as for hemodialysis*
Calcium	1,200-1,600 mg/day	Approximately 1,000-1,800 mg/day supplement as needed to maintain normal serum level	Same as for hemodialysis
Fat	None	Limit cholesterol to < 300 mg/day; emphasize use of polyunsaturated fats	Same as for hemodialysis

Adequacy: The CRI diet is deficient in calcium, iron, vitamin B_{12}, and zinc because of the low-phosphorus, low-protein intake. The need for vitamin and mineral supplementation should be assessed on an individual basis.[10] CRF diets containing less than 60 g of protein may be deficient in niacin, riboflavin, thiamin, and calcium for men and calcium and iron for women, according to the 1989 Recommended Dietary Allowances.

REFERENCES

1. Zeller, K.: N. Engl. J. Med., *324*:78–84, 1991.
2. Ihle, B. V.: N. Engl. J. Med., *321*:1773–1777, 1989.
3. Mitch, W. E.: *In* Nutrition and the Kidney. Edited by W. E. Mitch and S. Klahr. Boston, Little Brown, 1988.
4. Kopple, J. D.: *In* Modern Nutrition in Health and Disease. Edited by M. E. Shils and R. Young. Philadelphia, Lea & Febiger, 1988.
5. Blumen Krantz, M. J.: *In* Handbook of Dialysis. Edited by J. T. Daugirdas and T. S. Ing. Boston, Little Brown, 1988.
6. Alvestrand, A. S.: *In* Nutrition and the Kidney. Edited by W. E. Mitch and S. Klahr. Boston, Little Brown, 1988.
7. Diamond, S. M. Henrich, D. E.: *In* Nutrition and the Kidney. Edited by W. E. Mitch and S. Klahr. Boston, Little Brown, 1988.
8. Bergstrom, J.: Clin. Nephrol., *21*:29–35, 1984.
9. Hruska, A.: *In* Nutrition and the Kidney. Edited by W. E. Mitch and S. Klahr. Boston, Little Brown, 1988.
10. Wolkens, K., Schiro, K. (eds.): Suggested Guidelines for the Nutrition Care of Renal Patients. 2nd Ed. Chicago, The American Dietetic Association, 1992.
11. Renal Dietitians Dietetic Practice Group: National Renal Diet. Chicago, The American Dietetic Association, to be published.
12. Gillit, D., Stover, J., Spinozzi, N.S. (Eds.): A Clinical Guide to Nutrition Care in End-Stage Renal Disease. Chicago, American Dietetic Association, 1987.

*CAPD = continuous ambulatory peritoneal dialysis; CCPD = continuous cyclic peritoneal dialysis; IPD = intermittent peritoneal dialysis.
(Modified from The Manual of Clinical Dietetics. 4th Ed. Chicago, American Dietetic Association, 1992. With permission.)

TABLE A–26B-1. SAMPLE MENU FOR CHRONIC RENAL INSUFFICIENCY (70-kg man; 40 g protein, 2,000 kcal, 600 mg phosphorus)

BREAKFAST	LUNCH	DINNER
Orange juice (½ cup)	Roast beef (1 oz)	Baked chicken thigh (1 oz)
Cinnamon applesauce (½ cup)	Bread (2 slices)	White rice (½ cup)
Cornflakes (1 cup)	Mayonnaise (1 Tbsp)	Green beans (½ cup)
Toast (1 slice)	Lettuce salad (1 cup)	Low-sodium vegetable soup (½ cup)
Margarine (1 tsp)	Vinegar and oil dressing (1 Tbsp)	Dinner roll (1 small)
Jelly or jam (1 tsp)	Sliced canned peaches (1 cup)	Margarine (2 tsp)
Liquid nondairy creamer (½ cup)	Graham crackers (2)	Jelly
Coffee or tea with sugar	Lemon-lime soda (1 cup)	Strawberries (1 cup)
		Tea with sugar
		Lemonade (½ cup)
	SNACK	
	Apple pie (1 slice)	
	Tea with sugar	

APPROXIMATE NUTRIENT ANALYSIS

Energy (kcal)	2,057.2	Sodium (mg)	1,798.4
Protein (g) (7.9% of kcal)	40.6	Zinc (mg)	5.7
Carbohydrate (g) (61.8% of kcal)	317.6	Vitamin A (μg RE)	994.8
Total fat (g) (32.4% of kcal)	74.2	Vitamin C (mg)	180.2
Saturated fatty acids (g)	14.6	Thiamin (mg)	1.6
Monounsaturated fatty acids (g)	28.0	Riboflavin (mg)	1.4
Polyunsaturated fatty acids (g)	26.7	Niacin (mg)	19.1
Cholesterol (mg)	64.7	Folate (μg)	309.0
Calcium (mg)	258.1	Vitamin B_6 (mg)	1.3
Iron (mg)	12.5	Vitamin B_{12} (μg)	1.0
Magnesium (mg)	172.9	Dietary fiber (g)	17.7
Phosphorus (mg)	549.3	Water-insoluble fiber (g)	11.4
Potassium (mg)	2,138.0		

(From The Manual of Clinical Dietetics. 4th Ed. Chicago, American Dietetic Association, 1992. With permission.)

TABLE A–26B-2. SAMPLE MENU FOR HEMODIALYSIS (70-kg man; 85 g protein, 2 g sodium, 2 g potassium, 1,000 mg phosphorus, 1,000 ml fluid)

BREAKFAST	LUNCH	DINNER
Cranberry juice (½ cup)	Low-sodium vegetable soup (½ cup)	Broiled chicken (3 oz)
Grapefruit (½)	Unsalted crackers (4)	White rice (½ cup)
Cornflakes (¾ cup)	Lean hamburger patty (3 oz)	Green beans (½ cup)
White toast (2 slices)	Hamburger bun (1)	Hard dinner roll (1)
Margarine (2 tsp)	Unsalted mayonnaise (1 Tbsp)	Margarine (2 tsp)
Jelly (1 tbsp)	Lettuce	Lettuce salad (1 cup)
Hard-boiled egg (1)	Canned pears (½ cup)	Salt-free vinegar and oil dressing (1 Tbsp)
Coffee (½ cup)	Graham crackers (4)	Baked apple with sugar (1)
Sugar (4 tsp)	Lemonade (½ cup)	2% milk (½ cup)
Liquid nondairy creamer (½ cup)		
	SNACK THROUGHOUT DAY	
	Hard candy (6 pieces)	
	Lollipop (1 small)	
	Ginger ale (1 cup)	

APPROXIMATE NUTRIENT ANALYSIS

Energy (kcal)	2,618.4	Sodium (mg)	1,901.7
Protein (g) (12.6% of kcal)	82.2	Zinc (mg)	9.7
Carbohydrate (g) (58.4% of kcal)	382.3	Vitamin A (μg RE)	860.3
Total fat (g) (30% of kcal)	87.2	Vitamin C (mg)	132.0
Saturated fatty acids (g)	21.8	Thiamin (mg)	1.6
Monounsaturated fatty acids (g)	32.7	Riboflavin (mg)	1.7
Polyunsaturated fatty acids (g)	25.0	Niacin (mg)	26.4
Cholesterol (mg)	347.8	Folate (μg)	235.0
Calcium (mg)	458.0	Vitamin B_6 (mg)	1.8
Iron (mg)	15.4	Vitamin B_{12} (μg)	3.0
Magnesium (mg)	196.5	Dietary fiber (g)	17.9
Phosphorus (mg)	946.4	Water-insoluble fiber (g)	11.9
Potassium (mg)	2,069.4		

(From The Manual of Clinical Dietetics. 4th Ed. Chicago, American Dietetic Association, 1992. With permission.)

TABLE A–26B-3. SAMPLE MENU FOR PERITONEAL DIALYSIS (70-kg man; 105 g protein, 3 g sodium, 1.4 g phosphorus, 3–4 g potassium)

BREAKFAST	LUNCH	DINNER
Cranberry juice (½ cup)	Low-sodium vegetable soup (1 cup)	Green salad (3½ oz)
Cornflakes (¾ cup)	Lean hamburger patty (3 oz)	Vinegar and oil dressing (1 Tbsp)
Banana (½)	Hamburger bun	Broiled chicken breast (4 oz)
White toast (2 slices)	Sliced tomato (2 oz) and lettuce	Herbed white rice (½ cup)
Margarine (2 tsp)	Fresh fruit salad (½ cup)	Broccoli spears (2)
Skim milk (½ cup)	Graham crackers (4)	Hard dinner roll (1)
Coffee/tea	Coffee/tea	Margarine (2 tsp)
		Fresh strawberries (¾ cup)
		Coffee/tea
	SNACK	
	Unsalted crackers (5)	
	Tuna salad (½ cup)	
	Orange (1 medium)	

APPROXIMATE NUTRIENT ANALYSIS

Energy (kcal)	2,125.6	Sodium (mg)	1,964.8
Protein (g) (20.2% of kcal)	107.6	Zinc (mg)	10.2
Carbohydrate (g) (46.8% of kcal)	248.8	Vitamin A (μg RE)	1,077.0
Total fat (g) (33.4% of kcal)	78.8	Vitamin C (mg)	278.4
Saturated fatty acids (g)	19.3	Thiamin (mg)	1.9
Monounsaturated fatty acids (g)	28.2	Riboflavin (mg)	1.9
Polyunsaturated fatty acids (g)	24.3	Niacin (mg)	40.0
Cholesterol (mg)	193.6	Folate (μg)	340.3
Calcium (mg)	549.9	Vitamin B_6 (mg)	2.9
Iron (mg)	16.5	Vitamin B_{12} (μg)	3.9
Magnesium (mg)	280.5	Dietary fiber (g)	18.7
Phosphorus (mg)	1,069.6	Water-insoluble fiber (g)	10.9
Potassium (mg)	3,170.0		

Note: Calories provided may need to be adjusted based on calories absorbed from the dialysate exchanges.
(From The Manual of Clinical Dietetics. 4th Ed. Chicago, American Dietetic Association, 1992. With permission.)

TABLE A–26C. AVERAGE CALCULATION FIGURES FOR PLANNING CRI AND CRF DIETS*

FOOD EXCHANGES	kcal	Pro (g)	Na (mg)	K (mg)	Phos (mg)
Milk	120	4.0	80	185	110
Milk substitutes†	140	0.5	40	80	30
Meat	65	7.0	25	100	65
Starches	90	2.0	80	35	35
Vegetables‡					
Low K	25	1.0	15	70	20
Medium K	25	1.0	15	150	20
High K	25	1.0	15	270	20
Fruits					
Low K	70	0.5	Trace	70	15
Medium K	70	0.5	Trace	150	15
High K	70	0.5	Trace	270	15
Fats	45	Trace	55	10	5
High-calorie choices§	100	Trace	15	20	5
Beverages	Varies	Varies	Varies	Varies	Varies
Salt choices	—	—	250	—	—

*Serving sizes for each food choice are shown in the following renal exchange lists (Table A–26d).
†Milk substitute choices are nondairy products that can be used in lieu of milk and milk products.
‡Average sodium level values do not include canned vegetables. Add 250 mg sodium for canned vegetables with added salt.
§High-calorie choices are foods high in carbohydrates that contain only a trace of protein and minimal electrolytes. These should be used to raise calorie intake to the desired level.

TABLE A–26D. RENAL EXCHANGE LISTS

MILK EXCHANGES FOR CRI AND CRF PATIENTS (Average per choice: 4 g protein, 120 kcal, 80 mg sodium, 185 mg potassium, 110 mg phosphorus)	
Milk (nonfat, low-fat, whole)	½ cup
Alterna	1 cup
Buttermilk, cultured	½ cup
Chocolate milk	½ cup
Light cream or half and half	½ cup
Ice milk or ice cream	½ cup
Yogurt, plain or fruit-flavored	½ cup
Evaporated milk	¼ cup
Cream cheese	3 Tbsp
Sour cream	4 Tbsp
Sherbet	1 cup
Sweetened condensed milk	¼ cup
NONDAIRY MILK SUBSTITUTES FOR CRI AND CRF PATIENTS (Average per choice: 0.5 g protein, 140 kcal, 40 mg sodium, 80 mg potassium, 30 mg phosphorus)	
Dessert, nondairy frozen	½ cup
Dessert topping, nondairy frozen	½ cup
Liquid nondairy creamer, polyunsaturated	½ cup
MEAT EXCHANGES FOR CRI AND CRF PATIENTS (Average per ounce: 7 g protein, 65 kcal, 25 mg sodium, 100 mg potassium, 65 mg phosphorus)	
Prepared without added salt	
Beef	
Round, sirloin, flank, cubed, T-bone, and porterhouse steak; tenderloin, rib, chuck, and rump roast; ground beef or ground chuck	1 oz
Pork	
Fresh ham, tenderloin, chops, loin roast, cutlets	1 oz
Lamb	
Chops, leg, roasts	1 oz
Veal	
Chops, roasts, cutlets	1 oz
Poultry	
Chicken, turkey, Cornish hen, domestic duck, and goose	1 oz
Fish	
All fresh and frozen fish	1 oz
Lobster, scallops, shrimp, clams	1 oz
Crab, oysters	1½ oz
Canned tuna, canned salmon (unsalted)	1 oz
Sardines (unsalted)*	1 oz
Wild game	
Venison, rabbit, squirrel, pheasant, duck, goose	1 oz
Egg	
Whole	1 large
Egg white or yolk	2 large
Low-cholesterol egg product	¼ cup
Chitterlings	2 oz
Organ meats*	1 oz
Prepared with added salt	
Beef	
Deli-style roast beef†	1 oz
Pork	
Boiled or deli-style ham†	1 oz
Poultry	
Deli-style chicken or turkey†	1 oz
Fish	
Canned tuna, canned salmon†	1 oz
Sardines†	1 oz
Cheese	
Cottage†	¼ cup
High in sodium, phosphorus, and/or saturated fat (should be used in limited quantities)	
Bacon	
Frankfurters, bratwurst, Polish sausage	
Lunch meats, including bologna, braunschweiger, liverwurst, picnic loaf, salami, summer sausage	
All cheese except cottage cheese	

TABLE A–26D. CONTINUED

STARCH EXCHANGES FOR CRI AND CRF PATIENTS (Average per choice: 2 g protein, 90 kcal, 80 mg sodium, 35 mg potassium, 35 mg phosphorus)	
Breads and rolls	
Bread (French, Italian, raisin, light rye, sourdough white)	1 slice (1 oz)
Bagel	½ small (1 oz)
Bun, hamburger or hot dog	½
Danish pastry or sweet roll, no nuts	½ small
Dinner roll or hard roll	1 small
Doughnut	1 small
English muffin	½
Muffin, no nuts, bran or whole-wheat	1 small (1 oz)
Pancake‡§	1 small
Pita or pocket bread, 6″	½
Tortilla, corn, 6″	2
Tortilla, flour, 6″	1
Waffle‡§	1 small (1 oz)
Cereals and grains	
Cereals, ready-to-eat, most brands§	¾ cup
Puffed rice	2 cups
Puffed wheat	1 cup
Cooked cereal	
Cream of rice or wheat, farina, Malt-O-Meal	½ cup
Oat bran or oatmeal, Ralston	⅓ cup
Corn meal, cooked	¾ cup
Grits, cooked	½ cup
Flour, all-purpose	2½ Tbsp
Pasta (noodles, macaroni, spaghetti), cooked	½ cup
Pasta made with egg (egg noodles), cooked	⅓ cup
Rice, white or brown, cooked	½ cup
Crackers and snacks	
Crackers (saltines, round butter)	4
Graham crackers	3 squares
Melba toast	3 oblong
RyKrisp§	3
Popcorn, plain	1½ cups popped
Tortilla chips	¾ oz (9 chips)
Pretzels,§ sticks or rings	¾ oz (10 sticks)
Desserts	
Cake, angelfood	1/20 cake or 1 oz
Cake, 2″ × 2″	1 square or 1½ oz
Sandwich cookies‡§	4
Shortbread cookies	4
Sugar cookies	4
Sugar wafers	4
Vanilla wafers	10
Fruit pie (apple, berry, cherry, peach)	⅛ pie
Sweetened gelatin	½ cup
High in poor-quality protein and phosphorus (should be used rarely and in limited quantities)	
Bran cereal or muffins, Grape-Nuts, granola cereal or bars	
Boxed, frozen, or canned meals, entrees, or side dishes	
Pumpernickel, dark rye, whole-wheat or oatmeal breads	
Whole-wheat crackers	
Whole-wheat cereals	
Starchy vegetables for CRI PATIENTS	
Corn	⅓ cup or ½ ear
Green peas	¼ cup
Potatoes, boiled, mashed	½ cup
Potatoes, baked, white or sweet	1 small (3 oz)
Potatoes, french fried	½ cup or 10 small
Potatoes, hashed brown	½ cup
Squash, butternut, mashed	½ cup
Squash, winter, baked (all other varieties), cubed	1 cup

TABLE A–26D. CONTINUED

VEGETABLE EXCHANGES FOR CRI PATIENTS

(Average per choice: 1 g protein, 25 kcal, 15 mg sodium, 20 mg phosphorus. See Starch List for other vegetables. Prepared or canned without added salt.‖)

1 cup serving	
Alfalfa sprouts	Escarole
Cabbage	Lettuce, all varieties
Celery	Pepper, green, sweet
Cucumber (or ½ whole)	Radishes, sliced (or 15 small)
Eggplant	Turnips
Endive	Watercress
½ cup serving	
Artichoke	Onions
Bamboo shoots	Parsnips¶
Bean sprouts	Pumpkin
Beans, green or wax	Rutabagas¶
Beets	Squash, summer
Carrots (or 1 small)	Tomato (or 1 medium)
Cauliflower	Tomato juice, unsalted
Chard	Tomato juice, regular#
Chinese cabbage	Tomato puree
Collard greens	Turnip greens
Kale	Vegetable juice cocktail, unsalted
Kohlrabi	
Mushrooms, fresh (or 4 medium)	Vegetable juice cocktail, regular#
¼ serving	
Asparagus (or 2 spears)	Mushrooms, cooked
Avocado (¼ whole)	Mustard greens
Beet greens	Okra
Broccoli	Snow peas
Brussels sprouts	Spinach
Chili pepper	Tomato sauce

VEGETABLE EXCHANGES FOR CRF PATIENTS

(Average per choice: 1 g protein, 25 kcal, 15 mg sodium, 20 mg phosphorus. ½ cup per choice unless otherwise indicated. Prepared or canned without added salt.‖)

Low potassium (0–100 mg)	
Alfalfa sprouts (1 cup)	Cucumber, peeled
Bamboo shoots, canned	Endive
Bean sprouts	Lettuce, all varieties (1 cup)
Beans, green or wax	Escarole
Cabbage, raw	Pepper, green, sweet
Chard, raw	Watercress
Chinese cabbage, raw	Water chestnuts, canned
Medium potassium (101–200 mg)	
Artichoke	Mushrooms, canned¶ or fresh
Broccoli	Mustard greens
Cabbage, cooked	Onions
Carrots (1 small raw)	Peas, green¶
Cauliflower	Radishes
Celery, raw (1 stalk)	Snow peas¶
Collards	Spinach, raw
Corn (or ½ ear)¶	Squash, summer
Eggplant	Turnip greens
Kale	Turnips
High potassium (201–350 mg)	
Asparagus¶ (5 spears)	Potato,** hash browned
Avocado (¼ whole)	Potato chips** (1 oz or 14 chips)
Bamboo shoots,** fresh cooked	Pumpkin
Beet greens** (¼ cup)	Rutabagas
Beets	Spinach, cooked¶**
Brussels sprouts¶	Sweet potato¶**
Celery, cooked	Tomato (1 medium)
Chard**	Tomato juice, unsalted
Kohlrabi	Tomato juice, regular#
Mushrooms,¶ fresh cooked	Tomato paste¶ (2 Tbsp)
Okra¶	Winter squash¶ (¼ cup)
Parsnips¶	
Pepper, chili	
Potato,** baked (½ medium)	
Potato,¶ boiled or mashed	

TABLE A–26D. CONTINUED

FRUIT EXCHANGES FOR CRI PATIENTS
(Average per choice: 0.5 g protein, 70 kcal, 15 mg phosphorus)

1 cup serving
Apple (1 medium)
Apple juice
Applesauce
Cranberries
Cranberry juice cocktail
Papaya nectar
Peach nectar
Pear nectar
Pear, canned or fresh (1 medium)
Tangerine (1 medium)

½ cup serving
Apricot nectar
Banana (½ small)
Blueberries
Figs, canned
Fruit cocktail
Grape juice
Grapefruit (½ medium)
Grapefruit juice
Grapes (15 small)
Gooseberries
Kiwifruit (½ medium)
Lemon (½ medium)
Lemon juice
Mango (½ medium)
Nectarine (½ medium)
Orange (½ medium)
Peach, canned or fresh (½ medium)
Pineapple
Plums, canned or fresh (1 medium)
Rhubarb
Strawberries
Watermelon

¼ cup serving
Apricots (2 halves)
Apricots, dried (2)
Blackberries
Cantaloupe (⅛ small)
Cherries
Dates (2 Tbsp)
Figs, dried (1 whole)
Honeydew melon (⅛ small)
Orange juice
Papaya (¼ medium)
Prune juice
Prunes, cooked (5)
Raisins (2 Tbsp)
Raspberries

FRUIT EXCHANGES FOR CRF PATIENTS
(Average per choice: 0.5 g protein, 70 kcal, 15 mg phosphorus, ½ cup per choice unless otherwise indicated)

Low potassium (0–100 mg)
Applesauce
Blueberries
Cranberries (1 cup)
Cranberry juice cocktail (1 cup)
Grape juice
Lemon (½)
Papaya nectar
Peach nectar
Pear nectar
Pears, canned

Medium potassium (101–200 mg)
Apple (1 small, 2½″ diameter)
Apple juice
Apricot nectar
Blackberries
Cherries, sour or sweet
Fruit cocktail
Gooseberries
Grapefruit (½ small)
Grapefruit juice
Grapes (15 small)
Lemon juice
Mango
Papaya
Peach, canned
Peach, fresh (1 small, 2″ diameter)
Pineapple, canned or fresh
Plums, canned or fresh (1 medium)
Raisins (2 Tbsp)
Raspberries
Rhubarb
Strawberries
Tangerine (2½″ diameter)
Watermelon (1 cup)

High potassium (201–350 mg)
Apricots, canned or fresh (2 halves)
Apricots, dried (5)
Banana** (½ medium)
Cantaloupe (⅛ small)
Dates (¼ cup)
Figs, dried (2 whole)
Honeydew melon (⅛ small)
Kiwifruit (½ medium)
Nectarine (1 small, 2″ diameter)
Orange (1 small, 2½″ diameter)
Orange juice
Pear, fresh (1 medium)
Prune juice**
Prunes,** dried or canned (5)

TABLE A–26D. CONTINUED

FAT EXCHANGES FOR CRI AND CRF PATIENTS (Average per choice: trace protein, 45 kcal, 55 mg sodium, 10 mg potassium, 5 mg phosphorus)	
Unsaturated fats	
Margarine	1 tsp
Reduced-calorie margarine	1 Tbsp
Mayonnaise	1 tsp
Low-calorie mayonnaise	1 Tbsp
Oil	
Safflower, sunflower, corn, soybean, olive, peanut, canola	1 tsp
Salad dressing, mayonnaise-type	2 tsp
Salad dressing, oil-type	1 Tbsp
Low-calorie salad dressing (mayonnaise-type)††	2 Tbsp
Low-calorie salad dressing†† (oil-type)	2 Tbsp
Tartar sauce	1½ tsp
Saturated fats	
Butter	1 tsp
Coconut	2 Tbsp
Powdered coffee whitener	1 Tbsp
Solid shortening	1 tsp

HIGH CALORIE CHOICES FOR CRI AND CRF PATIENTS (Average per choice: trace protein, 100 kcal, 15 mg sodium, 20 mg potassium, 5 mg phosphorus)			
Beverages (count within fluid allowance)		Fruit-flavored drink	1 cup
Carbonated beverages	1 cup	Kool-Aid	1 cup
Fruit flavors, root beer, colas,‡‡ or pepper type		Limeade	1 cup
Cranberry juice cocktail	1 cup	Lemonade	1 cup
Frozen desserts (count within fluid allowance)		Tang	1 cup
Fruit ice	½ cup	Wine§§	½ cup
Juice bar (3 oz)	1 bar		
Candy and sweets		Popsicle (3 oz)	1 bar
Candy corn	20 or 1 oz	Sorbet	½ cup
Gumdrops	15 small		
Hard candy	4 pieces	Butter mints	14
Jellybeans	10	Fruit chews	4
LifeSavers or cough drops	12	Chewy fruit snacks	1 pouch
Marshmallows	5 large	Fruit Roll-Ups	2
Honey	2 Tbsp	Cranberry sauce or relish	¼ cup
Sugar, brown or white	2 Tbsp		
Jam or jelly	2 Tbsp		
Sugar, powdered	3 Tbsp		
Marmalade	2 Tbsp		
Syrup	2 Tbsp		
Special low-protein products for CRI PATIENTS			
Low-protein gelled dessert	½ cup		
Low-protein bread	1 slice		
Low-protein cookies	2		
Low-protein pasta	½ cup		
Low-protein rusk	2 slices		

TABLE A–26D. CONTINUED

SALT CHOICES FOR CRI AND CRF PATIENTS (Average per choice: 250 mg sodium)	
Salt	1/8 tsp
Seasoned salts (onion, garlic)	1/8 tsp
Accent	1/4 tsp
Barbecue sauce	2 Tbsp
Bouillon	1/3 cup
Catsup	1 1/2 Tbsp
Chili sauce	1 1/2 Tbsp
Dill pickle	1/6 large or 1/2 oz
Mustard	4 tsp
Olives, green	2 medium or 1/3 oz
Olives, black	3 large or 1 oz
Soy sauce	3/4 tsp
Steak sauce	2 1/2 tsp
Sweet pickle relish	2 1/2 Tbsp
Taco sauce	2 Tbsp
Tamari sauce	3/4 tsp
Teriyaki sauce	1 1/4 tsp
Worcestershire sauce	1 Tbsp

BEVERAGE CHOICES FOR CRF PATIENTS

The following beverages may be used as desired within daily fluid allowance.
Carbonated beverages (except Moxie, colas, and pepper-type)
Ice
Lemonade
Limeade
Mineral water
Water
The following beverages contain moderate amounts of potassium and/or phosphorus and should be used in limited quantities.
Beer and wine§§
Coffee, regular or decaffeinated
Coffee substitute (cereal grain beverage)
Fruit-flavored drinks with added vitamin C
Tea
Thirst quencher beverages
The following liquids are very high in sodium and/or potassium and should only be used as advised by a physician or dietitian.
Bouillon
Broth
Consomme
Salt-free broth or bouillon containing potassium chloride (KCl)
Remember: anything *that is liquid* or melts at room temperature must also be counted in fluid allowance (for example, ice cream, Popsicles, sherbet, gelatin).

*High phosphorus—≥ 100 mg/serving.
†High sodium—each serving counts as 1 meat choice and 1 salt choice.
‡High phosphorus—≥ 70 mg/serving.
§High sodium—each serving counts as 1 starch choice and 1 salt choice.
||For vegetables canned with salt, add 250 mg sodium and count as 1 vegetable choice and 1 salt choice.
¶High phosphorus—≥ 40 mg/serving.
#Very high sodium—each serving counts as 1 vegetable choice and 2 salt choices.
**Very high potassium—≥ 300 mg/serving.
††High sodium—each serving counts as 1 fat choice and 1 salt choice.
‡‡High phosphorus—≥ 20 mg/serving.
§§Check with physician for recommendation regarding alcohol.

Alterna, Ross Laboratories; Malt-O-Meal, Malt-O-Meal Co; Ralston, RyKrisp, Ralston Purina Co; Grape-Nuts, Kool-Aid, Tang, General Foods Corp; Popsicle, Popsicle Industries Inc; LifeSavers, Nabisco Brands, Inc; Fruit Roll-Ups, General Mills, Inc; Accent, Pet Inc; Moxie, Monarch Co, Atlanta GA 30341.

(Modified from Renal Dietitians Dietetic Practice Group: National Renal Diet. Chicago, The American Dietetic Association. In press. With permission.)

TABLE A—27A. SODIUM-CONTROLLED DIETS

Purpose: The goal of sodium restriction is to manage hypertension in sodium-sensitive individuals and promote the loss of excess fluids in edema and ascites.

General Rules

1. Avoid the use of all salt, baking soda, and/or baking powder in cooking and for table use.
2. Avoid medicines, laxatives, and salt substitutes unless prescribed by a physician.
3. Read labels carefully for sodium or salt content of packaged foods.

Modifications

1. *3,000 mg sodium (130 mEq).* Eliminate high-sodium processed foods and beverages, such as fast foods; salad dressings; smoked, salted, and koshered meats; regular canned food; pickled vegetables; luncheon meats; and commercially softened water. Allow up to 0.25 tsp table salt in cooking or at the table.
2. *2,000 mg sodium (87 mEq).* Eliminate processed and prepared foods and beverages high in sodium. Do not allow any salt in the preparation of foods or at the table. Limit milk and milk products to 16 fl oz daily. Check labels of canned and instant grain products for high-sodium sources.
3. *1,000 mg sodium (45 mEq).* Eliminate processed and prepared foods and beverages high in sodium. Omit regular canned foods, many frozen foods, deli foods, fast foods, cheeses, margarines, and regular salad dressings. Limit regular breads to 2 servings per day. Limit milk and milk products to 16 fl oz daily. Do not allow any salt in food preparation or for table use.
4. *500 mg sodium (22 mEq).* Omit canned or processed foods containing salt. Do not use any salt in food preparation or at the table. Omit vegetables containing high amounts of natural sodium. Limit meat to 6 oz daily, and milk and milk products to 8 fl oz daily. Use low-sodium bread in place of regular, and distilled water for cooking and drinking. This meal plan is used on a short-term basis only.
5. *250 mg sodium (11 mEq).* Use this meal plan for short terms only. Include the same foods as those in the 500-mg sodium diet, but use low-sodium milk in place of regular milk.

Adequacy: Based on the individual's food choices, the diets are adequate in all nutrients according to the 1989 National Research Council's Recommended Dietary Allowances. Unless carefully planned, however, the 250-mg and the 500-mg sodium diets can be inadequate in some nutrients.

(From The Manual of Clinical Dietetics. 4th Ed. Chicago, American Dietetic Association, 1992. With permission.)

TABLE A–27B-1. SAMPLE MENU FOR 3,000-MG SODIUM DIET*

BREAKFAST	LUNCH	DINNER
Orange juice (½ cup)	Low-sodium vegetable soup (1 cup)	Green salad (3½ oz)
Whole-grain cereal (¾ cup)	Unsalted crackers (4)	Vinegar and oil dressing (1 Tbsp)
Banana (½)	Lean beef patty (3 oz)	Broiled skinless chicken breast (3 oz)
Whole-wheat toast (2 slices)	Hamburger bun (1)	Herbed brown rice (½ cup)
Margarine (2 tsp)	Mustard (1 Tbsp)	Steamed broccoli (½ cup)
Jelly or jam (1 Tbsp)	Catsup (1 Tbsp)	Whole-grain roll (1)
2% milk (1 cup)	Sliced tomato (2 oz) and lettuce	Margarine (2 tsp)
Coffee/tea	Fresh fruit salad (½ cup)	Low-fat frozen yogurt (½ cup)
	Graham crackers (4)	Medium apple (1)
	2% milk (1 cup)	Coffee/tea
	Coffee/tea	

APPROXIMATE NUTRIENT ANALYSIS

Energy (kcal)	2,144.7	Sodium (mg)	2,334.8
Protein (g) (19.2% of kcal)	103.1	Zinc (mg)	13.3
Carbohydrate (g) (54.1% of kcal)	290.2	Vitamin A (μg RE)	1,409.2
Total fat (g) (29.2% of kcal)	69.6	Vitamin C (mg)	167.1
Saturated fatty acids (g)	22.6	Thiamin (mg)	1.8
Monounsaturated fatty acids (g)	25.0	Riboflavin (mg)	2.4
Polyunsaturated fatty acids (g)	15.0	Niacin (mg)	31.1
Cholesterol (mg)	186.6	Folate (μg)	400.3
Calcium (mg)	1,147.8	Vitamin B_6 (mg)	2.9
Iron (mg)	16.9	Vitamin B_{12} (μg)	4.3
Magnesium (mg)	459.8	Dietary fiber (g)	24.2
Phosphorus (mg)	1,604.3	Water-insoluble fiber (g)	17.2
Potassium (mg)	4,056.5		

*May use up to ¼ tsp salt per day in cooking and at the table.

(From The Manual of Clinical Dietetics. 4th Ed. Chicago, American Dietetic Association, 1992. With permission.)

TABLE A–27B-2. SAMPLE MENU FOR 2,000-MG SODIUM DIET

BREAKFAST	LUNCH	DINNER
Orange juice (½ cup)	Low-sodium vegetable soup (1 cup)	Green salad (3½ oz)
Whole-grain cereal (¾ cup)	Unsalted crackers (4)	Salt-free vinegar and oil dressing (1 Tbsp)
Banana (½)	Lean beef patty (3 oz)	Broiled skinless chicken breast (3 oz)
Whole-wheat toast (2 slices)	Hamburger bun (1)	Herbed brown rice (½ cup)
Margarine (2 tsp)	Mustard (1 Tbsp)	Steamed broccoli (½ cup)
Jelly or jam (1 Tbsp)	Low-sodium mayonnaise (1 Tbsp)	Whole-grain roll (1)
2% milk (1 cup)	Sliced tomato (2 oz) and lettuce	Margarine (2 tsp)
Coffee/tea	Fresh fruit salad (½ cup)	Italian fruit ice (½ cup)
	Graham crackers (4)	Medium apple (1)
	2% milk (1 cup)	Coffee/tea
	Coffee/tea	

APPROXIMATE NUTRIENT ANALYSIS

Energy (kcal)	2,239.7	Sodium (mg)	1,749.0
Protein (g) (17.5% of kcal)	98.1	Zinc (mg)	12.3
Carbohydrate (g) (53.2% of kcal)	297.8	Vitamin A (μg RE)	1,393.9
Total fat (g) (31.5% of kcal)	78.5	Vitamin C (mg)	165.2
Saturated fatty acids (g)	22.9	Thiamin (mg)	1.8
Monounsaturated fatty acids (g)	27.8	Riboflavin (mg)	2.2
Polyunsaturated fatty acids (g)	20.8	Niacin (mg)	30.7
Cholesterol (mg)	190.9	Folate (μg)	388.9
Calcium (mg)	989.5	Vitamin B_6 (mg)	2.9
Iron (mg)	16.2	Vitamin B_{12} (μg)	3.9
Magnesium (mg)	422.8	Dietary fiber (g)	23.3
Phosphorus (mg)	1,462.2	Water-insoluble fiber (g)	16.4
Potassium (mg)	3,751.4		

(From The Manual of Clinical Dietetics. 4th Ed. Chicago, American Dietetic Association, 1992. With permission.)

TABLE A–27B-3. SAMPLE MENU FOR 1,000-MG SODIUM DIET

BREAKFAST	LUNCH	DINNER
Orange juice (½ cup)	Low-sodium vegetable soup (1 cup)	Green salad (3½ oz)
Shredded wheat cereal (¾ cup)	Unsalted crackers (4)	Salt-free vinegar and oil dressing (1 Tbsp)
Banana (½)	Lean beef patty (3 oz)	Broiled skinless chicken breast (3 oz)
Low sodium whole-wheat toast (2 slices)	Low-sodium bread (2 sices)	Herbed brown rice (½ cup)
Unsalted margarine (2 tsp)	Low-sodium mayonnaise (1 Tbsp)	Steamed broccoli (½ cup)
Jelly or jam (1 Tbsp)	Sliced tomato (2 oz) and lettuce	Whole-grain roll (1)
2% milk (1 cup)	Fresh fruit salad (½ cup)	Unsalted margarine (2 tsp)
Coffee/tea	Graham crackers (4)	Italian fruit ice (½ cup)
	2% milk (1 cup)	Medium apple (1)
	Coffee/tea	Coffee/tea

APPROXIMATE NUTRIENT ANALYSIS

Energy (kcal)	2,255.1	Sodium (mg)	1,040.7
Protein (g) (17.9% of kcal)	100.9	Zinc (mg)	13.4
Carbohydrate (g) (54% of kcal)	304.2	Vitamin A (μg RE)	1,111.9
Total fat (g) (31.1% of kcal)	78.0	Vitamin C (mg)	153.9
Saturated fatty acids (g)	22.7	Thiamin (mg)	1.5
Monounsaturated fatty acids (g)	27.5	Riboflavin (mg)	1.9
Polyunsaturated fatty acids (g)	20.8	Niacin (mg)	28.2
Cholesterol (mg)	191.1	Folate (μg)	336.4
Calcium (mg)	952.5	Vitamin B_6 (mg)	2.6
Iron (mg)	14.6	Vitamin B_{12} (μg)	3.9
Magnesium (mg)	469.6	Dietary fiber (g)	26.7
Phosphorus (mg)	1,563.6	Water-insoluble fiber (g)	19.7
Potassium (mg)	3,863.0		

(From The Manual of Clinical Dietetics. 4th Ed. Chicago, American Dietetic Association, 1992. With permission.)

TABLE A–27B-4. SAMPLE MENU FOR 500-MG SODIUM DIET

BREAKFAST	LUNCH	DINNER
Orange juice (½ cup)	Low-sodium vegetable soup (1 cup)	Green salad (3½ oz)
Shredded wheat cereal (¾ cup)	Unsalted crackers (4)	Salt-free vinegar and oil dressing (1 Tbsp)
Banana (½)	Lean beef patty (3 oz)	Broiled skinless chicken breast (3 oz)
Low sodium whole-wheat toast (2 slices)	Low-sodium bread (2 sices)	Herbed brown rice (½ cup)
Unsalted margarine (2 tsp)	Low-sodium mayonnaise (1 Tbsp)	Steamed broccoli (½ cup)
Jelly or jam (1 Tbsp)	Sliced tomato (2 oz) and lettuce	Low-sodium bread (1 slice)
2% milk (1 cup)	Unsalted pretzels (1 oz)	Unsalted margarine (2 tsp)
Coffee/tea	Fresh fruit salad (½ cup)	Italian fruit ice (½ cup)
	Fruit juice (1 cup)	Medium apple (1)
	Coffee/tea	Coffee/tea

APPROXIMATE NUTRIENT ANALYSIS

Energy (kcal)	2,220.8	Sodium (mg)	594.7
Protein (g) (17.3% of kcal)	96.0	Zinc (mg)	12.3
Carbohydrate (g) (57.2% of kcal)	317.4	Vitamin A (μg RE)	1,109.7
Total fat (g) (28.5% of kcal)	70.3	Vitamin C (mg)	232.0
Saturated fatty acids (g)	18.6	Thiamin (mg)	1.6
Monounsaturated fatty acids (g)	24.8	Riboflavin (mg)	1.6
Polyunsaturated fatty acids (g)	20.2	Niacin (mg)	28.7
Cholesterol (mg)	170.3	Folate (μg)	347.2
Calcium (mg)	652.5	Vitamin B_6 (mg)	2.6
Iron (mg)	15.3	Vitamin B_{12} (μg)	3.0
Magnesium (mg)	438.1	Dietary fiber (g)	26.6
Phosphorus (mg)	1,316.2	Water-insoluble fiber (g)	19.2
Potassium (mg)	3,552.3		

(From The Manual of Clinical Dietetics. 4th Ed. Chicago, American Dietetic Association, 1992. With permission.)

TABLE A–27C. GUIDELINES FOR FOOD SELECTION

FOOD CATEGORY	FOODS RECOMMENDED	FOODS EXCLUDED FOR 3,000-MG SODIUM DIET	ADDITIONAL FOODS EXCLUDED FOR 2,000-MG SODIUM DIET*	ADDITIONAL FOODS EXCLUDED FOR 1,000-MG SODIUM DIET*
Beverages	Milk Eggnog Buttermilk (limit to 1 cup per week) Low-sodium or salt-free vegetable juices Regular vegetable or tomato juice (limit to ½ cup per day)	Greater than ½ cup regular vegetable or tomato juice Commercially softened water for drinking or cooking	Buttermilk (>½ cup), malted milk, chocolate milk, milkshake Regular milk (>2 cups) Regular vegetable or tomato juice	No additional restrictions
Vegetables (2–4 servings per day)	Fresh and frozen vegetables Low-sodium canned, drained vegetables	Sauerkraut Pickled vegetables and others prepared in brine Vegetables seasoned with bacon, ham, or pork	Regular canned vegetables Frozen vegetables prepared in sauce	Frozen peas, frozen lima beans, frozen mixed vegetables
Fruits (2 or more servings per day)	All fruits and fruit juices	No additional restrictions	Fruits processed with salt or sodium-containing compounds	No additional restrictions
Breads and cereals (4 or more servings per day)	Enriched white, wheat, rye, and pumpernickel Most cereals, hard rolls, and dinner rolls Crackers Unsalted snack crackers Breadsticks Biscuits, muffins, cornbread, pancakes, and waffles	Breads and rolls with salted tops Instant hot cereals	Quick breads Instant hot cereals Cooked dry cereals with added sodium Crackers with salted tops Self-rising flour and biscuit mixes Regular bread crumbs or cracker crumbs Commercial bread stuffing	Sweet rolls, crackers, and other products containing salt, baking powder, or self-rising flour Dry cereals
Potato or substitute	White or sweet potatoes Squash Enriched rice, barley, noodles, spaghetti, macaroni, and other pastas Homemade bread stuffing	Commercially prepared potato, rice, and pasta mixes Commercial stuffing	No additional restrictions	Instant potatoes

TABLE A—27C. CONTINUED

FOOD CATEGORY	FOODS RECOMMENDED	FOODS EXCLUDED FOR 3,000-MG SODIUM DIET	ADDITIONAL FOODS EXCLUDED FOR 2,000-MG SODIUM DIET*	ADDITIONAL FOODS EXCLUDED FOR 1,000-MG SODIUM DIET*
Meat or substitute	Fresh or fresh-frozen meats (beef, lamb, pork, veal, and game) Fresh or fresh-frozen poultry (chicken, turkey, Cornish hen, and others) Fresh-water or fresh-frozen unbreaded fish Most shellfish Canned tuna, rinsed Canned salmon, rinsed Eggs and egg substitutes Cheese in limited amounts Low-sodium cheese as desired Ricotta cheese and cream cheese (limit 2 oz per day) Cottage cheese, drained Regular yogurt Regular peanut butter (3 times per week) Dried peas and beans Frozen dinners (<600 mg sodium)	Any meat, fish, or poultry that is smoked, cured, salted, koshered, or canned (bacon, chipped beef, coldcuts, ham, hot dogs, and sausages) Sardines, anchovies, marinated herring, and pickled meats Pickled eggs Frozen breaded meats Processed cheese, cheese spreads, and sauces Salted nuts	Crab Lobster Regular hard and processed cheese Regular peanut butter Frozen dinner entrees (<500 mg sodium)	All shellfish Egg substitutes
Fats	Butter or margarine Vegetable oils Low-sodium salad dressing as desired Regular salad dressing in limited amounts Light, sour, and heavy cream	Salad dressings containing bacon, bacon fat, bacon bits, and salt pork Snack dips made with instant soup mixes and/or processed cheese	No additional restrictions	Nondairy cream (≤1 fl oz allowed per day) Salted butter or margarine Regular mayonnaise
Soups	Commercial canned and dehydrated soups, broth, and bouillon Homemade soups without added salt, made with allowed vegetables Homemade broth Low-sodium canned soups and broths	Excessive amounts of canned or dehydrated soups (>1 cup per week)	Regular canned or dehydrated commercial soups, broths, or bouillon	No additional restrictions

TABLE A–27C. CONTINUED

FOOD CATEGORY	FOODS RECOMMENDED	FOODS EXCLUDED FOR 3,000-MG SODIUM DIET	ADDITIONAL FOODS EXCLUDED FOR 2,000-MG SODIUM DIET*	ADDITIONAL FOODS EXCLUDED FOR 1,000-MG SODIUM DIET*
Sweets and desserts	Any sweets and desserts allowed	No additional restrictions	Desserts and sweets made with milk exceeding allowance	All candies made with sweet chocolate, nuts, or coconut Desserts make with rennin, rennin tablets Sherbets and flavored gelatin (>½ cup per day) Salted bakery foods, homemade or commercial
Miscellaneous	Limit added salt to ¼ tsp per day used at the table or in cooking Salt substitute with physician's approval Pepper, herbs, and spices Vinegar Lemon or lime juice Hot pepper sauce Low-sodium soy sauce Unsalted tortilla chips, pretzels, potato chips, popcorn	Any seasoning containing salt (garlic salt, celery salt, onion salt, and seasoned salt) Sea salt, rock salt, and kosher salt Any other seasoning containing salt and sodium compounds (meat tenderizers, monosodium glutamate [MSG: Accent]) Regular soy sauce Teriyaki sauce Most flavored vinegars Regular snack chips	Regular catsup, chili sauce, mustard, pickles, relishes, olives, and horseradish Barbecue, Worcestershire, and steak sauce Canned gravies and mixes	No additional restrictions

Guidelines for food selection for 500-mg sodium diet. Use the 1000-mg sodium diet guidelines with the following modifications:

- Use low sodium bread only.
- Omit sherbet and flavored gelatin.
- Limit meat to 6 oz per day. One egg may be used per day in place of 1 oz of meat.
- Omit the following vegetables: beets, beet greens, carrots, kale, spinach, celery, white turnips, rutabagas, mustard greens, chard, peas, and dandelion greens.
- Use distilled water.
- Limit milk and milk products to 8 oz per day.

*The foods listed under the 2 "Additional Foods Excluded" categories represent additions to the foods already excluded either in the preceding column (for 2,000-mg diet) or in the preceding 2 columns (for 1,000-mg diet).

(Adapted from The Manual of Clinical Dietetics. 4th ed. Chicago, American Dietetic Association, 1992. With permission.)

TABLE A—28A. RECOMMENDED DIET MODIFICATIONS TO LOWER BLOOD CHOLESTEROL

Purpose: The general aim of dietary therapy is to reduce elevated cholesterol levels while maintaining a nutritionally adequate eating pattern.

Use: Dietary therapy should occur in two steps, the Step-One and Step-Two Diets, that are designed to progressively reduce intakes of saturated fatty acids and cholesterol and to promote weight loss in patients who are overweight by eliminating excess total calories. The Step-One Diet should be prescribed and explained by the physician and his or her staff. This diet involves an intake of total fat less than 30% of calories, saturated fatty acids less than 10% of calories, and cholesterol less than 300 mg/day. The Step-Two Diet, used if the response to the Step-One Diet is insufficient, calls for a further reduction in saturated fatty acid intake to less than 7% of calories and in cholesterol to less than 200 mg/day. The Step-One Diet calls for the reduction of the major and obvious sources of saturated fatty acids and cholesterol in the diet; for many patients this can be achieved without a radical alteration in dietary habits. The Step-Two Diet requires careful attention to the whole diet to reduce intake of saturated fatty acids and cholesterol to a minimal level compatible with an acceptable and nutritious diet. Involvement of a registered dietitian is useful, particularly for intensive dietary therapy, such as the Step-Two Diet.

After starting the Step-One Diet, the total serum cholesterol level should be measured and adherence to the diet assessed at 4 to 6 weeks and at 3 months. If the total cholesterol monitoring goal is met, the LDL-cholesterol level should be measured to confirm that the LDL goal has been achieved. If this is the case, the patient enters a long-term monitoring program and is seen quarterly for the first year and twice yearly thereafter. At these visits total cholesterol level should be measured, and dietary and behavior modifications reinforced.

If the cholesterol goal has not been achieved with the Step-One Diet, the patient should generally be referred to a registered dietitian. With the aid of the dietitian, the patient should progress to the Step-Two Diet, or to another trial on the Step-One Diet (with progression to the Step-Two Diet if the response is still not satisfactory). On the Step-Two Diet, total cholesterol levels should again be measured and adherence to the diet assessed after 4 to 6 weeks and at 3 months of therapy. If the desired goal for total cholesterol (and for LDL-cholesterol) lowering has been attained, long-term monitoring can begin. If not, drug therapy should be considered. A minimum of 6 months of intensive dietary therapy and counseling should usually be carried out before initiating drug therapy; shorter periods can be considered in patients with severe elevations of LDL-cholesterol (> 225 mg/dl) or with definite coronary heart disease. Drug therapy should be added to, and not substituted for, dietary therapy.

Adequacy: Based on the individual's food choices, the diets are adequate in all nutrients according to the National Research Council's Recommended Dietary Allowances.

NATIONAL CHOLESTEROL EDUCATION PROGRAM: STEP-ONE AND STEP-TWO DIETS

	RECOMMENDED INTAKE	
NUTRIENT	Step-One Diet	Step-Two Diet
Total fat	Less than 30% of total calories	
Saturated fatty acids	Less than 10% of total calories	Less than 7% of total calories
Polyunsaturated fatty acids	Up to 10% of total calories	
Monounsaturated fatty acids	10% to 15% of total calories	
Carbohydrates	50% to 60% of total calories	
Protein	10% to 20% of total calories	
Cholesterol	Less than 300 mg/day	Less than 200 mg/day
Total calories	To achieve and maintain desirable weight	

(With permission from The National Cholesterol Education Program, Report of the Expert Panel on Detection, Evaluation, and Treatment of High Blood Cholesterol in Adults. U.S. Department of Health and Human Services, Public Health Service National Institutes of Health Publication No. 89-2925, 1989.)

TABLE A–28B. STEP-ONE DIET

FOOD CATEGORY	CHOOSE	DECREASE
Fish, chicken, turkey, and lean meat	Fish; poultry without skin; lean cuts of beef, lamb, pork or veal; shellfish	Fatty cuts of beef, lamb, pork; spare ribs; organ meats; regular cold cuts; sausage; hot dogs; bacon; sardines; roe
Skim and low-fat milk, cheese, yogurt, and dairy substitutes	Skim or 1% fat milk (liquid, powdered, evaporated); buttermilk	Whole milk (4% fat) (regular, evaporated, condensed); cream; half and half; 2% milk; imitation milk products; most nondairy creamers; whipped toppings
	Nonfat (0% fat) or low-fat yogurt	Whole-milk yogurt
	Low-fat cottage cheese (1% or 2% fat)	Whole-milk cottage cheese (4% fat)
	Low-fat, farmer, or pot cheeses (all of these should be labeled no more than 2 to 6 g fat/oz)	All natural cheeses (e.g., blue, roquefort, camembert, cheddar, swiss)
	Low-fat or "light" cream cheese, low-fat or "light" sour cream	Cream cheeses, sour cream
	Sherbet or sorbet	Ice cream
Eggs	Egg whites (2 whites = 1 whole egg in recipes), cholesterol-free egg substitutes	Egg yolks
Fruits and vegetables	Fresh, frozen, canned, or dried fruits and vegetables	Vegetables prepared in butter, cream, or other sauces
Breads and cereals	Homemade baked goods using unsaturated oils sparingly, angel food cake, low-fat crackers, low-fat cookies	Commercial baked goods: pies, cakes, doughnuts, croissants, pastries, muffins, biscuits, high-fat crackers, high-fat cookies
	Rice, pasta	Egg noodles
	Whole-grain breads and cereals (oatmeal, whole-wheat, rye, bran, multigrain, etc.)	Breads in which eggs are major ingredient
Fats and oils	Baking cocoa	Chocolate
	Unsaturated vegetable oils: corn, olive, rapeseed (canola oil), safflower, sesame, soybean, sunflower	Butter, coconut oil, palm oil, palm kernel oil, lard, bacon fat
	Margarine or shortening made from one of the unsaturated oils listed above	
	Diet margarine	
	Mayonnaise, salad dressings made with unsaturated oils listed above	Dressings made with egg yolk
	Low-fat dressings	
	Seeds and nuts	Coconut

TABLE A–28C-1. SAMPLE MENU FOR STEP-ONE DIET

BREAKFAST	LUNCH	DINNER
Orange juice (½ cup)	Vegetable soup (1 cup)	Green salad (3½ oz)
Whole-grain cereal (¾ cup)	Saltine crackers (4)	Vinegar and oil dressing (1 tbsp)
Banana (½)	Lean beef patty (3 oz)	Broiled skinless chicken breast (3 oz)
Whole-wheat toast (2 slices)	Hamburger bun (1)	Herbed brown rice (½ cup)
Diet margarine (2 tsp)	Mustard (1 tbsp)	Steamed broccoli (½ cup)
Jelly or jam (1 tbsp)	Low-fat mayonnaise (2 tsp)	Whole-grain roll (1)
1% milk (1 cup)	Sliced tomato (2 oz) and lettuce	Diet margarine (2 tsp)
Coffee/tea	Fresh fruit salad (½ cup)	Low-fat frozen yogurt (½ cup)
	Graham crackers (4)	Medium apple (1)
	1% milk (1 cup)	Coffee/tea
	Coffee/tea	

APPROXIMATE NUTRIENT ANALYSIS

Energy (kcal)	2,054.7	Iron (mg)	16.5	Thiamin (mg)	1.8
Protein (g) (19.9% of kcal)	102.1	Magnesium (mg)	456.4	Riboflavin (mg)	2.4
Carbohydrate (g) (55.5% of kcal)	285.3	Phosphorus (mg)	1,610.8	Niacin (mg)	29.0
Total fat (g) (27.1% of kcal)	61.8	Potassium (mg)	3,978.0	Folate (μg)	400.6
Saturated fatty acids (g)	19.4	Sodium (mg)	3,190.1	Vitamin B_6 (mg)	2.8
Monounsaturated fatty acids (g)	21.1	Zinc (mg)	14.4	Vitamin B_{12} (μg)	4.4
Polyunsaturated fatty acids (g)	14.8	Vitamin A (μg RE)	1,378.8	Dietary fiber (g)	24.1
Cholesterol (mg)	167.8	Vitamin C (mg)	165.2	Water-insoluble fiber (g)	17.0
Calcium (mg)	1,126.4				

(From The Manual of Clinical Dietetics. Chicago, American Dietetic Association, 1992. With permission.)

TABLE A–28C-2. SAMPLE MENU FOR STEP-TWO DIET

BREAKFAST	LUNCH	DINNER
Orange juice (½ cup)	Vegetable soup (1 cup)	Green salad (3½ oz)
Whole-grain cereal (¾ cup)	Saltine crackers (4)	Vinegar and oil dressing (1 tbsp)
Banana (½)	Sliced turkey (3 oz)	Broiled skinless chicken breast (3 oz)
Whole-wheat toast (2 slices)	Whole-wheat bread (2 slices)	Herbed brown rice (½ cup)
Diet margarine (2 tsp)	Mustard (1 tbsp)	Steamed broccoli (½ cup)
Jelly or jam (1 tbsp)	Low-fat mayonnaise (2 tsp)	Whole-grain roll (1)
Skim milk (1 cup)	Sliced tomato (2 oz) and lettuce	Diet margarine (2 tsp)
Coffee/tea	Fresh fruit salad (½ cup)	Low-fat frozen yogurt (½ cup)
	Graham crackers (4)	Medium apple (1)
	Skim milk (1 cup)	Coffee/tea
	Coffee/tea	

APPROXIMATE NUTRIENT ANALYSIS

Energy (kcal)	1,892.5	Iron (mg)	15.6	Thiamin (mg)	1.7
Protein (g) (21.6% of kcal)	102.3	Magnesium (mg)	471.0	Riboflavin (mg)	2.1
Carbohydrate (g) (61.2% of kcal)	289.7	Phosphorus (mg)	1,734.4	Niacin (mg)	32.6
Total fat (g) (20.4% of kcal)	42.9	Potassium (mg)	4,024.4	Folate (μg)	413.5
Saturated fatty acids (g)	10.6	Sodium (mg)	3,565.7	Vitamin B_6 (mg)	2.8
Monounsaturated fatty acids (g)	13.3	Zinc (mg)	12.4	Vitamin B_{12} (μg)	3.1
Polyunsaturated fatty acids (g)	14.7	Vitamin A (μg RE)	1,392.5	Dietary fiber (g)	25.3
Cholesterol (mg)	126.5	Vitamin C (mg)	165.3	Water-insoluble fiber (g)	18.0
Calcium (mg)	1,129.9				

(From The Manual of Clinical Dietetics. Chicago, American Dietetic Association, 1992. With permission.)

TABLE A–29A. GUIDELINES FOR FOOD SELECTION FOR FAT-RESTRICTED DIET (25 g or 50 g of FAT)

FOOD CATEGORY	RECOMMENDED	MAY CAUSE DISTRESS
Beverages	Skim milk; skim buttermilk; powdered and evaporated skim milk; coffee; tea; soda; other nondairy drinks	1%, 2%, whole milks; buttermilk made with whole milk; chocolate milk; evaporated milk; cream
Breads and cereals	Whole-grain breads; enriched breads; saltines; soda crackers; cold and cooked cereals; whole-grain cereal except granola-type; unbuttered popcorn; plain corn or flour tortillas	Biscuits; breads containing egg or cheese; sweet rolls; pancakes; French toast; doughnuts; waffles; fritters; buttered popcorn; muffins; granola-type cereals and breads to which extra fat is added; popovers; snack crackers with added fat; snack chips; stuffing; fried tortillas
Desserts	Sherbet; fruit ice; gelatin; angel food cake; vanilla wafers; graham crackers; meringues; pudding made with skim milk; fat-free commercial baked products; nonfat ice cream and frozen yogurt	All other cakes, cookies, pies, and pastries; puddings made with whole milk or eggs; cream puffs
Fats Amount listed equals 1 fat equivalent; 3 to 5 equivalents/day allowed for 50-g fat diet. (Unsaturated fats are recommended.	*Unsaturated* Margarine (1 tsp) Diet margarine (1 Tbsp) Mayonnaise reduced-calorie (1 Tbsp) regular (1 tsp) Creamy salad dressings reduced-calorie (1 Tbsp) regular (2 tsp) Other salad dressings reduced-calorie (2 Tbsp) regular (1 Tbsp) Vegetable oils (1 tsp) Nuts almonds (6 whole) cashews (1 Tbsp or 2 whole) peanuts (20 small or 10 large) peanut butter (2 tsp) cashew butter (2 tsp) walnuts (2 whole) pistachios (18 whole) other nuts (1 Tbsp) Seeds sesame (1 Tbsp) sunflower (1 Tbsp) pumpkin (2 tsp) Olives (10 small or 5 large) *Saturated* Bacon (1 slice) Bacon fat (1 tsp) Butter (1 tsp) Whipped butter (2 tsp) Chitterlings (½ oz) Shredded coconut (2 Tbsp) Cream light, coffee, table (2 Tbsp) heavy whipping (1 Tbsp) Sour cream (2 Tbsp) Cream cheese (1 Tbsp) Coffee whitener liquid (2 Tbsp) powder (4 tsp) Lard (1 tsp) Oil coconut (1 tsp) palm (1 tsp) Shortening (1 tsp) Sour cream (2 Tbsp) Salt pork (¼ oz)	Any in excess of amounts prescribed on diets and all others

TABLE A–29A. CONTINUED

FOOD CATEGORY	RECOMMENDED	MAY CAUSE DISTRESS
Fruits	Fresh, frozen, canned, or dried fruit; fruit juices	Avocado
Meats and meat substitutes For 50-g fat diet, 6 oz/day For 25-g fat diet, 5 oz/day (Recommended preparation methods are broiling, roasting, grilling, or boiling; weigh meat after cooking.)	Poultry breast meat without skin Veal all cuts Lean beef USDA good or choice cuts (i.e., round, sirloin, flank steak, tenderloin, and chopped beef); roast (rib, chuck, rump); steak (cube, Porterhouse, T-bone); meatloaf made with ground beef (95% lean) Lean pork fresh, canned, cured, or boiled ham; Canadian bacon; tenderloin; chops; loin roast; Boston butt; cutlets Lean lamb chops, leg, or roast Fish all fresh, frozen, or canned in water: crab, lobster, scallops, shrimp, clams, oysters, tuna; herring (uncreamed or smoked); sardines (canned, drained); salmon (canned in water) Luncheon meats 95% fat-free; lean ham, turkey, or beef Legumes cooked, canned, without added fat Tofu, tempeh, natto Cheese skim-milk cheeses; cottage cheese; parmesan cheese Low-fat yogurt; non-fat yogurt as desired Eggs poached; soft or hard cooked; scrambled, not fried in fat; count 1 egg as 1 oz of meat in daily meat allowance; egg substitutes as desired	Any fried, fatty, or heavily marbled meat, fish, or poultry Poultry duck, goose Beef most USDA prime cuts of beef, ribs, corned beef Pork spareribs; ground pork sausage (patty or link); ham hocks; pigs' feet; chitterlings Lamb patties (ground lamb) Fish tuna (packed in oil) salmon (packed in oil) Luncheon meats most, including bologna, salami, pimento loaf Sausage Polish; Italian; knockwurst; smoked bratwurst; frankfurter Legumes (cooked with added fat)
Potatoes and potato substitutes	Potatoes; rice; barley; noodles; spaghetti, macaroni, and other pastas	Fried potatoes; fried rice; potato chips; chow mein noodles
Soups	Fat-free broth; fat-free vegetable soup; cream soup made with skim milk and allowed fat; packaged dehydrated soups	All others
Sweets	Sugar; honey; jelly; jam; marmalade; molasses; maple syrup; sourballs; gumdrops; jelly beans; marshmallows; hard candy; cocoa powder	Butter, coconut, chocolate, and cream candies
Vegetables	All fresh, frozen, or canned vegetables prepared without fats, oil, or fat-containing sauces	Buttered, au gratin, creamed, or fried vegetables unless made with allowed fat allowance
Miscellaneous	Catsup; chili sauce; vinegar; pickles; vanilla; unbuttered popcorn; white sauce made with skim milk and allowed fat; mustard; all herbs and seasonings; apple butter	Olives and nuts in excess of specified portions; cream sauces; gravies; buttered popcorn

(From The Manual of Clinical Dietetics. 4th Ed. Chicago, American Dietetic Association, 1992. With permission.)

TABLE A—29B-1. SAMPLE MENU FOR FAT-RESTRICTED DIET (25 g of FAT)

BREAKFAST	LUNCH	DINNER
Orange juice (1 cup)	Fat-free vegetable soup (1 cup)	Green salad (3½ oz)
Whole-grain cereal (¾ cup)	Saltine crackers (4)	Fat-free dressing (1 Tbsp)
Banana (1)	Sliced turkey (2 oz)	Broiled skinless chicken breast (2 oz)
Whole-wheat toast (2 slices)	Whole-wheat bread (2 slices)	Herbed brown rice (½ cup)
Jelly or jam (2 Tbsp)	Mustard (1 Tbsp)	Steamed broccoli (½ cup)
Skim milk (1 cup)	Fat-free mayonnaise (1 Tbsp)	Whole-grain roll (1)
Coffee/tea	Sliced tomato (2 oz) and lettuce	Jelly or jam (1 Tbsp)
SNACK	Fresh fruit salad (½ cup)	Fruit ice or sorbet (½ cup)
Canned or fresh fruit (1 cup)	Graham crackers (4)	Medium apple (1)
Skim milk (½ cup)	Skim milk (1 cup)	Coffee/tea
	Coffee/tea	

APPROXIMATE NUTRIENT ANALYSIS

Energy (kcal)	2,016.4	Sodium (mg)	3,259.9
Protein (g) (18.8% of kcal)	94.7	Zinc (mg)	11.6
Carbohydrate (g) (75.6% of kcal)	380.9	Vitamin A (μg RE)	1,261.1
Total fat (g) (9.8% of kcal)	22.0	Vitamin C (mg)	271.7
Saturated fatty acids (g)	6.8	Thiamin (mg)	1.8
Monounsaturated fatty acids (g)	6.4	Riboflavin (mg)	2.2
Polyunsaturated fatty acids (g)	5.2	Niacin (mg)	28.7
Cholesterol (mg)	110.7	Folate (μg)	493.2
Calcium (mg)	1,169.7	Vitamin B_6 (mg)	3.3
Iron (mg)	16.6	Vitamin B_{12} (μg)	2.9
Magnesium (mg)	512.5	Dietary fiber (g)	29.3
Phosphorus (mg)	1,672.1	Water-insoluble fiber (g)	20.2
Potassium (mg)	4,681.4		

(From The Manual of Clinical Dietetics. 4th Ed. Chicago, American Dietetic Association, 1992. With permission.)

TABLE A—29B-2. SAMPLE MENU FOR FAT-RESTRICTED DIET (50 g of FAT))

BREAKFAST	LUNCH	DINNER
Orange juice (½ cup)	Fat-free vegetable soup (1 cup)	Green salad (3½ oz)
Whole-grain cereal (¾ cup)	Saltine crackers (4)	Fat-free dressing (1 Tbsp)
Banana (½)	Lean beef patty (3 oz)	Broiled skinless chicken breast (3 oz)
Whole-wheat toast (2 slices)	Hamburger bun (1)	Herbed brown rice (½ cup)
Margarine (1 tsp)	Mustard (1 Tbsp)	Steamed broccoli (½ cup)
Jelly or jam (1 Tbsp)	Reduced-calorie mayonnaise (1 Tbsp)	Whole-grain roll (1)
Skim milk (1 cup)	Sliced tomato (2 oz) and lettuce	Margarine (1 tsp)
Coffee/tea	Fresh fruit salad (½ cup)	Fruit ice or sorbet (½ cup)
SNACK	Graham crackers (4)	Medium apple (1)
Canned peaches (½ cup)	Skim milk (1 cup)	Coffee/tea
Skim milk (½ cup)	Coffee/tea	

APPROXIMATE NUTRIENT ANALYSIS

Energy (kcal)	2,053.2	Sodium (mg)	3,016.8
Protein (g) (20.1% of kcal)	103.3	Zinc (mg)	14.2
Carbohydrate (g) (60.7% of kcal)	311.7	Vitamin A (μg RE)	1,373.5
Total fat (g) (21.6% of kcal)	49.3	Vitamin C (mg)	171.7
Saturated fatty acids (g)	15.2	Thiamin (mg)	1.8
Monounsaturated fatty acids (g)	18.6	Riboflavin (mg)	2.3
Polyunsaturated fatty acids (g)	9.4	Niacin (mg)	29.7
Cholesterol (mg)	159.0	Folate (μg)	400.4
Calcium (mg)	1141.8	Vitamin B_6 (mg)	2.9
Iron (mg)	16.3	Vitamin B_{12} (μg)	4.5
Magnesium (mg)	440.4	Dietary fiber (g)	24.4
Phosphorus (mg)	1,642.1	Water-insoluble fiber (g)	16.9
Potassium (mg)	4,170.9		

(From The Manual of Clinical Dietetics. 4th Ed. Chicago, American Dietetic Association, 1992. With permission.)

TABLE A–30A. RESTRICTED-FIBER DIET

Purpose: The fiber- and residue-restricted diet is designed to prevent blockage of a stenosed gastrointestinal tract and to reduce the frequency and volume of fecal output while prolonging intestinal transit time.

Suggested General Guidelines:

1. Limit milk and milk products to 2 cups daily. If lactose intolerant, see lactose-controlled diet.
2. Limit fruits to the following: juices without pulp (excluding prune), canned fruit, and ripe bananas. Most raw fruits should be avoided, such as dates, figs, prunes, apples, blackberries, boysenberries, peaches, grapes, pears, pineapple, rhubarb, and fresh grapefruit and orange sections.
3. Limit vegetables to the following: vegetable juices without pulp, lettuce, and cooked/canned vegetables without seeds, such as asparagus, beets, green beans, seedless tomatoes, spinach, eggplant, and acorn squash.
4. Use only white or refined bread and cereal products, or baked products using refined flour. Cooked white and sweet potatoes without skin, white rice, and refined pasta are allowed.
5. Avoid tough fibrous meats with gristle: Allow ground or well-cooked tender beef, lamb, ham, veal, pork, poultry, fish, and organ meats. Eggs and cheese are acceptable.
6. Avoid peanuts, coconut, nuts, seeds, popcorn, dried beans, peas, legumes, and lentils.

Modifications: A low-fiber diet is not synonymous with a low-residue diet. The term residue refers to both the indigestible content of a food that acts as a laxative and the total postdigestive luminal contents that increase fecal output.[1,2] A low-fiber diet also can be a low-residue diet if milk and products that contain milk are limited to 2 cups or less per day, prune juice is omitted, and meat and shellfish with tough connective tissue are avoided. Milk, prune juice, and connective tissue from meats are low in fiber but may increase colonic residue and stool weight by mechanisms other than dietary fiber.[1]

Adequacy: Based on the individual's food choices, the diet is adequate in all nutrients according to the National Research Council's Recommended Dietary Allowances, 1989. Vitamin and mineral supplementation may be indicated, however, when illness results in suboptimal intakes and increased requirements. The benefit of long-term restriction of dietary fiber remains controversial. Strict reductions in milk products, vegetables, and fruit intake may necessitate calcium, ascorbic acid, and folate supplementation. Individual response, particularly in patients with ulcerative colitis and Crohn's disease, must be monitored to avoid an overly restrictive regimen and to determine continued indication for this diet.

References

1. Kramer, P.: The meaning of high and low residue diets. *Gastroenterology, 47*:649, 1964.
2. Connell, A.M.: The role of fibre in the gastrointestinal tract. *In* The Clinical Role of Fibre. Edited by P.E. Bowen, A.M. Connell, et al. Toronto, Ontario, Canada, Medical Education Services, 1985.

(From The Manual of Clinical Dietetics. 4th Ed. Chicago, American Dietetic Association, 1992. With permission.)

TABLE A—30B. HIGH-FIBER DIET

Purpose: The diet is designed to be high in dietary fiber. It is useful for decreasing intraluminal colonic pressure, increasing gastrointestinal motility and increasing the volume and weight of material that reaches the distal colon. Both soluble and insoluble fibers exert these physiologic effects, whereas only soluble fibers exert metabolic effects, such as delayed glucose absorption, increased sensitivity to insulin, altered intestinal enzyme activity, binding of bile acids, and decrease in serum cholesterol and triglyceride levels.

General Guidelines

1. The reported positive effects of fiber are derived from a diet high in fiber-rich foods. Increased fiber intake should come from a variety of food sources rather than dietary fiber supplements. This approach is more likely to ensure increased intake of minerals and other nutrients.
2. Consumption of adequate amounts of liquids (eight 8-fluid-ounce glasses per day) in conjunction with high-fiber intake is recommended.
3. Prior to recommending a twofold increase in dietary fiber consumption, an assessment of current fiber intake should be made. Estimates of fiber content of household portions of foods are shown in Table A—30c.
4. Advise gradual increase of dietary fiber intake to minimize potential side effects.

Fiber Components and Food Sources

Water-soluble fibers are hydrated, resulting in gel-like or viscous substances, and are fermented by colonic bacteria.

Water-soluble fibers:	Foods containing water-soluble fibers include:
Gum Mucilages Pectin Some hemicellulose	Fruits, vegetables, barley, legumes, oat, and oat bran

Water-insoluble fibers remain essentially unchanged during digestion.

Water-insoluble fibers:	Foods containing water-insoluble fibers include:
Cellulose Lignin Some hemicellulose	Fruits, vegetables, cereals, whole-wheat products, and wheat bran

Adequacy: Depending on individual food selection, the high-fiber diet is adequate in all nutrients according to the National Research Council's Recommended Dietary Allowances, 1989.

The adequacy of the high-fiber diet may be questionable for individuals whose mineral intake is marginal because of poor dietary practices or for "at-risk" groups (children, pregnant or lactating women, elderly or chronically ill persons). Some studies indicate that excessive intakes of some dietary fiber sources may bind and interfere with the absorption of the following minerals: calcium, copper, iron, magnesium, selenium, and zinc.[1] It is hypothesized, however, that long-term high-fiber diet would not by itself cause mineral or nutrient imbalances in the general population.[2,3] Intake of adequate fluids is necessary because of hygroscopic nature of fiber.

The American Dietetic Association recommends a daily dietary fiber intake of 20 to 35 g from a variety of sources combined with a low-fat, high-carbohydrate diet.[4]

References

1. Walter, A.: Mineral metabolism. *In Dietary Fibre, Fibre-Depleted Foods and Disease.* Edited by H. Trowell, D. Burkitt, and K. Heaton. Orlando, Academic Press, 1985.
2. Gordon, D.T.: Total dietary fiber and mineral absorption. *In Dietary Fiber Chemistry, Physiology and Health Effects.* Edited by D. Kritchevsky, C. Bonfield, and J.W. Anderson. New York, Plenum Press, 1990.
3. Slavin, J.L.: Dietary fiber: classification, chemical analyses and food sources. J. Am. Diet. Assoc., *87:*1164, 1987.
4. Position of The American Dietetic Association: Health implications of dietary fiber. Technical support paper. J. Am. Diet. Assoc., *88:*216, 1988.

Further Reading

Anderson, J.W.: Fiber and health: an overview. *Am. J. Gastroenterol, 82:*892, 1986.

Judd, P., Truswell, S.: Dietary fibre and blood lipids in man. *In Dietary Fibre Perspectives, Reviews and Bibliography.* Edited by A. Leeds. London, John Libbey, 1985.

Klurfeld, D.M.: The role of dietary fiber in gastrointestinal disease. *J. Am. Diet. Assoc., 87:*1178, 1987.

Lanza, E., and Batrum, R.: A critical review of fiber analysis and data. *J. Am. Diet. Assoc., 86:*732, 1986.

(Modified from The Manual of Clinical Dietetics. 4th Ed. Chicago, American Dietetic Association, 1992. With permission.)

TABLE A–30C. DIETARY FIBER CONTENT OF FOODS IN COMMONLY SERVED PORTIONS

FOOD GROUP	<1 g	1–1.9 g	2–2.9 g	3–3.9 g	4–4.9 g	5–5.9 g	> 6 g
Breads (1 slice)	Bagel White French	Whole-wheat	Bran muffin (1)	NA*	NA	NA	NA
Cereals (1 oz)	Rice Krispies Special K Cornflakes	Oatmeal Nutri-Grain Cheerios	Wheaties Shredded Wheat	Most Honey Bran	Bran Chex 40% Bran Flakes Raisin Bran	Corn Bran	All-Bran Bran Buds 100% Bran
Pasta (1 cup)	NA	Macaroni Spaghetti	NA	Whole-wheat spaghetti	NA	NA	NA
Rice (½ cup)	White	Brown	NA	NA	NA	NA	NA
Legumes (½ cup cooked)	NA	NA	NA	Lentils	Lima beans Dried peas	NA	Kidney beans Baked beans Navy beans
Vegetables (½ cup unless otherwise stated	Cucumber Lettuce (1 cup) Green pepper	Asparagus Green beans Cabbage Cauliflower Potato without skin (1) Celery	Broccoli Brussels sprouts Carrots Corn Potato with skin (1) Spinach	Peas	NA	NA	NA
Fruits (1 medium unless otherwise stated)	Grapes (20) Watermelon (1 cup)	Apricots (3) Grapefruit (½) Peach with skin Pineapple (½ cup)	Apple, without skin Banana Orange	Apple, with skin Pear, with skin Raspberries (½ cup)	NA	NA	NA

*Not applicable.

(Slavin, J.L.: Dietary fiber: Classification, chemical analyses, and food sources. J. Am. Diet. Assoc., *87*:1164, 1987. Reprinted with permission.)

TABLE A–30D-1. SAMPLE MENU FOR FIBER- AND RESIDUE-RESTRICTED DIET

BREAKFAST	LUNCH	DINNER
Strained orange juice (½ cup)	Vegetable broth (1 cup)	Strained tomato juice (½ cup)
Puffed rice cereal (¾ cup)	Saltine crackers (4)	Broiled skinless chicken breast (3 oz)
Canned peaches (½ cup)	Lean beef patty (3 oz)	White rice (½ cup)
White bread toast (2 slices)	Hamburger bun without seeds (1)	Cooked spinach (½ cup)
Margarine (2 tsp)	Mustard (1 Tbsp)	White roll (1)
Jelly (1 Tbsp)	Catsup (1 Tbsp)	Margarine (2 tsp)
2% milk (1 cup)	Canned fruit cocktail (½ cup)	Low-fat frozen yogurt (½ cup)
Coffee/tea	Vanilla wafer cookies (2)	Applesauce (½ cup)
	2% milk (1 cup)	Coffee/tea
	Coffee/tea	

APPROXIMATE NUTRIENT ANALYSIS

Energy (kcal)	1,857.2	Sodium (mg)	2,954.5
Protein (g) (20.9% of kcal)	97.0	Zinc (mg)	11.7
Carbohydrate (g) (52.1% of kcal)	241.9	Vitamin A (μg RE)	1,398.2
Total fat (g) (27.6% of kcal)	53.0	Vitamin C (mg)	132.1
Saturated fatty acids (g)	20.3	Thiamin (mg)	1.4
Monounsaturated fatty acids (g)	21.3	Riboflavin (mg)	2.0
Polyunsaturated fatty acids (g)	9.2	Niacin (mg)	25.4
Cholesterol (mg)	181.8	Folate (μg)	274.2
Calcium (mg)	1,138.7	Vitamin B_6 (mg)	1.7
Iron (mg)	13.2	Vitamin B_{12} (μg)	4.2
Magnesium (mg)	346.5	Dietary fiber (g)	14.3
Phosphorus (mg)	1,315.6	Water-insoluble fiber (g)	9.0
Potassium (mg)	3,482.6		

(From The Manual of Clinical Dietetics. 4th Ed. Chicago, American Dietetic Association, 1992. With permission.)

TABLE A—30D-2. SAMPLE MENU FOR HIGH-FIBER DIET*

BREAKFAST	LUNCH	DINNER
Orange juice (½ cup)	Split pea soup (1 cup)	Green salad (3½ oz)
Whole-grain cereal (¾ cup)	Whole-wheat crackers (4)	Vinegar and oil dressing (1 Tbsp)
Raisins (2 Tbsp)	Lean beef patty (3 oz)	Broiled skinless chicken breast (3 oz)
Whole wheat toast (2 slices)	Hamburger bun (1)	Herbed brown rice (½ cup)
Margarine (2 tsp)	Mustard (1 Tbsp)	Steamed broccoli (½ cup)
Jelly or jam (1 Tbsp)	Catsup (1 Tbsp)	Whole-grain roll (1)
2% milk (1 cup)	Sliced tomato (2 oz) and lettuce	Margarine (2 tsp)
Coffee/tea	Fresh fruit salad (½ cup)	Low-fat frozen yogurt (½ cup)
	Bran muffin (1)	Medium pear (1)
	2% milk (1 cup)	Coffee/tea
	Coffee/tea	

APPROXIMATE NUTRIENT ANALYSIS

Energy (kcal)	2,195.0	Sodium (mg)	3,175.6
Protein (g) (19.4% of kcal)	106.4	Zinc (mg)	14.4
Carbohydrate (g) (54.0% of kcal)	296.0	Vitamin A (μg RE)	1,381.1
Total fat (g) (29.6% of kcal)	72.1	Vitamin C (mg)	160.4
Saturated fatty acids (g)	23.0	Thiamin (mg)	1.8
Monounsaturated fatty acids (g)	25.7	Riboflavin (mg)	2.4
Polyunsaturated fatty acids (g)	16.0	Niacin (mg)	28.6
Cholesterol (mg)	190.9	Folate (μg)	425.4
Calcium (mg)	1,241.8	Vitamin B_6 (mg)	2.4
Iron (mg)	18.4	Vitamin B_{12} (μg)	4.3
Magnesium (mg)	511.7	Dietary fiber (g)	30.8
Phosphorus (mg)	1,763.0	Water-insoluble fiber (g)	21.1
Potassium (mg)	4,328.5		

*For further fat restriction, decrease servings of margarine and salad dressing. Use skimmed or 1% milk and milk products.

(From The Manual of Clinical Dietetics. 4th Ed. American Dietetic Association, 1992. With permission.)

TABLE A—31A. SOFT DIET

Purpose: The soft diet is designed for patients who are physically or neurologically unable to tolerate a general diet.
Adequacy: Based on the individual's food choice, the diet is adequate in all nutrients according to the National Research Council's Recommended Dietary Allowances, 1989.

TABLE A—31B. GUIDELINES FOR FOOD SELECTION FOR SOFT DIET

FOOD CATEGORY	RECOMMENDED	MAY CAUSE DISTRESS
Beverages	Milk and milk products; all other beverages	Alcoholic beverages
Breads and cereals	White, refined-wheat, or light-rye enriched breads, soft rolls and crackers; cooked or ready-to-eat cereals	Coarse cereals (e.g., bran); whole-grain breads or crackers with seeds; bread or bread products with nuts or dried fruits
Desserts	Cakes, cookies, pies, pudding, custard, ice cream, sherbet, and gelatin made with allowed foods; fruit ice and frozen pops	All sweets and desserts containing nuts, coconut, or dried fruits not allowed; fried pastries (e.g., doughnuts)
Fats	Butter or fortified margarine; salad dressings; all fats and oils	Highly seasoned salad dressings
Fruits	All fruit juices; cooked or canned fruit; avocado, banana, grapefruit, and orange sections without membrane; soft fruits (e.g., melons, strawberries)	Other fresh and dried fruits
Meats and meat substitutes	All lean, tender meats, poultry, fish, and shellfish; crisp bacon; eggs; mild-flavored cheeses; creamy peanut butter; soybean and other meat substitutes; plain or flavored yogurt	Strong-smelling or highly seasoned meats, cheeses, or fish (e.g., luncheon meats, frankfurters, sausage); yogurt with nuts or dried fruits
Potato or substitute	Potatoes; enriched rice, barley, spaghetti, macaroni, and other pasta	Potato chips, fried potatoes
Soups	Soups made with allowed foods	Highly seasoned soups and soups made with gas-producing vegetables
Sweets	Sugar; syrup; honey; jelly and seedless jam; hard candies; plain chocolate candies; molasses; marshmallows	Any with nuts or coconut
Vegetables	All vegetable juices; cooked vegetables and lettuce as tolerated; salads made from allowed foods	Raw and fried vegetables; whole kernel corn; gas-producing vegetables (eg, broccoli, Brussels sprouts, cabbage, onions, leeks, cauliflower, cucumber, green pepper, rutabagas, turnips, sauerkraut, dried peas, dried beans)
Miscellaneous	Iodized salt; flavorings; mildly flavored gravies and sauces; pepper, herbs, spices, catsup, mustard, and vinegar in moderation	Strongly flavored seasonings and condiments (e.g., garlic, chili sauce, chili pepper, horseradish); pickles; popcorn; nuts and coconut

(From The Manual of Clinical Dietetics. 4th Ed. Chicago, American Dietetic Association, 1992. With permission.)

TABLE A–31C. SAMPLE MENU FOR SOFT DIET

BREAKFAST	LUNCH	DINNER
Orange juice (½ cup)	Vegetable soup (1 cup)	Tomato juice (6 oz)
Refined cold cereal (¾ cup)	Saltine crackers (4)	Broiled skinless chicken breast (3 oz)
Banana (½ cup)	Lean beef patty (3 oz)	Enriched rice (½ cup)
White toast (2 slices)	Hamburger bun (1)	Steamed green beans (½ cup)
Margarine (2 tsp)	Mustard (1 Tbsp)	Soft dinner roll (1)
Jelly or jam (1 Tbsp)	Mayonnaise (1 Tbsp)	Margarine (2 tsp)
2% milk (1 cup)	Lettuce leaf	Low-fat frozen yogurt (½ cup)
Coffee/tea	Canned fruit cocktail (½ cup)	Applesauce (½ cup)
	Graham crackers (4)	Coffee/tea
	2% milk (1 cup)	
	Coffee/tea	

APPROXIMATE NUTRIENT ANALYSIS

Energy (kcal)	2,142.6	Sodium (mg)	3,581.9
Protein (g) (17.9% of kcal)	96.0	Zinc (mg)	12.5
Carbohydrate (g) (57.1% of kcal)	305.8	Vitamin A (μg RE)	944.5
Total fat (g) (25.5% of kcal)	60.8	Vitamin C (mg)	118.3
Saturated fatty acids (g)	21.8	Thiamin (mg)	2.0
Monounsaturated fatty acids (g)	23.0	Riboflavin (mg)	2.4
Polyunsaturated fatty acids (g)	9.9	Niacin (mg)	30.9
Cholesterol (mg)	185.9	Folate (μg)	327.2
Calcium (mg)	1,038.7	Vitamin B_6 (mg)	2.5
Iron (mg)	15.4	Vitamin B_{12} (μg)	4.4
Magnesium (mg)	308.9	Dietary fiber (g)	16.5
Phosphorus (mg)	1,319.1	Water-insoluble fiber (g)	11.1
Potassium (mg)	3,389.7		

(From The Manual of Clinical Dietetics. 4th Ed. Chicago, American Dietetic Association, 1992. With permission.)

TABLE A—32. DYSPHAGIA DIET

Stage I—Dysphagia puree, no liquids
Stage II—Dysphagia puree plus thick liquids
Stage III—Dysphagia puree plus thin liquids
Stage IV—Dysphagia mechanical soft foods, no liquids
Stage V—Dysphagia mechanical soft foods plus thick liquids
Stage VI—Dysphagia mechanical soft foods plus thin liquids

STAGE I—DYSPHAGIA PUREE, NO LIQUIDS

No liquids are provided unless specified by physician's order. Includes smooth, moist, and pureed foods that require little or no chewing but form a moist, cohesive bolus.

Food Group	Foods Allowed	Foods Avoided
Milk products	Pudding, custard, ice cream, plain or flavored yogurt (without fruit)	All others
Meat, poultry, and eggs	Pureed meat, chicken, fish; soufflés, soft cooked or poached eggs	All others
Vegetables and fruits	Pureed vegetables, fruits; applesauce, frozen fruit juices	All others
Breads and cereals	Thick cooked cereals, mashed potato	All others
Fats	Butter, margarine, sour cream	All others
Miscellaneous	Salt, pepper, ketchup, mustard, jelly, gelatin dessert	None

STAGE II—DYSPHAGIA PUREE PLUS THICK LIQUIDS

Includes all foods allowed in stage I with the addition of the following *thick liquids.*

Food Group	Liquids Allowed	Liquids Avoided
Milk products	Thickened eggnog, Carnation Instant Breakfast, milk shakes	All others
Soups	Thick creamed soups	Broth
Fruits	Thinned pureed fruits, nectar, vegetable juice	All others

STAGE III—DYSPHAGIA PUREE PLUS THIN LIQUIDS

Includes all foods allowed in stage II with the addition of the following *thin liquids.*

Food Group	Liquids Allowed	Liquids Avoided
Milk products	Eggnog, Carnation Instant Breakfast, milk	None
Soup	Thin creamed soups, broth	None
Beverages	Coffee, tea, soda, fruit juices	None

Note: Once a patient has mastered stage III, the diet can be either progressed in consistency (i.e., to stage V) or changed to puree.

STAGE IV—DYSPHAGIA MECHANICAL SOFT FOODS, NO LIQUIDS

No liquids are provided unless specified by physician's order. Includes minced and soft foods that require little or no chewing but form a soft, cohesive bolus.

Food Group	Liquids Allowed	Liquids Avoided
Milk products	Pudding, custard, ice cream, cream pies; plain, flavored, fruited yogurt	All others
Cheeses	Small-curd cottage cheese, ricotta cheese, American cheese, grated cheese	All others
Eggs	Soft scrambled eggs, crustless quiche, soufflés, egg salad	All others
Meat, fish, and poultry	Ground meat or poultry with gravy; chicken or tuna salad (without celery); meat loaf; hamburger; baked or broiled fish; salmon loaf; pasta casseroles	

TABLE A—32. CONTINUED

Food Group	Foods Allowed	Foods Avoided
Vegetables	Cooked and diced carrots, beets, chopped or creamed spinach, butternut or acorn squash	Raw vegetables, other cooked vegetables
Potatoes, rice, and noodles	Mashed or baked (without skin) potatoes, macaroni and cheese, egg noodles, spaghetti with gravy or sauce	Rice, coarse grain (kasha, buckwheat, bran)
Fruit	Mashed banana, canned or cooked fruits cut into small pieces	Fruits with pits, raisins; all others
Breads and cereals	Bread, soft rolls, muffins, soft French toast, pancakes, cooked cereal, dry cereals soaked in milk, cakes without nuts	Dry crackers, breads with seeds, raisins, nuts
Fats	Butter, margarine, sour cream, gravy, mayonnaise	Nuts, seeds

STAGE V—DYSPHAGIA MECHANICAL SOFT FOODS PLUS THICK LIQUIDS

Includes all food from stage IV with the addition of *thick liquids* as outlined in stage II.

STAGE VI—DYSPHAGIA MECHANICAL SOFT FOODS PLUS THIN LIQUIDS

Includes all food from stage IV with the addition of *thin liquids* as outlined in stage III.

Note: Once a patient has mastered stage VI, the diet can be either progressed in consistency (i.e., to regular) or changed to mechanical soft foods.

Patients at stages I and IV need to have fluid status monitored and fluid requirements met by alternate means.

Milk products may not be tolerated by individuals who are susceptible to increased mucus production probably secondary to casein, a milk protein. If this becomes a problem, substitutes should be found.

Suggestions for dietitians:

1. A member of the medical or nursing staff or dysphagia team should be present at the bedside when a patient initially receives a dysphagia diet or advances to a higher stage to evaluate the patient's tolerance of the stage.
2. The dietitian should work closely with medical and nursing staff for continued evaluation of the patient's diet tolerance and progression.
3. Calorie counts are indicated to evaluate adequacy of intake and to justify the need for supplementation or nutrition support.
4. The dietitian should work closely with the dysphagia team for physiologic evaluation of the patient's ability to chew and swallow to select the correct diet stage.
5. The dietitian should encourage small, frequent meals, particularly in the first stages of the diet.
6. As a guide, the following list gives a progression of food consistencies in order of increasing swallowing difficulty:
   - stiff jelled consistency
   - standard jelled consistency
   - thick purees
   - applesauce consistency
   - thick soup consistency
   - nectar consistency
   - standard thin liquids
   - chunk consistency (ground or diced)

Eating tips:

1. Food should be taken in small portions (½ tsp at a time).
2. The patient should sit upright with hips flexed at a 90° angle.
3. If possible, the neck should be at a 90° angle and flexed slightly forward.
4. The patient should sit up for 15 to 30 minutes both before and after meals.
5. Food should be placed on the unaffected side when possible.
6. Cold or hot foods may be better tolerated than foods at room temperature.

(From Antiaspiration-dysphagia Diet. *In* Diet Manual. New York, Memorial Sloan-Kettering Cancer Center, 1989. Reprinted by permission; and Bloch, A.S.: Nutrition Management of the Cancer Patient. Aspen, Rockville, MD, 1990. With permission.)

TABLE A—33A. ANTIDUMPING (POSTGASTRECTOMY) DIET

Purpose: This diet is designed to provide adequate calories and nutrients to support tissue healing and prevent weight loss and dumping syndrome after gastric surgery.[1–6]

Modifications: The diet limits beverages and liquids at meals, limits the intake of simple carbohydrates, and is high in protein and moderate in fat. Small, frequent feedings should be provided daily.[1,2] If no complications occur, additional foods are added as tolerated. Some patients are able to advance to a general diet within 2 to 3 weeks.[1]

After surgery, the diet generally progresses as follows:[1,2]

1. Ice chips held in mouth or small sips of water. Some people tolerate warm water better than ice chips or cold water.
2. Low-carbohydrate, clear liquids, such as broth, bouillon, unsweetened gelatin, or diluted unsweetened fruit juices, are given next.
3. The postgastrectomy diet then begins, with gradual progression to a general diet as tolerated.

It is important to note that the stated guidelines must be tailored to each patient's surgery, food tolerances, and nutrition problems and deficiencies.

General Guidelines[1,2,4,5,7,8]

1. Liquids should be given 30 to 60 minutes after meals and limited to 0.5-to 1-cup servings. At least 6 cups of fluid, however, should be consumed daily to replace losses resulting from diarrhea. Carbonated beverages and milk are not recommended initially.
2. Small, frequent feedings should be provided. The number of feedings depends on the patient's tolerance to specific portions of food. Foods should be eaten slowly and chewed well.
3. The diet should be low in simple carbohydrates, high in complex carbohydrates and protein, and moderate in fat.
4. All food and drink should be moderate in temperature. Cold drinks tend to cause increased gastric motility.
5. If "dumping" is a problem, the patient should lie down 20 to 30 minutes after meals to retard transit to the small bowel.
6. Introduce small amounts of milk to determine tolerance. If milk intolerance is found to be caused by a lactase deficiency, a lactose-restricted diet may be necessary (see Table A—35).
7. If adequate caloric intake cannot be provided because of steatorrhea, use of medium-chain triglyceride products may be needed.
8. Pectin, a dietary fiber found in fruits and vegetables, may be helpful for treating dumping syndrome. Pectin delays gastric emptying, slows carbohydrate absorption, and reduces the glycemic response.

Adequacy: The adequacy of the diet depends on the extent of surgery, as well as on individual food tolerances. With careful selection, this diet is adequate in all nutrients. After gastric surgery some patients experience malabsorption, which may be specific for macronutrients (e.g., carbohydrates, proteins, and fats) or micronutrients (e.g., folate, vitamin B_{12}, iron, vitamin D, and calcium).[2] Vitamin and mineral supplementation may be necessary depending on the extent of surgery and on whether the symptoms of dumping syndrome persist.[1,2]

References

1. Zeman, F.J.: *Clinical Nutrition and Dietetics.* 2nd Ed. New York, Macmillan, 1991.
2. Desai, M. Jeejeebhoy, K.N. *In* Modern Nutrition in Health and Disease. 7th Ed. Edited by M.E. Shils and V.R. Young. Philadelphia, Lea & Febiger, 1988.
3. Braga, M., Zuliani, L., Foppa, L., et al.: Br. J. Surg., *75*:477, 1988
4. Jordan, P. *In* Hardy's Textbook of Surgery. 2nd Ed. Edited by J. Hardy. Philadelphia, J.B. Lippincott, 1988.
5. Williams, S.R.: Nutrition and Diet Therapy. 6th Ed. St. Louis, Times Mirror/Mosby College Publishing, 1989.
6. Meyer, J.H. *In* Gastrointestinal Disease: Pathophysiology, Diagnosis, and Management. 4th Ed. Edited by M.H. Sleisenger, J.S. Fordtran. Philadelphia, W.B. Saunders, 1989.
7. Sawyers, J.L.: Am. J. Surg., *159*:8–13, 1990.
8. Alpers, D., Crouse, R., Stenson, W.: Manual of Nutritional Therapeutics. 2nd Ed. Boston, Little Brown, 1988.

TABLE A—33B. GUIDELINES FOR FOOD SELECTION FOR ANTIDUMPING (POSTGASTRECTOMY) DIET

FOOD CATEGORY	RECOMMENDED	MAY CAUSE DISTRESS*
Beverages†	Milk as tolerated; coffee; tea; unsweetened or diluted fruit drinks; unsweetened carbonated beverages	Alcohol; chocolate milk drinks; milkshakes; sweetened fruit drinks; sweetened carbonated beverages
Breads and cereals	Whole-grain or enriched breads and cereals; English muffins and bagels; unsweetened, cooked cereals	Breads made with dried fruits, nuts, and seeds; pastries; donuts; muffins
Cereals	Unsweetened dry and cooked cereals	Sugar-coated cereals, coarse cereals (e.g., bran)
Desserts	Plain cakes and cookies; sugar-free pudding, gelatin dessert, custard, yogurt, and frozen yogurt	All sweets and desserts made with chocolate or dried fruits; sweetened gelatin dessert; fried pastries; ice cream; ice milk; regular fruited or frozen yogurt
Fats	Butter; margarine; salad dressings; mayonnaise; vegetable oils; sour cream; cream cheese as tolerated	None
Fruits	Unsweetened canned fruits and fruit juice†; fresh fruits	All dried fruits; sweetened fruit juice; fruits canned in heavy syrup
Meats and meat substitutes	Lean tender meats; fish; poultry; shellfish; eggs; peanut butter; cottage cheese; mild cheeses; highly seasoned and spicy meats	Fried meats or eggs
Potato and potato substitutes	Potatoes; enriched rice; barley; noodles; spaghetti, macaroni, and other pastas	Any to which sugar has been added (e.g., candied sweet potatoes)
Soups	Soups made with allowed foods; spicy soups as tolerated	Soups prepared with heavy cream or high-fat ingredients
Sweets	Sugar substitutes and sweets made with sugar substitutes	Sugar; syrup; honey; jelly; jam; molasses; marshmallows
Vegetables	Cooked (fresh, frozen, canned) vegetables or vegetable juice†; raw vegetables as tolerated	Any to which sugar has been added
Miscellaneous	Iodized salt; pepper; mildly flavored sauces and gravies; strongly flavored seasonings as tolerated	None

*If no adverse symptoms occur, these foods can be added as tolerated.
†All fluids should be consumed 30 to 60 minutes after meals and limited to ½- to 1-cup servings.
(From The Manual of Clinical Dietetics. 4th Ed. Chicago, American Dietetic Association, 1992. With permission.)

TABLE A–33C. SAMPLE MENU FOR ANTIDUMPING (POSTGASTRECTOMY) DIET*

BREAKFAST	LUNCH	DINNER
Grapefruit (½)	Lean hamburger patty (2 oz)	Broiled skinless chicken breast (3 oz)
Oatmeal (½ cup)	Hamburger bun (1)	Herbed brown rice (½ cup)
Whole-wheat toast (1 slice)	Mayonnaise (1 Tbsp)	Steamed broccoli (½ cup)
Margarine (1 tsp)	Sliced tomato (2 oz) and lettuce	Margarine (2 tsp)
2% milk† (½ cup)	Fresh fruit salad (½ cup)	Unsweetened applesauce (½ cup)
Coffee/tea† (½ cup)	2% milk† (½ cup)	2% milk† (½ cup)
	Coffee/tea† (½ cup)	Coffee/tea† (½ cup)
MIDMORNING SNACK	**MIDAFTERNOON SNACK**	**BEDTIME SNACK**
Cheese (1 oz)	Roast beef (1 oz)	Peanut butter (2 Tbsp)
Saltine crackers (4)	Bread (1 slice)	Graham crackers (4)
Banana (½)	Mustard (1 tsp)	2% milk† (½ cup)
	Vegetable soup† (1 cup)	

APPROXIMATE NUTRIENT ANALYSIS

Energy (kcal)	2,055.9	Sodium (mg)	3,016.3
Protein (g) (20.9% of kcal)	107.4	Zinc (mg)	14.1
Carbohydrate (g) (41.7% of kcal)	214.1	Vitamin A (μg RE)	823.3
Total fat (g) (39.4% of kcal)	90.0	Vitamin C (mg)	136.2
Saturated fatty acids (g)	29.8	Thiamin (mg)	1.4
Monounsaturated fatty acids (g)	33.5	Riboflavin (mg)	1.9
Polyunsaturated fatty acids (g)	19.3	Niacin (mg)	27.1
Cholesterol (mg)	215.2	Folate (μg)	240.5
Calcium (mg)	1,035.6	Vitamin B_6 (mg)	2.3
Iron (mg)	12.0	Vitamin B_{12} (μg)	4.3
Magnesium (mg)	409.9	Dietary fiber (g)	21.6
Phosphorus (mg)	1,652.2	Water-insoluble fiber (g)	14.0
Potassium (mg)	3,270.6		

*The sample menu incorporates six (6) meals per day. The number of feedings depends on the patient's tolerance to food portions and therefore should be adjusted accordingly.

†Liquid should be given 30 to 60 minutes after the meal and limited to ½ cup to 1 cup servings.

(From The Manual of Clinical Dietetics. 4th Ed. Chicago, American Dietetic Association, 1992. With permission.)

TABLE A–34. GLUTEN-RESTRICTED AND GLIADIN- AND PROLAMIN-FREE (Wheat-, Rye-, Oat, and Barley-Free) DIET INSTRUCTION

This menu pattern is designed to provide adequate nutrition while eliminating wheat, rye, oats, and barley from the diet. The fraction of gluten protein in wheat that injures the intestine of susceptible persons is gliadin. The equivalent toxic protein fractions in barley, rye, and oats are prolamins. When all sources of gliadin and prolamin are removed from the diet, the intestine is able to regenerate, and normal function is usually restored.

Gliadin and prolamin may be either present in foods as a basic ingredient (i.e., listed as wheat, rye, oats, or barley) or added as a derivative when a food is processed or prepared. Thus, *reading labels carefully is very important!* A great deal of confusion occurs about the presence of gliadin- and prolamin-containing additives in foods. This table includes lists of both nebulous ingredients and common additives.

Since flour and cereal products are quite often used in the preparation of foods, it is important to be aware of the methods of preparation used as well as the foods themselves. This is especially true when dining out.

FOOD GROUP WITH SUGGESTED DAILY INTAKE	FOODS ALLOWED	FOODS TO AVOID
Milk (2 or more cups)	Fresh, dry, evaporated, or condensed milk; cream; sour cream;* whipping cream; yogurt*	Malted milk; some commercial chocolate drinks; some nondairy creamers.†
Meat, fish, poultry	All kinds of fresh meats, fish, other seafood, poultry; fish canned in oil, brine, or vegetable broth; some meat products, such as hot dogs and lunch meats†	Prepared meats containing wheat, rye, oats, or barley, such as some sausages,† hot dogs,† bologna†; luncheon meats†; ground beef and pork with oat bran added in the form of "Oatrim" or "LeanMaker"; chili con carne†; bread-containing products, such as swiss steak, meat loaf, and croquettes; tuna canned with hydrolyzed protein†; turkey with hydrolyzed vegetable protein (HVP) injected as part of the basting solution; "imitation Crab" containing wheat starch or other unacceptable filler.
Cheeses (Can be used for meat and milk groups)	All aged cheeses, such as cheddar, swiss, edam, parmesan; cottage cheese;* cream cheese;* pasteurized processed cheese*†	Any cheese product containing *oat gum* as an ingredient.
Eggs	Plain or in cooking.	Eggs in sauce made from wheat, rye, oat, or barley. Usually wheat flour is used in white sauce.
Potato or other starch	White and sweet potatoes; yams; hominy; rice; wild rice; special pasta made from rice, soy, or corn‡; some oriental rice and bean thread noodles.	Regular noodles; spaghetti or macaroni (semolina = wheat); most packaged rice mixes and frozen rice side dishes; frozen potato products with wheat starch or wheat flour added.
Vegetables (2 or more servings)	All plain, fresh, frozen, or canned; dried peas, beans, and lentils; some commercially prepared vegetables†	Creamed vegetables†; vegetables canned in sauce†; some canned baked beans†; commercially prepared vegetables and salads†
Fruits	All fresh, frozen, canned, or dried; all fruit juices; some canned pie fillings	Thickened or prepared fruits; some pie fillings†
Breads (3 or more servings)	Specially prepared breads using only allowed flours. Breads may be purchased ready-to-eat or as mixes to prepare at home. Recipes have been developed for home use and for use in automatic bread machines.‡	Those containing wheat, rye, oats, and/or barley flours. Avoid those with buckwheat, millet, amaranth, quinoa, spelt, or teff.§ *Beware: wheat-free* does not always mean gliadin- and prolamin-free! Breads made from "carob-soy flour" may contain 80% wheat flour!
Cereals (1 or more servings)	*Hot cereals* Corn meal Cream of Rice Hominy Rice *Cold cereals* Puffed Rice Corn Pops Fruity and Choc. Pebbles Kenmei Sun Flakes (corn & rice) Special cereals made without malt or malt flavoring.	Those containing wheat, rye, oats, barley, graham, wheat germ, malt or malt flavoring, kasha, bulgar, buckwheat,§ millet,§ amaranth,§ quinoa,§ spelt,§ teff.§ New products with "unusual" grains are constantly being introduced. Do not use them until you can clear them with a reliable source.

TABLE A–34. CONTINUED

FOOD GROUP WITH SUGGESTED DAILY INTAKE	FOODS ALLOWED	FOODS TO AVOID
Crackers and snack foods	Rice wafers; rice crackers; plain corn and potato chips; rice cakes†; pure cornmeal tortillas; popcorn; caramel corn†	Those with wheat, rye, barley, oats, or other questionable (grain-like) ingredients. *Read labels carefully.* Some coating mixes used on chips contain wheat flour! If the product shows "brown rice syrup," contact the manufacturer to check for "barley malt enzymes" used in processing.
Soups	Homemade broth and soup using allowed ingredients; a few canned soups;† specialty dry soup mixes‡	Most canned soups† and soup mixes†; bouillon and bouillon cubes with hydrolyzed vegetable protein (HVP). HVP may appear as "flavoring" or "natural flavoring" ingredient.
Flours and thickening agents	Arrowroot starch (A) Corn bean (B) Corn flour‡ (B, C, D) Corn germ (B) Corn meal (B, C, D) Potato flour (B, C, E) Potato starch flour (B, C, E) Rice bran (B) Rice flours Plain (B, C, D, E) Brown (B, C, D, E) Sweet (A, B, C, F) Rice polish‡ (B, C, G) Rice starch (A) Soy flour‡ (B, C, G) Tapioca starch (A)	Wheat starch Wheat germ, bran Wheat flour Rye Oats Barley Buckwheat§ Amaranth§ Quinoa§ Spelt§ Teff§ "Carob-soy" flour containing 80% wheat flour (made by Sterling Foods Co., Seattle)
A = good thickening agent; B = good combined with other flours; C = best combined with milk and eggs in baked products; D = grainy-textured products; E = drier product than with other flours; F = moister product than with other flours; G = adds distinct flavor to product, use with moderation.		
Fats	Butter; margarine; vegetable oil; hydrogenated vegetable oil; nuts; peanut butter; some salad dressings†; mayonnaise† (mayonnaise made with cider or wine vinegar is found at Kosher delis)	Some commercial salad dressings†‖
Desserts	Cakes; quick breads; pastries; puddings made with allowed ingredients; Cornstarch; tapioca; rice puddings; gelatin desserts; cook and serve puddings; "expensive" ice cream with a few simple ingredients; sorbet; frozen Yogurt†; sherbet†	Commercial cakes, cookies, pies, made with wheat, rye, oats, barley, millet, amaranth, buckwheat, quinoa, spelt, teff; Jello "instant" pudding; products containing brown rice syrup made with barley malt enzyme.
Beverages	Instant and ground coffee; instant tea; carbonated beverages†; pure cocoa powder; wines made in United States; rums; some root beers†; vodka distilled from grapes or potatoes.	Ovaltine; malted milk; ale; beer; gin; whiskeys‖; vodka distilled from grain; flavored coffees†; some herbal teas with barley or barley malt added†
Sweets	Jelly; jam; honey; brown and white sugar; molasses; most syrups†; some candy†; chocolate; pure cocoa; coconut; marshmallows†	Some commercial candies; foods with malt/malt flavoring or "natural flavoring"†; See's Molasses Chews; chocolate-coated nuts, which may be rolled in wheat flour†; brown rice syrup made with barley malt enzyme†
Miscellaneous	Spices (salt, pure pepper, cloves, ginger, nutmeg, cinnamon, allspice, etc.); herbs (oregano, rosemary, etc.); food coloring; alcohol-free extracts; yeast; baking soda; baking powder; cream of tartar; dry mustard; cider, rice and wine vinegars; olives; monosodium glutamate (MSG) made in United States	Condiments made with wheat-derived distilled white vinegar‖; alcohol-based extracts‖; some curry powders†; some dry seasoning mixes†; some gravy extracts†; some meat sauces†; most soy sauces†; some chewing gum†; communion wafers/bread#

TABLE A–34. CONTINUED

*Check vegetable gum used.
†Consult label and contact manufacturer to clarify questionable ingredients.
‡See Special Products List for availability and ordering information.
§Additional information is needed before this product can be cleared.
||Distilled white vinegar uses grain as a starting material. Most often the grain mash includes wheat. Whiskies, including "corn whiskey," use wheat, rye, oats, or barley in their mash. According to chemistry professors consulted, in large-scale distillation processes, such as those used in the manufacture of whiskey and vinegar, it is possible that a very small amount of protein may be carried over into the distillate. The presence of such a small amount of gliadin and/or prolamin must be tested via immunoassay. Currently, we are advising gliadin- and prolamin-intolerant individuals to use cider, wine, or rice vinegar in such food preparation as making salad dressings, pickles, and in cooking. To be 100% safe, purchase or make condiments with cider, wine or rice vinegar. These condiments (ketchup, mustard, mayonnaise, pickles) are usually available in kosher delis. Foods with nongrain vinegars are produced for Passover.
#Contact the Gluten Intolerance Group of North America to obtain instructions for making communion wafers from acceptable ingredients. Note: In Catholic communion, host crumbs are often added to the wine before it is served. A workable solution is to arrange to use a goblet of your own.

NEBULOUS INGREDIENT	INCLUDE	AVOID
"Hydrolyzed vegetable protein" or "hydrolyzed protein"	Those from soy, corn, or milk	Mixtures of wheat, corn, and soy*
"Flour" or "cereal products"	Rice flour, corn flour, corn meal, potato flour, soy flour	Wheat, rye, oats, barley, amaranth, quinoa, spelt, teff, millet, buckwheat
'Vegetable protein"	Soy, corn	Wheat, rye, oats, barley
"Vegetable broth"	In the United States, this must contain two or more of the following: beans, cabbage, carrots, celery, garlic, onions, parsley, peas, potatoes, green bell pepper, red bell pepper, spinach, or tomatoes. It cannot contain any other ingredients. *It can be used.*	
"Malt" or "malt flavoring"	Those derived from corn.	Those derived from barley or barley malt syrup.
"Brown rice syrup"	Rice only.	Rice plus barley malt enzyme.
"Starch"	In the United States, it must be *cornstarch.*	
"Modified starch" or "modified food starch"	Arrowroot, corn, potato waxy maize, maize.	Wheat starch
"Vegetable gum"	Carob bean, locust bean, cellulose, guar, gum arabic, gum acacia, gum tragacanth, xanthan gum	Oat gum.
"Soy sauce" or "soy sauce solids"	Those that *do not* contain wheat *(soy only)*	Those brewed from wheat and soy.
"Mono-" and "diglycerides"	Those using *non*wheat-based carrier.	Those using a wheat starch carrier.

These questionable ingredients must be cleared with the manufacturer before they are eaten. A sample letter requesting information on starting materials and packaging and processing ingredients is available at the end of this table.
*Hydrolyzed vegetable protein: A combination of wheat, corn, and soy is primarily used as starting material for hydrolyzed vegetable protein (HVP). When wheat protein is "hydrolyzed," its large amino acid chains are broken down into smaller chains. Some protein reseachers believe the same sequence of amino acids found in these smaller chains contain the same toxicity as the intact gliadin subfraction of the gluten protein. Thus, HVP made from wheat is not recommended for use on a gliadin-free diet.

ADDITIVES THAT ARE GLIADIN- AND PROLAMIN-FREE*

Adipic acid
Ascorbic acid

BHA
BHT
Beta carotene
Biotin

Calcium chloride
Calcium pantothenate
Calcium phosphate
Carboxymethylcellulose
Carrageenan
Citric acid
Corn sweetener
Corn syrup solids

Demineralized whey
Dextrimaltose
Dextrose–dextrins
Dioctyl sodium sulfosuccinate

Folic acid–folacin
Fructose
Fumaric acid

Gums: acacia, arabic, carob bean, cellulose, guar, locust bean, tragacanth, xanthan

Invert sugar

Lactic acid
Lactose
Lecithin

Magnesium hydroxide
Malic acid
Microcrystallin cellulose
Monosodium glutamate (MSG) made in United States

Niacin–niacinamide

Polyglycerol
Polysorbate 60; 80
Potassium citrate
Potassium iodide
Propylene glycol monostearate
Propylgallate
Pyridoxine hydrochloride

Riboflvin

Sodium acid pyraphosphate
Sodium ascorbate
Sodium benzoate
Sodium caseinate
Sodium citrate
Sodium hexametaphosphate
Sodium nitrate
Sodium silaco aluminate
Sorbitol–mannitol
Sucrose
Sulfosuccinate

Tartaric acid
Thiamine hydrochloride
Tri-calcium phosphate

Vanillan
Vitamin A (palmitate)
Vitamins and minerals

*The above is not an exhaustive list.

TABLE A—34. CONTINUED

MEDICATIONS	
All medications have fillers/dispersing agents added. These are usually lactose or corn starch. Wheat starch may also be used. *Before you take any medication, take the following precautions.* *Over-the-Counter Drug:* Read the list of active and inactive ingredients carefully. Use the list of "Nebulous Ingredients" in this table to spot potential problems. Ask your pharmacist to "translate" the terms you do not know. *Prescription Drug:* Inactive ingredients are *not* listed. Even your pharmacist must call the drug company to obtain this information! When the pharmaceutical company is contacted, they will need the lot number of the product so they can check the formulation of the batch you will be taking. A list of drug companies with addresses and phone numbers can be found in the Physicians' Desk Reference. *Liquid Cold and Flu Medications:* These medications often contain alcohol. Check source.	
SPECIAL PRODUCTS LIST	
AlpineAire Foods P.O. Box 926 Nevada City, CA 95959 916-272-1971	Freeze-dried foods for backpacking. Vacuumed packed. No preservatives, no added sugar, no artificial flavors or colors. Note: The "vegetable pasta" in Pasta Roma and Vegetable Pasta Stew *contains wheat flour.* Mail orders accepted.
Bickford Laboratories 282 S. Main Street Akron, OH 44308 216-762-4666	Forty-nine varieties of alcohol-free flavorings. Selection ranges from common flavorings, like vanilla and almond, to exotic. Mail orders accepted.
DeBoles Garden City Park, NY 11040	Corn pasta products, including ribbon noodles, macaroni, and spaghetti.
Dietary Specialties P.O. Box 227 Rochester, NY 14601 1-800-544-0099	A wide assortment of mixes, crackers, cookies, and pasta. Many exclusive imported items. Mail orders accepted.
Ener-G Foods, Inc. P.O. Box 84487 Seattle, WA 98124-5787 1-800-331-5222	Excellent assortment of flours and flour mixes. Will ship in bulk (20# boxes). Variety of baked products, dry soup mixes, flavorings. Mail orders accepted.
Lundberg Family Farms Box 369 Richvale, CA 95974 916-882-4551	Interesting variety of combination rices. Brown rice cereals and rice cakes. Note: Sweet Dreams Brown Rice Syrup is made using barley malt enzyme. Products made with this syrup should be avoided. Soups contain wheat-derived soy sauce. Mail orders accepted.
Med-Diet Inc. 3050 Ranchview Lane Plymouth, MN 55447 1-800-med-diet	Carries various brands of breads, crackers, cookies, cake and muffin mixes, and pasta. Note: Their order blank is not designed for those who must eliminate gliadin and prolamin. Request their list of "wheat/gluten-free foods that contain no wheat starch" so you'll know what to order!
Red Mill Farms, Inc. 290 S. 5th Street Brooklyn, NY 11211 718-384-2150	Three suitable products that are also lactose free: Dutch Chocolate Cake, Banana-Nut Cake, and Coconut Macaroons. All vacuumed packed. Mail orders accepted.
Tad Enterprizes 9356 Pleasant Tinley Park, IL 60477 708-429-2101	Carry a variety of flours for gliadin- and prolamin-free baking. Mail orders accepted.
Van Brode's Milling Clinton, MA 01510	Carries some cold breakfast cereals (malt free). Write for complete product information.

TABLE A—34. CONTINUED

WRITING EFFECTIVE LETTERS TO FOOD MANUFACTURERS*

Clarifying questionable ingredients on product labels and in medications is essential for those following this diet. Manufacturers are usually courteous and prompt when answering questions regarding their products. The usefulness of their reply, however, often depends on how the question is posed. Use the following letter format when you need to contact a a manufacturer.

Your Address
Date

Dear Sir/Madam:

I am on a gluten-restricted, gliadin- and prolamin-free diet for the treatment of celiac sprue (dermatitis herpetiformis). I must avoid the protein found in wheat, rye, oats, and barley, since they cause an immune response which damages the lining of my intestine.

Although I would like to use your product, (insert name), your ingredient listing does not give adequate information for me to determine if it would be suitable. Specifically, I need to know

examples would be:

the source of your "food starch modified"
whether your "soy sauce solids" are derived from wheat
what "natural flavorings" you use in this product
from what source your "vegetable gum" is derived
the inacive ingredients used in the medication, including those used in the coatings and capsules

Another likely source of gliadin and prolamin contamination is the incidental ingredients which are used in the packaging and processing of your product. Since these incidental ingredients are not listed on the packaging, I am relying on your thoroughness to clarify these substances.

If it would be possible, I would appreciate a copy of your response to be forwarded to: The Gluten Intolerance Group of North America
P.O. Box 23053
Seattle, WA 98102-0353

This will allow your efforts to be shared with others through our national organization which reaches health-care personnel as well as persons with celiac sprue and dermatitis herpetiformis. If you have questions regardiing these disorders and the required dietary restrictions, please direct them to our national office.

Thank you for your efforts on my behalf.

Sincerely,
Your Signature

*Additional information on celiac sprue and dermatitis herpetiformis may be obtained from The Gluten Intolerance Group of North America, P.O. Box 23053, Seattle WA 98102-0353.

TABLE A–35A. LACTOSE-CONTROLLED DIET

Purpose: The lactose-controlled diet is designed to prevent or reduce bloating, flatulence, cramping, and diarrhea associated with ingesting lactose-containing products.

Modifications: The diet is a general one that restricts or eliminates lactose-containing foods and beverages. Since tolerance of lactose may vary, the diet is usually administered on a trial-and-error basis.[1] Individual tolerance determines the amount of lactose allowed; many patients may be able to tolerate 5 to 8 g of lactose at a given time, especially if they consume it with a meal.[2]

Labels should be read carefully, and foods containing milk, lactose, milk solids, whey, curds, skim milk powder, and skim milk solids should be avoided. In addition to dairy products, the following food categories may contain lactose: breads, candy and cookies; cold cuts, hot dogs, and bologna; commercial sauces and gravies; cream soups; dry cereals; frostings; frozen breaded fish and chicken; prepared and processed foods; salad dressings containing milk or cheese; sugar substitutes; and instant drink mixes. Moreover, some medications and vitamins may contain lactose as a carrier. Lactate, lactalbumin, lactulate, and calcium compounds are salts of lactic acid and do not contain lactose.

Patients should be encouraged to experiment with the lactose-reduced or lactose-free products currently available. In addition, lactase enzyme is available in droplet form for use with lactose-containing beverages and in tablet form for ingestion prior to consuming a lactose-containing meal. Lactobacillus acidophilus milk is not equivalent to lactase-treated milk.

Tolerance to lactose is variable; if a patient is asymptomatic, no restrictions are necessary. If the patient experiences adverse reactions to lactose, cessation of symptoms should occur within 3 to 5 days on a lactose-controlled diet. Further testing may be necessary if symptoms persist.[2] Small amounts of lactose-containing food (approximately 3 g) several times a day may be tolerated better than a large amount of lactose ingested at one time.[3] Studies have shown that yogurt is significantly better tolerated than milk because of its high lactase activity.[3,4] Different brands and processing methods, however, may affect tolerance to yogurt.

Adequacy: Depending on individual food choices, the diet can provide adequate amounts of all essential nutrients. Calcium, vitamin D, and riboflavin may be deficient if all dairy products are avoided. Use of lactose-hydrolyzed milk and milk products could satisfy these nutrient needs; otherwise, supplementation may be necessary.

References

1. Shils, M.E., Young, V.R. (Eds.): Modern Nutrition in Health and Disease. 7th Ed. Philadelphia, Lea & Febiger, 1988.
2. Martini, M. Savaiano, D.: Am. J. Clin. Nutr., *47*:57–60, 1988.
3. Onwulata, C.I., Rao, D.R., Vankineni, P.: Am. J. Clin. Nutr., *49*:1233–1237, 1989.
4. Wytock, D.H., DiPalma, J.A.: Am. J. Clin. Nutr., *47*:454–457, 1988.

Further Reading

Burlant, A.: Lactose-Free Cooking. Wayne, NJ, Lockley Publishing, 1990.
Dobler, M.L.: Lactose Intolerance. Chicago, The American Dietetic Association, 1991, catalog no. 0881.
Martens, R.A., Martens, S.: The Milk Sugar Dilemma. 2nd Ed. Lansing, Medi-Ed Press, 1987.
Zukin, J.: Dairy-Free Cookbook. Rocklin, CA, Prima Publishing and Communications, 1989.

Special Product Information

Lactaid can be purchased in tablets, drops, or as lactase-treated milk and cheese products.

Lactaid Hotline
800-257-8650
9 AM–4 PM Eastern time
Monday through Friday
In Canada: 800-387-5711

Lactaid, Inc.
P.O. Box 111
Pleasantville, NJ 08232

Lactase tablets are produced by:

Kremers-Urban Company
P.O. Box 2038
Milwaukee, WI 53201

Dairy Ease tablets and lactose-treated milk (skim, 1%, and 2% fat) are produced by:

Winthrop Consumer Products
Glenbrook Laboratories
Division of Sterling Drug, Inc.
90 Park Ave.
New York, NY 10016

(From The Manual of Clinical Dietetics. 4th Ed. Chicago, American Dietetic Association, 1992. With permission.)

TABLE A—35B. GUIDELINES FOR FOOD SELECTION FOR LACTOSE-CONTROLLED DIET*

FOOD CATEGORY	RECOMMENDED	MAY CAUSE DISTRESS*
Beverages	All beverages with allowed ingredients; soybean milks; other lactose-free supplements; lactase-hydrolyzed milk	Milk, milk products, or acidophilus milk as tolerance dictates
Breads and cereals	Whole-grain or enriched breads and cereals	Depending on tolerance, some breads and cereals prepared with milk or milk products may need to be avoided
Desserts	Cakes, cookies, pies; flavored gelatin desserts; water ices made with allowed foods	Any prepared with milk or milk products (e.g., sherbet, ice cream, ice milk, custard, pudding, commercial desserts, and mixes)
Fats	Butter or margarine; salad dressings; nondairy creamer; all oils	Any prepared with lactose-containing ingredients
Fruits	All fruits and juices	None
Meats and meat substitutes	All meats, poultry, fish; eggs; peanut butter; dried peas and beans; hard, aged, and processed cheese, if tolerated; yogurt as tolerated	Cold cuts and frankfurters that contain lactose filler; cottage cheese
Potatoes and potato substitutes	Potatoes; enriched rice; barley; noodles, spaghetti, macaroni, and other pastas	Potatoes or substitutes prepared with milk or milk products; mixes prepared with lactose-containing ingredients
Soups	Broth; bouillon; soups made with allowed ingredients	Soups prepared with milk or milk products
Sweets	Sugar; corn syrup; pure maple syrup; honey; jellies; jams; pure sugar candies; marshmallows	Chocolate; caramels; any candies made with lactose-containing ingredients
Vegetables	All	Vegetables prepared with milk or milk products
Miscellaneous	All spices, seasonings, flavorings	Any prepared with milk or milk products

*A lactose-free diet, from which virtually all known sources of lactose are eliminated, may be indicated for patients with severe intolerance or a congenital lactase deficiency.

(From The Manual of Clinical Dietetics. 4th Ed. American Dietetic Association, 1992. With permission.)

TABLE A–35C. SAMPLE MENU FOR LACTOSE-CONTROLLED DIET*

BREAKFAST	LUNCH	DINNER
Orange juice (½ cup)	Vegetable soup (1 cup)	Green salad (3½ oz)
Whole-grain cereal (¾ cup)	Saltine crackers (4)	Oil and vinegar dressing (1 Tbsp)
Banana (½)	Lean beef patty (3 oz)	Broiled skinless chicken breast (3 oz)
Whole-wheat toast (2 slices)	Hamburger bun (1)	Herbed brown rice (½ cup)
Margarine (2 tsp)	Catsup (1 Tbsp)	Steamed broccoli (½ cup)
Jelly or jam (1 Tbsp)	Mustard (1 Tbsp)	Whole-grain roll (1)
Lactose-reduced 2% milk (1 cup)	Sliced tomato (2 oz) and lettuce	Margarine (2 tsp)
Coffee/tea	Fresh fruit salad (½ cup)	Fruit ice (½ cup)
	Graham crackers (4)	Medium apple (1)
	Lactose-reduced 2% milk (1 cup)	Coffee/tea
	Coffee/tea	

APPROXIMATE NUTRIENT ANALYSIS

Energy (kcal)	2,157.2	Sodium (mg)	3,069.8
Protein (g) (15.6% of kcal)	83.9	Zinc (mg)	11.7
Carbohydrate (g) (56.8% of kcal)	306.3	Vitamin A (μg RE)	1,111.5
Total fat (g) (30.1% of kcal)	72.1	Vitamin C (mg)	256.8
Saturated fatty acids (g)	18.3	Thiamin (mg)	1.7
Monounsaturated fatty acids (g)	27.3	Riboflavin (mg)	1.4
Polyunsaturated fatty acids (g)	19.4	Niacin (mg)	29.0
Cholesterol (mg)	144.4	Folate (μg)	471.0
Calcium (mg)	1,413.5	Vitamin B_6 (mg)	2.5
Iron (mg)	16.1	Vitamin B_{12} (μg)	2.2
Magnesium (mg)	380.2	Dietary fiber (g)	23.5
Phosphorus (mg)	1,121.7	Water-insoluble fiber (g)	16.4
Potassium (mg)	3,580.2		

*If lactose-reduced milk is not tolerated, substitute ½ cup nondairy creamer at breakfast and fruit juice at lunch. A calcium supplement should also be provided.

(From The Manual of Clinical Dietetics. 4th Ed. Chicago, American Dietetic Association, 1992. With permission.)

TABLE A—35D. LACTOSE CONTENT OF SELECTED MILK, MILK PRODUCTS, AND SUBSTITUTES*

PRODUCT		LACTOSE (APPROX. g/UNIT)
Milk	1 cup—244 g	11
Low-fat milk (2% fat)	1 cup—244 g	9–13
Skim milk	1 cup—244 g	12–14
Chocolate milk	1 cup—244 g	10–12
Sweetened condensed whole milk	1 cup—306 g	35
Dried whole milk	1 cup—128 g	48
Nonfat dry milk, instant	1½ cup—91 g	46
Buttermilk fluid	1 cup—245 g	9–11
Whipped cream topping	1 Tbsp—3 g	0.4
Light Cream	1 Tbsp—15 g	0.6
Half and Half	1 Tbsp—15 g	0.6
Low-fat yogurts†	8 oz—227–258 g	11–15
Cheese:		
Blue, cream, Parmesan, Colby	1 oz—28 g	0.7–0.8
Camembert, Limburger	1 oz—28 g	0.1
Cheddar, Gouda	1 oz—28 g	0.4–0.6
Cheese, pasteurized, processed:		
American	1 oz—28 g	0.5
Pimento	1 oz—28 g	0.5–1.7
Swiss	1 oz—28 g	0.4–0.6
Cottage cheese	1 cup—210 g	5–6
Cottage cheese, low-fat (2% fat)	1 cup—226 g	7–8
Butter	2 pats—10 g	0.1
Oleomargarine	2 pats—10 g	0
Ice cream		
Vanilla, regular	1 cup—133 g	9
French, soft	1 cup—173 g	9
Ice milk, vanilla	1 cup—131 g	10
Sherbet, orange	1 cup—193 g	4
Ice, orange	100 g	0

*Lactaid milk and other dairy products have lactose reduced by 70%. With further treatment, these products can be 100% lactose-free.

†Bacterial lactase in unpasteurized yogurt survives transit through the stomach, thus allowing digestion of the lactose present in yogurt. This process enables lactase-deficient individuals to consume these dairy products in moderate amounts (from ½ to 1 pint) with fewer or no symptoms. Data from Kolars, J.C., Levitt, M.D., Aouji, M., et al.: N. Engl. J. Med., *310*:1–3, 1984.

Lactase-deficient patients have been reported to experience no gastrointestinal distress after consuming pasteurized yogurt (500 g) even though the lactase activity is significantly destroyed by pasteurization. In contrast, cultured milk does result in gastrointestinal distress for lactose-intolerant individuals. Data from Savaiano, D.A., AbouElAnouar, A., Smith, D.E., et al.: Am. J. Clin. Nutr., *40*:1219–1223, 1984.

(From Walsh, J.D.: Am. J. Clin. Nutr., *31*:592–596, 1978. With permission of the author and publisher.)

TABLE A–36. OXALATE CONTENT OF SELECTED FOODS AND FOOD GROUPS

FOODS TO USE: THESE CONTAIN SMALL AMOUNTS OF OXALATE
0–2 mg OXALATE PER SERVING

Vegetables	Fruits	Beverages	Miscellaneous
Broccoli	Avocados	Apple juice	Butter
Brussels sprouts	Bananas	Barley water	Cheese, cheddar
Cabbage	Cherries	Beer, bottled	Chicken noodle soup
Cauliflower	Grapes, Thompson seedless	Cider	Cornflakes
Chives	Mangoes	Coca-Cola	Eggs
Cucumbers	Melons	Grapefruit juice	Egg noodle (chow mein)
Lettuce	Nectarines	Lemon squash drink (lemonade)	Fish (except sardines)
Mushrooms	Peaches, canned	Lucozade, bottled	Jelly with allowed fruit
Onions	Hiley	Milk	Lemon juice
Peas	Stokes	Orange juice	Lime juice
Potatoes, white	Pineapples	Pepsi-Cola	Macaroni
Radishes	Plums, golden gage, green gage	Pineapple juice	Margarine
Rice		Sherry, dry	Meats
Turnips		Wine	Oatmeal, porridge
			Oxtail soup
			Poultry
			Red plum jam
			Sweets, boiled

FOODS TO AVOID: THESE CONTAIN LARGE AMOUNTS OF OXALATE
>15 mg OXALATE PER SERVING

Vegetables	Fruits	Beverages	Miscellaneous
Beans in tomato sauce	Blackberries	Beer, lager	Chocolate
Beets	Blueberries	Tuborg Pilsner	Cocoa
Celery	Currants, red	Ovaltine (24 mg/8 oz)	Grits (white corn)
Chard, Swiss	Gooseberries, green	Tea (132–181.2 mg/8 oz)	Peanuts
Collards	Grapes, Concord		Pecans
Dandelion greens	Lemon peel		Soybean crackers
Eggplant	Lime peel		Wheat germ
Escarole	Raspberries, black		
Leeks	Rhubarb		
Okra			
Parsley			
Peppers, green			
Pokeweed			
Potatoes, sweet			
Rutabagas			
Spinach			
Squash, summer			

LOW-OXALATE MEAL PLAN
(40–50 mg)

Foods	Little or No Oxalate Content <2 mg Oxalate/Serving Eat as Desired	Moderate Oxalate Content 2–10 mg Oxalate/Serving Limit: 2 (½ cup) Servings/Day	High Oxalate Content >10 mg Oxalate/Serving Avoid Completely
Beverages/Juices	Apple juice	Coffee, any kind (8 oz serving)	Beer: draft
	Beer, bottled	Cranberry juice (4 oz)	Stout, Guinness Draft
	Coca-Cola (12 oz limit/day)	Grape juice (4 oz)	Lager, Tuborg Pilsner
	Distilled alcohol	Orange juice (4 oz)	Juices containing berries
	Grapefruit juice	Tomato juice (4 oz)	Ovaltine and other mixed beverage mixes
	Lemonade or limeade without peel	Nescafé powder	Tea, cocoa
	Wine, red, rosé		
	Pepsi-Cola (12 oz limit/day)		
	Pineapple juice		
	Tap water (prefered for extra calcium)		
Milk (2 or more cups)	Buttermilk		
	Low-fat milk		
	Low-fat yogurt with allowed fruit		
	Skim milk		

TABLE A–36. CONTINUED

LOW-OXALATE MEAL PLAN
(40–50 mg)

Foods	Little or No Oxalate Content <2 mg Oxalate/Serving Eat as Desired	Moderate Oxalate Content 2–10 mg Oxalate/Serving Limit: 2 (½ cup) Servings/Day	High Oxalate Content >10 mg Oxalate/Serving Avoid Completely
Meat Group	Eggs	Sardines	Baked beans canned in tomato sauce
	Cheese, cheddar		Peanut butter
	Lean lamb, beef, or pork		Soybean curd (Tofu)
	Poultry		
	Seafood		
Vegetables	Brussels sprouts	Asparagus	Beans, green, wax, dried
	Cauliflower	Broccoli	Beets, tops, root, greens
	Cabbage	Carrots	Celery
	Mushrooms	Corn, sweet white, sweet yellow	Chard, Swiss
	Onions	Cucumbers, peeled	Chives
	Peas, green	Green peas, canned	Collards
	Potatoes (Irish)	Lettuce, iceberg	Dandelion greens
	Radishes	Lima beans	Eggplant
		Parsnips	Escarole
		Tomato, 1 small	Kale
		Turnips	Leeks
			Mustard greens
			Okra
			Parsley
			Peppers, green
			Pokeweed
			Potatoes, sweet
			Rutabagas
			Spinach
			Squash, summer
			Watercress
Fruits	Avocados	Apples	Blackberries
	Banana	Apricots	Blueberries
	Cherries, Bing	Cherries, edible portion	Currants, red
	Grapefruit	Currants, black	Dewberries
	Grapes, Thompson seedless	Oranges, edible portion	Fruit cocktail
	Mangoes	Peaches, Alberta	Gooseberries
	Melons	Pears	Grapes, Concord
	cantaloupe	Pineapples	Lemon peel
	casaba	Plums, Damson	Lime peel
	honeydew	Prunes, Italian	Orange peel
	watermelon		Raspberries
	Nectarines		Rhubarb
	Peaches, Hiley		Strawberries
	Plums, green or Golden Age		Tangerines
Bread Starches	Cornflakes	Cornbread	Fruit cake
	Macaroni	Sponge cake	Grits, white corn
	Noodles	Spaghetti, canned in tomato sauce	Soybean crackers
	Oatmeal		Wheat germ
	Rice		
	Spaghetti		
	White bread		
Fats and Oils	Bacon		Peanuts
	Mayonnaise		Pecans
	Salad dressing		
	Vegetable oils		
Miscellaneous	Jelly or preserves (made with allowed fruits)	Chicken noodle soup, dehydrated	Chocolate, cocoa
	Lemon, lime juice		Pepper (in excess of 1 tsp/day)
	Salt, pepper (1 tsp/day)		Vegetable soup
	Soups with ingredients allowed		Tomato soup
	Sugar		

(From The Low Oxalate Diet Book, General Clinical Research Center, University of California at San Diego Medical Center and San Diego Chapter of National Foundation for Ileitis and Colitis, 1981. With permission.)

TABLE A—37. COMMERCIAL NUTRITION FORMULATIONS FOR ORAL AND TUBE FEEDING

The sixth and seventh editions included numerous tables providing detailed nutrient composition of a variety of available commercial formulas. In more recent years, the companies making these formulas have uniformly provided updated information in reprints that are widely distributed. These reprints often contain the composition of formulas produced by other companies as well as their own. Additionally, new and revised commercial preparations appear on the market in increasing numbers, whereas some older formulas have been removed. These commercial reference guides make the continued publication of detailed formulations unnecessary and actually undesirable in this volume. Thus, outdated information can be avoided.

A list is provided below of the companies currently producing and marketing such formulations. Address and telephone numbers are included to help the reader to obtain the most current information on a specific product. Each company also produces an enteral product reference list that provides nutrient analysis on each product, as well as other relevant information needed to make informed choices. They may be contacted for such publications or for other educational materials they provide. In addition, a list is included of the names of current formulations by dietary use characteristics.

COMPANY LISTS WITH IDENTIFICATION CODE

CLINTEC Nutrition Company (C)
Affiliated with Baxter Healthcare Corporation and Nestles S.A.
Three Parkway North, Suite 500
P.O. Box 760
Deerfield, IL 60015-0760
1-800-422-2752

KENDALL McGAW (K)
2525 McGaw Avenue
P.O. Box 19791
Irvine, CA 92713
714-660-2000
1-800-854-6851 (Technical Assistance)

MEAD JOHNSON ENTERAL NUTRITIONALS (M)
Mead Johnson Nutrition Group
A Bristol Myers Squibb Company
Evansville, IN 47721
1-800-457-3550

ELAN PHARMA (E)
320 Charles Street
Cambridge, MA 02141
617-868-6400
1-800-237-3535

ROSS LABORATORIES (R)
Division of Abbott Laboratories
625 Cleveland Avenue
Columbus, OH 43215
614-227-3333
1-800-544-7495

SANDOZ NUTRITION (S)
5300 West 23rd Street
Minneapolis, MN 55416
1-800-999-9978

SHERWOOD MEDICAL (SH)
1915 Olive Street
St. Louis, MO 63103-1642
314-621-7788
1-800-428-4400

TABLE A—37. CONTINUED

CURRENT LIST OF FORMULATIONS FOR ORAL AND/OR ENTERAL FEEDING BY DIETARY USE CHARACTERISTICS

Complete Diet Formulations Containing Some Natural Foods with Varying Residue

- Carnation Instant Breakfast (C)
- Carnation Instant Breakfast, no sugar (C)
- Compleat Regular (S)
- Compleat Modified (S)
- Meritene Powder (S)
- Sustagen (M)
- Vitaneed (SH)

Complete Defined-formula Diets with Intact Purified Protein, Low Residue, and No Lactose

- Attain (SH)
- CitriSource (S)
- Citrotein (S)
- Comply (SH)
- Ensure (R)
- Ensure HN (R)
- Ensure Plus (R)
- Ensure Plus HN (R)
- Entrition 0.5 (C)
- Entrition HN (C)
- Fortical (SH)
- Fortison (SH)
- Fortison, L.S. (SH)
- Introlan (E)
- Introlite (R)
- Isocal (M)
- Isocal HCN (M)
- Isocal HN (M)
- Isolan (E)
- Isosource (S)
- Isosource HN (S)
- Isotein HN (S)
- Magnacal (SH)
- Nitrolan (E)
- Nutren 1.0 (C)
- Nutren 1.5 (C)
- Nutren 2.0 (C)
- Nutrilan (E)
- Osmolite (R)
- Osmolite HN (R)
- Portagen (M)
- Pre-Attain (SH)
- Pre-Fortison (SH)
- Promote (R)
- Replete Oral (C)
- Resource Liquid (S)
- Resource Plus Liquid (S)
- Ross SLD (R)
- Susta II (M)
- Sustacal (M)
- Sustacal HC (M)
- Sustacal 8.8 (M)
- Travasorb MCT (C)
- Two Cal HN (R)
- Ultralan (E)

TABLE A–37. CONTINUED

Complete Defined Formula Diets with Intact Purified Protein, No Lactose-Containing Fiber
Ensure with Fiber (R)
Fiberlan (E)
Fibersource (S)
Fibersource HN (S)
Jevity (R)
Nutren with Fiber (C)
Profiber (SH)
Replete with Fiber (C)
Sustacal with Fiber (M)
Ultracal (M)
Defined Formula Diets with Hydrolyzed Protein or Amino Acids, Low Residue, and No Lactose
Accupep HPF (SH)
Alitraq (R)
Criticare HN (M)
Peptamen (C)
Reabilan (E)
Reabilan HN (E)
Tolerex (S)
Travasorb HN (C)
Travasorb (C)
Vital HN (R)
Vivonex T.E.N. (S)
Disease-Specific Formulations
Alterna (R)
Aminess Essential Amino Acid Tablets (C)
Amin-Aid (K)
Glucerna (R)
Hepatic-Aid II (K)
Immun-Aid (K)
Impact (S)
Impact with Fiber (S)
Lipisorb (M)
Nepro (R)
Nutri Hep (C)
Nutrivent (C)
Perative (R)
Protain XL (SH)
Pulmocare (R)
Replena (R)
Replete (C)
Stresstein (S)
Suplena (R)
Traum-Aid HBC (K)
TraumaCal (M)
Travasorb Hepatic (C)
Travasorb Renal (C)

( ) = Company identification, see preceding list.

*O'Brien KMI is now Elan Pharma. The Newtrition product line is now the Elan product line.

TABLE A–37. CONTINUED

Complete Defined Formula Diets with Intact Purified Protein, No Lactose-Containing Fiber
- Ensure with Fiber (R)
- Fiberlan (E)
- Fibersource (S)
- Fibersource HN (S)
- Jevity (R)
- Nutren with Fiber (C)
- Profiber (SH)
- Replete with Fiber (C)
- Sustacal with Fiber (M)
- Ultracal (M)

Defined Formula Diets with Hydrolyzed Protein or Amino Acids, Low Residue, and No Lactose
- Accupep HPF (SH)
- Alitraq (R)
- Criticare HN (M)
- Peptamen (C)
- Reabilan (E)
- Reabilan HN (E)
- Tolerex (S)
- Travasorb HN (C)
- Travasorb (C)
- Vital HN (R)
- Vivonex T.E.N. (S)

Disease-Specific Formulations
- Alterna (R)
- Aminess Essential Amino Acid Tablets (C)
- Amin-Aid (K)
- Glucerna (R)
- Hepatic-Aid II (K)
- Immun-Aid (K)
- Impact (S)
- Impact with Fiber (S)
- Lipisorb (M)
- Nepro (R)
- Nutri Hep (C)
- Nutrivent (C)
- Perative (R)
- Protain XL (SH)
- Pulmocare (R)
- Replena (R)
- Replete (C)
- Stresstein (S)
- Suplena (R)
- Traum-Aid HBC (K)
- TraumaCal (M)
- Travasorb Hepatic (C)
- Travasorb Renal (C)

( ) = Company identification, see preceding list.

*O'Brien KMI is now Elan Pharma. The Newtrition product line is now the Elan product line.

INDEX

Page numbers in *italics* indicate figures; numbers followed by "t" indicate tables.